The Avery Complete Guide to
MEDICINES

The Avery Complete Guide to MEDICINES

Ian Morton, PhD and Judith Hall, PhD

Avery

a member of

Penguin Putnam Inc.

New York

Most Avery books are available at special quantity discounts for bulk purchases for sales promotions, premiums, fund-raising, and educational needs. Special books or book excerpts also can be created to fit special needs. For details, write Putnam Special Markets, 375 Hudson Street, New York, NY 10014.

AVERY

a member of
Penguin Putnam Inc.
375 Hudson Street
New York, NY 10014
www.penguinputnam.com

Morton, Ian.
    The Avery complete guide to medicines / Ian Morton and Judith Hall.
    p. cm.
    Includes index.
    ISBN 1-58333-105-0
    1. Drugs—Handbooks, manuals, etc. 2. Materia medica—Handbooks, manuals, etc. I. Hall, Judith II. Title.

RM301.12.M656 2001   2001041236
615'.1—dc21

Printed in the United States of America
10 9 8 7 6 5 4 3 2 1

Editors in Chief: Judith Hall BSc PhD; Ian Morton BSc PhD MIBiol

US Senior Consulting Editor: Cheryl Burlett MS PHARM, PhC, BCPP

Contributors: Judith Hall BSc PhD; Pamela Mason BSc PhD MRPharmS; Sheena Meredith MB BS MRCS Eng LRCP Lond;
          Ian Morton BSc PhD MIBiol; John Wilkinson BSc PhD DIC MRSC C CHEM

US Editors: Jim Glenn; Jean Searcy

Design and copyediting: Sam Merrell; Louise Bostock Lang

Database editing and typesetting: Martin Griffiths; Neville Mooney

US Publishing Consultant: John Kelly

Publishing Director: Hal Robinson

Database technology: David Wilcockson (Librios Research Ltd, UK).

Contents

Introduction

The Avery Complete Guide to Medicines is designed to provide vitally important and easily accessible information for anyone who uses any kind of medication. At the heart of the book is information about drugs that may be prescribed by your doctor. But this book provides you with far more than that; it also gives information about over-the-counter products and medications as well as herbal remedies and nutritional supplements available at most drugstores. It is the only book currently available that provides such comprehensive and integrated information on such a wide range of products. It also has an A-to-Z section of disorders that explains them and lists drugs, herbal remedies, and supplements that may be used to treat them.

All the products described in this book can help treat illness, relieve symptoms, or provide other benefits to health. With so many different products available, it is increasingly difficult to know which one to choose. One of the aims of The Avery Complete Guide to Medicines is to give you the information you need to make a choice or to ask the right questions of your doctor or pharmacist.

It is important to realize that many of these powerful healing products can also have strong, sometimes unpleasant, and occasionally dangerous effects. In particular, you should be aware of the possible dangers of taking a combination of different medications. One piece of advice you will come across throughout this book is that you must consult a doctor or pharmacist before taking two or more different medications, whether over-the-counter drugs, herbal remedies, or supplements. To address this point specifically, the articles on drugs in their generic form—the fundamental active ingredient—list warnings about the possible dangers associated with each drug and describe common side effects. Additionally, and crucially, each article explains how that drug may interact with other drugs.

In providing all this information in one clearly written and extensively cross-referenced book, The Avery Complete Guide to Medicines presents detailed and often technical information in an accessible way. It will empower you to take an active and informed role in achieving and maintaining good health.

The authors and contributors

The team of writers who researched and wrote this book is among the first to integrate information about conventional and complementary medications in one book. They have included information on the latest drug treatments, on traditional herbal remedies, and up-to-date research on nutrition in health care. The encyclopedic guide to disorders brings these three strands together, making The Avery Complete Guide to Medicines a unique publication in its field.

Led by Dr. Ian Morton and Dr. Judith Hall, the team of authors and contributors approached the book with a clear and far-reaching vision—to provide the most up-to-date and accurate information possible, with a strictly scientific perspective. Drs. Morton and Hall hold to this scientific criterion with a passion.

They developed their keen interest in explaining modern medical practice to the general public, with a special interest in drugs, disorders, and treatments, while working together at the department of pharmacology at King's College, London. Since 1988, they have written and edited more than a dozen books for a general readership. One principle they have adhered to, in addition to that of scientific discipline, is that full and authoritative information, presented clearly, is what lay readers respect most and find most reassuring.

Dr. Morton, the author of more than 100 research papers, books, and monographs, is now a consultant editor and writer in pharmacology. Dr. Hall, after obtaining her doctorate in pharmacology from King's College, London, worked as a research fellow at King's College and at the University of Surrey, and in 1995 was awarded a Wellcome Trust

Medical Research Fellowship. She has written more than 50 research papers, reviews, books, and monographs, and was an editor of the *British Journal of Pharmacology*. Both Dr. Morton and Dr. Hall now devote their energies entirely to writing.

In creating this book, they were helped by Dr. John Wilkinson, senior lecturer in Pharmocognosy and head of the Phytochemistry Discovery Group at Herbal Research Laboratories, Middlesex, who provided the information about herbal remedies; by Dr. Pamela Mason, a former dispensing pharmacist and now a full-time writer on nutrition, diet, and medicines for a family readership; by a strong research and advisory team from the United States, including Jim Glenn, Jean Searcy, and Cheryl Burlett, currently Clinical Pharmacy Services Co-ordinator at St. Vincent Hospital, Santa Fe, New Mexico, who were responsible for the US research and in particular for the OTC brand entries; and Sheena Meredith, a former doctor and now a professional medical writer and editor, who has an active interest in the whole spectrum of health care in the world today and who advised on and researched the disorder entries.

The result is an invaluable reference book that includes intriguing insights into what illnesses are and how they can now be treated (or even how they may be treated in the future), with explanations on how drugs work, and with an overview of the fascinating world of herbalism. *The Avery Complete Guide to Medicines* is a source of information that will be relevant and interesting to everyone.

How to Use This Book

The Avery Complete Guide to Medicines is organized in four main sections, so that you can find all the information you need in the quickest possible way. These sections are linked together with cross-references, which appear in bold type with symbols placed in front of each to indicate in which section the information you are looking for can be found. The four sections are called **Disorders, Directory of Drugs**, **Herbal Remedies**, and **Vitamins, Minerals and Supplements**.

In the **Disorders** section, articles describe common illnesses and indicate how they are usually treated, and include whether this can be by orthodox drugs obtained from a physician or a drugstore, by herbal remedies, or by nutritional treatment in the form of vitamins, minerals or supplements. The structure of a typical article in the Disorders section is explained below.

Disorder article

Key

1 Name of a disorder or condition.

2 Description of the condition, including symptoms, causes, risk factors, and incidence.

3 Cross-reference to another entry. The symbol indicates the section of the book that contains the entry, in this case the Disorders section.

4 Methods of treatment and how they are administered.

5 The most common drugs and drug classes used in treatment.

6 Common herbal remedies used to treat the condition.

7 Vitamins, minerals, and supplents used to treat or prevent the condition.

Key to sections:

✪ = Disorder Section   ℞ = Drug Section

♣ = Herbal Section   ⚖ = Supplement Section

Key to drugs:

Ⓓ = Drug type/group   Ⓖ = Generic name   Ⓑ = Brand name

---

① **diabetes mellitus**
Diabetes mellitus is a condition in which the body is not able to efficiently utilize the sugar glucose, and is due to an inadequacy in the secretion, or effect, of the hormone ℞ **insulin**. Insulin is normally ② produced by the islets of Langerhans in the pancreas and normally enables the utilization of glucose as an energy source, and tissue building block, by virtually every cell in the body. In the absence of proper insulin release, or tissue reaction to it, glucose is wasted and passes out in the urine taking water with it. This causes the characteristic frequent urination, body wastage and weight loss, and leads to the metabolism of alternative sources of energy, particularly fats, which form toxic by-products.

There are two main types of diabetes mellitus. The first condition, type 1 diabetes mellitus, occurs most frequently in children and is consequently known as juvenile-onset diabetes (insulin-dependent diabetes mellitus; IDDM); the second, type 2 diabetes mellitus, arises more often in adults and is thus known as adult-onset diabetes mellitus (non-insulin-dependent diabetes mellitus; NIDDM).

Blood sugar levels must be carefully controlled, as they can quickly ③ become too high (✪ **hyperglycemia**), leading to chemical changes in which the blood may contain toxic ketones (which can sometimes be smelled on the breath); coma may follow.

④ **Treatment**
Type 1 diabetes mellitus is treated with careful dietary control and doses of ℞ **insulin**. Expert counseling, initial training, and blood-glucose monitoring are required because a stable blood-glucose level over long periods must be maintained.

For further information

⑤ ℞ DIRECTORY OF DRUGS:
antidiabetic treatment • insulin analog • (sulfonylurea) oral hypoglycemic (acetohexamide, chlorpropamide, glimepiride, glipizide, glyburide, tolazamide, tolbutamide) • (biguanide) oral hypoglycemic (metformin), other oral hypoglycemic drugs (acarbose, diazoxide, repaglinide, miglitol, rosiglitazone, pioglitazone) • glucagon • glucose

⑥ ♣ HERBAL REMEDIES:
artichoke • bilberry • fenugreek • garlic • holy basil • yucca

⑦ ⚖ VITAMINS, MINERALS, AND SUPPLEMENTS:
alpha-lipoic acid • chromium • conjugated linoleic acid • magnesium • manganese • niacin • vitamin E

In the **Directory of Drugs**, three kinds of articles about drugs are listed alphabetically. One kind of article describes approximately 3,000 of the most common **brands**, indicating the characteristics that identify it and also listing what the active ingredients are. These are **generic** drugs, and the second kind of article describes them in detail. These are the most important articles in this section, because generics are the basic building blocks of pharmacology. The third kind of article provides a general view of the main types, groups or classes of drugs, referred to as **drug type/group** articles, in order to give a more complete picture of what the broad categories of drugs are, how they work and what they are used for. The structure of brand articles and generic articles are explained below.

Generic article

Key

1 Symbol indicating this entry is about a generic drug.
2 Name of a generic drug.
3 List of the classes of drug that include this generic drug.
4 Common brands that contain this generic drug.
5 The way in which the drug may be administered, for example, oral or intravenous.
6 Information about the most common uses of the drug in treatment, and their mechanisms.
7 Warnings about the use of the drug.
8 Information about possible interactions that may occur with other drugs or types of drug.
9 Information about possible side effects that may result from taking the drug.

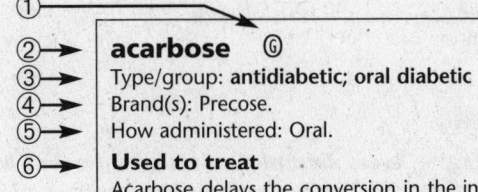

acarbose Ⓖ

Type/group: **antidiabetic; oral diabetic**
Brand(s): Precose.
How administered: Oral.

Used to treat
Acarbose delays the conversion in the intestine of starch and sucrose (sugar) to glucose, and subsequent absorption. It is used in treatment of type 2 ✪ **diabetes mellitus** (non-insulin-dependent diabetes mellitus, or NIDDM), sometimes in combination with other drugs. It may be of value in those where other drugs, or diet control, have not been successful, so is useful in people who are obese.

Warnings
• It should not be given to people with known hypersensitivity or allergy to this drug, cirrhosis, intestinal obstruction, or chronic intestinal disease, or inflammatory bowel disease.
• It should be used during pregnancy only if clearly needed.
• It should be given with caution to people with kidney impairment.
• It is not known whether acarbose is present in breast milk. Breast-feeding women should discontinue using this drug or stop breast-feeding.
• Blood glucose and liver enzymes are monitored.

Interactions
• Charcoal and digestive enzymes may reduce effectiveness of acarbose.
• Digoxin levels are lowered, decreasing its effect.

Side effects
• Gastrointestinal disturbances, including diarrhea, flatulence, bloating, distension, and abdominal pain (which becomes less with time).

Key to sections: ✪ = Disorder Section   ℞ = Drug Section   ♣ = Herbal Section   ♨ = Supplement Section
Key to drugs: Ⓓ = Drug type/group   Ⓖ = Generic name   Ⓑ = Brand name

Brand article

Key

1 Symbol of a drug brand entry.

2 Brand name of a drug.

3 Brief description, cross-referring to the generic (active drug) it contains, where detailed information about its action can be found.

4 The form in which it is used.

5 Its availability.

6 Warnings about its use, and any possible side effects it may have.

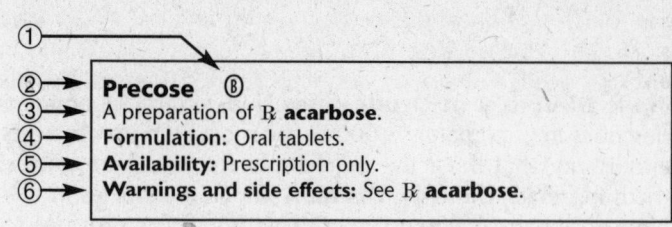

Precose Ⓑ
A preparation of ℞ **acarbose**.
Formulation: Oral tablets.
Availability: Prescription only.
Warnings and side effects: See ℞ **acarbose**.

Brand articles do not list disorders they may be used to treat, because this information is provided by the physician prescribing the drug, the pharmacist dispensing it or the manufacturer in documentation provided with it.

The third section of the **Avery Complete Guide to Herbal Medicines** is on **Herbal Remedies**. This section includes articles on herbs that can be used therapeutically and described with confidence in a scientific way. The structure of a typical article in this section is explained below.

Herbal Remedy article

Key

1 Common name of the herb.

2 The scientific or Latin name or names. In the case of some herbs, the active parts of the plant are also listed here.

3 Other common names of the herb. A list of many of these alternative names is provided at the end of the introduction to the Herbal Remedies section.

4 Description of the herb.

5 Information about preparation of the herb and the parts of the plant used.

6 The active ingredients of the plant and their biological action.

7 Traditional and other possible uses and indi-cations of the plant.

8 Warnings, information about interactions with other drugs, potential side effects, and other information of which users should be aware.

agrimony
(*Agrimonia eupatoria*)
Other common names: church steeples, cocklebur, common agrimony, liverwort, philanthropos, sticklewort, stickwort.
Agrimony is a faintly aromatic perennial herb, which grows from an underground rhizome to a height of approximately 3 feet (90 centimeters). The plant generally grows in damp conditions, such as marshes, wet fields, and patches of wasteground. The hairy stems of the plant bear three to five pairs of downy leaves, and in summer racemes of small yellow flowers.
Forms of preparation and parts used
The aerial parts of agrimony are used, usually as a tincture, infusion, or simply as the dried herb.
Active components
Agrimony contains a number of flavonoids and tannins, as well as phytosterols and vitamins.
Uses in treatment
Agrimony is traditionally used to staunch blood flow, and as a general digestive tonic, and especially for ✪ **diarrhea**. It has also been used for ✪ **cystitis**, ✪ **arthritis**, and as a gargle for sore throats (see ✪ **pharyngitis**). It is approved by some authorities for use in the treatment of skin inflammation (see ✪ **skin conditions**), mouth and pharynx inflammation, and diarrhea. Research suggests that agrimony infusions could be used for cutaneous porphyria, and that blood coagulation can be increased using the herb. Other studies have shown that agrimony extracts also have hypotensive activity.
Warnings, interactions, and side effects
• Although there are no reported toxic effects of agrimony with correct use and dosage, prolonged or excessive use of the herb is not recommended for anyone on medication for high or low blood pressure.
• Anyone taking an ℞ **anticoagulant** should avoid the herb.

Key to sections: ✪ = Disorder Section   ℞ = Drug Section   ♣ = Herbal Section   ⚯ = Supplement Section
Key to drugs: Ⓓ = Drug type/group   Ⓖ = Generic name   Ⓑ = Brand name

The fourth section of this book contains articles on the **Vitamins, Minerals, and Supplements** you are most likely to find in a drugstore, where some specific benefit in the treatment of disorders is known, whether this is to help prevent illness, or to support the body during the healing process. The structure of a typical article in this section is explained below.

Vitamins, Minerals, and Supplements article

Key

1 Name of vitamin, mineral, or supplement.

2 Information about the vitamin, mineral, or supplement and its sources.

3 The form(s) in which the vitamin, mineral, or supplement may be prepared, for example, tablets or capsules.

4 Brief description of the product's action.

5 Information about uses of the vitamin, mineral, or supplement with cross-references to other relevant entries.

6 Warnings about potential side effects or other information about which users should be aware.

7 Information about possible interactions that may occur with drugs or types of drug, including references to other relevant entries.

8 Information about possible side effects that may result from taking the supplement.

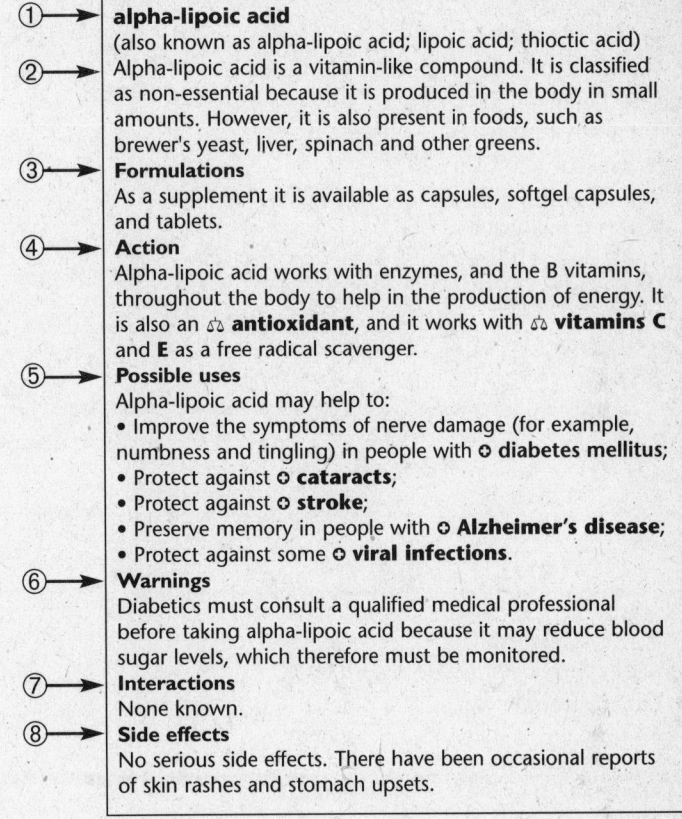

① **alpha-lipoic acid**
(also known as alpha-lipoic acid; lipoic acid; thioctic acid)
② Alpha-lipoic acid is a vitamin-like compound. It is classified as non-essential because it is produced in the body in small amounts. However, it is also present in foods, such as brewer's yeast, liver, spinach and other greens.

③ **Formulations**
As a supplement it is available as capsules, softgel capsules, and tablets.

④ **Action**
Alpha-lipoic acid works with enzymes, and the B vitamins, throughout the body to help in the production of energy. It is also an ⚖ **antioxidant**, and it works with ⚖ **vitamins C** and **E** as a free radical scavenger.

⑤ **Possible uses**
Alpha-lipoic acid may help to:
• Improve the symptoms of nerve damage (for example, numbness and tingling) in people with ✪ **diabetes mellitus**;
• Protect against ✪ **cataracts**;
• Protect against ✪ **stroke**;
• Preserve memory in people with ✪ **Alzheimer's disease**;
• Protect against some ✪ **viral infections**.

⑥ **Warnings**
Diabetics must consult a qualified medical professional before taking alpha-lipoic acid because it may reduce blood sugar levels, which therefore must be monitored.

⑦ **Interactions**
None known.

⑧ **Side effects**
No serious side effects. There have been occasional reports of skin rashes and stomach upsets.

Important points to remember when taking medicine

It is important to know why you are taking a medicine, and how to use your medicine properly. Medicines are used for several different reasons. Some are used for preventing illness (for example, vaccines); some for curing diseases (for example, antibacterials); some for controlling medical conditions (for example, antihypertensives); and some for alleviating symptoms while the condition gets better on its own (for example, painkillers). Special instructions apply to each. Therefore if you are at all unsure of any aspect of your treatment, or if they are not clearly explained in the Patient Information Leaflet, it is essential that you check with either your physician or pharmacist before taking any medication at all.

Key to sections: ✪ = Disorder Section   ℞ = Drug Section   ♣ = Herbal Section   ⚖ = Supplement Section
Key to drugs: Ⓓ = Drug type/group   Ⓖ = Generic name   Ⓑ = Brand name

PART 1

DISORDERS

Disorders

At the start of the twentieth century, even in countries in the Western world, most people died before the age of 50, and fewer than half the children born lived beyond the first year of their lives. Diseases such as smallpox and measles were commonplace and often fatal. Fortunately, due to huge advances in medicine, nutrition, and hygiene, the majority of people in the developed world today, live longer and enjoy a healthier life than their predecessors. However, many disease states are still prevalent in our society, and some "modern" disorders (for example, AIDS, and major obesity) are emerging, even though they were rare or unknown in previous generations. Health and disease is partly determined by your genes—indeed, individual chances of developing many disorders are largely determined at conception or within the first few months of life. However, the health of a person is also closely linked to their lifestyle and the environment.

Fortunately, for many common disorders, and increasingly for rarer conditions, medical treatment is available—whether with conventional or alternative medical approaches, surgical procedures, or eventually with genetic manipulation. Even if you are born with a genetic susceptibilty to a disorder, you can reduce your chances of developing it by taking control of the way you live—for example by living a healthy lifestyle, including taking nutritional supplements if required, and seeking appropriate early medical treatment if any problems do arise.

The role of complementary medicine

The increasing interest in alternative medicines, including herbal remedies and food supplements, is a trend in health care that is certain to continue. The reasons for this are not clearly defined, but probably include dissatisfaction with synthetic or orthodox treatments, coupled with a widely held belief that naturally derived products are both healthier and safer than synthetic agents. A desire to move towards self-medication and preventive approaches to disease management is likely to be another factor. However, there are considerable dangers in embracing this philosophy too fully. If you suffer from a serious complaint such as a heart arrhythmia or a blood clot, only promptly used front-line orthodox drugs offer a solution, and delay may be fatal. Similarly, many types of cancer, if dealt with promptly, respond to modern treatments. On the other hand, some other complaints do seem to be ameliorated by some herbal remedies. Also, in relation to a healthy lifestyle, there is good evidence that supplementation of the diet—for instance, with free radical scavengers—may help to reduce the incidence of some diseases.

Nevertheless, whether for orthodox or alternative medicines, it must be emphasized that, even if a little is good, more is not necessarily better. All substances, including vitamins, can be poisonous at higher doses, or in susceptible individuals, or in combination with other substances. Because of this, anyone taking any medication of any kind must always read the instructions supplied with it, and must seek advice from a physician, pharmacist, or other qualified specialist, about medicines of any description. As a basic principle, all medication must be regarded with caution.

How to use this section

The Disorders section of the book is emphatically not designed as a reference aid to self-diagnosis. It is intended to provide some background information about a condition once it has been medically diagnosed. It is also designed to be used as an entry point to the book in the search for further information on a possible therapy that may be suitable. But when exploring these options, always consult your healthcare professional who is familiar with your medical history.

This section describes nearly 350 medical disorders that can be prevented, given symptomatic relief, or cured by some form of medical procedure. Reference is made to available orthodox medicines, herbal remedies or minerals/vitamins/supplements.

The disorders are arranged in alphabetical order, with extensive cross-indexing from related or alternative terms. The disorders selected include most of the more common conditions such as influenza and diabetes mellitus, and also some rarer conditions—for example the autoimmune muscle weakness disorder myasthenia gravis and the pituitary tumor condition known as acromegaly—where drug therapy is now available and details are included in the generic drug entries section of the book.

Although not disorders in the strictest sense, some common conditions such as nausea, vomiting, pain, diarrhea and constipation, are also included because determination of the underlying cause of the symptoms and their control plays a significant role in medicine. Indeed, symptomatic relief represents the largest proportion of the market in short-term non-prescription, or over-the-counter (OTC), and herbal self-medication. Conditions or disorders treated predominantly by other approaches, including surgery, psychotherapy, and chiropractic manipulation, are not included.

A proper understanding of a medical condition lies in discovering its causative factors (often referred to as its etiology), and this is a first essential step towards an effective treatment or cure. This principle should apply irrespective of whether treatment is with a conventional medicine, herbal remedy or dietary supplement. For this reason, articles generally define the condition and its symptoms, outline some causes (for instance salmonella bacterial infection for food poisoning), identify factors that predispose an individual to the illness (such as age and family history), and then go on to discuss possible treatments. There are extensive cross-references to similar disorders, related disorders, and alternative names for conditions. Unusual and technical terms used in the text are explained in the **Glossary** section at the end of the book.

While most disorder entries describe specific conditions (for instance, asthma) and their drug treatment (in this case, antiasthmatic), there are also some more general entries such as skin conditions, brain-motor disorders and digestive system disorders. These general articles are included because they will be particularly helpful for readers who are unsure of their precise condition and who want to be directed to a more specific disorder (perhaps with an unfamiliar or difficult name). They will also be of interest to those who want to read more about conditions related to their specific disorder. These entries may also be of value for those interested in alternative herbal remedies and supplements, many of which are advocated for use in more collective upsets of body systems (for instance tonics for the digestive system), rather than for specific medical conditions.

Articles are structured with a general introduction to the subject, followed by several subsections. These are categorized under the headings Treatment, and For further information. Subheadings of the latter are Directory of Drugs, Herbal Remedies, and Vitamins, Minerals and Supplements.

TREATMENT of each disorder explains some of the common medical approaches to dealing with that disorder, whether by drugs or other interventions such as surgery.

FOR FURTHER INFORMATION lists treatments grouped under three subheadings relating to the main sections of this book: Directory of Drugs; Herbal Remedies; and Vitamins, Minerals, and Supplements. **Directory of Drugs** lists drug groups and/or individual generic drugs used for that particular disorder. **Herbal remedies** lists herbs that have traditional or approved uses relating to a particular disorder or group of disorders. **Vitamins, Minerals and Supplements** lists those products that are commonly used to help in the prevention or treatment of the disorder.

abdominal discomfort

see ✪ digestive system disorders.

abnormal puberty

Abnormal puberty is the abnormally early or late development of sexual maturity. Puberty in boys usually begins between ages 10 and 15, and in girls between ages 10 and 14. Abnormal puberty is when puberty occurs before or after these ages. In girls, early or precocious puberty is usually marked by early breast development and ovulation before age 8, and in boys, the production of sperm before age 10. Delayed or late puberty in girls is when menstruation has not started by the age of 16 or breast development before age 14. Abnormal puberty is usually due to a hormonal imbalance. For example, in boys with congenital adrenal hyperplasia, the adrenal glands produce excessive amounts of the male sex hormones, which can lead to precocious puberty; and in girls, it may be caused by an ovarian cyst developing in childhood, which may produce sex hormones resulting in early puberty. Chromosomal disorders, a tumour of the hypothalamus, or of the pituitary gland or damage to the pituitary gland (for example, due to head injury or meningitis) can also be a cause of abnormal puberty. Excessive weight loss or exercise, or prolonged illness can sometimes be a cause of delayed puberty.

Treatment

Treatment of abnormal puberty depends on the underlying cause, and it is this that will be treated. For example, if precocious puberty is due to an ovarian cyst in girls, this may be surgically removed. For drug treatment of precocious puberty, drugs that block the production of sex hormones or inhibit their action may be useful. Reduction of sex hormone secretion in both sexes may be achieved indirectly by reducing their release, which is caused by gonadotropins, through treatment with synthetic analogs of the hypothalamic hormone, gonadotropin-releasing hormone, (including ℞ **nafarelin** and leuprolide). In delayed puberty in boys, puberty can be induced by giving injections of androgen sex hormones (including ℞ **testosterone**, ℞ **methyltestosterone**, and ℞ **fluoxymesterone**) or drugs that stimulate the production of testosterone, or in girls by other hormonal treatments to promote sexual development. Alternatively, dopamine receptor stimulant drugs may be used (for instance bromocriptine) and these work by an indirect action on the pituitary gland.

For further information

℞ DIRECTORY OF DRUGS:

androgen • dopamine-receptor stimulant • hypothalamic hormone • sex hormone

abscess

An abscess is the accumulation of pus anywhere in the body; where it is walled off by inflamed tissue, and is usually caused by ✪ **bacterial infection** (for example, a ✪ **boil** or ✪ **carbuncle**, or tooth abscess (gumboil); abscesses may also occur within the body. They usually cause pain and often-visible swelling or other symptoms, depending on where they are.

Treatment

The release of the pus, as when a boil bursts, or is lanced, is necessary for healing. In the case of abscesses within the body, surgery may be required to drain the pus. Drug treatment may also be required, such as an ℞ **antibiotic** or ℞ **antibacterial**, if there is any infection. Many herbal remedies are available for ✪ **skin conditions** including abscesses.

For further information

℞ DIRECTORY OF DRUGS:
antibacterial • antibiotic
♣ HERBAL REMEDIES:
flax • marshmallow

aches

see ✪ musculoskeletal disorders.

acid indigestion

see ✪ indigestion.

acidosis

Acidosis is a condition in which the acidity of the fluids and tissues of the body is abnormally high (indicated by a blood pH below the normal range of 7.35–7.45), because of a failure to maintain the correct acid-base equilibrium (pH chemical balance). It occurs if respiration is impaired and the lungs cannot remove sufficient carbon dioxide from the blood (for example, in near drowning), or if the kidneys fail to retain enough bicarbonate in the blood. It may also be a complication of ✪ **diabetes mellitus**, liver failure, shock, or prolonged ✪ **diarrhea**. The person will usually be, and feel, extremely ill, and may have difficulty breathing.

Treatment

Treatment depends on the cause. Restoration of normal breathing, where this is the problem, is a matter of urgency. In other cases, treatment aims to restore the proper balance of blood chemistry, by giving certain ℞ **electrolytes** (usually sodium bicarbonate), which act as alkalinizing fluids—in emergency through an intravenous drip—then dealing with the underlying problem.

For further information

℞ DIRECTORY OF DRUGS:
electrolyte (rehydration solutions)

acne

Acne (also called acne vulgaris) is a skin condition, common in adolescence, resulting in pimples and blackheads, mostly on the face, neck, and back, which are unsightly and may be irritating. It is caused by hormonal changes that stimulate overactivity of the sebaceous glands, whose oily secretion (sebum) blocks the pores, particularly at hair follicles. Bacteria may also be present. A plug of keratin (the protein that forms hair and nails and adds protection to the skin) forms in the pores, causing pimples or darkening into a blackhead. In some cases acne may be linked to a mild deficiency of ⏃ **zinc**. See also ✪ **rosacea**.

Treatment

Mild cases can be treated by skin lotions such as ℞ **benzoyl peroxide**. More severe cases are often treated orally with an

℞ **antibacterial** antibiotic, or sometimes a ℞ **retinoid** such as ℞ **isotretinoin** (a drug related to vitamin A). Women can use a special form of the contraceptive pill. Of the herbal remedies available, ♣ **brewer's yeast** is considered to be one of the most useful.

For further information

℞ DIRECTORY OF DRUGS:

acne treatment

♣ HERBAL REMEDIES:

brewer's yeast • chaste tree • myrrh • tea tree

⚖ VITAMINS, MINERALS, AND SUPPLEMENTS:

vitamin B$_6$ • zinc

acne rosacea

see ✪ rosacea.

acquired immunodeficiency syndrome

see ✪ AIDS.

acromegaly

Acromegaly is a rare noncancerous tumor of the anterior part of the pituitary gland, resulting in overproduction of growth hormone (GH; also called somatotropin, somatropic hormone). The symptoms normally appear over time and include gradual, excessive growth of parts of the body (especially the bones of the face, jaw, and extremities), menstrual disturbances (such as absent or irregular periods) and infertility in women, or impotence, enlarged breasts, and leakage of fluid from the nipples in men. Pressure on adjacent areas of the brain may cause changes in the field of vision, ✪ **headaches** or ✪ **hypopituitarism**. In children, it can cause the condition called gigantism. Diagnosis includes measurement of hormone levels in the blood, and also confirmation that the side effects of certain ℞ **antipsychotic** drugs are not the cause.

Treatment

Drugs that mimic the actions of the hypothalamic hormone somatostatin (alternatively called growth hormone-release-inhibiting factor, and which physiologically controls the release of growth hormone) are very effective at reducing the release of growth hormone. ℞ **dopamine-receptor stimulants** can be used to control the symptoms of acromegaly (because dopamine is also a hypothalamic factor that controls the release of anterior pituitary hormones). Drugs are usually used short-term; later surgical removal of the tumor, or radiotherapy, is often necessary. See also ✪ **pituitary gland disorders and tumors**.

For further information

℞ DIRECTORY OF DRUGS:

dopamine-receptor stimulant (bromocriptine, pergolide) • **hypothalamic hormone** (such as **octreotide**)

ADD

see ✪ attention deficit disorder.

addiction

see ✪ drug dependency.

Addison's disease

Addison's disease (also called Addison's syndrome) is characterized by a group of symptoms caused by the failure of the adrenal gland to secrete ℞ **corticosteroid** hormones. It is usually caused by damage to an adrenal gland by an ✪ **autoimmune disorder**. A less common cause is as a complication of ✪ **tuberculosis**. Symptoms include weight loss, lethargy, low blood pressure (hypotension), and dark pigmentation of the skin and mucous membranes. Addison's disease is twice as common in women and sometimes runs in families. It is named after the English physician Thomas Addison (1793-1860), who first described it in 1855.

Treatment

Treatment is by hormone replacement therapy with corticosteroids.

For further information

℞ DIRECTORY OF DRUGS:

corticosteroid

Addison's syndrome

see ✪ Addison's disease.

ADHD

see ✪ attention deficit disorder.

affective disorders

Affective disorders (mood disorders) are types of ✪ **mental illness** that are characterized by marked affect (mood) changes. The term tends to be used somewhat differently by different authorities, but generally is used in contrast to ✪ **psychotic disorders**. It is similar in meaning to the term neurotic disorder, and encompasses ✪ **anxiety**-related conditions. Mood may be abnormally low as in clinical ✪ **depression**, abnormally elevated as in mania, or alternate between the two as in ✪ **bipolar disorder** (manic-depressive illness)—although unremitting manic behavior is regarded as psychotic, and treated accordingly with antipsychotic drugs. Anxiety is also considered an affective disorder. There are many states characterized by mood changes, though the actual cause varies greatly, for instance ✪ **obsessive-compulsive disorder**, panic disorder, trichotillomania, post-stroke emotional lability, premenstrual dysphoric disorder (PMDD) (see ✪ **premenstrual syndrome**), ✪ **anorexia nervosa**, kleptomania, post-traumatic stress disorder.

Treatment

Treatment depends on the diagnosis and may include psychotherapy as well as drugs. Most of the states mentioned above may respond to ℞ **antidepressants** (largely of the SSRI class), though some of these uses are on an "off-label", largely experimental basis. The manic phase of bipolar disorder is usually treated with ℞ **antimanic** drugs, predominantly lithium. Anxiety is treated with ℞ **antianxiety** drugs (anxiolytics). Many herbal remedies are available, some with proven efficacy for certain affective disorders (for example, ♣ **St. John's wort** for depression and anxiety), and some supplements including ⚖ **omega-3 fatty acids**, ⚖ **phenylalanine**, ⚖ **tyrosine**, ⚖ **vitamin B$_1$** (thiamine), and ⚖ **vitamin B$_6$** (pyridoxine) are considered to be helpful in preventing depression. See individual affective disorder entries for more information.

aging

Aging occurs as a result of the natural effects that take place in the body as one gets older. Obvious external effects include the loss of pigment from the hair or the loss of hair altogether (✪ **alopecia**), and the loss of elasticity in the skin, which leads to the formation of wrinkles. The gradual loss of calcium from the bones causes them to shrink slightly, resulting in a curvature to the spine and a stooped posture. Loss of accommodation (focusing ability) and other changes in the eyes may affect vision, and the senses of hearing and taste may also deteriorate. There is usually also a gradual loss in the sex drive (libido). Degenerative changes in the body may result in ✪ **arthritis** and ✪ **rheumatism**, but, although a person as a whole may "slow down", there is usually no change in intellectual capacity. The study of the disorders of the elderly is called geriatrics.

Treatment

The cellular changes that accumulate during the aging process, and possible ways of arresting or even reversing them, remain the subject of intensive research. Some supplements are claimed, though with limited evidence, to help slow some aspects of the aging process.

For further information

⚕ VITAMINS, MINERALS, AND SUPPLEMENTS:
coenzyme Q$_{10}$ • phosphatidylserine

AIDS

AIDS (acquired immunodeficiency syndrome) is a viral disease that causes failure of the body's normal immune response (defense system) by destroying a vital type of lymphocyte (white blood cell) called helper T-cells. The virus (one of two varieties of the human immunodeficiency virus, or HIV) is passed on in body fluids. Because AIDS can be passed on in semen it is a sexually transmitted disease that may be contracted through both heterosexual and homosexual intercourse. HIV can also be passed on in contaminated blood. In Western countries, where sterile needles are used in medical procedures and blood or blood products are carefully screened, transmission of HIV by this route is only a risk for drug users who share hypodermic needles. However, in many countries such precautions are inadequate and travelers who need medical treatment abroad may be at risk. HIV can also be transmitted from a mother to her baby either at birth or during breast-feeding.

Someone who has HIV may have no symptoms, yet still be infectious to others. Symptoms, which may not develop for years, include loss of weight, fever, diarrhea, and swelling of the lymph nodes. AIDS itself involves failure of the body to combat infections, especially a type of ✪ **pneumonia** called pneumocystic pneumonia (caused by the protozoan *Pneumocystic carinii*), which can be fatal. People with AIDS are also at risk of ✪ **tuberculosis** and of tumors, especially an otherwise rare cancer called ✪ **Kaposi's sarcoma**, which causes pigmented nodules on the skin. There can also be psychological problems such as ✪ **anxiety** and ✪ **depression**.

Treatment

Treatment with a combination of ℞ **antiviral** drugs can slow the progression of the symptoms of AIDS and its complications, sometimes considerably so, and new drugs are continually being developed. Considerable resources are being put into research efforts to find an effective vaccine against HIV. In addition to taking drug therapy, some supplements are purported as being helpful as additional therapy (glutamine), or in slowing the progression (selenium) of AIDS. Symptoms such as anxiety and depression can be controlled with antianxiety drugs and antidepressants.

For further information

℞ DIRECTORY OF DRUGS:
antiviral

⚕ VITAMINS, MINERALS, AND SUPPLEMENTS:
amino acid (glutamine) • **selenium**

alcoholism

Alcoholism is the physical dependence on (addiction to) alcohol. It affects mental functions such as judgment and memory, and causes physical skills to deteriorate. As well as the brain, other organs affected include the liver (✪ **cirrhosis**), heart (cardiomyopathy), and nerves (neuritis). Sudden deprivation of alcoholic drinks causes withdrawal symptoms of ✪ **anxiety**, tremor ("the shakes"), hallucinations, and delusions (delirium tremens, the "DTs").

Treatment

The main treatment for alcoholism is psychotherapy, possibly including group therapy and the use of substance-dependence drug treatment. One drug that is used to provide an incentive to discontinue drinking is ℞ **disulfiram** (Antabuse), which makes the subject vomit and experience other very unpleasant effects if he or she drinks alcohol. Some other drugs help reduce the craving for alcohol (for example, ℞ **clonidine hydrochloride**, ℞ **naloxone**, ℞ **naltrexone**). In detoxification treatment, a number of types of drug can be used to control withdrawal symptoms. These include sedative/hypnotic/antianxiety/antipsychotic group drugs. Beta-blockers can help to control some of the withdrawal symptoms. Other drugs used include ℞ **carbamazepine** and ℞ **lithium**. ⚕ **Vitamin B$_1$** (thiamine) is often given to help reverse the chronic neurological deficits that often accompany alcoholism and its associated dietary deficiencies.

For further information

℞ DIRECTORY OF DRUGS:
substance-dependence treatment (clonidine hydrochloride, disulfiram, naloxone hydrochloride, naltrexone hydrochloride) • **sedatives, antianxiety/antipsychotic** drugs (for example, chloral hydrate, chlordiazepoxide, clorazepate dipotassium, hydroxyzine, lorazepam, mesoridazine, thioridazine) • **beta-blocker** (acebutolol, atenolol, bisoprolol fumarate, labetalol hydrochloride, metoprolol tartrate, nadolol, propranolol hydrochloride, pindolol) • **lithium**

⚕ VITAMINS, MINERALS, AND SUPPLEMENTS:
vitamin B$_1$ (thiamine)

aldosteronism

see ✪ hyperaldosteronism.

alkalosis

Alkalosis is a condition in which body fluids have an abnormally high alkalinity (indicated by a pH above 7.45), because of a failure of the mechanism that maintains the acid-base equilibrium (pH

Key to symbols: ✪ = Disorder Section ℞ = Drug Section ♣ = Herbal Section ⚕ = Supplement Section

chemical balance). It may be caused by an excessive intake of alkali (in the form of bicarbonate or other ℞ **antacid**), by a loss of acidic digestive juices through excessive vomiting, by overbreathing (hyperventilating; as occurs in certain diseases), and occasionally by drugs. Symptoms include inappropriately deep breathing, and muscle weakness or cramp.

Treatment

Treatment depends on the cause. It may include correcting the disturbance of blood chemistry by giving fluids through a drip, drug treatment for particular symptoms (for instance ℞ **ammonium chloride** for acidification), or counteracting overbreathing, plus treatment of the underlying problem.

For further information

℞ DIRECTORY OF DRUGS:
ammonium chloride

allergic asthma

see ✚ asthma.

allergic conjunctivitis

see ✚ conjunctivitis.

allergic contact dermatitis

see ✚ dermatitis.

allergic dermatitis

see ✚ dermatitis.

allergy

Allergy is a bodily reaction, caused by hypersensitivity, to an allergen, a substance—a food (for example, nuts), medication (for example, penicillin), an animal product (for example, a bee ✚ **sting**), dust, or pollen, which the body treats as foreign, provoking a form of immune reaction. Symptoms range from ✚ **hay fever** or skin ✚ **rashes** to ✚ **asthma** and ✚ **anaphylactic reaction**, which in anaphylactic shock, can lead to potentially fatal collapse. One in seven Americans has a severe allergy. See also ✚ **hypersensitivity reaction**.

Treatment

Various creams and drugs, particularly the ℞ **antihistamine** group, which counteract the effects of histamine, are used to treat minor reactions. With an established allergy, the best course of action is to avoid the allergen where possible. In severe allergic reactions which may result in a collapse with anaphylaxis (anaphylactic shock), emergency treatment with the ℞ **sympathomimetic** ℞ **epinephrine** may be life-saving. It is thought that vitamin C may be beneficial in some disorders that have an allergic component. See individual disorder entries for more details.

alopecia

Alopecia is the medical term for baldness, although more often it is applied to the unusual loss of hair caused by a disease, drug side effects (for example, chemotherapy), or the puzzling disorder alopecia areata (in which hair falls out in patches for no known reason) than to natural hair loss with aging.

Treatment

Wigs and hairpieces may be used to disguise hair loss. For male-pattern balding, various forms of hair "transplants" have been attempted, and the drug ℞ **minoxidil** may be applied to the scalp to prevent further loss and stimulate regrowth.

For further information

℞ DIRECTORY OF DRUGS:
hair-growth promoter (minoxidil)

Alzheimer's disease

Alzheimer's disease is the most common form of ✚ **dementia**, where there is a progressive deterioration in mental ability, occurring in middle age or later. Its cause is unknown but various changes in brain structure and function have been found, including alterations in transmitter chemicals (especially acetylcholine). Some forms may be inherited. Symptoms include memory loss, especially for recent events; impaired intellectual performance and learning capacity; behavior changes, and defective judgment. Alzheimer's disease currently affects approximately 4 million Americans. The disease was named after the German neurologist Alois Alzheimer (1864–1915).

Treatment

There is no cure, but drugs that maintain levels of brain chemicals, which would be reduced as a result of the disease, may improve symptoms. There are many supplements that are claimed to have some beneficial effect.

For further information

℞ DIRECTORY OF DRUGS:
anticholinesterase • **dementia treatment**
♣ HERBAL REMEDIES:
ginkgo
⚗ VITAMINS, MINERALS, AND SUPPLEMENTS:
alpha-lipoic acid • **amino acid** (tyrosine) • **coenzyme Q$_{10}$** • **lecithin** • **phosphatidylserine** • **vitamin E**

amebiasis

see ✚ amebic dysentery.

amebic dysentery

Amebic dysentery (also called amebiasis) is a type of ✚ **dysentery** caused by the amoeba *Entamoeba histolytica* (a type of parasitic organism), common in tropical regions. It is usually caught by drinking water contaminated with human feces. The chief symptom is repeated attacks of ✚ **diarrhea** containing blood and mucus. ✚ **anemia**, liver abscess, or ✚ **hepatitis** may be complications.

Treatment

Treatment is with ℞ **tetracyclines** or other drugs that will kill the amoeba.

For further information

℞ DIRECTORY OF DRUGS:
amebicide and antiprotozoal (metronidazole) • **tetracycline**

amyotrophic lateral sclerosis

Amyotrophic lateral sclerosis (ALS) is a degenerative ✚ **brain-motor disorder**, a disease of the motor neurons (also called wasting palsy or Lou Gehrig's disease) where there is progressive weakening and atrophy, initially of the muscles of the forearms and legs but progressing to the face, and rest of the body. It is caused by the degeneration of neurons within the central nervous system. It generally appears in middle life, and results in death within about five years.

Treatment

There is no cure but the drug ℞ **riluzole** extends survival and/or time to tracheostomy.

For further information

℞ DIRECTORY OF DRUGS:
brain-motor disorder treatment (riluzole)

anaphylactic reaction

Anaphylactic reaction is a severe allergic reaction (✪ **hypersensitivity reaction**) to a foreign substance to which the body has previously become sensitized. In anaphylactic shock this reaches a life-threatening state with a massive release of histamine and other inflammatory mediators, causing hypotensive shock and cardiovascular collapse, severe bronchoconstriction (narrowing of the airways), swelling of the tongue and throat, raised (nettle-like) rash, abdominal pain, and diarrhea. These reactions can be triggered by insect bites or stings, drug reactions (for example, penicillin, local anesthetics, immunoglobulin serums), to varying degrees of severity. See also ✪ **allergy**.

Treatment

Anaphylactic shock is a medical emergency, and may require a tube to be inserted in the airways to facilitate breathing. The immediate treatment is injection with ℞ **epinephrine**, ℞ **antihistamines** and ℞ **steroids**. People who have a known hypersensitivity (for example, to bee or wasp stings) may carry a syringe preloaded with epinephrine. Hyposensitizing injections with diluted allergenic protein are sometimes successful. People with known hypersensitivity should avoid known triggers.

For further information

℞ DIRECTORY OF DRUGS:
antihistamine (chlorpheniramine maleate, **cyproheptadine hydrochloride, diphenhydramine hydrochloride**) • corticosteroid (for example, **methylprednisolone**) • desensitizing enzyme • sympathomimetic (for example, **epinephrine**)

anemia

Anemia is a blood condition involving a deficiency of hemoglobin (the oxygen-carrying pigment in red blood cells: the normal range is 12–16 grams/deciliter of blood for women or 13.5–18 grams/deciliter for men). The deficiency may be due to too few red blood cells (erythrocytes). Symptoms include pallor, tiredness, and breathlessness or ✪ **fatigue** after exertion. Among the many causes are blood loss (through hemorrhage), deficiency of iron (essential for the production of hemoglobin; iron deficiency anemia), over-rapid destruction of red blood cells (hemolytic anemia, usually caused by Rhesus factor incompatibility), damage to the bone marrow where red cells are produced (aplastic anemia), distorted red cells (as in ✪ **sickle-cell anemia**) and deficiency of vitamin B_{12}

(✪ **pernicious anemia**), a megaloblastic anemia (where there is production of large immature dysfunctional red blood cells). Anemia is therefore a symptom of another disorder.

Treatment

Treatment depends on the cause. For example, the drugs used to treat iron deficiency anemia are mainly salts of iron; for some megaloblastic anemias, certain B vitamins may be used. Supplements are available that can help prevent certain types of anemia (for example, ⚖ **iron** for iron deficiency anemia). Severe cases may require blood transfusion.

For further information

℞ DIRECTORY OF DRUGS:
anemia treatment
⚖ VITAMINS, MINERALS, AND SUPPLEMENTS:
iron • vitamin B_{12}

angina pectoris

Angina pectoris (also called angina of effort) is a chest pain that comes on during exertion, or sometimes emotional excitement or upset, and goes away when the person rests, or calms down. It is caused by an inability of the coronary arteries to supply enough blood to the heart muscle during periods of increased demand. This is usually due to ✪ **arteriosclerosis** within the coronary arteries but may also result from a spasm (sudden narrowing) of the arteries.

Treatment

Nitrate drugs such as ℞ **nitroglycerin**—taken by mouth spray or by dissolving a tablet under the tongue—usually relieve an attack rapidly. Longer-acting forms can be taken to prevent attacks, and are available as tablets, ointments, or patches. Other drugs may also be used (see ℞ **antianginal**). In more severe cases, surgery may be required to widen the narrowed arteries (coronary angioplasty) or to replace them (coronary artery bypass graft). Supplements are said to be beneficial, for example, by improving heart function and circulation (such as ⚖ **coenzyme Q_{10}**), and a traditional herbal remedy that may be of some benefit is ♣ **florists' chrysanthemum**. However, angina pectoris always requires professional medical treatment.

For further information

℞ DIRECTORY OF DRUGS:
antianginal
♣ HERBAL REMEDIES:
florists' chrysanthemum • red sage
⚖ VITAMINS, MINERALS, AND SUPPLEMENTS:
amino acid (lysine) • coenzyme Q_{10}

angioedema

Angioedema is an acute painless swelling of body tissues, often around the face and sometimes the genitals. It is usually due to an allergic reaction to, for example, a type of food (such as strawberries, nuts, seafood). It can be caused by an ✪ **allergy** to a drug or to an insect bite. There is also a rare, inherited form of angioedema, hereditary angioedema. There may be an itchy rash (✪ **urticaria**) on areas not swollen. If the larynx is affected, it can be life threatening, and it may be necessary to inject epinephrine. It may occur at the same time as anaphylaxis.

Treatment

Severe angioedema requires an urgent injection of ℞ **epinephrine**. A variety of other drugs can be used to treat milder cases. It is important to identify the causative agent, and take measures to avoid it.

For further information

℞ DIRECTORY OF DRUGS:

androgen (danazol, stanozolol) • antihistamine (for example, diphenhydramine hydrochloride, trimipramine hydrochloride, cyproheptadine hydrochloride) • corticosteroid (for example, hydrocortisone, prednisolone, prednisone) • epinephrine • tricyclic (nortriptyline hydrochloride)

angioneurotic edema

see ✪ angioedema.

ankylosing spondylitis

Ankylosing spondylitis is a disorder of the spine in which the vertebrae gradually fuse together, causing pain and stiffness. It is caused by inflammation of the synovial joints (synovitis) and may result in curvature of the spine (kyphosis). It most commonly affects men under age 30.

Treatment

There is no cure, but symptoms may be eased with drugs, rest, physiotherapy, or a spinal support. Occasionally, surgery may be required.

For further information

℞ DIRECTORY OF DRUGS:

non-narcotic analgesic • NSAID

anogenital wart

see ✪ wart.

anorexia nervosa

Anorexia nervosa is a psychological, ✪ anxiety-related disorder, usually affecting adolescent girls, in which those affected falsely believe themselves to be fat, or have a morbid fear of becoming fat. Usually their body image is distorted and they often develop an obsessive desire to lose weight. A background of family problems is common and there is often an underlying anxiety about developing sexuality. Those affected either eat little or no food, or attempt to counteract or purge what they do eat by inducing vomiting or abusing laxatives. Sometimes they will have periods of binge eating interspersed with purging (✪ bulimia). Symptoms include severe weight loss and the stopping of menstruation (amenorrhea). Without treatment, malnutrition eventually can lead to death.

Treatment

Anorexia nervosa always requires professional medical treatment. Treatment, which is difficult, is predominantly by psychotherapy to address underlying emotional disturbances and attempt to persuade the person to eat. See also ✪ appetite loss.

For further information

℞ DIRECTORY OF DRUGS:

appetite stimulant • antidepressant (SSRI)

♣ HERBAL REMEDIES:

blessed thistle • yellow gentian

anterior uveitis

see ✪ uveitis.

antibiotic-associated colitis

see ✪ pseudomembranous colitis.

anxiety

In general terms, anxiety is a feeling of fear and apprehension, anticipation of impending disaster or feeling of death, leading to restlessness and tension, often with physical symptoms such as difficulty in breathing and increased heart rate. In psychology, the term is used more specifically, and if deep and lasting, anxiety is regarded as a form of neurosis or neurotic disorder (in contrast to psychosis, or ✪ psychotic disorder). A central feature is that the anxiety has no specific or apparent cause, or that the reaction is out of proportion to the perceived cause. Free-floating anxiety is where there is generalized, persistent, pervasive fear that cannot be attributed to any specific object or event. What is sometimes called performance anxiety occurs for example prior to performing in a concert, prior to a job interview or public speaking. There are a number of mood disorders sometimes described as anxiety-related disorders, including panic disorder, where there are recurrent panic attacks of intense anxiety and alarming physical symptoms, obsessive-compulsive disorder and phobias. See also ✪ affective disorders.

Treatment

Psychotherapy can be very effective, but anxiety that interferes with a person's lifestyle can also be treated with ℞ antianxiety drugs (anxiolytics; sometimes called minor tranquilizers), most of which are ℞ benzodiazepines. Easing of the physical manifestations of anxiety such as hand tremor and heart palpitations can be very effective, for example, in treating anxiety prior to a job interview, public speaking or performing, and ℞ beta-blockers or the herbal remedy ♣ motherwort may be of use. There are many herbal remedies that can be tried that are traditionally used to relieve anxiety; some (for example, ♣ kava kava, ♣ St. John's wort) for which there is good evidence of efficacy.

For further information

℞ DIRECTORY OF DRUGS:

antianxiety drug (including **benzodiazepine**) • beta-blocker

♣ HERBAL REMEDIES:

bugleweed • hops • kava kava • lemon balm • motherwort • passionflower • St. John's wort • valerian • water hyssop

aortic aneurysm

see ✪ peripheral vascular disorders.

aortic incompetence

see ✪ heart valve disorders.

aortic stenosis

see ✿ heart valve disorders.

aplastic anemia

see ✿ anemia.

appetite loss

Appetite loss is the loss of the desire to eat. Appetite is the pleasurable sensation caused by the production of digestive juices in the mouth and stomach and which lead to the desire to eat. Appetite, along with hunger (which is a physical sensation stimulated by the body's need for food and involves contraction of the stomach caused by nervous and hormonal influences) determines how much we eat, and how often. Appetite loss is a characteristic of certain illnesses (such as ✿ **cancer**, ✿ **AIDS**), of childhood ("fussy eaters") and the elderly and debilitated and can be a side effect of some drugs. In severe cases of appetite loss where not enough food is consumed to meet the nutritional needs of the body, deficiencies (such as ✿ **vitamin deficiency**) may result. Appetite loss is not the same as ✿ **anorexia nervosa**.

Treatment

The underlying cause of the loss of appetite should be corrected if possible. Many herbal remedies are advocated as appetite stimulants. In severe cases of appetite loss where nutritional deficiencies may be a consequence of reduced eating, vitamin and mineral supplements can be useful, and ℞ **appetite stimulants** may be required.

For further information

℞ DIRECTORY OF DRUGS:

appetite stimulant

♣ HERBAL REMEDIES:

aloe • angelica • anise • blessed thistle • brewer's yeast • cardamom • centaury • chicory • cinnamon • cinnamon, Chinese • colombo • condurango • coriander • curcuma • dandelion • devil's claw • fenugreek • galangal • ginger • grains of paradise • haronga • hibiscus • horehound • horseradish • Iceland moss • immortelle • juniper • onion • radish • rosemary • sage • star anise • sweet orange • yarrow • yellow gentian

⚖ VITAMINS, MINERALS, AND SUPPLEMENTS:

minerals • vitamins

arrhythmia

Arrhythmia (dysrhythmia) of the heart is a ✿ **cardiovascular disorder** where there is an abnormality of the rate or rhythm of the heartbeat. In some cases there may be bradycardia (slower heartbeat than normal) or tachycardia (faster heartbeat than normal). Irregularities in the heartbeat are sometimes called ectopic beats. The reasons for arrhythmias are many and diagnosis is made by a specialist, initially from an EKG (electrocardiogram). There are many ways in which the heartbeat can falter—atrial tachycardia, supraventricular arrhythmias, ventricular arrhythmias, ventricular tachycardia, atrial flutter or fibrillation and the severe heartbeat irregularity that may follow a heart attack (✿ **myocardial infarction**).

Treatment

The treatment of abnormal heart rhythm is intended to strengthen and regularize a heartbeat that has become unsteady, and that is not showing its usual pattern of activity. There are a variety of drugs available, each for a fairly specific use. The treatment of arrhythmias requires careful diagnosis as to the type of arrythmia. Herbal remedies have traditional uses in arrhythmia and some supplements may be beneficial, however, arrhythmia always requires professional medical treatment.

For further information

℞ DIRECTORY OF DRUGS:

antiarrhythmic including **cardiac glycoside**, **calcium-channel blocker**, **local anesthetic**-related drugs, certain **beta-blockers**, a number of other drugs, including: **amiodarone hydrochloride** • **bretylium tosylate** • **mexiletine hydrochloride** • **moricizine hydrochloride** • **phenytoin** • **propafenone hydrochloride** • **quinidine** • and **magnesium sulfate**

♣ HERBAL REMEDIES:

lily of the valley

⚖ VITAMINS, MINERALS, AND SUPPLEMENTS:

omega-3 fatty acid • coenzyme Q_{10}

arteriosclerosis

Arteriosclerosis is a condition in which the walls of arteries become narrowed or less elastic, impairing blood flow to the areas they supply. It is also known as "hardening of the arteries." The most common form occurs when fatty deposits accumulate and damage the arterial wall, which then seriously impedes blood flow (✿ **atherosclerosis**). A major component of the fatty deposits is cholesterol, which is found in animal fats and dairy products. People with a high risk of atherosclerosis include those with high cholesterol levels, who are obese (see ✿ **obesity**), smokers, those who take little exercise, and those with a family history of the disorder. Arteriosclerosis may also occur due to minerals such as calcium being deposited in the arterial walls over time, or to general thickening and loss of elasticity in the small arteries with age or as a reaction to high blood pressure. There are no symptoms from arteriosclerosis itself, but if the coronary arteries supplying part of the heart muscle are affected, it can lead to ✿ **angina pectoris** due to poor circulation at times of increased demand, or may cut off blood flow altogether and cause a ✿ **myocardial infarction** (heart attack). A similar situation affecting the arteries supplying blood to the brain may lead to a ✿ **stroke**. Arteriosclerosis in an artery supplying blood to the legs may cause pain on walking and even ✿ **gangrene** due to the impaired blood supply.

Treatment

A healthy diet, containing low levels of animal fats and sugar but plenty of fruit and vegetables, combined with regular exercise and no smoking, can help prevent the disorder or avert complications. Some supplements rich in ⚖ **omega-3 fatty acids** are considered to be beneficial and the herbal remedies, evening primrose, flax, garlic, and soybean can be used to lower blood cholesterol. Drug treatment to lower high cholesterol levels may be recommended. Once symptoms have developed, further drug treatment and/or surgery may be needed to attempt to restore blood flow.

For further information

℞ DIRECTORY OF DRUGS:

lipid-regulating drug

♣ HERBAL REMEDIES:

evening primrose • flax • garlic • hawthorn • mistletoe • soybean

♉ VITAMINS, MINERALS, AND SUPPLEMENTS:

acidophilus • (amino acid) arginine • chromium • garlic • niacin • omega-3 fatty acid • vitamin E

arteritis

Arteritis is an inflammatory condition of the outer coat or inner layers of an artery. It can occur alone, or as a complication of another disorder, for example ✪ rheumatoid arthritis and systemic ✪ lupus ethythematosus (SLE). There are various types including infantile arteritis, rheumatic arteritis, Takayasu's arteritis and Buerger's disease. Temporal arteritis, also called giant cell arteritis, is where there is inflammation of the blood vessels around the head and scalp. In some cases it is an ✪ autoimmune disorder.

Treatment

Treatment depends on the type, but might include ℞ corticosteroids to reduce the inflammation.

For further information

℞ DIRECTORY OF DRUGS:

corticosteroid

arthralgia

see ✪ musculoskeletal disorders.

arthritis

Arthritis is inflammation in one or more joints, which causes pain, swelling, and warmth and stiffness in the joint. It is a ✪ musculoskeletal disorder, and is a feature of many diseases, some of which also affect other body tissues. Causes include wear and tear, an inherited tendency, and sometimes infections. The most common form is ✪ osteoarthritis (also called osteoarthrosis), in which joint linings degenerate either spontaneously or following trauma or overuse. The cartilage lining the joint is first eroded, typically in the hip, knee, or thumb, followed by damage to the bone. It gives a characteristic appearance on X-rays.

The next most common form is ✪ rheumatoid arthritis, an ✪ autoimmune disorder (where the body attacks its own tissues). This occurs more often in women than in men and typically first affects the ankles, feet, fingers, and wrists, then later the hips, knees, and shoulders. It is diagnosed with a blood test, and damage to the bone in the joint may show up on X-rays. Usually, rheumatoid arthritis has periods of remission and relapse during which progressive joint damage accumulates. Sometimes it resolves spontaneously but may leave deformity.

A similar joint disease accompanied by fever and other symptoms in children is juvenile rheumatoid arthritis, known as Still's disease. Arthritis may also occur as a complication of ✪ gout, ✪ psoriasis, and some forms of ✪ tuberculosis.

Treatment

What treatment is used will depend on the type of arthritis. The pain of most forms of arthritis can be eased with painkillers (℞ analgesic drugs) and ℞ anti-inflammatory drugs. In osteoarthritis, reducing the load on joints by losing weight (if appropriate) often helps, and surgery is sometimes carried out, including the use of artificial replacement joints, particularly for the hips and knees. Rheumatoid arthritis requires specialist treatment and it may be treated by drugs, physiotherapy (to keep the joints mobile), or surgery (to replace severely damaged joints). There are many supplements and herbal remedies available that can be tried in order to prevent or relieve some of the symptoms of arthritis.

For further information

℞ DIRECTORY OF DRUGS:

anti-inflammatory • antirheumatic • corticosteroid • NSAID

♣ HERBAL REMEDIES:

agrimony • angelica • blackcurrant • black horehound • boneset • cayenne • celery • devil's claw • feverfew • guelder rose • juniper • parsley • willow • yucca

♉ VITAMINS, MINERALS, AND SUPPLEMENTS:

boron • chondroitin • conjugated linoleic acid • copper • glucosamine and chondroitin • niacin • omega-3 fatty acid • pantothenic acid • S-adenosylmethionine

ascariasis

see ✪ worms.

aspergillosis

see ✪ fungal infections.

asthma

Asthma is an obstructive airways disease. It is a disorder of the bronchial tubes that carry air to the lungs, and which go into spasm and become narrower during an asthmatic attack. The linings of the airways become swollen and inflamed, which can then block the smaller airways. This causes difficulty in breathing (especially exhaling), coughing, or wheezing. Asthma usually begins in childhood and is often part of a hereditary tendency (atopy) to allergic reactions (✪ allergy), including ✪ eczema, and ✪ hay fever. Asthma may be provoked by drugs, cold air, pollen, dust, animal dander, infections, exercise, emotional stress, and occasionally some foods.

Treatment

Asthma requires professional attention. Immediate treatment during an attack is usually with ℞ bronchodilator drugs that expand the air passages. These include ℞ beta-adrenergic stimulant drugs such as ℞ salbutamol and ℞ xanthine derivatives such as ℞ theophylline, which are generally inhaled through an inhaler or nebulizer. The aim of long-term treatment is to manage the disorder so that there are fewer attacks, and to reduce the severity of the symptoms during an attack. Drugs for this include inhaled ℞ corticosteroids, and some newer ℞ antiasthmatic and ℞ antiallergic drugs such as the ℞ leukotriene receptor antagonists, ℞ lipoxygenase inhibitors, also sometimes mast cell stabilizers such as ℞ cromolyn sodium and ℞ nedocromil sodium.

Identifying and then avoiding the allergens (triggers) which cause attacks is also an important part of the process. Vitamins C and B$_6$ have possible uses in alleviating asthma, and many herbal remedies are available that are reported to help.

For further information

℞ DIRECTORY OF DRUGS:

antiallergic • antiasthmatic • beta-adrenergic stimulant • bronchodilator • corticosteroid • leukotriene receptor antagonist • lipoxygenase inhibitor • xanthine

♣ HERBAL REMEDIES:

anise • bloodroot • cowslip • elecampane • evening primrose • horehound • lemon verbena • lobelia • onion • passionflower • pill-bearing spurge • senega snakeroot • skunk cabbage • spikenard • squill • sweet cicely • thyme

♒ VITAMINS, MINERALS, AND SUPPLEMENTS:

vitamin B$_6$ • vitamin C

atherosclerosis

Atherosclerosis is a common arterial disorder characterized by an accumulation of cholesterol and other fatty substances in the inner layers of large and medium sized arteries, which causes the arteries to narrow. It is a type of ✪ **arteriosclerosis**. Blood flow to the organs supplied by the affected artery is reduced. The condition is a major cause of ✪ **stroke**, ✪ **myocardial infarction**, ✪ **coronary artery disease**, and ✪ **angina pectoris**. The disorder usually occurs with ✪ **aging** and is associated with smoking, ✪ **hypertension**, a high fat diet and lack of exercise, and people with inherited ✪ **hyperlipidemia** and ✪ **diabetes mellitus** are at particular risk.

Treatment

A healthy, active lifestyle with a low-fat diet and no smoking is the best prevention. In addition, many vitamins and supplements are available that are thought to be beneficial, for example, by reducing levels of LDL-cholesterol (♒ **vitamin E**). For those at risk, drugs may be prescribed to regulate blood lipids, and the risk of thrombus formation can be reduced by taking ℞ **antiplatelets** or ℞ **anticoagulants**. Surgery may become necessary, for instance balloon angioplasty to open up blocked blood vessels, bypass operations when there is atherosclerosis of the coronary artery. ✪ **diabetes mellitus** and ✪ **hypertension**, if present, must be carefully controlled. See also ✪ **cardiovascular disorders**.

For further information

℞ DIRECTORY OF DRUGS:

lipid-regulating drug (including, **fibrate**, **statin**) • anticoagulant (for example, **warfarin sodium**) • antiplatelet drug (for example, aspirin)

♣ HERBAL REMEDIES:

celery • wolfberry, Chinese • evening primrose • flax • garlic • guelder rose • gutta percha • hawthorn • mistletoe • onion • soybean • yarrow

♒ VITAMINS, MINERALS, AND SUPPLEMENTS:

acidophilus • (amino acid) arginine • chromium • niacin • omega-3 fatty acid • vitamin E

athlete's foot

Athlete's foot (✪ **tinea** pedis) is a highly contagious type of ringworm. It is a ✪ **fungal infection** that affects the skin between the toes, and which blisters, splits, and scales.

Treatment

Treatment is with ℞ **antifungal** drugs in the form of powders or creams, together with thorough drying between the toes after bathing. A tincture of cloves may be beneficial.

For further information

℞ DIRECTORY OF DRUGS:

antifungal

♣ HERBAL REMEDIES:

clove • myrrh

atopic dermatitis

see ✪ **dermatitis**.

attention deficit disorder

Attention deficit disorder is a recently recognized condition, often abbreviated to ADD. It usually occurs in children and may include a range of symptoms such as poor concentration, impaired learning ability, and behavioral problems. It is often accompanied by extreme overactivity and an inability to sit still (hyperactivity or hyperkinesis), so the two together are sometimes called attention deficit hyperactivity disorder (ADHD). Such children need little sleep and are prone to continual fidgeting, impulsiveness, and little understanding of risk. They are hard to parent and difficult to teach, and may become frustrated and sometimes aggressive. In some cases, affected children have impaired intelligence or mild brain damage, but usually the label is applied to disruptive children with learning problems. The disorder is sometimes hereditary. Diagnosis should be made by an expert.

Treatment

Behavior or family therapy can help in many cases. Increasingly, CNS stimulant drugs that are amphetamine derivatives such as ℞ **methylphenidate** (Ritalin) are given, which, paradoxically, calm the child's behavior. Affected families sometimes report dramatic improvements by eliminating food additives from the child's diet, although few doctors suggest this approach.

For further information

℞ DIRECTORY OF DRUGS:

CNS stimulant

attention deficit hyperactivity disorder

see ✪ **attention deficit disorder**.

autoimmune disorder

An autoimmune disorder is one of a group of disorders caused by a reaction that is mediated by the body's immune system acting against tissue or organs within the individual's own body. There are a number of important diseases with at least some autoimmune component, including ✪ **rheumatoid arthritis**, systemic ✪ **lupus** erythematosus, type 2 (insulin-dependent) ✪ **diabetes mellitus**, some forms of ✪ **Addison's disease**, Graves' disease of the thyroid gland (✪ hyperthyroidism), ✪ myasthenia gravis, ✪ vitiligo, ✪ Sjögren's syndrome, and ✪ pernicious anemia.

There is a ✪ **hypersensitivity reaction** as the body attacks itself instead of attacking invading micro-organisms as is its normal task. The reason why the body becomes unable to tell "self" from "non-self" is not clear, but a predisposition (which sometimes is genetic) may be triggered, for instance following treatment by certain drugs, or often by a virus. Sometimes there is a specific reaction in just one type of tissue or organs, but other times it is less specific. The types of reaction vary, but generally there is destruction of one sort of tissue, interference with normal function, and sometimes excess growth. Tissues most affected include all blood elements, gland tissue, and connective tissue.

Treatment

The general principle is to try to correct abnormal function, and for this many different drugs and treatments are used, for instance administered ℞ **hormones** such as insulin and thyroxine, or blood transfusions to replace missing factors. Drugs that down-moderate the immune system are valuable in many autoimmune disorders, especially ℞ **corticosteroids**. If sufficiently serious, ℞ **immunosuppressant** drugs may be used. In rheumatoid conditions, anti-inflammatory drugs such as ℞ **NSAIDs** are taken. See individual disorder entries for more information.

For further information

℞ DIRECTORY OF DRUGS:

corticosteroid • hormone (insulin analog, thyroid hormone)• immunosuppressant • NSAID

avitaminosis

see ✪ vitamin deficiency.

backache

Backache is a common condition, a ✪ **musculoskeletal disorder**, with many possible causes. Most backache results from strain, either of the ligaments or the muscles, or is related to some misalignment of an intervertebral disk (the disks between the vertebrae of the spine). Occasionally, a nerve is pinched and this may cause fibrositis or more severe symptoms. ✪ **arthritis** may be a cause. If there is persistent or sharp pain, consult a doctor for diagnosis.

Treatment

Often rest, or adjustment of posture, may relieve mild ✪ **pain**. Pain-killers, massage, or gentle exercises can also help with short-term strains. Some forms of complementary medicine (such as chiropractic or osteopathy) can be beneficial in treating long-term backache. In severe cases of slipped disk, surgery may be the best option if other methods do not control the pain. Some herbal remedies (for example, ♣ **juniper oil**) used externally may give some relief. See also ✪ **pain**.

For further information

℞ DIRECTORY OF DRUGS:

narcotic analgesic • non-narcotic analgesic • NSAID

♣ HERBAL REMEDIES:

juniper

bacterial infections

"Germs" are the root cause of a substantial proportion of human disease, both acute and chronic. Bacteria are microscopic single-celled organisms, larger than viruses but smaller than protozoan parasites.

Based on form, pathogenic (disease-causing) bacteria can be divided into a number of families of which the main three are bacilli (rod-shaped), cocci (spherical) and spirochetes or spirilla (spiral-shaped). The bacilli are responsible for botulism (such as paralytic ✪ **food poisoning**), ✪ **diphtheria**, ✪ Legionnaires' disease, ✪ **pertussis** (whooping cough), salmonellosis (for example, food poisoning), shigellosis (bacterial ✪ **dysentery**), ✪ **tetanus**, ✪ **tuberculosis** (TB), ✪ **typhoid fever**. The cocci are responsible for bacterial ✪ **endo-carditis**, bacterial ✪ **meningitis**, ✪ **pneumonia**, ✪ **tonsillitis**, ✪ **toxic shock syndrome**, and many ✪ **skin conditions**. Spirochetes are a small group responsible for ✪ **leptospirosis**, ✪ **Lyme disease**, ✪ **syphilis** and yaws (a tropical infectious disease). Though the form of pathogenic bacteria is important in their identification, there are a number of other clinically important properties. Some are aerobic (they require oxygen to multiply) so are most commonly found in the respiratory system and the skin, while others are anaerobic (do not require oxygen) so can thrive in deep wounds, internal organs, and in soil (and can therefore form spores in soil infecting wounds and cause tetanus and botulism). They are divided in another way in the pathology laboratory according to how they stain with a procedure known as Gram's stain. Those bacteria that stain in one way are called Gram-positive (including several *Streptococcus* and *Staphylococcus* species responsible for a range of serious infections, and many *Clostridium* species) and those that do not are Gram-negative (many *Salmonella* and *Vibrio cholerae*, which causes ✪ **cholera**). The body is well equipped to deal with minor bacterial infections, and the immune system recognizes that the potentially pathogenic organisms are "foreign". They are engulfed by white blood cells called neutrophils, while other white blood cells, lymphocytes, secrete antibodies that attack the bacteria. Sometimes a first infection will cause the body to produce antibodies, and these may resist further attack.

Treatment

Bacterial infections are treated with ℞ **antibacterial** drugs, of which some are ℞ **antibiotic** agents. For certain infections, the immune system can be primed so as to be ready for many bacterial infections by the process of vaccination (immunization with a vaccine). Some herbal remedies (such as ⚕ **garlic**) and supplements (such as ⚕ **vitamin C**) are promoted as being beneficial in preventing, treating or reducing tendency to ✪ **infection** in general. See specific disorder entries for more details.

balanitis

Balanitis is inflammation of the glans penis (head of the penis) and foreskin. Symptoms include soreness, and sometimes a discharge and rash. In diabetic balanitis, it is caused by the sugar content of the urine. Other causes include ✪ **bacterial infections**, ✪ **fungal infections** (for example, ✪ **candidiasis**) or ✪ **allergy**.

Treatment

Treatment depends on the underlying cause, but might include drugs to treat the infective component.

For further information

℞ DIRECTORY OF DRUGS:
antibacterial • antifungal

baldness

see ✪ alopecia.

basal cell carcinoma

see ✪ cancer.

Becker's muscular dystrophy

see ✪ muscular dystrophy.

bedsore

Bedsores are painful ulcerations of the skin and damage to the underlying tissues caused by constant pressure. They usually occur in bedridden people so ill or old that they cannot move themselves, or in unconscious individuals. The blood supply to the area may be seriously reduced, and the nerves affected, so that the person may not even be aware of the condition, which in severe cases can lead to ✪ gangrene. The condition is known technically as a decubitus ulcer or a pressure sore.

Treatment

Treatment is primarily by prevention: individuals should be turned regularly and be well cushioned. If a sore develops, dressings and good nursing care are vital. If these procedures do not work, then treatment with ℞ **antibacterials**, locally or systemically, may be necessary to treat any infection.

For further information

℞ DIRECTORY OF DRUGS:
antibacterial

bed-wetting

Bed-wetting is the involuntary passing of urine at night (the technical term is nocturnal enuresis). This is abnormal only after a child has definitely learned bladder control, which, on average, occurs around age 4. However, there are wide variations and many children are not dry at night until age 7 or later. Persistent bed-wetting often runs in families. Occasionally, there may be an underlying urinary tract problem, such as ✪ infection, or ✪ diabetes mellitus. More often the problem is behavioral (for example, it may occur after a stressful experience such as a divorce), and usually resolves itself with age.

Treatment

Patience and the avoidance of criticism are essential. Practical measures include a mattress cover, not having a drink just before bedtime, and encouragement to pass urine just before sleeping. Behavioral techniques such as rewarding dry nights, or alarm systems (a bell and pad), which wake the child just as urination starts, can be successful. Drug treatment may be offered for persistent bed-wetting.

For further information

℞ DIRECTORY OF DRUGS:
antidiuretic (for example, **desmopressin**) • **antispasmodic** (for example, **oxybutynin**) • **sympathomimetic** (for example, **ephedrine**) • **antidepressant** (tricyclic type, for example, **imipramine, nortriptyline hydrochloride**)
♣ HERBAL REMEDIES:
thyme

bee sting

see ✪ sting.

Behçet's syndrome

Behçet's syndrome is a rare and sometimes severe inflammatory disorder (see ✪ **inflammation**) characterized by recurrent mouth ✪ ulcers and genital ulcers, ✪ uveitis, and other effects including on the nervous system and blood. Its cause is unknown, but it is more common in men.

Treatment

Topical corticosteroids may be prescribed for ulcers and eye-drops for inflamed eyes. For more severe cases, drugs taken orally may be necessary. Some herbal remedies may relieve symptoms of uveitis and ulcers.

For further information

℞ DIRECTORY OF DRUGS:
corticosteroid

benign prostatic hyperplasia

see ✪ benign prostatic hypertrophy.

benign prostatic hypertrophy

Benign prostatic hypertrophy (BPH; also called benign prostatic hyperplasia) is where there is enlargement of the prostate gland. It is a common, noncancerous disorder among men over the age of 50. It is a progressive disorder that can lead to obstruction of the urethra and difficulty in passing urine.

Treatment

In mild cases, limiting fluid intake in the evening can provide relief of symptoms. In more serious cases, drug treatment may be necessary; commonly ℞ **alpha-adrenoceptor blockers** and sometimes antiandrogen drugs, or even surgery to remove part of the gland. There is good evidence that some herbal remedies (such as ♣ saw palmetto) are effective in treating some of the symptoms (such as any urination problems) of benign prostatic hypertrophy.

For further information

℞ DIRECTORY OF DRUGS:
alpha-adrenoceptor blocker (doxazosin mesylate, prazosin hydrochloride, tamsulosin hydrochloride, terazosin) • antiandrogen (finasteride)
♣ HERBAL REMEDIES:
saw palmetto • stinging nettle

beriberi

Beriberi is a ✪ **vitamin deficiency** disorder caused by a lack of ⚕⚕ **vitamin B$_1$** (thiamine). It occurs most commonly in areas where the diet consists mainly of polished rice. In Western countries it is prevalent among alcoholics (see ✪ **alcoholism**). Symptoms are those of muscle disorders, especially of the heart muscle, accompanied by the degeneration of nerves (peripheral neuritis), causing numbness and weakness. This condition by itself is dry beriberi; wet beriberi involves additional ✪ **fluid retention** in the tissues, causing swelling (edema).

Treatment
Treatment is to make up the vitamin deficiency.

For further information
⚖ VITAMINS, MINERALS, AND SUPPLEMENTS:
vitamin B$_1$ (thiamine)

bilharzia
see ✪ **schistosomiasis**.

biliary colic
see ✪ **colic**.

binge eating
see ✪ **bulimia**.

bipolar affective disorder
see ✪ **bipolar disorder**.

bipolar disorder
Also known as bipolar affective disorder or manic-depressive illness, bipolar disorder is a severe ✪ **mental illness** in which the person experiences extreme ✪ **depression** that alternates with bouts either of relative normality or of mania. During manic phases the person may appear elated or frenetic, with euphoria or irritability, incoherent speech, impulsiveness, extravagance, and poor judgment, sometimes becoming violent if grandiose plans are thwarted. Changes between moods may or may not be triggered by external factors, but the extremes of apathy reached in depressive phases, and the extremes of activity and violence reached in manic phases (if they occur) mean that hospitalization is often necessary. Some authorities regard bipolar disorder as a ✪ **psychotic disorder**, and certainly antipsychotic drugs, sometimes by acute injection, may be required to control manic phases, but the disorder as a whole is perceived by others as an ✪ **affective disorder** (that is to say, a mood disorder). There may be a hereditary predisposition to bipolar disorder.

Treatment
Treatment is with psychiatric intervention and the use of specialist drugs. The manic phase may require acute initial treatment with a markedly sedative ℞ **antipsychotic** such as ℞ **haloperidol** or ℞ **chlorpromazine**. Maintenance treatment to reduce the frequency of manic episodes is generally with lithium, but if this is not effective other drugs may be tried (for example, ℞ **carbamazepine** or ℞ **valproate sodium** (also used in other forms including valproic acid ℞ **divalproex sodium**). ℞ **Antidepressants** drugs may help reduce the severity or incidence of the depressive phase.

For further information
℞ DIRECTORY OF DRUGS:
antidepressant • antimanic • antipsychotic

bladder cancer
see ✪ **cancer**.

bleeding
see ✪ **hemorrhage**; ✪ **bleeding disorder**.

bleeding disorder
Bleeding or blood disorders are a group of conditions characterized by bleeding in the absence of injury, or tendency to prolonged or excessive bleeding after tissue injury. These disorders are grouped according to the root cause, generally some defect in the blood coagulation system, in platelet aggregation, or in the wall of the blood vessels themselves.

Coagulation of blood is a complex cascade of interacting biochemical processes mediated by a number of enzymes and coagulation factors. There are a number of coagulation factors that may be defective or absent, often due to a sex-linked genetic disorder, including deficient factor VIII (causing ✪ **hemophilia**), and factor IX (causing the Christmas factor disorder (Christmas disease)). A further Factor VIII defect is thought to cause von Willebrand's disease. Apart from inherited disorders, there are a number of further causes of coagulation defects, including a deficiency of vitamin K ("Koagulation" vitamin, essential to the blood-clotting process) due to diet or absorption problems, or liver disease. A further disorder is disseminated intravascular coagulation (DID), where various triggers cause clotting and platelet aggregation in small blood vessels, which uses up blood factors, so paradoxically results in an increased and severe tendency to bleed.

Platelet aggregation has an important role in preventing hemorrhage by plugging damaged blood vessels and forming an important part of a blood thrombus or clot. A shortage is called thrombocytopenia, when there may be multiple purple ✪ **bruises** caused by bleeding into the tissues. A number of drugs cause thrombocytopenia or interfere with the aggregation process (for example, aspirin).

Blood vessel defects may cause a tendency to bleed, and these may be seen in ✪ **scurvy** and after long-term corticosteroid treatment. There are a number of conditions of increased friability ("crumbliness") of small blood vessels or capillaries (for example, ✪ **menorrhagia**). ✪ **hemorrhage**, commonly called bleeding, is a loss of blood from the cardiovascular circulatory system. See also ✪ **hemorrhoids**.

Treatment
Treatment, where possible, is rectification of the cause. The missing blood factors may be replaced by an infusion of concentrated preparation of the factors prepared from human blood (see ℞ **hemostatic**). Blood transfusions may be necessary. Any dietary deficiencies need to be corrected. ⚖ **vitamin K** may be given by mouth or injection. A variety of specialized drugs are used for specific indications including ℞ **hematopoietic** agents or ℞ **hemostatics** agents (including antifibrinolytics and blood coag-

ulation factors), vitamin K (℞ **phytonadione**). The herbal remedies ♣ **plantain** and ♣ **smartweed** are used to manage bleeding or relieve bruising.

blepharitis

Blepharitis is an inflammatory condition of the margin of one or both eyelids. Symptoms of this ✪ **inflammation** include swelling, redness, itching, and crusts of dried mucus on the eyelids. Ulcerative blepharitis is caused by a ✪ **bacterial infection**, non-ulcerative blepharitis by ✪ **seborrhea**, ✪ **psoriasis**, or an ✪ **allergy**.

Treatment

Holding a warm, damp cloth against the eyelids can relieve symptoms. Topical ℞ **antibacterial** antibiotics to treat infection, and ℞ **corticosteroids** to reduce inflammation may be necessary.

For further information

℞ DIRECTORY OF DRUGS:
antibacterial (**bacitracin, gentamicin, tobramycin**) • corticosteroid (for example, **dexamethasone, prednisolone**)

blood disorders

see ✪ **bleeding disorder**; ✪ **hemorrhage**.

blood poisoning

see ✪ **septicemia**.

boil

A boil (furuncle) is a rounded, red, and painful swelling on the skin, containing pus. It is a smaller version of an ✪ **abscess**. Boils develop when *Staphylococcus* bacteria get into a hair follicle, a sebaceous duct, or an open wound.

Treatment

In general, boils heal spontaneously, but they may heal more quickly if the pus is released in aseptic conditions. Local heat may encourage them to "come to a head" and release the pus. Lancing a boil without antiseptic preparations or squeezing it usually will only spread the infection.

For further information

℞ DIRECTORY OF DRUGS:
antibacterial • antiseptic
♣ HERBAL REMEDIES:
arnica • brewer's yeast • devil's claw • marshmallow • myrrh • slippery elm

botulism

see ✪ **food poisoning**.

boulimia

see ✪ **bulimia**.

brain attack

see ✪ **stroke**.

brain-motor disorders

Brain-motor disorder is a term used here for a loose aggregation of neurological disorders of the central nervous system (CNS), which are characterized by disruption of such motor functions of the body as fine control of hand, leg, eye, and facial movements, and eventually the ability to move and walk. They can be caused by the degeneration of nerve centers in the brain and spinal cord that are involved in muscle control. Such degenerative diseases include ✪ **Huntington's disease** (chorea), ✪ **Parkinson's disease**, ✪ **Creutzfeldt-Jakob disease**, ✪ **multiple sclerosis**, Wernicke-Korsakoff syndrome, ✪ **motor neuron disease**, ✪ **amyotrophic lateral sclerosis**, Tourette syndrome and related choreas. There are other central nervous system degenerative disorders where motor degeneration is not a major or necessary characteristic, and these are not discussed here, but under their own headings (✪ **Alzheimer's disease**, ✪ **dementia**). Other motor disorders arise primarily not because of degenerative neurological disease, but from physical damage due to the lack of oxygen following hemorrhage (for example, subarachnoid hemorrhage, subdural hemorrhage, ✪ **stroke**) or other accidents. In a few instances there is a known cause for the condition, for instance vitamin B_1 deficiency and alcohol abuse in Wernicke-Korsakoff syndrome, and in these instances a reversal of the condition may be possible by eliminating the causal factors. Yet other motor disorders arise not through dysfunction in the CNS, but in the peripheral nervous system. For instance the muscle weakness disorder ✪ **myasthenia gravis**, is caused by impaired transmission between nerve and skeletal muscle.

Treatment

Most of these conditions are treated with physiotherapy and specialized medical treatment together with appropriate drug regimens. In some instances, it is possible to identify the cause as a deficiency or imbalance of certain neurotransmitters involved in CNS motor control, and then to use drugs to mimic neurotransmitter action, or to increase or decrease neurotransmitter release and actions; thus in Parkinson's disease, the action of dopamine is enhanced and that of acetylcholine suppressed (℞ **antiparkinsonism** drugs). In many cases the mood of the person is supported with ℞ **antidepressant** drugs (for example, Creutzfeldt-Jakob disease, Tourette syndrome). If there is an inflammatory component to the disorder, ℞ **corticosteroids** or ℞ **immunomodulators** drugs such as ℞ **interferons** may be useful (for example, multiple sclerosis). In many cases, especially for involuntary muscular tics and choreas, specialist drugs (including drugs also used as antipsychotic drugs) have been found to suppress such motor symptoms (℞ **haloperidol** and ℞ **pimozide** in Tourette's syndrome and related choreas; ℞ **fluphenazine** in Huntington's disease). Some drugs help improve outcome, for instance in amyotrophic lateral sclerosis, ℞ **riluzole** extends survival time and time to tracheostomy (see ℞ **brain-motor disorder treatment**). If muscle contractions are a problem (for example, Creutzfeldt-Jakob disease), ℞ **skeletal muscle relaxant** drugs may provide relief. For more information, see individual disorder entries.

brain syndrome

see ✪ **psychotic disorders**.

breast cancer

Breast cancer is a malignant tumor of breast tissue. The most common serious form of ⊙ **cancer** in women, it can also occur in men. The underlying cause is still unclear, but it is thought that the female sex hormone estrogen is an important factor. Some cases are hereditary (approximately 1 in 20), and certain people are more at risk than others (for example, those who are obese, or who have delayed or avoided pregnancy). The risk increases with age. The usual initial symptom is a lump in the breast, or, rarely, bleeding or discharge from the nipple. Undetected it may spread to adjacent lymph nodes, causing a lump in the armpit. The earlier treatment is begun, the better the chances are of a complete recovery. For this reason, women are encouraged to examine their breasts regularly (palpation) for lumps and to consult a doctor immediately for further tests (for example, mammography, ultrasound scanning) if any are found.

Treatment

Women with a high risk of breast cancer, especially those with an adverse family history of the condition, may take the estrogen-antagonist ℞ **tamoxifen** to reduce the risk. The usual treatment is surgery to remove the tumor (lumpectomy) or the whole breast (mastectomy). Sometimes radiotherapy and cytotoxic (cancer-killing) drugs may be prescribed, or tamoxifen may be taken to reduce the risk of estrogen-dependent secondary metastasis. A woman who has had a mastectomy may be fitted with an artificial breast (prosthesis) or have reconstructive surgery to construct a new breast mound.

For further information

℞ DIRECTORY OF DRUGS:
anticancer • antiestrogen (including **tamoxifen**)

brittle bones

see ⊙ **osteoporosis**.

bronchial congestion

Bronchial congestion is the accumulation of fluid (mucus) in the bronchi. It is a common symptom of ⊙ **respiratory tract disorders** such as ⊙ **colds**.

Treatment

℞ **Expectorants**, included in a lot of cough and cold cures and herbal remedies can be used to aid the coughing up of mucus. See also ⊙ **catarrh**.

For further information

℞ DIRECTORY OF DRUGS:
cold and cough preparation • expectorant
♣ HERBAL REMEDIES:
horehound • senega snakeroot • wood sage

bronchiectasis

Bronchiectasis is a ⊙ **respiratory tract disorder** characterized by a persistent ⊙ **cough** with large amounts of sputum. It is caused by the abnormal widening of the bronchi and the destruction of their linings. It often starts in childhood as a result of a lung infection, but there are other causes. Symptoms include cough, yellow or dark green sputum, coughing up blood, bad breath, shortness of breath and wheezing, and finger clubbing.

Treatment

Treatment consists of avoiding smoky atmospheres, chest physiotherapy, and drugs to widen the airways, and to treat any infection.

For further information

℞ DIRECTORY OF DRUGS:
antibacterial • bronchodilator

bronchitis

Bronchitis is a ⊙ **respiratory tract disorder** characterized by inflammation of the bronchi (the main airways that lead to the lungs). It often affects the bronchioles (smaller airways) as well as the throat and larynx. The acute form of the disorder is caused usually by a ⊙ **viral infection**, and results in a ⊙ **fever** with narrowing of the airways and coughing up of pus-containing sputum. It may be caused by the spread of another infection, for example, a respiratory tract infection, or a ⊙ **cold** that has spread to the sinuses. Chronic bronchitis, associated with a disorder of the upper respiratory tract, heavy cigarette smoking, or breathing of polluted air, also causes a persistent, productive ⊙ **cough** and possibly breathlessness.

Treatment

Acute viral bronchitis usually lasts only a few days. A bacterial infection may be treated with ℞ **antibacterials**, and an expectorant/mucolytic may be helpful in loosening the mucus; steam inhalations and cough remedies may also be beneficial. Many herbal remedies are available, which can be used for symptomatic relief in bronchitis, for example, to ease an irritating cough or relieve ⊙ **bronchial congestion** and ⊙ **catarrh**.

For further information

℞ DIRECTORY OF DRUGS:
antibacterial • bronchodilator • corticosteroid • expectorant • mucolytic
♣ HERBAL REMEDIES:
angelica • anise • black cherry • bloodroot • brewer's yeast • cardamom • chamomile, German • Chinese cinnamon (*Cinnamomum cassia*) **• cowslip • echinacea • elecampane • eucalyptus • fennel • ground ivy • hempnettle • horehound • horseradish • Iceland moss • ivy, English • Japanese mint • licorice • linden • lobelia • maidenhair fern • mallow • marshmallow • mullein • nasturtium • oak • pill-bearing spurge • pimpinella • pleurisy root • sanicle • senega snakeroot • skunk cabbage • soap bark • soapwort • squill • star anise • thyme • watercress • wild thyme • wood sage**

bronchopneumonia

see ⊙ **pneumonia**.

bronze diabetes

see ⊙ **hemochromatosis**.

brucellosis

Brucellosis (also called undulant fever) is caused by a ⊙ **bacterial infection** of cattle that can be passed to humans through contact or by drinking unpasteurized milk. Human symptoms include fatigue, weakness, and headache, then alternating fever and chills with enlargement of the spleen and lymph nodes (in the neck and armpits).

Treatment

Treatment is with prolonged courses of ℞ **antibacterial** drugs. Left untreated, the disorder may persist for years.

For further information

℞ DIRECTORY OF DRUGS:
antibacterial

bruise

Bruises (contusion) are the discoloration of the skin and swelling that are caused by a blow or excessive pressure. The color, caused by leakage of blood from damaged blood vessels, is pink at first, turning blue then yellowish. Unexplained bruising can be a sign of a ✪ **bleeding disorder**.

Treatment

A minor bruise can be relieved with cold compresses and will resolve spontaneously. Severe bruising should be examined by a doctor in case there is internal injury (such as a bone fracture) that may need treatment. If bruising appears and there is no obvious cause, it could be a sign of a ✪ **bleeding disorder** and should be examined by a doctor. Many herbal remedies, used externally, are considered to be beneficial in relieving bruises.

For further information

♣ HERBAL REMEDIES:
arnica • comfrey • plantain • shepherd's purse • witch hazel

Buerger's disease

see ✪ peripheral vascular disorders.

bulimia

Bulimia is compulsive binge overeating, often followed by measures to induce weight loss, for instance when associated with ✪ **anorexia nervosa**. The disorder typically appears in young women with poor self-image. There may also be symptoms of ✪ **anxiety** or ✪ **depression**. The physical symptoms of bulimia include abdominal pain and eroded teeth (the latter caused by gastric acid from induced vomiting).

Treatment

Specialist medical treatment is required. Normally, psychotherapy, especially cognitive therapy is recommended for bulimia associated with anorexia. Some antidepressant drugs seem to be helpful, for instance ℞ **fluoxetine** (Prozac) and also ℞ **lithium** are sometimes tried.

For further information

℞ DIRECTORY OF DRUGS:
antidepressant • lithium

burn

Burns are the damage or destruction of tissue caused by extreme heat, caustic chemicals, radiation, or high-voltage electricity. Similar damage caused by hot liquids or steam is called a scald. Burns are classified as first, second, or third degree. A first-degree burn damages only the outer layer of skin (the epidermis), causing reddening but no blisters; a second-degree burn is accompanied by blistering, and may damage the second layer of skin (the dermis); and a third-degree burn penetrates deeper, and destroys all the skin and possibly the tissues below—although, because nerve endings are also destroyed, it may be less painful than the other types. The seriousness of a burn, however, depends more on the extent of the area affected than the depth of the burn. See also ✪ **sunburn**.

Treatment

Any burn that involves more than 10% of the body's surface needs emergency treatment for shock (preferably in a specialist hospital burns unit) and to reduce the risk of infection. A skin graft may also be required. Minor burns should be placed under cold running water (to remove heat) for at least 10 minutes and then covered with a dry antiseptic dressing. Several herbal remedies are said to be useful in treating burns, however, in general cream or ointments should not be used.

For further information

℞ DIRECTORY OF DRUGS:
antiseptic (dry)

♣ HERBAL REMEDIES:
acanthus • aloe • cajuput • chamomile, German • echinacea • marigold • St. John's wort • white lily

bursitis

Bursitis is the ✪ **inflammation** of a bursa (a fluid-filled sac located in areas subject to friction, such as joints). It is caused by infection, pressure, or injury. Housemaid's knee, for example, affects the bursa of the knee. The bursa becomes swollen, causing pain and tenderness, and restricts the movement of the joint.

Treatment

Housemaid's knee is prevented by avoiding kneeling for long periods, particularly on hard surfaces. Once symptoms arise you should avoid kneeling at all. In any sort of bursitis, resting the affected joint, and taking painkilling drugs, may help. In severe cases, a doctor may drain off the excess fluid or inject ℞ **corticosteroid** drugs. Bursitis due to infection may be treated with an ℞ **antibacterial**.

For further information

℞ DIRECTORY OF DRUGS:
analgesic • corticosteroid • NSAID

calculus

Calculi are abnormal stones formed from an accumulation of mineral salts. Dental calculi take the form of a crust-like deposit on the crown and roots of teeth. Biliary calculi (✪ **gallstone**) are formed in the gallbladder or biliary tract. Urinary tract calculi are stones in the kidneys (renal), ureters, and bladder. The incidence of urinary tract calculi varies greatly geographically, and is, in part, related to diet. They are much more common in men than women, are commoner in the summer (possibly related to increased sweating and hence concentration of urine), and tend to reoccur in individuals. They may accompany urinary infection, ✪ **gout**, hyperparathyroidism or other ✪ **metabolic disorder**. Symptoms of renal calculi include renal ✪ **colic**; and of bladder calculi, difficulty in passing urine.

Treatment

Renal colic is treated immediately with bed rest and analgesics, with plenty of fluid in order to facilitate the passing of the stone. Larger stones need surgical intervention, though lithotripsy—disintegration of the stone with shock waves generated outside the body—has greatly aided treatment. Where stones are generated by metabolic disorders (for example, ✪ **cystinuria**), this may sometimes be corrected with drugs. Gallstones are sometimes treated with choliolythics, drugs that help dissolve the stones. Many herbal remedies are claimed to help, but evidence of their efficacy is often lacking.

For further information

℞ DIRECTORY OF DRUGS:
gallstone treatment (choliolythics including **ursodiol, monoctanoin**) • **narcotic analgesic** • **NSAIDs** (for example, **diclofenac**)

♣ HERBAL REMEDIES:
arenaria rubra • **asparagus** • **beans** (*Phaseolus vulgaris*) • **boldo** • **couchgrass** (*Agropyron repens*) • **goldenrod** • **horseradish** • **horsetail** • **hydrangea** • **Java tree** • **lovage** • **parsley** • **spiny rest harrow** • **stinging nettle** • **wild carrot**

cancer

Cancer (medically called neoplasm) is any of a large group of malignant diseases, which result in the presence of a malignant tumor formed by the abnormal and uncontrolled growth of cells. The cells then attach to other tissues, and may destroy them in the process. A cancer can form in any organ of the body, particularly in connective tissue, including bone and cartilage (sarcoma), or in the epithelium (membrane) that lines many internal organs and is present in quantity in the skin (carcinoma). Another form of cancer is ✪ **leukemia**, which affects the blood-producing bone marrow, and leads to the formation of cancerous white blood cells.

Part of the condition of malignancy is that cancers may spread around the body (by metastases), conveyed by the blood or lymphatic system. Initial symptoms of cancer depend on where in the body it develops, but may include skin ulceration, unexpected hemorrhage (bleeding) or discharge, a palpable lump under the skin, unusual difficulty in swallowing or defecating, an increase in the size of a skin marking (such as a mole), or blood in the sputum. In the US, the most common bodily sites for cancer are the skin, lung, prostate gland, breast, and colon. Cancer is the second biggest killer (heart disease is number one) in the US and the most common cause of death in children between ages 3 and 14.

Genetic (hereditary) factors (including ethnic background) increase the risk of many cancers, as do age, gender, and even where you live. Other influences such as smoking, radiation, and some ✪ **viral infections** are linked with the development of certain tumors; such cancer-promoting factors are called carcinogens. See also ✪ **breast cancer**; ✪ **prostate cancer**; ✪ **leukemia**.

Treatment

Treatment depends on where the cancer is, but often includes surgery, radiotherapy, and chemotherapy (cancer-killing drugs). In general, the earlier the treatment, the more likely it is to be successful. Prevention of some forms of cancer is, to an extent, possible by avoidance of substances (and associated activities, such as avoiding exposure to the sun to reduce the risk of skin cancer) known to be potential carcinogens. A traditional herbal remedy is ♣ **lapacho**, which is claimed to have a beneficial effect on some cancers. A number of dietary supplements are claimed to have properties that help protect against some cancers.

For further information

℞ DIRECTORY OF DRUGS:
anticancer • **cytotoxic**

♣ HERBAL REMEDIES:
garlic • **lapacho**

⚖ VITAMINS, MINERALS, AND SUPPLEMENTS:
amino acid (**glutamine**) • **antioxidant** • **calcium** • **carotenoid** (including **lycopene**) • **coenzyme Q**$_{10}$ • **conjugated linoleic acid** • **DHEA** • **folic acid** • **isoflavone** • **selenium** • **spirulina and other algae** • **vitamin C** • **vitamin D** • **vitamin E**

candida albicans

see ✪ **candidiasis**.

candidiasis

Candidiasis (also called moniliasis; thrush) is a ✪ **fungal infection** by a yeast-like fungus, some species of which live normally (and harmlessly) on the body. It occurs in moist, enclosed areas, such as the mouth, bronchial passages, and vagina, and in folds of skin. It appears as white blotches on red, inflamed tissue, and may itch. The fungus causes infection mainly when there is some change or abnormality in the external or internal environment, for example, fluctuating hormonal levels, a course of antibacterials, or an impaired immune system (for example, in ✪ **AIDS**). As an infection it can also be transmitted fairly easily to others by direct contact.

Treatment

Treatment is with ℞ **antifungal** drugs given as creams, tablets, or vaginal pessaries. The dietary supplement ⚖ **acidophilus** is also thought to be useful in preventing and treating candidiasis.

For further information

℞ DIRECTORY OF DRUGS:
antifungal

⚖ VITAMINS, MINERALS, AND SUPPLEMENTS:
acidophilus

canker sore

see ✪ **mouth ulcer**.

carbuncle

A carbuncle is a pus-filled swelling on the skin surface, caused by a ✪ **bacterial infection**. It has multiple heads or is formed in a cluster of swellings, and effectively represents a collection of ✪ **boils** with several drainage channels. Common sites are the back of the neck, buttocks, and thighs.

Treatment

Treatment is with an ℞ **antibacterial**. Occasionally, it may be necessary to lance the swelling to release the pus.

Key to symbols: ✪ = Disorder Section ℞ = Drug Section ♣ = Herbal Section ⚖ = Supplement Section

For further information
℞ DIRECTORY OF DRUGS:
antibacterial
♣ HERBAL REMEDIES:
arnica • brewer's yeast • devil's claw • marshmallow • myrrh • slippery elm

cardiac arrhythmia
see ✿ arrhythmia.

cardiac disease
see ✿ heart disease.

cardiac insufficiency
see ✿ cardiovascular disorders; ✿ heart disease.

cardiovascular disease
see ✿ cardiovascular disorders.

cardiovascular disorders
Cardiovascular disorders is a general term, which includes ✿ **heart disease**, for any of the many disorders of the heart and/or circulation including ✿ **angina pectoris**, ✿ **heart failure**, ✿ **heart valve disorders**, ✿ **hypertension** (high blood pressure), ✿ **coronary artery disease**, coronary thrombosis, hypertrophy of the heart, bacterial ✿ **endocarditis**, bradycardia (a slowing of the heart), tachycardia (speeding of the heart), heart block; ✿ **atherosclerosis**, ✿ **arteriosclerosis**, ✿ **myocardial infarction**, ✿ **arrhythmias**, ✿ **peripheral vascular disorders**, ✿ **Raynaud's disease**, ✿ **varicose veins**, ✿ **venous insufficiency**, and cardiac insufficiency (inability of the heart to pump efficiently). Some cardiovascular disorders (for example, atherosclerosis) predispose to others (such as hypertension). See individual disorder entries for further details.
Treatment
For some cardiovascular disorders (such as hypertension), risk factors include smoking, being overweight, an unhealthy diet, and lack of exercise; and life-style changes such as giving up smoking, weight loss, and exercise can result in significant improvements in symptoms. Treatment depends on the disorder and its cause, and may include surgery and drugs such as ℞ **antiarrhythmics**, ℞ **cardiac glycosides**, ℞ **antianginals**, ℞ **vasodilators**, ℞ **heart failure treatment**, ℞ **diuretics**, ℞ **ACE inhibitors**, ℞ **beta-blockers** and other ℞ **antihypertensives** drugs; also ancillary ℞ **lipid-regulating drugs** treatment together with drugs of the ℞ **anticoagulants** and ℞ **antiplatelet** agents types. A number of dietary supplements (including ⚕ **amino acids** (arginine, taurine), ⚕ **antioxidants**, ⚕ **carotenoids**, ⚕ **coenzyme Q$_{10}$**, ⚕ **conjugated linoleic acid**, ⚕ **DHEA**, ℞ **folic acid**, ⚕ **isoflavones**, ⚕ **magnesium**, ⚕ **omega-3 fatty acid**, ⚕ **S-adenosylmethionine**, ⚕ **selenium**, ⚕ **vitamin B$_6$**, ⚕ **vitamin B$_{12}$**, ⚕ **vitamin C**, ⚕ **vitamin E**) are claimed to protect against cardiovascular disease by, for example, lowering blood cholesterol levels or reducing free radicals, and many herbal remedies are claimed to be of use (including ♣ **hawthorn**, ⚕ **garlic**, ♣ **soybean**, ♣ **horse**

chestnut, ♣ **witch hazel**, ♣ **bilberry**, ♣ **butcher's broom**, ♣ **rosemary**). See individual disorder entries for more details.

carpal tunnel syndrome
Carpal tunnel syndrome is a set of symptoms caused by the compression of the median nerve between the carpal bones of the wrist and the band of strong fibrous tissue over them. The nerve normally serves the muscles of the ball of the thumb and transmits sensory information from all the fingers except the little finger. When it is compressed it results in tingling and numbness in all the areas to which it is connected. It may occur for no apparent reason, or following trauma, overuse of the wrist, in ✿ **diabetes mellitus**, in ✿ **pregnancy-related disorders**, or ✿ **hypothyroidism**. It is sometimes associated with ✿ **arthritis**.
Treatment
Treatment may include rest, splinting, or ℞ **corticosteroid** injections; in persistent cases, surgery may be undertaken to loosen the fibrous band. Treatment of any underlying condition may be necessary. ⚕ **vitamin B$_6$** is considered by some to be useful in the treatment of carpal tunnel syndrome.
For further information
℞ DIRECTORY OF DRUGS:
corticosteroid
⚕ VITAMINS, MINERALS, AND SUPPLEMENTS:
vitamin B$_6$

catarrh
Catarrh is the ✿ **inflammation** of the mucous membranes of the air-passages of the nose (✿ **rhinitis**) and trachea, with a discharge. It is a symptom of many respiratory tract disorders such as ✿ **coughs** and ✿ **colds**.
Treatment
℞ **decongestant** drugs can be used to relieve the symptoms of catarrh. Alternatively, some herbal remedies also have decongestant properties and can be used.
For further information
℞ DIRECTORY OF DRUGS:
cold and cough preparation • decongestant (for example, sympathomimetic)
♣ HERBAL REMEDIES
angelica • blessed thistle • boneset • cowslip • eucalyptus • eyebright • fennel • goldenseal • horseradish • licorice • linden • marshmallow • mullein • myrrh • pill-bearing spurge • peppermint • plantain • pokeroot • thyme • watercress • wild thyme • willow • wood sage

causalgia
Causalgia is a sharp burning or tingling ✿ **pain** in a limb, which is caused by nerve damage. Such damage is usually the result of an injury that has caused thinning (or some other deformity) of the skin surface and abnormal sensitivity of the sensory nerves within it. This condition is one of a group of disorders causing so-called neuropathic pain, which may be long-term, and which can be highly distressing.

Treatment

Neuropathic pains often do not respond well to drugs, though sometimes (opioid) ℞ **narcotic analgesic** may be given to temporally relieve the pain. Surgery may be necessary to sever nerves to the region altogether (sympathectomy).

For further information

℞ DIRECTORY OF DRUGS:
narcotic analgesic

celiac disease

Celiac disease (also known as gluten-sensitive enteropathy) is a ✪ **malabsorption disorder** where there is malabsorption of food, probably caused by an abnormal sensitivity (possibly due to damage) of the lining of the small intestine to the protein gluten (which is found in wheat, rye, and barley, and sometimes oats). The condition occurs mostly in young children and can run in families. The symptoms are all the signs of malnutrition, including deficiency disorders and ✪ **vitamin deficiency**. In adults (in whom the condition is also called sprue), symptoms are fatigue, cramps, and breathlessness.

Treatment

Under the supervision of a dietary expert a strict gluten-free diet must be followed, with supplements of vitamins and minerals to deal with any deficiency symptoms.

For further information

℞ DIRECTORY OF DRUGS:
vitamin and mineral supplement

⚖ VITAMINS, MINERALS, AND SUPPLEMENTS:
vitamins

cellulitis

Cellulitis is a ✪ **bacterial infection** of the skin and underlying tissues, usually with redness, swelling, pain, and local heat. There may also be malaise, headache, and chills. The elderly, diabetics, intravenous drug users, and those with HIV are at most risk.

Treatment

Antibacterials are prescribed to treat the infection, in severe cases by intravenous injection.

For further information

℞ DIRECTORY OF DRUGS:
antibacterial including **cephalosporin**s (for example, **cefazolin sodium**) • **macrolide** (for example, **erythromycin, azithromycin, clarithromycin**) • **penicillin** (penicillinase-resistant • for example, **dicloxacillin sodium, oxacillin sodium**)

cerebral hemorrhage

see ✪ stroke.

cerebral thrombosis

see ✪ stroke.

cerebrovascular accident

see ✪ stroke.

cervical cancer

see ✪ cancer.

change of life

see ✪ menopause.

chickenpox

Chickenpox is a highly infectious disease, which occurs mainly in children and is caused by a ✪ **herpes** virus, and transmitted by airborne droplets (in coughing or sneezing). The initial symptoms are those of a cold, with a high temperature, followed, a day later, by a characteristic rash of itchy blisters, which appear first on the chest and back, and then all over the body. The blisters turn into scabs, which last for up to two weeks before dropping off. Scratching them should be avoided as this may occasionally leave scars. Chickenpox is infectious from the start of symptoms until all the spots disappear. The individual may feel tired and unwell for a week or so afterward. Sometimes the spots become infected from scratching, and rarely there are more general complications. In people with vulnerable immune systems, such as those with ✪ **AIDS**, chickenpox can be very serious. The same virus (herpes zoster) causes ✪ **shingles** in adults, which may occur when the virus reactivates in later life.

Treatment

The aim of treatment is to alleviate the symptoms and this may include soothing lotions to relieve the itching (℞ **antipruritic** preparations or ♣ **witch hazel**) and plenty of liquids and medications to reduce fever. People at risk of complications, such as those with AIDS, may be given ℞ **antiviral** drugs.

For further information

℞ DIRECTORY OF DRUGS:
antiviral (for example, **acyclovir**) • **antipruritic**

♣ HERBAL REMEDIES:
witch hazel (for itching)

chilblain

Chilblains (also called pernio) are painful, reddened, swollen areas of tissue on the ears, toes, or fingers, accompanied by sensations of itching and burning. They are the result of an extreme response to cold, which is caused by an abnormally strong contraction of the blood vessels of the skin in order to conserve heat. The contraction is strong enough to deplete the flow of oxygen and nutrients in the blood to the areas affected. A tendency to develop chilblains often runs in families.

Treatment

The best treatment is prevention, which means keeping warm. In severe or persistent cases, drugs to improve blood flow to the extremities may be given (usually applied externally to the affected area).

For further information

℞ DIRECTORY OF DRUGS:
vasodilator

♣ HERBAL REMEDIES:
cayenne

chlamydial infections

Chlamydia are a group of tiny bacteria-like microorganisms that cause a range of diseases due to ✪ **bacterial infection**. For example, one form causes the eye disease ✪ **trachoma**, another the lung disease ✪ **psittacosis** (transmitted from birds), while other strains cause sexually transmitted diseases such as inflammation of the urethra (✪ **urethritis**) or vagina (✪ **vaginitis**). If vaginal infection spreads it may lead to ✪ **pelvic inflammatory disease** with blockage of the fallopian tubes, which is a common cause of ✪ **infertility** in women.

Treatment

Episodes of infection can be treated with ℞ **antibacterial** drugs. If vaginal infections remain untreated and lead to pelvic inflammatory disease, surgery may be needed.

For further information

℞ DIRECTORY OF DRUGS:
antibacterial

cholelithiasis

see ✪ **gallbladder disorders**.

cholera

Cholera is a potentially dangerous ✪ **bacterial infection** of the small intestine caused by *Vibrio cholerae*. It is contracted through eating or drinking material contaminated by the feces of an infected person. It is therefore common only in areas of poor sanitation. Symptoms are massive loss of fluid from the body through ✪ **vomiting** and ✪ **diarrhea**, and the consequent effects of dehydration (cramp and shock), which may be serious enough to cause death.

Treatment

The most important treatment is to replace the lost fluids and electrolytes by copious drinking of solutions of salted sugar or rice water, although treatment with the ℞ **antibacterial** drug ℞ **doxycycline** can speed recovery and also reduce dehydration. A vaccine is available, but its effectiveness is uncertain.

For further information

℞ DIRECTORY OF DRUGS:
doxycycline • **electrolyte** (rehydration solutions)

Christmas disease

see ✪ **hemophilia**; ✪ **bleeding disorder**.

Christmas factor disorder

see ✪ **bleeding disorder**.

chronic fatigue syndrome

Chronic fatigue syndrome is a condition of disabling fatigue that may last many months or even years. Slight exertion may make the person exhausted. Other symptoms include muscle weakness and aching, joint pains, changes in sleep patterns including an excessive need for sleep, intermittently raised temperature, swollen lymph nodes, sore throat, and ✪ **depression**. The cause is unknown but it often follows a ✪ **viral infection** (frequently respiratory or gastrointestinal), which is why it is sometimes known as "postviral fatigue syndrome." It has also, inappropriately, been called myalgic encephalomyelitis (ME).

Treatment

There is no specific treatment. Various medications or herbal remedies may be given to improve symptoms such as muscle pain, sore throat (for example, ℞ **non-narcotic analgesics** drugs) or depression (℞ **antidepressants**) if these are present. Graded exercise regimes or behavioral therapy may be helpful in some cases. Herbal remedies, such as evening primrose, have been suggested to be helpful but claims have not yet been evaluated scientifically.

chronic obstructive pulmonary disease

Chronic obstructive pulmonary disease (COPD) is a progressive, irreversible ✪ **respiratory tract disorder**. It is usually caused by smoking and results in wheezing, and shortness of breath. It is more common in men and in people over age 40. People with COPD usually have two separate lung disorders—chronic ✪ **bronchitis** and ✪ **emphysema**.

Treatment

It is important to stop smoking. Inhaled drugs to open the airways, and even oxygen may be necessary. Other drugs may be needed to treat any infection (for example, ℞ **antibacterials**) or symptoms (for example, ℞ **diuretics** for fluid retention causing swollen ankles). Many herbal remedies are purported to relieve symptoms of bronchitis.

For further information

℞ DIRECTORY OF DRUGS:
bronchodilator including **beta-adrenergic stimulant** (for example, **albuterol, bitolterol mesylate, isoetharine, isoproterenol, metaproterenol, pirbuterol, terbutaline sulfate**) • **xanthine** (for example, **theophylline**) • **anticholinergic** (**ipratropium bromide, atropine sulfate**) • also **corticosteroid** (for example, **budesonide**) • **antibacterial** • sometimes **diuretic** • **expectorant** (for example, **guaifenesin, potassium iodide**).

♣ HERBAL REMEDIES:

for some manifestations of bronchitis: **angelica** • **anise** • **black cherry** • **bloodroot** • **brewer's yeast** • **cardamom** • **chamomile, German** • **cinnamon, Chinese** • **cowslip** • **elecampane** • **eucalyptus** • **fennel** • **ground ivy** • **hempnettle** • **horehound** • **horseradish** • **Iceland moss** • **ivy, English** • **Japanese mint** • **licorice** • **linden** • **lobelia** • **maidenhair fern** • **mallow** • **marshmallow** • **mullein** • **nasturtium** • **oak** • **pill-bearing spurge** • **pimpinella** • **pleurisy root** • **sanicle** • **senega snakeroot** • **skunk cabbage** • **soap bark** • **soapwort** • **squill** • **star anise** • **thyme** • **watercress** • **wild thyme** • **wood sage**

circulatory disorders

see ✪ **cardiovascular disorders**.

cirrhosis

Cirrhosis is a ✪ **liver disorder** in which strands of fibrous scar tissue and abnormal nodular growths form in the liver, which loses its color and is characteristically misshapen. Liver function gradually fails as more of its cells are incapacitated and die. Causes include unknown factors (in more than half of all cases), ✪ **heart failure**,

○ **alcoholism**, viral ○ **hepatitis**, blockage of the common bile duct (draining bile from the gallbladder, a ○ **gallbladder disorder**), and ○ **autoimmune disorder** (where the immune system attacks the body's own tissues). Often cirrhosis produces no obvious symptoms; if there are, they include weight loss and poor appetite, nausea, and yellowing (jaundice) of the whites of the eyes and skin.

Treatment
Liver damage is irreversible; treatment aims to halt the damaging process, according to diagnosis of the cause, and may include drugs, a special diet, or surgery. Diuretic drugs are used to reduce ascites (accumulation of fluid in the peritoneal cavity); bile acid sequestrants help reduce the pruritis (itching) associated with obstruction of the biliary tract due to cirrhosis-induced damage; phytonadione (phytomenadione/vitamin K$_1$) administration may be necessary (sometimes by injection) because this vitamin is not well absorbed where bile-salt secretion is impaired, this sometimes being a consequence of damage to the gallbladder—which lies behind the liver—in cirrhosis.

For further information
℞ DIRECTORY OF DRUGS:
cholestyramine • diuretic • phytonadione
♣ HERBAL REMEDIES:
milk thistle

climacteric
see ○ **menopause**.

cluster headache
Cluster headaches are severe, brief episodes of often-intense ○ **pain** experienced in one part of the head and that recur over a few days. There may be gaps of months or years between each group of headaches. Symptoms, which often occur suddenly in the morning, include severe pain around one eye or temple, drooping eyelid, watering or redness of the eye, flushing and running or stuffy nostril. Smoking and drinking alcohol increase the risk of an attack in susceptible people.

Treatment
Drugs may be taken to reduce the frequency of the attacks (for example, ℞ **lithium**), to relieve the pain (℞ **NSAID** analgesics) or during attacks to shorten their intensity or duration (℞ **vasoconstrictor** ℞ **antimigraine** drugs). In severe attacks, oxygen inhalation can relieve symptoms.

For further information
℞ DIRECTORY OF DRUGS:
antimigraine drug (sumatriptan succinate, naratriptan, rizatriptan benzoate, zolmitriptan, dihydroergotamine mesylate) • lithium • NSAID

cold
A cold is a very common ○ **viral infection** of the mucous membranes of the nose, throat, and bronchial passages. Any of more than 200 viruses can cause the common cold. Colds are transmitted by droplets coughed or sneezed into the air or by direct contact with infected secretions (for example, by shaking hands with an infected person) that are readily transferred to the face. Initial

symptoms are generally a sore throat and a ○ **cough**, followed by a stuffy nose or painful breathing, and then a running nose; there may also be ○ **headache**, high temperature, and watering eyes.

Treatment
Affected people will usually be able to alleviate the worst symptoms by taking OTC ℞ **antipyretic** drugs such as ℞ **acetaminophen** to treat any fever, OTC ℞ **non-narcotic analgesics** (including ℞ **aspirin**, ℞ **ibuprofen**, and acetominophen) for headache and other pain, OTC ℞ **decongestants** to relieve congested airways, OTC ℞ **expectorants** to help the coughing-up of phlegm, and OTC ℞ **antitussives** to relieve dry unproductive cough. Alternatively, many herbal remedies are available to treat the symptoms of a cold. Some people think that supplements to the diet of vitamins (especially ♧ **vitamin C** in large doses) and ♧ **zinc** to boost the immune system help avoid or treat colds.

For further information
℞ DIRECTORY OF DRUGS:
cold and cough preparation • antipyretic (acetaminophen) • non-narcotic analgesic • antitussive • expectorant
♣ HERBAL REMEDIES:
angelica • anise • blackcurrant • brewer's yeast • cardamom • catnip • chamomile, German • cinnamon • cinnamon, Chinese • couch grass (*Elymus repens*) • echinacea • garlic • hibiscus • horseradish • Iceland moss • Japanese mint • larch • linden • marjoram • meadowsweet • mustard • myrrh • oak • onion • peppermint • premorse • radish • Scotch pine • southern bayberry • spruce • tea tree • weeping forsythia • wild thyme • willow • yarrow
♧ VITAMINS, MINERALS, AND SUPPLEMENTS:
vitamin A • vitamin C • zinc

cold sore
Cold sores are characteristic blisters that occur on the skin or mucous membranes due to ○ **viral infection** with a type of ○ **herpes** virus (herpes simplex). The virus type that causes cold sores around the lips and nose is closely related to the one causing genital herpes, and occasionally either type may cause blisters in their non-preferred area. Cold sores on the face are highly infectious and may be painful or itchy. They tend to recur. Occasionally they may infect the conjunctiva and cause eye complications.

Treatment
Treatment with ℞ **antiviral** drugs such as ℞ **acyclovir** can speed healing but does not affect the tendency to recur.

For further information
℞ DIRECTORY OF DRUGS:
antiviral
♣ HERBAL REMEDIES:
peppermint
♧ VITAMINS, MINERALS, AND SUPPLEMENTS
amino acid (lysine)

colic
Colic can be described as intense abdominal ○ **pain** originating, for instance, in the intestines or ureter, and which occurs in short cycles that peak and fade. In adults, causes include constipation,

intestinal obstruction, gallstones in the bile duct (biliary colic), and kidney stones (which are especially painful). In babies, so-called infantile colic is common in the first three or four months. The baby has periods of prolonged crying, often in the evenings, which are not related to the usual causes of crying such as hunger or discomfort. It is thought that this may be caused by gas in the intestines though emotional upheaval has been suggested as a cause.

Treatment

In adults medical assessment is advisable if colic persists. Sometimes drugs or herbal remedies acting on the smooth muscle of the affected organs can help ease the pain, but in some cases surgery may be required to treat the underlying cause. Infantile colic may be soothed by walking around with the baby, and episodes usually fade spontaneously after about four months of age.

For further information
℞ DIRECTORY OF DRUGS:
antispasmodic • anticholinergic
♣ HERBAL REMEDIES:
angelica • anise • catnip • cayenne • cinnamon • juniper • peppermint

colitis

Colitis can be any of several inflammatory conditions of the large intestine, most of which are of unknown cause. Symptoms may include diarrhea, bleeding, weight loss, and pain. One form of colitis is caused by antibiotic treatment (see ✪ **pseudomembranous colitis**). See also ✪ **ulcerative colitis**, ✪ **Crohn's disease**, ✪ **digestive system disorders**.

Treatment

The form of treatment depends on the cause, with different forms of colitis requiring differing therapies. But drug treatment for gut inflammation is often needed along with fluid and electrolyte replacement.

For further information
℞ DIRECTORY OF DRUGS:
aminosalicylate • antibacterial • corticosteroid • electrolyte
♣ HERBAL REMEDIES:
bilberry • witch hazel

colon cancer
see ✪ cancer.

colorectal cancer
see ✪ cancer.

common cold
see ✪ cold.

common wart
see ✪ wart.

conjunctivitis

Conjunctivitis is ✪ **inflammation** of the conjunctiva (the delicate membrane covering the front of the eyeball) of one or both eyes. Causes are local ✪ **infection** (infective conjunctivitis, sometimes called pink eye or red eye) when the disorder commonly occurs as a result of irritation by fumes or dust, or ✪ **allergy** (allergic conjunctivitis). Symptoms are a red and swollen eyelid, watering of the eye, and discomfort; there may also be a discharge of pus. Vision, however, is usually undisturbed.

Treatment

Most cases get better spontaneously within one or two weeks. If bacterial infection is responsible, antibacterial eyedrops may be given, and if due to allergy, antihistamines and antiallergic drugs may be taken for symptomatic relief. The herbal remedy raspberry has been used for conjunctivitis, but with little scientific evidence for its effectiveness.

For further information
℞ DIRECTORY OF DRUGS:
antiallergic • antibacterial • antihistamine
♣ HERBAL REMEDIES:
raspberry

Conn's disease
see ✪ hyperaldosteronism.

Conn's syndrome
see ✪ hyperaldosteronism.

constipation

Constipation can be defined as difficult, infrequent, or painful defecation, or abnormal hardness of the feces within the colon or rectum. Causes range from disruption of the circadian rhythm (normal daily rhythms) or a lack of dietary fiber, to ✪ **digestive system disorders** or the use of certain drugs. If constipation represents a definite change in bowel habit, or if simple measures fail to ease the problem, medical advice should be sought.

Treatment

In general the condition is temporary and, if necessary, can be remedied by taking a laxative (a food, supplement or drug that promotes defecation). Increasing the amount of fiber in the diet often helps in persistent cases. Treatment in cases of intestinal disorders depends on the underlying cause. Many herbal remedies are available to relieve constipation in the short term. If constipation persists, medical advice must be sought.

For further information
℞ DIRECTORY OF DRUGS:
laxative
♣ HERBAL REMEDIES:
aloe • black root • buckthorn • butternut • embelia • flax • frangula • Indian plantago • mallow • mountain flax • rhubarb, Chinese • tamarind • walnut • yellow dock

contact dermatitis
see ✪ dermatitis.

contusion
see ✪ bruise.

Key to symbols: ✪ = Disorder Section   ℞ = Drug Section   ♣ = Herbal Section   ⬥⬥ = Supplement Section

COPD

see ✪ chronic obstructive pulmonary disease.

corn

see ✪ wart.

coronary artery disease

Coronary artery disease (CAD), also called coronary heart disease, results from a narrowing of the coronary arteries, the blood vessels that supply the heart with blood. This causes damage to the heart muscle (myocardium). CAD in turn causes heart attacks (✪ **myocardial infarction**) and the chest pains characteristic of ✪ **angina pectoris**. It is a major cause of death. Mostly, CAD is a consequence of ✪ **atherosclerosis**, a narrowing and hardening of the coronary arteries due to the deposition of fatty deposits on the inner walls. This deposition is more common where there is high blood cholesterol due to a fatty diet. Other contributory factors include ✪ **hypertension,** ✪ **diabetes mellitus,** smoking, and lack of exercise. Some other diseases may inflame and so narrow the coronary arteries including the autoimmune disorder polyarteritis. The symptoms include palpitations, pain in the chest on exertion (angina pectoris), or a heart attack. There may be abnormal heart rhythms (arrhythmias), the development of chronic ✪ **heart failure** and edema (see ✪ **fluid retention**).

Treatment

Surgery, such as coronary angioplasty may be necessary to improve the blood supply to the heart. Drugs used depend on symptoms, but may include ℞ **lipid-regulating drugs** (whether or not blood cholesterol is high), ℞ **vasodilators** to improve blood supply to the myocardium, ℞ **beta-blockers** as vasodilators and to regulate heart rate, or ℞ **antiarrhythmics** to correct abnormal heart rhythms. Life-style changes are important and include stopping smoking, more exercise, and a low-fat diet.

For further information

℞ DIRECTORY OF DRUGS:

antiarrhythmic • beta-blocker •lipid-regulating drug • vasodilator (nitrate, for example, nitroglycerin, isosorbide dinitrate, isosorbide mononitrate)

⚖ VITAMINS, MINERALS, AND SUPPLEMENTS:

omega-3 fatty acid • vitamin E

coronary heart disease

see ✪ coronary artery disease.

cough

A cough is a sudden noisy expulsion of air from the lungs, which is essentially a protective reflex to clear secretion and irritants from the airways. The process is coordinated by a system of neurons in the brain, sometimes referred to as the "cough center." Generally coughing is beneficial, especially in chesty coughs where phlegm is being cleared upwards from the bronchioles of the lung. However, in disease, there may be a prolonged and painful cough that is unproductive. Chronic cough may accompany ✪ **lung cancer,** environmental allergies, many respiratory tract disorders, and chronic states such as ✪ **emphysema** and ✪ **bronchitis** (see also ✪ chronic obstructive pulmonary disease (COPD)).

Treatment

The cause of the cough should be established, as it may be a symptom of a serious underlying condition. Many OTC remedies for cough contain ℞ **expectorants** (usually ℞ **guaifenesin**), but clinical evidence for their appreciable efficacy is lacking. Cough suppressants that act on the cough center of the brain (℞ **antitussives**) such as the opioid drugs ℞ **codeine phosphate** and ℞ **dextromethorphan** should be reserved for dry cough. Some other types of drug, including certain sedating ℞ **antihistamines**, are incorporated into OTC cold and cough preparations, and may give symptomatic relief to cough by drying up secretions in the airways, and by aiding sleep. A large number of herbal remedies are promoted as helping cough in the short term, some by increasing resistance to colds.

For further information

℞ DIRECTORY OF DRUGS:

antihistamine • antitussive • cold and cough preparation • expectorant

♣ HERBAL REMEDIES:

anise • avocado • bitter milkwort • black cherry • blackcurrant • brewer's yeast • cardamom • chamomile, German • couch grass (*Elymus repens*) **• cowslip • echinacea • elecampane • eucalyptus • fennel • garden cress • hempnettle • horseradish • ivy, English • Japanese mint • lactucarium • linden • mallow • marshmallow • moneywort • mullein • mustard • nasturtium • oak • peppermint • pimpinella • premorse • radish • sanicle • senega snakeroot • soap bark • soapwort • spruce • star anise • thyme • watercress • white dead nettle • wolfberry, Chinese**

crab lice

see ✪ lice and mite infestation.

cretinism

see ✪ hyperthyroidism.

Creutzfeldt-Jakob disease

Creutzfeldt-Jakob Disease (CJD) is a fatal brain disease, formerly rare and occurring mostly in older people, but recently appearing in young people in Europe (New Variant CJD), and linked with a similar disease, bovine spongiform encephalopathy (BSE; "mad cow disease"), in cattle. Both conditions are caused by infectious agents called prions. These newly recognized agents survive normal methods of decontamination by heat, chemicals, or radiation. In some people, the source of the ✪ **infection** can be traced to earlier treatment with products derived from human tissue, mainly growth hormone before it was made synthetically (called somatropin), and also blood coagulation factors. In the 1980s, cattle became infected through the use of animal ingredients in their feedstuffs, a practice that has now been stopped. However, it is believed that material from infected cattle may have entered the human food supply, or have been used in the production of drugs, vaccines, and cosmetics, before controls were introduced to stop this. Because the incubation period (the time between infection and symptoms) of this new form of CJD can be many years, scientists are still unsure how many people may be at risk of developing the disease. Symptoms include twitching, ✪ **depression**, loss of balance and coordination, and rapidly progressing ✪ **dementia**. The disease is ultimately fatal.

Treatment

There is no treatment other than to keep individuals as comfortable as possible. Symptoms such as depression and muscle contractions can be helped with ℞ **antidepressant** and ℞ **skeletal muscle relaxant** drugs.

Crohn's disease

Crohn's disease is a serious ✪ **digestive system disorder** of the small intestine, particularly of the ileum where it joins the cecum. Parts of the intestinal wall become inflamed and may ulcerate; where folds of the intestine touch each other, small fissures break through from one fold to another. In an acute form, the condition may appear similar to appendicitis; in a chronic form, there may be partial intestinal obstruction, leading to ✪ **diarrhea**, pain, and the malabsorption of food. The cause is unknown but may be an infectious agent related to the mycobacterium that causes tuberculosis. The condition is named for the American gastroenterologist Burrill B. Crohn (1884–1983), who first described it in 1932. Crohn's disease and ✪ **ulcerative colitis**, are the two main disorders described as inflammatory bowel disease (IBD), a general term for chronic inflammatory diseases affecting the small or large intestine.

Treatment

Treatment is to relieve the symptoms, and generally includes drugs of the aminosalicylate group, which have been developed specially to treat this disorder; also metronidazole. To help suppress the inflammatory symptoms, ℞ **corticosteroids**, and sometimes ℞ **immunosuppressants** (including ℞ **cyclosporine**, ℞ **azathiaprine** and ℞ **infliximab**) are used. Bed rest helps, and surgery may also be necessary to remove the affected segment of the intestine. Barley is a traditional herbal remedy for irritable bowel conditions.

For further information

℞ DIRECTORY OF DRUGS:
aminosalicylate • corticosteroid • immunosuppressant

♣ HERBAL REMEDIES:
barley

⚕ VITAMINS, MINERALS, AND SUPPLEMENTS:
omega-3 fatty acid

croup

Croup is caused by inflammation of the larynx (the part of the throat containing the vocal cords), which, in young children (aged between 6 and 30 months), leads to partial obstruction of the air passages. Breathing becomes labored and noisy; there is a high temperature and a barking ✪ **cough**. The cause is usually a ✪ **viral infection**, but this may be complicated by secondary ✪ **bacterial infection**.

Treatment

Treatment is generally by humidifying the environment. Inhaled ℞ **corticosteroids** may be required and in the event of secondary

bacterial infection, antibacterials may be required. Very rarely, obstruction of the airways may necessitate surgery to restore proper breathing.

For further information

℞ DIRECTORY OF DRUGS:
antibacterial • corticosteroid

cryptococcosis

see ✪ **fungal infections**.

cryptosporidosis

see ✪ **protozoal infection**.

Cushing's syndrome

Cushing's syndrome indicates a group of disorders that result from excessive amounts of corticosteroids in the body. It can be due to disorders of the adrenal glands—endocrine glands located just above the kidneys—so that excessive amounts of corticosteroid hormones are released into the bloodstream. Other causes include prolonged treatment with ℞ **corticosteroid** drugs (for instance prednisolone taken for ✪ **rheumatoid arthritis**), a benign or cancerous tumor in the adrenal glands, a tumor in the anterior pituitary gland (which secretes the hormone, ACTH, that stimulates the adrenal glands into production; see ✪ **pituitary gland disorders and tumors**), or unknown factors. Symptoms include fatness of the face, neck, and torso (although the limbs remain thin), increased hair growth, weakness, and ✪ **fatigue**; there are also usually striations (stripes) on the skin and a reduced libido (sexual drive). Complications include ✪ **hypertension**, bone thinning and occasionally mental changes. The condition is named for the American surgeon Harvey Cushing (1869–1939).

Treatment

Treatment depends on the cause. If a tumor is responsible, this is usually removed by surgery, sometimes also with radiotherapy and hormone supplements. Excess corticosteroid secretion can be treated with ℞ **hormone antagonists** including drugs such as ℞ **aminoglutethimide** and ℞ **ketoconazole**, which work by blocking synthesis of steroids. If the symptoms appear when you are taking a long-term course of corticosteroids, it may be necessary to "taper-off" the dose; but you should not do this without your doctor's supervision.

For further information

℞ DIRECTORY OF DRUGS:
hormone antagonist (aminoglutethimide)

cutaneous leishmaniasis

see ✪ **leishmaniasis**.

cuts

see ✪ **wound**.

cystic fibrosis

Cystic fibrosis is a hereditary disease that causes exocrine glands (mucus- and sweat-producing glands) to produce abnormally thick mucus. The cause is a recessive gene carried by about 1 in 20 people. This means that both parents must carry the gene to produce an affected child. Only those with two defective genes, one from each parent, have symptoms; those with one defective gene are symptomless carriers of the condition. Organs affected include the liver, lungs, gut, and pancreas. It has the result that passages in which mucus is normally present may then become congested. Symptoms include the malabsorption of food and recurrent respiratory problems (see ✪ **malabsorption disorders.**)

Treatment

Treatment is to relieve the symptoms as far as possible and to slow the progression of lung disease, and maintain adequate nutrition. It may include replacement pancreatic digestive enzyme (℞ **pancreatin**), and physiotherapy and drugs (℞ **mucolytics** including ℞ **dornase alfa**) to help clear mucus from the lungs, and sometimes bronchodilators to widen the airway passages. In severe cases, a heart-lung transplant may be offered. Genetic counselling is offered to carrier parents. In future, gene therapy may be able to correct the underlying problem.

For further information

℞ DIRECTORY OF DRUGS:
bronchodilator • digestive enzyme • mucolytic

cystic mastitis

see ✪ **mastitis.**

cystinuria

Cystinuria is a condition where there is an abnormal presence of the amino acid cystine in the urine. One form is caused by an inherited disorder of the kidney. It can cause kidney or bladder stones (✪ **calculus**).

Treatment

Treatment consists of having a large fluid intake, and drugs aimed at preventing the formation of stones (for instance ℞ **penicillamine** reduces cystine levels in the urine), or by taking certain ℞ **electrolytes** (usually sodium bicarbonate), which have the effect of alkalinizing urine and so increasing the solubility of cystine.

For further information

℞ DIRECTORY OF DRUGS:
electrolyte (sodium bicarbonate) • penicillamine

cystitis

Cystitis is inflammation of the (urinary) bladder lining, most commonly caused by ✪ **bacterial infection** (bacterial cystitis), often *E. coli*. The condition is less common in men than in women (who have a shorter urethra—the passage from the bladder to the outside—for bacteria to penetrate). Symptoms are an increased frequency of urination, cloudy urine, and usually pain or a burning sensation on passing urine; there may also be a high temperature, abdominal cramp, and blood in the urine. Postmenopausal women and people with ✪ **diabetes mellitus** are prone to bacterial cystitis. Interstitial cystitis is a distinct and rare long-term condition of unknown cause, clinically given specialist treatment.

Treatment

Treatment may consist solely of flushing the infection out by drinking large volumes of water. Alternatively, antibacterial antibiotic or sulphonamide drugs may be prescribed to treat the infection. Certain urinary alkalinizer preparations available OTC (including sodium bicarbonate and sodium citrate) alkalinize the urine and reduce the burning sensation. There are many herbal preparations with mild ℞ **diuretic** or ℞ **antibacterial** properties, which may help relieve symptoms. While the condition lasts, special care with hygiene should be observed.

For further information

℞ DIRECTORY OF DRUGS:
antibacterial • diuretic • urinary alkalinizer
♣ HERBAL REMEDIES:
agrimony • arenaria rubra • bearberry • boldo • hydrangea • juniper • marshmallow • parsley • saw palmetto • uva-ursi

dandruff

Dandruff is the greasy scaling of the scalp in which flakes of dead skin accumulate among the hairs and may brush or fall off. About half of all individuals have troublesome dandruff, which has been linked with the presence of a yeast, *Malassezia ovalis* (previous name *Pityrosporum ovale*), a type of ✪ **fungal infection**, on the scalp. The medical name is pityriasis capitis.

Treatment

Treatment is with antidandruff lotions or shampoos containing ℞ **antiseborrheics** such as selenium sulphide and coal tar, or ℞ **antifungal** drugs.

For further information

℞ DIRECTORY OF DRUGS:
antifungal • antiseborrheic • skin preparation
♣ HERBAL REMEDIES:
henna

deafness

Deafness is a serious impairment, or total failure, of the sense of hearing. There are two main types of deafness. Conductive deafness arises when there is a blockage or failure in the conduction of sound vibrations from the outer ear to the auditory nerve (which leads from the inner ear to the brain), as may be caused by ✪ **otitis media** (infection of the middle ear) or certain degenerative conditions of the inner ear. Perceptive (or nerve) deafness (also called sensorineural deafness) is caused by damage to the cochlea, auditory nerve (the inner ear or nerve from the ear to the brain), or to the interpretative center in the brain, as may be caused by infection with ✪ **rubella** (German measles) before birth, injury, long-term noise, or disease (such as ✪ **Ménière's disease**). The type of deafness is diagnosed by various tests using tuning forks; testing of severity is by means of an audiogram, which measures the ability to hear different sound frequencies.

Treatment

The cause is treated where possible. Both types of deafness can sometimes be alleviated with a hearing aid. In some types of severe deafness, hearing can now be partially restored by means of a cochlear implant, an artificial hearing device surgically inserted into the ear.

decubitus ulcer

see ✪ **bedsore**.

deep vein thrombosis

Deep vein thrombosis (DVT) is the formation of a blood clot within a deep lying vein, for example a blood clot that forms in the calf veins when blood flow is sluggish or the blood's tendency to clot is increased. It is a type of phlebothrombosis; any condition where there is clot formation in a vein. Causes include impaired circulation to the legs from prolonged immobility (such as long-haul air flights), resulting from a surgical operation or a period of bed rest, as well as heart failure, pregnancy, and the contraceptive pill. The leg becomes swollen and sore, and there is a risk that the clot may break off, travel through the bloodstream (embolize), and become lodged in the lungs (pulmonary embolus, see ✪ **pulmonary embolism**), which can be fatal.

Treatment

Anticoagulant drugs are given to treat an established thrombosis, and occasionally surgery may be required to remove a large clot. ℞ **anticoagulant** drugs, which reduce clotting, may be given prior to a prolonged operation to reduce the risk, and sometimes ℞ **thrombolytic** drugs are used to dissolve clots. Recovering individuals are encouraged to become mobile or to do leg exercises to stimulate blood flow.

For further information

℞ DIRECTORY OF DRUGS:
anticoagulant • thrombolytic

dehydration

Dehydration is an excessive loss of water from the body tissues, which may follow prolonged ✪ **vomiting**, ✪ **fever**, ✪ **diarrhea**, or ✪ **acidosis**. Loss of excess water in turn leads to a loss of electrolytes, which causes flushed, dry skin, poor skin elasticity, failure to pass urine, dry mucous membranes and a coated tongue, drowsiness, and confusion. It can be especially dangerous in the elderly and young.

Treatment

Treatment aims to restore the normal fluid volume and replace lost electrolytes with dehydration solutions.

For further information

℞ DIRECTORY OF DRUGS:
electrolyte (rehydration solution)

delayed puberty

see ✪ **abnormal puberty**.

dementia

Dementia is a progressive deterioration in mental ability due to an underlying brain disorder. Dementia eventually results in complete disruption of the mental processes so that rational thought is no longer possible. The condition is generally reached gradually, but progressively, as a result of organic changes in brain tissue, usually in the form of cellular degeneration. Such changes may be caused by "old age" (senile dementia) at any age from about 60 onward, or by unknown factors prior to that age (presenile dementia,

including ✪ **Alzheimer's disease**) from about age 40 onward. It can also be caused by injury, infection (for example, ✪ **Creutzfeldt-Jakob disease**), poisoning, or any disease that results in a reduced blood supply to the brain over a long period. Other degenerative diseases which cause dementia include ✪ **Huntington's disease** and ✪ **Parkinson's disease**.

Treatment

In a few cases the condition is reversible. Most of those affected will undergo a progressive decline, although modern drug treatments may slow this and alleviate some of the symptoms. Vitamin B_{12} is considered by some to reduce the risk of dementia.

For further information

℞ DIRECTORY OF DRUGS:
dementia treatment
♣ HERBAL REMEDIES:
ginkgo
⚖ VITAMINS, MINERALS, AND SUPPLEMENTS:
vitamin B_{12}

dental caries

see ✪ **tooth decay**.

depression

Depression is an ✪ **affective disorder**, or mood disorder characterized by a state of mind that is dominated by feelings of despair and worthlessness. This may be accompanied by lethargy and disinterest in either eating or sleeping. The condition is natural in certain circumstances (such as the recent loss of a loved one, or the final frustration of long-held hopes) but is abnormal in the absence of such circumstances or if it is prolonged for an undue time (for instance after childbirth—postnatal depression). Untreated, severe depression may lead to suicide. Other effects may include neurotic changes in behavior and, in some people, ✪ **bipolar affective disorder** (formerly called manic-depressive illness) where periods of depression alternate with manic phases during which the person is elated, impulsive, and sometimes takes irrational risks.

Treatment

Tests may be carried out to see if there is an underlying physical cause (for example, Cushing's syndrome, Parkinson's disease). Treatment is with ℞ **antidepressant** drugs; psychotherapy, particularly behavioral (cognitive) therapy may be beneficial; occasionally a person may undergo electroconvulsive therapy (ECT). Some dietary supplements are said to be beneficial for depression, and several herbal remedies are available; some such as St. John's wort, have established antidepressant properties.

For further information

℞ DIRECTORY OF DRUGS:
antidepressant drugs • SSRI and related uptake inhibitor antidepressants (including **citalopram, fluvoxamine, fluoxetine, paroxetine, sertraline**) • MAOI and related (including **isocarboxazid, phenelzine, tranylcypromine**) • tricyclic and related (including **amitriptyline hydrochloride, amoxapine, clomipramine hydrochloride, desipramine hydrochloride, doxepin, imipramine, maprotiline hydrochloride, nortriptyline hydrochloride, protriptyline hydrochloride, trimipramine**

hydrochloride) • other antidepressants (including **bupropion hydrochloride, mirtazapine hydrochloride, methylphenidate, nefazodone hydrochloride, trazodone hydrochloride, venlafaxine**)

♣ HERBAL REMEDIES:

cola • **damiana** • **maté** • **St. John's wort** • **vervain**

⚕ VITAMINS, MINERALS, AND SUPPLEMENTS:

amino acid (phenylalanine, tyrosine) • **S-adenosylmethionine** • **omega-3 fatty acid** • **vitamin B$_1$ (thiamine)** • **vitamin B$_6$ (pyridoxine)** • **vitamin B$_{12}$ (cobalamin)**

dermatitis

Dermatitis is a ⊕ **skin condition** where there is inflammation of the skin surface, with redness and itching, caused by external agents (unlike ⊕ **eczema**, in which similar skin changes occur as a result of an internal tendency; both terms are, however, often used interchangeably). Primary irritant dermatitis is due to substances that irritate the skin, such as detergents or caustic substances, to which anyone exposed to a sufficient degree is vulnerable. Allergic contact dermatitis (allergic dermatitis) is due to individual sensitivity to particular substances, for example, nickel and poison ivy. Other types include atopic dermatitis and seborrheic dermatitis (see ⊕ **seborrhea**).

Treatment

The best treatment is to cease exposure to the cause. Where this is not possible, scrupulous drying of the hands and the use of ℞ **skin preparations** such as barrier-creams may avoid flare-ups. Dryness of the skin may be relieved with ℞ **emollient** lotions. In severe cases ℞ **corticosteroid** preparations may need to be applied to the skin. There are numerous herbal remedies available for inflammatory skin conditions.

For further information

℞ DIRECTORY OF DRUGS:

corticosteroid • **skin preparation** (including **emollient**)

♣ HERBAL REMEDIES:

brewer's yeast • **chamomile, German** • **cnidium** • **evening primrose** • **goldenseal** • **heartsease** • **henna** • **moneywort** • **oats** • **purple loosestrife** • **stinging nettle**

⚕ VITAMINS, MINERALS, AND SUPPLEMENTS:

gamma-linolenic acid (GLA)

dhobie itch

see ⊕ **dermatitis**.

diabetes insipidus

Diabetes insipidus is a rare disorder that is usually caused by a failure of the pituitary gland (the gland in the brain that controls the actions of most other glands) to produce or secrete enough antidiuretic hormone (ADH; vasopressin). ADH controls the amount of water reabsorbed by the kidneys. Symptoms of diabetes insipidus are a copious excretion of urine and an excessive thirst. A failure of the kidney to respond to ADH is also sometimes involved in diabetes insipidus.

Treatment

The main treatment of diabetes insipidus is to replace deficient ADH levels with vasopressin and analogues, most of which have to be injected but some are now available as a nasal spray (for example, ℞ **desmopressin**). Alternatively, in some varieties of diabetes insipidus (nephrogenic, and partial pituitary, diabetes insipidus) thiazide diuretics paradoxically relieve symptoms (for example, ℞ **chlortalidone**, ℞ **hydrochlorothiazide**). ℞ **carbamazepine** is sometimes tried as an "off-label" use.

For further information

℞ DIRECTORY OF DRUGS:

carbamazepine • **(thiazide) diuretic** (for example, **chlorthalidone, hydrochlorothiazide**) • **posterior pituitary hormone (vasopressin, lypressin, desmopressin)**

diabetes mellitus

Diabetes mellitus is a condition in which the body is not able to efficiently utilize the sugar glucose, and is due to an inadequacy in the secretion, or effect, of the hormone ℞ **insulin**. Insulin is normally produced by the islets of Langerhans (special cells in the pancreas) and normally enables the utilization of glucose as an energy source, and tissue building block, by virtually every cell in the body. In the absence of proper insulin release, or tissue reaction to it, glucose is wasted and passes out in the urine taking water with it. This causes the characteristic frequent urination, body wastage and weight loss, and leads to the metabolism of alternative sources of energy, particularly fats, which form toxic by-products. There are two main types of diabetes mellitus. The first condition, type 1 diabetes mellitus, occurs most frequently in children and is consequently known as juvenile-onset diabetes (insulin-dependent diabetes mellitus; IDDM); the second, type 2 diabetes mellitus, arises more often in adults and is thus known as adult-onset diabetes mellitus (non-insulin-dependent diabetes mellitus; NIDDM). The cause is generally unknown, although there may be a family tendency toward it; sometimes an infection or ⊕ **alcoholism** seems to contribute to its development in adults. In either case, diet, and blood sugar levels must be carefully controlled, as the latter can quickly become too high (hyperglycemia), leading to chemical changes in which the blood may contain toxic ketones (which can sometimes be smelled on the breath); coma may follow. However, coma may also follow an overly rapid lowering of blood sugar levels, from an imbalance between the diet and insulin dose. Long-term complications of diabetes mellitus include damage to small arteries, including those in the back of the eye, which can cause blindness, cardiovascular disorders, neuropathy, and kidney disease.

Treatment

Type 1 diabetes mellitus is treated with careful dietary control and doses of ℞ **insulin**. Insulin is commonly taken twice-daily by self-administered injection, of one or more of a range of insulin preparations, with different durations of action, and other characteristics. Expert counseling, initial training, and blood-glucose monitoring is required because a stable blood-glucose level over long periods must be maintained. Choice of suitable preparations, or combinations of preparations, may take some time to establish. Treatment for type 2 diabetes mellitus may require dietary change only, or drugs taken by mouth to help reduce blood sugar levels (℞ **oral hypoglycemics**). Diabetics should be aware of the symptoms of hypoglycemia ("hypoglycemic aware"). These include fatigue, weakness, confusion, headache, convulsions, hunger, nausea, pallor, sweating, and rapid breathing. Diabetics are advised to carry glucose that they can take by mouth if they feel the onset of blood glucose levels that are too low (hypoglycemia); otherwise the hormone glucagon, which has the opposite action to insulin, can be administered by injection in hypoglycemic emergency. There are many supplements and herbal remedies that are considered to be beneficial in controlling diabetes mellitus by lowering blood sugar (such as ♣ **fenugreek** and ♣ **artichoke**), or preventing or relieving some of the symptoms or possible consequences of diabetes mellitus (for example, ⚛ **alpha-lipoic acid** for nerve damage).

For further information

℞ DIRECTORY OF DRUGS:
antidiabetic treatment • **insulin analog (sulfonylurea)** • **oral hypoglycemic (acetohexamide, chlorpropamide, glimepiride, glipizide, glyburide, tolazamide, tolbutamide)** • **(biguanide) oral hypoglycemic (metformin)**, other **oral hypoglycemic** drugs (**acarbose, diazoxide, repaglinide, miglitol, rosiglitazone maleate, pioglitazone**) • **glucagon** • **glucose**

♣ HERBAL REMEDIES:
artichoke • bilberry • fenugreek • garlic • holy basil • yucca

⚛ VITAMINS, MINERALS, AND SUPPLEMENTS:
alpha-lipoic acid • chromium • conjugated linoleic acid • magnesium • manganese • niacin • vitamin E

diabetic vascular disease

see ⊙ peripheral vascular disorders.

diaper dermatitis

see ⊙ dermatitis.

diarrhea

Diarrhea is abnormally frequent defecation, or passing abnormally liquid feces. The urge to defecate may continue even after the rectum is empty. Loss of liquids in this fashion—especially in young children—may lead to dehydration. Causes of diarrhea range from stress, an over-rich diet, and mild ⊙ **gastritis** (inflammation of the stomach) and ⊙ **gastroenteritis**, to ⊙ **food poisoning**, ⊙ **otitis** media, chemical poisoning, infection of the intestines or of the lungs, infestation with ⊙ **worms**, and (rarely) ⊙ **cancer**.

Treatment

Treatment depends on diagnosis of the cause, but should include ℞ **electrolytes** in the form of rehydration solutions (℞ **electrolytes**) to replace lost liquid. If prolonged, and following medical advice ℞ **antidiarrheal** drugs can be taken. Many herbal remedies are available that can be used to treat diarrhea in the short term. However, if diarrhea persists, consult your doctor as it may be a symptom of an underlying serious disorder.

For further information

℞ DIRECTORY OF DRUGS:
antidiarrheal • electrolyte (rehydration solution)

♣ HERBAL REMEDIES:
agrimony • angostura • arrowroot • barley • bilberry • blackberry • cinnamon • cocoa • coffee • cola • elm bark • geum • jambul • lady's mantle • lemon verbena • logwood • lotus • meadowsweet • nutmeg • oak • plantain • poplar • potentilla • psyllium • purple loosestrife • raspberry • rhatany • rhubarb, Chinese • salep • sloe • southern bayberry • tormentil • wild mint • witch hazel • yarrow • yellow willowherb

digestive system disorders

Digestive system disorders are a large group of conditions that affect some part of the digestive (gastrointestinal) tract. Some disorders result in disruption of the digestive process itself, for example, by obstructing the passage of food down the gastrointestinal tracts (such as tumors), others interfere with the absorption of nutrients (for example, ⊙ **malabsorption disorders**, which is sometimes due to digestive enzyme deficiencies in ⊙ **pancreatitis** or ⊙ **cirrhosis**, or ⊙ **gallstones**). Other disorders may have little effect on the absorption of nutrients but have marked gastrointestinal tract symptoms (for example, ⊙ **peptic ulcer**, ⊙ **gastroesophageal reflux**, ⊙ **heartburn**, ⊙ **hiatus hernia**, ⊙ **indigestion**, and ⊙ **gastritis**). A number of important digestive tract disorders are due to ⊙ **food poisoning**. Symptoms depend on the particular disorder, but gastrointestinal disturbances may include abdominal discomfort or pain, heartburn, ⊙ **flatulence**, ⊙ **diarrhea** or ⊙ **constipation**. See also ⊙ **ulcerative colitis**, ⊙ **Crohn's disease**, ⊙ **colitis**, ⊙ **diverticular disease**, ⊙ **enteritis**, ⊙ **dysentery**.

Treatment

Treatment depends on the cause, and is dealt with under the specific disorder. Many herbal remedies have traditional uses as "digestive tonics" and as general treatments for gastrointestinal disturbances or digestive disorders. These include ♣ **jewel weed**, ♣ **honeysuckle**, ♣ **magnolia**, ♣ **horsemint, English**, ♣ **spearmint**, ♣ **lotus**, ♣ **reed herb**, ♣ **bistort**, ♣ **lavender cotton**, ♣ **hartstongue**, ♣ **cup plant**, and ♣ **broomcorn**. Vitamins and mineral supplements can be useful if the absorption of nutrients is affected, and many supplements are beneficial in specific digestive system disorders. See specific disorder entry for more details.

diphtheria

Diphtheria is a potentially dangerous—but now rare due to widespread immunization of children—contagious ⊙ **bacterial infection** that generally affects the throat but may also attack other areas of mucous membrane (such as in the nasal cavity and larynx) or the tissues of the skin. Some (human) carriers of the disease are not themselves affected. Symptoms are a sore throat, general malaise, and high temperature; weakness, and the appearance of a painful white "crust" at the back of the throat. Breathing may become labored.

Treatment

Treatment is isolation and bed rest in hospital, with ℞ **antibacterial** antibiotics and ℞ **antitoxin**. A ℞ **vaccine** is available (and usually administered during the first year of life).

For further information

℞ DIRECTORY OF DRUGS:

antibacterial • antitoxin • vaccine

discoid lupus erythematosus

see ✪ lupus.

disseminated intravascular coagulation

see ✪ bleeding disorder.

diverticular disease

Diverticular disease is so named because of the presence of small pouches called diverticula, in the wall of the gut, usually in the colon (the last part of the large intestine leading to the rectum and then the anus). Diverticula form in areas of weakness of the gut wall and become increasingly common with age. Usually they cause no symptoms, but when infected and inflamed (called diverticulitis) they can result in lower abdominal pain with ✪ constipation or ✪ diarrhea, and sometimes bleeding from the rectum. There may be a high temperature and other signs of infection. Sometimes an abscess may form.

Treatment

Treatment is to alleviate symptoms, sometimes with ℞ laxatives or ℞ antidiarrheal drugs, and rest, until the acute symptoms subside. A high-fiber diet with plenty of fluids will be recommended. If the condition recurs, or if an abscess forms, surgery may be necessary. Antibacterial drugs may be prescribed if the diverticula become infected.

For further information

℞ DIRECTORY OF DRUGS:

antibacterial • antidiarrheal • laxative

♣ HERBAL REMEDIES:

flax

diverticulitis

see ✪ diverticular disease.

Down's syndrome

Down's syndrome; also called trisomy 21 (formerly mongolism), is a congenital abnormality that most commonly results from the presence of an extra chromosome—a triad of the 21st chromosome instead of the normal pair—in the cell nuclei. The result is the characteristic formations of the skull and face, the tongue and the hands, and often mental retardation; stature may be squat. The condition may be accompanied by other congenital disorders, particularly heart malformations and deafness. Affected people may need special care all their lives. Statistically, the chances of giving birth to a Down's syndrome child grow with increasing maternal age.

Treatment

There is no treatment other than to correct associated deformities where possible. Various tests are offered to older mothers that can help to predict the risk of Down's syndrome, including ultrasound scanning, a teratogenetic blood test (the triple marker test—"triple test"), chorionic villus sampling, and amniocentesis (where fetal cells are sampled and their chromosomes analyzed), which may be followed by termination of affected pregnancies. Long-term support and medical care is needed for children to develop as much as possible. Genetic counseling may be appropriate.

dropsy

see ✪ fluid retention.

drug allergy

see ✪ allergy.

drug dependency

Drug dependence is a dependence on a particular drug, arising from either drug abuse or from its medical use. Non-medical use of self-administered drugs—that is for recreational or similar purposes without intent to prevent, cure, or treat disease—is commonly to provide a state of temporary euphoria or other psychedelic effect. Most such abused drugs eventually produce dependence or habituation (physical or psychological need to continue taking the drug). They include social drugs such as nicotine and alcohol (see ✪ alcoholism), as well as many drugs taken illicitly such as opiates, cocaine, amphetamines, etc., but also some prescribed drugs, for example, barbiturates, benzodiazepines.

Treatment

Treatment of dependence on drugs of abuse is extremely difficult, since it relies on the person wanting to stop their drug habit, and is based on psychological support during withdrawal and afterwards. Sometimes drugs are used to alleviate symptoms, to replace the drug of abuse with a less harmful substitute, or to enforce abstinence by causing unpleasant symptoms should the person lapse.

For further information

℞ DIRECTORY OF DRUGS:

substance-dependence treatment

dry eyes

Dry eyes occur as a result of a dryness of the cornea and conjunctiva of the eyes and are caused by a deficiency of tear production. They can be caused by a foreign body in the eye, or as the result of a disease such as ✪ Sjögren's syndrome, or keratoconjunctivitis sicca, where there is damage to the lacrimal glands (tear producing glands) of the eye.

Treatment

The underlying cause of any disease will be treated, and ℞ eye treatments in the form of ℞ artificial tears may relieve symptoms.

For further information

℞ DIRECTORY OF DRUGS:

eye treatment • artificial tears

Duchenne's muscular dystrophy

see ✪ muscular dystrophy.

duodenal ulcer

see ✪ peptic ulcer.

dysentery

Dysentery is a severe form of intestinal (gut) infection, which can spread elsewhere in the body. The main symptom is violent ✪ **diarrhea**, passing blood, and mucus. Dysentery has two main forms: ✪ **amebic dysentery** (amebiasis) and bacillary dysentery. The infective organisms of both forms—a protozoan in the first case, a bacterium in the second—are spread in food or water that are contaminated with the feces of a carrier, and thus occur mostly in areas of poor (or no) sanitation. Bacillary dysentery (shigellosis) has much milder symptoms—diarrhea, nausea, high temperature, and cramps; there may also be intestinal hemorrhage. It lasts for about 10 days.

Treatment

Treatment is with ℞ **electrolytes** as rehydration fluids, and ℞ **antibacterials** of various types; including for the bacterial forms ℞ **sulfonamides**, ℞ **azoles**, and ℞ **antibiotics**; and for the protozoal form, drugs of the ℞ **amebicide and antiprotozoal** class such as ℞ **metronidazole** and iodoquinol. There are several herbal remedies that, traditionally, are thought to be of some benefit, particularly in treating symptoms such as diarrhea.

For further information

℞ DIRECTORY OF DRUGS:
amebicide and antiprotozoal • antibacterial • electrolyte (rehydration solution)

♣ HERBAL REMEDIES:
cola • jambul • walnut • yarrow • yellow willowherb

dysmenorrhea

Dysmenorrhea is the ✪ **pain** experienced with menstruation. There are two forms: primary dysmenorrhea occurs in young women when the periods first start (at the menarche), when cramping abdominal pain during menstruation may be accompanied by general feelings of being unwell, nausea, and headache. This is believed to be due to hormonal disturbances. Secondary dysmenorrhea occurs in older women, who may experience aching or cramping pains prior to menstruation. This form may be a symptom of ✪ **endometriosis**, fibroids, or ✪ **pelvic inflammatory disease** (a result of infection ascending from the vagina to the uterus and Fallopian tubes); it can also be as a result of an intrauterine contraceptive device (IUD).

Treatment

In primary dysmenorrhea treatment aims to alleviate symptoms, and the problem usually settles down with age. Smooth muscle relaxants (℞ **antispasmodics**) may help, as may ℞ **non-narcotic analgesics**, especially of the **NSAID** type. In the secondary form, treatment is directed toward identifying and treating the underlying cause of the pain. A form of the ℞ **contraceptive** pill may be prescribed. If there is excessive blood loss, other approaches such as ℞ **anemia treatment** in the form of iron salts may be necessary (see ✪ **menorrhagia**). Many herbal remedies have traditional uses in relieving dysmenorrhea and menstrual disturbances in general.

For further information

℞ DIRECTORY OF DRUGS:
antispasmodic • contraceptive • NSAID

♣ HERBAL REMEDIES:
black cohosh • blue cohosh • chaste tree • false unicorn root • goldenseal • Jamaica dogwood • lactucarium • myrrh • pasque flower • skullcap • white peony • wild yam

dyspepsia

see ✪ **indigestion**.

dyspeptic conditions

see ✪ **indigestion**.

early puberty

see ✪ **abnormal puberty**.

eclampsia

Eclampsia is a dangerous condition, which represents a complication of toxemia of ✪ **pregnancy-related disorders** (pre-eclampsia), and affects women either in the last weeks of pregnancy or shortly after childbirth. Symptoms are high blood pressure (✪ **hypertension**), edema (swelling of the tissues because of accumulated fluid), protein in the urine (albuminuria or proteinuria), and convulsions leading to coma. If still pregnant at this stage, the mother is in danger of losing both the baby and her own life.

Treatment

Treatment is to relieve the symptoms—to prevent further convulsions (℞ **magnesium sulfate** given intravenously) and to lower blood pressure (℞ **antihypertensives** such as ℞ **labetalol**)—but may include the precautionary induction of labor, or a Cesarean section to deliver the baby.

For further information

℞ DIRECTORY OF DRUGS:
antihypertensive • magnesium sulfate

ectopic beats

see ✪ **arrhythmia**.

eczema

Eczema is a skin condition where there is inflammation of the outer layer (epidermis) of the skin. It causes a reddish, itching rash with blisters, which may weep and crust over. Marks or different textures in the skin may be left as a result. Unlike ✪ **dermatitis**, eczema is mainly due to an internal, often inherited, tendency and need not involve a reaction to external substances; both terms are, however, often used interchangeably. There are a number of distinct eczema disorders, and these may have different causes. Atopic eczema, which can appear anywhere on the body, is the most common form. It usually starts in childhood and is linked with a family tendency toward eczema, asthma, and hay fever (atopy). Seborrheic eczema (also called seborrheic dermatitis; see ✪ **seborrhea**) is also common, and involves the face and scalp. It is linked with a yeast organism and also ✪ **dandruff**. Another form is discoid eczema, which has round skin lesions in adults.

Treatment

Treatment depends on the diagnosis, but includes ℞ **emollient** skin lotions, and often one of a wide range of ℞ **corticosteroids** that are used for this purpose, usually as skin preparations but sometimes by mouth. A number of other drugs may be tried, in order to treat some aspect of eczema, including topical anti-infectives such as ℞ **clioquinol**, and ℞ **doxepin** for ✪ **pruritis**. In some cases special UV light therapy may be helpful. Many herbal remedies and supplements, applied to the skin or by mouth, are believed to benefit aspects of eczema.

For further information
℞ DIRECTORY OF DRUGS:
corticosteroid • emollient • skin preparation
♣ HERBAL REMEDIES:
brewer's yeast • chamomile, German • cnidium • evening primrose • goldenseal • heartsease • henna • moneywort • oats • purple loosestrife • stinging nettle
♒ VITAMINS, MINERALS, AND SUPPLEMENTS:
gamma-linolenic acid (GLA) • omega-3 fatty acid

edema
see ✪ **fluid retention**.

embolism
see ✪ **peripheral vascular disorders**.

emphysema
Emphysema is a term most often applied to the special case of pulmonary emphysema. This is where tissue degeneration in the lungs results in the overexpansion of the air sacs (alveoli). Further degeneration of the thin alveolar walls through which the respiratory exchange of gases takes place also occurs. Breathing becomes labored and difficult, especially if the person contracts a respiratory infection. The precise cause of pulmonary emphysema is uncertain, but it occurs mostly in men, is increasingly common with age, and is linked with chronic ✪ **bronchitis** and smoking. See also ✪ **chronic obstructive pulmonary disease** (COPD).

Treatment
The only treatment for chronic pulmonary emphysema is oxygen therapy to aid breathing. Treatment for associated bronchospasm includes several ℞ **bronchodilator** drugs, usually taken by inhalation.

For further information
℞ DIRECTORY OF DRUGS:
bronchodilator

encephalitis
Encephalitis is the inflammation of brain tissue. This is a dangerous condition caused by ✪ **viral infection** (for example, a complication of ✪ **measles**) or ✪ **bacterial infection**, or by an allergic reaction (especially to certain vaccines; see ✪ **allergy**), or metal ✪ **poisoning** (lead). The viral form is more common in the tropics, and may occur as a complication of several other viral diseases (particularly ✪ **herpes** infections). Symptoms are high temperature, vomiting, headache, and neck stiffness; there is mental confusion, which may lead to coma (in which breathing may become severely labored) and sometimes death. A worldwide epidemic of encephalitis lethargica, or "sleeping sickness," occurred in the 1920s, characterized

by headache, drowsiness, and coma, for which no specific cause has been identified.

Treatment
Treatment follows a diagnosis of the specific cause, and includes supportive measures and sometimes antibacterial, antiviral, or antiallergic medication.

For further information
℞ DIRECTORY OF DRUGS:
antiallergic • antibacterial • antiviral

endocarditis
Endocarditis is the ✪ **inflammation** of the endocardium (the lining of the heart cavity) and the heart valves. It is almost always caused by the presence of bacteria and sometimes fungi, carried in the bloodstream. It is sometimes a complication of ✪ **rheumatic fever** during childhood, but occurs, most often, following minor surgery (such as a tooth extraction) or childbirth. Symptoms are ✪ **fatigue** and bouts of fever; ✪ **anemia** and weight loss follow. "Blood spots" may appear on the skin, representing small clots (emboli). The heart valves may become damaged, sometimes leading to long-term problems.

Treatment
Treatment involves hospitalization, rest and ℞ **antibacterial** or ℞ **antifungal** therapy for several weeks; surgery may be required to repair or replace damaged heart valves (see ✪ **heart valve disorders**).

For further information
℞ DIRECTORY OF DRUGS:
antibacterial • antifungal

endometrial cancer
see ✪ **cancer**.

endometriosis
Endometriosis is the presence of small areas of tissue, of the same type as the endometrium (uterus-lining), not lining the uterus (womb) as normal, but elsewhere in the abdomen (such as on an ovary). The tissue goes through the same cycle as the rest of the endometrium, even bleeding at menstruation. If there is no immediate escape for the blood, the pain that follows may be severe for several days. The cause is usually a retrograde (backward) displacement of endometrial cells along a Fallopian tube (the tubes that connect the uterus with each ovary) into the abdomen. This occurs during menstruation. It is a common condition, affecting 1 in 5 women of childbearing age. Severe endometriosis can cause problems with fertility. Symptoms include ✪ **dysmenorrhea**, irregular (oligomenorrhea) and heavy menstrual bleeding (✪ **menorrhagia**), pain during intercourse, and lower abdominal pain on urination.

Treatment
Treatment is usually with ℞ **hypothalamic hormone** drugs (℞ **gonadorelin** analogs such as ℞ **danazol**), which alter the levels of pituitary hormones, or ℞ **progestin**-containing forms of the ℞ **contraceptive** pill. Severe cases may require surgery. The condition usually resolves during pregnancy and ceases after the

menopause. ♣ **cotton** oil has been used as a traditional treatment for endometriosis.

For further information
℞ DIRECTORY OF DRUGS:
contraceptive • hypothalamic hormone • antiestrogen

♣ HERBAL REMEDIES:
cotton

enteritis

Enteritis is an inflammation of the small intestine. Infectious enteritis is often due to a protozoan such as in ✪ **giardiasis** (lambliasis), although it can also be caused by a bacterium (for example, the myco-bacterium that causes ✪ **tuberculosis**). It usually causes ✪ **diarrhea**. See also ✪ **gastroenteritis**, ✪ **digestive system disorders**.

For further information
℞ DIRECTORY OF DRUGS:
amebicide and antiprotozoal • antibacterial • electrolyte (rehydration solution)

♣ HERBAL REMEDIES:
flax • peppermint

enterobiasis
see ✪ worms.

enterogastritis
see ✪ gastroenteritis.

enuresis
see ✪ bed-wetting.

epiglotitis
see ✪ inflammation.

epilepsy

Epilepsy is a general term for a type of seizure disorder that is char-acterized by seizures involving uncoordinated and vigorous electri-cal activity in the brain. Symptoms correspond both with the area, or areas, of the brain involved, and with the specific form of the disorder. The most serious form is grand mal epilepsy, in which a person falls unconscious, perhaps simultaneously uttering a cry; the muscles stiffen and then jerk and twitch; there may be bladder incontinence and the tongue may be bitten. After several minutes, the individual may drift peacefully into a deep sleep or enter a trance-like state. Seizures in Jacksonian epilepsy may also reach these extremes, but build progressively from localized twitching of the limbs. In absence seizures (typically petit mal epilepsy) there may be no more than a brief, temporary, period of loss of con-sciousness. In most forms there may, or may not, be an initial aura, a warning that a seizure is imminent. Causes may be unknown, a head injury, a disease in the cerebral cortex (which may produce additional hallucinations), a very high temperature, drug allergy, an electric shock, or asphyxia—and anyone at all, at any time of life, can be subject to a seizure.

Treatment
Treatment is generally with ℞ **antiepileptic**/℞ **anticonvulsant** drugs, and is aimed at reducing the frequency of seizures without causing inhibiting side effects. Individuals must not drive or operate dangerous machinery until the seizures are well controlled.

For further information
℞ DIRECTORY OF DRUGS:
anticonvulsant • antiepileptic

epistaxis
see ✪ **nosebleed**.

erysipelas

Erysipelas is a contagious ✪ **bacterial infection** of the skin, partic-ularly of the face and scalp, which can causes severe symptoms. Affected areas of skin become inflamed and swollen, and the per-son suffers a high temperature and vomiting.

Treatment
Treatment is with antibacterials, but the condition may recur.

For further information
℞ DIRECTORY OF DRUGS:
antibacterial

esophageal ulcer
see ✪ peptic ulcer.

esophagitis
see ✪ inflammation.

exfoliative dermatitis
see ✪ dermatitis.

exhaustion
see ✪ fatigue.

familial hyperlipidemia
see ✪ hyperlipidemia.

fatigue

Fatigue is physical—and to some extent mental—tiredness, felt mostly as a lack of inner energy, muscular weariness, and a strong desire for rest or sleep. Fatigue becomes a medical problem when the person is unable to carry out routine tasks or work due to a lack of energy. That fatigue has mental aspects is evident from the dif-ference that mood makes: absorbing interest or success can both drive away fatigue. Causes of fatigue include inadequate diet, ✪ **anemia**, unaccustomed stress, disease (such as ✪ **chronic fatigue syndrome**), and high environmental temperature.

Treatment
Treatment is to rest, if possible, and remedy the cause. Several herbal remedies are described as, and are traditionally used as, energy tonics and restoratives, and can be beneficial in fatigue.

For further information
♣ HERBAL REMEDIES:
cola • ginseng • ginseng, Siberian • green tea • guarana • maté

⚖ VITAMINS, MINERALS, AND SUPPLEMENTS
green tea

favism

Favism is a disorder that is characterized by an intolerance to fava beans (broad beans; *Vicia faba*). These contain a chemical that, in affected individuals, causes rapid destruction of red blood cells (hemolytic ✪ **anemia**), due to the person having biochemically abnormal red blood cells. Symptoms include ✪ **headache**, dizziness, ✪ **vomiting**, ✪ **jaundice**, ✪ **fever**, ✪ **diarrhea**, and white blood cell abnormalities. It can occur on inhalation of pollen from the plant, but is generally more severe when fresh fava beans are eaten raw, and in children. It is a genetically inherited condition, relatively common in populations originating from most parts of Africa, most parts of Asia, some Pacific Islands, and from southern (Mediterranean) areas of Europe (for example, southern Italians). Its biochemical cause is an enzyme deficiency disorder (✪ **G6PD-deficiency**; glucose 6-phosphate dehydrogenase deficiency), which also predisposes to serious adverse drug reactions (for example, to the ℞ **antimalarial** drug ℞ **primaquine**).

Treatment

It can be treated by blood transfusions and the avoidance of fava beans, pollen, and certain drugs. Those who have the disorder should avoid herbal remedies or supplements derived from the fava bean family, and should take expert advice before taking any OTC or prescribed medicines.

fever

Fever is classed as a body temperature that is higher than normal (normal is 37°C or about 98.6°F, measured in the mouth; 37.2°C or 99°F in the rectum). It is often associated with shivering and ✪ **headache**, thirst, and muscular aches; in addition there may be nausea, and either ✪ **diarrhea** or ✪ **constipation**. The medical term is pyrexia and the cause is almost always an infection—although, rarely, fever results from a blood disorder or cancer. Medical diagnosis should be sought, especially in young babies, if the fever lasts for more than a day, if vomiting occurs, or if the temperature rises as high as 39.4°C (104°F). A temperature higher than 40.5°C (105°F) may cause delirium. Certain infections (such as malaria) are accompanied by specific cycles of temperature variation.

Treatment

Treatment depends on the cause, and may include ℞ **antibacterial** drugs to treat a bacterial infection. ℞ **antipyretic** drugs, including some available OTC, such as ℞ **acetaminophen** can help to reduce fever. Many herbal remedies are said to have fever-reducing properties.

For further information

℞ DIRECTORY OF DRUGS:
antipyretic • antibacterial

♣ HERBAL REMEDIES:
angelica • anise • angostura • ash • cardamom • chamomile, German • chiretta • cinnamon, Chinese • couch grass (*Elymus repens*) • devil's claw • feverfew • geum • horseradish • Japanese mint • larch • lemon verbena • mustard • onion • pipsissewa •

radish • rehmannia • safflower • southern bayberry • spruce • vervain • weeping forsythia • willow • wolfberry, Chinese • yarrow

fibroid

Fibroids are benign (non-cancerous) growths of the fibrous muscular wall of the uterus (womb) or sometimes the vagina. The presence of a fibroid (or fibroids) is a common condition, generally without any symptoms. Rarely, however, they become so large as to press on other abdominal organs or to cause pain (✪ **dysmenorrhea**) and heavy menstrual bleeding (✪ **menorrhagia**); in this state they might cause infertility or—in pregnancy—cause miscarriage.

Treatment

Treatment is unnecessary unless symptoms are troublesome. If they are, fibroids can sometimes be removed by surgery, although in severe cases hysterectomy (removal of the womb) may be necessary. ℞ **Non-narcotic analgesics**, mainly of the NSAID group, may help manage pain.

For further information

℞ DIRECTORY OF DRUGS:
non-narcotic analgesic • NSAID

fibromyalgia

see ✪ **musculoskeletal disorders**.

flatulence

Flatulence is the intestinal discomfort or feeling of abdominal fullness that is relieved by belching or passing gas. It is a feature of a number of intestinal disorders such as dyspepsia, ✪ **indigestion**, ✪ **irritable bowel syndrome**, and sometimes poor fat absorption due to biliary disorders (see ✪ **malabsorption disorders**).

Treatment

The underlying cause will be treated. Drugs that help include ℞ **antifoaming agents** (sometimes incorporated into antacid preparations), which lower surface tension allowing small bubbles of froth to coalesce into large bubbles. The most effective are silicone polymers such as ℞ **dimethicone**, and absorbents such as ℞ **activated charcoal** may help in absorbing gases. Some herbal remedies have traditional uses in relieving flatulence.

For further information

℞ DIRECTORY OF DRUGS:
antiflatulence agents (including antifoaming agents, for example, dimethicone) and (absorbents, for example, activated charcoal)

♣ HERBAL REMEDIES:
angelica • anise • cinnamon • dandelion • fennel • horehound • gentian • juniper • oswego tea • parsley • peppermint • spearmint • spikenard

flu

see ✪ **influenza**.

fluid retention

Fluid retention (water retention) is the accumulation of excess fluid in the body. The medical term edema (dropsy) is generally used when there is accumulation of fluid in body tissues, which causes swelling of a part of the body; but the terms fluid retention or water retention are often used as lay words for much the same thing (especially when there is a subjective feeling of bloating). Water intake and output from the body is in constant flux, being taken in as food and when drinking, and being lost in urine, feces, sweat, and exhaled vapor. The amount in the body needs to be controlled in narrow limits for optimal health. In practice, much water is lost in balancing levels of electrolytes in the body, principally sodium. Thus if excess salt is taken in the diet, the only effective way to excrete it is in the urine. The kidney has the task of excreting salts and water, but is under the control of ADH (antidiuretic hormone; also called vasopressin), which is secreted by the posterior pituitary gland according to the osmolarity of the blood. Edema or fluid retention is a symptom with many possible causes, including heart and vascular disorders such as ✪ **coronary artery disease**, ✪ **heart failure**, ✪ **hypertension**, or ✪ **kidney disorders** such as ✪ **nephritis**, ✪ **hyperaldosteronism**, lymphatic system disorders, injury, corticosteroid therapy, or local infection. A feeling of water retention and bloating—due to the action of estrogens—is a common feature of the menstrual cycle, and may contribute to ✪ **premenstrual syndrome**. Idiopathic edema is fluid retention of unknown cause.

Treatment

Treatment focuses on correcting the underlying cause if known (for example, ℞ **antihypertensives** and ℞ **heart failure treatment**). Fluid retention and edema are normally treated with ℞ **diuretics**. A wide range of diuretic drugs with different modes of action is available to increase the amount of urine passed. If relevant, the edematous part of the body should be protected from injury and if a limb is edematous, elevating the extremity and applying an elastic stocking can help in some cases. For less serious cases of fluid retention, mild OTC preparations containing ammonium chloride can be used. There are numerous herbal remedies that have, to varying degrees, diuretic properties, and many are available that can be used to relieve feelings of bloating.

For further information
℞ DIRECTORY OF DRUGS:
diuretic

♣ HERBAL REMEDIES:

asparagus • blackcurrant • boldo • buchu • buckbean • butcher's broom • coffee • cola • corn silk • couchgrass (*Agropyron repens*) • dandelion • embelia • figwort • fringed pink • goldenrod • hibiscus • horse chestnut • horsetail • Java tree • juniper • lily of the valley • lichwort • maté • quassia • spiny rest harrow • stinging nettle • turmeric (*Curcuma zedoria*) • uva-ursi • watercress

food poisoning

Food ✪ **poisoning** is a sudden illness caused by the consumption of food contaminated by bacteria (such as *Salmonella*, *Campylobacter*, *Listeria*, *E. coli*) or their toxins (as with botulism), by chemical poisoning (for instance with insecticides not washed off), or by natural poisoning (for instance with poisonous berries or fungi). Food poisoning due to infection can be transmitted by contamination at source, as with vegetables contaminated with animal feces, or shellfish caught in sewage-polluted waters, by poor hygiene among food handlers, or by inadequate storage conditions, or food preparation that allows bacteria to multiply. Inadequately cooked, or cooked then reheated, meals are particular culprits. Symptoms in most cases are restricted to ✪ **vomiting**, ✪ **diarrhea**, abdominal pain, and collapse. Every day in the United States, it is estimated that 200,000 people are sickened by a foodborne disease, 900 are hospitalized, and 14 die. It is a ✪ **digestive system disorder**.

Treatment

Treatment depends on the cause but may only aim at alleviating the symptoms until recovery; rehydration solutions to replace water (℞ **electrolytes**), and sometimes antibacterials may be necessary.

For further information
℞ DIRECTORY OF DRUGS:

antibacterial • electrolyte (rehydration solution)

fungal infections

Fungal infections (also called mycoses) are usually relatively minor under normal conditions, but tend to thrive in hot, damp conditions, in the gut during antibiotic treatment (✪ **candidiasis**), and in the immunocompromised (for example, in ✪ **AIDS**) when they can become life-threatening. A number of conditions involving fungal infections are dealt with in individual articles: see ✪ **athlete's foot**, ✪ **balanitis**, ✪ **dandruff**, ✪ **otitis**, ✪ **pneumonia**, ✪ **skin conditions**, ✪ **superinfections**, ✪ **tinea**, and ✪ **vaginitis**.

Treatment

In most cases the infection is superficial, and a wide range of topical preparations containing ℞ **antifungal** agents are available, some OTC. Systemic or deep-seated infections (such as aspergillosis or cryptococcosis) are more of a problem, since antifungals tend to be toxic when given systemically. Some systemic antifungal antibiotics are used (for example, ℞ **amphotericin B** is reserved for a range of life-threatening infections), ℞ **griseofulvin** for tinea (ringworm) infections of the nails, or some azoles (for example, ℞ **fluconazole**). For more information, see the specific fungal infection. Some herbal remedies (such as garlic) are promoted as being beneficial in preventing, or reducing tendency to ✪ **infections** in general, and ⚕⚕ **acidophilus** is beneficial in ✪ **candidiasis**. See individual disorders for more details.

G6PD-deficiency

G6PD-deficiency (glucose 6-phosphate dehydrogenase enzyme deficiency) is an inherited condition that is relatively common in populations genetically originating from most parts of Africa and Asia, some of the Pacific Islands, and from southern (Mediterranean) areas of Europe (for example, southern Italians). In affected people, serious adverse reactions occur if they take certain drugs; for instance, the antimalarial drug ℞ **primaquine** causes red blood-cell hemolysis in 5-10% of men of African ancestry, leading to severe anemia. Adverse reactions also occur to certain foodstuffs; see ✪ **favism**. Individuals vary in the severity of their reactions, but the risk and severity of hemolysis is dose-related. Common drugs with some, but very individual, risk of red blood cell damage include antimalarials (pamaquin; primaquine; sometimes chloroquine, quinine; quinidine); sulphone drugs (for example, dapsone); sulphonamides; antibacterials (quinolones); vitamin K and derivatives (for example, phytonadione); succimer; methylene blue; nitrofurantoin and probenecid. Mothballs may contain naphthalene, which also causes red blood cell hemolysis in people with G6PD-deficiency.

Treatment

Severe adverse reactions can be treated by blood transfusion. A biochemical test is available to test for G6PD-deficiency but individuals can vary unpredictably in the severity of their reactions to the various drugs. Care should be taken to avoid herbal remedies or supplements that are derived from certain foodstuffs including the fava bean family.

galactorrhea

Galactorrhea is the spontaneous or persistent production of milk, when a woman is not pregnant or is lactating postpartum. It also happens, rarely, in men, where there is a watery exudate. The usual cause is an increase in the release into the bloodstream of the hormone prolactin, which is produced and secreted by the anterior pituitary gland. The most common cause is ✪ **prolactinoma**, a noncancerous tumor of the pituitary, but the condition can also be caused as a side effect of certain antipsychotic drugs (for example, chlorpromazine) or as a result of some infections such as ✪ **meningitis**. Diagnosis includes measurement of hormone levels in the blood.

Treatment

The physiological release of prolactin into the bloodstream is controlled by a hypothalamic factor called prolactin-release inhibiting factor (PRIF), now thought to be identical to the neurotransmitter dopamine. Therefore drugs of the dopamine receptor stimulant type are used as indirect prolactin antagonists to control symptoms of prolactinoma, and are often very effective. Sometimes surgical removal of the tumor, or radiotherapy, may be necessary. (See also ✪ **pituitary gland disorders and tumors**; ✪ **prolactinoma**).

For further information

℞ DIRECTORY OF DRUGS:
dopamine-receptor stimulant (bromocriptine, cabergoline, pergolide)

gallbladder disorders

Gallbladder complaints/disorders commonly involve ✪ **gallstone** formation (✪ **calculus**) and inflammation of the gallbladder (cholecsytitis), which is often a consequence of the blockage. A common symptom of gallbladder or gall duct blockage is ✪ **jaundice** and/or ✪ **colic** (which in this case can be a very intense stabbing pain). Sometimes ✪ **pancreatitis** or ✪ **cirrhosis** are associated conditions. See also ✪ **digestive system disorders**.

Treatment

In most cases treatment centers on the use of drugs to dissolve the stones (choliolythics, including ℞ **monoctanoin** and ℞ **ursodiol**); breaking up the stones using ultrasound therapy, or may be by surgical removal of the stones (cholelithotomy) or of the entire gallbladder (cholecystectomy) (see ℞ **gallstone treatment**). Pain

relief with ℞ **narcotic analgesics** or ℞ **NSAIDs** (for example, ℞ **diclofenac**) is usually necessary. Many herbal remedies are claimed to help dissolve stones or prevent their formation, but evidence of their efficacy is often lacking. There are many herbal remedies traditionally used for gallbladder complaints. These include: ♣ **black root**, ♣ **cardamom**, ♣ **celandine**, ♣ **chicory**, ♣ **curcuma**, ♣ **dandelion**, ♣ **haronga**, ♣ **immortelle**, ♣ **Japanese mint**, ♣ **Java tree**, ♣ **milk thistle**, ♣ **peppermint**, ♣ **tamarind**.

gallstone

Gallstones are composed of ✪ **calculus** (stone) made up of bile pigments (biliary calculus), cholesterol (derived mainly from animal fats in the diet), and calcium salts. They are located in the gallbladder or, less commonly but with more severe results, in the common bile duct. Formation of gallstones (cholelithiasis) occurs when the chemical structure of bile changes to make cholesterol less soluble. Symptoms may be absent, or there may be acute pain (biliary colic), jaundice, and inflammation of the gallbladder (cholecystitis) and the common bile duct.

Treatment

Treatment is only necessary if the stones cause symptoms, and may be by surgical removal, of the stones (cholelithotomy) or of the entire gallbladder (cholecystectomy), or by breaking up the stones using ultrasound therapy. ℞ **gallstone treatment** also includes drugs to dissolve the stones (choliolythics, including ℞ **ursodiol**).

For further information

℞ DIRECTORY OF DRUGS:
gallstone treatment • narcotic analgesic • NSAID (for example, diclofenac)

gangrene

Gangrene occurs when the blood supply to a tissue is cut off, which results in the death and decay of the affected tissue. It can be caused by any condition that interrupts the arterial blood flow, including injury (as might result from frostbite, ✪ **burns**, crushing, or a ✪ **wound**), infected ✪ **bedsores**, ✪ **arteriosclerosis**, ✪ **Raynaud's disease**, a strangulated ✪ **hernia**, ✪ **diabetes mellitus**, or ✪ **thrombosis**. Gangrene is classified as either "dry" (without bacterial invasion) or "moist" (with additional bacterial invasion). In both conditions, a red line on the skin surface may demarcate the edges of affected tissue. Dry gangrene causes painful withering of the tissue, loss of sensation, and a change of color in the skin surface, gradually to black. Moist gangrene produces red blistering of the skin, with heat, before showing the same symptoms. It is accompanied by a putrefactive smell. Another form of moist gangrene (gas gangrene) is caused by direct bacterial invasion of a wound.

Treatment

In all cases treatment involves surgical removal of the affected tissue, with ample doses of ℞ **antibacterial** drugs to prevent infection.

For further information

℞ DIRECTORY OF DRUGS:
antibacterial

gas

see ✪ flatulence.

gastric ulcer

see ✪ peptic ulcer.

gastric upset

see ✪ digestive system disorders.

gastritis

A common ✪ **digestive system disorder** that is caused by inflammation of the stomach lining. Acute gastritis, which has symptoms of ✪ **nausea**, ✪ **vomiting**, ✪ **appetite loss**, and discomfort after eating may be caused by severe burns, NSAIDs such as aspirin or ibuprofen, excessive alcohol consumption, food allergens or bacterial, viral, or chemical toxins. Chronic gastritis, which develops over months or years is usually a sign of an underlying disorder such as ✪ **Zollinger-Ellison syndrome**, ✪ **peptic ulcer** or stomach ✪ **cancer** and may occur in ✪ **Crohn's disease** or as a result of long term use of NSAIDs, alcohol or tobacco. There may be bleeding from the damaged stomach lining, which can lead to iron-deficient ✪ **anemia**.

Treatment

The treatment of gastritis depends on the cause. It usually improves with life-style changes and symptoms may be relieved by eating small, regular meals, reducing alcohol intake, and giving up smoking. The symptoms of mild gastritis can be treated with OTC antacids, which neutralize the stomach acid. If the cause of the gastritis is a peptic ulcer, ulcer-healing drugs may be prescribed.

For further information

℞ DIRECTORY OF DRUGS:
antacid • ulcer-healing drug
♣ HERBAL REMEDIES:
licorice • marshmallow • plantain • thyme

gastroenteritis

Gastroenteritis is the inflammation of the stomach lining and part of the small intestine, which results in, often severe, ✪ **diarrhea** and ✪ **vomiting**. Causes include ✪ **bacterial infection** (including *Salmonella* or *E. coli*) or ✪ **viral infection**, and toxins (causing ✪ **food poisoning**).

Treatment

Most cases resolve within a few days and all that is necessary is the maintenance of fluid intake. In severe cases and in infants, the person may become dehydrated and rehydration solutions containing ℞ **electrolytes** through a drip may be needed.

For further information

℞ DIRECTORY OF DRUGS:
electrolyte (rehydration solution)

gastroesophageal reflux

Gastroesophageal reflux, or acid reflux, is a common cause of acid ✪ **indigestion**. It results from the regurgitation of acid juices, from the stomach into the esophagus (gullet), the tube that joins the throat to the stomach. It can lead to harmful erosion since the esophagus does not have natural protection against acid. The inflammation and associated pain is sometimes referred to as heartburn. See also ✪ **digestive system disorders**.

Treatment

℞ **Antacids** are commonly used for the symptomatic relief of occasional problems, as are some antispasmodic drugs that reduce muscle spasms. Ulcer-healing drugs (℞ **H_2-antagonist**; ℞ **proton-pump inhibitors**) that actually decrease acid production in the stomach can be very effective, and may be used to treat continuing problems. In some cases, special gut ℞ **motility stimulants** that speed up stomach emptying may be used.

For further information

℞ DIRECTORY OF DRUGS:
antacid • antispasmodic, including anticholinergic • motility stimulant (metoclopramide hydrochloride) • H_2-antagonist • proton-pump inhibitor

gastrointestinal disorders

see ✪ digestive system disorders.

gastrointestinal disturbances

see ✪ digestive system disorders.

gastrointestinal tract disorders

see ✪ digestive system disorders.

genital warts

see ✪ wart.

German measles

see ✪ rubella.

giant cell arteritis

see ✪ arteritis.

giardiasis

Giardiasis (giardiosis) is an inflammatory intestinal condition caused by the protozoan *Giardia lamblia* and is caught from drinking water contaminated with cysts. It usually occurs in developing countries where hygiene is poor. Infection is most serious in people who have reduced immunity. Symptoms include ✪ **diarrhea**, bloating, ✪ **flatulence**, belching, ✪ **nausea**, and abdominal pain. If the condition continues there may be additional complications, which include damage to the lining of the small intestine and poor absorption of food. It is one of the causes of "traveler's diarrhea."

Treatment

Prevention is best; good personal hygiene (for example, washing hands) and the boiling of water. ℞ **Amebicide and antiprotozoal** drugs (for example, metronidazole) may be prescribed to destroy any protozoa.

For further information

℞ DIRECTORY OF DRUGS:
amebicide and antiprotozoal

gingivitis

Gingivitis is the inflammation of the gums, especially where the teeth meet the gums. The cause is almost always plaque (bacteria-containing deposits on the teeth), but it can occasionally be due to ill-fitting or dirty dentures, ✪ **diabetes mellitus**, ✪ **pregnancy-related disorders**, or gum overgrowth due to certain drugs. Symptoms are pain, swelling of the gums, and a tendency for them to bleed. Periodontitis (inflammation of the tissues that support the teeth) may develop, and the teeth may become loose in their sockets. If gingivitis develops suddenly, it is called ulcerated gingivitis ("trench mouth") and may require immediate treatment including ℞ **antibacterials**.

Treatment
Early stages are easily treated by an improvement in dental hygiene. Periodontitis may require more intensive dental treatment. Antibacterials may be required.

For further information
℞ DIRECTORY OF DRUGS:
antibacterial • antiseptic
♣ HERBAL REMEDIES:
myrrh

glandular fever

Glandular fever is an infectious disease (medically called infectious mononucleosis), a ✪ **viral infection** caused by the Epstein-Barr virus. It produces swelling of the lymph nodes in the neck, armpits, and groin, with lethargy, high temperature, headache, and sore throat; there may also be weight loss. The condition mostly affects adolescents and young adults. Possible complications include enlargement of the spleen and kidney malfunction. Symptoms may persist for some weeks and some of those affected develop ✪ **chronic fatigue syndrome**, which may last for many months afterward. It is also called "kissing disease."

Treatment
Treatment is with drugs including ℞ **antipyretics** and ℞ **non-narcotic analgesics** to alleviate the symptoms, and to rest when necessary. The herbal remedy ♣ **myrrh** has been used traditionally.

For further information
℞ DIRECTORY OF DRUGS:
antipyretic • non-narcotic analgesic • NSAID
♣ HERBAL REMEDIES:
myrrh

glaucoma

Glaucoma is a condition in which an increase in the fluid pressure within the eyeball (intraocular pressure) causes visual disturbances such as blurring, auras around light sources, and tunnel vision and, if left untreated, leads to eventual blindness. It may occur secondary to other eye diseases that impair the flow of fluid (aqueous humor) within the front part of the eye, but most cases occur without other forms of eye disease. Acute glaucoma results from the sudden blockage of the drainage of aqueous humor from the angle of the eye, and results in pain and marked blurring. It requires urgent treatment. In chronic simple glaucoma the build-up of pressure is gradual and usually occurs without pain. Symptoms only slowly become apparent. Glaucoma becomes increasingly frequent after middle age. The cause of the pressure increase is usually unknown—although it is more common in farsighted people, and there may be hereditary factors; occasionally glaucoma arises as a complication of ✪ **diabetes mellitus** or eye infection.

Treatment
Early treatment with eyedrops or drugs by mouth, to improve fluid outflow from the eye or to reduce the production of fluid, is essential. Surgical drainage may, however, be necessary.

For further information
℞ DIRECTORY OF DRUGS:
glaucoma treatment

glomerulonephritis

see ✪ **nephritis**.

glossitis

Glossitis is an ✪ **inflammation** of the tongue. Causes include a general infection of the mouth and throat (for instance ✪ **candidiasis** or ✪ **herpes** simplex) through poor oral hygiene, damage due to scalding liquids, cigarette smoking, alcohol consumption, ✪ **anemia**, malnutrition, ill-fitting dentures, and the use of certain antibiotics. Symptoms are pain, commonly a smooth red surface to the tongue, and difficulty in swallowing; the saliva may also be thicker than normal.

Treatment
Treatment depends on the cause and usually requires correcting the underlying problem. Relief may be obtained with ℞ **antifungal** mouthwashes (if due to candidiasis) in very mild cases of glossitis.

For further information
℞ DIRECTORY OF DRUGS:
antifungal

glue ear

Glue ear is the accumulation of fluid in the middle ear cavity, due to a repeated or persistent middle ear infection (✪ **otitis** media); often a result of recurring respiratory infections. It most commonly occurs during childhood, due to a failure of the Eustachian tube, which connects the middle ear with the back of the nose, to drain fluid accumulated during chronic inflammation. Symptoms are pain and temporarily impaired hearing. Sometimes the eardrum ruptures, releasing pus.

Treatment
Many cases improve spontaneously, and most children grow out of the problem. Where symptoms are severe, the fluid may be drained during surgery, and by the use of grommets—small tubes—inserted into the eardrum to allow the fluid to drain. An underlying infection may be treated with ℞ **antibacterial** drugs.

For further information
℞ DIRECTORY OF DRUGS:
antibacterial

gluten-sensitive enteropathy

see ✪ **celiac disease**.

gonorrhea

Gonorrhea is a contagious ✪ **bacterial infection** of the mucous membranes of the genitalia (and occasionally the anus, mouth, or eyes). It is a ✪ **sexually transmitted disease**. In men, symptoms are a thick yellowish discharge from the infected site (generally the penis), and inflammation of the urethra (the tube conducting urine and semen through the penis), leading to pain and difficulty in urination. Rarely, in an infected man, there are no symptoms, but he is still infectious. There are seldom symptoms in women. Women who do have symptoms experience a discharge from the infected site (generally the vagina), and pain. Women may pass the infection on to their baby during childbirth, causing eye infection (ophthalmia neonatorum). Diagnosis may require examination of the bacteria in a culture medium. If untreated, the condition can spread throughout the reproductive organs, resulting in sterility, and may cause complications in the eyes, heart, and joints.

Treatment

Treatment, which must be of both sexual partners to be effective, is with ℞ **penicillins** or other ℞ **antibacterial** drugs, mainly ℞ **antibiotics**.

For further information

℞ **DIRECTORY OF DRUGS:**
antibacterial

gout

Gout is a condition of exceedingly painful ✪ **inflammation** in specific joints, and in the skin. It is caused by the presence of excess uric acid in the blood. This is converted to sodium urate crystals, which become deposited in the joints. Uric acid is normally excreted in the urine; gout occurs when there is excess acid or when excretion is impaired, as may be the case after abnormal quantities of food and drink, following certain injuries, or during a course of diuretic drugs. There is also a hereditary factor. Often it affects one joint (usually that of the big toe), which swells with the skin surface turning red and shiny. Untreated or recurrent gout may lead to permanent joint and kidney damage.

Treatment

Treatment is with ℞ **antigout** drugs, which increase uric acid excretion. Bed rest is also advised. Several herbal remedies are traditionally used to treat gout.

For further information

℞ **DIRECTORY OF DRUGS:**
antigout

♣ **HERBAL REMEDIES:**

blackcurrant • black horehound • celery • devil's claw • guaiac • juniper • parsley • spiny rest harrow

grand mal

see ✪ epilepsy.

Grave's disease

see ✪ hyperthyroidism.

griping pain

see ✪ colic.

Guillain-Barré syndrome

Guillain-Barré syndrome is a neurological disorder (a polyneuritis) caused by an abnormal reaction in the peripheral nervous system. It typically appears 2–3 weeks after a minor infection of the respiratory tract or intestine (usually viral infections, or rarely following immunization). Symptoms include weakness in the limbs and sometimes paralysis, which may spread to include the muscles that control breathing. Recovery may take many months, and a few individuals are left with permanent disability.

Treatment

Treatment of early symptoms with intravenous ℞ **immune globulins** can hasten recovery. In cases where respiratory muscles are affected, artificial respiration on a ventilator, with physiotherapy may be needed. Plasmapheresis (the removal of plasma from blood, and subsequent reinfusion of that blood to replace red cells) may be used.

For further information

℞ **DIRECTORY OF DRUGS:**
immune globulin

halitosis

Halitosis is bad breath. Causes include poor dental hygiene and ✪ **tooth decay**, ✪ **infection** of the mouth, nose, or throat, stomach or lung disorders, and breathing through the mouth instead of the nose. More serious causes include liver disease and ✪ **diabetes mellitus**.

Treatment

Treatment depends on the cause—but unless that is medically diagnosed, it is generally dealt with by disguising the symptoms. ℞ **antiseptic** mouthwashes may be useful.

For further information

℞ **DIRECTORY OF DRUGS:**
antiseptic

Hansen's disease

see ✪ leprosy.

Hashimoto's thyroiditis

see ✪ hypothyroidism.

hay fever

Hay fever is an allergic response (an ✪ **allergy**) to the presence of pollen, grass dust, spores, or similar airborne plant particles. It is known medically as seasonal allergic ✪ **rhinitis**. Symptoms include a runny nose, sneezing, and watering eyes—due to inflammation of the nasal lining and conjunctiva (the membrane covering the eye), mainly caused by the release of histamine in the tissues.

Treatment

Treatment of the symptoms with ℞ **antihistamines**, either by mouth or nose-drops, is often effective, and many OTC preparations are available. Various ℞ **antiallergic** drugs—in serious cases ℞ **corticosteroids**—may be prescribed and used as nose-drops. If a specific allergen (a substance provoking the allergy) is identified, possibly by a patch test, desensitization (a method for reducing allergic responses by gradually building up tolerance to the allergen) may be possible.

For further information

℞ DIRECTORY OF DRUGS:

antiallergic • antihistamine • corticosteroid • decongestant

headache

Headache is a pain felt inside the head. Causes range from ✪ **fatigue** and ✪ **anxiety**, alcohol or other drug abuse, ear and eye disorders, ✪ **migraine**, ✪ **cluster headache**, and referred toothache, to serious infections such as ✪ **otitis** media (or interna), ✪ **meningitis**, ✪ **stroke**, various tumors (for example, pituitary tumors), concussion and other forms of injury, and disease of the brain itself. In general, however, most headaches are not serious.

Treatment

Treatment of most non-serious headaches is with non-narcotic analgesics (painkillers), many of which are available OTC including ℞ **aspirin** and ℞ **acetaminophen**. There are also some OTC preparations that contain small amounts of ℞ **codeine phosphate** and other ℞ **narcotic analgesics**. Many herbal remedies are available and can be taken to relieve mild headaches, tension headaches, and also ✪ **migraine**. These include ♣ **cola** and ♣ **feverfew**. Any headache that is not relieved by painkillers or if it is unusually severe, should be medically diagnosed. ⚗ **vitamin B$_2$** is thought to help some sufferers of migraine.

For further information

℞ DIRECTORY OF DRUGS:

narcotic analgesic • non-narcotic analgesic • NSAID

♣ HERBAL REMEDIES:

cola • feverfew • horsemint, English • maté • pasque flower • rosemary • willow

⚗ VITAMINS, MINERALS, AND SUPPLEMENTS:

vitamin B$_2$

headlice

see ✪ **lice and mite infestation**.

heart arrhythmia

see ✪ **arrhythmia**.

heart attack

see ✪ **myocardial infarction**.

heartburn

see ✪ **indigestion**.

heart disease

Heart disease is a general term for any of the many disorders of the heart, including ✪ **angina pectoris**, ✪ **heart failure**, ✪ **heart valve disorders**, ✪ **hypertension** (high blood pressure), ✪ **coronary artery disease**, coronary thrombosis, hypertrophy of the heart, bacterial ✪ **endocarditis**, bradycardia (a slowing of the heart), tachycardia (speeding of the heart), and heart block. See also ✪ **cardiovascular disorders**.

Treatment

Treatment depends on the cause and may include surgery and/or diverse drugs including: ℞ **diuretics**, ℞ **ACE inhibitors**, ℞ **beta-blockers**, and other ℞ **antihypertensives**, ℞ **cardiac glycosides**, ℞ **anticoagulants**, ℞ **antiplatelet** agents, ℞ **lipid-regulating drugs**, and heart failure treatments. A number of dietary supplements are claimed to protect against heart disease by, for example, lowering blood cholesterol levels or reducing free radicals. These include **amino acids** (arginine, taurine), ⚗ **antioxidant**, ⚗ **carotenoid**, ⚗ **coenzyme Q$_{10}$**, ⚗ **conjugated linoleic acid**, ⚗ **DHEA**, ℞ **folic acid**, ⚗ **garlic**, ⚗ **isoflavone**, ⚗ **magnesium**, ⚗ **omega-3 fatty acid**, ⚗ **S-adenosylmethionine**, ⚗ **selenium**, ⚗ **vitamin B$_6$**, ⚗ **vitamin B$_{12}$**, ⚗ **vitamin C**, ⚗ **vitamin E**. Many herbal remedies are claimed to be of use, such as ♣ **hawthorn**, ⚗ **garlic**, and ♣ **soybean**. See individual disorders for more information.

heart failure

Heart failure is a condition where the heart cannot pump enough blood to meet the metabolic demands of the body (especially for oxygen).

In acute heart failure there is a sudden deterioration, often due to severe heart attack (✪ **myocardial infarction**), and generally affecting the left side where fresh blood is pumped from the lungs. If not corrected, fluid accumulates in the lungs (pulmonary edema), presenting a potentially life-threatening situation. Other causes of acute heart failure are infections that stress the heart (for example, ✪ **pneumonia**), a specific infection of the heart valves (for example, infective ✪ **endocarditis**), or as a development of chronic heart failure. Although right-sided acute heart failure is uncommon, it may follow ✪ **pulmonary embolism** where a blood clot has blocked the blood supply from the lungs via the pulmonary artery.

In chronic heart failure there is a long-term difficulty in pumping blood around the body. This leads to a build-up of fluid (edema) in the lungs and tissues. This form of heart failure is most common in those over 65. Either left-sided or right-sided heart failure may develop initially, depending on the cause. In most cases, initial left-sided chronic heart failure follows a diminished blood supply to the heart as a result of ✪ **coronary artery disease** or, failing this, persistent hypertension, which makes the heart work harder. Initial right-sided chronic heart failure is commonly the result of a chronic lung disease, particularly ✪ **chronic obstructive pulmonary disease** (COPD). Other causes or risk factors of chronic heart failure include ✪ **anemia**, ✪ **heart valve disorders**, cardiomyopathy (see ✪ **heart disease**), ✪ **hyperthyroidism**, extreme ✪ **obesity** or as a risk factor in ✪ **diabetes mellitus**. Symptoms include edema, swelling of veins in the neck, breathlessness, and congestion of the lungs and the liver with blood.

Treatment

Treatment is mostly through diet and bed rest or the avoidance of extreme exercise. Surgery, including heart transplant, may be required depending on the cause. ℞ **Diuretics** will be prescribed to reduce edema. A variety of other drugs may also be prescribed, including a number of ℞ **antihypertensive** agents. Some vitamins, minerals, and supplements are said to be beneficial in protecting against heart failure.

For further information
℞ DIRECTORY OF DRUGS:
heart failure treatment
♣ HERBAL REMEDIES:
hawthorn
⚕ VITAMINS, MINERALS, AND SUPPLEMENTS:
amino acid (carnitine, taurine) • coenzyme Q$_{10}$

heart valve disorders

Heart valve disorders are problems with one or more of the four valves in the heart. The heart valves ensure that pumped blood flows in the right direction. Impaired valves affect the efficiency of the heart, so severe disorder may cause chronic ○ **heart failure** or ○ **arrhythmias** of heartbeat. Heart valve defects may be present at birth, be caused by infections of the lining of the heart (for example, ○ **rheumatic fever**) or by a heart attack (○ **myocardial infarction**). Conversely, damaged valves are more susceptible to infection (for example, infective ○ **endocarditis**). There are several types of disorder (for example, mitral stenosis, aortic stenosis, mitral incompetence, aortic incompetence). Diagnosis is made by a specialist, using EKG analysis.

Treatment
Where the valves are badly damaged, surgical replacement may be the best course. Alternatively, heart drugs are used to strengthen the beat or to correct irregularities of rhythm. Because of the risk of bacterial endocarditis, your doctor may recommend a single dose of ℞ **antibacterial** antibiotics before having dental extractions (which are known to release potentially dangerous bacteria into the bloodstream).

For further information
℞ DIRECTORY OF DRUGS:
ACE inhibitor • antiarrhythmic • antibacterial (for example, amoxicillin, metronidazole, vancomycin) **• anticoagulant • antiplatelet • cardiac glycoside • diuretic**

heatstroke

Heatstroke is the failure of the body's internal temperature-regulating mechanism, following continuous exposure to unaccustomed heat, such as in sunstroke. Symptoms include very high temperature, often above 104°F (40°C) without perspiration, ○ **headache**, ○ **nausea**, weakness, and eventual unconsciousness. The condition (also called sunstroke) may cause convulsions or be fatal if left untreated.

Treatment
The person's body should be kept cool by covering with damp cloths; drinks, especially drinks containing salt, should be administered to compensate for fluid loss. In severe cases rehydration fluids (℞ **electrolytes**)—through a drip—may be required.

For further information
℞ DIRECTORY OF DRUGS:
electrolyte (rehydration solution)

Helicobactor pylori
see ○ **peptic ulcer.**

helminth infestation
see ○ **worms.**

hemochromatosis

Hemochromatosis (also called "bronze diabetes") is a genetic condition, which causes iron to be excessively absorbed and deposited in body tissues, damaging them in the process. Iron is therefore dangerous to those affected (more than one million American men have this condition). In middle life it may cause ○ **impotence**, damage to the pancreas (resulting in ○ **diabetes mellitus**), liver ○ **cirrhoses**, liver ○ **cancer** and heart ○ **arrhythmias**. There is a bronzed appearance to the skin due to the deposition of iron pigment.

Treatment
Treatment involves the removal of blood. Drugs are used that bind (chelate) iron and hasten its elimination from the body. It is important that people suffering from hemochromatosis do not take iron supplements.

For further information
℞ DIRECTORY OF DRUGS:
antidote • chelating agent (for example, **desferoxamine mesylate**)

hemolytic anemia
see ○ **anemia.**

hemophilia

Hemophilia is an inherited ○ **bleeding disorder**. It is caused by an insufficiency in one of the clotting factors in the blood, most often Factor VIII (antihemophilic factor) and sometimes Factor IX (Christmas factor). In general, females are genetic carriers of the disorder, and males actually suffer from it (it is an X-linked disorder; that is, one carried on the X-chromosome). Symptoms are prolonged bleeding from even a slight injury, and sometimes spontaneous internal ○ **hemorrhages**, most often affecting muscles or joints.

Treatment
Treatment is with blood products that are comprised of blood or plasma (the fluid component of blood, with the blood cells removed) containing the missing factor or antihemophilic factor. The missing factor or antihemophilic factor is obtained either as an extract from blood or, as is now more possible, manufactured synthetically using recombinant molecular techniques. For mild to moderate cases, ℞ **desmopressin**, an analog of the posterior pituitary hormone vasopressin, can be used to boost factor VIII levels.

For further information
℞ DIRECTORY OF DRUGS:
antihemophilic factor • hemostatic (desmopressin)

hemorrhage

Hemorrhage, commonly called bleeding, is a loss of blood from the cardiovascular circulatory system. It may have many causes, such as physical damage or a bleeding disorder (for example, hemophilia); or it may result as a consequence of another disorder (for example, ⊙ **hemorrhoids**, ⊙ **nosebleed**, ⊙ **peptic ulcer**, and cerebrovascular hemorrhage (cerebral hemorrhage, subarachnoid hemorrhage, subdural hemorrhage)). Bleeding following minor trauma is often an unavoidable consequence and, in some cases, it may be necessary to treat people with a tendency to form blood clots with anticoagulant drugs (for example, after ⊙ **stroke** or ⊙ **myocardial infarction**). Substantial amounts of blood may be lost during menstruation (⊙ **menorrhagia**); and this excess bleeding may need to be corrected.

Treatment

If the hemorrhage is due to a ⊙ **bleeding disorder** such as hemophilia, it is necessary to replace missing coagulation factors by transfusion. Other diseases are corrected by an appropriate therapy, and blood or plasma transfusion can be life saving, where loss of blood is substantial or fast. Hemorrhagic disease of the newborn and some vitamin K malabsorption states are treated with injections of ℞ **phytonadione** (vitamin K_1 in drug form). A chronic tendency to bleed may sometimes be corrected by supplementing the diet with one of the forms of vitamin K used for this purpose. Iron deficiency may cause ⊙ **anemia**, which needs correcting. Various ℞ **hemostatic** drugs are available for correcting excess bleeding, and several herbal remedies have been traditionally used to treat different types of hemorrhage.

For further information

℞ DIRECTORY OF DRUGS:

anemia treatment • hemostatic drugs • **phytonadione**

♣ HERBAL REMEDIES:

garlic • geum • logwood • lotus • purple loosestrife • shepherd's purse • smartweed

⚖ VITAMINS, MINERALS, AND SUPPLEMENTS:

vitamin K

hemorrhoids

Hemorrhoids, or piles, are painfully distended veins in the walls of the anus. First-degree hemorrhoids remain inside the anus and may bleed at the end of defecation, but have no other symptoms. Second-degree hemorrhoids may appear at the entrance of the anus or outside and may cause discomfort but return spontaneously, whereas third-degree hemorrhoids require manual pressure to return them inside. The cause is usually prolonged ⊙ **constipation**.

Treatment

Treatment is generally by increasing fiber levels in the diet, in order to defeat constipation. Drugs may be given to soften the feces and reduce discomfort. Severe or persistent hemorrhoids can be treated by injections of ℞ **anorectal preparation** in the form of sclerosing agents that harden the tissue, infrared coagulation or ligation (tying off). Third-degree hemorrhoids may require surgical removal. Herbal remedies can help with the symptoms of piles by, for example, softening the stools, or astringents can be taken that tone the blood vessels and reduce bleeding (such as ♣ **pilewort**).

For further information

℞ DIRECTORY OF DRUGS:

anorectal preparation • sclerosing agent

♣ HERBAL REMEDIES:

bilberry • butcher's broom • chamomile, German • ground ivy • pilewort • plantain • poplar • purple loosestrife • smartweed • sweetclover • witch hazel • yellow toad flax

hepatitis

Hepatitis is an inflammation of the liver. In the case of infectious hepatitis it is caused by a ⊙ **viral infection** with one (or more) of a variety of hepatitis viruses. Non-infectious hepatitis is caused by certain drugs, poisons, chemicals, and ⊙ **alcoholism**, or may occur as a result of an ⊙ **autoimmune disorder** (in which the immune system attacks the body's own tissues). Acute viral hepatitis may be transmitted through food and drink in areas of poor hygiene and sanitation, and is caused mostly by hepatitis A or hepatitis B viruses. Symptoms are high temperature, ⊙ **nausea**, ⊙ **vomiting**, and loss of appetite; all these are followed by ⊙ **jaundice**, which may last for three weeks. At this stage the hepatitis is over but may in turn be followed by ⊙ **depression**. Thereafter recovery is usually complete. Hepatitis B virus infection, formerly called serum hepatitis, is transmitted in blood or blood products (such as treatment with antihemophilic factor), contaminated hypodermic or tattooing needles, sexual contact, or contact with other body fluids such as breast milk. Those with drug habits and male homosexuals are particularly at risk. Symptoms, which may take many months to develop, include ⊙ **headache**, ⊙ **fever**, malaise, and jaundice. Sometimes the hepatitis D virus is found along with hepatitis B, making the infection more severe. A similar form of hepatitis is caused by the hepatitis C virus (which has infected about 3% of people worldwide). All forms of viral hepatitis, but particularly those caused by hepatitis viruses B, C, and D, may progress to a chronic condition with long-term liver damage including ⊙ **cirrhosis** and tumors of the liver; such complications may be fatal. A chronic condition of hepatitis also results from ⊙ **alcoholism**, in which the alcohol causes liver cells to fill with fats. The cells then burst, and die. The dead cells inflame adjacent cells, and ⊙ **cirrhosis** may follow.

Treatment

Treatment of acute viral hepatitis is generally with bed rest, and then only initially. Alcohol must usually be avoided for a prolonged period to prevent further liver damage. Those in close contact with a person with hepatitis B may be injected with ℞ **immune globulin** as a precaution. Chronic hepatitis C can now be treated with ℞ **immunomodulator** drugs (certain ℞ **interferons**), and the ℞ **antiviral** drug ℞ **ribavirin**. Autoimmune hepatitis (chronic active hepatitis) may respond to ℞ **corticosteroid** or ℞ **immunosuppressant** drugs. Vaccines are available against hepatitis A (often given to travelers) and hepatitis B (given to medical staff and others at high risk). The herbs ♣ **bupleurum** and ♣ **green tea** have been shown to have some beneficial effects.

For further information

℞ DIRECTORY OF DRUGS:

antiviral • immune globulin • immunomodulator (interferons) • immunosuppressant • vaccine

♣ HERBAL REMEDIES:

bupleurum • green tea • milk thistle

hernia

A hernia, also called a rupture, is an abnormal protrusion of part of an organ, usually the intestine, through a gap in adjacent tissues. Most commonly, part of the intestine works its way through a weakened spot in the lower part of the abdominal wall (inguinal hernia), causing a swelling in the groin and some pain. A ✪ **hiatus hernia** occurs when part of the stomach rides up through the gap in the diaphragm meant for the esophagus (gullet); symptoms may be no more than regurgitation, but can be more problematic. In babies or following abdominal surgery in adults, a hernia may appear at the navel (umbilicus)—umbilical hernia. Rarely, other tissues—such as the peritoneum or part of the bladder—may be the protruding tissue.

Treatment

Most types of hernia can be reduced (replaced) fairly simply by manipulation, and kept in place if necessary by using a truss. Those that cannot may have to be dealt with surgically before they become strangulated (before the blood supply to the protruding portion is cut off by pressure and the tissue dies). Symptoms of hiatus hernia can be relieved with ℞ **antacids**.

herpes

Herpes is a localized infection of the skin or mucous membranes by the herpes viruses (spelt herpesviruses in medical circles). It results in clusters of small blisters (see ✪ **cold sore**). The herpes simplex virus has two forms, type I typically causing cold sores around the lips and nose; and type II usually causing genital herpes, a sexually transmitted disease. Occasionally, either type may cause blisters in their non-preferred area. The blisters are painful and, when they burst, highly contagious. Another herpes virus, called the varicella-zoster virus, causes ✪ **chickenpox** and, if the virus reactivates in later life, ✪ **shingles**.

Treatment

All forms of herpes virus infection may be treated with antiviral drugs such as ℞ **acyclovir**. In herpes simplex infections these can speed healing but do not affect the tendency to recur. Treatment is only necessary in chickenpox, for those at risk of complications. In shingles, strong painkillers may also be required.

For further information

℞ DIRECTORY OF DRUGS:
antiviral • narcotic analgesic
⚗ VITAMINS, MINERALS, AND SUPPLEMENTS:
amino acid (lysine)

hiatus hernia

Hiatus hernia is a fairly common type of ✪ **hernia** in which part, or all, of the stomach works its way upward through the gap in the diaphragm (the muscular sheet dividing the chest from the abdominal cavity) meant solely for the esophagus (gullet). Symptoms are generally minor and consist of indigestion, and a tendency toward regurgitation of acidic stomach contents at least as far as the throat.

Treatment

Treatment may be no more than a change of diet and sleeping with the head higher than the feet; and may be helped by drugs such

as ℞ **antacids**. However, if inflammation of the esophagus (esophagitis) occurs, surgery may be recommended.

For further information

℞ DIRECTORY OF DRUGS:
antacid

HIV

HIV (human immunodeficiency virus) is the cause of ✪ **AIDS**, a condition in which the body's normal immune defenses are severely impaired. HIV occurs in several forms and may be transmitted through contaminated blood, unsterile needles (including needles shared by drug addicts, those used in tattooing, and contaminated medical instruments), sexual activity (so causing a ✪ **sexually transmitted disease**), or passed from mother to infant either at birth or during breast-feeding. The symptoms of AIDS may take many years to develop.

Treatment

Treatment with ℞ **antiviral** drugs may delay the development or progression of AIDS. Considerable research is being expended to find an effective vaccine against HIV. The amino acid supplement ⚗ **glutamine** is considered by some to be helpful as additional therapy.

For further information

℞ DIRECTORY OF DRUGS:
antiviral
⚗ VITAMINS, MINERALS, AND SUPPLEMENTS:
amino acid (glutamine)

hives

see ✪ **urticaria**.

Hodgkin's disease

Hodgkin's disease is ✪ **cancer** of the lymphatic tissue. It generally originates in one or more lymph nodes, spreading to the spleen and liver, and possibly to the bones and bone marrow. Its symptoms are an enlargement of the lymph nodes ("glands") in the neck, armpits, or abdomen, ✪ **fatigue**, and malaise; there may also be high temperature, sweating at night, and itching. The condition is named for the English pathologist Thomas Hodgkin (1798–1866), who first described it in 1832.

Treatment

In early stages of the disease, cytotoxic (℞ **anticancer**, also called antineoplastic) drugs are very effective, although treatment has to be continued over many months. Later, however, surgery or radiotherapy—or both—may be required.

For further information

℞ DIRECTORY OF DRUGS:
anticancer • cytotoxic

hookworm

see ✪ **worms**.

housemaid's knee

see ✪ **bursitis**.

Huntington's chorea

see ✪ Huntington's disease.

Huntington's disease

Huntington's disease is a rare hereditary neurological disorder passed on as a dominant characteristic, meaning that any child who inherits the defective gene will develop the disorder—children of an affected parent have a 50% risk of getting the gene. The disease, which affects the basal ganglia of the brain (the parts involved with voluntary movement), was formerly called Huntington's chorea because it features involuntary jerks of the limbs, the muscles of the hips, shoulders, and face. It is named after the American physician George S. Huntington (1851-1916). Symptoms develop in middle age or later and also include behavior changes, a gradual dulling of the intellect, and personality change, due to progressive degeneration of the nerve cells of the brain. Progressive ✪ dementia is likely. See also ✪ brain-motor disorders.

Treatment

There is, as yet, no cure, but symptoms such as jerks and spasms can be relieved with drugs such as the ℞ **phenothiazine** drug ℞ **fluphenazine**. Affected individuals often need institutional care. The gene responsible has now been identified, which enables screening tests to detect affected (adult) children of those with the disease, so that they can plan ahead before symptoms develop and receive genetic counseling about the risk to offspring.

For further information
℞ DIRECTORY OF DRUGS:
phenothiazine (fluphenazine)

hyperacidity

see ✪ indigestion.

hyperaldosteronism

Hyperaldosteronism (aldosteronism) is a condition caused by an excess of the adrenal gland hormone aldosterone. Symptoms may include ✪ **hypertension**, ✪ **headache**, muscle weakness and cramps, thirst, and an increase in the frequency of urination and the volume of urine passed. Primary aldosteronism, also called Conn's disease, is caused by a disease of the adrenal cortex (for instance a non-cancerous tumor); secondary aldosteronism is a consequence of another underlying disorder, for example, congestive ✪ **heart failure** or ✪ **nephrotic syndrome**.

Treatment

Treatment usually involves drugs to block the action of excess aldosterone, mainly the aldosterone antagonist ℞ **spironolactone**, which also acts as a ℞ **diuretic** and ℞ **antihypertensive**.

For further information
℞ DIRECTORY OF DRUGS:
spironolactone

hypercalcemia

Hypercalcemia is an abnormally high blood calcium level. It is most commonly due to hyperparathyroidism, a state of overactivity of the parathyroid gland and its secretion of parathyroid hormone, which helps control calcium levels in the body. It can also be due

to bone ✪ **cancer**, where calcium is released into the blood from bone; by certain types of cancer of hormonal tissues; by an excessive intake of vitamin D, or by certain inflammatory states including sarcoidosis. Diagnosis is by measurement of blood calcium levels, followed by further investigation of cause.

Treatment

Treatment mainly consists of rectifying the cause. If there is carcinoma, ℞ **calcitonin-salmon** (a type of thyroid hormone) may help reduce blood calcium levels (the anticancer agent plicamycin also has a specific use for bone cancer). In some conditions ℞ **corticosteroids** may be useful. Certain diuretics may be tried on an "off-label" basis.

For further information
℞ DIRECTORY OF DRUGS:
thyroid hormone (calcitonin-salmon) • calcium-metabolism modifier (bisphosphonate) • corticosteroid • diuretic

hypercholesterolemia

see ✪ hyperlipidemia.

hyperemesis gravidarum

see ✪ morning sickness.

hyperhidrosis

Hyperhidrosis is frequent and excessive sweating. It can be in specific areas, or all over, and is common between the ages of 15–30. It can be a symptom of an underlying disorder such as ✪ **hyperthyroidism**, and is commonly seen in ✪ **Parkinson's disease**.

Treatment

Treatment is normaly by the topical application of aluminum-containing astringent salts, most commonly aluminum chloride (as hexahydrate). This is combined with careful washing; dusting powders may be useful to dry the skin. In Parkinson's disease, ℞ **anticholinergic** drugs are sometimes used. ♣ **sage** and ♣ **walnut** are available as herbal alternatives to reduce sweating.

For further information
℞ DIRECTORY OF DRUGS:
antiperspirant (aluminum chloride) • anticholinergic (for example, **hyoscyamine**)
♣ HERBAL REMEDIES:
sage • walnut

hyperlipidemia

Hyperlipidemia (hypercholesterolemia) is a term that covers a group of disorders that are characterized by high fat (lipid) levels in the blood. There are a number of types, some of which are highly genetically determined metabolic disorders (familial hyperlipidemia). Lipid is carried in the blood in the form of cholesterol, triglycerides, and lipoproteins. The lipoproteins are formed of a fat-protein combination, either high-density lipoprotein (HDL) or low-density lipoprotein (LDL). High levels of the LDL form ("bad cholesterol") relative to the HDL ("good cholesterol")—expressed as an LDL:HDL ratio—are detrimental to cardiovascular health. They predispose the individual to ✪ **coronary artery disease** and ✪ **stroke** due to ✪ **atherosclerosis** (build-up of fatty deposits in the arteries).

In addition to genetic and life-style factors, a number of other diseases may tend to cause hyperlipidemia, including ✪ **diabetes mellitus**, ✪ **Cushing's syndrome**, ✪ **hypothyroidism**, ✪ **kidney failure**, and ✪ **alcoholism**.

Treatment

Familial hyperlipidemia, especially if a double-dose of the gene has been inherited, must be treated as a matter of medical necessity. Several prescription lipid-regulating drugs are effective, and OTC agents such as ℞ **psyllium** reduce lipid absorption from the gut. Herbal remedies are available that are said to have lipid-regulating properties. For less severe hyperlipidemia, dietary modification in favor of a lower saturated fat intake may suffice. Several vitamins, minerals, and supplements are considered to be beneficial for maintaining a healthy lipid balance.

For further information

℞ DIRECTORY OF DRUGS:

lipid-regulating drug groups including **statin** agents (**atorvastatin, cerivastatin sodium, lovastatin, pravastatin sodium, simvastatin**) • **fibrate** agents (**gemfibrozil, fenofibrate, clofibrate**) • bile acid sequestrant agents (**cholestyramine**) nicotinic acid derivative (**niacin**) • **psyllium**

♣ HERBAL REMEDIES:

evening primrose • flax • garlic • soybean

⚗ VITAMINS, MINERALS, AND SUPPLEMENTS:

acidophilus • (amino acid) arginine • chromium • garlic • niacin • omega-3 fatty acid • vitamin E

hypersensitivity reaction

Hypersensitivity reaction is an excessive and inappropriate reaction of the immune system to an antigen (a foreign substance), occurring on a second or subsequent exposure to the sensitizing allergen; antibodies having been developed on first exposure. There can be a number of reasons for the exaggerated response, including genetic predisposition, the route of entrance to the body (airways reactions often being severe), and the site of reaction. The response itself is the same as the protective mechanisms of immunity, but can be so exaggerated as to lead to tissue damage and disease.

There are several main types of hypersensitivity reaction, differing in their cellular mediators and time-scale. Type I (anaphylactic or immediate hypersensitivity) is the basis of ✪ **allergy**, and involves the disintegration of sensitized mast cells. These release mediators including histamine, which lead to symptoms of ✪ **allergy** such as ✪ **asthma**, ✪ **urticaria** (nettle rash), allergic ✪ **rhinitis**, and, if extreme, acute ✪ **anaphylactic reaction** (called anaphylactic shock), and other allergic states. Care should be taken when using herbal remedies as hypersensitivity reactions are common (for example, to the daisy family). Type II hypersensitivity involves antibodies that react with antigens on cell surfaces, with resultant cell death, a form of reaction thought to be responsible for ✪ **autoimmune disorders**, and for the destruction of red blood cells (hemolysis), which is caused by certain drugs.

Treatment

Avoiding contact with the allergen is the only sure solution. Chronic reactions can be ameliorated through the use of ℞ **immunosuppressant** drugs. Symptomatic relief may be provided by ℞ **antihistamines** (℞ **chlorpheniramine**, ℞ **cyproheptadine**, dexchlorpheniramine, ℞ **diphenhydramine**), ℞ **sympathomimetics** (for example, ℞ **epinephrine**), ℞ **corticosteroids** (for example, ℞ **methylprednisolone**), and ℞ **antiallergics** (including mast cell stabilizers such as ℞ **cromolyn sodium**; ℞ **nedocromil sodium**).

hypertension

Hypertension is high blood pressure; above the levels expected at any particular age (blood pressure generally increases with age). The cause may be unknown (essential hypertension), or it may result from ✪ **kidney disorders**, hormonal disorders, heart or arterial disease, or any condition or drug that constricts (narrows) the blood vessels. People who drink excessive amounts of alcohol, or who are under long-term psychological stress may be at increased risk, and there is often a family history of hypertension, ✪ **obesity**, or heart disease. Most of those affected have no symptoms, although occasionally there may be headaches and audio or visual disturbances, until resultant complications arise, such as ✪ **heart failure**, a ✪ **stroke**, ✪ **myocardial infarction** (heart attack), ✪ **kidney failure**, ✪ **arteriosclerosis**, or cerebral hemorrhage. In pregnancy, hypertension can lead to pre-eclampsia and ✪ **eclampsia**. These are potentially dangerous if left untreated. It is estimated that there are about 50 million hypertensives in the US. Short-term hypertension may be caused by some OTC drugs, especially nasal ℞ **decongestants**, and "street" drugs such as cocaine.

Treatment

Treatment of hypertension, if diagnosed before complications develop, can often avoid permanent damage. If a specific cause is known, treatment may resolve the high blood pressure. In other cases, and in essential hypertension, treatment generally consists of long-term drug therapy with ℞ **diuretics**, and other antihypertensive drugs to decrease edema, in order to keep pressure down. Lifestyle changes, particularly weight-reduction, may also be advised, sometimes with ℞ **lipid-regulating drugs** when there is raised blood cholesterol. Additionally, some supplements and herbal remedies are considered to be beneficial in maintaining a healthy cardiovascular system.

For further information

℞ DIRECTORY OF DRUGS:

antihypertensive • diuretic • lipid-regulating drug

♣ HERBAL REMEDIES:

broom • celery • garlic • guelder rose • gutta percha • hawthorn • mistletoe • onion • wolfberry, Chinese • yarrow

⚗ VITAMINS, MINERALS, AND SUPPLEMENTS:

calcium • coenzyme Q$_{10}$ • garlic • magnesium • omega-3 fatty acid • potassium • zinc

hyperthyroidism

Hyperthyroidism is an excessive production and secretion of thyroid hormones by the thyroid gland in the neck, leading to symptoms of thyrotoxicosis, including rapid heartbeat, sweating, ✪ **anxiety**, sensitivity to heat, hunger, weight loss, and tremors.

Key to symbols: ✪ = Disorder Section ℞ = Drug Section ♣ = Herbal Section ⚗ = Supplement Section

The cause may be overactivity or overgrowth of the gland, a tumor of the thyroid, or a corresponding excess of thyroid-stimulating hormone (TSH) from the pituitary gland. There may be protruding eyes and neck swelling (goiter). A common cause is the ✪ **autoimmune disorder** Graves' disease, where the body produces antibodies that attack the thyroid gland, and which runs in families.

Treatment

Treatment may be with ℞ **antithyroid** drugs or radioactive iodine to decrease hormone production, but often involves the surgical removal of part of the thyroid gland. ♣ **motherwort** is a herbal remedy sometimes used as an additional treatment for hyperthyroidism.

For further information
℞ DIRECTORY OF DRUGS:
antithyroid
♣ HERBAL REMEDIES:
motherwort

hypocalcemia

Hypocalcemia (low blood calcium) is an abnormally low blood level of calcium. It is most commonly due to a vitamin D deficiency or little exposure to sunlight, but can be caused by ✪ **kidney failure** leading to poor calcium absorption, or ✪ **hypoparathyroidism**— under activity of the parathyroid gland (which helps control calcium levels in the body). Deficiency due to inadequate dietary intake is rare. Symptoms of severe hypocalcemia include tetany (painful twitches of the muscles). Chronic hypocalcemia may lead to low bone density with bone weakness, known as ✪ **rickets** in children, and osteomalacia in adults. Deficiency may increase the risk of ✪ **osteoporosis**.

Treatment

Treatment depends on cause. Vitamin D analogs (see ℞ **ergocalciferol**) correct the deficiency. Sometimes, parathyroid hormone analogs are used for hypoparathyroidism.

For further information
℞ DIRECTORY OF DRUGS:
hormone • ergocalciferol
⚖ VITAMINS, MINERALS, AND SUPPLEMENTS:
calcium • vitamin D

hypogonadism

Hypogonadism is a state of underactivity of the sexual organs, the gonads (testes and ovaries). Hypogonadism may be caused by a variety of disorders of the pituitary gland, which has an important role in controlling sexual development and function (see ✪ **pituitary gland disorders and tumors**). It may also be caused by disorders in the gonads themselves.

Treatment

Hormone deficiencies in men are treated with ℞ **androgens** (testosterone-derivatives). In women, it is usually an estrogen deficiency, which may be treated with oral ℞ **estrogens**, such as (for example, diethylstilbestrol, estradiol, estrone, estropipate, and estrogens, conjugated), or ℞ **androgens** (for example, testosterone, methyltestosterone, and fluoxymesterone).

For further information
℞ DIRECTORY OF DRUGS:
androgen • estrogen • sex hormone

hyponatremia

Hyponatremia is an abnormally low blood level of sodium. It is caused by either an excessive intake, or an excessive excretion, of water. It can lead to water intoxication, confusion, lethergy, muscle excitabilty, convulsions, and eventually coma.

Treatment

It can be treated by giving salt, either by mouth or infusion, to correct the balance.

For further information
℞ DIRECTORY OF DRUGS:
electrolyte (sodium chloride)

hypoparathyroidism

Hypoparathyroidism is a condition where there is an underproduction of parathyroid hormone (parathormone) by the parathyroid glands. This hormone regulates calcium levels in the body, and works in conjunction with calcitonin (produced by the adjacent thyroid glands) and vitamin D. Reasons for hypoparathyroidism include absence of the gland at birth, cessation of function and, more commonly, inadvertent surgical removal during surgery for hyperthyroidism. Symptoms of low calcium levels include tetany (painful spasms of skeletal muscles).

Treatment

For acute hypoparathyroidism with tetany, calcium chloride may be taken by slow intravenous injection. In chronic hypoparathyroidism, various preparations of calcium salts may be prescribed for the duration, usually in combination with vitamin D (which increases calcium absorption). For general good health (especially to avoid ✪ **osteoporosis**), not necessarily associated with clinical hypoparathyroidism, ⚖ **vitamin D** and ⚖ **calcium** supplements are available.

For further information
℞ DIRECTORY OF DRUGS:
calcium carbonate • vitamin preparations (vitamin D and derivatives: **calcitriol, ergocalciferol**)
⚖ VITAMINS, MINERALS, AND SUPPLEMENTS:
calcium • vitamin D (vitamin D_2, cholecalciferol/vitamin D_3)

hypopituitarism

Hypopituitarism is a group of conditions, commonly progressive, where there is underproduction of hormones produced and released by the pituitary gland (located near the base of the brain). The pituitary is divided into an anterior and posterior part; each of which secretes different hormones. Hypopituitarism may be caused by a tumor in the pituitary pressing on part of the gland, and so interfering with hormone release (see ✪ **pituitary gland disorders and tumors**). Since the release of pituitary hormones is, in turn, controlled by hypothalamic hormones, which is situated above the pituitary, problems with this brain area may be the root cause. On occasion the cause is physical damage or an interference in the blood supply to the gland. Since the main physiological role of the pituitary is the control of other hormone-secreting glands, the outcome of hypopituitarism is generally an underfunctioning of these glands, especially the sex glands, and the adrenal cortex. Symptoms of hypopituitarism vary with the cause, but often include sexual manifestations including lack of menstruation in women, shrinking of testes, and loss of facial hair in men, loss or pubic and underarm hair, and a decrease in libido. There may be other symptoms such as nausea and vomiting, dizziness, pale skin, tiredness, weight gain, and intolerance to cold. Diagnosis involves measurement of blood hormone levels, and pituitary function tests.

Treatment
Hypopituitarism is a serious condition requiring the substitution of synthetic hormones, administered as drugs in place of the natural hormones. These may be pituitary hormones (for example, growth hormone) or those of other affected glands (for example, ℞ **sex hormones**, ℞ **corticosteroids**).

For further information
℞ DIRECTORY OF DRUGS:
corticosteroid • anterior pituitary hormone • sex hormone

hypotension
Hypotension is lower than normal blood pressure, which can be due to a variety of causes. These include blood or fluid loss (as in ✪ **hemorrhage**, ✪ **burns**, severe ✪ **diarrhea**, and ✪ **vomiting**); severe allergic reactions, infections or abdominal emergencies; ✪ **myocardial infarction** (heart attack), ✪ **heart failure**, heart ✪ **arrhythmia**, hormonal imbalance, fainting, and certain drugs. There may be no symptoms. In some cases (for example, as a side effect of some drugs) blood pressure falls rapidly on standing too quickly (orthostatic hypotension; postural hypotension). This can lead to dizziness, sweating, and a feeling of light-headedness. Very rarely, a person may become semiconscious or undergo a state of extreme shock with circulatory failure.

Treatment
Treatment depends on the cause. In temporary falls of blood pressure, as in simple fainting, lying flat with the legs elevated usually produces relief. Severe acute cases associated with major medical problems may require antihypotensive drugs (such as the ℞ **sympathomimetics**, mephentermine, ℞ **metaraminol**, ℞ **methoxamine**, and ℞ **norepinephrine** (by infusion), ℞ **phenylephrine** (systemically), and ℞ **midodrine** (systemically for longer-term action), oxygen treatment, and electrolyte and rehydration fluid through an intravenous drip. ♣ **florists' chrysanthemum** is a traditional herbal remedy that may be of some benefit.

For further information
℞ DIRECTORY OF DRUGS:
alpha-adrenergic stimulant • electrolyte (rehydration solution) • sympathomimetic
♣ HERBAL REMEDIES:
broom • florists' chrysanthemum

hypothermia
Hypothermia is a condition of dangerously low body temperature (below 95°F; 35°C). This may result if the usual body mechanism for creating heat—shivering—is ineffective. It occurs most commonly in the elderly and the very young, during weather that is exceptionally cold for an exceptionally long time. It is also common in climbers and walkers, who are inadequately dressed for the cold conditions. The term is used also for a therapeutic reduction in a person's temperature as part of surgical procedure.

Treatment
Treatment is by gradual rewarming.

hypothyroidism
Hypothyroidism is an insufficient production and secretion of thyroid hormones by the thyroid gland, which is situated in the neck. This may be the result of a disease within the thyroid itself, over treatment of hyperthyroidism with antithyroid drugs, surgical removal of parts, or all, of the gland, or a corresponding lack of thyroid-stimulating hormone (TSH; ℞ **thyrotropin**) from the anterior pituitary gland. The most common cause is thyroiditis, particularly Hashimoto's thyroiditis, which is where the body produces antibodies that attack the thyroid gland, damaging it permanently (it can run in families).

Symptoms in adults, collectively called myxedema, include lethargy, weight gain, thickening of the skin, and coarsening of facial features, constipation, and general mental and physical slowness. There may be goiter (neck swelling). If untreated, complications may include heart failure, arterial disease, mental confusion, and even coma. Undetected failure of thyroid development in newborn babies may lead to cretinism (failure of mental development with a characteristic expression and cry).

Treatment
Treatment is usually with ℞ **thyroid hormone** supplements. Early treatment in babies can avoid the effects of cretinism. For the prevention of hypothyroidism due to iodine deficiency, there should be adequate iodine in the diet (usually as iodized salt).
If iodine deficiency is the cause of hypothyroidism (extremely rare in the US), ᪲ **kelp**, a rich source of iodine, may be beneficial.

For further information
℞ DIRECTORY OF DRUGS:
thyroid hormone
♣ HERBAL REMEDIES:
bladderwrack
᪲ VITAMINS, MINERALS, AND SUPPLEMENTS:
iodine • spirulina and other algae (kelp)

IBD
see ✪ inflammatory bowel disease (IBD).

IBS
see ✪ irritable bowel syndrome.

immunodeficiency disorder
Immunodeficiency disorders are any of a group of disorders caused by a defect in the body's normal immune response, which increases susceptibility to ✪ **infections**, including infection by micro-organisms that would not cause disease in healthy individuals (opportunistic infection). Immunodeficiency can be present at birth or may be acquired, as in ✪ **AIDS**, or due to various drugs.

Treatment

Treatment depends on the cause but generally involves a combination of avoidance of infections and treatment of those that do arise, where possible. The immune system may be helped by some drugs such as ℞ **interferons**, which are ℞ **immunomodulators**, and possibly encouraged to respond by ℞ **immunostimulants** (which include some herbal remedies).

For further information

℞ DIRECTORY OF DRUGS:
immunomodulator (interferons) • immunostimulant

♣ HERBAL REMEDIES:
astragalus • echinacea • mistletoe

impetigo

Impetigo is a ✪ **skin condition** often localized to regions such as the face, nose, and mouth. After an initial rash, fluid-filled blisters develop with crusting of the skin. It is normally due to ✪ **bacterial infection** (for example, streptococcal, staphylococcal) through a cut, abrasion or cold sore. The blisters tend to burst, and the condition is highly contagious.

Treatment

Treatment is with topical or oral ℞ **antibacterial** drugs including antibiotics, washing with warm salt solutions (with scrupulous hygiene).

For further information

℞ DIRECTORY OF DRUGS:
antibacterial • antibiotic

impotence

Impotence is the inability of a man to obtain, or to sustain, an erection of the penis, or failure to achieve ejaculation or orgasm during sexual intercourse. It may be due to physical problems, such as arterial disease or ✪ **diabetes mellitus**, or to psychological causes.

Treatment

Treatment with the drug ℞ **sildenafil** (Viagra) can give a viable erection provided there is normal sexual desire. Older treatments include injections of ℞ **vasodilator** drugs into the base of the penis, and prostheses that maintain hardness.

For further information

℞ DIRECTORY OF DRUGS:
impotence treatment • vasodilator

incontinence

Incontinence is a lack of control over the sphincters (valve-like rings of muscle) and other muscles that hold back urine in the bladder (urinary incontinence), or feces in the rectum (fecal incontinence)—or both. Causes range from muscular weakness (sometimes following childbirth), disease, and drug abuse (including alcoholism), to injury, stress, and excitement (stress incontinence).

Treatment

Treatment depends on the cause and may include ℞ **anticholinergic** drugs, exercises to strengthen the muscles of the pelvic floor or, in some cases, surgery or an implant.

For further information

℞ DIRECTORY OF DRUGS:
anticholinergic

indigestion

Indigestion is any form of disordered digestion that causes pain or discomfort in the lower chest or upper abdomen that is related to eating. The medical name is dyspepsia. Other symptoms may include a bloated feeling around the diaphragm, belching, and sometimes regurgitation of the liquid contents of the stomach up at least as far as the throat, causing heartburn, ✪ **flatulence**, ✪ **nausea**, or even ✪ **vomiting**. The cause of indigestion is usually overeating, eating too quickly, or eating food that is too rich, or that the stomach has difficulty in dealing with. Overindulgence in alcoholic drinks can also cause indigestion. Temporary indigestion is extremely common, and may be promoted by stress, ✪ **obesity**, or a ✪ **hiatus hernia**. Heartburn, a symptom of indigestion is characterized by a burning sensation at the bottom of the esophagus (gullet). It is caused by the rising of partly digested acidic contents of the stomach, which may result in inflammation of the lower part of the esophagus (esophagitis). However, symptoms that do not settle or that persist for a long period should be medically assessed, as occasionally they may suggest a more serious disorder, such as ✪ **peptic ulcer**, hiatus hernia, cholecystitis (inflammation of the gallbladder) or, rarely, cancer of the stomach or esophagus. See also ✪ **digestive system disorders**.

Treatment

Treatment of occasional indigestion is with antacids and lifestyle changes, such as weight loss, dietary modification, and the avoidance of stress. Many herbal remedies are considered to be beneficial in the short-term for the treatment of indigestion and related dyspeptic complaints. Persistent indigestion sould be medically assessed, and prescribed treatment depends on your doctor's diagnosis.

For further information

℞ DIRECTORY OF DRUGS:
antacid • H$_2$-antagonist

♣ HERBAL REMEDIES:
angelica • anise • artichoke • blessed thistle • boldo • brewer's yeast • caraway • cayenne • centaury • chamomile, German • chicory • cinnamon • cinnamon, Chinese • condurango • coriander • dandelion • devil's claw • embelia • fennel • galangal • ginger • grains of paradise • haronga • horehound • immortelle • jewel weed • lemon verbena • meadowsweet • onion • peppermint • quassia • radish • rosemary • St. John's wort • salep • sweet orange • thyme • turmeric • wild iris • yarrow • yellow gentian • zedoary

infantile arteritis

see ✪ arteritis.

infantile colic

see ✪ colic.

infection

Infection is an invasion of the body by pathological microorganisms (microbes; commonly known as germs) that reproduce and multiply causing disease. Infections are the most common cause of disease, and can be caused by bacteria, fungi, protozoa, viruses, and prions. Infections can be localized (for example, an infected cut or a boil, conjunctivitis, or respiratory tract infection) or can cause more widespread problems (such as ✪ **septicemia** or ✪ **AIDS**). Some types of infection (for example, ✪ **influenza**) can spread rapidly throughout a community. The control of infection in the community as a whole (by bodies such as the Centers for Disease Control) is a major policy of the healthcare service, in order to try and minimize the risk of infection in the community by immunization and public education (food hygiene). In the developed world, most infections can be prevented or effectively treated. However, in the developing world, many infectious diseases (such as ✪ **measles**) can be fatal, and in the tropics, disorders such as ✪ **cholera** and ✪ **malaria** are frequent causes of ill-health and death. Infectious diseases can spread rapidly and globally; AIDS and influenza are examples, and some diseases are re-emerging, such as ✪ **tuberculosis**, which have become resistant to drug treatment. Viral infections include: ✪ **chickenpox**, ✪ **glandular fever**, ✪ **herpes**, ✪ **mumps**, ✪ **poliomyelitis**, ✪ **HIV** and AIDs, yellow fever, bacterial infections (including ✪ **diphtheria**, ✪ **listeriosis**, ✪ **typhoid fever**, ✪ **cholera**, ✪ **scarlet fever**, ✪ **tetanus**, ✪ **Lyme disease**, and ✪ **Rocky Mountain spotted fever**), protozoal infections (including ✪ **malaria**, ✪ **giardiasis**, and ✪ **amebiasis**), fungal infections (including ✪ **candidiasis**, ✪ **cryptococcosis**, and ✪ **athlete's foot**, and prion infections (including ✪ **Creutzfeldt-Jakob disease**). For further information, see the specific disease; ✪ **bacterial infection**, ✪ **viral infection**, ✪ **fungal infection**, and ✪ **protozoal infection**.

Treatment

Routine immunization, drugs such as ℞ **antibiotics**, and improvements in diet and hygiene in the last century have all made great advances in infection control. Treatment of infection depends on the type of microorganism that is causing the infection, the site or location of the infection, and other factors, but includes ℞ **antivirals**, ℞ **antibacterials**, ℞ **antifungals**, ℞ **antiprotozoals**, and antibiotics. Symptoms of infection can also be treated (for example, fever with ℞ **antipyretics** and pain with ℞ **analgesics**). Some supplements (such as ♉ **carotenoid**, and ♉ **vitamins A** and ♉ **C**) and herbal remedies (such as ♣ **boneset**, ♣ **cajuput**, ♣ **cardamom**, ♣ **clove**, ♣ **couch grass** (*Elymus repens*), ♣ **echinacea**, ♣ **eucalyptus**, ♉ **garlic**, ♣ **chamomile, German**, ♣ **giant hyssop**, ♣ **larch**, ♣ **lungmoss**, ♣ **onion**, ♣ **Scotch pine**, ♣ **sea buckthorn**, and ♣ **withania**) are promoted as being useful in preventing or treating certain infections or a tendency to infection. See individual disorders for more information.

infectious mononucleosis

see ✪ **glandular fever**.

infective endocarditis

see ✪ **endocarditis**.

infective parotitis

see ✪ **mumps**.

infertility

Infertility is an inability to have children. In women, this can be the result of physical causes such as a failure of the ovaries to produce ova, an obstruction of the Fallopian tubes, or disease or injury in the uterus (womb) or vagina, or even psychological causes. In males this is usually due to the quantity or quality of the sperm produced, or to problems in successfully completing sexual intercourse.

Treatment

Treatment for some of these causes, in women and men, is possible. Drug ℞ **infertility treatment** using a number of hormones and their analogs may be used to stimulate ovulation; or surgery may be used to repair physical defects. In other cases, modern reproductive technology such as *in vitro* fertilization (IVF, to produce "test-tube babies") may be used. For some types of infertility, ♉ **zinc** is considered to be helpful.

For further information

℞ DIRECTORY OF DRUGS:
infertility treatment
♉ VITAMINS, MINERALS, AND SUPPLEMENTS:
zinc

inflammation

Inflammation is a local protective reaction of body tissues to injury (including bites and stings), irritation (including an allergic response), or infection. It occurs as a defensive mechanism, and results in redness and swelling, heat, pain, and sometimes loss of function. An increased blood supply is diverted to the area to assist in healing, and white blood cells (leukocytes) accumulate in order to entrap and neutralize infective organisms or material. Inflammation can occur in almost any part of the body. For example, a bacterial throat infection may cause inflammation with redness and swelling, causing difficulty in swallowing, pain, and loss of the voice, and pus from accumulated dead white blood cells (see ✪ **laryngitis**, ✪ **pharyngitis**). Inappropriate inflammation, may lead to often chronic inflammatory disease such as ✪ **lupus** or ✪ **Crohn's disease**.

Treatment

Inflammation itself is the body's normal defensive mechanism and is not treated. However, some symptoms (such as pain) can be relieved. If the inflammation is inappropriate (in inflammatory disease for example), it can be reduced by drug treatment. Treatment may include various ℞ **anti-inflammatory** drugs, including ℞ **corticosteroids** and ℞ **NSAIDs**, to suppress inflammation or relieve pain. Many herbal remedies are available, which are said to be beneficial in the treatment of different types of inflammation (such as respiratory tract infections or local skin inflammation). Herbal remedies that are available to treat inflammation include ♣ **arnica**, ♣ **bilberry**, ♣ **blackberry**, ♣ **bupleurum**, ♣ **cinnamon, Chinese**, ♣ **cardamom**, ♣ **clove**, ♣ **coffee**, ♣ **couch grass** (*Elymus repens*), ♣ **eyebright**, ♣ **flax**, ♣ **chamomile, German**, ♣ **herb Robert**, ♣ **Iceland moss**, ♣ **jambul**, ♣ **Japanese mint**, ♣ **larch**, ♣ **mallow**, ♣ **marigold**, ♣ **marshmallow**, ♣ **oak**, ♣ **onion**,

♣ **peppermint**, ♣ **plantain**, ♣ **potentilla**, ♣ **radish**, ♣ **rhatany**, ♣ **rose**, ♣ **sage**, ♣ **slippery elm**, ♣ **spruce**, ♣ **tormentil**, ♣ **white dead nettle**, ♣ **witch hazel**, ♣ **white lily**, ♣ **horseradish**, ♣ **willow**, ♣ **sloe**, ♣ **wood sage**, ♣ **bladderwort**, and ♣ **heartsease**. See individual entries for more details.

inflammatory bowel disease (IBD)
see ✪ **Crohn's disease**; ✪ **ulcerative colitis**.

inflammatory bowel disorders
see ✪ **ulcerative colitis**; ✪ **Crohn's disease**.

influenza
Influenza (also called "flu") is a highly infectious viral disease that attacks the upper respiratory tract. Symptoms are ✪ **headache**, muscle weakness, shivering with chills, high temperature—which may at times reach 40°C (104°F)—a sore throat, and a ✪ **cough**; all may last for about a week. The usual treatment is with bed rest and medications to relieve ✪ **fever** and discomfort. Secondary infections may occur as complications, especially infections of the ear, nose, and throat.

Treatment
Treatment is usually to alleviate symptoms while the person recovers. Complications due to secondary bacterial infection may be treated with ℞ **antibacterial** antibiotics. A ℞ **vaccine** is available for those at high risk of complications. Various OTC drugs including antipyretics such as ℞ **acetaminophen** to control fever, and ℞ **non-narcotic analgesic** drugs to relieve discomfort will usually be taken. ℞ **antiviral** drugs may be prescribed for people at risk, including ℞ **amantadine**, oseltamivir, ℞ **ribavirin**, ℞ **rimantadine**, and ℞ **zanamivir** (used to speed recovery and reduce the risk of complications). Vitamins A and C may help to fight colds and influenza.

For further information
℞ DIRECTORY OF DRUGS:
antipyretic • antiviral • non-narcotic analgesic • NSAID
♣ HERBAL REMEDIES:
cinnamon • echinacea • eucalyptus • pleurisy root • vervain • weeping forsythia • willow
⚕ VITAMINS, MINERALS, AND SUPPLEMENTS:
vitamin A • vitamin C

insomnia
Insomnia is a sleep disorder characterized by a chronic inability to fall—or to remain—asleep. Sleep requirements vary with circumstances (often being greater when recovering from illness or exertion), with age (being greatest in infants), and from person to person—but prolonged irregular or too short sleep periods are detrimental to health. Many factors may give rise to insomnia, including physical problems such as ✪ **pain**, ✪ **indigestion**, physical discomfort, or itching. Some diseases such as ✪ **hyperthyroidism**, ✪ **asthma**, obstructive sleep apnea, and various carcinomas commonly cause insomnia. Often sleep disorders may be associated with mood states such as ✪ **anxiety**, excitement or ✪ **depression**; or sometimes external factors such as a noise, waking to nurse

infants, etc. A temporary sleep disorder may be caused by ✪ **jet lag** where there is a displacement of the person's inherent circadian rhythm.

Treatment
Treatment depends on cause. As much as possible should be done to ensure quiet comfortable surroundings without bright light. A routine at bedtime including moderate exercise, a milky drink, avoidance of stimulants (for example, ℞ **caffeine** drinks or smoking) or excess alcohol, may help. Where depression or anxiety is involved, appropriate drugs may be prescribed—and this approach is increasingly being found to be beneficial in long-term management of insomnia. Pain may be treated with ℞ **analgesics** or specific drugs that ameliorate symptoms of disease at night (for example, long-acting ℞ **bronchodilators** for asthmatics; ℞ **antacids** for dyspeptics). Sleeping pills (℞ **hypnotics**) may be taken, but are prescribed much less than they used to be because of the risk of habituation. They are usually reserved for short-term use, when medically necessary or during emergencies (for example, following the loss of a loved one). However, the old barbiturate group of drugs (℞ **amobarbital**, ℞ **butabarbital**, ℞ **quazepam**, and ℞ **secobarbital sodium**)—which has only a small margin of safety on overdose and is highly habituating—has been largely replaced by ℞ **benzodiazepines** (including for example, ℞ **diazepam**, ℞ **estazolam**, ℞ **flurazepam**, ℞ **lorazepam**, ℞ **temazepam**, and ℞ **triazolam**), and more recent drugs (for instance ℞ **zolpidem**), which are significantly safer. A number of other hypnotics are used in special circumstances, including chloral hydrate, glutethimide, and meprobamate. Some mild OTC ℞ **sleep-aid products** (usually ℞ **promethazine** or ℞ **diphenhydramine**) are available, as are several herbal remedies that have long-established traditional uses for insomnia. For sleep disturbances including insomnia in ✪ **jet lag**, there is evidence that ⚕ **melatonin** speeds up a return to an appropriate circadian rhythm.

For further information
℞ DIRECTORY OF DRUGS:
antidepressant • barbiturate • hypnotic (including benzodiazepine) • sleep-aid product
♣ HERBAL REMEDIES:
black horehound • bugleweed • celery • chamomile, German • gotu kola • hops • Jamaica dogwood • kava kava • wild lettuce • lemon balm • passionflower • St. John's wort • tarragon, French • valerian
⚕ VITAMINS, MINERALS, AND SUPPLEMENTS:
melatonin

interstitial cystitis
see ✪ **cystitis**.

interstitial nephritis
see ✪ **nephritis**.

intertrigo
Intertrigo is an ✪ **inflammation** of the skin in areas where two surfaces rub together, such as underneath the breasts or in the groin, especially in obese people. Friction plus sweating causes the surface

of the skin to chafe, leading to irritation and soreness. Sometimes infection occurs, especially with *Candida* yeasts, making the symptoms worse (see ✪ **candidiasis**; ✪ **skin conditions**).

Treatment

Treatment is with emollient and other ℞ **skin preparations** including some herbal remedies. These are applied externally to soothe the area and treat any infection. Scrupulous hygiene and drying of the area, and attempts at weight loss, may help to prevent recurrence.

For further information

℞ DIRECTORY OF DRUGS:
emollient • skin preparation

♣ HERBAL REMEDIES:
aloe • marshmallow

intracerebral hemorrhage

see ✪ stroke.

iron deficient anemia

see ✪ anemia.

irritable bladder conditions

see ✪ urinary tract disorders.

irritable bowel syndrome

Irritable bowel syndrome (IBS) is characterized by bouts of abdominal pain occurring in spasms, sometimes with ✪ **diarrhea** or ✪ **constipation**, or alternating between the two. Sometimes also called mucous colitis or spastic colon, it may be due to abnormal contractions of the muscles of the intestinal wall, or to abnormal sensitivity to the presence of food in the intestines, but is not linked with any physical changes in the gut. The cause of this ✪ **digestive system disorder** is unknown but it may follow intestinal infection and is sometimes precipitated by stress. It can be a long-term disorder and may seriously interfere with a person's lifestyle, but does not lead to serious disease. Medical diagnosis is essential to rule out other conditions (such as ✪ **ulcerative colitis**, ✪ **Crohn's disease**, ✪ **lactose intolerance**, and ✪ **dysentery**).

Treatment

Treatment may include ℞ **anticholinergic** drugs (including atropine, dicyclomine, hyoscyamine, oxybutynin, propantheline, clidinium, and mepenzolate) to reduce spasm and associated pain, or agents such as bulk laxatives (for example, ℞ **psyllium**) to promote peristalsis and modify feces. Dietary changes, acidophilus supplements, and relaxation techniques may also help relieve symptoms. Relief may be gained from some herbal remedies.

For further information

℞ DIRECTORY OF DRUGS:
anticholinergic • laxative

♣ HERBAL REMEDIES:
flax • kava kava • peppermint • plantain • poplar

♒ VITAMINS, MINERALS, AND SUPPLEMENTS:
acidophilus

ischemic attack

see ✪ stroke.

itching

see ✪ pruritis.

jaundice

Jaundice (called medically icterus) is a yellow coloration of the skin, mucous membranes, and "whites" of the eyes. It is caused by excess blood levels of the bile pigment bilirubin. The excess may result from obstruction of the bile ducts, as with ✪ **gallstones** (obstructive jaundice); from ✪ **liver disorders** (such as ✪ **hepatitis** or ✪ **cirrhosis**), which cause a failure to dispose of bile normally (hepatocellular jaundice), or from the formation of too much bilirubin, due to an increased destruction of red cells in the blood in various conditions (hemolytic jaundice). Jaundice is often accompanied by itching, and the passing of dark urine.

Treatment

Treatment depends on diagnosis of the cause.

For further information

♣ HERBAL REMEDIES:
milk thistle • turmeric • yellow dock

jejunal ulcer

see ✪ peptic ulcer.

jet lag

Jet lag is a physical disorientation of the body when its circadian rhythms (daily variations driven by the "body clock") are not paralleled by the environmental time of day. It happens after traveling by air through several time zones, and causes disruption not only of the sleep and alertness patterns but also of body temperature mechanisms, and some glandular functions. Over wide time differences, the body may take up to a week to adapt fully to the new time zone. See also ✪ **insomnia**.

Treatment

Planning of flight times and activities, and the avoidance of alcohol in-flight, can reduce the effects. A doctor could prescribe a short-acting ℞ **hypnotic** (sleeping tablet) to enable sleep during the flight. Some mild OTC ℞ **sleep-aid products** (usually ℞ **promethazine** or ℞ **diphenhydramine hydrochloride**) are available. In the US, ♒ **melatonin**—a hormone that regulates body cycles—is available as a supplement and may help to combat jet lag. Herbal remedies that have sedative properties may also be useful.

For further information

℞ DIRECTORY OF DRUGS:
hypnotic • sleep-aid product

♣ HERBAL REMEDIES:
black horehound • bugleweed • celery • chamomile, German • gotu kola • hops • Jamaica dogwood • kava kava • wild lettuce • lemon balm • passionflower • St. John's wort • tarragon, French • valerian

♒ VITAMINS, MINERALS, AND SUPPLEMENTS:
melatonin

joint disease

see ✪ musculoskeletal disorders.

joint pain

see ✪ musculoskeletal disorders.

juvenile rheumatoid arthritis

see ✪ arthritis.

kala-azar

see ✪ leishmaniasis.

Kaposi's sarcoma

Kaposi's sarcoma is a form of malignant skin tumor—a cancer—arising from blood vessels close to the skin surface, and causing dark patches or nodules. It is relatively common in Mediterranean races and Jews, and among people with ✪ AIDS.

Treatment

Treatment may be with radiotherapy or, in advanced disease, chemotherapy (℞ **anticancer** drugs).

For further information

℞ DIRECTORY OF DRUGS:
anticancer • cytotoxic

keratitis

Keratitis is the inflammation of the cornea of the eye (the membrane covering the front surface of the eye), causing pain, blurred vision, and watery eyes. It may be due to ✪ **bacterial infection** or ✪ **viral infection**, injury to the eye, or exposure to irritants such as dust or chemicals.

Treatment

Treatment depends on the cause, but may include the removal of any irritants and covering the eye until the cornea heals, sometimes with the use of drugs (given as eyedrops) to treat inflammation, and possibly drugs to treat any infection.

For further information

℞ DIRECTORY OF DRUGS:
corticosteroid • anti-inflammatory

kidney cancer

see ✪ cancer.

kidney disease

see ✪ kidney disorder.

kidney disorder

Kidney disorders are any of a range of disorders that affect the tissues or the operation of the kidneys (urine-producing organs). Symptoms commonly include an increase or decrease in the passing of urine, abdominal pain, edma (accumulation of fluid in the tissues; see ✪ **fluid retention**), and the appearance of blood or other substances in the urine. Diseases that directly affect the kidney include ✪ **nephritis** (inflammation), ✪ **nephrolithiasis** (kidney stone), and ✪ **cancer**; many other diseases affect the kidneys indirectly.

Treatment

Treatment depends on the cause. Failure of both kidneys to function requires immediate emergency treatment. The herbs ♣ **club moss** and ♣ **fringed pink** are traditional remedies for general minor kidney-related problems and may be of some benefit.

For further information

♣ HERBAL REMEDIES:
club moss • fringed pink

kidney failure

Kidney failure is the complete breakdown in the function of one or both kidneys (the urine-producing organs). One kidney, provided that it is in good condition, can usually carry out the work of two if necessary. Failure of both, however, demands emergency treatment before poisonous wastes begin to accumulate catastrophically in the body.

Treatment

A dialysis machine (kidney machine) can perform the same filtration processes as the natural kidney, but requires time in training and in psychological adjustment. If available, a kidney transplant is generally the best option. Chronic kidney failure can be treated with drugs depending on the cause.

For further information

℞ DIRECTORY OF DRUGS:
antihypertensive • corticosteroid

kissing disease

see ✪ glandular fever.

kwashiorkor

Kwashiorkor is a type of malnutrition resulting from severe dietary deficiency, especially of protein; it is common among children in tropical Africa. Symptoms include malaise and apathy, diarrhea, a protuberant abdomen, pallor of the skin, and discoloration (reddening) of the hair. There may also be edema or deformity in the legs and feet.

Treatment

Treatment is to remedy the deficiency, where possible.

labyrinthitis

see ✪ otitis.

lactose intolerance

Lactose intolerance is an inability to digest lactose (the natural sugar found in milk; "milk sugar"; lactin). This is due to the absence or low activity of an enzyme (lactase) required by the intestines to break down lactose into simpler sugars (glucose and galactose). Drinking milk then produces diarrhea, abdominal pain, and bloating. The inherited condition is common among Asian and African peoples.

Treatment

Treatment is to avoid milk and milk products. ᎯᎯ **acidophilus** can help alleviate symptoms such as diarrhea and stomach cramps, and ᎯᎯ **calcium** may be useful in those who are unable to eat dairy products in order to prevent possible calcium deficiency.

For further information

⚗ VITAMINS, MINERALS, AND SUPPLEMENTS:
acidophilus • calcium

laryngitis

Laryngitis is the inflammation of the larynx (the part of the throat containing the vocal cords), particularly on the vocal cords. It is usually a result of the spread of a respiratory infection, such as a ✛ **cold**, or of ✛ **tonsillitis**, or may be due to irritation by fumes or chemicals, or to overuse of the voice. It is most common in heavy smokers and heavy drinkers. Symptoms are extreme hoarseness or the inability to talk at all, with pain on trying to do so. Breathing may also be difficult, and there may be a painful cough. In extreme cases, especially in children (when it is known as ✛ **croup**), the air passage may become obstructed.

Treatment

Treatment depends on the cause, but normally includes resting the voice for at least a couple of days, humidifying the environment, and steam inhalations. If ✛ **bacterial infection** is suspected, ℞ **antibacterials** may be administered, especially for treating young children, who sometimes develop complications. Very rarely, obstruction of the airways may necessitate surgery to restore proper breathing. The condition may become chronic. Some herbal remedies, such as ♣ **thyme**, have been used traditionally for laryngitis.

For further information

℞ DIRECTORY OF DRUGS:
antibacterial

♣ HERBAL REMEDIES:
Iceland moss • poplar • thyme

Lassa fever

Lassa fever is a serious viral disease, a hemorrhagic fever caused by an adenovirus, most common in West Africa, where it is carried by rodents. Symptoms of this ✛ **viral infection** include very high temperature, muscle pains, ✛ **headache**, slow heartbeat, and appetite loss. There may also be pain on swallowing, and tests may show a low white blood cell count. Some people recover, slowly; others deteriorate into confusion and coma.

Treatment

Treatment is to isolate the individual and to alleviate the symptoms as far as possible; injections of gamma globulin from a recently recovered person may help. The ℞ **antiviral** drug ℞ **ribavirin** may help combat the causative virus.

For further information

℞ DIRECTORY OF DRUGS:
antiviral • immune globulin

late puberty

see ✛ abnormal puberty.

lead poisoning

Lead poisoning is a form of ✛ **poisoning** caused by swallowing or inhaling lead and lead compounds. Acute and chronic forms seriously affect the normal functioning of parts of the body, although the symptoms may be different. Acute or sudden lead poisoning, often through inhalation, causes severe abdominal pain with cramps, ✛ **vomiting**, delirium, convulsions, and coma; tests show ✛ **anemia** and the presence of lead in the blood and urine. Chronic or long-term poisoning is indicated by a characteristic blue coloration of the gums ("lead line"), ✛ **fatigue**, ✛ **headache**, irritability, and breathlessness. There may also be abdominal pain and digestive disorders, with gradual signs of nerve damage (including loss of intellectual capacity).

Treatment

Treatment in both cases is with ℞ **chelating agents**, which are drugs that bind to metals, enabling their excretion (including ℞ **edetate calcium disodium**, ℞ **dimercaprol (BAL)**, succimer, and ℞ **penicillamine**). Any nerve damage must be diagnosed and treated, if possible, by a specialist.

For further information

℞ DIRECTORY OF DRUGS:
antidote • chelating agent

Legionnaires' disease

Legionnaires' disease is a ✛ **bacterial infection** of the lungs (a type of acute bacterial ✛ **pneumonia**), which caught the attention of the world when 29 of 182 people known to have contracted the disease (then unidentified) at, or near, the 1976 American Legion convention in Philadelphia, Pennsylvania, died from it. The bacterium (*Legionella pneumophila*) tends to reside in moist places, especially in ventilation systems that have humidifiers. Symptoms are lethargy and muscle pain, followed by high temperature and respiratory distress; kidney failure may also occur, as may the extreme symptoms of pneumonia.

Treatment

Treatment is with ℞ **antibacterials**, especially the antibiotic antibacterial ℞ **erythromycin**.

For further information

℞ DIRECTORY OF DRUGS:
antibacterial • antibiotic

leishmaniasis

Leishmaniasis is a group of ✛ **protozoal infection** caused by a protozoan parasite (genus *Leishmania*) that is carried by sandflies. There are three main forms: kala-azar, cutaneous leishmaniasis and American leishmaniasis (found in Central and South America). With kala-azar—a serious disorder—the parasite attacks the cells of the bone marrow, spleen, and lymphatic system. Symptoms include enlargement of, and damage to, the spleen and liver, recurrent high temperature, anemia, and weight loss; tests may show a low white blood cell count. Cutaneous leishmaniasis involves local ulcerative sores.

Treatment

Treatment of the disease is with ℞ **amebicide and antiprotozoals**, drugs containing antimony (for instance ℞ **pentamidine**) and ℞ **ketoconazole**, sometimes in conjunction with other drugs that prolong their action.

For further information

R DIRECTORY OF DRUGS:
amebicide and antiprotozoal • azole • pentamidine isethionate

leprosy

Leprosy (also called Hansen's disease) is a slow and progressively destructive ✪ **bacterial infection** that may be transmitted by direct contact or by air-borne droplets; children seem to contract it more readily than adults. The infection centers on the skin, mucous membranes, and nerves. There may be small areas of pale, disfigured skin that lose sensation (tuberculoid leprosy). Or there may be reddened nodules on the skin, loss of sensation over wide areas, eye inflammation, and recurrent bouts of fever (lepromatous leprosy), which can lead to deformity and paralysis. Some people suffer both types of symptoms.

Treatment

The course of the disease can be halted, but not reversed, through long-term (up to two years) treatment with a combination of anti-leprosy drugs (multidrug therapy). In some cases surgery may be able to repair some of the damage. A potential R **vaccine** is under development.

For further information

R DIRECTORY OF DRUGS:
antileprosy

leptospirosis

Leptospirosis is an infectious disease caused by types of the spiral-shaped bacterium *Leptospira interrogans*. The bacteria are carried by rats and dogs, and the disease transmitted in the animal's urine. Humans contract the ✪ **bacterial infection** by contact with contaminated soil or water—sewage workers and people who participate in water sports are at risk. In most cases, it causes a flu-like illness, but in severe forms (for example, Weil's disease) it can be life threatening.

Treatment

Treatment is with antibacterial antibiotics.

For further information

R DIRECTORY OF DRUGS:
antibacterial • penicillin • tetracycline

leukemia

Leukemia is a form of malignant disease, a ✪ **cancer**, which affects the organs that produce blood (mostly the bone marrow). It causes the production of far too many, and misshapen, white blood cells (leukocytes), thus also inhibiting the formation of other blood cells. The result is ✪ **anemia**, bleeding (through lack of the clotting factors), and extreme susceptibility to infections (through lack of much of the normal immune system in the bloodstream). There are a number of different types of leukemia.

Treatment

Treatment depends on the type of white cell being overproduced and on the rate at which the disease advances, but usually includes R **cytotoxic** (cancer-killing) drugs and radiotherapy; treatment is also necessary for any infections contracted.

For further information

R DIRECTORY OF DRUGS:
anticancer • cytotoxic

lice and mite infestation

Lice and mite infestations are caused by similar insects—both types infest the skin and cause intense itching. Lice of the genus *Pediculus* infest different regions of the body: *P. humanus capitis* infesting the head, *P. humanus corporis* infesting the body, and *P. humanus pubis* infesting the pubic region. They all cause intense itching, and subsequent scratching tends to damage the skin surface, and may eventually cause weeping lesions with bacterial infection. ✪ **scabies** is an infestation by the itch-mite *Sarcoptes scabiei*. The female mite tunnels into the top surface of the skin in order to lay her eggs, causing severe irritation as she does so. Newly hatched mites, also causing irritation with their secretions, then pass easily from person to person on direct contact.

Treatment

Similar drugs are used in pediculicidal and scabicidal treatment. Every member of an infected household should be treated, and clothing and bedding should be disinfected. Lice are treated with what are called pediculicide or pediculicidal drugs, whereas mites are treated with what are called scabicide or scabicidal drugs. Treatment is usually with local application of a cream, lotion or shampoo. R **Antipruritics** including R **antihistamines** may be given to relieve itching. ♣ **anise** and ♣ **quassia** are herbal alternatives.

For further information

R DIRECTORY OF DRUGS:

scabicide and pediculicide (for example, **lindane, malathion, permethrin**) • antipruritic (for example, **antihistamine**)

♣ HERBAL REMEDIES:
anise • quassia

listeriosis

Listeriosis ✪ **food poisoning** is caused by eating foods contaminated with a bacterium (*Listeria monocytogenes*) that is widespread in the soil and common in many animals. Infection may cause few symptoms, or a flu-like syndrome, but sometimes leads to serious complications including ✪ **septicemia** and ✪ **encephalitis** (especially in those with reduced immunity). It can also cause fetal death, miscarriage, or serious infection of the newborn; pregnant women are advised to avoid high-risk foods—soft cheeses (such as brie) and meat pâté.

Treatment

Treatment is with R **antibacterials**, sometimes given intravenously to those at risk (such as pregnant women).

For further information

R DIRECTORY OF DRUGS:
antibacterial

liver cancer

see ✪ **cancer**.

liver disorders

Liver disorders may arise from a number of causes. The liver is a very important organ, involved in metabolism of foods, drugs, and foreign chemicals, and also in the production of bile, which is stored in the gallbladder. Defective functioning may arise from ✪ **bacterial infection**, ✪ **viral infection**, and more rarely ✪ **worms** or ✪ **protozoal infection** (see ✪ **malaria**, ✪ **schistosomiasis**). Inflammation of the liver is called ✪ **hepatitis**, and infectious hepatitis is a common and relatively serious disorder. Non-infectious hepatitis is caused by certain drugs, poisons, chemicals, and ✪ **alcoholism**. Prolonged hepatitis may give way to ✪ **cirrhosis** of the liver, with actual tissue destruction. In many cases a symptom of liver disorder is ✪ **jaundice**, yellowing of the whites of the eyes and skin, and can be caused by the accumulation in the body of bile pigments due to their slow excretion as bile (as well as excess red blood cell breakdown). Other liver disorders include liver metastases, which are cancerous tumors of the liver that originate from ✪ **cancer** in other areas of the body (for example, lung, pancreas, and stomach).

Treatment

Treatment depends on the cause; and may include ℞ **antiviral**, ℞ **antibacterial**, ℞ **antimalarial**, ℞ **immunomodulators** (℞ **interferons**), ℞ **immunosuppressant**, ℞ **immune globulin**, ℞ **vaccine**, and ℞ **anticancer** drugs. Many herbal remedies are used to treat liver disorders or are taken as "liver tonics" and these include ♣ **black root**, ♣ **boldo**, ♣ **cardamom**, ♣ **celandine**, ♣ **chicory**, ♣ **curcuma**, ♣ **dandelion**, ♣ **haronga**, ♣ **immortelle**, ♣ **Japanese mint**, ♣ **Java tree**, ♣ **milk thistle**, ♣ **tamarind**, ♣ **wild iris**. See individual disorders for more information.

lobar pneumonia

see ✪ pneumonia.

Lou Gehrig's disease

see ✪ amyotrophic lateral sclerosis.

lumbago

Lumbago is a general term for ✪ **pain** in the lumbar region—the lower back. Causes include muscular strain (from lifting or carrying), a prolapsed intervertebral disk (more commonly known as a slipped disk), which may be accompanied by ✪ **sciatica**, curvature of the spine through disorder or long-term bad posture, or kidney or gynecological disorders. See also ✪ **musculoskeletal disorders**.

Treatment

Treatment, where possible, depends on the cause, but may include ℞ **non-narcotic analgesic** drugs to relieve pain or sometimes surgery.

For further information

℞ DIRECTORY OF DRUGS:

non-narcotic analgesic • NSAID

♣ HERBAL REMEDIES:

devil's claw • juniper

lung cancer

Lung cancer is ✪ **cancer** in a bronchial passage or in a lung. There are several types. A dangerous disorder, it may not be diagnosed until the cancer has already spread (by metastasis) elsewhere in the body. Symptoms are at first only a mild cough, becoming progressively worse, with blood in the sputum and increasing breathlessness. There may then be the collapse of a lung, or ✪ **pneumonia**. Weight loss and lethargy are common. The great majority of people who contract lung cancer are or have been heavy cigarette smokers. It is essentially incurable.

Treatment

Treatment is usually too late for removal of the lung to be totally successful; radiotherapy and anticancer drugs of the ℞ **cytotoxic** type may be used.

For further information

℞ DIRECTORY OF DRUGS:

anticancer • cytotoxic

lupus

Lupus is a term that covers a group of disorders that may or may not be interrelated, but all of which can produce scaly or disfiguring lesions on the skin. Lupus erythematosus, of which there are two forms, is thought to be an ✪ **autoimmune disorder** (in which the immune system attacks the body's own tissues). The lesser form, discoid lupus erythematosus, produces symptoms of reddened scaly areas of skin made worse by sunlight but fading over time; treatment generally involves ℞ **antimalarial** drugs. Systemic lupus erythematosus has the additional symptoms of ✪ **rheumatoid arthritis**, and may also affect the kidney and other functions. Lupus vulgaris is a rare condition not related to lupus erythematosus but corresponding to ✪ **tuberculosis** (bacillary invasion) of the skin, which, untreated, may cause severe scarring. An adverse reaction to certain drugs can cause a lupus-like syndrome.

Treatment

Treatment of lupus erythematosus is with corticosteroids or ℞ **immunosuppressant** drugs, which may prevent further attacks for long periods. The supplement DHEA is advocated as being beneficial in controlling some symptoms of lupus. Lupus vulgaris treatment is as for tuberculosis.

For further information

℞ DIRECTORY OF DRUGS:

antimalarial • antituberculosis • immunosuppressant

⚗ VITAMINS, MINERALS, AND SUPPLEMENTS:

DHEA

Lyme disease

Lyme disease is an infectious ✪ **bacterial** disease caused by the bacterium *Borrelia burgdorferi*. It is transmitted by tick bites (typically carried by deer), which, in most of those affected, causes a characteristic expanding, red skin rash up to a month after the bite. It was originally described in the community of Old Lyme, Connecticut. Other symptoms include ✪ **fever**, ✪ **headache**, and joint pains, and there may be later complications including ✪ **arthritis** and heart and nerve damage, especially if untreated.

Treatment

Treatment is with ℞ **antibacterial** drugs (including tetracyclines, macrolides, and penicillins), and ℞ **non-narcotic analgesic** (℞ **NSAID**) drugs to relieve symptoms. For people at risk, there is a vaccination (Lyme disease vaccine) available.

For further information

℞ DIRECTORY OF DRUGS:
antibacterial (**tetracycline**, **macrolide**, and **penicillin**) • **NSAID** •
non-narcotic analgesic • **vaccine**

lymphoma

Lymphoma is a term used to describe any of several types of ✪ **cancer** arising in the lymphatic system, including ✪ **Hodgkin's disease** and non-Hodgkin's lymphomas. Progressive lymph node enlargement, widespread or confined to a particular area, may be accompanied by symptoms such as fever, weight loss, lethargy, and sweating. The progress of the disease may be rapid or slow, with the prognosis varying accordingly.

Treatment

Treatment with ℞ **anticancer** drugs (chemotherapy) can be very successful, particularly if started early in the course of the disease. In some cases radiotherapy is also given. Surgery may be used in Hodgkin's disease, and bone marrow transplants in non-Hodgkin's lymphomas.

For further information

℞ DIRECTORY OF DRUGS:
anticancer • cytotoxic

macular degeneration

Macular degeneration is the progressive deterioration of the macula, which is the area near the center of the light-sensitive retina. The condition results in a progressive loss of central and detailed vision, although peripheral vision is unaffected. It is common in women and sometimes runs in families. It usually occurs in people over age 70. Excessive exposure to sunlight and smoking increase the risk of macular degeneration, and it can occur in some diseases such as retinitis pigmentosa.

Treatment

Some types (wet macular degeneration) can be treated by laser surgery. ⚖ **Carotenoids** and ⚖ **zinc** are considered by some to help protect against macular degeneration.

For further information

⚖ VITAMINS, MINERALS, AND SUPPLEMENTS:
carotenoid (for example, **beta-carotene**) • **zinc**

malabsorption disorders

Malabsorption disorders are a diverse group of disorders characterized by the poor absorption of substances in the diet from the gut into the bloodstream. They generally are a symptom or consequence of another illness. Some of these states are also referred to as malabsorption syndrome. Often the failure is in respect of a specific substance—commonly fats, but also perhaps certain vitamins or trace elements. In ✪ **celiac disease**, the small intestine is damaged by a reaction to gluten, so some nutrients are not properly absorbed. Less commonly, similar problems are seen in other intestinal complaints including ✪ **Crohn's disease**, ✪ **giardiasis**, ✪ **lymphoma**. Similarly, when surgical removal of parts of the intestine has been necessary, there may be impaired absorption. When there are disorders of the bile duct and gallbladder (for example, biliary cirrhosis, obstructed bile duct, and Crohn's disease), the outcome of the impaired secretion of bile salts is poor absorption and the breakdown of fats in the diet. In lactase deficiency, there is a deficiency of the enzyme that is responsible for the breakdown and absorption of the milk sugar lactose, resulting in an inability to digest this sugar. There is also ✪ **lactose intolerance**. In ✪ **pancreatitis** and ✪ **cystic fibrosis**, there is impaired production of pancreatic enzyme, which is necessary for the breakdown and absorption of fats and other nutrients in food. Malabsorption commonly results in diarrhea, anemia, edema, weight loss, and other signs of deficiency and malnutrition. See also ✪ **vitamin deficiency**.

Treatment

Generally the cause of the malabsorption disorder is investigated and corrected where possible. Where this is not possible, dietary supplements and restrictions may control the symptoms. Some ℞ **digestive enzymes** (for instance pancreatic enzymes including ℞ **pancrelipase**) can be added to the diet. There are a number of vitamins and minerals that can be valuable, depending on circumstances.

For further information

℞ DIRECTORY OF DRUGS:
digestive enzyme

⚖ VITAMINS, MINERALS, AND SUPPLEMENTS:
minerals • vitamins

malabsorption syndrome

see ✪ **malabsorption disorders**.

malaria

Malaria is a serious infection caused by protozoan parasites transmitted through the bites of *Anopheles* mosquitoes. It is relatively common in tropical and subtropical regions. It is one of the greatest public health problems in the world. Symptoms may develop from a few days up to a year after a mosquito bite. It can also be spread by blood transfusion from an infected person or by the use of an infected hypodermic needle. Once in a person's bloodstream, the young protozoans congregate in the internal organs (especially the liver) before taking again to the bloodstream and invading the red blood cells where they mature, reproduce, and periodically burst out. The resulting destruction of red blood cells in sufficient quantity causes anemia, and a fever that peaks and vanishes—only to recur regularly as waves of protozoans mature and invade the bloodstream. The details of the disease vary according to which of the four species of protozoan parasites is involved, as their life cycles vary. One rarer form of malaria, also called malignant malaria or blackwater fever, causes red blood cell destruction and kidney damage, and is sometimes fatal; in other, benign forms, fever may recur after intervals of three days (tertian fever) or four (quartan fever), each bout preceded by shivering and accompanied by headache, vomiting, and, often, delirium. It is a ✪ **protozoal infection**.

Treatment

Treatment is with ℞ **antimalarial** drugs, which should also be taken as a preventive measure by people traveling to areas where malaria is endemic (widespread). Medical advice is needed to determine the drug most effective at the time for a particular area, and drugs do not provide complete protection: precautions against being bitten by mosquitoes are also vital. Medical research is attempting to find a ℞ **vaccine** that is effective against malaria. ♣ **Solomon's seal**, a herbal remedy, is said to be useful in malaria. However, professional medical treatment is required for this serious illness.

For further information

℞ DIRECTORY OF DRUGS:
antimalarial
♣ HERBAL REMEDIES:
Solomon's seal

male pattern baldness

see ✪ **alopecia**.

malignant disease

see ✪ **cancer**.

manic depression

see ✪ **bipolar disorder**.

mastalgia

see ✪ **pain**.

mastitis

Mastitis is the inflammation of a woman's breast. It is generally caused by ✪ **bacterial infection** (typically *Staphylococcus aureus*), often after childbirth when the nipples may have become slightly damaged through suckling. Unless there are signs that an abscess is forming, the condition should not interrupt breast-feeding. Cystic (or chronic) mastitis, however, is not inflammation but the presence of small cysts in the breast tissues. Symptoms include tender red areas that spread away from the nipple, swelling, and pain. Resulting from hormonal imbalance, it occurs particularly just before menstruation, and particularly again just before the ✪ **menopause**.

Treatment

Treatment of infection is with ℞ **antibacterials**, usually ℞ **antibiotics**, which generally produce rapid relief.

For further information

℞ DIRECTORY OF DRUGS:
antibacterial

measles

Measles is a highly infectious ✪ **viral infection**, with the alternative medical names rubeola and morbilli. It occurs most commonly in children. Initial symptoms, after an incubation period of 8–15 days, are a ✪ **fever** and a catarrhal sore throat with a ✪ **cough**; the condition is infectious from this point on. Two days later, small spots, red with a white center, appear inside the cheeks (Koplik's spots), tending to fade a further two days later when a rash develops. The blotchy orange-pink rash typically originates behind the ears, spreads to the face, and then travels down the neck to the whole body. The rash lasts for five or six days, during which time the disease remains infectious. The cough may persist for 10 days or so afterward, and complications may include ✪ **pneumonia**, middle ear infections, and ✪ **encephalitis**.

Treatment

Treatment is to alleviate the symptoms (especially ℞ **antipyretic** drugs to control fever) and prevent complications. A vaccine is available and is usually given in infancy, along with rubella vaccine (MR) or more often with both mumps and rubella vaccine (℞ **MMR**). Contracting the disease usually confers lifelong immunity.

For further information

℞ DIRECTORY OF DRUGS:
antipyretic • vaccine

megaloblastic anemia

see ✪ **anemia**.

melanoma

Melanoma is a rare but serious type of skin ✪ **cancer** that centers on an area of melanocytes—the cells that produce the dark pigment melanin. They thus occur mostly in the skin (especially where the skin is pigmented with a mole), but also occasionally on the surface of the eye, and even in the mucous membranes of the mouth. Indications that a melanoma is forming include a change in color or size, bleeding or itching of a birthmark or mole. The main cause is over-exposure to sunlight.

Treatment

Treatment is usually with surgery and, if necessary, ℞ **anticancer** chemotherapy.

For further information

℞ DIRECTORY OF DRUGS:
anticancer • cytotoxic

Ménière's disease

Ménière's disease is a disorder of the inner ear that affects the functions of hearing and balance. It is believed to be caused by a build-up of fluid in the inner ear, leading to increased pressure in the fluid within the semicircular canals (which control sensations of balance). Symptoms are recurrent bouts of ✪ **tinnitus** (ringing in the ears) and ✪ **vertigo** (dizziness), with ✪ **nausea**, and temporary ✪ **deafness**. With repeated attacks, hearing may be permanently impaired.

Treatment

Treatment is to alleviate the symptoms as far as possible, including ℞ **antiemetic** (antinauseant) drugs (including ℞ **dimenhydrinate**, ℞ **meclizine**, and ℞ **scopolamine**) to reduce nausea, vertigo, and dizziness during attacks. In persistent cases, long-term drug treatment may be necessary as a preventive measure. Some-

     Key to symbols: ✪ = Disorder Section   ℞ = Drug Section   ♣ = Herbal Section   ♋ = Supplement Section

times injections into the inner ear or surgery are used for symptoms not controlled by drugs.

For further information

℞ DIRECTORY OF DRUGS:
antiemetic • antinauseant

meningeal cancer

see ✪ cancer.

meningitis

Meningitis is inflammation of the meninges (the membranes surrounding the brain and spinal cord), usually as a result of ✪ **infection** by various bacteria, viruses and, rarely, fungi. Symptoms are those of a heavy cold, followed by severe headache, very high temperature, vomiting, sensitivity to light and sound, and muscular spasm (especially involving a stiff neck). There may be confusion and, in extreme cases, convulsions. In meningococcal meningitis there is a characteristic rash with bleeding under the skin. Meningitis is a medical emergency as without treatment it may cause permanent brain damage or death.

Treatment

Treatment depends on diagnosis of the infective organism. Most forms of viral meningitis do not respond to antiviral drugs, although these are occasionally used. Otherwise the only treatment is bed rest. Fortunately, viral meningitis rarely causes serious damage. Bacterial meningitis requires urgent ℞ **antibacterial** treatment with antibiotics. Immunization is now possible against certain, but not all, forms of meningitis (℞ **meningococcal polysaccharide vaccine** against type C, ℞ **Haemophilus b conjugate vaccine**).

For further information

℞ DIRECTORY OF DRUGS:
antibacterial • antiviral • vaccine

menopause

The menopause is the cessation of ovulation and, thus, of childbearing capacity in a woman. It is accompanied by the cessation of menstruation (periods). The exact age at which it occurs (any time between the mid-30s and the later 50s, average age 51) depends on hormonal changes in the body, and generally follows a pattern in which menstrual periods gradually become either irregular or more widely spaced. A span of four to six years, known as the perimenopause, precedes the menopause when menstrual cycles and blood flow may be irregular, and may be associated with ✪ **depression** as estrogen levels decline. The menopause is popularly known as the "change of life"; the medical term is the climacteric, and it is only diagnosed when a woman has had no menstrual periods for a year. Rarely, periods may stop abruptly. The hormonal changes involved may also lead to hot flushes, minor disturbances of the heartbeat (palpitations), and dryness of the vagina, which may cause discomfort during intercourse.

Treatment

Many symptoms can be alleviated by hormone supplements (hormone replacement therapy, HRT), which also reduce the increased risk of ✪ **osteoporosis** to which postmenopausal women are liable.

Several herbal remedies (such as ♣ **black cohosh**) and supplements are available that also have beneficial effects.

For further information

℞ DIRECTORY OF DRUGS:
hormone replacement

♣ HERBAL REMEDIES:
black cohosh • blue cohosh • chaste tree • St. John's wort

⚖ VITAMINS, MINERALS, AND SUPPLEMENTS:
gamma-linolenic acid (GLA)

menorrhagia

Menorrhagia is unusually heavy menstruation and/or a prolonged duration of menstrual periods. Its causes are many, and include inflammation of the lining of the womb (endometritis), the presence of fibroids, ✪ **pelvic inflammatory disease**, ✪ **cancer** of the uterus, uterine polyps or ✪ **endometriosis**. Some cases are linked with hormonal imbalances, when the condition is known as dysfunctional uterine bleeding. Heavy periods may also occur when an intrauterine contraceptive device (IUD) is in place. If menorrhagia is severe and prolonged, iron-deficiency ✪ **anemia** may result.

Treatment

Treatment depends on the cause but may include drugs or surgery. If anemia is a problem, ⚖ **iron** supplements can be taken.

For further information

℞ DIRECTORY OF DRUGS:
anemia treatment • hemostatic • NSAID (mefenamic acid) • progestin

♣ HERBAL REMEDIES:
cotton • shepherd's purse • white peony

⚖ VITAMINS, MINERALS, AND SUPPLEMENTS:
iron (for anemia)

menstrual disorders

see ✪ dysmenorrhea; ✪ menorrhagia; ✪ premenstrual syndrome.

mental illness

Mental illness is a group of conditions in which the normal functions of the mind (generally of an adult) are disturbed. It affects thinking, emotions, memory, or perception. Causes may include injury to the brain (as by trauma, disease, or ✪ **poisoning** with drugs—including alcohol—or with certain heavy metals), long-term stress, acute emotion, or may be unknown. Mental illness may be categorized into various types including personality disorders, neuroses (✪ **affective disorders**; neurotic disorders, and mood disorders), and psychoses (✪ **psychotic disorder**). Of these, personality disorders, featuring maladaptive behaviors, generally most approach (and overlap with) normality. People with neuroses are aware of—and distressed by—their behavioral oddities, which may take the form of extreme ✪ **anxiety**, ✪ **depression**, or exaggerated behavior; whereas those with psychoses are unaware of them, having lost contact with reality and insight into their condition, for instance in ✪ **schizophrenia**.

Treatment

Treatment depends on the diagnosis but may include counseling, various forms of therapy, or drugs such as ℞ **antipsychotic**, ℞ **antidepressant**, ℞ **antianxiety**, and ℞ **antimanic** drugs. Some herbal remedies: ♣ **cola**, ♣ **damiana**, ♣ **maté**, ♣ **St. John's wort**, ♣ **vervain**, ♣ **bugleweed**, ♣ **hops**, ♣ **kava kava**, ♣ **lemon balm**, ♣ **passionflower**, ♣ **valerian**, ♣ **water hyssop**) can help alleviate the symptoms of anxiety and/or depression. Individuals with severe psychoses may require hospitalization to protect themselves or others. For specific treatments, see the individual disorder.

mercury poisoning

Mercury ✪ **poisoning** (also called Minamata disease) presents a collection of symptoms, due to the inhalation of mercury vapors or the ingestion or absorption of mercury through the skin, and from contaminated seafood and grain. Acute poisoning causes abdominal pain, ✪ **vomiting**, and ✪ **diarrhea**, sometimes with bleeding. It may lead to ✪ **kidney failure**. Chronic poisoning with smaller doses over a prolonged period causes digestive and urinary disturbances, ✪ **mouth ulcer**, and dental problems. Late effects include ✪ **anemia** and nerve damage.

Treatment

Treatment is first to remove the source of exposure, which may require extensive decontamination procedures. Thereafter it involves supportive measures to try to alleviate the symptoms. Sometimes treatment aims to counteract kidney damage and anemia. Severe acute poisoning can be treated with a ℞ **chelating agent** (which removes the toxic metal from the bloodstream).

For further information

℞ DIRECTORY OF DRUGS:
antidote • chelating agent

metabolic disorders

Metabolic disorders are deficiencies in the biochemistry of the body, normally due to inadequate levels of abnormal forms of essential enzymes in the body. Often when there is an abnormal enzyme form this is due to a familial factor, often a fault in the gene of one or both parents. There are now several hundred disorders linked to deficiency in a specific enzyme, and many more are expected to be discovered as a result of our increasing knowledge of the human genome, and the production of proteins, including enzymes, that it controls.

Treatment

In the future, treatment may be by correcting the deficient gene, but as yet this process is technically very difficult. Another approach in treating enzyme deficiencies is by administration of the missing enzyme as a drug, but there are a number of difficulties in using enzymes in therapeutics. A major one is that enzymes must normally be given by injection since, because they are proteins, they are broken down by digestive enzymes in the stomach or intestine. Another difficulty in the past, was the major problem of isolating enzymes from plant or animal tissues. Now they can be made by recombinant DNA technology, though the cost of such drugs is likely to be great. However, the enzyme imiglucerase, in a form manufactured by recombinant DNA technology, is used as a

replacement in the specialist treatment of Type 1 Gaucher's disease (a genetically determined enzyme deficiency disease affecting the spleen, liver, bone marrow, and lymph nodes).

In other cases, the biochemical consequences of the deficiency are treated. In many of the known cases of inborn errors of metabolism, such enzyme deficiencies may lead to a shortage in the body of an amino acid (for instance carnitine deficiency; treated with a dietary supplement of carnitine as levocarnitine), or of high levels of a precursor (a well known instance being phenylketanuria, where failure of conversion of phenylalanine into tyrosine leads to a build up of excess of the former which causes the disorder; treated by a special diet containing low levels of phenylalanine). Sodium phenylbutyrate is a soluble salt of the amino acid phenylbutyric acid, and is used as a treatment for urea cycle disturbances due to specific enzyme deficiencies, which cause a build-up of ammonia in the body. Where the enzyme deficiency causes a toxic product to accumulate, this can sometimes be treated by using chelating agent chemicals that work by chemically binding to certain metallic ions and other substances, making them less toxic and allowing their excretion (for instance of copper in Wilson's disease, for which the chelator penicillamine is used).

For further information

℞ DIRECTORY OF DRUGS:
chelating agent (penicillamine) • **enzyme (imiglucerase)** • **levocarnitine** • **sodium phenylbutyrate**

migraine

Migraines are severe one-sided ✪ **headaches**, with a characteristic throbbing nature, usually accompanied by ✪ **nausea** and ✪ **vomiting**, and sometimes by photophobia (intense dislike of light). Some people have an aura warning that the migraine is about to start, which may consist of visual disturbances such as tunnel vision or zigzag light patterns, or limb symptoms such as tingling, numbness, or weakness. A group of symptoms (mood changes such as ✪ **anxiety**, altered sense of smell, and a change in energy) called a prodrome may precede the migraine. These symptoms usually resolve before the headache starts. The cause is an abnormality in the blood flow within the brain or skull, with arterial spasm followed by dilation. Various factors such as certain foods (chocolate or cheese), low blood sugar, lack of sleep or stress, may trigger attacks. The migraine may last for hours or even days and makes normal activities impossible.

Treatment

℞ **antimigraine** drug treatment can be problematic, and to find a therapy from the wide range now available, which is effective in a given person may require a trial-and-error investigation, possibly with an input from a migraine clinic. Two types of therapy are required, one with a fast-onset of action to treat acute attacks, another for long-term prophylaxis. In acute attacks, antimigraine ℞ **vasoconstrictor** drugs may be taken (including ℞ **sumatriptan succinate**, ℞ **naratriptan**, ℞ **rizatriptan benzoate**, ℞ **zolmitriptan**, and ℞ **dihydroergotamine mesylate**), some preparations of which may be self-injected or taken by nasal spray (℞ **sumatriptan succinate**) to more quickly relieve an attack. Some other vasoconstrictor antimigraine drugs are also available that can be taken orally to prevent frequent attacks, including the older ergot-derived drugs (℞ **ergonovine**, ℞ **dihydroergotamine**, ℞ **methysergide**, and ℞ **ergoloid mesylates**). Other types of drugs taken by mouth in prophylaxis against attacks include ℞ **beta-blockers** (including atenolol, metoprolol, bisoprolol, penbutolol, and timolol) and ℞ **calcium-channel blockers** (℞ **amlodipine** and ℞ **nifedipine**). Some other drugs that may be tried in difficult types of vascular headache (see also ✪ **cluster headache**) include ℞ **valproic acid** and derivatives, ℞ **phenytoin**, ℞ **imipramine**, ℞ **chlorpromazine**, ℞ **isometheptene**, and ℞ **cyproheptadine**. Antinauseant drugs (℞ **antiemetics**) may also be taken to give relief from nausea (for instance ℞ **metoclopramide**).

For relief of pain, a number of OTC ℞ **non-narcotic analgesics** (some containing small amounts of ℞ **narcotic analgesics** such as ℞ **codeine phosphate**) are available, but tend not to be very effective in migraine headaches. Herbal remedies such as ♣ **feverfew** are beneficial in some sufferers and ⚕ **vitamin B$_2$** is considered to be useful by some. Herbal remedies such as ♣ **Jamaican dogwood** and ♣ **fumitory** for additional symptoms of migraine can be beneficial. Identifying what triggers an attack may help in prevention.

For further information
℞ DIRECTORY OF DRUGS:
antiemetic • antimigraine • antinauseant • narcotic analgesic • non-narcotic analgesic
♣ HERBAL REMEDIES:
cola • feverfew • fumitory • Jamaica dogwood
⚕ VITAMINS, MINERALS, AND SUPPLEMENTS:
vitamin B$_2$

miliaria
see ✪ prickly heat.

milk intolerance
see ✪ lactose intolerance.

mitral incompetence
see ✪ heart valve disorders.

mitral stenosis
see ✪ heart valve disorders.

moniliasis
see ✪ candidiasis.

mood disorder
see ✪ affective disorders.

morbilli
see ✪ measles.

morning sickness
Morning sickness is the ✪ **nausea**, and possibly ✪ **vomiting**, that is experienced by as many as half of all women during the early months of pregnancy, often, but not always, on rising in the mornings. It is a ✪ **pregnancy-related disorder**. It usually stops by the fourth month, and is believed to help protect the fetus against possibly harmful ingredients in food. Severe sickness during pregnancy (hyperemesis gravidarum) is uncommon but can indicate toxemia of pregnancy, a serious condition, which may lead to dehydration and sometimes to liver damage. Severe or persistent morning sickness should be reported to a doctor.

Treatment
For many women, a simple countermeasure is to frequently eat small easily digested snacks. Avoiding rich or greasy foods and ensuring adequate rest can reduce nausea. Antinausea drugs are not normally prescribed because of the risk of danger to the fetus and in general, no medications (including herbal) should be taken during pregnancy without professional medical advice.

motion sickness
Motion sickness (also called travel sickness, car sickness, air sickness and seasickness) is the ✪ **nausea**, and possibly ✪ **vomiting** and ✪ **headache**, caused by the movement of the vehicle in which the person is traveling. The effect results from the abnormally constant demands such movements make, both on the organs of balance in the inner ear, and on the eyes in adjusting to a persistently moving objective. An aura (one of various sensations that act as a warning) may precede an attack, consisting of yawning or a slight rise in temperature. Ginger is a popular herbal alternative.

Treatment
Treatment may include drugs with antinauseant properties, usually referred to as ℞ **antiemetics** (antisickness drugs) of which most are ℞ **antihistamines**. The drugs are best taken before a journey to prevent motion sickness.

For further information
℞ DIRECTORY OF DRUGS:
antiemetic • antinauseant
♣ HERBAL REMEDIES:
chamomile, German • ginger

motor neuron disease
Motor neuron disease is any of several rare disorders where there is progressive degeneration of the nerves, in the brain and spinal cord, which control muscular activity. The causes are unknown, but some forms are inherited. Onset is usually in middle age or later. Symptoms include increasing muscle weakness and wasting, from the extremities inward. Progressive muscular atrophy may take up to 20 years to develop fully and cause death; ✪ **amyotrophic lateral sclerosis** (Lou Gehrig's disease) around 2–5 years; and progressive bulbar paralysis (which attacks the throat) usually two. For a greater range of motor degenerative disorders, see also ✪ **brain-motor disorders**.

Treatment
Treatment is to alleviate the symptoms as far as possible; physiotherapy may help. The drug ℞ **riluzole** may reduce symptoms in some forms (amyotrophic lateral sclerosis) of motor neuron disease, but does not represent a cure.

For further information
℞ DIRECTORY OF DRUGS:
brain-motor disorder treatment

mouth ulcer

Mouth ulcers are painful sores in the lining of the mouth. In most cases, the cause is not known, but sometimes mouth ulcers are due to anemia, folic acid or vitamin B$_1$ deficiency, or certain disorders such as ✪ **herpes** simplex infection, ✪ **celiac disease**, ✪ **Crohn's disease** or ✪ **Behçet's syndrome**. Mouth ulcers tend to occur in people who are run down or under stress.

Treatment

Mouth ulcers usually disappear without treatment in two weeks. Drugs are available, some OTC, to apply topically. A number of herbal remedies can be used topically for symptomatic relief. Supplements of ⚛ **folic acid** and ⚛ **vitamin B$_1$** may help to prevent mouth ulcers.

For further information

℞ DIRECTORY OF DRUGS:
corticosteroid • local anesthetic
♣ HERBAL REMEDIES:
achyranthes • kava kava • sage
⚛ VITAMINS, MINERALS, AND SUPPLEMENTS:
folic acid• vitamin B$_1$

MRSA

see ✪ **superinfections**.

mucous colitis

see ✪ irritable bowel syndrome.

multiple sclerosis

Multiple sclerosis (MS) is a serious progressive ✪ **autoimmune disorder** caused by damage and hardening (sclerosis) to the myelin sheaths (demyelination) around the nerves. It occurs in scattered areas of the brain and spinal cord and this affects the function of the nerves involved. The onset is usually in young adults. Initial symptoms are muscular weakness and tingling or numbness in one or two limbs; there may also be blurred vision, bladder incontinence, or vertigo. Later symptoms may include all of these and other more serious effects of neural damage, depending on the actual nerves affected, which may include spastic paralysis (weakness accompanied by increased tone and spasm of the muscles), shaking, speech disorders, and visual loss. In the most common form of the disorder, there are periods of relapse and remission, when some or all of the symptoms resolve. In time, more deficits may remain after each relapse, leading to progressive disability. The advance of the disease may be slow or rapid. Some cases show a steady deterioration from the outset. A few people recover spontaneously; many endure decades of problems and remissions before stabilizing; those who do not stabilize are at risk of pulmonary or urinary complications.

Treatment

Treatment is to relieve the symptoms as far as possible, and may include physiotherapy and drug treatment of spasticity and incontinence. ℞ **Corticosteroids** may be used during relapses. Treatment with beta-interferon can be used in some types of MS, where it reduces the relapse rate and may lessen eventual disability.

♣ **evening primrose** and ⚛ **vitamin B$_{12}$** are considered by some to have beneficial effects.

For further information

℞ DIRECTORY OF DRUGS:
brain-motor disorder treatment • corticosteroid • immunomodulator (interferons)
♣ HERBAL REMEDIES:
evening primrose
⚛ VITAMINS, MINERALS, AND SUPPLEMENTS:
vitamin B$_{12}$

mumps

Mumps (called medically *infectious parotitis*) is a ✪ **viral infection** of the parotid salivary gland, most common in children. Initial symptoms are malaise and ✪ **nausea**, with a ✪ **headache** and ✪ **fever**. The person is already infectious at this stage. The temperature then soars even higher—probably to somewhere around 40°C (104°F)—and the salivary glands on one or both sides of the cheeks (the parotid glands) swell painfully, remaining sensitive to the touch. There may be difficulty in opening the mouth. After three to six days the symptoms fade, but the child remains infectious until the swelling has completely gone. In adults, mumps may cause further infections of the pancreas, brain, testes, or the ovaries, and in males after puberty testicular involvement can cause infertility.

Treatment

Treatment is isolation of the individual and alleviation of the symptoms as far as possible, and may include ℞ **non-narcotic analgesic** drugs. A vaccine is available, and is usually given in childhood along with measles and rubella immunization (MMR vaccine).

For further information

℞ DIRECTORY OF DRUGS:
non-narcotic analgesic • vaccine

muscle cramps

Muscle cramps are sudden and painful skeletal muscle spasms, commonly in the legs. Often called "a stitch" when abdominal muscles are concerned. They are a normal occurrence after vigorous or prolonged exercise, when the normal cause is a build-up of lactic acid in the muscles (which soon dissipates). In hot weather or exercise a loss of sodium in sweat may predispose to cramps. Night cramps may be caused by poor circulation in the limbs (for example, in ✪ **peripheral vascular disorders**). Writer's cramp in the muscles of the hand may be due to awkward posture or too prolonged activity. For cramping in menstruation (not skeletal muscle but uterine smooth muscle cramping) see ✪ **dysmenorrhea**, and for other internal smooth muscle cramping, see ✪ **colic**.

Treatment

If the cramps are in the limbs, the limbs can be stretched and rubbed to relieve the pain. Salts of ℞ **quinine** and replacement salt (electrolyte) solutions may be used if the problem persists. A number of types of drug are used to treat ✪ **peripheral vascular disorders**, mainly ℞ **vasodilators**.

For further information

℞ DIRECTORY OF DRUGS:
electrolyte • quinine • vasodilator

♣ HERBAL REMEDIES:
guelder rose

muscle pain

see ✪ musculoskeletal disorders.

muscular dystrophy

Muscular dystrophy represents any of a group of potentially severe disorders that almost exclusively affect males. The muscles progressively waste away although the nerves supplying them remain functional. The affected muscle fibers degenerate and are gradually replaced by fatty tissue. Almost all of the disorders in the group have hereditary factors—which may aid diagnosis. Other pointers toward diagnosis include age of onset and the progress of the disease; a muscle biopsy (tissue sample taken for testing) or electromyographic testing of muscle function may be useful. The most common form is Duchenne's muscular dystrophy, in which the muscles of the pelvis and back in boys under the age of four waste away. Another rarer form is Becker's muscular dystrophy.

Treatment

Treatment is to alleviate the symptoms and the difficulties associated with them as far as possible, and may include physiotherapy. The gene responsible for Duchenne's muscular dystrophy has now been identified, so screening and gene therapy may be possible in future.

For further information

℞ DIRECTORY OF DRUGS:
brain-motor disorder treatment

musculoskeletal disorders

Musculoskeletal disorders encompass a wide variety of conditions affecting skeletal muscle joints, ligaments, and bones. In some, there are marked manifestations, particularly ✪ **pain**, in the muscles and joints. Generally they involve a number of different structures and represent a range of aches referred to as ✪ **rheumatism**, ✪ **arthritis**, arthralgia, fibromyalgia, tendinitis, tennis elbow, rheumatoid diseases, ✪ **rheumatoid arthritis**, ✪ **lumbago**, ✪ **backache**, and ✪ **muscle cramps**. In some musculoskeletal disorders, the main problem is in the nerves supplying the muscle, including ✪ **sciatica**, ✪ **multiple sclerosis**, and ✪ **myasthenia gravis**. Other diseases affect primarily the muscles, for instance ✪ **muscular dystrophy**.

Treatment

Treatment depends on cause. In many of the disorders, some remission of symptoms can be gained by treatment with ℞ **anti-inflammatory** drugs including ℞ **corticosteroids**. Where there is an ✪ **autoimmune** component, ℞ **immunosuppressant** drugs may be used where symptoms are severe. To alleviate the symptoms and increase the movement of joints and mobility, physiotherapy may be especially valuable. In day-to-day management of pain, ℞ **non-narcotic analgesics** of the ℞ **NSAID** group are used extensively. Herbal remedies are available and many can be applied externally to relieve minor muscle aches and pains, and muscle spasms. Musculoskeletal disorders such as ✪ **arthritis** can be treated with a wide range of herbs (including ♣ **agrimony**, ♣ **angelica**, ♣ **arnica**, ♣ **balsam fir**, ♣ **blackcurrant**, ♣ **black horehound**, ♣ **bladderwrack**, ♣ **blue cohosh**, ♣ **black cohosh**, ♣ **boldo**, ♣ **boneset**, ♣ **buckbean**, ♣ **cajuput**, ♣ **cayenne**, ♣ **celery**, ♣ **dandelion**, ♣ **devil's claw**, ♣ **eucalyptus**, ♣ **mistletoe**, ♣ **feverfew**, ♣ **gotu kola**, ♣ **guaiac**, ♣ **guelder rose**, ♣ **horseradish**, ♣ **juniper**, ♣ **larch**, ♣ **laurel**, ♣ **lemon**, ♣ **meadowsweet**, ♣ **northern prickly ash**, ♣ **parsley**, ♣ **peppermint**, ♣ **pokeroot**, ♣ **rosemary**, ♣ **sarsaparilla**, ♣ **southern prickly ash**, ♣ **spiny rest harrow**, ♣ **stinging nettle**, ♣ **wild yam**, ♣ **willow**, ♣ **yucca**). Supplements (including ♒ **boron**, ♒ **chondroitin**, ♒ **copper**, ♒ **glucosamine and chondroitin**, ℞ **niacin**, ♒ **pantothenic acid**, ♒ **omega-3 fatty acid**, ♒ **conjugated linoleic acid**, and ♒ **S-adenosylmethionine**) are useful in some conditions. See individual disorder entries for further details.

myalgic encephalomyelitis

see ✪ chronic fatigue syndrome.

myasthenia gravis

Myasthenia gravis is a rare disorder caused by a reduction in the capacity of the neurotransmitter acetylcholine (one of the chemicals that enable nerve transmission) to effect muscle contractions in certain muscles of the body. It is an ✪ **autoimmune disorder** (caused by the immune system attacking the body's own tissues) and affects women more often than men, in which muscles become fatigued very easily, sometimes to the extent that they are effectively paralyzed. The muscles affected most commonly are those of the face and neck, giving symptoms of drooping, of one or both, upper eyelids (ptosis), blurred or double vision, and mispronounced speech.

Treatment

Treatment is with rest and ℞ **anticholinesterase** drugs, which can alleviate symptoms. In some cases where the disorder is caused by a tumor of the thymus gland, surgical removal of the thymus (a gland in the neck that is part of the immune system) may be beneficial. In extreme cases ℞ **corticosteroid** drugs or plasma exchange treatment are used.

For further information

℞ DIRECTORY OF DRUGS:
anticholinesterase • corticosteroid

mycoses

see ✪ fungal infections.

myocardial infarction

Myocardial infarction—popularly called "heart attack"—is the death of part of the heart muscle following the cessation of its blood supply. The usual cause is coronary thrombosis (a blood clot in one of the arteries supplying the heart muscle) due to ✪ **arteriosclerosis** in the coronary arteries (✪ **coronary artery disease**). The left ventricle is usually the center of infarction, causing sudden severe pain in the chest that may spread to the jaw or left arm, and which is often accompanied by sweating, nausea, or vomiting. The heart-beat may become ragged, and even stop. Emergency hospitalization is required to avoid complications, which can include shock, rupture of the heart muscle, ✪ **heart failure**, ✪ **pulmonary embolism** (a clot that travels to the lung blood vessels, see ✪ **thromboembolism**) or ✪ **heart valve disorders**. However, in many cases recovery, although slow, is complete. Risk factors include smoking, high fat diet, lack of exercise, and being overweight.

Treatment
Early treatment with ℞ **thrombolytic** ("clot-busting") drugs lessens the risk of fatal complications. People require intensive nursing and monitoring, sometimes with resuscitation in cases of cardiac arrest. Later drug treatment or surgery may be required depending on the individual; on the extent of the damage, and the risk of further attacks. Drugs that may play a part in prevention or treatment include: ℞ **antiplatelet** agents (including low-dose ℞ **aspirin**), ℞ **anticoagulants** (for example, oral ℞ **warfarin sodium**, ℞ **dicumarol**; injected ℞ **heparin**), ℞ **lipid-regulating drugs**, and ℞ **antihypertensives** including ℞ **beta-blockers**, ℞ **ACE inhibitors**, and ℞ **calcium-channel blockers**. Red sage and vitamin E are considered by some to have preventive properties. See also ✪ **cardiovascular disorders**, ✪ **heart disease**.

For further information
℞ DIRECTORY OF DRUGS:
ACE inhibitor • anticoagulant (warfarin sodium, dicumarol, heparin) • antihypertensive • antiplatelet • beta-blocker • calcium-channel blocker • lipid-regulating drug • thrombolytic
♣ HERBAL REMEDIES:
red sage
⚕ VITAMINS, MINERALS, AND SUPPLEMENTS:
vitamin E

napkin rash
see ✪ **dermatitis**.

narcolepsy
Narcolepsy is the tendency to fall asleep suddenly at any time during the day, whether convenient or not—while eating, driving, or having sex, for example. Narcolepsy produces bouts of shallow sleep that do not contribute to established circadian fatigue or sleep patterns. Sleep bouts are sometimes preceded by an extraordinarily vivid dream in which the sufferer feels awake but, often, paralysed (called a hypnagogic hallucination). Narcolepsy is occasionally associated with another condition (cataplexy) that causes people to collapse as if fainting, but with no loss of consciousness.

Treatment
There is no cure, but ℞ **CNS stimulant** drugs (including ℞ **modafinil**, ℞ **amphetamine sulfate**, ℞ **dextroamphetamine**, ℞ **ephedrine**, ℞ **methylphenidate**, and pemoline) may be given once the diagnosis—which is often missed—is made, and may counteract some of the symptoms. New drugs that act more specifically are being tested.

For further information
℞ DIRECTORY OF DRUGS:
CNS stimulant

nausea
Nausea is the feeling that one is about to vomit. Depending on the strength of the stimulus, and its interpretation by the brain, ✪ **vomiting** may or may not actually follow. Nausea may be caused by a disgusting sight or smell, or may be a symptom of various disorders. It is most commonly experienced as a result of severe indigestion, of traveling in an unsteady vehicle (✪ **motion sickness**), or of pregnancy (✪ **morning sickness**).

Treatment
The cause of the nausea should be established. Treatment (except morning sickness) is with ℞ **antiemetic** (antisickness) drugs, sometimes called ℞ **antinauseants**. Several herbal remedies (such as ♣ turmeric and ♣ ginger) are reported to relieve nausea, and can be used in the short term but not during pregnancy.

For further information
℞ DIRECTORY OF DRUGS:
antiemetic • antinauseant
♣ HERBAL REMEDIES:
anise • artichoke • ginger • turmeric • wild iris

nephritis
Nephritis is the inflammation of one or both kidneys. It usually centers either on the part of the kidney that filters blood (the glomeruli, thus glomerulonephritis); on the part that differentiates between reusable water and urine (the tubules, thus interstitial nephritis); or on the part that collects the urine for disposal via the ureter (the renal pelvis, thus pyelonephritis). The cause is often obscure, and in some cases may be an allergic reaction to a streptococcal throat infection. Symptoms can include blood or protein in the urine and often edema (fluid accumulation in the tissues).

Treatment
Treatment depends on diagnosis, but if the kidney is seriously incapacitated, dialysis (artificial filtration of the blood, taking over the functions of the kidney) or kidney transplant may be necessary. ℞ **antibacterial** drugs to treat infection may be prescribed.

For further information
℞ DIRECTORY OF DRUGS:
antibacterial

nephrolithiasis
Nephrolithiasis is the presence of one or more ✪ **calculi** (stones) in a kidney, caused by an excess of calcium, uric acid, or magnesium and other salts in the bloodstream. Symptoms are generally caused only when the stone moves from where it was lodged, or when it obstructs the flow within the kidney. There may then be severe pain (renal ✪ **colic**) and ✪ **vomiting**; sometimes blood appears in the urine.

Treatment
Treatment is with ℞ **non-narcotic analgesics** and large volumes of liquids. Ultrasound may be used to shatter the stone so that the

pieces pass out naturally; surgical intervention may be necessary to crush or remove large calculi.

For further information
℞ DIRECTORY OF DRUGS:
non-narcotic analgesic

nephrotic syndrome

Nephrotic syndrome is a disorder of the kidneys that results in severe ✪ **fluid retention** in the tissues (edema). It may be a symptom of various ✪ **kidney disorders**, such as glomerulonephritis (see ✪ **nephritis**). The immediate cause is the filtering off by the kidney of too much protein, channeling it to the urine instead of into the bloodstream. It can be a complication of many systemic diseases such as systemic lupus erythematosus (✪ **lupus**), ✪ **diabetes mellitus**, and multiple myeloma. Diagnosis may be complicated by the fact that some symptoms—such as high blood pressure (hypertension)—are themselves potential root causes. Other symptoms include general malaise and fatigue. The outlook is variable.

Treatment
Treatment depends on the cause, but can include ℞ **corticosteroid** drugs and ℞ **diuretics**.

For further information
℞ DIRECTORY OF DRUGS:
corticosteroid • diuretic

nervous tension

see ✪ anxiety.

neuralgia

Neuralgia is ✪ **pain** originating from a nerve of the peripheral nervous system (those outside the brain and spinal cord), commonly the trigeminal nerve in the face (trigeminal neuralgia). All pain is felt by means of the nerves, but some pains result from disorders of the nerves themselves, as when a nerve is pinched or is damaged through disease or injury. Sometimes the cause may remain unknown. Such pain may be severe and result in distress over long periods.

Treatment
Treatment depends on the nerve affected but may include drugs, herbal remedies or, as a last resort, surgery. Some herbal remedies have traditional uses in relieving nerve-pain.

For further information
℞ DIRECTORY OF DRUGS:
narcotic analgesic • non-narcotic analgesic • others including carbamazepine, phenytoin, imipramine, capsaicin (topical)
♣ HERBAL REMEDIES:
balsam fir • cajuput • hops • Jamaica dogwood • peppermint • St. John's wort

neuropathic pain

see ✪ pain.

nocturnal enuresis

see ✪ bed-wetting.

nonulcer dyspepsia

see ✪ **digestive system disorders**; ✪ **indigestion**.

nosebleed

A nosebleed (called medically epistaxis) is bleeding (✪ **hemorrhage**) from the nose, most commonly caused by injury or by continuous sneezing, and generally the result of the breaking of a minor blood vessel. However, nosebleed can happen spontaneously, especially in children and the elderly (whose blood vessels may be subject to some deterioration), in boys at puberty, and in people with high blood pressure or who have ✪ **bleeding disorder** (for instance thrombocytopenia).

Treatment
Pinching the nostrils together, packing them with gauze, or applying an ice pack to the bridge of the nose may help stem the flow. Cauterizing (destroying by heat) the bleeding vessel is a quick and effective treatment in severe cases. Seek medical advice if bleeding lasts longer than 30 minutes. Some herbal remedies have traditional uses for nosebleed.

For further information
♣ HERBAL REMEDIES:
achyranthes • shepherd's purse • yellow willowherb

obesity

Obesity is a general description for somebody who is very overweight. People are considered medically obese if their weight is 20% more than their maximum healthy weight for their height, build, age, and sex. Such an accumulation of fat in the body usually results simply from eating more food than the body needs to supply its daily energy requirements. Obesity runs in families, and there may be a genetic element, although poor eating habits often begin in childhood. Untreated, obesity may lead to cardiovascular problems, joint disorders, and other serious medical conditions.

Treatment
Reduction of calorie input through carefully controlled dieting is usually the best treatment. In extreme cases, drug treatment or even surgery may be considered.
♣ **bladderwrack** is a traditional herbal remedy, which is thought to help someone trying to lose weight.

For further information
℞ DIRECTORY OF DRUGS:
appetite suppressant
♣ HERBAL REMEDIES:
bladderwrack
⚕ VITAMINS, MINERALS, AND SUPPLEMENTS:
chitosan • chromium

obsessive-compulsive disorder

Obsessive-compulsive disorder is an ✪ **anxiety**-related disorder where uncontrollable thoughts, ideas, and feelings of compulsions or obsessions are severe enough to cause distress or interfere with a person's life. Obsessive thoughts are often accompanied by a compulsive ritual such as handwashing.

Treatment
Psychotherapy and ℞ **antidepressants** drugs are used.

For further information
℞ DIRECTORY OF DRUGS:
antidepressant (**tricyclic** (for example, **clomipramine hydrochloride**) • **SSRI** and related (**citalopram, fluoxetine, fluvoxamine, paroxetine, sertraline**, and **venlafaxine**)

opioid addiction
see ✪ drug dependency.

oral thrush
see ✪ candidiasis.

orchitis
Orchitis is the inflammation of one or both testes (the male sex organs inside the scrotum that produce sperm). It is often caused by general ✪ **viral** or ✪ **bacterial infection**; as, for example, with ✪ **mumps**, ✪ **tuberculosis**, and ✪ **syphilis**. Symptoms are local swelling and pain; there may also be nausea. Orchitis affecting both testes and caused by mumps may lead to sterility.

Treatment
Treatment is with painkillers and sometimes ℞ **corticosteroids**, and by support of the scrotum, together with treatment of any other contributory infection.

For further information
℞ DIRECTORY OF DRUGS:
antibacterial • antiviral • corticosteroid • non-narcotic analgesic

osteoarthritis
Osteoarthritis is the degeneration of the cartilaginous layer over the bones at a joint, which leads to friction and deformity of the actual bone surfaces. It is a ✪ **musculoskeletal disorder** that is more common in women than in men. There are several disorders that may cause such degeneration—including ✪ **obesity**—but injury and long-term stress at the joint (for instance in athletes and ballet dancers) may have the same effect. In addition, old age may retard the normal processes of healing. Main symptoms are local ✪ **pain** and loss of mobility; the joint may become visibly deformed. See also ✪ **arthritis**.

Treatment
Treatment of the symptoms is with analgesic and anti-inflammatory drugs (NSAIDs such as ℞ **aspirin** or ℞ **ibuprofen**), and rest. Reducing the load on the joint by weight loss or a walking stick may help in the long-term. Surgery may be necessary if simple measures do not succeed, and may include replacement of the affected joint with an artificial substitute, or locally acting ℞ **corticosteroid** injections. Several herbal remedies and supplements are considered to relieve some of the symptoms of arthritis.

For further information
℞ DIRECTORY OF DRUGS:
antirheumatic • corticosteroid • NSAID
♣ HERBAL REMEDIES:
agrimony • angelica • black horehound • blackcurrant • boneset • cayenne • celery • devil's claw • feverfew • guelder rose • juniper • parsley • willow • yucca

⚕⚕ VITAMINS, MINERALS, AND SUPPLEMENTS:
boron • chondroitin • conjugated linoleic acid • copper • glucosamine and chondroitin • niacin • omega-3 fatty acid • pantothenic acid • S-adenosylmethionine

osteomalacia
see ✪ rickets.

osteomyelitis
Osteomyelitis is an infection (normally a ✪ **bacterial infection**) of bone and bone marrow. It is seen more frequently in children, often in the long bones of the legs, arms, and vertebrae and is characterized by pain and other signs of infection. Diagnosis is by X-ray and blood cultures. With better hygiene and resistance to infection, the disease is now much less common in Western countries, but if left untreated it develops into bone fractures and deformity, and requires surgery.

Treatment
Acute osteomyelitis is treated with high dosage ℞ **antibacterial** antibiotics.

For further information
℞ DIRECTORY OF DRUGS:
antibacterial

osteoporosis
Osteoporosis is the degeneration of bone caused by the loss of both calcium salts and other structural elements. It is sometimes referred to as "brittle bones." To some extent part of the normal ✪ **aging** process, the condition may also result from injury, infection, hormonal imbalance, or prolonged treatment with corticosteroids. Women become much more liable to osteoporosis after the ✪ **menopause**. Symptoms are pain, a tendency toward fractures, and shrinking of the body stature (through shortening of the spine).

Treatment
Treatment depends on the cause but may include ℞ **calcium-metabolism modifier** drugs and rarely ℞ **anabolic steroids** to reduce further bone loss. Preventive measures include a diet with sufficient calcium and ⚕⚕ **vitamin D**, or supplements, and exercise from an early age to build up bone mass. In women, hormone replacement therapy (HRT), which is taken to alleviate menopausal symptoms also reduces the risk of osteoporosis.

For further information
℞ DIRECTORY OF DRUGS:
anabolic steroid • calcium-metabolism modifier • hormone replacement
⚕⚕ VITAMINS, MINERALS, AND SUPPLEMENTS:
boron • calcium • copper • isoflavone • magnesium • manganese • vitamin D • vitamin K

otitis
Otitis is an inflammation of the ear (otitis externa/media/interna is inflammation of the outer/middle/inner ear; inflammation of the inner ear is also called labyrinthitis). Symptoms of the three forms differ, although the cause in every case is a bacterial, viral, or fungal

✚ **infection**. Otitis externa usually takes the form of a local infection of the skin surface, and there may be itching and earache, with a possible discharge. Otitis media is often spread from infection of the mouth, throat, sinuses, or bronchial tubes, and causes severe pain, high temperature, and temporary ✚ **deafness**; occasionally the eardrum ruptures, releasing pus. Repeated infections in children can lead to ✚ **glue ear**. Otitis interna is a serious condition with symptoms including pain, vomiting, deafness, and constant vertigo, which may undermine the person's sense of reality.

Treatment
In otitis externa, dressings and ℞ **antibacterial** and other ℞ **anti-infective** eardrops generally eliminate the problem. Treatment of otitis media is aimed at alleviating the symptoms but may include anti-infective drugs or surgical drainage of accumulated fluid. Otitis interna requires specialist treatment that may last for several months.

For further information
℞ DIRECTORY OF DRUGS:
antibacterial • antifungal • antiviral

otitis externa
see ✚ **otitis**.

otitis interna
see ✚ **otitis**.

otitis media
see ✚ **otitis**.

ovarian cancer
see ✚ **cancer**.

overweight
see ✚ **obesity**.

Paget's disease (of the bone)
Paget's disease (bone) is a disorder of bone that occurs in old age involving thickening and disorganization of bone structure, especially in the skull, long bones of the limbs, spine, and pelvis. The medical name is osteitis deformans. There may be no symptoms, or the changes may cause pain or deformity; where the skull is affected the senses of sight and hearing may be impaired.

Treatment
Treatment is with ℞ **calcium-metabolism modifier** drugs to halt bone damage.

For further information
℞ DIRECTORY OF DRUGS:
calcium-metabolism modifier

Paget's disease (of the nipple)
Paget's disease (nipple) is ulceration and irritation around the nipple, representing the outward sign of an underlying form of ✚ **breast cancer**. It is also called nipple cancer.

Treatment
Treatment is usually by surgery, sometimes radiotherapy, and, in extensive cases, ℞ **anticancer** chemotherapy.

For further information
℞ DIRECTORY OF DRUGS:
anticancer

pain
Pain is a subjective sensation that tends to be localized and can vary over a scale of severity from mild discomfort through to unbearable. Though pain tends to be perceived as a disease or disorder, it is principally a symptom that warns the body of trauma, has the effect of immobilizing damaged parts of the body, and encourages the person to seek help. It is a characteristic symptom of many disorders ranging from indigestion to heart attacks. How serious the pain is perceived to be depends remarkably on circumstances, so on the battlefield the soldier may not in the short-run even be aware of serious physical damage, whereas an anxious individual in quite normal surroundings may believe the pain of a minor abrasion to indicate a serious injury. The subjective processing of pain in the nervous system depends greatly on experience and expectation, and for this reason pain clinics and other services can help the individual prepare for pain (as in pregnancy) or deal with excruciating pain (as in advanced cancer). Different descriptions of pain include earache (ear pain), mastalgia (breast pain), teething pain (pain when babies cut new teeth), dysuria (pain on urination), ✚ **dysmenorrhea** (pain on menstruation), and post-operative pain (pain following surgical operations).

Treatment
There are various types of pain, often described as throbbing, aching, dull, sharp, burning, searing, gripping, colicky, and so on. To some extent, this helps the physician diagnose a cause and treatment. In all cases the primary course is to try and deal with the cause of the pain. Thus a colicky pain might suggest intestinal discomfort that can be relieved with ℞ **antispasmodic** drugs and warmth. When there is clearly an inflammatory component to the origin of the pain, then ℞ **anti-inflammatory** drugs of various types are available. Pain-killing drugs (℞ **analgesics**) are indicated to help the individual deal with the pain while the condition rights itself or is treated. The physician has to make a choice as to whether it is necessary to prescribe ℞ **narcotic analgesics** (available only on prescription), which have quite serious side effects and run a risk of leading to drug-dependency, or to use ℞ **non-narcotic analgesics**, which generally have less disadvantages and may actually work better where there is an inflammatory component to the origin of the pain, for instance arthritis and rheumatic pain (most are of the ℞ **NSAID** class). The OTC analgesic ℞ **acetaminophen** does not have appreciable anti-inflammatory activity, but is safe except in overdose, and has very useful ℞ **antipyretic** activity, so deals with the fever as well as the discomfort of the common cold and similar ailments.

Some types of serious pain, such as ✚ **neuralgia** (especially trigeminal neuralgia), are paradoxical in origin and often do not respond to analgesics, so specialist drugs of other types are tried (for example, ℞ **carbamazepine**, ℞ **phenytoin**, ℞ **imipramine**, and topical

℞ **capsaicin**). Short-lasting potentially severe pain, for instance sutures and dental extraction, can be minimized through injection, near the site, of local anesthetics, or certain ℞ **benzodiazepines** given intravenously. For more involved procedures, general anesthetics can be used. A variety of herbal remedies and OTC medicines can be tried to alleviate different types of pain, although it should always be remembered that pain is a symptom ond overuse of painkillers (herbal or otherwise) may mask the progression of an underlying serious disorder. See individual disorder entries.

For further information

℞ DIRECTORY OF DRUGS:

antimigraine • benzodiazepine (for example, **midazolam**) • general anesthetic • local anesthetic • narcotic analgesic • non-narcotic analgesic • others including **carbamazepine, phenytoin, imipramine,** and **capsaicin** (topical)

♣ HERBAL REMEDIES:

boneset • cajuput • cayenne • clove • corydalis • feverfew • Japanese mint • lactucarium • meadowsweet • parsley • passionflower • St. John's wort • wild lettuce • wild yam • willow

♠♠ VITAMINS, MINERALS, AND SUPPLEMENTS:

glucosamine and chondroitin • pantothenic acid

pancreatic cancer

see ✪ cancer.

pancreatitis

Pancreatitis is an acute or chronic ✪ **inflammation** of the pancreas (the enzyme- and insulin-producing gland lying at the back of the abdominal cavity). Symptoms of the acute condition are severe pain in the upper abdomen, shock, ✪ **vomiting**, and high temperature. The cause may be an injury but often remains unknown, although it is associated with ✪ **alcoholism** and ✪ **gallstones.** Complications include cyst formation. It may recur. It is commonly due to long-term alcohol abuse, though there are other causes. Chronic pancreatitis may be symptomless or may cause similar but less severe symptoms; however, it leads on to pancreatic failure, which causes ✪ **diabetes mellitus** due to lack of insulin and malabsorption of foods. Certain drugs can cause pancreatitis as a side effect; these include ℞ **immunosuppressants** and (thiazide) ℞ **diuretics.**

Treatment

Diagnosis and treatment of acute pancreatitis demand urgent hospitalization. The person must have no food or drink by mouth and requires intravenous feeding. The pain may be severe and require ℞ **narcotic analgesics.** The diabetes mellitus following from chronic pancreatitis requires treatment with **insulin,** and ℞ **digestive enzyme** supplements (℞ **pancrelipase**) are given to correct the malabsorption; a low-fat diet will also have to be followed. No alcohol must be taken.

For further information

℞ DIRECTORY OF DRUGS:

insulin analog • digestive enzyme (pancreatin) • narcotic analgesic

panic attack disorder

see ✪ anxiety.

panic disorder

see ✪ anxiety; ✪ affective disorders.

paranoid illness

see ✪ psychotic disorders.

paranoid schizophrenia

see ✪ schizophrenia.

paratyphoid

see ✪ typhoid fever.

Parkinson's disease

Parkinson's disease is a disorder that affects the basal ganglia of the brain (involved with controlling movements), producing distressing physical symptoms. There is a deficiency in the neurotransmitter dopamine, which acts with acetylcholine, another neurotransmitter, to fine-tune muscle control. In Parkinson's disease, there are changes in these two neurotransmitters. Symptoms include tremors in the limbs (particularly when at rest), lack of facial expression, a monotonous voice, increasingly stooped posture, and a shuffling gait. The disease most commonly affects middle-aged or elderly people. The cause of the degeneration in the brain in Parkinson's disease is not known, although similar symptoms are seen in a syndrome (parkinsonism; parkinsonian extrapyramidal side effects) that may be provoked by certain drugs especially ℞ **antipsychotic** drugs, by carbon monoxide ✪ **poisoning**, metal poisoning (manganese), chemical poisoning (notably MPTP, a neurotoxin found as an impurity in certain "street" drugs), by cerebrovascular disease, damage to the CNS, or ✪ **encephalitis.**

Treatment

There is no cure, although symptoms may be relieved to some extent by various ℞ **antiparkinsonian** drugs, some of which (such as ℞ **levodopa**) enhance or mimic the effects of dopamine in the brain. Others (℞ **anticholinergics**) decrease the affects of acetylcholine. ℞ **Amantadine** is used in some situations. Physiotherapy may help, and surgery may be carried out in some cases to reduce tremor. Several supplements are promoted for their claimed benefits in Parkinson's disease.

For further information

℞ DIRECTORY OF DRUGS:

amantadine • anticholinergic • antiparkinsonian

♠♠ VITAMINS, MINERALS, AND SUPPLEMENTS:

antioxidant • coenzyme Q_{10} • octacosanol

parrot fever

see ✪ psittacosis.

pattern baldness

see ✪ alopecia.

Key to symbols: ✪ = Disorder Section ℞ = Drug Section ♣ = Herbal Section ♠♠ = Supplement Section

pellagra

Pellagra is a deficiency disease caused by a lack of vitamin B$_3$, niacin (nicotinic acid) or the amino acid tryptophan, from which niacin can be synthesized in the body. It can also occur as a result of a metabolic defect that interferes with the conversion of tryptophan to niacin. The condition may occur with ✪ **cirrhosis** of the liver (perhaps through ✪ **alcoholism**), with a severe gastric disorder, or where maize (corn), which is deficient in tryptophan, forms the staple diet. Symptoms are serious: ✪ **nausea,** ✪ **vomiting,** a sore mouth and red tongue, scaly discoloration of the skin on the neck, chest, and hands, and ✪ **depression.**

Treatment

Treatment is with vitamin supplements. ℞ **niacin** may be used in other forms including ℞ **niacinamide.**

For further information

℞ DIRECTORY OF DRUGS:
niacin

♋ VITAMINS, MINERALS, AND SUPPLEMENTS:
amino acid (tryptophan) • **niacin**

pelvic inflammatory disease

Pelvic inflammatory disease (PID) is a term that covers any inflammatory condition of the female pelvic organs (the reproductive organs). It is a common cause of pain in the pelvic region and usually results from bacterial infection, usually a ✪ **sexually transmitted disease** such as ✪ **gonorrhea,** ✪ **chlamydia,** or after abortion or childbirth. It can lead to ✪ **infertility** due to damage to the Fallopian tubes. Other symptoms may include fever, abnormal vaginal discharge, menstrual problems, and pain during sexual intercourse.

Treatment

Treatment is to treat the infection usually with ℞ **antibacterials** of an unusually wide range (because of the varied causes of the condition), also painkillers (℞ **NSAIDs**).

For further information

℞ DIRECTORY OF DRUGS:
aminoglycoside (for example, **gentamicin**) • **antibacterial** including **penicillin** (for example, **ampicillin, piperacillin, ticarcillin**) • **azole** (**metronidazole**) • **cephalosporin** (for example, **cefotetan, cefoxitin, ceftriaxone**) • **clindamycin** • **NSAID** • **quinolone** and related (for example, **ofloxacin**) • **tetracycline** (for example, **doxycycline**)

peptic ulcer

A peptic ulcer is an area of erosion in the lining (mucosa) of the stomach (gastric ulcer), in the first part of the duodenum (duodenal ulcer), the jejunum (jejunal ulcer) or, rarely, in the esophagus (esophageal ulcer). The immediate cause is the action of the combination of pepsin and hydrochloric acid, which are present naturally in gastric juices, either in concentration or upon a particularly weak spot in the lining. What might cause such concentration or weakness—and the observed relationship with ✪ **anxiety** or other forms of stress—is not fully understood, although aspirin, NSAIDs, and corticosteroids may predispose to the erosion. Duodenal and gastric ulcers have also been strongly linked with the presence of a bacterium called *Helicobacter pylori.* The main symptom is ✪ **pain,** sometimes linked to eating, especially after consuming alcohol, aspirin, and certain foods, or sometimes provoked by hunger. There may also be nausea and vomiting. Complications include bleeding, obstruction, and perforation, the last being a medical emergency.

Treatment

Symptoms may be relieved by ℞ **antacids** (for example, magaldrate) and by ℞ **anticholinergic** drugs. Various drugs are used to promote ulcer-healing (℞ **bismuth subsalicylate,** ℞ **sucralfate**), and where *H. pylori* infection is suspected, combination therapy with ℞ **antibacterials** is used. Many herbal remedies are considered to be effective in the treatment of peptic ulcer. Sometimes prostaglandin treatment may help healing. Occasionally surgery may be required, and is vital to treat severe complications such as hemorrhaging or perforation (rupture).

For further information

℞ DIRECTORY OF DRUGS:
antacid (for example, **magaldrate**) • **anticholinergic** (for example, **glycopyrrolate, propantheline bromide**) • **ulcer-healing drug** including **H$_2$-antagonist** (for example, **cimetidine, famotidine, nizatidine, ranitidine hydrochloride, bismuth subsalicylate, sucralfate**) • **Helicobacter pylori eradication regime** • **prostaglandin** (**misoprostol**) • **proton-pump inhibitor** (for example, **lansoprazole, omeprazole, pantoprazole sodium, rabeprazole sodium**)

♣ HERBAL REMEDIES:
licorice • **marshmallow** • **meadowsweet** • **slippery elm**

perennial allergic rhinitis

see ✪ **rhinitis.**

performance anxiety

see ✪ **anxiety.**

perimenopause

see ✪ **menopause.**

periodontitis

Periodontitis is an inflammation of the tissues that attach the teeth to the jaw (the periodontal tissues)—not just of the gums (✪ **gingivitis**), but also of the membranous ligament around the roots and the hard material that cements the roots in their sockets. It usually stems from plaque deposits on teeth due to poor oral hygiene; however, some people are predisposed to it. Chronic periodontitis causes gaps between gums and teeth, and loss of some fibrous and bony material that would otherwise support the teeth; often there is tooth loss. The condition is common in older people.

Treatment

Cleaning of the teeth by a dentist may help prevent progression in the early stages, and ℞ **antiseptic** mouthwashes may be effective. Later, more complicated dental procedures may be needed.

For further information

℞ DIRECTORY OF DRUGS:
antiseptic

♋ VITAMINS, MINERALS, AND SUPPLEMENTS:
coenzyme Q_{10}

period pain

see ✪ **dysmenorrhea.**

peripheral vascular disorders

Peripheral vascular disorders are conditions where there is dysfunction of the peripheral blood vessels that carry blood from the heart to the tissues and back.

Some of these diseases are life threatening and acute, including aortic aneurysm, which is a weakening and enlargement (and sometimes rupture) of a section of the wall of the main artery—the aorta—carrying blood from the heart to the lower body.

✪ **thrombosis** is the formation of a blood clot (known as a thrombus) in a blood vessel, blocking blood supply to part of the body. It is fairly common for the thrombus to form within the large veins of the leg—when it is called ✪ **deep vein thrombosis.** Thrombosis is similar in symptoms and effect to embolism, where a plug of any sort of material—known as an embolus—travels through the bloodstream until it becomes stuck in a blood vessel, usually an artery. Diabetic vascular disease is a complication of long-standing ✪ **diabetes mellitus,** causing damage to both small and large blood vessels throughout the peripheral blood circulation. If there is inadequate blood supply to an area, tissue death (✪ **gangrene)** develops. ✪ **varicose veins** appear when the valves of the veins, usually superficial veins of the leg, fail to allow blood to return to the heart and become swollen and distorted. Buerger's disease is a rare inflammatory (probably autoimmune) condition found in peripheral blood vessels, which is largely confined to men who smoke. Raynaud's phenomenon is a narrowing of the small arteries of the hands or feet seen in attacks, and accompanied by a tingling feeling and blanching of the skin. This phenomenon can be caused by a number of underlying complaints, including Buerger's disease and a number of autoimmune conditions. When the underlying cause is not clear, the condition is often referred to as ✪ **Raynaud's disease.** ✪ **thrombophlebitis** is inflammation in a vein and may cause a blood clot to lodge, causing damage. The compound condition ✪ **hypertension,** which also involves peripheral blood vessels, is discussed in a separate article.

Treatment

A wide variety of treatments are used to deal with this range of disorders. A number may require surgical intervention (aortic aneurysm, embolism, deep vein thrombosis, thrombophlebitis, varicose veins). In several cases, drugs that thin the blood (℞ **anticoagulant** and ℞ **antiplatelet** drugs) may have beneficial effects on the outcome of the condition. Raynaud's disease is often treated with ℞ **vasodilator** drugs. A number of natural and herbal remedies are thought to have beneficial effects on the circulation, some by having anticoagulant properties, others by topical rubefacient properties. Varicose veins are sometimes treated with ℞ **sclerosing agents.** Herbal remedies that may be useful, by promoting circulation or other effects, include ♣ **angelica,** ♣ **cayenne,** ♣ **gotu kola,** ♣ **cinnamon,** ♋ **garlic,** ♣ **hawthorn,** and ♣ **rosemary,** and

for Raynauld's disease, the vitamin ℞ **niacin** and the herbal remedy ♣ **ginkgo.**

peritonitis

Peritonitis is the ✪ **inflammation** of the peritoneum (the membranes lining the abdominal cavity and surrounding the organs of the abdomen), which may be due to infection spread from elsewhere in the body via the bloodstream (primary peritonitis) or to perforation (rupture) of an abdominal organ, such as may occur in peptic ulcer or with an inflamed appendix (secondary peritonitis). In both cases symptoms are abdominal pain and fever with, in the case of primary peritonitis, weight loss and fluid accumulation in the abdomen. In the case of secondary peritonitis, contamination by digestive juices or bacteria causes sudden, severe pain and shock.

Treatment

In primary peritonitis treatment is sometimes possible with ℞ **antibacterial** drugs, mainly ℞ **antibiotics,** and intravenous fluids, along with treatment of the cause; for instance, repair of perforated peptic ulcer. In secondary peritonitis surgery to repair the perforation is usually urgently required.

For further information

℞ DIRECTORY OF DRUGS:
antibacterial

pernicious anemia

Pernicious anemia is a deficiency disorder caused by the body's failure to absorb vitamin B_{12} (cyanocobalamin) or, rarely, through lack of the vitamin in the diet. Normally, an "intrinsic factor" secreted by the stomach catalyzes the absorption of vitamin B_{12}. If the factor is absent, as for instance in ✪ **autoimmune disease** where antibodies are produced that damage the stomach lining and prevent intrinsic factor being formed, the result is the onset of megaloblastic anemia, where large abnormal red blood cells (megaloblasts) are produced—with further symptoms of lassitude, difficulties in the sense of balance, and a sore tongue. In severe cases neurological symptoms may also occur. See also ✪ **anemia.**

Treatment

Treatment is by vitamin B_{12} injections (as ♋ **cyanocobalamin** or ℞ **hydroxocobalamin**), which may need to be continued for life in the case of intrinsic factor deficiency.

For further information

℞ DIRECTORY OF DRUGS:
cyanocobalamin • hydroxocobalamin
♋ VITAMINS, MINERALS, AND SUPPLEMENTS:
vitamin B_{12}

pernio

see ✪ **chilblain.**

pertussis

Pertussis (also called whooping cough) is a highly infective potentially serious ✪ **bacterial infection** of the membranous lining of the throat and bronchial passages, most common in young children. Symptoms appear in two stages: first there are the catarrhal symptoms of a heavy cold in which the dry, breathless cough with a high-pitched "whoop" when the infected person inhales, for which the disease is named, becomes more pronounced; then there are paroxysms of coughing, possibly with bleeding from the nose and mouth, which is caused by coughing and subsequently breaking blood vessels, and vomiting. Complications such as ✪ **pneumonia** may arise from this stage. Eventually the paroxysms subside and the symptoms gradually vanish, but full recovery may take several months.

Treatment

Drug treatment with ℞ **antibacterials** during the first stage may prevent the onset of the second; treatment otherwise is isolation and drugs to alleviate the symptoms. Vaccination is available, and is commonly administered (with ℞ **vaccines** against diphtheria and tetanus in the combined DTP vaccine) in three stages to infants in their first year of life. Several herbal remedies have traditional uses in pertussis.

For further information

℞ DIRECTORY OF DRUGS:
antibacterial • vaccine

♣ HERBAL REMEDIES:
horehound • red clover • senega snakeroot • squill • thyme

petit mal

see ✪ epilepsy.

pharyngitis

Pharyngitis is the ✪ **inflammation** of the pharynx (the region of the throat connecting the mouth and nose with the esophagus and airway). It involves a sore throat and difficulty or pain in swallowing. A common disorder, often associated with ✪ **tonsillitis**, the common ✪ **cold**, or other infections of the throat, mouth, or nose, it may also follow heavy cigarette smoking or alcohol consumption.

Treatment

Those affected should drink plenty of fluids and avoid cold or smoky atmospheres. Other treatment depends on the cause, if determined, and may include ℞ **antibacterials** if ✪ **bacterial infection** is suspected. Many herbal remedies have uses in mainly relieving symptoms of mouth and throat inflammation.

For further information

℞ DIRECTORY OF DRUGS:
antibacterial

♣ HERBAL REMEDIES:
agrimony • anise • bilberry • blackberry • blackcurrant • cardamom • chamomile, German • clove • coffee • echinacea • Iceland moss • jambul • Japanese mint • larch • maidenhair fern • mallow • marigold • marshmallow • myrrh • oak • onion • potentilla • radish • rhatany • rose • sage • senega snakeroot • southern bayberry • tormentil • weeping forsythia • white dead nettle • witch hazel • wood sage

phenylketonuria

Phenylketonuria (PKU) is an inherited condition characterized by the presence of phenylketone and other metabolites in the urine. It is due to an inborn error of metabolism (a ✪ **metabolic disor**der), which causes a deficiency of the enzyme phenylalanine hydroxylase. This enzyme metabolizes the natural amino acid phenylalanine to tyrosine. Phenylalanine is a constituent of protein in many foodstuffs. Accumulation of phenylalanine causes damage to the brain. It is relatively rare (about one case in 16,000 births) but screening tests are routinely carried out in newborns.

Treatment

The condition is characterized by severe mental handicap and other physical changes unless the diet of affected infants is switched to special foods free of this amino acid.

pheochromocytoma

Pheochromocytoma is an uncommon tumor of the adrenal medulla (core of the adrenal gland), which causes an excess secretion of epinephrine and norepinephrine. It can sometimes occur at other sites including the brain. Only a small proportion of pheochromocytoma become cancerous. Symptoms include ✪ **hypertension**, palpitations, ✪ **headache**, sweating, ✪ **nausea**, ✪ **vomiting**, nervousness, hyperglycemia and fainting, and heart symptoms such as palpitations and rapid pulse.

Treatment

In some cases the tumor can be surgically removed. Drugs such as ℞ **antihypertensives** and others can be taken to control the symptoms caused by an excess of norepinephrine and epinephrine.

For further information

℞ DIRECTORY OF DRUGS:
alpha-adrenoceptor blocker (for example, **phenoxybenzamine, phentolamine mesylate, prazosin hydrochloride**) • antihypertensive • antisympathetic • beta-blocker (for example, **propranolol hydrochloride**) • metyrosine

phlebitis

Phlebitis is the inflammation of the tubular wall of a vein. It occurs most often in the legs in association with ✪ **varicose veins**. Other causes include damage to the vein wall (for instance irritation due to an intravenous catheter), infection, ✪ **autoimmune disorder** (in which the immune system attacks the body's own tissues), or even ✪ **cancer** elsewhere in the body. Symptoms are pain, tenderness, and local redness in the skin. Clotting of the blood at the site (thrombophlebitis) may follow.

Treatment

Treatment is with elasticated support of the area, and anti-inflammatory (℞ **NSAID**) analgesics. If hypercoagulability of blood is a factor, ℞ **anticoagulant** drugs to prevent blood clotting may be taken.

For further information

℞ DIRECTORY OF DRUGS:
anticoagulant • NSAID • thrombolytic

PID

see ✪ pelvic inflammatory disease.

piles

see ✪ hemorrhoids.

pink eye

see ✪ **conjunctivitis**.

pin worms

see ✪ **worms**.

pituitary gland disorders and tumors

Pituitary gland disorders and tumors are an important group of complaints. Pituitary tumors are abnormal growths in the pituitary gland (located near the base of the brain). The pituitary gland is divided into an anterior and posterior part, each of which secretes different sorts of hormones. Tumors are relatively rare, and symptoms depend on the type of tumor. Some tumors cause excessive amounts of hormone to be released; others do not themselves release hormone but disrupt the function of parts of the pituitary gland. Examples of anterior pituitary tumors include those that cause an increase in the level of the hormone prolactin (see ✪ **prolactinoma**). Others cause ✪ **acromegaly** (overproduction of growth hormone, somatotropin), or ✪ **Cushing's syndrome**. Pressure on adjacent areas of the brain may cause changes in the field of vision, ✪ **headaches** or decreased pituitary function. Tumors that cause the release of posterior pituitary hormones (oxytocin and vasopressin) are less common, though a tumor that presses on the posterior pituitary may cause ✪ **diabetes insipidus**. In some pituitary disorders, the effects are seen on other glands, for instance the adrenal cortex, thyroid or sex glands.

Treatment

Sometimes involves surgical removal of the tumor or radiotherapy. Drugs to control symptoms include agents of the ℞ **dopamine-receptor stimulant** and somatostatin analog types, both of which mimic the actions of important endogenous release-inhibiting factors.

For further information

℞ DIRECTORY OF DRUGS:
dopamine-receptor stimulant • hypothalamic hormone (octreotide)

pityriasis capitis

see ✪ **dandruff**.

pityriasis rosea

Pityriasis rosea is a common, mild, generalized ✪ **skin condition** characterized by round or oval scaly-edged dark pink spots, affecting the upper arms and trunk. It is not known how it is caused and is not infectious, but may be associated with a ✪ **viral infection**. The diffuse rash is preceded by a round spot on the trunk.

Treatment

There may be itching; drugs to relieve this can be applied locally.

For further information

℞ DIRECTORY OF DRUGS:
antihistamine • antipruritic
♣ HERBAL REMEDIES:
see ✪ **skin conditions**

plantar wart

see ✪ **wart**.

pleurisy

Pleurisy is the inflammation of the pleura (the membranes around the lungs). It is usually caused by ✪ **infection** (such as ✪ **pneumonia**) but can be due to structural damage (such as injury or cancer). Symptoms are pain and shallow breathing. The fluid between the pleural layers loses consistency, and the resultant friction between the layers causes a characteristic "pleural rub" heard through a stethoscope.

Treatment

Treatment corresponds to the cause, but commonly includes pain-killing drugs (℞ **non-narcotic analgesic** and sometimes ℞ **narcotic analgesic**) and ℞ **antibacterial** antibiotics.

For further information

℞ DIRECTORY OF DRUGS:
antibacterial • narcotic analgesic • non-narcotic analgesic
♣ HERBAL REMEDIES:
angelica • pleurisy root

pneumonia

Pneumonia is inflammation of one or more lobes of the lung. The most common cause is ✪ **bacterial infection** (often *Streptococcus pneumoniae*)—although viral, fungal, and protozoan forms occur—and the primary effect is to clog the alveoli (air sacs) with pus so that no exchange of gases takes place and the lung becomes solid. Symptoms depend on how far the infection spreads. Lobar pneumonia affects one or more lobes of a lung; bronchopneumonia affects also the bronchioles (smaller airways) and the bronchi (major airways). Depending on the cause of the pneumonia, the person may suffer chest pain, high temperature, and rapid heartbeat. They may also cough up thick (often reddish) sputum, though in some cases (for instance viral pneumonia), symptoms may be less specific, and develop more slowly. ✪ **pleurisy** may occur, and the individual may become confused (especially the elderly).

Treatment

Treatment depends on identification of the infective organism, but generally includes drugs to treat the infection, and therapies to assist breathing.

For further information

℞ DIRECTORY OF DRUGS:
antibacterial • antifungal

poisoning

Poisoning can have many causes including accidental ingestion of chemicals, pesticides, weed-killers, industrial and environmental chemicals, food poisoning, insect and other animal stings and bites, toxic plants, and drug or herbal remedy overdose. Poisoning is responsible for a very considerable number of medical cases annually and its treatment presents a considerable technical challenge. Identification of the likely cause is generally the first step, and in emergency treatment of oral ingestion as the cause of the poisoning, a decision needs to be taken as to whether to induce vomiting. This is not done where the substance is caustic or corrosive, or where there is a risk of blocking the airways, for instance where breathing is depressed (as is the case with some drugs of abuse). When the poisoned individual is hospitalized, it may be possible to run chemical tests to identify the poison.

Treatment

Immediate medical advice is essential, for example from a specialist poisons unit. In some instances there are available specific ℞ **antidotes**, which are used to counteract poisons or overdose with other drugs. They can work in many ways. Where the poison works by stimulating, or over-stimulating, a distinct pharmacological receptor, an appropriate receptor antagonist can be used to reduce or completely block the effects of the poison; for instance naloxone hydrochloride is an ℞ **opioid antagonist** used for an overdose of a ℞ **narcotic analgesic** drug, such as morphine sulfate (or illicit heroin), and being quick-acting, it effectively reverses the respiratory depression and other symptoms of such an overdose. There are similar antagonists, used as antidotes, including the benzodiazepine antagonist ℞ **flumazenil** to counteract the effects of ℞ **benzodiazepine** drugs when taken in deliberate or accidental overdose, and similarly ℞ **anticholinergic** drugs (for example, atropine sulfate) are used to counteract the effects of ℞ **parasympathomimetic** drugs (for example, ℞ **anticholinesterase** insecticides).

Poisoning by some chemicals is best counteracted by using an antidote that binds to the poison, rendering it relatively inert and facilitating its excretion from the body. For example, a ℞ **chelating agent** is used as an antidote to toxic metal poisoning because it chemically binds to certain metallic ions and other substances (including arsenic, gold, mercury, lead, plutonium, uranium, and thorium).

To treat overdose poisoning by the ℞ **non-narcotic analgesic** drug ℞ **acetaminophen**, use can be made of ℞ **acetylcysteine** in treatment immediately after overdose, when the antidote works by chemically preventing the production of toxic products by the liver after poisoning with by excessive amounts of the analgesic.

Some of the serious effects of poisoning by drugs or chemicals that in themselves are not very toxic, but are metabolized in the body to toxic products, can be avoided by slowing down this metabolism. The very serious effects of methanol (methyl alcohol; wood alcohol—a contaminant of illicit spirits, and an additive to methylated spirits) are due to its metabolism in the body to the much more active chemical, formic acid, which kills nerve cells and the optic nerve, so blinding its victims. If ethanol (ordinary alcohol) is given acutely for a period in quite high quantities, it slows the metabolism of methanol and can protect against damage. A similar principle applies for use of fomepizole, a recently introduced drug, which is used to treat poisoning by ethylene glycol (antifreeze).

For use in the emergency treatment of cyanide poisoning, a combination of ℞ **sodium thiosalicylate** and sodium nitrite can be used, because the latter chemicals change the form of the blood pigment hemoglobin to one that is not affected by cyanide.

An ℞ **antivenin** is an antidote to the poison in a snakebite, a scorpion's sting, or a bite from any other poisonous creature (such as a spider), and is injected into the bloodstream for immediate relief.

The above examples are more-or-less specific remedies, but these are only available for a few of the many poisons that may affect the individual. In most of the remaining cases supportive therapy is appropriate, including ℞ **electrolyte** perfusion, warmth, maintenance of blood pressure, and other measures. Where respiration is severely depressed, ℞ **respiratory stimulant** drugs (analeptics; for instance doxapram) may be used. For many poisons an ℞ **adsorbent** chemical agent may be used, which binds other chemicals to their surfaces, so reducing the activity of the latter (for instance activated charcoal and kaolin).

poliomyelitis

Poliomyelitis (also called polio) is an infectious disease of the central nervous system caused by any of three polio viruses. Most common in hot climates, it particularly affects residents in areas of poor sanitation. Initial symptoms are high temperature, sore throat, and headaches, with gastric upset. Most people recover with no further problems; others, however, go on to experience muscle stiffness, and some then proceed to weakness and paralysis of one or more muscles, which may be permanent (hence the alternative name of the disease: infantile paralysis). It is a ✪ **viral infection**.

Treatment

There is no treatment other than drugs to relieve the symptoms including pain; modern oral or injected ℞ **vaccines** provide good protection.

For further information

℞ DIRECTORY OF DRUGS:

vaccine

polycystic ovary syndrome

Polycystic ovary syndrome is a disorder of the endocrine system where the ovaries develop numbers of fluid-filled cysts, and there is a failure of ovulation, amenorrhea, ✪ **infertility**, and sometimes growth of hair (hirsutism). It is a common disorder in women of reproductive age and sometimes runs in families. There is usually an imbalance in the secretion of sex hormones, including increased levels of testosterone and luteinizing hormone (LH), and decreased levels of follicle-stimulating hormones (FSH). This results from a major imbalance in the hypothalamic-pituitary gland-ovarian axis. Women affected may become resistant to the hormone insulin and develop ✪ **diabetes mellitus**. They are also more susceptible to a number of ✪ **cardiovascular disorders**.

Treatment

Infertility may be treated with infertility drugs including those that inhibit estrogens (for example, ℞ **clomiphene citrate**). Alternatively, irregular periods may be corrected through the use of the oral ℞ **contraceptive** pill (combined). Tendency to diabetes mellitus may be treated with oral ℞ **antidiabetic** agents.

For further information

℞ DIRECTORY OF DRUGS:

antidiabetic agent (for example, **metformin**) • **antiestrogen** (for example, **clomiphene citrate**) • **oral contraceptive**

porphyria

Porphyria is a group of hereditary conditions in which the nitrogenous compounds (porphyrins) that normally combine with iron and the protein globin to produce the red blood pigment hemoglobin are formed in excess. It affects either the liver or the composition of the blood as formed in the blood marrow. Symptoms include discoloration of the urine (to pink or purple) when it is left to stand, skin blistering with sensitivity to sunlight, neuritis, abdominal pain—and, usually, mental disturbance. In susceptible people, porphyria may be triggered by a number of different types of drugs.

Treatment

It is possible to prevent attacks to some degree by avoiding conditions or substances known to be triggering factors—such as sunlight or certain drugs. Treatment otherwise is to relieve symptoms, where drugs may sometimes be used (℞ **chlorpromazine**; ℞ **desmopressin**).

For further information

℞ DIRECTORY OF DRUGS:
chlorpromazine • desmopressin

posterior uveitis

see ✪ uveitis.

post-herpatic neuralgia

see ✪ neuralgia.

post-natal depression

see ✪ depression.

post-operative pain

see ✪ pain.

post-traumatic stress disorder

see ✪ affective disorders.

post viral syndrome

see ✪ chronic fatigue syndrome.

precocious puberty

see ✪ abnormal puberty.

pregnancy

see ✪ pregnancy-related disorders.

pregnancy-related disorders

Pregnancy is the period from conception to the birth of the baby. There are many physiological changes during the interval between the implantation of the ovum and delivery. Though a natural process, there are various medical interventions that may be of benefit to the mother and the child. Increasingly it is realized that the health of the mother before and during pregnancy can have lasting effects on the health and life expectancy of the child as an adult. Most of the common complaints that occur during pregnancy are not serious, and are caused by the normal changes of pregnancy such as changes in sex hormone level and extra weight. They include breast tenderness, ✪ **morning sickness**, ✪ **constipation**, skin changes (for example, pigmentation), heartburn, and ✪ **indigestion**. In later pregnancy there may be ✪ **varicose veins**, swollen ankles, ✪ **musculoskeletal disorders** (for example, ✪ **backache**), ✪ **anemia**, and ✪ **hemorrhoids**. Some women develop temporary ✪ **diabetes mellitus** during pregnancy, and in some women pre-eclampsia is a problem that if left untreated can lead to the serious condition, ✪ **eclampsia**. Following birth, some women experience ✪ **depression** (post natal depression), which may require treatment. Unvaccinated pregnant women should avoid contact with people with ✪ **rubella**.

Treatment

Avoidance of undue stress is beneficial, but adequate balanced nutrition is of paramount importance. It is now held by most medical authorities that it is necessary to give ℞ **folic acid** before, and during, pregnancy in order to minimize the risk of neural tube defects (for example, ✪ **spina bifida**). Sometimes folic acid is taken as an oral preparation, incorporating iron salts to guard against ✪ **anemia** for mothers at risk of iron deficiency. As well as from medical sources, iron and other minerals, folic acid, and vitamins are available OTC, but it is important to take advice on appropriate dosage, since many dietary supplements are toxic to the fetus in overdose. Similarly, many herbal preparations warn against use in pregnancy. Since the thalidomide tragedy, medical drugs are screened in an attempt to estimate the risks when used by pregnant mothers, and now generic drugs are rated, according to perceived risk, on a FDA (Federal Drugs Administration) scale running in five categories from A (controlled studies show no risk) through B, C, D to X (definitely contraindicated in pregnancy). However, physicians will often recommend that any drug that does not definitely need to be taken in pregnancy should not be taken. Exceptions have to be made, or considered, where the mother suffers from disorders that have to be treated such as ✪ **diabetes mellitus**, ✪ **epilepsy** or ✪ **AIDS**. In the case of epilepsy it seems likely that there is indeed a risk of antiepileptic drugs damaging the fetus. It is clear that children born of mothers who smoke (or are exposed to tobacco smoke), drink excess alcohol or take illegal drugs such as heroin, tend to be born with a low birth-weight, or develop recognized medical syndromes (for example, fetal alcohol syndrome; FAS) or a greater chance of diseases such as asthma. Screening for some fetal abnormalities (for example ✪ **Down's syndrome**) is now routine.

For further information

℞ DIRECTORY OF DRUGS:
anemia treatment (iron salts) • **folic acid** • **vitamin**
⚗ VITAMINS, MINERALS, AND SUPPLEMENTS:
folic acid • iron

premenstrual dysphoric disorder

see ✪ premenstrual syndrome.

premenstrual syndrome

Premenstrual syndrome (PMS) is a collection of symptoms that may be experienced by a woman in the last few days before the onset of each menstrual period. Such symptoms include tiredness,

✪ **headache**, abdominal tenderness, or bloating, and clumsiness. Some women also report ✪ **depression** or irritability, and emotional unease (premenstrual tension; PMT). Symptoms usually disappear as soon as menstruation starts. A distinction is sometimes made between premenstrual syndrome and a further syndrome called premenstrual dysphoric disorder (PMMD/PMDD), where the latter condition begins one or two weeks before menstruation, but otherwise is similar (see ✪ **affective disorders**).

Treatment
Treatment may involve ℞ **diuretic** drugs (to relieve bloating) and ℞ **progestin** preparations (derivatives of progesterone, one of the "female" hormones); ℞ **antidepressants** may also be prescribed. Many women gain relief from essential fatty acids, such as ♧ **gamma-linolenic acid (GLA)** (in supplement form or as the herbal remedy ♧ **evening primrose oil**). A number of other herbal remedies are available for ✪ **water retention**.

For further information
℞ DIRECTORY OF DRUGS:
antidepressant • diuretic • non-narcotic analgesic • NSAID • progestin
♣ HERBAL REMEDIES:
black cohosh • bugleweed • chaste tree • evening primrose • false unicorn root • lavender cotton • motherwort • oswego tea • potentilla
♧ VITAMINS, MINERALS, AND SUPPLEMENTS:
calcium • gamma-linolenic acid (GLA) • magnesium • vitamin B_6

premenstrual tension
see ✪ **premenstrual syndrome**.

pressure sore
see ✪ **bedsore**.

prickly heat
Prickly heat is a ✪ **skin condition**, medically called miliaria, which is characterized by an itchy ✪ **rash** made up of very small blisters surrounded with red skin. It occurs in hot weather and is caused by the blockage of sweat glands by dead bacteria or skin cells. It most generally occurs in overweight adults, and children and infants where it is commonly found in the diaper area.

Treatment
Treatment is by staying in a cooler environment and wearing loose clothing. Dusting powders, colloidal baths or herbal remedies to relieve the itching may be soothing; if persistent, topical ℞ **corticosteroids** may be prescribed.

For further information
℞ DIRECTORY OF DRUGS:
antipruritic • corticosteroid • skin preparation
♣ HERBAL REMEDIES:
heartsease • oats • peppermint

proctitis
Proctitis is ✪ **inflammation** of the rectum and anus. It causes soreness and bleeding, and sometimes has a discharge of mucus or pus.

It is often a feature of ✪ **Crohn's disease**, ✪ **ulcerative colitis** or ✪ **dysentery**. It can be caused by infection, radiation injury, trauma, ✪ **allergy**, and as a reaction to drugs.

Treatment
The treatment depends on the cause, but ℞ **corticosteroids** such as ℞ **hydrocortisone**; also ℞ **aminosalicylates** such as mesalamine can be used.

For further information
℞ DIRECTORY OF DRUGS:
corticosteroid • aminosalicylate

progressive bulbar paralysis
see ✪ **motor neuron disease**.

progressive muscular atrophy
see ✪ **motor neuron disease**.

prolactinoma
Prolactinoma is a noncancerous tumor of the anterior part of the pituitary gland, resulting in overproduction of the hormone prolactin. This type comprises about half of all pituitary tumors. The symptoms normally appear gradually and include amenorrhea or oligomenorrhea (absent or irregular periods), and ✪ **infertility** in women, or ✪ **impotence**, enlarged breasts, and leakage of fluid from the nipples in men. Pressure on adjacent areas of the brain may cause changes in the field of vision, headaches or ✪ **hypopituitarism**. Diagnosis includes measurement of hormone levels in the blood, and elimination of the effects of certain antipsychotic drugs (for example, chlorpromazine) or infections (for example, meningitis) as a cause. See ✪ **pituitary gland disorders and tumors**.

Treatment
The physiological release of prolactin into the bloodstream is controlled by a hypothalamic factor called prolactin-release inhibiting factor (PRIF), now thought to be identical to the neurotransmitter dopamine. Therefore drugs of the ℞ **dopamine-receptor stimulant** type are used as indirect prolactin antagonists to control symptoms of prolactinoma, and are often very effective. Sometimes surgical removal of the tumor, or radiotherapy, may be necessary (see also ✪ **pituitary gland disorders and tumors**).

For further information
℞ DIRECTORY OF DRUGS:
dopamine-receptor stimulant (for example, **bromocriptine, pergolide**)

prolapsed uterus
A prolapsed uterus is the displacement of the uterus (womb) downward, due to weakness in its supporting tissues, most often due to damage during childbirth. Sometimes the cervix (the neck of the womb) is visible at the vaginal opening; in severe cases, the uterus and vagina may protrude externally through the labia. Symptoms include pain, discomfort, and urinary difficulties or incontinence.

Treatment
Treatment usually requires surgery to replace the uterus and shorten stretched supporting ligaments, where necessary also

repairing the vagina or narrowing the opening. Post-menopausal women may be prescribed ℞ **estrogens**.

For further information
℞ DIRECTORY OF DRUGS:
estrogen

prostate cancer

Prostate cancer is a malignant tumor (carcinoma) of the prostate gland (the gland lying below the bladder, which secretes part of the seminal fluid) in men. It becomes increasingly common with age, and is the third leading cause of ✪ **cancer** death, with 120,000 new cases reported each year in the US. It is generally slow growing and may cause no symptoms, although as it enlarges it can cause difficulties with urination and may spread, especially to bone, causing pain. The tumor is dependent on male hormones (androgens) for its growth. Because the tumor increases secretion of an enzyme called prostate specific antigen (PSA), a screening test for PSA in the blood is possible.

Treatment
Treatment, where a tumor is discovered, may include hormone therapy with ℞ **antiandrogens**, such as ℞ **flutamide** and ℞ **goserelin**, which are examples of drugs that work in different ways to reduce androgen stimulation. Alternatively, surgery may be used to remove the tumor or, sometimes, the testicles (to stop hormone secretion). The supplement lycopene is said to protect against prostate cancer.

For further information
℞ DIRECTORY OF DRUGS:
antiandrogen • anticancer
⚕ VITAMINS, MINERALS, AND SUPPLEMENTS:
carotenoid (lycopene)

prostatic enlargement
see ✪ benign prostatic hypertrophy.

prostatitis

Prostatitis is ✪ **inflammation** of the prostate gland (the gland lying below the bladder, which secretes part of the seminal fluid) in men. It is often due to ✪ **bacterial infection**. In acute prostatitis symptoms are pain in the groin, and sometimes on urination, pain during bowel movements, with a high temperature. In chronic prostatitis difficulty in urination may progress to complete obstruction, with inability to urinate at all.

Treatment
Acute prostatitis, if due to infection, is usually treated with ℞ **antibacterial** drugs including ℞ **quinolones** and ℞ **antibiotics** such as the ℞ **cephalosporins** and ℞ **penicillins**. In chronic prostatitis surgery may be necessary to remove the prostate (prostatectomy). Other drugs may be used to relive symptoms.

For further information
℞ DIRECTORY OF DRUGS:
antibacterial
♣ HERBAL REMEDIES:
hydrangea • stinging nettle

protozoal infection

Protozoal infections are infections by simple unicellular organisms that are microscopic in size though bigger than bacteria. They are similar to amebae, which until recently were classified as a sub-class of the protozoa family, and for convenience are still generally grouped under protozoa. The most important protozoa, in terms of illness and death, are those of the genus *Plasmodium*, which cause ✪ **malaria**. Other major protozoal diseases found most commonly in countries with a hot, humid environment, are ✪ **leishmaniasis**, amebic ✪ **dysentery** (amebiasis); also ✪ **toxoplasmosis**, ✪ **trichomoniasis**, trypanosomiasis and ✪ **giardiasis** (lambliasis). A form of ✪ **pneumonia** is caused in immunosuppressed individuals (including those suffering from ✪ **AIDS**) by the protozoan *Pneumocystis carinii* (which has some features of both protozoa and fungi).

Treatment
Infection can be treated with gut or systemically active drugs (see ℞ **amebicide and antiprotozoal** entry) depending on which disease and at what stage. Sometimes ℞ **antibacterial** antibiotics are used concurrently to prevent opportunist infections (for example, tetracycline). See individual conditions for further details.

pruritis

Pruritis is the symptom of itching—an uncomfortable sensation leading to the urge to scratch. It is a symptom common to many ✪ **skin conditions** such as ✪ **urticaria**, ✪ **eczema**, ✪ **scabies**, or to an insect ✪ **sting** or bite, or drug ✪ **allergy**. It can also be a sign of an underlying disorder such as ✪ **liver disorder** or chronic ✪ **kidney disorder**. Scratching can lead to infection. Pruritis ani is a common condition of itching of the skin around the anus and can be caused by ✪ **candidiasis**, pinworms, or external ✪ **hemorrhoids**. Pruritis vulvae is the itching of the female external genitalia and can be caused by candidiasis, contact ✪ **dermatitis** or ✪ **trichomoniasis**.

Treatment
Drugs to relieve the itching can be applied locally.

For further information
℞ DIRECTORY OF DRUGS:
antihistamine • antipruritic
♣ HERBAL REMEDIES:
brewer's yeast • chamomile, German • cnidium • evening primrose • goldenseal • heartsease • henna • moneywort • oats • peppermint • purple loosestrife • stinging nettle

pruritis ani
see ✪ pruritis.

pruritis vulvae
see ✪ pruritis.

pseudomembranous colitis

Pseudomembranous colitis is an intestinal condition characterized by severe ✪ **diarrhea**. It is frequently caused by ℞ **antibacterial** antibiotic treatment that results in an overgrowth of the spore-forming bacterial organism *Clostridium difficile*. It is sometimes referred to as a ✪ **superinfection**. Symptoms include watery diarrhea, fever, and cramping. If allowed to progress, or antidiarrheals are used, it can continue into the serious condition toxic megacolon. It generally requires hospital treatment, but great care is necessary in order to prevent transmission between people due to inadequate hygiene.

Treatment

Treatment is with specialized ℞ **antibacterial** drugs active against this type of organism (anerobes).

For further information

℞ DIRECTORY OF DRUGS:
antibacterial (oral **vancomycin**, injected **metronidazole**)

⚖ VITAMINS, MINERALS, AND SUPPLEMENTS:
acidophilus

psittacosis

Psittacosis (also called ornithosis or parrot fever) is an infective illness caused by a bacterium (*Chlamydia psittaci*; see ✪ **chlamydial infections**) transmitted to humans by birds (especially parrots), and characterized by pneumonia-like symptoms in the respiratory system. It can be difficult to make a diagnosis, and antibody tests are used.

Treatment

Treatment is with ℞ **antibacterial** drugs active against this type of organism.

For further information

℞ DIRECTORY OF DRUGS:
oral **antibacterial** including **tetracyclines** (such as **demeclocycline, doxycycline, minocycline, oxytetracycline**, and **tetracycline**)

psoriasis

Psoriasis is a common noncontagious ✪ **skin condition**. Symptoms are scaly oval lesions upon patches of reddened skin anywhere on—or all over—the body, but especially on the elbows, knees, and scalp, often with brittle fingernails. The lesions are neither painful nor particularly irritating, but they are unsightly and may seriously interfere with individuals' lifestyles. The cause is unknown, but it runs in families and there are probably hereditary factors. Once contracted, usually in adolescence, the disease tends to peak and wane recurrently for the rest of the person's life; periods of complete remission are seldom longer than two years. Stress, injury, or prescribed drugs may trigger symptoms. Some affected individuals also develop a particular form of ✪ **arthritis**.

Treatment

Treatment is to alleviate the symptoms as far as possible: ℞ **skin preparations** (including ℞ **emollients**, ℞ **barrier creams**), ℞ **keratolytics** (including ℞ **salicylic acid** and ℞ **anthralin**), drugs related to vitamin D (for instance ℞ **calcipotriene** used topically); drugs related to vitamin A, most used topically (℞ **retinoids** including ℞ **isotretinoin**, etretinate, ℞ **acitretin**, ℞ **tazarotene**), topical ℞ **corticosteroids**, and ultraviolet radiation treatment. In severe cases stronger drugs including ℞ **immunosuppressants** such as ℞ **cyclosporine** and ℞ **methotrexate** can be taken. Several herbal remedies are considered to be beneficial, as are ⚖ **zinc** and

⚖ **omega-3 fatty acids**. If the disease leads to psychological problems, some form of counseling may be advised.

For further information

℞ DIRECTORY OF DRUGS:
barrier cream • corticosteroid • emollient • keratolytic • immunosuppressant • psoriasis treatment • retinoid • skin preparation

♣ HERBAL REMEDIES:
evening primrose • gotu kola • Oregon grape • sarsaparilla

⚖ VITAMINS, MINERALS, AND SUPPLEMENTS:
omega-3 fatty acid • zinc

psychosis

see ✪ **psychotic disorders**.

psychotic disorders

Psychotic disorders (psychoses) are major mental disorders characterized by a severe impairment of the sense of reality. They are usually contrasted with ✪ **affective disorders** (neurotic), which are not generally so severe, and where the subject is aware that they are ill. In psychotic illness the subject is not generally aware of the extent or even the nature of the problem—in other words a state traditionally perceived as "madness." The most common psychosis is ✪ **schizophrenia**, a group of illnesses with marked disturbances of behavior and emotional reactions, and delusions; sometimes called "split personality." Some other disorders that are regarded by some authorities as psychotic include ✪ **bipolar disorder**, but grouped by others (and in this book) with ✪ **affective disorders**. Similarly, paranoid illness is sometimes regarded as a psychotic disorder. The origin of psychosis is not fully understood, but often involves abnormal functioning of neurotransmitters in the brain, especially dopamine, serotonin, and acetylcholine. There is a strong familial or genetic tendency to develop schizophrenia. Sometimes there is an obvious organic, rather than psychiatric, origin of psychotic behavior, termed brain syndrome. This may be a degenerative condition (for example, ✪ **Alzheimer's disease**), chemical or environmental poisoning, a brain tumor or brain damage.

Treatment

Treatment depends on the cause. Management of schizophrenia and gross manic states is with psychiatric help combined with ℞ **antipsychotic** drugs—once referred to as major tranquilizers or neuroleptics in view of their ability to calm and tranquilize excitable individuals. There are currently many antipsychotic drugs available, of several different classes. Although most do have quite marked side effects, they are often successful enough at suppressing psychotic manifestations that people receiving medication are able to rejoin the community.

For further information

℞ DIRECTORY OF DRUGS:
antipsychotic

puberty

see ✪ **abnormal puberty**.

pubic lice

see ✪ lice and mite infestation.

pulmonary embolism

A pulmonary embolism is an obstruction of the pulmonary artery (the main artery supplying the lungs) or one of its branches, by an embolus, usually a blood clot or other material originating from blood vessels in the leg or lower body, sometimes called a thromboembolism. Sometimes the embolus is formed during periods of inactivity of the body, especially the lower lungs, as in cramped air travel. If the clot is big enough to block the main artery, the condition is life threatening. The symptoms depend on the size of the clot, and vary from a shortness of breath with low blood pressure, chest pains, coughing up of blood, and rapid pulse, to sudden death. Small emboli may produce unnoticed symptoms, but these may be recurrent, in which case the condition may progress to the condition called pulmonary hypertension.

Treatment

Treatment depends on the size of the embolus. Small emboli will dissolve with time but to aid this process, and with a risk of more emboli forming, ℞ **anticoagulants** are taken. In acute emergencies, ℞ **thrombolytic** ("clot-buster") drugs may be taken.

For further information

℞ DIRECTORY OF DRUGS:

anticoagulant (for example, **heparin, warfarin sodium**) • **thrombolytic**

pulmonary emphysema

see ✪ emphysema.

pulmonary hypertension

see ✪ pulmonary embolism.

pyelonephritis

see ✪ nephritis.

pyloric stenosis

Pyloric stenosis is a constriction of the final part of the stomach (pylorus) up to the pyloric sphincter; the muscular valve that allows partly digested food through to the next section of the alimentary canal. Such constriction in adults may be caused by a peptic ulcer or tumor growth; in infants it is due to a nodule on the pyloric muscle that tends to cause symptoms around four weeks after birth. In either case, consequent obstruction to the passage of food causes persistent vomiting, especially of fluids, and possible distension of the stomach; weight loss, and dehydration follow. Diagnosis may involve a barium meal (a special X-ray examination of the stomach) or direct vision with an endoscope (a fiber-optic tube passed into the stomach).

Treatment

Treatment depends on the cause, and may include ℞ **ulcer-healing drugs** in adults, or surgery.

For further information

℞ DIRECTORY OF DRUGS:

ulcer-healing drug

rabies

Rabies (also called hydrophobia) is a dangerous ✪ **viral infection** of the nervous system caught through contact with the saliva of an infected animal (commonly a dog or fox, or sometimes bat), for instance a bite or a lick over a skin abrasion. Symptoms may take from three weeks to a year to appear, and treatment taken before they become apparent is usually successful; once symptoms are present, recovery is unlikely. The symptoms take the form of a high temperature and depression, followed by manic excitement, violent agitation, and spasms of the throat that with an overproduction of saliva cause the classic "frothing at the mouth," especially if the person attempts to drink. Death usually follows.

Treatment

Treatment before symptoms appear includes isolation of the individual and an intensive course of rabies ℞ **vaccine** injections. ℞ **Rabies immune globulin** is available to give immediate passive immunity. Preventive vaccination is available for travelers.

For further information

℞ DIRECTORY OF DRUGS:

rabies • **immune globulin** • **vaccine**

rash

A rash is a temporary skin eruption, generally a group of spots or an area of inflamed skin, sometimes localized and sometimes over much of the body. Doctors describe rashes by appearance; blistered (large blisters), vesicular (small blisters), pustular (pus-filled blisters), macular (level and a different color to the skin), or papular and nodular (raised bumps) are just some of the terms used. Rashes may be associated with itching and fever, and though they are helpful in warning, or in diagnoses, of disease states, most rashes do not indicate a serious disorder. Causes may include a range of infectious diseases, including common childhood ailments (for example, ✪ chickenpox, ✪ rubella, ✪ scarlet fever), ✪ meningitis, ✪ typhoid fever, and many others (for example, ✪ Rocky Mountain spotted fever). A number of parasitic infestations cause skin eruptions (for example, ✪ Lyme disease, ✪ scabies), as do many insect and other animal bites. The type of rash characteristic of nettle stings is described as ✪ urticaria (hives), but may have many causes. Other diseases characterized by rash-like syndromes include: ✪ scurvy and ✪ pellagra (vitamin deficiency diseases), and systemic ✪ lupus erythematosus (SLE). Skin reactions are the main characteristic of many skin conditions (notably ✪ eczema, ✪ psoriasis, and acne ✪ rosacea). Some rashes are part of an immune reaction, including contact dermatitis (for example, rash where metal jewellery or fastenings touch the skin), reaction to appreciable numbers of drugs (for example, antibiotics especially penicillins, barbiturates, ACE inhibitors, NSAIDs, opiates, antivirals, and local anesthetics), reactions to toxic, caustic chemicals and sprays, to some foodstuffs (for example, peanuts, shellfish, strawberries, and eggs), ultraviolet light or plants (for example, nettles, poison ivy, poison oak). These allergic rashes may indicate a reaction more serious than simply skin eruptions, and a more generalized reaction (as in anaphylactic shock) may be life threatening and require emergency medical intervention.

Key to symbols: ✪ = Disorder Section ℞ = Drug Section ♣ = Herbal Section ⌘ = Supplement Section

Treatment

Treatment depends on cause, and often no intervention apart from soothing lotions (for example, ℞ **calamine**) or ℞ **antihistamine** preparations is necessary. For more serious conditions other ℞ **skin preparations** such as corticosteroid creams or lotions may be required. Infections or infestations are treated with specific remedies (for example, ℞ **antibacterial** drugs, ℞ **scabicide and pediculicidal** agents), and depending on the cause, herbal remedies such as ♣ **yellow toad flax** are available. See ✪ **skin conditions** and individual skin conditions for further information.

Raynaud's disease

Raynaud's disease is the constriction or spasm of blood vessels in the fingers, and sometimes other extremities, on exposure to cold, causing numbness, tingling, pain, and color changes. Typically, the fingertips turn white, then blue, then red on rewarming. After two years of having symptoms, if there is no apparent cause, it is known as Raynaud's disease. In about half of those with the condition, it is due to an underlying disorder called Raynaud's phenomenon, which can occur due to ✪ **arteriosclerosis** and various other diseases, such as ✪ **autoimmune disorders**, systemic lupus erythematosus (SLE), ✪ **lupus**, ✪ **rheumatoid arthritis** or scleroderma. It may also be caused by certain drugs (for instance some ℞ **ACE inhibitors**) or the prolonged use of vibrating tools. Very rarely the damage from restricted blood supply is so severe that ✪ **gangrene** ensues.

Treatment

Individuals are advised to keep the hands (and feet, ears, or nose, if affected) warm whenever possible. Sometimes ℞ **vasodilator** drugs are taken to relieve the blood vessel spasm, and in severe cases surgery to sever the nerves that control the response may be necessary.

For further information

℞ DIRECTORY OF DRUGS:
vasodilator

♣ HERBAL REMEDIES:
ginkgo

⚖ VITAMINS, MINERALS, AND SUPPLEMENTS:
niacin (as derivative such as **niacinamide**)

Raynaud's phenomenon

see ✪ **Raynaud's disease**.

red eye

see ✪ **conjunctivitis**.

renal colic

see ✪ **colic**; ✪ **calculus**.

renal disease

see ✪ **kidney disorder**.

renal stones

see ✪ **calculus**.

repetitive strain injury

Repetitive strain injury (RSI) is pain and inability to use part of a limb, often the muscles of the arms and hands, due to prolonged overuse. It generally involves repeated performance of a particular movement, or sometimes pressure application or weight bearing on a specific area. It classically affects computer operators, and may necessitate a change of job.

Treatment

Treatment may be with rest, strapping to reduce the load on the affected joint, and ℞ **NSAID** analgesics.

For further information

℞ DIRECTORY OF DRUGS:
NSAID

respiratory tract disorders

Respiratory tract disorders is a broad term that is used to describe any of a number of disorders that affect the airways, and includes ✪ **infections** of the upper respiratory tract leading to ✪ **common cold**, ✪ **influenza**, ✪ **laryngitis**, ✪ **pharyngitis**, ✪ **sinusitis**, ✪ **rhinitis**, and ✪ **tonsillitis**; and of the lower respiratory tract causing ✪ **bronchitis**, ✪ **pneumonia**, and tracheitis. ✪ **asthma** is an obstructive airways disease where the bronchial tubes that carry air to the lungs go into spasm and become narrower during an attack, while the linings of the airways become swollen and inflamed which can then block the smaller airways. ✪ **lung cancer** is a serious, essentially incurable respiratory tract disorder where the great majority of people who contract the disease are or have been heavy cigarette smokers. Symptoms of respiratory tract disorders depend on the cause and the specific disorder in question but can include difficulty breathing, ✪ **cough**, ✪ **bronchial congestion**, and wheezing. Respiratory problems are a characteristic of ✪ **cystic fibrosis**. See also ✪ **croup**, ✪ **emphysema**, ✪ **chronic obstructive pulmonary disease**, and ✪ **pertussis**.

Treatment

This depends on the specific disorder but for symptomatic relief, drugs, many of which are available OTC (for example, in cough and cold preparations) may include antitussives, which may help if there is cough, expectorants (to help cough up phlegm), nasal decongestants (to relieve symptoms of a blocked nose), and analgesics (to relive pain) may also give relief. If ✪ **bacterial infection** is present antibacterials including antibiotics may be prescribed. Many herbal remedies are said to be of value in respiratory tract disorders in general, including ♣ **soap bark**, ♣ **lungmoss**, ♣ **bitter milkwort**, and ♣ **Malabar nut**. ♣ **echinacea** and ⚖ **garlic** in particular, but also ♣ **Scotch pine** and ♣ **boneset** are considered valuable for respiratory tract infections. ♣ **lobelia** as an expectorant, ♣ **myrrh** to relieve respiratory ✪ **catarrh**, and ♣ **eucalyptus**, ♣ **radish**, ♣ **wild thyme**, and ♣ **pill-bearing spurge** amongst others are advocated for use in bronchitis and/or asthma. Numerous herbal remedies including ♣ **marshmallow**, ♣ **horseradish**, ♣ **licorice root**, Echinacea, ♣ **elecampane**, and ♣ **chamomile, German** have antitussive properties and can be used to relieve cough. Of the vitamins, minerals, and supplements available, ⚖ **vitamin B$_6$** and ⚖ **vitamin C** are both thought by some to be of value in alleviating asthma, and ⚖ **N-acetylcysteine** may be helpful in respiratory illnesses in general. See individual disorder entries for more details.

respiratory tract infections

see ✪ **infection**.

Reye's syndrome

Reye's syndrome is a rare disorder with brain inflammation (✪ **encephalitis**) and liver failure that occurs in children. The cause is unknown but it often follows a ✪ **viral infection** (for instance ✪ **chickenpox**) and has been linked with the use of ℞ **aspirin**, so it is now recommended that aspirin should never be given to children under the age of 12 without medical supervision. Other preparations containing salicylates, and herbal salicylates should be avoided.

Treatment

Hospitalization with intensive supervision and drug treatment is usually needed.

rheumatic fever

Rheumatic fever is the ✪ **inflammation** of the heart, joints, and skin following ✪ **bacterial infection**. It is a complex response by the body to an attack of ✪ **tonsillitis** or similar bacterial infection of the upper respiratory tract. Rheumatic fever may also affect the valves of the heart, causing rheumatic heart disease. Symptoms other than those of the original infection include pain and stiffness of the joints, which swell and redden (✪ **arthritis**) in sequence, and a skin ✪ **rash** with outbreaks of tender nodules. If the heart is affected, there is chest pain and breathlessness. Sometimes there is also inflammation of the brain tissue, resulting in chorea (writhing movements of the head and limbs). Despite the severity of these symptoms, lasting effects are uncommon, although heart valve damage may persist (see ✪ **heart valve disorders**). The symptoms are those of an ✪ **autoimmune disorder**, which is triggered by an infection.

Treatment

Treatment is with rest, systemic ℞ **corticosteroids** (for instance cortisone, prednisolone or dexamethasone), ℞ **NSAIDs** (including aspirin, salsalate, and choline salicylate), and a course of ℞ **antibacterial** drugs (antibiotics such as penicillin or erythromycin) may be continued for some years afterward.

For further information

℞ DIRECTORY OF DRUGS:
antibacterial • antibiotic • corticosteroid • NSAID

rheumatism

see ✪ **musculoskeletal disorders**.

rheumatoid arthritis

Rheumatoid arthritis is a form of ✪ **arthritis**, a ✪ **musculoskeletal disorder** that results in deformity through the degeneration of the synovial membrane that lines the joints, later affecting the bones, tendons, and surrounding tissues. It may also cause Raynaud's phenomenon (see ✪ **Raynaud's disease**). The disorder tends to attack joints symmetrically across the body, especially in the fingers,

wrists, and feet. It is an ✪ **autoimmune disorder** (meaning that the immune system starts to attack the body's own tissues) and is more common in women than men. There may be a heredity component. Most affected individuals possess a characteristic rheumatoid factor that is revealed by blood tests. The disease often eventually burns itself out, but the deformity remains.

Treatment

Specialist treatment is required and is with a wide variety of disease-modifying drugs. Treatment should be commenced early to avoid deformity. Many types of anti-inflammatory drugs are used, including ℞ **NSAIDs**, ℞ **corticosteroids**, ℞ **aminosalicylates**, ℞ **gold compounds**, also ℞ **immunosuppressants**. Many of these are reserved for use in dealing with flare-ups. Rest, and physiotherapy can also help to alleviate the pain, swelling, and stiffness. Surgery is sometimes required and may include joint replacements. See also ✪ **arthritis**.

For further information

℞ DIRECTORY OF DRUGS:
aminosalicylate • antirheumatic • corticosteroid • gold compound • immunomodulator • immunosuppressant • NSAID

♣ HERBAL REMEDIES:
evening primrose

♌ VITAMINS, MINERALS, AND SUPPLEMENTS:
gamma-linolenic acid (GLA)

rheumatoid disease

see ✪ **musculoskeletal disorders**.

rhinitis

Rhinitis is inflammation of the mucous membranes lining the nose. It is usually accompanied by swelling of the mucosa and a nasal discharge. Rhinitis is a symptom of colds and may be complicated with sinusitis. Allergic rhinitis affects people who experience an allergic reaction after they inhale airborne substance (allergens, such as pollen). If it occurs only in the spring and summer when pollen counts are high, it is known as seasonal allergic rhinitis (✪ **hay fever**). If it occurs all year round, it is known as perennial allergic rhinitis. Allergic rhinitis is more common in people who have other allergic disorders, such as asthma. The symptoms of both types of allergic rhinitis are an itchy sensation in the nose, blocked runny nose, sneezing, and itchy, red watery eyes.

Treatment

In allergic rhinitis, a skin prick test may be carried out to identify the allergen that causes the allergic rhinitis and treatment of the symptoms with **antihistamines** by mouth or nose-drops—many available OTC—is often effective. Various antiallergic drugs, in serious cases **corticosteroids**, may be prescribed and used as nose-drops. If a specific allergen (a substance provoking the allergy) is identified, possibly by a patch test, desensitization (a method for reducing allergic responses by gradually building up tolerance to the allergen) may be possible. Nasal **decongestants**, some available OTC, can be used for relief of symptoms of rhinitis.

For further information
℞ DIRECTORY OF DRUGS:
antiallergic • antihistamine • corticosteroid • nasal decongestant
♣ HERBAL REMEDIES:
marjoram

rickets

Rickets is a childhood condition that is caused by a deficiency of vitamin D (calciferol), resulting in turn in a calcium deficiency that leads to poor formation or deformity of the bones. Vitamin D deficiency is usually caused either by an inadequate diet or by lack of sunlight, and is particularly common among Asian children. It can occasionally be due to a ✪ kidney disorder (renal rickets), which has an increased mineral loss in urine. A similar condition is osteomalacia in adults.

Treatment
Treatment is to make up the deficiency with ⚖ vitamin D (⚖ cholecalciferol) and derivatives (℞ ergocalciferol). Calcium supplements (typically ℞ calcium carbonate and calcium acetate) can also be taken. If treatment is early enough, any deformity tends to disappear.

For further information
℞ DIRECTORY OF DRUGS:
calcium carbonate • ergocalciferol
⚖ VITAMINS, MINERALS, AND SUPPLEMENTS:
calcium • vitamin D

Rocky Mountain spotted fever

Rocky Mountain spotted fever (RMSF; also called spotted fever, tick fever, mountain fever) is a serious infectious illness caused by ✪ bacterial infection (*Rickettsia rickettsii*), which is carried by ticks in temperate regions of North and South America. It is characterized by ✪ fever, chills, bad ✪ headache, confusion, and ✪ rash. Prevention includes the use of insecticides and protective clothing, or vaccination of those at risk. It has similarities to other infections caused by *Rickettsia*, including the closely related rickettsialpox, and also the typhus group of diseases.

Treatment
Treatment includes careful nursing because of possible mortality from shock or renal failure, and the use of ℞ antibacterial antibiotic drugs.

For further information
℞ DIRECTORY OF DRUGS:
oral antibacterial drugs including the tetracycline group (such as doxycycline, tetracycline) and chloramphenicol

rosacea

Rosacea is a ✪ skin condition, an inflammation of the skin on the face. It is caused by a disorder of the sebaceous glands that secrete natural oils within the tissues. Symptoms are a redness of the skin, and lumps and spots similar to those of ✪ acne (rosacea is sometimes called acne rosacea). More women suffer from it than men. Its ultimate cause is unknown, though there may be a genetic link.

Treatment
Treatment is with ℞ antibacterial drugs, including (oral) ℞ tetracyclines, topical ℞ sulfonamides, and ℞ metronidazole.

For further information
℞ DIRECTORY OF DRUGS:
antibacterial (tetracycline, sulfonamide, and metronidazole)

round worms
see ✪ worms.

rubella

Rubella (commonly called German measles) is a highly infectious ✪ viral infection—contagious even before the appearance of symptoms, and for some time after they have gone. The initial symptoms are raised temperature, ✪ headache, and a sore throat, with swelling of the lymph glands at the back of the neck. The classic ✪ rash of reddish pink spots starts on the face and then spreads all over the body. It lasts up to about seven days, and confers natural life-long immunity. If it is contracted in the early stages of pregnancy, rubella can cause severe defects in a developing fetus, so unvaccinated pregnant women should keep well away from anyone with rubella.

Treatment
There is no cure; treatment is to alleviate symptoms, including ℞ antipyretics and non-narcotic analgesics (℞ NSAID). A ℞ vaccine is available and is usually given in infancy, along with measles (MR vaccine) or also with mumps immunization (MMR vaccine).

For further information
℞ DIRECTORY OF DRUGS:
antipyretic • non-narcotic analgesic • NSAID • vaccine (MMR (measles-mumps-rubella virus vaccine, live))

rubeola
see ✪ measles.

scabies

Scabies is an infestation of the skin by the itch-mite (*Sarcoptes scabiei*), which burrows into the skin to lay its eggs. A contagious condition, its symptoms are severe itching and rash, both caused by an allergic reaction to the mites and their larva in the skin tissues. Main sites affected are the finger webs, feet, nipples, and pubic region. See ✪ lice and mite infestations.

Treatment
Treatment is with a ℞ scabicide drug applied to the whole body except the face: the entire household should be treated. ℞ Antipruritics including ℞ antihistamines may be given to relieve itching.

For further information
℞ DIRECTORY OF DRUGS:
antipruritic (crotamiton and some antihistamine drugs) • scabicide and pediculicide agent (for example, lindane, malathion, permethrin)
♣ HERBAL REMEDIES:
cnidium • henna

scalds
see ⊕ wound.

scarlatina
see ⊕ scarlet fever.

scarlet fever
Scarlet fever (or scarlatina in its milder form) is a toxic manifestation of a ⊕ **bacterial infection** with the hemolytic streptococcal bacterium (*Streptococcus pyrogens*), which also causes ⊕ **tonsillitis**. Symptoms are a high temperature, sore throat, headache, vomiting, and, sometimes, diarrhea. A bright red ⊕ **rash** spreads from the neck all over the body; the tongue turns white and also has a rash-like covering of spots (strawberry tongue). The condition lasts for about four days—but the person may be contagious for at least another two weeks. After-effects may include flaking skin and temporary hair loss, and sometimes complications of ⊕ **otitis** or kidney inflammation.

Treatment
Treatment is with antibacterial drugs, usually ℞ **penicillin** or ℞ **erythromycin** class ℞ **antibiotics**.

For further information
℞ DIRECTORY OF DRUGS:
antibacterial • antibiotic • erythromycin • penicillin

schistosomiasis
Schistosomiasis (also called bilharzia or bilharziasis) is a disorder that is caused by an infestation by parasitic flukes of the genus *Schistosoma* (types of flat ⊕ **worm**). It is contracted by swimming in water contaminated both by human excreta and by the snails that nurture the larva of the fluke. Penetrating the skin, the flukes travel to the intestine and bladder. There they mature, and then release eggs. The eggs cause anemia and destroy surrounding tissue. Initial symptoms are high temperature, muscle pain, skin irritation ("swimmer's itch"), and coughing. ⊕ **dysentery**, enlargement of the spleen, and ⊕ **cirrhosis** of the liver may follow; tissue damage in the bladder may lead to cancer.

Treatment
Treatment is with highly powerful ℞ **anthelmintics** drugs toxic to the flukes (and potentially toxic to the individual); surgery may be necessary to repair tissue damage.

For further information
℞ DIRECTORY OF DRUGS:
anthelmintic

schizophrenia
Schizophrenia is a functional ⊕ **psychotic disorder** in which thought processes are disrupted, delusions and hallucinations deprive the person of part or all reality, and behavior may become violently antisocial. Hereditary factors may contribute toward a schizophrenic predisposition, and stress can precipitate exacerbations. Several types or stages have been observed. Simple schizophrenia merely describes an individual's increasing withdrawal into a closed world; paranoid schizophrenia is characterized by the frequency or prominence of delusions; and catatonic schizophrenia produces overagitated movements and excitement, alternately with extreme withdrawal.

Treatment
Treatment is with ℞ **antipsychotic** drugs and intensive support, both psychologically and socially, aiming to reduce the need for hospitalization or institutional care, and allow some integration into the community.

For further information
℞ DIRECTORY OF DRUGS:
antipsychotic

sciatica
Sciatica is a pain in the area of distribution of the sciatic nerve, from the buttock down the back of the leg to the foot. The condition is usually caused by the pinching of the nerve near its junction with the spinal cord, often as a result of displacement (prolapse) of an intervertebral disk (and is thus a type of referred pain—pain felt at a site distant to the one really affected). The immediate cause may be from lifting a heavy weight, a sudden twisting, or during the last few months of pregnancy because of change in posture—or there may be some more serious problem. Persistent sciatica should be medically diagnosed. It is a ⊕ **musculoskeletal disorder**.

Treatment
Treatment is with rest and ℞ **NSAID** drugs until the pain subsides. Persistent symptoms may require surgery.

For further information
℞ DIRECTORY OF DRUGS:
NSAID

scurvy
Scurvy is a disease caused by a serious ⊕ **vitamin deficiency** of vitamin C (ascorbic acid). Because the body can store enough vitamin C to prevent the manifestations of scurvy for about three months, the generally healthier diets eaten today mean that it is rarely seen, except in people such as explorers or as part of serious malnutrition. The symptoms of scurvy are a notable degeneration of connective tissue, which causes effects such as a weakness of blood vessels, poor wound healing, and bleeding gums. It is serious if found in children since bleeding in the membrane of the long bones interferes with their growth. Other symptoms include ⊕ **anemia**.

Treatment
Treatment consists of large oral doses of ᐺ **vitamin C**.

For further information
℞ DIRECTORY OF DRUGS:
vitamin
♣ HERBAL REMEDIES:
garden cress• lime • scurvy grass
ᐺ VITAMINS, MINERALS, AND SUPPLEMENTS:
vitamin C

sea sickness
see ⊕ motion sickness.

seasonal allergic disorder
see ⊕ hay fever.

seasonal allergic rhinitis

see ✪ hay fever.

seborrhea

Seborrhea is a ✪ **skin condition** caused by overproduction of the oily secretion (sebum) of the sebaceous glands. The glands themselves swell, especially on the face, and the skin takes on the oily texture that predisposes to ✪ **acne**. Scaling of the skin occurs, causing ✪ **dandruff**. A similar disorder—seborrheic ✪ **dermatitis**—causes the appearance of scaly plaques (patches) over areas of skin where sebaceous glands are most concentrated.

Treatment

In both cases, medicated ℞ **skin preparations** may help. Shampoos containing coal tar, sulfur or selenium sulfide may be effective. Where there is an infective component, preparations containing antibacterials (such as ℞ **sulfonamides**) or ℞ **antifungals** (℞ **ketoconazole**) may be used. Sometimes topical ℞ **corticosteroids** (for example, ℞ **hydrocortisone**) may be used.

For further information

℞ DIRECTORY OF DRUGS:
antibacterial • antifungal • antiseborrheic • corticosteroid • skin preparation

seborrheic dermatitis

see ✪ **dermatitis**.

septicemia

Septicemia (also called blood poisoning) is a condition due to the presence of bacteria in the blood circulation, which then multiply (and may gain access through a dirty wound). It is a dangerous condition because blood travels all over the body; an infection, therefore, can originate from anywhere in the body. It can be a complication of almost all types of serious infectious disease. ✪ **infection** can enter the blood of intravenous illegal drug users from contaminated needles. The result may be the destruction of whole areas of tissue if emergency treatment is not carried out. Symptoms are ✪ **fever** with rigors, and possibly a ✪ **rash** and abscesses (both externally and internally). The condition is most likely to occur in people with reduced immunity, for instance in ✪ AIDS or ✪ **diabetes mellitus**.

Treatment

The usual treatment is with large doses of ℞ **antibacterial** ℞ **antibiotics**.

For further information

℞ DIRECTORY OF DRUGS:
antibacterial • antibiotic

sexually transmitted disease

Sexually transmitted diseases (STD) are any of several infectious diseases, formerly known as venereal diseases, which may be transmitted by sexual intercourse or other sexual contact. They include ✪ **gonorrhea**, ✪ **syphilis**, genital ✪ **herpes**, genital ✪ **warts**, some ✪ **chlamydial infections**, and ✪ AIDS. They are treated by specialists in genito-urinary medicine. Symptoms vary but may include discharge from the penis or vagina, pain on urination, and ulcer-

ation on the sexual organs, mouth, or anus. Complications include ✪ **pelvic inflammatory disease** and sometimes infertility in women; some types of genital warts have been linked with the development of cervical cancer.

Treatment

Treatment depends on the cause but often includes ℞ **antibacterial** antibiotics.

For further information

℞ DIRECTORY OF DRUGS:
antibacterial • antiviral

sexually transmitted infections

see ✪ **sexually transmitted disease**.

shigellosis

see ✪ **dysentery**.

shingles

Shingles (medical name ✪ **herpes** zoster) is an acute ✪ **viral infection** of nerve tracts near the skin. It occurs most commonly in older adults, although it is caused by the same virus (varicella zoster virus/ VZV) that causes ✪ **chickenpox** in children; it is due to the reactivation of the latent virus. Shingles is characterized by a very sensitive, red, blistering rash over the area of skin in which the nerves are affected—commonly the chest, but sometimes the face and eyes. The blisters fill with pus, form scabs, and gradually disappear. Although the symptoms generally decrease of their own accord within four weeks, some effects (especially pain) may continue for months afterward.

Treatment

Treatment is to alleviate the symptoms as much as possible, and may require strong painkillers in the form of ℞ **narcotic analgesics** or ℞ **non-narcotic analgesics**. ℞ **Antiviral** drugs (including topical valacyclovir or famciclovir) may also be given, especially if the eye is affected, or in people who have reduced immunity (for instance in ✪ AIDS).

For further information

℞ DIRECTORY OF DRUGS:
antiviral • narcotic analgesic • non-narcotic analgesic

sickle-cell anemia

Sickle-cell anemia (also called sickle-cell disease) is a hereditary type of ✪ **anemia** that mainly affects people of African or Mediterranean ancestry. Only those who inherit both of a pair of sickle-cell genes, one from each parent, develop the disease (those with only one gene are carriers, meaning they are themselves healthy but will pass the gene to about half of their children; called "sickle trait"). The condition is caused by an abnormality of hemoglobin (the oxygen-carrying molecule) in red blood cells, which causes the cells to be shaped like crescents ("sickle shaped" rather than disks), a process known as sickling. As a result, the cells have difficulty in circulating through narrow blood capillaries, and tend to be broken down instead, leading to anemia and ✪ **jaundice**. Alternatively, there may be widespread thrombosis where the blood cells congregate because they become lodged in small vessels. As an unexpected form of compensation, the disease confers immunity to certain forms of ✪ **malaria** (a common tropical disease transmitted by mosquitoes), which perhaps accounts for the genetic continuance of the trait.

Treatment

There is as yet no cure, and treatment is directed at alleviating symptoms.

sideroblastic anemia

see ✪ **anemia**.

sinusitis

Sinusitis is the ✪ **inflammation** of one or more of the air-filled cavities of the bones of the skull over the eyes, and each side of the nose. All of the sinuses connect with the nasal cavity, and an infection there may spread into the sinuses causing an accumulation of mucus and pus, which, until it drains, may give rise to ✪ **pain** and tenderness. It can be caused by a complication or upper respiratory tract infection, dental extraction, and/or changes in atmospheric pressure such as in air travel.

Treatment

The condition often resolves spontaneously, but treatment with ℞ **decongestant** nose-drops or tablets, ℞ **non-narcotic analgesics** and sometimes ℞ **antibacterial** antibiotics may be needed if ✪ **bacterial infection** is present. A few cases where this fails may require treatment by minor surgery.

For further information

℞ DIRECTORY OF DRUGS:

antibacterial • antibiotic • decongestant • non-narcotic analgesic

Sjögren's syndrome

Sjögren's syndrome is a condition in which there is lack of tear fluid and saliva, resulting in dry eyes and mouth, and sometimes accompanied by joint problems and other symptoms. It is an ✪ **autoimmune disorder**, meaning that the immune system attacks the body's own tissues. Sometimes it occurs in association with other disorders, such as ✪ **rheumatoid arthritis**. It is more common in women than in men.

Treatment

Treatment is to deal with symptoms, including ℞ **eye treatments** in the form of eyedrops—"artificial tears"—containing saline and such substances as ℞ **hydroxypropyl methylcellulose**, which help prevent drying. Also ℞ **NSAIDs** may be used as painkillers for joint pains. The dry mouth may be helped by ℞ **parasympathomimetic** drugs such as pilocarpine.

For further information

℞ DIRECTORY OF DRUGS:

eye treatment • NSAID • parasympathomimetic

skin conditions

Skin is the specialized outermost covering of the body. It acts both as a barrier between the internal organs and the environment, and also as an organ in its own right through functions such as sweating (mediating heat loss in hot environments). It also contains sensory nervous structures that respond to pressure, touch, temperature, itching, and pain; these functions helping the body respond appropriately to the external environment. Skin is composed of a relatively tough and thick outer layer (epidermis) covering a more delicate inner layer (dermis). Beneath these is the fatty subcutaneous layer. The dermis and subcutaneous layers have an abundant blood supply. Projecting through the epidermis from the dermis are other structures such as the sweat glands, hairs cells (surrounded by the sebaceous glands), and nails. The skin takes on a form depending on its function, and within the mouth and cavities of the body is called the mucous membrane. There are many skin conditions and diseases affecting these various structures.

Some skin conditions are generalized conditions affecting many or most skin areas. These include ✪ **psoriasis**, ✪ **eczema** of a number of types, ✪ **dermatitis** of different characteristics (contact, seborrheic), erythema multiforme, ✪ **pityriasis rosea**, ✪ **rashes** with a wide variety of causes, purpura (reddish-purple spots on the skin due to small areas of bleeding from capillaries); due to deficient platelets (for example, thrombocytopenic purpurea—which can be caused by drugs) or as found in old age (senile purpurea).

Some conditions are more localized, and these include ✪ **acne**, ✪ **rosacea**, ✪ **hyperhidrosis**, ✪ **vitiligo**, moles, various neoplasms, ✪ **lupus** (lupus erythematosus), erythema nodosum, seborrheic keratosis, corn(s) and calluses, chapped hands, ✪ **prickly heat**, and cradle cap in babies. A number of skin conditions have principally infectious causes, and these include ringworm, ✪ **scabies**, ✪ **warts**, ✪ **impetigo**, ✪ **athlete's foot**, ✪ **cold sores**(s), and ✪ **dandruff**.

Treatment

Treatment depends on cause. With many conditions often no intervention apart from soothing lotions (for example, ℞ **calamine**) may be indicated. Infections or infestations are treated with specific anti-infective remedies (for example, ℞ **antibacterial** antibiotics, ℞ **scabicide and pediculicidal** agents, ℞ **antifungal** drugs, and ℞ **antiviral** drugs). Where there is an inflammatory component, ℞ **NSAIDs** (topical or oral), ℞ **antihistamine** preparations (topical or oral), topical ℞ **corticosteroids**, and other ℞ **antiallergics** may sometimes be used. For more serious conditions corticosteroid creams or lotions may be required. For the relief of itch, ℞ **antipruritics** may be used (for example, ℞ **crotamiton**, and ℞ **antihistamines**) though are rarely very effective. Many emollient or astringent herbal remedies are promoted for their ability to treat specific, or general skin conditions (agrimony, aloe, cnidium, evening primrose, fenugreek, figwort, gotu kola, heartsease, horehound, Indian mallow, jambul, myrrh, oak, oats, pokeroot, red clover, sea buckthorn, fumitory, stinging nettle, tea tree, walnut, white dead nettle, wild iris, witch hazel, yellow toad flax, German chamomile, yellow dock, linden, bladderwort, Oregon grape, sarsaparilla, golden seal, henna, moneywort, purple loosestrife), and minerals (for example, zinc), vitamins (for example, vitamin A, vitamin B_6, niacin) and supplements (biotin, folic acid, and gammalinolenic acid) are thought to have beneficial or preventive effects. Cradle cap in babies is sometimes helped by shampoos containing the supplement biotin or herbal heartsease. See ℞ **skin preparations** and individual skin conditions for further information.

SLE

see ✪ lupus.

sleep disorders

see ✪ insomnia.

smoking dependency

Smoking dependency is a strong compulsion to continue with the habitual use of tobacco, most often in the form of cigarettes, with an intense craving and irritability if it is suddenly withdrawn. Although smoking represents a means of relieving stress or of boosting concentration, it is also linked with the development of many different diseases, including ✪ **heart disease** and various ✪ **cancers**, especially lung cancer. The nicotine inhaled in cigarette smoke—which is the component responsible for dependence on smoking—causes the release in the body of epinephrine and norepinephrine, which in turn causes a rise in blood pressure by narrowing the blood vessels, and encourages the increase of free fatty acids in the blood. The carbon monoxide inhaled prevents the full exchange of gases in the lungs, depriving the body of oxygen. Other substances inhaled (such as tar) irritate the mucous membrane lining the bronchial passages and may cause lung cancer. Pregnant women and people with heart, blood or breathing disorders are particularly at risk. It has been calculated that for every person who dies in a road accident, four die from smoking-related disorders. It is a type of ✪ **drug dependency**.

Treatment

A huge number of methods for giving up smoking are available, ranging from counseling and support groups to acupuncture and ℞ **substance-dependence treatments** such as nicotine substitutes. The latter, available in various forms including skin patches, give a dose of nicotine without the other harmful ingredients of tobacco smoke, tiding the person over until the habit of smoking is broken. Nevertheless, quitting is extremely difficult and many people take several attempts before they succeed. Lobelia, which contains chemicals similar to nicotine, was formerly used as an anti-smoking aid, and although it is not available as such in the US for this purpose, it can be obtained in the form of a herbal remedy. However, there are potentially dangerous side effects associated with the use of ♣ **lobelia** and its use is not recommended.

For further information

℞ DIRECTORY OF DRUGS:
substance-dependence treatment

snakebite

A snakebite is the bite of a snake, normally resulting in pain and sometimes redness and swelling at the site, with other symptoms according to the type of venom and degree of ✪ **poisoning**, which, in severe cases, may be fatal. People who travel in remote areas of the countryside where poisonous snakes are common are advised to carry a supply of ℞ **antivenin**.

Treatment

If somebody is bitten, the snake should be identified if possible (or killed and kept) to assist a doctor in prescribing as an antidote the appropriate antivenin (an antivenom containing antibodies capable of reacting with, and neutralizing, proteinous toxins in the snake's venom). Otherwise, therapy is supportive.

For further information

℞ DIRECTORY OF DRUGS:
antivenin

sore throat

see ✪ pharyngitis.

sour stomach

see ✪ indigestion.

spastic colon

see ✪ irritable bowel syndrome.

spina bifida

Spina bifida is a relatively common (10–20 per 1000 births) congenital spinal defect in which one or more vertebra (backbones) fail to develop properly, or at all. As a result, a section of the spinal cord is unprotected and may buckle; associated nerves and other tissues may also bulge out of the gap in the spine or be displaced. It is a form of neural tube defect, a group of conditions in which the spine fails to develop properly in the fetus. The condition causes paralysis, potential deformity of areas supplied by affected nerves, and incontinence. There may or may not also be mental retardation. The condition is associated with high levels of a protein, called alpha fetoprotein, in the amniotic fluid surrounding a developing fetus. This enables its detection by a blood test at around the 16th week of pregnancy, with confirmation by amniocentesis and ultrasound if high levels are suspected. The parents will be offered genetic counseling, and a termination of pregnancy (✪ **abortion**) may be an option.

Treatment

Surgical treatment is possible in some cases. The risk of spina bifida is reduced if the intending mother takes ℞ **folic acid** supplements from before the time of conception.

For further information

℞ DIRECTORY OF DRUGS:
folic acid

⚖ VITAMINS, MINERALS, AND SUPPLEMENTS:
folic acid

sprain

Sprains are stretching or partial tearing of one or more ligaments or other tissues around joints, particularly in the ankle. See ✪ **musculoskeletal disorders**.

Treatment

Treatment includes immediate ice packs, ℞ **NSAID** analgesics, and long-term rest. Full healing may take months.

For further information

℞ DIRECTORY OF DRUGS:
NSAID

♣ HERBAL REMEDIES:
comfrey

status asthmaticus

see ✪ asthma.

status epilepticus

see ✪ epilepsy.

stiffness

see ✪ musculoskeletal disorders.

Still's disease

see ✪ arthritis.

sting

A sting is the injection of poison by an insect, especially a wasp, bee, jellyfish, scorpion, sea urchin, or shellfish. Unless the sting causes an allergic reaction, is in a highly sensitive area of the skin, or in a hypersensitive (allergic) person, or is multiple, there is usually no danger.

Treatment

The site should be checked to make sure that the sting (poison sac) is not still in the skin; if it is, it should be scraped out with a fingernail or blunt edge, not pulled out or removed with tweezers (which can squeeze more poison into the skin). Ice can be used to soothe any type of sting. Various OTC topical preparations are available that may alleviate the pain. For severe stings, drugs that may be used include ℞ **NSAIDs**, ℞ **antihistamines**, ℞ **corticosteroids**, and ℞ **local anesthetics**. For those who are liable to ✪ **hypersensitivity reaction**, anaphylaxis treatment may be required (and suitable kits are available for self-injection for bee or for wasp stings).

For further information

℞ DIRECTORY OF DRUGS:
antihistamine • corticosteroid • local anesthetic • NSAID

stomach cancer

see ✪ cancer.

stomach disorders

see ✪ digestive system disorders.

stomach upset

see ✪ indigestion.

strep throat

Strep throat is a ✪ **bacterial infection** of the oral pharynx and tonsils, caused by a strain of *Streptococcus*. Symptoms, which begin abruptly a few days after infection, include chills, fever, sore throat, swollen lymph nodes in the neck, and there can be nausea and vomiting. It is caught after exposure to the bacteria in airborne droplets or after direct contact with an infected person. Complications of strep throat include ✪ **sinusitis**, ✪ **scarlet fever**, and ✪ **otitis** media.

Treatment

A swab may be taken to confirm the diagnosis. Treatment is with **antibacterials** such as penicillin or erythromycin, which may be given by injection. Relatives and carers may be treated to prevent them contracting the infection. Pain relief with analgesics may be necessary.

For further information

℞ DIRECTORY OF DRUGS:
antibacterial • antibiotic • analgesic

Streptococcal sore throat

see ✪ strep throat.

stress

Stress is physical or mental overexertion. Physical stress may aggravate an already existing condition or injury. Mental stress— ✪ **anxiety**, grief, constant pain, and so on—may cause not only behavioral problems but also physical symptoms. Long-term stress may affect the body's hormone balance. Some physical conditions, if not actually caused by mental stress, are certainly made worse by it (such as ✪ **peptic ulcer**, ✪ **migraine**, and some types of ✪ **allergy**). Attempts to remove stress are therefore an important part of the treatment of such disorders.

Treatment

Treatment depends on the source of stress, and will usually include attempts to avoid or reduce lifestyle factors that provoke stress and sometimes training in mental coping skills to deal with stress more effectively. Drugs that may help in the management of stress include ℞ **antidepressant** and ℞ **antianxiety** agents.

There are various herbal remedies, which may be of some benefit in reducing or coping with stress.

For further information

℞ DIRECTORY OF DRUGS:
antianxiety • antidepressant

♣ HERBAL REMEDIES:
codonopsis • ginseng, Siberian • hops • kava kava • oats

stroke

Stroke, which is referred to medically as cerebrovascular accident (CVA) is primarily a vascular condition. However, it is usually followed by neurological damage due to the lack of oxygen (ischemia) in part of the brain. In stroke, there is a disruption in the blood flow to part of the brain, caused either by a thrombus (blood clot) or an embolus (a plug of any sort of material) in an artery supplying the brain (these together are sometimes called ischemic stroke), or alternatively by the bursting of a blood vessel anywhere in the brain. About a half of all strokes follow the formation of blood clots in the arteries of the brain, called cerebral thrombosis. A further third of strokes are caused by bursting of blood vessels in cerebrovascular hemorrhage, called according to where it occurs, subarachnoid hemorrhage (SAH), subdural hemorrhage, or intracerebral (cerebral) hemorrhage. Further causes of stroke are cerebral embolism, which occurs when fragments of a blood clot or other material are carried up to the arteries of the brain from where they originally formed. This is often associated with thrombi formation in heart diseases including ✪ **heart valve disorders**, ✪ **arrhythmias**, and recent ✪ **myocardial infarction** (heart attack). Overall, the risk of thrombi being carried to the brain circulation, or blood clots being formed in vessels, is increased if blood vessel walls are damaged as in ○ **arteriosclerosis**, a disorder in term associated with ○ **hyperlipidemia** and high fat diet, ○ **hypertension**, ○ **diabetes mellitus**, and smoking. The result of these types of interruption of blood supply to the brain is a lack of oxygen in areas of neuronal tissue affected (generally on one side of the brain only). This results in the sudden paralysis of one side of the body (weak and temporary, strong and permanent, or any intermediate form), numbness on one side, slurred speech, clumsiness and loss of fine control; visual disturbances, vomiting, and headache. A mild stroke may precede a more serious one, and if the symptoms persist for less than 24 hours, it is referred to as a transient ischemic attack. Diagnosis and treatment of one event may reduce the chance of a second. The nature of the resulting paralysis depends on the area of the brain affected: very often the weakness is only partial but speech may be affected (if the victim is conscious); sometimes there is incontinence. Some people make a full recovery, but others retain a variety of handicaps (including loss of speech or partial paralysis), which improve only very slowly, if at all. Stroke is the third most common cause of death, and the second most common cause of brain disability in the Western world (after Alzheimer's disease). An old term for a stroke is apoplexy, and today it is sometimes called a "brain attack", serving as a reminder of the speed required in treating it.

Treatment

Short- and long-term treatment depends on the cause of the stroke. Where investigation reveals the likelihood of a blood clot as the cause, intravenous injection of "clot-buster" (℞ **thrombolytic**) drugs is sometimes used, and commonly ℞ **anticoagulant** drugs are used both short-term by injection and long-term by mouth. These are supplemented by drugs that inhibit platelet aggregation, all to reduce the risk of further clots. On the other hand, if the cause is thought to be a bleed, ℞ **nimodipine**, a calcium-channel blocker that has vasodilator actions on the cerebral arteries, may be given because it reduces ischemic damage to the brain tissue following subarachnoid hemorrhage and transient ischemic attacks. Long-term drug treatment of stroke aims to reduce the chance of further strokes by correcting factors that predispose to it; especially lowering blood pressure with ℞ **antihypertensive** drugs, correcting high blood lipids with ℞ **lipid-regulating drugs**, and making lifestyle changes such as taking moderate exercise, and giving up smoking. Physiotherapy (and, if necessary, speech therapy) is necessary mostly to achieve rehabilitation. Depending on the underlying cause, surgery may occasionally be recommended to reduce the risk of a second stroke.

For further information

℞ DIRECTORY OF DRUGS:

anticoagulant (for example, oral **warfarin sodium, dicumarol**; injected **heparin**) • **antiplatelet** agents (for example, **aspirin, clopidogrel, ticlopidine**) • **calcium-channel blocker** (**nimodipine**) • **lipid-regulating drug** (for example, **simvastatin**) • **thrombolytic** (for example, **alteplase, recombinant**) • **vasodilator**

⚖ VITAMINS, MINERALS, AND SUPPLEMENTS:

alpha-lipoic acid • potassium • vitamin E

subarachnoid hemorrhage

see ○ **stroke**.

subdural hemorrhage

see ○ **stroke**.

sunburn

Sunburn is the overheating of the skin by the ultraviolet radiation of the sun. A genuine form of burn, extreme sunburn may cause swelling, blistering, and shock symptoms (○ **heatstroke**). People with fair skin and red hair are more at risk as their skin type is more sensitive. Recurrent sunburn or long-term exposure to the sun over a long period, may cause the skin to age prematurely, and can cause serious skin disorders including ○ **cancer**. Severe sunburn in children increases the risk of malignant melanoma in later life.

Treatment

Treatment is to protect against the excess effects of sun with ℞ **sunscreens** or to avoid further sun exposure, and ease the symptoms with soothing skin preparations.

For further information

℞ DIRECTORY OF DRUGS:

skin preparation • sunscreen

♣ HERBAL REMEDIES:

poplar

superinfections

Superinfections are secondary superimposed infections that occur when another infection is being treated with antimicrobial drugs. In the gut, it normally reflects a change in the normal flora leading to atypical, though not necessarily pathogenic (disease-causing) species, which are resistant to that antimicrobial. They can replicate to become dominant: for instance, yeast organisms may flourish when penicillins are being used during bacterial infection. Yeasts that may do this include *Candida* species, which can cause ○ **candidiasis** (thrush) of the mouth, anus, or vagina. Sometimes the superinfection is an antibiotic-resistant strain of the original pathogenic bacterium, for instance MRSA (methoxycillin-resistant *Staphylococcus aureus*), which are pathogenic staphylococcal superinfections resistant to all regular members of the penicillin family. One form of colitis, ○ **pseudomembranous colitis**, is caused by antibiotic superinfection (for example, bacterial organism *Clostridium difficile*).

Treatment

In the case of MRSA infections, reserved antibiotics (for example, ℞ **vancomycin**) or antibacterial antibiotics unrelated to any other antibiotics (topical ℞ **mupirocin**) have to be used. However, vancomycin-resistant infections (for example, vancomycin-resistant *Enterococcus faecium*; VRE) have now developed. A recently introduced synthetic ℞ **antibacterial** antibiotic, ℞ **linezolid** has been introduced for treatment. In the case of yeast infections, ℞ **antifungals** active against the superinfection are used. Healthy intestinal flora is believed to be encouraged by taking cultures of friendly bacteria as food supplements (for example, ⚖ **acidophilus** and bifidus).

For further information

℞ DIRECTORY OF DRUGS:

antibiotic (linezolid, rifampin, topical **mupirocin**, **vancomycin**) • **antifungal** (for example, amphotericin, ketoconazole)

⚕ VITAMINS, MINERALS, AND SUPPLEMENTS:

acidophilus

sweating, excess

see ✪ **hyperhidrosis**.

syphilis

Syphilis is a contagious ✪ **sexually transmitted disease** (STD) that is caused by ✪ **bacterial infection**. Technically there are three stages of syphilis; it is now rare, however, for the third stage to appear, thanks to modern treatments. Primary syphilis involves the formation of a chancre (hard painless and highly infective sore) at the site of the infection, on a mucous membrane (in the vagina, urethra, mouth, or anus) 1–12 weeks after contact with the infected person. It secretes a highly infectious fluid and persists for between two and six weeks before healing spontaneously. Secondary syphilis appears after a further interval of about 6–24 weeks. Symptoms are headache, high temperature, muscle pain, fatigue, and a rash. Ulcers form in the site of the infection and are again highly infectious; this stage may last for several months. Tertiary syphilis develops in 3–15 years or more, and may affect any part of the body and appear in almost any extreme form—severe heart disease, severe skin or bone disorder, or severe disease of the brain and spinal cord. Symptoms and tissue damage correspond to location.

Treatment

℞ **penicillin** forms the basis of all treatments for syphilis, including ℞ **antibacterial** treatment for those born with the disease (congenital syphilis) due to the mother having the infection.

For further information

℞ DIRECTORY OF DRUGS:

antibacterial

systemic lupus erythematosus

see ✪ **lupus**.

tapeworm

Tapeworms are parasitic ✪ **worms** that may infest the intestines. Flat worm species involved are all of the *Cestoda* class, so they are sometimes called cestodes, and notably include various *Taenia* species. The larvae are consumed in undercooked contaminated beef, pork or fish (for example, raw fish—sushi) and mature into the adult worms once in the intestine. Tapeworms have a hooked head that attaches to the intestinal wall, with a flat, segmented body dangling beneath. Eggs form in the segments, which break off and pass out of the body. The major symptom is the appearance of these segments in the feces; there may also be abdominal pain. Tapeworms can also cause the formation of intestinal cysts, containing more larvae (see also ✪ **worms**).

Treatment

Treatment is with ℞ **anthelmintic** (antihelminthic; antiworm) drugs.

For further information

℞ DIRECTORY OF DRUGS:

anthelmintic

♣ HERBAL REMEDIES:

cotton • lavender cotton

teething

Teething is the period when babies cut their first set of teeth, and is generally during the period from six months to three years old. The eruption of the teeth may produce swollen and inflamed gums, salivation, ✪ **pain**, and fretful behavior in the baby. Sometimes there is high temperature, vomiting or loss of appetite, diarrhea, earache, cough, and rash in the diaper area.

Treatment

Something firm to chew on, painkilling local anesthetic gels, and drugs to lower body temperature (℞ **antipyretics** such as ℞ **acetaminophen**). ℞ **NSAID** analgesics such as ℞ **ibuprofen** may be used in young children on your doctor's advice; ℞ **aspirin** is avoided because of a risk of ✪ **Reye's syndrome**. Topical gels containing local anesthetic such as benzocaine are available OTC for short term use.

For further information

℞ DIRECTORY OF DRUGS:

antipyretic • local anesthetic • NSAID

temporal arteritis

see ✪ **arteritis**.

tendinitis

see ✪ **musculoskeletal disorders**.

tennis elbow

see ✪ **musculoskeletal disorders**.

tension headache

see ✪ **headache**.

testicular cancer

see ✪ **cancer**.

tetanus

Tetanus is a serious central nervous system (CNS: brain and spinal cord) condition that is caused by infection with spores of the bacterium *Clostridium tetani*. This causative organism lives in soil, manure, and sometimes the human gut, and tends to infect through open cuts and wounds. In developing countries it can kill newborns through ✪ **bacterial infection** of the umbilical stump. Symptoms include stiffness of the jaw (lockjaw; trismus), back, abdomen, and muscles of the face. Eventually these effects on the muscles may stop the subject breathing, resulting in death.

Treatment

Normally this is by vaccination to prevent the infection in all likely to contract it, either with single vaccines or combined with others. In the event of contracting tetanus, a human ℞ **immune globulin** may be used to neutralize the bacterial toxin liberated. If there are convulsions or excessive muscle tetanus, ℞ anticonvulsant drugs of various types may be used, sometimes by intravenous injection. Specialized supportive nursing, including the use of oxygen, is required.

For further information
℞ DIRECTORY OF DRUGS:

anticonvulsant (including **benzodiazepine (diazepam)** • **barbiturate (secobarbital sodium)** • **immune globulin (tetanus immune globulin)** • **phenothiazine (chlorpromazine)** • **skeletal muscle relaxant (methocarbamol)** • **vaccine (diphtheria and tetanus toxoid, adsorbed (DT; Td), tetanus toxoid, adsorbed)**

threadworm
see ✪ **worms.**

thrombocytopenia
see ✪ **bleeding disorder.**

thromboembolism
A thromboembolism is the presence of a blood clot that has become detached from its site of origin and traveled around the bloodstream (embolized) to lodge elsewhere. Causes are those of ✪ **thrombosis**, and symptoms may be similar. However, the most common site for an embolus to lodge is in the lungs (✪ **pulmonary embolism**); a large embolus here may cause sudden death, smaller ones may cause ✪ **heart failure** or lung symptoms including coughing up of blood.

Treatment
Treatment depends on the site but may include ℞ **thrombolytic** drugs to dissolve the clot (thrombolysis) or, particularly with a pulmonary embolus, surgery to remove the obstruction. Long-term, ℞ **anticoagulant** and ℞ **antiplatelet** drugs may be taken to reduce the risk of further incidents.

For further information
℞ DIRECTORY OF DRUGS:

anticoagulant • antiplatelet • thrombolytic

thrombophlebitis
Thrombophlebitis is the clotting of blood (✪ **thrombosis**) that occurs at the site of an inflammation in the wall of a vein (✪ **phlebitis**). Pregnant women are particularly at risk, and it typically occurs in the leg veins, producing pain, tenderness, and swelling, with local redness in the skin if superficial veins are involved. If deep veins of the calf are involved (✪ **deep vein thrombosis**), complications can include thromboembolism. See also ✪ **peripheral vascular disorders.**

Treatment
Treatment of superficial thrombophlebitis is with elasticated support of the area, and ℞ **anti-inflammatory** and ℞ **analgesic** drugs. Treatment where deep veins are involved may require drugs to prevent thromboembolism, including long-term ℞ **anticoagulant** and ℞ **antiplatelet** drugs.

For further information
℞ DIRECTORY OF DRUGS:

anticoagulant • thrombolytic

thrombosis
Thrombosis is characterized by the presence of one or more blood clots in a blood vessel. It may be caused either by disease or deformity of the blood vessel, or by a disturbance of the blood clotting mechanism—or by a combination of both. There may be associated inflammation. The result of thrombosis in an artery is a deficiency in blood circulation to the tissues supplied by the blood vessel. If this is the heart or the brain, symptoms of ✪ **myocardial infarction** or ✪ **stroke** may follow, and emergency treatment is necessary. If the clot (thrombus) becomes detached from its original site, it may travel (as an embolus) around the circulation until it lodges elsewhere—which may be equally dangerous.

Treatment
Treatment depends on diagnosis and location, but may include ℞ **thrombolytic** drugs to dissolve the clot (thrombolysis) or, sometimes, surgery. Long-term, ℞ **anticoagulant** and ℞ **antiplatelet** drugs may be given to reduce the risk of further incidents.

For further information
℞ DIRECTORY OF DRUGS:

anticoagulant • antiplatelet • thrombolytic

thrush
see ✪ **candidiasis.**

thyroid cancer
see ✪ **cancer.**

thyroiditis
see ✪ **hypothyroidism.**

thyrotoxicosis
see ✪ **hyperthyroidism.**

tinea
Tinea is a term that covers any of a group of ✪ **fungal infections**, usually of the skin, nails or hair. Medically the second part of the name denotes the area affected, thus tinea pedis is ✪ **athlete's foot** and tinea cruris affect the groin, tinea capitis affects the head, tinea corporis affects most of the body; tinea unguium affects the nails, tinea versicolor affects the skin and causes tan-colored patches. Many of the fungi are from a group called dermatophytes, and some forms are called ringworm.

Treatment
Treatment is with ℞ **antifungal** drugs in the form of powders or creams, together with thorough drying of the areas affected after washing. Some stronger oral agents are reserved for deep-seated infections, for instance ℞ **griseofulvin** for nail infections.

For further information
℞ DIRECTORY OF DRUGS:

antifungal drugs including **antibiotic** agents (for example, **griseofulvin**), many **azole** agents (for example, **clotrimazole, econazole, ketoconazole, miconazole, oxiconazole, sulconazole nitrate**) • **benzoic acid** • **clioquinol** • **haloprogin** • **naftifine** • **selenium sulfide** • **terbinafine** • **tolnaftate** • **undecylenic acid**

♣ HERBAL REMEDIES
clove • myrrh (athlete's foot)

tinnitus

Tinnitus is noises heard in the ear not caused by external sounds. Often the cause is not discovered, but the condition may result from an excess of wax, high blood pressure, infections of the eardrum or inner ear, the use of certain drugs (such as ℞ **aspirin** and ℞ **quinine**) or disorders such as ✪ **Ménière's disease**, ✪ **anemia**, and ✪ **hyperthyroidism**.

Treatment

Treatment depends on the cause; any underlying condition should be corrected, if possible, and any hearing loss alleviated with a hearing aid. Otherwise, relaxation techniques and masking with a white noise machine may be helpful in reducing the distress caused by the sounds.

For further information
♣ HERBAL REMEDIES:
ginkgo

tonsillitis

Tonsillitis is the ✪ **inflammation** of the tonsils (the bulging tissues at either side of the back of the mouth) that may be caused by (often streptococcal) ✪ **bacterial infection** or ✪ **viral infection**. Symptoms are a sore throat, high temperature, headache, and difficulty in swallowing. Young children may additionally suffer stomach cramps and abdominal pain, and are particularly vulnerable to repeated attacks. Acute tonsillitis may accompany ✪ **scarlet fever**.

Treatment

Treatment depends on diagnosis of the infective organism but also concentrates on alleviating the symptoms; ℞ **antibacterial** antibiotics may be used in cases of bacterial infection. The practice of surgically removing the tonsils (tonsillectomy) is now rare except in cases of excessively recurrent tonsillitis.

For further information
℞ DIRECTORY OF DRUGS:
antibacterial • antibiotic
♣ HERBAL REMEDIES:
thyme

toothache

see ✪ **pain**.

tooth decay

Tooth decay (medically called dental caries) is caused by the bacterial invasion—promoted by sugary and acidic foods and drinks—of the plaque (layer of debris) that adheres to the surface enamel of a tooth. This can cause the gradual decomposition of the enamel and erosion of the dentine that comprises the substance of the tooth. Untreated, the destruction of the tooth eventually reaches the pulp, causing toothache, and potentially forming an abscess. Tooth decay can be prevented to a great degree by minimizing the intake of sugary foods and fruit drinks, by regular oral hygiene, and by the application of fluoride salts (an ingredient of many tooth-

pastes). Fluoride is present in drinking water in many communities or is added (in the developed world).

Treatment

Dental repair involves the removal of any decay (using a drill), and the stopping up of the resultant hole with a filling material. Dental preparations containing fluoride salts (for example, sodium fluoride) can be used in mouthwashes or tooth gels, as well as in toothpastes.

For further information
℞ HERBAL REMEDIES:
clove • green tea • kava kava

Tourette syndrome

see ✪ **brain-motor disorders**.

toxic shock syndrome

Toxic shock syndrome is a severe acute condition in which shock develops as a result of ✪ **bacterial infection**, usually *Staphylococcus aureus*. There is a sudden collapse of blood pressure, and the person will be weak, pale, and sweaty. It is most often linked to the use of tampons, which can provide a site for bacterial growth in the vagina.

Treatment

Treatment involves ℞ **antibacterial** antibiotics and often a drip to rebalance body fluids.

For further information
℞ DIRECTORY OF DRUGS:
antibacterial • antibiotic

toxocariasis

see ✪ **worms**.

toxoplasmosis

Toxoplasmosis is a potentially dangerous ✪ **protozoal infection** resulting from infestation by a parasitic protozoan (*Toxoplasmosis gondii*), which can use almost any mammal (for example, cats) or bird as its host. People ordinarily contract toxoplasmosis by eating undercooked meat that contains the protozoan larvae, possibly by contamination from animal feces. Symptoms are usually relatively mild—muscle pains, slight lymph node enlargement—but may sometimes be severe, especially in people with reduced immunity (as in ✪ **AIDS**). More severe symptoms can involve secondary inflammations and, in pregnant women, abnormalities in the fetus or a miscarriage.

Treatment

Treated early, the condition responds quickly to drugs that are active against ℞ **amebicide and antiprotozoal** infections, including ℞ **sulfonamides** and drugs also used as ℞ **antimalarials**.

For further information
℞ DIRECTORY OF DRUGS:
amebicide and antiprotozoal • antimalarial • sulfonamide

tracheitis

see ✪ **respiratory tract disorders**.

Key to symbols: ✪ = Disorder Section ℞ = Drug Section ♣ = Herbal Section ⚕ = Supplement Section

trachoma

Trachoma is an infectious disease, a ○ **chlamydial infection** that affects the cornea and conjunctiva of the eye. The organism responsible for this persistent infection is one of the virus-like bacterial organisms called ○ **chlamydia** (*Chlamydia trachomatis*), and is transmitted by direct contact and by flies. The infection causes ○ **conjunctivitis**, photophobia (an aversion to light) and watering eyes, and eventual damage to the mucus and tear glands resulting in dry eye (keratoconjunctivitis sicca). Unless treated, trachoma may cause blindness.

Treatment

℞ **antibacterial** antibiotic drugs used topically or by mouth are used to eradicate infection. Surgery may be necessary to treat scarring.

For further information

℞ DIRECTORY OF DRUGS:
antibacterial (**macrolide, sulfonamide,** and **tetracycline** drugs)

transient ischemic attack

see ○ **stroke**.

traveler's diarrhea

see ○ **giardiasis**.

travel sickness

see ○ **motion sickness**.

trench mouth

see ○ **gingivitis**.

trichomoniasis

Trichomoniasis (trichomoniosis) is a ○ **protozoal infection** caused by the protozoan *Trichomonas vaginalis*, which is a unicellular organism. It is a common cause of troublesome ○ **vaginitis** in women, and is usually transmitted sexually. It may also, less commonly, cause urethral infection in men, when it is often symptomless. Diagnosis may involve taking swabs for laboratory analysis.

Treatment

℞ **antibacterial** ℞ **antiprotozoal** drugs by mouth are used to eradicate infection.

For further information

℞ DIRECTORY OF DRUGS:
amebicide and **antiprotozoal** (**azole** drugs including **metronidazole**)

trichotillomania

Trichotillomania is the habit of constantly pulling at the hair by the person with the condition. It is seen in children, psychotic individuals, and those with developmental metal handicap. See ○ **affective disorders**.

Treatment

This depends on the cause, and may involve psychotherapy, ℞ **antipsychotic** drugs and certain ℞ **antidepressants** (for example, ℞ **fluoxetine**).

For further information

℞ DIRECTORY OF DRUGS:
antidepressant • antipsychotic

trigeminal neuralgia

Trigeminal neuralgia is a disorder of the trigeminal nerve (fifth cranial nerve, a sensory neuron), which causes episodic, often severe, stabbing pain in regions of the face including the cheek, chin, and gums. It is generally quite incapacitating for the duration of the attack, seconds to minutes, and causes a wincing (which gives it the alternative name tic douleux meaning painful twitch). It is generally seen in middle life or later, but in the young may be associated with ○ **multiple sclerosis**. The cause of the hyperexcitability of the trigeminal nerve is not known, and often simply touching the cheek, shaving, eating, or drinking may bring on an attack. It may even be caused just by talking. See ○ **neuralgia**.

Treatment

No treatment is sure to be affective, but a number of drugs usually prescribed for other purposes may be tried ("off-label"), often alternated because resistance to a single drug tends to develop. Conventional analgesics are rarely effective.

For further information

℞ DIRECTORY OF DRUGS:
carbamazepine • clonidine hydrochloride • imipramine • phenytoin • topical **capsaicin**

tuberculosis

Tuberculosis is a potentially serious ○ **bacterial infection** caused by a bacillus (*Mycobacterium tuberculosis*) that may attack any part of the body and cause tissue damage. It is usually transmitted by the inhalation or ingestion of infected droplets. The primary site of infection is the lungs and associated lymph nodes, at which point the disease may halt temporarily or permanently. Diagnosis may be difficult. It may show no real symptoms or it may cause weight loss, high temperature, and blood in the sputum. If the disorder spreads into the bloodstream, the effects are widespread and may be catastrophic, causing long-term ill health. It can be fatal.

Treatment

Treatment is with a combination of ℞ **antituberculosis** drugs (often certain ℞ **antibiotics** in combination with other ℞ **antibacterial** drugs including ℞ **sulfonamide**-related drugs), and is usually symptomatically rapidly effective, although the drug course will have to be maintained for many months to prevent recurrence. It always requires medical attention.

For further information

℞ DIRECTORY OF DRUGS:
antibacterial • antibiotic • antituberculosis • sulfonamide
♣ HERBAL REMEDIES:
myrrh • Solomon's seal

tumor

A tumor, or neoplasm, is a new and anomalous growth of cells where there should be none. Some tumors are harmless (benign), while others continue to grow and are liable to have parts that detach and drift elsewhere and start new tumors (termed malignant), through a process called metastasis. Malignant tumors are called ✪ **cancers** and are categorized by the type of cells of which they are composed. Hollow swellings filled with liquid, however, especially on the skin surface, are much more likely to be abscesses (filled with pus) or cysts (fluid-filled swellings.) Any unexpected lump, detected internally (perhaps by palpation—examination by feeling), should be immediately diagnosed by a doctor.

Treatment

Treatment depends on the type of tumor but may involve surgery to remove the lump and, for cancerous tumors, radiotherapy or ℞ **anticancer** (antineoplastic) chemotherapy.

For further information

℞ DIRECTORY OF DRUGS:
anticancer • cytotoxic

typhoid fever

Typhoid fever is a ✪ **bacterial infection** caused by a species of *Salmonella* (*S. typhi*) bacteria. Other species cause milder forms of the disease including paratyphoid (*S. paratyphi*). Typhoid is usually contracted by eating or drinking something contaminated with infected human urine or excreta. The bacteria multiply in the intestines and travel through the wall of the small intestine into the bloodstream, where they are carried to other organs throughout the body. Symptoms are very high temperature, slow heartbeat, nosebleed, and abdominal pain; there is usually a rash on the front of the body. Delirium may follow. Complications may include ✪ **pneumonia** or intestinal bleeding. Symptoms abate after two weeks, and the disease clears by the fourth week. Diagnosis may require culture tests.

Treatment

Treatment is with ℞ **antibiotics** and other ℞ **antibacterial** drugs, if necessary, transfusions. A ℞ **vaccine** is available. Good hygiene is the best protection.

For further information

℞ DIRECTORY OF DRUGS:
antibacterial • vaccine

ulcer

An ulcer is an open lesion (sore) on the skin or a mucous membrane that results from necrosis (destruction and death) of tissue due to causes such as ✪ **inflammation**, ✪ **infection** or physical damage or pressure (pressure ulcer; see ✪ **bedsore**). As a site, the lower leg is common and leg ulcers are often slow to heal. On mucous membranes, ulcers are commonly seen in the mouth (see ✪ **mouth ulcers**), but can extend to most sites within the digestive tract (see ✪ **ulcerative colitis**, ✪ **peptic ulcer**.) Genital ulcers are relatively common, and there can also be corneal ulcers of the eye. Tissue ulcers are a feature of many inflammatory disorders (for example, ✪ **Behçet's syndrome**) and infections.

Treatment

If infection is a component, ℞ **antibacterial** drugs may be used topically or orally. Inflammatory conditions sometimes require ℞ **corticosteroids**. The pain of mouth ulcers may be relieved with ℞ **local anesthetics**. Skin ulcers require careful bandaging. Often, dietary improvement and possibly vitamin supplementation helps

persistent ulcers. A number of herbal remedies are promoted as being beneficial for skin and other superficial ulcers. (See also ✪ **peptic ulcer**).

For further information

℞ DIRECTORY OF DRUGS:
antibacterial • corticosteroid • local anesthetic • ulcer-healing drug

♣ HERBAL REMEDIES:
Superficial ulcers: aloe • blessed thistle • chamomile, German • devil's claw • hops • horse chestnut • kava kava • myrrh • plantain • sage • white lily
Peptic ulcers: marshmallow • yarrow

⚖ VITAMINS, MINERALS, AND SUPPLEMENTS:
Superficial ulcers: vitamin A

ulcerative colitis

Ulcerative colitis is the inflammation and ulceration of the part of the large intestine called the colon, and, usually, the rectum. Ulcerative colitis occurs mostly in young adults, without evident cause. Symptoms are attacks of diarrhea, bleeding from the anus, pain, and internal spasm. In the long term, the condition may eventually result in perforation (rupture) of the intestine, and ✪ **peritonitis**. It makes up, with ✪ **Crohn's disease**, one of the two main disorders described as inflammatory bowel disease (IBD), a general term for chronic inflammatory diseases affecting the small or large intestine.

Treatment

Treatment is generally with drugs of several different types, including ℞ **aminosalicylates** (for example, ℞ **mesalamine**), ℞ **antidiarrheals** (℞ **loperamide**, ℞ **diphenoxylate**), ℞ **corticosteroids**, and sometimes ℞ **immunosuppressants** (℞ **cyclosporine**, ℞ **azathiaprine**). Surgery may also be necessary; recurrent bouts may require a colostomy (diversion of part of the intestine to open through the abdominal wall into a bag).

For further information

℞ DIRECTORY OF DRUGS:
aminosalicylate • antidiarrheal • corticosteroid • immunosuppressant

♣ HERBAL REMEDIES:
barley

ulcerative gingivitis

see ✪ **gingivitis**.

undulant fever

see ✪ **brucellosis**.

urethritis

Urethritis is the ✪ **inflammation** of the urethra (the tube conveying urine from the bladder to the outside). It is caused by sexually transmitted infection that may be specific (such as ✪ **gonorrhea**) or non-specific (non-specific urethritis), or by lesser local infection spread, for example, from the bladder (✪ **cystitis**). Symptoms are frequent and uncomfortable urination and a painful discharge.

Treatment

Treatment, following diagnosis, is usually with ℞ **antibacterial** antibiotics.

For further information

℞ DIRECTORY OF DRUGS:

antibacterial • antibiotic

♣ HERBAL REMEDIES:

marshmallow • uva-ursi

urinary retention

see ✪ urinary tract disorders.

urinary tract disorders

The urinary system includes all systems from production of urine in the kidneys, passage in the ureters to the bladder, and thence via the urethra to expulsion from the body. There are many potential disorders to these systems.

Urinary tract infections are relatively common, and if untreated there is always a risk that the infection will regress to the kidneys and cause serious damage. ✪ **bacterial infections** can cause ✪ **cystitis** (inflammation of the bladder), ✪ **urethritis** (inflammation of the ureter), and pyelonephritis (inflammation of the kidney). Some forms of urethritis are caused by ✪ **sexually transmitted diseases**, including ✪ **gonorrhea** and non-specific urethritis (NSU). Factors that predispose to infection include any condition that impairs drainage, including enlarged prostate as in ✪ **benign prostatic hypertrophy** (BPH) or ✪ **prostatitis**, urethral stricture, pregnancy, urinary tract stones (✪ **calculus**), bladder tumor, problems with nervous control (for example, in spinal injury and ✪ **spina bifida**), also infrequent urination or inadequate fluid intake.

Urination (micturition) difficulties, either too frequent or not sufficiently frequent, also painful micturition, may in turn be related to a number of disorders, including urinary tract infections, ✪ **diabetes insipidus**, or uncontrolled ✪ **diabetes mellitus**. Urinary incontinence in the elderly or women who have had children, can be due to physical changes, lowered tone in the muscle controlling the urethra and associated structure, of problems in the nerve supply (including after surgery, especially for BPH or ✪ **prostate cancer**). Nocturnal enuresis (✪ **bed-wetting**) is common in children but may continue in adulthood where there are physical or emotional problems.

Treatment

Treatment depends on cause. Most infections can be treated with ℞ **antibacterial** drugs of an unusually wide range, especially those that are excreted unchanged into the urine, including ℞ **antibiotics**, ℞ **sulfonamides** and derivatives, and ℞ **quinolone** antibacterials. Urinary retention of physical origin is sometimes treated with parasympathomimetic drugs that stimulate bladder smooth muscle tone directly. Conversely, urinary frequency, particularly in BPH, can be treated with drugs that affect the actions of either the sympathomimetic nervous system or the parasympathomimetic nervous system (which together control emptying of the bladder) or by drugs that relax bladder smooth muscle tone, or herbal remedies such as saw palmetto or stinging nettle. ℞ **Parasympathomimetic** drugs include: ℞ **bethanechol chlo-**

ride, ℞ **alpha-adrenergic blocker** agents, ℞ **doxazosin,** ℞ **phenoxybenzamine,** ℞ **prazosin hydrochloride,** ℞ **tamsulosin hydrochloride,** ℞ **terazosin,** and (antimuscarinic) ℞ **anticholinergic** agents including: ℞ **atropine sulfate,** ℞ **hyoscyamine,** ℞ **oxybutynin,** and ℞ **tolterodine tartrate.** ℞ **anticholinesterase** agents (℞ **neostigmine methylsulfate**) are also used. Phenazopyridine and phenyl salicylate can be used as topical analgesics to alleviate irritation of the urinary tract and bladder. ℞ **Citrates** of sodium and potassium are available in OTC remedies as alkalizing agents for the relief of discomfort of mild urinary tract infection by making the urine less acid. If there is infection, then ℞ **antibiotic,** ℞ **sulfonamide,** and ℞ **quinolones** drugs may be necessary. Herbal remedies for urinary tract disorders in general include ♣ **angelica,** ♣ **arenaria rubra,** ♣ **asparagus,** ♣ **beans,** ♣ **birch,** ♣ **bladderwort,** ♣ **celery,** ♣ **corn silk,** ♣ **couchgrass** (*Agropyron repens*), ♣ **dandelion,** ♣ **echinacea,** ♣ **fringed pink,** ♣ **goldenrod,** ♣ **hartstongue,** ♣ **horseradish,** ♣ **horsetail,** ♣ **Java tree,** ♣ **lichwort,** ♣ **lovage,** ♣ **nasturtium,** ♣ **parsley,** ♣ **pipsissewa,** ♣ **poplar,** ♣ **sandalwood,** ♣ **spiny rest harrow,** ♣ **stinging nettle,** ♣ **uva-ursi,** ♣ **yarrow,** ♣ **saw palmetto,** ♣ **stinging nettle,** ♣ **pumpkin,** and ♣ **juniper.** See individual disorders for more information.

urticaria

Urticaria (also called hives or nettle rash) is a ✪ **skin condition** due to a minor allergic reaction of the skin, involving an itching rash or area of round wheals; occasionally there are also raised lumps or swelling. Symptoms may last from a couple of hours to several months. The triggering factor is usually dietary (particularly shellfish, eggs, or strawberries), but may occasionally be an infection. See also ✪ **angioedema**.

Treatment

Treatment usually involves topical application of ℞ **antihistamine** preparations.

For further information

℞ DIRECTORY OF DRUGS:

antihistamine

♣ HERBAL REMEDIES:

peppermint

uveitis

Uveitis is inflammation of the uveal tract of the eye. Causes include ✪ **allergy,** ✪ **diabetes mellitus,** trauma, ✪ **infection,** ✪ **autoimmune disorders** (for example, juvenile chronic arthritis), and some inflammatory disorders (for example, sarcoidosis). The symptoms of anterior uveitis include red and watery eyes, blurred vision, eye ache, sensitivity to bright light, and a small irregular pupil. In posterior uveitis, there may be blurred vision and also spots or haziness in the visual field. If left untreated, some types of uveitis can lead to ✪ **glaucoma** and seriously impaired vision.

Treatment

℞ **mydriatic** (atropine sulfate, scopolamine hydrobromide) eyedrops are given to dilate the pupil and to stop the iris from sticking to the lens. ℞ **anti-inflammatory** drugs including ℞ **corticosteroids** (for example, dexamethasone, hydrocortisone, and prednisolone acetate) and ℞ **NSAIDs** (for example, flurbiprofen) may be prescribed to treat any inflammation.

For further information

℞ DIRECTORY OF DRUGS:
corticosteroid • mydriatic • NSAID

vaginal thrush

see ✪ **candidiasis**.

vaginitis

Vaginitis is the inflammation of the vagina, causing pain and discharge. It is commonly caused by a change that affects the normally harmless bacteria ordinarily present in the vagina—for example, a new method of contraception, having sexual intercourse for the first time or changing sexual partner, or starting a regimen of antibacterials. The bacteria then cause an ✪ **infection**. Vaginitis can occur after the ✪ **menopause** as a result of a lack of female sex hormones. It may also be a symptom of a ✪ **sexually transmitted disease** such as the ✪ **fungal infection** ✪ **candidiasis** (thrush) or ✪ **protozoal infection** such as ✪ **trichomoniasis**.

Treatment

Treatment depends on the cause but may involve ℞ **antibacterial**, ℞ **antifungal** or ℞ **amebicide and antiprotozoal** drugs; often the sexual partner should also receive treatment.

For further information

℞ DIRECTORY OF DRUGS:
amebicide and antiprotozoal • antibacterial • antifungal
♣ HERBAL REMEDIES:
cnidium • uva-ursi

varicose veins

Varicose veins are distended and twisted veins, blue when close to the skin surface, caused through internal pressure—for instance on the pelvic veins during pregnancy (see ✪ **pregnancy-related disorders**)—or damage to the valves that would normally control the blood back-flow. There may be some hereditary predisposition. They occur most commonly in the legs, where damage to the valves and veins may cause ✪ **phlebitis** and venous thrombosis, but are also found fairly often at the anus (as ✪ **hemorrhage**). Symptoms, apart from appearance, are pain and local swelling.

Treatment

Treatment consists largely of supportive pressure, the artificial creation of thrombosis in the vein to occlude (close) it (sclerotherapy) including with ℞ **sclerosing agents** (for example, ℞ **ethanolamine oleate**, ℞ **sodium tetradecyl sulfate**), or surgery to repair or remove it.

For further information

℞ DIRECTORY OF DRUGS:
sclerosing agent
♣ HERBAL REMEDIES:
horse chestnut • witch hazel

vascular disease

see ✪ **cardiovascular disorders**.

venereal disease

see ✪ **sexually transmitted disease**.

venous insufficiency

This is an abnormal circulatory condition characterized by a decreased return of the venous blood from the legs to the trunk of the body. Symptoms of venous insufficiency include edema (see ✪ **fluid retention**) and ✪ **pain**, and ulceration may follow.

Treatment

This usually consists of elevation of the legs and use of elastic hose. The underlying cause of the condition will be treated appropriately. Many herbal remedies are said to be beneficial in treating symptoms.

For further information

℞ DIRECTORY OF DRUGS:
diuretic
♣ HERBAL REMEDIES:
bilberry • butcher's broom • horse chestnut • witch hazel

verruca

A verruca is a type of ✪ **wart**, which when it occurs on the soles of the feet is sometimes referred to as a plantar wart. Projecting from the skin surface, verrucas are naturally subject to great pressure on standing and walking, and may become callused over and cause pain. They are caused by the common ✪ **wart** virus and are highly contagious, to the extent that epidemics in schools and sports changing-rooms are not uncommon.

Treatment

Treatment is to remove them by freezing with liquid nitrogen, application (under careful medical supervision) of caustic solutions (including ℞ **salicylic acid** available OTC), cauterization, or surgery.

For further information

℞ DIRECTORY OF DRUGS:
keratolytic (formaldehyde, imiquimod, podofilox, salicylic acid)

vertigo

Vertigo is extreme dizziness, in which the immediate environment is falsely perceived to be spinning round at high speed or tilting at an angle. The result of a disorder of the mechanism that regulates balance (in the inner ear or the auditory nerve and its center in the brain), it may be caused by infection, low or high blood pressure, or drug abuse. The disabling effect may be accompanied by ✪ **nausea** and ✪ **vomiting**; also, occasionally, other difficulties in vision and hearing. Medical diagnosis is essential.

Treatment

Treatment depends on the cause but may include ℞ **antiemetic** (antinauseant) drugs to alleviate the symptoms.

For further information

℞ DIRECTORY OF DRUGS:
antiemetic
♣ HERBAL REMEDIES:
ginkgo

Key to symbols: ✪ = Disorder Section ℞ = Drug Section ♣ = Herbal Section ⚕ = Supplement Section

vestibular disorder

Vestibular disorders are any of a group of disorders that affect the vestibular apparatus (semicircular canals and related structures) of the inner ear. Infection of these organs results in ✪ **vertigo**, dizziness, nausea, and impaired hearing. A longer-term disorder is ✪ **Ménière's disease**, which affects the functions of hearing and balance, and is believed to be caused by fluid build-up in the inner ear, with symptoms including recurrent bouts of ✪ **tinnitus** (ringing in the ears), ✪ **nausea**, and temporary ✪ **deafness**.

Treatment

Infections of the inner ear are treated with oral ℞ **antibacterial** antibiotics. Symptoms of infection and of Ménière's disease may be helped by ℞ **antiemetics** with ℞ **antinauseant** properties, and some of these help the feelings of vertigo and dizziness.

For further information

℞ DIRECTORY OF DRUGS:
antibacterial • **antiemetic/antinauseant** (for example, **dimenhydrinate, meclizine hydrochloride, scopolamine hydrobromide**)

viral enchephalitis

see ✪ encephalitis.

viral infection

Viral infections include relatively trivial diseases such as ✪ **warts**, everyday infections such as the common ✪ **cold**, through to more serious complaints such as ✪ **influenza**, to often-lethal conditions such as ✪ **Lassa fever**, ✪ **rabies**, and ✪ **HIV**. Viruses differ from bacteria in that they are smaller and simpler—being unable to grow or reproduce outside the body of the host organism. They reproduce by inserting their genetic machinery—their genome—into the cellular machinery of the host, causing it to replicate viral genetic material. There are two main sorts of virus: DNA viruses where the nucleic acid genetic material is in the form of two intertwined strands of DNA, and the RNA viruses, which are comprised of a single strand. Some viral infections are linked to ✪ **cancer**.

Treatment

There are various antiviral strategies including improvements in public hygiene to reduce the chance of infection, natural or induced immunity, and drug intervention. The body uses its immune system to produce antibodies that "recognize" the virus and cause it to be engulfed by macrophages carried in the bloodstream. When this is successful there will be immunity against a second attack of infection. Immunization with specific vaccines aimed at a given type of virus is normally a highly effective procedure, and has lead to the elimination of smallpox, the near elimination of poliomyelitis, and effective control of chickenpox, mumps, measles, hepatitis A and B, yellow fever, rabies, and some others. This approach is most effective with DNA viruses and some RNA viruses, which are relatively stable in form. However, RNA viruses can readily mutate into new forms sufficiently different so as not to be recognized by the host. It is for this reason that vaccination is more difficult against, for instance influenza, the common cold, and HIV (human immunodeficiency virus). Antiviral drugs have been developed that target various stages in viral movement within the body, viral attachment to the host cell, or replication within it. For instance, some effective anti-HIV drugs utilize the fact that HIV is an RNA retrovirus containing an enzyme called reverse transcriptase, which it must use to make a DNA copy of the viral RNA. This copy is incorporated into the host genome. Thus, the reverse transcriptase inhibitor group of antiviral drugs (for example, ℞ **zidovudine** and ℞ **didanosine**) are inhibitors of this key viral enzyme, and so prevent replication of the virus. Because of mutations of the HIV virus conferring resistance to individual drugs, it has now become common to use multidrug therapy, where combinations of two or more drugs are used (for example, reverse transcriptase inhibitors with protease inhibitors) for long periods to prevent HIV developing into full-blown AIDS. Thus, some antiviral drugs can be lifesavers in immunocompromised individuals. Serious cytomegaloviral infections may also be contained by treatment with ℞ **ganciclovir**. Infections due to the ✪ **herpes** viruses (for example, cold sores, genital herpes, shingles, and chickenpox) may be prevented or contained by early treatment with ℞ **acyclovir**. Some herbal remedies (such as ⚕ **garlic**) and supplements (such as ⚕ **vitamin C** and ⚕ **alpha-lipoic acid**) are promoted as being beneficial in preventing, treating or reducing tendency to ✪ **infections** in general.

vitamin deficiency

Vitamin deficiencies (also called avitaminosis) are conditions that result from a deficiency or lack of absorption, or use by the body, of one or more vitamins. Symptoms depend on the vitamin concerned, for instance vitamin C deficiency can result in ✪ **scurvy**, vitamin D deficiency can result in ✪ **rickets** in children and ✪ **osteomalacia** in adults. Young children and the elderly, and those with ✪ **malabsorption disorders** are particularly prone.

Treatment

Treatment of the underlying cause and supplementation with the vitamin concerned.

For further information

℞ DIRECTORY OF DRUGS:
the vitamin concerned

♣ HERBAL REMEDIES:

alfalfa (many vitamins) • **blackcurrant** • **brewer's yeast** (B vitamins) • **garden cress** (vitamin C) • **lime** (vitamin C) • **scurvy grass** (vitamin C) • **sea buckthorn** (vitamin C) • **watercress** (vitamin C)

⚕ VITAMINS, MINERALS, AND SUPPLEMENTS:
the vitamin concerned

vitiligo

Vitiligo is a hypopigmentation condition in which patches of surface skin lose all melanin (skin pigment) pigmentation, and become white. Beginning anywhere in the body, the patches may expand to cover most of it—or may gradually disappear as pigmentation is somehow restored. It is an ✪ **autoimmune disorder** (one in which the immune system attacks the body's own tissues), which especially affects dark-skinned races.

Treatment

Treatment may be with plant-derived photosensitizing drugs (for example, methoxsalen, trioxsalen) combined with ultraviolet light (UVA) radiation therapy. This may help especially if the person has darker skin coloring. The depigmenting agent monobenzone may be used in the final stage of depigmentation of excessive vitiligo. In other cases camouflage make-up is often recommended. Exposure to sun should be regulated.

vomiting

Vomiting is the forcible ejection of the contents of the stomach through the mouth, an involuntary act that is a symptom of many disorders. There are usually other accompanying symptoms including the subjective symptom of ✪ **nausea**, salivation, sweating, pallor of the skin, and other cardiovascular changes. Sometimes there is an overpowering sense of nausea but with no actual vomiting. The nervous impulses that cause the reflex response originate in the so-called "vomiting center"—a chemoreceptor trigger zone in the brainstem. Activation of the trigger zone can be caused by toxins released in food poisoning (for example, ✪ **cholera**), radiation therapy, and many drugs including opiates such as morphine, general anesthetics, many cancer chemotherapeutic agents, and some antibiotics. Vomiting is a characteristic symptom of many separate diseases or states, notably ✪ **Ménière's disease**, ✪ **Addison's disease**, ✪ **food poisoning**, ✪ **gastroenteritis**, ✪ **hepatitis**, ✪ **pancreatitis**, ✪ **peptic ulcer**, various brain and neuroendocrine tumors, as well as ✪ **motion sickness**, and ✪ **pregnancy-related disorders** (✪ **morning sickness**).

Treatment

Vomiting is a symptom so its method of treatment depends on the cause and the individual concerned. Where possible, the cause of the vomiting should be corrected. Any treatment of vomiting in pregnancy requires expert medical advice and in general no medicines or herbal remedies should be taken without advice. Of the drugs used for emetic symptoms, there are ℞ **antiemetic** drugs that prevent vomiting (emesis) and also drugs that are ℞ **antinauseant**, which are used to reduce or prevent the sensation of nausea that very often precedes the physical process of vomiting. In practice, there is considerable overlap between the two drug types, and the terms are mainly used interchangably. Antiemetics are used to help reduce the vomiting that accompanies radiotherapy and chemotherapy, and certain types may work by actually preventing vomiting, and helping the passage of food out of the stomach into the gut; that is, they act as gastrointestinal motility stimulants. Some of these drugs act at the chemoreceptor trigger-zone in the brain. Generally, where nausea and subsequent vomiting can be anticipated, treatment in advance is more effective, for instance in motion sickness (travel sickness), also in the treatment of cancer by radiotherapy, and chemotherapy. For these latter purposes, cannabis derivatives (for example, nabilone) are on trial for treating difficult cases.

For further information

℞ DIRECTORY OF DRUGS:
anticholinergic drug (for example, **scopolamine hydrobromide**) • **antiemetic/antinauseant**—including **serotonin-receptor**

antagonist agents (**dolasetron mesylate, granisetron, ondansetron**) • **antihistamine** (for example, **dimenhydrinate, meclozine hydrochloride**) • **motility stimulant** (**metoclopramide hydrochloride**) • **phenothiazine** (for example, **chlorpromazine, perphenazine, trientine hydrochloride** • others (for example **droperidol, haloperidol**)

♣ HERBAL REMEDIES:
black horehound • clove • galangal • nutmeg • wild iris

von Willebrands' disease

see ✪ **bleeding disorder**.

wart

Warts are columnar growths on the skin. Usually painless, harmless and small, warts constitute the first type of (usually benign) tumor definitively known to be caused by a virus, the human papillomavirus (papavirus group). Pigmented or not, they may appear virtually anywhere on the skin—but particularly on the hands, elbows, and knees—and may disappear as quickly and spontaneously. They are named according to their appearance and the different sites on the body on which they occur, and include plantar warts, common warts, and verrucas. Some around the genital region are sexually transmitted, and some types of the papavirus, which cause genital warts may be linked with the development of cervical cancer. Others on the soles of the feet may be painful because of the pressure constantly put on them. Corns can look similar but are on the skin of a foot joint or toe, and are caused by pressure due to ill-fitting shoes.

Treatment

Treatment is generally only necessary for genital warts and verrucas, although it may be administered elsewhere for cosmetic purposes. Removal of a skin wart is by application of caustic solutions (℞ **keratolytics** available OTC), or by cauterization or freezing under medical supervision. Genital warts require specialist treatment and, for women, regular smear tests thereafter. Treatment of corns is also with keratolytic agents.

For further information

℞ DIRECTORY OF DRUGS:
keratolytic

♣ HERBAL REMEDIES:
heartsease • oats • willow

wasp sting

see ✪ **sting**.

wasting palsy

see ✪ **amyotrophic lateral sclerosis**.

water retention

see ✪ **fluid retention**.

Weil's disease

see ✪ **leptospirosis**.

Wernicke-Korsakoff syndrome

see ✪ brain-motor disorders.

whipworm

see ✪ worms.

whooping cough

see ✪ pertussis.

Wilson's disease

Wilson's disease is a rare inherited ✪ metabolic disorder caused by a deficiency of the protein that carries copper in the blood. It leads to copper deposits in the liver, which on release cause liver and brain disease. It is named for Samuel Wilson (1878–1937), an English neurologist. The person may have jaundice, mental retardation, and parkinsonism (see ✪ Parkinson's disease), and often has a characteristic brown ring in the eyes due to copper deposits.

Treatment

Drug treatment with ℞ chelating agents aims to mop up excess copper, and can prevent mental retardation and other symptoms if started early enough.

For further information

℞ DIRECTORY OF DRUGS:
chelating agent (penicillamine, trientine hydrochloride)

wind

see ✪ flatulence.

worms

The term worms refers to a parasitic infestation by any of various types of primitive legless animals, particularly by a type that attacks the intestines. Symptoms may include diarrhea, abdominal pain, and sometimes fever; untreated infection may lead to anemia, malabsorption of food, and complications such as intestinal ✪ ulcers, liver abscesses, or lung disease. There are a number of types of parasitic worms. Infestation by roundworms (also called hookworms, pinworms, threadworms, or seaworms): the species involved is commonly *Enterobius vermicularis*, which causes enterobiasis; or *Strongyloides stercoralis*, which casues strongyloidiasis. Infestation by ✪ tapeworms (*Cestoda* class) is mainly of the intestines, although tapeworms can also affect the liver. Infestation by flukes tends to affect the blood vessels, bladder, liver, or lungs: diseases caused include ✪ schistosomiasis.

Treatment

Treatment in all cases is with ℞ anthelmintics (antiworm) drugs or, if necessary, surgery.

For further information

℞ DIRECTORY OF DRUGS:
ulcer-healing drug including H$_2$-antagonist (for example, cimetidine, famotidine, nizatidine, ranitidine hydrochloride) • proton-pump inhibitor (for example lansoprazole, omeprazole, pantoprazole sodium, rabeprazole sodium)

♣ HERBAL REMEDIES:
elecampane • lavender cotton • quassia • thyme

wound

A wound is any trauma to the skin and sometimes underlying tissues by mechanical damage, including surgery. There are various types of wound, including abrasion (graze), laceration, contusion, and penetrating wounds.

Treatment

Wounds that are not too serious can be treated by normal first-aid measures, including cleaning and dressing the wound. More serious wounds may need suturing (stitching), and if contaminated may need antibacterial treatment rather than simple antiseptics. Many herbal remedies are available to apply externally to aid wound healing.

For further information

℞ DIRECTORY OF DRUGS:
antibacterial • antiseptic

♣ HERBAL REMEDIES:
aloe • bistort • blessed thistle • cajuput • chamomile, German • echinacea • elm bark • horsetail • marigold • poplar • rosemary • selfheal • shepherd's purse • smartweed • St. John's wort • raspberry

⚖ VITAMINS, MINERALS, AND SUPPLEMENTS:
royal jelly and bee products (propolis) • vitamin C

Zollinger-Ellison syndrome

Zollinger-Ellison syndrome is an uncommon condition where there is recurrent ✪ peptic ulcer formation in the stomach and duodenum. The cause is over-secretion of the gut hormone gastrin (usually because of a tumor in the gastric region consisting of cells of the type normally found in the pancreas gland), which causes secretion of large amounts of acid in the stomach leading to ulceration. Because of the acid, there may also be ✪ diarrhea and abnormal fatty feces.

Treatment

Usually the tumor is removed surgically, but ℞ ulcer-healing drugs may be used to control acid secretion prior to surgery.

For further information

℞ DIRECTORY OF DRUGS:
ulcer-healing drug including H$_2$-antagonist (for example, cimetidine, famotidine, nizatidine, ranitidine hydrochloride) • clotrimazole, econazole, ketoconazole, miconazole, oxiconazole) • proton-pump inhibitor (for example, lansoprazole, omeprazole, pantoprazole sodium)

PART 2

DIRECTORY OF DRUGS

Directory of Drugs

The drugs industry is one of the most rapidly expanding areas of commerce. Although pharmaceutical companies are increasingly international in their organization, many (whether US- or foreign-owned) have a strong base in the USA. In research and development, scientists in the USA have an enviable record of innovation. Also, in the later stages of drug development, which involve clinical trials and ultimately the approval and continuing licensing of drugs for use in patients, the FDA (Food and Drug Administration) sets world standards for authoritative assessment of safety and efficacy of drugs. The USA currently has one of the most restrictive and safety-motivated legislation policies in the world, which limits the majority of drugs to prescription-only use.

The fuel for this success story in the pharmaceutical industry over the last two or three decades, has come from the discovery and development of some hundreds of new generic drugs, often representing entirely new classes of drugs. The first of the relatively recent, completely new, and massively successful classes of drugs include the beta-blocker "heart-drugs" and the ulcer-healing H_2-antagonists. These drugs were not discovered by chance. They were developed by making logical, and extensive, chemical variations on the natural neurotransmitter or hormone involved, in order to obtain useful drugs that work by blocking recognition areas (receptors) on the cell membrane.

Similar logic has been applied in discovering drugs that target important enzymes and selectively inhibiting them. For example, the antihypertensive angiotensin-converting enzyme (ACE) inhibitors, phosphodiesterase inhibitor vasodilator drugs used as heart drugs and in impotence treatment (for example, sildenafil, the generic drug in the brand Viagra), and cholinesterase inhibitors for dementia treatments (for example, donepezil, in the brand Aricept, and rivastigmine, in the brand Exelon). There have been many other notable advances in recent years, including "best-selling" drugs for depression, for example, the SSRI antidepressant fluoxetine (the generic drug in the brand Prozac), a number of antiviral drugs used in the treatment of HIV/AIDS, and proton-pump inhibitors for ulcer treatment. More advances most certainly will come with new methods of manufacturing complex new drugs using gene technology, as discussed below.

Drugs from plants

Many new drugs have come from and will continue to come from nature. Indeed, before World War II, herbal medications were listed side-by-side with "chemical drugs" in the US Pharmacopeia. The Herbal Remedies section of this book confirms the considerable potential there is for identifying and developing active components found in traditional herbal remedies and incorporating them into modern healthcare programs.

Pharmacology and medicinal chemistry have a long history of discovering lead compounds in plant and other natural organisms. In the second half of the twentieth century, hundreds of valuable antibiotics were developed from ferments of fungal molds. Chemicals isolated from such ferments are used not only for treating infections by microorganisms but also as cytotoxic agents in cancer treatment, and as starting chemicals in the discovery of drugs for a variety of further purposes.

Notable recent examples of natural chemicals developed for therapeutic use include the taxane group of chemically complex alkaloids (for instance, paclitaxel/Taxol), which have a central place in the treatment of ovarian and breast cancer. Drugs of this type were originally isolated from the bark of the rare Pacific yew tree, but there are now several such drugs manufactured semisynthetically from needles of the common yew. It should be noted, as discussed in the introduction to the Herbal Remedies section of this book, that modern commercial drugs tend to be single active compounds with one clearly defined pharmacological activity. Herbal remedies, in contrast, can contain dozens, or even hundreds, of biologically active compounds, which can have multiple pharmacological targets. In orthodox medicine, the isolation of a single active compound is regarded as important, or necessary, for two good reasons.

First, both safety and efficacy of a drug depends on reliability and careful control of dose. For all chemical remedies, orthodox or herbal, there is a limited margin of safety between the dose that is effective for the therapeutic purpose, and the higher dose at which serious adverse toxic effects may be encountered. For some medicines the ratio of these two doses, sometimes called the therapeutic ratio, is worryingly small. For digitalis glycosides found in the foxglove (*Digitalis purpurea*), and still used to treat heart failure, this ratio can be less than twofold. Over the years when medical preparations were manufactured directly from extracts of foxglove leaves, different batches of leaves were found to vary greatly in pharmacological effect, so elaborate biological standardization procedures were necessary to ensure safety. In use today, pure preparations of the isolated cardiac glycosides—the active chemicals are digoxin and digitoxin—are available, so it is easier to ensure consistent therapeutic effect and a greatly reduced risk of adverse toxicity. This principle of ensuring safety through controlling dose, applies to all forms of medication. In a similar way it has been necessary to isolate and purify other natural products, such as hormones of animal origin (including insulin and growth hormone), to ensure reliability and safety of dosing. The purity of medications is important, because all too often impurities in natural products have proved to be a major cause of toxicity.

Second, the isolation of a single active compound from natural medicines has the advantage that it allows synthetic chemical variations to be made, with a view to improving some aspects of the drug, such as potency, specificity, duration of action, ease of absorption, and other important properties. While it is true that many prescribed drugs have their origins in natural substances from fungi, higher plants, or animals, in many cases it is not the original chemical that is used, but some semisyn-

thetic or synthetic analog. In some cases the original pure plant chemical (for example, the opiate morphine extracted from crude opium) coexists in orthodox medical use alongside some dozens of newer narcotic analgesic drugs made by a small or large chemical modification of the original molecule. In other cases, the original plant compounds (for instance, drugs like the classic skeletal muscle relaxant, tubocurarine, which was once used during the majority of operations) have been completely supplanted by newer synthetic drugs.

The manufacture of complex drugs

A major reason for using natural products has been that, purely as chemicals, they are often very complex molecules that would be difficult to make entirely synthetically. Some drugs have to be manufactured semisynthetically using plant chemicals which may in themselves be pharmacologically inactive. For instance, steroid hormones are chemically complex, but since the basic steroid structure occurs in many plants, there is the opportunity to use their steroids as a source. For example, "natural" estrogen and progestin hormones—used in hormone therapy and contraception—are manufactured from a sterol found wild in Mexican yams.

Although many sorts of alkaloid and steroid drugs can be manufactured semisynthetically from plants and fungal molds, this leaves many types of drug inaccessible by this route. Many hormones (for example, insulin and growth hormone) and natural factors (including the cytokines and blood formation and coagulation factors) in the body are peptides or small proteins, and drugs required to replace or supplement them, or modify their actions, are too complex to be made by conventional chemical means. In the past, where practicable, these proteins have been extracted from animal tissues. However, they may not be available in adequate amounts, and there are purity and safety concerns.

The role of gene technology

The recent development of genetic engineering applied to drug manufacture has changed all this. It is now possible to manufacture even large proteins and related chemicals, including those normally present in the animal body in tiny amounts. Drugs that can now be manufactured include such vital drugs as hormones (especially human insulin and human growth hormone). A new form of drug called monoclonal antibodies can now be manufactured. These are pure protein molecules of human form, which in principle might work as a sort of specific "magic bullet," targeting only certain sites in the body so as to deliberately modify function. Such antibodies (for example, daclizumab, basiliximab, palivizumab, and rituximab) are already proving valuable as new types of immunosuppressants for use in organ transplantation. Other genetically engineered drugs appearing in this book include enzymes (dornase alfa and imiglucerase), a number of hemostatic, hematopoietic, and antihemophilic factors (including erythropoietin, Factor VIII), vaccines (notably hepatitis B vaccine), and cytokines (interferons and interleukins).

In this way, life-prolonging novel treatment, for example, for cancer, AIDS, bleeding and hormone-deficiency diseases, is becoming economically as well as theoretically possible. A bonus of these biosynthetically manufactured drugs is their enhanced safety, especially in preventing infection, immune reactions and other biological complications. For example, human growth hormone, which is used to treat short stature (dwarfism) in children, was at one time isolated from the pituitary glands of cadavers and so brought with it the risk of acquiring Creutzfeldt-Jakob disease due to infecting contamination. However, it has now been replaced in the USA by somatropin, which is a biosynthetic human form that has no risk of contamination.

Future developments

Will this rapid progress continue? Some people within the industry are not optimistic because of escalating costs of drug development—to produce just one new drug can take years and cost millions. However, new research strategies involving the emerging science of molecular biology and genetic engineering, may prove cheaper and more effective, and allow the development of amazing new sorts of drugs.

Progress in the chemotherapy of infection in the past few decades has not be smooth. In the fight against bacterial and some other infections there were several decades of enormous optimism and progress, and we now have over 100 generic antibiotic drugs in use in the USA alone (and detailed in this book), and these can be used in treating a very wide range of bacterial infections. Additionally, several chemical families of entirely synthetic agents have been developed, for example, quinolones against bacterial infection and azoles against fungal and protozoal infections. But, at the same time, there has been worldwide over-use of antibiotics, and strains of bacteria resistant to all but a few "reserve" antibiotics, especially infections by MRSA (methoxycillin-resistant *Staphylococcus aureus*), are becoming all too common. The pharmaceutical industry has to look again for sources of new antibacterial drugs.

Turning to the search for chemotherapeutic drugs active against viruses rather than bacteria, initial progress was slow, partly because no antibiotics are effective against viruses. About two decades ago virtually no antiviral drugs were known, but then the spread of AIDS infection proved a catalyst in terms of research expenditure, and there are now over two dozen antiviral agents available in the USA (and detailed in this book), and more are emerging all the time. Most of these drugs were developed in logical ways from studying differences in the biochemistry of the virus compared to their animal hosts, and devising drugs that could inhibit growth or kill viruses without doing too much damage to the human host. In fact, many of these antiviral drugs are relatively simple chemicals, many being nucleoside analogs that resemble cellular molecules necessary to viral function or replication, and often working as enzyme inhibitors against an essential virus-specific enzyme.

In terms of the development of resistance by pathogenic (disease-causing) organisms, the moral from the treatment of tuberculosis and other very serious infections has been that multidrug treatment often proves better in the long run. The concurrent use of two or three different classes of antiviral drugs in the treatment of AIDS (for example, protease inhibitors together with reverse transcriptase inhibitors) has proved to be of great benefit to the patient (and also to a child born to a mother with the disease).

The next revolutionary advance is expected to be the development of "individualized" medications, which are tailored to the particular person being treated. This may be one of the spin-offs of the Human Genome Project now that the entire human genetic code has been sequenced. It is now technically possible to examine the genome of an individual and identify areas within the chromosomes that make that person genetically susceptible to particular diseases (but who may not yet have symptoms), or likely to be at risk of an adverse reaction from certain drugs. Early attempts are already being made to delete, replace, or prevent expression of defective genetic material (for example, by transfer of DNA in gene therapy for cystic fibrosis). These future approaches can be regarded as a special extension of drug therapy.

How are drugs prescribed and used?

Successful medical therapy has always depended on a partnership between the patient and medical professionals—pharmacists, doctors, and nursing staff. Everyone is different and requires individual treatment, which is a truth that is often easy to forget in a world where the mass-production and standardization of products and practice is regarded as the norm. Medicines are prepared and tested according to the most rigorous criteria of standardization, for the sake of safety as well as for economic efficiency. But because people are all likely to be different to some degree, either in their basic genetic make-up or in the circumstances surrounding the condition they are seeking to treat, an individual's response to a certain drug must therefore be taken into account.

Where prescribed medicines are concerned, the doctor has the information and knowledge to allow him or her to help interpret specific needs and situations, and prescribe accordingly. But an increasing number of medicines are now becoming available without prescription and can be bought directly from a pharmacy (OTC, or over-the-counter).

Associated with this is a growing trend to give an increasing share of the advisory role to the pharmacist. However, the doctor will know important details of a patient's history and present condition, which is privileged information that will not be available to the pharmacist. Consequently, this trend towards making more medicines available without prescription places a substantial responsibility for choosing the correct medication on the individual, or on carers in the case of children, the elderly, and those who are too ill to cooperate. This book contains much of the information necessary for making sensible choices.

The FDA and licensing medicines

In the USA, virtually all aspects of the use of drugs is the responsibility of the federal agency the FDA (Food and Drug Administration), which enforces federal regulations on the manufacture and distribution of drugs, foods, and cosmetics, and which has the task of preventing the sale of impure or dangerous substances. As explained in the introduction to the Vitamins, Minerals, and Supplements part of this book, for legislative and operational purposes, drugs are separated under the Dietary Supplement Health and Education Act (DSHEA), 1994, from vitamins, minerals, herbs or other botanicals, and amino acids. All of this latter group are treated as dietary substances, and are regulated in a similar manner to food products, and they cannot be marketed as medicines or food additives.

This means that it is only in the case of drugs can claims be made in relation to the suitability or otherwise of a drug product in relation to disease. The present position of the FDA in relation to drug safety and efficacy can best be understood by looking at its development from its origins. Under early drug regulation in the USA, as in the first Federal Food and Drug Act of 1906, there were no requirements to establish drug safety and efficacy (it was mainly concerned with the interstate transport of misbranded or adulterated food and drugs). This act was amended in 1938 following the deaths of about 100 children resulting from the marketing of a sulfonamide drug dissolved in a toxic solvent, and the FDA was entrusted with enforcing the act which now required truthful labeling and safety of drugs. For the first time toxicity studies were required and new medicines had to receive approval through a new drug application (NDA), but efficacy was not defined and so it was still possible to market a drug with extravagant claims. Following a period of rapid expansion of marketed drugs, there was a further check due to the thalidomide disaster of the 1960s, which resulted in a worldwide concern about possible teratogenic (causing abnormalities in fetal development) and other toxicity of new drugs. For the first time, the use of drugs was debated publicly, and it became clear that many unnecessary drugs were being marketed worldwide.

In the USA concern led to amendments to the 1962 Food, Drug and Cosmetics Act in 1962, called the Harris-Kefauver Amendments. This modification of working practice meant that the FDA required proof from pharmacological and toxicological research, submitted as an application for an investigational new drug (IND) before clinical studies in people could begin. For drugs introduced after 1962, proof of efficacy and documentation of toxicity was required so that the new drug could be evaluated in terms of risks-to-benefit ratio for the disease that was to be treated. This is still basically the scheme today, although there have been a number of alterations and amendments to it in practice. Closely associated with the FDA is the Center for Drug Evaluation and Research (CDER), which examines drugs both for safety and therapeutic effectiveness. Similar schemes have come into being in other countries, and examples include organizations such as the Committee on Safety of Medicines (CSM) and the Drugs Control Agency (DCA) in the UK, and the European Medicines Evaluation Agency (EMEA).

This degree of legislation has both increased the cost involved in bringing a drug to the market (about $500 million per drug) and delays the introduction (the average drugs takes 10 to 12 years to develop). Although the FDA employs about 8,000 people, the complexity of the review process means that the number of approvals of some categories of drug fell to an all time low in spite of increased applications. Last year, in the category for new molecular entities, the number fell from 35 to 27.

The slow progress of new drugs becoming available reflects a conflict between the right of the consumer and consumer groups to have prescribed only drugs with evidence of a high risks-to-benefit ratio, and the need of manufacturers to develop and market new drugs quickly and effectively. In practice, the delay means that patients at risk are not getting new and effective medication in a timely manner. The delay has been brought to a head by the needs of people with AIDS. A new short-cut procedure has been brought into play in such cases, where for life-threatening diseases new drugs can be used with limited evidence with regard to efficacy and safety.

For mainline medications, the present FDA arrangements regulate all aspects of the manufacture and distribution of drugs. One important end result is that individual brand preparations of generic drugs have approval for specific diseases or conditions, when administered by a specific route, and with other limitations. When a drug is marketed there is an approved package insert, a patient information leaflet or product information leaflet provided by the drug manufacturer in cooperation with the FDA, which is intended to be read by the patient or carer. It includes clearly stated information about special care or precautions to be taken when using a particular drug.

Clinical trials submitted as evidence for approval cover only limited circumstances. It is a provision of the relevant act that the FDA cannot interfere with the practice of medicine, and once the efficacy of a drug has been established, this allows the physician to determine appropriate use. In practice, drugs are often used in a number of "off-label" or "unlabeled" uses. Some of these uses are quite routine, others may not be as well established or may reflect more recent research. This book mentions common off-label uses in generic drug articles.

Since the thalidomide disaster, there has been much greater awareness of the possibility of damage to the fetus, and also the growing infant, by drug action, however rare this may be. Largely on the basis of animal data, the FDA classifies drugs into five categories. The use-in-pregnancy rating system (A, B, C, D, X) weighs the degree to which available information has ruled out risk to the fetus against the drug's potential benefit to the patient. They range from category A, where controlled studies in pregnant women show no risk to the fetus, to category X, where the drug is contraindicated in pregnancy because of positive evidence of fetal abnormalities or a degrees of risk that clearly outweighs any possible benefit to the patient. The categories are used uniformly, however, the precautionary language used by individual manufacturers for individual drugs can vary.

The move to non-prescription drugs

The process of moving towards non-prescription rather than prescription drugs is referred to as "the switch process" or the "Rx-to-OTC switch." The number of drugs switched each year from prescription-only to an OTC (over-the-counter or non-prescription) status has been substantial in the last two decades. More than 80 ingredients, dosage-forms, and strengths have been switched from Rx status or introduced as new OTC drugs since 1976, accounting for over 700 marketed products. This switch has had a great effect on the marketing of proprietary medicines. For example, the analgesic drug ibuprofen was one of the prescription drugs that changed status comparatively recently, and now there are 20 major OTC proprietary preparations of it listed in this book alone. For acetaminophen, which switched much earlier, there are over 240 major preparations listed.

Members of several major drug groups have quite recently had their status changed from Rx to OTC. For example, members of the ulcer-healing H_2-antagonist group (for example, ranitidine, used in the brand Zantac) are now available OTC (although only for the treatment of dyspepsia/indigestion rather than ulcers), a number of OTC corticosteroid preparations (for topical (external) use for certain skin conditions), and antifungal treatments (for thrush infections) have all become available without prescription.

However, there is controversy as to whether these common OTC preparations (especially the common analgesics—acetaminophen, aspirin, and ibuprofen) should be available from general retail outlets such as grocery stores, discount stores, and other convenient retail outlets. Some believe that the sale of some or all OTC preparations should be restricted to sales supervised by a qualified pharmacist (normally in a pharmacy). But others argue that this is a druggists' monopoly and will only serve to maintain high prices.

As more medicines become readily available without prescription, authorities in the USA expect people to become more skilled at knowing when they should seek expert advice. For much the same reasons, the list of drugs that may be prescribed by ancillary health workers has also been extended, and it is likely that various healthcare workers will be empowered in future either to prescribe or to recommend medication.

Controlled Substances Act

The non-medical and illicit use of drugs is an increasing problem. Controlled substances come under the jurisdiction of the Controlled Substances Act (1970). Such drugs are categorized according to their potential for abuse: the greater the potential, the more strict the limitations on their prescription. Category I covers substances that are deemed to have no medical use (for example, heroin or LSD). Categories II to V regulate certain medical drugs, from morphine (Category II), with high addictive potential, to low-dosage codeine (Category V), with negligible addictive potential. The kinds of drugs covered in the schedules are mostly opioids, tranquilizers, hallucinogens, stimulants (for example, amphetamine), and anabolic steroids.

Drugs and the traveler

Anyone traveling abroad should be aware that the generic names of drugs differ little between countries. This book lists generic drugs under American standard names (United States Adopted Name; USAN), but in most cases gives major European or International ones (International Non-proprietary Name; rINN), so it should be valuable for use when traveling. One of the best-known examples is acetaminophen, which is called paracetamol in the UK.

Proprietary names used by a manufacturer for the same generic drug are today less likely to be totally different according to the country in which it is marketed, although there may be minor variations in spelling to accommodate local requirements. It is important to note that some medicines available abroad, both OTC and prescription, may not have been rigorously tested or approved in the USA. A pharmacist should always be consulted in cases of doubt.

Drugs and the Internet

There is now quite wide availability of medicines (and medical advice) on the Internet, and much of this is essentially unregulated and unverified. Some of the medicines offered for sale (notably Viagra) are actually prescription-only in the USA. Clearly this is yet another set of circumstances where the individual needs access to impartial and accurate information of the type that this book can offer. To determine whether a web site is a licensed pharmacy in good standing, the reader can check with the *National Association of Boards of Pharmacy* (NABP) (www.nabp.net; 847 698-6227), who issue a certification called *Verified Internet Pharmacy Practice Sites*™ (VIPPS™) to approved sites.

Using medicines

How are medicines taken? Medicines have to be able to get to the place where they are to work. How they are given to do this is called the "route of administration." They can be applied directly to the site of action (topically), by mouth (orally), by injection (parenterally), by rectum (rectally), via the lungs (by inhalation), and through the skin (transdermally). There are good reasons why different routes of administration are chosen for different purposes.

For example, when a medicine is being used to treat a skin, vaginal, ear, nose, mouth, or eye condition, the best way to achieve this is by preparing (formulating) the medicine in a form that can be applied directly (such as a cream, pessary, or drops). When a medicine is applied directly to the site at which it acts, it is called a topical medicine; and because, in general, very little of the medicine enters the body, systemic side effects are likely to be few and minor. Inhalation is another way of delivering a medicine to the site where it is to have its therapeutic effect (the bronchioles (small airways) of the lungs), and again this route of administration limits side effects if it is a drug that is little absorbed from there into the bloodstream. However, some drugs are inevitably absorbed in small amounts so act systemically (for example, corticosteroids when inhaled in asthma prophylaxis).

Often, however, medicines need to be inside the body in order to reach the tissue of an organ that needs to be treated (for example, kidney, heart, or blood vessels). This is mainly achieved by allowing the drug to travel to the relevant tissue or organ in the bloodstream. So when a medicine is taken by mouth (orally), it is absorbed from the stomach or intestine, enters the bloodstream of the body in much the same way as nutrients do from food, and is then transported to its site of action. After transdermal application, the medicine enters the body through the skin (for instance, hormone therapy in the menopause, nicotine patches for quitting smoking). Injection is another way of introducing a medicine into the body, and is a useful route of administration when a drug needs to act quickly (and avoids the drug getting broken down by the gastrointestinal tract). Sometimes "depot" injections are used where the medicine is released slowly into the blood from a "pool" injected under the skin. These systemic routes of administration, where the medicine is conveyed in the bloodstream, mean that the drug reaches most tissues and organs in the body, in addition to the ones it is being used to treat, and for this reason drugs taken systemically may have quite extensive side effects. Sometimes a medicine may have to be taken rectally, in the form of an enema, suppository, or solution. This may be because the person is too ill to take the medicine by mouth (in particular if the person is vomiting), or because the medicine would be broken down by the stomach.

Why do side effects occur?

One of the biggest problems associated with taking medicines relates to their possible side effects.

Drugs act by having specific effects on the body, usually to attack the cause or relieve the symptoms of an illness. However, while dealing with the conditions they were designed to treat, many drugs also affect the body in other, undesirable ways that are incidental to their primary purpose. These adverse reactions, or side effects, may be so mild as to be barely noticeable, or so severe as to be life-threatening, depending both on the drug and on the individual.

Adverse reactions that result in side effects can be categorized into one of two main kinds, Type A reactions and Type B reactions.

Type A reactions are inherent in the way the drug acts pharmacologically, and are largely inevitable and very difficult to circumvent. For instance, the side effects of drowsiness and sedation (due to actions on the brain) are so common with antihistamines that they are accepted by most people as inevitable. However, the pharmaceutical industry is well aware of the inconvenience of side effects, and attempts are continually being made to minimize them. For example, newer antihistamines are altered chemically to restrict the drug's access to the brain. It is important to be aware that such developments are occurring so that, where undesirable side effects are experienced, discussion with a physician may result in finding a more individually acceptable treatment.

Type B reactions are less predictable, and are often referred to as "idiosyncratic." A major cause of these idiosyncratic reactions is a true allergic reaction to a drug by the body's immune system. A sensitivity reaction of this kind can be a serious threat, and the dangers can only be minimized if the person is aware of the danger because of an earlier reaction to a drug of that class. Physicians routinely ask whether a person is allergic to antibiotics or local anesthetics before prescribing them—and everyone must know his or her own idiosyncratic (allergic) responses. After immunizations with vaccines, such as those using egg products in their manufacture, the person is asked to stay afterwards for at least 20 minutes because of possible allergic reactions. However, some antibiotics, local anesthetics, and other drugs that cause allergic reactions are now available over-the-counter for non-prescription use, so it is vitally important to read the patient information leaflet that comes with the medicine, and be aware of the warning signs of reaction. In particular, some medicines contain arachis oil (peanut oil) to which many are now allergic.

Post-marketing surveillance by the manufacturer and direct reporting, means that new drugs in particular are monitored for all suspected adverse drug reactions. If the FDA has sufficient concern then there may be specific warnings about the type of patient for whom the drug should not be prescribed, and sometimes the early withdrawal of that drug from the market.

Are drugs really safe?

Questions about drug safety only make sense on a risk-to-benefit basis. In other words, does the severity of the condition warrant risking certain known side effects? At one end of the scale, for example, is a certain individual's headache sufficiently severe that it is worth risking the known side effects of aspirin? If the individual is in good health with no history of intolerance to NSAID (non-steroidal anti-inflammatory drugs), and no form of stomach upset, then the answer may well be Yes. On the other hand if the individual is a child under 12 years, or a person who has a predisposition towards gastric ulcers or asthma, then the answer will be No.

At the other end of the risks-to-benefit scale is the person who has a life-threatening infection, or a disorder as serious as cancer. Then the physician may discuss with him or her whether to prescribe a treatment with drugs that would be too toxic to use for a less serious condition.

In terms of risks-to-benefit, vaccination is an extremely valuable precaution. It can, by treating the most vulnerable sectors of the population, completely eliminate some infectious diseases. Smallpox infection no longer exists in the world population, and poliomyelitis may soon be eliminated; both as a result of global vaccination programs. MMR vaccination of children has been introduced with the intention of eliminating mumps, measles, and rubella (German measles).

Although there may be very rare incidences of serious adverse reactions, most people accept that these risks are far outweighed by the considerable threat to children of contracting the infections themselves. And in any vaccination program, it is important that all children, rather than just a selection, are vaccinated, or the diseases may regenerate in the unvaccinated group and so become re-established in the population.

When interpreting the side-effects of individual drugs listed in this book, it is important to understand that the longer the period a drug has been in use, the longer the list of possible side effects is likely to be. Conversely, new drugs may appear to be free of side effects because relatively little is known about them as they are still going through the reporting processes. In the listings provided in this book, generally the most frequently experienced side effects appear first, while those at the end of the list are likely to be seen less often, often with some comment.

Similarly, the "warnings" are based on experience that doctors accumulate in using that drug, and some drugs may not be used by certain people (they are "contraindicated"), so an alternative drug may be tried.

It can also be seen that the majority of the drugs in this book should be avoided by women who are pregnant or breast-feeding, because, although it is not always known that they are dangerous to the baby, the lessons of the thalidomide disaster have not been forgotten.

Individuals at risk of adverse reaction

People suffering from the following conditions are particularly susceptible to certain drugs or forms of drug treatment. Although the conditions are generally rare, it is very important to be aware of them, and reminders to this effect appear throughout the book under the lists of "warnings."

Inherited conditions

Porphyria appears as a "should not be given" warning in many entries. This fairly rare inherited condition, which causes abnormal metabolism of blood pigments, is serious in its own right, but is potentially lethal in combination with a wide range of drugs—some of which are commonly available and otherwise harmless. Normally, people who have porphyria know so, but the condition is sufficiently serious that relatives of patients should also be screened.

G6PD deficiency (glucose 6-phosphate dehydrogenase enzyme deficiency) is a genetically inherited condition, and is relatively common in African, Indian, and some Mediterranean peoples. Serious adverse reactions occur in those affected when they take any of a range of drugs; for example, the antimalarial drug primaquine causes red blood cell hemolysis in five to ten percent of black men, leading to severe anemia.

Slow acetylators are people in a similar situation to G6PD deficiency. Slow acetylators describes an inherited condition where an enzyme that breaks down drugs within the body has low activity, and so it is therefore important that lower doses of such drugs (for example, isoniazid) are taken by people with this disorder.

Non-inherited conditions

Age needs to be taken into account as a factor in drug doses. The elderly metabolize drugs slowly so lower doses usually need to be used. The elderly are also more likely to become confused with drugs that act on the brain. Children are especially at risk, and doctors have special ways of working out appropriate doses when it is necessary to prescribe for the young. The manufacturers of OTC medicines always take care to indicate the age groups and doses for those of their products appropriate for children, and the labeling should be read carefully. It is important to remember that only the current labeling on these OTC products is definitive.

Certain conditions or disorders are particularly likely to have an adverse effect on the action of medication, and these include the following.

Kidney disorders slow down the excretion of drugs, so that active constituents may remain in the body for longer than is intended; because of this, doses should be adjusted.

Liver disorders slow down the body's metabolism of drugs, so lower doses may be needed.

Alcoholism is likely to have caused damage to the liver, so the same considerations apply as to liver disorders—the slowing down of the body's metabolism of drugs so that lower doses than usual may be required.

Heart disease requires special care when drugs are prescribed, and people suffering heart conditions usually need special advice about the safe use of medicines.

Pregnancy and breast-feeding

Pregnancy requires special care and, as mentioned already, it is probably best to avoid taking any drugs during pregnancy if this is possible. Even before becoming pregnant it is a good idea to stop using some drugs (including, in particular, cigarette smoking and alcohol) to avoid any residual effects. Not all drugs are damaging in pregnancy, and indeed some may be beneficial—supplements of the vitamin folic acid, for example, help prevent neural tube defects (for example, spinal bifida) when taken before and during the first three months of pregnancy. As noted above, FDA pregnancy categories (A, B, C, D and X) ascribed to each drug are a general classification by the degree of hazard they may pose if taken during pregnancy. A table of the FDA categories and the generic drugs to which each relates is provided at the end of this introduction to the Directory of Drugs. It is extremely important to consult your doctor before taking any medication during pregnancy, including herbal remedies, supplements, and any form of alternative remedy.

For breast-feeding, specific information is available on which drugs should be avoided because they pass to the baby through the mother's milk or because they affect milk production. Here, too, as a general rule it is best to avoid all drugs if possible (including smoking and taking any illicit drugs). If considering taking medicines while breast-feeding, a doctor should be consulted in every case.

Drug interactions

One of the greatest inherent dangers in the use of either prescription or non-prescription drugs lies in the unpredictability of the interaction between two or more different drugs, or even in the interaction between drugs, herbal remedies, minerals/vitamins/supplements, foodstuffs, or environmental factors. It is very important to be aware of them, and reminders to this effect appear throughout the book listed under "Interactions." When buying, or being prescribed a medicine, always tell your doctor or pharmacist if you are taking any other medication—including herbal remedies or minerals/vitamins/supplements—because of possible interactions (and vice-versa).

The risk of serious interactions between monoamine-oxidase inhibitor (MAOI) antidepressants and certain foodstuffs, herbal remedies, and decongestants is well known. Most people will be aware of the additive or potentiating action that alcohol has on the sedative or sleep-enhancing effects of many drugs, such as benzodiazepine anxiolytics, antihistamines, and components of "cold cures." It is an important legal requirement that medicines are labeled in standard ways to warn the user of such hazards.

There is a widely held belief that antibiotics and alcohol "do not mix." This is true for some but not for all. For example, certain antibiotics (for instance, azole antimicrobials such as metronidazole) interfere with the metabolism of alcohol, so that it produces a toxic metabolite, called acetaldehyde, in the body, and this may make the subject feel very ill indeed (see the entry on disulfiram).

Details of some of the more worrying drug interactions are given in the individual generic entries. However, by no means all interactions are detrimental, and two drugs may be specifically prescribed to be taken together for a variety of reasons. For example, one of a pair of drugs may inhibit the break down or excretion of the other drug, so prolonging its beneficial effects (for example, clavulanic acid prolongs the duration of action of antibiotics such as amoxycillin by inhibiting bacterial penicillinase enzymes which break down many penicillin antibiotics). Another reason for taking two drugs simultaneously is where one drug counteracts the adverse effects of the other. This can occur in the treatment of Parkinson's disease and other diseases of the central nervous system.

In general, however, drug interactions are complex and sometimes difficult to predict, and depend on individual circumstances, and so full details of all possible interactions are not included in this book. Doctors and pharmacists will have detailed charts of known interactions which in all cases should be consulted, and expert opinion should always be taken if more than one drug is to be used at a time.

Guidelines and points to remember

It is important to know why you are taking a medicine, and how to use your medicine properly. Medicines are used to prevent (for example, vaccines), cure (for example, antibacterials), or control (for example, antihypertensives) medical conditions or to alleviate symptoms (for example, painkillers) while the condition gets better on its own. Some important things that you should know before taking your medicine are listed below. Each medicine has special instructions unique to itself—therefore if you are at all unsure of any of these points, or they are not clearly explained in the Patient Information Leaflet, it is imperative that you check with either your doctor or pharmacist (often the quickest and easiest approach is to contact your pharmacist first). The FDA has an informative website: www.fda.gov/cder/index/.

Remember, good medical therapy depends on a partnership between the patient and medical professionals, but deregulation is lowering the protective shield afforded by the prescription-only approach to drug therapy, and as a result greater responsibility is being thrown on the individual. We must therefore become conversant with some facts about our own individual reactions to the basic types of drugs. We must know when it is essential to seek advice from the healthcare professionals and what to ask them. This dictionary is **not** a guide to self-medication, but it is intended to help in this process by providing a comprehensive source of understandable information about the medicines themselves.

Dr. Judith Hall, BSc PhD
Dr. Ian Morton, BSc PhD MIBiol

Questions to ask about your medicine

This information should appear in the patient information leaflet that comes with your medicine. If you are unclear about any of the information-consult your doctor or pharmacist. Some questions you may ask are listed below.

- **Are there any important side effects that should be looked out for or reported?**
- **Do you have a pre-existing condition or allergy you should have told your doctor or pharmacist about?**
- **Are you pregnant, planning to become pregnant, or breast-feeding? Check with your doctor or pharmacist before taking any medicine.**
- **Are there other medications, herbal remedies, vitamins, minerals, and supplements that should not be taken at the same time?**
- **Should it be taken before, during, or after meals?**
- **What should you do if you miss a dose?**
- **Will the medicine make you drowsy or dizzy so that driving may be dangerous?**
- **Can you drink alcohol when taking the medicine?**
- **Should the whole course of medicine be taken even if you get better?**
- **How should the medicine be stored/ discarded?**

FDA Pregnancy Categories

The FDA designates five categories of caution for drugs in relation to pregnancy. Regardless of the designated category, however, no drug should be taken during pregnancy unless under the careful supervision of a physician, who will ensure that the benefits of it are greater than the potential risk. The most dangerous category is designated X. The least dangerous category—although this does not mean any drug is safe—is designated A. Categories B, C, and D indicate degrees of danger in between these two. A formal description of each FDA category is presented on the following pages, followed by a list of the generic drugs to which the category relates.

Some of the drugs listed pose more risk to the fetus at certain stages of pregnancy. For example, antihistamines are generally not used in the third trimester as newborns may have severe reactions to this class. For some drugs, this is reflected in the assigned FDA pregnancy category which changes depending on the stage of pregnancy. For example, the angiotensin-receptor antagonist drugs (losartan, candesartan, irbesartan, telmisartan, valsartan) and ACE inhibitor drugs (benazepril, captopril, enalapril, enalaprilat, fosinopril, lisinopril, moexipril, quinapril, ramipril, trandolapril) are classed as Category C in the first trimester of pregnancy (as listed), but rise to Category D risk in the second and third trimester. Medical advice must always be taken when taking any drug during pregnancy.

FDA Pregnancy Category X

Studies have demonstrated that fetal abnormalities or evidence of fetal risk are associated with generic drugs in this category, and the risk of use by a woman who is pregnant or who may become pregnant outweighs any possible benefit of use of the drug.

acetohydroxamic acid	disulfiram	isotretinoin	pravastatin sodium
acitretin	ergotamine tartrate	leflunomide	quazepam
anabolic steroid	estazolam	leuprolide acetate	quinine
anisindione	esterified estrogens	levonorgestrel	raloxifene
atorvastatin	estradiol	lovastatin	ribavirin
bicalutamide	estramustine phosphate	medroxyprogesterone	simvastatin
cerivastatin sodium	sodium	megestrol acetate	stanozolol
cetrorelix	estrogens, conjugated	menotropins	tazarotene
chorionic gonadotropin	estrone	mestranol	temazepam
clomiphene citrate	estropipate	methotrexate	testosterone
danazol	ethinyl estradiol	methyltestosterone	thalidomide
desogestrel	finasteride	mifepristone	triazolam
diclofenac	fluoxymesterone	misoprostol	urofollitropin
dicumarol	fluvastatin	nafarelin acetatenandrolone	warfarin sodium
dienestrol	follitropin alfa/beta	norethindrone	
diethylstilbestrol	goserelin	norgestrel	
dihydroergotamine mesylate	halofantrine hydrochloride	oxytocin	

FDA Pregnancy Category D

Studies have demonstrated positive evidence of fetal risk from the use of drugs in this category, but in certain cases of serious disease, for instance where it is life-threatening, it is possible that the risk may be regarded as acceptable by the responsible physician if safer drugs are found to be ineffective.

alprazolam	dacarbazine	letrozole	phenobarbital
altretamine	daunorubicin	lithium	phenytoin
aminoglutethimide	demeclocycline	lomustine	piroxicam
amiodarone hydrochloride	diazepam	lorazepam	potassium iodide
amobarbital	dihydrotachysterol	magnesium salicylate	procarbazine
anastrozole	divalproex sodium	mechlorethamine	progesterone
aspirin	docetaxel	hydrochloride	propylthiouracil
atenolol	doxorubicin hydrochloride	meclofenamate sodium	rofecoxib
azathiaprine	doxycycline	mefenamic acid	ropinirole
bleomycin	epirubicin hydrochloride	meloxicam	salsalate
bromocriptine	ergocalciferol	melphalan	secobarbital sodium
busulfan	ethosuximide	mephenytoin	sodium salicylate
butabarbital	etodolac	mephobarbital	sodium thiosalicylate
capecitabine	etoposide	meprobamate	streptomycin
carbamazepine	exemestane	mercaptopurine	sulindac
carboplatin	fenoprofen	methimazole	tamoxifen
carboprost	fludarabine phosphate	methsuximide	temozolomide
carmustine	fluorouracil	midazolam	tetracycline hydrochloride
celecoxib	flurazepam	minocycline	thioguanine
chlorambucil	flutamide	mitomycin	thiotepa
chlordiazepoxide	fosphenytoin	mitoxantrone	tobramycin
chlorpropamide	gemcitabine	nabumetone	tolmetin sodium
choline salicylate	halazepam	neomycin	topotecan
cisplatin	hydrocortisone	netilmicin	toremifene
cladribine	hydroxyprogesterone caproate	nicotine	tretinoin
clonazepam	hydroxyurea	nortriptyline hydrochloride	trimetrexate glucuronate
clorazepate dipotassium	idarubicin hydrochloride	oxaprozin	valproate sodium and
colchicine	ifosfamide	oxazepam	derivatives
cortisone	irinotecan hydrochloride	oxytetracycline	vinblastine sulfate
cyclophosphamide	kanamycin	paclitaxel	vincristine sulfate
cytarabine	ketoprofen	pentostatin	vinorelbine tartrate

FDA Pregnancy Category C

Drugs in this category have been shown to cause fetal damage in animal studies, but no specific evidence is available for a human fetus, although the risk of such damage must be considered a possibility, so these drugs should only be taken under the careful and considered supervision of a physician who is aware of the signficant factors.

abacavir
abciximab
acetazolamide
acetohexamide
acyclovir
adapalene
adenosine
albendazole
albuterol
alclometasone
aldesleukin
alendronate sodium
alfentanil
allopurinol
alteplase, recombinant
amantadine
ambenonium chloride
amifostine
amikacin
aminobenzoate potassium
aminocaproic acid
amitriptyline hydrochloride
amlodipine besylate
ammonium chloride
amoxapine
amphetamine sulfate
amprenavir
anagrelide hydrochloride
anistreplase
anthralin
antihemophilic factor
anti-inhibitor coagulant
 complex
apraclonidine
ascorbic acid
atovaquone
atovaquone-proguanil
atracurium besylate
atropine sulfate
auranofin
aurothioglucose
azelastine hydrochloride
bacitracin
baclofen
BCG intravesical
BCG vaccine
becaplermin
beclomethasone dipropionate
benazepril hydrochloride
bendroflumethiazide
benzocaine
benzoyl peroxide
benzthiazide
benztropine mesylate
bepridil hydrochloride
betamethasone
betaxolol hydrochloride
bethanechol chloride
biperiden
bismuth subsalicylate
bisoprolol fumarate
bitolterol mesylate
bretylium tosylate
brinzolamide
buclizine hydrochloride
budesonide
bumetanide
bupivacaine
buprenorphine hydrochloride
butoconazole
butorphanol tartrate
calcipotriene

calcitonin-salmon
calcitriol
candesartan cilexetil
capreomycin
capsaicin
captopril
carbachol
carbidopa
carisoprodol
carteolol
carvedilol
cascara sagrada
celecoxib
cevimeline hydrochloride
chloral hydrate
chloramphenicol
chloroprocaine hydrochloride
chloroquine
chlorpromazine
chlorzoxazone
cidofovir
cilostazol
citalopram
citrates
clarithromycin
clioquinol
clobetasol propionate
clocortolone pivalate
clofazimine
clofibrate
clomipramine hydrochloride
clonidine hydrochloride
coagulation Factor VIIa
 recombinant; rFVIIa
coal tar
cocaine
codeine phosphate
colistin
corticotropin
cosyntropin
crotamiton
cyanocobalamin;
 hydroxocobalamin
cyclopentolate hydrochloride
cycloserine
cyclosporine
daclizumab
dactinomycin
dantrolene sodium
dapsone
desensitizing products
desipramine hydrochloride
desoxymetasone
dexamethasone
dexrazoxane
dextroamphetamine
 (dexamphetamine sulfate)
diazoxide
dibucaine
dichlorphenamide
dicyclomine hydrochloride
diflunisal
digitoxin
digoxin
digoxin immune Fab
diltiazem hydrochloride
dinoprostone
diphenoxylate hydrochloride
diphtheria and tetanus toxoids
 (all forms)
esmolol hydrochloride
ethanolamine oleatepertussis

diphtheria antitoxin
dirithromycin
disopyramide
docusate sodium
donepezil
dopamine hydrochloride
dorzolamide
doxazosin mesylate
doxepin
droperidol
echothiophate iodide
econazole
edrophonium chloride
efavirenz
enalapril maleate
enoxacin
entacapone
ephedrine
epinephrine
epoetin alfa
eprosartan mesylate
ergonovine maleate
esmolol hydrochloride
ethanolamine oleate
etodolac
Factor IX; Factor IX complex
felodipine
fenofibrate
fenoprofen
fentanyl
fexofenadine hydrochloride
filgrastim
flecainide acetate
flucytosine
fludrocortisone
flumazenil
flunisolide
fluocinolone acetonide
fluocinonide
fluorescein sodium
fluorometholone
fluphenazine
flurandrenolide
flurbiprofen
fluticasone propionate
fluvoxamine
fomepizole
foscarnet sodium
fosinopril sodium
furosemide
gabapentin
ganciclovir
gemfibrozil
gentamicin
glimepiride
glipizide
glutethimide
glycerin
griseofulvin
guaifenesin
guanabenz acetate
guanethidine monosulfate
Haemophilus b conjugate
 vaccine
halcinonide
haloperidol
heparin
hepatitis A vaccine,
 inactivated
hepatitis B immune globulin
hepatitis B vaccine
hexachlorophene

homatropine hydrobromide
hyaluronidase
hydralazine hydrochloride
hydroflumethiazide
hydromorphone
 hydrochloride
hydroxychloroquine sulfate
hydroxyzine
hyoscyamine
idoxuridine
imiglucerase
imipenem-cilastatin
imipramine
immune globulin, human
inamrinone lactate
indinavir
infliximab
influenza virus vaccine
insulin aspart recombinant
insulin glargine
interferons
ipecac syrup
irbesartan
iron dextran
isocarboxazid
isoetharine
isoniazid
isoproterenol
isosorbide dinitrate
isosorbide mononitrate
isradipine
itraconazole
ivermectin
ketoconazole
ketoprofen
ketorolac tromethamine
ketotifen
labetalol hydrochloride
lamivudine
lamotrigine
latanoprost
leucovorin calcium
levalbuterol hydrochloride
levamisole hydrochloride
levetiracetam
levobunolol
levocabastine hydrochloride
levodopa
lidocaine
linezolid
lisinopril
losartan potassium
loxapine
Lyme disease vaccine
 (recombinant OspA)
mafenide
mannitol
mebendazole
mecamylamine hydrochloride
meclofenamate sodium
mefenamic acid
mefloquine
meloxicam
meningococcal
 polysaccharide vaccine
mepenzolate bromide
mepivacaine hydrochloride
mesoridazine
metaproterenol
metaraminol
methamphetamine
methantheline bromide

methazolamide
methenamine
methocarbamol
methotrimeprazine
methoxamine hydrochloride
methyclothiazide
methylergonovine
methylphenidate
methylprednisolone
metipranolol
metoprolol tartrate
metyrosine
mexiletine hydrochloride
miconazole
midodrine hydrochloride
milrinone
mineral oil
minoxidil
mirtazapine hydrochloride
mivacurium
MMR (measles-mumps-
    rubella virus vaccine, live)
modafinil
moexipril hydrochloride
molindone
mometasone
monoctanoin
morphine sulfate
muromonab-CD3
mycophenolate mofetil
nabumetone
nadolol
nalbuphine hydrochloride
naltrexone hydrochloride
naphazoline hydrochloride
naratriptan
nefazodone hydrochloride
neostigmine methylsulfate
nevirapine
nicardipine hydrochloride
nifedipine
nilutamide
nimodipine
nisoldipine
nitroglycerin
norepinephrine bitartrate
nystatin
olanzapine
olsalazine sodium
omeprazole
oprelvekin
orphenadrine
oxamniquine
oxaprozin
oxcarbazepine
oxymetazoline hydrochloride
oxymorphone hydrochloride
palivizumab
pamidronate disodium
pancreatin
pancuronium bromide
pantoprazole sodium
papaverine
paraldehyde
pegademase bovine
penbutolol sulfate
pentamidine isethionate

pentoxifylline
perindopril erbumine
perphenazine
phendimetrazine
phenelzine
phenoxybenzamine
phentermine
phentolamine mesylate
phenylephrine hydrochloride
phytonadione
pilocarpine
pimozide
pioglitazone
pirbuterol
piroxicam
pneumococcal vaccines
podofilox
poliovirus vaccines
polythiazide
pralidoxime chloride
pramipexole
pramoxine hydrochloride
prazosin hydrochloride
prilocaine hydrochloride
primaquine
primidone
procainamide hydrochloride
procaine
prochlorperazine
procyclidine
promazine
promethazine hydrochloride
propafenone hydrochloride
propantheline bromide
proparacaine
propoxyphene hydrochloride
propranolol hydrochloride
protamine sulfate
protirelin
protriptyline hydrochloride
pseudoephedrine
pyrantel
pyrazinamide
pyridostigmine bromide
pyrimethamine
quetiapine
quinapril hydrochloride
quinethazone
quinidine
rabies immune globulin,
    human (RIG)
rabies vaccines
ramipril
remifentanil
repaglinide
reserpine
reteplase, recombinant
Rh0(D) immune globulin
    (human)
rifampin
riluzole
rimantadine
rimexolone
risperidone
rituximab
rivastigmine
rizatriptan benzoate

rofecoxib
ropivacaine hydrochloride
rosiglitazone maleate
rubella vaccine, live
salmeterol
sargramostim
scopolamine hydrobromide
selegiline hydrochloride
selenium sulfide
senna
sermorelin
sibutramine
sirolimus
sodium chloride
sodium nitroprusside
sodium phenylbutyrate
sodium polystyrene sulfonate
sodium tetradecyl sulfate
sodium thiosulfate
somatropin
spironolactone
stavudine
streptokinase
succinylcholine chloride
sulconazole nitrate
sulfadiazine
sulfadoxine
sulfamethoxazole
sulfinpyrazone
sulfisoxazole
sulindac
sumatriptan succinate
tacrine hydrochloride
tacrolimus
telmisartan
tenecteplase
terazosin
terconazole
testolactone
tetanus immune globulin (TIG)
tetanus toxoid, adsorbed
tetracaine
tetrahydrozoline
    hydrochloride
theophylline
thiabendazole
thiethylperazine maleate
thioridazine
thiothixene
thyrotropin
tiagabine
tiludronate sodium
timolol maleate
tioconazole
tizanidine
tocainide hydrochloride
tolazamide
tolbutamide
tolcapone
tolmetin sodium
tolnaftate
tolterodine tartrate
topiramate
tramadol hydrochloride
trandolapril
tranylcypromine
trazodone hydrochloride

triacetin
triamcinolone
trichlormethiazide
trifluoperazine
triflupromazine hydrochloride
trifluridine
trihexyphenidyl
trimethaphan camsylate
trimethobenzamide
    hydrochloride
trimethoprim (TMP)
trimethoprim and
    sulfamethozazole
trimipramine hydrochloride
triple sulfa cream
tropicamide
tuberculin
typhoid vaccines
urea
valrubicin
valsartan
vancomycin
varicella virus vaccine, live
varicella-zoster immune
    globulin (human) (VZIG)
vasopressin
venlafaxine
verapamil hydrochloride
verteporfin
xylometazoline hydrochloride
yellow fever vaccine
zalcitabine
zanamivir
zileuton
zolmitriptan
zonisamide

FDA Pregnancy Category B

Although drugs in this category have been shown not to cause fetal damage in animal studies, no specific evidence is available for a human fetus, so these drugs cannot be considered safe and should only be taken under the careful and considered supervision of a physician, who is aware of the signficant factors.

acarbose
acebutolol
acetaminophen
acetylcysteine
acrivastine
alprostadil
amiloride
amoxicillin
amphotericin B
ampicillin
antithrombin III human
aprotinin
ardeparin sodium
azatadine maleate
azelaic acid
azithromycin
aztreonam
basiliximab
bisacodyl
brimonidine tartrate
brompheniramine maleate
bupropion hydrochloride
buspirone
cabergoline
carbenicillin
carbinoxamine maleate
cefaclor
cefadroxil
cefamandole
cefazolin sodium
cefepime
cefixime
cefotaxime
cefotetan
cefoxitin
cefpodoxime
cefprozil
ceftazidime
ceftriaxone
cefuroxime
cephalexin
cephradine
cetirizine hydrochloride
chlorhexidine
chlorothiazide
chlorpheniramine maleate
chlortetracycline
chlorthalidone
cholestyramine
cimetidine
cinoxacin
ciprofloxacin
cisatracurium
clemastine
clindamycin
clopidogrel
clotrimazole
cloxacillin sodium
clozapine

colesevelam
colestipol hydrochloride
cromolyn sodium
cyclizine
cyclobenzaprine
cyproheptadine
  hydrochloride
dalteparin sodium
danaparoid sodium
desmopressin
diclofenac
dicloxacillin sodium
didanosine
dimenhydrinate
diphenhydramine
dipivefrin hydrochloride
dipyridamole
dobutamine hydrochloride
dolasetron mesylate
dornase alfa
doxapram
doxylamine
dronabinol
emedastine
enoxaparin sodium
epoprostenol sodium
eptifibatide
erythromycin
etanercept
ethacrynic acid
ethambutol
etidocaine
etidronate disodium
famciclovir
famotidine
fenoldopam mesylate
flavoxate hydrochloride
fluconazole
fluoxetine
fosfomycin
furazolidone
gatifloxacin
glatiramer acetate
glucagon
glyburide
glycopyrrolate
gonadorelin
granisetron
guanadrel
guanfacine hydrochloride
haloprogin
hydrochlorothiazide
hydrocodone bitartrate
ibuprofen
imiquimod
indapamide
indomethacin
insulin analog lispro

insulin lispro and insulin lispro
  protamine
insulin zinc suspension lente
insulin, isophane suspension insulin, NPH
insulin, regular
insulin, regular and isophane
  mixture
ipratropium bromide
lactulose
lansoprazole
lepirudin
levobupivacaine
levocarnitine
levofloxacin
lindane
lodoxamide tromethamine
lomefloxacin
loperamide hydrochloride
loratadine
lypressin
malathion
maprotiline hydrochloride
meclizine hydrochloride
meclocycline sulfosalicylate
meperidine hydrochloride
meropenem
mesalamine
mesna
metformin
methadone hydrochloride
methyldopa
metoclopramide
metolazone
metronidazole
mezlocillin
miglitol
montelukast sodium
moricizine hydrochloride
moxifloxacin
mupirocin
nafcillin
naftifine
nalidixic acid
naloxone hydrochloride
naproxen
nedocromil sodium
nelfinavir
nitrofurantoin
nizatidine
norfloxacin
octreotide
ofloxacin
ondansetron
orlistat
oxacillin sodium
oxiconazole
oxybutynin
oxycodone

paregoric
paroxetine
penciclovir
penicillin G
penicillin V
pentazocine
pergolide
permethrin
pheniramine maleate
pindolol
piperacillin
polymyxin B sulfate
praziquantel
prednisolone
prednisone
probenecid
pyrilamine maleate
quinupristin-dalfopristin
rabeprazole sodium
ranitidine bismuth citrate
ranitidine hydrochloride
rifabutin
ritodrine hydrochloride
ritonavir
rocuronium bromide
saquinavir
sertraline
sildenafil
silver sulfadiazine
somatrem
sotalol hydrochloride
sparfloxacin
spectinomycin
sucralfate
sulfacetamide
sulfasalazine
tamsulosin hydrochloride
terbinafine
terbutaline sulfate
tetracycline hydrochloride
ticarcillin
ticlopidine
tinzaparin sodium
tirofiban
torsemide
tranexamic acid
tretinoin
triamterene
triprolidine hydrochloride
urokinase
ursodiol
valacyclovir
vecuronium bromide
zafirlukast
zidovudine
zolpidem

FDA Pregnancy Category A

Drugs in this category have not caused damage to a human fetus, so the risk of fetal damage from these drugs is considered to be unlikely.

ferrous fumarate
ferrous gluconate

ferrous sulfate
folic acid

levothyroxine sodium
liothyronine

magnesium sulfate
niacin

A+D Ointment with Zinc Oxide ℞

A preparation of dimethicone, ℞ **zinc oxide**, benzyl alcohol, ♻ **vitamins A**, and ♻ **D**, ℞ **cod-liver oil**, and ℞ **mineral oil**.
Formulation: Topical ointment.
Availability: OTC.
Warnings and side effects: See ℞ **simethicone**; ℞ **zinc oxide**; ♻ **vitamin A**; ♻ **vitamin D**; ℞ **cod-liver oil**; ℞ **mineral oil**.

A-200 ℞

A preparation of ℞ **pyrethrin**.
Formulation: Topical shampoo.
Availability: OTC.
Warnings and side effects: See ℞ **pyrethrin**.

A & D Medicated ℞

A preparation of ℞ **zinc oxide**, ℞ **petrolatum**, ℞ **cod-liver oil**, ℞ **mineral oil**, ♻ **vitamin A**, and ♻ **vitamin D**.
Formulation: Topical ointment.
Availability: OTC.
Warnings and side effects: See ℞ **zinc oxide**; ℞ **petrolatum**; ℞ **cod-liver oil**; ℞ **mineral oil**; ♻ **vitamin A**; ♻ **vitamin D**.

abacavir ⓖ

Type/Group: **antiviral**.
Brand(s): Ziagen. Combination: with *zidovudine* and *lamivudine*: Trizivir.
How administered: Orally.
Used to treat
HIV infection. This is a reverse transcriptase antiviral drug which is used as an antiretroviral for treatment of ✪ **HIV** infection, in combination with other antivirals.
Warnings
• It should not be given to people with known hypersensitivity to this drug or its metabolites.
• Abacavir should be used during pregnancy only if the potential benefit outweighs the possible risks to the fetus.
• Although it is not known whether abacavir is present in breast milk, the Centers for Disease Control and Prevention recommend that HIV-infected mothers do not breast-feed.
• It is a specialist drug, and there will be full assessment and patient monitoring throughout treatment. Unusual symptoms, such as fever, severe tiredness, achiness, nausea, or vomiting, should be reported to a doctor immediately and, if advised, treatment stopped.
• Abacavir belongs to class of antivirals that can cause liver damage, particularly if used for a long time, and more often in women than men.
Interactions
No drug interactions of significance are known.
Side effects
• There may be serious hypersensitivity reactions, dizziness, headache, insomnia, nausea and vomiting, diarrhea, abdominal pain, anorexia, fatigue and lethargy, fever, or blood changes.

abciximab ⓖ

Type/Group: **antiplatelet**.
Brand(s): ReoPro.
How administered: Intravenous injection or infusion.
Used to treat
Blood clotting. Abciximab is one of a relatively new class of drugs, a monoclonal antibody (a form of pure antibody produced by a type of molecular engineering). In this case the cloned antibody is one that inhibits platelet aggregation and thrombus formation. It is used by specialist doctors as an additional treatment alongside ℞ **heparin** and ℞ **aspirin** for the prevention of complications due to clot formation in high-risk patients undergoing certain types of coronary angioplasty operations.
Warnings
• It should not be given to people with known hypersensitivity to this drug or to any product prepared with mouse protein. It should not be used by anyone with a condition that would make internal bleeding more likely, for example, recent surgery or injury, current bleeding, uncontrolled high blood pressure, or taking a medication to slow blood clotting.
• It is used only in a hospital setting, under close supervision, and after a full medical assessment.
• Abciximab should be used during pregnancy only if it is clearly needed.
• Medical judgment is required if breast-feeding is being considered. It is not known whether it appears in breast milk.
• Antibodies to abciximab may form, and so that a second treatment may cause a significant hypersensitivity reaction (which may include anaphylaxis).
Interactions
• If used with ℞ **thrombolytic** agents and ℞ **anticoagulants**, there is an increased risk of bleeding.
Side effects
• Commonly, bleeding which may be a serious complication.
• Low blood pressure, slower pulse, nausea, swelling of the extremities, or anemia may also occur.

Abelcet ℞

A preparation of ℞ **amphotericin B**.
Formulation: Injection (intravenous).
Availability: Prescription only.
Warnings and side effects: See ℞ **amphotericin B**.

abortifacient ⓓ

Generics: **carboprost**; **dinoprostone**; **mifepristone**.
Actions and uses
Abortifacient drugs are used to induce ✪ **abortion** or miscarriage, as a medical alternative to surgical termination. A number of types of drug have been used to achieve this, but commonly the antiprogestin drug ℞ **mifepristone** is used (given orally) and/or a ℞ **prostaglandin** (for example, ℞ **carboprost**, ℞ **dinoprostone**) (given by pessary).
Limitations
See the individual drug entries.

Absorbine Athlete's Foot Cream; Absorbine Footcare ®

A preparation of ℞ **tolnaftate**.
Formulation: Topical cream, topical liquid spray (Footcare).
Availability: OTC.
Warnings and side effects: See ℞ **tolnaftate**.

acarbose ©

Type/Group: **antidiabetic; oral hypoglycemic**.
Brand(s): Precose.
How administered: Orally.

Used to treat

Diabetes mellitus. Acarbose delays the conversion in the intestine of starch and sucrose (sugar) to glucose, and subsequent absorption. It is used in treatment of type 2 ✪ **diabetes mellitus** (non-insulin-dependent diabetes mellitus, or NIDDM), sometimes in combination with other drugs. It may be of value in people where other drugs, or diet control, have not been successful, and so is useful in those who are obese.

Warnings

• It should not be given to people with known hypersensitivity or allergy to this drug, cirrhosis, intestinal obstruction, chronic intestinal disease or inflammatory bowel disease.
• It should be given with caution to people with kidney impairment.
• It should be used during pregnancy only if clearly needed.
• It is not known whether acarbose is present in breast milk. Breastfeeding women should discontinue using this drug or stop breastfeeding.
• Blood glucose and liver enzymes are monitored.
• People who are also taking ℞ **insulin, regular** or a ℞ **sulphonylurea**-class oral hypoglycemic drug, in addition to acarbose, need to carry glucose (to counteract hypoglycemia) rather than sucrose, since acarbose interferes with the conversion and absorption of sucrose.

Interactions

• ℞ **Activated charcoal** and ℞ **digestive enzymes** may reduce the effectiveness of acarbose.
• Lowers ℞ **Digoxin** levels, decreasing its effect.

Side effects

• Gastrointestinal disturbances, including diarrhea, flatulence, bloating, distension and abdominal pain (which becomes less with time).

Accolate ®

A preparation of ℞ **zafirlukast**.
Formulation: Oral tablets.
Availability: Prescription only.
Warnings and side effects: See ℞ **zafirlukast**.

Accupril ®

A preparation of ℞ **quinapril hydrochloride**.
Formulation: Oral tablets, available in 4 strengths.
Availability: Prescription only.
Warnings and side effects: See ℞ **quinapril hydrochloride**.

Accurbron ®

A preparation of ℞ **theophylline**.
Formulation: Oral syrup.
Availability: Prescription only.
Warnings and side effects: See ℞ **theophylline**.

Accuretic ®

A preparation of ℞ **hydrochlorothiazide** and ℞ **quinapril** or benzapril.
Formulation: Oral tablets, in several strengths.
Availability: Prescription only.
Warnings and side effects: See ℞ **hydrochlorothiazide**; ℞ **quinapril**.

Accutane ®

A preparation of ℞ **isotretinoin**.
Formulation: Capsules in 3 strengths.
Availability: Prescription only.
Warnings and side effects: See ℞ **isotretinoin**.

acebutolol ©

Type/Group: **beta-blocker; antiarrhythmic; antihypertensive**.
Brand(s): Sectral; various generic.
How administered: Orally.

Used to treat

High blood pressure (see ✪ **hypertension**), irregular heartbeat (see ✪ **arrhythmia**). Beta-blockers are generally not given to anyone with asthma or other bronchospastic disease (for example, chronic bronchitis or emphysema), but acebutolol may be used with caution if other blood-pressure lowering treatments have failed.

Warnings

• It should not be given to people with known hypersensitivity to any beta-blocking drug, who have certain heartbeat irregularities or heart failure. It should not be used in cardiogenic shock.
• It should be given with caution to people with hypoglycemia, hyperthyroidism, myasthenia gravis, congestive heart failure, peripheral vascular disease, or liver or kidney impairment.
• Acebutolol should be used during pregnancy only if the potential benefit outweighs the possible risk to the fetus.
• It appears in breast milk, and so nursing women should discontinue using this drug or stop breast-feeding.
• Abruptly stopping using a beta-blocker may have adverse effects, including on the heart.
• The use of this drug may mask signs of hyperthyroidism or hypoglycemia.
• Beta-blockers may intensify allergic responses to a variety of allergens in people with a history of severe anaphylactic reaction.
• No other medication (including OTCs, herbal remedies, and supplements) should be taken without consulting a doctor first. Some ℞ **nasal decongestants**, commonly available over the counter, contain ℞ **alpha-adrenergic stimulants** (for example, ℞ **phenylephrine**) which may cause a severe hypertensive reaction if taken with beta-blockers.

Key to symbols: ✪ = Disorder Section ℞ = Drug Section ♣ = Herbal Section ◊◊ = Supplement Section

Interactions

• A serious increase in blood pressure may occur after withdrawal from ℞ **clonidine**, or from both drugs at the same time.

• The effects of ℞ **alpha-adrenergic stimulants**, ℞ **ergot alkaloids**, ℞ **epinephrine**, and ℞ **lidocaine** may be increased, with the risk of serious adverse effects.

• ℞ **Calcium-channel blockers** (particularly ℞ **diltiazem** and ℞ **verapamil**), ℞ **guanethidine**, and ℞ **reserpine** have the potential for increasing undesirable effects, with exaggerated slowing of heartbeat or hypotension.

• The effects of nondepolarizing ℞ **skeletal muscle relaxants** may be variable, with the possible risk of significant adverse effects associated with major surgery.

• The effects of ℞ **insulin** and ℞ **sulfonylureas** may be reduced.

• ℞ **Antacids** (for example, ℞ **aluminum hydroxide**, ℞ **magnesium hydroxide**), ℞ **barbiturates**, ⚕ **calcium** salts, ℞ **cholestyramine**, ℞ **colestipol**, ℞ NSAIDs, ℞ **penicillins**, ℞ **rifampin**, and ℞ **salicylates** may reduce the levels and effectiveness of beta-blockers.

• If used with ℞ **diuretics** and other antihypertensive drugs, there are additive effects which are often used to therapeutic advantage.

Side effects

These are infrequent and may include:

• Dizziness, fatigue, gastrointestinal disturbances (for example, constipation, diarrhea, nausea), headache, slowing of the heart rate, hypotension, poor circulation, breathing difficulty, or urinary frequency;

• Less frequently, itching or rash, arthralgia (joint pain), edema, sleep disturbances, asthma-like symptoms and bronchospasm, or abnormal vision. Unusual antibodies often develop, though lupus-like symptoms (fever, myalgia, pleurisy, various inflammations) seldom occur;

• Heart failure, should it develop, generally requires withdrawal (gradually, if possible) of this drug.

ACE inhibitor ⓓ

(angiotensin-converting enzyme inhibitor)

Generics: **benazepril hydrochloride; captopril; enalapril maleate; fosinopril sodium; lisinopril; moexipril hydrochloride; perindopril erbumine; quinapril hydrochloride; ramipril; trandolapril.**

Actions and uses

The full name of ACE inhibitors is angiotensin-converting enzyme inhibitors. They are used in the treatment of ⊙ **hypertension** and ⊙ **heart failure**. They are enzyme inhibitors that work by inhibiting the conversion of the natural circulating hormone angiotensin I to angiotensin II. Because the latter is a powerful vasoconstrictor (narrows blood vessels), the overall effect is vasodilatation (see ℞ **vasodilator**) with an overall hypotensive (lowering blood pressure) effect. There has been a considerable increase recently in the use of ACE inhibitors in the treatment of moderate hypertension and of severe hypertension when other treatments are not suitable or successful. Some are also used as an antihypertensive in insulin-dependent ⊙ **diabetes mellitus** to protect the kidney. They are usually used in conjunction with other antihypertensive treat-

ments, especially ℞ **diuretics** and sometimes ℞ **calcium-channel blockers**, and with ℞ **digoxin** in the treatment of heart failure.

Limitations

ACE inhibitors should not be given to people with known hypersensitivity to this class of drugs, who have renovascular disease, and certain heart defects, or who are pregnant. They should be given with caution to people with peripheral vascular disease or severe atherosclerosis. ACE inhibitors can cause severe hypotension, especially when beginning treatment, if the person is also taking diuretics, is on a low-sodium diet, has heart failure, or is dehydrated. They can also cause kidney impairment. Other side effects include persistent dry cough, angioedema, rash (sometimes with itching and urticaria), pancreatitis, respiratory tract symptoms (for example, sinusitis, rhinitis) and sore throat, and gastrointestinal effects such as nausea and vomiting, indigestion, diarrhea, or constipation. There may be altered liver function, jaundice, hepatitis, and changes in blood counts. Occasionally, headache, dizziness, fatigue and malaise, taste disturbance, tingling in the extremities, and bronchospasm.

Acel-Imune ⓑ

A preparation of ℞ **diphtheria and tetanus toxoids and acellular pertussis vaccine, adsorbed (DTaP)**.

Formulation: Injection.

Availability: Prescription only.

Warnings and side effects: See ℞ **diphtheria and tetanus toxoids and acellular pertussis vaccine (DTaP)**.

Aceon ⓑ

A preparation of ℞ **perindopril erbumine**.

Formulation: Oral tablets, available in 3 strengths.

Availability: Prescription only.

Warnings and side effects: See ℞ **perindopril erbumine**.

Acephen Suppositories ⓑ

A preparation of ℞ **acetaminophen**.

Formulation: Rectal suppository, available in 3 strengths.

Availability: OTC.

Warnings and side effects: See ℞ **acetaminophen**.

acetaminophen ⓖ

(paracetamol)

Type/Group: **non-narcotic analgesic; antipyretic**.

Brand(s): Aceta, Aceta Elixir; Anacin Aspirin Free Maximum Strength Caplets, Gelcaps; Apacet Chewable Tablets, Drops; Dapacin Capsules; Dynafed Extra Strength Tablets, Children's Dynafed Jr.; Feverall Children's Sprinkles; Junior Strength Sprinkles; Genapap Tablets, Extra Strength Tablets, Caplets, Children's Chewable Tablets, Infants' Drops, Children's Elixir; Genebs Tablets, Extra Strength Tablets, Caplets; Halenol Children's Liquid; Liquiprin Drops for Children; Mapap Regular Strength, Extra Strength, Children's Chewable Tablets, Children's Elixir, Infant Drops; Maranox; Meda Cap, Meda Tab; Oraphen-PD Elixir; Panadol Tablets, Caplets, Children's Chewable Tablets; Junior Strength Caplets, Children's Liquid, Infants' Drops; Ridenol Elixir; Silapap

Children's Elixir, Silapap Infants' Drops; Tapanol Regular Strength Tablets, Extra Strength Tablets, Caplets, Gelcaps; Tempra Tablets, Tempra 1 (Drops), Tempra 2 (Syrup), Tempra 3 (Chewable Tablets); Tylenol Regular Strength Tablets, Caplets, Extra Strength Tablets, Caplets, Gelcaps, Adult Liquid, Arthritis Extended Relief Caplets, Junior Strength Soft-Chew Tablets, Coated Caplets, Children's Soft-Chew Tablets, Childrens' Elixir, Infants' Drops; Uni-Ace Drops. Topical (rectal suppositories): Acephen Suppositories; Acetaminophen Uniserts; Feverall Infants' Suppositories, Children's Suppositories, Junior Strength Suppositories; Neopap; Combinations: With various: APAP-Plus Tablets (*caffeine*); Flexaphen (*chlorzoxazone*); Excedrin Aspirin Free Caplets, Geltabs (*caffeine*); Fem-1 Tablets (*pamabrom*); Lobac Capsules (*salicylamide, phenyltoloxamine citrate*); Femback Caplets (*salicylamide, phenyltoloxamine citrate*); Flextra-DS Tablets (*phenyltoloxamine citrate*); Midol Maximum Strength Menstrual Caplets, Geltabs (*caffeine, pyrilamine maleate*); Midol Maximum Strength PMS Caplets, Geltabs (*pamabrom, pyrilamine maleate*); Pamprin Maximum Pain Relief Caplets (*magnesium salicylate, pamabrom*); Pamprin Multi-Symptom Maximum Strength Tablets, Caplets (*pamabrom, pyrilamine maleate*); Premsyn PMS Caplets (*pamabrom*); Vitelle Lurline PMS Tablets (*pamabrom, pyridoxine hydrochloride*). With aspirin: Goody's Body Pain Powder. (Plus) *caffeine*: Excedrin Migraine, Extra Strength Caplets, Tablets, Geltabs; Goody's Extra Strength Headache Powder; Saleto Tablets (has *salicylamide*); Summit Extra Strength Caplets; Vanquish Caplets (has *aluminum hydroxide* and *magnesium hydroxide*). With butalbital: Axocet Capsules; Bucet Capsules; Bupap Tablets; Butex Forte Capsules; Dolgic Tablets; Marten-Tab; Phrenilin Forte Capsules; Repan CF Tablets; Sedapap Tablets; Tencon Capsules. With butalbital and caffeine: Esgic Tablets, Capsules, Esgic-Plus Tablets, Capsules; Fioricet Tablets; Margesic Capsules; Medigesic Capsules; Repan Tablets; Triad Capsules. With codeine: Aceta w/ Codeine; Capital w/Codeine Suspension; Fioricet w/Codeine Capsules; Phenaphen w/Codeine Capsules; Tylenol w/Codeine Elixir; Tylenol w/Codeine Tablets. With dextromethorphan and pseudoephedrine: Alka-Seltzer Plus Cold & Flu Liqui-Gels; Contac Severe Cold & Flu Non-Drowsy Caplets; Thera-Flu Non-Drowsy Formula Maximum Strength; Robitussin Multi Symptom Honey Flu; Sudfed Severe Cold Formula Caplets, Tablets; Tylenol Flu Maximum Strength Non-Drowsy Gelcaps; Vicks Dayquil. (Plus) *chlorpheniramine maleate*: Alka-Selzer Plus Cold & Cough LiquiGels; Children's Tylenol Cold Plus Cough Chewable Tablets; Comtrex Maximum Strength Multi-Symptom Cold & Cough Relief Caplets, Tablets; Contac Severe Cold & Flu Caplets; Genacol Tablets; Kolephrin/DM Caplets; Medi-Flu Liquid; Multi-Symptom Tylenol Cold Caplets, Tablets; NightTime TheraFlu Powder; Robitussin Nighttime Honey Flu; Triaminic Severe Cold & Fever; Vicks 44M Cold & Flu Relief. (Plus) *doxylamine succinate*: Alka-Seltzer Plus NightTime Cold Liqui-Gels; Genite Liquid; Nytcold Medicine Liquid; Vicks NyQuil. (Plus) *guaifenesin*: Sudafed Cold & Cough Liquid Caps; Robitussin Cold Multi-Symptom Cold & Flu Liqui-Gels, Caplets; Vicks DayQuil LiquiCaps. (Plus) *pyrilamine maleate*: Robitussin Night Relief Liquid. With hydrocodone: Anexia Tablets; Bancap HC Capsules; Ceta-Plus Capsules; Co-Gesic Tablets;

Dolacet Capsules; Duocet Capsules; Hydrocet Capsules; Hydrogesic; Hy-Phen Tablets; Lorcet-HD Capsules, Lorcet Plus, Lorcet 10/500 Tablets; Lortab Elixir, Tablets; Margesic H Capsules; Norco Tablets; Oncet Capsules; Panacet Tablets; Stagesic Capsules; T-Gesic Capsules; Vicodin Tablets, ES, HP, Vicoprofen Tablets; Zydone Tablets. (Plus) *chlorpheniramine maleate, phenylephrine, acetaminophen, caffeine*: Hycomine Compound Tablets. With phenylephrine: (Plus) *brompheniramine maleate*: Dimetane Decongestant Tablets. (Plus) *chlorpheniramine maleate*: Aclophen Tablets; Covangesic Tablets (has *pyrilamine maleate*); Dristan Cold Multi-Symptom Formula Tablets; Gendecon Tablets; Histagesic Modified Tablets; Histex SR; ND-Gesic Tablets (has *pyrilamine maleate*). With pseudoephedrine: Alka-Seltzer Plus Cold & Sinus Capsules; Allerest No Drowsiness Tablets, Caplets; Children's Cepacol Liquid; Coldrine Tablets; Dristan Cold Caplets; Maximum Strength Dynafed Tablets; Maximum Strength Sine-Aid Tablets, Caplets, Gelcaps; Maximum Strength Sudafed Sinus Tablets, Caplets; Maximum Strength Tylenol Tablets, Caplets, Gelcaps, Geltabs; No Drowsiness Sinarest Tablets; Ornex Caplets, Max Strength Caplets; Sine-Off Maximum Strength No Drowsiness Formula Caplets; Sinutab Without Drowsiness Tablets, Caplets; Sinus Excedrin Extra Strength Tablets, Caplets; Vicks DayQuil Sinus Pressure & Pain Relief Caplets. (Plus) *brompheniramine maleate*: Drixoral Cold & Flu Tablets; Maximum Strength Dristan Cold Caplets. (Plus) *chlorpheniramine maleate*: Alka-Seltzer Plus Allergy Liqui-Gels; Allerest Sinus Pain Formula Tabs; Children's Tylenol Cold Liquid, Tablets; Codimal Capsule, Tablets; Co-Hist Tablets; Comtrex Allergy-Sinus Tablets, Caplets; Kolephrin Caplets; Maximum Strength Tylenol Allergy Sinus Caplets, Gelcaps; Sinarest Sinus Tablets, Extra Strength Tablets; Sine-Off Sinus Medicine Caplets; Sinutab Maximum Strength Sinus Allergy Caplets, Tablets; TheraFlu Flu and Cold Medicine Powder. (Plus) *diphenhydramine*: Actifed Sinus Daytime/Nighttime Caplets, Tablets; Benadryl Allergy/Cold Tablets; Contac Day & Night Allergy/Sinus Caplets; Tylenol Flu Night Time Maximum Strength Powder (has *phenylalanine*). (Plus) *triprolidine*: Actifed Plus Caplets, Tablets. Other Combinations: With *oxycodone*: Endocet Tablets; Percocet Tablets, Roxicet Tablets, 5/500 Caplets, Oral Solution; Tylox Capsules. With *pentazocine*: Talacen. With *propoxyphene*: Darvocet-N; Propacet; Wygesic; various generic. (Most combinations available as generic.)

How administered: Orally; topically (suppositories).

Used to treat

All forms of mild to moderate pain, especially ✪ **headache** (including ✪ **migraine**). It can be used to reduce fever and raised body temperature, including following immunization in babies, and in brief febrile convulsions. In many ways it is similar to ℞ **aspirin**, except that it does not cause gastric irritation or relieve inflammation. It is not associated with ✪ **Reye's syndrome**, does not possess ℞ **antiplatelet**/℞ **antithrombotic** properties, and causes sensitivity reactions less frequently than aspirin, and so it is often used in circumstances where aspirin should be avoided.

Warnings

• It should not be used by people with known hypersensitivity to this drug.

Key to symbols: ✪ = Disorder Section ℞ = Drug Section ♣ = Herbal Section ⚕⚕ = Supplement Section

• It should be used with caution by people with impaired liver or kidney function, or who suffer from alcoholism (which causes liver damage).

• Except in high dosage, acetaminophen is considered safe for use during pregnancy.

• It does appear in breast milk, but has no known adverse effects in infants.

• The risk of liver damage is increased in people who use acetaminophen and who take three or more alcohol-containing drinks per day.

Interactions

• If taken with alcohol, ℞ **anticonvulsants** (for example, phenytoin, carbamazepine, barbiturates), ℞ **isoniazid**, ℞ **rifampin**, and ℞ **sulfinpyrazone**, there is a higher risk of liver damage.

• The therapeutic effects of loop ℞ **diuretics**, ℞ **lamotrigine**, and ℞ **zidovudine** may be reduced by acetaminophen.

• ℞ **activated charcoal** when administered soon after acetaminophen overdose may block further absorption and limit toxic effects.

Side effects

These depend on how it is administered and use.

• There are few side effects if dosage is low, though there may be rashes.

• After prolonged use there may be acute pancreatitis and blood disorders.

• High overdosage or prolonged use may result in liver or kidney dysfunction.

Acetaminophen Uniserts ⑧

A preparation of ℞ **acetaminophen**.
Formulation: Rectal suppository, available in 3 strengths.
Availability: OTC.
Warnings and side effects: See ℞ **acetaminophen**.

Aceta Tablets; Elixir ⑧

A preparation of ℞ **acetaminophen**.
Formulation: Oral liquid; tablets, available in two strengths.
Availability: OTC.
Warnings and side effects: See ℞ **acetaminophen**.

Aceta w/Codeine Tablets ⑧

A preparation of ℞ **codeine phosphate** and ℞ **acetaminophen**.
Formulation: Oral tablets.
Availability: Prescription only.
Warnings and side effects: See ℞ **codeine phosphate**; ℞ **acetaminophen**.

acetazolamide Ⓖ

Type/Group: **carbonic anhydrase inhibitor; anticonvulsant; antiepileptic; diuretic**.
Brand(s): Diamox; various generic.
How administered: Orally; injection.

Used to treat

Acetazolamide is mainly used in ℞ **glaucoma treatment** to treat several forms of the disorder (for example, narrow angle and open angle ✪ **glaucoma**), because it reduces the formation of aqueous humor in the eye. It acts as a diuretic and is sometimes used to treat edema (for example, in congestive ✪ **heart failure**), though it has been largely replaced by ℞ **thiazides**. It has also been used as an antiepileptic to assist in the prevention of certain types of epileptic seizures (petit mal, grand mal, mixed), especially in children. Additionally, it is sometimes used to treat the symptoms of ✪ **premenstrual syndrome** and to prevent and treat acute mountain sickness.

Warnings

• Avoid its use in people with known hypersensitivity to this drug, or with cirrhosis, severe kidney or liver impairment, low sodium or potassium levels, or adrenocortical insufficiency. Use with caution if there is known ℞ **sulfonamide** sensitivity or hypercalciuria.

• There may be a risk of birth defects, so do not use in pregnancy, especially in the first trimester, unless potential benefit outweighs potential risk to the fetus.

• Acetazolamide appears only in trace amounts in breast milk, but medical judgment is required if breast-feeding is being considered.

• A doctor must be notified if sore throat, fever, unusual bleeding or bruising, skin rash, flank pain, or tingling of hands or feet occurs.

• There is risk of bone marrow depression, anemia, other blood abnormalities, kidney impairment and electrolyte imbalances, thus regular medical monitoring is necessary.

• This drug may cause elevated glucose levels in those with diabetes mellitus and so should be used with caution.

• This drug may cause drowsiness and so driving or any hazardous activity should be avoided.

Interactions

• Acetazolamide increases the likelihood of toxic effects if used with ℞ **cyclosporine**.

• It decreases the levels of ℞ **primidone**.

• It can interact with ℞ **salicylates** to intensify the side effects of both.

• It may increase the side effects of ℞ **diflunisal** and cause a significant decrease in intraocular pressure.

Side effects

• There may be nausea and vomiting, and diarrhea.

• Taste disturbances; loss of appetite.

• Tingling in the extremities, flushing, headache, dizziness.

• Fatigue, depression, irritability.

• Thirst, increased urine production.

• Less frequently there may be reduced libido and changes in blood sugar.

• Hypersensitivity reactions may include fever, rash, and itching.

• Potentially serious side effects include seizures, blood cell disorders, skin, kidney, and liver disorders.

acetohexamide Ⓖ

Type/Group: **antidiabetic; oral hypoglycemic; sulfonylurea**.
Brand(s): Dymelor; various generic.
How administered: Orally.

Used to treat

Acetohexamide is used in the treatment for type 2 ⊙ **diabetes mellitus** (non-insulin-dependent diabetes mellitus; NIDDM).

Warnings

• It should not be given to people with juvenile diabetes or ketoacidosis.

• It should be given with caution to people with heart, thyroid, kidney, or liver disease, severe hypoglycemic reactions, and those over 65.

• It is inappropriate for use during pregnancy (insulin is the drug of choice).

• Medical judgment is required if breast-feeding is being considered, because there is a potential for adverse effects on the infant.

• Alcohol should be avoided while using this drug, as it can cause unpleasant symptoms and interfere with blood sugar control.

• There are potentially multiple drug interactions with acetohexamide, and a clinician must always be consulted before taking any other medication (including OTCs, herbal remedies, and supplements).

Interactions

• ℞ NSAIDs, ℞ **salicylates**, ℞ **sulfonamides**, ℞ **chloramphenicol**, coumarins, ℞ **probenecid**, ℞ MAOIs, and ℞ **beta-blockers** may enhance the hypoglycemic effect of sulfonylureas.

• ℞ **Thiazide** and other ℞ **diuretics**, ℞ **corticosteroids**, ℞ **phenothiazines**, ℞ **thyroid hormones**, ℞ **estrogens**, ℞ **oral contraceptives**, ℞ **phenytoin**, ℞ **niacin**, ℞ **sympathomimetics**, and ℞ **isoniazid** may lead to the loss of control of sugar levels.

• Oral ℞ **miconazole**, ℞ **diclofenac**, ℞ **ibuprofen**, ℞ **naproxen**, and ℞ **mefenamic acid** have the potential for severe hypoglycemia.

Side effects

• Frequently, dizziness, fatigue, headache, lethargy, weakness, and gastrointestinal effects.

• Uncommonly, ringing ears, jaundice, hypoglycemia, and allergic skin reactions.

• Rarely, liver damage and blood changes.

acetohydroxamic acid (AHA) Ⓖ

Type/Group: **urinary acidifier**.
Brand(s): Lithostat.
How administered: Orally.

Used to treat

Acetohydroxamic acid is used with other drugs in the treatment of chronic urinary tract infections due to certain organisms. It works by inhibiting the bacterial enzyme, urease, and so causes less conversion of urea to ammonia, and this decreases pH to a more acid level allowing other ℞ **antimicrobials** given at the same time to work better. It is not antibacterial itself and does not directly acidify the urine. It will only work when infection is caused by bacteria that use urease.

Warnings

• It should not be given to people with severe kidney disease.

• It should be used with caution by people with kidney or liver impairment.

• This drug must not be taken during pregnancy. It may cause harm to the fetus. Becoming pregnant while using this drug should be avoided.

• Not recommended for use while breast-feeding.

• Avoid alcohol as it can cause a rash.

Interactions

• This drug chelates (bonds with) heavy metals.

Side effects

• Nausea, vomiting, headache, phlebitis, nervousness, rash, and blood abnormalities.

acetylcholine chloride Ⓖ

Type/Group: **parasympathomimetic**.
Brand(s): Miochol-E.
How administered: Injection (intraocular).

Used to treat

Acetylcholine chloride is applied in solution to the eye for cataract surgery, iridectomy, and other types of surgery requiring rapid miosis (constriction of the pupil). It is rarely used therapeutically because it is rapidly broken down in the body.

Warnings

• It should not be given to people with known hypersensitivity to this drug, with inflammatory eye disease, or with certain kinds of glaucoma or asthma.

• Its safety in pregnancy and breast-feeding has not been studied, but caution is advised.

• Blurring of vision may affect the ability to perform skilled tasks such as driving.

• A thorough examination must be performed before using this drug if there is any reason to suspect retinal disease or retinal tearing. Retinal detachment is a risk in such people.

Interactions

No interactions are known when used topically.

Side effects

• It may cause headache, stinging in the eyes, cloudiness, slight swelling of the cornea, and decreased night vision.

• Although systemic side effects unrelated to the eyes or vision are quite rare, they can include sweating, breathing difficulties, flushing, a fall in blood pressure, and slow heartbeat.

acetylcysteine Ⓖ

(*N*-acetylcysteine)
Type/Group: **mucolytic; antidote**.
Brand(s): Mucomyst; Mucosil-10, Mucosil-20; various generic.
How administered: Inhalation; tracheal catheter (as mucolytic); orally; via gastric tube (as antidote).

Used to treat

Acetylcysteine liquefies mucus, thus relieving obstruction in such conditions as ⊙ **pneumonia**, chronic bronchopulmonary disease (⊙ **emphysema**, ⊙ **bronchitis**, tracheobronchitis), ⊙ **cystic fibrosis**, and ⊙ **tuberculosis**. It can also be used before a diagnostic scan of the lungs or after trauma to the lungs (including surgery). An unrelated use is as an antidote for overdose poisoning by the non-narcotic analgesic ℞ **acetaminophen**. The initial symptoms of poisoning, nausea and vomiting, usually settle within 24 hours, but give way to a serious toxic effect on the liver which takes some days to develop. It is to prevent these latter effects that treatment is directed and is required as soon as possible after overdose, normally in a hospital.

Warnings
• It should not be given to people with known hypersensitivity or allergy to this drug, but when used as an antidote the need to prevent liver damage outweighs other considerations.
• It should be given with caution to people with asthma.
• It should be used during pregnancy only when clearly needed.
• Medical judgment is required if breast-feeding is being considered. It is not known whether this drug is present in breast milk.
• If the large volume of liquefied secretions cannot be efficiently expelled, because of obstruction or inadequate cough, the airway may have to be kept open with a tube and suction.
• In the case of acetaminophen overdose, severe vomiting can occur. People who already have conditions such as peptic ulcer or esophageal varices are at greater risk of hemorrhage. As acetylcysteine may aggravate vomiting, the risks of its use in such cases must be weighed against the likelihood of liver damage without it.

Interactions
None of significance have been reported.

Side effects
• Irritation of the throat and airways, occasionally with blood in the sputum, bronchospasm (sudden constriction of the airways), mouth sores, nausea, vomiting, fever, runny nose, drowsiness, and tightness in the chest.
• Hives is a rare but significant allergic reaction, and if it occurs, use of the drug should be stopped except when administration as an antidote is judged more important.

Achromycin ℬ
A preparation of ℞ **tetracycline hydrochloride**.
Formulation: Ointment.
Availability: OTC.
Warnings and side effects: See ℞ **tetracycline hydrochloride**.

aciclovir Ⓖ
see ℞ **acyclovir**.

Aciphex ℬ
A preparation of ℞ **rabeprazole**.
Formulation: Oral tablets, delayed release.
Availability: Prescription only.
Warnings and side effects: See ℞ **rabeprazole**.

acitretin Ⓖ
Type/Group: psoriasis treatment; retinoid.
Brand(s): Soriatane.
How administered: Orally.

Used to treat
Acitretin is taken over a period of weeks to relieve severe ✪ **psoriasis** that is resistant to other treatments and for other ✪ **skin conditions** (including severe Darier's disease). It is chemically a retinoid (it is a metabolite of etretinate, which is a derivative of retinol or ⚕ **vitamin A**) and has a marked effect on the cells that make up the skin epithelium.

Warnings
• It should not be given to people with certain liver or kidney disorders.
• It must not be used by pregnant women. Women of childbearing potential are given special counseling before acitretin is prescribed, and must agree to continue using two reliable contraceptive means for three years after ending treatment. It will be prescribed after obtaining a report of a negative pregnancy test and once the woman concerned has started her menstrual period. (Some kinds of contraceptives fail during and after acitretin therapy.) Alcohol worsens and prolongs the probability of serious effects on the fetus, so women of childbearing potential are warned not to ingest any products containing alcohol.
• Acitretin should not be used by nursing women.
• This is a specialist drug prescribed only by expert doctors and a full assessment for suitability will be made, and monitoring (for example, liver function and blood glucose) is generally required.
• Anyone taking this drug must not donate blood during treatment or for three years after discontinuing use.
• Exposure to sunlight or any other UV source must be minimized.
• The full benefit of treatment may take two to three months.
• Vitamin A supplements beyond the minimum recommended daily dose should be avoided, as there is a possibility of an increased toxic effect in combination with retinoids, such as acitretin.

Interactions
• If taken with ℞ **glyburide**, this may affect blood glucose levels.
• Methotrexate may increase the risk of liver damage.
• alcohol enhances the conversion of acitretin to longer-lived etretinate, with potentially severe effects in pregnancy.
• Acitretin may cause failure of contraception, such as progestin-only, "minipill" ℞ **contraceptives**.

Side effects
• Inflammation and cracking lips (cheilitis), dry skin, eyes, or mucous membrane, muscle and joint ache, hair loss, reversible visual disturbances, nausea, headache, sweating, changes in liver function, blood disorders, mood changes, drowsiness, and others.

Aclophen Tablets ℬ
A preparation of ℞ **phenylephrine hydrochloride**, ℞ **acetaminophen**, and ℞ **chlorpheniramine maleate**.
Formulation: Oral tablets, long acting.
Availability: Prescription only.
Warnings and side effects: See ℞ **phenylephrine hydrochloride**; ℞ **acetaminophen**; ℞ **chlorpheniramine maleate**.

Aclovate ℬ
A preparation of ℞ **alclometasone**.
Formulation: Cream; ointment.

Availability: Prescription only.
Warnings and side effects: See ℞ **alclometasone**.

Acne Lotion 10 ⑧

A preparation of ℞ **sulfur**.
Formulation: Topical lotion.
Availability: OTC.
Warnings and side effects: See ℞ **sulfur**.

acne treatment ⑩

Generics: adapalene; aluminum acetate; azelaic acid; benzoic acid; benzoyl peroxide; chlortetracycline; clindamycin; coal tar; demeclocycline; doxycycline; erythromycin; ichthammol; isotretinoin; meclocycline sulfosalicylate; metronidazole; minocycline; oxytetracycline; resorcinol; salicylic acid; sulfacetamide; sulfur; tazarotene; tretinoin.

Actions and uses

Drugs for treating ✪ **acne** are used to deal with several different aspects of this difficult condition (also called ✪ **acne** vulgaris). The characteristic eruptions, which are caused by a plug of keratin in the pores that pimples and darkens, may be helped by various ℞ **skin preparation** treatments, especially lotions containing ℞ **keratolytic** and similar agents. Keratolytics include ℞ **benzoyl peroxide**, ℞ **salicylic acid**, ℞ **benzoic acid**, ℞ **resorcinol**, ℞ **azelaic acid**, ℞ **coal tar**, and ℞ **ichthammol**. They may be used with ℞ **sulfur** and ℞ **astringent** preparations containing ℞ **zinc oxide** or ℞ **astringent** agents (℞ **aluminum acetate**).

The site of the acne often becomes infected and some antiacne drugs (for example, ℞ **azelaic acid**) do have ℞ **antibacterial** action. Severe cases can be treated by mouth with ℞ **antibacterial** drugs, including ℞ **antibiotic** agents, mainly of the tetracycline group (notably ℞ **chlortetracycline**, ℞ **demeclocycline**, ℞ **doxycycline**, ℞ **meclocycline**, ℞ **minocycline**, and ℞ **oxytetracycline**), ℞ **erythromycin**, and ℞ **clindamycin**. In some cases ℞ **retinoid** drugs—vitamin-A derivatives—may be used topically (externally), for example, ℞ **tretinoin**, ℞ **adapalene**, and ℞ **tazarotene**, or in severe cases (including severe recalcitrant cystic acne) they may be taken by mouth, for example, ℞ **isotretinoin** and ℞ **tretinoin**.

Acne is common in adolescence and ℞ **sex hormone** changes may stimulate overactivity of the sebaceous glands. In women, a special form of the ℞ **oral contraceptive** pill may be prescribed to deal with the problem. In some cases acne may be linked to a mild deficiency of ♒ **zinc**.

A related condition is ✪ **rosacea** (also called acne rosacea) and for this, too, ℞ **antibacterial** drugs, such as ℞ **erythromycin**, topical ℞ **metronidazole** and topical ℞ **sulfonamide** agents (℞ **sulfacetamide**, as sodium sulfacetamide) are used.

Limitations

The evaluation of acne-type conditions is best made by a specialist. Dietary and hygiene advice may help rectify the condition. Simple acne preparations are effective in many cases, but antibacterial or hormonal treatment may be required in others. Oral retinoids are rather toxic and are reserved for severe cases. See the individual drug entries (particularly with regard to pregnancy).

Acnomel ⑧

A preparation of ℞ **sulfur** and ℞ **resorcinol**.
Formulation: Topical cream.
Availability: OTC.
Warnings and side effects: See ℞ **sulfur**; ℞ **resorcinol**.

Acnotex ⑧

A preparation of ℞ **sulfur** and ℞ **resorcinol**.
Formulation: Topical lotion.
Availability: OTC.
Warnings and side effects: See ℞ **sulfur**; ℞ **resorcinol**.

acrivastine ⑥

Type/Group: antihistamine; antiallergic.
Brand(s): Semprex-D Capsules (also contains *pseudoephedrine hydrochloride*).
How administered: Orally.

Used to treat

Acrivastine has only recently been developed and has less sedative side effects than some of the older antihistamines. In the US it is available only in combination with ℞ **pseudoephedrine**. It can be used for the symptomatic relief of allergic conditions, such as ✪ **hay fever** (seasonal allergic rhinitis) and ✪ **urticaria**.

Warnings

• It should not be given to people with known hypersensitivity to this drug or with known sensitivity to antihistamines such as ℞ **triprolidine**.
• Antihistamines should be given with caution to people with heart disease, hypertension, hyperthyroidism, increased intraocular pressure (pressure in the eyeball, as in glaucoma), enlarged prostate, or certain cardiovascular, obstructive bladder or gastrointestinal conditions, kidney impairment, porphyria, epilepsy, or liver disease.
• Acrivastine should be used during pregnancy only if it is clearly needed.
• Medical judgment is required if breast-feeding is being considered. It is not known whether this drug appears in breast milk.
• Side effects are more frequent in the elderly.

Interactions

• ℞ **MAOI** antidepressants may prolong and intensify the ℞ **anticholinergic** (see Side effects below) and sedative effects of antihistamines.
• If used with ℞ **tricyclic** antidepressants, other antihistamines, ℞ **skeletal muscle relaxants**, ℞ **opioids**, ℞ **barbiturates**, ℞ **hypnotics**, ℞ **sedatives**, or ℞ **antianxiety** drugs, there is a risk of intensified side effects.
• Alcohol may intensify side effects such as drowsiness and impaired mental alertness.

Side effects

• These depend on how it is administered. Principally there is drowsiness, but compared with other antihistamines there are far fewer sedative, psychomotor, and anticholinergic effects (dry mouth, blurred vision, urinary retention, gastrointestinal disturbances).

• This type of antihistamine may also cause headache, dizziness, impaired muscular coordination, rashes, photosensitivity (abnormal sensitivity to light), palpitations, blood disorders, sleep disturbances, liver disturbances, and hypotension.

ACT Ⓑ

see ℞ dactinomycin.

Actagen-C Cough Syrup Ⓑ

A preparation of ℞ codeine phosphate; ℞ pseudoephedrine, and ℞ triprolidine.
Formulation: Oral syrup.
Availability: May or may not require a prescription.
Warnings and side effects: See ℞ codeine phosphate; ℞ pseudoephedrine; ℞ triprolidine.

Acthar; H.P. Acthar Gel Ⓑ

A preparation of ℞ corticotropin.
Formulation: Injection in several strengths. Gel is a repository injection for extended release.
Availability: Prescription only.
Warnings and side effects: See ℞ corticotropin.

ActHib Ⓑ

A preparation of ℞ Haemophilus b conjugate vaccine.
Formulation: Injection.
Availability: Prescription only.
Warnings and side effects: See ℞ Haemophilus b conjugate vaccine.

Acticin Ⓑ

A preparation of ℞ permethrin.
Formulation: Topical cream.
Availability: Prescription only.
Warnings and side effects: See ℞ permethrin.

Acticort 100 Ⓑ

A preparation of ℞ hydrocortisone.
Formulation: Lotion.
Availability: Prescription only.
Warnings and side effects: See ℞ hydrocortisone.

Actidose-Aqua Ⓑ

A preparation of ℞ activated charcoal.
Formulation: Liquid.
Availability: OTC.
Warnings and side effects: See ℞ activated charcoal.

Actidose with Sorbitol Ⓑ

A preparation of ℞ activated charcoal and ℞ sorbitol.
Formulation: Liquid.
Availability: OTC.
Warnings and side effects: See ℞ activated charcoal; ℞ sorbitol.

Actifed Plus Caplets, Tablets Ⓑ

A preparation of ℞ pseudoephedrine, ℞ triprolidine hydrochloride, and ℞ acetaminophen.
Formulation: Oral tablets.
Availability: OTC.
Warnings and side effects: See ℞ pseudoephedrine; ℞ triprolidine hydrochloride; ℞ acetaminophen.

Actifed Allergy Tablets Ⓑ

A preparation of ℞ pseudoephedrine and ℞ diphenhydramine hydrochloride.
Formulation: Oral tablets.
Availability: OTC.
Warnings and side effects: See ℞ pseudoephedrine; ℞ diphenhydramine hydrochloride.

Actifed Cold & Allergy Tablets Ⓑ

A preparation of ℞ pseudoephedrine and ℞ triprolidine hydrochloride.
Formulation: Oral tablets.
Availability: OTC.
Warnings and side effects: See ℞ pseudoephedrine; ℞ triprolidine hydrochloride.

Actifed Sinus Daytime/Nighttime Caplets; Tablets Ⓑ

A preparation of ℞ pseudoephedrine, ℞ acetaminophen, and ℞ diphenhydramine hydrochloride.
Formulation: Oral tablets.
Availability: OTC.
Warnings and side effects: See ℞ pseudoephedrine; ℞ acetaminophen; ℞ diphenhydramine hydrochloride.

Actifed w/Codeine Cough Syrup Ⓑ

A preparation of ℞ codeine phosphate, ℞ pseudoephedrine, and ℞ triprolidine.
Formulation: Oral syrup.
Availability: May or may not require a prescription.
Warnings and side effects: See ℞ codeine phosphate; ℞ pseudoephedrine; ℞ triprolidine.

Actigall Ⓑ

A preparation of ℞ ursodiol.
Formulation: Oral capsules.
Availability: Prescription only.
Warnings and side effects: See ℞ ursodiol.

Actimmune Ⓑ

A preparation of ℞ interferons (interferon gamma-1b).
Formulation: Injection.
Availability: Prescription only.
Warnings and side effects: See ℞ interferons.

actinomycin D Ⓖ

see ℞ dactinomycin.

Actiq ℞

A preparation of ℞ **fentanyl**.
Formulation: Lozenges on a stick; five strengths, all high dosage, to be used only by those who are already on opioid tolerant.
Availability: Prescription only.
Warnings and side effects: See ℞ **fentanyl**.

Actisite ℞

A preparation of ℞ **tetracycline hydrochloride**.
Formulation: Periodontal fiber.
Availability: Prescription only.
Warnings and side effects: See ℞ **tetracycline hydrochloride**.

Activase ℞

A preparation of ℞ **alteplase, recombinant**.
Formulation: Intravenous injection or infusion.
Availability: Prescription only.
Warnings and side effects: See ℞ **alteplase, recombinant**.

activated charcoal Ⓖ

(charcoal)
Type/Group: antidote; adsorbent; antidiarrheal; antiflatulence.
Brand(s): Actidose-Aqua; Liqui-Char; various generic. With *simethicone*: Charcoal Plus; Flatulex. With *sorbitol*: Actidose with Sorbital; CharcoAid; CharcoAid 2000.
How administered: Orally.

Used to treat

Activated charcoal is used for soaking up poisons in the stomach or small intestine, especially drug overdoses in cases where only a small quantity of the drug may be extremely toxic (for example, some ℞ **antidepressants**). It is an adsorbent material and can help prevent the effects of drug overdose by increasing the elimination of certain drugs even after they have been absorbed (for example, ℞ **phenobarbital** and ℞ **theophylline**). It can also be used in preparations for treating ✪ **diarrhea** (it is effective in binding together fecal matter) and can relieve ✪ **flatulence**.

Warnings

• It should not be used to treat overdose of mineral acids and alkalis, and it is not particularly effective in treating overdose of alcohol or iron salts.
• There are no adverse effects known when used during pregnancy.
• When used as an antidote, vomiting must be induced first to clear the stomach of most of the contents.
• It must be given to conscious people only.
• It is not recommended for children under one year of age.

Interactions

• Activated charcoal adsorbs the emetic ℞ **ipecac syrup**, so nullifying its effect.
• Some dairy foods (milk, ice cream, and sherbet) weaken the adsorptive ability of activated charcoal.
• When used regularly to treat flatulence or diarrhea, it may reduce the absorption of many other drugs, for example, ℞ **acetaminophen**, ℞ **aspirin**, ℞ **barbiturates**, ℞ **carbamazepine**, ℞ **digitoxin**, ℞ **hydantoins**, ℞ **phenothiazines**, ℞ **quinine**, ℞ **sulfonylureas**, ℞ **tetracyclines**, ℞ **tricyclic** antidepressants, and ℞ **theophylline**. It may adsorb vitamins, minerals, enzymes, and other nutrients.

Side effects

• High doses, taken quickly, may cause vomiting, but it is regarded as safe in normal use.
• Stools may be colored black and there may be gastrointestinal disturbances, nausea, and vomiting.

Activella ℞

A preparation of ℞ **ethinyl estradiol** and ℞ **norethindrone**.
Formulation: Oral tablets.
Availability: Prescription only.
Warnings and side effects: See ℞ **ethinyl estradiol**; ℞ **norethindrone**.

Actos ℞

A preparation of ℞ **pioglitazone**.
Formulation: Oral tablets in several strengths.
Availability: Prescription only.
Warnings and side effects: See ℞ **pioglitazone**.

Acular ℞

A preparation of ℞ **ketorolac tromethamine**.
Formulation: Ophthalmic solution.
Availability: Prescription only.
Warnings and side effects: See ℞ **ketorolac tromethamine**.

acyclovir Ⓖ

(aciclovir)
Type/Group: **antiviral**.
Brand(s): Zovirax; various generic.
How administered: Orally; topically; injection or intravenous infusion.

Used to treat

Acyclovir is used specifically to treat infection by the herpes viruses (for example, ✪ **shingles**, ✪ **chickenpox**, ✪ **cold sores**, genital ✪ **herpes**, and herpes infections of the eye and mouth). It works by inhibiting the action of enzymes in human cells that are used by the virus to replicate itself. To be effective, however, treatment must begin early. It can be valuable in immunocompromised people. It can also be used to prevent individuals at risk from contracting a herpes disease.

Warnings

• It should not be given to people who become hypersensitive to the drug.
• It should be given with caution to people with liver or kidney disorders, or who are dehydrated.
• Acyclovir should be used during pregnancy only if the potential benefit outweighs the possible risks to the fetus.
• Medical judgment is required if breast-feeding is being considered. When given orally or intravenously, it appears in breast milk. The effects of topical (external) application are not presently known, but caution should still be exercised.

• Kidney function may be impaired by this drug, and so dosage must be adjusted for patients with existing kidney dysfunction, or who are taking other drugs that may adversely affect the kidneys.
• It is essential to maintain fluid intake when receiving acyclovir intravenously, so that the drug cannot concentrate in the kidneys and cause damage.
• Although neurologic adverse reactions to the intravenous form of this drug are uncommon, they can be severe. Medical judgment is necessary when any neurologic abnormality is known to be present, when there has been a prior reaction to a cytotoxic drug, or when given concurrently with ℞ **methotrexate** or ℞ **interferon**.

Interactions
• ℞ **Probenecid** increases the levels of intravenous acyclovir.
• ℞ **Zidovudine** may cause extreme drowsiness and lethargy.

Side effects
• When applied topically (externally), there may be a temporary burning or stinging sensation. Some people experience a localized drying of the skin.
• When taken orally, it may give rise to gastrointestinal disturbance (for example, nausea, vomiting) and various blood-cell deficiencies. There may also be fatigue, rash, headache, tremor, and effects on mood.
• When injected there may be hallucinations, sleepiness, and severe local inflammation at the injection site.

Adagen Ⓑ
A preparation of ℞ **pegademase bovine** and ℞ **interferons**.
Formulation: Injection.
Availability: Prescription only.
Warnings and side effects: See ℞ **interferons**; ℞ **pegademase bovine**.

Adalat Ⓑ
A preparation of ℞ **nifedipine**.
Formulation: Oral capsules, available in two strengths.
Availability: Prescription only.
Warnings and side effects: See ℞ **nifedipine**.

Adalat CC Ⓑ
A preparation of ℞ **nifedipine**.
Formulation: Oral tablets, sustained release, available in 3 strengths.
Availability: Prescription only.
Warnings and side effects: See ℞ **nifedipine**.

adapalene Ⓖ
Type/Group: **acne treatment; retinoid**.
Brand(s): Differin.
How administered: Topically (external).

Used to treat
Adapalene is used for the topical treatment of ✪ **acne**. It is chemically a retinoid (a derivative of retinol, or ⚬⚬ **vitamin A**).

Warnings
• It should not be given to people with known hypersensitivity to this drug.
• Adapalene should be used during pregnancy only if the potential benefit outweighs the possible risk to the fetus.
• Medical judgment is required if breast-feeding is being considered. It is not known whether it appears in breast milk.
• Sunburned, eczematous or broken skin, mucous membranes, severe acne, and the eyes must be avoided.
• It should not be applied over large areas.
• Ultraviolet light must be avoided.
• Sometimes acne may appear to get worse at first, but improvement should be noticed after 8 to 12 weeks.

Interactions
• Skin irritation is more likely if adapalene is used with other topical preparations such as alcohol, ℞ **astringents**, ℞ **resorcinol**, ℞ **salicylic acid**, strong soaps, and products containing ℞ **sulfur**.

Side effects
• There may be skin irritation and other skin reactions, but side effects usually subside after one month.

Adapin Ⓑ
A preparation of ℞ **doxepin**.
Formulation: Oral tablets in several strengths.
Availability: Prescription only.
Warnings and side effects: See ℞ **doxepin**.

Adenocard Ⓑ
A preparation of ℞ **adenosine**.
Formulation: Injection.
Availability: Prescription only.
Warnings and side effects: See ℞ **adenosine**.

adenosine Ⓖ
Type/Group: **antiarrhythmic**.
Brand(s): Adenocard.
How administered: Injection.

Used to treat
Adenosine is used to correct certain abnormal heart rhythms (primarily, a kind of fast atrial rhythm; see ✪ **arrhythmia**). It has been used, as well, to help in the diagnosis of certain heart conditions and to relieve symptoms of some complications of ✪ **varicose veins**.

Warnings
• It should not be given to people with known hypersensitivity to this drug, or with certain heart arrhythmias.
• It should be given with caution to people with asthma.
• Adenosine should be used during pregnancy only if it is clearly needed.
• Its effects in breast-feeding have not been studied. Consult your doctor if you plan to breast feed.
• It should be used only after other appropriate (and simpler) non-drug measures have failed to restore regular atrial rhythm.

Interactions

• ℞ **carbamazepine** and ℞ **dipyridamole** may intensify adenosine's effects.
• ℞ **digoxin** and ℞ **verapamil** may have the potential to cause serious arrhythmias.
• ℞ **caffeine** and ℞ **theophylline** may decrease adenosine's effects.

Side effects

• Frequently, facial flushing, shortness of breath, and the sensation of pressure on the chest.
• Other effects may include nausea, lightheadedness, headache, sweating, palpitations, and tingling in the arms.

Adipex-P Ⓑ

A preparation of ℞ **phentermine**.
Formulation: Oral capsules in several strengths.
Availability: Prescription only.
Warnings and side effects: See ℞ **phentermine**.

Adipost Ⓑ

A preparation of ℞ **phendimetrazine**.
Formulation: Sustained release capsules.
Availability: Prescription only.
Warnings and side effects: See ℞ **phendimetrazine**.

Adprin-B; Extra Strength Adprin-B Ⓑ

A preparation of ℞ **aspirin** buffered with ℞ **calcium carbonate**, ℞ **magnesium carbonate**, and magnesium oxide.
Formulation: Oral tablets.
Availability: OTC.
Warnings and side effects: See ℞ **aspirin**; ℞ **calcium carbonate**; ℞ **magnesium carbonate**; ℞ **magnesium hydroxide**.

adrenaline Ⓖ

see ℞ **epinephrine**.

adrenergic-neuron blocker Ⓓ

Generics: bretylium tosylate; guanabenz acetate; guanethidine monosulfate.

Actions and uses

Adrenergic-neuron blockers act to prevent the release of norepinephrine (noradrenaline) from the adrenergic nerves of the sympathetic nervous system, which is involved in controlling involuntary functions such as blood pressure, heart rate, and the activity of muscles of internal organs (such as blood vessels, intestines) and glandular secretions. Norepinephrine is the main neurotransmitter of the sympathetic nervous system and therefore adrenergic-neuron blockers cause an overall ℞ **antisympathetic** action with a fall in blood pressure. The main use of such drugs, therefore, is as ℞ **antihypertensives** in the treatment of ✪ **hypertension**.

Limitations

Because they have quite severe side effects (see individual generics), they are not drugs-of-choice in the treatment of moderate to severe high blood pressure.

adrenergic-neurone blocker Ⓓ

see ℞ **adrenergic-neuron blocker**.

adrenocorticosteroid Ⓓ

see ℞ **corticosteroid**.

Adriamycin RDF; Adriamycin PFS Ⓑ

A preparation of ℞ **doxorubicin**.
Formulation: Powder for injection.
Availability: Prescription only.
Warnings and side effects: See ℞ **doxorubicin**.

Adrucil Ⓑ

A preparation of ℞ **fluorouracil**.
Formulation: Oral tablets; Injection.
Availability: Prescription only.
Warnings and side effects: See ℞ **fluorouracil**.

adsorbent Ⓓ

Generics: activated charcoal; kaolin.

Actions and uses

Adsorbents are chemical agents that bind other chemicals to their surfaces, so reducing the activity of the latter. ℞ **activated charcoal** (charcoal) is widely used to bind chemicals and gases. It may be used as an ℞ **antidote** to bind poisons in the stomach or small intestine, or drugs in overdose and so helping their safe removal from the body (for example, ℞ **antidepressants**, ℞ **barbiturates**, and ℞ **theophylline**). It can also be used in ℞ **antiflatulence** to relieve ✪ **flatulence**, and also in ℞ **antidiarrheal** preparations to bind fecal matter and possibly toxins and relieve ✪ **diarrhea**. ℞ **kaolin** is a purified white clay used as an adsorbent in antidiarrheal preparations.

Limitations

Adsorbents may reduce the absorption of many other drugs and also may adsorb vitamins, minerals, enzymes, and other nutrients, so reducing their amounts in the blood.

Adsorbocarpine Ⓑ

A preparation of ℞ **pilocarpine**.
Formulation: Ophthalmic solution in several strengths.
Availability: Prescription only.
Warnings and side effects: See ℞ **pilocarpine**.

Adsorbonac Ⓑ

A preparation of ℞ **sodium chloride**, ℞ **povidone**, ℞ **hydroxyethylcellulose**, and ℞ **poloxamer 188**.
Formulation: Ophthalmic solution.
Availability: OTC.
Warnings and side effects: See ℞ **sodium chloride**; ℞ **povidone**; ℞ **hydroxyethylcellulose**; ℞ **poloxamer 188**.

Advil Junior Strength Tablets, Chewable Tablets Ⓑ

A preparation of ℞ **ibuprofen**.
Formulation: Oral tablets, chewable.

Availability: OTC.

Warnings and side effects: See ℞ ibuprofen. These chewable tablets contain the sweetener aspartame, which should be avoided by individuals with phenylketonuria.

Advil Children's Oral Suspension; Pediatric Drops ⓑ

A preparation of ℞ ibuprofen.
Formulation: Oral liquid.
Availability: OTC.
Warnings and side effects: See ℞ ibuprofen.

Advil Cold & Sinus Caplets ⓑ

A preparation of ℞ pseudoephedrine and ℞ ibuprofen.
Formulation: Oral tablets.
Availability: OTC.
Warnings and side effects: See ℞ pseudoephedrine; ℞ ibuprofen.

Advil Tablets; Liqui-Gels ⓑ

A preparation of ℞ ibuprofen.
Formulation: Oral tablets; capsules (Liqui-Gels).
Availability: OTC.
Warnings and side effects: See ℞ ibuprofen.

Aerosporin ⓑ

A preparation of ℞ polymyxin B.
Formulation: Injection.
Availability: Prescription only.
Warnings and side effects: See ℞ polymyxin B.

Afrin; Afrin Sinus; Afrin Children's Nose Drops ⓑ

A preparation of ℞ oxymetazoline hydrochloride.
Formulation: Nasal spray; drops.
Availability: OTC.
Warnings and side effects: See ℞ oxymetazoline hydrochloride.

Afrin Moisturizing Saline Mist ⓑ

A preparation of ℞ sodium chloride.
Formulation: Nasal mist.
Availability: OTC.
Warnings and side effects: See ℞ sodium chloride.

Afrin Tablets ⓑ

A preparation of pseudoephedrine sulfate.
Formulation: Oral tablets, available as immediate or extended release.
Availability: OTC.
Warnings and side effects: See ℞ pseudoephedrine.

Aftate for Athlete's Foot; Aftate for Jock Itch ⓑ

A preparation of ℞ tolnaftate.

Formulation: Topical gel; topical spray powder; topical spray liquid (athlete's foot only).
Availability: OTC.
Warnings and side effects: See ℞ tolnaftate.

Agenerase ⓑ

A preparation of ℞ amprenavir.
Formulation: Oral capsules; oral suspension.
Availability: Prescription only.
Warnings and side effects: See ℞ amprenavir.

Aggrastat ⓑ

A preparation of ℞ tirofiban.
Formulation: Intravenous infusion.
Availability: Prescription only.
Warnings and side effects: See ℞ tirofiban.

Aggrenox ⓑ

A preparation of ℞ aspirin and ℞ dipyridamole.
Formulation: Oral capsules.
Availability: Prescription only.
Warnings and side effects: See ℞ aspirin; ℞ dipyridamole.

Agoral ⓑ

A preparation of ℞ senna.
Formulation: Oral liquid.
Availability: OTC.
Warnings and side effects: See ℞ senna.

Agrylin ⓑ

A preparation of ℞ anagrelide hydrochloride.
Formulation: Oral capsules, available in two strengths.
Availability: Prescription only.
Warnings and side effects: See ℞ anagrelide hydrochloride.

AH-Chew D Tablets ⓑ

A preparation of ℞ phenylephrine hydrochloride.
Formulation: Oral tablets, chewable.
Availability: OTC.
Warnings and side effects: See ℞ phenylephrine hydrochloride.

AH-Chew Tablets ⓑ

A preparation of methscopolamine nitrate, ℞ chlorpheniramine maleate, and ℞ phenylephrine.
Formulation: Oral tablets.
Availability: Prescription only.
Warnings and side effects: See ℞ scopolamine; ℞ chlorpheniramine maleate; ℞ phenylephrine.

AHF ⓖ

see ℞ antihemophilic factor.

A-Hydrocort ⓑ

A preparation of ℞ hydrocortisone.
Formulation: Injection in several strengths.

Availability: Prescription only.
Warnings and side effects: See ℞ hydrocortisone.

Airet ⓑ

A preparation of ℞ albuterol.
Formulation: Solution for inhalation.
Availability: Prescription only.
Warnings and side effects: See ℞ albuterol.

Akarpine ⓑ

A preparation of ℞ pilocarpine.
Formulation: Ophthalmic solution, available in three strengths.
Availability: Prescription only.
Warnings and side effects: See ℞ pilocarpine.

AK-Chlor ⓑ

A preparation of ℞ chloramphenicol.
Formulation: Eye drops; ointment.
Availability: Prescription only.
Warnings and side effects: See ℞ chloramphenicol.

AK-Cide ⓑ

A preparation of ℞ prednisolone, sodium sulfate, and sodium sulfacemide.
Formulation: Eye drops; ophthalmic ointment.
Availability: Prescription only.
Warnings and side effects: See ℞ prednisone.

AK-Con ⓑ

A preparation of ℞ naphazoline hydrochloride.
Formulation: Eye drops.
Availability: Prescription only.
Warnings and side effects: See ℞ naphazoline hydrochloride.

AK-Dex ⓑ

A preparation of ℞ dexamethasone.
Formulation: Eye drops.
Availability: Prescription only.
Warnings and side effects: See ℞ dexamethasone.

AK-Dilate ⓑ

A preparation of ℞ phenylephrine hydrochloride.
Formulation: Eye drops, available in two strengths.
Availability: Prescription only.
Warnings and side effects: See ℞ phenylephrine hydrochloride.

AK-Fluor ⓑ

A preparation of ℞ fluorescein sodium.
Formulation: Injection.
Availability: Prescription only.
Warnings and side effects: See ℞ fluorescein sodium.

Akineton ⓑ

A preparation of ℞ biperiden.
Formulation: Oral tablets; solution for injection.

Availability: Prescription only.
Warnings and side effects: See ℞ biperiden.

AK-Nefrin ⓑ

A preparation of ℞ phenylephrine hydrochloride.
Formulation: Eye drops.
Availability: OTC.
Warnings and side effects: See ℞ phenylephrine hydrochloride.

Akne-mycin ⓑ

A preparation of ℞ erythromycin.
Formulation: Topical solution; ointment.
Availability: Prescription only.
Warnings and side effects: See ℞ erythromycin.

AK-Neo-Dex ⓑ

A preparation of ℞ dexamethasone and ℞ neomycin.
Formulation: Ophthalmic solution.
Availability: Prescription only.
Warnings and side effects: See ℞ dexamethasone; ℞ neomycin

AK-Pentolate ⓑ

A preparation of ℞ cyclopentolate hydrochloride.
Formulation: Ophthalmic solution.
Availability: Prescription only.
Warnings and side effects: See ℞ cyclopentolate hydrochloride.

AKPro ⓑ

A preparation of ℞ dipivefrin hydrochloride.
Formulation: Eye drops.
Availability: Prescription only.
Warnings and side effects: See ℞ dipivefrin hydrochloride.

AK-Spore H.C. (Otic) ⓑ

A preparation of ℞ hydrocortisone, ℞ neomycin, and ℞ polymyxin B.
Formulation: Ear drops.
Availability: Prescription only.
Warnings and side effects: See ℞ hydrocortisone; ℞ neomycin; ℞ polymyxin B.

AK-Spore Ophthalmic Ointment ⓑ

A preparation of ℞ neomycin, ℞ polymyxin B, and ℞ bacitracin.
Formulation: Topical ointment.
Availability: Prescription only.
Warnings and side effects: See ℞ neomycin; ℞ polymyxin B; ℞ bacitracin.

AK-Spore Ophthalmic Solution ⓑ

A preparation of ℞ neomycin, ℞ polymyxin B, and ℞ gramicidin.
Formulation: Eye drops.
Availability: Prescription only.
Warnings and side effects: See ℞ neomycin; ℞ polymyxin B; ℞ gramicidin.

AK-Sulf Ⓑ

A preparation of ℞ **sulfacetamide**.
Formulation: Eye drops, ophthalmic ointment.
Availability: Prescription only.
Warnings and side effects: See ℞ **sulfacetamide**.

AK-Trol Ophthalmic Solution Ⓑ

A preparation of ℞ **neomycin**, ℞ **dexamethasone**, and benzalkonium hydrochloride.
Formulation: Eye drops.
Availability: Prescription only.
Warnings and side effects: See ℞ **neomycin**; ℞ **dexamethasone**.

AK-Trol Suspension Ⓑ

A preparation of ℞ **dexamethasone**, ℞ **neomycin**, and ℞ **polymyxin B**.
Formulation: Opthalmic solution.
Availability: Prescription only.
Warnings and side effects: See ℞ **dexamethasone**; ℞ **neomycin**; ℞ **polymyxin B**.

Akwa Tears Ⓑ

A preparation of ℞ **polyvinyl alcohol**.
Formulation: Ophthalmic solution.
Availability: OTC.
Warnings and side effects: See ℞ **polyvinyl alcohol**.

Ala-Cort Ⓑ

A preparation of ℞ **hydrocortisone**.
Formulation: Cream; lotion.
Availability: Prescription only.
Warnings and side effects: See ℞ **hydrocortisone**.

Ala-Quin Ⓑ

A preparation of ℞ **hydrocortisone** and ℞ **clioquinol**.
Formulation: Cream.
Availability: Prescription only.
Warnings and side effects: See ℞ **hydrocortisone**; ℞ **clioquinol**.

Ala-Scalp Ⓑ

A preparation of ℞ **hydrocortisone**.
Formulation: Lotion.
Availability: Prescription only.
Warnings and side effects: See ℞ **hydrocortisone**.

Albalon Ⓑ

A preparation of ℞ **naphazoline hydrochloride**.
Formulation: Eye drops.
Availability: Prescription only.
Warnings and side effects: See ℞ **naphazoline hydrochloride**.

albendazole Ⓖ

Type/Group: **anthelmintic**.
Brand(s): Albenza Tablets.

How administered: Orally.

Used to treat

Albendazole is a synthetic drug used to provide cover during surgery for the removal of cysts caused by the dog ✪ **tapeworm** *Echinococcus granulosus*, as treatment when surgery is not possible, and also to treat active cysts of the pork tapeworm *Taenia solium*.

Warnings

• It should not be given to people with known hypersensitivity to this drug.

• It should not be used during pregnancy unless there is no alternative, and pregnancy, if planned, should be delayed one month after completing therapy with albendazole.

• Medical judgment is required if breast-feeding is being considered. It is not known whether breast milk is affected.

• Liver function must be monitored, and if enzyme levels rise significantly, albendazole should be discontinued until levels return to normal.

• Blood disorders have been reported, and blood counts will be monitored.

Interactions

• ℞ **Dexamethasone**, ℞ **praziquantel**, and ℞ **cimetidine** may raise levels of albendazole.

Side effects

• There may be headache, dizziness, gastrointestinal disturbances, hair loss, rash, fever, and liver disorders.

• Blood disorders have been reported, and blood counts will be monitored.

Albenza Tablets Ⓑ

A preparation of ℞ **albendazole**.
Formulation: Oral tablets.
Availability: Prescription only.
Warnings and side effects: See ℞ **albendazole**.

albuterol Ⓖ

(salbutamol)
Type/Group: **antiasthmatic; sympathomimetic; beta-adrenergic stimulant**.
Brand(s): Airet; Proventil; Ventolin; Volmax; various generic.
Combinations: with *ipratropium*: Combivent.
How administered: Orally; inhalant.

Used to treat

Albuterol is mainly used as a ℞ **bronchodilator** in reversible obstructive airways disease, as an antiasthmatic treatment in severe acute and chronic ✪ **asthma**, and for exercise-induced bronchospasm. It is also available in another chemical form, as ℞ **levalbuterol hydrochloride**, one of its isomers (it is a racemic mix of isomers).

Warnings

• It should not be given to people with known hypersensitivity to albuterol, heart arrhythmias, or severe heart disease.

• It should be given with caution to people with certain heart diseases, hyperthyroidism, diabetes mellitus, hypertension, or prostatic hypertrophy.

• It should be used in pregnancy only if it is clearly needed because it may cross the placenta and inhibit uterine contractions.

• Medical judgment is required if breast-feeding is being considered. It is not known if it appears in breast milk.

• Rarely, may have adverse effects on heart and blood pressure, or may lead to paradoxical bronchoconstriction.

Interactions

• ℞ **Beta-blockers** decrease the effects of albuterol.

• If used with ℞ **furosemide**, there is a risk of enhancing furosemide's potassium-lowering effect.

Side effects

• Frequently, headache, nausea, restlessness, nervousness, trembling, dizziness, throat dryness, irritation or inflammation.

• Occasionally, insomnia, weakness, altered taste or smell.

• With inhalation, coughing and bronchial irritation.

• Rarely, drowsiness, diarrhea, dry mouth, flushing, sweating, loss of appetite.

alclometasone Ⓖ

Type/Group: **corticosteroid; anti-inflammatory.**
Brand(s): Aclovate.
How administered: Topically.

Used to treat

Alclometasone is used for the topical (applied externally) treatment of ✪ **psoriasis**, ✪ **eczema**, and contact ✪ **dermatitis**, and for itching in ✪ **skin conditions.**

Warnings

• It should not be used by people with known hypersensitivity to corticosteroids, or with fungal infections.

• It should be used with caution by anyone with a bacterial or viral infection, or by children, who may be more susceptible to systemic side effects (that is, affecting the whole body).

• Corticosteroids can cross the placenta. It is unknown whether external application could result in sufficient systemic absorption to create a hazard to the fetus. Alclometasone, therefore, should be used during pregnancy only if it is medically judged that the benefits outweigh potential risk to the fetus.

• Medical judgment is also required if breast-feeding is being considered. When taken internally, corticosteroids are excreted in breast milk and may suppress growth and interfere with production of natural corticosteroids in the infant. It is unknown whether external application could result in sufficient systemic absorption to produce detectable amounts in breast milk.

• Topical corticosteroids can be absorbed in sufficient amounts to produce systemic effects. Do not use over large surface areas or for a prolonged period, to minimize the risk of systemic absorption.

• It is not usually recommended for use on the groin, armpits, or face.

• Bandages or dressings must not be placed over the treated area unless directed by a doctor, as this may increase the risk of adverse skin reactions.

• Weeping, denuded, or infected areas must be avoided.

• A doctor must be notified and use of alclometasone stopped if local irritation or fever develops.

Interactions

No significant interactions have been reported when used topically.

Side effects

• Occasionally, irritation and itching.

• Rarely, allergic rash.

• There may be systemic side effects if alclometasone is absorbed (symptoms of Cushing's syndrome, high blood sugar).

Alconefrin Ⓑ

A preparation of ℞ **phenylephrine hydrochloride.**
Formulation: Drops.
Availability: OTC.
Warnings and side effects: See ℞ **phenylephrine hydrochloride.**

Aldactazide Ⓑ

A preparation of ℞ **hydrochlorothiazide** and ℞ **spironolactone.**
Formulation: Oral tablets, available in two strengths.
Availability: Prescription only.
Warnings and side effects: See ℞ **hydrochlorothiazide;** ℞ **spironolactone.**

Aldactone Ⓑ

A preparation of ℞ **spironolactone.**
Formulation: Oral tablets.
Availability: Prescription only.
Warnings and side effects: See ℞ **spironolactone.**

Aldara Ⓑ

A preparation of ℞ **imiquimod.**
Formulation: Topical cream.
Availability: Prescription only.
Warnings and side effects: See ℞ **imiquimod.**

aldesleukin Ⓖ

Type/Group: **immunomodulator; anticancer.**
Brand(s): Proleukin.
How administered: Intravenous infusion.

Used to treat

Aldesleukin (recombinant interleukin-2), is one of the cytokine inflammatory mediators called interleukins, produced naturally by cells of the immune system in response, for example, to infection. Synthetic (recombinant) versions can be used as biological response modifiers (℞ **immunomodulators** or ℞ **immunostimulants**). Aldesleukin can be used mainly for treating metastatic renal cell carcinoma. It has been investigated, with some success, for the treatment of ✪ **melanoma**, colorectal (large intestine) cancer, non-Hodgkin's ✪ **lymphoma**, and ✪ **Kaposi's sarcoma.**

Warnings

• It should not be given to people with known hypersensitivity to this drug, or who show impaired heart or lung response to certain tests, who have significant liver, kidney or central nervous system (CNS) impairment. This is a specialist drug and is used only after a full medical assessment.

• The specific effects of aldesleukin on the fetus are not known, but because of its often severe adverse effects it should be used in pregnancy only with extreme caution, weighing the potential benefit against the possible risk to the women and the fetus.

• Medical judgment is required if breast-feeding is being considered.

• Aldesleukin is used only in a hospital setting and under qualified supervision, with frequent monitoring of the blood and heart and lung function. Hypersensitivity reactions (including hypotension, bronchospasm, and allergic swelling) and serious heart disturbances have occurred.

• A syndrome of seepage bleeding through blood capillaries may occur (called capillary leak syndrome), which can be very serious and requires special medical management.

• Autoimmune disease (for example, certain thyroid disorders) may be worsened by aldesleukin.

Interactions

• A number of drug interactions are known, and will be evaluated by specialist doctors.

Side effects

Side effects are frequent, often serious, and sometime fatal. They include:

• Fever and chills, nausea, diarrhea and vomiting, pain, fatigue and malaise, lung congestion, difficulty in breathing, changes in urinary output, loss of appetite, gastrointestinal bleeding, and jaundice. Changes in blood values may be dramatic and serious. Heart, kidney, and thyroid function may be affected, with potentially serious consequences. Irritability, mental confusion, or depression may also occur.

Aldoclor-150; Aldoclor-250 Tablets Ⓑ

A preparation of ℞ **chlorothiazide** and ℞ **methyldopa**.
Formulation: Oral tablets, in two (chlorothiazide) strengths.
Availability: Prescription only.
Warnings and side effects: See ℞ **chlorothiazide**; ℞ **methyldopa**.

Aldomet Tablets; Oral Suspension; Injection Ⓑ

A preparation of ℞ **methyldopa**.
Formulation: Oral tablets (three strengths); oral liquid; injection (methyldopa).
Availability: Prescription only.
Warnings and side effects: See ℞ **methyldopa**; Injectable form contains sodium bisulfite, which may cause allergic reaction in a few people.

Aldoril-15; Aldoril-25; D30; D50 Tablets Ⓑ

A preparation of ℞ **hydrochlorothiazide** and ℞ **methyldopa**.
Formulation: Oral tablets, in four strengths.
Availability: Prescription only.
Warnings and side effects: See ℞ **hydrochlorothiazide**; ℞ **methyldopa**.

alendronate sodium Ⓖ

(alendronic acid)
Type/Group: **bisphosphonate; calcium-metabolism modifier**.
Brand(s): Fosamax.
How administered: Orally.

Used to treat

Alendronate is used to treat and prevent postmenopausal ⊕ **osteoporosis** and to prevent bone fractures in postmenopausal women. It is also used to treat osteoporosis due to hormonal disorders and ⊕ **Paget's disease (of the bone)**.

Warnings

• It should not be given to people with known hypersensitivity to bisphosphonates, kidney impairment, esophageal abnormalities, or hypocalcemia (low blood levels of calcium).

• It should be given with caution to people with gastrointestinal diseases (as it may worsen these conditions), or uncorrected vitamin or mineral deficiencies (for example, vitamin-D deficiency).

• Alendronate sodium might affect bone development in the fetus or delay delivery. It should be used during pregnancy only if clearly needed.

• It is not recommended for use while breast-feeding.

• It is is very poorly absorbed and should be taken first thing in the morning before any food or beverage to maximize absorption. Take with a glass of plain water only, as mineral water, coffee, tea, or any kind of juice will interfere with absorption.

• Do not lie down for at least 30 minutes after taking medicine and until eating the first food of the day, in order to speed absorption and minimize irritation to the esophagus.

• It is not recommended for use along with ℞ **HRT** (hormone replacement therapy for menopause).

Interactions

• ℞ **aspirin** may increase gastrointestinal disturbance.
• ℞ **Antacids** reduce absorption.

Side effects

• Frequently, back pain, and abdominal pain.
• Occasionally, nausea, constipation, diarrhea, and flatulence.
• Rarely, skin rash, and esophageal irritation.

alendronic acid Ⓖ

see ℞ **alendronate sodium**.

Alenic Alka Liquid; Extra Strength Tablets Ⓑ

A preparation of ℞ **aluminum hydroxide** and ℞ **magnesium carbonate**.
Formulation: Oral tablets, chewable; liquid.
Availability: OTC.
Warnings and side effects: See ℞ **aluminum hydroxide**; ℞ **magnesium carbonate**.

Alesse Ⓑ

A preparation of ℞ **ethinyl estradiol**, and ℞ **levonorgestrel**.
Formulation: Calendar pack of oral tablets.
Availability: Prescription only.

Warnings and side effects: See ℞ **ethinyl estradiol**; ℞ **levonorgestrel**.

Aleve Tablets; Capsules; Gelcaps ⑧

A preparation of ℞ **naproxen**.
Formulation: Oral tablets; capsules; gelcaps.
Availability: OTC.
Warnings and side effects: See ℞ **naproxen**.

Alfenta ⑧

A preparation of ℞ **alfentanil**.
Formulation: Injection.
Availability: Prescription only.
Warnings and side effects: See ℞ **alfentanil**.

alfentanil ⑥

Type/Group: narcotic analgesic; opioid; general anesthetic.
Brand(s): Alfenta.
How administered: Injection.

Used to treat

Alfentanil is used for short surgical operations, induction of anes-thesia, minor surgery, in combination to enhance the effect of a ℞ **general anesthetic**, and to suppress breathing in patients on artificial ventilation.

Warnings

• It should not be given to people with known hypersensitivity to this drug. Opioids (even the weaker ones) should not be given to people with asthma, seriously depressed breathing disorders, prostatic hypertrophy, convulsive disorders, raised intracranial pressure, or a head injury.
• Depending on use and dose, opioids should be given with caution to the elderly, to anyone with hypotension, certain liver, kidney or adrenal disorders, hypothyroidism (under-activity of the thyroid gland), alcoholism, or a history of drug abuse. This is a specialist hospital drug used under strict supervised conditions following a full medical assessment.
• Alfentanil should be used during pregnancy only if the benefits outweigh the possible risks.
• Because of its potential to cause withdrawal symptoms in nursing infants, it should not be used while breast-feeding.
• Alfentanil is a Schedule II controlled substance.
• Prolonged use of narcotics can lead to physical dependence (addiction), although this rarely happens in routine medical use.
• Treatment by injection may cause pain and tissue damage at the site of the injection.
• Drowsiness may affect the performance of skilled tasks such as driving.
• The effects of alcohol may be enhanced (including a higher risk of respiratory depression).

Interactions

• If the following drugs are used with alfentanil, then effects may be enhanced with potentially serious results: ℞ **barbiturates**; inhalant ℞ **anesthetics**; ℞ **MAOIs**; ℞ **opioids**; protease inhibitors (for example, ℞ **nelfinavir**, ℞ **ritonavir**, ℞ **saquinavir**); alcohol;

℞ **chlorpromazine**; ℞ **thioridazine**; ℞ **cimetidine**; ℞ **erythromycin**; ℞ **diazepam**.
• ℞ **Buprenorphine**, ℞ **butorphanol**, ℞ **nalbuphine**, and ℞ **pentazocine** may trigger withdrawal symptoms in people dependent on opioids.

Side effects

• Depending on use and dose, there may be nausea and vomiting, drowsiness, loss of appetite, urinary retention, and constipation. There is commonly sedation and occasionally euphoria, which may lead to a state of mental detachment or confusion. Also, there may be a dry mouth, flushing of the face, sweating, headache, palpitations, changes in heart rate, postural hypotension (a lowering of blood pressure on standing), rashes, miosis (pupil constriction), mood change, and hallucinations.
• An overdose of alfentanil may cause rigidity of skeletal muscles, particularly of the chest, and respiratory depression.

alginic acid ⑥

Type/Group: demulcent.
Brand(s): Gaviscon Extra Strength Relief Formula Tablets; Genaton Tablets.
How administered: Orally.

Used to treat

Alginic acid, usually in the form of magnesium alginate or sodium alginate, is used in certain ℞ **antacid** preparations to protect against esophageal reflux. It is extracted from seaweed and has a viscous, sticky consistency.

Warnings

None significant.

Interactions

None significant.

Side effects

None significant.

Alka-Seltzer Effervescent Tablets, Gold ⑧

A preparation of ♌ **potassium bicarbonate** and ℞ **sodium bicar-bonate** and ℞ **sodium citrate**.
Formulation: Effervescent tablets.
Availability: OTC.
Warnings and side effects: See ♌ **potassium bicarbonate**; ℞ **sodium bicarbonate**; ℞ **sodium citrate**.

alkaloid ⑩

Generics: atropine sulfate; bromocriptine; codeine phosphate; dextromethorphan; ephedrine; ergonovine maleate; ergotamine tartrate; hyoscine hydrobromide; hyoscyamine; ipecac syrup; methylergonovine maleate; methysergide; morphine sulfate; nalbuphine hydrochloride; nicotine; oxycodone; papaverine; pentazocine; pergolide; pilocarpine; quinidine; quinine; vinblastine sulfate; vincristine sulfate; vinorelbine tartrate.

Actions and uses

Alkaloid is a chemical name for a group of chemically similar com-pounds that are used as drugs. The majority of alkaloids were orig-inally extracted from plants and are chemically heterocyclic, often complex, organic compounds with basic (alkali) properties, and in medicine they are usually administered in the form of their salts (for example, hydrochloride or sulfate). Many synthetic drugs are of a similar chemical structure and so technically are also alkaloids. Examples of plant alkaloids in medical use include: several of the ℞ **belladonna alkaloid** compounds from *Atropa belladonna* and related plant species (for example, ℞ **atropine sulfate**, ℞ **hyoscyamine**, and ℞ **scopolamine hydrobromide**); the alkaloids of opium from the poppy *Papaver somniferum* (for example ℞ **codeine phosphate**, ℞ **morphine sulfate**, and ℞ **papaverine**); ℞ **ergot alkaloids** (for example, ℞ **ergonovine maleate** and ℞ **ergotamine tartrate**); the ℞ **cinchona alkaloids** (℞ **quinidine** and ℞ **quinine**) from the bark of the cinchona tree; the ℞ **vinca alkaloids** (for example, ℞ **vinblastine sulfate** and ℞ **vincristine sulfate**); ℞ **ephedrine** from Chinese plants of the *Ephedra* species; ℞ **nicotine** from *Nicotiana tabacum;* ℞ **pilocarpine** from a South American *Pilocarpus* shrub; and ℞ **ipecac syrup**, which contains emetine and cephaeline from ipecac ("Brazil root").

Limitations

Plant alkaloids are used in medicine both for reasons of tradition, and also because many are complex chemical compounds that would be expensive to manufacture synthetically. Nevertheless, with time, some have been replaced with semi-synthetic derivatives that have improved properties such as potency, absorption, duration of action, selectivity, safety, or cost (for example, ℞ **bromocriptine**, ℞ **dextromethorphan**, ℞ **methylergonovine maleate**, ℞ **methysergide**, ℞ **nalbuphine hydrochloride**, ℞ **oxycodone**, ℞ **pentazocine**, ℞ **pergolide**, and ℞ **vinorelbine tartrate**.

Alka-Mints ®

A preparation of ℞ **calcium carbonate**.
Formulation: Oral tablets, chewable.
Availability: OTC.
Warnings and side effects: See ℞ **calcium carbonate**.

Alka-Seltzer Plus Allergy Liqui-Gels ®

A preparation of ℞ **pseudoephedrine**, ℞ **acetaminophen**, and ℞ **chlorpheniramine maleate**.
Formulation: Oral capsules.
Availability: OTC.
Warnings and side effects: See ℞ **pseudoephedrine**; ℞ **acetaminophen**; ℞ **chlorpheniramine maleate**.

Alka-Seltzer Plus Cold & Cough Liqui-Gels ®

A preparation of ℞ **dextromethorphan**, ℞ **acetaminophen**, ℞ **chlorpheniramine maleate**, and ℞ **pseudoephedrine**.
Formulation: Oral gel capsules.
Availability: OTC.
Warnings and side effects: See ℞ **dextromethorphan**; ℞ **acetaminophen**; ℞ **chlorpheniramine maleate**; ℞ **pseudoephedrine**.

Alka-Seltzer Plus Cold & Sinus Capsules ®

A preparation of ℞ **pseudoephedrine** and ℞ **acetaminophen**.
Formulation: Oral capsules.
Availability: OTC.
Warnings and side effects: See ℞ **pseudoephedrine**; ℞ **acetaminophen**.

Alka-Seltzer Plus NightTime Cold Liqui-Gels ®

A preparation of ℞ **dextromethorphan**, ℞ **acetaminophen**, pseudoephedrine, and ℞ **doxylamine**.
Formulation: Oral gel capsules.
Availability: OTC.
Warnings and side effects: See ℞ **dextromethorphan**; ℞ **acetaminophen**; ℞ **pseudoephedrine**; ℞ **doxylamine**.

Alka-Seltzer with Aspirin; Extra Strength with Aspirin ®

A preparation of ℞ **aspirin** buffered with ℞ **sodium bicarbonate**.
Formulation: Effervescent tablets, to be dissolved.
Availability: OTC.
Warnings and side effects: See ℞ **aspirin**; ℞ **sodium bicarbonate**.

Alkeran ®

A preparation of ℞ **melphalan**.
Formulation: Oral tablets; powder for injection.
Availability: Prescription only.
Warnings and side effects: See ℞ **melphalan**.

Alkets Tablets; Antacid Extra Strength Tablets ®

A preparation of ℞ **calcium carbonate**.
Formulation: Oral tablets, chewable.
Availability: OTC.
Warnings and side effects: See ℞ **calcium carbonate**.

Allegra-D ®

A preparation of ℞ **pseudoephedrine** and ℞ **fexofenadine**.
Formulation: Oral tablets, sustained release.
Availability: Prescription only.
Warnings and side effects: See ℞ **pseudoephedrine**; ℞ **fexofenadine**.

Allegra Tablets; Capsules ®

A preparation of ℞ **fexofenadine hydrochloride**.
Formulation: Oral capsules; tablets, available in three strengths.
Availability: Prescription only.
Warnings and side effects: See ℞ **fexofenadine hydrochloride**.

Allent Capsules ®

A preparation of ℞ **pseudoephedrine** and ℞ **brompheniramine maleate**.
Formulation: Oral capsules, extended relase.
Availability: Prescription only.

Warnings and side effects: See ℞ pseudoephedrine; ℞ brompheniramine maleate.

Aller-Chlor Tablets; Syrup ⑱

A preparation of ℞ chlorpheniramine maleate.
Formulation: Oral tablets; syrup.
Availability: OTC.
Warnings and side effects: See ℞ chlorpheniramine maleate.

Allercon Tablets ⑱

A preparation of ℞ pseudoephedrine and ℞ triprolidine hydrochloride.
Formulation: Oral tablets.
Availability: OTC.
Warnings and side effects: See ℞ pseudoephedrine; ℞ triprolidine hydrochloride.

Allerest 12 Hour Nasal ⑱

A preparation of ℞ oxymetazoline hydrochloride.
Formulation: Nasal spray.
Availability: OTC.
Warnings and side effects: See ℞ oxymetazoline hydrochloride.

Allerest No Drowsiness, Caplets ⑱

A preparation of ℞ pseudoephedrine and ℞ acetaminophen.
Formulation: Oral tablets.
Availability: OTC.
Warnings and side effects: See ℞ pseudoephedrine; ℞ acetaminophen.

Allerest Eye Drops ⑱

A preparation of ℞ naphazoline hydrochloride.
Formulation: Eye drops.
Availability: OTC.
Warnings and side effects: See ℞ naphazoline hydrochloride.

Allerest Maximum Strength Tablets ⑱

A preparation of ℞ pseudoephedrine and ℞ chlorpheniramine maleate.
Formulation: Oral tablets.
Availability: OTC.
Warnings and side effects: See ℞ pseudoephedrine; ℞ chlorpheniramine maleate.

Allerest Sinus Pain Formula Tablets ⑱

A preparation of ℞ pseudoephedrine, ℞ acetaminophen, and ℞ chlorpheniramine maleate.
Formulation: Oral tablets.
Availability: OTC.
Warnings and side effects: See ℞ pseudoephedrine; ℞ acetaminophen; ℞ chlorpheniramine maleate.

Allerfrim Tablets, Syrup ⑱

A preparation of ℞ pseudoephedrine and ℞ triprolidine hydrochloride.
Formulation: Oral tablets; syrup.
Availability: OTC.
Warnings and side effects: See ℞ pseudoephedrine; ℞ triprolidine hydrochloride.

Allerfrin w/Codeine Cough Syrup ⑱

A preparation of ℞ codeine phosphate, ℞ pseudoephedrine and ℞ triprolidine.
Formulation: Oral syrup.
Availability: May or may not require a prescription.
Warnings and side effects: See ℞ codeine phosphate; ℞ pseudoephedrine; ℞ triprolidine.

Allergy ⑱

A preparation of ℞ chlorpheniramine maleate.
Formulation: Oral tablets.
Availability: OTC.
Warnings and side effects: See ℞ chlorpheniramine maleate.

Allergy Drops; Maximum Strength Allergy Drops ⑱

A preparation of ℞ naphazoline hydrochloride.
Formulation: Eye drops.
Availability: OTC.
Warnings and side effects: See ℞ naphazoline hydrochloride.

AllerMax Caplets; Allergy & Cough Formula Liquid ⑱

A preparation of ℞ diphenhydramine hydrochloride.
Formulation: Oral tablets; liquid.
Availability: OTC.
Warnings and side effects: See ℞ diphenhydramine hydrochloride.

Allermed Capsules ⑱

A preparation of ℞ pseudoephedrine.
Formulation: Oral capsules.
Availability: OTC.
Warnings and side effects: See ℞ pseudoephedrine.

Allerphed Syrup ⑱

A preparation of ℞ pseudoephedrine and ℞ triprolidine hydrochloride.
Formulation: Oral syrup.
Availability: OTC.
Warnings and side effects: See ℞ pseudoephedrine; ℞ triprolidine hydrochloride.

AlleRx Day ⑱

A preparation of methscopolamine nitrate and ℞ pseudoephedrine.
Formulation: Oral tablets.

Key to symbols: ✪ = Disorder Section ℞ = Drug Section ♣ = Herbal Section ☡ = Supplement Section

Availability: Prescription only.
Warnings and side effects: See ℞ **scopolamine**;
℞ **pseudoephedrine**.

AlleRx Night ⑧

A preparation of methscopolamine nitrate and
℞ **chlorpheniramine maleate**.
Formulation: Oral tablets.
Availability: Prescription only.
Warnings and side effects: See ℞ **scopolamine**;
℞ **chlorpheniramine maleate**; ℞ **pseudoephedrine**.

allopurinol ⑥

Type/Group: **uricosuric; xanthine-oxidase inhibitor; antigout**.
Brand(s): Aloprim; Zyloprim; various generic.
How administered: Orally; injection.

Used to treat

Allopurinol blocks the action of the enzyme xanthine-oxidase, which produces uric acid and so can be used to treat excess uric acid in the blood (hyperuricemia) by reducing its synthesis. It is used to prevent attacks of ✪ **gout** and to treat uric acid and calcium oxalate stones in the urinary tract (kidney stones: see ✪ **calculus**). Although not labeled for such use, it is also prescribed as a mouthwash to treat stomatitis (mouth sores) induced by certain drug treatments.

Warnings

• It should not be given to people with known hypersensitivity to the drug.
• It should be given with caution to people with kidney or liver disease.
• Allopurinol's safety during pregnancy is not established. It should be used only when clearly needed.
• Medical judgment is required if breast-feeding is being considered. It is not known whether this drug appears in breast milk.
• It may cause drowsiness and so impair the performance of skilled tasks such as driving.

Interactions

• If used with ℞ **ampicillin**, there is an increased risk of rash.
• The effects of oral ℞ **anticoagulants** may be increased.
• The toxicity of ℞ **azathiaprine**, ℞ **mercaptopurine**, ℞ **cyclosporine**, ℞ **cyclophosphamide**, and ℞ **tacrolimus** is increased.
• ℞ **theophylline** levels may be increased when used with large doses of allopurinol.
• If used with ℞ **thiazide** diuretics or ℞ **ACE inhibitors**, there is an increased risk of a hypersensitivity reaction to allopurinol.
• Aluminum salts may reduce the response to allopurinol.

Side effects

• Rash (which may mean that treatment should be stopped), gastrointestinal disorders, fever, and skin reactions.
• Rarely, malaise, headache, vertigo, drowsiness, hypertension, taste disturbance, hair loss, liver toxicity, peripheral nerve disorders, and kidney and blood disorders.

Almacone Liquid ⑧

A preparation of ℞ **aluminum hydroxide** and ℞ **simethicone**.
Formulation: Oral liquid.
Availability: OTC.
Warnings and side effects: See ℞ **aluminum hydroxide**;
℞ **simethicone**.

Almacone Tablets; Almacone II Double Strength Liquid ⑧

A preparation of ℞ **aluminum hydroxide**, ℞ **magnesium hydroxide**, and ℞ **simethicone**.
Formulation: Oral tablets, chewable; liquid.
Availability: OTC.
Warnings and side effects: See ℞ **aluminum hydroxide**;
℞ **magnesium hydroxide**; ℞ **simethicone**.

Almag Plus Suspension ⑧

A preparation of ℞ **aluminum hydroxide**, ℞ **magnesium hydroxide**, and ℞ **simethicone**.
Formulation: Oral liquid.
Availability: OTC.
Warnings and side effects: See ℞ **aluminum hydroxide**;
℞ **magnesium hydroxide**; ℞ **simethicone**.

Almag Suspension ⑧

A preparation of ℞ **aluminum hydroxide** and ℞ **magnesium hydroxide**.
Formulation: Oral liquid.
Availability: OTC.
Warnings and side effects: See ℞ **aluminum hydroxide**;
℞ **magnesium hydroxide**.

Alomide ⑧

A preparation of ℞ **lodoxamide tromethamine**.
Formulation: Ophthalmic solution.
Availability: Prescription only.
Warnings and side effects: See ℞ **lodoxamide tromethamine**.

Aloprim ⑧

A preparation of ℞ **allopurinol**.
Formulation: Injection.
Availability: Prescription only.
Warnings and side effects: See ℞ **allopurinol**.

Alora ⑧

A preparation of ℞ **estradiol**.
Formulation: Transdermal patch in several strengths.
Availability: Prescription only.
Warnings and side effects: See ℞ **estradiol**.

Alor Tablets ⑧

A preparation of ℞ **hydrocodone** and ℞ **aspirin**.
Formulation: Oral tablets.
Availability: Prescription only.
Warnings and side effects: See ℞ **hydrocodone**; ℞ **aspirin**.

alpha-adrenergic blocker ⓓ

(alpha-adrenoceptor blocker; alpha-adrenoceptor antagonist)
Generics: **dihydroergotamine mesylate; doxazosin mesylate; ergoloid mesylates; phenoxybenzamine; phentolamine mesylate; prazosin hydrochloride; tamsulosin hydrochloride; terazosin.**

Actions and uses

Alpha-adrenergic blockers act at alpha-adrenoceptors to inhibit some actions of alpha receptor-stimulant natural mediators and drugs, such as ℞ **epinephrine** (adrenaline, a hormone released from the adrenal gland) and the neurotransmitter norepinephrine (noradrenaline, which is released from sympathetic nerves). They also inhibit some actions of the ℞ **sympathomimetic** drugs.

Selective alpha-adrenoceptor blocking drugs work by blocking only the receptor sites called alpha-adrenoceptors (but not beta-adrenergic receptors), thereby preventing part of the spectrum of actions of epinephrine-like agents. A major use of alpha-blockers is in ℞ **antihypertensive** treatment (often in conjunction with other drugs), because they lower blood pressure when it is raised in ✪ **hypertension** by preventing the ℞ **vasoconstrictor** actions of norepinephrine and epinephrine (including in the treatment of ✪ **pheochromocytoma**) (for example, ℞ **doxazosin mesylate,** ℞ **phenoxybenzamine,** ℞ **phentolamine mesylate,** ℞ **prazosin hydrochloride,** ℞ **terazosin**). They are also used to treat urinary retention in ✪ **benign prostatic hypertrophy** (BPH) through an action on the blood circulation within the prostate (for example, ℞ **doxazosin mesylate,** ℞ **terazosin**), to increase blood flow in ✪ **Raynaud's disease,** in ℞ **impotence treatment** for erectile dysfunction (for example, ℞ **phentolamine mesylate**), and sometimes as nootropics for ✪ **dementia** to improve cognition (for example, ℞ **ergoloid mesylates**). Some members which are not typical of the class are sometimes used for migraine (for example, ℞ **dihydroergotamine mesylate**).

Limitations

Most alpha-adrenergic blockers have rather widespread actions, largely because alpha-adrenergic receptors are very widely distributed in the body. For this and other reasons, they are now less extensively used in the treatment of hypertension (other drugs having proved to be more acceptable). On the other hand, they now have a well-established role in the treatment of the symptoms of benign prostatic hypertrophy (BPH).

alpha-adrenergic stimulant ⓓ

(alpha-adrenoceptor stimulant; alpha-agonist)
Generics: **apraclonidine; clonidine hydrochloride; epinephrine; metaraminol; methoxamine hydrochloride; midodrine hydrochloride; naphazoline hydrochloride; norepinephrine bitartrate; oxymetazoline hydrochloride; phenylephrine hydrochloride; tetrahydrozoline hydrochloride; xylometazoline hydrochloride.**

Actions and uses

Alpha-adrenergic stimulant drugs act at alpha-adrenoceptors, which, along with beta-adrenoceptors, are the sites that recognize and respond to the natural hormones and neurotransmitters of the sympathetic nervous system (such as epinephrine and norepineph-

rine). Drugs that activate this system, by whatever mechanism, are called ℞ **sympathomimetics.** There are two types of alpha-adrenoceptors. Stimulants acting at the alpha$_1$-subtype of receptor on blood vessels are ℞ **vasoconstrictor** drugs and are widely used for their nasal ℞ **decongestant** actions (for example, ℞ **phenylephrine hydrochloride,** ℞ **naphazoline hydrochloride,** ℞ **oxymetazoline hydrochloride,** ℞ **xylometazoline hydrochloride**). Because they raise blood pressure, they are used to treat cases of acute ✪ **hypotension** or circulatory shock, particularly in emergency situations, such as bleeding, allergic drug reactions, brain injury, or surgical complications (for example, ℞ **metaraminol,** ℞ **norepinephrine bitartrate,** ℞ **methoxamine hydrochloride,** ℞ **phenylephrine hydrochloride,** ℞ **midodrine hydrochloride**). Some of these drugs also have ℞ **beta-adrenergic stimulant** properties, and so both raise blood pressure and have ℞ **cardiac stimulant** actions. They can be used in emergency situations such as cardiac arrest (for example, ℞ **norepinephrine bitartrate**). Some of the alpha-adrenergic stimulant vasoconstrictor drugs are used locally for ophthalmological (eye) examination (for example, phenylephrine hydrochloride) and together with a ℞ **local anesthetic** to prolong the duration of action of the anesthetic, or are incorporated into preparations for ✪ **hemorrhoids.**

The second type of receptors at which some alpha-adrenergic stimulants act are the alpha$_2$-subtype of receptor, and although drugs selective for this subtype are not yet extensively used in medicine, recently such agents (for example, ℞ **apraclonidine**) have been introduced into ℞ **glaucoma treatment,** especially to control or prevent postoperative elevation of intraocular pressure (pressure in the eyeball) after laser surgery, and as a short-term additional treatment in people who require further reduction of intraocular pressure. Also, it is likely that some ℞ **antihypertensive** drugs, such as ℞ **clonidine hydrochloride,** work through acting on this type of receptor in the brain.

Limitations

Most of these drugs do not have a selective action, largely because alpha-adrenergic receptors are found throughout the body, and so they have many potential side effects. In emergency use this is not a significant limitation, but otherwise their side effects are extensive. Where the drugs can be applied locally, such as eyedrops or by local injection, the side effects are less extensive. Those used as nasal decongestants are best used by nosedrops or as a spray, but their main disadvantage is that there may be "rebound congestion" when they are used for too long. Although some nasal decongestants are incorporated into many over-the-counter remedies of the ℞ **cold and cough preparation** type, their use is potentially risky because widespread systemic vasoconstriction (narrowing of blood vessels) may raise blood pressure to dangerous levels and even cause a hypertensive crisis.

alpha-adrenoceptor antagonist ⓓ

see ℞ **alpha-adrenergic blocker.**

alpha-adrenoceptor blocker ⓓ

see ℞ **alpha-adrenergic blocker.**

alpha-adrenoceptor stimulant Ⓓ

see ℞ alpha-adrenergic stimulant.

alpha-agonist Ⓓ

see ℞ alpha-adrenergic stimulant.

alpha-blocker Ⓓ

see ℞ alpha-adrenergic blocker.

Alphagan Ⓑ

A preparation of ℞ brimonidine.
Formulation: Eye drops.
Availability: Prescription only.
Warnings and side effects: See ℞ brimonidine.

Alphanate Ⓑ

A preparation of ℞ antihemophilic factor (Factor VIII).
Formulation: Intravenous infusion.
Availability: Prescription only.
Warnings and side effects: See ℞ antihemophilic factor.
Contains a small amount of ℞ heparin.

AlphaNine SD Ⓑ

A preparation of ℞ Factor IX complex.
Formulation: Intravenous infusion.
Availability: Prescription only.
Warnings and side effects: See ℞ Factor IX complex (also
contains Factors II, VII, X). Contains a small amount of ℞ heparin.

Alphatrex Ⓑ

A preparation of ℞ betamethasone.
Formulation: Ointment; cream; lotion.
Availability: Prescription only.
Warnings and side effects: See ℞ betamethasone.

alprazolam Ⓖ

Type/Group: antianxiety; benzodiazepine.
Brand(s): Xanax; various generic.
How administered: Orally.

Used to treat

Alprazolam is used in the treatment of ✪ anxiety, panic disorder,
and anxiety with depressive symptoms. Although not stated by the
manufacturer for such treatment, it may be prescribed for agoraphobia with social phobia, ✪ depression, or ✪ premenstrual syndrome.

Warnings

• It should not be given to people with known hypersensitivity to
benzodiazepines, with untreated open-angle glaucoma, acute
narrow-angle glaucoma, or psychosis. It should not be used while
taking ℞ itraconazole, ℞ ketoconazole, or ℞ nefazodone.
• It should be given with caution to people with liver, lung or kidney
disease, who are over 65, or in a weakened condition (debilitated).
• Alprazolam is not recommended for use during pregnancy. Its use
in the first trimester should almost always be avoided. A doctor

must be contacted if pregnancy occurs while alprazolam is being
taken.
• It should not normally be used by nursing mothers.
• It may cause drowsiness and judgment, thinking, and the
performance of skilled tasks may be impaired (such as driving).
• Alcohol should be avoided, because side effects may be increased.
• Psychotropic medications should not be used unless prescribed
by a doctor.
• A doctor must be consulted before stopping or increasing dosage,
because benzodiazepines may cause psychological and physical
dependence and withdrawal symptoms.
• Grapefruit juice may increase the effects of alprazolam.

Interactions

• ℞ carbamazepine, ℞ phenytoin, and ℞ rifampin reduce the
effects of benzodiazepines.
• ℞ cimetidine, ℞ ciprofloxacin, ℞ clarithromycin, delavirdine,
℞ disulfiram, ℞ erythromycin, ℞ fluconazole, ℞ fluoxetine,
℞ fluvoxamine, ℞ isoniazid, ℞ metoprolol, ℞ omeprazole,
℞ quinolones, and troleandomycin may increase the effects of
alprazolam.
• ℞ itraconazole, ℞ ketoconazole, and ℞ nefazodone increase
effects of alprazolam and and must not be used at the same.
• Alcohol enhances some side effects.

Side effects

• Depending on use, there may be dizziness, drowsiness, postural
hypotension (lowered blood pressure on standing), and blurred
vision.
• Less frequently, anxiety, confusion, impaired movement and
coordination (particularly in older individuals), mental changes,
headache, insomnia, changes in heart rate, elevated blood
pressure, enlarged pupils, ringing in the ears (tinnitus), loss of
appetite, gastrointestinal problems, dry mouth, liver disorders, and
skin reactions.

alprostadil Ⓖ

Type/Group: impotence treatment; prostaglandin.
Brand(s): Caverject; Edex; Muse; Prostin VR Pediatric.
How administered: Intracavernosal injection into the penis; direct
urethral application; intravenous injection (babies).

Used to treat

Alprostadil is a prostaglandin (PGE_1) used to maintain babies born
with congenital heart defects (to maintain patency of ductus arteriosus), while emergency preparations are being made for corrective surgery and intensive care. In men, it is used to treat erectile
dysfunction (see ✪ impotence).

Warnings

• It should not be given to babies with respiratory distress
syndrome, to men with conditions predisposing to prolonged
erection (for example, sickle-cell anemia), anatomical
deformations of the penis (for example, Peyronie's disease), or
penile implants.
• It should be given with caution to men with severe liver disease
or blood-clotting disorders.
• It should not be given to women.

• A condom must be used if the woman partner is pregnant or intends to become pregnant.

Interactions

• In men, ℞ **anticoagulants**, ℞ **heparin**, and ℞ **thrombolytic** agents may increase the risk of bleeding after intracavernosal injection.

• In men, alprostadil may reduce the levels of cyclosporine.

Side effects

• Babies: Medical personnel will provide careful control and constant monitoring to minimize side effects and other difficulties.

• Men: Prolonged erection, painful penis, testicular pain, and swelling during erection, dizziness, headache, effects on the cardiovascular system, fainting, dry mouth, weakness, rash, swelling, warmth, burning sensation, and effects on urination. Also, effects on the heart and blood.

Altace ®

A preparation of ℞ **ramipril**.
Formulation: Oral capsules, available in four strengths.
Availability: Prescription only.
Warnings and side effects: See ℞ **ramipril**.

alteplase, recombinant ©

(tissue-type plasminogen activator; rt-PA)
Type/Group: **thrombolytic; fibrinolytic**.
Brand(s): Activase.
How administered: Intravenous injection, infusion.

Used to treat

Alteplase is a synthesized (recombinant DNA technology) type of enzyme with the property of breaking up blood clots. It is used in serious conditions such as ✪ **myocardial infarction** (heart attack), ✪ **stroke**, and ✪ **pulmonary embolism**.

Warnings

• It will be administered by experienced personnel after a full medical assessment. It should not be given to people with active internal bleeding, uncontrolled high blood pressure, a history of stroke, or injury, surgery or bleeding involving the nervous system (brain or spine) within the previous 2 months.

• It should be given with caution to people with cerebrovascular disease, who have had recent major surgery, recent injury or internal bleeding (for example, in the gastrointestinal tract, urinary tract), bacterial endocarditis or acute pericarditis, indwelling catheters, high blood pressure, severe diabetes mellitus, significant liver or kidney impairment, or any condition (for example, taking anticoagulant drugs, low platelet count) or disorder that would make bleeding more likely.

• Alteplase should be used during pregnancy only when it is clearly needed.

• Medical judgment is required if breast-feeding is being considered.

• Although reported rarely, thrombolytics may free bits of plaque that may lodge (usually) in the smaller blood vessels. This may result in abrupt, sharp pain in a leg, foot, the toes, back, or flank. ("Purple toes syndrome" appears as mottled, purplish discoloration of the toes.) More serious obstructions are possible, which may cause kidney failure, pancreatitis, hypertension, heart attack, stroke, and other serious obstructive events.

Interactions

• If taken with ℞ **heparin**, there is an increased risk of bleeding, with potentially life-threatening adverse effects.

• If taken with drugs that act against ⚖ **vitamin K** (for example, ℞ **warfarin sodium**), there is an increased risk of bleeding.

• ℞ **abciximab**, ℞ **aspirin**, and ℞ **dipyridamole**, may lower platelet activity and increase the risk of bleeding when used with alteplase.

Side effects

• The chief complication is hemorrhage (although major bleeding is not frequent), which may occur at virtually anywhere in the body.

• Other side effects may include slowed heart rate and other arrhythmias, shock, heart failure, fluid in the lungs or brain, or events associated with new embolism. Mild allergic reaction has occurred.

AlternaGEL ®

A preparation of ℞ **aluminum hydroxide**.
Formulation: Oral liquid.
Availability: OTC.
Warnings and side effects: See ℞ **aluminum hydroxide**.

altretamine ©

(hexamethylmelamine)
Type/Group: **anticancer; cytotoxic**.
Brand(s): Hexalen.
How administered: Orally; intravenous injection.

Used to treat

Altretamine is a synthetic cytotoxic drug used in the treatment of advanced ovarian ✪ **cancer**.

Warnings

• It should not be given to people with known hypersensitivity to altretamine.

• It should be given with caution to people with pre-existing bone marrow depression or decreased neurological function. This is a specialist drug which will be used following a full evaluation by specialist physicians.

• Altretamine is not recommended for use during pregnancy unless it is medically judged to be essential, because it may cause birth defects. Becoming pregnant while using this drug must be avoided.

• It should not be used if breast-feeding.

• It can have adverse neurological effects and monitoring will be necessary.

• Drugs that work in a similar way to altretamine have been associated with the development of secondary malignancies (new cancers).

Interactions

• ℞ **cimetidine** may increase the effects of altretamine.

• ℞ **MAOIs** may cause severe postural hypotension (low blood pressure on standing).

Key to symbols: ✪ = Disorder Section ℞ = Drug Section ♣ = Herbal Section ⚖ = Supplement Section

Side effects

• Frequently, nausea and vomiting, mild to moderate myelosuppression (reduced production of blood cells), mild peripheral nerve disorders, blood changes, neurologic effects (confusion, depression), unusual bleeding, and bruising.

• Occasionally, diarrhea, loss of appetite, abdominal cramps, skin rash, and itching. It may impair fertility.

Alu-Cap; Alu-Tab ®

A preparation of ℞ **aluminum hydroxide**.
Formulation: Oral tablets; capsules.
Availability: OTC.
Warnings and side effects: See ℞ **aluminum hydroxide**.

Aludrox Suspension ®

A preparation of ℞ **aluminum hydroxide**, ℞ **magnesium hydroxide**, and ℞ **simethicone**.
Formulation: Oral liquid.
Availability: OTC.
Warnings and side effects: See ℞ **aluminum hydroxide**; ℞ **magnesium hydroxide**; ℞ **simethicone**.

aluminum acetate ⑥

Type/Group: astringent.
Brand(s): Buro-Sol; Bluboro Powder; Boropak Powder; Domeboro; Pedi-Boro; Bite-Rx; various generic (Burrow's or Modified Burrow's Solution).
How administered: Topically (external).

Used to treat

Aluminum acetate is used primarily to clean sites of infection and inflammation such as poison ivy, ✪ **athlete's foot**, ✪ **acne**, and particularly weeping or suppurating wounds or sores.

Warnings

• It should not be given to people with known hypersensitivity to aluminum or any component of the products.

• Avoid contact with eyes.

• A doctor must be consulted if irritation develops or the inflammation spreads.

• The affected area must not be covered with plastic or any other impervious material.

Interactions

• If taken with collagenase, enzyme activity may be inhibited.

Side effects

None significant.

aluminum chloride ⑥

Type/Group: antiperspirant; astringent.
Brand(s): Drysol.
How administered: Topically (external).

Used to treat

Aluminum chloride can be used to treat ✪ **hyperhidrosis** (excessive sweating).

Warnings

None significant.

Interactions

None significant.

Side effects

None significant.

aluminum hydroxide ⑥

Type/Group: antacid.
Brand(s): AlternaGEL; Alu-Tab, Alu-Cap; Amphogel Tablets, Suspension; Dialume; various generic. Combinations: With *magnesium carbonate*: Alenic Alka Liquid, Extra Strength Tablets; Gaviscon Liquid, Extra Strength Relief Formula Liquid (also has *simethicone*); Genaton Liquid. (Plus): *sodium bicarbonate*: Gaviscon Extra Strength Relief Formula Tablets; Genaton Extra Strength Tablets. With *magnesium hydroxide*: Almag Suspension; Maalox Suspension, Therapeutic Concentrate; Magnalox Liquid; Magnox Suspension; Mintox Tablets, Suspenion; Rulox Tablets, Suspension. (Plus): *simethicone*: Almag Plus Suspension; Almacone Tablets, Almacone II; Aludrox; Gas Ban DS Liquid; Gelusil; Kudrox Double Strength; Maalox Extra Strength Suspension; Mi-Acid II; Mintox Plus, Extra Strength; Mygel II; Mylagen II; Mylanta Tablets, Double Strength Tablets, Liquid; Rulox Plus Tablets, Suspension; Simaal Gel 2 Liquid; Tempo Tablets (also has *calcium carbonate*). With *magnesium trisilicate, sodium bicarbonate*: Foamicon; Gaviscon Tablets, Gaviscon-2 Double Strength Tablets; Genaton Tablets. With *mineral oil*: Nephrox Liquid. With *simethicone*: Almacone Liquid; Di-Gel Liquid; Mi-Acid Liquid; Mylagen Liquid; Mygel Suspension; Mylanta Liquid; Simaal Gel Liquid.
How administered: Orally.

Used to treat

Aluminum hydroxide (often prepared as aluminum hydroxide gel) has a long duration of action because it is relatively insoluble in water. It can be used for the symptomatic relief of ✪ **indigestion**, hyperacidity, gastritis, ✪ **peptic ulcer**, and esophageal reflux. In an unrelated use, because it binds phosphates in the gastrointestinal tract and promotes their excretion, it can also be used to treat elevated levels of phosphates in the blood (hyperphosphatemia), for instance in kidney failure.

Warnings

• It should not be used by people with hypophosphatemia (low blood phosphates) or kidney disease.

• It should be used with caution by people with impaired kidney or intestinal function, porphyria, who are taking certain drugs, are on sodium-restricted diets, or are dehydrated.

• No ill-effects during pregnancy have been associated with aluminum hydroxide, but a doctor should always be consulted before taking any drug during pregnancy.

• Medical judgment is required if breast-feeding is being considered.

• Overusing antacids may cause "acid rebound," which is an increase in stomach acid secretion. Aluminum hydroxide, therefore, should not be used for more than two weeks continuously.

• It should not be used when there is abdominal pain, nausea, or vomiting, unless directed by a doctor.

• Anyone taking any medication, including OTCs, herbal remedies, and supplements, should consult a doctor before using an antacid, because antacids may alter the absorption of a wide range of drugs.

• Stools may appear white or speckled.

Interactions

• ℞ **Sodium polystyrene sulfonate** resins must not be taken with magnesium or aluminum antacids, because there is potential for systemic ✪ **alkalosis**.

• Buffered ℞ **aspirin**/antacid combinations should not be used in any long-term treatment, for example, for rheumatic inflammation.

• The following drugs may have their absorption and actions impaired: ℞ **ACE inhibitors** (for example, ℞ **captopril**); ℞ **allopurinol**; ℞ **atenolol**; ℞ **chloroquine**; ℞ **corticosteroids** (for example, ℞ **dexamethasone**), ℞ **diflunisal**, ℞ **digoxin**; ℞ **ethambutol**; ℞ **H$_2$-antagonists** (for example, ℞ **cimetidine**; ℞ **ranitidine**); ℞ **hydantoins**; ℞ **indomethacin**; ℞ **isoniazid**; ℞ **ketoconazole**; ℞ **nitrofurantoin**; ℞ **penicillamine**; ℞ **phenothiazines**; ℞ **quinolones**; ℞ **tetracyclines**; ℞ **thyroid hormones**; and ℞ **ticlopidine**. Doses of these drugs should be taken several hours apart from doses of the antacid (a doctor should be consulted for full instructions and cautions).

• ℞ **Benzodiazepines**, ℞ **dicumarol**, ℞ **quinidine**, ℞ **sulfonylureas**, and ℞ **valproate** may have their absorption increased and so there is a higher potential for adverse effects.

Side effects

• There may be constipation.

• Occasionally, nausea and vomiting, and low phosphate levels.

Alupent ℞

A preparation of ℞ **metaproterenol**.

Formulation: Oral tablets; oral syrup; aerosol inhaler; solution for inhalation.

Availability: Prescription only.

Warnings and side effects: See ℞ **metaproterenol**.

Alzheimer's treatment ✪

see ℞ **dementia treatment**.

amantadine Ⓖ

Type/Group: **antiparkinsonism; antiviral**.

Brand(s): Symmetrel; various generic.

How administered: Orally.

Used to treat

Amantadine is a treatment for ✪ **Parkinson's disease** and parkinsonism caused by drugs, carbon monoxide poisoning, encephalitis, and arteriosclerosis. It is also used to prevent and treat viral infection by ✪ **influenza** type A.

Warnings

• It should not be used by people with known hypersensitivity to this drug, or infants less than one year of age.

• It should be used with caution by those with seizure disorder, congestive heart failure, psychiatric disorders, liver or kidney disorders, peripheral edema (swelling of the ankles, legs, or feet), recurrent eczema, cerebrovascular disease, or gastric ulcers.

• Amantadine should be used during pregnancy only if clearly needed and if the benefits outweigh the potential risk to the fetus.

• It appears in breast milk and so medical judgment is required whether or not to breast-feed.

• Anyone taking CNS (central nervous system) stimulants, such as ℞ **methylphenidate** (Ritalin), should be aware that these drugs may increase CNS effects.

• To avoid insomnia, it should not be taken near bedtime.

• Side effects such as dizziness, confusion, and blurred vision are possible, so caution is advised when carrying out skilled tasks such as driving.

• Withdrawal of treatment for Parkinson's disease must be gradual.

Interactions

• ℞ **tricyclic** antidepressants, ℞ **antihistamines**, ℞ **phenothiazines**, and ℞ **anticholinergics** may increase anticholinergic side effects (such as dry mouth, blurred vision, increased heart rate, dry skin, and so on).

Side effects

• Frequently, nausea, dizziness, poor concentration, insomnia, and nervousness.

• Occasionally, postural hypotension (lowered blood pressure on standing), loss of appetite, headache, livedo reticularis (reddish blue blotching of the skin), blurred vision, urinary retention, dry mouth.

• Rarely, vomiting, depression, irritation or swelling of eyes, skin rash, blood disorders, seizures, and effects on the heart.

Amaryl ℞

A preparation of ℞ **glimepiride**.

Formulation: Oral tablets.

Availability: Prescription only.

Warnings and side effects: See ℞ **glimepiride**.

ambenonium chloride Ⓖ

Type/Group: **anticholinesterase**.

Brand(s): Mytelase.

How administered: Orally.

Used to treat

Ambenonium chloride enhances the effects of the neurotransmitter ℞ **acetylcholine**, and is used to treat ✪ **myasthenia gravis**, particularly in people sensitive to pyridostigmine bromide.

Warnings

• It should not be used by people with known hypersensitivity to anticholinesterases, or with urinary or intestinal obstruction.

• It should be given with caution to anyone with seizure disorder, asthma, certain heart conditions, hyperthyroidism, peptic ulcer, or hypotension.

• Medical judgment is required if pregnant. It is not known whether or not this drug can harm the fetus, but it would not be expected to cross the placenta or be excreted into breast milk. It may cause transient muscle weakness in newborns. It should be given with caution to breast-feeding mothers.

• It must not be used with any other cholinergic medication except under a doctor's supervision.

Key to symbols: ✪ = Disorder Section   ℞ = Drug Section   ♣ = Herbal Section   ⚖ = Supplement Section

• A doctor must be contacted at once if side effects occur (see below).

• It should be taken on an empty stomach.

Interactions

• ℞ **Tacrine** and other anticholinesterases may increase cholinergic effects.

• ℞ **Aminoglycoside** antibiotics (such as, ℞ **neomycin**, ℞ **streptomycin**) may increase the effects of ambenonium.

• ℞ **Corticosteroids**, ⚤ **magnesium**, and ℞ **local anesthetics** may interfere with the action of ambenonium.

Side effects

A doctor must be contacted if any of the following occur:

• Nausea, vomiting, diarrhea, sweating, increased salivation, irregular heartbeat, muscle weakness, severe abdominal pain, and difficulty in breathing.

• Other possible effects include urinary urgency, frequency, or incontinence, abdominal cramps, changes in vision, dizziness, drowsiness, headache, and incoordination.

Ambenyl Cough Syrup Ⓑ

A preparation of ℞ **codeine phosphate** and bromodiphenhydramine.

Formulation: Oral syrup.

Availability: May or may not require a prescription.

Warnings and side effects: See ℞ **codeine phosphate**.

Ambenyl-D Liquid Ⓑ

A preparation of ℞ **dextromethorphan**, ℞ **pseudoephedrine**, and ℞ **guaifenesin**.

Formulation: Oral liquid.

Availability: OTC.

Warnings and side effects: See ℞ **dextromethorphan**; ℞ **pseudoephedrine**; ℞ **guaifenesin**.

Ambien Ⓑ

A preparation of ℞ **zolpidem**.

Formulation: Oral tablets in several strengths.

Availability: Prescription only.

Warnings and side effects: See ℞ **zolpidem**.

Amcort Ⓑ

A preparation of ℞ **triamcinolone**.

Formulation: Suspension for injection.

Availability: Prescription only.

Warnings and side effects: See ℞ **triamcinolone**.

amebicide and antiprotozoal ⒟

(antiamebicidal; amoebicide; antiprotozoal)

Generics: chloroquine; furazolidone; ipecac syrup; metronidazole; sulfamethoxazole; trimethoprim (TMP); trimetrexate glucuronate.

Actions and uses

Amebicidal drugs are ℞ **antimicrobial** drugs used to treat infection by the microscopic organisms (microorganisms, microbes) known as amebae (or amoebae). Until recently they were classified as a subclass of the protozoa family, and for convenience are still generally grouped under protozoa. Amebae cause such disorders as ✪ **amebic dysentery** and hepatic amebiasis. The best-known and most-used amebicidal is the ℞ **azole**. Others include ℞ **chloroquine**, emetine (contained in ipecacuanha; ipecac syrup), iodoquinol, and paromycin.

Antiprotozoal drugs are used to treat or prevent infections caused by microorganisms called protozoa. These are simple unicellular organisms that are microscopic in size but bigger than bacteria. The most important protozoa, in terms of illness and death, are those of the genus *Plasmodium*, which cause ✪ **malaria** (see ℞ **antimalarial**). Other major diseases caused by ✪ **protozoal infections**—found most commonly in countries with a hot, humid climate—are ✪ **leishmaniasis**, ✪ **toxoplasmosis**, ✪ **trichomoniasis**, trypanosomiasis, and ✪ **giardiasis** (lambliasis). In immunosuppressed individuals (including those suffering from ✪ **AIDS**), a form of ✪ **pneumonia** is caused by the protozoan *Pneumocystis carinii* (which has some features of both protozoan and fungi).

For most of these, ℞ **metronidazole** (or the related azole ℞ **furazolidone**) is effective. For *Pneumocystis carinii* infection, ℞ **trimetrexate glucuronate** and the ℞ **trimethoprim and sulfamethoxazole** (co-trimoxazole) combination may be taken.

Limitations

Prevention—in terms of clean drinking water and good food and personal hygiene—is better than treatment for these infections. Where disease is endemic, some of the less toxic drugs (particularly oral metronidazole) may be recommended as a preventive treatment to avoid contracting the disease.

Amen Ⓑ

A preparation of ℞ **medroxyprogesterone**.

Formulation: Oral tablets.

Availability: Prescription only.

Warnings and side effects: See ℞ **medroxyprogesterone**.

Amerge Ⓑ

A preparation of ℞ **naratriptan**.

Formulation: Oral tablets, available in two strengths.

Availability: Prescription only.

Warnings and side effects: See ℞ **naratriptan**.

Americaine Ⓑ

A preparation of ℞ **benzocaine**.

Formulation: Topical ear drops.

Availability: Prescription only.

Warnings and side effects: See ℞ **benzocaine**.

Americaine Anesthetic Spray Ⓑ

A preparation of ℞ **benzocaine**.

Formulation: Topical spray.

Availability: OTC.

Warnings and side effects: See ℞ **benzocaine**.

A-Methapred Ⓑ

A preparation of ℞ **methylprednisolone**.

Formulation: Powder for injection.
Availability: Prescription only.
Warnings and side effects: See ℞ **methylprednisolone**.

amfebutamone Ⓖ

see ℞ **bupropion hydrochloride**.

Amicar Tablets; Syrup; Injection Ⓑ

A preparation of ℞ **aminocaproic acid**.
Formulation: Oral tablets; syrup; intravenous infusion.
Availability: Prescription only.
Warnings and side effects: See ℞ **aminocaproic acid**.

amifostine Ⓖ

Type/Group: **cytoprotectant**.
Brand(s): Ethyol.
How administered: Intravenous infusion.
Used to treat
Amifostine is used to reduce cumulative kidney damage due to treatment of certain cancers with repeated doses of ℞ **cisplatin**. It is also used to prevent xerostomia (dry mouth) during radiotherapy for head and neck cancer.
Warnings
• It should not be given to people with known hypersensitivity to this drug (or to other aminothiol compounds), who are hypotensive, or dehydrated. This is a specialist drug and is used only after a full medical assessment.
• The effects of amifostine in pregnancy are not known, but adverse effects on the fetus are thought possible. It should be used only if the potential benefit outweighs the possible risk to the fetus.
• Medical judgment is required if breast-feeding is being considered.
• It is a specialist hospital drug and there will be monitoring of various functions such as blood pressure and calcium levels.
• An ℞ **antiemetic** should be given before and during administration of amifostine.
Interactions
• If taken with ℞ **antihypertensives**, there is a possibility of additive effect in producing a fall in blood pressure during infusion of amifostine.
Side effects
• Nausea and vomiting occur frequently and may be severe.
• Other side effects may include hypotension, flushing, chills, dizziness, sleepiness, hiccups, and sneezing. Rarely, convulsions.

Amigesic Tablets; Caplets; Capsules Ⓑ

A preparation of ℞ **salsalate**.
Formulation: Oral tablets; capsules.
Availability: Prescription only.
Warnings and side effects: See ℞ **salsalate**.

amikacin Ⓖ

Type/Group: **aminoglycoside; antibiotic; antibacterial**.
Brand(s): Amikin; various generic.
How administered: Injection.

Used to treat
Amikacin is used primarily against serious ⊕ **bacterial infections** caused by Gram-negative bacteria that prove to be resistant to the more widely used aminoglycoside ℞ **gentamicin**.
Warnings
• It should not be given to people with known hypersensitivity to amikacin or other aminoglycosides, or with severe kidney disease.
• It should be given with caution to people with mild kidney disease, hearing deficits or vertigo, dehydration, muscular disorders such as myasthenia gravis or parkinsonism, and those over 65.
• Medical judgment is required when giving to young infants.
• It should be used during pregnancy only if medically judged to be clearly needed and if the potential benefits outweigh the risks to the fetus (it crosses the placenta and could cause damage to ears or kidneys).
• Medical judgment is required if breast-feeding is being considered.
• Aminoglycosides are associated with nephrotoxicity (damage to the kidneys) and ototoxicity (damage in the ears). Irreversible vestibular impairment can occur, resulting in vertigo and difficulty maintaining balance. Permanent hearing loss in one or both ears can also occur. The risk is greatest in those with pre-existing impairments, with high doses, and with prolonged use.
• A doctor must be contacted if there are problems with hearing, vision, balance, urination, or headaches, even after the course of treatment is completed.
• The use of antibiotics may result in superinfection due to bacterial imbalance.
Interactions
• ℞ **Atracurium**, ℞ **succinylcholine**, ℞ **vecuronium**, or neuromuscular blocking agents taken with amikacin increases respiratory depression.
• ℞ **ethacrynic acid** and ℞ **carboplatin** increase the risk of ear damage.
• ℞ **Amphotericin B**, ℞ **cephalosporins**, ℞ **cyclosporine**, methoxyflurane, and ℞ **NSAIDs** may increase the risk of kidney damage.
• ℞ **carboplatin**, ℞ **cisplatin**, and ℞ **vancomycin** increase the risk of ear or kidney damage.
• ℞ **carbenicillin**, ℞ **penicillins**, ℞ **piperacillin**, and ℞ **ticarcillin** could inactivate amikacin in people with kidney failure.
Side effects
• Frequently, gastrointestinal upsets.
• Occasionally, rash, fever, hives, and itching.
• Rarely, hair loss, elevated blood pressure, and weakness.
• Additional serious effects include neurotoxicity (nerve damage), ototoxicity, deafness, and kidney damage.

Amikin Ⓑ

A preparation of ℞ **amikacin**.
Formulation: Injection in adult and pediatric strengths.
Availability: Prescription only.
Warnings and side effects: See ℞ **amikacin**.

amiloride Ⓖ

Type/Group: **diuretic; antihypertensive; heart failure treatment.**
Brand(s): Midamor. Combinations: With *hydrochlorothiazide*: Moduretic.
How administered: Orally.

Used to treat

Amiloride is a weak, potassium-sparing diuretic which retains potassium in the body and is therefore used as an alternative to, or commonly in combination with, other diuretics such as the thiazide and loop diuretics (which normally cause a loss of potassium from the body). It can be used to treat congestive ✪ **heart failure** and ✪ **hypertension** (combined with other drugs, for example, ℞ **beta-blockers**).

Warnings

• It should not be given to people with known hypersensitivity to this drug, with impaired kidney function, high potassium levels, who are already receiving potassium supplements or drugs to reduce potassium loss, or with diabetes mellitus.
• It should be given with caution to the elderly and people with cardiopulmonary disease or severe liver impairment.
• Amiloride should be used in pregnancy only if it is clearly needed.
• Medical judgment is required if breast-feeding is being considered.
• If symptoms such as paresthesia (tingling sensations), muscular weakness, or fatigue occur, treatment must be stopped immediately and a doctor notified.
• It should not be used together with other potassium-sparing diuretics, such as ℞ **spironolactone** or ℞ **triamterene**.
• Electrolytes should be monitored periodically.
• It may cause dizziness, headache, or visual disturbances, and so may impair the performance of skilled tasks such as driving.
• Foods rich in potassium should not be consumed in large quantities, for example, bananas, oranges, and salt substitutes.

Interactions

• Potassium-containing preparations (for example, certain drugs, salt substitutes, low-salt milk), spironolactone, and triamterene should be avoided, because of the risk of severe hyperkalemia (high blood potassium), with the potential of serious heart irregularities or arrest.
• ℞ **ACE inhibitors** may also raise potassium levels and cause possible heart arrhythmias.
• The levels of ℞ **lithium** may rise, with the risk of lithium toxicity.
• The levels and effects of ℞ **digoxin** may be lowered.
• ℞ **NSAID**s may reduce the effects of amiloride and raise potassium levels.

Side effects

• Gastrointestinal upsets, skin rashes, headache, or dizziness.
• Less frequently, dry mouth, muscle cramps, confusion (particularly in the elderly), postural hypotension (fall in blood pressure on standing), raised blood potassium, and lowered blood sodium.
• Rarely, serious blood disorders.

aminobenzoate potassium Ⓖ

Type/Group: **vitamin.**
Brand(s): Potaba.
How administered: Orally.

Used to treat

Aminobenzoate potassium is a derivative of para-aminobenzoic acid (PABA), considered to be a vitamin (vitamin H), and is used as an antifibrotic in the treatment of disorders associated with excess fibrous tissue, such as scleroderma and Peyronie's disease. There is uncertainty about how it works and how well.

Warnings

• It should not be given to people who are taking ℞ **sulfonamides** or who have a history of allergy to this drug.
• It should be given with caution to people with kidney function impairment.
• Its safety in pregnancy has not been established and it should be used only when the potential benefits outweigh the possible risk to the fetus.
• Medical judgment is required if breast-feeding is being considered. It is not known whether this drug appears in breast milk.
• Take with food and plenty of liquid to avoid upset stomach.

Interactions

No significant interactions specific to this drug are known.

Side effects

• Nausea or anorexia and rash (your doctor may recommend you to discontinue treatment if these occur).

aminobenzoic acid (PABA) Ⓖ

Type/Group: **sunscreen.**
Brand(s): Original Eclipse Sunscreen; Tropical Gold Dark Tanning; Hawaiian Dark Tanning Oil.
How administered: Topically (external).

Used to treat

Aminobenzoic acid is an unusual drug, sometimes classed as one of the B-complex vitamins, that helps to protect the skin from ultraviolet radiation and is present in some ℞ **sunscreens**, although it is used less than it once was.

Warnings

• It should not be given to people with known hypersensitivity to aminobenzoic acid or related drugs.
• A doctor should be consulted before using while pregnant or breast-feeding.
• Protection is temporary, and so creams and lotions must be reapplied periodically.
• Preparations containing aminobenzoates may cause photosensitivity (abnormal sensitivity to sunlight) reactions.
• It may permanently stain clothes or upholstery yellow or brown.

Interactions

None significant are known.

Side effects

• Irritation and rash.

aminocaproic acid ⓖ

Type/Group: **hemostatic**.
Brand(s): Amicar; various generic.
How administered: Orally; intravenous infusion.

Used to treat

Aminocaproic acid inhibits the activation of plasminogen, an enzyme in the blood that dissolves blood clots, which means that it is antithrombolytic. It is used to control excessive bleeding, particularly in life-threatening situations. Other uses, although not stated by the manufacturer, have included prevention of recurrence of subarachnoid hemorrhage, management of certain bleeding disorders, and bleeding resulting from certain surgical procedures (heart bypass, prostate) or cancer.

Warnings

• It should not be given to people with a normal clotting process or with uncontrolled generalized clotting (disseminated intravascular coagulation; DIC).
• It should be given with caution to people with heart, liver, or kidney disease. It will be used only after a full medical assessment.
• Aminocaproic acid should be used during pregnancy only if the potential benefit outweighs the possible risk to the fetus.
• Medical judgment is required if breast-feeding is being considered.
• In cases where bleeding is from the upper urinary tract (kidneys, ureters) aminocaproic acid may cause obstruction (by clot formation). It will only be used where the benefits outweigh the risks.

Interactions

• ℞ **Oral contraceptives** and ℞ **estrogen** may intensify the coagulation effect of aminocaproic acid.

Side effects

• These may include gastrointestinal disturbances (for example, nausea, cramps, diarrhea), malaise, dizziness, reddening of the conjunctiva (inside of the eyelid), nasal stuffiness, rash, ringing in the ears, and headache.
• Infrequently, delirium, kidney damage, phlebitis and hypotension, weakness, and fatigue.

aminoglutethimide ⓖ

Type/Group: **hormone antagonist**.
How administered: Orally
Brand(s): Cytadren.

Used to treat

Aminoglutethimide is used to suppress adrenal function in ✪ **Cushing's syndrome**, a disease in which the adrenal gland releases excessive corticosteroid hormones. Although not stated by the manufacturer for such use, it may also be prescribed to treat advanced cancer of the breast or prostate. It is an enzyme inhibitor and in treating these disorders it is thought to work as an indirect hormone antagonist, by inhibiting the synthesis of steroid hormones in the body.

Warnings

• It should not be used by people with known hypersensitivity to glutethimide or aminoglutethimide.

• It should be given with caution to people with abnormally low adrenal function.
• It should not be used during pregnancy if possible, as there is a risk of harming the fetus.
• It should not be used by breast-feeding mothers.
• It may cause adrenal cortical hypofunction at times of stress.
• There will be medical monitoring throughout treatment (such as thyroid function, blood pressure, blood count).

Interactions

• The effectiveness of ℞ **anticoagulants**, ℞ **dexamethasone**, ℞ **digitoxin**, ℞ **medroxyprogesterone**, ℞ **theophylline**, and ℞ **tamoxifen** may be reduced.

Side effects

• Most frequently, drowsiness, dizziness, skin rash and itching, nausea and loss of appetite, hair growth (hirsutism), effects on the heart and liver.
• It may cause an abnormal reduction in adrenal function (adrenal insufficiency), hypotension, and blood-cell disorders,

aminoglycoside ⓓ

Generics: **amikacin**; **gentamicin**; **kanamycin**; **neomycin**; **netilmicin**; **streptomycin**; **tobramycin**.

Actions and uses

Aminoglycosides make up a chemical class of ℞ **antibiotic** drugs that have ℞ **antibacterial** activity—they are all bactericidal (that is, they kill bacteria rather than merely inhibiting their growth). They are used to treat ✪ **bacterial infections**. Although they can be used against some Gram-positive bacteria, they are used primarily to treat serious infections caused by Gram-negative bacteria. Infections treated include ✪ **septicemia**, ✪ **meningitis**, infections of the heart (✪ **endocarditis**; sometimes in conjunction with ℞ **penicillin** antibiotics), the biliary and urinary tracts, the eyes and skin, and ✪ **pneumonia** in hospital patients. ℞ **streptomycin** is an original member of the aminoglycoside family and is used in combination with other antibiotics for ℞ **antituberculosis** chemotherapy, where treatment for ✪ **tuberculosis** takes many months.
Aminoglycosides are not absorbed from the undamaged gut, so they must normally be administered by injection, or by topical application (externally) in the case of the more toxic members (for example, ℞ **neomycin**). However, because they are not absorbed, it does mean they can be used to reduce levels of bacteria in the colon prior to intestinal surgery or examination.

Limitations

The disadvantage of this group of antibiotics is that they all share a number of common toxic properties (adverse side effects). They are removed from the body via the kidneys, which can result in a potentially dangerous accumulation in people with impaired kidney function. Toxic effects are related to the dose and one of the most serious is ototoxicity (impaired hearing and balance), and the previously mentioned kidney toxicity. See also the individual drug entries.

aminosalicylate ⓓ

(5-aminosalicylate; gastrointestinal anti-inflammatory agent)

Generics: **balsalazide disodium; mesalamine; olsalazine sodium; sulfasalazine.**

Actions and uses

Aminosalicylates are a chemical class that contains a 5-aminosalicylic acid component. They are used to maintain remission of the symptoms of inflammatory bowel disease and ⊙ **ulcerative colitis**, and to treat active ⊙ **Crohn's disease**, proctitis, and proctosigmoiditis. They can also be taken to treat cases of ⊙ **rheumatoid arthritis** which have not responded to other drugs.

The drugs in this group include ℞ **mesalamine**, which is 5-aminosalicylic acid itself, ℞ **olsalazine sodium**, which is two molecules of 5-aminosalicylic acid joined together, ℞ **sulfasalazine**, which combines within the one chemical both 5-aminosalicylic acid and the (℞ **sulfonamide**) ℞ **antibacterial** drug sulfapyridine, and ℞ **balsalazide disodium**, which is a prodrug of 5-aminosalicylic acid.

Limitations

The aminosalicylate component of these drugs causes side effects such as diarrhea, salicylate hypersensitivity, and effects on the kidney (interstitial nephritis). Sulfasalazine also has sulfonamide-related side effects, including rashes, photosensitivity, serious allergic reactions, liver failure, and serious blood disorders. The sensitivity of individual patients to one or other chemical component partly determines the most suitable treatment. People taking aminosalicylates should tell their doctor if they have any unexplained bruising, bleeding, sore throat, fever, or malaise. Any such symptoms may indicate possible effects on the blood and so treatment should probably be stopped. See also the individual drug entries.

amiodarone hydrochloride ⓖ

Type/Group: **antiarrhythmic.**

Brand(s): Cordarone; Pacerone; generic.

How administered: Orally; injection.

Used to treat

Amiodarone is a toxic drug used to treat certain life-threatening irregularities of the heartbeat (see ⊙ **arrhythmia**), especially in cases where, for one reason or another, alternative drugs cannot be used.

Warnings

• It should not be given to people with known hypersensitivity to this drug, or with certain conduction disorders.

• This is a specialist hospital drug which will be administered by clinicians experienced in treating life-threatening arrhythmias and who are thoroughly familiar with this drug. Extensive medical checks will be carried out, including close monitoring of lung function and periodic evaluation of thyroid, liver, eyes, heart, and electrolytes.

• Amiodarone should be used during pregnancy only when the potential benefit outweighs the possible risk to the fetus.

• It is present in breast milk and nursing women should discontinue using this drug or stop breast-feeding.

• Precautions, such as sunscreens and protective clothing, should be used to minimize exposure to sunlight or ultraviolet light.

Interactions

• ℞ cimetidine and ℞ ritonavir may intensify the effects of amiodarone.

• The levels and effects of other antiarrhythmic drugs (for example, ℞ disopyramide, ℞ flecainide, ℞ lidocaine, ℞ procainamide, ℞ quinidine), ℞ anticoagulants, ℞ beta-blockers, ℞ calcium-channel blockers, ℞ dextromethorphan, ℞ digoxin, ℞ fentanyl, ℞ hydantoins, ℞ methotrexate, and ℞ theophylline may be increased, with potential for adverse effects.

• ℞ cholestyramine and ℞ hydantoins may reduce the levels and effects of amiodarone.

Side effects

These are many and affect a high proportion of people. They include:

• Pulmonary effects (fibrosis and pneumonitis, which may be life-threatening), blood, liver or thyroid changes, arrhythmias and other heart disorders, and effects on the central nervous system, symptoms may include gastrointestinal disturbances (for example, nausea, vomiting, constipation, loss of appetite), photosensitivity, visual disturbances (sometimes severe), inflammation of the lungs, incoordination, dizziness, tingling sensations, sleep disturbances, unusual taste or smell sensations, edema, or flushing;

• Hypotension occurs commonly when amiodarone is given by injection.

Amitone ⓑ

A preparation of ℞ **calcium carbonate**.

Formulation: Oral tablets, chewable.

Availability: OTC.

Warnings and side effects: See ℞ calcium carbonate.

amitriptyline hydrochloride ⓖ

Type/Group: **antidepressant; tricyclic.**

Brand(s): Elavil; various generic. Combinations: With *perphenazine*: Triavil; Etrafon. With *chlordiazepoxide*: Limbitrol.

How administered: Orally; injection.

Used to treat

Amitriptyline can be used to treat ⊙ **depression**. It has very marked sedative properties, which may be of benefit to agitated or violent patients. Although not stated by the manufacturer for such treatment, it is sometimes used with ℞ **analgesics** for ⊙ **pain** of many kinds, including cancer, migraine, and arthritis, as well as for the treatment of bulimia and panic disorder, and of certain skin conditions. As is the case with other antidepressants, this drug is also being evaluated for other uses.

Warnings

• It should not be given to people with known hypersensitivity to this drug, if they are just recovering from myocardial infarction, or are taking or who have stopped taking ℞ **MAOI** antidepressants within the previous 14 days (see Interactioins below).

• It should be given with caution to people with a history of cardiovascular disorders, seizures, urinary retention, elevated intraocular pressure (pressure in the eyeball), with heart or thyroid disease, pheochromocytoma, diabetes mellitus, prostatic hypertrophy, angle-closure glaucoma, or kidney or liver disease.

• Amitriptyline should be used during pregnancy only if the benefits clearly outweigh the possible risk to the fetus.

• It should not be used by nursing mothers.

• Other symptoms of a psychiatric illness may worsen.

• Episodes of mania or hypomania may occur, especially in people with bipolar affective disorder (manic depression).

• There may be photosensitization, so exposure to sunlight should be minimized.

• Treatment should be stopped gradually, lowering the dose over a period of time.

• It is not generally given to children less than 12 years of age.

• It may be two to three weeks before there are any signs of improvement.

• It may impair the performance of skilled tasks, such as driving.

• Alcohol, grapefruit juice, and smoking can all affect tricyclics (see Interactions below).

Interactions

• Serious or even fatal reactions can occur if ℞ **MAOI** antidepressants are taken at the same time as tricyclics.

• The effects of ℞ **epinephrine**, ℞ **norepinephrine**, and ℞ **phenylephrine** on blood pressure are intensified.

• Grapefruit juice increases the levels of tricyclics.

• ℞ **clonidine hydrochloride** should not be used with tricyclics, because a dangerous increase in blood pressure and hypertensive crisis is possible.

• The effects of ℞ **guanethidine monosulfate**, ℞ **levodopa**, and ℞ **sympathomimetics** may be reduced by tricyclics.

• The effects of ℞ **anticholinergics**, dicumarol, ℞ **quinolones**, grepafloxacin, and sparfloxacin may be enhanced by tricyclics.

• ℞ **Barbiturates**, ℞ **activated charcoal**, and rifamycin-related antibiotics may reduce the effectiveness of tricyclics.

• ℞ **Cimetidine**, ℞ **SSRIs**, ℞ **haloperidol**, ℞ **bupropion**, ℞ **valproate sodium** (and other valproic acid derivatives), and histamine ℞ **H2-antagonists** may increase the levels of tricyclics in the blood.

• The levels of ℞ **carbamazepine** may increase, while blood levels of tricyclics decrease.

• Smoking may affect the metabolism of tricyclics.

• The effects of alcohol may be enhanced.

Side effects

• These can be many and include, along with other members of this class, pronounced ℞ **anticholinergic** side effects, such as dizziness, drowsiness, difficulty in concentrating, dry mouth, blurred vision, constipation and other gastrointestinal symptoms, postural hypotension (lowered blood pressure on standing), irregular heartbeat, white blood cell and platelet disorders, and urinary retention, photosensitivity (abnormal sensitivity to sunlight), and skin reactions.

• Tricyclics can also cause weight gain, changes in appetite and libido, liver disorders, and convulsions.

amlodipine besilate ⑥

see ℞ **amlodipine besylate**.

amlodipine besylate ⑥

(amlodipine besilate)

Type/Group: **calcium-channel blocker; antianginal; antihypertensive**.

Brand(s): Norvasc. Combinations: With *benazepril hydrochloride*: Lotrel.

How administered: Orally.

Used to treat

Amlodipine besylate can be used to treat ✪ **hypertension** and in the prevention of ✪ **angina pectoris** attacks.

Warnings

• It should not be given to people with known hypersensitivity to this drug, or with certain heart arrhythmias.

• It should be given with caution to people with congestive heart failure or impaired liver function.

• It should be used during pregnancy only if the potential benefits outweighs the risks to the fetus.

• Breast-feeding women should either discontinue using this drug or stop breast-feeding.

• If amlodipine is given to replace a ℞ **beta-blocker**, then withdrawal of the beta-blocker should not be abrupt. Calcium-channel blockers, also, should not be discontinued abruptly.

Interactions

No interactions of significance are known.

Side effects

• These are generally mild and may include edema, facial flushing, palpitations, drowsiness, dizziness, fatigue, nausea, or abdominal pain.

ammonium chloride ⑥

Type/Group: **diuretic; expectorant; electrolyte; urinary acidifier**.

Brand(s): (OTC oral diuretics): Aqua-Ban. (Injection): Various generic.

How administered: Orally; injection (infusion).

Used to treat

Ammonium chloride is used in some OTC preparations for the relief of premenstrual water retention. Also, it can cause metabolic ✪ **acidosis** and so can be used to correct metabolic ✪ **alkalosis**. It has some use in the therapeutic acidification of urine, which increases the rate of the excretion of some drugs and poisons, and is therefore effectively an antidote. Occasionally it is used in OTC cough treatments as an expectorant, although evidence of its beneficial effects is lacking.

Warnings

• It should not be given to people with significantly impaired kidney or liver function.

• It should be given with caution to people with pulmonary insufficiency.

• Ammonium chloride should be used during pregnancy only when it is clearly needed.

• No problems are known when used while breast-feeding.

• Large doses may cause metabolic acidosis, with symptoms such as nausea, vomiting, hyperventilation, and progressive drowsiness.

Pallor, sweating, slow heart beat, arrhythmias, or generalized twitching may indicate a serious overdose and ammonia toxicity.

Interactions

No interactions of significance are known.

Side effects

• There may be stomach irritation, nausea, or vomiting.

amobarbital Ⓖ

(amylobarbitone)

Type/Group: **sedatives; hypnotic; barbiturate.**
Brand(s): Amytal. Combinations: With *secobarbital sodium*: Tuinal.
How administered: Orally, injection.

Used to treat

Amobarbital is used only when absolutely necessary, and in the short term only, to treat severe and difficult-to-treat ✪ **insomnia.** Although not stated by the manufacturer for such use, it may be prescribed as an ℞ **antiepileptic** for severe episodes in specialized epilepsy centers and as an additional treatment in psychiatry.

Warnings

• It should not be given to people with known hypersensitivity to barbiturates, respiratory depression, severe liver impairment, or porphyria.
• It should be given with caution to people with anemia, addiction to barbiturates, liver disease, chronic obstructive pulmonary disease (COPD), emphysema, kidney disease, high blood pressure, acute or chronic pain, mental depression, or a history of drug abuse. Caution is also recommended for anyone over the age of 65.
• Amobarbital should not be used during pregnancy if possible. A doctor must be contacted if pregnancy occurs while using this drug.
• Medical judgment is required if breast-feeding is being considered.
• There is a high risk for dependence (addiction) and abuse.
• It loses its effectiveness for treating insomnia after about two weeks.
• Avoid driving or other activities requiring alertness.
• Do not drink alcohol.
• Do not stop using this drug abruptly after long-term use.
• It is very dangerous in overdose.
• Amobarbital is a Schedule II controlled substance.

Interactions

• Amobarbital decreases the response to oral ℞ **anticoagulants** (for example, ℞ **warfarin sodium**).
• If used with ℞ **acetaminophen**, there is an increased risk of toxic effects on the liver.
• The levels and beneficial effects of the following drug are reduced: ℞ **antidepressants;** ℞ **beta-blockers;** ℞ **calcium-channel blockers;** ℞ **corticosteroids;** ℞ **cyclosporine;** ℞ **digitoxin;** ℞ **disopyramide,** ℞ **doxycycline,** ℞ **estrogens,** ℞ **griseofulvin;** ℞ **oral contraceptives;** ℞ **propafenone;** ℞ **quinidine;** ℞ **tacrolimus;** ℞ **theophylline.**
• ℞ **MAOI** antidepressants prolong the effects of barbiturates.
• If amobarbital is used with an ℞ **antipsychotic**, the effects of both drugs are reduced.

• The levels of ℞ **chloramphenicol** are reduced, while those of the barbiturate are increased.
• If used with methoxyflurane, the adverse effects on the kidneys are increased.
• The effects of ℞ **narcotic analgesics** may be altered, with increased central nervous system (CNS) depression.
• ℞ **Valproic acid** increases the levels of barbiturate.
• If used with alcohol, there is excessive central nervous system (CNS) depression.

Side effects

• Depending on the dose, use, and type, there may be hangover with drowsiness, lack of energy, or rash.
• Less frequently, CNS depression, dizziness, headache, lightheadedness, mental depression, physical dependence, slurred speech, excitement in children and those over 65, vertigo, slowed heartbeat, lowered blood pressure, gastrointestinal upset, or hives.
• Rare but serious side effects include blood cell disorders, breathing stoppages, respiratory depression, spasms of the bronchi or larynx, and Stevens-Johnson syndrome (a severe skin disorder).

amoebicide Ⓓ

see ℞ amebicide and antiprotozoal.

Amosan Ⓑ

A preparation of ℞ **sodium perborate.**
Formulation: Topical liquid.
Availability: OTC.
Warnings and side effects: See ℞ sodium perborate.

amoxapine Ⓖ

Type/Group: **antidepressant; tricyclic.**
Brand(s): Ascendin; various generic.
How administered: Orally.

Used to treat

Amoxapine can be used to treat ✪ **depression**, particularly when the depression is accompanied by ✪ **anxiety.**

Warnings

• It should not be given to people with known hypersensitivity to this drug, if they are just recovering from myocardial infarction, or are taking or have stopped taking ℞ **MAOI** antidepressants within the previous 14 days.
• It should be given with caution to people with a history of seizures, cardiovascular disorders, urinary retention, elevated intraocular pressure (pressure in the eyeball), heart or thyroid disease, pheochromocytoma, diabetes mellitus, prostatic hypertrophy, angle-closure glaucoma, or kidney or liver disease.
• Amoxapine should be used during pregnancy only if the benefits outweigh the possible risk to the fetus.
• It should not be used by nursing mothers.
• Other symptoms of a psychiatric illness may worsen.
• Episodes of mania or hypomania may occur, especially in people with bipolar affective disorder (manic depression).
• There may be photosensitization, so exposure to sunlight should be minimized.

• Treatment should be stopped gradually by lowering the dose over a period of time.

• It is not generally given to children less than 16 years of age.

• It may be two to three weeks before there are any signs of improvement.

• It may impair the performance of skilled tasks, such as driving.

• Alcohol, grapefruit juice, and smoking can all affect tricyclics (see Interactions below).

Interactions

• Serious or even fatal reactions can occur if ℞ **MAOI** antidepressants are taken at the same time as tricyclics.

• The effects of ℞ **epinephrine**, ℞ **norepinephrine**, and ℞ **phenylephrine** on blood pressure are intensified.

• Grapefruit juice increases the levels of tricyclics.

• ℞ **clonidine hydrochloride** should not be used with tricyclics, because a dangerous increase in blood pressure and hypertensive crisis is possible.

• The effects of ℞ **guanethidine monosulfate**, ℞ **levodopa**, and ℞ **sympathomimetics** may be reduced by tricyclics.

• The effects of ℞ **anticholinergics**, dicumarol, ℞ **quinolones**, grepafloxacin, and sparfloxacin may be enhanced by tricyclics.

• ℞ **Barbiturates**, ℞ **activated charcoal**, and rifamycin-related antibiotics may reduce the effectiveness of tricyclics.

• ℞ **Cimetidine**, ℞ **SSRIs**, ℞ **haloperidol**, ℞ **bupropion**, ℞ **valproate sodium** (and other valproic acid derivatives), and histamine ℞ **H2-antagonists** may increase the levels of tricyclics in the blood.

• The levels of ℞ **carbamazepine** may increase, while blood levels of tricyclics decrease.

• Smoking may affect the metabolism of tricyclics.

• The effects of alcohol may be enhanced.

Side effects

• These can be many and include, along with other members of this class, pronounced ℞ **anticholinergic** side effects, such as drowsiness, difficulty in concentrating, dry mouth, blurred vision, constipation, postural hypotension (lowered blood pressure on standing), urinary retention, photosensitivity (abnormal sensitivity to sunlight), and skin reactions.

• Tricyclics can also cause weight gain, changes in appetite and libido, liver disorders, and convulsions.

• Rarely, amoxapine may also cause tardive dyskinesia (abnormal movement), and has been linked with neuroleptic malignant syndrome (a serious disorder caused by neuroleptic drugs), and in women, menstrual irregularities, breast enlargement, and galactorrhoea.

amoxicillin Ⓖ

Type/Group: **antibiotic; penicillin; antibacterial; Helicobacter pylori eradication regime**.

Brand(s): Amoxil; Moxillin; Trimox; Wymox; various generic.

Combinations: With *clavulanic acid*: Augmentin.

How administered: Orally; injection.

Used to treat

Amoxicillin is a broad-spectrum penicillin-type drug used to treat ⊙ **bacterial infections** of the respiratory tract and soft tissues, bac-

terial ⊙ **meningitis**, ⊙ **septicemia**, and ⊙ **gonorrhea**, as well as for the prevention of bacterial ⊙ **endocarditis**. It is also used in combination with the beta-lactamase inhibitor ℞ **clavulanic acid** (which helps combat antibiotic resistance due to bacteria by developing an enzyme called beta-lactamase that breaks down penicillins), to treat infections of the skin and skin structures, and gynecological and intra-abdominal infections. It is also used in *Helicobacter pylori* eradication regimes for duodenal ulcers (see ⊙ peptic ulcer).

Warnings

• It should not be given to people with known hypersensitivity to penicillins.

• It should be given with caution to people with allergies to ℞ **cephalosporins** or ℞ **imipenem**, with impaired kidney function, or with mononucleosis (may cause rash). It should also be used with caution in newborn babies.

• Penicillins cross the placenta and should be used in pregnancy only if medically judged to be needed.

• Medical judgment is also required for breast-feeding mothers.

• Serious and occasionally fatal hypersensitivity reactions can occur. Notify the doctor if skin rash, itching, hives, severe diarrhea, shortness of breath, black tongue, sore throat, nausea, fever, swollen joints, or any unusual bleeding or bruising occurs.

• Take on an empty stomach (one hour before or two hours after eating).

• The full course of treatment prescribed must be completed or infection may return.

• Superinfections from the altered bacterial balance created by antibiotic treatment may occur, and may result in ⊙ **pseudomembranous colitis**. A doctor must be contacted if there is severe abdominal pain, or moderate to severe diarrhea.

Interactions

• Amoxicillin taken with ℞ **allopurinol** may increase the risk of rash.

• The effectiveness of ℞ **oral contraceptives** may be reduced.

• ℞ **Tetracyclines**, ℞ **chloramphenicol**, and ℞ **macrolide** antibiotics may reduce the effectiveness of amoxicillin.

• The effects of ℞ **atenolol** may be reduced.

• The effects of ℞ **methotrexate** may be increased.

• ℞ **Probenecid** may increase the levels of penicillins.

Side effects

• Frequently, gastrointestinal disturbances (nausea, vomiting, diarrhea).

• Occasionally, rash and hives.

Amoxil Ⓑ

A preparation of ℞ **amoxicillin**.

Formulation: Oral capsules, chewable tablets, oral suspension, each in several strengths, pediatric drops.

Availability: Prescription only.

Warnings and side effects: See ℞ **amoxicillin**.

amphetamine sulfate Ⓖ

Type/Group: **CNS stimulant**.

Brand(s): Combinations: With *dextroamphetamine*: Adderall.

How administered: Orally.

Used to treat

Amphetamine sulfate is a drug that works directly on the brain as a stimulant. It is currently available only in combination with the similar drug, ℞ **dextroamphetamine**, in a product that may be prescribed to treat ✪ **narcolepsy** (a condition involving irresistible attacks of sleep during the daytime) and ✪ **attention deficit disorder** in children. Although not stated by the manufacturer for such use, it may also be prescribed as an additional treatment in the short-term treatment of ✪ **obesity**

Warnings

• It should not be given to people with known hypersensitivity to sympathomimetic amines, advanced arteriosclerosis, symptomatic heart disease, hypertension, hyperthyroidism, glaucoma, agitated states, or a history of drug abuse.

• It is not known whether this drug can harm the fetus. It should be used during pregnancy only if it is clearly needed.

• It should not be used by nursing mothers.

• It may impair ability to perform tasks requiring alertness, such as driving.

• This drug has a high abuse potential. Do not use in larger doses or for a longer period than prescribed. Tolerance, extreme psychological dependence, and severe social disability may occur.

• Amphetamine is a Schedule II controlled substance.

Interactions

• Amphetamine sulfate must not be used along with, or within two weeks of discontinuing, an ℞ **MAOI** antidepressant. Severe and even fatal reactions can occur.

• If used with ℞ **selegiline** or ℞ **furazolidone**, severe hypertensive reactions are possible.

• ℞ **tricyclic** antidepressants and urinary acidifiers may reduce the levels of amphetamines.

• ℞ **sodium bicarbonate** may increase the effects of amphetamines.

Side effects

• Frequently, headache, nervousness, dizziness, hypersalivation, nausea diarrhea, and dry mouth.

• Occasionally, depression, anxiety, insomnia, delayed sleep, euphoria, restlessness, and changes in heartbeat.

Amphocin ⑧

A preparation of ℞ **amphotericin B**.
Formulation: Injection (intravenous).
Availability: Prescription only.
Warnings and side effects: See ℞ **amphotericin B**.

Amphojel Tablets; Suspension ⑧

A preparation of ℞ **aluminum hydroxide**.
Formulation: Oral tablets (2 strengths); liquid.
Availability: OTC.
Warnings and side effects: See ℞ **aluminum hydroxide**.

Amphotec ⑧

A preparation of ℞ **amphotericin B**.
Formulation: Injection (intravenous).

Availability: Prescription only.
Warnings and side effects: See ℞ **amphotericin B**.

amphotericin ⑥

see ℞ **amphotericin B**.

amphotericin B ⑥

(amphotericin)
Type/Group: **antifungal; antibiotic**.
Brand(s): Abelcet; Amphocin; Amphotec; Fungizone.
How administered: Intravenous infusion; topically (external).

Used to treat

Amphotericin B is a broad-spectrum antifungal, one of the polyene antibiotics, and is an extremely important drug in the treatment of serious and potentially fatal systemic ✪ **fungal infections**, when it is given by intravenous infusion. However, it is a toxic drug and side effects are common. It is not to be used to treat noninvasive fungal infections such as oral thrush or vaginal candidiasis. There have been recent attempts to minimize toxicity (particularly to the kidney) by making a lipid formulation (encapsulated in liposomes) and a colloidal dispersion (with sodium cholesteryl sulfate). Amphotericin B is also used topically (externally) to treat infections caused by *Candida albicans*.

Warnings

• It should not be given to people with known hypersensitivity to amphotericin B.

• It should be given with caution to people with kidney disease and those who are undergoing anticancer treatment.

• It is not known whether it harms the fetus. It should be used during pregnancy only if clearly needed.

• Because of the possibility of serious reactions in infants, breast-feeding is not recommended.

• Kidney damage is a serious factor. Alternatives to the conventional form of the drug are less toxic.

• Contact with the eyes must be avoided.

• Adverse reactions during infusion are frequent (chills, fever, reduced blood pressure, vomiting, nausea, headache, panting), and other drugs may be given to minimize these.

• Long-term treatment may be needed to clear infection.

Interactions

• ℞ **Aminoglycosides** and ℞ **cyclosporine** may increase kidney toxicity.

• If taken with neuromuscular blocking agents, muscle relaxation may be prolonged due to decreased potassium levels.

Side effects

These depend on how it is administered, dose, and use, and can be severe.

• May cause fever, headache, vomiting, diarrhea, loss of appetite, abdominal pain, muscle and joint pain.

• Rarely, heart, hearing, liver, kidney and blood disorders, seizures, and allergic reactions.

• There may be reactions at the injection site, and contact dermatitis, stinging and other skin reactions when used topically.

ampicillin ⑥

Type/Group: **antibiotic; penicillin; antibacterial**.
Brand(s): Principen; Totacillin; Marcillin; various generic.
Combinations: With *sulbactam*: Unasyn. With *probenecid*: Principen with Probenecid; Polycillin PRB; Probampicin.
How administered: Orally; injection.

Used to treat

Ampicillin is a broad-spectrum penicillin-type drug used to treat ✪ **bacterial infections** of the respiratory tract and soft tissues, bacterial ✪ **meningitis**, ✪ **septicemia**, and ✪ **gonorrhea**, as well as for the prevention of bacterial ✪ **endocarditis**. In combination with the beta-lactamase inhibitor sulbactam sodium, it is used to treat skin and skin-structure infections, and certain intra-abdominal and gynecological infections.

Warnings

• It should not be used by people with known hypersensitivity to penicillins.
• It should be given with caution to people with allergies to ℞ **cephalosporins** or ℞ **imipenem**, with kidney function impairment, or with mononucleosis (may cause rash). It should also be used with caution in newborn babies.
• Penicillins cross the placenta and should be used in pregnancy only if medically judged to be needed.
• Medical judgment is also required for breast-feeding mothers.
• Serious and occasionally fatal hypersensitivity reactions can occur. A doctor must be contacted if skin rash, itching, hives, severe diarrhea, shortness of breath, black tongue, sore throat, nausea, fever, swollen joints, or any unusual bleeding or bruising occurs.
• Take on an empty stomach (one hour before or two hours after eating).
• The full course of treatment prescribed must be completed or infection may return.
• Superinfections from the altered bacterial balance created by antibiotic treatment may occur and may result in ✪ **pseudomembranous colitis**. A doctor must be contacted if severe abdominal pain, or moderate to severe diarrhea occurs.

Interactions

• Ampicillin taken with ℞ **allopurinol** may increase the risk of rash.
• ℞ **Tetracyclines** ℞ **chloramphenicol**, and ℞ **macrolide** antibiotics may reduce the effectiveness of ampicillin.
• The effects of ℞ **atenolol** may be reduced.
• The effects of ℞ **methotrexate** may be increased.

Side effects

• Frequently, gastrointestinal disturbances (nausea, vomiting, diarrhea), oral or vaginal candidiasis (thrush).
• Occasionally, rash, hives, and headache.
• Rarely, dizziness or seizure.

amprenavir ⑥

Type/Group: **antiviral**.
Brand(s): Agenerase.
How administered: Orally.

Used to treat

Amprenavir is a protease inhibitor that is used in combination with other drugs to treat ✪ **HIV** infection.

Warnings

• It should not be given to people with known hypersensitivity to amprenavir.
• It should be given with caution to people with blood coagulation defects related to vitamin-K deficiency, diabetes mellitus, hemophilia, liver insufficiency, or hypersensitivity to other protease inhibitors or sulfonamides. Medical judgment is also required for children under 4 years old.
• Amprenavir's safety during pregnancy has not been established. It should be used during pregnancy only when the potential benefits outweigh the possible riks to the fetus.
• The Centers for Disease Control and Prevention recommend that HIV-infected mothers do not breast-feed.
• It is a specialist drug, and there will be full assessment and patient monitoring throughout treatment.
• Do not take vitamin E supplements with this drug because its capsules and solution contain high doses of vitamin E.
• Severe, possibly life-threatening rash (Stevens-Johnson syndrome; a skin disorder) has been reported.
• A doctor must be consulted before taking any other drug with amprenavir (including OTCs, herbal remedies, and supplements) to avoid potentially serious interactions.
• The effectiveness of ℞ **oral contraceptives** may be reduced.

Interactions

These are many and include:
• ℞ **triazolam**, ℞ **ergot alkaloids**, ℞ **midazolam**, and ℞ **bepridil** must not be taken with amprenavir to avoid potentially life-threatening problems;
• ℞ **rifampin** must not be taken with amprenavir, because rifampin substantially reduces its effectiveness;
• ℞ **abacavir**, ℞ **ritonavir**, and ℞ **nevirapine** may increase the effects of amprenavir.
• If taken with ℞ **barbiturates**, ℞ **carbamazepine**, ℞ **phenytoin**, or ℞ **rifabutin**, the effects of amprenavir are reduced while the other drug's are increased.
• ℞ **erythromycin** increases the effects of both drugs.
• The levels of ℞ **lovastatin**, ℞ **saquinavir**, ℞ **sildenafil**, and ℞ **simvastatin** may be increased.
• The effectiveness of ℞ **oral contraceptives** may be reduced.

Side effects

• Commonly, gastrointestinal effects, rash, and a tingling sensation around the mouth.
• Frequently, depression or mood disorder, headache, changes in blood levels of sugar and triglycerides.

amylobarbitone ⑥

see ℞ amobarbital.

Amytal ⑧

A preparation of ℞ amobarbital.
Formulation: Oral tablets; injection.
Availability: Prescription only.
Warnings and side effects: See ℞ amobarbital.

anabolic Ⓓ

see ℞ anabolic steroid.

anabolic steroid Ⓓ

(anabolics; "steroids")
Generics: **nandrolone; stanozolol; testolactone.**
Actions and uses
Anabolic steroids are agents (chemically derived from the ℞ **androgen** testosterone) that generally promote body growth, promote masculinization, and oppose ℞ **estrogen** hormones in the body. In practice, all agents have mixed androgen and anabolic actions.
℞ **stanozolol** is a ℞ **steroid** with enhanced anabolic activity that can be used to treat hereditary ✪ **angioedema** and certain other conditions by assisting the metabolic synthesis of protein in the body.
Limitations
The anabolic steroids have very pronounced actions on muscle growth and are subject to abuse for the enhancement of athletic performance or physical appearance. ℞ **stanozolol** is a Schedule III controlled substance.
The side effects of androgen/anabolic agents are marked (see ℞ **androgen** and ℞ **stanozolol**). In particular, effects on the liver can be very serious. The use of anabolic steroids may increase the risk of arteriosclerosis and coronary artery disease. Stanozolol should not be taken while pregnant because of the potential masculinization of the fetus (a doctor must be contacted if pregnancy occurs while taking this drug).

Anacin Aspirin Free Maxiumum Strength Gel Caplets; Tablets Ⓑ

A preparation of ℞ **acetaminophen.**
Formulation: Oral tablets; gelcaplets.
Availability: OTC.
Warnings and side effects: See ℞ **acetaminophen.**

Anacin Tablets; Caplets Ⓑ

A preparation of ℞ **aspirin** and ℞ **caffeine.**
Formulation: Oral tablets and caplets.
Availability: OTC.
Warnings and side effects: See ℞ **aspirin;** ℞ **caffeine.**

Anafranil Ⓑ

A preparation of ℞ **clomipramine hydrochloride.**
Formulation: Oral capsules in several strengths.
Availability: Prescription only.
Warnings and side effects: See ℞ **clomipramine hydrochloride.**

anagrelide hydrochloride Ⓖ

Type/Group: **antiplatelet.**
Brand(s): Agrylin.
How administered: Orally.
Used to treat
Anagrelide is an antiplatelet (℞ **antithrombotic**) drug which is used to treat symptoms of a condition called essential thromb-ocythemia, in which platelet counts—and risk of thrombosis—are high. Its action is not completely understood, but it appears to interfere with the maturation of the parent cell (megakaryocyte) that produces platelets.
Warnings
• It should be given with caution to people with cardiovascular disease, or liver or kidney impairment.
• It should be used during pregnancy only if the potential benefit outweighs the possible risk to the fetus.
• Medical judgment is required if breast-feeding is being considered. It is not known whether this drug appears in breast milk.
• Anagrelide is used only under close medical supervision (especially when beginning treatment), with monitoring of blood, liver, and kidney functions.
• This drug has some effect on heart action (similar to the effects of ℞ **cardiac glycosides**) and a cardiovascular examination is recommended before beginning treatment.
Interactions
• ℞ **sucralfate** may reduce the absorption and levels of anagrelide.
Side effects
• The most common are headache, palpitations or rapid heartbeat, weakness, gastrointestinal disturbances (for example, diarrhea, abdominal pain, nausea, gas), edema, dizziness, shortness of breath, rash and tingling sensations.
• Although infrequent, serious cardiac events, stroke, pulmonary conditions (infiltrates, fibrosis), pancreatitis, gastrointestinal ulcer, and seizure have been reported.

Ana-Guard Ⓑ

A preparation of ℞ **epinephrine.**
Formulation: Injection.
Availability: Prescription only.
Warnings and side effects: See ℞ **epinephrine.**

analeptic Ⓓ

see ℞ **respiratory stimulant.**

analgesic Ⓓ

(painkillers)
Generics: *Narcotic analgesics* (opioid): **alfentanil; buprenorphine hydrochloride; codeine phosphate; dextromethorphan; fentanyl; hydrocodone bitartrate; meperidine hydrochloride; methadone hydrochloride; morphine sulfate; nalbuphine hydrochloride; oxycodone; pentazocine; propoxyphene hydrochloride; remifentanil; tramadol hydrochloride.**
Generics: *Non-narcotic analgesics* (NSAIDs): **aspirin; celecoxib; choline salicylate; diclofenac; diflunisal; etodolac; fenoprofen; flurbiprofen; ibuprofen; indomethacin; ketoprofen; ketorolac tromethamine; magnesium salicylate; meclofenamate sodium; mefenamic acid; meloxicam; methyl salicylate; nabumetone; naproxen; oxaprozin; piroxicam; rofecoxib; salsalate; salicylic acid; sodium salicylate; sodium thiosalicylate; sulindac; tolmetin sodium; (acetaminophen).**

Generics: *Counter-irritants*: **camphor; capsaicin; menthol; methyl salicylate; turpentine oil.**

Actions and uses

Analgesic is a term used for drugs that relieve ✪ **pain**. These pain-killers can work in a number of ways, and the choice of analgesic depends on a number of factors. In this book the term analgesic is restricted to two main classes of drug.

First, the ℞ **narcotic analgesic** morphine-like drugs which have powerful actions on the central nervous system (CNS) and alter the perception of pain. Because of the numerous possible side effects, the most important of which is drug dependence (habituation or addiction), this class is usually used under strict medical supervision and preparations are normally available only on prescription. Narcotic analgesics are used for different types and severities of pain, but where there is severe pain (for example, after surgery, due to injury, or terminal cancer) there is little choice but to use this class. They all work by mimicking actions of the natural ℞ **opioid** neurotransmitters (enkephalins, endorphins, dynorphins) in the brain, and most members are chemically ℞ **opiate** drugs. They are discussed in more detail in the narcotic analgesic entry.

Second, the ℞ **non-narcotic analgesic** ℞ **aspirin**-like agents, which are drugs that have no tendency to produce dependence, but are by no means free of side effects (mainly gastrointestinal upsets). This class is referred to by many names, including weak analgesics (slightly misleading given their powerful actions in treating inflammatory pain) and, in medical circles, a very large number are referred to as non-steroidal, anti-inflammatory drugs, abbreviated to ℞ **NSAID**. These have valuable anti-inflammatory actions, and can be used for a variety of purposes, ranging from mild aches and pains (at lower dosages) due to ✪ **musculoskeletal disorders**), to the treatment of ✪ **rheumatoid arthritis** (at higher dosages). They work by inhibiting enzymes of cyclo-oxygenase system resulting in changes in the synthesis and metabolism of the natural ℞ **prostaglandin**, thromboxane and related inflammatory local hormones. An exception is ℞ **acetaminophen**, which does not have strong anti-inflammatory actions, but along with NSAIDs has ℞ **antipyretic** effects (the ability to lower raised body temperature when there is ✪ **fever**). All these drugs are discussed in more detail in the non-narcotic analgesic, NSAID, and individual drug entries.

Apart from these two main classes, there are other drugs that are sometimes referred to as analgesic because of their ability to relieve pain. Some agents (for example, ℞ **capsaicin**, ℞ **methyl salicylate**) are applied topically (externally) as local analgesics in the form of rubbing creams to treat muscle and joint aches and sprains (see ℞ **counter-irritant** and rubefacient). Many other drugs may relieve pain in specific disease states, but by convention are not generally referred to as analgesics. Examples include ℞ **antimigraine** drugs, such as sumatriptan, which work through a vasoconstrictor action on blood vessels (narrowing blood vessels) in the skull (see ✪ **migraine**), and also ℞ **carbamazepine** which relieves the pain of trigeminal ✪ **neuralgia** (but not other pain) by an action on nerve cells. Local anesthetics applied topically can dull the sensation of pain for example of ✪ **teething** or ✪ **hemorrhoids**. Also, an injection into an inflamed and painful joint (as for example in tendinitis) with ℞ **corticosteroids** can lead to dramatic pain relief.

Limitations

See the individual drug entries and drug groups.

Analpram-HC ⑧

A preparation of ℞ **hydrocortisone** and ℞ **pramoxine hydrochloride.**
Formulation: Cream in two strengths.
Availability: Prescription only.
Warnings and side effects: See ℞ **hydrocortisone;** ℞ **pramoxine hydrochloride.**

Anamine T.D. Capsules; Syrup ⑧

A preparation of ℞ **pseudoephedrine** and ℞ **chlorpheniramine maleate.**
Formulation: Oral capsules, sustained release; syrup.
Availability: Prescription only.
Warnings and side effects: See ℞ **pseudoephedrine;** ℞ **chlorpheniramine maleate.**

Anaplex HD Syrup ⑧

A preparation of ℞ **hydrocodone,** ℞ **pseudoephedrine,** and ℞ **brompheniramine maleate.**
Formulation: Oral syrup.
Availability: Prescription only.
Warnings and side effects: See ℞ **hydrocodone;** ℞ **pseudoephedrine;** ℞ **brompheniramine maleate.**

Anaplex Liquid ⑧

A preparation of ℞ **pseudoephedrine** and ℞ **chlorpheniramine maleate.**
Formulation: Oral liquid.
Availability: Prescription only.
Warnings and side effects: See ℞ **pseudoephedrine;** ℞ **chlorpheniramine maleate.**

Anaprox; Anaprox DS ⑧

A preparation of ℞ **naproxen.**
Formulation: Oral tablets.
Availability: Prescription only.
Warnings and side effects: See ℞ **naproxen.**

Anaspaz ⑧

A preparation of ℞ **hyoscyamine.**
Formulation: Oral tablets.
Availability: Prescription only.
Warnings and side effects: See ℞ **hyoscyamine.**

anastrozole Ⓖ

Type/Group: **anticancer; hormone antagonist.**
Brand(s): Armidex.
How administered: Orally.

Used to treat

Anastrozole is used to treat advanced breast cancer in postmeno-pausal women whose disease has progressed following ℞ **antiestrogen** (for example, tamoxifen) treatment. It is an aromatase inhibitor that works by inhibiting the conversion of androgens (male sex hormones) into estrogens.

Warnings

• It should not be used by people with known hypersensitivity to this drug or whose disease is not responsive to antiestrogen therapy.

• Anastrozole should not be used during pregnancy. A doctor must be contacted if pregnancy occurs while taking this drug.

• Medical judgment is required if breast-feeding is being considered.

• It may increase cholesterol levels.

• Infrequently, it may cause vaginal bleeding, mainly during the first few weeks of therapy.

Interactions

There are no reported interactions attributed to anastrozole.

Side effects

• Weakness, nausea, headache, hot flashes, pain of various kinds, shortness of breath, gastrointestinal effects, cough or sore throat, dizziness, rash, dry mouth, edema, depression, and sleepiness.

Anatuss DM Tablets; Syrup ⑧

A preparation of ℞ **dextromethorphan**, ℞ **pseudoephedrine**, and ℞ **guaifenesin**.

Formulation: Oral tablets; syrup.

Availability: OTC.

Warnings and side effects: See ℞ **dextromethorphan**; ℞ **pseudoephedrine**; ℞ **guaifenesin**.

Anatuss LA Tablets ⑧

A preparation of ℞ **pseudoephedrine** and ℞ **guaifenesin**.

Formulation: Oral tablets, long acting.

Availability: Prescription only.

Warnings and side effects: See ℞ **pseudoephedrine**; ℞ **guaifenesin**.

Anbesol ⑧

A preparation of ℞ **benzocaine** and ℞ **povidone-iodine**.

Formulation: Topical liquid.

Availability: OTC.

Warnings and side effects: See ℞ **benzocaine**; ℞ **iodine**; **povidone-iodine**.

Ancef ⑧

A preparation of ℞ **cefazolin sodium**.

Formulation: Injection in several strengths.

Availability: Prescription only.

Warnings and side effects: See ℞ **cefazolin sodium**.

Ancet Liquid ⑧

A preparation of ℞ **sodium lauryl sulfate**.

Formulation: Topical liquid.

Availability: OTC.

Warnings and side effects: See ℞ **sodium lauryl sulfate**.

Ancobon ⑧

A preparation of ℞ **flucytosine**.

Formulation: Oral capsules in two strengths.

Availability: Prescription only.

Warnings and side effects: See ℞ **flucytosine**.

Androderm ⑧

A preparation of ℞ **testosterone**.

Formulation: Transdermal patch in two strengths.

Availability: Prescription only.

Warnings and side effects: See ℞ **testosterone**.

androgen ⑩

(male sex hormone)

Generics: fluoxymesterone; methyltestosterone; testosterone.

Actions and uses

Androgens are a group of predominantly male (℞ **steroid**) ℞ **sex hormones**, which stimulate the development of male sex organs and male secondary sexual characteristics.

In men they are produced primarily by the testes. The main form is called ℞ **testosterone**. Androgens are, however, produced in both men and women by the adrenal glands, and in women small quantities are also secreted by the ovaries. An excessive amount in women causes masculinization.

Synthetic forms of the natural hormone and of a number of synthetic androgen analogs are used in medicine (such as ℞ **fluoxymesterone** and ℞ **methyltestosterone**) to correct hormonal deficiency, as replacement therapy in testicular failure to treat male hypogonadism (subnormal secretion of sex hormones), and delayed puberty in boys (see ⊙ **abnormal puberty**). In women they are used as therapy for advanced metastatic ⊙ **breast cancer**, and sometimes for postpartum (after childbirth) breast pain and engorgement, or for menopausal women as part of ℞ **hormone replacement** (see ⊙ **menopause**).

Testolactone is somewhat different in that as well as having androgen activity it inhibits the synthesis of the natural ℞ **estrogen** hormone estrone, effectively acting as an indirect ℞ **antiestrogen**, and so can be used to help reduce proliferation of hormone-dependent breast cancer. ℞ **stanozolol** is an androgen and ℞ **anabolic steroid** which can be used to treat hereditary ⊙ **angioedema** by assisting the metabolic synthesis of protein in the body. Drugs that inhibit the actions of androgens are called ℞ **antiandrogen** agents and are also used in medicine.

Limitations

These drugs have marked side effects and their dosage needs to be carefully controlled. In men, there may be impotence and testicular atrophy, and a wide range of other effects including mood changes. In women, there is frequently virilization (deepening voice, growth of body hair, acne, and so on). Prolonged use of high doses may cause serious liver disease, and, rarely, cancer in women. See the individual drug entries.

A number of androgens are Schedule III controlled substances (because of misuse, especially stanozolol, for the enhancement of athletic performance or physical appearance).

androgen antagonist Ⓓ

see ℞ **antiandrogen**.

Android Ⓑ

A preparation of ℞ **methyltestosterone**.
Formulation: Oral tablets in several strengths.
Availability: Prescription only.
Warnings and side effects: See ℞ **methyltestosterone**.

Andro L.A. Ⓑ

A preparation of ℞ **testosterone**.
Formulation: Injection.
Availability: Prescription only.
Warnings and side effects: See ℞ **testosterone**.

Andropository-200 Ⓑ

A preparation of ℞ **testosterone**.
Formulation: Injection.
Availability: Prescription only.
Warnings and side effects: See ℞ **testosterone**.

Anectine; Anectine Flo-Pack Ⓑ

A preparation of ℞ **succinylcholine chloride**.
Formulation: Injection (powder for infusion).
Availability: Prescription only.
Warnings and side effects: See ℞ **succinylcholine chloride**.

anemia treatment Ⓓ

Generics: cyanocobalamin; epoetin alfa; ferrous fumarate; ferrous gluconate; ferrous sulfate; folic acid; hydroxocobalamin.

Actions and uses

℞ **anemia treatment** involves the use of drugs to correct a deficiency of the oxygen-carrying capacity of red blood cells. The type of treatment used depends on the cause of the anemia. For example, the drugs given to treat iron-deficient Ⓞ **anemia** are mainly salts of iron and are used where there is deficiency of iron which is needed to synthesize hemoglobin, the oxygen carrying red blood cell pigment in blood and a similar oxygen-carrier in muscles. Dietary deficiency of iron in the diet, blood loss (for example, due to disorders of menstruation, such as menorrhagia, or childbirth), and diseases that reduce the proper absorption of other nutrients (for example, folic acid and vitamin B_{12} needed for red blood-cell production), can all lead to forms of anemia.

☄ **iron** supplements may be taken by mouth in one of several forms, as iron-rich salts such as ℞ **ferrous fumarate**, ℞ **ferrous gluconate** or ℞ **ferrous sulfate** (and others). There are also forms of iron—*parenteral iron*—for use by injection or intravenous infusion. Iron supplements are used where there is or is likely to be a deficiency of iron during pregnancy.

℞ **folic acid** is a vitamin of the B complex and is used to treat certain forms of anemia (specifically certain forms of megaloblastic anemia). Good food sources of folic acid include liver and vegetables, and its consumption is particularly necessary during the first few months of pregnancy. Folic acid supplements are recommended before and during pregnancy to help prevent neural tube defects such as spina bifida.

☄ **cyanocobalamin** and ℞ **hydroxocobalamin** (two forms of ☄ **vitamin B_{12}**) are used to treat vitamin B_{12} deficiency, pernicious anemia, and vitamin B_{12} malabsorption syndrome as well as to meet increased vitamin B_{12} requirements in pregnancy and certain diseases. Vitamin B_{12} is readily found in most normal, well-balanced diets (for example, in fish, eggs, liver, and red meat). Vegans, who eat no animal products at all, may eventually suffer from deficiency of this vitamin. A deficiency of vitamin B_{12} will cause megaloblastic anemia where large deformed red blood cells are produced, and this leads to degeneration of nerves in the central and peripheral nervous systems and abnormalities of epithelia (particularly the lining of the mouth and gut). Apart from poor diet, deficiency can also be caused by the lack of an intrinsic factor necessary for absorption in the stomach (pernicious anemia) and by various malabsorption syndromes in the gut (sometimes due to drugs). Hydroxocobalamin is preferred to cyanocobalamin for initial treatment, but either may be used in maintenance treatment. Cyanocobalamin is used to treat nutritional vitamin B_{12} deficiency. Different routes of administration (oral, injection, and so on) are used for different purposes.

The natural body growth factor erythropoietin (EPO) is now available in a form of human erythropoietin synthesized by recombinant (DNA technology) techniques as ℞ **epoetin alfa**. It is used as a ℞ **hematopoietic** drug when anemia is due to the kidneys' failure to stimulate red blood-cell production in the bone marrow (and after some forms of cancer chemotherapy).

Limitations

See the individual drug entries.

Anergan 50 Ⓑ

A preparation of ℞ **promethazine hydrochloride**.
Formulation: Injection, intramuscular only.
Availability: Prescription only.
Warnings and side effects: See ℞ **promethazine hydrochloride**.

Anestacon Ⓑ

A preparation of ℞ **lidocaine**.
Formulation: Topical jelly.
Availability: Prescription.
Warnings and side effects: See ℞ **lidocaine**.

anesthetic Ⓓ

(anaesthetic)

Actions and uses

Anesthetic drugs are used to reduce sensation, especially pain. There are two main types, ℞ **local anesthetic** drugs and ℞ **general anesthetic** drugs.

Limitations

See the ℞ **local anesthetic** and ℞ **general anesthetic** entries.

Anexsia Tablets ⓑ

A preparation of ℞ **hydrocodone bitartrate** and
℞ **acetaminophen**.
Formulation: Oral tablets, available in 3 strengths.
Availability: Prescription only.
Warnings and side effects: See ℞ **hydrocodone bitartrate**;
℞ **acetaminophen**.

angina treatment ⓓ

see ℞ **antianginal**.

angiotensin-converting enzyme inhibitor ⓓ

see ℞ **ACE inhibitor**.

angiotensin II receptor antagonist ⓓ

see ℞ **angiotensin-receptor blocker**.

angiotensin-receptor antagonist ⓓ

see ℞ **angiotensin-receptor blocker**.

angiotensin-receptor blocker ⓓ

(angiotensin-receptor antagonist; angiotensin II receptor
antagonist)
**Generics: candesartan cilexetil; eprosartan mesylate;
irbesartan; losartan potassium; telmisartan; valsartan**.

Actions and uses

Angiotensin-receptor blockers are recently introduced drugs that
work by blocking angiotensin receptors. Angiotensin II is a circulating ℞ **hormone** that is a powerful ℞ **vasoconstrictor** (narrows
blood vessels) and so blocking its effects leads to a fall in blood pressure. Drugs of this type can be used in the treatment of
❍ **hypertension** as ℞ **antihypertensive** agents, and their use in
the treatment of ❍ **heart failure** is under evaluation. Their general
actions and uses are similar to those of ℞ **ACE inhibitors**, but unlike
some earlier ACE inhibitors they do not cause a persistent dry
cough, and so are given to people who had to stop taking ACE
inhibitors because of this cough.

Limitations

Angiotensin-receptor blockers in general appear to cause few and
infrequent side effects (often indistinguishable from placebo
effects).

anisindione ⓖ

Type/Group: **anticoagulant**.
Brand(s): Miradon.
How administered: Orally.

Used to treat

Anisindione can be used to prevent the formation of clots in certain
heart disorders or after heart surgery (especially following implantation of prosthetic heart valves), and to treat or prevent venous
❍ **thrombosis** and ❍ **pulmonary embolism**, especially after a
heart attack. Although its action is very similar to the coumarins
(℞ **dicumarol**, ℞ **warfarin sodium**), anisindione belongs to a different chemical family and is generally used for people who cannot
tolerate coumarins.

Warnings

• It should not be given to people with known hypersensitivity to
this drug, with active bleeding, a tendency to bleed or blood-
forming disorders, pericarditis or bacterial endocarditis,
uncontrolled high blood pressure, injury or surgery that is still
healing, or recent surgery involving the eye or nervous system. It
will be administered by experts and only after a full medical
assessment.

• It should be given with caution to people with vascular disease
or congestive heart failure, indwelling catheters, gastrointestinal
infection, high blood pressure, severe diabetes mellitus, serious
vitamin C deficiency, polycythemia vera, recent traumatic injury,
or liver or kidney impairment.

• Anisindione is not used by women who are or may become
pregnant.

• Medical judgment is required if breast-feeding is being
considered.

• It should not be given to anyone who may not be able to cope
with self-administration (for example, who are senile, alcoholic,
psychotic, or uncooperative), nor should it be used where there are
no facilities for performing periodic blood testing.

• A doctor should be contacted immediately if any unusual
symptoms or bleeding occur, such as pain, swelling or discomfort,
prolonged bleeding from a cut, nosebleeds or bleeding gums from
brushing, increased menstrual flow, bruising, dark urine, red or tar
black stools, headache, dizziness, or weakness.

• A doctor must be notified of any illness.

• Activities that might cause traumatic injury (such as sports) should
be avoided.

• Diet should be normal and balanced. Significant changes in the
amount of vitamin K in the diet (as from eating large amounts of
green leafy vegetables) can alter the anticoagulant effect of
anisindione.

• Anisindione may free tiny bits of plaque that may lodge (usually)
in the smaller blood vessels, which may result in abrupt, sharp pain
in a leg, foot, the toes, back, or flank. ("Purple toes syndrome"
appears as mottled, purplish discoloration of the toes.) More
serious obstructions are possible, and may cause kidney
insufficiency, pancreatitis, penile gangrene, hypertension,
paralysis, or stroke. Use of anisindione should be stopped if any of
these occur.

Interactions

• The following drugs may increase the levels and effects of
anisindione, with an increased risk of bleeding: ℞ **acetaminophen**;
℞ **allopurinol**; ℞ **amiodarone hydrochloride**; ℞ **androgens**;
℞ **beta-blockers**; ℞ **chloral hydrate**; ℞ **chloramphenicol**;
℞ **chlorpropamide**; ℞ **cimetidine**; ℞ **clofibrate**;
℞ **corticosteroids**; ℞ **cyclophosphamide**; ℞ **disulfiram**;
℞ **erythromycin**; ℞ **fluconazole**; ℞ **gemfibrozil**; ℞ **glucagon**;
℞ **hydantoins**; ℞ **ifosfamide**; ℞ **influenza virus vaccine**;
℞ **isoniazid**; ℞ **ketoconazole**; loop ℞ **diuretics**; ℞ **lovastatin**;

℞ metronidazole; ℞ miconazole; ℞ moricizine; ℞ nalidixic acid; ℞ omeprazole; ℞ propafenone; ℞ propoxyphene; ℞ quinidine; ℞ quinine; ℞ quinolones; ℞ streptokinase; ℞ sulfinpyrazone; ℞ sulfonamides; ℞ tamoxifen; ℞ thyroid hormones; ℞ trimethoprim and sulfamethoxazole; and ℞ urokinase. Use of streptokinase or urokinase with anisindione may be hazardous.

• ℞ **Aminoglycosides**, ℞ **mineral oil**, ℞ **tetracyclines**, and ⚕ **vitamin E** interfere with vitamin K and may cause an increased risk of bleeding when taken with anisindione.

• ℞ **Cephalosporins**, ℞ **diflunisal**, ℞ **NSAID**s, ℞ **penicillins**, and ℞ **salicylates** may have various effects that make bleeding more likely when used with anisindione.

• The following drugs may reduce the levels and effects of anisindione: alcohol; ℞ **aminoglutethimide**; ℞ **barbiturates**; ℞ **carbamazepine**; ℞ **cholestyramine**; ℞ **oral contraceptives**; ℞ **dicloxacillin**; ℞ **estrogens**; etretinate; ℞ **glutethimide**; ℞ **griseofulvin**; ℞ **nafcillin**; ℞ **rifampin**; ℞ **spironolactone**; ℞ **sucralfate**; ℞ **thiazide** diuretics; ℞ **trazodone**; ⚕ **vitamin C** (at high doses); ⚕ **vitamin K.**

Side effects

• The chief complication is hemorrhage, which may occur at virtually any site in the body.

• Infrequently, dermatitis, headache, gastrointestinal disturbances, sore throat or blurred vision. Urine may be colored pink or orange. There may also be hypersensitivity reactions, including rashes and fever, blood disorders, and kidney or liver damage.

anisoylated plasminogen streptokinase activator complex ⓖ

see ℞ anistreplase.

anistreplase ⓖ

(anisoylated plasminogen streptokinase activator complex; APSAC)
Type/Group: **thrombolytic; fibrinolytic.**
Brand(s): Eminase.
How administered: Intravenous injection, infusion.

Used to treat

Anistreplase provides enzyme activity in a complex way, resulting in the breaking up blood clots. It is used in ✚ **myocardial infarction** (heart attack) to reduce the risk of heart failure and improve survival.

Warnings

• It should not be given to people with known hypersensitivity to this drug (or to ℞ **streptokinase**), or with active internal bleeding, uncontrolled high blood pressure, a history of stroke, or injury, surgery or bleeding involving the nervous system (brain or spine) within the previous two months. It will be given by experienced personnel after a full medical assessment.

• It should be given with caution to people with cerebrovascular disease, who have had recent major surgery, recent injury or internal bleeding (for example, in the gastrointestinal tract or urinary tract), bacterial endocarditis or acute pericarditis, high blood pressure, severe diabetes mellitus, significant liver or kidney impairment, or any condition (for example, taking anticoagulant

drugs, low platelet (thrombocyte) count or disorder that would make bleeding more likely.

• Anistreplase should be used during pregnancy only when it is clearly needed.

• Medical judgment is required if breast-feeding is being considered.

• Although reported rarely, thrombolytics may free bits of plaque that may lodge (usually) in the smaller blood vessels, which may result in abrupt, sharp pain in a leg, foot, the toes, back, or flank. ("Purple toes syndrome" appears as mottled, purplish discoloration of the toes.) More serious obstructions are possible, which may cause kidney failure, pancreatitis, hypertension, heart attack, stroke, and other serious obstructive events.

Interactions

• If taken with ℞ **anticoagulants**, there is an increased risk of bleeding (although despite some increased risk, ℞ **heparin** may have some benefit when given afterwards, as levels of anistreplase fall).

Side effects

• The chief complication is hemorrhage (although major bleeding is not frequent), which may occur at virtually any site in the body. Arrhythmias and hypotension occur commonly.

• Other side effects may include headache, shock, events associated with a new embolism, joint pain, dizziness, shortness of breath and fluid in the lungs. Allergic symptoms may occur, with symptoms such as fever and chills, hives, itching, flushing, allergic swelling, shortness of breath, or bronchospasm.

anorectal preparation ⓓ

(haemorrhoid/hemorrhoid preparation; rectoanal preparation)
Generics: **glycerin; lactulose; mineral oil; sodium tetradecyl sulphate.**

Actions and uses

Anorectal preparations are used to treat or lessen the symptoms of conditions affecting the anus or rectum. The most common complaint is probably ✚ **hemorrhoids** (piles), painfully distended, sometimes bleeding veins in the walls of the anus. The cause is often prolonged constipation. Treatment is generally through increasing levels of fiber in the diet to defeat constipation, sometimes with ℞ **laxative** drugs (for instance ℞ **mineral oil**, ℞ **glycerin**, and ℞ **lactulose**) to soften the feces and reduce discomfort. Severe or persistent hemorrhoids may be treated by procedures that include injections with ℞ **sclerosing agent** preparations (℞ **sodium tetradecyl sulphate**) which harden the tissue, infrared coagulation, or ligation (application of a ligature).

Other agents that help treat inflammation in the perianal area include such ℞ **anti-inflammatory** agents as the ℞ **corticosteroid** drugs (including ℞ **hydrocortisone**), ℞ **astringent** agents (℞ **aluminum acetate**), ℞ **emollient** agents (for instance ℞ **petrolatum**), and ℞ **vasoconstrictor** drugs (including ℞ **phenylephrine hydrochloride**, ℞ **ephedrine**), all in topical (external) or hemorrhoid preparations. Itching is helped by ℞ **local anesthetic** agents (including ℞ **lidocaine** and ℞ **dibucaine**) used topically. Certain ℞ **keratolytic** agents can be used to treat and dissolve warts of the external genital and perianal areas (for instance ℞ **podofilox** and ℞ **imiquimod**).

Limitations

See the individual drug entries.

anorectic Ⓓ

see ℞ **appetite suppressant**.

Ansaid Ⓑ

A preparation of ℞ **flurbiprofen**.
Formulation: Oral tablets, available in two strengths.
Availability: Prescription only.
Warnings and side effects: See ℞ **flurbiprofen**.

Antabuse Ⓑ

A preparation of ℞ **disulfiram**.
Formulation: Oral tablets.
Availability: Prescription only.
Warnings and side effects: See ℞ **disulfiram**.

antacid Ⓓ

Generics: alginic acid; aluminum hydroxide; calcium carbonate; magaldrate; magnesium carbonate; magnesium hydroxide; magnesium trisilicate; sodium bicarbonate; sucralfate;

Actions and uses

Antacid preparations are used to neutralize the hydrochloric acid (gastric acid) that the stomach produces as part of the normal digestion of food. Overproduction of acid (hyperacidity) can cause the symptoms of dyspepsia (✪ **indigestion**), which can be exacerbated by alcohol and ℞ **NSAID** drugs. Antacids give symptomatic relief of the dyspepsia and ✪ **gastritis** associated with ✪ **peptic ulcers** (gastric or duodenal ulcer), but do not allow actual healing of ulcers unless taken in sufficient quantities over long periods. A further painful condition is the regurgitation of acid and enzymes into the esophagus (✪ **gastroesophageal reflux**), which in the short term causes heartburn and in the long term can cause inflammation (reflux esophagitis: which is common in ✪ **hiatus hernia** and pregnancy).

Antacids used include salts of aluminum (℞ **sucralfate** and ℞ **aluminum hydroxide**), salts of magnesium (℞ **magnesium carbonate** and ℞ **magnesium trisilicate**), combinations of both (℞ **magaldrate**), other basic salts (℞ **calcium carbonate** and ℞ **sodium bicarbonate**), and other agents (for instance ℞ **alginic acid**, usually in the form of magnesium alginate or sodium alginate, which has ℞ **demulcent** actions and is used in preparations to protect against gastroesophageal reflux).

Limitations

Antacids do have side effects. Bicarbonates and carbonates tend to cause flatulence and belching, and some aluminum-containing antacids cause constipation, while magnesium-containing antacids can cause diarrhea (so are often used in combination to cancel out their effects). ℞ **Magaldrate** comprises a chemical mixture of basic salts of aluminum and magnesium (actually it is aluminum magnesium hydroxide sulfate), and this mixture of the two is considered sometimes to be an advantage. Some preparations contain high

concentrations of sodium, and so should not be used by anyone on a sodium-restricted diet. Some antacids last for a short period of time, especially ℞ **sodium bicarbonate**, but ℞ **magnesium trisilicate** has the advantage of a long duration of action.

Although antacids can effectively reduce acidity, they are commonly combined with other drugs (for example, ℞ **antifoaming agent**, ℞ **demulcent**, and ℞ **ulcer-healing drug** treatment.) See also the individual drug entries.

antazoline Ⓖ

Type/Group: antihistamine; antiallergic.
Brand(s): (In combination with ℞ **naphazoline**): Vasocon-A; various generic.
How administered: Topical (ophthalmic).

Used to treat

Antazoline is used for the relief of allergic symptoms such as allergic ✪ **conjunctivitis** in the eye.

Warnings

None significant.

Interactions

None significant.

Side effects

None significant.

anterior pituitary hormone Ⓓ

Generics: corticotropin; gonadotropin; somatropin; thyrotropin.

Actions and uses

Anterior pituitary hormones constitute one of the two classes of endocrine (blood-borne) hormones secreted by the pituitary gland, situated as a projection of the brain at the base of the skull. On release into the bloodstream, these hormones generally act on other glands (for example, thyroid glands, adrenal glands, sex glands) within the body to control release of further hormones that, in turn, act on organs and cells within the body. In this respect they differ from the other class, the ℞ **posterior pituitary hormones**, which are able to act directly. Chemically, both classes are peptides, that is, short sequences of amino acids arranged as in proteins.

Anterior pituitary hormones, which include adrenocorticotropic hormone (ACTH; in drug form it is called ℞ **corticotropin** or corticotrophin); growth hormone (GH, somatotropin or somatotrophin; the synthetic drug form is called ℞ **somatropin**); prolactin; thyroid-stimulating hormone (TSH, thyrotropin hormone; the drug form is ℞ **thyrotropin** or thyrotrophin); or the gonadotropins (gonadotropins, follicle-stimulating hormone (FSH), and luteinizing hormone (LH), which are also produced by the chorionic tissue of the placenta). The release of these hormones is controlled, in turn, by factors that travel, in a specialized system of portal blood vessels, the short distance from the hypothalamus (an adjacent brain area: see ℞ **hypothalamic hormone**).

Some of the anterior pituitary hormones, or their analogs, are used in medicine, sometimes as ℞ **diagnostic agents**. Growth hormone (somatotropin) is used in an identical but synthetic form called somatropin, to treat growth failure due to growth hormone deficiency and a number of related conditions. Thyrotropin can be used as a diagnostic agent to identify cases of thyroid failure. A number of ℞ **gonadotrophins** are used in various treatments.

Limitations

Since all the pituitary hormones are chemically peptides, they cannot be given by mouth because they would be digested in the same way as dietary protein, and instead have to be injected This limits their use (although this does not matter when they are used as diagnostic agents), however, it is possible to develop synthetic analogs that are more stable. The group most used are the gonadotropins which are glycoproteins and this means they are relatively stable (they are produced also by the chorionic tissue of the placenta).

anthelminthic ⓘ

see ℞ **anthelmintic.**

anthelmintic ⓘ

(anthelminthic; antihelminthic)

Generics: **albendazole; pyrantel; ivermectin; mebendazole; oxamniquine; piperazine; praziquantel; thiabendazole.**

Actions and uses

Anthelmintic drugs are used to treat infestation by parasitic organisms of the helminth (✪ **worm**) family, including roundworm, pinworm, whipworm, and hookworm. Various species cause a number of specific disorders (see ✪ **worms**), including ✪ **enterobiasis** (*Enterobius vermicularis*: common pinworm), strongyloidiasis (*Strongyloides*: roundworms), onchocerciasis (*Onchocerca volvulus*: nematode) and ✪ **schistosomiasis** (flukes of the genus *Schistosoma*). Particularly in warmer regions of the world, worms infest the intestines, and drugs can be given to kill the worms or anesthetize them so that they can then be excreted. Complications arise if the worms migrate within the body, in which case the treatment becomes very unpleasant.

A number of drugs are available and which one is used depends both on the species of worm involved, and whether a nematode has moved from the intestine to the tissues, but typically ℞ **mebendazole**, ℞ **thiabendazole**, ℞ **albendazole**, and ℞ **ivermectin** are used. Cestodes (tapeworms) are typically treated with ℞ **praziquantel** or ℞ **albendazole**. Trematodes (flukes) usually respond to ℞ **praziquantel.**

Limitations

Prevention is better than treatment. Personal and food hygiene is important, as is avoiding areas known to be infested (for instance, some flukes can penetrate a person's skin while he or she is swimming). Of all these drugs, ℞ **praziquantel** is particularly well tolerated when taken by mouth. Thiabendazole should be used during pregnancy only if the potential benefits outweigh the possible risks to the fetus.

Anthra-Derm ⓑ

A preparation of ℞ **anthralin.**
Formulation: Topical ointment in two strengths.
Availability: Prescription only.
Warnings and side effects: See ℞ **anthralin.**

anthralin ⓖ

(dithranol)
Type/Group: **psoriasis treatment.**
Brand(s): Anthra-Derm; Drithocreme; Micanol.
How administered: Topically (external).

Used to treat

Anthralin is the most powerful drug presently used to treat chronic or milder forms of ✪ **psoriasis** in topical application and is incorporated into a number of preparations. Lesions are covered for a period with a dressing on which there is a preparation of anthralin in weak solution. The concentration is adjusted to suit individual response and tolerance of the associated skin irritation. It is thought to work by inhibiting skin (epidermal) cell division (antimitotic) and may be used in combination with ℞ **keratolytics** or with agents that have a moisturizing effect (such as ℞ **urea**).

Warnings

• It should not be given to people with known hypersensitivity to anthralin or any component of the products.
• It is not known whether anthralin can harm the fetus, and so it should be used only during pregnancy if clearly needed.
• Although it is not known whether this drug appears in breast milk, because there is a potential for harm to the infant, use while nursing is not recommended.
• Contact with the eyes or sensitive areas of the skin must be avoided.
• It may stain fabrics, skin, fingernails, or hair. It must be applied sparingly and carefully.

Interactions

• Topical ℞ **corticosteroids** should not be used with anthralin.

Side effects

• Irritation of normal skin and allergic reaction.

antiallergic ⓘ

Generics: **acrivastine; antazoline; azatadine maleate; azelastine hydrochloride; brompheniramine maleate; cetirizine hydrochloride; chlorphenamine maleate; clemastine; cromolyn sodium; cyproheptadine hydrochloride; dexamethasone; diphenhydramine hydrochloride; fexofenadine hydrochloride; fluticasone propionate; hydrocortisone; hydroxyzine; ketotifen; loratadine; montelukast sodium; nedocromil sodium; pheniramine maleate; prednisolone; prednisone; promethazine hydrochloride; pyrilamine maleate; triamcinolone; triprolidine hydrochloride; zafirlukast; zileuton.**

Actions and uses

℞ **antiallergic** drugs relieve the symptoms of an allergic reaction that follows exposure to specific substances to which a person is allergic. These substances may be endogenous (in the person's body) or exogenous (present in the environment). Because allergic reactions generally cause the release of the natural local hormone histamine within the body, drugs of the ℞ **antihistamine** class (including ℞ **antazoline**, ℞ **emedastine**, and ℞ **ketotifen**) are often very effective for providing symptomatic relief. For example, allergic skin reactions to foreign proteins, contact dermatitis, and insect stings and bites, show characteristic symptoms—including pruritis (itching), urticaria (an itchy skin rash), and erythema (reddening of the skin)—and these often respond well to treatment with antihistamines (including local application in a cream).

However, because allergic responses cause an inflammatory effect, many antiallergic drugs are also ℞ **anti-inflammatory**. One major group used for both purposes are the ℞ **corticosteroid** agents (including ℞ **dexamethasone**, ℞ **fluticasone propionate**, ℞ **hydrocortisone**, ℞ **prednisolone**, ℞ **prednisone**, ℞ **triamcinolone**) and drugs of this group are used for a wide variety of purposes. They can be used for the treatment of rheumatic disorders such as ✪ **arthritis** and ✪ **osteoarthritis**, allergic states, collagen diseases, liver disorders, allergic and inflammatory disorders of the intestinal tract, liver and kidney disorders, and respiratory diseases (such as bronchial ✪ **asthma**). They are particularly used for inflammation associated with skin conditions, such as ✪ **eczema** and ✪ **psoriasis**, and of the eyes, ears or nose.

A further class of drugs, sometimes called *mast-cell stabilizers*, also give anti-inflammatory protection from the symptoms of allergic asthma, and allergic symptoms in the eye (for example, allergic ✪ **conjunctivitis**), nose (for example, environmental allergy symptoms including ✪ **hay fever**), intestine (for example, food allergy), and elsewhere. This may be achieved by topical (external) application, oral administration, or inhalation (as appropriate) of ℞ **cromolyn sodium** and ℞ **nedocromil sodium**. These drugs are thought to work by preventing the release of histamine and other substances (from mast-cell stores).

Two new classes of anti-inflammatory drugs that can be used to treat the symptoms of allergic reactions work by preventing the release of inflammatory mediators called leukotrienes, which are increasingly thought to be important, especially in the lungs. ℞ **lipoxygenase inhibitor** drugs (also called *5-lipoxygenase inhibitor* agents) work by blocking enzymes involved in the production of leukotrienes, and the first such drug in use, ℞ **zileuton**, is used by mouth in the chronic treatment and prevention of asthma. Drugs of the ℞ **leukotriene receptor antagonist** class (including ℞ **montelukast sodium** and ℞ **zafirlukast**), are used to prevent the actions of leukotrienes at their receptors, and can be used as an add-on therapy for individuals not adequately controlled by inhaled corticosteroids and short-acting ℞ **beta-adrenergic stimulant** drugs to prevent mild to moderate asthma attacks (including, along with other drugs, exercise-induced bronchospasm), but not to treat acute attacks.

Limitations
In general, the corticosteroids will suppress or mask inflammatory responses at most sites (including the skin), but these drugs have quite marked and serious side effects, and are only taken by mouth in serious conditions and are normally used topically (externally) only for short-term relief of symptoms.

antiamebicidal ⓓ
see ℞ amebicide and antiprotozoal.

antiandrogen ⓓ
Generics: **bicalutamide; flutamide; nilutamide; gonadorelin; nafarelin acetate; leuprolide acetate.**

Actions and uses
Antiandrogen (androgen antagonist) agents are a class of drugs with ℞ **hormone antagonist** activity, which act directly or indirectly to reduce the effect of the male sex hormone testosterone on its target tissues. They can do this in a number of ways.

First, some drugs act directly by blocking androgen receptors (for example, ℞ **bicalutamide**, ℞ **flutamide** and ℞ **nilutamide**) and may combine this with blocking testosterone uptake into the cell (for example, flutamide).

Second, a group of hormone antagonist drugs also sometimes referred to as antiestrogen, work more indirectly. For instance, the ℞ **hypothalamic hormone** called gonadotropin-releasing hormone (LH-RH), used in its synthetic drug form, ℞ **gonadorelin**, or as synthetic chemical analogs (for example, ℞ **goserelin**, ℞ **nafarelin acetate**, and ℞ **leuprolide acetate**) is used therapeutically, in the treatment of ✪ **cancer** and sex hormone disorders. They work by suppressing the formation or inhibiting the release of sex hormones including both estrogens and androgens, but they do this via their initial action on the anterior pituitary gland, which in turn affects the sex glands that release these sex hormones.

Limitations
Drugs that are used to modify hormone actions or release tend to have widespread side effects, and these are generally regarded as acceptable unless the condition being treated warrants otherwise. The majority of these drugs are used for modifying sex hormones activity in the body when it is involved in a number of serious disorders that require intervention. Some of these are disorders of sexual development including precocious puberty (see ✪ **abnormal puberty**); but probably most are used in ℞ **anticancer** therapy in men to help treat hormone-dependent tumors of the prostate (see ✪ **prostate cancer**).

Future development toward developing more acceptable hormone antagonists may be expected to feature receptors antagonists, since such drugs generally are relatively specific in their actions and effects.

antianginal ⓓ
Generics: **sodium nitroprusside; nitroglycerin; isosorbide dinitrate; isosorbide mononitrate; atenolol; metoprolol tartrate; nadolol; propranolol hydrochloride; amlodipine besylate; nicardipine hydrochloride; diltiazem hydrochloride; nicardipine hydrochloride; nifedipine; verapamil hydrochloride; bepridil hydrochloride.**

Actions and uses
Antianginal drugs are used to relieve the pain of ✪ **angina pectoris**, which is an intense pain originating from the heart and is due to ischemia (insufficient blood supply to the heart muscle). It occurs particularly when the heart is working hard as in "exercise angina," although in "unstable angina" it can even occur when the person is resting. The disorder often results from atheroma, which is a disease state of the lining of the arteries of the heart where there is a build up of fatty deposits. The objective of drug treatment is to reduce the heart's workload and to prevent spasm or to dilate the arteries of the heart (the coronary arteries).

Commonly, direct-acting ℞ **vasodilator** (widen blood vessels) drugs are used, such as the ℞ **nitrate** agents (including ℞ **nitroglycerin**, ℞ **isosorbide dinitrate**, ℞ **isosorbide mononitrate**). The ℞ **beta-blocker** group of drugs prevent the normal increase in heart rate seen in exercise by blocking the effect of epinephrine and norepinephrine on the heart, and are very effective in preventing anginal pain. Examples of beta-blockers used include ℞ **atenolol**, ℞ **metoprolol tartrate**, ℞ **nadolol** and ℞ **propranolol hydrochloride**. More recently, ℞ **calcium-channel blocker** drugs (for example, ℞ **amlodipine besylate**, ℞ **nicardipine hydrochloride**, ℞ **diltiazem hydrochloride**, ℞ **nicardipine hydrochloride**, ℞ **nifedipine**, ℞ **verapamil hydrochloride**, and ℞ **bepridil hydrochloride**) have become more widely used in the treatment of angina to prevent attacks (as well as being ℞ **antihypertensive**).

Limitations

The various drugs discussed here have direct or indirect vasodilator properties and may act on the coronary arteries, peripheral small arteries, and other blood vessels, and this helps to reduce the workload on the heart. If drug treatment is not sufficient, then a coronary bypass operation may be needed.

Given that the general cause of angina is atheroma, drugs to help this are now regarded as supportive therapy. Therefore, treatment with a ℞ **lipid-regulating drug** may be of benefit, along with ℞ **antiplatelet** (and sometimes ℞ **anticoagulant**) drugs to prevent thrombus formation, which would pose a risk of myocardial infarction (heart attack) and stroke.

antianxiety ⓓ
(anxiolytic)

Generics: **atenolol; buspirone; chlordiazepoxide; clonazepam; diazepam; estazolam; halazepam; hydroxyzine; lorazepam; meprobamate; oxazepam; propranolol hydrochloride; nadolol.**

Actions and uses

Antianxiety drugs are used to relieve medically diagnosed ⊕ **anxiety** states. Drugs of this class are sometimes, somewhat misleadingly, referred to as minor tranquilizers. They are often used as an additional, supportive treatment to psychotherapy. Antianxiety drugs are prescribed in the short-term treatment of anxiety disorders, preoperative apprehension, and sometimes for tremors, tension headache, and panic disorders, also, in conjunction with other drugs, in the treatment of acute alcohol withdrawal symptoms. Treatment is at the lowest dose effective and is not to be prolonged, because psychological dependence and physical dependence (addiction) readily occurs and may make withdrawal difficult. The best-known and most-used is the ℞ **benzodiazepine** group, for example, ℞ **alprazolam**, ℞ **chlordiazepoxide**, ℞ **clonazepam**, ℞ **diazepam**, ℞ **estazolam**, ℞ **halazepam**, ℞ **lorazepam**, and ℞ **oxazepam**. Other drugs such as ℞ **meprobamate** and some of the ℞ **antipsychotic** drugs (at low doses), and some drugs from the ℞ **antihistamine** group (including ℞ **hydroxyzine**) may also be used. The novel drug ℞ **buspirone**, which is not chemically related to other antianxiety drugs, is thought to work as a ℞ **serotonin-receptor stimulant** in the brain (probably acting at the 5-HT$_{1A}$-receptor subtype). Additionally, ℞ **beta-blocker** drugs (for example, ℞ **atenolol** and ℞ **propranolol hydrochloride**) are sometimes used to treat anxiety by preventing the physical symptoms such as palpitations of the heart, sweating and tremor, which helps the patient to stop the chain reaction of worry to fear to panic. Some people in the performing arts use these drugs to control stagefright (performance anxiety). Some of these drugs take time to work and careful adjustment of the dose will probably be necessary.

Limitations

See individual drug entries.

antiarrhythmic ⓓ
(antidysrhythmic)

Generics: **acebutolol; amiodarone hydrochloride; bretylium tosylate; digitoxin; digoxin; diltiazem hydrochloride; disopyramide; esmolol hydrochloride; flecainide acetate; mexiletine hydrochloride; moricizine hydrochloride; procainamide hydrochloride; propafenone hydrochloride; propranolol hydrochloride; quinidine; sotalol hydrochloride; tocainide hydrochloride; verapamil hydrochloride.**

Actions and uses

Antiarrhythmic drugs strengthen and regularize a heartbeat that has become unsteady and is not showing its usual pattern of activity. But because there are many ways in which the heartbeat can falter—atrial tachycardia, supraventricular arrhythmias, ventricular arrhythmias, ventricular tachycardia, atrial flutter or fibrillation (see ⊕ **arrhythmia**), and the severe heartbeat irregularity that may follow a heart attack (⊕ **myocardial infarction**)—there is a variety of drugs available, each for a fairly specific use. The treatment of arrhythmias requires careful diagnosis as to the type of arrhythmia, including an electrocardiogram (ECG), which helps determine which type of drug is likely to benefit the particular complaint. Drugs are put into various groups according to their type of use in treating particular types of antiarrhythmic, including in resuscitation. Group I drugs include ℞ **quinidine**, ℞ **procainamide**, ℞ **lidocaine**, and ℞ **phenytoin**; Group II drugs include ℞ **propranolol hydrochloride**, ℞ **esmolol hydrochloride**, ℞ **acebutolol**, and ℞ **acebutolol**; Group III includes ℞ **bretylium tosylate**, ℞ **amiodarone hydrochloride**, and ℞ **sotalol hydrochloride**; and Group IV includes ℞ **verapamil hydrochloride**, ℞ **digoxin**, and ℞ **digitoxin**.

Some of these drugs have other actions, additional to their antiarrhythmic properties. The ℞ **cardiac glycoside** agents (℞ **digoxin** and ℞ **digitoxin**) are also used for their ℞ **cardiac stimulant** properties. Others are also ℞ **beta-blocker** drugs (including ℞ **acebutolol**, ℞ **esmolol hydrochloride**, ℞ **propranolol hydrochloride**, ℞ **sotalol hydrochloride**), ℞ **calcium-channel blocker** drugs (℞ **diltiazem hydrochloride**, ℞ **verapamil**), ℞ **local anesthetic**-related (℞ **lidocaine**, ℞ **tocainide hydrochloride**, and ℞ **procainamide hydrochloride**). A number of other specialist drugs are used in special circumstances, but are not detailed here.

Limitations

These drugs are prescribed and used by specialists, and treatment is often begun in a hospital. See also the individual drug entries.

antiasthmatic Ⓓ

Generics: **albuterol; bitolterol mesylate; beclomethasone dipropionate; budesonide; cromolyn sodium; ipratropium bromide; isoetharine; levalbuterol hydrochloride; montelukast sodium; nedocromil sodium; pirbuterol; triamcinolone; salmeterol; terbutaline sulfate; theophylline; zafirlukast; zileuton.**

Actions and uses

Antiasthmatic drugs relieve the symptoms of bronchial ✪ **asthma** or prevent recurrent attacks. The symptoms of asthma include bronchoconstriction (a narrowing of the bronchioles of the airways in the lungs, which makes it difficult to exhale), often with over-secretion of fluid by glands within the bronchioles, with coughing, wheezing, and breathing difficulties (dyspnoea). Two main types of drugs are used to treat this condition: one group treats acute attacks; the other prevents attacks (prophylaxis).

℞ **bronchodilator** drugs are in the first group and they are ℞ **smooth muscle relaxant** agents, which work by dilating and relaxing the muscle of the bronchioles. The most commonly used bronchodilators are the ℞ **beta-adrenergic stimulant** class (which are ℞ **sympathomimetic** drugs). They act by stimulating beta-adrenergic receptors located on the smooth muscle of the airways. Importantly, differences in receptors at different sites allows selectivity of action, and this selectivity means safer drugs. Therefore the beta$_2$-receptor stimulants used in asthma (inhaled from an aerosol) do not significantly stimulate the beta$_1$-receptors of the heart (which would cause speeding of the heart and other symptoms). Examples of beta$_2$-stimulant drugs that are used to cause bronchodilation are ℞ **albuterol**, ℞ **levalbuterol** (another chemical form of albuterol), ℞ **terbutaline**, ℞ **bitolterol**, ℞ **isoetharine**, and ℞ **pirbuterol**. ℞ **salmeterol** is different in that it too has beta$_2$-receptor selectivity—and is generally similar to albuterol—but its effects last for much longer. Therefore it may be used to prevent asthma attacks throughout the night after inhalation before going to bed. The beta-adrenergic stimulants, normally inhaled, are mostly used for treating acute attacks (or immediately before exertion in exercise asthma).

Other bronchodilator drugs that work directly on the bronchioles, and may be used both to treat and prevent attacks, include the ℞ **xanthine** compounds (℞ **theophylline** and its derivatives aminophylline, dyphylline, and oxtriphylline), and these are used for the treatment of asthma, and chronic ✪ **bronchitis** and ✪ **emphysema** (as in COPD, ✪ **chronic obstructive pulmonary disease**). They are not inhaled but are taken by mouth, rectal suppository, or injection in emergencies.

The second group of antiasthmatic drugs do not directly cause bronchodilation, but because of their ℞ **anti-inflammatory** action, they prevent the release of local inflammatory mediators, which contribute to attacks, and so prevent asthma attacks and provide symptomatic relief. Of these anti-inflammatory prophylactic (preventive) drugs, the ℞ **corticosteroid** group (including ℞ **beclomethasone dipropionate**, ℞ **budesonide**, and sometimes ℞ **triamcinolone**) is extensively used by inhalation at low doses to reduce the incidence of attacks. Other anti-inflammatory drugs include the mast-cell stabilizers (℞ **cromolyn sodium** and ℞ **nedocromil sodium**), ℞ **leukotriene receptor antagonists** (including ℞ **montelukast** and ℞ **zafirlukast**), and the ℞ **lipoxygenase inhibitor** agents (℞ **zileuton**), which are all taken by mouth to prevent attacks.

There are a number of other drugs that act on the airways which are occasionally used. ℞ **ipratropium bromide**, for example, is an ℞ **anticholinergic** drug with bronchodilator properties which is mainly used (by inhalation) for maintenance treatment of bronchospasm in chronic obstructive pulmonary disease (COPD), including bronchitis and emphysema. It may sometimes also be used to prevent exercise-induced asthma.

Limitations

These drugs are inhaled where possible in order to deliver the drug more precisely to where it is required and this preciseness helps to limit side effects. A great deal of research has been carried out to design devices that are able to more efficiently deliver the inhaled droplets, or particles, of bronchodilator or anti-inflammatory drugs into the airways, particularly in an attempt to reach the narrower bronchioles. See also the individual drug entries.

antibacterial Ⓓ

Actions and uses

Antibacterials are drugs used to treat ✪ **bacterial infections** caused by bacteria on which they have a selective toxic action.

Most of these agents are ℞ **antibiotic** in origin, but some useful antibacterial drugs are entirely synthetic in origin, including ℞ **quinolone**, ℞ **sulfonamide** and ℞ **sulfone** agents.

Antibacterial drugs can be used both topically (for example, on the skin or the eye) to treat infections of superficial tissues or systemically (carried by the blood to the site of infection after being swallowed or injected). A distinction can be made between bacteriostatic drugs, which act primarily by arresting bacterial growth (for example, ℞ **tetracycline**, ℞ **sulphonamide** and chloramphenicol-like drugs) and the *bactericidal* agents, which act primarily by killing bacteria (for example, ℞ **aminoglycoside**, ℞ **cephalosporin** and ℞ **penicillin** classes; also ℞ **isoniazid** and ℞ **rifampicin**). As bacteria are the largest and most diverse group of pathogenic (disease-causing) microorganisms, antibacterials form the major constituent group of ℞ **antimicrobial** drugs. The modes of action of the antibiotics are discussed in that entry.

Limitations

See individual class entries.

AntibiOtic Ⓑ

A preparation of ℞ **hydrocortisone**, ℞ **neomycin**, and ℞ **polymyxin B sulfate**.
Formulation: Ear drops.
Availability: Prescription only.
Warnings and side effects: See ℞ **hydrocortisone**; ℞ **neomycin**; ℞ **polymyxin B sulfate**.

antibiotic Ⓓ

Actions and uses

Antibiotics are, strictly speaking, natural products secreted by microorganisms into their environment where they inhibit the growth of competing microorganisms of different types. But in common usage the term is often applied to any drug, natural or synthetic, that has a selectively toxic action on bacteria or similar non-nucleated, single-celled microorganisms (including chlamydia, rickettsia, and mycoplasma), that is, they are ℞ **antibacterial** (see ✪ **bacterial infections**). None are effective against viruses (see ℞ **antiviral**), but some are effective against some of the pathogenic (disease-causing) molds and yeasts (see ℞ **antifungal** agents; ✪ **fungal infections**). So the more accurate and specific term—antibacterial, antifungal, and so forth—is to be preferred.

In fact, most modern antibiotics are either completely synthetic or semi-synthetic (manufactured by a, sometimes elaborate, chemical alteration of a natural substance), but many are generally modeled on natural antibiotic substances. Some modern agents, for instance the ℞ **quinolone** antibacterials, are often referred to as antibiotics even though they are entirely synthetic and not based on natural molecules.

Apart from these considerations, many families of antibiotic molecules are not used for any antimicrobial actions that they may have, but instead are used for their toxic actions on cancer cells, that is, they are used as ℞ **cytotoxic** agents in ℞ **anticancer** chemotherapy, or as ℞ **immunosuppressant** drugs. Others again, because of their great chemical complexity, are used as starting points for the semi-synthetic development of drugs with a wide spectrum of actions—a trend that is developing.

There are important differences between the various antibacterial antibiotic families and these dictate their use in medicine. When administered by an appropriate route, such as topically (to the skin or eyes, for example), by mouth, by injection, or by infusion, antibiotics kill microorganisms such as bacteria—bactericidal action—or inhibit their growth—bacteriostatic action. Their selectively toxic action on an invading microorganisms exploits differences between bacteria and their human host cells. Major target sites are the bacterial cell wall located outside the cell membrane (animal cells have only a cell membrane) or the bacterial ribosome (the protein-synthesizing organelle within its cell), which in microorganisms is different from human cells. Antibiotic families such as the ℞ **penicillin** and ℞ **cephalosporin** groups (collectively known as ℞ **beta-lactam** antibiotics) attack the bacterial cell wall, whereas antibiotics of the ℞ **aminoglycoside** and ℞ **tetracycline** groups attack the bacterial ribosomes within the cell. However, viruses, because they lack both cell walls and ribosomes, are resistant to these and other types of antibiotic.

See also ℞ **polymyxin**.

Limitations

Unfortunately, because of the widespread use of antibiotics, certain strains of common bacteria have developed resistance to antibiotics that were once effective against them, and this has become a major problem. A mechanism by which bacteria become resistant is by the development of enzymes called penicillinases, which break down penicillins and so limit an antibiotic's action. It has proved possible both to use drugs that inhibit these enzymes and, more directly, to develop penicillinase-resistant antibiotics.

Another problem is the occurrence of ✪ **superinfections**, in which the use of a broad-spectrum antibiotic disturbs the normal, harm-less bacterial population in the body, as well as the pathogenic ones. In mild cases this may allow, for example, an existing but latent oral or vaginal thrush infection to become worse, or mild diarrhea to develop. In rare cases the superinfection that develops is more serious than the disorder for which the antibiotic was administered (for example, ✪ **pseudomembranous colitis**).

anticancer ⓪

Generics: **interferons; tamoxifen; cisplatin; carboplatin; cytotoxic**.

Actions and uses

Anticancer drugs are used to treat ✪ **cancer** and most of them are ℞ **cytotoxic** drugs. Cytotoxics work by interfering with cell replication or production, so preventing the growth of new cancerous tissue. Inevitably, this means that normal cell production is also affected, which causes serious side effects. They are usually given in combination in a group of treatments known collectively as chemotherapy, sometimes in combination with radiotherapy and/or surgery.

However, cytotoxic drugs are not always necessary in some types of cancer, for example, where the growth of a tumor is dependent on sex hormone levels (as with some cases of ✪ **breast cancer** or ✪ **prostate cancer**), and here treatment with a ℞ **sex hormone** opposite to the patient's own sex, or ℞ **hormone** antagonist drugs (for example, ℞ **tamoxifen** at estrogen receptors), can be extremely beneficial (although, again, the side effects of some may be quite severe). Other drugs used directly or indirectly as additional, supportive (adjunctive) treatments include ℞ **corticosteroid** drugs and other ℞ **immunosuppressant** agents and also ℞ **immunomodulator** agents such as the ℞ **interferons** (for example, interferon alfa-2a, interferon alfa-2b, and interferon alfacon-1).

Recently, there have been significant advances in drug adjunctive therapy which is used to reduce side effects of chemotherapy and radiotherapy. In particular, the recently introduced ℞ **antiemetic/** ℞ **antinauseant** drugs, such as ℞ **ondansetron**, have revolutionized anticancer treatment that involves the platinum-containing group of drugs (℞ **carboplatin** and ℞ **cisplatin**), which are particularly prone to cause nausea and vomiting. Inevitably, as mentioned, many anticancer drugs—particularly cytotoxic drugs—cause extensive side effects. During chemotherapy, which will be carried out by specialists, there will be extensive monitoring of blood counts and, depending on the type of anticancer drug, other body systems and vital signs.

Increasingly, genetic knowledge obtained using the new techniques of molecular biology is highlighting factors in people which predispose them to certain types of cancers. In the case of familiar breast cancer, the use of tamoxifen as a preventive agent in those at risk is being explored.

Limitations

See the individual drug entries.

anticholinergic ⓪

(antimuscarinic)

Generics: **atropine sulfate; benztropine mesylate; biperiden; cyclopentolate hydrochloride; dicyclomine hydrochloride; flavoxate hydrochloride; glycopyrrolate; homatropine hydrobromide; hyoscyamine; ipratropium bromide; oxybutynin; procyclidine; propantheline bromide; scopolamine hydrobromide; tolterodine tartrate; trihexyphenidyl; trimethobenzamide hydrochloride; tropicamide.**

Actions and uses

Anticholinergic drugs inhibit the action, release, or production of the neurotransmitter acetylcholine, which plays an important role in the nervous system. The term is commonly used instead of the more precise term antimuscarinic (drugs that block the actions of acetylcholine at muscarinic receptors). Anticholinergic drugs (of the antimuscarinic type) tend to relax smooth (involuntary) muscle, reduce the secretion of saliva, digestive juices and sweat, and dilate the pupil of the eye (mydriasis). They can therefore be used as ℞ **antispasmodic** drugs in the treatment of intestinal ✪ **colic** for urinary frequency (for instance ℞ **oxybutynin**, ℞ **propantheline bromide**, ℞ **tolterodine tartrate**; see ✪ **urinary tract disorders**), in ℞ **antiparkinsonism** therapy for symptomatic relief of symptoms (see ✪ **Parkinson's disease**), as an additional treatment with an ℞ **ulcer-healing drug** for ✪ **peptic ulcer**, as ℞ **antinauseant** or ℞ **antiemetic** drugs in the treatment of ✪ **motion sickness** (℞ **scopolamine hydrobromide**), and as ℞ **mydriatic** drugs to dilate the pupil for ophthalmic examinations (for instance ℞ **cyclopentolate hydrochloride**, ℞ **homatropine hydrobromide**, ℞ **tropicamide**, and sometimes ℞ **atropine sulfate**). Other uses include as ℞ **antidote** agents to reverse the adverse effects of overdose with ℞ **anticholinesterase** agents (agricultural accidental ✪ **poisoning** or warfare) and in routine use in medicine (for instance ℞ **glycopyrrolate**).

The original members of this group were ℞ **belladonna alkaloid** drugs (℞ **atropine sulfate**, ℞ **hyoscyamine**, ℞ **scopolamine hydrobromide**), but later members are synthetic chemical analogs or new structures.

The other main groups of anticholinergic drugs work at sites where acetylcholine interacts with nicotinic receptors (such as in the autonomic ganglia, skeletal neuromuscular junction, and central nervous system) and have quite different actions. See ℞ **ganglion-blocker** and ℞ **skeletal muscle relaxant** drugs.

Limitations

The systemic use of these drugs is usually accompanied by side effects that include: dry mouth, dry skin, blurred vision, increased heart rate, constipation, and difficulty in urinating. A number of other types of drug, for instance, most members of the ℞ **antihistamine** group, can also cause anticholinergic side effects.

anticholinesterase Ⓓ

(cholinesterase inhibitor)

Generics: **ambenonium chloride; donepezil; edrophonium chloride; neostigmine methylsulfate; pyridostigmine bromide; rivastigmine; tacrine hydrochloride.**

Actions and uses

Anticholinesterase drugs are enzyme inhibitors that act on certain enzymes (called cholinesterases) which are normally involved in the rapid break down of the natural neurotransmitter acetylcholine, and so anticholinesterases stop it being broken down. Acetylcholine is released from cholinergic nerves and has many actions in the body. Consequently, since anticholinesterase drugs enhance the effects of acetylcholine following its release from these nerves, they may have a very wide range of actions and can be used for a variety of purposes. But this comes with the disadvantage of a variety of side effects.

Because of their actions at the junction of nerves with skeletal (voluntary) muscles, anticholinesterases (for example, ℞ **edrophonium chloride**, ℞ **pyridostigmine bromide**, ℞ **ambenonium chloride**) are used in the diagnosis and treatment of the muscle-weakness disease ✪ **myasthenia gravis**. At the end of surgical operations in which certain ℞ **skeletal muscle relaxants** have been used, the anaesthetist is able to reverse the muscle paralysis by injecting an anticholinesterase (for example, ℞ **neostigmine methylsulfate**, ℞ **pyridostigmine bromide**). In organs supplied by parasympathetic division of the autonomic nervous system, anticholinesterases cause an exaggeration of the nerves' actions (known as ℞ **parasympathomimetic** actions) and they can be used for a number of purposes, such as stimulation of the bladder in urinary retention (for example, ℞ **neostigmine methylsulfate**: see ✪ **urinary tract disorders**).

Recently, some anticholinesterases (for example, ℞ **donepezil**, ℞ **rivastigmine**, ℞ **tacrine hydrochloride**) have been introduced for the treatment of impaired mental cognition in ✪ **Alzheimer's disease** (see ℞ **dementia treatment**).

Limitations

Because cholinesterase enzymes are very widely distributed (including within the brain), anticholinesterases have widespread and generally undesirable side effects, such as slowing of the heart, constriction of the airways with excessive production of secretions, and actions on the brain.

In anticholinesterase poisoning, their diverse actions can be life-threatening. Chemicals with anticholinesterase properties are used as insecticides (and in chemical warfare), so the use of ℞ **antidotes** may be required (for example, ℞ **pralidoxime chloride** with ℞ **atropine sulphate**) if there is poisoning or overdose.

anticoagulant Ⓓ

(antithrombotic)

Generics: **anisindione; antithrombin III human; ardeparin sodium; dalteparin sodium; dicumarol; enoxaparin sodium; heparin; lepirudin; warfarin sodium.**

Actions and uses

Anticoagulants help prevent the formation of blood clots. Blood clots—called thrombi when formed in blood vessels—are formed by the action of a natural blood element called thrombin, which acts as an enzyme in forming the fibrin web-like elements in the thrombus. Anticoagulants prevent this process and so are sometimes called antithrombotic drugs. A second essential element of the thrombus is the platelets (thrombocytes). These become entangled in the fibrin web, so allowing the thrombus to plug vessels and stop hemorrhage. This second process is prevented by ℞ **antiplatelet** agents (such as ℞ **aspirin**), so occasionally anticoagulant and antiplatelet agents are prescribed together when there is a particular risk of thrombus formation. In general, anticoagulants prevent thrombi forming or enlarging within veins or within the heart, whereas antiplatelet agents work better to prevent thrombi forming in arteries. A third class of drugs, ℞ **fibrinolytic** agents, can be used to dissolve thrombi once they have formed. Neither anticoagulant nor antiplatelet drugs dissolve thrombi, although they may help prevent the extension of blood clots that have already formed.

Anticoagulants are used for a number of purposes, including the prevention or treatment of venous ✪ **thrombosis** (especially deep-vein thrombosis after surgery), prevention of clotting in arterial or cardiac surgery (for example, following implantation of prosthetic heart valves), and prevention of ✪ **embolism** (including that which may be associated with atrial fibrillation). They also reduce the risk of ischemic complications in certain acute heart conditions, and are used in blood transfusions, dialysis, and blood samples.

Anticoagulants fall into two groups, those that must be injected or infused, and those that can be taken by mouth—these differences in part influence their uses.

The blood's own natural anticoagulant is ℞ **heparin**. It is produced by the liver, leukocytes (white blood cells), and in some other sites, including mast cells. It inhibits the action of the enzyme thrombin, which is needed for the final stages of blood coagulation. In medicine, it is purified after extraction from bovine lungs and porcine intestinal mucosa. It is probably still the most effective anticoagulant known, but must be injected and so is termed a parenteral anticoagulant. There are semisynthetic versions of heparin, called low molecular weight heparins (℞ **ardeparin sodium**, ℞ **dalteparin sodium**, ℞ **enoxaparin sodium**), and these have similar uses to heparin but have a longer duration of action.

℞ **lepirudin** is another parenteral anticoagulant, a synthetic (recombinant, DNA technology process) version of natural hirudin from the salivary glands of the medicinal leech. It can be used for anticoagulation where antithrombotic treatment is needed, but where the individual concerned has an adverse reaction to heparin (for instance, in thrombocytopenia).

℞ **antithrombin III** is a natural anticoagulant found in the body. It inhibits the action of several clotting enzymes that activate thrombin. In people with a hereditary deficiency of this thrombin inhibitor, antithrombin III is used parenterally, in surgical or obstetrical procedures, to lower the risk of thrombosis, and to treat pulmonary embolism.

Oral anticoagulants, include the synthetic agents ℞ **warfarin sodium** and ℞ **dicumarol** (called coumarins), and ℞ **anisindione**, which is a synthetic anticoagulant that belongs to a different chemical family (anisindone), but which has similar actions to the coumarins. They work by antagonizing the action of vitamin K, the natural blood coagulation vitamin, and take days to reach full action—unlike the heparins. Because their actions are long-lasting, and the drugs can be taken by mouth, they can be prescribed for

long-term use—if necessary for life—to lessen the risk of further thrombotic episodes.

Limitations

All anticoagulants will be prescribed by specialists following a full medical assessment. There are a number of conditions when they must be used with caution, especially those where there is a risk of bleeding. Some people are sensitive to a particular group, for example, people who are allergic to porcine products, in which case a substitute will be found from another group. For instance, ℞ **anisindione** is generally reserved for treatment in people who cannot tolerate coumarins.

A doctor must be contacted if there is bleeding, bruising, dizziness, itching, rash, lightheadedness, swelling, or breathing problems. Some of these drugs cannot be used in pregnancy, for example, ℞ **warfarin sodium** and dicumarol are placed in the Food and Drug Administration's Pregnancy Category X, which means that they should not be used by women who are or may become pregnant.

anticonvulsant ⓓ

Generics: **acetazolamide; carbamazepine; clonazepam; clorazepate dipotassium; diazepam; divalproex sodium; ethosuximide; fosphenytoin; gabapentin; lamotrigine; levetiracetam; magnesium sulfate; mephenytoin; mephobarbital; methsuximide; phenytoin; primidone; tiagabine; topiramate; valproate sodium; zonisamide.**

Actions and uses

Anticonvulsant drugs are used to control or prevent convulsions. Their primary use is to control seizures caused by one or other form of ✪ **epilepsy**, and so they are often called ℞ **antiepileptics**, although there are some distinct differences in the treatment of epileptic seizures as compared to non-epileptic convulsive states. Some anticonvulsant drugs may also be used to treat, for instance, drug or chemical poisoning, and some of these (for example, ℞ **clonazepam**, ℞ **diazepam**, ℞ **magnesium sulfate**, ℞ **paraldehyde**) are not necessarily effective or commonly used for treating epilepsy. Antiepileptic drugs and their uses are discussed the ℞ **antiepileptic** entry.

Limitations

See the individual drug entries.

antidepressant ⓓ

Generics: **amitriptyline hydrochloride; amoxapine; bupropion hydrochloride; citalopram; clomipramine hydrochloride; desipramine hydrochloride; doxepin; fluoxetine; fluvoxamine; imipramine; isocarboxazid; maprotiline hydrochloride; mirtazapine hydrochloride; nefazodone hydrochloride; nortriptyline hydrochloride; paroxetine; phenelzine; protriptyline hydrochloride; tranylcypromine; trazodone hydrochloride; trimipramine hydrochloride; venlafaxine.**

Actions and uses

Antidepressants are used to relieve the symptoms of the affective disorder ✪ **depression**. There are several different groups of antidepressants, but they all work by changing the levels of monoamine neurotransmitters (serotonin and norepinephrine) in areas of the brain that regulate mood. Some increase neurotransmitter levels by blocking monoamine reuptake into brain neurons after release in the normal process of neurotransmission. These include the ℞ **SSRI** group (selective serotonin reuptake inhibitors) and the ℞ **tricyclic** group (which are comprised of three chemical rings). The ℞ **MAOIs** (monoamine-oxidase inhibitors) block the metabolic breakdown of the monoamine neurotransmitters by inhibiting specific enzymes known as monoamine-oxidases. There are various other ways antidepressants can act, but all affect brain monoamine neurotransmitters in some way.

All these types of antidepressants may be used to elevate mood, help resume normal functioning, and reduce the frequency of depressive periods in those with long-term depression. They may also be given to help in more acute, short-term treatments, such as after a loss of a loved one or in postnatal depression. As well as being used to treat depression, sometimes drugs of this class are prescribed to help in the treatment of ✪ **insomnia**, substance-dependence treatment (for example, ℞ **bupropion hydrochloride** for someone trying to stop smoking), and for a wide range of affective disorders, including ✪ **anorexia nervosa**, ✪ **obsessive-compulsive disorder**, and social phobias. In ✪ **bipolar disorder** (manic-depressive illness), the manic phases are controlled with special ℞ **antimanic** drugs, but antidepressants may be used to help with the depressive phases.

Limitations

All antidepressants have significant side effects, although these do generally subside or lessen with time. All take some time to work, about 3 weeks before there is any marked improvement with SSRIs, but less with the tricyclics (which have an immediate sedative effect, which can be an advantage with highly anxious patients). The MAOI group has a serious limitation because there are strict dietary restrictions when taking most drugs of this group. Because the enzyme monoamine-oxidase also detoxifies the amine tyramine in the body, when certain foodstuffs that contain this amine (for example, cheese, fermented soybean products, meat or yeast extracts, and some alcoholic beverages) are ingested, or medicines that contain sympathomimetic amines are taken (for example, cough and cold remedies that contain ℞ **ephedrine** or ℞ **pseudoephedrine**) the outcome may be a hypertensive (high blood pressure) crisis. Drugs of the ℞ **amphetamine** class (for example, ℞ **dextroamphetamine**, ℞ **methamphetamine**) also have serious hypertensive interactions with MAOIs. In the search for the best treatment, switching between different groups is not easy because each one needs a quite long washout period before the next type can be tried, otherwise there can be potentially dangerous interactions. A doctor must always be consulted before taking any other medication (including OTC (over-the-counter) medication, herbal remedies, and supplements) while using antidepressants. Similarly, more than one type of antidepressant must never be taken at the same time, and this applies to herbal antidepressant remedies as well as more conventional antidepressants. Generally, the SSRI group has the least side effects, but the tricyclic group is very much cheaper.

Apart from their actions on brain monoamines, all the antidepressants have other (generally undesirable) effects in the body, notably anticholinergic side effects (for example, dry mouth, gastrointestinal disturbances, and sedation). Efforts to develop new antidepressants have been largely directed at reducing these and other side effects. See the drug group entries for more details: ℞ **MAOI**; ℞ **SSRI**; ℞ **tricyclic**.

Some more recent antidepressants have been developed from these groups in attempts to find antidepressants with fewer limitations. These drugs include ℞ **mirtazapine hydrochloride**, ℞ **nefazodone hydrochloride**, and ℞ **venlafaxine**, which are like SSRIs but affect norepinephrine as well as serotonin uptake (such drugs are sometimes referred to as a selective serotonin and noradrenaline uptake inhibitors or Snares). The recently introduced drug ℞ **trazodone hydrochloride** is like the tricyclics but has less anticholinergic side effects (for example, dry mouth, gastrointestinal disturbances, and sedation). ℞ **bupropion hydrochloride** also inhibits uptake of the brain amine ℞ **dopamine**, and has atypical properties; it is also used as a substance-dependence treatment to aid nicotine withdrawal in people trying to quit smoking.

antidiabetic ⓓ

Generics: acarbose; acetohexamide; chlorpropamide; glimepiride; glipizide; glyburide; insulin, regular; insulin analog (lispro); insulin aspart recombinant; insulin lispro and insulin lispro protamine; insulin, regular and isophane mixture; insulin, isophane suspension (insulin, NPH); insulin glargine; insulin zinc suspension (lente); metformin; miglitol; pioglitazone; repaglinide; tolazamide; tolbutamide.

Actions and uses

℞ **antidiabetic** drugs are used in the treatment of ✪ **diabetes mellitus**. There are two main forms of diabetic treatment.

The first form of treatment involves the use of ℞ **oral hypoglycemic** agents, which are synthetic drugs taken by mouth to reduce the levels of glucose (sugar) in the bloodstream, and these are used primarily in the treatment of type 2 diabetes (non-insulin-dependent diabetes mellitus; NIDDM; maturity-onset diabetes) when there is still some residual capacity in the pancreas for the production of the hormone insulin. Chemically, many of these are from the ℞ **sulphonylurea** group (for example, ℞ **chlorpropamide**, ℞ **glimepiride**, ℞ **tolazamide**, ℞ **tolbutamide**, ℞ **acetohexamide**, ℞ **glipizide**, ℞ **glimepiride**, and ℞ **glyburide**). Also used are ℞ **biguanide** agents (℞ **metformin**) and other newer synthetic drugs, including ℞ **rosiglitazone**, ℞ **pioglitazone**, ℞ **repaglinide**, ℞ **miglitol**, and ℞ **acarbose**.

The second form of treatment involves the use of insulin in the form of various ℞ **insulin analog** preparations, and this is mainly used for type 1 diabetes (insulin-dependent diabetes mellitus; IDDM; juvenile-onset diabetes) and must be injected. There are many insulin preparations available and the difference between them is mainly how long their effects last.

Details of the use of the two main drug groups are given in the ℞ **oral hypoglycemic** and ℞ **insulin analog** entries. For the unrelated disorder, diabetes insipidus, see ℞ **diabetes insipidus treatment**

Limitations

See the individual drug entries.

antidiarrheal ⓪

(antidiarrhoeal)

Generics: **activated charcoal; bismuth subsalicylate; citrates; codeine phosphate; diphenoxylate hydrochloride; kaolin; loperamide hydrochloride; morphine sulfate.**

Actions and uses

Antidiarrheal drugs prevent the onset of ✪ **diarrhea** or assist in its treatment. The main medical treatment while diarrhea lasts should always be the replacement of fluid and electrolytes (particularly sodium). ℞ **electrolyte** solutions (rehydration solutions) are available OTC (over-the-counter) for oral use, but are also given by intravenous infusion in medical emergencies. Rehydration solutions are salts made up into a dilute solution with water, and usually contain ℞ **sodium chloride**, potassium chloride, and ℞ **citrates** of sodium and potassium (which allow adjustment of pH), and often glucose.

The main antidiarrheals, which stop diarrhea once it has started are preparations containing ℞ **opioid** (℞ **opiate**) agents. These are antimotility drugs (motility refers to movement) and work by reducing peristalsis (the rhythmic movement of the intestine), which slows the movement of fecal material and also decreases fluid secretion in the intestines. Such drugs are ℞ **loperamide hydrochloride,** ℞ **codeine phosphate,** ℞ **morphine sulfate,** ℞ **diphenoxylate hydrochloride,** and ℞ **paregoric.** ℞ **bismuth subsalicylate** is another common OTC compound used for the relief of indigestion without causing constipation, the relief of nausea, and to control diarrhea, including "traveler's diarrhea."

Some antidiarrheal preparations contain adsorbent materials that bind fecal material into solid masses. They may be mixtures containing ℞ **kaolin** or sometimes ℞ **activated charcoal.** These may also be useful in controlling fecal consistency for people who have undergone colostomy or ileostomy.

Diarrhea caused by inflammatory disorders, such as ✪ **irritable bowel syndrome,** ✪ **ulcerative colitis,** and ✪ **Crohn's disease** may be relieved by treatment with ℞ **corticosteroid** or ℞ **aminosalicylate** drugs. When diarrhea is caused by a bacterial infection (for example, *Campylobacter*), if severe, this can be treated with ℞ **antibacterial** drugs (for example, an ℞ **antibiotic** such as ℞ **erythromycin** or ℞ **ciprofloxacin**).

Limitations

Opioid-type antidiarrheal preparations that give prompt relief are generally available without prescription. However, they may well be overused and the more important replacement of fluids or use of rehydration solutions may be omitted because of this.

antidiuretic ⓪

Generics: **desmopressin; lypressin; vasopressin.**

Actions and uses

Antidiuretic drugs decrease the formation of ✪ urine. The major use of compounds of this type is in ℞ **diabetes insipidus treatment,** where the natural ℞ **posterior pituitary hormone,** antidiuretic hormone (ADH) in either of its two natural forms (℞ **vasopressin** and ℞ **lypressin**), or a synthetic analog, ℞ **desmopressin,** may be used. Desmopressin has the advantage that, although it is a peptide, it does not have to be used by injection like the others, but

can be taken by mouth or by intranasal spray (it is absorbed into the bloodstream from the nasal mucosa). Apart from their use to treat pituitary-originated ✪ **diabetes insipidus,** some of these drugs may also be used to treat ✪ **bed-wetting,** or for temporary increased urination following head trauma or surgery in the pituitary region.

Aside from drugs that act as antidiuretics by mimicking the actions of ADH in the body, there is a drug available, ℞ **demeclocycline** (in an "off-label" use of this antibiotic) that has the opposite action, and it can be used as a ℞ **hormone antagonist** to treat over-secretion of ADH (through an action it has on the kidneys).

Limitations

See the individual drug entries.

antidote ⓪

Generics: **acetylcysteine; atropine sulfate; desferoxamine mesylate; dexrazoxane; digoxin immune Fab; dimercaprol; edetate calcium disodium; flumazenil; fomepizole; naloxone hydrochloride; pralidoxime chloride; protamine sulfate; sodium nitrite; sodium thiosulfate; trientine hydrochloride.**

Actions and uses

Antidotes are drugs used to counteract poisons or overdose with other drugs, including herbal remedies. They are used in a wide variety of circumstances and can work in many ways. First, the most straightforward and commonly used method is where the poison works by stimulating, or over-stimulating, a distinct pharmacological receptor, since here the appropriate receptor antagonist can be used to reduce or completely block the effects of the poison. For example, ℞ **naloxone hydrochloride** is an ℞ **opioid** receptor antagonist and can be used as an antidote to an overdose of an (opioid) ℞ **narcotic analgesic** drug, such as ℞ **morphine sulfate** (or illicit heroin) and being quick-acting it effectively reverses the respiratory depression, coma, or convulsions that result from such an overdose. It can also be used at the end of operations to reverse respiratory depression caused by narcotic analgesics, and in newborn babies where mothers have been given large amounts of opioid (such as ℞ **pethidine**) for pain-relief during labour. The same principle applies to the use of the benzodiazepine antagonist ℞ **flumazenil** to counteract the effects of ℞ **benzodiazepine** drugs when used in operative procedures or when taken in overdose. Similarly ℞ **anticholinergic** drugs (for example, ℞ **atropine sulfate**) are used to counteract the effects of ℞ **parasympathomimetic** drugs (for example, ℞ **anticholinesterase** insecticides).

Second, poisoning by some agents is best counteracted by using an antidote that binds to the poison, rendering it relatively inert and helping its excretion (removal) from the body. For example, a ℞ **chelating agent** is used as an antidote to toxic metal poisoning because it chemically binds to certain metallic ions and other substances, making them less toxic and allowing their excretion from the body. Chelating agents are used to treat too high levels of metals of external origin (accidental or environmental), in ✪ **metabolic disorders** (for example, high levels of copper in Wilson's disease) or other disease states (for example, ℞ **penicillamine** in ✪ **rheumatoid arthritis**). Examples of chelating agents are: ℞ edetate calcium disodium; ℞ desferoxamine mesylate; ℞ dexrazoxane; ℞ dimercaprol (BAL); ℞ trientine hydrochloride.

An ℞ **antivenin** is an antidote to the poison in a snakebite, a scorpion's sting, or a bite from any other poisonous creature (such as a spider). Normally, it is an antiserum and is injected into the bloodstream for immediate relief (although it has its own adverse side effects). Another approach is to manufacture antibody fragments that react with a drug to neutralize it, for example, ℞ **digoxin immune Fab** to react with ℞ **cardiac glycosides** for use in the emergency treatment of an overdose. To treat overdose poisoning by the ℞ **non-narcotic analgesic** drug ℞ **acetaminophen**, ℞ **acetylcysteine** can be used immediately after overdose. The antidote works by chemically preventing the production of toxic products by the liver after poisoning by excessive amounts of the analgesic.

A different principle is used with ℞ **anticholinesterase** poisoning. These enzyme inhibitor drugs are used in medicine, as insecticides, and in chemical warfare. ℞ **pralidoxime chloride** is an antidote that actually reactivates the cholinesterase enzyme after it has been poisoned by anticholinesterases and is highly effective (taken in conjunction with other drugs) in preventing the life-endangering chemical changes to certain anticholinesterases. In all cases of poisoning, prompt action in using an antidote is necessary.

Some of the serious effects of poisoning by drugs or chemicals that in themselves are not very toxic, but are metabolized in the body to toxic products, can be avoided by slowing down this metabolism. The very serious effects of methanol (methyl alcohol; wood alcohol: a contaminant of illicit spirits, and an additive to methylated spirits) are due to its metabolism in the body to the much more active chemical, formic acid, which kills nerve cells and the optic nerve, so blinding its victims. If ethanol (ordinary alcohol) is given acutely for a period in quite high quantities, it slows the metabolism of methanol and can protect against damage. A similar principle applies for ℞ **fomepizole**, a recently introduced drug, which is used to treat poisoning by ethylene glycol (antifreeze). The drug ℞ **protamine sulfate** can be used to treat an overdose of ℞ **heparin** because it binds to the latter so limiting its ℞ **anticoagulant** activity. For use in the emergency treatment of cyanide poisoning, ℞ **sodium thiosulfate** and ℞ **sodium nitrite** can be used, because the latter chemicals change to a form of the blood pigment hemoglobin to one that is not affected by cyanide.

Limitations
See the individual drug entries.

anti-D (Rh$_0$) immunoglobulin ⓖ
see ℞ Rh$_0$(D) immune globulin (human).

anti-D Rh$_0$ immunoglobulin ⓖ
see ℞ Rh$_0$(D) immune globulin (human).

antidysrhythmic ⓓ
see ℞ antiarrhythmic.

antiemetic ⓓ
Generics: **scopolamine hydrobromide; cyclizine; meclizine hydrochloride; dimenhydrinate; buclizine hydrochloride; promethazine hydrochloride; diphenhydramine hydrochloride; thiethylperazine maleate; prochlorperazine; chlorpromazine; trimethobenzamide hydrochloride; perphenazine; haloperidol; droperidol; metoclopramide hydrochloride; granisetron; ondansetron; dolasetron mesylate; dronabinol.**

Actions and uses
Antiemetic drugs that prevent vomiting (emesis), whereas ℞ **antinauseant** drugs are used to reduce or prevent the *sensation* of nausea that very often precedes the physical process of vomiting. In practice, there is considerable overlap between the two drug types, and the terms are often used interchangeably.

Drugs used mainly to prevent and treat the nausea, vomiting and dizziness of motion sickness, and for vertigo that may arise from disorders of the balance function of the inner ear, are discussed in more detail in the ℞ **antinauseant** entry.

Antiemetics are used especially to help reduce the vomiting that accompanies radiotherapy and chemotherapy and may help by actually preventing vomiting and helping the passage of food out of the stomach; that is, they act as gastric ℞ **motility stimulants** (for example, ℞ **metoclopramide hydrochloride**). Alternatively, there are some recently developed drugs that can also be very effective for helping prevent the vomiting that is a common side effect of chemotherapy, radiotherapy and sometimes after surgery. These are the ℞ **serotonin-receptor antagonist** drugs (acting at the 5-HT$_3$ receptor subtype) such as ℞ **granisetron**, ℞ **ondansetron**, and ℞ **dolasetron mesylate**. They probably owe part of their effectiveness to actions on the "chemoreceptor triggerzone" in the brain, and part to actions within the gut.

Limitations
See individual drug entries.

antiepileptic ⓓ
(epileptic treatment)
Generics: **acetazolamide; carbamazepine; clonazepam; clorazepate dipotassium; diazepam; divalproex sodium; ethosuximide; fosphenytoin; gabapentin; lamotrigine; levetiracetam; magnesium sulfate; mephenytoin; mephobarbital; methsuximide; paraldehyde; phenobarbital; phenytoin; primidone; tiagabine; topiramate; valproate sodium; zonisamide.**

Actions and uses
Antiepileptic drugs are used to prevent the occurrence of epileptic seizures. Some of these drugs work against other types of convulsion (non-epileptic convulsive disorders), so in the more general sense are termed ℞ **anticonvulsant** drugs.

In order to prevent the occurrence of epileptic seizures, often over many years, an effective concentration of the drug must be maintained according to each person's requirements. Establishing such an effective tolerated dose may take time.

Generally, only one drug is required at any one time and the drug of choice depends on the type and severity of the epilepsy.

℞ **carbamazepine**, ℞ **phenytoin** (and the similar drugs ℞ **fosphenytoin** and ℞ **mephenytoin**; all three are often referred to by their chemical name hydantoin), and ℞ **valproate sodium** (also used in other forms, including valproic acid and ℞ **divalproex sodium**) are the drugs of choice for tonic-clonic seizures (grand mal) as part of a syndrome of primary generalized epilepsy; ℞ **ethosuximide** and ℞ **valproate sodium** are used for absence seizures (petit mal); and ℞ **clonazepam**, ℞ **ethosuximide** and valproate sodium for myoclonic seizures.

For other types of seizure, such as atypical absence, atonic, and tonic seizures (often in childhood), phenytoin, sodium valproate, clonazepam, ℞ **phenobarbital**, or ℞ **ethosuximide** are often used. Other drugs used (see individual entries for details) include ℞ **acetazolamide**; ℞ **clorazepate dipotassium**, ℞ **clonazepam**, ℞ **diazepam**, ℞ **gabapentin**, ℞ **levetiracetam**, ℞ **magnesium sulfate**, ℞ **mephenytoin**, ℞ **mephobarbital**, ℞ **methsuximide**, ℞ **paraldehyde**, ℞ **primidone**, ℞ **topiramate**, ℞ **tiagabine**, and ℞ **zonisamide**. See also ℞ **anticonvulsants**.

Limitatons

Many of these drugs have quite appreciable side effects, and some are not recommended for use in women of childbearing age. Evaluation of appropriate therapy for individuals is often made by specialists. See also the individual drug entries.

antiestrogen ⓓ

(antioestrogen; estrogen antagonist; oestrogen antagonist)
Generics: **aminoglutethimide; anastrozole; clomifene citrate; exemestane; letrozole; tamoxifen; testolactone; toremifene**.

Actions and uses

Antiestrogen (estrogen antagonist) agents are a class of drugs with ℞ **hormone antagonist** activity, which act directly or indirectly to reduce the effect of female ℞ **estrogen** sex hormones (for example, estradiol and estriol) on their target tissues. They can do this in a number of ways.

First, some drugs used to treat ⊙ **cancer** act directly by blocking estrogen receptors (for example, ℞ **tamoxifen** and ℞ **toremifene**). Their actions tend to be relatively specific when used in ℞ **anticancer** therapy. A similar agent is clomifene citrate, which is used in ℞ **infertility treatment** (see ⊙ **infertility**).

Second, some drugs work more indirectly as aromatase inhibitors; that is, they inhibit an enzyme involved in the normal biochemical conversion of androgens to estrogens in the body, and thereby prevent the formation of estrogens (for example, ℞ **anastrozole**, ℞ **exemestane**, and ℞ **letrozole**).

Third, a group of hormone antagonist drugs, also sometimes referred to as antiestrogen, work even more indirectly. For instance, the natural ℞ **hypothalamic hormone** gonadotropin-releasing hormone (LH-RH), used in its synthetic drug form, ℞ **gonadorelin**, or as synthetic chemical analogs (for example, ℞ **goserelin**, ℞ **nafarelin acetate**, and ℞ **leuprolide acetate**) is used in the treatment of cancer and sex hormone disorders. These drugs suppress the formation, or inhibit the release, of sex hormones, including both estrogens and androgens, but they do this via their initial action on the anterior pituitary gland, which in turn affects the sex glands that release these sex hormones.

Fourth, ℞ **testolactone** is somewhat different in that as well as having ℞ **androgen** activity it inhibits the synthesis of the natural ℞ **estrogen** hormone estrone, effectively acting as an indirect antiestrogen, and so it can be used to help reduce proliferation of hormone-sensitive ⊙ **breast cancer**.

Limitations

Drugs that are used to modify hormone action or release tend to have widespread side effects. These are generally regarded as acceptable if the condition being treated warrants them. The majority of these drugs are used for modifying sex hormone activity in the body when it is involved in a number of serious disorders that require intervention. Some of these are disorders of sexual development or fertility, and endometriosis; but most are used in ℞ **anticancer** therapy, in women, to help treat hormone-dependent tumors of the breast or uterus.

Future development of more acceptable hormone antagonists may be expected to feature receptor antagonists, since such drugs are generally relatively specific in their actions and effects. For example, ℞ **tamoxifen** is sufficiently well tolerated that it is being taken by some relatively young, "at-risk," women (for example, where there is a family history of breast cancer) who have not yet developed the condition, but to prevent its early development.

antiflatulence ⓓ

(antifoaming agent)
Generics: **activated charcoal; dimeticone**.

Actions and uses

Antiflatulence preparations relieve ⊙ **flatulence** and can be divided into two main types.

First, are the antifoaming agents, which are chemicals commonly incorporated into ℞ **antacid** preparations in order to lower surface tension so that small bubbles of froth coalesce into large bubbles, which allows the remedy to pass more easily through the intestine. They are commonly used to treat flatulence and a feeling of fullness and bloating. The most effective are silicone polymers such as ℞ **dimeticone** (simethicone; dimethicone). Second, are drugs with an ℞ **adsorbent** action for gases, for example, ℞ **activated charcoal**.

Limitations

See the individual drug entries.

antifoaming agent ⓓ

see ℞ **antiflatulence**.

antifungal ⓓ

Generics: **amphotericin B; benzoic acid; butoconazole; clioquinol; clotrimazole; econazole; fluconazole; flucytosine; griseofulvin; haloprogin; ichthammol; itraconazole; ketoconazole; miconazole; naftifine; nystatin; oxiconazole; sulconazole nitrate; terbinafine; terconazole; tioconazole; tolnaftate; undecylenic acid**.

Actions and uses

Antifungal drugs are ℞ **antimicrobial** agents that are used to treat infections caused by fungal microorganisms. Some are

℞ **antibiotic** drugs that, chemically, are produced naturally or synthetically.

⊙ **fungal infections** are usually not a major problem in healthy, well-nourished people. However, superficial, localized infections such as ⊙ **thrush** (caused by *Candida albicans*), ⊙ **athlete's foot**, and ringworm (caused by fungi of the dermatophyte group) are common. Severe infections occur most frequently in situations where the host's immunity is low, for example, following immunosuppression for transplant surgery, or in AIDS. Under such conditions fungi that are not normally pathogenic (disease-causing) can exploit the person's altered state and cause infection. Some of the drugs used are chemically ℞ **antibiotic** agents, such as ℞ **nystatin**, ℞ **amphotericin B**, and ℞ **griseofulvin**, and for serious infections these may be used systemically (for instance, for ringworm infections of the skin, hair, and nails; also for general systemic infection). Others are synthetic ℞ **azole** drugs (imidazoles/triazoles), such as ℞ **clotrimazole**, ℞ **econazole**, ℞ **fluconazole**, ℞ **itraconazole**, ℞ **miconazole**, ℞ **butoconazole**, ℞ **terconazole**, ℞ **tioconazole**, ℞ **oxiconazole**, and ℞ **sulconazole nitrate**, ℞ **sulconazole**. These are generally used for local infections, especially *Candida* fungal infections (candidiasis) of the throat, mouth, vagina, esophagus, and fingernails, but some can be used for systemic treatment, for example, ℞ **ketoconazole**, ℞ **itraconazole**, ℞ **fluconazole**. There are a variety of other agents, including flucytosine, which are reserved for serious systemic fungal infections, for example, ℞ **undecylenic acid**, ℞ **haloprogin**, ℞ **naftifine**, ℞ **terbinafine**, and ℞ **tolnaftate** for topical use.

Limitations

Unfortunately, the most powerful antifungal drugs also tend to be highly toxic. The azole group is relatively safe when used topically (externally), but have a number of adverse effects when taken by mouth (orally). Some minerals, including ♾ **magnesium** and ♾ **calcium**, can reduce the effects of azoles taken orally, and supplements containing these minerals should be avoided when taking oral azole antifungals. See also the individual drug entries.

antigout ⓓ

Generics: **allopurinol; citrates; colchicine; naproxen; probenecid; sodium bicarbonate; diclofenac; sodium thiosalicylate; sulfinpyrazone; sulindac.**

Actions and uses

Antigout drugs are used to treat ⊙ **gout**, which is a type of arthritic condition with exceedingly painful inflammation in specific joints and in the skin. It is mainly caused by the presence of excess uric acid in the blood, which is deposited as sodium urate crystals in the joints. A number of different types of drugs are used in the management of this disorder.

To reduce the production of uric acid in the body, ℞ **xanthine-oxidase inhibitor** drugs (mainly ℞ **allopurinol**) are used. Such agents are enzyme inhibitors which work by inhibiting the enzyme (xanthine-oxidase) which produces uric acid and so can be used to reduce excess uric acid in the blood (hyperuricemia) by reducing its synthesis. Allopurinol is only administered for the long-term treatment of gout and not acute attacks (which would be made worse).

To increase the excretion of uric acid from the blood into the urine and hence out of the body, ℞ **uricosuric** agents are used. These agents are used in long-term prevention and the most commonly used is ℞ **probenecid**, but ℞ **sulfinpyrazone** may also be used. For short-term treatment, particularly as an introductory measure to prevent and relieve acute attacks, initial treatment may be with ℞ **colchicine**, a complex alkaloid derived from the autumn crocus. In gouty arthritis, colchicine specifically inhibits the action of certain white blood cells (neutrophils), where they would cause release of inflammatory mediators and pain.

To treat the pain and inflammation of gout, drugs of the ℞ **NSAID** group (including ℞ **naproxen**, ℞ **sulindac**, and ℞ **diclofenac**) may be used, but not ℞ **aspirin** because it can interfere with uric acid excretion. ℞ **sodium thiosalicylate** is sometimes used by injection. If the pain and inflammation is severe, ℞ **corticosteroid** drugs may be given, sometimes by injection into the joint. When taken orally, ℞ **urinary alkalinizer** agents cause the urine to become alkaline (that is, less acid) and may help in uric acid excretion. The agents mainly used are ℞ **citrates**, often a sodium citrate and citric acid solution (Shohl's solution), or potassium citrate combinations.

What exactly causes gout is not fully understood, although there may be a hereditary factor. It can be caused by the long-term use of ℞ **diuretic** drugs, and their use is restricted in people who already suffer from gout. The frequency of attacks may be reduced by avoiding those foods (such as liver) that generate a lot of uric acid in the body. Chronic gout sufferers may be prescribed allopurinol for life. The use of colchicine is limited to the treatment of acute attacks, since it is rather toxic (although usually very effective).

Limitations

See the individual drug entries.

antihelminthic ⓓ

see ℞ **anthelmintic.**

antihemophilic factor ⓖ

(Factor VIII; AHF)

Type/Group: **hemostatic.**

Brand(s): (Derived from human source): Alphanate; Hemofil M; Koate-HP; Monoclate-P. (Recombinant synthetic): Bioclate; Helixate; Kogenate, Kogenate FS; Recombinate.

How administered: Intravenous infusion.

Used to treat

Antihemophilic factor is used to prevent or control bleeding episodes in people with classical ⊙ **hemophilia** (hemophilia A), in which there is a deficiency of the clotting factor, Factor VIII. Some antihemophilic factor is prepared from human blood plasma, some from a porcine (pig) source, and some is synthesized by recombinant techniques.

Warnings

• It should not be given to people with known hypersensitivity to mouse, hamster, or bovine protein. Antihemophilic factor is not effective in controlling bleeding associated with von Willebrand's disease. It will be given by experienced personnel after a full medical assessment.

• It should be used during pregnancy only when it is clearly needed.

• Medical judgment is required if breast-feeding is being considered.

• As with most substances that are derived from human blood plasma, there is a risk of exposure to viral infection (for example, AIDS and hepatitis A, B, and C). Where possible, vaccination against hepatitis A and B will be recommended, but infection with hepatitis C is the more likely.

• Some people with hemophilia develop inhibitor substances to Factor VIII, and the response to antihemophilic factor may be greatly reduced.

• Hypersensitivity symptoms, such as hives, tightness of the chest or wheezing, should be reported to a doctor.

• Trace amounts of the proteins that distinguish the blood groups (ABO) may be present. With large or frequent doses, the possibility exists for blood-type incompatibility reactions (for example, hemolytic anemia) in persons with type A, B, or AB blood.

Interactions

No interactions of significance are known.

Side effects

• These may include headache, drowsiness, acute anemia, increased tendency to bleed, flushing, somnolence, diarrhea, dizziness, sore throat, cold feet, or rash.

antihistamine ⓓ

Generics: **acrivastine; antazoline; azatadine maleate; azelastine hydrochloride; brompheniramine maleate; buclizine hydrochloride; cetirizine hydrochloride; chlorphenamine maleate; clemastine; cyclizine; cyproheptadine hydrochloride; dimenhydrinate; diphenhydramine hydrochloride; doxylamine; fexofenadine hydrochloride; hydroxyzine; ketotifen; loratadine; meclizine hydrochloride; pheniramine maleate; promethazine hydrochloride; pyrilamine maleate; triprolidine hydrochloride.**

Actions and uses

Antihistamine drugs inhibit many of the effects of histamine in the body, particularly when it is released as the result of people coming into contact with substances (allergens) to which they are allergic. Consequently, antihistamines are often used for antiallergic purposes, particularly for the symptomatic relief of such symptoms of allergy as the rhinitis of ○ **hay fever**, and various skin reactions, including rashes and wheals (○ **urticaria**), and antipruritic treatment against ○ **pruritis** (itching). Sometimes antihistamines are prescribed for the acute emergency treatment of ○ **anaphylactic reaction**, notably life-threatening constriction of the airways. There can be many allergenic triggers of histamine release, including inhalation of pollen, insect bites and stings, contact with some metal objects, food constituents, food dye additives, many environmental factors, and a number of drugs (notably ℞ **penicillin**-type ℞ **antibiotic** drugs, ℞ **local anesthetic** drugs; also, potentially, all drugs of a protein or peptide nature, such as blood products, ℞ **vaccine** preparations, and ℞ **immune globulin** preparations).

In addition to their uses specifically to antagonize the effects of the allergic release of histamine, many drugs conventionally classed as antihistamines have other uses, not necessarily involving the actions of histamine. For instance, a number also have ℞ **antinauseant** properties and can be used in ℞ **antiemetic** treatment to help prevent vomiting associated with ○ **motion sickness**, ○ **vertigo** or the effects of chemotherapy (for example, ℞ **buclizine hydrochloride**, ℞ **dimenhydrinate**, ℞ **meclizine hydrochloride**, ℞ **pheniramine maleate**, and ℞ **promethazine hydrochloride**).

Limitations

All long-established antihistamines have marked side effects in that they all produce drowsiness. But this has been almost completely overcome in some recently developed antihistamines (for example, ℞ **acrivastine**, ℞ **fexofenadine hydrochloride**, and ℞ **loratadine**) by basing them on chemical structures that do not readily permeate from the bloodstream to the brain. However, although the ℞ **sedative** action of the older antihistamines is a disadvantage when they are used against allergies, this sedative property does allow them to be used as ℞ **hypnotic** drugs, sometimes in OTC (over-the-counter) ℞ **sleep-aid product** preparations (for example, ℞ **diphenhydramine hydrochloride** and ℞ **doxylamine**). A number of the antihistamine group are incorporated, along with other drugs, into ℞ **cold and cough preparation** remedies where they may help alleviate the symptoms of ○ **rhinitis**, help dry up secretions in the airways, and may help alleviate ○ **cough** (although some of these actions may well be due to their ℞ **anticholinergic** or sedative properties). One of the antihistamine group (diphenhydramine hydrochloride) can be used as an ℞ **antiparkinsonism** agent for certain people, such as the elderly, to alleviate some symptoms of parkinsonism, but this is probably by virtue of the anticholinergic (rather than antihistamine) activity which is a characteristic of this and some other of these chemicals.

The antihistamine group discussed above act only at one receptor type in the body, and technically are referred to as H_1-antagonists to distinguish them from the quite different ℞ H_2-**antagonist** group, which are used in the treatment of ulcers (see ℞ **ulcer-healing drug**).

antihypertensive ⓓ

Actions and uses

Antihypertensives reduce ○ **hypertension** (an elevation of arterial blood pressure above the normal range expected in a particular age group and sex) and so reduce the risk of heart attacks, kidney failure, or stroke. Their use may also be beneficial in the treatment of ○ **angina pectoris** (see ℞ **antianginal** drugs) and congestive ℞ **heart failure treatment** where the individual also has these complications. Because of the importance of hypertension as a very common disease, a large number of drugs classes have been developed in order to treat this disorder. Further details of the drugs will be found under the appropriate headings.

Most treatment includes the use of ℞ **diuretic** drugs, and often a mild diuretic may be all that is required. These drugs are useful in congestive ℞ **heart failure treatment** when this accompanies the

Key to symbols: ○ = Disorder Section ℞ = Drug Section ♣ = Herbal Section ⚕⚕ = Supplement Section hypertension, and will help reduce edema in most conditions. Frequently, diuretics are taken along with other drugs.

Groups of drugs very commonly used as antihypertensives include ℞ **beta-blocker**, ℞ **ACE inhibitor**, and ℞ **angiotensin-receptor blocker** drugs. Further groups used under certain conditions include ℞ **calcium-channel blocker**, ℞ **antisympathetic**, and ℞ **nitrate** drugs. Most of these drugs act in the end as ℞ **vasodilator** agents, widening blood vessels, decreasing peripheral resistance, and so lowering blood pressure. Further details about these drugs will be found at their entries.

Limitations

See the type/group and individual drug entries.

antihypoglycemic ⓓ

Generics: **diazoxide; glucagon; glucose.**

Actions and uses

Antihypoglycemics are drugs that raise blood glucose (sugar) when it is too low (hypoglycemia). The drug ℞ **diazoxide** can be used by mouth to treat chronic hypoglycemia, for example, where a pancreatic tumor causes excessive secretion of insulin. ℞ **glucagon** is a natural hormone produced and secreted by the pancreas in order to cause an increase in blood sugar levels; that is, it is a hyperglycemic agent. It is normally part of a balancing mechanism with insulin, which has the opposite effect (see ℞ **insulin analog**). Glucagon can be given by injection to people with low blood sugar levels in an emergency. Diabetics on certain hypoglycemic drugs need to carry ℞ **glucose** as an antihypoglycemic to take by mouth to deal with possible hypotensive crises caused by too low levels of blood sugar.

Limitations

See the individual drug entries.

anti-infective ⓓ

See ℞ **antibacterial;** ℞ **antifungal;** ℞ **antiviral.**

anti-inflammatory ⓓ

Generics: **aspirin; celecoxib; choline salicylate; cromolyn sodium; dexamethasone; diclofenac; diflunisal; etodolac; fenoprofen; flurbiprofen; ibuprofen; fluticasone propionate; hydrocortisone; indomethacin; ketoprofen; ketorolac tromethamine; magnesium salicylate; meclofenamate sodium; mefenamic acid; meloxicam; methyl salicylate; montelukast sodium; nabumetone; naproxen; nedocromil sodium; oxaprozin; piroxicam; prednisolone; prednisone; rofecoxib; salicylic acid; salsalate; sodium salicylate; sodium thiosalicylate; sulindac; tolmetin sodium; triamcinolone; zileuton; zafirlukast.**

Actions and uses

℞ **anti-inflammatory** drugs are used to reduce inflammation. Although inflammation is essentially a normal defensive mechanism—it is the body's response to injury (for example, a reaction to tissue injury, infection, or inhalation of foreign proteins)—the manifestations may be so serious and/or inappropriate, or involve such discomfort, that treatment with anti-inflammatory drugs is required. Inflammatory conditions can be acute (for example,

insect strings) or chronic (for example, chronic asthma, dermatitis, and other skin conditions).

The ℞ NSAID (non-steroidal anti-inflammatory) drugs, such as ℞ **aspirin**, ℞ **ibuprofen**, and ℞ **naproxen**, can give effective relief from inflammatory pain, tissue swelling, joint immobilization, and can also lower raised body temperature, which means that they are often the first choice of treatment. They work by inhibiting the production and release in the body of pro-inflammatory local hormone mediators (℞ **prostaglandin** and related compounds) and, used with care, can be relatively free of side effects.

For more serious conditions ℞ **corticosteroid** drugs may be required (for example ℞ **dexamethasone**, ℞ **fluticasone propionate**, ℞ **hydrocortisone**, ℞ **prednisolone**, ℞ **prednisone**, and ℞ **triamcinolone**). Drugs of this group can be used for a wide variety of purposes. They can be used for the treatment of rheumatic disorders such as ✪ arthritis and ✪ osteoarthritis, allergic states, collagen diseases, liver and kidney disorders, allergic and inflammatory disorders of the intestinal tract, respiratory diseases (such as bronchial ✪ asthma). However, they can cause so many complications that they are mainly given by local application as some forms of ℞ **skin preparation**, which are used for inflammation associated with conditions such as ✪ eczema and ✪ psoriasis, and of the eyes, ears, or nose. They are also safer to use when inhaled into the lungs for asthma, and only given in injection form for serious conditions and emergencies, such as ✪ anaphylactic reaction. A further class of drugs, sometimes called mast-cell stabilizers, such as ℞ **cromolyn sodium** and ℞ **nedocromil sodium**, also give anti-inflammatory protection from the symptoms of allergic asthma, and allergic symptoms in the eye (for example, allergic ✪ conjunctivitis), nose (such as, environmental allergy symptoms including allergic rhinitis), intestine (for example, food allergy), and elsewhere. They may be used by topical (external) application, taken by mouth, or inhaled, depending on the circumstances. They are thought to work by preventing the release of histamine and other substances (from mast-cell stores).

Two new classes of anti-inflammatory drugs work by preventing the release of inflammatory mediators called leukotrienes, which are increasingly thought to be important, especially in the lungs. ℞ **lipoxygenase inhibitor** drugs (also called *5-lipoxygenase inhibitor* agents) work by blocking enzymes involved in the production of leukotrienes, and the first such drug in use, ℞ **zileuton**, is taken by mouth in the long-term treatment and prevention of asthma. The second class, the ℞ **leukotriene receptor antagonist** (including ℞ **montelukast** and ℞ **zafirlukast**), prevent the actions of leukotrienes at their receptors, and can be used as an additional treatment in the management of asthma which is not adequately controlled by other methods.

Limitations

See individual drug and drug group entries.

anti-inhibitor coagulant complex ⓖ

(Factor VIII inhibitor bypassing fraction)

Type/Group: **hemostatic.**

Brand(s): Autoplex T; Feiba VH Immuno.

How administered: Injection (intravenous).

Used to treat

Anti-inhibitor coagulant complex is used to treat bleeding episodes, or before surgery, in persons with inhibitors to Factor VIII. It is prepared from human blood plasma and may contain various clotting factors, and their precursors, in varying proportion—it is standardized by the measure of its effect on clotting times.

Warnings

• It should not be given to people with signs of clots being broken up in the blood (fibrinolysis), uncontrolled generalized clotting (disseminated intravascular coagulation; DIC), or who have a normal coagulation mechanism. It will be given by experienced personnel after a full medical assessment.

• It should be given with caution to people with liver disease.

• It should be used during pregnancy only when it is clearly needed.

• Medical judgment is required if breast-feeding is being considered.

• As with most substances that are derived from human blood plasma, there is a risk of exposure to viral infection (for example, AIDS and hepatitis A, B, and C). Where possible vaccination against hepatitis A and B is recommended, but infection with hepatitis C is more likely.

• There is some risk of thrombosis when these clotting factors are used. If uncontrolled generalized clotting (disseminated intravascular coagulation; DIC) occurs, the use of this anti-inhibitor complex should stop immediately.

• Trace amounts of the proteins that distinguish the blood groups (ABO) may be present. With large or frequent doses, the possibility exists for blood-type incompatibility reactions (for example, hemolytic anemia) in persons with type A, B, or AB blood.

• There is frequently an increase in Factor VIII inhibitor after anti-inhibitor coagulant complex is used.

Interactions

• ℞ **aminocaproic acid** and ℞ **tranexamic acid** are not recommended for use with anti-inhibitor coagulant complex.

Side effects

• Rapid infusion may result in headache, flushing, changes in blood pressure or heart rate.

• Other side effects may include fever, chills, and allergic responses, which range from rashes to anaphylactoid reactions.

antimalarial Ⓓ

Generics: **chloroquine; hydroxychloroquine sulfate; doxycycline; quinidine; quinine.**

Actions and uses

Antimalarial drugs are used to treat or prevent ✪ **malaria**. Malaria is caused by infection of the red blood cells by a small organism called a protozoan (of the genus *Plasmodium*), which is carried by several species of mosquito of the genus *Anopheles*. Infection occurs as a result of a mosquito bite.

Prophylaxis to prevent, or treat, malarial infection has become somewhat difficult due to the emergence of strains of the infection in some parts of the world which are resistant to standard drugs. For this reason expert advice about medication is required before traveling.

The synthetic chemical class of drug that has most commonly been used to treat or prevent infection is the quinolines; both 4-aminoquinolines, of which ℞ **chloroquine** is the standard (other examples are ℞ **hydroxychloroquine sulfate** and mefloquine), and 8-aminoquinolines (for instance, primaquine). In certain areas of the world strains of *Plasmodium falciparum* and others have recently developed resistance to chloroquine. In this case, it may not be advisable to use the main alternative, mefloquine (it has adverse effects on the heart, can cause psychiatric disturbances, and is not recommended for pregnant women or children), so a regimen may be recommended where chloroquine and additionally ℞ **sulfadoxine** (always together with ℞ **pyrimethamine**) are taken in the event of a febrile (feverish) illness. Alternatively, the ℞ **antibiotic** drug ℞ **doxycycline** may be taken as a preventive measure.

Of the other drugs, ℞ **quinine**, the traditional ℞ **cinchona alkaloid** remedy for malaria, is used for treatment (but not for prevention) of ℞ **chloroquine**-resistant infection. Very occasionally, the closely related drug ℞ **quinidine** is used for life-threatening malaria caused by *Plasmodium falciparum*. Primaquine is now only recommend as a radical cure of *P. vivax* malaria or following other therapy where it is endemic.

Limitations

Although the prevention of malaria by drugs cannot be guaranteed, the use of antimalarial drugs before, during, and for a period after a trip to a region where malaria is endemic (constantly present) is recommended (and is required by some countries as a condition for entry) for protection. Availability of particular antimalarial drugs differs from country to country. Primary prophylaxis (prevention)—personal protection against being bitten—is very important. See also the individual drug entries.

antimania Ⓓ

(bipolar disorder treatment; manic-depressive treatment)
Generics: **carbamazepine; chlorpromazine; fluoxetine; haloperidol; lithium; valproate sodium.**

Actions and uses

Antimania (antimanic) drugs are used to treat ✪ **bipolar disorder** (manic-depressive illness), which is characterized by periods of mood normality punctuated by episodes of *mania* and bouts of ✪ **depression**. It is because of these mood swings around the norm, that one of the names for the disorder is bipolar disorder. The manic phase may require acute treatment and here, initially, ℞ **antipsychotic** drugs (for example, haloperidol and chlorpromazine) are often used. Maintenance treatment to reduce the frequency of manic episodes is generally with ℞ **lithium** (as carbonate or citrate), but if this is not effective, or tolerated, other drugs may be tried (for example, ℞ **carbamazepine** or ℞ **valproate sodium**, and other valproic acid derivatives). Also, ℞ **antidepressant** drugs (for instance ℞ **fluoxetine**) may help reduce the severity or incidence of the depressive phase.

Limitations

Lithium is a remarkably effective drug. Although it has significant side effects, its use is so successful that these effects (caused by its toxicity) are considered justifiable. The blood levels of lithium must be maintained within quite narrow margins to get the most effect without undue toxicity, which means regular blood-level measurements throughout the treatment.

antimanic Ⓓ

see ℞ antimania.

antimicrobial Ⓓ

Actions and uses

Antimicrobial drugs are used to treat infections caused by microbes (microorganisms), which include the major classes of pathogenic (disease-causing) microorganisms covered in this book—viruses, mycoplasma, mycobacteria, rickettsia, chlamydia, protozoa, bacteria, and fungi (but not helminths; worms). The term therefore covers ℞ antibacterial, ℞ antifungal, ℞ antimalarial, ℞ antiprotozoal, and ℞ antiviral drug classes. Many of the major antibacterial drugs are chemically of ℞ antibiotic origin.

Limitations

See the individual drug type/group entries.

antimigraine Ⓓ

(migraine treatment)

Generics: **acetaminophen; amitriptyline hydrochloride; aspirin; atenolol; chlorpromazine; codeine phosphate; cyclizine; cyproheptadine hydrochloride; fluoxetine; isometheptene mucate; metoclopramide hydrochloride; nadolol; naratriptan; nifedipine; propranolol hydrochloride; rizatriptan benzoate; sumatriptan succinate; timolol maleate; zolmitriptan.**

Actions and uses

Antimigraine drugs are used to treat ✪ migraine in two basic ways: first, they may be given on a long-term basis to prevent or reduce the frequency or severity of attacks; second, they may be given just before or during an attack to reduce its severity. Migraine is a specific, clinically recognized form of headache and not just a particularly severe headache. The symptoms of migraine commonly include a throbbing pain confined to one side of the head (unilateral headache), nausea and vomiting, intolerance of light, and disturbances of hearing, feeling and speech. A migraine attack is often preceded by a forewarning, called an "aura," up to 30 minutes before an attack, consisting of visual disturbances and weakness or numbness of the limbs, and which usually fades when the headache begins.

As mentioned, drugs are used in two different ways to treat migraine (and also the related condition called "cluster headache"): long-term and short-term. The drugs given chronically (that is, long-term) to help prevent attacks (prophylactic use) include ℞ **calcium-channel blockers** (for example, ℞ **nifedipine**), ℞ **beta-blockers** (for example, ℞ **atenolol**, ℞ **nadolol**, ℞ **propranolol hydrochloride**, ℞ **timolol maleate**). The second group may be used either at the aura stage or during the attack itself, and for maximum effect the speed of administration and subsequent absorption of the drug is the all-important factor. Drugs directly affecting blood vessels and which can be used during the attack stage include the recently introduced (5-HT$_1$-subtype) ℞ **serotonin-receptor stimulant** class of ℞ **vasoconstrictor** drugs (℞ **naratriptan**, ℞ **rizatriptan**, ℞ **sumatriptan**, ℞ **zolmitriptan**)

which can achieve a rapid onset of action, some by self-injection or administration by nasal spray. Older drugs that act directly on blood vessels include the ℞ **ergot alkaloid** (ergoloid) drugs (for example, ℞ **ergotamine tartrate**, ℞ **dihydroergotamine mesylate**, ℞ **ergonovine maleate**, and ℞ **methysergide**), which are sometimes used chronically.

Various other drugs are sometimes used in resistant cases to treat some aspect of migraine attacks (for example, ℞ **cyproheptadine hydrochloride**, ℞ **isometheptene mucate**, ℞ **amitriptyline hydrochloride**, ℞ **fluoxetine**, ℞ **chlorpromazine**). A number of ℞ **analgesics** can be used to deal with the pain of an attack and are often incorporated into compound preparations together with a variety of other drugs (for example, ℞ **aspirin**, ℞ **codeine phosphate**, ℞ **acetaminophen**). Sometimes drugs with ℞ **antinauseant** or ℞ **antiemetic** properties are included in migraine preparations to reduce the associated symptoms of ✪ nausea and ✪ vomiting (for example, ℞ **cyclizine**, ℞ **metoclopramide hydrochloride**).

The exact causes of migraine are not known but it seems most likely that it results from blood vessels in the head narrowing down and then expanding. This affects the blood flow to the brain, so triggering the perceptual disturbances (particularly vision) and the pain. This may be a consequence of raised levels of "vasoactive amines," which have an effect on blood vessels. Eating certain foods may cause these raised levels, or attacks may be provoked by stress, oral contraceptives, unaccustomed exercise, altered sleeping patterns, or low blood sugar levels. Foods such as chocolate, some dairy products, including ripe cheese, and yeast extracts contain tyramine, and all may precipitate attacks. Some migraine sufferers do not have the enzyme which breaks down tyramine, so a build-up of it may set off a series of biochemical events leading to a migraine. The primary treatment should be prevention, which involves identifying the factors that trigger an attack. Because there may be a number of factors that contribute to migraine, everyone should establish his or her own preventive strategy. For example, if particular foods are the cause, then some changes in diet may be enough to prevent attacks.

In all cases, the appropriate drug will vary from person to person. It is often worth having an evaluation carried out by a specialist clinic. The success rate of any individual drug may be less than 50 percent overall and yet be very effective for some individual sufferers. The vasoconstrictor drugs have effects on blood vessels other than in the skull, and may not be suitable for some people with certain risk factors.

Limitations

See the individual drug entries.

Antiminth Ⓑ

A preparation of ℞ **pyrantel**.

Formulation: Oral suspension.

Availability: OTC.

Warnings and side effects: See ℞ **pyrantel**.

antimuscarinic Ⓓ

see ℞ anticholinergic.

antinauseant ⓓ

Generics: **buclizine hydrochloride; chlorpromazine; cyclizine; dimenhydrinate; diphenhydramine hydrochloride; dolasetron mesylate; droperidol; granisetron; haloperidol; meclizine hydrochloride; metoclopramide hydrochloride; ondansetron; perphenazine; prochlorperazine; promethazine hydrochloride; scopolamine hydrobromide; thiethylperazine maleate; trimethobenzamide hydrochloride.**

Actions and uses

Antinauseant drugs are used to prevent or minimize the feeling of nausea and to reduce any subsequent vomiting. Most agents of this type are also classed as ℞ **antiemetic** drugs because of this similar use. Commonly, the term antinauseant is used interchangeably with antiemetic, but in some ways this is misleading because some of the latter drugs do indeed help prevent the act of emesis (vomiting), but the aim of antinauseant treatment is to prevent the emergence of the feeling of nausea—which normally precedes vomiting. However, there are many drugs that can be regarded as both antinauseant and antiemetic drugs.

The type of drug used as an antinauseant, and the likelihood of its success, depends on the mechanism and origin of the nausea, which can be triggered in a number of ways. ✪ **motion sickness**, or travel sickness, can often be prevented by taking before traveling antinauseants such as the ℞ **anticholinergic** drug ℞ **scopolamine hydrobromide**. This drug is also used to prevent and treat the ✪ **vertigo** and nausea associated with ✪ **Ménière's disease** and middle-ear surgery, but it does have marked ℞ **sedative** properties.

℞ **antihistamine** drugs of the sedative types are also extensively used to prevent and treat the nausea, vomiting, and dizziness of motion sickness, and for vertigo that may occur due to disorders of the balance function of the inner ear. Such drugs include ℞ **cyclizine**, ℞ **meclizine hydrochloride**, ℞ **dimenhydrinate**, ℞ **promethazine hydrochloride**, and ℞ **diphenhydramine hydrochloride**. Although these are, for convenience, usually referred to as antihistamines, with respect to their use in treating the conditions mentioned above, they are almost certainly working here as anticholinergic drugs, and indeed have most of the same side effects (dry mouth, sedation, and others) as do anticholinergics like ℞ **scopolamine hydrobromide**. All of the above antinauseants are available without prescription in forms suitable for motion sickness, but for inner ear and related conditions they may have to be prescribed.

A number of stronger antinauseant/antiemetic drugs are sometimes used for more serious conditions, including to reduce the incidence of nausea and vomiting in patients about to undergo surgery or diagnostic procedures, in the prevention of nausea caused by chemotherapy, radiotherapy, or by the vertigo and labyrinthine disorders, and vomiting in terminal illness. These include ℞ **buclizine hydrochloride**, ℞ **thiethylperazine**, ℞ **prochlorperazine**, ℞ **chlorpromazine**, ℞ **trimethobenzamide hydrochloride**, ℞ **perphenazine**, ℞ **haloperidol**, and ℞ **droperidol**.

Some of the drugs discussed, for instance, ℞ **droperidol**, can be used together with drugs that tend to cause, as a side effect, nausea and vomiting—notably ℞ **narcotic analgesic** agents—to reduce this, for example in surgery (but care is needed since both classes of drugs tend to depress respiration).

The nausea and vomiting that is caused by chemotherapy and radiotherapy can be difficult to treat. However, some ℞ **antiemetic** drugs, such as ℞ **motility stimulant** drugs (for example, ℞ **metoclopramide hydrochloride**), may be of some use by preventing vomiting and helping food out of the stomach. Alternatively, there are some recently developed drugs that can also be very effective for nausea relief in chemotherapy, radiotherapy and after surgery. These include the ℞ **serotonin-receptor antagonist** drugs (acting at the $5\text{-}HT_3$ receptor subtype) such as ℞ **granisetron**, ℞ **ondansetron**, and ℞ **dolasetron mesylate**. Recently, ℞ **dronabinol**, a psychoactive constituent of marijuana (*Cannabis sativa*) that both stimulates appetite and effectively suppresses nausea and vomiting, has been introduced as an antinauseant and ℞ **antiemetic**, used for the control of such symptoms in persons undergoing chemotherapy or radiotherapy for cancer.

Limitations

See the individual drug entries.

antioestrogen ⓓ

see ℞ antiestrogen.

antiparkinsonian ⓓ

see ℞ antiparkinsonism.

antiparkinsonism ⓓ

(antiparkinsonian; antiparkinson's; Parkinson's disease treatment)
Generics: **amantadine; benztropine mesylate; biperiden; carbidopa; entacapone; levodopa; pramipexole; procyclidine; ropinirole; selegiline hydrochloride; tolcapone; trihexyphenidyl.**

Actions and uses

Antiparkinsonism drugs are used to treat parkinsonism and ✪ **Parkinson's disease**. The term parkinsonism is used to describe the symptoms of several disorders of the central nervous system (CNS), including muscle tremor and rigidity (extrapyramidal symptoms), especially in the limbs. The parkinsonism syndrome is caused by an imbalance in the actions of the neurotransmitters acetylcholine and dopamine, which have generally opposing actions on motor control in the brain. Classic Parkinson's disease is a neurological degenerative disease where this imbalance is mainly due to degeneration of dopamine-containing neurons in a discrete brain area called the substantia nigra in the basal ganglia, which are concerned with motor control in the body. However, what are known as parkinsonian extrapyramidal side effects may also be caused by treatment with several types of drugs, especially ℞ **antipsychotic** drugs (for example, ℞ **haloperidol**), by carbon monoxide poisoning, cerebrovascular disease, encephalitis, and by damage to the CNS.

There are two main approaches to antiparkinsonian treatment: first, by increasing dopamine-like (dopaminergic) actions; second, by decreasing acetylcholine-like (cholinergic) actions.

The dopaminergic balance may be increased by giving ℞ **levodopa** (which is naturally converted into dopamine in the body), often with other drugs (for example, ℞ **carbidopa**, ℞ **entacapone**, ℞ **selegiline hydrochloride**, ℞ **tolcapone**) that prolong its action by inhibiting enzymes responsible for the breakdown of dopamine in the body. Alternatively, by using dopamine receptor stimulant drugs which mimic the actions of dopamine itself (℞ **bromocriptine**, ℞ **pergolide**, ℞ **pramipexole**, ℞ **ropinirole**). Unusually, ℞ **amantadine** is thought to work here by increasing dopamine release from neurons that are still intact.

Drugs that decrease cholinergic actions—℞ **anticholinergic** drugs (more accurately, antimuscarinics)—include ℞ **atropine**, ℞ **benztropine mesylate**, benzhexol hydrochloride, ℞ **biperiden**, ℞ **diphenhydramine hydrochloride**, ℞ **procyclidine**, and ℞ **trihexyphenidyl**.

Limitations

It is not normally possible to regain full control of movement and coordination for a long period. The normal drug of choice used first for people with moderate disability is levodopa, generally taken with carbidopa or enzyme inhibitors that prevent metabolism outside the brain, because this greatly reduces the dose necessary. Nevertheless, unfortunately the beneficial effect of levodopa on muscle rigidity and movements often gradually diminishes over about 5 years, and involuntary writhing movements appear. Also, there may be fluctuations in the state of the person, called "on-off states." When levodopa becomes less effective, then drugs with dopaminergic actions, or amantadine may be used. For controlling fine tremor and some other movement including that induced by antipsychotic drugs, the anticholinergic drugs may be used. However, they have quite marked side effects, including dry mouth, impaired vision, constipation, and difficulty in urination. For these reasons, often several drugs are used at once. It is a difficult and often lengthy process to achieve the optimum dose in each person and there are certain side effects (such as confusion in the elderly) that occur with all the treatments.

Treatments that are still experimental are aimed at directly replacing the missing neurons in the substantia nigra by implanting cells form outside the body, possibly stem cells or embryo cells, with the use of nerve-growth factors to encourage cell growth.

antiparkinson's Ⓓ

see ℞ antiparkinsonism.

antiperspirant Ⓓ

Generics: **aluminum chloride**.

Actions and uses

Antiperspirant preparations help to prevent sweating. Medically, they are required only in cases of severe ✪ **hyperhidrosis** (excessive sweating), when a disorder of the sweat glands causes constant and streaming perspiration. In such cases, ℞ **aluminum chloride** is an effective ℞ **astringent** with powerful antiperspirant properties.

Limitations

See the individual drug entry.

antiplatelet Ⓓ

Generics: **abciximab**; **anagrelide hydrochloride**; **aspirin**; **cilostazol**; **dipyridamole**; **epoprostenol sodium**; **eptifibatide**; **clopidogrel**; **ticlopidine**; **tirofiban**.

Actions and uses

Antiplatelet drugs (also known as *platelet aggregation inhibitors*) help prevent the clumping of platelets, which are components in the formation of blood clots. Clots formed within blood vessels are called thrombi, and are composed of two elements. First, activation of a natural blood element called *thrombin* acts as an enzyme in forming the web-like fibrin elements of the thrombus. Second, platelets (thrombocytes) can be activated so that they stick together and become entangled in the fibrin web. This allows the thrombus to plug vessels and stop bleeding. This second process is prevented by antiplatelet agents—the first by ℞ **anticoagulant** agents—and these two types of drugs are sometimes prescribed in combination when there is a particular risk of thrombus formation. In general, anticoagulants prevent thrombi forming, or enlarging, within veins or within the heart, whereas anticoagulants work to prevent thrombi forming in arteries.

Antiplatelet drugs (for example, ℞ **aspirin**, taken at low doses) can be used as a preventive treatment (prophylactic use) in people who are at risk, for instance, after a ✪ **heart attack**, ✪ **stroke**, or bypass operation. However, this same action may increase bleeding time and so people receiving anticoagulant drugs do not also take antiplatelet drugs unless it is medically necessary.

By decreasing platelet aggregation, antiplatelet drugs may beneficially stop thrombus formation on the arterial side of the circulation, where thrombi are formed mostly by platelet aggregation and so anticoagulant drugs would have little effect.

Other antiplatelet drugs include ℞ **dipyridamole**, which is used in heart procedures including insertion of artificial heart valves, and in coronary arteriography. ℞ **cilostazol** is used to reduce symptoms in intermittent claudication (poor circulation to the extremities). ℞ **ticlopidine** is used to reduce new blood-clotting complications, such as stroke, in people with a history of atherosclerotic disease (ischemic stroke, myocardial infarction, or peripheral arterial disease). ℞ **tirofiban** and ℞ **clopidogrel** are antiplatelet drugs, which can be used (together with ℞ **heparin**) to prevent thrombosis in acute cardiac conditions in which myocardial infarction (heart attack) has already occurred or is likely to occur. ℞ **eptifibatide** is used for similar purposes and has been used in combination with heparin and ℞ **aspirin**.

℞ **anagrelide** is used to treat symptoms of a condition called essential thrombocythemia, in which platelet counts—and risk of thrombosis—are high. Its action is not completely understood, but it appears to interfere with the maturation of the parent cell (megakaryocyte) which produces platelets.

℞ **abciximab** is one of a relatively new class of drug, a monoclonal antibody, which is a cloned antibody that inhibits platelet aggregation and thrombus formation. It is used by specialists as an additional treatment to heparin and aspirin for the prevention of complications due to clot formation in high-risk people undergoing certain types of coronary angioplasty operations. Similarly, ℞ **epoprostenol** (prostacyclin)—another specialist drug—is a

℞ **prostaglandin** naturally present in blood vessel walls, which has potent ℞ **vasodilator** and antiplatelet activity. When given by intravenous infusion it stops platelets sticking to each other, to surgically inserted tubes, or artificial heart valves. It is also used to treat pulmonary hypertension.

Limitations

There is currently great interest in the applications of ℞ **antiplatelet** drugs to the treatment of cardiovascular disease. Aspirin has the great advantage in that it is both cheap and has a long duration of action. The additional ℞ **antiplatelet** action of aspirin is not directly related to its analgesic (painkilling) action, and in this respect other ℞ **NSAID** drugs are not nearly so powerful and cannot be used instead of aspirin (it is due to inhibition of the COX-2 subtype of a cyclo-oxygenase enzyme—rather than inhibition of the COX-1 subtype—which is responsible for its anti-inflammatory action).

The disadvantage of aspirin is that in tablet form, it irritates the stomach lining and may cause bleeding and ulceration. This limits its combination with anticoagulants (for example, with ℞ **heparin** or ℞ **warfarin sodium**) to better prevent arterial thrombi formation, because this increases bleeding time and the risk of hemorrhage. A number of the newer antiplatelet agents do not have this disadvantage, and so may be combined. This is not to say that all new agents are safe, for example, ticlopidine may have depressive effects on levels of certain blood cells, and is usually reserved for cases where aspirin cannot be tolerated.

Neither anticoagulant nor antiplatelet drugs dissolve thrombi, although they may help prevent the extension of blood clots that have already formed. A third class of drugs, ℞ **fibrinolytic** agents, can be used to dissolve thrombi once they have formed. See also the individual drug entries.

antiprotozoal ⓓ

see ℞ **amebicide and antiprotozoal**.

antipruritic ⓓ

Generics: **crotamiton; diphenhydramine hydrochloride; hydroxyzine**.

Actions and uses

Antipruritic drugs are used to relieve ⊙ **pruritis**, which is the symptom of itching—an uncomfortable sensation leading to the urge to scratch. This is a common symptom of many skin disorders such as ⊙ **urticaria** (also called hives or nettle rash), ⊙ **eczema**, and ⊙ **scabies**, or to an insect ⊙ **sting** or bite, or drug allergy. It can also be a sign of an underlying disorder.

Drugs used include ℞ **crotamiton** and ℞ **antihistamine** drugs with sedative properties (for instance, ℞ **diphenhydramine hydrochloride** and ℞ **hydroxyzine**). Sometimes ℞ **corticosteroid** drugs (for example, ℞ **desoxymetasone**) are useful.

Limitations

Unfortunately, few drugs are very effective for relieving itching. Soothing lotions (especially ones containing ℞ **calamine**) may be as effective as specific drugs. Wherever possible, the underlying cause should be treated (for example, skin fungal infections).

antipsychotic ⓓ

Generics: **chlorpromazine; clozapine; haloperidol; loxapine; mesoridazine; molindone; olanzapine; perphenazine; prochlorperazine; promazine; quetiapine; risperidone; thioridazine; thiothixene; trifluoperazine**.

Actions and uses

℞ **antipsychotic** or neuroleptic, drugs calm and soothe people without impairing consciousness. They are used mainly to treat psychologically disturbed people, particularly those who manifest the complex behavioral patterns of ⊙ **schizophrenia**, and also those with brain damage, toxic delirium, and mania. In the short term, some can also be used as ℞ **anxiolytic** drugs to treat severe ⊙ **anxiety**. Because they can affect mood, in the short term some may worsen ⊙ **depression**, but in other cases there may be useful ℞ **antidepressant** actions with a beneficial elevation of mood.

Antipsychotics with markedly depressant side effects were at one time somewhat misleadingly, known as major tranquilizers, because, for example, in schizophrenics the tranquilizing effect is of secondary importance and for some even an undesirable effect.

Antipsychotics work by acting in the brain, principally as ℞ **dopamine-receptor blocker** agents, to change the balance of the effects there of the neurotransmitter dopamine, which is intimately involved in mood. Antipsychotic drugs differ in their characteristics and side effects. They are usually grouped and named according to their chemical structures, because this to a large extent determines a drug's pharmacological profile.

The biggest group of drugs, the ℞ **phenothiazine** agents, contains many different drugs (including some that are more commonly used for other disorders). Some phenothiazine-related antipsychotics are ℞ **chlorpromazine**, ℞ **promazine**, ℞ **perphenazine**, ℞ **prochlorperazine**, ℞ **trifluoperazine**, ℞ **thioridazine** and ℞ **mesoridazine**. Other chemical groups resemble phenothiazines in their actions and are often grouped with them, for example, thioxanthenes (℞ **thiothixene**), diphenylbutylpiperidines/butyrophenones (℞ **haloperidol**), indolones (℞ **molindone**), and dibenzoxazepines (℞ **loxapine**). Later, novel (often called "atypical") antipsychotics were developed from the dibenzepines (℞ **clozapine**, ℞ **olanzapine** and ℞ **quetiapine**) and benzisoxazoles (℞ **risperidone**). ℞ **reserpine**, an unrelated antipsychotic, is a plant alkaloid.

The earlier "typical" antipsychotics all have ℞ **dopamine-receptor blocker** actions (working particularly at the D_2-subtype of receptor) and this accounts for much of their antipsychotic actions, but also for many of their serious side effects (notably extrapyramidal side effects: see Limitations below). The later "atypical" antipsychotics, developed out of clozapine, tend to block different subtypes of dopamine receptor, and also have ℞ **serotonin-receptor antagonist** activity, and are often better tolerated because of greatly reduced extrapyramidal side effects (and less raised levels of the pituitary hormone prolactin, which is involved in lactation and explains the milk ejecting and other side effects affecting the breast).

Antipsychotic drugs may be given by mouth, by intravenous or intramuscular injection, or sometimes, in the form of special oily preparations, as a long-lasting deep-intramuscular "depot" injection.

Limitations

Because the balance of neurotransmitters in the brain is in a finely tuned state, there is a price to pay for interference with this, and drugs used to treat a neurological or psychological disorder inevitably have some undesirable side effects. The antipsychotic drugs are particularly bad in this respect. These side effects, collectively, are called extrapyramidal symptoms and divide into two main groups: the acute dystonias that develop in the first few weeks and reverse on stopping the drug; or tardive dyskinesia (tardive means "late"), which develops after months or years, and which does not reverse. Some of these acute dystonias resemble symptoms seen in ✪ **Parkinson's disease**, and are therefore termed "parkinsonian symptoms." These dystonias include tremor, slow movements and cog-wheel rigidity, akathisia ("restless-leg syndrome"), abnormal face movements (protruding tongue, head-turning, and wryneck), and other manifestations. Most or all of these dystonias are caused because antipsychotic drugs work by blocking dopamine receptors in the brain. Parkinson's disease is due largely to the depletion of dopamine in the brain, which leads to some similar symptoms. Some of these side effects can be controlled with other drugs or by careful control of dosage. However, the so-called "atypical" antipsychotics may have fewer side effects because they are more selective, more precise in which set of dopamine receptors are blocked. Tardive dyskinesia is a complex syndrome, characterized by sometimes disabling involuntary movements, and may resemble a worsening of the psychotic condition being treated. Although it develops only after the prolonged use of certain drugs, it is not usually reversible and is a major problem in antipsychotic treatment, and may even get worse if antipsychotic drug treatment is stopped. Its incidence depends greatly on dosage and the age of the person (being greater in those over 50), and the drug used ("atypical" antipsychotics are better in this respect). Further side effects of dopamine antagonists, including breast swelling, pain, and lactation in both sexes, are due to the blocking of certain subsets of dopamine receptors in the brain,.

Other side effects seen with certain antipsychotic drugs result from blocking of the actions of the neurotransmitter acetylcholine. These ℞ **anticholinergic** (antimuscarinic) side effects include a dry mouth, gastrointestinal upsets, and disturbances in vision, but are generally less marked with newer drugs.

For more details about side effects see the individual drug entries.

antipyretic ⓓ

Generics: **acetaminophen; aspirin; ibuprofen.**

Actions and uses

Antipyretic drugs are used to reduce raised body temperature, for example, in ✪ **fever**, but they do not lower normal body temperature. Most ℞ **NSAID** agents have antipyretic activity, but only some are used for this purpose. The best-known and most-used antipyretics (and ℞ **non-narcotic analgesics**) are ℞ **acetaminophen** (paracetamol), ℞ **aspirin**, and ℞ **ibuprofen**.

Limitations

Aspirin is no longer recommended for children because of a perceived risk of causing the rare, but serious, condition called ✪ **Reye's syndrome**. In general, where an ℞ anti-inflammatory analgesic and antipyretic is required for adults or children, ibuprofen is usually considered safe.

antirheumatic ⓓ

Generics: **aspirin; auranofin; aurothioglucose; azathiaprine; betamethasone; celecoxib; chloroquine; choline salicylate; cortisone; cyclosporine; dexamethasone; diclofenac; diflunisal; etodolac; fenoprofen; flurbiprofen; hydrocortisone; hydroxychloroquine sulfate; ibuprofen; indomethacin; infliximab; ketoprofen; ketorolac tromethamine; leflunomide; magnesium salicylate; meclofenamate sodium; mefenamic acid; meloxicam; methotrexate; methylprednisolone; nabumetone; naproxen; oxaprozin; penicillamine; piroxicam; prednisolone; prednisone; rofecoxib; salsalate; sodium salicylate; sulfasalazine; sulindac; tolmetin sodium; triamcinolone.**

Actions and uses

Antirheumatics are used to relieve the pain and inflammation of rheumatism and arthritis, particularly ✪ **rheumatoid arthritis** (antirheumatoid drugs) and ✪ **osteoarthritis**, and so they are also known as antiarthritic drugs (see also ✪ **musculoskeletal disorders**). The primary form of treatment is with ℞ **non-narcotic analgesic** drugs of the ℞ **NSAID** group (non-steroidal anti-inflammatory drugs), such as ℞ **aspirin**, ℞ **ibuprofen**, ℞ **fenoprofen**, ℞ **naproxen**, ℞ **indomethacin**, and ℞ **celecoxib**. Some members of the ℞ **corticosteroid** group can also be used because of their ℞ **anti-inflammatory** activity (for example, ℞ **prednisolone**, ℞ **triamcinolone**).

There are some drugs that act as disease-modifying arthritis drugs that halt the progression of certain musculoskeletal disorders, for example ℞ **gold compound** preparations (for example, ℞ **auranofin** and ℞ **aurothioglucose**). Some ℞ **immunosuppressant** drugs may be used (for example, ℞ **cyclosporine**, ℞ **leflunomide**, ℞ **methotrexate**), also the new ℞ **immunomodulator** agents ℞ **etanercept** and infliximab (used with methotrexate). Other disease-modifying drugs sometimes used include ℞ **penicillamine**, ℞ **sulfasalazine**, ℞ **chloroquine**, and ℞ **hydroxychloroquine sulfate**.

Limitations

Some of these drugs have unpleasant side effects and others can take up to 6 months to have any beneficial effect. Treatment should be supervised by specialists. See also ✪ **musculoskeletal disorders**.

antiseborrheic ⓓ

coal tar; ketoconazole; lithium; salicylic acid; selenium sulfide; sulfacetamide; sulfur; zinc sulfate.

Actions and uses

Antiseborrheic drugs are used to treat ✪ **seborrhea**, a disorder caused by overproduction of the oily secretion (sebum) of the sebaceous glands. These glands swell, especially on the face, and the skin becomes oily, which tends to cause ✪ **acne**. The skin also scales and this causes ○ **dandruff**. In a similar disorder—seborrheic dermatitis—there are scaly plaques over areas of skin where there are many sebaceous glands.

In both cases, medicated ℞ **skin preparations** may help. Shampoos containing ℞ **keratolytic** drugs (℞ **coal tar**) that dissolve away some of the outer layer of the skin may help, including drugs that combine antimicrobial and keratolytic activity (often ℞ **sulfur** or ℞ **selenium sulfide**). An infective component can be specifically treated with preparations containing an ℞ **antibacterial** such as a ℞ **sulfonamide** (℞ **sulfacetamide**) or other ℞ **antimicrobial** agent (℞ **ketoconazole**). Sometimes topical (external) ℞ **corticosteroid** preparations may be used.

Limitations

Most of these treatments are relatively free of side effects because they are applied externally, but they should not be used on broken skin or very inflamed areas. Some, for instance coal tar, may cause irritation and initially the condition may worsen. If the condition does not improve after regular use, the preparation should not be used any more.

antiseptic ⓓ

Generics: **cetylpyridinium chloride; chlorhexidine; chloroxylenol; gentian violet; glutaraldehyde; hexachlorophene; hexylresorcinol; hydrogen peroxide; iodine; povidone-iodine; phenol; silver sulfadiazine; sodium hypochlorite; sodium perborate; thymol; triclosan.**

Actions and uses

Antiseptic agents are used to destroy microorganisms or inhibit their activity to such an extent that they are less, or no longer, harmful to health. Antiseptics can be used to prevent ○ **infections** and to limit the spread of pathogenic (disease-causing) microorganisms. The term is often used synonymously with ℞ **disinfectant**. However, the latter term can also apply to agents used on inanimate objects (such as surgical equipment), as well as for agents used on the skin and other living tissue.

A number of antiseptics are sufficiently mild, or can be used at low enough concentrations, for use as a mouthwash for oral hygiene (because they inhibit odor-forming bacteria), for ○ **gingivitis**, the relief of minor oral inflammation such as canker sores (ulcers), denture irritation, and post-dental procedure irritation. Examples include ℞ **thymol**, ℞ **hydrogen peroxide**, ℞ **carbamide peroxide**, ℞ **hexylresorcinol**, ℞ **chlorhexidine**, ℞ **sodium perborate**, and ℞ **cetylpyridinium chloride**.

Other antiseptics are more commonly used by topical application to the skin. They can be used to prevent minor staphylococcal infections, and for cleaning and relief of pain from minor burns, insect bites or inflammation. Examples include, ℞ **silver sulfadiazine**, ℞ **chloroxylenol**, ℞ **triclosan**, ℞ **phenol**, ℞ **gentian violet**, ♧ **iodine**, and ℞ **povidone**.

Further agents are relatively strong and can be irritant. However, they can be used as disinfectants, and are used for such purposes as surgical scrubs and cleansers, for example, ℞ **hexachlorophene**, ℞ **sodium hypochlorite**, and ℞ **glutaraldehyde**.

Limitations

Even the mildest of these agents can cause irritation to sensitive skin, especially a baby's skin. Antiseptics, in general, are probably overused. Traditionally, they have been applied to abrasions and wounds in the belief that they will help healing. In fact the reverse is true; all these agents—if used in a strong enough solution to kill all germs—can inhibit the invasion of white blood cells, which help in dealing with pathogenic (disease-causing) microorganisms, and therefore inhibit subsequent wound-healing. In many circumstances, a sterile (dry for burns) dressing, after appropriate washing, is probably sufficient.

antiserum ⓓ

see ℞ **antitoxin**.

Antispas ⓡ

A preparation of ℞ **dicyclomine hydrochloride**.
Formulation: Injection.
Availability: Prescription only.
Warnings and side effects: See ℞ **dicyclomine hydrochloride**.

antispasmodic ⓓ

Generics: **atropine sulfate; dicyclomine hydrochloride; flavoxate hydrochloride; glycopyrrolate; hyoscyamine; oxybutynin; peppermint oil; tolterodine tartrate.**

Actions and uses

Antispasmodic (spasmolytic) drugs relieve spasm in smooth muscle (for example, muscles in the intestinal walls, the respiratory tract, and the uterus) and form part of the group of drugs known collectively as ℞ **smooth muscle relaxant** agents. Some are used to relieve abdominal pain due to intestinal ○ **colic**, some to help relieve the discomfort of ○ **dysmenorrhea**, and others as ℞ **bronchodilator** drugs, for example, in the treatment of ○ **asthma**. They can also be used, along with other drugs, as an additional treatment of non-ulcer dyspepsia (○ **indigestion**), ○ **diverticular disease**, and ○ **irritable bowel syndrome**. They include the ℞ **anticholinergic** drugs, such as ℞ **atropine sulfate**, ℞ **hyoscyamine**, ℞ **dicyclomine hydrochloride**, ℞ **flavoxate hydrochloride**, ℞ **mepenzolate bromide**, ℞ **methantheline bromide**, ℞ **glycopyrrolate**, and ℞ **dicyclomine hydrochloride**. Other agents include ℞ **peppermint oil**, which may be used to relieve ○ **colic** and the symptoms of irritable bowel syndrome.

Limitations

See the individual drug entries.

antisympathetic ⓓ

Generics: **clonidine hydrochloride; guanabenz acetate; guanethidine monosulfate; guanfacine hydrochloride; methyldopa; metirosine.**

Actions and uses

Antisympathetics act at particular sites within the sympathetic nervous system to reduce its overall effect. Since activity within this division of the (autonomic) nervous system controls blood pressure and heart rate, drugs that act to reduce its activity cause a fall in blood pressure. Their main use, therefore, is as ℞ **antihypertensive** drugs in the treatment of ⊙ **hypertension**.

There are a number of sites and mechanisms by which such drugs act. Some work within the central nervous system (CNS) to reduce the activity of the sympathetic nervous system. For instance, ℞ **clonidine hydrochloride**, ℞ **guanfacine hydrochloride** and ℞ **guanabenz acetate** are selective alpha$_2$-subtype ℞ **alpha-adrenergic stimulants**, and act within the brain to decrease neurotransmitter output. This in turn lowers blood pressure—and is, therefore, a useful way to reduce hypertension. Similarly, ℞ **methyldopa** is converted within the body to a metabolite with this action. ℞ **metirosine** inhibits one of the enzymes (tyrosine hydroxylase) that produce norepinephrine (the sympathetic neurotransmitter) within nerves. Another distinct class of drugs, the ℞ **adrenergic-neuron blocker** drugs (for example, ℞ **guanethidine monosulphate**) work to interfere with the storage and release of norepinephrine.

Limitations
All these drugs have quite marked side effects and some of them may be used at the same time as other classes of antihypertensives, for instance ℞ **diuretic** drugs. See the individual drug entries.

antithrombin III human ⑥
Type/Group: **anticoagulant**.
Brand(s): Thrombate III.
How administered: Intravenous infusion.

Used to treat
Antithrombin III is a natural anticoagulant in the body. It inhibits the action of several clotting enzymes that activate thrombin, which is needed for the final stages of blood coagulation. In people with hereditary deficiency of this thrombin inhibitor (an uncommon condition), antithrombin III is used in surgery or obstetrical procedures to lower the risk of ⊙ **thrombosis**, and to treat ⊙ **pulmonary embolism**.

Warnings
• There are no special cautions. It will be given by experienced personnel after a full medical assessment.
• It should be used during pregnancy only if it is clearly needed.
• Medical judgment is required if breast-feeding is being considered.
• As with most substances that are derived from human blood plasma, there is risk of exposure to viral infection (for example, AIDS and hepatitis A, B, and C). Infection with hepatitis C is the most likely.

Interactions
• The anticoagulant effect of ℞ **heparin** is enhanced, with the potential for bleeding (heparin dosage should be reduced).

Side effects
• These are uncommon and may include dizziness, chest tightness, nausea, foul taste in the mouth, chills or cramps. Rarely, fever, hives, and shortness of breath have been reported.

antithrombotic ⑩
see ℞ **anticoagulant**.

antithyroid ⑩
(thyroid antagonist)
Generics: **iodine; methimazole; propranolol hydrochloride; propylthiouracil; thyrotropin.**

Actions and uses
℞ **antithyroid** drugs are used in the treatment of an over-active thyroid gland (⊙ **hyperthyroidism**; thyrotoxicosis). In thyrotoxicosis there is an excess secretion of ℞ **thyroid hormone** and this results in an exaggeration of the normal activity of the gland, which causes increased metabolic rate, raised body temperature, sweating, increased sensitivity to heat, nervousness, tremor, raised heart rate, tendency to fatigue, and sometimes loss of body weight with an increased appetite.

How the disease is treated depends on its cause. However, if it is severe then surgical removal of part of the gland may be necessary, although more commonly the gland is treated with radioactive iodine (I^{131}) to reduce the number of cells. Drugs are used to either control the symptoms in the long term, or in the short term to prepare the gland for more radical intervention. For this purpose, ℞ **beta-blocker** drugs (usually ℞ **propranolol hydrochloride**) are used in the prevention of a number of the signs and symptoms of thyrotoxicosis. They work by blocking the effects of over-stimulation caused by the release of epinephrine and norepinephrine by ℞ **thyroid hormones**, but do not treat the cause of the problem in the thyroid gland itself.

Some other drugs, ℞ **methimazole** and ℞ **propylthiouracil**, act as indirect ℞ **hormone antagonist** agents by inhibiting the thyroid gland's production of thyroid hormones, so preventing an excess of thyroid hormone entering the blood, and are therefore useful in the treatment of the symptoms caused by excess thyroid hormones. They are also used to lessen hyperthyroidism in preparation for surgery or radiation therapy. Iodine, which is chemically incorporated into the two thyroid hormones thyroxine and triiodothyronine, can be given to suppress gland activity prior to thyroid surgery.

As a ℞ **diagnostic agent**, use can be made of ℞ **thyrotropin** (thyroid-stimulating-hormone; TSH), the ℞ **anterior pituitary hormone** that controls the release of thyroid hormones from the thyroid gland. It can be used as a drug to identify cases of thyroid failure and to establish a diagnosis of decreased thyroid reserve.

Limitations
See the individual drug entries.

antitoxin ⑩
(antiserum)
Generics: **diphtheria antitoxin.**

Actions and uses
Antitoxin refers to antibody material (generally called antiserum) that reacts with the toxin released by a bacterium (rather than to the bacterium itself), and the same term (antitoxin or more specifically ℞ **antivenin**) is used for antibodies raised to the toxins contained in snake or spider bites. The antiserum produced can be used to provide passive immunity to people who have been exposed, and works, in the short-term only, as a sort of ℞ **antidote** by neutralizing the toxin. However, since antitoxin material is gen-

erally produced in horses, hypersensitivity reactions are common (because the impure preparations contain "foreign" horse protein). For this reason, where there is a choice, ℞ **immune globulin** containing antibodies from human blood are generally preferred (for example, ✪ **tetanus** ℞ **immune globulin** (TIE)), even when it is technically possible to manufacture antitoxins in animals (this is generally true when the organism produces an exotoxin, a particularly potent toxin that is released from the parasite to work at a distance). Snake and spider venom antitoxins are available from special centers, along with ℞ **diphtheria antitoxin**.

Limitations
Local or systemic allergic hypersensitivity reactions can occur where the immune globulin has been prepared in an animal species (for example, horse for diphtheria antitoxin).

antitrichomonal ⑩
see ℞ amebicide and antiprotozoal.

antitubercular ⑩
see ℞ antituberculosis.

antituberculosis ⑩
(antitubercular)
Generics: **BCG vaccine; capreomycin; cycloserine; ethambutol; isoniazid; pyrazinamide; rifampicin; streptomycin.**

Actions and uses
Antituberculosis (or antituberculous) drugs are used, generally in combination, to treat ✪ **tuberculosis**.

Treatment is either primary (first round of treatment) or retreatment (a more serious return of infection, which might denote resistance to the usual drugs).

Primary drugs are ℞ **isoniazid**, ℞ **rifampicin**, ℞ **ethambutol**, ℞ **pyrazinamide**, and ℞ **streptomycin**. These are used in combinations of two or more (usually isoniazid and rifampicin) in order to tackle the disease as efficiently as possible, while reducing the risk of encountering bacterial resistance. Usually, bactericidal (destructive to organism) drugs (for instance, isoniazid/rifampicin, and pyrazinamide/streptomycin) and bacteriostatic (prevents growth of organism) drugs (for instance, ethambutol and cycloserine) are used in combination—the former to sterilize the lesions. The long-form regimen of treatment can last up to 24 months, while the short-form regimen is for 9 months.

Retreatment drugs include ℞ **cycloserine**, ℞ **capreomycin**, and, rarely, a number of more specialized drugs, including ℞ **kanamycin**, ethionamide, and ℞ **aminosalicylate** (p-amino-salicyclic acid; PAS).

Limitations
If treatment is not successful, for example, because the person suffers intolerable side effects or because the disease was resistant to treatment, then other drugs are used. Some unusual drugs, or agents that have fallen out of use, are used when there are difficult or resistant strains—which is an increasing problem.

Drug treatment of tuberculosis is necessary where the far more effective public health measure of vaccination has, for some reason, failed (see ℞ **BCG vaccine**).

antitussive ⑩
Generics: **codeine phosphate; dextromethorphan; hydrocodone bitartrate; hydromorphone hydrochloride; morphine sulfate; oxymorphone hydrochloride**. Expectorants include: **antihistamine; guaifenesin; ipecac syrup**. Demulcents: **glycerin**.

Actions and uses
Cough suppressants are antitussives that work on the coughing center in the brain. They include the (℞ **opioid**) ℞ **opiate** drugs ℞ **codeine phosphate**, ℞ **dextromethorphan**, ℞ **morphine sulfate**, ℞ **hydrocodone bitartrate**, and ℞ **oxymorphone hydrochloride**. They are very effective, but tend to cause constipation as a side effect and so should not be used for prolonged periods. Some of these are available as OTC (over-the-counter) preparations, but others are prescription-only.

Where the cough is "productive," other drugs are available, which are incorporated into cough preparations and ℞ **cold and cough preparation** remedies. These drugs, which are not strictly antitussives, include ℞ **expectorant** agents, which decrease the viscosity of mucus. They also increase the secretion of liquid mucus in dry, irritant, unproductive coughs. These include ℞ **guaifenesin** and ℞ **ipecac syrup** (ipecacuanha), although there is doubt about their effectiveness. In serious conditions where there may be coughing (for instance, in cystic fibrosis, pneumonia, or chronic bronchopulmonary disease) a more effective ℞ **mucolytic** drug may be needed.

Sedative members of the ℞ **antihistamine** group are incorporated into many proprietary cough preparations. These may work by drying up secretions or by virtue of their sedative actions, so allowing sleep and, therefore, some relief from coughing.

℞ **demulcent** agents are preparations that soothe or protect mucous membranes, and substances such as syrup, honey, and ℞ **glycerin** are sometimes incorporated into cough remedies.

Limitations
Because the physiological function of coughing is to clear phlegm and mucus from the airways, it is generally recommended that only dry coughs are treated with antitussives of the opioid type. Where the cough is "productive," the other drugs mentioned should be used. See also the individual drug entries.

Anti-Tuss Syrup ⑧
A preparation of ℞ **guaifenesin**.
Formulation: Oral syrup.
Availability: OTC.
Warnings and side effects: See ℞ **guaifenesin**.

antivenin ⑩
(antivenom)
Actions and uses
Antivenin (antivenom) is an ℞ **antidote** to the poison in a snakebite, a scorpion's sting, or a bite from any other poisonous creature (such as a black widow spider). Normally, it is an ℞ **antitoxin** that is injected into the bloodstream for immediate relief through passive immunization. Identification of the poisonous creature is important so that the right antidote can be selected. In the US the

most common venomous snakes are members of the family *Crotalidae* (rattlesnakes, copperheads, water moccasins), although venomous bites are also inflicted by the North American coral snake (*Microbus flurries*). Antivenins for these species are generally available, as well as for spider bites by the black widow (*Lactrodectus mactans*). Antivenins for more exotic species are available through the Centers for Disease Control (CDC). They are given by injection or intravenous infusion, and treatment is under specialist supervision.

Limitations

Because antivenoms are themselves foreign proteins (usually derived from horse serum), hypersensitivity reactions (including ✪ **anaphylactic reactions**) are not uncommon and may exacerbate the symptoms and distress caused by the bite itself, and so antivenoms are only used where symptoms are severe. There may be preliminary testing for hypersensitivity to horse serum.

antivenin (antivenom) Ⓖ

Type/Group: **antidote**.

How administered: Injection; intravenous infusion.

Used to treat

Antivenin is an antidote to the poison in a snakebite, a scorpion's sting, or a bite from any other poisonous creature (such as a spider). Normally, it is an ℞ **antitoxin** that is injected into the bloodstream for immediate relief through passive immunization. Identification of the poisonous creature is important so that the right antidote can be selected. In the US the most common venomous snakes are members of the family *Crotalidae* (rattlesnakes, copperheads, water moccasins), although venomous bites are also inflicted by the North American coral snake (*Micrurus fulvius*). Antivenins for these species are generally available, as well as for spider bites by the black widow (*Lactrodectus mactans*). Antivenins for more exotic species are available through the Centers for Disease Control (CDC).

Warnings

• Treatment is under specialist conditions.

• Because antivenoms are themselves foreign proteins (usually derived from horse serum) hypersensitivity reactions (including anaphylactic shock) are not uncommon and may exacerbate the symptoms and distress caused by the bite itself, therefore antivenoms are only used where symptoms are severe.

• There may be preliminary testing for hypersensitivity to horse serum.

antivenom Ⓓ

see ℞ **antivenin**.

Antivert; Antivert/25; Antivert/50 Ⓑ

A preparation of ℞ **meclizine hydrochloride**.

Formulation: Oral tablets, 3 strengths.

Availability: Prescription only.

Warnings and side effects: See ℞ **meclizine hydrochloride**.

antiviral Ⓓ

Generics: **abacavir; acyclovir; amantadine; amprenavir; cidofovir; didanosine (ddl); efavirenz; famciclovir; foscarnet sodium; ganciclovir (DHPG); idoxuridine; imiquimod; indinavir; interferons; lamivudine; nelfinavir; nevirapine; palivizumab; penciclovir; ribavirin; rimantadine; ritonavir; saquinavir; stavudine; trifluridine; valacyclovir; zalcitabine; zanamivir; zidovudine**.

Actions and uses

℞ **antiviral** drugs are used to treat infections caused by viruses, which are microorganisms much smaller than bacteria, so minute they cannot be seen under the normal (light) microscope. They can only replicate within the living cells of the host that they parasitize. Drugs of the ℞ **antibiotic** group have no effect against viruses, and treatment of infection is only possible with some relatively new antiviral drugs. In the recent past, the use of antivirals was restricted to preventive or disease-limitation treatment (for example, ℞ **acyclovir** against herpes viruses). However, some recently developed antiviral drugs can be lifesavers, or at least prolong life, especially in immunocompromised patients. A great deal of effort is currently being made to develop antivirals for use in the treatment of HIV infection, but ✪ **AIDS** treatment also relies heavily on drugs active against bacterial, fungal, or other opportunist microbial infections.

Antivirals can be divided into groups on the basis of how they work. Most currently used antiviral drugs are only effective when the viruses are replicating. Some are nucleoside analogs (or related compounds) which resemble cellular molecules necessary to viral function or replication, often working as ℞ **enzyme** inhibitors against essential viral enzymes because some viral enzymes are virus-specific, so antiviral drugs can target them without affecting the person too much. For example, the group of antivirals modeled on the natural nucleosides involved in cell division and replication, which work against the enzyme reverse transcriptase are termed reverse-transcriptase inhibitors (for example, ℞ **didanosine**, ℞ **lamivudine**, ℞ **stavudine**, and ℞ **zidovudine**). Some even later drugs (the non-nucleoside group) which chemically are not actually nucleosides (for example, ℞ **efavirenz**, ℞ **nevirapine**) but which also work as reverse-transcriptase inhibitors. Some other antivirals prevent viral cell replication by inhibiting nucleic acid synthesis (DNA polymerase inhibitors) and these include the first extensively used antiviral drug, ℞ **acyclovir**, and also ℞ **foscarnet sodium** and ℞ **ganciclovir**.

The most recently introduced group of antivirals, the protease inhibitors, work as enzyme inhibitors acting against an enzyme (HIV-1 protease) which is essential for the replication of viruses. Examples of this group include ℞ **indinavir**, ℞ **ritonavir**, ℞ **nelfinavir**, ℞ **amprenavir**, and ℞ **saquinavir**.

There are a number of other types of antivirals that work in a different ways. For instance, ℞ **palivizumab**, one of a relatively new class of drug, is a monoclonal antibody (a form of pure antibody produced by a type of molecular engineering) that neutralizes the respiratory syncytial virus (RSV), which is sometimes responsible for serious lower respiratory disease in infants. The ℞ **interferons** are ℞ **immunomodulator** agents that help the body's immunological defenses against infections and other diseases, and some drugs of this type are being tried against viral hepatitis infections (including interferon alfa-2b, interferon beta, and interferon alfacon-1).

In clinical practice, antivirals are often grouped by the types of infection against which they are effective (rather than by how they work). However, HIV infections are increasingly being treated by a combination of drugs chosen from several different drug groups, for instance protease inhibitors together with reverse-transcriptase inhibitors. Since protease inhibitor and reverse-transcriptase inhibitor drugs work against a retrovirus (a RNA virus), these drugs are sometimes referred to as antiretroviral agents.

Infections due to the ✪ **herpes** viruses (for example, cold sores, eye infections, genital herpes, shingles, and chickenpox) may be contained by early treatment with ℞ **acyclovir**, ℞ **famciclovir**, ℞ **idoxuridine** ℞ **penciclovir**, ℞ **trifluridine**, or ℞ **valaciclovir**. Serious cytomegaloviral (CMV) infections may be contained by treatment with ℞ **ganciclovir** and ℞ **foscarnet sodium**. ℞ **Ribavirin**, which inhibits a wide range of DNA and RNA viruses, can be used to treat respiratory syncytial virus (RSV) in infants and children, which causes severe lower respiratory tract infections. Some antiviral drugs are active against ✪ **influenza** A or B virus, including ℞ **amantadine**, ℞ **rimantadine**, and ℞ **zanamivir** (which works by inhibiting a viral neuraminidase enzyme essential for viral replication).

Limitations

Many of these antiviral drugs have major side effects and most of them are used under specialist supervision in hospital. Full assessment of a person's particular circumstances and suitability will be carried out, and an explanation of the possible side effects will be given. In terms of public health, prevention of viral infection is best achieved by ℞ **vaccination** (for example, against poliomyelitis, rubella, measles and mumps, and some types of rabies), but continual mutation of other viruses makes vaccination more difficult (for example, flu, the common cold, HIV). See also the individual drug entries.

Antizol Ⓑ

A preparation of ℞ **fomepizole**.
Formulation: Injection.
Availability: Prescription only.
Warnings and side effects: See ℞ **fomepizole**.

Antrizine Tablets Ⓑ

A preparation of ℞ **meclizine hydrochloride**.
Formulation: Oral tablets.
Availability: Prescription only.
Warnings and side effects: See ℞ **meclizine hydrochloride**.

Anturane Ⓑ

A preparation of ℞ **sulfinpyrazone**.
Formulation: Oral tablets; oral capsules.
Availability: Prescription only.
Warnings and side effects: See ℞ **sulfinpyrazone**.

Anumed HC Ⓑ

A preparation of ℞ **hydrocortisone**.
Formulation: Rectal suppository.
Availability: Prescription only.
Warnings and side effects: See ℞ **hydrocortisone**.

Anusol-HC Ⓑ

A preparation of ℞ **hydrocortisone**.
Formulation: Cream.
Availability: Prescription only.
Warnings and side effects: See ℞ **hydrocortisone**.

Anusol HC-1 Ⓑ

A preparation of ℞ **hydrocortisone** and ℞ **urea**.
Formulation: Cream; ointment.
Availability: Prescription only.
Warnings and side effects: See ℞ **hydrocortisone**; ℞ **urea**.

anxiolytic Ⓓ

see ℞ **antianxiety**.

Apacet Chewable Tablets; Solution Ⓑ

A preparation of ℞ **acetaminophen**.
Formulation: Chewable tablets; solution.
Availability: OTC.
Warnings and side effects: See ℞ **acetaminophen**.

APAP-Plus Tablets Ⓑ

A preparation of ℞ **acetaminophen** and ℞ **caffeine**.
Formulation: Oral tablets.
Availability: OTC.
Warnings and side effects: See ℞ **acetaminophen**; ℞ **caffeine**.

A.P.L. Ⓑ

A preparation of ℞ **chorionic gonadotropin**.
Formulation: Injection.
Availability: Prescription only.
Warnings and side effects: See ℞ **chorionic gonadotropin**.

appetite stimulant Ⓓ

Generics: **desipramine hydrochloride; fluoxetine; megestrol acetate**.

Actions and uses

Appetite stimulant treatment usually relies on treating an underlying disorder. However, the ℞ **progestin** agent ℞ **megestrol acetate** has been used as a treatment for ✪ **appetite loss**, emaciation, or unexplained serious weight loss in ✪ **AIDS** patients.

Where the apparent loss of appetite is thought to be due to ✪ **anorexia nervosa**, a number of antidepressants have been used, including some from the ℞ **tricyclic** group (including ℞ **desipramine**) and the newer ℞ **SSRI** group (including ℞ **fluoxetine**).

Recently, ℞ **dronabinol**, a psychoactive constituent of marijuana (*Cannabis sativa*) that stimulates appetite has been introduced for purposes that include the restoration of appetite where there is appetite loss in persons with AIDS.

Limitations

See the individual drug entries.

appetite suppressant ⓓ

(anorectic)

Generics: **karaya; methamphetamine; methylcellulose; phendimetrazine; phentermine; psyllium; sibutramine; sterculia gum.**

Actions and uses

Appetite suppressant (anorectic) drugs are used in ⊕ **obesity** (see ℞ **obesity treatment**) and fall into three main types.

The first type works by acting on the brain to reduce appetite, and a number of these drugs are related to amphetamine, and some ℞ **sympathomimetic** drugs of this class were once used extensively in appetite suppressant treatment (for example, dextroamphetamine and amphetamine), but there is a tendency for those who use stimulant drugs on a regular basis to become dependant and show a withdrawal syndrome when they stop taking them, so such preparations are no longer prescribed for this purpose. However, some amphetamine-related CNS (central nervous system) stimulants are sometimes used for the short-term treatment of obesity (occasionally ℞ **methamphetamine**, but usually ℞ **phentermine** and ℞ **phendimetrazine**).

The second type also works on the brain to modify appetite, and is represented by the newly introduced agent ℞ **sibutramine**, which works by inhibiting reuptake of norepinephrine, serotonin, and dopamine in the central nervous system (a similar activity to certain ℞ **antidepressant** drugs).

The third type works by bulking out the food eaten, so it feels that more has been eaten. ℞ **bulk-forming agent** OTC (over-the-counter) drugs include ℞ **methylcellulose**, ℞ **karaya** (sterculia gum), and ℞ **psyllium** (psyllium hydrophilic mucilloid). See also ℞ **obesity treatment**.

Limitations

Amphetamines have a considerable abuse potential, and they are placed in the Drug Enforcement Agency Schedule II category, which is reserved for drugs with a high abuse risk. Apart from the risk of habituation, there may be long-term personality changes, hypertensive crises, and damage to heart valves. Treatment with these drugs should be short term only, and there is also a growing doubt among experts over the medical value of such a treatment (for instance, there may be "rebound" weight gain once the treatment is over). The bulking agents tend to have ℞ **laxative** actions. A similar approach is to incorporate more fiber-containing foodstuffs (for example, vegetables and bran) into the diet. Both types of drug are intended to assist in the medical treatment of obesity, where the primary therapy is an appropriate diet.

apraclonidine ⓖ

Type/Group: **alpha-adrenergic stimulant.**
Brand(s): Iopidine.
How administered: Topically (eyes).

Used to treat

Apraclonidine is a derivative of ℞ **clonidine hydrochloride** and reduces the rate of production of aqueous humor (fluid) in the eyeball. It is used to control or prevent an increase of pressure in the eyeball (intraocular pressure) after laser surgery and as a short-term, additional treatment for people who require further reduction of intraocular pressure.

Warnings

• It should not be given to people with known hypersensitivity to apraclonidine or clonidine, or who are taking ℞ **MAOIs**.
• It should be given with caution to people with a history of vasovagal attack, severe cardiovascular disease, impaired kidney function, and depression.
• Apraclonidine's safety during pregnancy has not been established. It should be used only if the potential benefit outweighs the possible risk to the fetus.
• Medical judgment is required if breast-feeding is being considered. It is not known whether it appears in breast milk.
• Its effectiveness in lowering intraocular pressure may decrease over time in some people.
• If allergic-like symptoms in the eye occur (redness, itching, discomfort, swelling of eyelids and conjunctiva), treatment should be stopped.
• It can cause sleepiness and dizziness, and so impair the performance of skilled tasks, such as driving.

Interactions

• If taken with cardiovascular agents, apraclonidine may further reduce pulse rate and blood pressure.
• MAOIs should not be used with apraclonidine because their effects may be increased.

Side effects

• Occasionally, increased blood flow to the eye, itching, tearing, discomfort, swelling, dry mouth, and foreign body sensation.
• Since apraclonidine can be absorbed through the eye into the body, there could be systemic effects, for instance on the cardiovascular system (for example palpitations).

Apresazide 25/25; 50/50; 100/50 ⓑ

A preparation of ℞ **hydralazine hydrochloride** and ℞ **hydrochlorothiazide**.
Formulation: Oral tablets, in 3 (hydralazine/hydrochlorthiazide) strengths.
Availability: Prescription only.
Warnings and side effects: See ℞ **hydralazine hydrochloride**; ℞ **hydrochlorothiazide**.

Apresoline Tablets; Injection ⓑ

A preparation of ℞ **hydralazine hydrochloride**.
Formulation: Oral tablets (in four strengths); injection.
Availability: Prescription only.
Warnings and side effects: See ℞ **hydralazine hydrochloride**. The 100mg tablet contains tartrazine (FD&C yellow No. 5), a dye that may cause allergic reaction in a few people, but especially those with sensitivity to aspirin.

Aprodine Tablets; Syrup ®

A preparation of ℞ **pseudoephedrine** and ℞ **triprolidine hydrochloride**.
Formulation: Oral tablets; syrup.
Availability: OTC.
Warnings and side effects: See ℞ **pseudoephedrine**; ℞ **triprolidine hydrochloride**.

Aprodine w/Codeine Cough Syrup ®

A preparation of ℞ **codeine phosphate**, ℞ **pseudoephedrine**, and ℞ **triprolidine hydrochloride**.
Formulation: Oral syrup.
Availability: May or may not require a prescription.
Warnings and side effects: See ℞ **codeine phosphate**; ℞ **pseudoephedrine**; ℞ **triprolidine hydrochloride**.

aprotinin ©

Type/Group: hemostatic.
Brand(s): Trasylol.
How administered: Intravenous injection or infusion.

Used to treat

Aprotinin is a natural enzyme inhibitor that has antithrombolytic activity—it inhibits the proteolytic enzymes that normally dissolve blood clots. Medically, it can be used to reduce blood loss in people having repeated heart bypass surgery and in selected cases of a first bypass operation.

Warnings

• It should not be given to people with known hypersensitivity to this drug. It will be given by experienced personnel after a full medical assessment.
• Aprotinin should be used during pregnancy only when it is clearly needed.
• Medical judgment is required if breast-feeding is being considered.
• A small test dose is recommended before use, and if an allergic reaction occurs, it should not be used.

Interactions

• Aprotinin may block the hypotensive effect of ℞ **captopril**.
• It may inhibit the clot-dissolving effects of ℞ **thrombolytic** agents.
• If taken with ℞ **heparin**, clotting time may be prolonged.

Side effects

• Adverse reactions are uncommon and may include fever, asthma, shortness of breath or phlebitis. Although not frequent there may be hypersensitivity reactions (including anaphylaxis), effects on heart function or rhythm, an increase in blood-clotting time, and kidney or liver damage.

APSAC ©

see ℞ **anistreplase**.

Aqua-Ban; Aqua-Ban Plus ®

A preparation of ℞ **ammonium chloride**, ℞ **caffeine**, and ℞ **ferrous sulfate** (Aqua-Ban Plus).
Formulation: Oral tablets, available in two strengths.
Availability: OTC.
Warnings and side effects: See ℞ **ammonium chloride**; ℞ **caffeine**; ℞ **ferrous sulfate**.

Aquachloral ®

A preparation of ℞ **chloral hydrate**.
Formulation: Rectal suppositories.
Availability: Prescription only.
Warnings and side effects: See ℞ **chloral hydrate**.

AquaMEPHYTON ®

A preparation of ℞ **phytonadione**.
Formulation: Injection.
Availability: Prescription only.
Warnings and side effects: See ℞ **phytonadione**.

Aquaphyllin ®

A preparation of ℞ **theophylline**.
Formulation: Oral syrup.
Availability: Prescription only.
Warnings and side effects: See ℞ **theophylline**.

Aquatab DM ®

A preparation of ℞ **dextromethorphan** and ℞ **guaifenesin**.
Formulation: Oral tablets.
Availability: Prescription only.
Warnings and side effects: See ℞ **dextromethorphan**; ℞ **guaifenesin**.

Aqua Tar ®

A preparation of ℞ **coal tar**.
Formulation: Topical gel.
Availability: OTC.
Warnings and side effects: See ℞ **coal tar**.

Aquatensen ®

A preparation of ℞ **methyclothiazide**.
Formulation: Oral tablets.
Availability: Prescription only.
Warnings and side effects: See ℞ **methyclothiazide**.

Aralen Phosphate; Aralen Hydrochloride ®

A preparation of ℞ **chloroquine**.
Formulation: Oral tablets (Phospate); injection (Hydrochloride).
Availability: Prescription only.
Warnings and side effects: See ℞ **chloroquine**.

Aramine ®

A preparation of ℞ **metaraminol**.
Formulation: Injection (usually intravenous infusion).
Availability: Prescription only.
Warnings and side effects: See ℞ **metaraminol**. This drug contains sodium bisulfite, which may cause serious allergic reaction (eg, hives, wheezing, anaphylaxis) in susceptible individuals.

Arava ®

A preparation of ℞ **leflunomide**.
Formulation: Oral tablets, available in 3 strengths.
Availability: Prescription only.
Warnings and side effects: See ℞ **leflunomide**.

ardeparin sodium ©

Type/Group: **anticoagulant**.
Brand(s): Normiflo.
How administered: Injection (subcutaneous).

Used to treat

Ardeparin sodium is a low molecular weight heparin, an anticoagulant. It can be used to prevent ☉ **deep vein thrombosis** after knee replacement surgery, to lower the chance of complications from embolism.

Warnings

• It should not be given to people with known hypersensitivity to this drug or to pork products, with active major bleeding, or where lab testing shows antibodies to platelets when taking this drug. It will be administered by experienced personnel after a full medical assessment.

• It should be given with caution to people with an increased risk of hemorrhage (for example, uncontrolled hypertension, bleeding disorders, active ulcer, recent stroke, or surgery), and in those who have experienced a reduction of platelet (thrombocyte) levels after taking heparin. It should be given with caution to anyone with a tendency to bleed or recent gastrointestinal bleeding, with low thrombocyte levels or platelet defects, or with severe kidney or liver impairment.

• It should be used during pregnancy only if the potential benefit outweighs the possible risk to the fetus.

• Medical judgment is required if breast-feeding is being considered. It is not known whether this drug appears in breast milk.

Interactions

• If taken with other anticoagulants, ℞ **antiplatelet** agents, or ℞ **NSAIDs**, there is a higher potential for bleeding (caution is advised).

Side effects

• The most common are hematoma (a trapped accumulation of blood) at the injection site and post-operative bleeding, which may occasionally occur at non-surgical sites, particularly in the gastrointestinal tract. There may be changes in liver function, headache, dizziness, and allergic reactions (for example, rash, itching, fever).

Aredia ®

A preparation of ℞ **pamidronate disodium**.
Formulation: Injection.
Availability: Prescription only.
Warnings and side effects: See ℞ **pamidronate disodium**.

Arfonad ®

A preparation of ℞ **trimethaphan camsylate**.
Formulation: Intravenous infusion.

Availability: Prescription only.
Warnings and side effects: See ℞ **trimethaphan camsylate**.

Argesic Cream ®

A preparation of ℞ **methyl salicylate** and various.
Formulation: Topical cream.
Availability: OTC.
Warnings and side effects: See ℞ **methyl salicylate**.

Argesic-SA Tablets ®

A preparation of ℞ **salsalate**.
Formulation: Oral tablets.
Availability: Prescription only.
Warnings and side effects: See ℞ **salsalate**.

Aricept ®

A preparation of ℞ **donepezil**.
Formulation: Oral tablets.
Availability: Prescription only.
Warnings and side effects: See ℞ **donepezil**.

Aristocort; Aristocort A ®

A preparation of ℞ **triamcinolone**.
Formulation: Ointment; cream, both in several strengths. Aristocort A is in a water-washable base.
Availability: Prescription only.
Warnings and side effects: See ℞ **triamcinolone**.

Aristocort Intralesional; Aristocort Forte ®

A preparation of ℞ **triamcinolone**.
Formulation: Suspension for injection (Forte contains a higher concentration of the drug).
Availability: Prescription only.
Warnings and side effects: See ℞ **triamcinolone**.

Aristocort (Oral) ®

A preparation of ℞ **triamcinolone**.
Formulation: Oral tablets in two strengths.
Availability: Prescription only.
Warnings and side effects: See ℞ **triamcinolone**.

Aristospan Intralesional; Aristospan Intra-articular ®

A preparation of ℞ **triamcinolone**.
Formulation: Suspension for injection.
Availability: Prescription only.
Warnings and side effects: See ℞ **triamcinolone**.

Armidex ®

A preparation of ℞ **anastrozole**.
Formulation: Oral tablets.
Availability: Prescription only.
Warnings and side effects: See ℞ **anastrozole**.

Aromasin ⑧

A preparation of ℞ **exemestane**.
Formulation: Oral tablets.
Availability: Prescription only.
Warnings and side effects: See ℞ **exemestane**.

Artane; Artane Sequels ⑧

A preparation of ℞ **trihexyphenidyl**.
Formulation: Oral tablets; Artane Sequels are extended release.
Availability: Prescription only.
Warnings and side effects: See ℞ **trihexyphenidyl**.

Arth-G Tablets ⑧

A preparation of ℞ **salsalate**.
Formulation: Oral tablets.
Availability: Prescription only.
Warnings and side effects: See ℞ **salsalate**.

ArthriCare Triple-Medicated Gel ⑧

A preparation of ℞ **methyl salicylate**, ℞ **menthol**, methyl nicotinate and various.
Formulation: Topical gel.
Availability: OTC.
Warnings and side effects: See ℞ **methyl salicylate**; ℞ **menthol**.

Arthritis Foundation Pain Reliever ⑧

A preparation of ℞ **aspirin**.
Formulation: Oral tablets.
Availability: OTC.
Warnings and side effects: See ℞ **aspirin**.

Arthritis Pain Formula ⑧

A preparation of ℞ **aspirin**, buffered with ℞ **magnesium hydroxide** and ℞ **aluminum hydroxide**.
Formulation: Oral tablets.
Availability: OTC.
Warnings and side effects: See ℞ **aspirin**; ℞ **magnesium hydroxide**; ℞ **aluminum hydroxide**.

Arthropan Liquid ⑧

A preparation of ℞ **choline salicylate**.
Formulation: Oral liquid.
Availability: OTC.
Warnings and side effects: See ℞ **choline salicylate**.

Arthrotec ⑧

A preparation of ℞ **diclofenac** and ℞ **misoprostol**.
Formulation: Oral tablets, available in two strengths.
Availability: Prescription only.
Warnings and side effects: See ℞ **diclofenac**; ℞ **misoprostol**.

artificial saliva ⑩

Generics: **carboxymethylcellulose sodium; hydroxyethylcellulose; sodium chloride**.

Actions and uses
Artificial saliva is used to make up a deficiency of saliva in conditions that cause a dry mouth, including Sjögren's syndrome (which causes dry mouth and eyes), Sicca syndrome, certain drug treatments, and after radiotherapy. Common preparations used include viscous constituents such as ℞ **carboxymethlycellulose sodium** and various ℞ **electrolyte** salts (especially ℞ **sodium chloride** and salts of potassium).
Limitations
See the individual drug entries.

artificial tears ⑩

Generics: **carboxymethylcellulose sodium; petrolatum; polyvinyl alcohol; povidone**.
Actions and uses
Artificial tears are used where there is dryness of the eyes due to disease, such as Sjögren's syndrome (where there is also a dry mouth), and to relieve corneal edema. Eyedrops are available containing agents such as hydroxyethylcellulose, hydroxypropyl methylcellulose, carboxymethlycellulose sodium, povidone, and petrolatum.
Limitations
See the individual drug entries.

Artificial tears Plus ⑧

A preparation of ℞ **polyvinyl alcohol** and ℞ **povidone**.
Formulation: Eyedrops.
Availability: OTC.
Warnings and side effects: See ℞ **polyvinyl alcohol**; ℞ **povidone**.

Asacol ⑧

A preparation of ℞ **mesalamine**.
Formulation: Oral tablets, delayed release.
Availability: Prescription only.
Warnings and side effects: See ℞ **mesalamine**.

ascorbic acid ⑥

(vitamin C)
Type/Group: **vitamin**.
Brand(s): Cecon; Cevi-Bid; Dull-C; Vita-C; various generic.
How administered: Orally.

Used to treat
Ascorbic acid (vitamin C) is essential for the development and maintenance of cells and tissues. It cannot be made within the body and must be found in the diet (good food sources are vegetables and citrus fruits). Deficiency eventually leads to scurvy, but before that there is a lowered resistance to infection, and other disorders may develop, particularly in the elderly. However, vitamin C supplements are rarely necessary with a normal, well-balanced diet. It is an ⚕⚕ **antioxidant** and free radical scavenger. There have been claims that "pharmacological" (high) doses help prevent colds and because of this it is incorporated into a number of cold remedies (although, in fact, not at particularly high doses). It may increase

absorption of some other drugs (for example iron preparations). See also the vitamin C entry in the Supplements part.

Warnings

• It should not be given to people with known sensitivity to tartrazine, sulfites, or other components of the available ascorbic acid products.

• It should be given with caution to people on sodium restricted diets, taking daily salicylate treatment, using warfarin, with diabetes mellitus, G6PD deficiency, or a history of kidney stones.

• (at doses higher than RDA). Large doses in pregnancy may cause scurvy in newborns.

• Medical judgment is required if breast-feeding is being considered.

• Urine acidification may lead to hard crystals in the urine.

• Prolonged high doses may lead to scurvy upon discontinuance.

Interactions

None significant.

Side effects

• Rarely, gastrointestinal effects and increased urination. With injection, flushing, headache, dizziness, sleepiness, insomnia, and pain at the injection site.

Ascriptin Tablets; A/D; Extra Strength ®

A preparation of ℞ **aspirin**, buffered with ℞ **magnesium hydroxide**, ℞ **aluminum hydroxide**, and ℞ **calcium carbonate**.
Formulation: Oral tablets.
Availability: OTC.
Warnings and side effects: See ℞ **aspirin**; ℞ **magnesium hydroxide**; ℞ **aluminum hydroxide**; ℞ **calcium carbonate**.

Asendin ®

A preparation of ℞ **amoxapine**.
Formulation: Oral tablets in several strengths.
Availability: Prescription only.
Warnings and side effects: See ℞ **amoxapine**.

Asmalix ®

A preparation of ℞ **theophylline**.
Formulation: Oral elixir.
Availability: Prescription only.
Warnings and side effects: See ℞ **theophylline**.

A-Spas S/L ®

A preparation of ℞ **hyoscyamine**.
Formulation: Sublingual tablets.
Availability: Prescription only.
Warnings and side effects: See ℞ **hyoscyamine**.

Aspergum ®

A preparation of ℞ **aspirin**.
Formulation: Chewing gum.
Availability: OTC.
Warnings and side effects: See ℞ **aspirin**.

aspirin Ⓖ

(acetylsalicylic acid (ASA))

Type/Group: non-narcotic analgesic; antipyretic; anti-inflammatory; antirheumatic; antiplatelet.

Brand(s): Arthritis Foundation Pain Reliever; Aspergum; Bayer Genuine Aspirin Tablets, Caplets, Gelcaps, Extra Strength Tablets, Caplets, Gelcaps, Extra Strength Arthritis Pain Regimen, Bayer Aspirin Regimen Children's Chewable Aspirin, Bayer Aspirin Regimen Adult Low Strength, Regular Strength; Ecotrin Regular Strength Tablets, Low Strength Tablets, Maximum Strength Tablets; Empirin; Genprin; Halfprin 81, 1/2 Halfprin; Heartline; Norwich Extra-Strength; St. Joseph Adult Chewable Aspirin; ZORprin; various generic. Buffered aspirin: Adprin-B, Extra Strength Adprin-B; Alka-Seltzer with Aspirin, Extra Strength with Aspirin; Arthritis Pain Formula; Ascriptin Tablets, A/D, Extra Strength; Asprimox Tablets, Caplets, Extra Protection for Arthritis Pain Tablets, Caplets; Bayer Aspirin Regime with Calcium, Extra Strength Bayer Plus Caplets; Bufferin Tablets, Tri-Buffered Bufferin Tablets, Caplets; Buffex; Cama Arthritis Pain Reliever; Magnaprin Tablets, Arthritis Strength Captabs; various generic. Combinations: With acetaminophen: Goody's Body Pain Powder. (Plus) *caffeine*: Excedrin Migraine, Extra Strength Caplets, Tablets, Geltabs; Goody's Extra Strength Headache Powder; Saleto Tablets (has *salicylamide*); Summit Extra Strength Caplets; Vanquish Caplets (has *aluminum hydroxide* and *magnesium hydroxide*). With caffeine: Anacin Tablets, Caplets; BC Powder Original Formula, Arthritis Strength (both have *salicylamide*); P-A-C Analgesic Tablets. With other constituents: With *butalbital and caffeine*: Fiorinal; Fiortal. With *carisoprodol*: Soldol Compound; Soma Compound; Soma Compound w/Codeine (has *codeine*). With *codeine*: Empirin w/ Codeine; Fiorinal w/Codeine Capsules. With *diphenhydramine*: Bayer PM Extra Strength Aspirin Plus Sleep Aid Caplets. With *dipyridamole*: Aggrenox. With *hydrocodone*: Alor Tablets; Damason-P Tablets; Lortab ASA Tablets; Panasal Tablets. With *meprobamate*: Equagesic Tablets. With *methocarbamol*: Robaxisal. With *orphenadrine citrate, caffeine*: Norgesic. With *oxycodone*: Percodan Tablets; Roxiprin Tablets. With *pentazocine*: Talwin Compound. With *propoxyphene*: Darvon Compound-65 Pulvules; various generic. With *pseudoephedrine*: Ursinus Inlay-Tabs. (Many combinations available as generic.)

How administered: Orally.

Used to treat

Aspirin is a well-known and widely used ℞ **NSAID** (non-steroidal anti-inflammatory drug), non-narcotic analgesic (painkiller), and antirheumatic. As an analgesic it relieves mild to moderate pain, particularly ✚ **headache**, toothache, and ✚ **dysmenorrhea** (period pain). It is a useful antipyretic for reducing raised body temperature in the treatment of the common ✚ **cold**, ✚ **fever**, or ✚ **influenza**. Aspirin reduces platelet aggregation (it "thins" the blood), which allows its prophylactic (preventive) use, at a low dose, as an ℞ **antiplatelet** treatment in those at risk, such as people who have already suffered a heart attack or stroke, or following bypass surgery, as part of antiangina treatment (see ℞ **antianginal**) to avoid blood clots and so forth. However, this same action may also increase bleeding time, so those taking

℞ **anticoagulants** must avoid aspirin. In tablet form, aspirin irritates the stomach lining and may cause bleeding and ulceration, and so soluble aspirin is preferred.

Warnings

• It should not be used by people with known hypersensitivity to this drug or other ℞ **salicylates**, and or certain bleeding disorders or conditions (such as, hemophilia, vitamin K deficiency, low platelet levels), or where there is a tendency to, or active, peptic ulceration.

• It should be given with caution to people taking certain drugs for gout or diabetes mellitus, or who have allergic disorders (especially asthma and skin conditions), in the elderly, children or teenagers, and where there are certain liver or kidney disorders or asthma, or nasal polyps.

• Aspirin can adversely affect the health both of a pregnant woman and the fetus. It should not be used during pregnancy, and especially not in the third trimester, when risk to the fetus is highest.

• Breast-feeding mothers should either discontinue this drug or stop breast-feeding.

• Because of a link between aspirin and the rare, but serious, condition called ✪ **Reye's syndrome** (which causes inflammation of the brain and liver), aspirin should not be given to children or teenagers who have, or might have, chickenpox or influenza. As so many infections resemble flu in their initial symptoms, aspirin should not, as a general rule, be used to treat fever, ache, and malaise by anyone in this age group except on the advice of a doctor.

• If dizziness, changes in hearing, or ringing in the ears (tinnitus) occurs, stop using this drug. These are usually the first symptoms of overdose.

• Aspirin can produce the same allergic-like symptoms that may occur after taking other NSAIDs, including bronchospasm in "aspirin-sensitive" asthmatics.

• It should not be taken, if possible, for a week before any surgery.

Interactions

• ℞ **Anticoagulants** have an additive effect in prolonging bleeding time.

• There is generally no benefit in taking aspirin with other NSAIDs (in particular, ℞ **ketorolac**) or salicylates, but there is a higher risk of gastrointestinal upsets and bleeding. Alcohol increases the risk of bleeding, particularly of an existing ulcer.

• ℞ **Antacids**, ℞ **corticosteroids**, ℞ **urinary alkalinizers**, and ℞ **activated charcoal** may lower the abosrption or therapeutic effect of aspirin.

• ℞ **Carbonic-anhydrase inhibitors** (for example, ℞ **acetazolamide**) increase the risk of overdose symptoms for both aspirin and these drugs.

• The effects of the following drugs may be exaggerated: ℞ **phenytoin**; ℞ **nitroglycerin**; ℞ **valproate sodium** (and other valproic acid derivatives); ℞ **methotrexate**.

• Aspirin taken with ℞ **insulin** or ℞ **sulfonylureas** may cause a greater glucose-lowering effect.

• The therapeutic effects of the followng drugs may be reduced: ℞ **angiotensin-receptor blockers**; ℞ **beta-blockers**; loop ℞ **diuretics**; ℞ **spironolactone**.

• ℞ **Uricosuric** agents (used in the treatment of gout, for example, phenylbutazone, ℞ **probenecid**, and ℞ **sulfinpyrazone**) may lose their effectiveness.

• There is a risk of accidental overdose and toxic effects if aspirin is taken with OTC medications containing salicylates in some form (for example, some ℞ **antacids**).

• Foods with ℞ **antiplatelet** properties, such as ♣ **ginger** and ⚖ **garlic**, may enhance aspirin's antiplatelet effect.

• Foods high in salicylates, such as curry powder, gherkins, licorice, paprika, prunes, raisins, and tea, may increase the risk of side effects.

Side effects

These depend on how administered, dose, and use, and vary in severity and frequency.

• The most common are gastrointestinal upsets, nausea, heartburn, diarrhea, and prolonged bleeding time (with consequent risk of ulceration). (The gastrointestinal upsets may be minimized by taking aspirin with milk or food.)

• There may be hypersensitivity reactions, including hives, rash, bronchospasm, edema, headache, blood disorders, ringing in the ears, dizziness, and fluid retention.

• Reversible kidney failure, particularly in renal impairment, has occurred. Liver damage is rare.

• When aspirin is used topically (such as a gel or cream) most of these side effects and warnings do not apply. However, hypersensitivity reactions (for example, asthma-like symptoms) may occur in susceptible people if there is systemic absorption (that is, absorbed into the body).

Asprimox Tablets; Caplets; Extra Protection for Arthritis ℞

A preparation of ℞ **aspirin**, buffered with ℞ **magnesium hydroxide**, ℞ **aluminum hydroxide**, and ℞ **calcium carbonate**..
Formulation: Oral tablets.
Availability: OTC.
Warnings and side effects: See ℞ **aspirin**; ℞ **magnesium hydroxide**; ℞ **aluminum hydroxide**; ℞ **calcium carbonate**.

Astelin Nasal Spray ℞

A preparation of ℞ **azelastine hydrochloride**.
Formulation: Nasal spray.
Availability: Prescription only.
Warnings and side effects: See ℞ **azelastine hydrochloride**.

AsthmaHaler Mist ℞

A preparation of ℞ **epinephrine** bitartrate.
Formulation: Nasal spray aerosol.
Availability: OTC.
Warnings and side effects: See ℞ **epinephrine**.

AsthmaNefrin ℞

A preparation of racepinephrine.
Formulation: Solution for inhalation.
Availability: Prescription only.
Warnings and side effects: See ℞ **epinephrine**.

Astramorph PF Ⓑ

A preparation of ℞ morphine sulfate.
Formulation: Injection; available in two strengths.
Availability: Prescription only.
Warnings and side effects: See ℞ morphine sulfate.

astringent Ⓓ

Generics: **aluminum acetate; aluminum chloride; calamine; gentian violet; silver sulfadiazine; tannic acid; zinc oxide; zinc sulfate.**

Actions and uses

Astringent agents precipitate proteins and are used in lotions to harden and protect skin where there are minor abrasions. They can also be used in lozenges, mouthwashes, eyedrops, eardrops, and antiperspirants. Aluminum salts are effective astringents. ℞ **aluminum acetate** can be used to clean sites of ✪ **infection** and inflammation such as poison ivy, athlete's foot, acne, and particularly weeping or suppurating wounds or sores. ℞ **aluminum chloride** is an astringent with powerful antiperspirant properties and can be used to treat ✪ **hyperhidrosis** (excessive sweating). Zinc salts are also effective astringents. ℞ **zinc sulfate** can be used as an astringent and wound cleanser (also in eyedrops). ℞ **zinc oxide** is a mild astringent used primarily to treat ✪ **skin conditions**, such as diaper rash, urinary rash, and ✪ **eczema**. It is available OTC (over-the-counter) in many compound forms as a cream, an ointment, and dusting powder. The compound preparation ℞ **calamine** is a suspension containing zinc oxide as the active ingredient, and also ferrous oxide. It has a mild astringent action and is incorporated into several preparations, which are used to cool and soothe itching skin in conditions such as poison ivy, diaper rash, and insect bites. It is also used in some emollient preparations. ℞ **tannic acid** can be used to form a film over mouth sores, which protects the area from food and drink (and also to relieve the pain or itching of cold sores or fever blisters).

In some substances, astringent and ℞ **antiseptic** properties are combined. ℞ **silver sulfadiazine** is a compound combining the (sulfonamide) ℞ **sulfadiazine**, which has a broad spectrum of ℞ **antibacterial** activity with the astringent and antiseptic properties of the silver. It is used primarily to inhibit infection of burns. ℞ **gentian violet** is a dye with astringent and oxidizing properties, which is used as an antiseptic and is occasionally administered topically (externally) to treat fungal skin infections or abrasions and minor ✪ **wounds**.

Limitations

See the individual drug entries.

Atacand Ⓑ

A preparation of ℞ candesartan cilexetil.
Formulation: Oral tablets, available in 4 strengths.
Availability: Prescription only.
Warnings and side effects: See ℞ candesartan cilexetil.

Atarax Tablets; Syrup Ⓑ

A preparation of hydroxyzine hydrochloride.
Formulation: Oral syrup; tablets, available in 4 strengths.

Availability: Prescription only.
Warnings and side effects: See ℞ hydroxyzine.

atenolol Ⓖ

Type/Group: beta-blocker; antianginal; antihypertensive.
Brand(s): Tenormin; various generic. Combinations: With *chlorthalidone*: Tenoretic; various generic.
How administered: Orally; injection.

Used to treat

Atenolol can be used to lower blood pressure (see ✪ **hypertension**), to relieve symptoms and to improve exercise tolerance in ✪ **angina pectoris**, and sometimes to regularize heartbeat, to prevent migraine, alcohol withdrawal syndrome, and anxiety. It is also used after a heart attack to enhance recovery. Beta-blockers are generally not given to people with asthma or other bronchospastic disease (for example, chronic bronchitis or emphysema), but atenolol may be used with caution when other blood-pressure lowering treatments have failed.

Warnings

• It should not be given to people with known hypersensitivity to any beta-blocking drug, who have certain heartbeat irregularities or heart failure, or in cardiogenic shock.

• It should be given with caution to people with diabetes mellitus or hypoglycemia, hyperthyroidism, myasthenia gravis, congestive heart failure, peripheral vascular disease, or liver or kidney impairment.

• Atenolol can harm the fetus and it should not be used during pregnancy.

• Medical judgment is required if breast-feeding is being considered. It appears in breast milk and may cause adverse effects in breast-feeding infants.

• Abruptly stopping using a beta-blocker may have adverse effects, including on the heart.

• The use of this drug may mask signs of hyperthyroidism or hypoglycemia.

• Other medications (including OTCs, herbal remedies, and supplements) must not be used without consulting a doctor. Some ℞ **nasal decongestants**, commonly available over the counter, contain ℞ **alpha-adrenergic stimulants** (for example, ℞ **phenylephrine**) that may cause a severe hypertensive reaction if taken with beta-blockers.

Interactions

• A serious blood pressure increase may occur after withdrawal from ℞ **clonidine hydrochloride** or both drugs at the same time.

• The effects of ℞ **alpha-adrenergic stimulants**, ℞ **ergot alkaloids**, ℞ **epinephrine**, and ℞ **lidocaine** may be increased, with risk of serious adverse effects.

• If taken with ℞ **calcium-channel blockers**, ℞ **guanethidine monosulfate**, or ℞ **reserpine**, there is potential for undesirable additive effects, with exaggerated slowing of heartbeat or hypotension.

• The effects if taken with nondepolarizing ℞ **skeletal muscle relaxants** are variable, with the possible risk of significant adverse effects associated with major surgery.

• The effects of ℞ **insulin** and ℞ **sulfonylureas** may be reduced by atenolol.

• ℞ **Antacids** (for example, ℞ **aluminum hydroxide,** ℞ **magnesium hydroxide**), ℞ **barbiturates,** ⚕⚕ **calcium** salts, ℞ **cholestyramine,** ℞ **colestipol hydrochloride,** ℞ **NSAID**s, ℞ **penicillins,** and ℞ **rifampin** may reduce the levels and effectiveness of atenolol.

• If used with ℞ **diuretics** and other antihypertensive drugs, there are additive effects which are often used to therapeutic advantage.

Side effects

These are infrequent and may include:

• Dizziness, cold extremities, fatigue, lethargy, slowing of the heart rate, hypotension, breathing difficulty or wheezing, nausea, diarrhea, or mental depression;

• Less frequently, edema, sleep disturbances, mental confusion, abnormal vision, dry eyes, and rash or itching. Unusual antibodies may develop, though lupus-like symptoms (fever, myalgia, pleurisy, various inflammations) seldom occur;

• Heart failure, should it develop, generally requires withdrawal (gradually, if possible) of this drug.

Ativan ⑧

A preparation of ℞ **lorazepam.**
Formulation: Oral tablets in several strengths; oral solution; injectable solution.
Availability: Prescription only.
Warnings and side effects: See ℞ **lorazepam.**

atorvastatin ⑥

Type/Group: **lipid-regulating drug; statin.**
Brand(s): Lipitor.
How administered: Orally.

Used to treat

Atorvastatin is a (statin/HMG-CoA reductase inhibitor) lipid-regulating drug that can be used in ✪ **hyperlipidemia** to reduce the levels, or change the proportions, of various lipids in the bloodstream. It is usually given to people in whom a strict and regular dietary regime alone is not having the desired effect, and in familial hypercholesterolemia.

Warnings

• It should not be given to people with liver disease.

• Atorvastatin is considered hazardous to the fetus. It is given to women of childbearing age only when they are thought highly unlikely to conceive and have been informed of the risks.

• It should not be used while breast-feeding.

• It can cause destruction of muscle tissue with resulting damage to the kidneys and even kidney failure. When taking atorvastatin, any unusual muscle pain or tenderness should be reported to a doctor immediately and treatment discontinued.

• Potentially harmful changes in liver function may occur, so that periodic tests are necessary to evaluate the drug's effect.

Interactions

• ℞ **Azoles** (antifungals such as ℞ **itraconazole,** ℞ **ketoconazole**), mibefradil, ℞ **erythromycin,** ℞ **clarithromycin,** ℞ **nefazodone,** ℞ **cyclosporine,**

℞ **gemfibrozil,** and ℞ **niacin** (nicotinic acid, a B vitamin) may increase levels of atorvastatin.

• ℞ **warfarin sodium** may increase antiblood-clotting effects.

Side effects

• Constipation, abdominal pain, muscle cramps, rash, insomnia, headache, flatulence, and dyspepsia.

atovaquone ⑥

Type/Group: **amebicide and antiprotozoal.**
Brand(s): Mepron.
How administered: Orally.

Used to treat

Atovaquone is used to prevent and treat ✪ **pneumonia** caused by the protozoan (but fungal-like) microorganism *Pneumocystis carinii* in people whose immune system has been suppressed (either following transplant surgery or because of a disease such as ✪ **AIDS**).

Warnings

• It should not be given to people with known severe hypersensitivity to atovaquone, or gastrointestinal disorders that inhibit absorption.

• It should be given with caution to anyone over 65 or with severe liver impairment.

• Atovaquone may harm the fetus. It should be used during pregnancy only if the potential benefits justify the possible risks to the fetus.

• Medical judgment is required if breast-feeding is being considered. The drug may appear in breast milk.

• Any other medication, including herbal remedies or supplements, must not be taken without consulting a doctor first.

• Take with food as this helps the drug to be absorbed.

Interactions

• ℞ **rifampin** levels may be increased while levels of atovaquone are decreased.

Side effects

• Frequently, rash, gastrointestinal upsets, headache, fever, insomnia, and cough.

• Occasionally, thrush, loss of strength and energy, anemia, and blood changes.

atovaquone-proguanil ⑥

Type/Group: **antimalarial; amebicide and antiprotozoal.**
Brand(s): Malarone.
How administered: Orally.

Used to treat

Atovaquone-proguanil is an oral antimalarial combination (atovaquone and proguanil hydrochloride in a fixed dose combination). *Plasmodium falciparum* exhibits a high incidence of resistance to both atovaquone and proguanil as single agents for the treatment of ✪ **malaria**, but the combination has potent synergistic antimalarial activity.

Warnings

• It should not be given to people with known severe hypersensitivity to atovaquone or proguanil.

• It should be given with caution to people with kidney or liver impairment, or gastrointestinal disorders that inhibit absorption.

Key to symbols: ✪ = Disorder Section ℞ = Drug Section ♣ = Herbal Section ⚕⚕ = Supplement Section

• This drug may not be appropriate for people with severe and complicated malaria.

• Treatment may be less effective in black and Asian people because the drug is metabolized more slowly than in Caucasians.

• It should not be used during pregnancy or while nursing.

• A doctor must be contacted if fever develops.

• It may cause dizziness, so do not drive or perform other activities requiring alertness until the effects of drug are known.

• Take with meals to maximize absorption.

Interactions

• ℞ **rifampin** may decrease the levels of atovaquone.

• ℞ **tetracycline** and ℞ **metoclopramide hydrochloride** may reduce the effects of atovaquone.

• If used with ℞ **omeprazole**, the drugs may interfere with one another.

Side effects

• Dizziness, loss of appetite, mild diarrhea, nausea upset stomach, difficulty breathing or increased shortness of breath, fever or chills, severe diarrhea, skin rash, itching, unusual tiredness or weakness, and vomiting.

atracurium besilate ⓖ

see ℞ **atracurium besylate.**

atracurium besylate ⓖ

(atracurium besilate)
Type/Group: **skeletal muscle relaxant.**
Brand(s): Tracurium.
How administered: Injection.

Used to treat

Atracurium besylate is a non-depolarizing neuromuscular blocking agent used as a skeletal muscle relaxant to induce muscle paralysis during surgery.

Warnings

• It should not be used by people with known hypersensitivity to this drug.

• It should be given caution to people with certain heart and neuromuscular diseases, or with kidney, liver, or lung disorders. Atracurium besylate is for administration only by trained personnel in hospitals, and individuals will be fully assessed for suitability prior to use.

• It should be used during pregnancy only if the benefits outweigh the risk of harming the fetus.

• Medical judgment is required if breast-feeding is being considered.

Interactions

• This drug is for administration only by trained personnel in hospitals. Individual patient's current and future therapy regimes will be fully assessed in order to avoid potential drug interactions.

Side effects

• Hypotension, flushing, rash, hives, allergic reaction, and spasm of the bronchi or larynx.

Atretol ⓑ

A preparation of ℞ **carbamazepine.**

Formulation: Oral tablets.
Availability: Prescription only.
Warnings and side effects: See ℞ **carbamazepine.**

Atrohist Pediatric Capsules ⓑ

A preparation of ℞ **pseudoephedrine** and ℞ **chlorpheniramine maleate.**
Formulation: Oral capsules, sustained release.
Availability: Prescription only.
Warnings and side effects: See ℞ **pseudoephedrine;** ℞ **chlorpheniramine maleate.**

Atrohist Pediatric Suspension ⓑ

A preparation of phenylephrine tannate, chlorpheniramine tannate, and pyrilamine tannate.
Formulation: Oral liquid.
Availability: Prescription only.
Warnings and side effects: See ℞ **phenylephrine hydrochloride;** ℞ **chlorpheniramine maleate;** ℞ **pyrilamine maleate.**

Atromid S ⓑ

A preparation of ℞ **clofibrate.**
Formulation: Oral capsules.
Availability: Prescription only.
Warnings and side effects: See ℞ **clofibrate.**

atropine sulfate ⓖ

(atropine sulphate)
Type/Group: **anticholinergic; antispasmodic; belladonna alkaloid.**
Brand(s): Atropisol; Isopto Atropine; Sal-Tropine; various generic.
Combinations: With *phenobarbital, hyoscyamine* and *scopolamine*: Barbidonna Tablets; Donnatal Capsules, Elixir, Extentabs, Tablets; Hyosophen Elixir, Tablets. With *diphenoxylate hydrochloride*: Logen; Lomenate; Lomotil Liquid, Tablets; Lonox Tablets. With *difenoxin hydrochloride*: Motofen Tablets. With *digestive enzymes, hyoscyamine* and *phenobarbital*: Arco-Lase Plus Tablets. With *multiple analgesic/antibacterial agents*: Atrosept; Dolsed; Prosed/DS; Trac Tabs 2X; Urised Tablets.
How administered: Orally; injection; topically (eye).

Used to treat

Atropine depresses certain functions of the autonomic nervous system, which results in smooth muscle relaxation. It is used in a number of preparations with other drugs for gastrointestinal complaints. It is commonly used during operations to dry up secretions and protect the heart. It can also be used to cause a long-lasting dilation of the pupil of the eye for ophthalmic procedures. Atropine decreases the secretion of gastric acid, but it has too many side effects to make it suitable for routine treatment of ✪ **peptic ulcers.** It may also be used as an ℞ **antidote** in organophosphate (℞ **anticholinesterase** insecticide) poisoning. It can also be used for the rigidity and tremor of parkinsonism (see ℞ **antiparkinsonism**).

Warnings

• It should not be given to people with known hypersensitivity to belladonna alkaloids. Depending on route and dose, it should not be administered to anyone with closed-angle glaucoma, myasthenia gravis, prostate gland enlargement, or certain gastrointestinal disorders.

• It should be given with caution to people with urinary retention, ulcerative colitis, pyloric stenosis, kidney disease, hyperthyroidism, liver disease, and chronic obstructive pulmonary disease (COPD), or who have Down's syndrome or thyrotoxicosis. It may worsen gastroesophageal reflux and certain cardiovascular disorders.

• Atropine should be used during pregnancy only if it is clearly needed.

• Medical judgment is required if breast-feeding is being considered. As a general rule, nursing mothers should not use this drug.

• Long-term use in children is not recommended, as this is a powerful drug with potentially serious side effects that develop more quickly in children.

• In hot weather, heat prostration (fever and heat stroke due to reduced sweating) is more likely in people who are taking an anticholinergic drug, such as atropine sulfate.

Interactions

• ℞ **amantadine**, ℞ **tricyclic** antidepressants, and ℞ **rimantadine** may increase atropine's side effects.

• The effects of ℞ **atenolol** and ℞ **digoxin** may be increased.

• Atropine may reduce the antipsychotic effects of ℞ **phenothiazines**.

Side effects

• Depending on how it is administered, use, and dose, there may be dry mouth, difficulty in swallowing and thirst, dilation of the pupils and loss of ability to focus, increase in intraocular pressure (pressure in the eyeball), dry skin with flushing, slowing then speeding of the heart, urgency then difficulty in urination, constipation, palpitations, and heart arrhythmias.

• Rarely, there may be high temperature accompanied by delirium or hallucinations. When used as eyedrops, there may be other local side effects such as stinging, irritation, conjunctivitis, or contact dermatitis. Systemic side effects on using eyedrops are more common in the elderly and children.

atropine sulphate Ⓖ

see ℞ atropine sulfate.

Atropisol Ⓑ

A preparation of ℞ **atropine sulfate**.
Formulation: Eye drop solution.
Availability: Prescription only.
Warnings and side effects: See ℞ atropine sulfate.

Atrosept Ⓑ

A preparation of ℞ **atropine sulfate**, ℞ **hyoscyamine**, ℞ **methenamine**, methylene blue, phenyl ℞ **salicylate**, and ℞ **benzoic acid**.
Formulation: Oral tablets.
Availability: Prescription only.

Warnings and side effects: See ℞ **atropine sulfate**; ℞ **hyoscyamine**; ℞ **methenamine**; ℞ **salicylates**; ℞ **benzoic acid**.

Atrovent Ⓑ

A preparation of ℞ **ipratropium bromide**.
Formulation: Aerosol spray, solution for inhalation, nasal spray.
Availability: Prescription only.
Warnings and side effects: See ℞ **ipratropium bromide**.

A/T/S Ⓑ

A preparation of ℞ **erythromycin**.
Formulation: Topical solution; topical gel.
Availability: Prescription only.
Warnings and side effects: See ℞ **erythromycin**.

Atuss EX Syrup Ⓑ

A preparation of ℞ **hydrocodone bitartrate** and ℞ **guaifenesin**.
Formulation: Oral syrup.
Availability: Prescription only.
Warnings and side effects: See ℞ **hydrocodone bitartrate**; ℞ **guaifenesin**.

Atuss-G Syrup Ⓑ

A preparation of ℞ **hydrocodone bitartrate**, ℞ **guaifenesin**, and ℞ **phenylephrine hydrochloride**.
Formulation: Oral syrup.
Availability: Prescription only.
Warnings and side effects: See ℞ **hydrocodone bitartrate**; ℞ **guaifenesin**; ℞ **phenylephrine hydrochloride**.

Atuss MS Ⓑ

A preparation of ℞ **hydrocodone bitartrate**, ℞ **chlorpheniramine maleate**, and ℞ **phenylephrine hydrochloride**.
Formulation: Oral liquid; syrup.
Availability: Prescription only.
Warnings and side effects: See ℞ **hydrocodone bitartrate**; ℞ **chlorpheniramine maleate**; ℞ **phenylephrine hydrochloride**.

Augmentin Ⓑ

A preparation of ℞ **amoxicillin** and ℞ **clavulanic acid**.
Formulation: Oral capsules, chewable tablets, oral suspension, each in several strengths.
Availability: Prescription only.
Warnings and side effects: See ℞ **amoxicillin**; ℞ **clavulanic acid**.

auranofin Ⓖ

Type/Group: antirheumatic; anti-inflammatory; gold compound.
Brand(s): Ridaura.
How administered: Orally.

Used to treat

Auranofin is a chemical form in which gold may be used to aid the treatment of severe, progressive ✪ **rheumatoid arthritis** (and juve-

Key to symbols: ✪ = Disorder Section   ℞ = Drug Section   ♣ = Herbal Section   ⚬⚬ = Supplement Section

nile arthritis) when ℞ **NSAID**s alone are not adequate. It works extremely slowly and takes several months to have any beneficial effect.

Warnings

• It should not be used by people with known hypersensitivity to this drug, with blood disorders, bone marrow disease or porphyria, severe kidney or liver impairment, necrotizing enterocolitis, certain skin disorders, systemic lupus erythematosus (SLE), congestive heart failure, and certain other disorders.

• It should be used with caution in people with liver or kidney disease, skin rash, or inflammatory bowel disease.

• This drug poses risks both to the mother and fetus during pregnancy. Its use should be stopped if at all possible when pregnancy is discovered. If a pregnancy is planned, gold therapy should be stopped some time before pregnancy, as gold is cleared from the body's tissues only slowly.

• Breast-feeding mothers should either discontinue using this drug or stop breast-feeding.

• Regular blood counts and monitoring of a wide range of body functions during treatment is necessary.

• A doctor must be contacted if sore throat, infection, fever, unexplained bruising, bleeding or purple patches, mouth ulcers, metallic taste, rashes, cough, or breathlessness, conjunctivitis (eye inflammation), or hair loss occur.

Interactions

• The concentration of ℞ **phenytoin** may be increased by auranofin.

• ℞ **penicillamine** is used sometimes as an antirheumatic, but because it clears heavy metals from the body it should not be part of a treatment that includes auranofin.

Side effects

• Severe reactions in a few people and potentially serious skin and blood disorders.

• More commonly, a change in bowel habits, diarrhea, skin reactions, mouth sores, abdominal cramping or pain, nausea, and impaired kidney function.

• Rarely, peripheral nerve disorders, fibrosis, liver toxicity and jaundice, hair loss, and colitis.

Aureomycin Ⓑ

A preparation of ℞ **chlortetracycline**.
Formulation: Ointment.
Availability: OTC.
Warnings and side effects: See ℞ **chlortetracycline**.

Aurolate Ⓑ

A preparation of gold sodium thiomalate.
Formulation: Oral tablets.
Availability: Prescription only.
Warnings and side effects: See ℞ **gold compound**.

aurothioglucose Ⓖ

Type/Group: **antirheumatic; anti-inflammatory; gold compound**.
Brand(s): Aurolate; Myochrysine.

How administered: Injection (intramuscular only).

Used to treat

Aurothioglucose is a chemical form in which gold may be used to augment the management of severe, progressive Ⓞ **rheumatoid arthritis** (and juvenile arthritis), psoriatic arthritis, Felty's syndrome, and Sjögren's syndrome when ℞ **NSAID** treatment alone is not adequate. It works extremely slowly and takes several months to have any beneficial effect.

Warnings

• It should not be used by people with known hypersensitivity to this drug, with uncontrolled diabetes mellitus, blood disorders, bone marrow disease or porphyria, severe kidney or liver impairment, certain skin disorders, systemic lupus erythematosus (SLE), and certain other disorders.

• Aurothioglucose poses risks both to the mother and fetus. It should be discontinued if at all possible when pregnancy is discovered. If a pregnancy is planned, gold therapy should be stopped some time before pregnancy, as gold is cleared from the body's tissues only slowly.

• Breast-feeding mothers should either discontinue using this drug or stop breast-feeding.

• Regular blood counts and monitoring of a wide range of body functions during treatment is necessary.

• A doctor must be contacted if a sore throat, infection, fever, unexplained bruising, bleeding or purple patches, mouth ulcers, metallic taste, rashes, cough, or breathlessness occur.

Interactions

• ℞ **penicillamine** is used sometimes as an antirheumatic, but because it clears heavy metals from the body it should not be part of a treatment that includes aurothioglucose.

Side effects

• Commonly, skin reactions, mouth sores, and impaired kidney function.

• Infrequently, gastrointestinal symptoms or discomfort.

• A few people may experience severe reactions and blood disorders.

• Rarely, peripheral nerve disorders, fibrosis, liver toxicity and jaundice, hair loss, and colitis.

Autoplex T Ⓑ

A preparation of ℞ **anti-inhibitor coagulant complex**.
Formulation: Injection (intravenous).
Availability: Prescription only.
Warnings and side effects: See ℞ **anti-inhibitor coagulant complex**. Contains a small amount of ℞ **heparin**.

Avalide Ⓑ

A preparation of ℞ **hydrochlorothiazide** and ℞ **irbesartan**.
Formulation: Oral tablets, in two (irbesartan) strengths.
Availability: Prescription only.
Warnings and side effects: See ℞ **hydrochlorothiazide**; ℞ **irbesartan**.

Avandia Ⓑ

A preparation of ℞ **rosiglitazone maleate**.

Formulation: Oral tablets in several strengths.
Availability: Prescription only.
Warnings and side effects: See ℞ **rosiglitazone maleate.**

Avapro ⑧

A preparation of ℞ **irbesartan.**
Formulation: Oral tablets, available in 3 strengths.
Availability: Prescription only.
Warnings and side effects: See ℞ **irbesartan.**

Aveeno Anti-Itch ⑧

A preparation of ℞ **calamine;** ℞ **camphor;** ℞ **simethicone,** and
primoxine.
Formulation: Topical cream, topical lotion.
Availability: OTC.
Warnings and side effects: See ℞ **calamine;** ℞ **camphor;**
℞ **simethicone.**

Aveeno Cleansing for Acne-Prone Skin ⑧

A preparation of ℞ **salicylic acid;** ℞ **titanium dioxide,** and
℞ **glycerin.**
Formulation: Soap-free medicated bar.
Availability: OTC.
Warnings and side effects: See ℞ **salicylic acid;** ℞ **titanium
dioxide;** ℞ **glycerin.**

Avelox ⑧

A preparation of ℞ **moxifloxacin.**
Formulation: Oral tablets.
Availability: Prescription only.
Warnings and side effects: See ℞ **moxifloxacin.**

Aventyl ⑧

A preparation of ℞ **nortriptyline hydrochloride.**
Formulation: Oral capsules in several strengths.
Availability: Prescription only.
Warnings and side effects: See ℞ **nortriptyline hydrochloride.**

Avita ⑧

A preparation of ℞ **tretinoin.**
Formulation: Topical cream.
Availability: Prescription only.
Warnings and side effects: See ℞ **tretinoin.**

Avonex ⑧

A preparation of interferon beta-1a.
Formulation: Injection.
Availability: Prescription only.
Warnings and side effects: See ℞ **interferons.**

Axid AR; Axid Pulvules ⑧

A preparation of ℞ **nizatidine.**
Formulation: Oral tablets; capsules.
Availability: OTC; Pulvules are prescription only.
Warnings and side effects: See ℞ **nizatidine.**

Axocet Capsules ⑧

A preparation of ℞ **acetaminophen** and ℞ **butabarbital.**
Formulation: Oral capsules.
Availability: Prescription only.
Warnings and side effects: See ℞ **acetaminophen;**
℞ **butabarbital.**

Aygestin ⑧

A preparation of ℞ **norethindrone.**
Formulation: Oral tablets.
Availability: Prescription only.
Warnings and side effects: See ℞ **norethindrone.**

Azactam ⑧

A preparation of ℞ **aztreonam.**
Formulation: Injection.
Availability: Prescription only.
Warnings and side effects: See ℞ **aztreonam.**

azatadine maleate ⑥

Type/Group: **antihistamine; antiallergic.**
Brand(s): Optimine. Combinations: With *pseudoephedrine
hydrochloride*: Rynatan Tablets; Trinalin Repetabs.
How administered: Orally.

Used to treat
Azatadine can be used for the relief of allergic symptoms such as
✪ **hay fever** (seasonal allergic rhinitis), perennial allergic rhinitis
and chronic ✪ **urticaria.**

Warnings
• It should not be given to people with known hypersensitivity to
this drug (or with known sensitivity to other antihistamines).
• Antihistamines should be given with caution to people with
asthma or lower respiratory disease, renal disease, heart disease,
hypertension, hyperthyroidism, epilepsy, porphyria, increased
intraocular pressure (pressure in the eyeball, as in glaucoma),
enlarged prostate, urinary retention, or certain obstructive bladder
or gastrointestinal conditions.
• Azatadine should be used during pregnancy only if it is clearly
needed, but not in the third trimester, as newborns or premature
infants may have severe reactions, including convulsions, to
antihistamines.
• Nursing mothers should discontinue using this drug or
discontinue breast-feeding.
• This drug must not be given to infants, and for children under
the age of 12 medical or manufacturer's instructions must be
followed closely.
• Because of its sedative side effects, the performance of skilled
tasks, such as driving, may be impaired.
• Side effects are more frequent in the elderly.

Interactions
• ℞ MAOI antidepressants may prolong and intensify the
℞ **anticholinergic** (see Side effects below) and sedative effects of
antihistamines.
• If used with ℞ **tricyclic** antidepressants, other antihistamines,
℞ skeletal muscle relaxants, ℞ opioids, ℞ barbiturates,

R hypnotics, R sedatives, or R antianxiety drugs, there is a risk of intensified side effects.

• Alcohol may intensify side effects such as drowsiness and impaired mental alertness.

Side effects

• Side effects depend on how it is administered. For this type of antihistamine, there is commonly drowsiness, headache, impaired muscular coordination or dizziness, anticholinergic effects (dry mouth, blurred vision, urinary retention, gastrointestinal disturbances), occasional rashes and photosensitivity (abnormal sensitivity to light), palpitations, and heart arrhythmias.

• Rarely, there may be stimulation instead of sedation (paradoxical stimulation), especially in children (and convulsions in overdose), hypersensitivity reactions, blood disorders, liver disturbances, depression, sleep disturbances, and hypotension.

azathiaprine Ⓖ

Type/Group: **antirheumatic; immunosuppressant; cytotoxic.**
Brand(s): Imuran; various generic.
How administered: Orally; intravenous infusion.

Used to treat

Azathiaprine is mainly used to reduce tissue rejection in people who have had a transplant, but it can also be used to treat ✪ rheumatoid arthritis. It has been investigated (with varied success) for the treatment of ✪ ulcerative colitis, ✪ myasthenia gravis, ✪ Crohn's disease, and the rare disorder Behçet's syndrome (especially eye symptoms).

Warnings

• It should not be given to people with known hypersensitivity to this drug (and to mercaptopurine, if injected). This is a specialist drug and is used only after a full medical assessment.

• When used to treat rheumatoid arthritis, azathiaprine should not be given during pregnancy.

• Azathiaprine can harm the fetus and its use should be avoided, if at all possible, during pregnancy.

• Medical judgment is required if breast-feeding is being considered.

• Like other immunosuppressants, azathiaprine is a toxic drug and is used only under close medical supervision. Monitoring of blood values is necessary, as well as periodic checks for other signs of toxicity.

• Treatment with azathiaprine inevitably leaves the body vulnerable to infection.

• There may be a higher vulnerability to certain cancers, as well. The risk of cancer is increased in people with rheumatic arthritis who have previously received alkylating agents (for example, R chlorambucil, R melphalan) will be evaluated by specialists.

• Symptoms such as unusual bleeding or bruising, fever, sore throat, mouth sores, signs of infection, abdominal pain, pale stools, or darkened urine should be reported to a doctor.

Interactions

• Severe white blood cell deficiency (leukopenia) is possible if used with R ACE inhibitors.

• R allopurinol and R methotrexate may raise the levels of azathiaprine and intensify its effects, and so there would be a greater risk for toxicity.

• The effects of R anticoagulants and R cyclosporine may be reduced.

• The effects of R skeletal muscle relaxants (nondepolarizing; for example, R atracurium, R pancuronium, R vecuronium) may be reduced or reversed.

Side effects

• Hypersensitivity reactions, such as dizziness, malaise, nausea and vomiting, fever, muscular pains and shivering, joint pain, skin eruptions, hypotension with interstitial nephritis (inflammation of the kidneys), changes in liver function, jaundice, heart arrhythmias, low blood pressure (requiring withdrawal of treatment), symptoms of bone marrow suppression, which should be reported (for example, bleeding or bruising), or infection.

azelaic acid Ⓖ

Type/Group: **keratolytic; antibacterial; acne treatment.**
Brand(s): Azelex.
How administered: Topically (external).

Used to treat

Azelaic acid is used to treat ✪ acne.

Warnings

• It should not be given to people with known hypersensitivity to azelaic acid.

• It should be used during pregnancy only if clearly needed.

• Medical judgment is required if breast-feeding is being considered.

• There are a few reports of darkening of the skin.

Interactions

No significant interactions have been noted.

Side effects

• Occasionally, itching, burning, stinging, and tingling.

• Rarely, redness, dryness, rash, peeling, irritation, and rash.

azelastine hydrochloride Ⓖ

Type/Group: **antihistamine; antiallergic.**
Brand(s): Astelin Nasal Spray.
How administered: Topically (nasal spray; eye)

Used to treat

Azelastine can be used to treat the symptoms of allergic conditions such as ✪ hay fever (seasonal allergic rhinitis) and in the treatment of itching of the eye that occurs with allergic ✪ conjunctivitis.

Warnings

• It should not be given to people with known hypersensitivity to this drug (or with known sensitivity to other antihistamines).

• Antihistamines should be given with caution to people with asthma or lower respiratory disease, heart disease, hypertension, hyperthyroidism, epilepsy, porphyria, increased intraocular pressure (pressure in the eyeball, as in glaucoma), enlarged prostate, urinary retention, or certain obstructive bladder or gastrointestinal conditions.

• Azelastine should be used during pregnancy only if the potential benefit outweighs the risk to the fetus and not in the third trimester as newborns may have severe reactions to antihistamines.

• Nursing mothers should discontinue using this drug or discontinue breast-feeding.

• This drug must not be given to infants, and for children under the age of 12 the manufacturer's or medical instructions must be followed closely.

• Because of its sedative side effects, the performance of skilled tasks, such as driving, may be impaired.

• Side effects are more frequent in the elderly.

Interactions

• ℞ **MAOI** antidepressants may prolong and intensify the ℞ **anticholinergic** (see Side effects below) and sedative effects of antihistamines.

• If used with ℞ **tricyclic** antidepressants, other antihistamines, ℞ **skeletal muscle relaxants**, ℞ **phenothiazines**, ℞ **opioids**, ℞ **barbiturates**, ℞ **hypnotics**, ℞ **sedatives**, or ℞ **antianxiety** drugs, there is a risk of intensified side effects.

• ℞ **cimetidine** increases the levels of azelastine.

• Alcohol may intensify side effects such as drowsiness and impaired mental alertness.

Side effects

• Side effects depend on how it is administered. When taken as a nasal spray, it may cause headache, somnolence, bitter taste, and weight gain. As eyedrops, it may also cause burning and stinging of the eyes.

• For this type of antihistamine, side effects may include drowsiness, headache, impaired muscular coordination or dizziness, anticholinergic effects (dry mouth, blurred vision, urinary retention, gastrointestinal disturbances), occasional rashes and photosensitivity (abnormal sensitivity to light), palpitations, and heart arrhythmias.

• Rarely, there may be stimulation instead of sedation (paradoxical stimulation), especially in children (and convulsions in overdose), hypersensitivity reactions, blood disorders, liver disturbances, depression, sleep disturbances, and hypotension.

Azelex ℞

A preparation of ℞ **azelaic acid**.
Formulation: Topical cream.
Availability: Prescription only.
Warnings and side effects: See ℞ **azelaic acid**.

azidothymidine Ⓖ

see ℞ **zidovudine**.

azithromycin Ⓖ

Type/Group: **macrolide; antibiotic; antibacterial.**
Brand(s): Zithromax.
How administered: Orally; injection.

Used to treat

Azithromycin has more activity against Gram-negative organisms compared to ℞ **erythromycin** (although less against Gram-positive bacteria) and can be used to treat ✚ **bacterial infections** as an

alternative for people allergic to penicillin. It is used to treat infections of the middle ear, the respiratory tract (for example, ✚ **pharyngitis** and ✚ **tonsillitis**) (including *H. influenzae*), the skin and soft tissues, and certain genital infections. It has a long duration of action and so usually it can be taken once a day.

Warnings

• It should not be given to people with known hypersensitivity to any of the macrolide antibiotics.

• It should be given with caution to people with kidney, heart or liver dysfunction. (See also Interactions below.)

• It should be used during pregnancy only if it is clearly needed and if the potential benefits outweigh the possible risks to the fetus.

• Medical judgment is required if breast-feeding is being considered. It is unknown whether this drug appears in breast milk.

• Superinfections due to the altered bacterial balance created by the use of antibiotics may occur. A doctor must be contacted if there is severe abdominal pain, moderate to severe diarrhea, or any new or unusual symptoms.

• Rare, serious allergic reactions have occurred.

Interactions

• The effectiveness of ℞ **penicillins** may be reduced.

• There is a risk of a fatal reaction if macrolides are used with ℞ **pimozide**.

• If used with HMG-CoA reductase inhibitors, there is a risk of damage or destruction of muscle tissue.

Side effects

• Occasionally, gastrointestinal upsets (nausea, vomiting, diarrhea).

• Rarely, headache and dizziness.

Azmacort ℞

A preparation of ℞ **triamcinolone**.
Formulation: Aerosol inhalant.
Availability: Prescription only.
Warnings and side effects: See ℞ **triamcinolone**.

azole Ⓓ

Generics: **butoconazole; clotrimazole; econazole; fluconazole; itraconazole; ketoconazole; metronidazole; miconazole; oxiconazole; terconazole; thiabendazole; tioconazole.**

Actions and uses

Azoles are an important group of synthetic drugs mainly used for their broad-spectrum ℞ **antifungal** activity, and are active against most fungi and yeasts. Others have some useful ℞ **amebicide and antiprotozoal** (for example, ℞ **metronidazole**), or weak ℞ **antibacterial** activity (for example, ℞ **metronidazole**). They are therefore all ℞ **antimicrobial** drugs. Additionally, some have ℞ **anthelmintic** activity (for example, ℞ **mebendazole**, ℞ **thiabendazole**, and ℞ **albendazole**).

Azoles are thought to combat ✚ **fungal infections** (such as ✚ **candidiasis**) by damaging the fungal cell membrane. It is thought they inhibit an enzyme called demethylase at concentrations harmless to people. They form the mainstay of ✚ **candidiasis** treatment.

Conventionally, the azoles are put into further chemical subclasses: imidazoles, triazoles, and benzimidazoles. The imidazole chemical group includes ℞ **clotrimazole**, ℞ **econazole**, ℞ **ketoconazole**, ℞ **metronidazole**, ℞ **miconazole**, and ℞ **tioconazole**. The triazole group includes ℞ **fluconazole** and ℞ **itraconazole**. The benzimidazole group includes ℞ **tiabendazole**.

Limitations
See the individual drug entries.

AZT Ⓖ
see ℞ zidovudine.

aztreonam Ⓖ
Type/Group: **beta-lactam; antibacterial; antibiotic.**
Brand(s): Azactam.
How administered: Injection.

Used to treat
Aztreonam is the first of a new chemical type of beta-lactam antibiotic called a monolactam, and is used to treat severe ⊙ **bacterial infections** caused by Gram-negative bacteria, including *Pseudomonas aeruginosa* and *Haemophilus influenzae (Hib),* urinary and lower respiratory tract infections, skin and skin structures, muscle and bone infections, intra-abdominal septicemia infections, and gynecologic infections, as well as to manage infection from susceptible organisms during surgery.

Warnings
• It should not be given to people with known hypersensitivity to aztreonam.
• It should be given with caution to people with a history of allergy, particularly to antibiotics (penicillins, cephalosporins), and those with impaired liver or kidney function.
• Aztreonam's safety in pregnancy has not been established. It does cross the placenta and should be used only if the benefits outweigh the risk to the fetus.
• Medical judgment is required if breast-feeding is being considered. It does appear in breast milk.
• Superinfections due to the altered bacterial balance created by antibiotic treatment may occur. A doctor must be contacted if there is severe abdominal pain, or moderate to severe diarrhea.
• Rarely, there may be severe allergic reactions.

Interactions
• There is an increased risk of kidney disorders if used with ℞ **aminoglycosides.**
• ℞ **Cephalosporins** and ℞ **imipenem** may interfere with the effectiveness of aztreonam.

Side effects
• Occasionally, discomfort at injection site, nausea, vomiting, diarrhea, and rash.
• Rarely, thrombophlebitis at injection site, abdominal cramps, headache, or low blood pressure.

Azulfadine Tablets; EN-tabs Ⓑ
A preparation of ℞ **sulfasalazine.**
Formulation: Oral tablets; EN-tabs are delayed release.
Availability: Prescription only.

Warnings and side effects: See ℞ **sulfasalazine**.

Baciguent Ⓑ
A preparation of ℞ **bacitracin.**
Formulation: Topical ointment.
Availability: OTC.
Warnings and side effects: See ℞ **bacitracin.**

Baci-IM Ⓑ
A preparation of ℞ **bacitracin.**
Formulation: Injection.
Availability: Prescription only.
Warnings and side effects: See ℞ **bacitracin.**

bacitracin Ⓖ
Type/Group: **antibacterial; antibiotic.**
Brand(s): Systemic: Baci-IM; various generic. Topical: Baciguent; various generic. Combinations: With *polymyxin B:* Betadine First Aid Antibiotics and Moisturizer; Polysporin. With *polymyxin B* and *pramoxine hydrochloride:* Betadine First Aid Antibiotics and Pain Reliever. With *neomycin* and *polymyxin B:* AK-Spore Ophthalmic Ointment; Medi-Quick Ointment; Mycitracin Maximum; Mycitracin Plus; Neomixin Ointment; Neosporin Maximum Strength; Neosporin Ointment; Septa Ointment; Triple Antibiotic Ointment; Triple Antibiotic Ophthalmic; various generic. With *neomycin,* polymyxin *B,* and *lidocaine:* Campho-Phenique Antibiotic Plus Pain Reliever; Clomycin; Lanabiotic; Mycitracin; Neosporin Plus; Spectrocin Plus; Tribiotic Plus. With *neomycin, polymyxin B, diperodon:* Bactine First Aid Antibiotic Plus Anesthetic Ointment. With *hydrocortisone* and *polymyxin B:* Cortisporin; Neotricin-HC. With *hydrocortisone* and *polymyxin B* and *neomycin:* Neotricin HC Ophthalmic.
How administered: Injection; topically (eye; skin).

Used to treat
Bacitracin is a polypeptide that is commonly used for the treatment of ⊙ **bacterial infections** of the eye and skin and, usually in combination with other antibiotics, in the form of an ointment for topical application. It is also used to treat infants with ⊙ **pneumonia** and ⊙ **emphysema.**

Warnings
• It should not be given to people with known hypersensitivity to bacitracin, or with severe kidney disease.
• Avoid using it internally during pregnancy.
• Medical judgment is required if breast-feeding is being considered.
• Kidney damage and failure can occur with systemic use.
• The use of antibiotics can lead to overgrowth of nonsusceptible organisms, leading to a secondary infection.

Interactions
• ℞ **Aminoglycosides** increase the risk of kidney dysfunction and respiratory arrest.

Side effects
• Systemic: Frequently, severe pain, thrombophlebitis at injection site. Occasionally, fever, hives, nausea, vomiting, diarrhea, and kidney dysfunction.

• Topical: An allergic reaction, causing increased irritation and inflammation.

baclofen ⒢

Type/Group: **skeletal muscle relaxant**.
Brand(s): Lioresal; various generic.
How administered: Orally; implanted infusion (intrathecal).

Used to treat

Baclofen is used for relaxing muscles that are in spasm (spasticity), particularly when caused by an injury to, or a disease of, the central nervous system (for example, multiple sclerosis). It works by an action on the central nervous system (spinal cord). Although not stated by the manufacturer for such use, it may be prescribed for treatment of trigeminal neuralgia (a nerve disorder), of spasticity in children with cerebral palsy, and, along with antipsychotics, of tardive dyskinesia.

Warnings

• It should not be used by people with known hypersensitivity to baclofen, or with spasm due to rheumatic disorders, stroke, cerebral palsy, or Parkinson's disease (efficacy has not been established for these diseases).
• It should be given with caution to people with peptic ulcers, kidney or bladder disorders, liver or lung disorders, porphyria, seizure disorder, diabetes mellitus, and those over 65.
• The effects on fetus are unknown, and so should be used only if clearly needed.
• Medical judgment is required if breast-feeding is being considered. It is excreted in breast milk in small amounts.
• Stopping of treatment must be gradual, over one to two weeks, otherwise it may cause hallucinations or seizures.
• It may worsen psychotic disorders.
• It may impair the perfomance of skilled tasks, such as driving.
• Alcohol must be avoided.

Interactions

• The effects of baclofen and CNS depressants (for example, ℞ **antianxiety** drugs) are increased if taken together.
• There is an increased sedative effect with alcohol.
• There is an increase hypotensive effect with ℞ **diuretics**, ℞ **ACE inhibitors**, and ℞ **angiotensin-receptor blockers**.
• ℞ **NSAIDs** (for example, ℞ **ibuprofen**) reduce the excretion of baclofen and increase risk of toxicity.

Side effects

• Commonly, transient drowsiness, weakness, dizziness, lightheadedness, nausea, and vomiting.
• Occasionally, headache, tingling in hands or feet, constipation, loss of appetite, hypotension, confusion, and nasal congestion.
• Rarely, CNS excitement or restlessness, slurred speech, tremor, dry mouth, diarrhea, and painful or frequent urination.

Bactine First Aid Antibiotic Plus Anesthetic Ointment Ⓑ

A preparation of ℞ **neomycin**, ℞ **polymyxin B sulfate**, ℞ **bacitracin**, and diperodon.
Formulation: Topical ointment.
Availability: OTC.

Warnings and side effects: See ℞ **neomycin**; ℞ **polymyxin B sulfate**; ℞ **bacitracin**; diperodon.

Bactine Hydrocortisone; Bactine Maximum Strength Ⓑ

A preparation of ℞ **hydrocortisone**.
Formulation: Cream in two strengths.
Availability: OTC.
Warnings and side effects: See ℞ **hydrocortisone**.

Bactrim; Bactrim DS; Bactrim Pediatric, Bactrim IV Ⓑ

A preparation of ℞ **trimethoprim and sulfamethoxazole**.
Formulation: Oral tablets in regular and double strengths (DS); oral suspension (pediatric); injectable solution.
Availability: Prescription only.
Warnings and side effects: See ℞ **trimethoprim and sulfamethoxazole**.

Bactroban Ⓑ

A preparation of ℞ **mupirocin**.
Formulation: Topical cream, topical ointment, nasal ointment.
Availability: Prescription only.
Warnings and side effects: See ℞ **mupirocin**.

Bactrocill Ⓑ

A preparation of ℞ **oxacillin sodium**.
Formulation: Oral capsules.
Availability: Prescription only.
Warnings and side effects: See ℞ **oxacillin sodium**.

BAL in Oil Ⓑ

A preparation of ℞ **dimercaprol (BAL)**.
Formulation: Injection, intramuscular only.
Availability: Prescription only.
Warnings and side effects: See ℞ **dimercaprol (BAL)**. Only available as solution in peanut oil (hypersensitivity to peanuts contraindicates use).

Balmex Baby Ⓑ

A preparation of ℞ **zinc oxide**.
Formulation: Topical powder.
Availability: OTC.
Warnings and side effects: See ℞ **zinc oxide**.

Balnetar Ⓑ

A preparation of ℞ **coal tar**, ℞ **lanolin**, and ℞ **docusate sodium**.
Formulation: Bath oil.
Availability: OTC.
Warnings and side effects: See ℞ **coal tar**; ℞ **lanolin**; ℞ **docusate sodium**.

balsalazide disodium ⒢

Type/Group: **aminosalicylate; anti-inflammatory**.
Brand(s): Colazil.

How administered: Orally.

Used to treat
Balsalazide disodium is an 5-aminosalicylate, a drug related to ℞ **mesalamine** and a prodrug of 5-aminosalicylic acid, which can be used in the treatment of ✚ **ulcerative colitis**, particularly in patients sensitive to the ℞ **sulfonamide** content of other agents.

Warnings
• It should not be given to people with known hypersensitivity to ℞ **salicylates**, balsalazide metabolites, or any components of the product.
• It should be given with caution to people with impaired kidney function.
• There are no adequate and well-controlled studies of its use during pregnancy. It should be used only if it is clearly needed.
• Medical judgment is required if breast-feeding is being considered. It is not known whether it appears in breast milk.
• People with pyloric stenosis may have prolonged gastric retention of balsalazide.

Interactions
No interaction studies have been performed, although there is a possibility that the effects of oral ℞ **antibiotics** may be reduced.

Side effects
• Headache, gastrointestinal effects, respiratory infection, muscle pain, nasal inflammation, insomnia, and fatigue.

Bancap HC Capsules Ⓑ
A preparation of ℞ **hydrocodone bitartrate** and ℞ **acetaminophen**.
Formulation: Oral capsules.
Availability: Prescription only.
Warnings and side effects: See ℞ **hydrocodone bitartrate**; ℞ **acetaminophen**.

Banflex Ⓑ
A preparation of ℞ **orphenadrine**.
Formulation: Injection.
Availability: Prescription only.
Warnings and side effects: See ℞ **orphenadrine**.

Banophen Capsules; Caplets Ⓑ
A preparation of ℞ **diphenhydramine hydrochloride**.
Formulation: Oral capsules; tablets.
Availability: OTC.
Warnings and side effects: See ℞ **diphenhydramine hydrochloride**.

Banophen Decongestant Capsules Ⓑ
A preparation of ℞ **pseudoephedrine** and ℞ **diphenhydramine hydrochloride**.
Formulation: Oral Capsules.
Availability: OTC.
Warnings and side effects: See ℞ **pseudoephedrine**; ℞ **diphenhydramine hydrochloride**.

Barbidonna Tablets; Barbidonna No. 2 Tablets Ⓑ
A preparation of ℞ **atropine sulfate**, ℞ **hyoscyamine**, ℞ **scopolamine hydrobromide**, and ℞ **phenobarbital**.
Formulation: Oral tablets (No.2 Tablets are twice the dose of phenobarbital).
Availability: Prescription only.
Warnings and side effects: See ℞ **atropine sulfate**; ℞ **hyoscyamine**; ℞ **scopolamine hydrobromide**; ℞ **phenobarbital**.

barbiturate Ⓓ
Generics: **amobarbital; phenobarbital**.

Actions and uses
Barbiturates are a chemical class of drugs that are derived from barbituric acid. They have a wide range of essentially central nervous system (CNS) depressant actions.
In medicine, they are much less used than they once were. However, some are still used as ℞ **hypnotic**, ℞ **general anesthetic**, and ℞ **anticonvulsant**/℞ **antiepileptic** drugs. They work by a direct action on the brain, depressing specific areas, and may be slow- or fast-acting. All are extremely effective. ℞ **amobarbital**, ℞ **secobarbital**, sodium mephobarbital, and ℞ **butabarbital** are barbiturates used as ℞ **sedative** and ℞ **hypnotic** agents, but only when absolutely necessary, to treat severe and difficult to treat ✚ **insomnia**. Sometimes, they may be prescribed as ℞ **antiepileptic** drugs for severe episodes in specialized epilepsy centers, and as supportive, additional treatments in psychiatry. ℞ **phenobarbital** and ℞ **mephobarbital** are used as ℞ **anticonvulsant**/℞ **antiepileptic** agents in the prevention of most types of recurrent seizures in ✚ **epilepsy** and for status epilepticus. It is also used as a sedative and hypnotic to treat severe and intractable insomnia, and for sedation before an operation. Thiopental sodium is a specialist drug which is used as a short-acting ℞ **general anesthetic** mainly for inducing (bringing about) anesthesia at the start of operations before the use of a gaseous general anesthetic.

Limitations
Although very effective depressants, barbiturates rapidly cause tolerance, which may lead to both psychological and physical dependence (addiction), and so are used as infrequently as possible. Moreover, prolonged use, even in small doses, can have serious toxic side effects and in overdose they are lethal without specialist intervention. See also the individual drug entries.

Barc Ⓑ
A preparation of ℞ **pyrethrin**.
Formulation: Topical liquid.
Availability: OTC.
Warnings and side effects: See ℞ **pyrethrin**.

barrier cream Ⓓ
Generics: **petrolatum; simethicone**.

Actions and uses
Barrier creams can be used to protect the skin against irritants, chapping, urine, and feces (diaper rash: see ✚ **dermatitis**),

✪ hemorrhoids, bedsores, and toxic substances. They are normally applied as an ointment or cream, commonly in a petrolatum (petroleum jelly) base and often incorporating a specific water-repelling silicone compound (mostly simethicone, the activated form of dimethicone).

Limitations

See the individual drug entries.

basiliximab ⑥

Type/Group: **immunosuppressant**.
Brand(s): Simulect.
How administered: Intravenous infusion.

Used to treat

Basiliximab is one of a relatively new class of drug, a monoclonal antibody (a form of pure antibody produced by a type of molecular engineering). In this case the cloned antibody is one that prevents proliferation of the white blood cells, T-lymphocytes, which have an important role in immunity and cell rejection. It is used for prophylaxis (prevention) of rejection in kidney transplantation, and is used together with ℞ **cyclosporine** and ℞ **corticosteroids**.

Warnings

• It should not be given to people with known hypersensitivity to this drug or to any product prepared with mouse protein. This is a specialist drug and is used only after a full medical assessment.
• The effects of basiliximab in pregnancy are not known, but adverse effects on the fetus are thought possible. It should be used only if the potential benefit outweighs the possible risk to the fetus. Women of childbearing potential should use effective contraception during treatment and for two months afterwards.
• Medical judgment is required if breast-feeding is being considered.
• Basiliximab is used only by specialists in immunosuppressive therapy and under qualified supervision.
• It is not known whether this drug may have long-term effects on the immune system's response to new antigens (for example, viruses or bacteria that were not previously encountered by the body's defenses).
• People receiving immunosuppressive treatment may have a greater risk of opportunistic infection and lymphoproliferative disorders, although no higher risk is now associated with basiliximab.

Interactions

No drug interactions of significance are known.

Side effects

This drug is still under evaluation and side effects probably or possibly associated with it have not emerged. It is used in combination with cyclosporine and corticosteroids, and only in people undergoing major surgery, and so any immediate side effects it may have are difficult to distinguish.

Baycol ⑥

A preparation of ℞ **cerivastatin sodium**.
Formulation: Oral tablets.
Availability: Prescription only.
Warnings and side effects: See ℞ **cerivastatin sodium**.

Bayer Genuine Aspirin Tablets, Caplets ⑧

Also: **Extra Strength Enteric 500**
A preparation of ℞ **aspirin**.
Formulation: Oral tablets.
Availability: OTC.
Warnings and side effects: See ℞ **aspirin**.

Bayer Aspirin Adult Low Strength Tablets ⑧

A preparation of ℞ **aspirin**.
Formulation: Oral tablets; delayed release.
Availability: OTC.
Warnings and side effects: See ℞ **aspirin**.

Bayer Children's Aspirin ⑧

A preparation of ℞ **aspirin**.
Formulation: Oral tablets, chewable.
Availability: OTC.
Warnings and side effects: See ℞ **aspirin**.

Bayer PM Extra Strength Aspirin Plus Sleep Aid Caplet ⑧

A preparation of ℞ **aspirin** and ℞ **diphenhydramine hydrochloride**.
Formulation: Oral tablets.
Availability: OTC.
Warnings and side effects: See ℞ **aspirin**; ℞ **diphenhydramine hydrochloride**.

BayGam ⑧

A preparation of ℞ **immune globulin, human (IG)**.
Formulation: Intramuscular injection.
Availability: Prescription only.
Warnings and side effects: See ℞ **immune globulin, human (IG)**.

Bay-Hep B ⑧

A preparation of ℞ **hepatitis B immune globulin (HBIG)**.
Formulation: Intramuscular injection.
Availability: Prescription only.
Warnings and side effects: See ℞ **hepatitis B immune globulin (HBIG)**.

BayRho-D Full Dose, Mini-Dose ⑧

A preparation of ℞ $Rh_0(D)$ **immune globulin (human)**.
Formulation: Intramuscular injection.
Availability: Prescription only.
Warnings and side effects: See ℞ $Rh_0(D)$ **immune globulin (human)**.

BCG intravesical ⑥

Type/Group: **vaccine; anticancer; immunostimulant**.
Brand(s): Pacis; TheraCys; TICE BCG (for intravesical use).
How administered: Intravesical.

Key to symbols: ✪ = Disorder Section ℞ = Drug Section ♣ = Herbal Section ∿ = Supplement Section

Used to treat

BCG intravesical is used as a treatment *in situ* of bladder ✪ **cancer**. The drug was originally developed as a ✪ **tuberculosis** vaccine produced from a live attenuated strain of the tuberculosis bacillus, but can be used for this unrelated purpose.

Warnings

• It is a specialist drug and a full assessment for suitability will be carried out.

• Its safety during pregnancy is not established and should be avoided if possible.

• It should not be used by nursing mothers.

• Allergic reactions may occur.

• Serious systemic infection may occur. A doctor must be contacted if blood in urine, fever, chills, cough, skin rash, new urinary problems, or flu-like symptoms occur.

Interactions

• Bone marrow depressants, ℞ **immunosuppressants**, and radiation may impair response.

• Antimicrobial treatment for other infections may interfere with effectiveness.

Side effects

• Frequently, scanty urine, urinary frequency, blood in urine, and allergic reaction.

• Occasionally, cystitis, urinary urgency, anemia, nausea, vomiting, loss of appetite, diarrhea, and bone and joint aches.

• Rarely, urinary tract infection, urinary incontinence, and cramping.

BCG vaccine ⑥

Type/Group: **vaccine**.
Brand(s): TICE BCG.
How administered: Percutaneous injection.

Used to treat

BCG vaccine (bacillus Calmette-Guérin vaccine, or BCG) is produced from a live attenuated (weakened) strain of the ✪ **tuberculosis** bacillus *Mycobacterium bovis*, which no longer causes the disease in humans, but stimulates formation in the body of the specific antibodies that react also with the bacillus *Mycobacterium tuberculosis*, which causes tuberculosis (TB). It is used for vaccination of children and infants who are at risk of close, prolonged exposure to the bacteria. In general, vaccination with it is no longer recommended in the US for routine use except in adults with higher risk (such as health workers or others likely to come into contact with active respiratory tuberculosis) unless there is a change in reaction to ℞ **tuberculin** skin test. Visitors to countries where there is a high incidence of TB should consider vaccination if a tuberculin skin test results in little or no reaction, indicating lack of antibodies. BCG vaccine is also used as an ℞ **anticancer** drug for the specific treatment of carcinoma of the bladder.

Warnings

• It should not be used by people with known hypersensitivity to the vaccine, or with impaired immune response from whatever cause (for example, due to disease or cytotoxic drugs).

• It should be used during pregnancy only when it is clearly needed.

• Breast-feeding mothers should either not be vaccinated or stop breast feeding.

• This vaccine should be given with caution to people receiving ℞ **corticosteroids**, as they may facilitate an active infection.

• After administration, people will be required to wait for some time to ensure that there is no serious reaction (such as anaphylaxis).

Interactions

• ℞ **Antimicrobials** and ℞ **immunosuppressants** may reduce the effectiveness of the vaccine.

Side effects

• There may be swelling and irritation at the site of vaccination, which usually disappears in 10 to 14 days.

• Infrequently, other skin reactions, such as rash or hives, or swelling of lymph glands (near the injection site).

BCNU ⑥

see ℞ **carmustine**.

BC Powder Original Formula; Arthritis Strength ⑧

A preparation of ℞ **aspirin**, ℞ **caffeine**, and ℞ **salicylamide**.
Formulation: Soluble powder.
Availability: OTC.
Warnings and side effects: See ℞ **aspirin**; ℞ **salicylamide**; ℞ **caffeine**.

B-D Glucose ⑧

A preparation of ℞ **glucose**.
Formulation: Oral tablets, chewable.
Availability: OTC.
Warnings and side effects: See ℞ **glucose**.

becaplermin ⑥

Type/Group: **growth factor; skin preparation**.
Brand(s): Regranex.
How administered: Topically (external).

Used to treat

Becaplermin is used topically as an additional treatment of ulcers found in neuropathic diabetic disease. It is a recently introduced form of human platelet-derived growth factor (PDGF), manufactured by recombinant technology. Growth factors are proteins produced normally in tiny quantities by cells in the body, acting as a sort of local hormone to modulate cell growth.

Warnings

• It should not be given to people with known hypersensitivity to parabens, *m*-cresol, or any other component of the product, or those with known neoplasms (tumors) at the site of application.

• It should be given with caution to people with malignant disease, osteomyelitis, or diseased arteries.

• It is not known whether becaplermin can harm the fetus. It is used in pregnancy only if clearly needed.

• Medical judgment is required if breast-feeding is being considered. It is not known whether this drug appears in breast milk.

• Becaplermin should be given in a carefully measured quantity, which is determined by a doctor or other medical professional based upon the size of the ulcer.

• Safety and effectiveness in those under the age of 16 has not been established.

• It should not be used on infected skin.

Interactions

No interactions are known.

Side effects

• Irritation, sometimes rashes and edema.

beclomethasone dipropionate ⒢

Type/Group: **corticosteroid; antiasthmatic; anti-inflammatory.**
Brand(s): Beconase; Beclovent; Vancenase; Vanceril.
How administered: Inhalation; intranasal (nasal inhaler, nasal spray).

Used to treat

Beclomethasone dipropionate is prescribed as a respiratory inhalant for the treatment and prevention of bronchial ✪ asthma, and as a treatment for nasal inflammation from allergies, including seasonal allergic rhinitis and perennial allergic rhinitis and colds (vasomotor rhinitis).

Warnings

• It should not be used by people with known hypersensitivity to corticosteroids, or those with certain infections such as systematic fungal infections, or viral, bacterial, or fungal infections of the throat, mouth, or lungs.

• It should be given with caution to anyone with adrenal insufficiency.

• Corticosteroids can cross the placenta, and beclomethasone dipropionate, therefore, should be used during pregnancy only if it is medically judged that the benefits outweigh potential risk to the fetus.

• Medical judgment is also required if breast-feeding is being considered. When taken internally, corticosteroids are excreted in breast milk and may suppress growth and interfere with the production of natural corticosteroids in the infant. It is not known whether, or under what conditions, enough of the drug is absorbed from topical (inhaled or intranasal) use to create these risks.

• Localized fungal infections (thrush) have occurred in the mouths and throats of people using corticosteroid inhalants.

• Because corticosteroids suppress the immune system, anyone using long-term inhalant therapy is particularly susceptible to infections (for example, chickenpox, measles), and may become sicker than others, so risk of exposure must be minimized.

• Monitor growth in children and adolescents because there is evidence that oral corticosteroids may suppress growth with prolonged use or at high dosages. It is not known whether enough of the drug is absorbed from inhaled or intranasal use to create these risks.

• Special care and monitoring is required by asthmatics who are transferred from using systemically active to inhaled corticosteroids because serious reactions (even fatal) can occur during times of stress due to adrenal insufficiency. People will be advised of what to do (for example, resume systemic corticosteroids) during times of stress or severe asthma attacks, and a medic-alert bracelet/warning card should be carried explaining this.

Interactions

No significant interactions have been reported.

Side effects

These depend on how administered, dose, duration of treatment, and use.

• Inhalation: Frequently, throat irritation, dry mouth, hoarseness. Rarely, transient bronchospasm.

• Intranasal: Occasionally, mild nose or throat irritation, nosebleed, sore throat, and sneezing. Rarely, thrush, eye pain, bronchospasm, and systemic effects are possible (for example, adrenal insufficiency).

Beclovent Ⓑ

A preparation of ℞ **beclomethasone dipropionate.**
Formulation: Aerosol oral inhalent.
Availability: Prescription only.
Warnings and side effects: See ℞ **beclomethasone dipropionate.**

Beconase; Beconase AQ Ⓑ

A preparation of ℞ **beclomethasone dipropionate.**
Formulation: Aerosol nasal inhalent; nasal spray (AQ).
Availability: Prescription only.
Warnings and side effects: See ℞ **beclomethasone dipropionate.**

Beepen-VK Ⓑ

A preparation of ℞ **penicillin V.**
Formulation: Oral tablets in different strengths; oral solution.
Availability: Prescription only.
Warnings and side effects: See ℞ **penicillin V.**

Bellacane SR Ⓑ

A preparation of ℞ **ergotamine tartrate,** ℞ **belladonna alkaloid,** and ℞ **phenobarbital.**
Formulation: Oral tablets (sustained release).
Availability: Prescription only.
Warnings and side effects: See ℞ **ergotamine tartrate;** ℞ **belladonna alkaloid;** ℞ **phenobarbital.**

Bellacane Tablets Ⓑ

A preparation of ℞ **hyoscyamine** and ℞ **phenobarbital.**
Formulation: Oral tablets.
Availability: Prescription only.
Warnings and side effects: See ℞ **hyoscyamine;** ℞ **phenobarbital.**

belladonna alkaloid ⒟

Generics: **atropine sulfate; hyoscyamine; scopolamine hydrobromide.**

Actions and uses

Belladonna alkaloid drugs are derived from solanaceous plants such as *Atropa belladonna* (deadly nightshade) and are used in therapeutics in a number of chemical forms including hyoscyamine (the natural *l*-isomer) atropine sulfate (*dl*-hyoscyamine), and the closely related alkaloid scopolamine hydrobromide (hyoscine hydrobromide).

These drugs have *anticholinergic* (more accurately *antimuscarinic*) properties and are used for a variety of medical purposes; see ℞ **anticholinergic** entry for actions and uses. More recent anticholinergic drugs are synthetic chemical analogs or novel structures based on important parts of the atropine molecule.

Poisoning due to eating the berries of *Atropa belladonna* is not uncommon, particularly in children. Indeed, it has been one of the more popular poisons throughout history, from the time of Imperial Rome to the Borgias in 15th-century Italy. The name *belladonna* literally means "beautiful lady" and is thought to refer to the use of the plant as a cosmetic in ancient times, when it was used as eyedrops to dilate the pupils.

Limitations
See individual drug entries.

Bellergal-S ⑧
A preparation of ℞ **ergotamine tartrate**, ℞ **belladonna alkaloid**, and ℞ **phenobarbital**.
Formulation: Oral tablets.
Availability: Prescription only.
Warnings and side effects: See ℞ **ergotamine tartrate**; ℞ **belladonna alkaloid**; ℞ **phenobarbital**.

Bel-Phen-Ergot SR ⑧
A preparation of ℞ **ergotamine tartrate**, ℞ **belladonna alkaloid**, and ℞ **phenobarbital**.
Formulation: Oral tablets (sustained release).
Availability: Prescription only.
Warnings and side effects: See ℞ **ergotamine tartrate**; ℞ **belladonna alkaloid**; ℞ **phenobarbital**.

Benadryl Allergy/Cold Tablets ⑧
A preparation of ℞ **pseudoephedrine**, ℞ **acetaminophen**, and ℞ **diphenhydramine hydrochloride**.
Formulation: Oral tablets.
Availability: OTC.
Warnings and side effects: See ℞ **pseudoephedrine**; ℞ **acetaminophen**; ℞ **diphenhydramine hydrochloride**.

Benadryl Allergy Decongestant Tablets; Decongestant Liquid ⑧
A preparation of ℞ **pseudoephedrine** and ℞ **diphenhydramine hydrochloride**.
Formulation: Oral tablets; liquid.
Availability: OTC.
Warnings and side effects: See ℞ **pseudoephedrine**; ℞ **diphenhydramine hydrochloride**.

Benadryl Allergy Ultratabs ⑧
Also: **Kapseals; Chewables; Allergy Liquid; Liqui Gels**
A preparation of ℞ **diphenhydramine hydrochloride**.

Formulation: Oral tablets; capsules; liquid; liquigels.
Availability: OTC.
Warnings and side effects: See ℞ **diphenhydramine hydrochloride**. The chewable tablets contain the sweetener aspartame (with phenylalanine), which should be avoided by individuals with phenylketonuria.

Benadryl Itch Relief Stick ⑧
Also: **Itch Stopping Cream; Itch Stopping Spray**
A preparation of ℞ **diphenhydramine hydrochloride**; all but Gel contain zinc acetate.
Formulation: Topical aerosol, cream, gel, solid paste stick; Cream, Gel, and Spray available in two strengths. Childrens's formulations also available.
Availability: OTC.
Warnings and side effects: See ℞ **diphenhydramine hydrochloride**.

benazepril hydrochloride ⑥
Type/Group: **ACE inhibitor; antihypertensive; heart failure treatment; vasodilator.**
Brand(s): Lotensin. Combinations: With *amlodipine*: Lotrel. With *hydrochlorothiazide*: Lotensin HCT.
How administered: Orally.

Used to treat
Benazepril is used to treat ✪ **hypertension**, alone or with, especially, ℞ **thiazide** ℞ **diuretics** and also other drugs such as ℞ **calcium-channel blockers** (it is available with ℞ **amlodipine besylate**).

Warnings
• It should not be given to people with known hypersensitivity to this drug or to any other ACE inhibitor.

• It should be given with caution to people with severe congestive heart failure or certain other cardiovascular disorders, a history of anaphylaxis, collagen vascular disease (for example, systemic lupus erythematosus; SLE), diabetes mellitus, depressed immune response, or with impaired kidney function or on dialysis.

• Risk in pregnancy increases substantially from the first through to the second and third trimesters. ACE inhibitors can cause injury to the fetus, even death. The use of these drugs should stop as soon as pregnancy is detected.

• Medical judgment is required if breast-feeding is being considered. Benazepril appears in breast milk.

• Use of this drug should stop and a doctor notified immediately if signs of angioedema appear (swelling of the face, eyes, lips, tongue, larynx, or extremities; difficulty in breathing or swallowing). Swelling of the larynx, closing off the airway, can be life-threatening.

• Anyone taking an ACE inhibitor should not interrupt or discontinue treatment without first checking with a doctor.

• Any suspected infections (for example, fever, sore throat) should be reported to a doctor, because ACE inhibitors may cause blood changes which can affect immune response.

Key to symbols: ⑩ = Drug type/group   ⑥ = Generic name   ⑧ = Brand name

• ACE inhibitors generally have less effect on blood pressure in blacks than in non-blacks, and the likelihood of angioedema is higher among blacks, as well.

Interactions

• ACE inhibitors have apparently triggered life-threatening anaphylactoid reactions when used by people also receiving ℞ **desensitizing vaccines**.

• ℞ **Anesthetics** (for example, in surgery), ℞ **phenothiazines**, and ℞ **probenecid** may increase the levels or hypotensive effect of benazepril.

• Levels of ℞ **lithium** may be increased, with the potential for toxic effects.

• If used with potassium-sparing ℞ **diuretics** or other preparations containing potassium (for example, supplements and salt substitutes), levels of potassium may rise.

• ℞ **NSAIDs** may increase the risk of kidney damage or (in some cases) reduce the effects of ACE inhibitors.

• ℞ **Antacids** and ℞ **rifampin** may reduce the effects of benazepril. Antacids should not be used for several hours after a dose of an ACE inhibitor (a doctor should be consulted for full instructions and cautions).

• If used with other antihypertensives and diuretics, the effects of these drugs may be increased. This additive effect is sometimes used to advantage in combination treatments for high blood pressure.

Side effects

• Occasionally there may be headache, dizziness, fatigue, postural hypotension (lowered blood pressure on standing, usually causing dizziness), drowsiness, or persistent dry cough.

• Infrequently, fainting, weakness, palpitations, gastrointestinal disturbances (for example, nausea and vomiting, constipation), rash, angioedema, asthma, insomnia, tingling in the extremities, hair loss, or photosensitivity. Pancreatitis or changes in blood counts have also occurred.

• Although it is uncommon, ACE inhibitors can cause very marked hypotension (especially when beginning treatment) and kidney impairment.

bendroflumethiazide Ⓖ

Type/Group: **diuretic; thiazide; antihypertensive**.
Brand(s): Naturetin. Combinations: With *nadolol*: Corzide.
How administered: Orally.

Used to treat

Bendroflumethiazide is used in the treatment of ⊕ **hypertension** either alone or in conjunction with other types of diuretic or other drugs (for example, ℞ **beta-blockers**). It can also be used in the treatment of edema. Thiazide diuretics have also become a major part of the treatment for nephrogenic ⊕ **diabetes insipidus**.

Warnings

• It should not be given to people with known hypersensitivity to thiazides (or to ℞ **sulfonamide**-derived drugs), or severe kidney or liver disorders.

• It should be given with caution to elderly people, anyone with high cholesterol or triglyceride levels, or with liver or kidney impairment.

• Bendroflumethiazide should be used during pregnancy only when the potential benefit outweighs the possible risk to the fetus.

• Medical judgment is required if breast-feeding is being considered.

• Early symptoms of electrolyte imbalance may include muscle weakness or cramps, nausea, vomiting, restlessness or lethargy, dry mouth, excessive thirst, fast pulse or dizziness. A doctor must be contacted if such symptoms occur.

• Thiazides may aggravate symptoms of diabetes or gout, and worsen or activate lupus erythematosus.

• Periodic monitoring of electrolytes (particularly potassium, sodium, chloride, and bicarbonate) is needed.

• Photosensitivity may develop and so precautions such as protective clothing or sunscreens should be used.

• Thiazides interact with a number of drugs, including some over-the-counter preparations. A doctor must be consulted before taking any other medications (including OTCs, herbal remedies, and supplements).

Interactions

• There is a higher risk of a hypersensitivity reaction to ℞ **allopurinol**.

• The effects of ℞ **anesthetics**, ℞ **anticancer** drugs, other antihypertensives, ℞ **diazoxide**, ♎ **calcium** salts, ℞ **cardiac glycosides**, ℞ **lithium**, loop diuretics, ℞ **methyldopa**, nondepolarizing ℞ **skeletal muscle relaxants**, and ♎ **vitamin D** may be increased, with the potential for significant adverse effects or toxicity. An additive effect is sometimes used to advantage in combining thiazides with other antihypertensives.

• The effects of ℞ **anticoagulants** and antigout agents (for example, ℞ **probenecid**, ℞ **sulfinpyrazone**) may be lowered by thiazides.

• The doses of ℞ **insulin** and ℞ **sulfonylureas** may need to be adjusted, as thiazides may increase blood sugar levels.

• ℞ **Amphotericin B**, ℞ **anticholinergics**, ℞ **corticosteroids**, ℞ **corticotropin**, and ℞ **MAOIs** may increase the effects of thiazides, with the possibility of significant electrolyte loss, especially potassium.

• ℞ **cholestyramine**, ℞ **colestipol hydrochloride**, ℞ **methenamine**, and ℞ **NSAIDs** (especially ℞ **indomethacin**) may reduce the effectiveness of thiazide diuretics.

• There is an increased possibility of postural hypotension (lowered blood pressure on standing) if taken with alcohol, ℞ **barbiturates**, or ℞ **opioids**.

Side effects

• There may be dizziness, headache, muscle cramps, mild gastrointestinal upsets, postural hypotension, restlessness, reversible impotence, low blood levels of potassium, sodium, magnesium or chloride, raised blood urea, glucose and lipids, and gout.

• Rarely, photosensitivity, blood disorders, skin reactions, and pancreatitis.

Benefix Ⓡ

A preparation of ℞ **Factor IX** (recombinant).
Formulation: Intravenous infusion.

Availability: Prescription only.
Warnings and side effects: See ℞ Factor IX.

Benemid Ⓑ

A preparation of ℞ probenecid.
Formulation: Oral tablets.
Availability: Prescription only.
Warnings and side effects: See ℞ probenecid.

Ben-Gay Original Ointment Ⓑ

A preparation of ℞ methyl salicylate, ℞ menthol, and various.
Formulation: Topical ointment.
Availability: OTC.
Warnings and side effects: See ℞ methyl salicylate; ℞ menthol.

Ben-Gay Regular Strength Cream Ⓑ

Also: **Ultra Strength Cream; Arthritis Formula**
A preparation of ℞ methyl salicylate, ℞ menthol, and various.
Formulation: Topical cream.
Availability: OTC.
Warnings and side effects: See ℞ methyl salicylate; ℞ menthol.

Benoxyl Ⓑ

A preparation of ℞ benzoyl peroxide.
Formulation: Topical lotion in several strengths.
Availability: OTC.
Warnings and side effects: See ℞ benzoyl peroxide.

Bensal HP Ⓑ

A preparation of ℞ benzoic acid and ℞ salicylic acid.
Formulation: Topical ointment.
Availability: Prescription only.
Warnings and side effects: See ℞ benzoic acid; ℞ salicylic acid.

Bensulfoid Ⓑ

A preparation of ℞ sulfur and ℞ resorcinol.
Formulation: Topical cream.
Availability: OTC.
Warnings and side effects: See ℞ sulfur ℞ resorcinol.

Bentyl Tablets; Capsules; Syrup; Injection Ⓑ

A preparation of ℞ dicyclomine hydrochloride.
Formulation: Oral tablets; capsules; syrup; injection.
Availability: Prescription only.
Warnings and side effects: See ℞ dicyclomine hydrochloride.

Benylin Adult Formula; DM Cough Syrup Ⓑ

A preparation of ℞ dextromethorphan.
Formulation: Oral liquid; syrup.
Availability: OTC.
Warnings and side effects: See ℞ dextromethorphan.

Benylin Expectorant Liquid Ⓑ

A preparation of ℞ dextromethorphan and ℞ guaifenesin.

Formulation: Oral liquid.
Availability: OTC.
Warnings and side effects: See ℞ dextromethorphan; ℞ guaifenesin.

Benylin Multi-Symptom Liquid Ⓑ

A preparation of ℞ dextromethorphan, ℞ pseudoephedrine, and ℞ guaifenesin.
Formulation: Oral liquid.
Availability: OTC.
Warnings and side effects: See ℞ dextromethorphan; ℞ pseudoephedrine; ℞ guaifenesin.

Benylin Pediatric Ⓑ

A preparation of ℞ dextromethorphan.
Formulation: Oral liquid.
Availability: OTC.
Warnings and side effects: See ℞ dextromethorphan.

Benzac; Benzac AC; Benzac W: Benzac AC Wash: Ⓑ

A preparation of ℞ benzoyl peroxide.
Formulation: Topical gel in several strengths, various bases.
Availability: Prescription only.
Warnings and side effects: See ℞ benzoyl peroxide.

Benzagel Ⓑ

A preparation of ℞ benzoyl peroxide.
Formulation: Topical gel in several strengths.
Availability: Prescription only.
Warnings and side effects: See ℞ benzoyl peroxide.

Benzamycin Ⓑ

A preparation of ℞ erythromycin and ℞ benzoyl peroxide.
Formulation: Topical gel.
Availability: Prescription only.
Warnings and side effects: See ℞ erythromycin; ℞ benzoyl peroxide.

benzocaine Ⓖ

Type/Group: local anesthetic.
Brand(s): Americaine Anesthetic Spray; Americaine Otic; Anbesol Maximum Strength; Dermoplast; Lanacane Cream; Lanacane Spray; Orajel Mouth-Aid; Orabase Gel; Hurricane Gel, Hurricane Spray. Combinations: With *benzalkonium hydrochloride*: Orajel Mouth Sore; Tanac. With *resorcinol*: Bicozene. With *triclosan*: Solarcaine Spray; Solarcaine.
How administered: Topically (external).
Used to treat
Benzocaine is used to relieve ✪ **pain** in the skin surface or mucous membranes, particularly in or around the mouth (for example, mouth ulcers) and throat, or (in combination with other drugs) in the ears.

Warnings
• It should not be given to people with known hypersensitivity or methemoglobinemia (a serious blood disorder).
• Benzocaine should be used during pregnancy only if the potential benefits outweigh the possible risk to the fetus, particularly in the first trimester.
• Medical judgment is required if breast-feeding is being considered.
• It should not be used in infants younger than one year.
• Prolonged use should be avoided.

Interactions
• There are possible additive effects if taken with ℞ **antiarrhythmics** (for example, ℞ **tocainide**, ℞ **mexiletine**).

Side effects
• Some people may experience hypersensitivity reactions. Local burning, stinging, tenderness, and peeling may occur.

benzodiazepine ⓘ
Generics: **alprazolam; chlordiazepoxide; clonazepam; diazepam; estazolam; flumazenil; halazepam; lorazepam; midazolam; oxazepam; quazepam; temazepam; triazolam.**

Actions and uses
℞ **benzodiazepines** belong, chemically, to a large group of drugs that have a marked effect upon the central nervous system (CNS). Their effects—and so their uses—vary according to the level of dose, the frequency of dosage, and which member of the group is used. They have, to varying degrees, ℞ **sedative**, ℞ **antianxiety** (anxiolytic), ℞ **hypnotic**, ℞ **anticonvulsant**/℞ **antiepileptic**, ℞ **antiemetic**, and ℞ **skeletal muscle relaxant** actions. They can also cause amnesia, which, in addition to their other properties, is a reason why they may be used as a postoperative medication in order to allow patients to forget unpleasant procedures. Benzodiazepines are also used in the initial stages of ℞ **lithium** treatment of mania, and a variety of other purposes (some "off-label").
Benzodiazepines that are used as hypnotics to treat insomnia have virtually replaced earlier drugs, such as the ℞ **barbiturates** and ℞ **chloral hydrate**, because they are just as effective but much safer in overdose. Those used include some with a long duration of action, and so are only acceptable if some degree of sedation the next day is acceptable (or valuable, as in anxiety states), and these include ℞ **flurazepam** and ℞ **lorazepam**. Alternatively, there are some short-acting agents that are eliminated rapidly from the system compared to other benzodiazepines, but may cause withdrawal problems the day after use (and are only prescribed for very short courses), and these include ℞ **quazepam**, ℞ **temazepam**, and ℞ **triazolam**. Benzodiazepines used to treat anxiety include ℞ **alprazolam**, ℞ **chlordiazepoxide**, ℞ **clonazepam**, ℞ **diazepam**, ℞ **estazolam**, ℞ **halazepam**, lorazepam, and ℞ **oxazepam**. Benzodiazepines such as ℞ **diazepam** and ℞ **midazolam** can be used as sedatives in preoperative medication, because of their ability to cause amnesia (as mentioned), for induction of general anesthesia, as a sedative during diagnostic procedures such as endoscopy, and for dental procedures. Benzodiazepines used for anticonvulsant/antiepileptic purposes, include ℞ **clonazepam**, ℞ **diazepam**, and ℞ **lorazepam**. Those

used as skeletal muscle relaxants include diazepam. ℞ **lorazepam** is sometimes used as an antiemetic for chemotherapy-induced nausea and vomiting.
Although not chemically a benzodiazepine, ℞ **zolpidem** is a recently introduced drug which works in the same way as the benzodiazepines (at the same receptors in the brain). It can be used for the short-term treatment of ✪ **insomnia**.

Limitations
Benzodiazepine are remarkably safe in normal use, and overdose is rarely fatal. However, blood and liver function tests may be necessary during treatment. Benzodiazepines are cleared from the body faster in smokers, so they may require higher doses than normal. It is now realized that serious dependence may result from prolonged use of benzodiazepines, and there may be a paradoxical increase in hostility and aggression in anxious patients having long-term treatment. There are now antagonists, such as the benzodiazepine ℞ **flumazenil**, which can be used to reverse some of the central nervous system effects of benzodiazepines, for instance, at the end of operations. See also the individual drug entries.

benzoic acid ⓖ
Type/Group: **antifungal; keratolytic**.
Brand(s): Combinations: With *salicylic acid*: Whitfield's; Bensal HP.
How administered: Topically (external).

Used to treat
Benzoic acid is a treatment for ringworm infections, and is incorporated into non-proprietary and proprietary ointments and creams.

Warnings
• It should not be given to people with known hypersensitivity to benzoic acid.
• There is no indication that benzoic acid causes harm in pregnancy and breast feeding, but a doctor should be consulted before use.
• It is regarded as safe in normal topical use, but should not be ingested.
• When using on children, take care to prevent them from reaching the affected area with the mouth.

Interactions
None known.

Side effects
• Rarely, increased skin irritation, stinging, or inflammation.

benzoyl peroxide ⓖ
Type/Group: **keratolytic; antimicrobial; acne treatment**.
Brand(s): Combinations: Benzac; Benzagel; Benoxyl; Clearasil Maximum Strength; Desquam; Dryox; Fostex; Oxy; PanOxyl; Persa-Gel; Triaz. With *erythromycin*: Benzamycin. With *salicylic acid*: Bensal HP. With *sulfur*: Dryox S.; Sulfoxyl.
How administered: Topically (external).

Used to treat
Alone, or in combination with other drugs, benzoyl peroxide is used to treat ✪ **acne** and oily skin.

Warnings
• It should not be given to people with known hypersensitivity to benzoyl peroxide.

Key to symbols: ✪ = Disorder Section ℞ = Drug Section ♣ = Herbal Section ♊ = Supplement Section

• Topical application in pregnancy is generally considered safe.

• Medical judgment is required if breast-feeding is being considered.

• It should not be used to treat rosacea.

• When applying, avoid the eyes, inside the nose, mouth, and mucous membranes.

• It may bleach fabrics.

Interactions

• Benzoyl peroxide taken with ℞ **tretinoin** may cause skin irritation.

Side effects

• Occasionally, excessive drying, rash, irritation, scaling, stinging, redness, and swelling.

benzthiazide ⓖ

Type/Group: **diuretic; thiazide; antihypertensive.**

Used to treat

Benzthiazide is used to treat ✪ **hypertension** either alone or with other types of diuretic or other drugs (for example, ℞ **beta-blockers**). It can also be used in the treatment of edema. Thiazide diuretics have also become a major part of the treatment of nephrogenic ✪ **diabetes insipidus.**

Warnings

• It should not be given to people with known hypersensitivity to thiazides (or to ℞ **sulfonamide**-derived drugs), or severe kidney or liver disorders.

• It should be given with caution to elderly people, anyone with high cholesterol or triglyceride levels, or with liver or kidney impairment.

• Benzthiazide should be used during pregnancy only when the potential benefit outweighs the possible risk to the fetus.

• Medical judgment is required if breast-feeding is being considered.

• Early symptoms of electrolyte imbalance may include muscle weakness or cramps, nausea, vomiting, restlessness or lethargy, dry mouth, excessive thirst, fast pulse, or dizziness. A doctor must be contacted if such symptoms occur.

• Thiazides may aggravate symptoms of diabetes or gout, and worsen or activate lupus erythematosus.

• Periodic monitoring of electrolytes (particularly potassium, sodium, chloride, and bicarbonate) is needed.

• Photosensitivity may develop and so precautions such as protective clothing or sunscreens should be used.

• Thiazides interact with a number of drugs, including some over-the-counter preparations. A doctor must be consulted before taking any other medications (including OTCs, herbal remedies, and supplements).

Interactions

• There is a higher risk of a hypersensitivity reaction to ℞ **allopurinol.**

• The effects of ℞ **anesthetics**, ℞ **anticancer** drugs, other antihypertensives, ℞ **diazoxide**, ⚕ **calcium** salts, ℞ **cardiac glycosides**, ℞ **lithium**, loop diuretics, ℞ **methyldopa**, nondepolarizing ℞ **skeletal muscle relaxants**, and ⚕ **vitamin D** may be increased, with the potential for significant adverse effects

or toxicity. An additive effect is sometimes used to advantage in combining thiazides with other antihypertensives.

• The effects of ℞ **anticoagulants** and antigout agents (for example, ℞ **probenecid**, ℞ **sulfinpyrazone**) may be lowered by thiazides.

• The doses of ℞ **insulin** and ℞ **sulfonylureas** may need to be adjusted, as thiazides may increase blood sugar levels.

• ℞ **Amphotericin B**, ℞ **anticholinergics**, ℞ **corticosteroids**, ℞ **corticotropin**, and ℞ **MAOI**s may increase the effects of thiazides, with the possibility of significant electrolyte loss, especially potassium.

• ℞ **cholestyramine**, ℞ **colestipol hydrochloride**, ℞ **methenamine**, and NSAIDs (especially ℞ **indomethacin**) may reduce the effectiveness of thiazide diuretics.

• There is an increased possibility of postural hypotension (lowered blood pressure on standing) if taken with alcohol, ℞ **barbiturates**, or ℞ **opioids**.

Side effects

• There may be dizziness, headache, muscle cramps, mild gastrointestinal upsets, postural hypotension, reversible impotence, low blood levels of potassium, sodium, magnesium or chloride, raised blood urea, glucose and lipids, and gout.

• Rarely, photosensitivity, blood disorders, skin reactions, and pancreatitis.

benztropine mesylate ⓖ

Type/Group: **anticholinergic; antiparkinsonism.**
Brand(s): Cogentin; various generic.
How administered: Orally; injection.

Used to treat

Benztropine mesylate is an adjunctive (additional) treatment for all types of parkinsonism (see ℞ **antiparkinsonism**), and for extrapyramidal disorders (except tardive dyskinesia) caused by drugs, including ℞ **antipsychotic** drugs.

Warnings

• It should not be used in people with known hypersensitivity to this drug, narrow-angle glaucoma, gastrointestinal obstruction, stenosing peptic ulcers (ulcers located so as to narrow passage through some portion of the gastrointestinal system), prostatic hypertrophy or bladder neck obstructions, myasthenia gravis, or megacolon.

• Benztropine mesylate should be used with caution in children and in those with impaired kidney or liver function, or heart or blood pressure disorders.

• Anyone over 60 may be particularly sensitive to anticholinergic drugs, and they, as well as those with psychiatric disorders, should exercise caution when using this drug, because there have been isolated cases of susceptible individuals experiencing confusion, euphoria, or agitation.

• Benztropine mesylate should be used during pregnancy only if clearly needed and if the benefits outweigh the potential risk to the fetus.

• It is not known whether it appears in breast milk. However, infants are particularly sensitive to anticholinergic effects, and so medical judgment is also required if breast-feeding is being considered.

Key to symbols: Ⓓ = Drug type/group   ⓖ = Generic name   Ⓑ = Brand name

219

• Use with caution during hot weather as there is a risk of heat stroke due to decreased sweating.

• It may affect the performance of skilled tasks, such as driving.

• There is a possibility of addiction because this drug can cause euphoria.

• It may cause drowsiness, and when given by injection, it may cause hypotension.

Interactions

• The effectiveness of ℞ **levodopa** may be reduced.

• The effectiveness of ℞ **phenothiazines** may be reduced, while anticholinergic side effects may be increased.

• Benztropine mesylate taken with ℞ **haloperidol** and similar ℞ **antipsychotics** may cause a worsening of psychiatric symptoms and the development of tardive dyskinesia (abnormal movement).

• The likelihood of ℞ **anticholinergic** side effects may be increased if taken with anticholinergics or ℞ **amantadine**.

Side effects

• Dry mouth and constipation are common.

• Occasionally, there is urinary retention, blurred vision, dizziness, speeding of the heart, sensitivity reaction, or nervousness, effects on the eye and skin, sedation, or decreased sweating.

benzylpenicillin ⓖ

see ℞ penicillin G.

bepridil hydrochloride ⓖ

Type/Group: **calcium-channel blocker; antianginal.**
Brand(s): Vascor.
How administered: Orally.

Used to treat

Bepridil is used to prevent attacks of ✪ **angina pectoris**, sometimes in combination with ℞ **beta-blockers** or ℞ **nitrates**. It has the potential to cause more serious side effects than most other anti-anginals and is usually reserved for people who cannot be treated satisfactorily with other drugs.

Warnings

• It should not be given to people with known hypersensitivity to this drug, with a history of serious heart arrhythmias or certain other conduction abnormalities (or taking drugs that might cause such conditions), significant hypotension, uncompensated heart failure, or who have had a heart attack within 3 months previously to beginning treatment with this drug.

• It should be given with caution to elderly people, anyone with congestive heart failure, or significantly impaired liver or kidney function.

• Bepridil should be used during pregnancy only if the potential benefit outweighs the risk to the fetus.

• Medical judgment is required if breast-feeding is being considered. It appears in breast milk.

• It may cause new, serious arrhythmias.

• A doctor must be contacted if irregular heartbeat, shortness of breath, dizziness, hypotension, or constipation develops.

• Regular electrocardiograms and monitoring of potassium levels is necessary.

Interactions

• There is a risk of severe hypotension if used with ℞ **fentanyl**. Bepridil should be discontinued at least 36 hours before giving fentanyl.

• ℞ **Antiarrhythmics** (for example, ℞ **quinidine**, ℞ **procainamide**), ℞ **cardiac glycosides**, and ℞ **tricyclic** antidepressants may exaggerate certain effects on heart conduction.

• If used with ℞ **digoxin**, the effects are thought to be minimal, but caution is advised for people with conduction abnormalities.

• There are increased effects if used with ℞ **propranolol** or other ℞ **beta-blockers**, which may be useful, but caution is advised for people with conduction abnormalities.

Side effects

• The most frequent are dizziness, nervousness, gastrointestinal disturbances (for example, nausea, diarrhea, abdominal pain), palpitations, or headache. There may also be tremor, drowsiness, shortness of breath, ringing in the ears, dry mouth, tingling sensations, rash, or changes in heart rate.

• Significant changes in heart conduction may occur, but serious complications are uncommon.

• Infrequent side effects may include fluid in the lungs or changes in liver function.

beta-adrenergic blocker ⓓ

see ℞ beta-blocker.

beta-adrenergic stimulant ⓓ

albuterol; bitolterol mesylate; dobutamine hydrochloride; dopamine hydrochloride; epinephrine; pirbuterol; isoetharine; levalbuterol hydrochloride; metaproterenol; norepinephrine bitartrate; ritodrine hydrochloride; salmeterol; terbutaline sulfate.

Actions and uses

℞ **beta-adrenergic stimulant** (beta-adrenoceptor stimulants; beta-adrenoceptor agonists; beta-agonists; beta-stimulants) are drugs that act at beta-adrenergic receptors, which, along with alpha-adrenergic receptors, are the sites that recognize and respond to the natural hormones and neurotransmitters (epinephrine and norepinephrine) of the sympathetic nervous system. Drugs that activate this system, by whatever mechanism, are called ℞ **sympathomimetic** drugs.

Important actions of beta-adrenergic stimulants include bronchodilation, speeding and strengthening of the heartbeat, and relaxation of contraction of the uterus and intestine. The differences in receptors (called $beta_1$-receptor and $beta_2$-receptors) at different sites means that their action can be more precise and selective. For example, $beta_2$-receptor stimulant drugs are normally used as ℞ **bronchodilator** drugs in the treatment of reversible obstructive airways disease such as an ℞ **antiasthmatic** treatment in severe acute and chronic asthma, and for exercise-induced broncho-spasm. They are generally inhaled from an aerosol. They can act within the respiratory tract without also stimulating the heart (a $beta_1$-receptor site), which could be dangerous. Examples of $beta_2$-stimulant drugs used to cause bronchodilation are ℞ **albuterol**,

Key to symbols: ✪ = Disorder Section ℞ = Drug Section ♣ = Herbal Section ⚖ = Supplement Section

℞ **levalbuterol** (another chemical form of albuterol), ℞ **terbutaline**, ℞ **bitolterol**, ℞ **isoetharine**, and ℞ **pirbuterol**. ℞ **salmeterol** is different in that it too has beta$_2$-receptor selectivity—and is generally similar to albuterol—but its effects last longer. It may be used, therefore, to prevent asthma attacks throughout the night after inhalation before going to bed and also for long-duration prevention of exercise-induced bronchospasm. It is also used in maintenance treatment of bronchospasm associated with chronic ✪ **bronchitis** and ✪ **emphysema** (COPD, ✪ **chronic obstructive pulmonary disease**). Drugs that are not selective between the two beta-receptor types, for instance ℞ **metaproterenol** are now less used for their airways actions.

A further site in the body acted on by beta-adrenergic stimulant drugs is the uterus, which they relax. ℞ **Ritodrine** and sometimes ℞ **terbutaline** can be used to prevent or delay premature labor by relaxing the walls of the uterus when given towards term.

Drugs of the beta$_1$-receptor subtype (which stimulate the heart to beat more strongly and faster) are less used than the beta$_2$-receptor stimulant bronchodilator drugs. In emergencies ℞ **epinephrine** and ℞ **norepinephrine bitartrate** (which also have ℞ **alpha-adrenergic stimulant** actions), may be injected for their (beta$_1$-receptor mediated) ℞ **cardiac stimulant** actions in cardiac arrest, and for their hypertensive properties (alpha-receptor mediated) to treat circulatory collapse. Also, they are sometimes injected for emergency treatment of the bronchoconstriction of ✪ **anaphylactic reaction**, and in ✪ **angioedema**. Similarly, ℞ **dobutamine hydrochloride** and ℞ **dopamine hydrochloride**, which have ℞ **dopamine-receptor stimulant** actions as well as some the beta$_1$-receptor cardiac stimulant activity, can be variously used to treat serious heart emergencies, including cardiogenic shock, septic shock, and during open-heart surgery.

The development of selective beta$_2$-receptor stimulant drugs that can be used as bronchodilators without normally having adverse effects on the heart has been one of the success stories of medicinal chemistry. Earlier drugs without this high degree of selectivity (for instance ℞ **isoproterenol**) are now seldom used. They were linked with fatal adverse effects on the heart when they were the only drugs available. Of the modern generation beta$_2$-receptor stimulants, some such as ℞ **albuterol** do not necessarily have to be taken by inhalation, but are also available in forms to be taken by mouth (for those with no heart problems).

Limitations

There seems to be a growing overuse of this type of drug, especially in asthma, and the individual user becomes less responsive to a given dose, and tends to use the inhaler at more frequent intervals. ℞ **salmeterol** has the advantage that its long duration allows it to work for the length of a night—although overuse may exacerbate the problem. Taking inhaled low-dose ℞ **corticosteroid** drugs at the same time may help prevent overuse of inhaled beta-stimulants. See also the individual drug entries.

beta-adrenoceptor agonist Ⓓ

see ℞ **beta-adrenergic stimulant**.

beta-adrenoceptor antagonist Ⓓ

see ℞ **beta-blocker**.

beta-adrenoceptor stimulant Ⓓ

see ℞ **beta-adrenergic stimulant**.

beta-agonist Ⓓ

see ℞ **beta-adrenergic stimulant**.

beta-blocker Ⓓ

(beta-adrenergic blocker beta-adrenoceptor antagonist)
Generics: **acebutolol; atenolol; betaxolol hydrochloride; bisoprolol fumarate; carteolol; carvedilol; esmolol hydrochloride; labetalol hydrochloride; levobunolol; metipranolol; metoprolol tartrate; nadolol; penbutolol sulfate; pindolol; propranolol hydrochloride; sotalol hydrochloride; timolol maleate.**

Actions and uses

Beta-blockers inhibit some actions of the sympathetic nervous system by preventing the actions of ℞ **epinephrine** and norepinephrine (hormone and neurotransmitter mediators, respectively) by blocking the receptors, called beta-adrenoceptors, on which they act. Correspondingly, ℞ **alpha-adrenergic blocker** drugs inhibit the remaining actions by occupying the other main class of adrenoceptor, alpha-adrenoceptors. These two classes of receptors are responsible for the very widespread actions of epinephrine and norepinephrine in the body, both in normal physiology and in stress. For example, they speed the heart, constrict or dilate certain blood vessels (the overall effect is that they increase blood pressure) and suppress activity in the intestines. In general, they prepare the body for emergency action.

In disease, some of these actions may be inappropriate, exaggerated, and detrimental to health, so beta-blockers may be used to restore a more healthy balance. They may be used as ℞ **antihypertensive** drugs to lower blood pressure when it is abnormally raised in cardiovascular disease, as ℞ **antiarrhythmic** drugs to correct heartbeat irregularities, and as ℞ **antianginal** drugs to prevent the pain of ✪ **angina pectoris** during exercise and to treat ✪ **myocardial infarction** (damage to heart muscle) associated with heart attacks. Further uses are as ℞ **antimigraine** drugs to prevent migraine attacks (prophylaxis), as ✪ **anxiety** (anxiolytic) drugs to reduce anxiety, particularly tremor and a racing heart, as ℞ **antithyroid** drugs, specifically, shortly before surgery to correct thyrotoxicosis and, in the form of eyedrops, in ℞ **glaucoma treatment** to lower raised intraocular pressure (pressure in the eyeball). Different beta-blockers are used for different purposes, and there are a number of reasons for this. Some of them are relatively lipid-soluble (lipid is a type of fat in the blood) and some are relatively water-soluble, and the latter are less likely to enter the fat of the brain cells and so have less CNS (central nervous system) effects such as sleep disturbances and nightmares (for example ℞ **atenolol**, ℞ **bisoprolol fumarate**, ℞ **carteolol**, ℞ **esmolol hydrochloride**, ℞ **nadolol**, ℞ **sotalol hydrochloride**). Others have some ability to act on the heart, so cause less slowing of the heart or coldness in the extremities (for example, ℞ **acebutolol**,

℞ carteolol, ℞ penbutolol sulfate, ℞ pindolol). Others again are more active on the heart than other sites, such as the bronchioles, and so are called *cardioselective*. These drugs are more suitable for treating people who also have ✪ asthma than others that have quite marked effects on the bronchioles, when there is no alternative antiasthma drug suitable (for example, ℞ **acebutolol**, ℞ **atenolol**, ℞ **betaxolol hydrochloride**, ℞ **bisoprolol fumarate**, ℞ **metoprolol tartrate**).

Some beta-blockers are regarded as safe when given topically (externally) to the eye in glaucoma treatment as only a little of the drug is absorbed from eyedrops into the body, but side effects may still occur (℞ **betaxolol hydrochloride**, ℞ **carteolol**, ℞ **betaxolol hydrochloride**, ℞ **carteolol**, ℞ **levobunolol**, ℞ **metipranolol**, ℞ **timolol maleate**).

In general, recently introduced drugs are often only licensed for use in treating a single disorder (for example, ✪ **hypertension**), where they have been most extensively tested. But if they prove to be well tolerated by patients, they may eventually be licensed for use in treating a range of disorders. For example, the oldest beta-blocker, ℞ **propranolol hydrochloride**, is used for some 12 different purposes. Beta-blockers are commonly given with other antihypertensives such as ℞ **diuretic** and ℞ **calcium-channel blocker** drugs.

Limitations

There may be a price to pay when using beta-blockers for a given disorder, in as much as they will also block beta-receptors elsewhere in the body, so reducing the normal, beneficial actions of epinephrine and norepinephrine, and these side effects may well be undesirable. For instance, they may precipitate asthma attacks. Similarly, the blood flow in the extremities will often be reduced, so patients may complain of cold feet or hands.

Propranolol is the only one that is more widely used and sometimes for reducing symptoms of thyrotoxicosis. Beta-blockers can mask symptoms of hyperthyroidism leading to hyperthyroid storm on abrupt withdrawal. They may also mask the symptoms of low blood sugar in diabetic people, who should be aware of this. Abrupt discontinuance of a beta-blocker may have adverse effects on the heart. Beta-blockers also may intensify allergic responses to a variety of allergens in persons with a history of severe ✪ **anaphylactic reaction**.

See also the individual drug entries.

Betachron E-R   ⑧

A preparation of ℞ **propranolol hydrochloride**.
Formulation: Oral capsules, extended release, available in 4 strengths.
Availability: Prescription only.
Warnings and side effects: See ℞ **propranolol hydrochloride**.

Betadine   ⑧

A preparation of ℞ **povidone-iodine**.
Formulation: Shampoo, aerosol, cream, gel, mouthwash, ointment, swab stick, sponge brush, perianal wash, skin cleanser solution.
Availability: OTC.
Warnings and side effects: See ℞ **iodine; povidone-iodine**.

Betadine First Aid Antibiotics and Moisturizer   ⑧

A preparation of ℞ **polymyxin B sulfate** and ℞ **bacitracin**.
Formulation: Topical ointment.
Availability: OTC.
Warnings and side effects: See ℞ **polymyxin B sulfate**; ℞ **bacitracin**.

Betadine First Aid Antibiotics and Pain Reliever   ⑧

A preparation of ℞ **polymyxin B sulfate**, ℞ **bacitracin**, and ℞ **pramoxine hydrochloride**.
Formulation: Topical ointment.
Availability: OTC.
Warnings and side effects: See ℞ **polymyxin B sulfate**; ℞ **bacitracin**; ℞ **pramoxine hydrochloride**.

Betagan   ⑧

A preparation of ℞ **levobunolol**.
Formulation: Eye drops in two strengths.
Availability: Prescription only.
Warnings and side effects: See ℞ **levobunolol**.

beta-lactam   ⑩

Actions and uses

The beta-lactam class are chemically the group of ℞ **antibiotic** drugs that have a certain chemical structure called a lactam ring. They are used to treat ✪ **bacterial infections**. This extensive family includes the ℞ **penicillin** group (whose generic names usually end -cillin (for example ℞ **amoxicillin**, ℞ **ampicillin**), the ℞ **cephalosporin** group (whose names start with cef or ceph; for example, cefaclor and cephalexin), together with newer synthetic classes such as the carbapenem group (including ℞ **meropenem** and imipenem, used as ℞ **imipenem-cilastatin**), and also the monobactam group (for example, ℞ **aztreonam**).

Limitations

A notable adverse reaction to this family of antibiotics is an allergic drug response, which can be dangerous. Allergy to one class makes reaction to another likely, although not inevitable. See also the individual drug entries.

beta-lactamase inhibitor   ⑩

see ℞ **penicillinase inhibitor**.

betamethasone   ⑥

Type/Group: corticosteroid; anti-inflammatory; immunosuppressant.
Brand(s): Celestone. As betamethasone *sodium phosphate*: Celestoject; Cel-U-Jac. As betamethasone *dipropionate*: Alphatrex; Diprolene; Diprosone. As *betamethasone valerate*: Luxiq; Valisone; Beta-Val; Betatrex. As betamethasone *sodium phosphate* combined with betamethasone *acetate*: Celestone Soluspan. Combinations: With *clotrimazole*: Lotrisone.
How administered: Orally; injection; topically.

Used to treat

Betamethasone is used for the treatment of many kinds of inflammation, particularly inflammation associated with skin conditions, such as ✪ **eczema** and ✪ **psoriasis**, and of the eyes, ears, or nose. Like other corticosteroids, it has major and varied effects on metabolism, and modifies the operation of the immune system. Therefore, it may be used to treat a variety of conditions, including adrenal insufficiency, congenital adrenal hyperplasia, rheumatic disorders (such as ✪ **arthritis** and ✪ **osteoarthritis**), allergic states, collagen diseases, allergic and inflammatory eye disorders, intestinal tract, liver and kidney disorders, skin diseases, respiratory diseases (such as bronchial ✪ **asthma**), edemas, and malignancies.

Warnings

• It should not be used by people with known hypersensitivity to corticosteroids (or sulfites in the case of preparations that contain sodium bisulfite), or those with systemic fungal infections.

• It should be given with caution to anyone with low thyroid function, peptic ulcers, hepatitis, cirrhosis, ocular herpes simplex, history of tuberculosis, diabetes mellitus, glaucoma, seizure disorders, nonspecific colitis, congestive heart failure, myocardial infarction (heart attack), hypertension, psychosis, or kidney insufficiency, and by people over 65 and children. External use by those with marked circulation impairment should be undertaken with care.

• Corticosteroids can cross the placenta, and betamethasone, therefore, should be used during pregnancy only if it is medically judged that the benefits outweigh potential risk to the fetus.

• Medical judgment is also required if breast-feeding is being considered. Corticosteroids are excreted in breast milk and could suppress growth and interfere with the production of corticosteroids in the infant. It is not known whether, or under what conditions, enough of the drug is absorbed from topical use to create these risks.

• It may mask signs of infection and interfere with the body's ability to keep infection from spreading.

• Live vaccines must not be taken while using this drug.

• It may reactivate latent tuberculosis or amebiasis.

• It causes increased excretion of calcium and other minerals (a supplement may be needed).

• Prolonged use may lead to adrenal insufficiency. A doctor must be notified if there is unusual weight gain, swelling of the legs or feet, muscle weakness, black tarry stools, vomiting of blood, puffing of the face, menstrual irregularities, or prolonged sore throat, fever, cold, or infection.

• Those on chronic steroid therapy should wear medic-alert bracelet or the equivalent.

• Any other medication (including herbal remedies) must not be used without consulting a doctor.

• Discontinuing this drug must be down under medical supervision. Its use must be stopped gradually to avoid adverse reactions.

• The contraceptive effect of IUDs (intrauterine device) may be decreased.

• Dentists and other doctors must be informed of the use of this drug during, and for 12 months after discontinuing, treatment.

Supportive drugs may be required in the event of severe illness, surgery, or trauma.

• When using topically, in order to minimize the risk of systemic absorption and accompanying side effects, betamethasone must not be applied over large surface areas, for a prolonged period, or covered with bandages.

• It is not usually recommended for use on the groin, armpits or face.

Interactions

• Betamethasone taken with ℞ **amphotericin** or ℞ **diuretics** may further reduce potassium levels.

• The effects of ℞ **aspirin**, oral ℞ **hypoglycemics**, ℞ **insulin**, diuretics, and ෴ **potassium** supplements may be reduced.

• ℞ **Barbiturates**, ℞ **hydantoins**, and ℞ **rifampin** may reduce the effects of corticosteroids.

• ℞ **Ketoconazole**, ℞ **estrogens**, oral ℞ **contraceptives**, and nondepolarizing muscle relaxants may increase the effects of corticosteroids.

• Oral ℞ **anticoagulants** and ℞ **theophylline** may alter the effects of either corticosteroids or the other drug, or both.

• The effectiveness of ℞ **anticholinesterases**, ℞ **isoniazid**, ℞ **salicylates**, and ℞ **somatrem** may be reduced.

• ℞ **Cyclosporine** and digitalis may increase the risk of toxicity.

Side effects

These depend on how administered, dose, duration of treatment, and use.

• Systemic use: Frequently, increased appetite, abdominal tightness, nervousness, insomnia, and false sense of well-being. Occasionally, dizziness, flushing, increased sweating, decreased or blurred vision, mood swings. Rarely, allergic reaction, hallucinations, mental depression, Cushing's syndrome, muscle wasting, osteoporosis, and other potentially serious side effects such as seizures, congestive heart failure, hemorrhage, and pancreatitis.

• Topical use: Burning, stinging or itching, allergic contact rash, blisters, thinning of skin with easy bruising, and raised dark red spots on skin.

Betapace Tablets; Betapace AF ®

A preparation of ℞ **sotalol hydrochloride**.

Formulation: Oral tablets (four strengths); AF are also tablets (three strengths).

Availability: Prescription only.

Warnings and side effects: See ℞ **sotalol hydrochloride**.

Betaseron ®

A preparation of ℞ **interferon** beta-1b.

Formulation: Injection.

Availability: Prescription only.

Warnings and side effects: See ℞ **interferons**.

beta-stimulant ⑩

see ℞ **beta-adrenergic stimulant**.

Betatrex ®

A preparation of ℞ **betamethasone**.
Formulation: Ointment; cream; lotion.
Availability: Prescription only.
Warnings and side effects: See ℞ **betamethasone**.

Beta-Val ®

A preparation of ℞ **betamethasone**.
Formulation: Cream, lotion, and ointment.
Availability: Prescription only.
Warnings and side effects: See ℞ **betamethasone**.

betaxolol hydrochloride ©

Type/Group: beta-blocker; antihypertensive; glaucoma treatment.
Brand(s): Kerlone; Betoptic.
How administered: Orally; topically (as eyedrops).

Used to treat

Betaxolol can be used to lower blood pressure (see ✪ **hypertension**). In the form of eyedrops it may be used for chronic simple (open-angle) ✪ **glaucoma** and ocular hypertension.

Warnings

• It should not be given to people with known hypersensitivity to any beta-blocking drug, who have certain heartbeat irregularities or heart failure, or bronchial asthma, allergic bronchospasm or severe chronic obstructive pulmonary disease (COPD). It should not be used in cardiogenic shock.
• It should be given with caution to people with diabetes mellitus or hypoglycemia, hyperthyroidism, myasthenia gravis, congestive heart failure, peripheral vascular disease, moderate bronchospastic disease (for example, chronic bronchitis, emphysema), or liver or kidney impairment.
• Betaxolol's safety during pregnancy has not been established and it should be used only if the potential benefit outweighs the possible risk to the fetus.
• Medical judgment is required if breast-feeding is being considered. It is not known whether it appears in breast milk.
• Abruptly stopping betaxolol taken orally may have adverse effects, including on the heart.
• Ophthalmic preparations can be absorbed systemically, so systemic side effects may be observed (see below).
• The use of this drug may mask signs of hyperthyroidism or hypoglycemia.
• Other medications (including OTCs, herbal remedies, and supplements) must not be taken without consulting a doctor. Some ℞ **nasal decongestants**, commonly available over the counter, contain ℞ **alpha-adrenergic stimulants** (for example, ℞ **phenylephrine**) that may cause a severe hypertensive reaction if taken with beta-blockers.

Interactions

• A serious blood pressure increase may occur after withdrawal from ℞ **clonidine hydrochloride** or both drugs at the same time.
• Other ℞ **antiarrhythmics** (for example, ℞ **amiodarone**, ℞ **disopyramide**, ℞ **procainamide**, ℞ **quinidine**) and

℞ **tricyclics** have the potential for significant adverse effects on heart rhythm.
• The effects of ℞ **alpha-adrenergic stimulants**, ℞ **ergot alkaloids**, ℞ **epinephrine**, ℞ **lidocaine**, and ℞ **theophylline** may be increased, with the risk of serious adverse effects.
• ℞ **Calcium-channel blockers** (particularly ℞ **diltiazem hydrochloride** and ℞ **verapamil**), ℞ **guanethidine monosulfate**, and ℞ **reserpine** have the potential for increasing undesirable effects, with exaggerated slowing of heartbeat or hypotension.
• The effects of nondepolarizing ℞ **skeletal muscle relaxants** may be variable, with the possible risk of significant adverse effects associated with major surgery.
• The effects of ℞ **insulin** and ℞ **sulfonylureas** may be reduced by betaxolol.
• ℞ **Antacids** (for example, ℞ **aluminum hydroxide**, ℞ **magnesium hydroxide**), ℞ **barbiturates**, ⚬⚬ **calcium** salts, ℞ **cholestyramine**, ℞ **colestipol hydrochloride**, ℞ **NSAIDs**, ℞ **penicillins**, ℞ **rifampin**, and ℞ **salicylates** may reduce the levels and effectiveness of betaxolol. Antacids should not be taken within two hours of beta-blockers.
• If used with ℞ **diuretics** and other antihypertensive drugs, there are additive effects which are often used to therapeutic advantage.

Side effects

• Oral use: Effects may include dizziness, nausea, headache, fatigue, constipation or diarrhea. Occasionally, there may be insomnia, flatulence, urinary frequency, impotence, or decreased libido. Rarely, rash, arrhythmias, joint and muscle pain, confusion, or strange taste sensations.
• Ophthalmic (topical) use: Frequently, eye irritation or visual disturbances. Occasionally, increased light sensitivity or watering of eyes. Rarely, dry eyes, conjunctivitis, or eye pain.

bethanechol chloride ©

Type/Group: parasympathomimetic.
Brand(s): Myotonachol; various generic.
How administered: Orally.

Used to treat

Bethanechol chloride is used to treat urinary retention (particularly following surgery or childbirth).

Warnings

• It should not be given to people with known hypersensitivity to the drug, or those who suffer from urinary or intestinal obstruction, asthma, epilepsy, parkinsonism, thyroid or certain heart disorders, peritonitis, or who have peptic ulcers.
• It should be used during pregnancy only if it is clearly needed.
• Medical judgment is required if breast-feeding is being considered. It is not known whether this drug is appears in breast milk.
• It can cause postural hypotension (lowered blood pressure on standing).
• It should not be taken immediately before or after eating.

Interactions

• If used with cholinergic drugs or ℞ **tacrine**, there may be additive effects.

• If used with ℞ **beta-blockers**, there is an increased risk of bradycardia.
• ℞ **Quinidine** or ℞ **procainamide** may increase the effects of bethanechol chloride.

Side effects
• There may be sweating, malaise, nausea, diarrhea, intestinal colic, dizziness, fall in blood pressure, and a slow heart rate.
• Rarely, bronchial spasm and an asthmatic attack.

Betoptic; Betoptic S ⓑ
A preparation of ℞ **betaxolol hydrochloride**.
Formulation: Eye drops (solution; suspension).
Availability: Prescription only.
Warnings and side effects: See ℞ **betaxolol hydrochloride**.

Biaxin; Biaxin XL ⓑ
A preparation of ℞ **clarithromycin**.
Formulation: Oral tablets; extended release tablets (XL); oral suspension.
Availability: Prescription only.
Warnings and side effects: See ℞ **clarithromycin**.

bicalutamide ⓖ
Type/Group: hormone antagonist; antiandrogen; anticancer.
Brand(s): **Casodex.**
How administered: Orally.

Used to treat
Bicalutamide is used an anticancer drug, sometimes in combination with other drugs, for the treatment of ✪ **prostate cancer**.

Warnings
• It should not be used by people with known hypersensitivity to this drug.
• Bicalutamide is not indicated for use in women, and is contraindicated in women who are or may become pregnant.
• It should be given with caution to people with certain liver disorders (liver function may be monitored).
• Bicalutamide should not be used by pregnant or breast-feeding mothers.
• Feminization may occur during treatment.
• Use of this drug must not be stopped without consulting a doctor.

Interactions
• Bicalutamide may interfere with the effects of ℞ **anticoagulants** (for example, warfarin).

Side effects
• Hot flashes, growth and tenderness of breasts, weakness, itching, sleepiness, effects on the liver and cardiovascular system.
• Other effects (more common in older adults) include dizziness, insomnia, decreased libido, impotence, loss of appetite, shortness of breath, gastrointestinal problems (such as flatulence, constipation, and indigestion), hair loss, rashes, sweating, edema, dry mouth, chest and abdominal pain.

Bicillin ⓑ
A preparation of ℞ **penicillin G**, benzathine, and ℞ **procaine** combination.

Formulation: Injection.
Availability: Prescription only.
Warnings and side effects: See ℞ **penicillin G**; ℞ **procaine**.

Bicitra ⓑ
A preparation of ℞ **citrates**.
Formulation: Oral solution.
Availability: Prescription only.
Warnings and side effects: See ℞ **citrates**.

Bicozene ⓑ
A preparation of ℞ **benzocaine** and ℞ **resorcinol**.
Formulation: Topical cream.
Availability: OTC.
Warnings and side effects: See ℞ **benzocaine**; ℞ **resorcinol**.

Big Shot B 12 ⓑ
A preparation of ℞ **cyanocobalamin**.
Formulation: Oral tablets.
Availability: OTC.
Warnings and side effects: See ℞ **cyanocobalamin**

biguanide ⓓ
Generics: **metformin**.

Actions and uses
℞ **biguanide**s are a chemical class of ℞ **oral hypoglycemic drugs**—of which ℞ **metformin** is the only example currently available in the USA—which are used in ℞ **antidiabetic** treatment for type 2 ✪ **diabetes mellitus** (non-insulin-dependent diabetes mellitus; maturity-onset diabetes). Metformin has a different mode of action from the sulphonylurea group of oral hypoglycemics, and is not interchangeable with them. It is thought to work mainly by decreasing liver glucose production, decreasing absorption of glucose from the intestine, and improving sensitivity to insulin by increasing peripheral uptake and utilization of glucose. It only acts in the presence of endogenous insulin (that is, produced within the body) and is effective only in diabetics who still have some functioning pancreatic islet cells.
Metformin is not used as much as the ℞ **sulfonylurea** oral hypoglycemic drugs, but may be used as an alternative in people who have not responded satisfactorily to those drugs, or to diet alone. Some authorities consider it the drug of first choice in obese patients in whom strict dieting has failed to control diabetes. When the combination of strict diet and metformin treatment fails, other options which may be considered include combining it with ℞ **acarbose** or other oral hypoglycemics, or ℞ **insulin analog** agents by injection. Hypoglycemia is not a problem with metformin and other advantages are the lower incidence of weight gain.

Limitations
There is a possibility of gastrointestinal side effects. See also the individual drug entries.

Biltricide ⓑ
A preparation of ℞ **praziquantel**.
Formulation: Oral tablets.

Availability: Prescription only.
Warnings and side effects: See ℞ **praziquantel.**

Biocef ℬ

A preparation of ℞ **cephalexin.**
Formulation: Capsules; oral suspension.
Availability: Prescription only.
Warnings and side effects: See ℞ **cephalexin.**

Bioclate ℬ

A preparation of ℞ **antihemophilic factor** (recombinant).
Formulation: Intravenous infusion.
Availability: Prescription only.
Warnings and side effects: See ℞ **antihemophilic factor.**

Biohist-LA Tablets ℬ

A preparation of ℞ **pseudoephedrine** and ℞ **chlorpheniramine maleate.**
Formulation: Oral tablets, sustained release.
Availability: Prescription only.
Warnings and side effects: See ℞ **pseudoephedrine;**
℞ **chlorpheniramine maleate.**

biological response modifier Ⓓ

see ℞ **immunomodulator.**

biperiden Ⓖ

Type/Group: anticholinergic; antiparkinsonism.
Brand(s): **Akineton;** various generic.
How administered: Orally or by injection.

Used to treat

Biperiden is a treatment for all types of parkinsonism (see ℞ **antiparkinsonism**). It increases mobility and decreases rigidity. The tendency to produce an excess of saliva is also reduced, but it has only a limited effect on bradykinesia (slow, poor movement) and does not alleviate tardive dyskinesia (abnormal movement). Additionally, it is used to treat extrapyramidal symptoms in some cases where they are produced by drugs. It is thought to work by correcting the over-effectiveness of the neurotransmitter acetylcholine (cholinergic excess), which results from the deficiency of dopamine that occurs in parkinsonism.

Warnings

• It should not be used in people with known hypersensitivity to this drug, narrow-angle glaucoma, gastrointestinal obstruction, stenosing peptic ulcers (ulcers located so as to narrow passage through some portion of the gastrointestinal system), prostatic hypertrophy or bladder neck obstructions, myasthenia gravis, or megacolon.
• It should be used with caution by those with impaired kidney or liver function, or certain cardiovascular disorders.
• Anyone over 60 may be particularly sensitive to anticholinergic drugs, and they, as well as people with psychiatric disorders, should exercise caution when using this drug, because there have been isolated cases of susceptible people experiencing confusion, euphoria, or agitation.

• Biperiden should be used during pregnancy only if clearly needed and if the benefits outweigh the potential risks to the fetus.
• It is not known whether this drug is excreted in breast milk. However, infants are particularly sensitive to anticholinergic effects, and so medical judgment is also required if breast-feeding is being considered.
• Use with caution during hot weather as there is a risk of heat stroke due to decreased sweating.
• It may affect the performance of skilled tasks, such as driving.
• There is a possibility of addiction because this drug can cause euphoria.
• It may cause drowsiness, and when given by injection, it may cause hypotension.
• Treatment must be ended gradually and not abruptly.

Interactions

• The effectiveness of ℞ **levodopa** may be reduced.
• The effectiveness of ℞ **phenothiazines** may be reduced, while ℞ **anticholinergic** side effects may be increased.
• Biperiden taken with ℞ **haloperidol** and similar ℞ **antipsychotics** may cause a worsening of psychiatric symptoms and the development of tardive dyskinesia (abnormal movement).
• The likelihood of anticholinergic side effects may be increased if taken with anticholinergics or ℞ **amantadine.**

Side effects

• Dry mouth and constipation are common.
• Occasionally, there is urinary retention, blurred vision, dizziness, speeding of the heart, sensitivity reactions or nervousness, decreased sweating, sedation, and skin reactions.

biphosphonate Ⓓ

see ℞ **bisphosphonate.**

bipolar disorder Ⓓ

see ℞ **antimanic.**

Bisac-Evac Tablets; Suppositories ℬ

A preparation of ℞ **bisacodyl.**
Formulation: Oral tablets; rectal suppositories.
Availability: OTC.
Warnings and side effects: See ℞ **bisacodyl.**

bisacodyl Ⓖ

Type/Group: laxative.
Brand(s): **Bisac-Evac; Caroid; Correctol; Dulcolax; Feen-a-mint; Fleet Laxative Tablets, Suppositories, Bisacodyl Enema; Modane; Reliable Gentle Laxative; Women's Gentle Laxative;** various generic.
How administered: Orally; topically (rectal).

Used to treat

Bisacodyl is a (stimulant) laxative, used to promote defecation and relieve ✪ **constipation.** It seems to work by stimulating motility (movement) in the intestine (especially through stimulating the rectal mucosa), but some medical authorities do not approve of the frequent use of stimulant laxatives (as compared to the relatively benign bulking-agent laxatives, which help establish good bowel habit). Medically, bisacodyl can be used to evacuate the colon prior to rectal examination or surgery. With oral tablets, full effects are achieved after several hours, while suppositories achieve effects within an hour.

Warnings

• It should not be given to people with any form of intestinal obstruction and certain other gastrointestinal disorders.

• Bisacodyl should be avoided during pregnancy.

• Medical judgment is required if breast-feeding is being considered. It does appear in breast milk.

• It must not be used if there is abdominal pain, nausea, or vomiting, unless directed by a doctor.

• Rectal preparations should not be used in people with hemorrhoids or anal fissures.

• Chronic use of laxatives may cause fluid and electrolyte imbalances, vitamin and mineral deficiencies, and abnormal bowel function. Generally, they should not be used for more than a week.

• Do not take oral forms within one hour of drinking milk or using an ℞ **antacid**.

• A doctor must be consulted first before taking any other medication (including OTCs, herbal remedies, and supplements), because laxatives may alter the absorption of a wide range of drugs.

Interactions

• ℞ **Antacids** and milk may dissolve the coating of bisacodyl tablets, with the possibility of gastric irritation. Bisacodyl should not be taken orally within one hour of milk or antacids.

• Laxatives may alter the absorption of a wide range of drugs.

Side effects

• There may be abdominal cramps, nausea or vomiting, or appetite loss.

• Suppositories can sometimes cause local irritation, and with prolonged use inflammation and proctitis.

Bismatrol; Extra Strength Liquid ®

A preparation of ℞ **bismuth subsalicylate**.
Formulation: Oral liquid; tablets, chewable.
Availability: OTC.
Warnings and side effects: See ℞ **bismuth subsalicylate**.

bismuth salicylate ⑥

see ℞ **bismuth subsalicylate**.

bismuth subsalicylate ⑥

(bismuth salicylate)
Type/Group: **antidiarrheal; Helicobacter pylori eradication regime; ulcer-healing drug.**
Brand(s): Bismatrol; Pepto-Bismol; various generic. Combinations: With *metronidazole, tetracycline*: Helidac. With *kaolin, pectin*: Kaodene Non-Narcotic Liquid.
How administered: Orally.

Used to treat

Bismuth subsalicylate is a common OTC compound used for the relief of ✿ **indigestion** without causing constipation, relief of ✿ **nausea**, and to control ✿ **diarrhea**, including "traveler's diarrhea." It is also used as part of *Helicobacter pylori* eradication regimes in the treatment of ✿ **peptic ulcer**.

Warnings

• It should not be given to people with known sensitivity to ℞ **salicylates** (for example, ℞ **aspirin**).

• It should be used during pregnancy only if clearly needed. Salicylates may adversely affect the health both of a pregnant woman and the fetus. They should not, in general, be used during pregnancy, and especially not in the third trimester, when risk is highest to the fetus. Consult a physician before using bismuth subsalicylate during pregnancy.

• It may appear in breast milk and so should not be used by nursing mothers.

• Impaction (fecal mass in the rectum or colon) may occur in infants or debilitated persons.

• It should not be used together with other salicylates, as inadvertent overdose may result.

• If ringing in the ears occurs, discontinue all salicylate-containing medications.

• Bismuth subsalicylate should not be taken for more than two days, or if diarrhea is accompanied by fever over 101°F.

• Because of a link between aspirin, a salicylate, and the rare, but serious, condition called ✿ **Reye's syndrome**, other salicylates, including bismuth subsalicylate, should not be given to children or teenagers who have, or might have, chickenpox or flu. As so many infections resemble flu in their initial symptoms, they should not, as a general rule, be used to treat fever, ache, and malaise by anyone in this age group except on the advice of a doctor.

Interactions

• Other salicylates (for example, aspirin) or ℞ **NSAIDs** have additive effects.

• The absorption and effect of ℞ **tetracyclines** may be decreased.

• ℞ **Anticoagulants** increase bleeding time.

• ℞ **Carbonic-anhydrase inhibitors** (for example, ℞ **acetazolamide**) increase the likelihood of overdose symptoms for both aspirin and these drugs.

• The effects of ℞ **phenytoin**, ℞ **nitroglycerin**, ℞ **valproic acid**, and ℞ **methotrexate** may be exaggerated.

• Aspirin may cause a greater glucose-lowering effect if taken ℞ **insulin** or ℞ **sulfonylureas**.

• Uricosuric drugs (used in treatment of gout, for example, phenylbutazone, ℞ **probenecid**, ℞ **sulfinpyrazone**) may lose their effectiveness.

Side effects

• There may be darkened stools, also confusion, twitching, black tongue and gums, and ringing in the ears (tinnitus) if the salicylate doses are high.

• Very rarely, damage to nerves from absorption of bismuth.

bisoprolol fumarate ⑥

Type/Group: **beta-blocker; antihypertensive.**
Brand(s): Zebeta. Combinations: With *hydrochlorothiazide*: Ziac Tablets.
How administered: Orally.

Used to treat

Bisoprolol is used alone or in combination with other drugs to lower blood pressure (see ✿ **hypertension**). Beta-blockers are generally not given to people with asthma or other bronchospastic disease (for example, chronic bronchitis or emphysema), but bisoprolol may be used with caution when other blood-pressure lowering treatments have failed.

Warnings

• It should not be given to people with known hypersensitivity to any beta-blocking drug, who have certain heartbeat irregularities or heart failure. It should not be used in cardiogenic shock.

• It should be given with caution to people with diabetes mellitus or hypoglycemia, hyperthyroidism, myasthenia gravis, congestive heart failure, peripheral vascular disease, or liver or kidney impairment.

• It should be used during pregnancy only if the potential benefit outweighs the possible risk to the fetus.

• Medical judgment is required if breast-feeding is being considered. It is not known whether this drug appears in breast milk.

• Abruptly stopping using a beta-blocker may have adverse effects, including on the heart.

• The use of this drug may mask signs of hyperthyroidism or hypoglycemia.

• Other medications (including OTCs, herbal remedies, or supplements) must not be taken without consulting a doctor. Some ℞ **nasal decongestants**, commonly available over the counter, contain ℞ **alpha-adrenergic stimulants** (for example, ℞ **phenylephrine**) which may cause a severe hypertensive reaction if taken with beta-blockers.

Interactions

• A serious blood pressure increase may occur after withdrawal from ℞ **clonidine hydrochloride** or both drugs at the same time.

• Other ℞ **antiarrhythmics** (for example, ℞ **amiodarone hydrochloride**, ℞ **disopyramide**, ℞ **procainamide**, ℞ **quinidine**) and ℞ **tricyclics** have the potential for significant adverse effects on heart rhythm.

• The effects of ℞ **alpha-adrenergic stimulants**, ℞ **ergot alkaloids**, ℞ **epinephrine**, and ℞ **lidocaine** may be increased, with the risk of serious adverse effects.

• ℞ **Calcium-channel blockers**, ℞ **guanethidine monosulfate**, and ℞ **reserpine** have the potential for increasing undesirable effects, with exaggerated slowing of heartbeat or hypotension.

• The effects of nondepolarizing ℞ **skeletal muscle relaxants** may be variable, with the possible risk of significant adverse effects associated with major surgery.

• The effects of ℞ **insulin** and ℞ **sulfonylureas** may be reduced by bisoprolol.

• ℞ **Antacids** (for example, ℞ **aluminum hydroxide**, ℞ **magnesium hydroxide**), ℞ **barbiturates**, ♙ **calcium** salts, ℞ **cholestyramine**, ℞ **colestipol hydrochloride**, ℞ **NSAIDs**, ℞ **penicillins**, ℞ **rifampin**, and ℞ **salicylates** may reduce the levels and effectiveness of bisoprolol.

• If used with ℞ **diuretics** and other antihypertensive drugs, there are additive effects which are often used to therapeutic advantage.

Side effects

These are infrequent, usually mild, and may include:

• Fatigue, gastrointestinal disturbances (for example, diarrhea, nausea, vomiting), breathing difficulty, slowing of the heart rate or chest pain;

• Occasionally, dizziness, headache, cold extremities, dry mouth, arthralgia (joint pain), rash, sleep disturbances, and mental depression;

• Heart failure, should it develop, generally requires withdrawal (gradually, if possible) of this drug.

bisphosphonate ⓓ

Generics: **etidronate disodium; pamidronate disodium; tiludronate sodium; alendronate sodium.**

Actions and uses

Bisphosphonates are a chemical drug class used as ℞ **calcium-metabolism modifier** drugs to treat a number of conditions of disturbed calcium metabolism, including ✪ **Paget's disease (of the bone)**, to prevent and treat heterotropic ossification due to spinal cord injury or hip replacement, and to treat hormone-induced disorders of bone metabolism, to prevent postmenopausal ✪ **osteoporosis** and bone fractures in postmenopausal women, bone pain in prostate and breast cancer, and ✪ **hypercalcemia** due to malignancy.

These drugs (for example, ℞ **etidronate disodium**, ℞ **pamidronate disodium**, ℞ **tiludronate sodium**, ℞ **alendronate sodium**) are enzyme-resistant analogs of pyrophosphate, which is a natural physiological inhibitor of bone mineralization.

Limitations

Bisphosphonates are generally poorly absorbed when taken by mouth, and ℞ **alendronate sodium** must be taken first thing in the morning before any food. Others, such as ℞ **pamidronate disodium** and ℞ **etidronate disodium,** can be injected. They all have significant side effects, including nausea, diarrhea, headache, generalized body pain, and back pain. See also the individual drug entries.

Bite-Rx ⑧

A preparation of ℞ **aluminum acetate.**
Formulation: Topical solution.
Availability: OTC.
Warnings and side effects: See ℞ **aluminum acetate.**

bitolterol mesylate ⑥

Type/Group: **antiasthmatic; sympathomimetic; beta-adrenergic stimulant.**
Brand(s): Tornalate.
How administered: Inhalation.

Used to treat

Bitolterol is used to prevent and treat bronchial ✪ **asthma** and reversible bronchospasm.

Warnings

• It should not be given to people with known hypersensitivity to bitolterol or other sympathomimetics.

• It should be given with caution to people with certain heart diseases, hyperthyroidism, diabetes mellitus, hypertension, or prostatic hypertrophy.

• It should only be used in pregnancy if clearly needed. It is not known whether this drug crosses the placenta, but it may inhibit uterine contractions.

• Medical judgment is required if breast-feeding is being considered. It is not known if it appears in breast milk.

• Rarely, it may have adverse effects on the heart and blood pressure, or may lead to paradoxical bronchoconstriction.

Interactions

• ℞ **Beta-blockers** decrease the effects of bitolterol.

• If used with ℞ **furosemide**, there is a risk of enhancing furosemide's potassium-lowering effect.

Side effects

• Frequently, tremors and nervousness.

• Less frequently, dizziness, headache, mental changes, insomnia, chest discomfort, palpitations, speeded heart rate, throat irritation, gastrointestinal effects, muscle cramps, coughing, and shortness of breath.

Black Draught Syrup ®

A preparation of casanthranol, ℞ **methyl salicylate**, ♣ **rhubarb**, ℞ **senna**, and ℞ **menthol**.

Formulation: Oral syrup.

Availability: OTC.

Warnings and side effects: See ℞ **cascara sagrada**; ℞ **methyl salicylate**; ♣ **rhubarb**; ℞ **senna**; ℞ **menthol**. Syrup contains tartrazine (FD&C yellow No. 5), a dye that may cause allergic reaction in a few people, but especially those with sensitivity to aspirin.

Black Draught Tablets; Granules ®

A preparation of ℞ **senna**.

Formulation: Oral tablets; granules.

Availability: OTC.

Warnings and side effects: See ℞ **senna**. Granules contain tartrazine (FD&C yellow No. 5), a dye that may cause allergic reaction in a few people, but especially those with sensitivity to aspirin.

Blenoxane ®

A preparation of ℞ **bleomycin**.

Formulation: Powder for injection.

Availability: Prescription only.

Warnings and side effects: See ℞ **bleomycin**.

bleomycin ⑥

Type/Group: **anticancer; cytotoxic**.

Brand(s): Blenoxane.

How administered: Injection; intrapleural infusion.

Used to treat

Bleomycin is a cytotoxic drug (an antibiotic in origin) that has wide use as an anticancer treatment for ✪ **lymphomas**, testicular ✪ **cancer**, malignant pleural effusion (excess fluid in lung cavity), and squamous cell carcinoma.

Warnings

• It should not be given to people with known hypersensitivity to bleomycin.

• It should be given with caution to people with severe kidney or lung dysfunction. This is a specialist drug which will be used following a full evaluation by specialist physicians.

• Bleomycin is not recommended for use during pregnancy unless it is medically judged to be essential, because it may cause birth defects. Becoming pregnant while using this drug should be avoided.

• It should not be used if breast-feeding.

• It has adverse lung effects in around 10 percent of people, which sometimes progress into a serious disease (the risk may be dose-related).

• Infrequently, it may adversely affect the kidneys or liver.

• In common with many anticancer drugs, bleomycin can cause cancer or genetic mutations in cells.

Interactions

• The levels of ℞ **digoxin** and ℞ **phenytoin** may be decreased.

Side effects

• Frequently, loss of appetite and weight, skin reactions (redness, swelling, hives, streaking, small blisters, darkening), sores on lips or tongue, nausea, vomiting, hair loss, fever, chills.

• Occasionally, pain at tumor site, inflammation of mouth mucosa, and thrombophlebitis. Pneumonitis which can progress to pulmonary fibrosis is a serious adverse effect of bleomycin. A few lymphoma patients experience an unusual allergic reaction consisting of chills, fever, hypotension, mental confusion, and wheezing.

Bleph-10 ®

A preparation of ℞ **sulfacetamide**.

Formulation: Eye drops; ophthalmic ointment.

Availability: Prescription only.

Warnings and side effects: See ℞ **sulfacetamide**.

Blephamide ®

A preparation of ℞ **prednisolone**, ℞ **sodium phosphate** and sodium sulfacemide.

Formulation: Ophthalmic ointment.

Availability: Prescription only.

Warnings and side effects: See ℞ **prednisolone**; ℞ **sodium phosphate**.

Blistex Ointment ®

A preparation of ℞ **camphor**, ℞ **menthol**, and ℞ **phenol**.

Formulation: Topical ointment.

Availability: OTC.

Warnings and side effects: See ℞ **camphor**; ℞ **menthol**; ℞ **phenol**.

Blocadren ®

A preparation of ℞ **timolol maleate**.

Formulation: Oral tablets, available in 3 strengths.

Availability: Prescription only.

Warnings and side effects: See ℞ timolol maleate.

blood-thinning drug Ⓓ

see ℞ anticoagulant.

Bluboro Powder Ⓑ

A preparation of aluminum sulfate and calcium acetate.
Formulation: Powder packets.
Availability: OTC.
Warnings and side effects: See ℞ aluminum acetate.

Blue Ⓑ

A preparation of ℞ pyrethrin.
Formulation: Topical gel.
Availability: OTC.
Warnings and side effects: See ℞ pyrethrin.

Bonine Chewable Tablets Ⓑ

A preparation of ℞ meclizine hydrochloride.
Formulation: Oral tablets, chewable.
Availability: OTC.
Warnings and side effects: See ℞ meclizine hydrochloride.

Bontril PDM Ⓑ

A preparation of ℞ phendimetrazine.
Formulation: Oral tablets.
Availability: Prescription only.
Warnings and side effects: See ℞ phendimetrazine.

Borofax Skin Protectant Ⓑ

A preparation of ℞ petrolatum, ℞ zinc oxide, and ℞ lanolin.
Formulation: Topical ointment.
Availability: OTC.
Warnings and side effects: See ℞ petrolatum; ℞ zinc oxide; ℞ lanolin.

Boropak Powder Ⓑ

A preparation of aluminum sulfate and calcium acetate.
Formulation: Powder packets.
Availability: OTC.
Warnings and side effects: See ℞ aluminum acetate.

Bottom Better Ⓑ

A preparation of ℞ lanolin and ℞ petrolatum.
Formulation: Topical ointment.
Availability: OTC.
Warnings and side effects: See ℞ lanolin; ℞ petrolatum.

Boyal Salve Ⓑ

A preparation of ℞ ichthammol, ℞ benzocaine, ℞ lanolin, and ℞ petrolatum.
Formulation: Topical ointment.
Availability: OTC.
Warnings and side effects: See ℞ ichthammol; ℞ benzocaine; ℞ lanolin; ℞ petrolatum.

brain-motor disorder treatment Ⓓ

Generics: haloperidol; riluzole; fluphenazine.
Actions and uses
Brain-motor disorder treatment is a term used here for the treatment of neurological disorders of the central nervous system (CNS), which are characterized by a disruption of such motor functions of the body as fine control of the hand, for example, eye and facial movements, and eventually the ability to move and walk. The cause can be degeneration in nerve centers of the brain and spinal cord that are involved in muscle control. For example, ✪ Huntington's disease (chorea), ✪ Parkinson's disease, ✪ Creutzfeldt-Jakob disease, ✪ multiple sclerosis, ✪ motor neuron disease, ✪ amyotrophic lateral sclerosis, Tourette's syndrome and related choreas. Treatments for some of these disorders are discussed at their own entries. Further information about drug treatment of Parkinson's disease can be found at ℞ antiparkinsonism.

Yet other motor disorders arise not through dysfunction in the CNS, but in the peripheral nervous system, for instance, the muscle weakness disorder ✪ myasthenia gravis is caused by impaired transmission between nerve and skeletal muscle (its treatment is detailed under ℞ anticholinesterase).

In some instances it is possible to identify the cause as a deficiency or imbalance of certain neurotransmitters involved in CNS motor control. The aim of drug treatment is, therefore, to mimic neurotransmitter action, or to increase or decrease neurotransmitter release and action. For example, in Parkinson's disease, the action of dopamine is enhanced and that of acetylcholine suppressed. In many cases the mood of the patient is supported with ℞ antidepressant drugs (for example, in Creutzfeldt-Jakob disease and Gilles de la Tourette syndrome).

Where there is an inflammatory aspect to the disorder, ℞ corticosteroid drugs or ℞ interferons may be useful (for example, in multiple sclerosis). In many cases, especially for involuntary muscular tics and choreas, specialist drugs (including agents also used as ℞ antipsychotic drugs) have been found to suppress symptoms such as motor symptoms (for example, ℞ haloperidol and ℞ pimozide in Gilles de la Tourette syndrome and related choreas, and ℞ fluphenazine in Huntingdon's disease). Some drugs help improve outcome, for instance in amyotrophic lateral sclerosis, ℞ riluzole extends survival and time to tracheostomy. Where muscle contractions are a problem (for example, Creutzfeldt-Jakob disease), ℞ skeletal muscle relaxant drugs may provide relief.
Limitations
See the individual drug entries.

Breathe Free Ⓑ

A preparation of ℞ sodium chloride.
Formulation: Nasal mist.
Availability: OTC.
Warnings and side effects: See ℞ sodium chloride.

Breonesin Capsules Ⓑ

A preparation of ℞ guaifenesin.
Formulation: Oral capsules.

Availability: OTC.
Warnings and side effects: See ℞ guaifenesin.

Brethine ⓑ

A preparation of ℞ terbutaline sulfate.
Formulation: Oral tablets in two strengths; injection.
Availability: Prescription only.
Warnings and side effects: See ℞ terbutaline sulfate.

bretilium tosilate ⓖ

see ℞ bretylium tosylate.

bretylium tosylate ⓖ

(bretilium tosilate)
Type/Group: **antiarrhythmic; adrenergic-neuron blocker; antisympathetic.**
Brand(s): Various generic.
How administered: Injection.

Used to treat

Bretylium tosilate is used to treat abnormal heart rhythms in resuscitation (see ✪ **arrhythmia**), where other treatments have not been successful. It has ℞ **adrenergic-neuron blocker** actions, and as an ℞ **antisympathetic** prevents release of norepinephrine from sympathetic nerves.

Warnings

• It should be given with caution to people with conditions that restrict heart output (for example, aortic stenosis). It is a specialist drug and is used only under qualified medical supervision and in adequately equipped facilities (with the capability of constant monitoring).
• It should be used during pregnancy only if it is clearly needed.
• As this drug is used only in life-threatening circumstances, breast-feeding is not a consideration.
• Bretylium does suppress the activity of norepinephrine, but its initial, short-lasting effect is to release large amounts of norepinephrine. There may be, therefore, a transient increase in blood pressure and possible worsening of arrhythmias.

Interactions

• The effects of catecholamines (for example, ℞ **dopamine**, ℞ **norepinephrine**) may be intensified.
• Bretylium should not be used when arrhythmias may have been caused by an overdose of ℞ **digoxin**. Also, digoxin treatment should not be begun while bretylium is being used.
• The effects of other antiarrhythmic drugs may be unpredictable.

Side effects

• Hypotension is the most common, and nausea and vomiting may follow rapid injection.
• Other side effects may include nasal stuffiness, loose stools, diarrhea, and dizziness. There may be tissue damage at the site of injection.

Brevibloc ⓑ

A preparation of ℞ esmolol hydrochloride.
Formulation: Intravenous infusion.
Availability: Prescription only.

Warnings and side effects: See ℞ esmolol hydrochloride.

Brevicon ⓑ

A preparation of ℞ ethinyl estradiol and ℞ norethindrone.
Formulation: Calendar pack of oral tablets, 21 or 28 days.
Availability: Prescription only.
Warnings and side effects: See ℞ ethinyl estradiol; ℞ norethindrone.

Brexin L.A. Capsules ⓑ

A preparation of ℞ pseudoephedrine and ℞ chlorpheniramine maleate.
Formulation: Oral capsules, sustained release.
Availability: Prescription only.
Warnings and side effects: See ℞ pseudoephedrine; ℞ chlorpheniramine maleate.

Bricanyl ⓑ

A preparation of ℞ terbutaline sulfate.
Formulation: Oral tablets in two strengths.
Availability: Prescription only.
Warnings and side effects: See ℞ terbutaline sulfate.

brimonidine tartrate ⓖ

Type/Group: **alpha-adrenergic stimulant; glaucoma treatment.**
Brand(s): Alphagan.
How administered: Topically (eyes).

Used to treat

Brimonidine can be used to treat ✪ **glaucoma** (open-angle glaucoma and ocular hypertension), particularly when other drugs have not been effective or are not appropriate.

Warnings

• It should not be given to people with known hypersensitivity to brimonidine or who are taking ℞ **MAOIs.**
• It should be given with caution to people with severe cardiovascular disease, depression, cerebral or coronary insufficiency, Raynaud's phenomenon, or postural hypotension.
• Brimonidine's safety during pregnancy has not been established. It should be used only if the potential benefit outweighs the possible risk to the fetus.
• It should not be used by nursing mothers.
• Its effectiveness to lower pressure in the eyeball (intraocular pressure) may decrease over time in some people.
• It may cause drowsiness and so impair the performance of skilled tasks, such as driving.
• The preservative in the available forms of brimonidine may be absorbed onto soft contact lenses, and so it should be used 15 minutes before putting in the lenses.

Interactions

• The effects of CNS (central nervous system) depressants (for example, alcohol, ℞ **barbiturates**, ℞ **opiates**, ℞ **sedatives**, ℞ **anesthetics**), ℞ **beta-blockers**, ℞ **antihypertensives**, and ℞ **cardiac glycosides**) may be increased.
• ℞ **tricyclic** antidepressants can reduce the effects of brimonidine.

Key to symbols: ⓓ = Drug type/group   ⓖ = Generic name   ⓑ = Brand name

• ℞ **MAOI**s should not be used with brimonidine because their effects may be increased.

Side effects

• Frequently, drowsiness, fatigue, headache, blurred vision, burning, foreign body sensation, itching, stinging, tearing in eyes, and dry mouth.

• Occasionally, corneal staining, light sensitivity, swollen eyelids, and dizziness.

• Since brimonidine can be absorbed through the eye into the body, there could be systemic effects, for instance on the cardiovascular system (for example, palpitations).

brinzolamide ⓖ

Type/Group: **carbonic anhydrase inhibitor; glaucoma treatment.**
Brand(s): Azopt.
How administered: Topically (eyes).

Used to treat

Brinzolamide is used to treat ✪ **glaucoma**. It reduces the formation of aqueous humor (fluid) in the eye and thereby lowers pressure in the eyeball.

Warnings

• It should not be given to people with known hypersensitivity to brinzolamide or ℞ **sulfonamides**.

• It should be given with caution to people with severe kidney or liver impairment.

• Brinzolamide's safety in pregnancy has not been established. It should be used only if the potential benefit outweighs the possible risk to the fetus.

• Medical judgment is required if breast-feeding is being considered.

• Brinzolamide is a sulfonamide and is absorbed systemically, and so has the potential for producing the adverse reactions produced by this class of drug.

• The preservative in brinzolamide solution, benzalkonium chloride, may be absorbed by soft contact lenses.

Interactions

No significant interactions have been reported.

Side effects

• Frequently, blurred vision, bitter, sour or unusual taste.

• Less frequently, inflamed eyelid, dry eye, foreign body sensation, discharge, discomfort, inflammation, pain, or itching of the eye, and nasal inflammation.

Brofed Elixir ⓑ

A preparation of ℞ **pseudoephedrine** and ℞ **brompheniramine maleate**.
Formulation: Oral liquid.
Availability: Prescription only.
Warnings and side effects: See ℞ **pseudoephedrine**; ℞ **brompheniramine maleate**.

Bromadine-DM ⓑ

A preparation of ℞ **dextromethorphan**, ℞ **brompheniramine maleate**, and ℞ **pseudoephedrine**.

Formulation: Oral liquid.
Availability: Prescription only.
Warnings and side effects: See ℞ **dextromethorphan**; ℞ **brompheniramine maleate**; ℞ **pseudoephedrine**.

Bromanyl Syrup ⓑ

A preparation of ℞ **codeine phosphate** and bromodiphenhydramine.
Formulation: Oral capsules; syrup.
Availability: May or may not require a prescription.
Warnings and side effects: See ℞ **codeine phosphate**.

Bromarest DX Cough Syrup ⓑ

A preparation of ℞ **dextromethorphan**, ℞ **brompheniramine maleate**, and ℞ **pseudoephedrine**.
Formulation: Oral syrup.
Availability: Prescription only.
Warnings and side effects: See ℞ **dextromethorphan**; ℞ **brompheniramine maleate**; ℞ **pseudoephedrine**.

Bromatane DX Cough Syrup ⓑ

A preparation of ℞ **dextromethorphan**, ℞ **brompheniramine maleate**, and ℞ **pseudoephedrine**.
Formulation: Oral syrup.
Availability: Prescription only.
Warnings and side effects: See ℞ **dextromethorphan**; ℞ **brompheniramine maleate**; ℞ **pseudoephedrine**.

Bromfed DM Cough Syrup ⓑ

A preparation of ℞ **pseudoephedrine** sulfate and dexbrompheniramine maleate.
Formulation: Oral syrup.
Availability: Prescription only.
Warnings and side effects: See ℞ **brompheniramine maleate**; ℞ **pseudoephedrine**.

Bromfed Syrup ⓑ

A preparation of pseudoephedrine sulfate and dexbrompheniramine maleate.
Formulation: Oral syrup.
Availability: OTC.
Warnings and side effects: See ℞ **pseudoephedrine**; ℞ **brompheniramine maleate**.

Bromfed Tablets; Capsules; PD Capsules ⓑ

A preparation of ℞ **pseudoephedrine** and ℞ **brompheniramine maleate**.
Formulation: Oral tablets; capsules, sustained release.
Availability: Prescription only.
Warnings and side effects: See ℞ **pseudoephedrine**; ℞ **brompheniramine maleate**.

Key to symbols: ✪ = Disorder Section ℞ = Drug Section ♣ = Herbal Section ⚬⚬ = Supplement Section

Bromfenex Capsules; Bromfenex PD Capsules Ⓑ

A preparation of ℞ **pseudoephedrine** and ℞ **brompheniramine maleate**.

Formulation: Oral capsules, sustained release.

Availability: Prescription only.

Warnings and side effects: See ℞ **pseudoephedrine**; ℞ **brompheniramine maleate**.

bromocriptine Ⓖ

Type/Group: **dopamine-receptor stimulant; antiparkinsonism; ergot alkaloid.**

Brand(s): Parlodel.

How administered: Orally.

Used to treat

Bromocriptine is used to treat parkinsonism (but not the parkinsonian symptoms caused by certain drug therapies: see ℞ **antiparkinsonism**). It works by stimulating the dopamine receptors in the brain (it is a dopamine-receptor stimulant) and so is different to the more commonly used ℞ **levodopa**, which is converted to dopamine in the body. It is therefore useful for people who, for whatever reason, cannot tolerate levodopa. Occasionally, the two drugs are combined. Bromocriptine has alternative uses (some related to its ability to inhibit prolactin secretion by the pituitary gland): to treat delayed puberty caused by hormonal insufficiency; to relieve certain menstrual disorders, infertility, prolactinoma (tumor of the pituitary gland, leading to excess prolactin secretion); and sometimes for treating acromegaly (over-secretion of the anterior pituitary gland due to a tumor). Although not stated by the manufacturer for such use, it is sometimes also used to treat cyclical benign breast disease, to prevent lactation, for neuroleptic malignant syndrome, and cocaine addiction.

Warnings

• It should not be given to people with known hypersensitivity to any ergot alkaloid, or with severe ischemic disease or peripheral vascular disease (such as Raynaud's disease).

• It should be given with caution to people with menstrual disorders, liver and kidney disorders, porphyria, or cardiovascular disorders.

• Bromocriptine should not be used during pregnancy or while breast-feeding.

• Full and regular monitoring of various body systems is essential during treatment.

Interactions

• ℞ **erythromycin** may increase the levels of bromocriptine, causing overdose effects.

• ℞ **Sympathomimetics** may seriously intensify its side effects.

• ℞ **Amitriptyline**, ℞ **phenothiazines**, ℞ **imipramine**, ℞ **methyldopa**, and ℞ **reserpine** may block the prolactin-reducing effect of bromocriptine, and so the dose may have to be increased.

• If used with phenylpropanolamine, the risk of adverse reactions is increased (for example, seizures, hypertension).

Side effects

• There may be nausea, vomiting, constipation, headache, dizziness (especially on rising from sitting or lying down-postural hypotension), spasm in the blood vessels of the extremities, involuntary movements, and drowsiness.

• High dosage may cause hallucinations, a state of confusion, leg cramps, and a variety of rare disorders that may be serious, such as seizures, stroke, shock, changes in heart rhythm, and gastrointestinal bleeding.

Bromphen DX Cough Syrup Ⓑ

A preparation of ℞ **dextromethorphan**, ℞ **brompheniramine maleate**, and ℞ **pseudoephedrine**.

Formulation: Oral syrup.

Availability: Prescription only.

Warnings and side effects: See ℞ **dextromethorphan**; ℞ **brompheniramine maleate**; ℞ **pseudoephedrine**.

brompheniramine maleate Ⓖ

Type/Group: **antihistamine; antiallergic; cold and cough preparation.**

Brand(s): (all combinations): With phenylephrine: Dimetane Decongestant Elixir. (Plus) *acetaminophen*: Dimetane Decongestant Tablets. With pseudoephedrine: Allent Capsules; Brofed Elixir; Bromfed Capsules, Bromfed Tablets, PD Capsules; Bromfed Syrup; Bromfenex Capsules, PD Capsules; Dallergy-JR Capsules; Dexaphen-S.A. Tablets; Disobrom Tablets; Disophrol Tablets; Disophrol Chronotabs; Drixomed Tablets; Drixoral Cold & Allergy Tablets; Drixoral Syrup; Endafed Capsules; Iofed Capsules, PD Capsules; Lodrane LD Capsules; Respahist Capsules; Rondec Chewable Tablets; Touro A & H Capsules; ULTRAbrom Capsules, PD Capsules. (Plus) *acetaminophen*: Drixoral Cold & Flu Tablets; Maximum Strength Dristan Cold Caplets. (Plus) *dextromethorphan*: Bromadine-DM; Bromarest DX Cough Syrup; Bromatane DX Cough Syrup; Bromfed DM Cough Syrup; Bromphen DX Cough Syrup; Dimetane-DX Cough Syrup; Myphetane DX Cough Syrup. (Plus) *hydrocodone*: Anaplex HD Syrup. (Most combinations available as generics.)

How administered: Orally; injection.

Used to treat

Brompheniramine is used to treat the symptoms of allergic conditions such as ✪ **hay fever** (seasonal allergic rhinitis) and ✪ **urticaria**, and is also used, in combination with other drugs, for ✪ **colds** and ✪ **coughs**.

Warnings

• It should not be given to people with known hypersensitivity to this drug (or with known sensitivity to other antihistamines).

• Antihistamines should be given with caution to people with asthma (and never during an attack) or lower respiratory disease, heart disease, hypertension, hyperthyroidism, epilepsy, porphyria, increased intraocular pressure (pressure in the eyeball, as in glaucoma), enlarged prostate, urinary retention, or certain obstructive bladder or gastrointestinal conditions.

• Brompheniramine should be used during pregnancy only if it is clearly needed.

• Nursing mothers should discontinue using this drug or discontinue breast-feeding.

• This drug must not be given to infants, and for children under the age of 12 the manufacturer's or medical instructions must be followed closely.

• Because of its sedative side effects, the performance of skilled tasks, such as driving, may be impaired.

• Side effects are more frequent in the elderly.

Interactions

• ℞ **MAOI** antidepressants may prolong and intensify the ℞ **anticholinergic** (see Side effects below) and sedative effects of antihistamines.

• If used with ℞ **tricyclic** antidepressants, other antihistamines, ℞ **skeletal muscle relaxants**, ℞ **antipsychotics**, ℞ **opioids**, ℞ **barbiturates**, ℞ **hypnotics**, ℞ **sedatives**, or ℞ **antianxiety** drugs, there is a risk of intensified side effects.

• Alcohol may intensify side effects such as drowsiness and impaired mental alertness.

Side effects

• These depend on how it is administered. For this type of antihistamine, there is commonly drowsiness, headache, impaired muscular coordination or dizziness, anticholinergic effects (dry mouth, blurred vision, urinary retention, gastrointestinal disturbances), occasional rashes and photosensitivity (abnormal sensitivity to light), palpitations and heart arrhythmias.

• Rarely, there may be stimulation instead of sedation (paradoxical stimulation), especially in children (and convulsions in overdose), hypersensitivity reactions, blood disorders, liver disturbances, depression, sleep disturbances, and hypotension.

bronchodilator ⑩

Generics: **albuterol; bitolterol mesylate; ipratropium bromide; isoetharine; levalbuterol hydrochloride; metaproterenol; pirbuterol; salmeterol; terbutaline sulfate; theophylline.**

Actions and uses

Bronchodilators are ℞ **smooth muscle relaxant** agents which act on the bronchioles (air passages in the lungs), so allowing air to flow more easily in or out (the latter being the major problem in obstructive airways disease). There are a number of conditions that cause bronchospasm (spasm in the bronchial muscles) and increased secretion of mucus and so blockage, but the most common are ✪ **asthma** and ✪ **chronic obstructive pulmonary disease** (COPD), including ✪ **bronchitis**, and ✪ **emphysema**.

The type of drug mainly used to treat bronchospasm is a ℞ **beta-adrenergic stimulant** (℞ **sympathomimetic**) agent (mainly selective for $beta_2$-receptors). These drugs (including ℞ **albuterol**, ℞ **levalbuterol hydrochloride**, ℞ **terbutaline**, ℞ **bitolterol**, ℞ **isoetharine**, ℞ **pirbuterol**, ℞ **salmeterol**, ℞ **metaproterenol** and ℞ **salmeterol**) work by stimulating beta-adrenoceptors on the smooth muscle of the airways, which normally respond to adrenal hormones and sympathetic nerve neurotransmitters (epinephrine and norepinephrine).

℞ **xanthine** compounds (℞ **theophylline** and its derivatives aminophylline, dyphylline, and oxtriphylline) are entirely different, and work as bronchodilators by acting directly on the smooth muscle

of the bronchioles. They are mainly used as an ℞ **antiasthmatic**, and for the treatment of chronic bronchitis and emphysema (as in COPD). They are not inhaled but taken by mouth, by rectal suppository, or injection in emergencies. Also used as bronchodilators are inhaled (antimuscarinic) ℞ **anticholinergic** drugs (mainly ℞ **ipratropium bromide**), which are used for maintenance treatment of bronchospasm in chronic obstructive pulmonary disease (COPD), including bronchitis, and emphysema.

All these drugs (except the xanthines) are best administered directly to the airways (except in an emergency) by the use of aerosols, ventilator sprays, or nebulizing mists, because this minimizes side effects as less of the drug is absorbed into the bloodstream.

Bronchodilator treatment has become dominated by the selective $beta_2$-receptor stimulant drugs (see ℞ **beta-adrenergic stimulant**). The development of these drugs, which can be used as bronchodilators without normally having adverse effects on the heart, has been one of the success stories of medicinal chemistry. Of the modern generation $beta_2$-receptor stimulants, some (such as ℞ **albuterol**) are so selective they do not necessarily have to be taken by inhalation, but are also available in oral forms (for those with no heart problems).

Limitations

There seems to be individual overuse of this treatment, especially in asthma, and people become less responsive to a given dose and tend to use the inhaler more and more. See also the individual drug entries.

Broncholate Softgels; Syrup ⑧

A preparation of ℞ **ephedrine** and ℞ **guaifenesin**.

Formulation: Oral capsules; syrup.

Availability: Prescription only.

Warnings and side effects: See ℞ **ephedrine**; ℞ **guaifenesin**.

Bronkaid Dual Action Caplets ⑧

A preparation of ℞ **ephedrine** and ℞ **guaifenesin**.

Formulation: Oral tablets.

Availability: OTC.

Warnings and side effects: See ℞ **ephedrine**; ℞ **guaifenesin**.

Bronkotuss Expectorant Liquid ⑧

A preparation of ℞ **ephedrine**, ℞ **chlorpheniramine maleate**, and ℞ **guaifenesin**.

Formulation: Oral liquid.

Availability: Prescription only.

Warnings and side effects: See ℞ **ephedrine**; ℞ **chlorpheniramine maleate**; ℞ **guaifenesin**.

Brontex ⑧

A preparation of ℞ **codeine phosphate** and ℞ **guaifenesin**.

Formulation: Oral tablets.

Availability: Prescription only.

Warnings and side effects: See ℞ **codeine phosphate**; ℞ **guaifenesin**.

Bucet Capsules ®

A preparation of ℞ **acetaminophen** and ℞ **butabarbital**.
Formulation: Oral capsules.
Availability: Prescription only.
Warnings and side effects: See ℞ **acetaminophen**;
℞ **butabarbital**.

Bucladin-S Softabs ®

A preparation of ℞ **buclizine hydrochloride**.
Formulation: Oral tablets.
Availability: Prescription only.
Warnings and side effects: See ℞ **buclizine hydrochloride**.
Contains tartrazine (FD&C yellow No 5), a dye that may cause
allergic reaction in a few people, but especially those with
sensitivity to aspirin.

buclizine hydrochloride ©

Type/Group: **antihistamine; antinauseant**.
Brand(s): Bucladin-S Softabs.
How administered: Orally.

Used to treat

Buclizine is used to treat ✪ **motion sickness**, ✪ **nausea**, and
✪ **vomiting**.

Warnings

• It should not be given to people with known hypersensitivity to
this drug (or with known sensitivity to other antihistamines).
• Antihistamines should be given with caution to people with
asthma or lower respiratory disease, heart disease, hypertension,
hyperthyroidism, epilepsy, porphyria, increased intraocular
pressure (pressure in the eyeball, as in glaucoma), enlarged
prostate, urinary retention, or certain obstructive bladder or
gastrointestinal conditions.
• Buclizine should not be used during pregnancy.
• Nursing mothers should discontinue using this drug or
discontinue breast-feeding.
• Because of its sedative side effects, the performance of skilled
tasks, such as driving, may be impaired.
• Side effects are more frequent in the elderly.

Interactions

• ℞ **MAOI** antidepressants may prolong and intensify the
℞ **anticholinergic** (see Side effects below) and sedative effects of
antihistamines.
• If used with ℞ **tricyclic** antidepressants, other antihistamines,
℞ **skeletal muscle relaxants**, ℞ **opioids**, ℞ **barbiturates**,
℞ **hypnotics**, ℞ **sedatives**, or ℞ **antianxiety** drugs, there is a risk
of intensified side effects.
• Alcohol may intensify side effects such as drowsiness and
impaired mental alertness.

Side effects

• These depend on how it is administered. For this type of
antihistamine, there is commonly drowsiness, headache, impaired
muscular coordination or dizziness, anticholinergic effects (dry
mouth, blurred vision, urinary retention, gastrointestinal
disturbances; these are slightly more severe than with other
antihistamines), occasional rashes and photosensitivity (abnormal
sensitivity to light), palpitations and heart arrhythmias.
• Rarely, there may be stimulation instead of sedation (paradoxical
stimulation), especially in children (and convulsions in overdose),
hypersensitivity reactions, blood disorders, liver disturbances,
depression, sleep disturbances, and hypotension.

budesonide ©

Type/Group: **corticosteroid; antiasthmatic; decongestant**.
Brand(s): Pulmicort; Rhinocort.
How administered: Inhalation; intranasal.

Used to treat

Budesonide is prescribed as a treatment for nasal inflammation
from allergies (seasonal allergic rhinitis, perennial allergic rhinitis)
and as a respiratory inhalant for maintenance treatment of bronchial ✪ **asthma**. It is not for use in acute asthma attacks.

Warnings

• It should not be used by anyone with known hypersensitivity to
corticosteroids, systemic fungal infections, or who have persistent
positive sputum tests for *Candida albicans* (the organism causing
thrush).
• It should be given with caution to anyone with glaucoma, ocular
herpes simplex, latent or active tuberculosis, recent nasal trauma,
or who has undergone surgery.
• Corticosteroids can cross the placenta, and budesonide,
therefore, should be used during pregnancy only if it is medically
judged that the benefits outweigh potential risk to the fetus.
• Medical judgment is also required if breast-feeding is being
considered. When taken internally, corticosteroids are excreted in
breast milk and may suppress growth and interfere with the
production of natural corticosteroids in the infant. It is not known
whether, or under what conditions, enough of the drug is absorbed
from topical use to create these risks.
• Localized fungal infections (thrush) have occurred in the mouths
and throats of people using corticosteroid inhalants.
• Because corticosteroids suppress the immune system, those using
long-term inhalant therapy are particularly susceptible to infections
(for example, chickenpox, measles), and may become sicker than
others, so risk of exposure must be minimized.
• Growth in children and adolescents must be monitored because
there is evidence that oral corticosteroids may suppress growth
with prolonged use or at high dosages. It is not known whether
enough of the drug is absorbed from inhaled or intranasal use to
create these risks.
• Special care and monitoring is required by asthmatics who are
transferred from using systemically active to inhaled corticosteroids
because serious reactions (even fatal) can occur during times of
stress due to adrenal insufficiency. Patients will be advised of what
to do (for example, resume systemic corticosteroids) during times
of stress or severe asthma attacks and a medic-alert bracelet/
warning card should be carried explaining this.

Interactions

No significant interactions have been reported.

Side effects

These depend on how administered, dose, duration of treatment and use.

- Inhalation: Frequently, flu-like syndrome, headache, throat irritation, and difficulty swallowing. Occasionally, back pain, vomiting, altered taste, hoarseness, abdominal pain, nausea, and upset stomach.
- Intranasal: Most frequently, mild nose or throat irritation, burning, stinging, or dryness, headache, cough. Occasionally, dry mouth, upset stomach, rebound congestion, runny nose, and loss of sense of taste. Rarely, acute sensitivity reactions occur (hives, swelling, severe bronchospasm). Systemic effects are possible (for example, adrenal insufficiency).

Bufferin Tablets; Caplets; Tri-Buffered Bufferin Tablets ⑧

A preparation of ℞ **aspirin**, buffered with ♉ **magnesium oxide**, ℞ **magnesium carbonate**, ℞ **calcium carbonate**.
Formulation: Oral tablets.
Availability: OTC.
Warnings and side effects: See ℞ **aspirin**; ℞ **magnesium carbonate**; ℞ **magnesium hydroxide**; ℞ **calcium carbonate**.

Buffex ⑧

A preparation of ℞ **aspirin**, buffered with aluminum glycinate, ℞ **magnesium carbonate**.
Formulation: Oral tablets.
Availability: OTC.
Warnings and side effects: See ℞ **aspirin**; ℞ **magnesium carbonate**.

bulk-forming agent ⑩

Generics: **methylcellulose; psyllium**.

Actions and uses

Bulk-forming agents are substances that when taken by mouth absorb large amounts of water and swell up, becoming bulkier. For example, the vegetable gum ℞ **karaya** (sterculia gum), ℞ **psyllium** (psyllium hydrophilic mucilloid), and ℞ **methylcellulose**. They are used for two main purposes: first, as ℞ **laxative** agents in ✪ **constipation**; second, as ℞ **appetite suppressants** in ✪ **obesity** (see ℞ **obesity treatment**), because the body feels it has actually taken in more than it has. These agents are available over the counter.

Limitations

It is important to maintain adequate fluid intake when taking bulking agents. They may affect absorption of a wide range of drugs.

Bullfrog Sunblock ⑧

A preparation of ℞ **cinnamates** and other ingredients.
Formulation: Topical lotion, gel, stick.
Availability: OTC.
Warnings and side effects: See ℞ **cinnamates**.

bumetanide ⑥

Type/Group: **diuretic; antihypertensive**.

Brand(s): Bumex; various generic.
How administered: Orally; injection.

Used to treat

Bumetanide is a powerful diuretic of the loop class. It can be used to treat edema (including fluid build-up in the lungs), low urine production (oliguria) due to kidney failure, and also, alone or with other drugs, ✪ **hypertension**.

Warnings

- It should not be given to people with known hypersensitivity to this drug, with anuria (no urine), or in an electrolyte-depleted state.
- It should be given with caution to people with cirrhosis of the liver, or who have certain kidney disorders, gout, diabetes mellitus, an enlarged prostate gland, or porphyria.
- It should be used during pregnancy only if the potential benefit outweighs the possible risk to the fetus.
- Medical judgment is required if breast-feeding is being considered.
- Dehydration may result from too intense a diuretic effect, particularly in elderly people or anyone with a restricted sodium intake.
- Early symptoms of electrolyte imbalance may include muscle weakness or cramps, nausea, vomiting, restlessness or lethargy, dry mouth, excessive thirst, fast pulse, or dizziness. A doctor must be contacted if such symptoms occur.
- Loop diuretics may aggravate symptoms of diabetes mellitus or gout, and worsen or activate lupus erythematosus.
- Periodic monitoring of electrolytes, and kidney and liver function is needed.
- Photosensitivity may develop and so precautions such as protective clothing or sunscreens should be used.
- It may cause postural hypotension (lowered blood pressure on standing up), so get up slowly.

Interactions

- There is a risk of ℞ **lithium** toxicity, and so generally these two drugs should not be used together.
- The effects of ℞ **aminoglycosides**, ℞ **anticoagulants**, other antihypertensives, ℞ **cardiac glycosides**, ℞ **chloral hydrate**, and ℞ **propranolol** may be increased, with the potential of significant side effects or toxicity. An additive effect is sometimes used to advantage in combining loop diuretics with other antihypertensives.
- ℞ **Sulfonylureas** may raise blood sugar levels in diabetics with previously stabilized regimens.
- If taken with ℞ **cisplatin**, there is a potential for increased effects and toxicity.
- ℞ **Amphotericin B**, ℞ **corticosteroids**, and ℞ **corticotropin** may increase the effect of reducing potassium levels, with the possibility of severe depletion.
- The effects of nondepolarizing ℞ **skeletal muscle relaxants** and ℞ **theophylline** are unpredictable.
- ℞ **Activated charcoal**, ℞ **hydantoins**, ℞ **NSAIDs**, and antigout agents (for example, ℞ **probenecid**, ℞ **sulfinpyrazone**) may reduce the effects of bumetanide.

Side effects

• There may be abnormally low blood pressure (hypotension), gastrointestinal disturbances, raised levels of urea in the blood or gout, raised blood glucose, male sexual dysfunction, changes in fats in the blood, headache, dizziness, ringing in the ears and hearing loss. Electrolyte levels in the blood (for example, potassium, sodium, magnesium, and chloride) may be lowered. There may be skin rashes, photosensitivity, effects on bone marrow, blood changes, or pancreatitis. Many of these effects are only seen with high or prolonged dosage; hearing loss (usually reversible) is associated with rapid injection, high dosage, and use with other drugs that affect hearing.

Bumex ®

A preparation of ℞ **bumetanide**.
Formulation: Oral tablets (3 strengths); injection.
Availability: Prescription only.
Warnings and side effects: See ℞ **bumetanide**.

Bupap Tablets ®

A preparation of ℞ **acetaminophen** and ℞ **butabarbital**.
Formulation: Oral tablets.
Availability: Prescription only.
Warnings and side effects: See ℞ **acetaminophen**; ℞ **butabarbital**.

Buphenyl ®

A preparation of ℞ **sodium phenylbutyrate**.
Formulation: Oral tablets; powder.
Availability: Prescription only.
Warnings and side effects: See ℞ **sodium phenylbutyrate**.

bupivacaine ©

Type/Group: **local anesthetic**.
Brand(s): Marcaine; Sensorcaine.
How administered: Local injection.

Used to treat

Bupivacaine is an amide derivative of another local anesthetic ℞ **lidocaine** hydrochloride, and is particularly long-lasting. It is used for spinal anesthesia, including epidural injection (especially during labor), for nerve block, for oral and ophthalmic (eye) surgery, and by local infiltration.

Warnings

• It should not be given to people with known hypersensitivity to local anesthetics or para-aminobenzoic acid. It is a specialist drug and there will be a full medical assessment.

• Bupivacaine's safety in pregnancy has not been established. It should be used only if it is clearly needed.

• Medical judgment is required if breast-feeding is being considered. It is not known whether it appears in breast milk.

• Its use during labor may prolong delivery.

• It can cause cardiac depression, peripheral vasodilatation, or CNS (central nervous system) toxicity.

• Because bupivacaine has a long duration of action, its anesthetic effect may continue for some time after dental procedures have been carried out. Chewing solid foods or probing the anesthetized area should be avoided.

Interactions

• ℞ **Metoprolol**, ℞ **nadolol**, ℞ **propranolol**, and ℞ **cimetidine** increase the levels of bupivacaine.

Side effects

These vary with use and may include:

• Anxiety, disorientation, drowsiness, tremors, speeded heart rate, blood pressure changes, blurred vision, nausea, pupil dilation, vomiting, and allergic skin reactions.

Buprenex ®

A preparation of ℞ **buprenorphine hydrochloride**.
Formulation: Injection.
Availability: Prescription only.
Warnings and side effects: See ℞ **buprenorphine hydrochloride**.

buprenorphine hydrochloride ©

Type/Group: **narcotic analgesic; opioid**.
Brand(s): Buprenex.
How administered: Injection.

Used to treat

Buprenorphine hydrochloride is long-acting (its effects last longer than ℞ **morphine**) and it is used to treat moderate to severe ✪ **pain**, including during surgical operations.

Warnings

• It should not be given to people with known hypersensitivity to this drug. Opioids (even the weaker ones) should not be given to people with asthma, to anyone with seriously depressed breathing disorders, with prostatic hypertrophy, convulsive disorders, raised intracranial pressure, or a head injury.

• Depending on use and dose, they should be given with caution to the elderly, or to anyone with hypotension, certain liver, kidney, biliary tract or adrenal disorders, hypothyroidism (under-activity of the thyroid gland), alcoholism, or a history of drug abuse.

• Buprenorphine should be used during pregnancy only if the benefits outweigh the potential risks.

• Medical judgment is required if breast-feeding is being considered.

• It has some opioid antagonist properties and so it may be dangerous to use it with other narcotic analgesics, and can precipitate withdrawal symptoms in people habituated to, for instance, high doses of morphine or heroin (diamorphine).

• It is a Schedule V controlled substance.

• Prolonged use of narcotics can lead to physical dependence (addiction), although this rarely happens in routine medical use.

• Drowsiness may affect the performance of skilled tasks such as driving.

• The effects of alcohol may be enhanced (including a higher risk of respiratory depression).

• ℞ **Benzodiazepines** have caused serious respiratory side effects when used with this drug.

Interactions
• If used with ℞ **barbiturates**, ℞ **general anesthetics**, ℞ **opioids**, ℞ **tranquilizers** (for example, ℞ **phenothiazines**), ℞ **sedatives**, ℞ **benzodiazepines** (for example, ℞ **diazepam**, ℞ **lorazepam**), or alcohol, increased effects are possible.

Side effects
• Depending on use and dose, there may be nausea and vomiting, drowsiness, loss of appetite, urinary retention, and constipation. There is commonly sedation, and occasionally euphoria, which may lead to a state of mental detachment or confusion. Also, there may be dizziness, sweating, headache, palpitations, changes in heart rate, postural hypotension (a lowering of blood pressure on standing, causing dizziness), rashes, miosis (pupil constriction), dry mouth, flushing of the face, mood change, and hallucinations.
• Rare but serious reactions include respiratory depression and coma.

bupropion hydrochloride ⓖ
(amfebutamone)
Type/Group: **antidepressant; substance-dependence treatment.**
Brand(s): (Antidepressant): Wellbutrin. (Antismoking): Zyban.
How administered: Orally.

Used to treat
Bupropion hydrochloride can be used to treat depressive illness (see ⊙ **depression**) and as an aid to quit smoking (in combination with motivational support). It is chemically an aminoketone derivative, unrelated to other antidepressants (and differing in that it inhibits neuronal uptake of dopamine as well as the usual monoamines).

Warnings
• It should not be given to people with known hypersensitivity to this drug, a history of bulimia or anorexia nervosa, anyone using another product containing bupropion, or anyone taking or have stopped taking a ℞ **MAOI** antidepressant in the previous 14 days.
• It should be given with caution to people with a history of seizures, recent myocardial infarction (heart attack), head trauma, CNS (central nervous system) tumor, liver cirrhosis, diabetes, heart disease, liver disease, bipolar disorder (manic depression), or with drug or alcohol addiction; and with extreme caution to anyone taking CNS stimulants (over-the-counter or prescribed) or anorectics (which are CNS stimulants) because of an increased risk of seizure.
• Bupropion should be used in pregnancy only if the benefits outweigh the possible risk to the fetus.
• It should not be used by nursing mothers.
• Bupropion is associated with a small (0.4 percent) risk of seizure. The risk appears to increase as dosage increases, so doctors' instructions must be followed carefully.
• It may impair the performance of skilled tasks requiring mental alertness or physical skills, such as driving.
• Minimize or avoid alcohol consumption.
• A doctor should be consulted before taking any other medications, including OTC preparations, herbal remedies, supplements, or other natural or alternative products.

• Avoid direct exposure to sunlight or sunlamps.
• It may take two to four weeks before there are any signs of improvement.
• Treatment should be stopped gradually, lowering the dose over a period of time.

Interactions
• Serious or even fatal reactions can occur if ℞ **MAOI** antidepressants are taken at the same time, or within a period of a few weeks after the use of, other antidepressants.
• The effects of ℞ **tricyclic** antidepressants may be enhanced by bupropion.
• The effects of ℞ **levodopa** may be increased, with an increased risk of side effects.
• ℞ **ritonavir** may increase the effects of bupropion, with the potential for toxicity.
• The blood levels of ℞ **carbamazepine** may be decreased.
• There may be a dangerous interaction with ℞ **theophylline** and derivatives.
• ℞ **nicotine** (as patches) may lead to a higher rate of hypertension when used with bupropion.
• Bupropion has inhibitory effects on enzymes involved in the metabolism of a wide range of drugs, so there may be potentially dangerous interactions with a number of drugs apart from those listed above, including systemic ℞ **corticosteroids** and possibly some ℞ **antimalarials**.

Side effects
• Agitation, anxiety, confusion, headache/migraine/insomnia, nausea, vomiting, and dry mouth.
• Less frequently, dizziness, sweating, tremor, seizures, irregular heartbeat, changes in blood pressure, edema, auditory disturbances, blurred vision, appetite increase, constipation, indigestion, impotence, loss of libido, menstrual complaints, urinary frequency, effects on blood sugar levels, breast enlargement in men, arthritis, and skin reactions.

Burn-O-Jel ®
A preparation of ℞ **lidocaine**.
Formulation: Topical gel.
Availability: OTC.
Warnings and side effects: See ℞ **lidocaine**.

Buro-Sol ®
A preparation of ℞ **aluminum acetate**.
Formulation: Topical powder.
Availability: OTC.
Warnings and side effects: See ℞ **aluminum acetate**.

BuSpar ®
A preparation of ℞ **buspirone**.
Formulation: Oral tablets in several strengths.
Availability: Prescription only.
Warnings and side effects: See ℞ **buspirone**.

buspirone ⓖ
Type/Group: **antianxiety; serotonin-receptor stimulant.**

Brand(s): BuSpar.
How administered: Orally.

Used to treat

Buspirone is used to treat ✪ **anxiety**. Although not stated by the manufacturer for such use, it may be used for ✪ **premenstrual syndrome** (PMS).

Warnings

• It should not be given to people with known hypersensitivity to this drug, with epilepsy, or severe liver or kidney impairment.
• It should be given with caution to anyone over the age of 65.
• Buspirone should be used during pregnancy only if the benefits outweigh the risk to the fetus.
• Medical judgment is required if breast-feeding is being considered.
• It may impair the performance of skilled tasks such as driving.
• Avoid alcohol (see Interactions below).
• Treatment may take 3 to 4 weeks, although improvements may be seen earlier.

Interactions

• If used with ℞ **fluoxetine**, the beneficial effects of both drugs are reduced.
• ℞ **Erythromycin**, ℞ **itraconazole**, and ℞ **nefazodone** may increase levels of buspirone.
• The levels of ℞ **haloperidol** may be increased.
• If used with ℞ **trazodone**, there may be effects on the liver.
• ℞ **MAOI** antidepressants may cause a rise in blood pressure.
• Alcohol may enhance the depressant effect.

Side effects

• Nausea, dizziness, drowsiness, headache, nervousness, excitement, lightheadedness, tinnitus, and dream disturbances.
• Less frequently, movement disorders, headache, tingling sensation, tremor, effects on the heart, gastrointestinal effects, change in libido, urinary disorders, menstrual irregularity, muscle pain, cramps, or weakness, chest congestion, breathing irregularities, hair loss, skin reactions, fatigue, fever, sweating, and weight gain.

busulfan ⓖ

(busulphan)
Type/Group: **anticancer; cytotoxic**.
Brand(s): Myleran; Busulfex.
How administered: Orally; intravenous injection.

Used to treat

Busulfan is an (*alkylating agent*) anticancer drug, used particularly for chronic myelogenous ✪ **leukemias**. It works by direct interference with the DNA.

Warnings

• It should not be given to people with known hypersensitivity to busulfan. This is a specialist drug which will be used following a full evaluation by specialist physicians.
• Busulfan is not recommended for use during pregnancy unless it is medically judged to be essential, because it may cause birth defects. Becoming pregnant while using this drug should be avoided.
• It should not be used if breast-feeding.

• It depresses bone marrow, which may cause bleeding and a reduced resistance to infection (bone marrow function will be closely monitored).
• It can cause a syndrome resembling adrenal insufficiency (weakness, severe fatigue, weight loss) with prolonged use.
• Rarely, it may cause changes in lung cells, or cells of other organs, impair liver function, and cause seizures.
• It can impair fertility in men and women (which may be reversible).
• In common with many anticancer drugs, it is associated with the development of secondary malignancies (new cancers).

Interactions

• ℞ **Acetaminophen** and ℞ **itraconazole** may increase the effects of busulfan.
• ℞ **Cyclophosphamide** may increase the risk of heart reactions.
• ℞ **Phenytoin** may reduce the effects of busulfan.
• ℞ **Thioguanine** may increase the risk of liver problems.

Side effects

• Oral use: In addition to those listed under Warnings above, darkening of the skin, allergic skin reactions, cataracts, electrolyte changes, and others.
• Injection: Gastrointestinal effects, fever, headache, chills, pain, electrolyte changes, swelling, insomnia, anxiety, dizziness, depression, speeded heartbeat, elevated blood pressure, thrombosis, nasal inflammation, vasodilatation, and allergic reaction.

Busulfex ⓑ

A preparation of ℞ **busulfan**.
Formulation: Injection.
Availability: Prescription only.
Warnings and side effects: See ℞ **busulfan**.

busulphan ⓖ

see ℞ **busulfan**.

butabarbital ⓖ

(butobarbitone)
Type/Group: **hypnotic; sedatives; barbiturate**.
Brand(s): Butisal; various generic.
How administered: Orally.

Used to treat

Butabarbital is used only when absolutely necessary, and in the short term only, to treat severe and difficult to treat ✪ **insomnia**.

Warnings

• It should not be given to people with known hypersensitivity to barbiturates, respiratory depression, severe liver impairment, or porphyria.
• It should be given with caution to people with anemia, addiction to barbiturates, liver disease, chronic obstructive pulmonary disease (COPD), emphysema, high blood pressure, acute or chronic pain, mental depression, or a history of drug abuse. Caution is also recommended for anyone over the age of 65.

• Butabarbital should not be used during pregnancy if possible. A doctor must be contacted if pregnancy occurs while using this drug.

• Medical judgment is required if breast-feeding is being considered.

• There is a high risk for dependence (addiction) and abuse.

• It loses its effectiveness for treating insomnia after about two weeks.

• Avoid driving or other activities requiring alertness.

• Do not drink alcohol (see Interactions below).

• Do not stop using this drug abruptly after long-term use.

• It is very dangerous in overdose.

• Butabarbital is a Schedule III controlled substance.

Interactions

• Butabarbital decreases the response to oral ℞ **anticoagulants** (for example, ℞ **warfarin sodium**).

• If used with ℞ **acetaminophen**, there is an increased risk of toxic effects on the liver.

• The levels and beneficial effects of the following drug are reduced: ℞ **antidepressants**; ℞ **beta-blockers**; ℞ **calcium-channel blockers**; ℞ **corticosteroids**; ℞ **cyclosporine**; ℞ **digitoxin**, ℞ **disopyramide**, ℞ **doxycycline**, ℞ **estrogens**, ℞ **griseofulvin**; ℞ **oral contraceptives**; ℞ **propafenone**; ℞ **quinidine**; ℞ **tacrolimus**; ℞ **theophylline**.

• ℞ **MAOI** antidepressants prolong the effects of barbiturates.

• If butabarbital is used with an ℞ **antipsychotic**, the effects of both drugs are reduced.

• The levels of ℞ **chloramphenicol** are reduced, while those of the barbiturate are increased.

• If used with methoxyflurane, the adverse effects on the kidneys are increased.

• The effects of ℞ **narcotic analgesics** may be altered, with increased central nervous system (CNS) depression.

• ℞ **Valproic acid** increases the levels of barbiturate.

• If used with alcohol, there is excessive central nervous system (CNS) depression.

Side effects

• There may be hangover with drowsiness, lack of energy, or rash.

• Less frequently, central nervous system (CNS) depression, dizziness, headache, lightheadedness, mental depression, physical dependence, slurred speech, excitement in children and those over 65, vertigo, slowed heartbeat, lowered blood pressure, gastrointestinal upset, and hives.

• Rare but serious side effects include blood cell disorders, breathing stoppages, respiratory depression, spasms of the bronchi or larynx, and Stevens-Johnson syndrome (a severe skin disorder).

Butex Forte Capsules ⑧

A preparation of ℞ **acetaminophen** and ℞ **butabarbital**.
Formulation: Oral capsules.
Availability: Prescription only.
Warnings and side effects: See ℞ **acetaminophen**; ℞ **butabarbital**.

Butisol ⑧

A preparation of ℞ **butabarbital**.
Formulation: Oral tablets; elixir.
Availability: Prescription only.
Warnings and side effects: See ℞ **butabarbital**.

butobarbitone ⑥

see ℞ **butabarbital**.

butoconazole ⑥

Type/Group: **antifungal; azole**.
Brand(s): Femstat; Gynazole.
How administered: Topically (external).

Used to treat

Butoconazole is an imidazole/azole antifungal drug used to treat vaginal ✪ **candidiasis**.

Warnings

• It should not be given to people with known sensitivity to butoconazole.

• Its safety in pregnancy has not been established. It should not be used in the first trimester, and used in the second and third trimester only if clearly needed.

• Do not use while breast-feeding.

• Sexual intercourse should be avoided.

Interactions

No significant interactions have been reported when used topically.

Side effects

• Itching, pain, burning, genital or abdominal pain, and headache.

butorphanol tartrate ⑥

Type/Group: **narcotic analgesic; opioid**.
Brand(s): Stadol, Stadol NS.
How administered: Nasal spray; injection.

Used to treat

Butorphanol tartrate is used to treat moderate to severe ✪ **pain**, including use before surgery or labor and delivery. It is an opioid, but less likely to cause dependence than some others in this class of analgesics. However, it can trigger withdrawal symptoms if used by people dependent on opioids.

Warnings

• It should not be given to people with known hypersensitivity to this drug, or with certain cardiovascular complications. Opioids (even the weaker ones) should not be given to asthmatics, people with seriously depressed breathing disorders, prostatic hypertrophy, convulsive disorders, raised intracranial pressure or a head injury.

• Depending on use and dose, they should be given with caution to the elderly, or to those with hypotension, porphyria, certain liver, kidney or adrenal disorders, hypothyroidism (under-activity of the thyroid gland), or alcoholism.

• Butorphanol should be used during pregnancy only if the potential benefit outweighs the possible risk to the fetus. (It is used, however, during delivery—with caution if the fetus has an abnormal heart rhythm.)

Key to symbols: ✪ = Disorder Section ℞ = Drug Section ♣ = Herbal Section ⚕⚕ = Supplement Section

• Medical judgment is required if breast-feeding is being considered.

• Forms of butorphanol are Schedule IV controlled substances.

• With prolonged use, narcotics can lead to physical dependence (addiction), although this rarely happens in routine medical use.

• Treatment by injection may cause pain and tissue damage at the site of the injection.

• Drowsiness may affect the performance of skilled tasks such as driving.

• The effects of alcohol may be enhanced (with a higher risk of respiratory depression).

Interactions

• ℞ **Barbiturates**, ℞ **general anesthetics**, ℞ **opioids**, ℞ **tranquilizers** (for example, ℞ **phenothiazines**), ℞ **sedatives**, ℞ **benzodiazepines** (for example, ℞ **diazepam**, ℞ **lorazepam**), or alcohol taken with butorphanol are likely to enhance effects.

• If used with nasal ℞ **decongestants** (for example, ℞ **oxymetazoline**), butorphanol nasal spray may be absorbed more slowly, and so will have a slower pain-killing effect.

Side effects

• There may be sedation, dizziness, vomiting, nausea, and constipation. There is occasionally euphoria, which may lead to a state of mental detachment or confusion.

• Less frequently, there may be sweating, headache, palpitations, changes in heart rate, postural hypotension (a lowering of blood pressure on standing, causing dizziness), rashes, miosis (pupil constriction), dry mouth, flushing of the face, mood change, and hallucinations.

Byclomine Tablets; Capsules ⑧

A preparation of ℞ **dicyclomine hydrochloride**.
Formulation: Oral tablets; capsules.
Availability: Prescription only.
Warnings and side effects: See ℞ **dicyclomine hydrochloride**.

cabergoline ⑥

Type/Group: dopamine-receptor stimulant; antiparkinsonism.
Brand(s): Dostinex.
How administered: Orally.

Used to treat

Cabergoline has properties similar to ℞ **bromocriptine**. It is used in the treatment of hormonal disorders due to an excess secretion of the hormone prolactin. Although not stated by the manufacturer for such use, it is sometimes prescribed for the treatment of ⊙ Parkinson's disease.

Warnings

• It should not be given to people with known hypersensitivity to ergot derivatives, uncontrolled hypertension, or pregnancy-induced hypertension.

• It should be given with caution to people with liver impairment.

• Cabergoline should be used during pregnancy only if it is clearly needed.

• It is not recommended for use while breast-feeding. This drug interferes with milk production.

Interactions

• It should not be used with ℞ **phenothiazines**, butyrophenones, thioxanthenes, or ℞ **metoclopramide**.

Side effects

• Nausea, headache, constipation, dizziness, fatigue, and sleepiness.

Cafatine ⑧

A preparation of ℞ **ergotamine tartrate**, ℞ **caffeine**, and ℞ **belladonna alkaloids**.
Formulation: Oral tablets; suppositories (without belladonna alkaloids).
Availability: Prescription only.
Warnings and side effects: See ℞ **ergotamine tartrate**; ℞ **caffeine**; ℞ **belladonna alkaloids**.

Cafergot ⑧

A preparation of ℞ **ergotamine tartrate** and ℞ **caffeine**.
Formulation: Suppositories.
Availability: Prescription only.
Warnings and side effects: See ℞ **ergotamine tartrate**; ℞ **caffeine**.

Cafetrate ⑧

A preparation of ℞ **ergotamine tartrate** and ℞ **caffeine**.
Formulation: Suppositories.
Availability: Prescription only.
Warnings and side effects: See ℞ **ergotamine tartrate**; ℞ **caffeine**.

caffeine ⑥

Type/Group: xanthine; CNS stimulant; respiratory stimulant.
Brand(s): Anacin Tablets; Caplets; APAP-Plus Tablets; Aqua-Ban; Aqua-Ban Plus; Darvon Compound-65 Pulvules; Ercaf; Esgic Tablets, Capsules; Esgic-Plus Tablets, Capsules; Excedrin Aspirin Free Caplets, Geltabs; Excedrin Migraine; Extra Strength Caplets; Tablets; Geltabs; Fioricet Tablets; Fioricet w/Codeine Capsules; Fiortal Capsules; Goody's Extra Strength Headache Powder; Hycomine Compound Tablets; Margesic Capsules; Medigesic Capsules; Midol Maximum Strength Menstrual Caplets, Geltabs; Norgesic; Norgesic Forte; P-A-C Analgesic Tablets; Repan Tablets; Repan Tablets; Saleto Tablets; Scot-Tussin Original 5-Action Liquid; Syrup; Summit Extra Strength Caplets; Triad Capsules; Vanquish Tablets; Wigraine
How administered: Orally; injection.

Used to treat

Caffeine is a central nervous sytem (CNS) stimulant with antifatigue and antidrowsiness properties, and is a major constituent of a number of beverages of herbal origin, including tea, coffee, and chocolate, and is incorporated into cola and other soft drinks. It has weak respiratory stimulant properties, and is sometimes used (by injection) to treat overdose with respiratory depressant drugs in adults, or ("off-label") to treat breathing difficulty (apnea) in newborne infants. It is incorporated as an adjuvent in many analgesic preparations, where it is thought to act by enhancing absorption of the analgesic or by having weak analgesic actions itself. It is also incorporated into some antimigraine and antiheadache preparations, and may enhance the actions of other drugs or have a direct effect on the cerebral blood vessels. It has diuretic properties and is incorporated in some diuretic preparations, including those for premenstrual bloating due to fluid retention

Warnings

• It should not be given to people with known hypersensitivity to xanthines (including those experiencing dizziness, palpitations, and increased or abnormal heart rate), active peptic ulcer disease, or a seizure disorder that is uncontrolled by anticonvulsant medication.

• It should be used with caution in people with heart disease, hypoxemia, liver disease, hypertension, congestive heart failure, or alcoholism; it should also be used with caution in newborns.

• Excessive doses may cause severe toxicity; symptoms include insomnia, breathing difficulty (dyspnea), CNS excitement progressing to delirium with alternating states of consciousness and muscle twitching, heart arrhythmias, hyperglycemia, glucosuria and ketonuria, diuresis, raised blood potassium and lymphocytes.

• It should be used during pregnancy only when it is clearly needed.

• It should not be used when breast-feeding, as it is readily distributed in breast milk.

Interactions

• An increased dose is required for people who smoke.

• R **beta-blockers** may have their cardiac stimulation effects enhanced by caffeine.

• R **phenytoin** may reduce the levels of caffeine.

• Smoking may reduce the levels of caffeine.

• Regular consumption of caffeine may reduce clearance (removal) of R **theophylline** from the body and so increase its blood levels.

• Allopurinol inhibits the breakdown (metabolization) of caffeine in the body.

• R **oral contraceptives**, R **cimetidine**, R **disulfiram**, some R **quinolone** drugs, R **terbinafine**, phenylpropanolamine, and R **mexiletine hydrochloride** may increase the levels of caffeine.

• R **clozapine** may have its actions increased by caffeine.

• R **aspirin** and R **phenobarbital** may be metabolized more rapidly in habitual caffeine users.

Side effects

• Commonly, dizziness, restlessness, speeded heart rate.

• Occasionally, marked palpitations, gastrointestinal effects (including diarrhea, worsened ulcer symptoms), urinary frequency, and insomnia.

Caladryl; Caladryl for Kids ®

A preparation of R **calamine**.
Formulation: Topical cream, topical lotion.
Availability: OTC.
Warnings and side effects: See R **calamine**.

Calamatum ®

A preparation of R **calamine**, R **zinc oxide**, R **menthol**, and R **benzocaine**.
Formulation: Topical spray.

Availability: OTC.
Warnings and side effects: See R **calamine**; R **zinc oxide**; R **menthol**; R **benzocaine**.

calamine ⑥

Type/Group: skin preparation; astringent.
Brand(s): Ivarest; Caladryl; Resinol; Calamatum; Rhuli Spray; Aveeno Anti-Itch; various generic.
How administered: Topically (external).

Used to treat

Calamine is a suspension containing R **zinc oxide** (the active ingredient) and ferrous oxide, and has a mild astringent action. It is incorporated into several preparations that are used to cool and soothe itching skin in conditions such as poison ivy, diaper rash, and insect bites. It is also used in some R **emollient** preparations.

Warnings

• It should not be given to people with known hypersensitivity to any ingredient in the preparations.

• Do not use for longer periods or at higher dosages than recommended.

• Do not use on broken skin, deep or puncture wounds, or cuts.

Interactions

No significant interactions are known.

Side effects

Calamine is considered safe in normal topical use.

Calamycin Lotion ®

A preparation of R **pyrilamine maleate**, R **calamine**, R **benzocaine**, and R **chloroxylenol**.
Formulation: Topical lotion.
Availability: OTC.
Warnings and side effects: See R **pyrilamine maleate**; R **calamine**; R **benzocaine**; R **chloroxylenol**.

Calan Tablets; SR Tablets ®

A preparation of R **verapamil hydrochloride**.
Formulation: Oral tablets (3 strengths); sustained-release tablets (SR, 3 strengths).
Availability: Prescription only.
Warnings and side effects: See R **verapamil hydrochloride**.
Calan SR is only used for control of high blood pressure.

Calcidrine Syrup ®

A preparation of R **codeine phosphate** and calcium iodide anhydrous.
Formulation: Oral syrup.
Availability: May or may not require a prescription.
Warnings and side effects: See R **codeine phosphate**.

Calciferol ®

A preparation of R **ergocalciferol**.
Formulation: Oral liquid; injection.
Availability: Liquid is OTC; injection is prescription only.
Warnings and side effects: See R **ergocalciferol**.

Calcijex ®

A preparation of ℞ **calcitriol**.
Formulation: Injection.
Availability: Prescription only.
Warnings and side effects: See ℞ **calcitriol**.

calcipotriene ©

(calcipotriol)
Type/Group: **psoriasis treatment**.
Brand(s): Dovonex.
How administered: Topically (external).

Warnings

• It should not be given to people with hypercalcemia (high blood calcium) or evidence of vitamin D toxicity.
• It should be given with caution to children and those over 65.
• It should be used during pregnancy only if the potential benefit outweighs the possible risk to the fetus.
• Medical judgment is required if breast-feeding is being considered.
• It must not be used on the face.
• Excessive topical (external) use can cause systemic effects (effects within the body).

Interactions

No significant interactions are known.

Side effects

• Frequently, burning, itching, and skin irritation.
• Occasionally, reddened dry skin, peeling, rash, and worsening of psoriasis.
• Rarely, skin atrophy, darkening of the skin, and folliculitis (inflammation of hair follicles).

calcipotriol ©

see ℞ **calcipotriene**.

calcitonin-salmon ©

(salcatonin)
Type/Group: **thyroid hormone; calcium-metabolism modifier**.
How administered: Injection; intranasal.
Brand(s): Miacalcin; Salmonine.

Used to treat

Calcitonin is a thyroid hormone whose function is to lower levels of calcium in the blood (which increases deposits of calcium in the bones). It is used to lower abnormally high calcium levels (**⊙ hypercalcemia**), to treat **⊙ Paget's disease (of the bone)** and for postmenopausal **⊙ osteoporosis**. Calcitonin-salmon is a synthetic version of the form that is found in salmon and an analog of the human form.

Warnings

• It should not be used by people with known hypersensitivity (a skin test is recommended) to this drug.
• It should be given with caution to people with kidney impairment and heart failure.
• It should be used during pregnancy only if the benefits outweigh the risks to the fetus.

• Medical judgment is required if breast-feeding is being considered. In animals, calcitonin inhibits milk production.
• Antibodies to calcitonin may develop after long-term use, but treatment often remains effective.

Interactions

None have been noted.

Side effects

• For people using the nasal spray, nasal infection or irritation, and back pain.
• Following injection, infrequently there is nausea, vomiting, other gastrointestinal effects, flushing dizziness, tingling in the hands, and bad taste.

calcitriol ©

(1,25-dihydroxycolecalciferol)
Type/Group: **vitamin; osteoporosis treatment**.
Brand(s): Rocaltrol; Calcijex.
How administered: Orally; injection.

Used to treat

Calcitriol (1,25-dihydroxycholecalciferol) is a synthesized form of vitamin D that is used to make up vitamin D deficiency in the body, such as in the treatment of hypocalemia (low blood calcium) in dialysis patients with chronic renal failure and in individuals with hypoparathyroidism. It is also sometimes used to treat certain forms of osteoporosis.

Warnings

• It should not be given to people with known hypercalcemia (high blood calcium), hyperphosphatemia, or elevated levels of vitamin D, decreased kidney function, malabsorption syndrome, or abnormal sensitivity to the effects of vitamin D.
• It should be given with caution to people with kidney stones, kidney failure, or heart disease.
• (when dose exceeds RDA for vitamin D). Calcitriol should be used during pregnancy only if the potential benefit outweighs the possible risk to the fetus.
• Medical judgment is required if breast-feeding is being considered. Calcium levels in the infant should be monitored if pharmacologic doses are taken.
• Adequate dietary calcium is necessary for clinical response to treatment.

Interactions

• People on dialysis may develop raised serum levels of magnesium if calcitriol is used with magnesium-containing ℞ **antacids**.
• If used with digitalis glycosides or ℞ **verapamil**, there are adverse cardiac effects from hypercalcemia.
• ℞ **Cholestyramine**, ℞ **ketoconazole**, ℞ **mineral oil**, ℞ **phenytoin**, and ℞ **phenobarbital** may reduce vitamin D synthesis.
• If used with ℞ **thiazide** ℞ **diuretics**, there is an increased risk of hypercalcemia.

Side effects

• Infrequently, weakness, headache, somnolence, gastrointestinal effects, mental changes, weight loss, changes in urination, joint and muscle ache.

calcium carbonate ⑥

Type/Group: **antacid; electrolyte**.

Brand(s): Alka-Mints; Alkets Tablets, Antacid Extra Strength; Amitone; Calglycine Antacid; Chooz; Dicarbosil; Equilet; Maalox Antacid Caplets; Mallarmint; Mylanta Lozenges; Titralac Tablets, Extra Strength Tablets; Tums, Tums E-X, Tums Ultra; various generic. Combinations: With *magnesium carbonate*: Marblen Tablets, Liquid; Mi-Acid Gelcaps; Mylagen Gelcaps; Mylanta Gelcaps. With *magnesium hydroxide*: Mylanta Supreme; Rolaids Calcium Rich Tablets. (Plus): *simethicone*: Di-Gel Advanced Formula; Tempo Tablets (also has *aluminum hydroxide*). With *simethicone*: Gas Ban; Titrilac Plus Tablets, Liquid.

How administered: Orally.

Used to treat

Calcium carbonate, or chalk, is used as an antacid and ♌ **calcium** supplement. It is incorporated into many over-the-counter preparations used to relieve hyperacidity, ✪ **indigestion**, and for the symptomatic relief of ✪ **peptic ulcer**. It is also used as a source of calcium in conditions that deplete calcium levels in the body (for example, hypoparathyroidism, chronic diarrhea, sprue, pregnancy, osteoporosis, pancreatitis, alkalosis, and hyperphosphatemia).

Warnings

• It should be used with caution by people with hypertension, impaired kidney or heart function, or who are taking certain drugs.

• No ill-effects during pregnancy have been associated with calcium carbonate, but a doctor should always be consulted before taking any drug during pregnancy or if breast-feeding.

• Overusing antacids may cause "acid rebound," which is an increase in stomach acid secretion. Calcium carbonate, therefore, should not be used for more than two weeks continuously.

• Do not use when there is abdominal pain, nausea, or vomiting, unless directed by a doctor.

• Calcium carbonate, with prolonged use, may cause milk-alkali syndrome, a serious illness characterized by headache, nausea, vomiting, weakness, alkalosis, and the possibility of kidney damage.

• Anyone taking any medication, including OTCs, herbal remedies, and supplements, should consult a doctor before using an antacid, because antacids may alter the absorption of a wide range of drugs.

Interactions

• The absorption of ℞ **cardiac glycosides** (℞ **digoxin**, ℞ **digitoxin**) and ℞ **quinidine** may be increased, with the potential for cardiac effects.

• The absorption and action of ℞ **atenolol**, ℞ **hydantoins**, iron salts, ℞ **quinolones**, salicylates, and ℞ **tetracyclines** may be lowered. Doses of these drugs should be taken several hours apart from doses of calcium carbonate (a doctor should be consulted for full instructions and cautions).

• Buffered ℞ **aspirin**/antacid combinations should not be used in any long-term treatment, for example, for rheumatic inflammation.

Side effects

• There may be belching or flatulence, and less commonly constipation.

calcium-channel antagonist ⑩

see ℞ **calcium-channel blocker**.

calcium-channel blocker ⑩

(calcium-channel antagonist; calcium-entry blocker).

Generics: **amlodipine besylate; bepridil hydrochloride; diltiazem hydrochloride; felodipine; isradipine; nicardipine hydrochloride; nifedipine; nimodipine; nisoldipine; verapamil hydrochloride**.

Actions and uses

Calcium-channel blocker drugs are a fairly recently introduced class which are being increasingly used in medicine. They work by blocking entry of calcium through channels (specialized pores in a cell's membrane) that admit calcium ions from the fluid surrounding cells to the interior of the cell. Since calcium has very profound activities within cells (such as increasing muscle contraction and electrical excitability), these drugs have powerful effects on cell function.

Their main uses include: a direct ℞ **smooth muscle relaxant** action causing dilatation of blood vessels and effects on heart muscle, which has led to their widespread use as ℞ **antihypertensive** agents (for example, ℞ **amlodipine besylate**, ℞ **isradipine**, ℞ **nicardipine hydrochloride**, ℞ **nifedipine**, ℞ **nisoldipine**, and ℞ **verapamil hydrochloride**); as ℞ **antianginal** treatment (℞ **amlodipine besylate**, ℞ **diltiazem hydrochloride**, ℞ **nicardipine hydrochloride**, ℞ **nifedipine**, ℞ **verapamil hydrochloride**, and ℞ **bepridil hydrochloride**); as ℞ **antiarrhythmic** agents (including ℞ **verapamil hydrochloride** and ℞ **diltiazem hydrochloride**).

There are some more specialist uses including in the prevention of damage to the brain due to ischemia (lack of blood supply) following subarachnoid hemorrhage (a form of ✪ **stroke**, by reducing the risk of cerebral vasospasm which could lead to neurological damage) (for example, ℞ **nimodipine**); as a vasodilator in ✪ **Raynaud's disease** (including ℞ **nicardipine hydrochloride** and ℞ **nifedipine**), and after ✪ **myocardial infarction** (heart attack) when the use of a ℞ **beta-blocker** is not appropriate (℞ **verapamil hydrochloride**).

Limitations

This group of drugs has proved to be very useful, and the range of conditions that may be treated is growing. However, they are not without side effects. Grapefruit juice, for example, may prolong the action of some of them. They should not be taken with a high fat meal or grapefruit juice. See also the individual drug entries.

Calcium Disodium Versenate ℞

A preparation of ℞ **edetate calcium disodium**.

Formulation: Injection.

Availability: Prescription only.

Warnings and side effects: See ℞ **edetate calcium disodium**.

calcium-entry blocker ⑩

see ℞ **calcium-channel blocker**.

Key to symbols: ✪ = Disorder Section ℞ = Drug Section ♣ = Herbal Section ♌ = Supplement Section

calcium folinate Ⓖ

see ℞ leucovorin calcium.

calcium-metabolism modifier Ⓓ

Generics: **alendronate sodium; calcitonin-salmon; calcium carbonate; dihydrotachysterol (DHT); etidronate disodium; pamidronate disodium; ergocalciferol; calcitriol; tiludronate sodium.**

Actions and uses

℞ **calcium-metabolism modifier** drugs alter the metabolism and therefore the levels of calcium in the body. Calcium has an important role in most body processes and there are many ways in which it can be disrupted in disease.

In the normal physiology of the body, two important hormones regulate levels of calcium and related ions. The first is parathyroid hormone (parathormone; parathyrin; PTH) which is secreted by the parathyroid glands (which lie close to the thyroid glands in the neck). It increases the concentration of calcium (and decreases phosphate levels) in the blood, but is not currently used in medicine. The second hormone is calcitonin which is secreted from the thyroid gland, and is quite unrelated to thyroxine which is also produced in the thyroid gland but is secreted by different cells. Calcitonin lowers calcium levels in the blood, and its action is balanced in the body by corresponding opposite action of parathyroid hormone from the adjacent parathyroid gland.

Calcitonin is used in medicine to lower blood levels of calcium when they are abnormally high (✪ **hypercalcemia**), to treat ✪ **Paget's disease (of the bone)** and for postmenopausal ✪ **osteoporosis**. It works by reducing calcium uptake of bone and has effects on the kidney. Preparations for clinical use include synthetic ℞ **calcitonin-salmon** (salcatonin), although natural porcine (pig) calcitonin has been available and it is expected to become available more widely in the synthetic human form.

⚕ **vitamin D** acts with parathyroid hormone and increases the absorption of calcium (and, to a lesser extent, phosphorus) from the intestine, to deposit it in the bones. A deficiency of vitamin D therefore results in bone deficiency disorders, for example, ✪ **rickets** in children. Vitamin D occurs, or is used, in a number of natural forms, including synthetic ℞ **ergocalciferol** (natural calciferol, vitamin D_2), synthetic ℞ **calcitriol**, and ℞ **dihydrotachysterol** (a synthetic form related to D_2 and D_3). These forms are used to treat osteoporosis, refractory rickets, familial hypophosphatemia, and ✪ **hypoparathyroidism**.

Calcium forms used in medicine to counter too low levels include the mineral supplements ℞ **calcium carbonate**, calcium gluconate, calcium lactate, and calcium bicarbonate.

℞ **bisphosphonate** drugs (also called bisphosphonates or diphosphonates) are used as calcium-metabolism modifiers to treat a number of conditions of disturbed calcium metabolism, including Paget's disease of the bone, to prevent and treat heterotropic ossification due to spinal cord injury or hip replacement, hormone-induced disorders of bone metabolism, to prevent postmenopausal osteoporosis and bone fractures in postmenopausal women, bone pain in prostate and breast cancer, and hypercalcemia due to malignancy. These drugs are enzyme-resistant (so they are not broken down fast in the body) analogs of pyrophosphate (a natural inhibitor of bone mineralization), for example ℞ **etidronate disodium**, ℞ **pamidronate disodium**, ℞ **tiludronate sodium**, and ℞ **alendronate sodium**.

Diagnosis and treatment of disorders of calcium metabolism is a specialist procedure. Some of these drugs are being increasingly used to treat postmenopausal osteoporosis, especially where this does not respond adequately to ℞ **hormone replacement** with ℞ **estrogen** hormones.

Limitations

℞ **bisphosphonate** drugs are mainly poorly absorbed when taken by mouth, and ℞ **alendronate sodium** must be taken first thing in the morning before any food. Others, such as ℞ **pamidronate disodium** and ℞ **etidronate disodium**, can be injected. They all have significant side effects, including nausea, diarrhea, headache, generalized body pain, and back pain. See also the individual drug entries.

Caldecort Maximum Strength Ⓑ

A preparation of ℞ **hydrocortisone**.
Formulation: Cream.
Availability: OTC.
Warnings and side effects: See ℞ hydrocortisone.

Caldesene Ⓑ

A preparation of ℞ **cod-liver oil**, ℞ **zinc oxide**, and ℞ **lanolin**.
Formulation: Topical ointment.
Availability: OTC.
Warnings and side effects: See ℞ cod-liver oil; ℞ zinc oxide; ℞ lanolin.

Calglcycine Antacid Ⓑ

A preparation of ℞ **calcium carbonate**.
Formulation: Oral tablets.
Availability: OTC.
Warnings and side effects: See ℞ calcium carbonate.

Calm-X Ⓑ

A preparation of ℞ **dimenhydrinate**.
Formulation: Oral tablets.
Availability: OTC.
Warnings and side effects: See ℞ dimenhydrinate.

Cama Arthritis Pain Reliever Ⓑ

A preparation of ℞ **aspirin**, buffered with ℞ **aluminum hydroxide**, ⚕ **magnesium oxide**.
Formulation: Oral tablets.
Availability: OTC.
Warnings and side effects: See ℞ aspirin; ℞ aluminum hydroxide; ℞ magnesium hydroxide.

Campho-Phenique Ⓑ

A preparation of ℞ **camphor**, ℞ **phenol**, and eucalyptus oil.
Formulation: Topical liquid; topical gel.
Availability: OTC.

Warnings and side effects: See ℞ camphor; ℞ phenol; eucalyptus oil.

Campho-Phenique Antibiotic Plus Pain Reliever ®

A preparation of ℞ neomycin, ℞ polymyxin B sulfate, ℞ bacitracin, and ℞ lidocaine.
Formulation: Topical ointment.
Availability: OTC.
Warnings and side effects: See ℞ neomycin; ℞ polymyxin B sulfate; ℞ bacitracin; ℞ lidocaine.

camphor ©

Type/Group: counter-irritant.
Brand(s): Blistex; Chap Stix; Double Ice ArthriCare Gel; Lip Medex; MenthoRub Ointment; Methalgen Cream; Vick's Vapo-Rub.
How administered: Topically (external).

Used to treat

Camphor is an aromatic substance with mild counter-irritant, or rubefacient, properties. It is incorporated into a number of topical (external use) preparations that are used to help relieve itchiness, and to treat symptoms of muscular pains and rheumatism, arthritis, and similar conditions when the skin is intact. Aromatic vapors from some preparations are inhaled for relief of cough.

Warnings

• It should not be given to people with known hypersensitivity to camphor. Strong concentrations should not be used on children.
• Avoid eyes and mucous membranes.
• Avoid cuts and abraded skin.

Interactions

No significant drug interactions are known.

Side effects

• Temporary burning, stinging, and sneezing.

Camtosar ®

A preparation of ℞ irinotecan hydrochloride.
Formulation: Injection.
Availability: Prescription only.
Warnings and side effects: See ℞ irinotecan hydrochloride.

candesartan cilexetil ©

Type/Group: angiotensin-receptor blocker; antihypertensive; vasodilator.
Brand(s): Atacand.
How administered: Orally.

Used to treat

Candesarten cilexetil is a prodrug of candesartan, to which it is converted in the body. It can be used, alone or in combination with other drugs, to treat ✪ hypertension.

Warnings

• It should not be given to people with known hypersensitivity to this drug.
• It should be given with caution to people with severe congestive heart failure, severely impaired liver or kidney function, or renal stenosis. Any fluid- or salt-depleted condition (as from diuretic use) should be corrected before using this drug.
• Risk in pregnancy increases substantially from the first through to the second and third trimesters. Angiotensin-receptor blockers can cause injury to the developing fetus. The use of these drugs should stop as soon as pregnancy is detected.
• Medical judgment is required if breast-feeding is being considered.
• Blood pressure should be checked regularly.

Interactions

No drug interactions of significance are known.

Side effects

• Angiotensin-receptor blockers in general appear to cause few and infrequent side effects (often indistinguishable from placebo effects). The most common, with candesartan, may include dizziness, leg and back pain, upper respiratory infection, sore throat, and rhinitis.
• Uncommon side effects may include dry cough, fatigue, headache, gastrointestinal disturbances, chest pain or edema. Symptoms such as weakness, rash and effects on heart rhythm seldom occur. There may be changes in kidney function, and angioedema (an allergic swelling reaction, often of the face) has been reported.

candidiasis treatment ⑩

Generics: amphotericin B; butoconazole; clotrimazole; fluconazole; flucytosine; itraconazole; ketoconazole; miconazole; nystatin; terconazole; tioconazole.

Actions and uses

Candidiasis treatment is for an infection (also called moniliasis or thrush) by a yeast-like fungus, which occurs in moist, enclosed areas, such as the mouth, bronchial passages, and vagina, and also in folds of skin (see also ✪ candidiasis; ✪ skin conditions). Treatment is with ℞ antifungal drugs given as creams, tablets, or vaginal pessaries. Most are synthetic ℞ azole drugs (imidazoles/triazoles), such as ℞ butoconazole, ℞ clotrimazole, ℞ fluconazole, ℞ itraconazole, ℞ miconazole, ℞ terconazole, and ℞ tioconazole. These are generally applied topically (externally), but some can be used for systemic treatment (for example, ℞ itraconazole and ℞ fluconazole), as can the synthetic drug ℞ flucytosine. Some of the drugs used are chemically ℞ antibiotic agents, such as ℞ nystatin and ℞ amphotericin B, and for serious infections may be used systemically (often ℞ nystatin).

Limitations

People who are infected should be aware that the fungus causes infection mainly when there is some change or abnormality in the external or internal environment, for example, fluctuating hormonal levels, an impaired immune system (as in AIDS), or a course of antibacterials (especially the ℞ cephalosporin group). If someone is known to be susceptible to infection, then if antibiotics are required, the doctor prescribing them should be informed so a suitable choice can be made.

A number of the azole antifungal drug preparations are now available OTC (over-the-counter) for simple uncomplicated thrush, and although drugs of this group are generally safe, systemic

℞ **itraconazole** and ℞ **fluconazole** should be used during pregnancy or while nursing only if the benefits clearly outweigh the possible risks. See also the individual drug entries.

Capastat Sulfate ⑧

A preparation of ℞ **capreomycin**.
Formulation: Injection.
Availability: Prescription only.
Warnings and side effects: See ℞ **capreomycin**.

capecitabine ⑥

Type/Group: **anticancer**.
Brand(s): Xeloda.
How administered: Orally.

Used to treat

Capecitabine is a recently introduced drug that is used to treat metastatic ✪ **breast cancer** resistant to other treatments. Although not yet labeled for such use, it may also be used for colorectal cancer (cancer of the large intestine).

Warnings

• It should not be given to people with known hypersensitivity to 5-flourouracil (for which capecitabine is a prodrug).
• It should be given with caution to people with severely impaired liver or kidney function, or heart disease. This is a specialist drug which will be used following a full evaluation by specialist physicians.
• Capecitabine is not recommended for use during pregnancy unless it is medically judged to be essential, because it may cause birth defects. Becoming pregnant while using this drug should be avoided.
• It should not be used if breast-feeding.
• It can induce diarrhea, sometimes severe. Anyone over age 80 may experience a higher level of adverse gastrointestinal effects.
• In common with many anticancer drugs, capecitabine may cause mutations and impair fertility.
• It may cause blood problems that slow healing and increase the risk of infection.
• Adverse heart events may occur. These are more common in people with a history of coronary artery disease.
• If "hand-and-foot syndrome" (numbness, tingling, painful swelling, redness, blistering, ulceration, pain and discomfort) occurs, treatment with capecitabine may have to be stopped.
• A doctor must be contacted if fever, chills, or a sore throat develop.

Interactions

• ℞ **Leucovorin** and ℞ **antacids** may increase the effects of capecitabine.

Side effects

• Dehydration, infection, fever, loss of appetite, pain, swelling, redness or tingling in hands or feet, pain swelling redness, or sores in mouth or throat, severe nausea, headache, constipation, dry skin, itching, weakness, and hand-and-foot syndrome.

Capital w/Codeine Suspension ⑧

A preparation of ℞ **codeine phosphate** and ℞ **acetaminophen**.

Formulation: Oral liquid.
Availability: May or may not require a prescription.
Warnings and side effects: See ℞ **codeine phosphate**; ℞ **acetaminophen**.

Capoten ⑧

A preparation of ℞ **captopril**.
Formulation: Oral tablets, available in 4 strengths.
Availability: Prescription only.
Warnings and side effects: See ℞ **captopril**.

Capozide 25/15 ⑧

Also: **Capozide 25/25; Capozide 50/15; Capozide 50/25**
A preparation of ℞ **captopril** and ℞ **hydrochlorothiazide**.
Formulation: Oral tablets, in 4 (captopril/hydrochlorothiazide) strengths.
Availability: Prescription only.
Warnings and side effects: See ℞ **captopril**; ℞ **hydrochlorothiazide**.

capreomycin ⑥

Type/Group: **antibiotic; antituberculosis**.
Brand(s): Capastat.
How administered: Injection.

Used to treat

Capreomycin is a polypeptide antibiotic used specifically in the treatment of ✪ **tuberculosis** that is resistant to the first-line drugs, or in cases where those drugs are not tolerated.

Warnings

• It should not be given to people with known hypersensitivity to capreomycin.
• It should be given with caution to people with kidney or liver impairment, Parkinsonism or myasthenia gravis, or hearing loss.
• Well-controlled studies have not been performed, therefore, it should be used during pregnancy only if clearly needed and if potential benefits outweigh the risks to the fetus.
• Medical judgment is required if breast-feeding is being considered. It is not known whether capreomycin appears in breast milk.
• Capreomycin has been associated with nephrotoxicity (damage to the kidneys) and ototoxicity (damage in the ears).

Interactions

• ℞ **Aminoglycosides** may increase the risk of respiratory paralysis and kidney dysfunction.
• There is an increased risk of ototoxicity if taken with ethacrynic acid.
• Capreomycin may increase the effects of neuromuscular blocking agents.

Side effects

• Blood changes, allergic reactions, such as rash and hives, pain at injection site, fever, headache, hearing loss, tinnitus, ototoxicity, and kidney damage.

capsaicin ⑥

Type/Group: **counter-irritant; psoriasis treatment**.

Brand(s): Capsin; Capzasin-P; Dolorac; No Pain-HP; Pain Doctor; Pain-X; R-Gel; Rid-a-Pain HP; Zostrix.
How administered: Topically (external).

Used to treat

Capsaicin is the active principle of capsicum, which is often used medically in the form of the resin called capsicum oleoresin and is a pungent extract from capsicum peppers. Both capsicum resin and capsaicin are incorporated into medicines used to relieve pain from ✪ **rheumatoid arthritis**, ✪ **osteoarthritis**, and for the relief of neuralgias such as the pain following ✪ **shingles** or diabetic neuropathy. It has a rubefacient, or counter-irritant, action, and when rubbed in topically to the skin has an effect that is not completely understood, but which may block pain signals that would normally go to the pain centers in the brain. Capsaicin is also being investigated as a treatment for psoriasis, intractable itching, pain following mastectomy, trigeminal neuralgia, and phantom limb pain.

Warnings

• It should not be given to people with known hypersensitivity to this drug.
• Capsaicin's safety during pregnancy has not been established.
• Medical judgment is required if breast-feeding is being considered.
• Avoid contact with the eyes and broken or irritated skin.
• Transient burning may occur on application, but this usually diminishes with repeated use.

Interactions

No significant interactions are known.

Side effects

• Frequently, stinging and redness of skin.
• Rarely, cough and respiratory irritation.

Capsin Ⓡ

A preparation of ℞ **capsaicin**.
Formulation: Topical lotion in two strengths.
Availability: OTC.
Warnings and side effects: See ℞ **capsaicin**.

captopril ⓖ

Type/Group: **ACE inhibitor; vasodilator; antihypertensive; heart failure treatment**.
Brand(s): Capoten; various generic. Combinations: With *hydrochlorothiazide*: Capozide.
How administered: Orally.

Used to treat

Captopril is used in the treatment of ✪ **hypertension** and congestive ✪ **heart failure**. It is often used with other classes of drug, particularly ℞ **thiazide** ℞ **diuretics**. Additionally, it can be used following ✪ **myocardial infarction** (damage to heart muscle, usually after a heart attack) and in diabetic nephropathy (kidney disease) in type 1 insulin-dependent diabetes mellitus.

Warnings

• It should not be given to people with known hypersensitivity to this drug or to any other ACE inhibitor.
• It should be given with caution to people with severe congestive heart failure, or certain other cardiovascular disorders, a history of

anaphylaxis, collagen vascular disease (for example, systemic lupus erythematosus; SLE), diabetes mellitus, depressed immune response, or with impaired kidney function or on dialysis.
• Risk in pregnancy increases substantially from the first through to the second and third trimesters. ACE inhibitors can cause injury to the fetus, even death. The use of these drugs should stop as soon as pregnancy is detected.
• Medical judgment is required if breast-feeding is being considered. Captopril appears in breast milk.
• Use of this drug should stop and a doctor notified immediately if signs of angioedema appear (swelling of the face, eyes, lips, tongue, larynx, or extremities; difficulty in breathing or swallowing). Swelling of the larynx, closing off the airway, can be life-threatening.
• Anyone taking an ACE inhibitor should not interrupt or discontinue treatment without first checking with a doctor.
• Any suspected infections (for example, fever, sore throat) should be reported to a doctor. ACE inhibitors may cause blood changes which can affect immune response.
• ACE inhibitors generally have less effect on blood pressure in blacks than in non-blacks, and the likelihood of angioedema is higher among blacks, as well.

Interactions

• ACE inhibitors have apparently triggered life-threatening anaphylactoid reactions when used by people also receiving ℞ **desensitizing vaccines**.
• ℞ **Anesthetics** (for example, in surgery), ℞ **phenothiazines**, and ℞ **probenecid** may increase the levels or hypotensive effect of captopril.
• Levels of ℞ **lithium** may be increased, with the potential for toxic effects.
• If used with potassium-sparing ℞ **diuretics** or other preparations containing potassium (for example, supplements and salt substitutes), levels of potassium may rise.
• ℞ **NSAID**s may increase the risk of kidney damage or (in some cases) reduce the effects of ACE inhibitors.
• ℞ **Antacids** and ℞ **rifampin** may reduce the effects of captopril. Antacids should not be used for several hours after a dose of an ACE inhibitor (a doctor should be consulted for full instructions and cautions).
• If used with other antihypertensives and diuretics, the effects of these drugs may be increased. This additive effect is sometimes used to advantage in combination treatments for high blood pressure.

Side effects

• The most common are rash and an abnormal taste sensation.
• Occasionally there may be headache, dizziness, fatigue, insomnia, tingling in the extremities, tachycardia, or gastrointestinal disturbances (for example, nausea and vomiting, indigestion, diarrhea, constipation).
• Infrequently, weight loss, hair loss, or photosensitivity (abnormal sensitivity to light). Although it is uncommon, ACE inhibitors can cause very marked hypotension (especially when beginning treatment) and kidney impairment. They may also cause persistent dry cough.

• Rarely, there may be angioedema, altered liver function, jaundice, hepatitis, pancreatitis, or changes in blood counts.

Capzasin-·P Ⓑ

A preparation of ℞ **capsaicin**.
Formulation: Topical cream.
Availability: OTC.
Warnings and side effects: See ℞ **capsaicin**.

Carafate Tablets; Suspension Ⓑ

A preparation of ℞ **sucralfate**.
Formulation: Oral tablets; liquid.
Availability: Prescription only.
Warnings and side effects: See ℞ **sucralfate**.

carbachol Ⓖ

Type/Group: **parasympathomimetic; glaucoma treatment**.
Brand(s): Carbastat; Carboptic; Miostat; Isopto Carbachol.
How administered: Intraocular, topically (eyes).

Used to treat

Carbachol is used to treat ⊙ **glaucoma** and during eye surgery to lower pressure in the eyeball and constrict the pupil.

Warnings

• It should not be given to people with known hypersensitivity to carbachol, or to anyone with corneal abrasions.

• It should be given with caution to people with bradycardia, cardiac arrhythmia, hyperthyroidism, asthma, gastrointestinal or urinary tract obstruction, peptic ulcer, parkinsonism, epilepsy, peritonitis, or susceptibility to retinal detachment.

• Carbachol's safety during pregnancy has not been established. It should be used only if the potential benefit outweighs the possible risk to the fetus.

• Medical judgment is required if breast-feeding is being considered.

• Extra care must be taken when driving during the first few days of treatment.

• It may cause problems with adapting to poor light and the dark (for example, driving at night or performing tasks in poor light).

Interactions

• Topical (applied externally) ℞ **NSAIDs** may decrease the effect of carbachol.

Side effects

• Brow ache and headache, which may get worse in the weeks following treatment. There may also be blurred vision, itching, burning and smarting, and other effects on the eye.

• Since carbachol can be absorbed through the eye into the body, there could be systemic effects.

carbamazepine Ⓖ

Type/Group: **anticonvulsant; antiepileptic**.
Brand(s): Atretol; Carbatrol; Epitol; Tegretol, Tegretol-XR, Suspension; various generic.
How administered: Orally.

Used to treat

Carbamazepine is used in the preventive treatment of ⊙ **epilepsy** (such as tonic-clonic, complex-partial, and mixed seizures) and to relieve the pain of trigeminal neuralgia (a searing pain from the trigeminal nerve in the face). Although the manufacturer doesn't list such treatments, it is sometimes prescribed for the management of certain psychotic disorders, in the treatment of diabetes insipidus, alcohol withdrawal, restless legs syndrome, and sometimes for a variety of neurogenic pains (for example, phantom limb pain and pain of diabetic neuropathy).

Warnings

• Avoid its use in people with known hypersensitivity to this drug or to ℞ **tricyclic** antidepressants, who are taking ℞ **MAOI** antidepressants (see below), who have porphyria, or a history of bone marrow depression.

• Use with caution in people with glaucoma, impairment of liver, kidney, or heart function, or a history of blood reactions to other drugs.

• Carbamazepine is considered hazardous to the fetus and should not be used during pregnancy.

• Breast-feeding mothers should either discontinue using this drug or stop breast-feeding.

• Discontinue taking a monoamine-oxidase inhibitor (MAOI) antidepressant at least 14 days before taking carbamazepine.

• Medical advice must be sought if fever, bruising, bleeding, sore throat, rash, or mouth ulcers occur.

• Withdrawal should be gradual.

• Urine may turn pink-brown.

• Because of its sedative side effects, the performance of skilled tasks, such as driving, may be impaired.

Interactions

• Carbamazepine may increase the levels, with potential toxic effects, of the following drugs: ℞ **cimetidine**; ℞ **danazol**; ℞ **diltiazem hydrochloride**; ℞ **erythromycin**; ℞ **clarithromycin**; ℞ **fluoxetine**; ℞ **fluvoxamine**; ℞ **itraconazole**; ℞ **ketoconazole**; ℞ **loratadine**; ℞ **nicotinamide**; ℞ **propoxyphene**; ℞ **verapamil**.

• When taken with ℞ **isoniazid** it increases the risk of side effects (for both drugs).

• ℞ **lithium** may increase the risk of CNS (central nervous system) toxicity.

• The effects when taken with ℞ **valproate sodium** are unpredictable, though carbamazepine levels may rise and valproate fall.

• The levels of the following drugs may be reduced: ℞ **tricyclics** and succinimides, for example, ℞ **ethosuximide**, ℞ **methsuximide**); ℞ **acetaminophen**; ℞ **alprazolam**; ℞ **bupropion**; ℞ **clozapine**; ℞ **cyclosporine**; ℞ **dicumarol**; ℞ **doxycycline**; ℞ **felodipine**; ℞ **haloperidol**; ℞ **lamotrigine**; ℞ **phenytoin**; ℞ **theophylline**; ℞ **topiramate**; ℞ **warfarin sodium**.

• There is a possibility of increased toxicity with ℞ **calcium-channel blockers**.

• Bleeding and loss of contraceptive reliability are possible with hormonal ℞ **contraceptives**.

• The following drugs may lower levels of carbamazepine: ℞ **cisplatin**; ℞ **doxorubicin hydrochloride**; felbamate; ℞ **phenobarbital**; ℞ **phenytoin**; ℞ **primidone**; ℞ **rifampin**; ℞ **theophylline**.

Side effects

These are many and diverse, including:

• Water retention, skin disorders, sedation, nausea and vomiting;

• Dizziness, drowsiness, headache, unsteady gait, confusion, and agitation (particularly in seniors);

• Visual disturbances and double or blurred vision;

• Hair loss, cardiovascular, and gastrointestinal disturbances, mental disturbances;

• Blood and liver disorders, growth of breasts in men, impotence, aggression, and depression;

• Potentially serious side effects include congestive heart failure, blood, skin, and liver disorders.

carbamide Ⓖ

see ℞ **urea**.

carbamide peroxide Ⓖ

(urea peroxohydrate; urea peroxide)

Type/Group: **antiseptic; anti-infective**.

Brand(s): Gly-Oxide Liquid; Orajel Perioseptic; Proxigel.

How administered: Topically (external).

Used to treat

Carbamide peroxide is a a convenient source of hydrogen peroxide, and is used in preparations for the relief of minor oral inflammation such as canker sores, denture irritation, and post-dental procedure irritation. It may also be used to aid oral hygiene because it inhibits odor-forming bacteria.

Warnings

• It should not be given to people with known hypersensitivity to this drug, or to children under age 3 except under direction of a doctor or dentist.

• A doctor or dentist must be contacted and its use discontinued if irritation persists or inflammation worsens.

Interactions

When used topically (externally), none are known.

Side effects

• There may be some irritation and redness.

Carbastat Ⓑ

A preparation of ℞ **carbachol**.

Formulation: Intraocular solution.

Availability: Prescription only.

Warnings and side effects: See ℞ **carbachol**.

Carbatrol Ⓑ

A preparation of ℞ **carbamazepine**.

Formulation: Oral capsules, extended release.

Availability: Prescription only.

Warnings and side effects: See ℞ **carbamazepine**.

carbenicillin Ⓖ

Type/Group: **antibiotic; penicillin**.

Brand(s): Geocillin.

How administered: Orally.

Used to treat

Carbenicillin is a semisynthetic penicillin derivative used to treat urinary tract infections (see ☉ **urinary tract disorders**), bacteriuria, and ☉ **prostatitis**.

Warnings

• It should not be used by people with known hypersensitivity to penicillins, ℞ **cephalosporins**, or ℞ **imipenem**.

• It should be given with caution to anyone with severe kidney impairment.

• Penicillins cross the placenta and should be used in pregnancy only if medically judged to be needed.

• Medical judgment is also required for breast-feeding mothers.

• Serious and occasionally fatal hypersensitivity reactions can occur.

• Superinfections from the altered bacterial balance created by antibiotic treatment may occur and may result in ☉ **pseudomembranous colitis**. A doctor must be contacted if severe abdominal pain, or moderate to severe diarrhea occurs.

Interactions

• The effectiveness of ℞ **aminoglycosides** may be reduced.

• ℞ **Tetracyclines**, ℞ **chloramphenicol**, and ℞ **macrolide** antibiotics may reduce the effectiveness of carbenicillin.

• Large doses of penicillin may increase the levels of ℞ **methotrexate**.

• The effectiveness of ℞ **oral contraceptives** may be reduced.

• ℞ **Probenecid** may increase the levels of carbenicillin.

Side effects

• Occasionally, headache, itchy eyes, bad taste, gastrointestinal effects, vaginitis, blood changes, and skin reactions.

• Serious possible effects include bone marrow depression.

Carbex Ⓑ

A preparation of ℞ **selegiline hydrochloride**.

Formulation: Oral tablets.

Availability: Prescription only.

Warnings and side effects: See ℞ **selegiline hydrochloride**.

carbidopa Ⓖ

Type/Group: **antiparkinsonism**.

Brand(s): Sinemet.

How administered: Orally.

Used to treat

Carbidopa is administered only in combination with ℞ **levodopa** to treat ☉ **Parkinson's disease**, but not the parkinsonian symptoms induced by other drugs (see ℞ **antiparkinsonism**). It is levodopa that actually has the major effect, but carbidopa is an enzyme inhibitor that blocks the breakdown of levodopa to dopamine in the body before it reaches the brain where it carries out its function. The presence of carbidopa allows the dose of levodopa to be at a minimum and so minimizes potentially severe side effects and speeds the therapeutic response.

Key to symbols: ☉ = Disorder Section ℞ = Drug Section ♣ = Herbal Section ⚕ = Supplement Section

Warnings

• It should not be used by people with known sensitivity to this drug.

• The effects in pregnancy are unknown and so carbidopa should be used only if clearly needed and if the benefits outweigh the possible risk to the fetus.

• It should not be used by breast-feeding mothers.

• Those over 65 may need less carbidopa/levodopa due to an age-related decrease in the enzyme that carbidopa inhibits. It is therefore important not to exceed the established dosage.

• Treatment with levodopa/carbidopa must be ended gradually and not abruptly.

Interactions

• There are rare reports of hypertension and dyskinesia (abnormal movement) when levodopa/carbidopa is given at the same time as ℞ tricyclic antidepressants.

Side effects

None have been reported at recommended doses, but any adverse reactions to carbidopa/levodopa are generally attributed to ℞ **levodopa**.

carbinoxamine maleate ⓖ

Type/Group: **antihistamine; cold and cough preparation.**
Brand(s): Histex PD Liquid. Combinations: With *pseudoephedrine*: Carbiset Tablets, TR Tablets; Carbodec Tablets, TR Tablets, Syrup; Cardec-S Syrup; Palgic-D Tablets Extended Release; Rondec Tablets, TR Tablets, Syrup, Oral Drops. With *pseudoephedrine and dextromethorphan*: Carbodec DM Syrup, Drops; Cardec DM Syrup, Drops; Pseudo-Car DM Syrup; Rondamine-DM Drops; Rondec-DM Syrup, Drops; Sildec-DM Syrup, Pediatric Drops; Tussafed Syrup, Drops. With *pseudoephedrine and hydrocodone*: Histex HC.
How administered: Orally.

Used to treat

Carbinoxamine is used mostly in compound preparations for ✪ **colds** and ✪ **coughs**, and for allergy conditions such as ✪ **hay fever** (seasonal allergic rhinitis).

Warnings

• It should not be given to people with known hypersensitivity to this drug (or with known sensitivity to other antihistamines).

• Antihistamines should be given with caution to people with lower respiratory disease or asthma (and never during an attack), heart disease, hypertension, hyperthyroidism, epilepsy, porphyria, increased intraocular pressure (pressure in the eyeball, as in glaucoma), enlarged prostate, urinary retention, or certain obstructive bladder or gastrointestinal conditions.

• Carbinoxamine should be used during pregnancy only if it is clearly needed, but not in the third trimester, as newborns or premature infants may have severe reactions, including convulsions, to antihistamines.

• Nursing mothers should discontinue using this drug or discontinue breast-feeding.

• This drug must not be given to infants, and for children under the age of 12 the manufacturer's or medical instructions must be followed closely.

• Because of its sedative side effects, the performance of skilled tasks, such as driving, may be impaired.

• Side effects are more frequent in the elderly.

Interactions

• ℞ **MAOI** antidepressants may prolong and intensify the ℞ **anticholinergic** effects of antihistamines (see Side effects below).

• If used with ℞ **tricyclic** antidepressants, other antihistamines, ℞ **skeletal muscle relaxants**, ℞ **opioids**, ℞ **barbiturates**, ℞ **hypnotics**, ℞ **sedatives**, or ℞ **antianxiety** drugs, there is a risk of intensified side effects.

• Alcohol may intensify side effects such as drowsiness and impaired mental alertness.

Side effects

• These depend on how it is administered. For this type of antihistamine, there is commonly drowsiness, headache, impaired muscular coordination or dizziness, anticholinergic effects (dry mouth, blurred vision, urinary retention, gastrointestinal disturbances), occasional rashes and photosensitivity (abnormal sensitivity to light), palpitations and heart arrhythmias.

• Rarely, there may be stimulation instead of sedation (paradoxical stimulation), especially in children (and convulsions in overdose), hypersensitivity reactions, blood disorders, liver disturbances, depression, sleep disturbances, and hypotension.

Carbiset Tablets; TR Tablets ⓑ

A preparation of ℞ **pseudoephedrine** and ℞ **carbinoxamine maleate**.
Formulation: Oral tablets; TR tablets, sustained release.
Availability: Prescription only.
Warnings and side effects: See ℞ **pseudoephedrine**; ℞ **carbinoxamine maleate**.

Carbocaine ⓑ

A preparation of ℞ **mepivacaine hydrochloride**.
Formulation: Injection in several strengths.
Availability: Prescription only.
Warnings and side effects: See ℞ **mepivacaine hydrochloride**.

Carbodec DM Syrup; Drops ⓑ

A preparation of ℞ **dextromethorphan**, ℞ **carbinoxamine maleate**, and ℞ **pseudoephedrine**.
Formulation: Oral syrup; drops are pediatric, lower strength.
Availability: Prescription only.
Warnings and side effects: See ℞ **dextromethorphan**; ℞ **carbinoxamine maleate**; ℞ **pseudoephedrine**.

Carbodec Tablets; TR Tablets; Syrup ⓑ

A preparation of ℞ **pseudoephedrine** and ℞ **carbinoxamine maleate**.
Formulation: Oral tablets; TR tablets, sustained release; syrup.
Availability: Prescription only.
Warnings and side effects: See ℞ **pseudoephedrine**; ℞ **carbinoxamine maleate**.

carbolic acid ⑥

see ℞ **phenol**.

carbomer ⑥

(polyacrylic acid)

Type/Group: **emollient**.

Brand(s): Nivea After Tan; Icy Hot Cream.

How administered: Topically (external).

Used to treat

Carbomer is a synthetic agent that is used in emollient preparations.

Warnings

None significant.

Interactions

None significant.

Side effects

None significant.

carbonic anhydrase inhibitor ⑩

Generics: **acetazolamide; dichlorphenamide; dorzolamide; methazolamide**.

Actions and uses

Carbonic anhydrase inhibitors have enzyme-inhibitor actions against the enzyme carbonic anhydrase, which is present throughout the body and has an important role in the control of acid-base balance (pH).

Medical uses of carbonic anhydrase inhibitors include as weak ℞ **diuretic** drugs to treat systemic edema (see ✪ **fluid retention**; ℞ **acetazolamide**), in ℞ **glaucoma treatment** for various types of ✪ **glaucoma** and related disorders (by reducing the formation of aqueous humor and so reducing the pressure in the eyeball: ℞ **acetazolamide**, ℞ **dichlorphenamide**, and ℞ **methazolamide**), as ℞ **antiepileptic** drugs to assist in the treatment of ✪ **epilepsy** by preventing certain types of seizures (petit mal, grand mal, mixed) especially in children, to prevent and treat mountain sickness (acetazolamide, an unlicensed use), and sometimes to treat the symptoms of ✪ **premenstrual syndrome**.

Limitations

See the individual drug entries.

carboplatin ⑥

Type/Group: **anticancer; cytotoxic**.

Brand(s): Paraplatin.

How administered: Injection.

Used to treat

Carboplatin is a (platinum compound) cytotoxic drug (derived from ℞ **cisplatin**) that is used as a treatment specifically for ✪ **cancer** of the ovary.

Warnings

• It should not be given to people with a history of severe allergic reaction to carboplatin or other platinum compounds, or severe bone marrow depression.

• It should be given with caution to people with kidney function impairment. This is a specialist drug which will be used following a full evaluation by specialist physicians.

• Carboplatin is not recommended for use during pregnancy unless it is medically judged to be essential, because it may cause birth defects. Becoming pregnant while using this drug must be avoided.

• It should not be used if breast-feeding.

• It can produce depressed bone marrow function, which can lead to bleeding and a reduced resistance to infection.

• Peripheral nerve damage, although rare, may occur, particularly in people who are over 65 or have previously been treated with a related drug.

• In common with many anticancer drugs, carboplatin may cause cancer or genetic mutations in cells.

Interactions

• The effects of ℞ **phenytoin** may be reduced.

Side effects

• Frequently, vomiting (which can be severe), generalized pain, weakness, and tiredness.

• Occasionally, nausea, other gastrointestinal disturbances, and peripheral nerve effects (for example, tingling in hands or feet).

• Rarely, hair loss, visual disturbances, ear abnormalities, and allergic reaction.

carboprost ⑥

(prostaglandin F$_{2alpha}$)

Type/Group: **prostaglandin; abortifacient; uterine stimulant**.

Brand(s): Hemabate.

How administered: Injection.

Used to treat

Carboprost is primarily used to treat bleeding following childbirth, which is caused by the muscles of the uterus losing their tone. It is an analog of prostaglandin, a synthetic form related to PGF$_{2alpha}$, which is a local hormone naturally involved in controlling the muscles of the uterus. It is generally used in people who are unresponsive to other medications. It may also be used to induce abortion.

Warnings

• It should not be given to people with known hypersensitivity to carboprost or other prostaglandins, acute pelvic inflammatory disease, or active heart, lung, kidney or liver disease.

• It should be given with caution to people with a history of asthma, hypotension, hypertension, anemia, jaundice, diabetes mellitus, epilepsy, past uterine surgery uterus, or heart, adrenal or liver disease.

• The dose that affects the uterus puts the embryo or fetus at risk. It is therefore used only under specialist conditions.

• This is a specialist drug for hospital use only.

Interactions

• If used with ℞ **oxytocics** there are additive effects.

Side effects

• Frequently, nausea, vomiting, and diarrhea.

• Occasionally, fever, chills, facial flushing, chills, headache, and blood pressure changes.

• Rarely, wheezing, troubled breathing, or tightness in the chest.

　　　Key to symbols:　✪ = Disorder Section　℞ = Drug Section　♣ = Herbal Section　⟐ = Supplement Section

Carboptic ®

A preparation of ℞ **carbachol**.
Formulation: Eye drops.
Availability: Prescription only.
Warnings and side effects: See ℞ **carbachol**.

carboxymethlycellulose sodium ⓖ

(carmellose sodium)
Type/Group: **artificial saliva; artificial tears**.
Brand(s): Glandosane; Moi-Stir; Celluvisc; Refresh Plus.
How administered: Topically (external).

Used to treat

Carboxymethlycellulose sodium is a substance that is incorporated into mouth-spray preparations for dry mouth (for example, due to Sicca syndrome, certain drug treatments, and after radiotherapy) and into artificial tears.

Warnings

• It should not be given to people with known hypersensitivity to this agent.
• It may cause mild stinging or temporary blurred vision.

Interactions

None significant.

Side effects

None significant.

Cardec DM Syrup; Drops ®

A preparation of ℞ **dextromethorphan**, ℞ **carbinoxamine maleate**, and ℞ **pseudoephedrine**.
Formulation: Oral syrup; drops are pediatric, lower strength.
Availability: Prescription only.
Warnings and side effects: See ℞ **dextromethorphan**;
℞ **carbinoxamine maleate**; ℞ **pseudoephedrine**.

Cardene; Cardene SR; Injection ®

A preparation of ℞ **nicardipine hydrochloride**.
Formulation: Oral capsules (2 strengths); sustained-release capsules (SR, 3 strengths); injection.
Availability: Prescription only.
Warnings and side effects: See ℞ **nicardipine hydrochloride**.

cardiac glycoside ⓓ

Generics: **digitoxin; digoxin**.

Actions and uses

Cardiac glycoside drugs are a chemical class derived from the leaf of the *Digitalis* foxgloves. These drugs have a pronounced effect on a failing heart by increasing the force of contraction and so have been commonly used for their ℞ **cardiac stimulant** actions to increase the force in ℞ **heart failure treatment**. They can also correct certain abnormal heart rhythms (for example, atrial fibrillation and atrial flutter: see ⊙ **arrhythmia**) and are therefore used as an ℞ **antiarrhythmic** treatment.
Today, these drugs are used far less often, because doses that are useful therapeutically are close to those that are toxic, so dose must be carefully adjusted in the individual.

A digitalis ℞ **antidote**, ℞ **digoxin immune Fab**, is manufactured antibody fragments that react with a drug to neutralize it in emergency treatment.

Limitations

See the individual drug entries.

cardiac stimulant ⓓ

Generics: **digitoxin; digoxin; dobutamine hydrochloride; dopamine hydrochloride; epinephrine; inamrinone lactate; isoproterenol; midodrine hydrochloride; milrinone; norepinephrine bitartrate**.

Actions and uses

Cardiac stimulant drugs are used in medicine to stimulate the rate or the force of the heartbeat, but only when it is weak as a result of some disease state or in medical emergencies. ℞ **Cardiac glycoside** drugs (for example, ℞ **digoxin**, ℞ **digitoxin**) have a pronounced effect on the failing heart, increasing the force of contraction and so have been widely prescribed in ℞ **heart failure treatment**. A number of ℞ **sympathomimetic** agents can be used directly to stimulate the heart through their ℞ **beta-adrenergic stimulant** properties (for example, ℞ **epinephrine**, ℞ **norepinephrine bitartrate**, ℞ **isoproterenol**), also ℞ **dobutamine hydrochloride** and ℞ **dopamine hydrochloride**, which also have ℞ **dopamine-receptor stimulant** properties.
There is increased use of ℞ **phosphodiesterase inhibitor** agents, since drugs of this type (℞ **milrinone** and ℞ **inamrinone lactate**), have a stimulatory action on heart muscle (myocardium), and can be used in severe congestive heart failure. The ones used are relatively specific for the form of the phosphodiesterase enzyme (type III) in the heart compared to other tissues and organs, which limits their side effects.

Limitations

Most of these drugs tend to be reserved for emergencies, such as cardiogenic shock, septic shock, during heart surgery, and in cardiac infarction and cardiac arrest. See also the individual drug entries.

Cardizem; Cardizem SR, CD; Injection ®

A preparation of ℞ **diltiazem hydrochloride**.
Availability: Prescription only.
Warnings and side effects: See ℞ **diltiazem hydrochloride**.

Cardura ®

A preparation of ℞ **doxazosin mesylate**.
Formulation: Oral tablets, available in 4 strengths.
Availability: Prescription only.
Warnings and side effects: See ℞ **doxazosin mesylate**.

carisoprodol ⓖ

Type/Group: **skeletal muscle relaxant**.
Brand(s): Soma; various generic. Combinations: With *aspirin*: Sodol Compound; Soma Compound. With *aspirin* and *codeine*: Soma compound with Codeine.
How administered: Orally.

Used to treat

Carisoprodol is used as in addition to other treatments (such as rest, physical therapy) for the relief of acute muscle pain. It works by an action on the central nervous system (CNS).

Warnings

• It should not be used by people with known hypersensitivity to carisoprodol or related compounds, such as meprobamate, or with intermittent porphyria.

• It should be given with caution to people with kidney or liver disease, and those over 65.

• The effects on the fetus are unknown. It should be used in pregnancy only if clearly needed.

• Medical judgment is required if breast-feeding is being considered. Carisoprodol is excreted in breast milk.

• Rarely, an adverse reaction to this drug may occur within minutes or hours of taking the first dose. Symptoms include weakness, transient paralysis of the limbs, dizziness, temporary loss of vision, agitation, and euphoria.

• It may impair the performance of skilled tasks, such as driving.

• Stopping of treatment must be gradual, otherwise there may be mild withdrawal symptoms, such as insomnia, chills, and nausea.

Interactions

• If taken with CNS depressants (including alcohol), the effects are increased.

Side effects

• Commonly, dizziness, drowsiness, weakness, and nausea.

• Rarely, flushing, fever, rash, speeded heart beat, and skin disorders.

carmellose sodium ⓖ

see ℞ carboxymethlycellulose sodium.

Carmol HC ⓑ

A preparation of ℞ **hydrocortisone** and ℞ **urea**.
Formulation: Cream.
Availability: Prescription only.
Warnings and side effects: See ℞ **hydrocortisone**; ℞ **urea**.

carmustine ⓖ

(BCNU)
Type/Group: **anticancer; cytotoxic**.
Brand(s): BiCNU; Gliadel.
How administered: Intravenous injection.

Used to treat

Carmustine is a cytotoxic drug (an alkylating agent) that works by direct interference with DNA and so prevents normal cell replication. It is used to treat some myelomas, ✪ **lymphomas**, and brain ✪ **tumors**.

Warnings

• It should not be given to people with known severe hypersensitivity to carmustine.

• It should be given with caution to people with certain blood disorders. This is a specialist drug which will be used following a full evaluation by specialist physicians.

• Carmustine is not recommended for use during pregnancy unless it is medically judged to be essential, because it may cause birth defects. Becoming pregnant while using this drug must be avoided.

• It should not be used if breast-feeding.

• It can cause severe bone marrow suppression, which may lead to bleeding and a reduced resistance to infection.

• In common with many anticancer drugs, it is associated with the development of secondary malignancies (new cancers).

• It can impair fertility in men and women (which may be reversible).

• Damage to lungs, apparently dose-related, has been associated with this drug.

• It may impair kidney function, damage the eyes, and cause seizure, brain herniation, swelling in the brain, or infection inside skull.

Interactions

• ℞ **Cimetidine** and ℞ **mitomycin** may enhance side effects.

• The levels of ℞ **digoxin** and ℞ **phenytoin** may be reduced.

Side effects

• Frequently, pain at injection site, skin discoloration along veins, nausea and vomiting.

• Occasionally, diarrhea, irritated esophagus, loss of appetite, pain, and effects on the eye.

• Rarely, thrombophlebitis.

Carnitor ⓑ

A preparation of ℞ **levocarnitine**.
Formulation: Oral tablets; oral solution; injection.
Availability: Prescription only.
Warnings and side effects: See ℞ **levocarnitine**.

Caroid ⓑ

A preparation of ℞ **bisacodyl**.
Formulation: Oral tablets.
Availability: OTC.
Warnings and side effects: See ℞ **bisacodyl**.

carteolol ⓖ

Type/Group: **beta-blocker; antihypertensive; glaucoma treatment**.
Brand(s): (Oral): Cartrol. (Ophthalmic, topical): Ocupress; various generic.
How administered: Orally; topically (as eyedrops).

Used to treat

Carteolol can be used to lower blood pressure (see ✪ **hypertension**). In the form of eyedrops it may be used to treat chronic simple (open-angle) ✪ **glaucoma**. It is thought to work by slowing the rate of production of the aqueous humor in the eye.

Warnings

• It should not be given to people with known hypersensitivity to any beta-blocking drug, who have certain heartbeat irregularities or heart failure, or bronchial asthma, allergic bronchospasm or severe chronic obstructive pulmonary disease (COPD). It should not be used in cardiogenic shock.

• It should be given with caution to people with diabetes mellitus or hypoglycemia, hyperthyroidism, myasthenia gravis, congestive heart failure, peripheral vascular disease, moderate bronchospastic disease (for example, chronic bronchitis or emphysema), or liver or kidney impairment.

• Carteolol's safety during pregnancy has not been established and it should be used only if the potential benefit outweighs the possible risk to the fetus.

• Medical judgment is required if breast-feeding is being considered. It is not known whether it appears in breast milk.

• Abruptly stopping using a beta-blocker may have adverse effects, including on the heart.

• The use of this drug may mask signs of hyperthyroidism or hypoglycemia.

• Ophthalmic (eye) preparations can be absorbed systemically, so systemic side effects may be observed (see below).

• Other medications (including OTCs, herbal remedies, and supplements) must not be taken without consulting a doctor. Some ℞ **nasal decongestants**, commonly available over the counter, contain ℞ **alpha-adrenergic stimulants** (for example, ℞ **phenylephrine**) that may cause a severe hypertensive reaction if taken with beta-blockers.

Interactions

• A serious blood pressure increase may occur after withdrawal from ℞ **clonidine hydrochloride** or both drugs at the same time.

• Other ℞ **antiarrhythmics** (for example, ℞ **amiodarone**, ℞ **disopyramide**, ℞ **quinidine**, and ℞ **procainamide**) and ℞ **tricyclics** have the potential for significant adverse effects on heart rhythm.

• The effects of ℞ **alpha-adrenergic stimulants**, ℞ **ergot alkaloids**, ℞ **epinephrine**, ℞ **lidocaine**, and ℞ **theophylline** may be increased, with the risk of serious adverse effects.

• ℞ **Calcium-channel blockers** (particularly ℞ **diltiazem hydrochloride** and ℞ **verapamil**), ℞ **guanethidine monosulfate**, and ℞ **reserpine** have the potential for increasing undesirable effects, with exaggerated slowing of heartbeat or hypotension.

• The effects of nondepolarizing ℞ **skeletal muscle relaxants** may be variable, with the possible risk of significant adverse effects associated with major surgery.

• The effects of ℞ **beta-adrenergic stimulants** (for example, ℞ **albuterol**, ℞ **terbutaline**), ℞ **insulin**, and ℞ **sulfonylureas** may be reduced.

• The levels of ℞ **digoxin** may be increased and dose adjustment may be necessary.

• ℞ **Antacids** (for example, ℞ **aluminum hydroxide**, ℞ **magnesium hydroxide**), ℞ **barbiturates**, ⚕ **calcium** salts, ℞ **cholestyramine**, ℞ **colestipol hydrochloride**, ℞ **NSAIDs**, ℞ **phenytoin**, ℞ **penicillins**, ℞ **rifampin**, and ℞ **salicylates** may reduce the levels and effectiveness of beta-blockers. Antacids should not be taken within two hours of beta-blockers.

• If used with ℞ **diuretics** and other antihypertensive drugs, there are additive effects which are often used to therapeutic advantage.

Side effects

• Oral use: May include dizziness, nausea, headache, fatigue, constipation or diarrhea. Occasionally, insomnia, flatulence, urinary frequency, impotence or decreased libido. Rarely, rash, arrhythmias, joint and muscle pain, confusion, or strange taste sensations.

• Ophthalmic (topical) use: Frequently, eye irritation or visual disturbances. Occasionally, increased light sensitivity or watering of eyes. Rarely, dry eyes, conjunctivitis, or eye pain.

Cartrol Ⓑ

A preparation of ℞ **carteolol**.
Formulation: Oral tablets, available two strengths.
Availability: Prescription only.
Warnings and side effects: See ℞ **carteolol**.

carvedilol Ⓖ

Type/Group: **beta-blocker; alpha-adrenergic blocker; antihypertensive; heart failure treatment; vasodilator**.
Brand(s): Coreg.
How administered: Orally.

Used to treat

Carvedilol is an unusual drug that combines both beta-blocker and alpha-adrenergic blocker properties. It can be used, alone or in combination with other drugs, to reduce high blood pressure (see ⊕ **hypertension**), and to treat congestive ⊕ **heart failure**.

Warnings

• It should not be given to people with known hypersensitivity to any beta-blocking drug, who have certain heartbeat irregularities, severe heart failure, or bronchial asthma. It should not be used in cardiogenic shock.

• It should be given with caution to people with diabetes mellitus or hypoglycemia, hyperthyroidism, myasthenia gravis, peripheral vascular disease, or liver or kidney impairment. Beta-blockers are usually not given to anyone with a nonallergic bronchospastic disease (for example, chronic bronchitis or emphysema).

• Carvedilol should be used during pregnancy only if the potential benefit outweighs the possible risk to the fetus.

• It appears in breast milk, and so nursing women should discontinue using this drug or stop breast-feeding.

• Abruptly stopping using carvedilol, because it has beta-blocker properties, may have adverse effects, including on the heart.

• The use of this drug may mask signs of hyperthyroidism or hypoglycemia.

• Other medications (including OTCs, herbal remedies, and supplements) must not be taken without consulting a doctor. Some ℞ **nasal decongestants**, commonly available over the counter, contain ℞ **alpha-adrenergic stimulants** (for example, ℞ **phenylephrine**) that may cause a severe hypertensive reaction if taken with beta-blockers.

Interactions

• A serious blood pressure increase may occur after withdrawal from ℞ **clonidine hydrochloride** or both drugs at the same time.

• Other ℞ **antiarrhythmics** (for example, ℞ **amiodarone**, ℞ **disopyramide**, ℞ **quinidine**, ℞ **procainamide**) and ℞ **tricyclics** have the potential for significant adverse effects on heart rhythm.

• The effects of ℞ **alpha-adrenergic stimulants**, ℞ **ergot alkaloids**, ℞ **epinephrine**, ℞ **hydralazine hydrochloride**, ℞ **lidocaine**, and ℞ **theophylline** may be increased, with the risk of serious adverse effects.

• ℞ **Calcium-channel blockers** (particularly ℞ **diltiazem hydrochloride** and ℞ **verapamil**), ℞ **guanethidine monosulfate**, ℞ **MAOIs**, and ℞ **reserpine** have the potential for increasing undesirable effects, with exaggerated slowing of heartbeat or hypotension.

• The effects of nondepolarizing ℞ **skeletal muscle relaxants** may be variable, with the possible risk of significant adverse effects associated with major surgery.

• The effects of ℞ **beta-adrenergic stimulants** (for example, ℞ **albuterol**, ℞ **terbutaline**), ℞ **insulin**, and ℞ **sulfonylureas** may be reduced.

• ℞ **Fluoxetine**, ℞ **paroxetine**, and ℞ **propafenone** may increase the levels and effects of carvedilol.

• The levels of ℞ **digoxin** may be increased and dose adjustment may be necessary.

• ℞ **Cimetidine** may increase the effect of carvedilol.

• ℞ **Antacids** (for example, ℞ **aluminum hydroxide**, ℞ **magnesium hydroxide**), ℞ **barbiturates**, ⚐ **calcium** salts, ℞ **cholestyramine**, ℞ **colestipol hydrochloride**, ℞ **NSAIDs**, ℞ **phenytoin**, ℞ **penicillins**, ℞ **rifampin**, and ℞ **salicylates** may reduce the levels and effectiveness of beta-blockers. Antacids should not be taken within two hours of beta-blockers.

• If used with ℞ **diuretics** and other antihypertensive drugs, there are additive effects which are often used to therapeutic advantage.

Side effects

• Dizziness, slowing of heart rate, gastrointestinal disturbances (for example, diarrhea, nausea, vomiting), hyperglycemia (high blood sugar), edema, vision disturbances, postural hypotension (low blood pressure when standing up), weight gain, and arthralgia (joint pain);

• Less frequently, bronchitis, insomnia, headache, more frequent infection, fainting, and blood or liver changes;

• Heart failure, should it develop, generally requires withdrawal (gradually, if possible) of this drug.

Cascara Aromatic Liquid ®

A preparation of ℞ **cascara sagrada**.
Formulation: Oral liquid.
Availability: OTC.
Warnings and side effects: See ℞ **cascara sagrada**.

cascara sagrada ©

Type/Group: **laxative**.
Brand(s): Cascara Aromatic Liquid; Nature's Remedy Tablets; various generic. Combinations: With *docusate sodium:* Diocto C Syrup; DOK-Plus; Doxidan; Peri-Colace; Silace-C Syrup; various generic. With *methyl salicylate, rhubarb, senna:* Black Draught Syrup.
How administered: Orally.

Used to treat

Cascara sagrada is a traditional, powerful (*stimulant*) laxative which is still in fairly widespread use. It contains anthraquinones (cascarosides) that work by strongly stimulating muscular activity of the intestinal walls, and may take from 6 to 8 hours to have any relieving effect on ✪ **constipation**. It comes from the bark of *Rhamnus purshiana* sometimes (not commonly) called Cascara buckthorn, but is different from buckthorn (*Rhamnus catharticus*), whose fruit is also a laxative.

Warnings

• It should not be given to people with any form of intestinal obstruction and certain other gastrointestinal disorders.

• Generally, stimulant laxatives should be avoided during pregnancy, unless directed by a doctor.

• Medical judgment is required if breast-feeding is being considered. Cascara appears in breast milk and may cause a brown discoloration, and diarrhea in newborn babies.

• Do not use if there is abdominal pain, nausea, or vomiting, unless directed by a doctor.

• Chronic use of laxatives may cause fluid and electrolyte imbalances, vitamin and mineral deficiencies, and abnormal bowel function. Generally, they should not be used for more than a week.

• A doctor must be consulted first before taking any other medication (including OTCs, herbal remedies, and supplements), because laxatives may alter the absorption of a wide range of drugs.

• Urine may change color (pink, red, or brown).

Interactions

No interactions of significance are known.

• Laxatives may alter the absorption of a wide range of drugs.

Side effects

• There may be abdominal cramps, nausea, vomiting, or discolored urine.

• Suppositories can sometimes cause local irritation.

Casodex ®

A preparation of ℞ **bicalutamide**.
Formulation: Oral tablets.
Availability: Prescription only.
Warnings and side effects: See ℞ **bicalutamide**.

castor oil ©

Type/Group: **emollient**.
Brand(s): Hydrosinol; Kank-A; Seba-Nil Cleansing Mask; Sulfoil; Purge: Emulsoil; various generic.
How administered: Topically (external).

Used to treat

Castor oil is found in some skin preparations and barrier creams. It was once widely used as a (stimulant) laxative but is now largely obsolete.

Warnings

None significant.

Interactions

None significant.

Side effects

None significant.

Cataflam ⓑ

A preparation of ℞ **diclofenac**.
Formulation: Oral tablets.
Availability: Prescription only.
Warnings and side effects: See ℞ **diclofenac**.

Catapres Tablets; Catapres-TTS ⓑ

A preparation of ℞ **clonidine hydrochloride**.
Formulation: Oral tablets (3 strengths); transdermal patch (TTS, three strengths).
Availability: Prescription only.
Warnings and side effects: See ℞ **clonidine hydrochloride**.

cation-exchange resin ⓓ

Generics: **sodium polystyrene sulfonate**.

Actions and uses

Cation-exchange resin agents chemically bind specific cations (positively charged ions). Potassium-removing resin is used to treat excessively high levels of potassium in the blood (hyperkalemia), for example, in people who have kidney dialysis. Its action may require hours or days, so other methods are preferred in urgent situations.

Limitations

See the individual drug entries.

Caverject ⓑ

A preparation of ℞ **alprostadil**.
Formulation: Injection.
Availability: Prescription only.
Warnings and side effects: See ℞ **alprostadil**.

CCNU ⓖ

see ℞ **lomustine**.

Ceclor ⓑ

A preparation of ℞ **cefaclor**.
Formulation: Tablets; capsule; oral liquid.
Availability: Prescription only.
Warnings and side effects: See ℞ **cefaclor**.

Cecon ⓑ

A preparation of ℞ **ascorbic acid**.
Formulation: Oral solution.
Availability: Prescription only.
Warnings and side effects: See ℞ **ascorbic acid**.

CeeNu ⓑ

A preparation of ℞ **lomustine**.
Formulation: Oral capsules in several strengths.
Availability: Prescription only.
Warnings and side effects: See ℞ **lomustine**.

cefaclor ⓖ

Type/Group: **cephalosporin; antibacterial; antibiotic**.
Brand(s): Ceclor; various generic.

How administered: Orally.

Used to treat

Cefaclor is a "second-generation" cephalosporins used to treat Gram-positive and Gram-negative ⊙ **bacterial infections** of the respiratory and urinary tracts, skin and skin structures, and ears. It is used particularly for infections that do not respond to other drugs.

Warnings

• It should not be used in people with a history of hypersensitivity to cephalosporins.
• It should be given with caution to people with allergies to penicillins or other agents, or who have kidney disease.
• Cefaclor crosses the placenta and may have adverse effects on the fetus. Its use in pregnancy requires medical judgment to weigh the benefits against the risk of harming the fetus.
• Medical judgment is also required if breast-feeding is being considered, because there is evidence that small amounts of cephalosporins do appear in breast milk.
• A severe hypersensitivity reaction is possible, particularly in individuals who are allergic to penicillin.
• The drug must be taken for the full length of treatment, because infection can return.
• Superinfections from the altered bacterial balance created by antibiotic treatment may occur, and may result in pseudomembranous colitis (an intestinal disorder characterized by severe diarrhea). ℞ **antidiarrheal** must not be used as this can result in toxic megacolon, a life-threatening dilation of the bowel. A doctor must be contacted in cases of severe abdominal pain, or moderate to severe diarrhea.
• Rarely, this drug may cause kidney damage.

Interactions

• ℞ **Probenecid** increases the concentration of cefaclor.
• ℞ **Aminoglycosides** increase the risk of kidney damage.
• ℞ **warfarin sodium** activity may be increased.

Side effects

• Frequently, oral candidiasis (thrush), mild diarrhea, nausea, and vaginal yeast infections.
• Occasionally, serum sickness reaction (skin rash, joint pain, fever).
• Rarely, hemolytic anemia and other blood disorders, bone marrow suppression, kidney damage, and pseudomembranous colitis.

cefadroxil ⓖ

Type/Group: **cephalosporin; antibacterial; antibiotic**.
Brand(s): Duricef; various generic.
How administered: Orally.

Used to treat

Cefadroxil is a broad-spectrum, "first-generation" cephalosporin, which is used to treat ⊙ **bacterial infections** of the urinary tract and skin, and for some respiratory tract infections.

Warnings

• It should not be given to people with a history of hypersensitivity to cephalosporins.
• It should be given with caution to people with allergies to penicillins.

• The safety of cefadroxil in pregnancy is not established, and it readily crosses the placenta. Medical judgment is required to assess the benefits against the risk of harming the fetus.

• Medical judgment is also required if breast-feeding is being considered, because there is evidence that small amounts of cephalosporins do appear in breast milk.

• A severe hypersensitivity reaction is possible, particularly in anyone with a history of allergies, particularly allergy to penicillins.

• The drug must be taken for the full length of treatment, because infection can return.

• Superinfections from the altered bacterial balance created by antibiotic treatment may occur, and may result in pseudomembranous colitis (an intestinal disorder characterized by severe diarrhea). ℞ **antidiarrheal** drugs must not be taken as this can result in toxic megacolon, a life-threatening dilation of the bowel. A doctor must be contacted if there is severe abdominal pain, or moderate to severe diarrhea.

• Rarely, this drug may cause kidney damage.

Interactions
• ℞ **Probenecid** increases the concentration of cefadroxil.
• ℞ **Aminoglycosides** increase the risk of kidney damage.
• Loop ℞ **diuretics** increase the risk of damage to the kidneys.

Side effects
• Frequently, oral candidiasis (thrush), mild diarrhea, nausea, appetite loss, and vaginal yeast infections.
• Occasionally, serum sickness reaction (skin rash, joint pain, fever) and pseudomembranous colitis (an intestinal disorder characterized by severe diarrhea).
• Rarely, hemolytic anemia, erythema multiform (blistering, peeling, loosening of the skin), and kidney damage.

cefamandole Ⓖ
(cephamandole)
Type/Group: **cephalosporin; antibacterial; antibiotic.**
Brand(s): Mandol; various generic.
How administered: Injection.

Used to treat
Cefamandole is a broad-spectrum, "second-generation" cephalosporin, which is used to treat a broad range of Ⓞ **bacterial infections**. It is less susceptible to inactivation by bacterial penicillinase than others in its class, and is therefore effective against a greater range of Gram-negative bacteria, for example, penicillin-resistant *Neisseria gonorrhoeae* and *Haemophilus influenzae*. It can be used to treat infections of the lower respiratory tract, urinary tract, skin and skin structure, bones, and joints. It is also prescribed for Ⓞ **peritonitis**, Ⓞ **septicemia**, and to prevent infection during surgery.

Warnings
• It should not be given to people with a history of hypersensitivity to cephalosporins.
• It should be given with caution to people with allergies to penicillins, kidney impairment, or certain blood disorders.
• Cefamandole's safety in pregnancy is not established, and this drug readily crosses the placenta. Medical judgment is required to assess the benefits against the risk of harming the fetus.

• Medical judgment is also required if breast-feeding is being considered, because there is evidence that small amounts of cephalosporins do appear in breast milk.

• Drinking alcohol with, or within a few days after having used, cefamandole can cause acute alcohol intolerance, such as headache, nausea, vomiting, and other unpleasant effects.

• A severe hypersensitivity reaction is possible, particularly in those who are allergic to penicillins.

• Superinfections from the altered bacterial balance created by antibiotic treatment may occur, and may result in pseudomembranous colitis (an intestinal disorder characterized by severe diarrhea). ℞ **antidiarrheal** drugs must not be used, as this can result in toxic megacolon, a life-threatening dilation of the bowel. A doctor must be contacted if there is severe abdominal pain, or moderate to severe diarrhea.

• Rarely, cefamandole may cause kidney damage.

Interactions
• Cefamandole taken with oral ℞ **anticoagulants** increases anticlotting activity, so increasing the risk of bleeding.
• ℞ **Probenecid** increases the concentration of cefamandole.
• Loop ℞ **diuretics** increase the risk of damage to kidneys.
• ℞ **Aminoglycosides** may increase the risk of kidney damage.

Side effects
• Frequently, oral candidiasis (thrush), mild diarrhea, nausea, and vaginal yeast infections.
• Occasionally, serum sickness reaction (skin rash, joint pain, fever), and vomiting.
• Rarely, bleeding, hemolytic anemia and other blood disorders, bone marrow suppression, pseudomembranous colitis (an intestinal disorder characterized by severe diarrhea), and kidney damage.

cefazolin sodium Ⓖ
Type/Group: **cephalosporin; antibacterial; antibiotic.**
Brand(s): Ancef; Kefzol; Zolicef; various generic.
How administered: Injection.

Used to treat
Cefazolin is an antibacterial and (partially synthetic) antibiotic drug which is used to treat Ⓞ **bacterial infections** of the lower respiratory tract, urinary tract, biliary (gallbladder) tract, and genitourinary tract. It may also be prescribed to treat infections of the skin and skin structures, bones and joints, Ⓞ **endocarditis** (infection of the lining of the heart), Ⓞ **prostatitis**, Ⓞ **septicemia**, and to prevent infection during surgery.

Warnings
• It should not be given to people with a history of hypersensitivity to cephalosporins.
• It should be given with caution to people with allergies to penicillins, kidney impairment, or certain blood disorders.
• Cefazolin sodium's safety in pregnancy is not established, and it readily crosses the placenta. Medical judgment is required to assess the benefits against the risk of harming the fetus.
• Medical judgment is also required if breast-feeding is being considered, because there is evidence that small amounts of cephalosporins do appear in breast milk.

• Drinking alcohol with, or within a few days after having used, cefazolin can cause acute alcohol intolerance, such as headache, nausea, vomiting, and other unpleasant effects.

• Superinfections from the altered bacterial balance created by antibiotic treatment may occur, and may result in pseudomembranous colitis (an intestinal disorder characterized by severe diarrhea). ℞ **antidiarrheal** drugs must not be taken as this can result in toxic megacolon, a life-threatening dilation of the bowel. A doctor must be contacted if there is severe abdominal pain, or moderate to severe diarrhea.

• Rarely, this drug may cause kidney damage.

• A severe hypersensitivity reaction is possible, particularly in those with a history of allergy to penicillins.

Interactions

• Cefazolin taken with oral ℞ **anticoagulants** increases anticlotting activity, so increasing the risk of bleeding.

• ℞ **Probenecid** increases the concentration of cefazolin.

• Loop ℞ **diuretics** increase the risk of damage to the kidneys.

• ℞ **Aminoglycosides** may increase kidney damage.

• ℞ **Chloramphenicol** inhibits the antibacterial activity of cefazolin.

Side effects

• Frequently, oral candidiasis (thrush), mild diarrhea, nausea, and vaginal yeast infections.

• Occasionally, serum sickness reaction (skin rash, joint pain, fever), and vomiting.

• Rarely, bleeding, hemolytic anemia and other blood disorders, bone marrow suppression, pseudomembranous colitis (an intestinal disorder characterized by severe diarrhea), and kidney damage.

cefepime Ⓖ

Type/Group: **cephalosporin; antibacterial; antibiotic.**
Brand(s): Maxipime.
How administered: Injection.

Used to treat

Cefepime is a broad-spectrum, "fourth-generation" cephalosporin which is used to treat infections of the urinary tract (including kidney infections), lower respiratory tract (including ✪ **pneumonia**), and certain white cell disorders. It may also be prescribed to treat infections of the skin and skin structures, bacremia (blood infection), and certain white blood cell disorders in children. It has a low potential for resistance because it does not readily induce beta-lactamase enzymes, so less bacterial resistance is likely to develop.

Warnings

• It should not be given to people with a history of hypersensitivity to cephalosporins.

• It should be given with caution to people with allergies to penicillins, or decreased prothrombin (blood-clotting) activity.

• Cefepime's safety in pregnancy is not established, and it readily crosses the placenta. Medical judgment is required to assess the benefits against the risk of harming the fetus.

• Medical judgment is also required if breast-feeding is being considered, because there is evidence that small amounts of cephalosporins do appear in breast milk.

• A severe hypersensitivity reaction is possible, particularly in those with a history of allergy to penicillins.

• Superinfections from the altered bacterial balance created by antibiotic treatment may occur, and may result in pseudomembranous colitis (an intestinal disorder characterized by severe diarrhea). ℞ **antidiarrheal** drugs must not be taken as this can result in toxic megacolon, a life-threatening dilation of the bowel. A doctor must be contacted if there is severe abdominal pain, or moderate to severe diarrhea.

• Rarely, this drug may cause kidney damage.

Interactions

• Cefepime taken with oral ℞ **anticoagulants** increases anticlotting activity, so increasing the risk of bleeding.

• ℞ **Probenecid** increases the concentration of cefepime.

• Loop ℞ **diuretics** increase the risk of damage to the kidneys.

• ℞ **Aminoglycosides** may increase kidney damage.

Side effects

• Frequently, oral candidiasis (thrush), mild diarrhea, nausea, and vaginal yeast infections.

• Occasionally, serum sickness reaction (skin rash, joint pain, fever), and vomiting.

• Rarely, hemorrhage, hemolytic anemia and other blood disorders, bone marrow suppression, pseudomembranous colitis (an intestinal disorder characterized by severe diarrhea), and serious skin disorders, and kidney damage.

cefixime Ⓖ

Type/Group: **cephalosporin; antibacterial; antibiotic.**
Brand(s): Suprax.
How administered: Orally.

Used to treat

Cefixime is a broad-spectrum, "third-generation" cephalosporin. It is used to treat ear infections, ✪ **bronchitis**, infections of the throat and pharynx, uncomplicated urinary tract infections and uncomplicated ✪ **gonorrhea**. It has a longer duration of action than many other cephalosporins taken by mouth.

Warnings

• It should not be given to people with a history of hypersensitivity to cephalosporins.

• It should be given with caution to people with allergies to penicillins or other drugs, a history of gastrointestinal disease, or with kidney disease.

• Cefixime's safety in pregnancy is not established, and it readily crosses the placenta. Medical judgment is required to assess the benefits against the risk of harming the fetus.

• Medical judgment is also required if breast-feeding is being considered, because there is evidence that small amounts of some cephalosporins do appear in breast milk.

• A severe hypersensitivity reaction is possible, particularly in those with a history of allergy to penicillins.

• The drug must be taken for the full length of treatment, because infection can return.

• Superinfections from the altered bacterial balance created by antibiotic treatment may occur, and may result in pseudomembranous colitis (an intestinal disorder characterized by

severe diarrhea). ℞ **antidiarrheal** drugs must not be taken as this can result in toxic megacolon, a life-threatening dilation of the bowel. A doctor must be contacted if there is severe abdominal pain, or moderate to severe diarrhea.
• Rarely, this drug may cause kidney damage.

Interactions
• Cefixime taken with oral ℞ **anticoagulants** increases anticlotting activity, so increasing the risk of bleeding.
• ℞ **Probenecid** increases the concentration of cefixime.
• Loop ℞ **diuretics** increase the risk of damage to the kidneys.
• ℞ **Aminoglycosides** may increase kidney damage.

Side effects
• Frequently, oral candidiasis (thrush), mild diarrhea, nausea, and vaginal yeast infections.
• Occasionally, nausea, serum sickness reaction (skin rash, joint pain, fever), and kidney damage.

Cefotan ®
A preparation of ℞ **cefotetan**.
Formulation: Injection.
Availability: Prescription only.
Warnings and side effects: See ℞ cefotetan.

cefotaxime Ⓖ
Type/Group: **cephalosporin; antibacterial; antibiotic**.
Brand(s): Claforan.
How administered: Injection.

Used to treat
Cefotaxime is one of the "third-generation" cephalosporins, which can be used to treat a wide range of ✪ **bacterial infections**, including urinary tract and intra-abdominal infections, ✪ **meningitis**, and ✪ **gonorrhea**. It can also be used to prevent infection during surgery.

Warnings
• It should not be given to people with a history of hypersensitivity to cephalosporins.
• It should be given with caution to people with allergies to penicillins, kidney impairment, or a history of gastrointestinal disease.
• Cefotaxime's safety in pregnancy is not established, and it readily crosses the placenta. Medical judgment is required to assess the benefits against the risk to the fetus.
• Medical judgment is also required if breast-feeding is being considered, because there is evidence that small amounts of cephalosporins do appear in breast milk.
• A severe hypersensitivity reaction is possible, particularly in those with a history of allergy to penicillins.
• Superinfections from the altered bacterial balance created by antibiotic treatment may occur, and may result in pseudomembranous colitis (an intestinal disorder characterized by severe diarrhea). ℞ **antidiarrheal** drugs must not be taken as this can result in toxic megacolon, a life-threatening dilation of the bowel. A doctor must be contacted if there is severe abdominal pain, or moderate to severe diarrhea.

• The drug must be taken for the full length of treatment, because infection can return.
• In rare cases, it may cause kidney damage.

Interactions
• Cefotaxime taken with oral ℞ **anticoagulants** increases anticlotting activity, so increasing the risk of bleeding.
• ℞ **Probenecid** increases the concentration of cefotaxime.
• ℞ **chloramphenicol** inhibits the antibacterial activity of cefotaxime.
• ℞ **Aminoglycosides** may increase kidney damage.

Side effects
• Frequently, oral candidiasis (thrush), mild diarrhea, nausea, and vaginal yeast infections.
• Occasionally, nausea, serum sickness reaction (skin rash, joint pain, fever), and vomiting.
• Rarely, bleeding, bone marrow suppression, pseudomembranous colitis, hemolytic anemia, thrombophlebitis from injection, and kidney damage.

cefotetan Ⓖ
Type/Group: **cephalosporin; antibacterial; antibiotic**.
Brand(s): Cefotan.
How administered: Injection.

Used to treat
Cefotetan is a broad-spectrum, "second-generation" cephalosporin, which is used to treat a range of ✪ **bacterial infections**, including urinary tract, lower respiratory, intra-abdominal, and gynecologic infections, as well as to prevent infection during surgery.

Warnings
• It should not be given to people with a history of hypersensitivity to cephalosporins.
• It should be given with caution to people with allergies to penicillins, kidney impairment, or certain blood disorders.
• Cefotetan's safety in pregnancy is not established, and it readily crosses the placenta. Medical judgment is required to assess the benefits against the risk to the fetus.
• Medical judgment is also required if breast-feeding is being considered, because there is evidence that small amounts of cephalosporins do appear in breast milk.
• Drinking alcohol with, or within a few days after having used, cefotetan can cause acute alcohol intolerance, such as headache, nausea, vomiting, speeded heartbeat, and other unpleasant effects.
• A severe hypersensitivity reaction is possible, particularly in those who are allergic to penicillins.
• Superinfections from the altered bacterial balance created by antibiotic treatment may occur, and may result in pseudomembranous colitis (an intestinal disorder characterized by severe diarrhea). ℞ **antidiarrheal** drugs must not be taken as this can result in toxic megacolon, a life-threatening dilation of the bowel. A doctor must be contacted if there is severe abdominal pain, or moderate to severe diarrhea.
• Rarely, it may cause damage to the kidneys.

Key to symbols: ✪ = Disorder Section ℞ = Drug Section ♣ = Herbal Section ♒ = Supplement Section

Interactions

• Cefotetan taken with oral ℞ **anticoagulants** increases anticlotting activity, so increasing the risk of bleeding.

• ℞ **Probenecid** increases the concentration of cefotetan.

• ℞ **chloramphenicol** inhibits the antibacterial activity of cefotetan.

• Loop ℞ **diuretics** increase the risk of damage to the kidneys.

• ℞ **Aminoglycosides** may increase kidney damage.

Side effects

• Frequently, oral candidiasis (thrush), mild diarrhea, nausea, and vaginal yeast infections.

• Occasionally, nausea, unusual bruising or bleeding, and serum sickness reaction (skin rash, joint pain, fever).

• Rarely, thrombophlebitis at injection site, and kidney damage.

cefoxitin Ⓖ

Type/Group: **cephalosporin; antibiotic; antibacterial.**
Brand(s): Mefoxin.
How administered: Injection.

Used to treat

Cefoxitin is one of the "second-generation" cephalosporins, and can be used to treat a wide range of ⊘ **bacterial infections**, particularly abdominal sepsis, such as ⊘ **peritonitis**, urinary tract infections, ⊘ **gonorrhea**, and to prevent infection during operations. It is also prescribed for urinary tract, gynecological, bone and joint, and skin and skin structure infections.

Warnings

• It should not be given to people with known hypersensitivity to cephalosporins.

• It should be given with caution to people with hypersensitivity to penicillins or with kidney disease.

• Cefoxitin should be used during pregnancy only if it is clearly needed.

• Medical judgment is required if breast-feeding is being considered. It is not known whether this drug appears in breast milk.

• Superinfections due to the altered bacterial balance caused by antibiotic treatment may occur. A doctor must be contacted if there is severe abdominal pain, or moderate to severe diarrhea which may indicate ⊘ **pseudomembranous colitis** (a serious condition).

• Kidney toxicity may develop.

• A severe hypersensitivity reaction is possible, particularly in people who are allergic to penicillins.

Interactions

• If used with ℞ **aminoglycosides**, there is increased kidney toxicity.

• ℞ **chloramphenicol** may reduce the effects of cefoxitin.

• The anticoagulant effect of oral ℞ **anticoagulants** is enhanced.

Side effects

• Discomfort from injection, oral candidiasis, mild diarrhea, mild abdominal cramping, and vaginal candidiasis.

• Occasionally, nausea, unusual bruising or bleeding, joint pain, and fever.

• Rarely, allergic reaction and thrombophlebitis at injection site.

cefpodoxime Ⓖ

Type/Group: **cephalosporin; antibacterial; antibiotic.**
Brand(s): Vantin.
How administered: Orally.

Used to treat

Cefpodoxime is a broad-spectrum, "second-generation" cephalosporin, which is used to treat ⊘ **bacterial infections** of the respiratory tract, including ⊘ **bronchitis** and ⊘ **pneumonia**, skin and soft tissue infections, earache and ⊘ **tonsillitis**, infections of the urinary tract, ⊘ **gonorrhea**, and infections that are recurrent, chronic, or resistant to other drugs.

Warnings

• It should not be given to people with a history of hypersensitivity to cephalosporins.

• It should be given with caution to people with allergies to penicillins, kidney impairment, or a history of allergies or gastrointestinal disease.

• Cefpodoxime's safety in pregnancy is not established, and it readily crosses the placenta. Medical judgment is required to assess the benefits against the risk of harming the fetus.

• Medical judgment is also required if breast-feeding is being considered, because there is evidence that small amounts of cephalosporins do appear in breast milk.

• A severe hypersensitivity reaction is possible, particularly in those with a history of allergy to penicillins.

• The drug must be taken for the full length of treatment, because infection can return.

• Superinfections from the altered bacterial balance created by antibiotic treatment may occur, and may result in pseudomembranous colitis (an intestinal disorder characterized by severe diarrhea). ℞ **antidiarrheal** drugs must not be taken as this can result in toxic megacolon, a life-threatening dilation of the bowel. A doctor must be contacted if there is severe abdominal pain, or moderate to severe diarrhea.

• Rarely, it may cause kidney damage.

Interactions

• ℞ **Antacids** and ℞ **H₂-antagonist** may reduce the effectiveness of cefpodoxime.

• ℞ **Probenecid** increases the concentration of cefpodoxime.

• Loop ℞ **diuretics** increase the risk of damage to the kidneys.

• ℞ **Aminoglycosides** may increase kidney damage.

Side effects

• Frequently, oral candidiasis (thrush), mild diarrhea, nausea, and vaginal yeast infections.

• Occasionally, nausea, unusual bruising or bleeding, serum sickness reaction (skin rash, joint pain, fever), and kidney damage.

cefprozil Ⓖ

Type/Group: **cephalosporin; antibacterial; antibiotic.**
Brand(s): Cefzil
How administered: Orally.

Used to treat

Cefprozil is a broad-spectrum, "second-generation" cephalosporin, which is used to treat ⊘ **bacterial infections**, including pharyngitis (inflammation of the area between the mouth and esophagus),

✪ **tonsillitis**, bacterial infections related to acute or chronic ✪ **bronchitis**, uncomplicated skin and skin structure infections, and acute ✪ **sinusitis**.

Warnings
• It should not be given to people with a history of hypersensitivity to cephalosporins.
• It should be given with caution to people with allergies to penicillins, kidney impairment, or a history of allergies or gastrointestinal disease.
• Cefprozil's safety in pregnancy is not established, and it readily crosses the placenta. Medical judgment is required to assess the benefits against the risk of harming the fetus.
• Medical judgment is also required if breast-feeding is being considered, because there is evidence that small amounts of cephalosporins do appear in breast milk.
• A severe hypersensitivity reaction is possible, particularly in those with a history of allergy to penicillins.
• The drug must be taken for the full length of treatment, because infection can return.
• Superinfections from the altered bacterial balance created by antibiotic treatment may occur, and may result in pseudomembranous colitis (an intestinal disorder characterized by severe diarrhea). ℞ **antidiarrheal** drugs must not be taken as this can result in toxic megacolon, a life-threatening dilation of the bowel. A doctor must be contacted if there is severe abdominal pain, or moderate to severe diarrhea.
• Rarely, this drug may cause kidney damage.

Interactions
• Loop ℞ **diuretics** increase the risk of damage to the kidneys.
• ℞ **Aminoglycosides** may increase kidney damage.
• ℞ **Probenecid** increases the concentration of cefprozil.

Side effects
• Frequently, oral candidiasis (thrush), mild diarrhea, nausea, and vaginal yeast infections.
• Occasionally, nausea, unusual bruising or bleeding, and serum sickness reaction (skin rash, joint pain, fever).
• Potentially, hemolytic anemia, bone marrow suppression, pseudomembranous colitis (an intestinal disorder characterized by severe diarrhea), and kidney damage.

cefradine Ⓖ
see ℞ cephradine.

ceftazidime Ⓖ
Type/Group: **cephalosporin; antibacterial; antibiotic**.
Brand(s): Ceptaz; Fortaz; Tazicef.
How administered: Injection.

Used to treat
Ceftazidime is a broad-spectrum, "third-generation" cephalosporin which can be used to treat ✪ **bacterial infections** of the skin and soft tissues, the urinary and respiratory tracts, as well as gynecologic infections, intra-abdominal infections, such as ✪ **peritonitis**, ✪ **septicemia**, and ✪ **meningitis**. It is among the most effective of the cephalosporins against bacterial infections, and is particularly useful for infections due to *Pseudomonas aeruginosa*.

Warnings
• It should not be given to people with a history of hypersensitivity to cephalosporins, or in children under 12.
• It should be given with caution to people with allergies to penicillins or kidney disease.
• Ceftazidime's safety in pregnancy is not established, and it readily crosses the placenta. Medical judgment is required to assess the benefits against the risk of harming the fetus.
• Medical judgment is also required if breast-feeding is being considered, because there is evidence that small amounts of cephalosporins do appear in breast milk.
• A severe hypersensitivity reaction is possible, particularly in those with a history of allergy to penicillins.
• Superinfections from the altered bacterial balance created by antibiotic treatment may occur, and may result in pseudomembranous colitis (an intestinal disorder characterized by severe diarrhea). ℞ **antidiarrheal** drugs must not be taken as this can result in toxic megacolon, a life-threatening dilation of the bowel. A doctor must be contacted if there is severe abdominal pain, or moderate to severe diarrhea.
• Rarely, this drug may cause kidney damage.

Interactions
• Loop ℞ **diuretics** increase the risk of damage to the kidneys.
• ℞ **Aminoglycosides** may increase kidney damage.
• ℞ **Chloramphenicol** may decrease the effectiveness of ceftazidime.

Side effects
• Frequently, oral candidiasis (thrush), mild diarrhea, nausea, and vaginal yeast infections.
• Occasionally, serum sickness reaction (skin rash, joint pain, fever), and vomiting.
• Potentially, hemolytic anemia, bone marrow suppression, pseudomembranous colitis (an intestinal disorder characterized by severe diarrhea), and kidney damage.

Ceftin Ⓡ
A preparation of ℞ **cefuroxime**.
Formulation: Tablets; oral suspension.
Availability: Prescription only.
Warnings and side effects: See ℞ cefuroxime.

ceftriaxone Ⓖ
Type/Group: **cephalosporin; antibacterial; antibiotic**.
Brand(s): Rocephin.
How administered: Injection.

Used to treat
Ceftriaxone is a broad-spectrum, "third-generation" cephalosporin, which can be used to treat a wide range of Gram-negative ✪ **bacterial infections**, including ✪ **gonorrhea** and ✪ **meningitis**. It can also be used to treat ✪ **Lyme disease** and to prevent infections during surgery. It has a much longer duration of action than others of this class.

Warnings
• It should not be given to people with a history of hypersensitivity to cephalosporins, or in children under 12.

• It should be given with caution to people with allergies to penicillins or kidney disease.

• Ceftriaxone's safety in pregnancy is not established, and it readily crosses the placenta. Medical judgment is required to assess the benefits against the risk of harming the fetus.

• Medical judgment is also required if breast-feeding is being considered, because there is evidence that small amounts of cephalosporins do appear in breast milk.

• A severe hypersensitivity reaction is possible, particularly in those with a history of allergy to penicillins.

• Superinfections from the altered bacterial balance created by antibiotic treatment may occur, and may result in pseudomembranous colitis (an intestinal disorder characterized by severe diarrhea). ℞ **antidiarrheal** drugs must not be taken as this can result in toxic megacolon, a life-threatening dilation of the bowel. A doctor must be contacted if there is severe abdominal pain, or moderate to severe diarrhea.

• Rarely, this drug may cause kidney damage.

Interactions
• ℞ **warfarin sodium** may increase anticoagulant activity.
• ℞ **Probenecid** increases the concentration of ceftriaxone.
• Loop ℞ **diuretics** increase the risk of damage to the kidneys.
• ℞ **Aminoglycosides** could increase kidney damage.

Side effects
• Frequently, oral candidiasis (thrush), mild diarrhea, nausea, and vaginal yeast infections.
• Occasionally, serum sickness reaction (skin rash, joint pain, fever), and vomiting.
• Rarely, bleeding, hemolytic anemia and other blood disorders, bone marrow suppression, pseudomembranous colitis (an intestinal disorder characterized by severe diarrhea), and kidney damage.

cefuroxime Ⓖ
(cefuroxone)

Type/Group: **cephalosporin; antibacterial; antibiotic.**
Brand(s): *Cefuroxime* (as *axetil*): Ceftin (oral). *Cefuroxime sodium*: Kefurox; Zinacef (injection).
How administered: Orally; injection.

Used to treat
Cefuroxime is a broad-spectrum, "second-generation" cephalosporin, which can be used to treat a wide range of ✪ **bacterial infections** (such as, earache, sore throat, ✪ **bronchitis**, skin infections) and particularly Gram-negative infections of the urinary, respiratory, and genital tracts, ✪ **septicemia**, ✪ **meningitis**, and *Haemophilus influenzae* and *Neisseria gonorrhoeae*. It is also used to treat early ✪ **Lyme disease**. Cefuroxime comes in two different forms with slightly different indications.

Warnings
• It should not be used by people with history of hypersensitivity to cephalosporins.
• It should be given with caution to people with allergies to penicillins, or kidney disease.

• Cefuroxime's safety in pregnancy is not established, and it readily crosses the placenta. Medical judgment is required to assess the benefits against the risk of harming the fetus.

• Medical judgment is also required if breast-feeding is being considered, because there is evidence that small amounts of cephalosporins do appear in breast milk.

• A severe hypersensitivity reaction is possible, particularly in those with a history of allergy to penicillins.

• The drug must be taken for the full length of treatment, because infection can return.

• Superinfections from the altered bacterial balance created by antibiotic treatment may occur, and may result in pseudomembranous colitis (an intestinal disorder characterized by severe diarrhea). ℞ **antidiarrheal** drugs must not be taken as this can result in toxic megacolon, a life-threatening dilation of the bowel. A doctor must be contacted if there is severe abdominal pain, or moderate to severe diarrhea.

• Rarely, this drug may cause kidney damage.

Interactions
• ℞ **Antacids**, ℞ **H₂-antagonists**, ℞ **omeprazole**, and ℞ **lansoprazole** may reduce absorption of cefuroxime.
• ℞ **Probenecid** increases the concentration of cefuroxime.
• Loop ℞ **diuretics** increase the risk of damage to the kidneys.
• ℞ **Aminoglycosides** may increase kidney damage.

Side effects
• Frequently, oral candidiasis (thrush), mild diarrhea, nausea, and vaginal yeast infections.
• Occasionally, nausea, and serum sickness reaction (skin rash, joint pain, fever).
• Rarely, bleeding diarrhea and damage to the kidneys.

cefuroxone Ⓖ
see ℞ cefuroxime.

Cefzil Ⓑ
A preparation of ℞ cefprozil.
Formulation: Tablets; oral suspension.
Availability: Prescription only.
Warnings and side effects: See ℞ cefprozil.

Celebrex Ⓑ
A preparation of ℞ celecoxib.
Formulation: Oral capsules, available in two strengths.
Availability: Prescription only.
Warnings and side effects: See ℞ celecoxib.

celecoxib Ⓖ
Type/Group: **anti-inflammatory; antirheumatic; non-narcotic analgesic; NSAID.**
Brand(s): Celebrex.
How administered: Orally.

Used to treat
Celecoxib is used to treat pain and inflammation in ✪ **rheumatoid arthritis** and ✪ **osteoarthritis**. It is also used as an adjunct (additional treatment to enhance effectiveness), to reduce numbers of

polyps that may arise in the bowel in a disorder called FAP (familial adenomatous polyposis).

Warnings

• It should not be used by people with known hypersensitivity to this drug or to other NSAIDs (including ℞ **aspirin**), or to ℞ **sulfonamides**.

• It should not be given to anyone with chronic kidney disease, certain bleeding disorders or conditions (such as hemophilia, vitamin K deficiency, low blood-platelet levels), or who have a tendency to, or active, peptic ulceration.

• It should be given with caution to people with peripheral edema, congestive heart failure, high blood pressure, or allergic disorders (especially asthma and skin conditions), in the elderly, in those with any kind of kidney impairment, with certain liver disorders, or who are dehydrated.

• Celecoxib should be used during pregnancy only when it is medically judged to be clearly needed. In the third trimester, however, it should only be used if the benefits outweigh the potential harm to the fetus because risk to the fetus is higher at this time.

• Breast-feeding mothers should either discontinue this drug or stop breast-feeding.

• With regular use (as in the treatment of osteoarthritis), NSAIDs may cause gastrointestinal bleeding, ulceration, or perforation. Any signs of bleeding (for example, black stools) should be reported to a physician immediately.

• Most NSAIDs have the potential, particularly with regular use, to cause liver damage. Periodic evaluation of liver function is necessary in long-term therapy (more than two months).

• Side effects are more frequent in the elderly.

• Gastrointestinal upsets may be minimized by taking the drug with milk or food.

Interactions

• There is generally no added benefit in taking other NSAIDs or other ℞ **salicylates** at the same time, but there is a higher risk of gastrointestinal upsets and bleeding.

• Celecoxib taken with alcohol or ℞ **corticosteroids** increases the risk of bleeding, particularly if there is an existing ulcer.

• ℞ **Anticoagulants** (for example, ℞ **warfarin sodium**) should be used with caution, because they may make bleeding more likely.

• The effectiveness of ℞ **diuretics** and ℞ **ACE inhibitors** may be reduced.

• ℞ **Fluconazole** may raise the concentration of celecoxib.

• The effects of ℞ **cyclosporine** and ℞ **lithium** may be exaggerated, with potential for toxicity.

Side effects

These vary in severity and how often they occur.

• Commonly, gastrointestinal upsets, diarrhea, heartburn, nausea, high blood pressure, swelling of the extremities, and dehydration.

• Less frequently there may be vomiting, constipation, flatulence, headache, ringing in the ears (tinnitus), nervousness, and insomnia.

• Prolonged bleeding time (with consequent risk of ulceration) is possible with high dosage, and other blood changes can occur, including anemia.

• Hypersensitivity reactions may include symptoms such as hives, rash, chest tightness, asthma, or bronchospasm.

• Reversible kidney failure, particularly in people with impaired kidney function has occurred. Liver damage is rare.

Celestone ®

A preparation of ℞ **betamethasone**.
Formulation: Oral tablets; syrup.
Availability: Prescription only.
Warnings and side effects: See ℞ **betamethasone**.

Celestone Soluspan ®

A preparation of ℞ **betamethasone**, ℞ **sodium phosphate**.
Formulation: Injection.
Availability: Prescription only.
Warnings and side effects: See ℞ **betamethasone**; ℞ **sodium phosphate**.

Celexa ®

A preparation of ℞ **citalopram**.
Formulation: Oral tablets of varying strengths; oral suspension.
Availability: Prescription only.
Warnings and side effects: See ℞ **citalopram**.

CellCept ®

A preparation of ℞ **mycophenolate mofetil**.
Formulation: Oral tablets; capsules; oral liquid; injection (infusion).
Availability: Prescription only.

Celluvisc ®

A preparation of ℞ **carboxymethylcellulose sodium**.
Formulation: Ophthalmic solution.
Availability: OTC.
Warnings and side effects: See ℞ **carboxymethylcellulose sodium**.

Celontin Kapseals ®

A preparation of ℞ **methsuximide**.
Formulation: Oral capsules, available in two strengths.
Availability: Prescription only.
Warnings and side effects: See ℞ **methsuximide**.

Cel-U-Jec ®

A preparation of ℞ **betamethasone**, ℞ **sodium phosphate**.
Formulation: Injection.
Availability: Prescription only.
Warnings and side effects: See ℞ **betamethasone**; ℞ **sodium phosphate**.

Cenafed Plus Tablets ®

A preparation of ℞ **pseudoephedrine** and ℞ **triprolidine hydrochloride**.
Formulation: Oral tablets.
Availability: OTC.

Warnings and side effects: See ℞ pseudoephedrine; ℞ triprolidine hydrochloride.

Cenafed Tablets; Syrup ⓑ

A preparation of ℞ pseudoephedrine.
Formulation: Oral tablets; syrup.
Availability: OTC.
Warnings and side effects: See ℞ pseudoephedrine.

Cenestin ⓑ

A preparation of ℞ estrogens, conjugated.
Formulation: Injection.
Availability: Prescription only.
Warnings and side effects: See ℞ estrogens, conjugated.

Cepacol; Cepacol Throat ⓑ

A preparation of ℞ cetylpyridinium chloride.
Formulation: Mouthwash; Lozenges.
Availability: OTC.
Warnings and side effects: See ℞ cetylpyridinium chloride.

Cepacol Anesthetic ⓑ

A preparation of ℞ benzocaine and ℞ cetylpyridinium chloride.
Formulation: Lozenges.
Availability: OTC.
Warnings and side effects: See ℞ benzocaine; ℞ cetylpyridinium chloride.

Cepastat Cherry ⓑ

A preparation of ℞ menthol and ℞ phenol.
Formulation: Lozenges.
Availability: OTC.
Warnings and side effects: See ℞ menthol; ℞ phenol.

cephalexin ⓖ

Type/Group: **cephalosporin; antibacterial; antibiotic.**
Brand(s): Biocef; Keflex; Keftab; various generic.
How administered: Orally; injection.

Used to treat

Cephalexin is a broad-spectrum, "first-generation" cephalosporin, which is widely used to treat ✪ **bacterial infections**, particularly of the respiratory tract, skin, bone, and urinary tract.

Warnings

• It should not be given to people with a history of hypersensitivity to cephalosporins.
• It should be given with caution to people with allergies to penicillins, kidney impairment, or a history of allergies, or gastrointestinal diseases such as ulcerative colitis.
• Cephalexin's safety in pregnancy is not established, and it readily crosses the placenta. Medical judgment is required to assess the benefits against the risk of harming the fetus.
• Medical judgment is also required if breast-feeding is being considered, because there is evidence that small amounts of cephalosporins do appear in breast milk.

• A severe hypersensitivity reaction is possible, particularly in those with a history of allergy to penicillins.
• The drug must be taken for the full length of treatment, because infection can return.
• Superinfections from the altered bacterial balance created by antibiotic treatment may occur, and may result in pseudomembranous colitis (an intestinal disorder characterized by severe diarrhea). ℞ **antidiarrheal** drugs must not be taken as this can result in toxic megacolon, a life-threatening dilation of the bowel. A doctor must be contacted if there is severe abdominal pain, or moderate to severe diarrhea.
• Rarely, this drug may cause kidney damage.

Interactions

• ℞ **Aminoglycosides** may increase kidney damage.
• ℞ **Probenecid** increases the concentration of cephalosporins.
• Loop ℞ **diuretics** increase the risk of damage to the kidneys.

Side effects

• Frequently, oral candidiasis (thrush), mild diarrhea, nausea, and vaginal yeast infections.
• Occasionally, serum sickness reaction (skin rash, joint pain, fever), and vomiting.
• Rarely, hemolytic anemia, erythema multiform (blistering, peeling, loosening of the skin), and kidney damage.

cephalosporin ⓓ

Generics: **cefaclor; cefadroxil; cefamandole; cefazolin sodium; cefepime; cefixime; cefotaxime; cefotetan; cefpodoxime; cefprozil; ceftazidime; ceftriaxone; cefuroxime; cephalexin; cephradine.**

Actions and uses

Cephalosporins are ℞ **antibiotics** that are chemically of the ℞ **beta-lactam** group. They are broad-spectrum ℞ **antibacterial** agents that act against both Gram-positive and Gram-negative bacteria and are used to treat ✪ **bacterial infections**. Their chemical structure is similar to that of the ℞ **penicillin** group as they both contain a beta-lactam ring, hence their classification as beta-lactam antibiotics. The similarity in structure extends to how they act: both classes inhibit the synthesis of the bacterial cell wall, making it defective and unstable, so killing growing bacteria—they are bactericidal.

As a group, the cephalosporins are generally active against streptococci, staphylococci, and a number of Gram-negative bacteria, including many coliforms. Examples of the original, "first-generation" cephalosporins are ℞ **cephradine** and ℞ **cefadroxil**. Some "second-generation" cephalosporins (for example, ℞ **cefuroxime** and ℞ **cefamandole**) are resistant to bacterial penicillinase enzymes, which widens their range of action to include treating sensitive Gram-negative organisms, including *Haemophilus influenzae*.

Some of the latest, "third-generation," cephalosporins (for example, ℞ **cefotaxime**, ℞ **ceftazidime**) act as antibacterials against certain Gram-negative bacteria (for example, *Haemophilus influenzae*) and pseudomonal infections (for example, *Pseudomonas aeruginosa*). Many cephalosporins are actively excreted by the kidney and therefore reach considerably higher concentrations in the urine than in the blood. For this reason, they may be used to treat infections of the urinary tract while they are being excreted from the body.

Limitations

In general, cephalosporins are rarely the drug of first choice, but provide a useful alternative, or reserve option, in particular situations. The cephalosporins currently used are relatively non-toxic and only occasional blood-clotting problems, ✪ **superinfections**, and hypersensitivity reactions occur (only 10 percent of people allergic to penicillin show sensitivity to cephalosporins).

cephamandole ⓖ

see ℞ **cefamandole**.

cephradine ⓖ

(cefradine)
Type/Group: **cephalosporin; antibacterial; antibiotic.**
Brand(s): Velosef; various generic.
How administered: Orally.

Used to treat

Cephradine is a broad-spectrum, "first-generation" cephalosporin, which can be used to treat a wide range of ✪ **bacterial infections** of the upper respiratory tract, skin and skin structures, and urinary tract, and is also used to prevent infection during surgery.

Warnings

• It should not be given to people with a history of hypersensitivity to cephalosporins.
• It should be given with caution to people with allergies to penicillins or kidney impairment.
• Cephradine's safety in pregnancy is not established, and it readily crosses the placenta. Medical judgment is required to assess the benefits against the risk of harming the fetus.
• Medical judgment is also required if breast-feeding is being considered, because there is evidence that small amounts of cephalosporins do appear in breast milk.
• A severe hypersensitivity reaction is possible, particularly in those with a history of allergy to penicillins.
• The drug must be taken for the full length of treatment, because infection can return.
• Superinfections from the altered bacterial balance created by antibiotic treatment may occur, and may result in pseudomembranous colitis (an intestinal disorder characterized by severe diarrhea). ℞ **antidiarrheal** drugs must not be taken as this can result in toxic megacolon, a life-threatening dilation of the bowel. A doctor must be contacted if there is severe abdominal pain, or moderate to severe diarrhea.
• Rarely, this drug may cause kidney damage.

Interactions

• ℞ **Probenecid** increases the concentration of cephalosporins.
• Loop ℞ **diuretics** increase the risk of damage to the kidneys.
• ℞ **Aminoglycosides** increase the risk of damage to kidneys.

Side effects

• Frequently, oral candidiasis (thrush), mild diarrhea, nausea, and vaginal yeast infections.

• Occasionally, serum sickness reaction (skin rash, joint pain, fever), and vomiting.
• Rarely, hemolytic anemia, bone marrow suppression, bleeding, and kidney damage.

Cephulac ®

A preparation of ℞ **lactulose**.
Formulation: Oral liquid.
Availability: Prescription only.
Warnings and side effects: See ℞ **lactulose**.

Ceptaz ®

A preparation of ℞ **ceftazidime**.
Formulation: Injection.
Availability: Prescription only.
Warnings and side effects: See ℞ **ceftazidime**.

Cerebyx ®

A preparation of ℞ **fosphenytoin**.
Formulation: Injection.
Availability: Prescription only.
Warnings and side effects: See ℞ **fosphenytoin**.

Cerezyme ®

A preparation of ℞ **imiglucerase**.
Formulation: Powder for injection.
Availability: Prescription only.
Warnings and side effects: See ℞ **imiglucerase**.

cerivastatin sodium ⓖ

Type/Group: **lipid-regulating drug; statin.**
Brand(s): Baycol.
How administered: Orally.

Used to treat

Cerivastatin is a (statin/HMG-CoA reductase inhibitor) lipid-regulating drug that can be used in ✪ **hyperlipidemia** to reduce the levels, or change the proportions, of various lipids in the bloodstream. It is usually given to people in whom a strict and regular dietary regime alone is not having the desired effect.

Warnings

• It should not be given to people with active liver disease,
• It should be given with caution to people with liver dysfunction, kidney insufficiency, conditions predisposing to kidney failure, uncontrolled epilepsy, and heavy users of alcohol.
• Cerivastatin is considered potentially hazardous to the fetus. It is given to women of childbearing age only when they are thought highly unlikely to conceive and have been informed of the risks.
• It should not be used while breast-feeding.
• It might cause destruction of muscle tissue with resulting damage to the kidneys and even kidney failure. When taking cerivastatin, any unusual muscle pain or tenderness should be reported to a doctor immediately and treatment discontinued.
• Potentially harmful changes in liver function may occur, and so periodic tests are necessary to check the drug's effect.

Interactions

• ℞ **Azoles** (antifungals such as ℞ **itraconazole,** ℞ **ketoconazole**), **mibefradil,** ℞ **erythromycin,** ℞ **clarithromycin,** ℞ **nefazodone,** ℞ **cyclosporine,** ℞ **gemfibrozil,** and ℞ **niacin** (nicotinic acid, a B vitamin) may increase the levels of cerivastatin.

Side effects

• Constipation, abdominal pain, muscle cramps, rash, and insomnia.

Cerose-DM Liquid Ⓑ

A preparation of ℞ **dextromethorphan,** ℞ **chlorpheniramine maleate,** and ℞ **phenylephrine hydrochloride.**
Formulation: Oral liquid.
Availability: OTC.
Warnings and side effects: See ℞ **dextromethorphan;** ℞ **chlorpheniramine maleate;** ℞ **phenylephrine hydrochloride.**

Certiva Ⓑ

A preparation of ℞ **diphtheria and tetanus toxoids and acellular pertussis vaccine (DTaP).**
Formulation: Injection.
Availability: Prescription only.
Warnings and side effects: See ℞ **diphtheria and tetanus toxoids and acellular pertussis vaccine (DTaP).**

Cervidil Ⓑ

A preparation of ℞ **dinoprostone.**
Formulation: Vaginal insert.
Availability: Prescription only.
Warnings and side effects: See ℞ **dinoprostone.**

Ceta Ⓑ

A preparation of ℞ **sodium lauryl sulfate** and hydroxycellulose.
Formulation: Topical liquid.
Availability: OTC.
Warnings and side effects: See ℞ **sodium lauryl sulfate.**

Cetacort Ⓑ

A preparation of ℞ **hydrocortisone.**
Formulation: Lotion in two strengths.
Availability: Prescription only.
Warnings and side effects: See ℞ **hydrocortisone.**

Cetamide; Isopto Cetamide Ⓑ

A preparation of ℞ **sulfacetamide.**
Formulation: Eye drops (Isopto); ophthalmic ointment.
Availability: Prescription only.
Warnings and side effects: See ℞ **sulfacetamide.**

Ceta-Plus Capsules Ⓑ

A preparation of ℞ **hydrocodone bitartrate** and ℞ **acetaminophen.**
Formulation: Oral capsules.
Availability: Prescription only.
Warnings and side effects: See ℞ **hydrocodone bitartrate;** ℞ **acetaminophen.**

Cetapred Ⓑ

A preparation of ℞ **prednisolone** acetate and sodium sulfacemide.
Formulation: Ophthalmic ointment.
Availability: Prescription only.
Warnings and side effects: See ℞ **prednisolone.**

cetirizine hydrochloride Ⓖ

Type/Group: antihistamine; antiallergic.
Brand(s): Zyrtec Tables, Syrup.
How administered: Orally.

Used to treat

Cetirizine is a recently developed antihistamine with less side effects (such as sedation) than some of the older members of this class. It can be used for the symptomatic relief of allergic symptoms such as ⊙ **hay fever** (seasonal allergic rhinitis), perennial allergic rhinitis, and chronic ⊙ **urticaria.**

Warnings

• It should not be given to people with known hypersensitivity to this drug (or with known sensitivity to other antihistamines, but especially to ℞ **hydroxyzine**).
• Antihistamines should be given with caution to people with asthma or lower respiratory disease, heart disease, hypertension, hyperthyroidism, epilepsy, increased intraocular pressure (pressure in the eyeball, as in glaucoma), enlarged prostate, urinary retention, or certain obstructive bladder or gastrointestinal conditions.
• Cetirizine should be used during pregnancy only if it is clearly needed.
• Nursing mothers should discontinue using this drug or discontinue breast-feeding.
• Administer with caution to the elderly and to those with kidney or liver impairment.
• Because of possible sedative side effects, the performance of skilled tasks, such as driving, may be impaired.
• Side effects are more frequent in the elderly.

Interactions

• ℞ **MAOI** antidepressants may prolong and intensify the ℞ **anticholinergic** effects of antihistamines (see Side effects below).
• If used with ℞ **tricyclic** antidepressants, other antihistamines, ℞ **skeletal muscle relaxants,** ℞ **opioids,** ℞ **barbiturates,** ℞ **hypnotics,** ℞ **sedatives,** or ℞ **antianxiety** drugs, there is a risk of intensified side effects.
• Alcohol may intensify side effects such as drowsiness and impaired mental alertness.

Side effects

• These depend on how it is administered. The incidence of sedation and anticholinergic side effects is low. For this type of antihistamine, there is occasionally drowsiness, headache, impaired muscular coordination or dizziness, and anticholinergic effects (dry mouth, blurred vision, urinary retention, gastrointestinal disturbances).

• Rarely, there may be occasional rashes and photosensitivity (abnormal sensitivity to light), palpitations and heart arrhythmias, stimulation instead of sedation (paradoxical stimulation), especially in children (and convulsions in overdose), hypersensitivity reactions, blood disorders, liver disturbances, depression, sleep disturbances, and hypotension.

cetrorelix ⑥

Type/Group: **hormone antagonist**.
Brand(s): Cetrotide.
How administered: Injection.

Used to treat
Cetrorelix inhibits the release of gonadotrophins (LH & FSH). It is used in the treatment of ✪ **infertility** by assisted reproductive techniques (IVF) (see also ℞ **infertility treatment**).

Warnings
• It should not be given to people with known hypersensitivity to cetrorelix, extrinsic peptide hormones, mannitol, or gonadotropin-releasing hormones, or those over age 65. Cetrorelix should only be used under the supervision of a specialist physician.
• It is not for use during pregnancy or while breast-feeding. The possibility of pregnancy should be excluded before starting treatment.
• A doctor must be contacted immediately if overdose is suspected.

Interactions
No formal drug interaction studies have been performed.

Side effects
• Reddening, itching, swelling at injection site, nausea, and vomiting.

Cetrotide ⑧

A preparation of ℞ **cetrorelix**.
Formulation: Vial for injection.
Availability: Prescription only.
Warnings and side effects: See ℞ **cetrorelix**.

cetylpyridinium chloride ⑥

Type/Group: **antiseptic**.
Brand(s): Cepacol; Cepacol Anesthetic; Scope; Orajel Mouth Aid.
How administered: Orally/topically.

Used to treat
Cetylpyridinium chloride is used as a mouthwash or gargle for oral hygiene and minor throat infections.

Warnings
None significant.

Interactions
None significant.

Side effects
None significant.

Cevi-Bid ⑧

A preparation of ℞ **ascorbic acid**.
Formulation: Oral tablets.
Availability: Prescription only.
Warnings and side effects: See ℞ **ascorbic acid**.

cevimeline hydrochloride ⑥

Type/Group: **parasympathomimetic**.
Brand(s): Evoxac.
How administered: Orally.

Used to treat
Cevimeline is a (muscarinic) cholinergic agonist which is used for the treatment of dry mouth symptoms in ✪ **Sjögren's syndrome**.

Warnings
• It should not be given to people with uncontrolled asthma, known hypersensitivity to this drug, for those whom miosis (contraction of the pupil) is undesirable, or anyone with a history of cholelithiasis or nephrolithiasis.
• It should be used during pregnancy only if the potential benefits outweigh the possible risk to the fetus.
• It is not recommended for use while breast-feeding.
• Care must be taken while driving at night or performing hazardous activities in reduced lighting.

Interactions
• If used with ℞ **beta-blockers**, there may be conduction (nerve impulse) disturbances.
• If used with ℞ **parasympathomimetics**, effects are increased.
• Cevimeline may interfere with ℞ **anticholinergics**.

Side effects
• Constipation, sweating, tremor, abnormal vision, hypertonia, peripheral edema, chest pain, muscle aches, fever, loss of appetite, eye pain, earache, dry mouth, dizziness, salivary gland pain, itching, and flu-like symptoms.

Chap Stick Medicated Lip Balm ⑧

A preparation of ℞ **camphor**, ℞ **phenol**, ℞ **menthol**, ℞ **lanolin**, and ℞ **petrolatum**.
Formulation: Topical ointment, sticks.
Availability: OTC.
Warnings and side effects: See ℞ **camphor**; ℞ **phenol**; ℞ **menthol**; ℞ **lanolin**; ℞ **petrolatum**.

CharcoAid ⑧

A preparation of ℞ **activated charcoal** and ℞ **sorbitol**.
Formulation: Suspension.
Availability: OTC.
Warnings and side effects: See ℞ **activated charcoal**; ℞ **sorbitol**.

CharcoAid 2000 ⑧

A preparation of ℞ **activated charcoal**.
Formulation: Liquid or granules, liquid available with or without sorbitol.
Availability: OTC.
Warnings and side effects: See ℞ **activated charcoal**; ℞ **sorbitol**.

chelating agent ⑩

Generics: **desferoxamine mesylate**; **dexrazoxane**; **dimercaprol**; **edetate calcium disodium**; **trientine hydrochloride**.

Key to symbols: ✪ = Disorder Section ℞ = Drug Section ♣ = Herbal Section ◊◊ = Supplement Section

Actions and uses

Chelating agents are used in ℞ **antidote** treatment, mainly in metal ✪ **poisoning**. They work by chemically binding to certain metallic ions and other substances, making them less toxic and allowing the body to eliminate (excrete) them. Toxic substances that may be chelated include arsenic, gold, mercury, lead, chromium, manganese, nickel and zinc, plutonium, uranium, and thorium (depending on the specific chelating agent).

They are also used to reduce unacceptably high levels of metals in ✪ **metabolic disorder** treatment (for example, of copper in Wilson's disease by ℞ **trientine hydrochloride**), to treat disease states (for example, ℞ **penicillamine** in rheumatoid arthritis, to treat iron poisoning or an overload of iron in the tissues (for example, in aplastic anemia due to repeated blood transfusions, with ℞ **desferoxamine mesylate**), for the treatment of aluminum overload (for example, ℞ **desferoxamine mesylate** in people having kidney dialysis), and to reduce the severity of heart damage when using ℞ **cytotoxic** anticancer agents, such as ℞ **doxorubicin hydrochloride** (for example, ℞ **dexrazoxane**).

Limitations

See the individual drug entries.

Cheracol Cough Syrup ⑧

A preparation of ℞ **codeine phosphate** and ℞ **guaifenesin**.
Formulation: Oral syrup.
Availability: May or may not require a prescription.
Warnings and side effects: See ℞ **codeine phosphate**; ℞ **guaifenesin**.

Cheracol D Cough Liquid ⑧

A preparation of ℞ **dextromethorphan** and ℞ **guaifenesin**.
Formulation: Oral liquid.
Availability: OTC.
Warnings and side effects: See ℞ **dextromethorphan**; ℞ **guaifenesin**.

Cheracol Nasal ⑧

A preparation of ℞ **oxymetazoline hydrochloride**.
Formulation: Nasal spray.
Availability: OTC.
Warnings and side effects: See ℞ **oxymetazoline hydrochloride**.

Cheracol Sore Throat ⑧

A preparation of ℞ **phenol**.
Formulation: Throat spray.
Availability: OTC.
Warnings and side effects: See ℞ **phenol**.

Chibroxin ⑧

A preparation of ℞ **norfloxacin**.
Formulation: Eye drops.
Availability: Prescription only.
Warnings and side effects: See ℞ **norfloxacin**.

Children's Cepacol Liquid ⑧

A preparation of ℞ **pseudoephedrine** and ℞ **acetaminophen**.
Formulation: Oral liquid.
Availability: OTC.
Warnings and side effects: See ℞ **pseudoephedrine**; ℞ **acetaminophen**.

Children's Congestion Relief ⑧

A preparation of ℞ **pseudoephedrine**.
Formulation: Oral liquid.
Availability: OTC.
Warnings and side effects: See ℞ **pseudoephedrine**.

Children's Dramamine ⑧

A preparation of ℞ **dimenhydrinate**.
Formulation: Oral liquid.
Availability: OTC.
Warnings and side effects: See ℞ **dimenhydrinate**.

Children's Hold ⑧

A preparation of ℞ **dextromethorphan**.
Formulation: Lozenges.
Availability: OTC.
Warnings and side effects: See ℞ **dextromethorphan**.

Children's Silfedrine ⑧

A preparation of ℞ **pseudoephedrine**.
Formulation: Oral liquid.
Availability: OTC.
Warnings and side effects: See ℞ **pseudoephedrine**.

Children's Tylenol Cold Plus Cough Chewable Tablets ⑧

A preparation of ℞ **dextromethorphan**, ℞ **acetaminophen**, ℞ **chlorpheniramine maleate**, and ℞ **pseudoephedrine**.
Formulation: Oral tablets.
Availability: OTC.
Warnings and side effects: See ℞ **dextromethorphan**; ℞ **acetaminophen**; ℞ **chlorpheniramine maleate**; ℞ **pseudoephedrine**.

Children's Tylenol Cold Tablets; Liquid ⑧

A preparation of ℞ **pseudoephedrine**, ℞ **chlorpheniramine maleate**, and ℞ **acetaminophen**.
Formulation: Oral tablets, chewable; liquid.
Availability: OTC.
Warnings and side effects: See ℞ **pseudoephedrine**; ℞ **chlorpheniramine maleate**; ℞ **acetaminophen**. The chewable tablets contain the sweetener aspartame (with phenylalanine), which should be avoided by individuals with phenylketonuria.

Chirocaine ⑧

A preparation of ℞ **levobupivacaine**.
Formulation: Injection.
Availability: Prescription only.

Key to symbols: Ⓓ = Drug type/group   Ⓖ = Generic name   Ⓑ = Brand name

Warnings and side effects: See ℞ **levobupivacaine**.

Chlo-Amine ⑧

A preparation of ℞ **chlorpheniramine maleate**.
Formulation: Oral tablets, chewable.
Availability: OTC.
Warnings and side effects: See ℞ **chlorpheniramine maleate**.

Chlorafed Timecelles; H.S. Timecelles; Liquid ⑧

A preparation of ℞ **pseudoephedrine** and ℞ **chlorpheniramine maleate**.
Formulation: Oral capsules, sustained release; liquid.
Availability: Capsules prescription only; Liquid is OTC.
Warnings and side effects: See ℞ **pseudoephedrine**; ℞ **chlorpheniramine maleate**.

chloral hydrate ⑥

Type/Group: **sedatives; hypnotic**.
Brand(s): Aquachloral; Noctec.
How administered: Orally; rectal suppositories.

Used to treat

Chloral hydrate is a short-term sedative and hypnotic drug which used to be considered particularly useful in inducing sleep in children or older adults. It is used for nocturnal sedation, as well as pre-operative sedation, sedation prior to EEG evaluations, as an additional treatment to opiates and analgesics in postoperative care and pain control, as well as for alcohol withdrawal.

Warnings

• It should not be given to people with known hypersensitivity to this drug, severe kidney, liver or heart disease, or with stomach inflammation (gastritis).
• It should be given with caution to people with heart disease, certain gastrointestinal conditions, acute intermittent porphyria, a history of drug abuse, tartrazine sensitivity, or in anyone over the age of 65.
• Chloral hydrate should be used during pregnancy only if it is clearly needed.
• Medical judgment is required if breast-feeding is being considered.
• It may cause upset stomach, and should be taken with plenty of water or other liquid.
• Avoid alcohol.
• Avoid contact with skin or mucous membranes.
• Tolerance (addiction) can occur with prolonged use.

Interactions

• If used with ℞ **warfarin sodium**, there is a temporary increase in the response to warfarin.
• If used with ℞ **barbiturates** or other central nervous system (CNS) depressants, there are increased effects.
• If used with alcohol, there are increased depressant effects on the central nervous system (CNS).

Side effects

• Drowsiness, stomach irritation, abdominal distension, and flatulence.

• Occasionally, rashes, vertigo and lightheadedness, headache, unsteadiness and incoordination, confusion and excitement (for example, night terror, delirium).
• Rare but serious side effects include white blood cell disorders.

chlorambucil ⑥

Type/Group: **anticancer; cytotoxic**.
Brand(s): Leukeran.
How administered: Orally.

Used to treat

Chlorambucil is a cytotoxic drug (an alkylating agent) that is used particularly for chronic lymphocytic ✪ **leukemia**, ✪ **lymphomas**, and ✪ **Hodgkin's disease**. It works by interfering with the DNA and so preventing normal cell replication.

Warnings

• It should not be given to people with known hypersensitivity to chlorambucil. Those allergic to other alkylating agents may experience a rash. This is a specialist drug which will be used following a full evaluation by specialist physicians.
• Chlorambucil is not recommended for use during pregnancy unless it is medically judged to be essential, because it may cause birth defects. Becoming pregnant while using this drug must be avoided.
• It should not be used if breast-feeding.
• It can cause severe bone marrow depression, which may lead to bleeding and a reduced resistance to infection.
• In common with many anticancer drugs, it causes cancer and can interfere with fertility.
• It may cause seizures, particularly in children.
• A doctor must be contacted if unusual bleeding or bruising, fever, nausea, skin rash, chills, sore throat, shortness of breath, cough or wheezing, amenorrhea, unusual lumps, joint, stomach, flank pain, sores in mouth, or yellowing skin or eyes occur.

Interactions

No specific interactions of significance to this drug are known.

Side effects

• Frequently, gastrointestinal effects (depend on dosage).
• Occasionally, skin rash, irritation or itching, and cold sores.
• Rarely, hair loss, hives, reddening of skin, increased uric acid in blood, and significant blood changes.

chloramphenicol ⑥

Type/Group: **antibacterial; antibiotic**.
Brand(s): Cloromycetin; Chloroptic; AK-Chlor; various generic.
Combinations: With *polymyxin B* and *hydrocortisone*: Opthocort. With *desoxyribonuclease* and *fibrinolysin*: Elase-Chloromycetin.
How administered: Orally; injection; topically (eye).

Used to treat

Chloramphenicol is used to treat many forms of ✪ **bacterial infection**. However, the serious side effects caused by its systemic use mean that it is normally restricted to certain severe infections, such as typhoid fever, ✪ **Rocky Mountain spotted fever**, Q fever, ✪ **meningitis**, and, in particular, infections caused by *Haemophilus influenzae*. It is useful in treating conditions such as bacterial conjunctivitis, external ear canal infections, and many types of skin

Key to symbols: ✪ = Disorder Section ℞ = Drug Section ♣ = Herbal Section ♌ = Supplement Section

infection, because when it is applied topically (externally) to the eyes, ears or skin, its toxicity is rarely a concern.

Warnings

These depend on the route of administration.

• It should not be given to people with known hypersensitivity to chloramphenicol.

• It should be given with caution to people with allergies to penicillins or cephalosporins, with acute intermittent porphyria, G6PD deficiency (a genetic enzyme disorder), with impaired kidney or liver function, or anyone over the age of 65.

• Chloramphenical's safety in pregnancy has not been established. It does cross the placenta and should be used only if the benefits outweigh the possible risk to the fetus. It should not be used near term or during labor, as toxic reactions in newborn babies have occurred.

• Medical judgment is required if breast-feeding is being considered. It does appear in breast milk.

• It should not be used to treat trivial infections (for example, flu, colds, or throat infections) or infections other than those for which it is prescribed.

• Serious and fatal blood disorders may occur after systemic use. A doctor must be contacted if unusual bleeding or bruising occurs (though there will be monitoring).

• Superinfections due to the altered bacterial balance created by antibiotic treatment may occur. A doctor must be contacted if there is severe abdominal pain, or moderate to severe diarrhea.

Interactions

These depend on the route of administration.

• The anticoagulant effect of ℞ **warfarin sodium** may be increased.

• The effects of ℞ **barbiturates** may be increased, while the effects of chloramphenicol may be reduced.

• The antibacterial effects of ℞ **ceftazidime** and ℞ **penicillins** are reduced.

• There is an increased risk of certain blood disorders if taken with ℞ **cimetidine**.

• ℞ **Phenytoin** levels are increased, possibly to dangerous levels.

• If used with ℞ **rifampin**, the levels of chloramphenicol may be reduced.

• Anticoagulant effects are increased when taken with ℞ **sulfonylureas**.

Side effects

• Systemic use: Occasionally, nausea, vomiting, or diarrhea. Rarely, rash, shortness of breath, confusion, headache, numbness or weakness in hands or feet, and potentially serious blood disorders.

• Topical use: Occasionally, blurred vision, burning, stinging, and allergic reaction. Rarely, inflammation of the optic nerve. Aplastic anemia has been reported.

chlordiazepoxide ⓖ

Type/Group: **antianxiety; benzodiazepine.**
Brand(s): Librium; Librium for injection; various generic.
Combinations: With *amitriptyline hydrochloride*: Limbitrol. With *clidinium*: Clindex, Librax.
How administered: Orally, injectable solution.

Used to treat

Chlordiazepoxide can be used in the short-term treatment of ✪ **anxiety** disorders, preoperative apprehension and anxiety, and, in conjunction with other drugs, in the treatment of acute alcohol withdrawal symptoms. Although not stated by the manufacturer for such treatment, it may be prescribed for tremors, tension headache, and panic disorders.

Warnings

• It should not be given to people with known hypersensitivity to benzodiazepines, or with narrow-angle glaucoma or psychosis.

• It should be given with caution to people with porphyria, respiratory, liver or kidney disease, who are over 65, or in a weakened (debilitated) condition.

• Chlordiazepoxide is not recommended for use during pregnancy. Its use in the first trimester should almost always be avoided. A doctor must be contacted if pregnancy occurs while this drug is being taken.

• It should not normally be used by nursing mothers.

• It may cause drowsiness and so the performance of skilled tasks may be impaired, such as driving.

• Avoid alcohol consumption, because adverse side effects may be increased (see Side effects below).

• Avoid other psychotropic medications unless prescribed by a doctor.

• A doctor must be consulted before discontinuing use or increasing dosage, because benzodiazepines may produce psychological and physical dependence and withdrawal symptoms.

Interactions

• ℞ **cimetidine**, ℞ **disulfiram**, ℞ **fluconazole**, ℞ **itraconazole**, and ℞ **ketoconazole** may increase the effects of chlordiazepoxide.

• If used with ℞ **levodopa**, Parkinsonian symptoms could be increased.

Side effects

• Depending on dose, use, and how it is administered, there many be confusion and drowsiness.

• Less frequently, memory loss, impaired movement and coordination, mental changes, dizziness, headache, insomnia, slurred speech, elevated blood pressure, postural hypotension (lowered blood pressure on standing), changes in heart rate, auditory disturbances, blurred vision, eye changes, loss of appetite, dry mouth, gastrointestinal problems, changes in libido, menstrual irregularities, urinary incontinence or retention, and skin reactions. A rare but serious side effect is shock.

Chlordrine S.R. Capsules ⓑ

A preparation of ℞ **pseudoephedrine** and ℞ **chlorpheniramine maleate**.
Formulation: Oral capsules, sustained release.
Availability: Prescription only.
Warnings and side effects: See ℞ **pseudoephedrine**; ℞ **chlorpheniramine maleate**.

chlorhexidine ⓖ

Type/Group: **antiseptic; disinfectant.**

Brand(s): BactoShield; Betasept; Dyna-Hex; Exidine Scrub; Hibistat; Peridex; PerioChip PerioGard.
How administered: Topically (external).

Used to treat
Chlorhexidine is a constituent in many preparations and is used mainly as a mouthwash for oral hygiene and ✪ **gingivitis**. It can also be used as an insert to reduce gum pocket depth in adults with ✪ **periodontitis**, and as a surgical scrub and preoperative cleanser.

Warnings
• It should not be given to people with known sensitivity to chlorhexidine.
• Its safety in pregnancy has not been established. It should be used during pregnancy only if clearly needed.
• Medical judgment is required if breast-feeding is being considered. It is not known whether this drug appears in breast milk.
• It may increase calculus deposits on teeth.
• It may stain oral surfaces.

Interactions
No significant interactions have been reported when used topically.

Side effects
• Altered taste perception and minor irritation.
• Rarely, allergic reaction.

chlormethine hydrochloride ⑥
see ℞ mechlorethamine hydrochloride.

Chloromycetin; Chloromycetin Optic; Chloromycetin Otic ⑧
A preparation of ℞ **chloramphenicol**.
Formulation: Injection; Optic: eye drops; ointment. Otic: ear drops.
Availability: Prescription only.
Warnings and side effects: See ℞ **chloramphenicol**.

Chloromycetin-hydrocortisone ⑧
A preparation of ℞ **chloramphenicol** and ℞ **hydrocortisone**.
Formulation: Eye drops.
Availability: Prescription only.
Warnings and side effects: See ℞ **chloramphenicol**; ℞ **hydrocortisone**.

chloroprocaine hydrochloride ⑥
Type/Group: **local anesthetic**.
Brand(s): Nesacaine.
How administered: Local injection.

Used to treat
Chloroprocaine is used for peripheral and central nerve block.

Warnings
• It should not be given to people with known hypersensitivity to chloroprocaine. It is a specialist drug and there will be a full medical assessment.
• It should be used in pregnancy only when it is clearly needed.

• Medical judgment is required if breast-feeding is being considered.
• It can cause cardiac depression, peripheral vasodilatation, or CNS (central nervous system) toxicity.

Interactions
• There may be additive effects if used with ℞ **antiarrhythmics** (for example, ℞ **tocainide**, ℞ **mexiletine**).
• The effects of ℞ **sulfonamides** are reduced.

Side effects
• Occasionally, pain at injection site, burning, stinging, or tenderness where applied.
• Rarely (generally with a high dose), drowsiness, dizziness, disorientation, lightheadedness, tremors, apprehension, euphoria, sensation of heat, cold, or numbness, blurred or double vision, tinnitus, nausea, or allergic reactions.

Chloroptic; Chloroptic S.O.P. ⑧
A preparation of ℞ **chloramphenicol**.
Formulation: Eye drops; ointment.
Availability: Prescription only.
Warnings and side effects: See ℞ **chloramphenicol**.

chloroquine ⑥
Type/Group: **antimalarial; amebicide and antiprotozoal**.
Brand(s): Aralen Phosphate, Aralen Hydrochloride.
How administered: Orally; injection.

Used to treat
Chloroquine is a (4-aminoquinoline) drug used to treat and prevent contraction of ✪ **malaria**. In certain areas of the world strains of *Plasmodium falciparum* and other strains have recently exhibited resistance to chloroquine, so an alternative therapy is now advised. It is also effective in treating amebic infection in the body but is absorbed into the blood too quickly to treat infection of the intestinal lumen. Although not stated by the manufacturer for such treatments, it may be prescribed as an antirheumatic to slow the progress of rheumatic disease (for example, ✪ **rheumatoid arthritis** and lupus erythematosus (see ✪ **lupus**)).

Warnings
• It should not be used by anyone with known hypersensitivity to any 4-aminoquinoline drug, or with retinal damage from taking such a drug, or those who have psoriasis or porphyria (though cases may arise where potential benefit outweighs potential risk).
• Children should not take this drug in long-term therapy.
• It should be used with caution by anyone with G6PD deficiency, alcoholism, or who have impairment of kidney or liver function. (Which warnings apply depend on the proposed use of chloroquine.)
• Chloroquine should be used during pregnancy only when the benefits outweigh the potential risk to the fetus. Birth defects have been reported in cases where chloroquine was administered for lupus erythematosus, although not where it was used for prevention of malaria. Study and evaluation is incomplete.
• Breast-feeding mothers should either discontinue using this drug or stop breast-feeding.

Key to symbols: ✪ = Disorder Section ℞ = Drug Section ♣ = Herbal Section ⚕⚕ = Supplement Section

• Chloroquine is very toxic in overdose. In acute cases, seizures and death may occur within two hours.

• In long-term use, eye examinations, medical monitoring of liver function, and blood cell counts are necessary.

Interactions

• ℞ **cimetidine** may raise the concentration of chloroquine.

• If taken with mefloquine there is a greater risk of convulsions.

• Chloroquine may inhibit the immunizing effect of ℞ **rabies vaccine**.

• If taken with ℞ **amiodarone hydrochloride** or levacetylmethadol, there is a risk of disorders of heart rhythm.

Side effects

These depend on how administered, use, and dose.

• There may be nausea and vomiting, headache, or gastrointestinal disturbance;

• Occasionally, itching and rash;

• Susceptible people may suffer psychotic episodes, blood disorders, damage to the eyes, and effects to the hair.

Chloroserpine Tablets ⑧

A preparation of ℞ **chlorothiazide** and ℞ **reserpine**.
Formulation: Oral tablets.
Availability: Prescription only.
Warnings and side effects: See ℞ **chlorothiazide**; ℞ **reserpine**.

chlorothiazide ⑥

Type/Group: diuretic; thiazide; antihypertensive.
Brand(s): Diurigen; Diuril; various generic. Combinations: With *methyldopa*: Aldoclor-150, 250 Tablets. With *reserpine*: Chloroserpine Tablets, various generic.
How administered: Orally; injection.

Used to treat

Chlorothiazide is used in the treatment of ⊙ **hypertension**, either alone or along with other types of diuretic or other drugs (for example, ℞ **beta-blockers**). It can also be used in the treatment of edema. Thiazide diuretics have also become a major part of treatment for nephrogenic ⊙ **diabetes insipidus**. This is the only thiazide available as an injection, although this form is only used in an emergency or when medication cannot be given orally.

Warnings

• It should not be given to people with known hypersensitivity to thiazides (or to ℞ **sulfonamide**-derived drugs), or severe kidney or liver disorders.

• It should be given with caution to elderly people, anyone with high cholesterol or triglyceride levels, or liver or kidney impairment.

• It should be used in pregnancy only when the potential benefit outweighs the possible risk to the fetus.

• Medical judgment is required if breast-feeding is being considered.

• Early symptoms of electrolyte imbalance may include muscle weakness or cramps, nausea, vomiting, restlessness or lethargy, dry mouth, excessive thirst, fast pulse, or dizziness. A doctor must be contacted if such symptoms occur.

• Thiazides may aggravate symptoms of diabetes or gout, and worsen or activate lupus erythematosus.

• Periodic monitoring of electrolytes (particularly potassium, sodium, chloride, and bicarbonate) is needed.

• Photosensitivity may develop and so precautions such as protective clothing or sunscreens should be used.

• Thiazides interact with a number of drugs, including some over-the-counter preparations. A doctor must be consulted before taking any other medications (including OTCs, herbal remedies, and supplements).

Interactions

• There is a higher risk of a hypersensitivity reaction to ℞ **allopurinol**.

• The effects of ℞ **anesthetics**, ℞ **anticancer** drugs, other antihypertensives, ℞ **diazoxide**, ⚶ **calcium** salts, ℞ **cardiac glycosides**, ℞ **lithium**, loop diuretics, ℞ **methyldopa**, nondepolarizing ℞ **skeletal muscle relaxants**, and ⚶ **vitamin D** may be increased, with the potential for significant adverse effects or toxicity. An additive effect is sometimes used to advantage in combining thiazides with other antihypertensives.

• The effects of ℞ **anticoagulants** and antigout agents (for example, ℞ **probenecid**, ℞ **sulfinpyrazone**) may be lowered by thiazides.

• The doses of ℞ **insulin** and ℞ **sulfonylureas** may need to be adjusted, as thiazides may increase blood sugar levels.

• ℞ **Amphotericin B**, ℞ **anticholinergics**, ℞ **corticosteroids**, ℞ **corticotropin**, and ℞ **MAOI**s may increase the effects of thiazides, with the possibility of significant electrolyte loss, especially potassium.

• ℞ **cholestyramine**, ℞ **colestipol hydrochloride**, ℞ **methenamine**, and ℞ **NSAID**s (especially ℞ **Indomethacin**) may reduce the effectiveness of thiazide diuretics.

• There is an increased possibility of postural hypotension (lowered blood pressure on standing) if taken with alcohol, ℞ **barbiturates**, or ℞ **opioids**.

Side effects

• There may be dizziness, headache, muscle cramps, mild gastrointestinal upsets, postural hypotension, reversible impotence, low blood potassium, sodium, magnesium and chloride, raised blood urea, glucose and lipids, and gout.

• Rarely, photosensitivity, blood disorders, skin reactions, and pancreatitis.

chloroxylenol ⑥

Type/Group: **antiseptic**.
Brand(s): Foille; Unguentine Plus.
How administered: Topically (external).

Used to treat

Chloroxylenol is used for many purposes, including to prevent minor staphylococcal infections of the skin.

Warnings

None significant.

Interactions

None significant.

Side effects

None significant.

Chlorphed-LA ®

A preparation of ℞ **oxymetazoline hydrochloride**.
Formulation: Nasal spray.
Availability: OTC.
Warnings and side effects: See ℞ **oxymetazoline hydrochloride**.

Chlorphedrine SR Capsules ®

A preparation of ℞ **pseudoephedrine** and ℞ **chlorpheniramine maleate**.
Formulation: Oral capsules, sustained release.
Availability: Prescription only.
Warnings and side effects: See ℞ **pseudoephedrine**; ℞ **chlorpheniramine maleate**.

chlorphenamine maleate ⑥

see ℞ **chlorpheniramine maleate**.

chlorpheniramine maleate ⑥

(chlorphenamine maleate)
Type/Group: antihistamine; antiallergic; cold and cough preparation.
Brand(s): Aller-Chlor Tablets, Syrup; Allergy; Chlo-Amine; Chlor-Trimeton Allergy 4 Hour, 8 Hour, 12 Hour, 4 Hour Syrup; Polaramine Tablets, Repetabs, Syrup; various generic.
Combinations: With codeine: (Plus) *pseudoephedrine*: Codehist DH Elixir; Decohistine DH Liquid; Phenhist DH w/Codeine Liquid; Ryna-C Liquid. (Plus) *phenylephrine and potassium iodide*: Pediacof Syrup; Pedituss Cough Syrup. With dextromethorphan: Primatuss Cough Mixture 4 Liquid; Scot-Tussin DM Liquid; Tricodene Sugar Free Liquid. (Plus) *guaifenesin and phenylephrine*: Donatussin Syrup. (Plus) *phenylephrine*: Cerose-DM Liquid. (Plus) *pseudoephedrine*: Children's Vicks Nyquil; Rescon-DM Liquid; Rhinosyn-DM Liquid; Triaminic Night Time Maximum Strength. (Plus) *pseudoephedrine and acetaminophen*: Alka-Selzer Plus Cold & Cough LiquiGels; Children's Tylenol Cold Plus Cough Chewable Tablets; Comtrex Maximum Strength Multi-Symptom Cold & Cough Relief Caplets, Tablets; Contac Severe Cold & Flu Caplets; Genacol Tablets; Kolephrin/DM Caplets; Medi-Flu Liquid; Multi-Symptom Tylenol Cold Caplets, Tablets; NightTime TheraFlu Powder; Robitussin Nighttime Honey Flu; Triaminic Severe Cold & Fever; Vicks 44M Cold & Flu Relief. With guaifenesin: (Plus) *ephedrine*: Bronkotuss Expectorant Liquid. (Plus) *phenylephrine*: Donatussin Drops. (Plus) *pseudoephedrine*: Polaramine Expectorant Liquid (has *dexchlorpheniramine maleate*). With hydrocodone: S-T Forte-2 Liquid. (Plus) *phenylephrine*: Atuss MS, HD, HD Syrup, DM Syrup; ED-TLC Liquid; ED Tuss HC Liquid; Endagen-HD Liquid; Endal-HD Liquid, Plus Liquid; Hitussin HC Syrup; Histinex HC Syrup; Iodal HD; Iotussin HC Syrup; Tussanil DH Syrup; Vanex-HD Liquid. (Plus) *phenylephrine, acetaminophen, caffeine*: Hycomine Compound Tablets. (Plus) *pseudoephedrine*: Histinex PV Syrup; Hyphed; Pancof-HC Liquid; P-V-Tussin Syrup. With phenylephrine: Comhist Tablets, LA Capsules (have *phenyltoloxamine citrate*); Dallergy-D Syrup; ED A-Hist Tablets, Liquid; Histatab Plus Tablets; Histor-D Syrup; Rolatuss Plain Liquid; Ru-Tuss Liquid. (Plus) *acetaminophen*:

Aclophen Tablets; Covangesic Tablets (has *pyrilamine maleate*); Dristan Cold Multi-Symptom Formula Tablets; Gendecon Tablets; Histagesic Modified Tablets; Histex SR; ND-Gesic Tablets (has *pyrilamine maleate*). (Plus) *pyrilamine tannate*: Atrohist Pediatric Suspension; Gelhist Pediatric Suspension; Rhinatate Tablets; R-Tannamine Tablets, Pediatric Suspension; R-Tannate Tablets, Pediatric Suspension; Rynatan Pediatric Suspension; Triotann Tablets; Tri-Tannate Tablets, Pediatric Suspension. With pseudoephedrine: Allerest Maximum Strength Tablets; Anamine T.D. Capsules, Syrup; Anaplex Liquid; Atrohist Pediatric Capsules; Biohist-LA Tablets; Brexin L.A. Capsules; Chlorafed Timecelles, H.S. Timecelles, Liquid; Chlordrine S.R. Capsules; Chlorphedrine SR Capsules; Chlor-Trimeton 12 Hour Relief Capsules, 4 Hour Relief Tablets; Colfed-A Capsules; Cophene No. 2 Tablets; Copyronil 2 Pulvules; Deconamine SR Capsules, Tablets, Syrup; Duralex Capsules; Fedahist Tablets, Timecaps, Gyrocaps; Hayfebrol Liquid; Histalet Syrup; Klerist-D Capsules, Tablets; Kronofed-A Capsules; Jr. Capsules; ND Clear Capsules; Novafed A Capsules; Palgic DS Syrup; Pseudo-Gest Plus Tablets; Rescon Capsules, ED Capsules, JR Capsules; Rhinosyn-PD Liquid; Rinade B.I.D. Capsules; Ryna Liquid; Sudafed Plus Tablets; Tanafed. (Plus) *acetaminophen*: Alka-Seltzer Plus Allergy Liqui-Gels; Allerest Sinus Pain Formula Tabs; Children's Tylenol Cold Liquid, Tablets; Codimal Capsule, Tablets; Co-Hist Tablets; Comtrex Allergy-Sinus Tablets, Caplets; Kolephrin Caplets; Maximum Strength Tylenol Allergy Sinus Caplets, Gelcaps; Sinarest Sinus Tablets, Extra Strength Tablets; Sine-Off Sinus Medicine Caplets; Sinutab Maximum Strength Sinus Allergy Caplets, Tablets; TheraFlu Flu and Cold Medicine Powder. With other constituents: With *hydrocortisone and pyrilamine maleate*: HC Derma-Pax Liquid. With *pyrilamine maleate*: Derma-Pax Lotion. (Most combinations available as generic.)
How administered: Orally; injection; topically (external).

Used to treat

Chlorpheniramine is used to treat the symptoms of many allergic conditions, including ✪ **hay fever** (seasonal allergic rhinitis), perennial allergic rhinitis and ✪ **urticaria**, and also occasionally in emergencies to treat anaphylactic shock (see ✪ **anaphylactic reaction**. It is also incorporated in some preparations for ✪ **coughs** and ✪ **colds**. Some preparations may use a more active form of this drug, dexchlorpheniramine maleate.

Warnings

• It should not be given to people with known hypersensitivity to this drug (or with known sensitivity to other antihistamines).

• Antihistamines should be given with caution to people with lower respiratory disease or asthma (and never during an attack), heart and renal disease, hypertension, hyperthyroidism, epilepsy, increased intraocular pressure (pressure in the eyeball, as in glaucoma), enlarged prostate, urinary retention, or certain obstructive bladder or gastrointestinal conditions.

• Chlorpheniramine should be used during pregnancy only if it is clearly needed, but not in the third trimester, as newborns or premature infants may have severe reactions, including convulsions, to antihistamines.

• Nursing mothers should discontinue using this drug or discontinue breast-feeding.

• This drug must not be given to infants, and for children under the age of 12 the manufacturer's or medical instructions must be followed closely.

• Because of its sedative side effects, the performance of skilled tasks, such as driving, may be impaired.

• Side effects are more frequent in the elderly.

Interactions

• ℞ **MAOI** antidepressants may prolong and intensify the ℞ **anticholinergic** effects of antihistamines (see Side effects below).

• If used with ℞ **tricyclic** antidepressants, other antihistamines, ℞ **skeletal muscle relaxants**, ℞ **phenothiazines**, ℞ **opioids**, ℞ **barbiturates**, ℞ **hypnotics**, ℞ **sedatives**, or ℞ **antianxiety** drugs, there is a risk of intensified side effects.

• Alcohol may intensify side effects such as drowsiness and impaired mental alertness.

Side effects

• These depend on how it is administered. For this type of antihistamine, there is commonly drowsiness, headache, impaired muscular coordination or dizziness, anticholinergic effects (dry mouth, blurred vision, urinary retention, gastrointestinal disturbances), tinnitus, occasional rashes and photosensitivity (abnormal sensitivity to light), palpitations and heart arrhythmias.

• Rarely, there may be stimulation instead of sedation (paradoxical stimulation), especially in children (and convulsions in overdose), hypersensitivity reactions, blood disorders, liver disturbances, depression, sleep disturbances, and hypotension.

• Injections can be irritant, and may cause short-lasting hypotension and stimulation of the central nervous system.

chlorpromazine ⑥

Type/Group: **antipsychotic; antinauseant; antiemetic; phenothiazine.**
Brand(s): Thorazine; various generic. Combinations: With amitriptyline hydrochloride: Limbitrol.
How administered: Orally; injection; suppository.

Used to treat

Chlorpromazine is chemically an important member of the phenothiazines and has a number of actions and uses. It is used as an antipsychotic and has marked sedative effects that make it a useful treatment for ✪ schizophrenia and other psychoses (see ✪ psychotic disorders), particularly during violent behavioral disturbances. It is also used preoperatively for relaxation and to remedy intractable hiccups. Additionally, it has an important use as an antinauseant and antiemetic to relieve nausea and vomiting, particularly in terminal illness. It is also prescribed for intermittent ✪ porphyria, behavioral problems in children, and as an additional treatment for ✪ tetanus. Although not stated by the manufacturer for such use, it is sometimes prescribed for "angel dust" psychosis (form of psychosis caused by people misusing the hallucinogenic drug phencyclidine) and ✪ migraine.

Warnings

• It should not be given to people with known hypersensitivity to this drug, with circulatory collapse, liver damage, cerebral arteriosclerosis, coronary disease, severe high or low blood pressure, certain blood diseases, coma, brain damage, bone marrow depression, or alcohol and barbiturate withdrawal.

• It should be given with caution to people with certain conditions, including seizure disorders, high blood pressure, pheochromocytoma, glaucoma, liver disease, heart or kidney disease, and chronic obstructive pulmonary disease (COPD).

• Chlorpromazine should not be used during pregnancy unless it is essential. A doctor must be contacted if pregnancy occurs while taking this drug.

• It should not be used by nursing mothers.

• It may cause drowsiness and the performance of skilled tasks, such as driving, may be impaired.

• It may cause postural hypotension (lowered blood pressure on standing), so rise slowly from a reclining position. Older people in particular should exercise caution.

• It may increase susceptibility to heat stroke, so exercise caution in hot weather.

• Avoid alcohol consumption.

• It may cause sensitivity to sunlight (photosensitivity), so exposure should be minimized (use a sunscreen, sunglasses, and so on).

• If used for a long time, tardive dyskinesia (see ℞ **antipsychotics**) occasionally develops.

• Urine may turn red-brown or pink.

• Treatment must be stopped gradually.

Interactions

• Antipsychotics may reduce the ℞ **antiparkinsonian** effect of ℞ **levodopa.**

• If used with an ℞ **antidepressant** or ℞ **propranolol**, the levels of both drugs may be increased.

• If used with ℞ **lithium**, the levels of both drugs may be decreased.

• ℞ **Antimalarials** (amodiaquine, chloroquine, sulfadoxine, pyrimethamine) may increase the concentrations of chlorpromazine.

• ℞ **Anticholinergics**, ℞ **barbiturates**, ℞ **narcotic analgesics**, and ℞ **orphenadrine** lower the levels of an antipsychotic and/or increase the occurrence of anticholinergic and/or CNS (central nervous system) effects.

• Chlorpromazine reduces the effects of oral ℞ **anticoagulants.**

• If used with ℞ **clonidine hydrochloride**, ℞ **guanadrel** or ℞ **guanethidine monosulfate**, there is a risk of severe lowering of blood pressure.

• The response to ℞ **epinephrine** may be changed by antipsychotics.

• If used with alcohol, there is a risk of increased effects and hypotension.

Side effects

• These can be many and include drowsiness, postural hypotension, photosensitivity, loss of appetite and constipation.

• Less frequently, extrapyramidal symptoms (see ℞ **antipsychotics**) dry mouth, nasal constriction, difficulty in urination, blurred vision, cardiovascular effects, respiratory depression, changes in hormone function (irregular menstruation, growth of breasts, abnormal milk production, impotence, weight gain), sensitivity reactions, blood cell disorders, rashes, jaundice and alterations in liver function, and eye changes.

• Rarely, neuroleptic malignant syndrome (a potentially fatal condition characterized by very high fever, muscle rigidity, changes in mental status, and irregular pulse, blood pressure, and/or heart rhythm), seizure, and cardiac arrest. Intramuscular injection may be painful.

chlorpropamide Ⓖ
Type/Group: **antidiabetic; oral hypoglycemic; sulfonylurea; diabetes insipidus treatment.**
Brand(s): Diabinese; various generic.
How administered: Orally.

Used to treat
Chlorpropamide is used for type 2 ✪ **diabetes mellitus** (non-insulin-dependent diabetes mellitus; NIDDM). It works by augmenting what remains of insulin production in the pancreas and its effect lasts longer than that of most similar drugs. Unusually for a sulfonylurea, chlorpropamide can also be used for ✪ **diabetes insipidus** (although not stated by the manufacturer for such use), although only mild forms caused by pituitary or thalamic malfunction.

Warnings
• It should not be given to people with with type 1 diabetes mellitus, or ketoacidosis.
• It should be given with caution to people with heart, thyroid, kidney, or liver disease, severe hypoglycemic reactions, or who are over 65.
• It is inappropriate for use during pregnancy (insulin is the drug of choice).
• Medical judgment is required if breast-feeding is being considered.
• Alcohol should be avoided, as it can cause unpleasant symptoms and interfere with blood sugar control.
• There are potentially multiple drug interactions with chlorpropamide. A doctor should be consulted before taking any other medication (including OTCs, herbal remedies, and supplements).

Interactions
• ℞ NSAIDs, ℞ **salicylates**, ℞ **sulfonamides**, ℞ **chloramphenicol**, coumarins, ℞ **probenecid**, ℞ **MAOIs**, and ℞ **beta-blockers** may enhance the hypoglycemic effect of sulfonylureas.
• ℞ **Thiazide** and other ℞ **diuretics**, ℞ **corticosteroids**, ℞ **phenothiazines**, ℞ **thyroid hormones**, ℞ **estrogens**, ℞ **oral contraceptives**, ℞ **phenytoin**, ℞ **niacin**, ℞ **sympathomimetics**, and ℞ **isoniazid** may lead to the loss of control of sugar levels.
• Oral ℞ **miconazole**, ℞ **diclofenac**, ℞ **ibuprofen**, ℞ **naproxen**, and ℞ **mefenamic acid** have the potential for severe hypoglycemia.

Side effects
• Frequently, dizziness, drowsiness, weakness, and headache.
• Less commonly, gastrointestinal effects, metabolic disorders, allergic skin reactions (potentially serious), photosensitivity, and serious blood disorders.

chlortalidone Ⓖ
see ℞ **chlorthalidone**.

chlortetracycline Ⓖ
Type/Group: **tetracycline; antibiotic; antibacterial.**
Brand(s): Aureomycin.
How administered: Topically (external).

Used to treat
Chlortetracycline is a broad-spectrum antibiotic used to treat ✪ **acne.**

Warnings
• It should not be given to people with known hypersensitivity to tetracyclines or any component of the product.
• It should be given with caution to people with kidney or liver function impairment, as significant absorption through the skin may result from prolonged use.
• It should be used in pregnancy only if it is clearly needed and if the benefits outweigh the possible risk to the fetus.
• Medical judgment is required if breast-feeding is being considered.
• It is considered safe in topical (external) use.

Interactions
No significant interactions have been reported.

Side effects
Systemic effects are unlikely and there are no significant topical side effects, except on prolonged use.

chlorthalidone Ⓖ
(chlortalidone)
Type/Group: **diuretic; thiazide; antihypertensive.**
Brand(s): Hygroton; Thalitone; various generic. Combinations: With *atenolol*: Tenoretic; various generic. With *clonidine*: Combipres.
How administered: Orally.

Used to treat
Chlorthalidone is used in the treatment of ✪ **hypertension**, either alone or along with other types of diuretic or other drugs (for example, ℞ **beta-blockers**). It can also be used in the treatment of edema. Thiazide diuretics have also become a major part of the treatment for nephrogenic ✪ **diabetes insipidus.**

Warnings
• It should not be given to people with known hypersensitivity to thiazides (or to ℞ **sulfonamide**-derived drugs), or severe kidney or liver disorders.
• It should be given with caution to elderly people, or anyone with high cholesterol or triglyceride levels, or liver or kidney impairment.
• It should be used in pregnancy only when the potential benefit outweighs the possible risk to the fetus.
• Medical judgment is required if breast-feeding is being considered.
• Early symptoms of electrolyte imbalance may include muscle weakness or cramps, nausea, vomiting, restlessness or lethargy, dry mouth, excessive thirst, fast pulse, or dizziness. A doctor must be contacted if such symptoms occur.
• Thiazides may aggravate symptoms of diabetes or gout, and worsen or activate lupus erythematosus.
• Periodic monitoring of electrolytes (particularly potassium, sodium, chloride, and bicarbonate) is needed.

• Photosensitivity may develop and so precautions such as protective clothing or sunscreens should be used.
• Thiazides interact with a number of drugs, including some over-the-counter preparations. A doctor must be contacted before taking any other medications (including OTCs, herbal remedies, and supplements).

Interactions

• There is a higher risk of a hypersensitivity reaction to ℞ **allopurinol**.
• The effects of ℞ **anesthetics**, ℞ **anticancer** drugs, other antihypertensives, ℞ **diazoxide**, ⚘ **calcium** salts, ℞ **cardiac glycosides**, ℞ **lithium**, loop diuretics, ℞ **methyldopa**, nondepolarizing ℞ **skeletal muscle relaxants**, and ⚘ **vitamin D** may be increased, with the potential for significant adverse effects or toxicity. An additive effect is sometimes used to advantage in combining thiazides with other antihypertensives.
• The effects of ℞ **anticoagulants** and antigout agents (for example, ℞ **probenecid**, ℞ **sulfinpyrazone**) may be lowered by thiazides.
• The doses of ℞ **insulin** and ℞ **sulfonylureas** may need to be adjusted, as thiazides may increase blood sugar levels.
• ℞ **Amphotericin B**, ℞ **anticholinergics**, ℞ **corticosteroids**, ℞ **corticotropin**, and ℞ **MAOIs** may increase the effects of thiazides, with the possibility of significant electrolyte loss, especially potassium.
• ℞ **cholestyramine**, ℞ **colestipol hydrochloride**, ℞ **methenamine**, and ℞ **NSAIDs** (especially ℞ **indomethacin**) may reduce the effectiveness of thiazide diuretics.
• There is an increased possibility of postural hypotension (lowered blood pressure on standing) if taken with alcohol, ℞ **barbiturates**, or ℞ **opioids**.

Side effects

• There may be dizziness, headache, muscle cramps, mild gastrointestinal upsets, postural hypotension, reversible impotence, low blood potassium, sodium, magnesium and chloride, raised blood urea, glucose and lipids, and gout.
• Rarely photosensitivity, blood disorders, skin reactions, and pancreatitis.

Chlor-Trimeton 12 Hour Relief Capsules; 4 Hour Relief Tablet ⓑ

A preparation of ℞ **pseudoephedrine** and ℞ **chlorpheniramine maleate**.
Formulation: Oral tablets, sustained release.
Availability: OTC.
Warnings and side effects: See ℞ **pseudoephedrine**; ℞ **chlorpheniramine maleate**.

Chlor-Trimeton Allergy 4 Hour; 8 Hour; 12 Hour Tablets; 4 Ho ⓑ

A preparation of ℞ **chlorpheniramine maleate**.
Formulation: Oral syrup; tablets, 8 Hour and 12 Hour are time release.
Availability: OTC.
Warnings and side effects: See ℞ **chlorpheniramine maleate**.

chlorzoxazone ⓖ

Type/Group: skeletal muscle relaxant.
Brand(s): Paraflex; Remular-S; Parafon Forte DSC; various generic.
Combinations: With *acetaminophen*: Flexaphen.
How administered: Orally.

Used to treat

Chlorzoxazone can be used along with other treatments (such as rest, physical therapy) for the relief of acute muscle pain.

Warnings

• It should not be used by people with known hypersensitivity to chlorzoxazone.
• It should be given with caution to people with impaired liver function, or a history of drug allergies.
• The effects on the fetus are unknown. It should be used during pregnancy only if the benefits outweigh the potential risks.
• Medical judgment is required if breast-feeding is being considered.
• There is a potential for psychological dependence.
• It may impair the perfomance of skilled tasks, such as driving.
• It may discolor urine.

Interactions

None of significance have been reported.

Side effects

• Dizziness, and drowsiness.
• Infrequently, nausea, anemia, rash and itching, gastrointestinal disturbances, malaise or overstimulation.
• Rarely, gastrointestinal bleeding, allergic reactions, and blood disorders.

Cholac ⓑ

A preparation of ℞ **lactulose**.
Formulation: Oral liquid.
Availability: Prescription only.
Warnings and side effects: See ℞ **lactulose**.

Cholan-HMB ⓑ

A preparation of ℞ **dehydrocholic acid**.
Formulation: Oral tablets.
Availability: OTC.
Warnings and side effects: See ℞ **dehydrocholic acid**.

cholestyramine ⓖ

(colestyramine)
Type/Group: lipid-regulating drug.
Brand(s): Questran; Prevalite.
How administered: Orally.

Used to treat

Cholestyramine is a resin that binds bile acids in the gut, and thereby reduces absorption of bile salts from the gut, resulting in changed cholesterol metabolism in the liver. It can be used in the treatment of ⊙ **hyperlipidemia** to reduce the levels, or change the proportions, of various lipids in the bloodstream. Generally, it is given only to people in whom a strict and regular dietary regime alone is not having the desired effect. The drug is also used to relieve pruritus in partial biliary obstruction. Although not stated by the manufacturer for such use, it may also be prescribed to treat diarrhea due to bile acid and digitalis toxicity.

Warnings
• It should not be given to people with known hypersensitivity to cholestyramine or with complete biliary obstruction.
• It should be given with caution to people with gastrointestinal dysfunction, hemorrhoids, bleeding disorders, or osteoporosis.
• Cholestyramine's safety during pregnancy has not been established, but the drug is not absorbed systemically. It may interfere with maternal absorption of fat-soluble vitamins. It should be used only if the potential benefits outweigh the possible risk to the fetus.
• Medical judgment is required if breast-feeding is being considered, because of potential interference with vitamin absorption.
• A doctor must be contacted immediately if bleeding, constipation, or any new symptoms occur.
• Reduction of folic acid levels may occur with long-term use.
• Other medication must be taken one hour before or four hours after cholestyramine.

Interactions
• The levels of ℞ **acetaminophen**, ℞ **amiodarone hydrochloride**, ℞ **corticosteroids**, ℞ **diclofenac**, digitalis glycosides, ℞ **furosemide**, ℞ **methotrexate**, ℞ **metronidazole**, ℞ **thiazide** diuretics, ℞ **thyroid hormones**, and ℞ **valproic acid** may be reduced by cholestyramine.
• The effectiveness of oral ℞ **anticoagulants** may be reduced.

Side effects
• Frequently, constipation (may lead to fecal impaction) and abdominal pain, other gastrointestinal effects (such as nausea).
• Occasionally, headache and dizziness.
• Rarely, gallstones, peptic ulcer, or malabsorption syndrome.

choline salicylate ©
Type/Group: **antipyretic; anti-inflammatory; antirheumatic; non-narcotic analgesic.**
Brand(s): Arthropan Liquid. Combinations: With *magnesium salicylate*: Tricosal Tablets; Trilisate Tablets, Liquid; various generic. How administered: Orally.

Used to treat
Choline salicylate has similar properties to ℞ **aspirin**, although usually with less marked gastrointestinal side effects. It is used to relieve mild to moderate pain and in the treatment of ✪ **osteoarthritis**, ✪ **rheumatoid arthritis**, and related rheumatic conditions. Choline and other ℞ **salicylates** generally do not have aspirin's degree of ℞ **antiplatelet** activity, and so should not be used as an aspirin substitute when aspirin's preventive ℞ **antithrombotic** effects are required.

Warnings
• Avoid its use in people with known hypersensitivity to this drug or to other salicylates (including aspirin), who have chronic kidney disease, certain bleeding disorders or conditions (such as, hemophilia, vitamin K deficiency, low platelet levels), or who have a tendency to, or active, peptic ulceration.

• It should be given with caution to people taking certain drugs for gout or diabetes mellitus, or with allergic disorders (especially asthma and skin conditions), in the elderly, children or teenagers, in those with any kind of kidney impairment, or with certain liver disorders.
• Salicylates can adversely affect the health both of a pregnant woman and the fetus, and so should not be used during pregnancy, and especially not in the third trimester, when risk to the fetus is at its highest.
• Breast-feeding mothers should either discontinue this drug or stop breast-feeding.
• Because of a link between salicylates and the rare, but serious, condition called ✪ **Reye's syndrome** (which causes inflammation of the brain and liver), salicylates should not be given to children or teenagers who have, or might have, chickenpox or influenza. As so many infections resemble flu in their initial symptoms, salicylates should not, as a general rule, be used to treat fever, aches, or malaise by anyone in this age group except on the advice of a doctor.
• Excessive use of salicylates in babies for teething upsets has resulted in poisoning.
• If dizziness, change in hearing, or ringing in the ears (tinnitus) occurs, stop using this drug. These are usually the first symptoms of overdose.
• Salicylates can produce the same allergic-like symptoms (including bronchospasm) that may occur after taking other NSAIDs, including bronchospasm in "aspirin-sensitive" asthmatics.

Interactions
• ℞ **Anticoagulants** have an additive effect in prolonging bleeding time.
• There is generally no added benefit in taking other NSAIDs or other salicylates at the same time, but there is a higher risk of gastrointestinal upsets and bleeding.
• If taken with alcohol, there is an increased risk of bleeding, particularly of an existing ulcer.
• ℞ **Antacids**, ℞ **corticosteroids**, ℞ **urinary alkalinizers**, and ℞ **activated charcoal** may lower the absorption or therapeutic effect of salicylates.
• ℞ **Carbonic-anhydrase inhibitors** (for example, ℞ **acetazolamide**) increase the risk of overdose symptoms for both aspirin and these drugs.
• The effects of the following drugs may be exaggerated: ℞ **phenytoin**; ℞ **nitroglycerin**; ℞ **valproate sodium** (and other valproic acid derivatives); ℞ **methotrexate**.
• Choline taken with ℞ **insulin** or ℞ **sulfonylureas** may cause a greater glucose-lowering effect.
• The therapeutic effects of ℞ **angiotensin-receptor blockers**, ℞ **beta-blockers**, loop ℞ **diuretics**, and ℞ **spironolactone** may be reduced by salicylates.
• ℞ **Uricosuric** agents (used in the treatment of gout, for example, phenylbutazone, ℞ **probenecid**, and ℞ **sulfinpyrazone**) may lose their effectiveness.
• There is a risk of accidental overdose and toxic effects if taken with OTC medications containing salicylates in some form (for example, some ℞ **antacids**).

• Foods high in salicylates, such as curry powder, gherkins, licorice, paprika, prunes, raisins, and tea, may increase the risk of side effects.

Side effects

These vary in severity and frequency.

• The most common are gastrointestinal upsets, nausea, heartburn, diarrhea, and prolonged bleeding time (with consequent risk of ulceration). (The gastrointestinal upsets may be minimized by taking the drug with milk or food.)

• There may be hypersensitivity reactions, including hives, rash, bronchospasm, edema, headache, blood disorders, ringing in the ears, dizziness, and fluid retention.

• Reversible kidney failure, particularly in renal impairment, has occurred. Liver damage is rare.

cholinesterase inhibitor Ⓓ

see ℞ **anticholinesterase**.

Chooz Ⓑ

A preparation of ℞ **calcium carbonate**.
Formulation: Oral tablets, in gum form.
Availability: OTC.
Warnings and side effects: See ℞ **calcium carbonate**.

chorionic gonadotropin Ⓖ

(human chorionic gonadotropin; HCG)
Type/Group: **sex hormone; gonadotropin; infertility treatment**.
Brand(s): A.P.L; Novarel; Pregnyl; Profasi; various generic.
How administered: Injection.

Used to treat

Chorionic gonadotropin is secreted by the chorionic tissue of the placenta, and is obtained from the urine of pregnant women. It can be used in women whose failure to ovulate is not due to primary ovarian failure and who have been pretreated with ℞ **menotropins** or a ℞ **follitropin**. It can also be used for selected cases of hypogonadotropic hypogonadism (caused by subnormal secretion of sex hormones) in males, and to induce testicular descent (usually temporary) in young males.

Warnings

• It should not be used by people with precocious puberty, prostate cancer or other androgen-dependent cancer, prior allergic reactions.

• It should be given with caution to people with epilepsy, migraine, or asthma, or with heart or kidney disease.

• Chorionic gonadotropin should not be used by women who are pregnant.

• Medical judgment is required if breast-feeding is being considered.

• Risk of multiple births is increased by infertility treatment.

Interactions

There are no reported significant interactions attributed to chorionic gonadotropin.

Side effects

• Headache, irritability, edema, restlessness, depression, fatigue, precocious puberty, breast growth in males, pain at injection site,

aggressive behavior, ovarian hyperstimulation (sudden ovarian enlargement), enlargement of pre-existing ovarian cysts and possible rupture, arterial thromboembolism.

• Rarely, ovarian cancer.

Chronulac Ⓑ

A preparation of ℞ **lactulose**.
Formulation: Oral liquid.
Availability: Prescription only.
Warnings and side effects: See ℞ **lactulose**.

Cibalith-S Ⓑ

A preparation of ℞ **lithium**.
Formulation: Syrup.
Availability: Prescription only.
Warnings and side effects: See ℞ **lithium**.

ciclosporin Ⓖ

see ℞ **cyclosporine**.

Cidex; Cidex Plus 28 Ⓑ

A preparation of ℞ **glutaraldehyde**.
Formulation: Solution.
Availability: OTC.
Warnings and side effects: See ℞ **glutaraldehyde**.

cidofovir Ⓖ

Type/Group: **antiviral**.
Brand(s): Vistide.
How administered: Orally; intravenous infusion.

Used to treat

Cidofovir is used in the treatment of cytomegalovirus (CMV) retinitis infections in people with ⊕ **AIDS**. It is always given with the drug ℞ **probenecid** to prolong its action.

Warnings

• It should not be given to people with known hypersensitivity to cidofovir.

• It should be given with caution to people with kidney impairment or diabetes mellitus.

• Cidofovir should be used during pregnancy only when it is clearly needed and when the potential benefits outweigh the possible risks to the the fetus.

• HIV-infected women are advised not to breast-feed.

• There is a serious risk of kidney damage.

• It is a specialist drug, and there will be full assessment and patient monitoring throughout treatment.

Interactions

• ℞ **Aminoglycosides**, ℞ **amphotericin B**, ℞ **foscarnet**, and ℞ **pentamidine** increase the risk and degree of the adverse effects on the kidneys.

Side effects

• Frequently, nausea, vomiting, fever, unusual tiredness, rash, diarrhea, headache, hair loss, chills, loss of appetite, shortness of breath, abdominal pain, and blood-cell disorders.

cilostazol Ⓖ

Type/Group: **antiplatelet**.
Brand(s): Pletal.
How administered: Orally.

Used to treat

Cilostazol is used to prevent ✪ **thrombosis** (blood-clot formation), but does not have an ℞ **anticoagulant** action. It works by stopping platelets sticking to one another or to the walls of blood vessels. It is used to reduce symptoms in intermittent claudication—an atherosclerotic restriction of blood supply to the extremities that usually results in pain, cramps, or tiredness when walking.

Warnings

• It should not be given to people with known hypersensitivity to this drug, or with congestive heart failure of any severity.
• Complete studies have not been done and it should be used during pregnancy only if the potential benefit outweighs the possible risk to the fetus.
• Medical judgment is required if breast-feeding is being considered.
• This drug has effects on heart action and rhythm that are especially undesirable in people with any degree of heart failure. Information is not currently available concerning any effects this drug may have if used by people with severe heart disease.
• Relief of symptoms may occur as soon as 2 to 4 weeks after beginning cilostazol treatment, but it may take longer, up to 12 weeks, before results are seen.

Interactions

• ℞ **azole** antifungals (for example, ℞ **ketoconazole**, ℞ **miconazole**), ℞ **diltiazem hydrochloride**, ℞ **fluoxetine**, ℞ **fluvoxamine**, ℞ **macrolide** antibiotics (for example, ℞ **erythromycin**), ℞ **nefazodone**, ℞ **omeprazole**, and ℞ **sertraline** may increase the levels and effect of cilostazol.
• Grapefruit juice should be avoided, because it may increase levels of this drug.
• Cilostazol should be taken a half hour before or two hours after eating (a high-fat meal can greatly increase absorption and levels of this drug).
• Smoking may decrease the levels and effect of cilostazol.
• The effects of using cilostazol with other antiplatelets (for example, ℞ **clopidogrel**) are unknown.

Side effects

• The most common are headache and gastrointestinal disturbances (for example, diarrhea, abnormal stools, indigestion). Other side effects may include rhinitis, sore throat, swelling of the extremities or infection.
• Less frequently, effects on the heart or blood pressure, changes in kidney or liver function, blood abnormalities, bleeding (particularly of the gastrointestinal tract), and effects on the eyes (blurred vision, conjunctivitis, blindness, retinal bleeding).
• Asthma and hypersensitivity, with facial swelling, fever, rash or hives, has occurred.

Ciloxan Ⓑ

A preparation of ℞ **ciprofloxacin**.
Formulation: Eye drops.

Availability: Prescription only.
Warnings and side effects: See ℞ **ciprofloxacin**.

cimetidine Ⓖ

Type/Group: **H₂-antagonist; ulcer-healing drug**.
Brand(s): Tagamet; Tagamet HB; various generic.
How administered: Orally; injection; infusion.

Used to treat

Cimetidine is used to assist in the treatment of benign ✪ **peptic ulcers** (gastric and duodenal), to relieve heartburn in cases of reflux esophagitis, ✪ **Zollinger-Ellison syndrome**, and a variety of conditions where reduction of acidity is beneficial. It is now also available without prescription (in a limited amount and for short-term uses only) for the relief of heartburn, ✪ **indigestion** and acid indigestion/hyperacidity and sour stomach. It works by reducing the secretion of gastric acid (by acting as a histamine receptor—H₂-receptor—antagonist), so reducing erosion and bleeding from peptic ulcers and allowing them a chance to heal. However, treatment with cimetidine should not be given before full diagnosis of gastric bleeding or serious pain has been carried out, because its action in restricting gastric secretions may possibly mask the presence of other serious disorders such as stomach cancer.

Warnings

• It should not be given to people with known hypersensitivity to this drug.
• It should be given with caution to people with kidney or liver impairment.
• It should be used during pregnancy only if clearly needed.
• It may appear in breast milk and so should be avoided by nursing mothers.
• A doctor must be consulted before using cimetidine over-the-counter if already taking, or planning to take, other medications, particularly nifedipine, phenytoin, theophylline, tricyclic antidepressants, warfarin, or herbal remedies (see Interactions below).
• Although infrequent, confusional states (depression, anxiety, psychosis, hallucinations) have occurred; the risk is highest among those who are severely ill or have existing kidney or liver disease. These conditions clear up within a few days of discontinuing the drug.
• H₂-antagonists, like this one, may mask symptoms of gastric cancer, and this possibility must be eliminated with particular care in persons who have reached middle-age.
• Frequency and severity of side effects is higher in the elderly.

Interactions

• Cimetidine (but not the other available H₂-antagonists) inhibits some enzymes (such as the microsomal oxidative system of the liver), and because of this it can intensify the effects of a number of other drugs. This is of special importance for people stabilized on the drugs ℞ **warfarin sodium**, ℞ **theophylline**, ℞ **tricyclic** antidepressants, ℞ **nifedipine**, and ℞ **phenytoin**. Serious toxic reactions are possible.
• Cimetidine may slow the breakdown of many drugs, including the following: alcohol; ℞ **carbamazepine**; ℞ **carmustine**; ℞ **chlordiazepoxide**; most ℞ **benzodiazepines**; ℞ **caffeine**;

℞ **calcium-channel blockers**; ℞ **flecainide**; ℞ **fluorouracil**; ℞ **labetalol**; ℞ **lidocaine**; ℞ **metoprolol**; ℞ **metronidazole**; ℞ **moricizine**, ℞ **procainamide**; ℞ **propafenone**; ℞ **propranolol**; ℞ **quinidine**; ℞ **quinine**; ℞ **sulfonylureas**; tacrine; ℞ **triamterene**; ℞ **valproic acid**. The levels and effects of these drugs may, therefore, be increased (in some cases with potential for toxicity) and adjustments of dosage may be necessary.

• ℞ **Narcotic (opioid) analgesics** and ℞ **succinylcholine** increase the risk of reparatory depression.

• The levels and effects of ℞ **digoxin**, iron salts (⚬⚬ **iron** supplements), ℞ **fluconazole**, ℞ **indomethacin**, ℞ **ketoconazole**, ℞ **tetracyclines**, and ℞ **tocainide** may be decreased. (Ketoconazole should be taken at least two hours before cimetidine.)

• ℞ **Antacids**, ℞ **anticholinergics**, and ℞ **metoclopramide** may decrease the absorption of cimetidine, reducing its effects. Doses of antacids and cimetidine should be staggered.

• Cigarette smoking reverses some of the effects of cimetidine, so interfering with ulcer healing.

Side effects

• Infrequently, headache, dizziness, drowsiness, or diarrhea.

• Rarely, pancreatitis, arthralgia (joint pain), hair loss, hypersensitivity reactions (including fever, inflammation of blood vessels, anaphylaxis), blood disorders, seizures, effects on the liver and the heart.

• There have been occasional reports of impotence and the growth of breasts in men.

• Confusional states occur predominantly in those who are severely ill.

cinchocaine Ⓖ

see ℞ **dibucaine**.

cinchona alkaloid Ⓓ

Generics: **quinidine**; **quinine**.

Actions and uses

Cinchona alkaloids are chemically complex substances extracted from the bark of the cinchona tree (also known as Peruvian, Jesuit's bark or Cardinal's bark). The best-known cinchona alkaloid is ℞ **quinine**, which has been used for many centuries to treat fevers and is still sometimes used as an ℞ **antimalarial** in the treatment of certain forms of ⚬ **malaria**. The other main cinchona alkaloid is ℞ **quinidine** (which is chemically similar to quinine, but is its other isomer), which is used as an ℞ **antiarrhythmic** to treat heartbeat irregularities (supraventricular ⚬ **arrhythmias**).

Limitations

Quinine has a bitter taste and is incorporated into certain non-medicinal drinks. People who are sensitive to it or who consume large quantities of "tonic water" may experience one of its more marked side effects, which is tinnitus (a ringing in the ears). Quinidine is rather toxic and is less used than at one time.

cinnamates Ⓖ

Type/Group: **sunscreen**.

Brand(s): Bullfrog Sunblock; Coppertone Shade Sunblock; Coppertone Oil Free; Neutrogena Sunblock Stick; PreSun Ultra; Shade; Vaseline Intensive Care Moisturizing Sunblock.
How administered: Topically (external).

Used to treat

Cinnamates are a class of constituents which include octyl methoxycinnamate; ethylhexyl *p*-methoxycinnamate, and octocrylene. They are effective primarily against the UVB spectrum.

Warnings

None significant.

Interactions

None significant.

Side effects

None significant:

Cinobac Ⓑ

A preparation of ℞ **cinoxacin**.
Formulation: Oral capsules.
Availability: Prescription only.
Warnings and side effects: See ℞ **cinoxacin**.

cinoxacin Ⓖ

Type/Group: **quinolone**; **antibacterial**.
Brand(s): Cinobac.
How administered: Orally.

Used to treat

Cinoxacin is used primarily to treat infections of the urinary tract.

Warnings

• It should not be given to people with known hypersensitivity to cinoxacin or other quinolones, or a history of convulsive disorders.

• It should be given with caution to people over 65, with kidney disease, liver disease, CNS (central nervous system) damage, or severe cerebral arteriosclerosis.

• Cinoxacin's use in pregnancy or while breast-feeding is not recommended. Other quinolones cross the placenta. Some quinolones appear in breast milk and might pose a risk to the infant.

• Seizure and other CNS effects have occurred, usually from overdosage or individual susceptibility to such effects.

• Serious allergic reactions have occurred, and any adverse reactions should be reported to a doctor.

Interactions

• ℞ **Probenecid** increases the effect of cinoxacin.

Side effects

• Frequently, dizziness, headache, and gastrointestinal upsets.

• Occasionally, effects on the eyes, ringing in the ears, light sensitivity, rash, itching, and hives.

Cipro Ⓑ

A preparation of ℞ **ciprofloxacin**.
Formulation: Oral tablets in several strengths; oral suspension; injection.
Availability: Prescription only.
Warnings and side effects: See ℞ **ciprofloxacin**.

Key to symbols: Ⓓ = Drug type/group   Ⓖ = Generic name   Ⓑ = Brand name

ciprofloxacin Ⓖ

Type/Group: **quinolone; antibacterial**.
Brand(s): Cipro; Ciloxan. With *hydrocortisone*: Cipro HC.
How administered: Orally; injection; topically (eye).

Used to treat

Ciprofloxacin is used to treat ✚ **bacterial infections**, especially in people who are allergic to ℞ **penicillin** or whose strain of bacterium is resistant to standard antibiotics. It is active against many Gram-negative bacteria, including *salmonella, Shigella, campylobacter* and, *Neisseria,* and against Gram-positive bacteria including members of the staphylococcus and streptococcal family (for example *Streptococcus pneumoniae* and *Enterococcus faecalis*). It is used to treat infections of the urinary, gastrointestinal and respiratory tracts, and gonorrhea, but usually only when these cases are resistant to more conventional agents. It can also be used topically (externally) for eye infections.

Warnings

• It should not be given to people with known a history of hypersensitivity to ciprofloxacin or other quinolones, or to children under 18, as there is a possibility of damage to joints and cartilage in growing children.
• It should be given with caution to people over 65, with kidney disease, liver disease, CNS (central nervous system) damage, or severe cerebral arteriosclerosis.
• It should be avoided during pregnancy or while breast-feeding if possible. Ciprofloxacin appears in breast milk at relatively high concentrations and could harm the infant. Allow 48 hours from last dose before resuming breast-feeding.
• Superinfections due to the altered bacterial balance caused by antibiotic treatment may occur. A doctor must be contacted if there is severe abdominal pain, or moderate to severe diarrhea.
• Adequate fluid intake should be maintained.
• Rare, but serious, side effects of quinolones include seizure and other CNS effects, and severe, occasionally fatal, allergic reactions.
• Photosensitivity reactions (abnormal sensitivity to light) have occurred, and so excessive exposure to sun or ultraviolet light must be avoided.
• Dairy products, zinc, magnesium, and iron reduce the absorption or effects of ciprofloxacin and so should be avoided (including supplements).

Interactions

• ℞ **Antacids,** ♨ **calcium,** ℞ **didanosine (ddI),** ♨ **iron** preparations, ♨ **magnesium,** ℞ **sodium bicarbonate**, and ♨ **zinc** reduce the effects of ciprofloxacin and should not be taken within 4 hours (before or after) of a dose.
• The levels of ℞ **theophylline,** antipyrine, ℞ **caffeine,** ℞ **diazepam,** ℞ **metoprolol,** ℞ **pentoxifylline,** ℞ **phenytoin,** ℞ **propranolol,** ℞ **ropinirole,** ℞ **xanthine,** and ℞ **warfarin sodium** may be increased.
• The effects of oral ℞ **anticoagulants** may be increased.
• If used with ℞ **foscarnet**, the risk of seizure is increased.

Side effects

• Systemic use: Frequently, gastrointestinal upsets, confusion, and crystalluria (mineral crystals in urine). Occasionally, abdominal pain, headache, and rash. Rarely, dizziness, confusion, tremors, hallucinations, insomnia, dry mouth, tingling sensations, and effects on the heart.
• Topical use: Frequently, burning and crusting in the corner of the eye. Occasionally, bad taste in the mouth, a sense of something in the eye, redness of eyelids, and eyelid itching.

Cipro HC Ⓑ

A preparation of ℞ **hydrocortisone** and ℞ **ciprofloxacin**.
Formulation: Ear drops.
Availability: Prescription only.
Warnings and side effects: See ℞ **hydrocortisone**; ℞ **ciprofloxacin.**

cisatracurium Ⓖ

Type/Group: **skeletal muscle relaxant**.
Brand(s): Nimbex.
How administered: Injection.

Used to treat

Cisatracurium is a nondepolarizing skeletal muscle relaxant (and is a form of atracurium) used to induce muscle paralysis (of medium duration) during surgery.

Warnings

• It should not be used by people with known hypersensitivity to this drug.
• It should be given with caution to people with certain heart and neuromuscular diseases, or with kidney, liver, or lung disorders.
• This drug is for administration only by trained personnel in hospitals. Individual patients will be fully assessed for suitability prior to use.
• It should be used during pregnancy only if the benefits outweigh the risks to the fetus.
• Medical judgment is required if breast-feeding is being considered.

Interactions

• This drug is for administration only by trained personnel in hospitals. An individual patient's current and future therapy regimes will be fully assessed in order to avoid potential drug interactions.

Side effects

• Rarely, hypotension, bradycardia, flushing, and spasm of the bronchi.

cisplatin Ⓖ

Type/Group: **anticancer; cytotoxic**.
Brand(s): Platinol-AQ; generic.
How administered: Injection.

Used to treat

Cisplatin is a (platinum compound) cytotoxic drug (an organic complex of platinum) that works by damaging the DNA of replicating cells and so can be used in the treatment of certain solid tumors, including ovarian ✚ **cancer** and testicular teratoma, and advanced bladder cancer.

Warnings

• It should not be given to people with a known history of severe allergic reaction to cisplatin or other platinum compounds, or with

Key to symbols: ✚ = Disorder Section ℞ = Drug Section ♣ = Herbal Section ♨ = Supplement Section

bone marrow depression, kidney impairment, or hearing impairment.

• It should be given with caution to people who have had previous treatment with other anticancer agents. This is a specialist drug which will be used following a full evaluation by specialist physicians.

• Cisplatin is not recommended for use during pregnancy unless it is medically judged to be essential, because it may cause birth defects. Becoming pregnant while using this drug must be avoided.

• It should not be used if breast-feeding.

• It can produce severely depressed bone marrow function.

• Adverse effects on the kidneys may occur.

• Ear damage (ringing, loss of high frequency hearing, occasionally deafness) is a potential adverse effect, which may be more likely in children.

• Severe allergic reactions have occurred.

• In common with many anticancer drugs, cisplatin may cause cancer or genetic mutations in cells.

• Severe neurologic effects can occur, but rarely at usual doses.

• Effects on the eyes, largely reversible by drug discontinuation, have occurred.

Interactions

• If taken with ℞ **aminoglycosides** there is an increased risk of kidney damage.

• The effects of ℞ **phenytoin** may be reduced.

• Loop ℞ **diuretics** increase the risk of adverse effects on ears.

Side effects

• Frequently, nausea, vomiting, and bone marrow depression.

• Occasionally, numbness, tingling of fingers, toes or face, pain or redness at injection site, loss of taste or appetite.

• Rarely, hemolytic (destruction of red blood cells) anemia, blurred vision, inflamed mouth mucosa.

citalopram Ⓖ

Type/Group: **antidepressant; SSRI.**
Brand(s): Celexa.
How administered: Orally.

Used to treat

Citalopram is used to treat ✪ **depression** and has the advantage over some earlier antidepressants because it has relatively less sedative and ℞ **anticholinergic** side effects. Although not stated by the manufacturer for such treatment, it is sometimes used for panic disorder, ✪ **obsessive-compulsive disorder**, post-stroke emotional lability, premenstrual dysphoric syndrome, alcohol abuse, and ✪ **dementia**. It may take some weeks to reach full effect and the decline of its effects after ending treatment is also slow. As is the case with other antidepressants, this drug is also being evaluated for other uses.

Warnings

• It should not be given to people with known hypersensitivity to this type of drug or to anyone taking a ℞ **MAOI** antidepressant (see Interactions below).

• It should be given with caution to people with liver or severe kidney impairment, cardiovascular disease, seizure disorder,

diabetes mellitus, psychosis, or bipolar disorder (manic-depressive illness), as well as to anyone receiving electroconvulsive therapy.

• Citalopram should be used during pregnancy only if the benefits outweigh the the possible risk to the fetus.

• Medical judgment is required if breast-feeding is being considered.

• A doctor must be consulted before taking any other medication, including OTC preparations, herbal remedies (especially ♣ **St. John's wort**), supplements (for example the ⚭ **amino acids** tryptophan and tyramine), or any other natural or alternative products.

• Avoid or minimize alcohol consumption.

• Judgment, thinking, and physical skills may be impaired, so use caution when first taking the drug.

• It may cause sensitivity to sunlight.

• Treatment should be stopped gradually, lowering the dose over a period of time.

• It may be 5 to 6 weeks before there are any signs of improvement.

Interactions

• Serious and even fatal reactions have occurred when ℞ **MAOI** antidepressants are taken with other antidepressants. There should be at least a 14-day gap between discontinuing one and starting the other.

• ℞ **buspirone** and ℞ **sibutramine** increase the risk of adverse effects due to excessive serotonin.

• The levels of ℞ **imipramine** and other ℞ **tricyclics**, and ℞ **metoprolol** may be increased.

• ℞ **cimetidine** may increase the effect of citalopram.

• If used with certain ℞ **antimigraine** medications (for example, ℞ **naratriptan**, ℞ **sumatriptan**), there is an increased risk of weakness and incoordination.

Side effects

• Headache/migraine, effects on taste and smell, difficulty in concentration and memory loss, speeding of the heart, changes in weight, cough, nausea, vomiting, sleepiness, tingling in the extremities, loss of emotion, gastrointestinal symptoms, dry mouth, change in sense of taste, frequent or painful urination, abnormal ejaculation.

• Less frequently, insomnia, confusion, restlessness, hypotension, postural hypotension (lowered blood pressure on standing), palpitations, muscle pain, changes in appetite, lack of menstruation, sweating, and rash.

• Rare but serious side effects include seizures.

Citanest Plain Ⓑ

A preparation of ℞ **prilocaine hydrochloride**.
Formulation: Injection.
Availability: Prescription only.
Warnings and side effects: See ℞ **prilocaine hydrochloride**.

citrates Ⓖ

(citric acid; potassium citrate; sodium citrate)
Type/Group: **urinary alkalinizer; electrolyte; antigout.**
Brand(s): Bicitra; Cytra-2; Cytra-3; Citra-K; Cytra-LC; Oracit; Polycitra.

How administered: Orally.

Used to treat

Citrates make the urine alkaline instead of acid, which is an action that is useful for relieving pain in some infections of the urinary tract or the bladder (see ✪ **urinary tract disorders**), in the treatment of ✪ **gout** and to treat chronic metabolic ✪ **acidosis**, such as that caused by renal tubular acidosis.

Warnings

• It should not be given to people with severe kidney impairment along with certain urinary disorders, untreated Addison's disease, acute dehydration, heat cramps, hereditary episodic muscular weakness, severe myocardial damage, or hypokalemia (low levels of blood potassium).

• It should be given with caution to people with heart disease or impaired kidney function.

• Citrates should be used during pregnancy only if the potential benefit outweighs the possible risk to the fetus.

• Medical judgment is required if breast-feeding is being considered.

• Dilute with water and take after meals to minimize gastrointestinal effects of potassium salts.

Interactions

• The levels of ℞ **chlorpropamide**, ℞ **lithium**, ℞ **methenamine**, ℞ **methotrexate**, ℞ **salicylates**, and ℞ **tetracyclines** may be reduced.

• The levels of ℞ **anorectics**, ℞ **flecainide**, mecamylamine, ℞ **quinidine**, and ℞ **sympathomimetics** may be increased.

Side effects

• Occasionally, gastrointestinal effects, weakness, listlessness, mental confusion, and tingling of the extremities.

• Rarely, metabolic alkalosis, hyperkalemia (high levels of blood potassium), and hypernatremia (high levels of blood sodium).

citric acid   Ⓖ

see ℞ **citrates**.

Citrucel; Citrucel Sugar Free   Ⓑ

A preparation of ℞ **methylcellulose**.
Formulation: Oral powder.
Availability: OTC.
Warnings and side effects: See ℞ **methylcellulose**. The sugar-free powder contains the sweetner aspartame (with phenylalanine), which should be avoided by individuals with phenylketonuria.

cladribine   Ⓖ

Type/Group: **anticancer; cytotoxic**.
Brand(s): Leustatin.
How administered: Intravenous infusion.

Used to treat

Cladribine is a cytotoxic drug (an antimetabolite) that is used for hairy cell ✪ **leukemia**, and, although not stated by the manufacturer for such use, may be prescribed for chronic lymphocytic leukemia in some people.

Warnings

• It should not be given to people with known hypersensitivity to cladribine.

• It should be given with caution to people with impaired kidney function or liver insufficiency, or pre-existing bone marrow suppression. This is a specialist drug which will be used following a full evaluation by specialist physicians.

• Cladribine is not recommended for use during pregnancy unless it is medically judged to be essential, because it may cause birth defects. Becoming pregnant while using this drug must be avoided.

• It should not be used if breast-feeding.

• It can cause bone marrow depression, which may lead to bleeding and a reduced resistance to infection.

• High doses may produce acute adverse effects on the kidneys or nervous system.

• In common with many anticancer drugs, cladribine might cause genetic mutations in cells or impair fertility.

• Some people have experienced high fever which may have been associated with infection.

Interactions

No interactions specific to this drug are known.

Side effects

• Frequently, fever, injection site reactions, fatigue, headache, rash, gastrointestinal disturbance, and marked decrease in bone marrow cells.

• Occasionally, local bleeding under the skin, abnormal breath or chest sounds, chills, weakness, insomnia, peripheral edema, cough, and sweating.

Claforan   Ⓑ

A preparation of ℞ **cefotaxime**.
Formulation: Injection.
Availability: Prescription only.
Warnings and side effects: See ℞ **cefotaxime**.

clarithromycin   Ⓖ

Type/Group: **macrolide, antibiotic, antibacterial, Helicobacter pylori eradication regime**.
Brand(s): Biaxin.
How administered: Orally.

Used to treat

Clarithromycin is a derivative of ℞ **erythromycin**, and is usually given to people who are allergic to penicillin. It can be used to treat ✪ **bacterial infections**, including skin, soft tissue and respiratory tract infections, otitis media infections (see ✪ **otitis**), and for *Helicobacter pylori* infection (see ℞ **Helicobacter pylori eradication regimes**). It may also be given to prevent and treat disseminated (throughout the body) mycobacterial infections in advanced ✪ **HIV** infection.

Warnings

• It should not be given to people with known hypersensitivity to any of the macrolide antibiotics.

• It should be given with caution to people with kidney or liver dysfunction, and to children.

• Clarithromycin should be used during pregnancy only if there are no alternatives.

• Medical judgment is required if breast-feeding is being considered. It is unknown whether this drug appears in breast milk.

• Superinfections due to the altered bacterial balance created by the use of antibiotics may occur. A doctor must be contacted if there is severe abdominal pain, moderate to severe diarrhea, or any new or unusual symptoms.

• Alcohol must be avoided because it reduces the levels of clarithromycin.

Interactions

• Clarithromycin must not be used with astemizole, ℞ **fexofenadine**, cisapride, or ℞ **pimozide** because of the risk of serious heart-rate disorders.

• There is the possibility of ergotism if used with ℞ **ergotamine**.

• The effects of ℞ **alfentanil**, ℞ **atorvastatin**, ℞ **bromocriptine**, ℞ **buspirone**, ℞ **carbamazepine**, ℞ **clozapine**, ℞ **colchicine**, ℞ **cyclosporine**, ℞ **diazepam**, ℞ **digoxin**, ℞ **disopyramide**, ℞ **felodipine**, ℞ **itraconazole**, ℞ **lovastatin**, ℞ **methylprednisolone**, ℞ **midazolam**, ℞ **quinidine**, ℞ **sildenafil**, ℞ **simvastatin**, ℞ **tacrolimus**, ℞ **theophylline**, ℞ **triazolam**, ℞ **valproic acid**, ℞ **warfarin sodium**, and zopiclone may be increased.

• The levels of ℞ **amprenavir**, ℞ **indinavir**, ℞ **nelfinavir**, ℞ **ritonavir**, and ℞ **saquinavir**, and of clarithromycin, may be increased.

• The effects of ℞ **penicillin** and ℞ **zafirlukast** may be decreased.

Side effects

• Frequently, gastrointestinal upsets (diarrhea, nausea, indigestion, abdominal discomfort), altered taste, and rash.

• Occasionally, headache.

• Rarely, allergic reaction or liver damage.

Claritin-D 24-hour Tablets ®

A preparation of ℞ **pseudoephedrine** and ℞ **loratadine**.
Formulation: Oral tablets.
Availability: Prescription only.
Warnings and side effects: See ℞ **pseudoephedrine**; ℞ **loratadine**.

Claritin Tablets; Reditabs; Syrup ®

A preparation of ℞ **loratadine**.
Formulation: Oral syrup; tablets; Reditabs are placed on the tongue and dissolve rapidly.
Availability: Prescription only.
Warnings and side effects: See ℞ **loratadine**.

clavulanic acid Ⓖ

(potassium clavulanate)
Type/Group: penicillinase inhibitor.
Brand(s): Combinations: With *amoxicillin*: Augmentin. With *ticarcillin*: Timentin.
How administered: Orally; injection.

Used to treat

Clavulanic acid is used to combat bacterial resistance to ℞ **penicillin**. It works as an enzyme inhibitor by inhibiting the penicillinase enzymes ("beta-lactamases") that are produced by some bacteria. These enzymes can inactivate many antibiotics of the penicillin family. It is only used in combination with penicillins.

Warnings

There are no contraindications for clavulanic acid.
There is no information on the effects of clavulanic acid in pregnancy or breast-feeding.

Interactions

There are no reported interactions.

Side effects

• Side effects from the combination are attributed to penicillin.

• Some liver disorders are more common with ℞ **amoxicillin** when combined with clavulanic acid, than when taken alone.

Clearasil Clearstick Regular Strength ®

Also: **Double Clear Pads Regular Strength**
A preparation of ℞ **salicylic acid** and various.
Formulation: Topical liquid; medicated pad.
Availability: OTC.
Warnings and side effects: See ℞ **salicylic acid**.

Clearasil Daily Face Wash ®

A preparation of ℞ **triclosan**.
Formulation: Topical liquid.
Availability: OTC.
Warnings and side effects: See ℞ **triclosan**.

Clearasil Maximum Strength ®

A preparation of ℞ **benzoyl peroxide**.
Formulation: Topical lotion.
Availability: OTC.
Warnings and side effects: See ℞ **benzoyl peroxide**.

Clearasil Medicated Deep Cleanser ®

Also: **Acne Fighting Pads; Double Textured Pads**
A preparation of ℞ **salicylic acid** and various.
Formulation: Topical liquid; medicated pads.
Availability: OTC.
Warnings and side effects: See ℞ **salicylic acid**.

Clear Eyes; Clear Eyes ACR ®

A preparation of ℞ **naphazoline hydrochloride**.
Formulation: Eye drops.
Availability: OTC.
Warnings and side effects: See ℞ **naphazoline hydrochloride**.

Clear Tussin 30 Liquid ®

A preparation of ℞ **dextromethorphan** and ℞ **guaifenesin**.
Formulation: Oral liquid.
Availability: OTC.
Warnings and side effects: See ℞ **dextromethorphan**; ℞ **guaifenesin**.

clemastine Ⓖ

Type/Group: **antihistamine; antiallergic**.
Brand(s): Tavist Tablets, Syrup.
How administered: Orally.

Used to treat

Clemastine is used for the symptomatic relief of allergic symptoms, such as ✪ **hay fever** (seasonal allergic rhinitis), perennial rhinitis, and ✪ **urticaria**.

Warnings

• It should not be given to people with known hypersensitivity to this drug (or with known sensitivity to other antihistamines).
• Antihistamines should be used given with caution to people with lower respiratory disease or asthma (and never during an attack), heart disease, hypertension, hyperthyroidism, epilepsy, porphyria, increased intraocular pressure (pressure in the eyeball, as in glaucoma), enlarged prostate, urinary retention, or certain obstructive bladder or gastrointestinal conditions, liver or kidney disease.
• Clemastine should be used during pregnancy only if it is clearly needed, but not in the third trimester, as newborns or premature infants may have severe reactions, including convulsions, to antihistamines.
• Nursing mothers should discontinue using this drug or discontinue breast-feeding.
• This drug must not be given to infants, and for children under the age of 12 the manufacturer's or medical instructions must be followed closely.
• Because of its sedative side effects, the performance of skilled tasks, such as driving, may be impaired.
• Side effects are more frequent in the elderly.

Interactions

• ℞ **MAOI** antidepressants may prolong and intensify the ℞ **anticholinergic** effects of antihistamines (see Side effects below).
• If used with ℞ **tricyclic** antidepressants, other antihistamines, ℞ **skeletal muscle relaxants**, ℞ **opioids**, ℞ **barbiturates**, ℞ **hypnotics**, ℞ **sedatives**, or ℞ **antianxiety** drugs, there is a risk of intensified side effects.
• Alcohol may intensify side effects such as drowsiness and impaired mental alertness.

Side effects

• These depend on how it is administered. For this type of antihistamine, there is commonly drowsiness, headache, impaired muscular coordination or dizziness, anticholinergic effects (dry mouth, blurred vision, urinary retention, gastrointestinal disturbances), occasional rashes and photosensitivity (abnormal sensitivity to light), palpitations and heart arrhythmias.
• Rarely, there may be stimulation instead of sedation (paradoxical stimulation), especially in children (and convulsions in overdose), hypersensitivity reactions, blood disorders, liver disturbances, depression, sleep disturbances, and hypotension.

Cleocin; Cleocin Pediatric Ⓑ

A preparation of ℞ **clindamycin**.

Formulation: Oral capsules in several strengths; oral solution (Pediatric); injection; vaginal cream; vaginal suppository.
Availability: Prescription only.
Warnings and side effects: See ℞ **clindamycin**. Some capsules contain tartrazine, which may cause an allergic reaction in susceptible individuals. Although the incidence of allergy is low, it is more frequent in those who are allergic to aspirin.

Cleocin T Ⓑ

A preparation of ℞ **clindamycin**.
Formulation: Topical gel; topical lotion; topical solution.
Availability: Prescription only.
Warnings and side effects: See ℞ **clindamycin**.

Climara Ⓑ

A preparation of ℞ **estradiol**.
Formulation: Transdermal patch in several strengths.
Availability: Prescription only.
Warnings and side effects: See ℞ **estradiol**.

Clinda-Derm Ⓑ

A preparation of ℞ **clindamycin**.
Formulation: Topical solution.
Availability: Prescription only.
Warnings and side effects: See ℞ **clindamycin**.

clindamycin Ⓖ

Type/Group: **antibiotic; antibacterial**.
Brand(s): Cleocin; Cleocin T; Clinda-Derm; Clindets; C/T/S; various generic.
How administered: Orally; intravenous infusion; intravaginal; topically (external).

Used to treat

Clindamycin is used to treat ✪ **bacterial infections** of bones and joints, ✪ **peritonitis** (inflammation of the peritoneal lining of the abdominal cavity), serious respiratory tract infections, ✪ **septicemia**, and infections of the female pelvis and genital tract. It is active against many anaerobic bacteria (including *Bacteroides fragilis*) and Gram-positive cocci (including penicillin-resistant Staphylococci). It can also be used to treat ✪ **acne** and vaginal infections. It is not widely used systemically because of its serious side effects.

Warnings

• It should not be given to people with known hypersensitivity to clindamycin or lincomycin.
• It should be given with caution to people with a history of gastrointestinal disease, severe kidney or liver disease, allergy, and anyone over 65.
• It should be used during pregnancy only if clearly needed and if the potential benefits outweigh the risks to the fetus.
• It can be used when breast-feeding, but it appears in breast milk and so medical judgment is required.
• It can cause severe and possibly fatal colitis, characterized by severe persistent diarrhea, severe abdominal cramps, and possibly the passage of blood and mucus. Any such symptoms must be reported to a doctor.

• When used to treat vaginal infections, intercourse should be avoided during treatments.

• The use of antibiotics may result in superinfection from nonsusceptible organisms, especially yeasts.

• Diet foods containing sodium cyclamate may decrease the effect of clindamycin.

Interactions

• Adsorbent ℞ **antidiarrheals** (for example, ℞ **kaolin**-pectin) may delay absorption.

• ℞ **chloramphenicol** and ℞ **erythromycin** may reduce the effects of clindamycin.

Side effects

• Systemic: Frequently, gastrointestinal upset. Occasionally, abscess at injection site when used intravenously. Rare but serious effects are blood disorders, kidney damage, and hypotension.

• Vaginal: Headache, dizziness, gastrointestinal upset, and, rarely, allergic reaction.

• Topical: Rash, abdominal pain, mild diarrhea, stinging or burning.

Clindets ⑧

A preparation of ℞ **clindamycin**.
Formulation: Topical solution (swab).
Availability: Prescription only.
Warnings and side effects: See ℞ **clindamycin**.

Clinoril ⑧

A preparation of ℞ **sulindac**.
Formulation: Oral tablets, available in two strengths.
Availability: Prescription only.
Warnings and side effects: See ℞ **sulindac**.

clioquinol ⑥

(iodochlorhydroxyquin)
Type/Group: **antifungal; antimicrobial**.
Brand(s): Generic only. Combinations: With hydrocortisone: Ala-Quin; Corque; Hysone; Pedi-Cort V; Zone-A-Forte. With *hydrocortisone* and *pramoxine*: 1 + 1-F Creme.
How administered: Topically (external).

Used to treat

Clioquinol is chemically an iodine-containing member of the 8-hydroxyquinoline group. Its primary use is for ✪ **eczema**, ✪ **athlete's foot**, and other ✪ **fungal infections**.

Warnings

• It should not be given to people with known sensitivity to clioquinol, or very young children.

• It is not known whether clioquinol harms the fetus. It should be used during pregnancy only if clearly needed.

• Medical judgment is required if breast-feeding is being considered. It is not known if the drug appears in breast milk.

• Systemic absorption can lead to serious nerve damage.

• It must not be used for diaper rash.

• Bandages must not be placed over the treated area unless directed by a doctor.

Interactions

No significant interactions have been reported.

Side effects

• Burning, rash, redness, itching, staining of hair and skin, and hives.

clobetasol propionate ⑥

Type/Group: **corticosteroid; anti-inflammatory**.
Brand(s): Temovate; Cormax; Embeline E; various generics.
How administered: Topically.

Used to treat

Clobetasol propionate is used to treat severe, non-infective inflammation of the skin caused by conditions such as ✪ **eczema**, ✪ **pruritis**, contact ✪ **dermatitis** and ✪ **psoriasis**, especially in cases where less powerful steroid treatments have failed.

Warnings

• It should not be used by people with known hypersensitivity to corticosteroids, or those with fungal infections.

• It should be given with caution to anyone with bacterial or viral infections, and to children, who may be more susceptible to systemic side effects.

• It must not be applied to the face, groin, or armpits.

• Corticosteroids can cross the placenta. It is unknown whether external application could result in sufficient systemic absorption to create a hazard to the fetus. Clobetasol, therefore, should be used during pregnancy only if it is medically judged that the benefits outweigh potential risk to the fetus.

• Medical judgment is also required if breast-feeding is being considered. When taken internally, corticosteroids are excreted in breast milk and may suppress growth and interfere with the production of natural corticosteroids in the infant. It is unknown whether external application could result in sufficient systemic absorption to produce detectable amounts in breast milk.

• Topical corticosteroids can be absorbed in sufficient amounts to produce systemic effects. Clobetasol, therefore, must not be used over large surface areas or for a prolonged period to minimize the risk of systemic absorption.

• Bandages or dressings must not be placed over the treated area unless directed by a doctor, as this may increase the risk of adverse skin reactions.

• Avoid weeping, denuded, infected areas, and the eyes.

• A doctor must be notified and use of clobetasol stopped if local irritation or fever develops.

Interactions

No significant interactions have been reported.

Side effects

• Occasionally, irritation and itching.

• Rarely, allergic rash, systemic effects are possible (for example, adrenal insufficiency), reversible liver changes, reduced glucose tolerance, and white blood cell disorders.

clocortolone pivalate ⑥

Type/Group: **corticosteroid; anti-inflammatory**.
Brand(s): Cloderm.
How administered: Topically.

Used to treat

Clocortolone pivalate is used in the treatment of severe inflammation of the skin caused by conditions such as ✪ **eczema**, ✪ **pruritis**, ✪ **psoriasis** and contact ✪ **dermatitis**.

Warnings

• It should not be used by people with known hypersensitivity to corticosteroids, or those with fungal infections.

• It should be given with caution to anyone with bacterial or viral infections, and to children, who may be more susceptible to systemic side effects.

• It must not be applied to the face, groin, or armpits.

• Corticosteroids can cross the placenta. It is unknown whether external application could result in sufficient systemic absorption to create a hazard to the fetus. Clocortolone, therefore, should be used during pregnancy only if it is medically judged that the benefits outweigh potential risk to the fetus.

• Medical judgment is also required if breast-feeding is being considered. When taken internally, corticosteroids are excreted in breast milk and may suppress growth and interfere with production of natural corticosteroids in the infant. It is unknown whether external application could result in sufficient systemic absorption to produce detectable amounts in breast milk.

• Topical corticosteroids can be absorbed in sufficient amounts to produce systemic effects. Do not use over large surface areas or for a prolonged period, to minimize risk of systemic absorption.

• Bandages or dressings must not be placed over the treated area unless directed by a doctor, as this may increase the risk of adverse skin reactions.

• Weeping, denuded, or infected areas, and the eyes must be avoided.

• A doctor must be notified and use of clocortolone stopped if local irritation or fever develops.

Interactions

No significant interactions have been reported.

Side effects

• Occasionally, irritation and itching.

• Rarely, allergic rash, systemic effects are possible (for example, adrenal insufficiency), reversible liver changes, reduced glucose tolerance, and white blood cell disorders.

Cloderm ℗

A preparation of ℞ **clocortolone pivalate**.
Formulation: Ointment.
Availability: Prescription only.
Warnings and side effects: See ℞ **clocortolone pivalate**.

clofazimine Ⓖ

Type/Group: **antibacterial**.
Brand(s): Lamprene.
How administered: Orally.

Used to treat

Clofazimine is used in combination with other drugs in the treatment of the major form of ✪ **leprosy**. The fact that the treatment requires multiple drugs is due to the increasing resistance shown by the leprosy bacterium.

Warnings

• It should not be given to people with known hypersensitivity to clofazimine.

• It should be given with caution to people with abdominal pain, diarrhea, or mental depression.

• Clofazimine should be used during pregnancy only if it is clearly needed and if the potential benefits outweigh the possible risks to the fetus.

• Medical judgment is required if breast-feeding is being considered. It does appear in breast milk.

• Severe abdominal symptoms can occur.

• Frequently, it may discolor skin from pink to brownish black (also discolors tears, sweat, sputum, urine, and feces). Some people find the skin discoloration very disturbing. Although it is reversible, it may take some months or years to disappear after treatment has ended.

Interactions

• If at the same time as receiving ℞ **BCG vaccine** (bacillus Calmette-Guérin vaccine), clofazimine may interfere with the development of an immune response.

Side effects

• Scaling, dryness, rash, itching, redness of skin; dizziness, drowsiness, fatigue, burning, irritated eyes, liver disorders, and metabolic changes.

clofibrate Ⓖ

Type/Group: **lipid-regulating drug; fibrate**.
Brand(s): Atromid-S.
How administered: Orally.

Used to treat

Clofibrate is used in ✪ **hyperlipidemia** to reduce the levels, or change the proportions, of various lipids in the bloodstream. Generally, it is given only to people in whom a strict and regular dietary regime alone is not having the desired effect.

Warnings

• It should not be given to people with severe kidney or liver disease, or primary biliary cirrhosis.

• It should be given with caution to people with peptic ulcer.

• It should be used during pregnancy only if the potential benefits outweigh the possible risks to the fetus.

• It should not be used while breast-feeding.

• Rarely, it can cause heart dysrhythmias.

Interactions

• ℞ **Antidiabetics** may enhance the effects of clofibrate.

• If taken with ℞ **furosemide**, the effects of both drugs are enhanced.

• There is an increased risk of adverse effects with ℞ **lovastatin**.

• The effects of oral ℞ **anticoagulants** are increased.

Side effects

• Dizziness, drowsiness, fatigue, gastrointestinal effects, decreased libido, urinary problems, impotence, muscle and joint pain, rash, itching, hives, hair loss, and blood changes.

Clomid ℗

A preparation of ℞ **clomiphene citrate**.

Formulation: Oral tablets.
Availability: Prescription only.
Warnings and side effects: See ℞ **clomiphene citrate.**

clomifene citrate ⓖ

see ℞ **clomiphene citrate.**

clomiphene citrate ⓖ

(clomifene citrate)
Type/Group: antiestrogen; infertility treatment.
Brand(s): Clomid; Milophene; Serophene; various generic.
How administered: Orally.

Used to treat

Clomiphene citrate is a sex hormone antagonist (an antiestrogen) used in women whose infertility is linked to the persistent presence of estrogens and a consequent failure to ovulate (characterized by sparse or infrequent periods). Clomiphene citrate prevents the action of estrogens and this increases secretion of gonadotrophins, which cause ovulation. Although not stated by the manufacturer for such treatment, it may be prescribed for male infertility.

Warnings

• It should not be used by people with ovarian cysts, certain liver disorders, or abnormal uterine bleeding.
• It should be given with caution to women with certain gynecological conditions, high blood pressure, depression, or diabetes mellitus.
• Clomiphene citrate must not be used during pregnancy but note, it is an infertility treatment.
• Medical judgment is required if breast-feeding is being considered.
• The risk of multiple births is increased.
• Prolonged use may increase the risk of ovarian cancer. It is not recommended for use over more than 3 cycles.
• Blurring or other visual symptoms occasionally occur; use caution when driving or operating machinery, particularly in variable lighting conditions.

Interactions

The interactions for clomiphene citrate have not been documented.

Side effects

• Hot flashes, abnormal ovarian enlargement, nausea, vomiting, dizziness and insomnia, breast tenderness, weight gain, rashes, and hair loss.

clomipramine hydrochloride ⓖ

Type/Group: tricyclic.
Brand(s): Anafranil; various generic.
How administered: Orally.

Used to treat

Clomipramine hydrochloride can be used to treat ✪ **obsessive-compulsive disorder** (OCD). Although not stated by the manufacturer for such treatment, it is sometimes used for ✪ **depression,** panic disorder, premenstrual symptoms, or to assist in the treatment aimed at reducing the incidence of catalepsy in narcoleptic patients (those who fall asleep in quiet or monotonous periods: see

✪ **narcolepsy**). As with other drugs in its class, it is also being evaluated for other uses.

Warnings

• It should not be given to people with known hypersensitivity to this drug, just recovering from myocardial infarction (heart attack), or anyone taking or stopped taking ℞ **MAOI** antidepressants within the previous 14 days.
• It should be given with caution to people with a history of seizures, urinary retention, elevated intraocular pressure (pressure in the eyeball), heart or thyroid disease, diabetes mellitus, angle-closure glaucoma, or kidney or liver disease.
• Clomipramine should be used during pregnancy only if the benefits outweigh the possible risk to the fetus.
• It should not be used by nursing mothers.
• Other symptoms of a psychiatric illnesses may worsen.
• Episodes of mania or hypomania may occur, especially in people with bipolar disorder (manic depression).
• Exposure to sunlight should be minimized because of possible photosensitization (sensitivity to light).
• Treatment should be stopped gradually by lowering the dose over a period of time.
• It is not generally given to children under the age of 10.
• It may be two to three weeks before there are any signs of improvement.
• It may impair the performance of skilled tasks, such as driving.
• Alcohol, grapefruit juice, and smoking can all affect tricyclics (see Interactions below).

Interactions

• Serious or even fatal reactions can occur if ℞ **MAOI** antidepressants are taken at the same time as tricyclics.
• The effects of ℞ **epinephrine,** ℞ **norepinephrine,** and ℞ **phenylephrine** on blood pressure are intensified.
• Grapefruit juice increases the levels of tricyclics.
• ℞ **clonidine hydrochloride** should not be used with tricyclics, because a dangerous increase in blood pressure and hypertensive crisis is possible.
• The effects of ℞ **guanethidine monosulfate,** ℞ **levodopa,** and ℞ **sympathomimetics** may be reduced by tricyclics.
• The effects of ℞ **anticholinergics,** dicumarol, ℞ **quinolones,** grepafloxacin, and sparfloxacin may be enhanced by tricyclics.
• ℞ **Barbiturates,** ℞ **activated charcoal,** and rifamycin-related antibiotics may reduce the effectiveness of tricyclics.
• ℞ **Cimetidine,** ℞ **SSRIs,** ℞ **haloperidol,** ℞ **bupropion,** ℞ **valproate sodium** (and other valproic acid derivatives), and histamine ℞ **H_2-antagonists** may increase the levels of tricyclics in the blood.
• The levels of ℞ **carbamazepine** may increase, while blood levels of tricyclics decrease.
• Smoking may affect the metabolism of tricyclics.
• The effects of alcohol may be enhanced.

Side effects

• Although uncommon, there may be a risk of seizure. Sexual dysfunction, particularly among males, has occurred at a high rate among those taking clomipramine. There may be dizziness and headache. Along with other members of this class, it has pronounced ℞ **anticholinergic** side effects, notably drowsiness and difficulty in concentrating, dry mouth, blurred vision, constipation, postural hypotension (lowered blood pressure on standing) and urinary retention. It may also cause weight gain.

Clomycin ⑧

A preparation of ℞ **neomycin**, ℞ **polymyxin B sulfate**, ℞ **bacitracin**, and ℞ **lidocaine**.
Formulation: Topical ointment.
Availability: OTC.
Warnings and side effects: See ℞ neomycin; ℞ polymyxin B sulfate; ℞ bacitracin; ℞ lidocaine.

clonazepam ⑥

Type/Group: anticonvulsant; antianxiety; benzodiazepine; antiepileptic.
Brand(s): Klonopin; various generic.
How administered: Orally.
Used to treat
Clonazepam is used for treatment of certain seizure and panic disorders. Although not stated by the manufacturer for such use, it may be prescribed for ○ **anxiety**, restless legs, Parkinsonian slurred speech, multifocal tic disorders, acute manic episodes in people with ○ **bipolar disorder**, certain neurological pain syndromes, and as an additional treatment in the management of ○ **schizophrenia**.
Warnings
• It should not be given to people with known hypersensitivity to benzodiazepines, or with narrow-angle glaucoma or severe liver disease.
• It should be given with caution to people with chronic obstructive pulmonary disease (COPD), impaired kidney function, status epilepticus, or who are over 65.
• Clonazepam is not recommended for use during pregnancy. Its use in the first trimester should almost always be avoided. A doctor must be contacted if pregnancy occurs while this drug is being taken.
• Medical judgment is required if breast-feeding is being considered.
• It may cause drowsiness and so impair the performance of skilled tasks such as driving.
• Avoid alcohol, because side effects may be increased (see Side effects below).
• Avoid other psychotropic medications unless prescribed by a doctor.
• A doctor must be consulted before discontinuing use or increasing dosage, because benzodiazepines may produce psychological and physical dependence and withdrawal symptoms.
Interactions
• ℞ **disulfiram** may increase the levels of clonazepam.
• If used with valproic acid, the occurrence of absence seizures may increase.
• If used with alcohol, side effects may be increased.

Side effects
• Commonly, drowsiness. Other effects include unsteadiness and incoordination, headache, insomnia, slurred speech, suicidal tendencies, tremor, hypotension, changes in heartbeat such as palpitations, eye abnormalities, gastrointestinal effects, changes in appetite, urinary problems, congestion, shortness of breath, respiratory depression, rash, sore gums, and dry mouth.
• Rare but serious side effects include blood cell disorders.

clonidine hydrochloride ⑥

Type/Group: antisympathetic; analgesic; antihypertensive.
Brand(s): Catapres, Catapres-TTS; Duraclon; various generic.
How administered: Orally; transdermal (adsorbed through the skin); injection.
Used to treat
Clonidine decreases the release of norepinephrine (noradrenaline) from sympathetic nerves. Alone, or in combination with ℞ **diuretics** or other antihypertensive drugs, it is used to treat ○ **hypertension**. A separate use, in combination with ℞ **opioids** and taken under specialist conditions, is as an analgesic to treat severe ○ **pain** (for example, in cancer patients). Although not stated by the manufacturer for such treatments, it may be prescribed for a range of therapeutic uses, including prevention of ○ **migraine** attacks, relieving menstrual and menopausal complaints (for example, "hot flashes"), management of diarrhea (for example, in diabetes mellitus), reduction of intraocular pressure (pressure in the eyeball) in open-angle ○ **glaucoma**, treating the symptoms (tics) of Tourette's syndrome, as a temporary aid in drug detoxification, and for acute symptoms (for example, psychosis) in certain mental illnesses. Its effectiveness, however, has not been well established for some of these purposes.
Warnings
• It should not be given to people with known hypersensitivity to this drug.
• It should be given with caution to people with severe heart function insufficiency, conduction disturbances, recent heart attack, cerebrovascular disease, peripheral circulation disorders (for example, Raynaud's disease), mental depression, or impaired kidney function.
• Clonidine should be used during pregnancy only if it is clearly needed.
• Medical judgment is required if breast-feeding is being considered.
• Abruptly discontinuing using this drug or missing regular doses may cause a "rebound" rise in blood pressure.
• Other medications, including OTCs, herbal remedies, supplements, or other alternative remedies, must not be taken without consulting a doctor first.
• When used as an analgesic, it will be prescribed under specialist conditions after a full medical assessment.
• Because of possible sedative side effects, caution is advised for potentially hazardous activities, such as driving, that require mental alertness.

Interactions

• If taken with ℞ **verapamil**, there may be significantly increased effects, with the risk of severe hypotension (lowered blood pressure) and heart effects.

• ℞ **Beta-blockers**, ℞ **calcium-channel blockers**, ℞ **cardiac glycosides**, and ℞ **guanethidine monosulfate** may slow heart rate excessively or cause other heart disturbances.

• There is a general potential for increased or intensified effects if used with alcohol other ℞ **analgesics**, ℞ **anesthetics**, ℞ **barbiturates**, ℞ **benzodiazepines**, ℞ **opioids**, ℞ **phenothiazines**, and ℞ **sedatives**.

• The effectiveness of ℞ **levodopa** may be reduced.

• ℞ **prazosin** and ℞ **tricyclic** antidepressants may reduce the antihypertensive effect of clonidine.

• If used with other antihypertensives and diuretics, the effects of these drugs may be increased. This additive effect is sometimes used to advantage in combination treatments for high blood pressure.

Side effects

• Dry mouth, drowsiness or sedation are fairly common. Other frequent side effects may include dizziness, constipation, headache, fatigue, nausea, vomiting, postural hypotension (lowered blood pressure on standing up, usually causing dizziness), or sexual dysfunction.

• Less frequently, mental changes (for example, restlessness, vivid dreams, anxiety, depression or euphoria, hallucinations), fluid retention, rashes, slow heart rate or poor circulation in the extremities. Some side effects may occur less often when clonidine is used in transdermal form, although there may be various skin reactions (for example, itching and inflammation) where the patch is attached.

• Clonidine used for migraine may cause insomnia and aggravate depression.

clopidogrel ⑥

Type/Group: **antiplatelet**.
Brand(s): Plavix.
How administered: Orally.

Used to treat

Clopidogrel is used to prevent ✪ **thrombosis** (blood-clot formation), but does not have an ℞ **anticoagulant** action. It works by stopping platelets sticking to one another or to the walls of blood vessels. It is used to reduce new blood-clotting complications, such as stroke, in persons with a history of atherosclerotic disease (ischemic stroke, myocardial infarction, or peripheral arterial disease).

Warnings

• It should not be given to people with known hypersensitivity to this drug, or with active bleeding (for example, peptic ulcer, intracranial hemorrhage).

• It should be given with caution to people with any condition or disorder that would make bleeding more likely (for example, injury, surgery) or severe liver impairment.

• Complete studies have not been done and it should be used during pregnancy only if it is clearly needed.

• Medical judgment is required if breast-feeding is being considered. It is not known whether this drug appears in breast milk.

• When using this drug, bleeding takes longer to stop, but unusual bleeding should be reported to a doctor. Also, any doctor or dentist should be advised that clopidogrel is being used before any surgery is performed or any new drug prescribed.

Interactions

• ℞ **fluvastatin**, many ℞ **NSAIDs**, ℞ **phenytoin**, ℞ **tamoxifen**, ℞ **tolbutamide**, and ℞ **torsemide** and other drugs which are broken down in a similar way in the body may have an increased effect. NSAIDs (for example, ℞ **naproxen**) additionally have a greater risk of causing gastrointestinal bleeding.

• If taken with ℞ **warfarin sodium**, clopidogrel prolongs bleeding time, and so the two should be used together with caution.

Side effects

• These are generally no different from those of ℞ **aspirin**, and may include gastrointestinal disturbances (for example, abdominal pain, indigestion, diarrhea, nausea, bleeding), rash and itching, bruising, joint pain, leg cramps, headache, dizziness, upper respiratory infection, and nosebleed.

• Allergic reaction, liver and biliary disorders, and anemia or other blood changes are uncommon. Intracranial bleeding or hemorrhage of wounds, or within the eyes, lungs, and so on, occur no more frequently than with aspirin.

Clopra ⑧

A preparation of ℞ **metoclopramide hydrochloride**.
Formulation: Oral tablets.
Availability: Prescription only.
Warnings and side effects: See ℞ **metoclopramide hydrochloride**.

clorazepate dipotassium ⑥

(dipotassium clorazepate)
Type/Group: **antianxiety; anticonvulsant; benzodiazepine**.
Brand(s): Gen-Xene; Tranxene; various generic.
How administered: Orally.

Used to treat

Chlorazepate is used in the short-term treatment of ✪ **anxiety**, to treat acute alcohol withdrawal, and as adjunctive treatment (additional treatment to enhance effectiveness) for partial seizures.

Warnings

• It should not be given to people with known hypersensitivity to this or similar drugs, or those with narrow-angle glaucoma or psychosis.

• It should be given with caution to people over 65, in a weakened (debilitated) condition, or anyone with liver or kidney disease or a history of drug abuse.

• Clorazepate crosses the placenta and may produce withdrawal symptoms or CNS (central nervous system) depression in newborns. It should be used in pregnancy only if the benefits are medically judged to outweigh the potential of harm to the fetus.

• It is excreted into breast milk and should not be used by breast-feeding mothers.

• Clorazepate dipotassium is a Schedule IV controlled substance.
• Treatment must not be ended abruptly following long-term use.
• It may cause drowsiness or dizziness and so impair the performance of skilled tasks, such as driving.
• It should not be used for everyday stress or for longer than 4 months, because drug dependence could develop.
• Alcohol or other CNS depressants must be avoided.

Interactions
• ℞ **cimetidine** and ℞ **disulfiram** may increase the effects of clorazepate.
• ℞ **rifampin** may reduce the effects of clorazepate.

Side effects
• Frequently, drowsiness.
• Occasionally, dizziness, gastrointestinal disturbance, nervousness, blurred vision, dry mouth, headache, confusion, unsteadiness or incoordination, rash, irritability, slurred speech, and cardiovascular effects.
• Rarely, hyperactivity or nervousness in children, debilitated individuals, and those over 65.

clotrimazole ⑥

Type/Group: **antifungal; antimicrobial; azole**.
Brand(s): Cruex; Desenex; Lotrimin; Mycelex. Combinations: With *betamethasone*: Lotrisone.
How administered: Topically (external); buccal.

Used to treat
Clotrimazole is an azole/imidazole drug that works by interfering with amino acid transport in the invading organisms. It can be used in topical (external) application to treat ✪ **fungal infections** (including *Candida* organisms) of the skin and mucous membranes (especially the vagina, throat, and mouth) and to prevent fungal infection of the mouth and throat in some immunosuppressed people.

Warnings
• It should not be given to people with known sensitivity to clotrimazole.
• It should be given with caution to people with liver disorders and when using the buccal (mouth) form.
• It is unknown whether clotrimazole harms the fetus. It should be used during pregnancy only if clearly needed, and especially vaginal application should be avoided in the first trimester.
• Medical judgment is required if breast-feeding is being considered. It is not known if the drug appears in breast milk.
• Contact with the eyes must be avoided.

Interactions
• The levels of ℞ **cyclosporine** and ℞ **tacrolimus** may be increased.

Side effects
These depend on how it is administered.
• Abdominal cramps, bloating, urinary pain and frequency, blistering, burning, peeling of skin, rash, and hives.
• With buccal topical use, there may be some absorption into the body with consequent systemic drug interactions and side effects.

cloxacillin sodium ⑥

Type/Group: **antibiotic; penicillin; antibacterial**.
How administered: Orally.

Used to treat
Cloxacillin sodium is a semisynthetic penicillinase-resistant penicillin used to treat ✪ **bacterial infections** of the respiratory tract, skin and skin structures, bones and joints.

Warnings
• It should not be used by people with known hypersensitivity to penicillins.
• It should be given with caution to people with allergies to ℞ **cephalosporins** or ℞ **imipenem**, or with impaired kidney function.
• Penicillins cross the placenta and should be used in pregnancy only if medically judged to be needed.
• Cloxacillin should not be used while breast-feeding.
• Serious and occasionally fatal hypersensitivity reactions can occur. A doctor must be contacted if skin rash, itching, hives, severe diarrhea, shortness of breath, black tongue, sore throat, nausea, fever, swollen joints, or any unusual bleeding or bruising occurs.
• Superinfections from the altered bacterial balance created by antibiotic treatment may occur and may result in ✪ **pseudomembranous colitis**. A doctor must be contacted if there is severe abdominal pain, or moderate to severe diarrhea.
• Take on an empty stomach (one hour before or two hours after eating).
• The full course of treatment prescribed must be completed or infection may return.

Interactions
• ℞ **Tetracyclines** may reduce the effectiveness of penicillins.

Side effects
• Frequently, gastrointestinal disturbances (nausea, vomiting, diarrhea), headache, oral or vaginal candidiasis (thrush).
• Occasionally, fever, rash, and itching. Serious possible effects include bone marrow depression.

Cloxapen ⑧

A preparation of ℞ **cloxacillin sodium**.
Formulation: Oral capsules in several strengths.
Availability: Prescription only.
Warnings and side effects: See ℞ **cloxacillin sodium**.

clozapine ⑥

Type/Group: **antipsychotic**.
Brand(s): Clozaril; various generic.
How administered: Orally.

Used to treat
Clozapine is one of a group sometimes termed "atypical" antipsychotics, which can be used for the treatment of ✪ **schizophrenia** in people who do not respond to, or who cannot tolerate, conventional antipsychotic drugs. Because clozapine can cause serious blood disorders, it is used only through a patient management system that requires compliance with safety monitoring procedures, including regular blood counts.

Warnings

• It should not be given to people with known hypersensitivity to clozapine, with certain blood cell disorders, severe CNS (central nervous system) depression, comatose states, narrow-angle glaucoma, or uncontrolled epilepsy.

• It should be given with caution to people with cardiovascular, heart, lung, kidney or liver disease, prostatic enlargement, seizure disorders (epilepsy), or anyone over 65.

• Clozapine should be used during pregnancy only if it is clearly needed.

• It should not be used by nursing mothers.

• There is a risk of developing a potentially life-threatening blood disorder. A doctor must be contacted immediately if any symptoms of infection, such as lethargy, weakness, fever, or sore throat, develop.

• It causes sedation and so the performance of skilled tasks, such as driving, may be impaired.

• The dose must be reduced gradually when discontinuing.

• If used for a long time, tardive dyskinesia (see ℞ **antipsychotics**) occasionally develops.

• Avoid alcohol.

Interactions

• If used with ℞ **fluvoxamine**, there is a marked increase in the levels of clozapine and its side effects.

• ℞ **carbamazepine**, ℞ **phenytoin**, ℞ **primidone**, and ℞ **valproic acid** reduce the effects of clozapine.

• ℞ **cimetidine**, ℞ **clarithromycin**, troleandomycin, and ℞ **erythromycin** increase the effects of clozapine.

• There have been isolated reports of cardiorespiratory collapse when used with ℞ **diazepam**.

• If used with alcohol, there is a risk of increased effects (sedative) with antipsychotics.

Side effects

• Drowsiness dizziness, vertigo, postural hypotension (lowered blood pressure on rising), fainting, speeded heart rate, increased salivation, and seizure.

• Less frequently, agitation, confusion, depression, disturbed sleep, heart or chest pain, heart abnormality, ECG change, blurred vision, speeded heartbeat, changes in blood pressure, abdominal discomfort, loss of appetite, constipation, diarrhea, dry mouth, heartburn, nausea or vomiting, abnormal ejaculation, urinary urgency, frequency, incontinence or retention, rash, fever, and weight gain.

• Rarely, neuroleptic malignant syndrome (a potentially fatal condition characterized by very high fever, muscle rigidity, changes in mental status, and irregular pulse, blood pressure and/ or heart rhythm), seizures, and potentially serious blood cell disorders.

Clozaril ⓑ

A preparation of ℞ **clozapine**.
Formulation: Oral tablets in several strengths.
Availability: Prescription only.
Warnings and side effects: See ℞ **clozapine**.

CNS stimulant ⓓ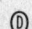

Generics: **caffeine; dextroamphetamine; methamphetamine; methylphenidate; modafinil; phendimetrazine; phentermine.**

Actions and uses

CNS stimulant drugs stimulate the central nervous system (CNS) in various ways. They can be used to treat people suffering from ✪ **narcolepsy**(an extreme tendency to fall asleep when engaged in monotonous activities or when in quiet surroundings), for example, ℞ **modafinil**, ℞ **methylphenidate**, and ℞ **dextroamphetamine**. Some ℞ **sympathomimetic** drugs of this class were once used extensively as ℞ **appetite suppressants** (for example, dextroamphetamine and amphetamine), but there is a tendency for those who use stimulant drugs on a regular basis to become drug-dependant and show a withdrawal syndrome when they stop taking the drug, so such preparations are no longer prescribed for this purpose. However, some amphetamine-related CNS stimulants are sometimes (℞ **methamphetamine**) or generally (℞ **phentermine** and ℞ **phendimetrazine**) prescribed for short-term treatment of ✪ **obesity**.

Some amphetamine-related drugs are also prescribed in the treatment of attention deficit disorder in children (℞ **dextroamphetamine**, ℞ **methamphetamine**, ℞ **methylphenidate**).

℞ **caffeine** and related ℞ **xanthine** compounds are mild stimulants (see ✪ **fatigue**) and for medical purposes ℞ **caffeine** is incorporated into several proprietary OTC (over-the-counter) analgesic preparations and ℞ **cold and cough preparations**.

Limitations

Amphetamines have a very high potential for abuse and they are placed in the Drug Enforcement Agency Schedule II category. Apart from the risk of habituation, there may be long-term personality changes, hypertensive (high blood pressure) crises, and damage to heart valves.

There is growing doubt among experts over the medical value of CNS stimulant drugs in the treatment of obesity, for instance, there may be a weight relapse once that treatment has finished. Taking any CNS stimulants regularly, in combination or in high doses (including herbal remedies) is not advisable. See also the herbal remedies: ♣ **coffee**; ♣ **cola**; ♧ **ginseng**; ♣ **green tea**; ♣ **guarana**; ♣ **maté**; ♣ **ginseng, Siberian**.

coagulation Factor VIIa recombinant; rFVIIa ⓖ

Type/Group: **antihemophilic factor; hemostatic.**
Brand(s): NovoSeven.
How administered: Injection.

Used to treat

Coagulation Factor VIIa is a hemostatic and antihemophilic agent used to treat bleeding episodes in persons with ✪ **hemophilia** A or B with inhibitors to Factor VIII or Factor IX. It is synthesized by recombinant techniques, using no human serum or proteins.

Warnings

• It should not be given to people with known hypersensitivity to mouse, hamster, or bovine proteins. It will be administered by experienced personnel after a full medical assessment.

• It should be given with caution to people with advanced cardiovascular disease, "crush" injuries (that may make thrombosis more likely), or with kidney impairment.

• It should be used during pregnancy only if the potential benefit outweighs the possible risk to the fetus.

• Medical judgment is required if breast-feeding is being considered.

• There is some risk of thrombosis when coagulation factors are used. If signs of thrombosis or intravascular coagulation appear, dosage of Factor VIIa should be reduced or stopped.

• Hypersensitivity symptoms, such as hives, tightness of the chest or wheezing, should be reported to a doctor.

Interactions

• Coagulation factor concentrates (for example, ℞ **Factor IX complex**) are not recommended for combined use with this drug.

Side effects

• There may be fever, bleeding, changes in blood pressure, allergic reaction, slowing of heartbeat, coagulation abnormalities, edema, or headache.

coal tar Ⓖ

Type/Group: **keratolytic; psoriasis treatment; acne treatment**.
Brand(s): Shampoos: Creamy Tar; Denorex; DHS Tar; Doak Tar; Doctar; Duplex T; High Potency Tar; Iocon; Ionil T Plus; MG 217 Medicated Tar; Neutrogena T/Gel; Packer's Pine Tar; Pentrax; Polytar; Protar Protein; Tegrin; Trotar; TVC-2 Dandruff; Zetar. Bath Preparations: Balnetar; Cutar; Doak Tar Oil; Polytar Bath. Other preparations: AquaTar; Doak Tar; Estar; Fototar; Medotar; MG217 Medicated Tar; Neutrogena T/Derm; Oxipor VHC; Packer's Pine Tar; P & S Plus; PsoriGel; Taraphilic; Tegrin for Psoriasis.
How administered: Topically (external).

Used to treat

Coal tar is a black, viscous liquid obtained by the distillation of coal. It is used on the skin to reduce inflammation and itching and also has some keratolytic properties. It is used to treat ✪ **psoriasis** and chronic atopic ✪ **eczema**, and as an ℞ **antiseborrheic** for seborrheic ✪ **dermatitis**, where it is used in solution at a concentration determined by a person's condition and response.

Warnings

• It should not be given to people with known hypersensitivity to coal tar or any component of the products.

• It should be used during pregnancy only if it is clearly needed.

• Medical judgment is required if breast-feeding is being considered. It is not known whether it appears in breast milk.

• Avoid contact with eyes, and acutely inflamed or broken skin.

• Stop using it if irritation develops or if the condition worsens or does not improve after regular use.

• Minimize exposure to sunlight and avoid sunlamps because it may increase tendency to sunburn.

• Do not use for prolonged periods without consulting a doctor.

• It may discolor skin or hair.

Interactions

No significant interactions are known.

Side effects

None significant.

cocaine Ⓖ

Type/Group: **local anesthetic; CNS stimulant; sympathomimetic**.
Brand(s): Generic only.
How administered: Topically (external).

Used to treat

Cocaine can be used as a local anesthetic for topical (external) application for procedures to the ears, nose, and larynx.

Warnings

• It should not be given to people with known hypersensitivity to cocaine.

• It should be given with caution to people with severely traumatized mucous membranes.

• It must not be applied to the eyes.

• Cocaine should be used during pregnancy only when it is clearly needed. It increases the risk of premature delivery, miscarriage, and life-threatening complications.

• Medical judgment is required if breast-feeding is being considered.

• Although it does not produce true physical dependence, cocaine can create a very strong psychological dependence, and its use is limited to supervised and surgical procedures.

• It is a Schedule II controlled substance.

Interactions

• There may be additive effects if used with ℞ **antiarrhythmics** (for example, ℞ **tocainide**, ℞ **mexiletine**).

Side effects

• It can be absorbed systemically (into the body) and cause systemic side effects. Slowed heart rate at small doses, increased heart rate after larger doses. May also be excitatory CNS (central nervous system) reactions (nervousness, restlessness, euphoria, excitement, tremors) followed by CNS depression.

Codehist DH Elixir Ⓑ

A preparation of ℞ **codeine phosphate**, ℞ **pseudoephedrine**, and ℞ **chlorpheniramine maleate**.
Formulation: Oral liquid.
Availability: May or may not require a prescription.
Warnings and side effects: See ℞ **codeine phosphate**; ℞ **pseudoephedrine**; ℞ **chlorpheniramine maleate**.

codeine phosphate Ⓖ

Type/Group: **narcotic analgesic; opioid; antitussive; antidiarrheal**.
Brand(s): Various generic. Combinations (for cold and cough relief): With pseudoephedrine: Nucofed. (Plus) *guaifenesin*: Cycofed Pediatric Syrup; Deconsal Pediatric Syrup; Deproist Expectorant with Codeine Liquid; Guiatussin DAC Syrup; Isoclor Expectorant Liquid; Mytussin DAC Liquid; Novagest Expectorant Liquid; Nucofed Expectorant Syrup; Nucofed Pediatric Expectorant Syrup; Nucotuss Expectorant Codeine Liquid; Nucotuss Pediatric Expectorant Syrup; Phenhist Expectorant Liquid; Robafen DAC Syrup; Robitussin-DAC Syrup; Ryna-CX Liquid. (Plus) *chlorpheniramine*: Codehist DH Elixir; Decohistine DH Liquid; Phenhist DH w/Codeine Liquid; Ryna-C Liquid. (Plus) *triprolidine*:

Actagen-C Cough Syrup; Actifed w/Codeine Cough Syrup; Allerfrin w/Codeine Syrup; Aprodine w/Codeine Syrup; Triafed w/Codeine Syrup. With phenylephrine: (Plus) *chlorpheniramine and potassium iodide*: Pediacof Syrup; Pedituss Cough Syrup. (Plus) *promethazine*: Phenergan VC with Codeine Syrup; Pherazine VC w/Codeine Syrup; Promethist with Codeine Syrup. (Plus) *pyrilamine*: Codimal PH Syrup. With other constituents: With *bromodiphenhydramine*: Ambenyl Cough Syrup; Bromanyl Syrup. With *promethazine*: Phenergan with Codeine Syrup; Pherazine w/Codeine Syrup. With *pyrilamine*: Tricodene Cough & Cold Liquid. With *guaifenesin*: Brontex; Cheracol Cough Syrup; Gani-Tuss NR; Guiatussin w/ Codeine Expectorant Liquid; Halotussin AC; Mytussin AC Cough Syrup; Robitussin A-C Syrup; Romilar AC; Tussi-Organidin-S NR Liquid. With *calcium iodide*: Calcidrine Syrup. Combinations (for pain relief or muscle relaxant): With *aspirin*: Empirin w/Codeine; Fiorinal w/Codeine Capsules. With *acetaminophen*: Aceta w/ Codeine; Capital w/Codeine Suspension; Fioricet w/Codeine Capsules (also butalbital and caffeine); Phenaphen w/Codeine Capsules; Tylenol w/Codeine Elixir; Tylenol w/Codeine Tablets. With *carisoprodol*: Soma Compound w/Codeine. (Most combinations available as generics.

How administered: Orally; injection.

Used to treat

Codeine is a common but often minor constituent of drug brands intended to relieve mild to moderate pain. It is also an antitussive and is used with other drugs (for example ℞ **acetaminophen**, ℞ **guaifenesin**, ℞ **caffeine**) in a number of cough-and-cold preparations. Codeine can also reduce intestinal motility (rhythmic movement of the gut) and so can be used as an ℞ **antidiarrheal** and antimotility treatment. Codeine phosphate tablets (that is, codeine alone without the addition of other constituents) are available only on prescription, and travelers going abroad may require a doctor's letter explaining why they are required.

Warnings

• It should not be given to people with known hypersensitivity to this drug, or to premature infants, or anyone in labor when a premature delivery is expected. Opioids (even the weaker ones) should not be given to people with asthma, with seriously depressed breathing disorders, prostatic hypertrophy, convulsive disorders, raised intracranial pressure, or a head injury.

• Depending on use and dose, they should be given with caution to the elderly, or to anyone with hypotension, certain liver, kidney, or adrenal disorders, hypothyroidism (under-activity of the thyroid gland), alcoholism, or a history of drug abuse.

• Codeine should be used during pregnancy only if it is clearly needed.

• Medical judgment is required if breast-feeding is being considered. Codeine appears in breast milk.

• Prolonged use of narcotics can lead to physical dependence (addiction), although this rarely happens in routine medical use.

• Codeine is a Schedule II controlled substance, but in defined doses in combination with other drugs it may be classed as III or IV.

• Drowsiness may affect the performance of skilled tasks such as driving.

• The effects of alcohol may be enhanced (including a higher risk of respiratory depression).

Interactions

• If used with ℞ **barbiturates**, ℞ **general anesthetics**, ℞ **opioids**, ℞ **tranquilizers** (for example, ℞ **phenothiazines**), ℞ **sedatives**, ℞ **benzodiazepines** (for example, ℞ **diazepam**, ℞ **lorazepam**), alcohol, or ℞ **antihistamines** increased effects are possible.

Side effects

• Depending on use, how it is administered, and dose, there may be dizziness, nausea and vomiting, drowsiness, loss of appetite, urinary retention, and constipation. There is commonly sedation, and occasionally euphoria, which may lead to a state of mental detachment or confusion. Also, there may be sweating, headache, palpitations, changes in heart rate, postural hypotension (a lowering of blood pressure on standing, causing dizziness), rashes, miosis (pupil constriction), dry mouth, flushing of the face, mood change, and hallucinations.

• Tolerance occurs readily, although dependence (addiction) is relatively unusual. Serious adverse effects with the doses of codeine contained in cough-and-cold preparations are relatively rare.

co-dergocrine mesilates ⓖ

see ℞ ergoloid mesylates.

Codiclear DH Syrup ⓑ

A preparation of ℞ **hydrocodone bitartrate** and ℞ **guaifenesin**.
Formulation: Oral syrup.
Availability: Prescription only.
Warnings and side effects: See ℞ **hydrocodone bitartrate**; ℞ **guaifenesin**.

Codimal Capsules; Tablets ⓑ

A preparation of ℞ **pseudoephedrine**, ℞ **acetaminophen**, and ℞ **chlorpheniramine maleate**.
Formulation: Oral tablets; capsules.
Availability: OTC.
Warnings and side effects: See ℞ **pseudoephedrine**; ℞ **acetaminophen**; ℞ **chlorpheniramine maleate**.

Codimal DM Syrup ⓑ

A preparation of ℞ **dextromethorphan**, ℞ **pyrilamine maleate**, and ℞ **phenylephrine hydrochloride**.
Formulation: Oral syrup.
Availability: OTC.
Warnings and side effects: See ℞ **dextromethorphan**; ℞ **pyrilamine maleate**; ℞ **phenylephrine hydrochloride**.

Codimal PH Syrup ⓑ

A preparation of ℞ **codeine phosphate**, ℞ **phenylephrine hydrochloride**, and ℞ **pyrilamine maleate**.
Formulation: Oral syrup.
Availability: May or may not require a prescription.
Warnings and side effects: See ℞ **codeine phosphate**; ℞ **phenylephrine hydrochloride**; ℞ **pyrilamine maleate**.

cod-liver oil ⓖ

Type/Group: **emollient; vitamin.**
Brand(s): Caldesene; Desitin.
How administered: Topically (external).

Used to treat

Cod-liver oil is one of the constituents of some diaper rash treatments and other topical ointments. At one time it was commonly used as a source of ⚐ **vitamin A** and ⚐ **vitamin D**, but now other sources are preferred.

Warnings

None significant.

Interactions

None significant.

Side effects

None significant.

Cogentin ⓑ

A preparation of ℞ **benztropine mesylate.**
Formulation: Oral tablets; injection.
Availability: Prescription only.
Warnings and side effects: See ℞ **benztropine mesylate.**

Co-Gesic Tablets ⓑ

A preparation of ℞ **hydrocodone bitartrate** and ℞ **acetaminophen.**
Formulation: Oral capsules.
Availability: Prescription only.
Warnings and side effects: See ℞ **hydrocodone bitartrate;** ℞ **acetaminophen.**

Cognex ⓑ

A preparation of ℞ **tacrine hydrochloride.**
Formulation: Oral capsules.
Availability: Prescription only.
Warnings and side effects: See ℞ **tacrine hydrochloride.**

Co-Hist Tablets ⓑ

A preparation of ℞ **pseudoephedrine,** ℞ **acetaminophen,** and ℞ **chlorpheniramine maleate.**
Formulation: Oral tablets.
Availability: OTC.
Warnings and side effects: See ℞ **pseudoephedrine;** ℞ **acetaminophen;** ℞ **chlorpheniramine maleate.**

Colace Capsules, Liquid, Syrup ⓑ

A preparation of ℞ **docusate sodium.**
Formulation: Oral capsules (2 strengths); liquid; syrup.
Availability: OTC.
Warnings and side effects: See ℞ **docusate sodium.**

Colace Suppositories ⓑ

A preparation of ℞ **glycerin.**
Formulation: Rectal suppositories.
Availability: OTC.
Warnings and side effects: See ℞ **glycerin.**

Colazal ⓑ

A preparation of ℞ **balsalazide disodium.**
Formulation: Oral capsules.
Availability: Prescription only.
Warnings and side effects: See ℞ **balsalazide disodium.**

colchicine ⓖ

Type/Group: **uricosuric; antigout.**
Brand(s): Generic only. Combinations: With *probenecid*: Proben-C; Colbenemid.
How administered: Orally.

Used to treat

Colchicine is a drug derived from the autumn crocus *Colchicum autumnale* and is used in the treatment of ⚙ **gout,** particularly as a short-term, introductory measure to prevent acute attacks during initial treatment with other drugs (for example, ℞ **allopurinol**) that reduce uric acid levels in the blood.

Warnings

• It should not be given to people with known hypersensitivity to this drug or any of its constituents, or with serious gastrointestinal, kidney, liver, heart, or blood disorders.
• It should be given with caution to people over 65 or in a debilitated condition.
• Colchicine may harm the fetus. It should be used during pregnancy only when the potential benefits outweigh the possible risks to the fetus.
• Medical judgment is required if breast-feeding is being considered. It is not known whether this drug appears in breast milk.
• It may impair fertility in men.

Interactions

• The levels of ℞ **cyclosporine** and ℞ **tacrolimus** may be increased.
• There is a risk of serious toxicity from colchicine if used with ℞ **erythromycin,** ℞ **clarithromycin,** or troleandomycin.

Side effects

• Nausea, vomiting and abdominal pain.
• Rarely, peripheral nerve disorders, loss of hair, or blood disorders. High or excessive dosage may lead to gastrointestinal bleeding and diarrhea, rashes, and liver or kidney damage.

cold and cough preparation ⓓ

Actions and uses

Cold and cough preparations aim to treat the variety of symptoms associated with the common cold, coughs, fever, nasal congestion, catarrh associated with influenza, sore and inflamed throat, and congestion of the upper airways and sinuses. There is a vast range of such products and they are generally available OTC (over-the-counter). The drugs classes incorporated into these remedies are as follows.

Analgesics (painkillers) of the ℞ **non-narcotic analgesic** group which also have ℞ **antipyretic** properties—℞ aspirin, ℞ **acetaminophen,** ℞ **ibuprofen**—are frequently used. They may be combined with low-dose (OTC) forms of ℞ **narcotic analgesic** drugs (including ℞ **codeine phosphate** and ℞ **dextromethorphan**) which also have useful ℞ **antitussive** activity when used for dry cough. Some preparations intended for the relief of a "productive" cough, include an expectorant, usually ℞ **guaifenesin**. It is common to incorporate nasal ℞ **decongestant** drugs in cough and cold preparations taken by mouth and these can be used instead of taking decongestants intranasally. Most decongestants are ℞ **sympathomimetic** agents with a ℞ **vasoconstrictor** action (constrict blood vessels), and work by constricting blood vessels in the mucous membranes of the airways and nasal cavity, so reducing the thickness of this nasal lining, improving drainage, and possibly decreasing mucous and fluid secretions. Some of these drugs are direct acting ℞ **alpha-adrenergic stimulant** agents (including ℞ **epinephrine**, ℞ **naphazoline hydrochloride**, ℞ **oxymetazoline hydrochloride**, ℞ **phenylephrine hydrochloride**). Others are indirect sympathomimetics that release norepinephrine from sympathetic nerve-endings (for instance ℞ **pseudoephedrine**, ℞ **ephedrine**).

Compound preparations often contain an ℞ **antihistamine** (such as ℞ **promethazine hydrochloride**, ℞ **brompheniramine maleate**, ℞ **chlorpheniramine maleate**, ℞ **diphenhydramine hydrochloride**). Although these agents are most useful against allergic symptoms of head and chest infections, such as hay fever and allergic rhinitis, they are also "dry-up" secretions in the common cold. Further, since the antihistamines incorporated into these cold and cough remedies are of the sedative type, they may help people sleep. Some preparations contain the ℞ **CNS stimulant** ℞ **caffeine**. There may be numerous minor agents incorporated such the aromatics ℞ **thymol**.

Limitations

There is very extensive use of these compound preparations, because of a perceived need by the public. They are generally relatively safe, except where someone has some other disorder. The biggest danger lies in taking vasoconstrictor decongestants by mouth, rather than as nosedrops or a spray, since these drugs have a tendency to cause side effects such as raised blood pressure. However, most people are unaware of this, but it is important to realize that the vasoconstriction, speeding of the heart, and hypertension often caused by sympathomimetic drugs are detrimental and potentially dangerous in people who have certain cardiovascular disorders. Further, sympathomimetics can have serious interactions with a number of other drug classes, especially (℞ **MAOI**) ℞ **antidepressant** drugs. Therefore it is better to use topical preparations (applied externally) of vasoconstrictor drugs, including decongestants, to minimize systemic side effects.

Coldrine Tablets ®

A preparation of ℞ **pseudoephedrine** and ℞ **acetaminophen**.
Formulation: Oral tablets.
Availability: OTC.
Warnings and side effects: See ℞ **pseudoephedrine**; ℞ **acetaminophen**. Tablets contain sodium metabisulfite, which may cause allergic reaction, sometimes serious, in a few people.

colesevelam ©

Type/Group: **lipid-regulating drug**.

Brand(s): WelChol.
How administered: Orally.

Used to treat

Colesevelam is a recently introduced LDL-cholesterol-lowering agent, a bile acid sequesterer, that can be used, either alone or with other drugs (for example ℞ **lovastatin**) when changes in diet and exercise alone have not proven effective.

Warnings

• It should not be given to people with known hypersensitivity to the drug or any component of the product, or to anyone with bowel obstruction.

• It should be given with caution to people with certain gastrointestinal disorders, with susceptibility to vitamin A, D, E, or K deficiencies, and those with very high triglyceride levels.

• There are no adequate and well-controlled studies in pregnant women, and so it should be used only if clearly needed.

• Medical judgment is required if breast-feeding is being considered.

• Must be taken with liquid or food.

Interactions

• The effects of ℞ **verapamil** may be reduced.

Side effects

• Occasionally, constipation and upset stomach.

Colestid ®

A preparation of ℞ **colestipol hydrochloride**.
Formulation: Oral tablets; oral granules.
Availability: Prescription only.
Warnings and side effects: See ℞ **colestipol hydrochloride**.

colestipol hydrochloride ©

Type/Group: **lipid-regulating drug**.
Brand(s): Colestid.
How administered: Orally.

Used to treat

Colestipol is a resin that binds bile acids in the gut to form an insoluble complex, and thereby reduces absorption of bile salts from the gut, resulting in changed cholesterol metabolism in the liver. It can be used as a lipid-regulating drug in ○ **hyperlipidemia** to reduce the levels, or change the proportions, of various lipids in the bloodstream. Generally, it is given only to people in whom a strict and regular dietary regime alone is not having the desired effect. Although not stated by the manufacturer for such use, it may also be prescribed to treat diarrhea due to digitalis toxicity.

Warnings

• It should not be given to people with known hypersensitivity to colestipol, or with complete biliary obstruction.

• It should be given with caution to people with gastrointestinal dysfunction, hemorrhoids, bleeding disorders, or osteoporosis.

• Colestipol's safety during pregnancy has not been established, but the drug is not absorbed systemically. It may interfere with maternal absorption of fat-soluble vitamins. It should be used only if the potential benefits outweigh the possible risks to the fetus.

• Medical judgment is required if breast-feeding is being considered, because of the potential interference with vitamin absorption.

• A doctor must be contacted immediately if bleeding, constipation, or any new symptoms occur.

• A reduction of folic acid levels may occur with long-term use.

• Other medication must be taken one hour before or four hours after colestipol.

Interactions

• The levels of ℞ **acetaminophen**, ℞ **amiodarone hydrochloride**, ℞ **corticosteroids**, ℞ **diclofenac**, digitalis glycosides, ℞ **furosemide**, ℞ **methotrexate**, ℞ **metronidazole**, ℞ **thiazide** diuretics, ℞ **thyroid hormones**, and ℞ **valproic acid** may be reduced.

• The effectiveness of oral ℞ **anticoagulants** may be reduced.

Side effects

• Frequently, constipation (may lead to fecal impaction) and other gastrointestinal effects.

• Occasionally, headache and dizziness.

• Rarely, gallstones, peptic ulcer, and malabsorption syndrome (due to reduced absorption of vitamins A, D, E, and K).

colestyramine Ⓖ

see ℞ **cholestyramine**.

Colfed-A Capsules Ⓑ

A preparation of ℞ **pseudoephedrine** and ℞ **chlorpheniramine maleate**.

Formulation: Oral capsules, sustained release.

Availability: Prescription only.

Warnings and side effects: See ℞ **pseudoephedrine**; ℞ **chlorpheniramine maleate**.

colistimethate sodium Ⓖ

see ℞ **colistin**.

colistin Ⓖ

(colistimethate sodium)

Type/Group: **polymyxin; antibiotic; antibacterial.**

Brand(s): Coly-Mycin-M.

How administered: Injection; topically (external).

Used to treat

Colistin (polymyxin E) may be given by injection (in the form colistimethate sodium (colistin sulfomethate sodium)) to treat infection by Gram-negative bacteria, including *Pseudomonas aeruginosa*. It is a comparatively toxic member of the polymyxin family, but is used externally as an ingredient in a fixed combination with other drugs that can be prescribed to treat infections of the external ear canal.

Warnings

• It should not be given to people with known hypersensitivity to colistin.

• It should be given with caution to people with kidney impairment, porphyria, or myasthenia gravis.

• It crosses the placenta and effects on the fetus have not been established, and so it should be used during pregnancy only if clearly needed and if the potential benefits outweigh the risks to the fetus.

• Breast-feeding should be stopped while this drug is being taken.

• Neurological effects (tingling or numbness, dizziness, slurred speech) can occur transiently. Do not drive or perform other tasks requiring physical skills or mental alertness while being treated.

• Kidney dysfunction may rarely occur, and is generally reversed by lowering dosage or discontinuing use.

• Respiratory arrest has occurred following intramuscular injection.

Interactions

• ℞ **Aminoglycosides** increase the risk of kidney dysfunction and respiratory arrest.

• Cephalothin may increase the risk of kidney dysfunction.

• Nondepolarizing ℞ **muscle relaxants** may increase neurological side effects.

Side effects

These depend on how it is administered. There may be:

• Tingling or burning sensation, generalized itching or hives, fever, gastrointestinal upset; dizziness, slurred speech, kidney and respiratory dysfunction.

Collyrium Fresh Ⓑ

A preparation of ℞ **tetrahydrozoline hydrochloride**.

Formulation: Eye drops.

Availability: OTC.

Warnings and side effects: See ℞ **tetrahydrozoline hydrochloride**.

colony-stimulating factor Ⓓ

see ℞ **hematopoietic**.

Coly-Mycin M Ⓑ

A preparation of ℞ **colistin**.

Formulation: Injection.

Availability: Prescription only.

Warnings and side effects: See ℞ **colistin**.

Combipres 0.1; 0.2; 0.3 Ⓑ

A preparation of ℞ **chlorthalidone** and ℞ **clonidine hydrochloride**.

Formulation: Oral tablets, available in 3 (clonidine) strengths.

Availability: Prescription only.

Warnings and side effects: See ℞ **chlorthalidone**; ℞ **clonidine hydrochloride**.

Combivent Ⓑ

A preparation of ℞ **albuterol** and ℞ **ipratropium bromide**.

Formulation: Inhalant.

Availability: Prescription only.

Warnings and side effects: See ℞ **albuterol**; ℞ **ipratropium bromide**.

Combivir ⑧

A preparation of ℞ **lamivudine** and ℞ **zidovudine**.
Formulation: Oral tablets.
Availability: Prescription only.
Warnings and side effects: See ℞ lamivudine; ℞ zidovudine.

Comfort Eye Drops ⑧

A preparation of ℞ **naphazoline hydrochloride**.
Formulation: Eye drops.
Availability: OTC.
Warnings and side effects: See ℞ naphazoline hydrochloride.

Comfort Tears ⑧

A preparation of ℞ **hydroxyethylcellulose**.
Formulation: Ophthalmic solution.
Availability: OTC.
Warnings and side effects: See ℞ hydroxyethylcellulose.

Comhist Tablets; LA Capsules ⑧

A preparation of ℞ **phenylephrine hydrochloride**,
℞ **chlorpheniramine maleate**, and phenyltoloxamine citrate.
Formulation: Oral tablets; capsules, long acting.
Availability: Prescription only.
Warnings and side effects: See ℞ phenylephrine hydrochloride;
℞ chlorpheniramine maleate.

Compazine Tablets; Spansule ⑧

A preparation of ℞ **prochlorperazine**.
Formulation: Oral tablets; extended release capsules (Spansule);
syrup; rectal suppositories; injectable solution.
Availability: Prescription only.
Warnings and side effects: See ℞ prochlorperazine.

Compound W Liquid; Gel ⑧

A preparation of ℞ **salicylic acid**, ℞ **camphor**, ℞ **castor oil**, and
various.
Formulation: Topical liquid; gel.
Availability: OTC.
Warnings and side effects: See ℞ salicylic acid; ℞ camphor;
℞ castor oil.

Comtan ⑧

A preparation of ℞ **entacapone**.
Formulation: Oral tablet.
Availability: Prescription only.
Warnings and side effects: See ℞ entacapone.

Comtrex Allergy-Sinus Tablets; Caplets ⑧

A preparation of ℞ **pseudoephedrine**, ℞ **acetaminophen**, and
℞ **chlorpheniramine maleate**.
Formulation: Oral tablets.
Availability: OTC.
Warnings and side effects: See ℞ pseudoephedrine;
℞ acetaminophen; ℞ chlorpheniramine maleate.

Comtrex Maximum Strength Cold & Cough Relieft Caplets ⑧

Also: Tablets
A preparation of ℞ **dextromethorphan**, ℞ **acetaminophen**,
℞ **chlorpheniramine maleate**, and ℞ **pseudoephedrine**.
Formulation: Oral tablets; caplets.
Availability: OTC.
Warnings and side effects: See ℞ dextromethorphan;
℞ acetaminophen; ℞ chlorpheniramine maleate;
℞ pseudoephedrine.

Comvax ⑧

A preparation of ℞ **hepatitis B vaccine**.
Formulation: Intramuscular injection.
Availability: Prescription only.
Warnings and side effects: See ℞ hepatitis B vaccine.

Condylox ⑧

A preparation of ℞ **podofilox**.
Formulation: Topical solution (external genital warts); topical gel
(external and periananl warts).
Availability: Prescription only.
Warnings and side effects: See ℞ podofilox.

Congess SR Capsules; Jr. Capsules ⑧

A preparation of ℞ **pseudoephedrine** and ℞ **guaifenesin**.
Formulation: Oral capsules, sustained release.
Availability: Prescription only.
Warnings and side effects: See ℞ pseudoephedrine;
℞ guaifenesin.

Congestac Caplets ⑧

A preparation of ℞ **pseudoephedrine** and ℞ **guaifenesin**.
Formulation: Oral tablets.
Availability: OTC.
Warnings and side effects: See ℞ pseudoephedrine;
℞ guaifenesin.

Congestion Relief Tablets ⑧

A preparation of ℞ **pseudoephedrine**.
Formulation: Oral tablets.
Availability: OTC.
Warnings and side effects: See ℞ pseudoephedrine.

congestive heart failure treatment ⑩

see ℞ heart failure treatment.

Constulose ⑧

A preparation of ℞ **lactulose**.
Formulation: Oral liquid.
Availability: Prescription only.
Warnings and side effects: See ℞ lactulose.

Contac Day & Night Allergy/Sinus Caplets ℞

A preparation of ℞ **pseudoephedrine**, ℞ **acetaminophen**, and ℞ **diphenhydramine hydrochloride** (night only).
Formulation: Oral tablets.
Availability: OTC.
Warnings and side effects: See ℞ **pseudoephedrine**; ℞ **acetaminophen**; ℞ **diphenhydramine hydrochloride**.

Contac Severe Cold & Flu Caplets ℞

A preparation of ℞ **dextromethorphan**, ℞ **acetaminophen**, ℞ **chlorpheniramine maleate**, and ℞ **pseudoephedrine**.
Formulation: Oral caplets.
Availability: OTC.
Warnings and side effects: See ℞ **dextromethorphan**; ℞ **acetaminophen**; ℞ **chlorpheniramine maleate**; ℞ **pseudoephedrine**.

contraceptive ⊙

Generics: **levonorgestrel**.

Actions and uses

Contraceptives can be used to prevent pregnancy in a number of ways. ℞ **oral contraceptive** preparations are discussed in their appropriate articles. See also ℞ **hormone replacement**.

Contraceptive sex hormones can also be given by injection or implant, and as intrauterine devices (IUD). For example, the ℞ **progestogen** drug ℞ **levonorgestrel** is available as a subdermal implant (under the skin) and as an IUD. Other methods include mechanical intrauterine contraceptive devices. These are not normally regarded as drugs (and are not within the scope of this book), but some have a copper wire incorporated, which is thought to be pharmacologically active in changing production of local mediators (probably prostaglandins), which effect implantation. Spermicidal contraceptive chemicals are available as topical preparations (external application), but their effectiveness when used alone is low.

Limitations

See individual drug entry.

Copaxone ℞

A preparation of ℞ **glatiramer acetate**.
Formulation: Subcutaneous injection.
Availability: Prescription only.
Warnings and side effects: See ℞ **glatiramer acetate**.

Cophene No. 2 Tablets ℞

A preparation of ℞ **pseudoephedrine** and ℞ **chlorpheniramine maleate**.
Formulation: Oral tablets, sustained release.
Availability: Prescription only.
Warnings and side effects: See ℞ **pseudoephedrine**; ℞ **chlorpheniramine maleate**.

Cophene XP Liquid ℞

A preparation of ℞ **hydrocodone bitartrate**, ℞ **pseudoephedrine**, and ℞ **guaifenesin**.
Formulation: Oral syrup.
Availability: Prescription only.
Warnings and side effects: See ℞ **hydrocodone bitartrate**; ℞ **pseudoephedrine**; ℞ **guaifenesin**.

Coppertone Oil Free ℞

A preparation of ℞ **cinnamates**, other ingredients.
Formulation: Topical lotion.
Availability: OTC.
Warnings and side effects: See ℞ **cinnamates**.

Coppertone Shade Sunblock ℞

A preparation of ℞ **cinnamates**, other ingredients.
Formulation: Topical lotion.
Availability: OTC.
Warnings and side effects: See ℞ **cinnamates**.

Co-Pyronil 2 Pulvules ℞

A preparation of ℞ **pseudoephedrine** and ℞ **chlorpheniramine maleate**.
Formulation: Oral tablets.
Availability: OTC.
Warnings and side effects: See ℞ **pseudoephedrine**; ℞ **chlorpheniramine maleate**.

Cordarone ℞

A preparation of ℞ **amiodarone hydrochloride**.
Formulation: Oral tablets; injection.
Availability: Prescription only.
Warnings and side effects: See ℞ **amiodarone hydrochloride**. Injection contains benzyl alchohol, which may cause hypersensitivity reaction ("gasping syndrome") in susceptible individuals.

Cordran; Cordran SP ℞

A preparation of ℞ **flurandrenolide**.
Formulation: Cream; ointment; lotion; all in several strengths; tape.
Availability: Prescription only.
Warnings and side effects: See ℞ **flurandrenolide**.

Coreg ℞

A preparation of ℞ **carvedilol**.
Formulation: Oral tablets, available in 4 strengths.
Availability: Prescription only.
Warnings and side effects: See ℞ **carvedilol**.

Corgard ℞

A preparation of ℞ **nadolol**.
Formulation: Oral tablets, available in five strengths.
Availability: Prescription only.
Warnings and side effects: See ℞ **nadolol**.

Corlopam ®

A preparation of ℞ **fenoldopam mesylate**.
Formulation: Intravenous infusion.
Availability: Prescription only.
Warnings and side effects: See ℞ **fenoldopam mesylate**.
Contains sodium metabisulfite, which may cause hypersensitivity reaction in a few individuals-more frequently in those with asthma.

Cormax ®

A preparation of ℞ **clobetasol propionate**.
Formulation: Ointment.
Availability: Prescription only.
Warnings and side effects: See ℞ **clobetasol propionate**.

Corque ®

A preparation of ℞ **hydrocortisone** and ℞ **clioquinol**.
Formulation: Cream.
Availability: Prescription only.
Warnings and side effects: See ℞ **hydrocortisone**; ℞ **clioquinol**.

Correctol ®

A preparation of ℞ **bisacodyl**.
Formulation: Oral tablets.
Availability: OTC.
Warnings and side effects: See ℞ **bisacodyl**.

Cortaid; Intensive Therapy; Maximum Strength Fastick ®

A preparation of ℞ **hydrocortisone**.
Formulation: Cream; spray; roll-on stick.
Availability: OTC.
Warnings and side effects: See ℞ **hydrocortisone**.

Cortaid with Aloe; Maximum Strength Cortaid Cream ®

A preparation of ℞ **hydrocortisone**.
Formulation: Cream; ointment.
Availability: OTC.
Warnings and side effects: See ℞ **hydrocortisone**.

Cortastat ®

A preparation of ℞ **dexamethasone**, ℞ **sodium phosphate**.
Formulation: Injection.
Availability: Prescription only.
Warnings and side effects: See ℞ **dexamethasone**; ℞ **sodium phosphate**.

Cort-Dome; Cort-Dome High Potency ®

A preparation of ℞ **hydrocortisone**.
Formulation: Cream in two strengths.
Availability: Prescription only.
Warnings and side effects: See ℞ **hydrocortisone**.

Cortef ®

A preparation of ℞ **hydrocortisone**.
Formulation: Oral suspension.
Availability: Prescription only.
Warnings and side effects: See ℞ **hydrocortisone**.

Cortef Feminine Itch ®

A preparation of ℞ **hydrocortisone**.
Formulation: Cream.
Availability: OTC.
Warnings and side effects: See ℞ **hydrocortisone**.

Cortenema ®

A preparation of ℞ **hydrocortisone**.
Formulation: Retention enema.
Availability: Prescription only.
Warnings and side effects: See ℞ **hydrocortisone**.

Corticaine ®

A preparation of ℞ **hydrocortisone**, ℞ **menthol**, and ℞ **glycerin**.
Formulation: Cream.
Availability: OTC.
Warnings and side effects: See ℞ **hydrocortisone**; ℞ **menthol**; ℞ **glycerin**.

Corticosporin Suspension ®

A preparation of ℞ **hydrocortisone** and ℞ **neomycin**.
Formulation: Eye drops.
Availability: Prescription only.
Warnings and side effects: See ℞ **hydrocortisone**; ℞ **neomycin**.

corticosteroid ⓓ

(adrenocorticosteroid)
Generics: **alclometasone; beclomethasone dipropionate; betamethasone; budesonide; clobetasol propionate; clobetasol propionate; clocortolone pivalate; cortisone; cosyntropin; desoxymetasone; dexamethasone; fludrocortisone; flunisolide; fluocinolone acetonide; fluocinonide; fluorometholone; flurandrenolide; fluticasone propionate; halcinonide; hydrocortisone; methylprednisolone; mometasone; prednisolone; prednisone; triamcinolone.**

Actions and uses

Corticosteroids are steroid hormones secreted by the cortex (outer part) of the adrenal glands, or are synthetic substances that closely resemble the chemical structure and actions of the the natural forms. There are two main types of corticosteroids, glucocorticoids and mineralocorticoids. The latter assist in maintaining the salt-and-water balance of the body.

Corticosteroids such as the glucocorticoid ℞ **hydrocortisone** and the mineralocorticoid ℞ **fludrocortisone** can be given to people for replacement therapy where there is a deficiency, in Addison's disease or following adrenalectomy or hypopituitarism.

The glucocorticoids are potent ℞ **anti-inflammatory** and ℞ **antiallergic** drugs and are widely used, for example, to treat inflammatory and/or allergic reactions of the skin (see ⊕ **skin conditions**) and airways, for neoplastic (⊕ **cancer**) disease in combination with ℞ **cytotoxic** ℞ **anticancer** drugs, and in anti-inflammatory/℞ **immunosuppressive** treatment of chronic illnesses such as ✪ **rheumatoid arthritis** and other connective tissue disorders (for example, ✪ **lupus** and inflammatory bowel disease (IBD) (✪ **Crohn's disease**; ✪ **ulcerative colitis**)). Corticosteroids form a major part of ℞ **antiasthmatic** treatment, when they are generally inhaled for the prevention of ✪ **asthma** attacks.

Compound preparations containing a number of active principles are available that contain ℞ **antibacterial** or ℞ **antifungal** drugs with an anti-inflammatory corticosteroid. They can be used in conditions where an infection is also present, especially applied topically (externally) for skin and eye conditions.

The release of corticosteroids from the adrenal gland can be induced by the (peptide) ℞ **anterior pituitary hormone** ℞ **corticotropin** (adrenocorticotrophic hormone; ACTH) and its analog ℞ **cosyntropin**, and these may be used for ℞ **diagnostic agent** purposes or to treat some diseases.

Limitations

Although glucocorticoid corticosteroids are one of the most widely used families of drugs, they do have some major drawbacks. If used on a long-term basis, the cortex of the adrenal gland becomes adapted to the corticosteroid drug, and sudden withdrawal must be avoided because of the risk of a crisis due to adrenal insufficiency. People on corticosteroid treatment carry warning cards or wear a medic alert bracelet indicating that they need supplementary steroid therapy during the management of crises. Full withdrawal from treatment is slow, and it may take up to 12 months for the adrenal glands to return to normal function.

Since corticosteroids vary widely in potency (efficacy or maximum effect)—being divided into four or more classes (ranging from "low potency" to "very high potency")—wherever possible people are treated initially with the lowest potency corticosteroid at the lowest dose that will improve symptoms. Because there is a tendency for the effects of steroids to "wear-off", for instance, when used for chronic skin conditions such as ✪ **eczema** and ✪ **psoriasis**, this approach allows for increases in the strength of corticosteroid preparations over a period of time.

All corticosteroid preparations must be used with caution because the corticosteroid component diminishes a person's natural immune response to infection. Systemic use, or absorption of a high dose of topical corticosteroid over a period of time, causes a wide range of undesirable systemic side effects (see individual drug entries).

corticotropin Ⓖ

(adrenocorticotropic hormone (ACTH))

Type/Group: **hormone; anterior pituitary hormone; diagnostic agent**.

Brand(s): Acthar; various generic.

How administered: Injection.

Used to treat

Corticotropin is used for diagnostic testing of adrenocortical function, to treat hypercalcemia (abnormally high calcium levels) of cancer, multiple sclerosis, and certain thyroid infections. Although not stated by the manufacturers for such use, it may also be prescribed for treatment of spasms in infants. Corticotropin is not a

℞ **corticosteroid**, being produced and secreted by the anterior pituitary gland, but has some actions in the body like those of a corticosteroid because its physiological role is to stimulate and control the production and secretion of corticosteroids from the adrenal gland.

Warnings

• It should not be used by people with known hypersensitivity to corticosteroids, systemic fungal infections, ocular herpes simplex, scleroderma (local or general hardening of the skin), or primary adrenocortical insufficiency/hyperfunction.

• It should be given with caution to anyone with a peptic ulcer, clotting disorder, a history of tuberculosis, thyroid disorder, liver cirrhosis, nonspecific ulcerative colitis, hypertension, psychosis, kidney insufficiency, seizures, or osteoporosis.

• Adverse fetal effects can occur, and it should be used in pregnancy only if medically judged that it is needed.

• Medical judgment is also required if breast-feeding is being considered.

• Long-term therapy may have adverse effects, including cataracts and glaucoma, electrolyte imbalances, muscle wasting, osteoporosis, and cessation of menstruation.

• Prolonged use in children will inhibit skeletal growth, so growth must be monitored.

• It may mask signs of infection and chronic disease.

• Those who have had tuberculosis may experience a reactivation of the disease.

• Live virus vaccines must not be taken while using this drug.

• The dosage must be reduced gradually upon discontinuation, which must be under medical supervision.

Interactions

• ℞ **corticotropin** taken with ℞ **amphotericin** or ℞ **diuretics** may further reduce potassium levels.

• The effects of ℞ **aspirin**, ℞ **oral hypoglycemics**, ℞ **insulin**, ℞ **diuretics**, and ⚕ **potassium** supplements may be reduced.

Side effects

• Frequently, insomnia, heartburn, nervousness, abdominal tightness, increased sweating, acne, mood swings, increased appetite, facial flushing, delayed wound healing, increased susceptibility to infection, and diarrhea or constipation.

• Occasionally, headache, edema, change in skin color, and frequent urination.

• Rarely, speeded heartbeat, allergic reaction, and psychic changes.

• Potentially serious side effects include seizures and pancreatitis.

Cortifoam Ⓑ

A preparation of ℞ **hydrocortisone**.

Formulation: Intrarectal foam.

Availability: Prescription only.

Warnings and side effects: See ℞ **hydrocortisone**.

cortisone Ⓖ

Type/Group: **corticosteroid; anti-inflammatory; immunosuppressant**.

Brand(s): Cortrosyn; Cortone Acetate; various generic..

How administered: Injection; orally.

Used to treat

Cortisone is used for the treatment of many kinds of inflammation. It has major and varied effects on metabolism, and modifies the operation of the immune system, and so it may be used to treat a range of conditions, including adrenal insufficiency, congenital adrenal abnormalities, rheumatic disorders, such as ✪ **arthritis** and ✪ **osteoarthritis**, allergic states, collagen diseases, allergic and inflammatory eye disorders, intestinal tract, liver and kidney disorders, skin diseases, respiratory diseases (such as bronchial ✪ **asthma**), edemas, and malignancies.

Warnings

• It should not be used by people with known hypersensitivity to corticosteroids, or those with systemic fungal infections.

• It should be given with caution to anyone with low thyroid function, diabetes mellitus, glaucoma, esophagitis, peptic ulcers, hepatitis, cirrhosis, ocular herpes simplex, history of tuberculosis, nonspecific colitis, congestive heart failure, myocardial infarction (heart attack), hypertension, psychosis, or kidney insufficiency. Also, it should be given with caution to anyone over 65 and children.

• Corticosteroids can cross the placenta, and cortisone, therefore, should be used during pregnancy only if it is medically judged to be essential.

• Medical judgment is also required if breast-feeding is being considered. Cortisone is excreted in breast milk and could suppress growth and interfere with the production of corticosteroids in the infant. It is not known whether, or under what conditions, enough of the drug is absorbed from topical use to create these risks.

• It may mask signs of infection and interfere with the body's ability to keep infection from spreading.

• Live vaccines must not be taken while using this drug.

• It may reactivate latent tuberculosis or amebiasis.

• It causes increased excretion of calcium and other minerals, and so supplements may be needed.

• Prolonged use may lead to adrenal insufficiency. A doctor must be notified of unusual weight gain, swelling of the legs or feet, muscle weakness, puffing of the face, menstrual irregularities, or prolonged infections such as sore throat, fever, or colds (signs/ symptoms of adrenal insufficiency).

• Those on chronic steroid therapy should wear a medic-alert bracelet or the equivalent.

• The contraceptive effect of IUDs (intrauterine device) may be decreased.

• No other medication (including herbal remedies and supplements) must be taken without consulting a doctor.

• Discontinuation of treatment must be gradual and under medical supervision to avoid adverse reactions.

• Dentists and other doctors must be informed of the use of this drug during, and for 12 months after discontinuing, treatment. Supportive drugs may be required in the event of severe illness, surgery, or trauma.

Interactions

• Cortisone taken with ℞ **amphotericin** or ℞ **diuretics** may further reduce potassium levels.

• The effects of ℞ **aspirin**, ℞ **oral hypoglycemics**, ℞ **insulin**, ℞ **diuretics**, and ♐ **potassium** supplements may be reduced.

• The effects of ℞ **barbiturates**, ℞ **hydantoins**, and ℞ **rifampin** may be reduced.

• ℞ **ketoconazole**, ℞ **estrogens**, ℞ **oral contraceptives**, and nondepolarizing muscle relaxants may increase the effects of corticosteroids.

• Oral ℞ **anticoagulants** and ℞ **theophylline** may alter the effects of either corticosteroids or the other drug, or both.

• The effectiveness of ℞ **anticholinesterases**, ℞ **isoniazid**, ℞ **salicylates**, or ℞ **somatrem** may be reduced.

• ℞ **cyclosporine** and digitalis may increase the risk of toxicity.

Side effects

• Frequently, insomnia, heartburn, nervousness, abdominal tightness, increased sweating, acne, mood swings, increased appetite, facial flushing, delayed wound healing, increased susceptibility to infection, diarrhea, or constipation.

• Occasionally, headache, edema, change in skin color, and frequent urination.

• Rarely, speeded heartbeat, allergic skin reaction, psychosis, hallucinations, and depression. Potentially serious side effects include seizures and platelet disorders.

Cortisporin ⓑ

A preparation of ℞ **hydrocortisone**, ℞ **neomycin**, ℞ **bacitracin**, and ℞ **polymyxin B**.
Formulation: Ointment.
Availability: Prescription only.
Warnings and side effects: See ℞ **hydrocortisone**; ℞ **neomycin**; ℞ **bacitracin**; ℞ **polymyxin B**

Cortisporin Cream ⓑ

A preparation of ℞ **hydrocortisone**, ℞ **polymyxin B sulfate**, and ℞ **neomycin** sulfate.
Formulation: Cream.
Availability: Prescription only.
Warnings and side effects: See ℞ **hydrocortisone**; ℞ **polymyxin B sulfate**; ℞ **neomycin**.

Cortisporin Ointment ⓑ

A preparation of ℞ **hydrocortisone**, ℞ **bacitracin**, ℞ **neomycin**, and ℞ **polymyxin B sulfate**.
Formulation: Cream.
Availability: Prescription only.
Warnings and side effects: See ℞ **hydrocortisone**; ℞ **bacitracin**; ℞ **neomycin**; ℞ **polymyxin B sulfate**.

Cortisporin Otic ⓑ

A preparation of ℞ **hydrocortisone**, ℞ **neomycin**, and ℞ **polymyxin B sulfate**.
Formulation: Ear drops.
Availability: Prescription only.
Warnings and side effects: See ℞ **hydrocortisone**; ℞ **neomycin**; ℞ **polymyxin B sulfate**.

Cortizone·5; 10 ®
A preparation of ℞ **hydrocortisone**.
Formulation: Ointment in two strengths, cream.
Availability: OTC.
Warnings and side effects: See ℞ **hydrocortisone**.

Cortizone for Kids ®
A preparation of ℞ **hydrocortisone**.
Formulation: Cream.
Availability: OTC.
Warnings and side effects: See ℞ **hydrocortisone**.

Cortone Acetate ®
A preparation of ℞ **betamethasone**.
Formulation: Oral tablets; syrup.
Availability: Prescription only.
Warnings and side effects: See ℞ **betamethasone**.

Cortrosyn ®
A preparation of ℞ **cosyntropin**.
Formulation: Injection.
Availability: Prescription only.
Warnings and side effects: See ℞ **cosyntropin**.

Corzide 40/5; Corzide 80/5 ®
A preparation of ℞ **nadolol** and ℞ **bendroflumethiazide**.
Formulation: Oral tablets, available in two (nadolol) strengths.
Availability: Prescription only.
Warnings and side effects: See ℞ **nadolol**;
℞ **bendroflumethiazide**.

Cosmegen ®
A preparation of ℞ **dactinomycin**.
Formulation: Powder for injection.
Availability: Prescription only.
Warnings and side effects: See ℞ **dactinomycin**.

Cosopt Ocumeter ®
A preparation of ℞ **dorzolamide** and ℞ **timolol maleate**.
Formulation: Eye drops.
Availability: Prescription only.
Warnings and side effects: See ℞ **dorzolamide**; ℞ **timolol maleate**.

cosyntropin ⑥
Type/Group: **hormone; anterior pituitary hormone; diagnostic agent**.
Brand(s): Cortrosyn.
Formulation: Injection.
Used to treat
Cosyntropin is a synthetic derivative of ℞ **corticotropin**, or adrenocorticotrophic hormone (ACTH), and is used for diagnostic testing of adrenocortical function.

Warnings
• It should not be used by people with known hypersensitivity to cosyntropin or corticotropin.
• Adverse fetal effects can occur. Cosyntropin, therefore, should be used during pregnancy only if it is medically judged to be essential.
• It should not be used by breast-feeding mothers.
• The short duration for diagnostic use does not produce effects of long-term corticotropin therapy.
Interactions
No significant interactions have been reported.
Side effects
• Occasionally, nausea and vomiting.
• Rarely, allergic reaction (fever, itching).

Cotazyme Capsules; Cotazym-S ®
A preparation of ℞ **pancreatin** (amylase, lipase, protease).
Formulation: Oral capsules, two strengths.
Availability: Prescription only.
Warnings and side effects: See ℞ **pancreatin**.

Cotrim; Cotrim DS; Cotrim Pediatric ®
A preparation of ℞ **trimethoprim and sulfamethoxazole**.
Formulation: Oral tablets in regular and double strengths (DS); oral suspension (pediatric).
Availability: Prescription only.
Warnings and side effects: See ℞ **trimethoprim and sulfamethoxazole**.

co-trimoxazole ⑥
see ℞ **trimethoprim and sulfamethoxazole**.

Coumadin ®
A preparation of ℞ **warfarin sodium**.
Formulation: Oral tablets (nine strengths); injection.
Availability: Prescription only.
Warnings and side effects: See ℞ **warfarin sodium**.

counter-irritant ⑩
Generics: **camphor; capsaicin; menthol; methyl salicylate; turpentine oil**.
Actions and uses
Counter-irritant substances are topical preparations that when rubbed onto the skin relieve pain in underlying muscles and joints. Most of these substances are also called rubefacient agents, which is a name derived from the fact that they redden the skin by causing the blood vessels of the skin to dilate, which gives a soothing feeling of warmth—and is one explanation of how they work. The term counter-irritant refers to the idea that local irritation of the sensory nerve endings (where they act selectively) alters or offsets pain in the underlying muscle or joints, possibly by blocking pain signals that would normally go to the pain centers in the central nervous system. However, it is now known that the rubefacient actions of some of the substances are also due to stimulation of sensory nerves in the skin, causing them to release vasodilator (widens blood vessels) substances. The two explanations of how these drugs work

may add up to much the same thing. Some of the counter-irritants are rubbed onto the gums (for example, in ◯ **teething** babies) where they have some sort of ℞ **local anesthetic** or local painkilling action. A number of these substances are aromatic or volatile oils.

The most thoroughly studied of this group is ℞ **capsaicin**, the active principle of capsicum, which is often used medically in the form of the resin capsicum oleoresin, and is a pungent extract from capsicum peppers (it is also used as a herbal remedy, see ♣ **cayenne**). Both capsaicin and capsicum resin are incorporated into medicines used to relieve ◯ **pain** from ◯ **rheumatoid arthritis**, ◯ **osteoarthritis**, and of the pain following ◯ **shingles** or diabetic neuropathy. It has evident rubefacient action when applied to the skin and rubbed in. Capsaicin is also being investigated as a treatment for ◯ **psoriasis**, intractable itching, pain following mastectomy, trigeminal neuralgia, and phantom limb pain.

℞ **turpentine oil** is both a counter-irritant and a rubefacient, and is included in some compound preparations that are used by external application for the symptomatic relief of pain associated with rheumatism, ◯ **neuralgia**, fibrosis, and sprains and stiffness of the joints.

℞ **menthol** is a white, crystalline substance derived from peppermint oil (an essential oil extracted from a plant of the mint family), and is chemically a ℞ **terpene**. It is available in several specific chemical forms, of which levomenthol is one preferred isomer. It is included in some preparations, which are rubbed into the skin to relieve muscle or joint pain. It and similar aromatic oils are commonly used in inhalants intended to clear the nasal or catarrhal congestion associated with colds, rhinitis, or sinusitis. But whether it works in a similar way here is not known. ℞ **camphor** is an aromatic substance with mild counter-irritant properties, and is incorporated into a number of preparations used to help relieve itchiness. It is also used to treat symptoms of muscular pains and rheumatism, arthritis, and similar conditions. Aromatic vapors from some preparations are inhaled for relief of cough.

Limitations

All of these agents can irritate the skin, and may burn or sting temporarily. Some people show hypersensitivity reactions. Strong concentrations should not be used on children. The eyes and mucous membranes should be avoided, also avoid cuts and abraded skin. Consult a doctor before using during pregnancy or while breastfeeding. Preparations are toxic if inadvertently taken by mouth. See also the individual drug entries.

Covangesic Tablets   ®

A preparation of ℞ **phenylephrine hydrochloride**, ℞ **acetaminophen**, ℞ **chlorpheniramine maleate**, and ℞ **pyrilamine maleate**, and phenylpropanolamine.

Formulation: Oral tablets.

Availability: OTC.

Warnings and side effects: See ℞ **phenylephrine hydrochloride**; ℞ **acetaminophen**; ℞ **chlorpheniramine maleate**; ℞ **pyrilamine maleate**.

Covera-HS   ®

A preparation of ℞ **verapamil hydrochloride**.

Formulation: Oral tablets, extended-release tablets, available in two strengths.

Availability: Prescription only.

Warnings and side effects: See ℞ **verapamil hydrochloride**.

Cozaar   ®

A preparation of ℞ **losartan potassium**.

Formulation: Oral tablets, available in 3 strengths.

Availability: Prescription only.

Warnings and side effects: See ℞ **losartan potassium**.

Creamy Tar   ®

A preparation of ℞ **coal tar**.

Formulation: Shampoo.

Availability: OTC.

Warnings and side effects: See ℞ **coal tar**.

Creon 5, 10, 15 Minimicrospheres   ®

A preparation of ℞ **pancreatin** (amylase, lipase, protease).

Formulation: Oral capsules, containing coated microspheres.

Availability: Prescription only.

Warnings and side effects: See ℞ **pancreatin**.

Creo-Terpin   ®

A preparation of ℞ **dextromethorphan**.

Formulation: Liquid.

Availability: OTC.

Warnings and side effects: See ℞ **dextromethorphan**. Contains tartrazine (FD&C yellow No 5), a dye that may cause allergic reaction in a few people, but especially those with sensitivity to aspirin.

Crixivan   ®

A preparation of ℞ **indinavir**.

Formulation: Oral tablets in several strengths.

Availability: Prescription only.

Warnings and side effects: See ℞ **indinavir**.

Crolom   ®

A preparation of ℞ **cromolyn sodium**.

Formulation: Ophthalmic solution.

Availability: Prescription only.

Warnings and side effects: See ℞ **cromolyn sodium**.

cromolyn sodium   Ⓖ

(sodium cromoglicate; disodium cromoglycate)

Type/Group: **antiasthmatic; antiallergic.**

Brand(s): Crolom; Gastrocrom; Intal; Nasalcrom; Opticron; generic.

How administered: Inhalation; intranasal; topically (eye); orally.

Used to treat

Cromolyn sodium is used to prevent recurrent ◯ **asthma** and allergic symptoms in the eye (for example, allergic ◯ **conjunctivitis**), nose (for example, environmental allergy symptoms including allergic rhinitis), intestine (for example, food allergy), and elsewhere. It is not clear how it works, but its anti-inflammatory activity appears to involve a reduction in the release of inflammatory mediators.

Warnings
• It should not be given to people with known hypersensitivity or allergy to this drug.
• It should be given with caution to people with impaired kidney or liver function.
• It should only be used in pregnancy when medically judged to be clearly needed.
• Medical judgment is required if breast-feeding is being considered. It is not known whether this drug is present in breast milk.
• It is not effective against acute asthma attacks.
• Its effects in treating asthma may take up to 4 weeks.
• Rarely, acute allergic reactions have occurred.

Interactions
No significant interactions have been reported.

Side effects
• Inhalation: Frequently, cough, dry mouth and throat, stuffy nose, throat irritation, unpleasant taste. Occasionally, bronchospasm, hoarseness, watering eyes. Rarely, dizziness, painful urination, muscle or joint pain, skin rash.
• Nasal: Frequently, burning, stinging, irritation of the nose, increased sneezing. Occasionally, cough, headache, unpleasant taste, postnasal drip. Rarely, nose bleeds, skin rash.
• Ophthalmic: Frequently, burning, stinging of the eyes. Occasionally, increased watering or itching of the eye. Rarely, edema of the eye, and eye irritation.
• Oral: Headache, gastrointestinal effects, itching, unusual tiredness (it is not known whether these effects of oral use are drug-induced, as they are similar to the symptoms of the underlying disease).

crotamiton ⓖ
Type/Group: **scabicide and pediculicide; antipruritic.**
Brand(s): Eurex.
How administered: Topically (external).

Used to treat
Crotamiton is used to relieve pruritus (itching) of the skin (although its beneficial effect has been questioned). It also has scabicidal (acaricide) activity and is used sometimes to eliminate the ⊙ **scabies** infestation (although there are more effective agents) and to treat the itching after elimination.

Warnings
• It should not be given to people with known hypersensitivity to this drug.
• It is not known whether it can harm the fetus, and should be used in pregnancy only if clearly needed.
• Medical judgment is required if breast-feeding is being considered. It is not known whether it appears in breast milk.
• Do not apply to acutely inflamed, raw or weeping skin, or to the eyes or mouth.

Interactions
No significant interactions are known.

Side effects
• Contact dermatitis irritation, itching, and rash.

Cruex; Cruex Aerosol ⓑ
A preparation of ℞ **undecylenic acid.**
Formulation: Topical cream; topical powder; aerosol spray powder.
Availability: OTC.
Warnings and side effects: See ℞ **undecylenic acid.**

crystal violet ⓖ
see ℞ **gentian violet.**

Crystamine ⓑ
A preparation of ⚖ **cyanocobalamin.**
Formulation: Injection.
Availability: Prescription only.
Warnings and side effects: See ⚖ **cyanocobalamin.**

Crysti 1000 ⓑ
A preparation of ⚖ **cyanocobalamin.**
Formulation: Injection.
Availability: Prescription only.
Warnings and side effects: See ⚖ **cyanocobalamin.**

Crystodigin ⓑ
A preparation of ℞ **digitoxin.**
Formulation: Oral tablets.
Availability: Prescription only.
Warnings and side effects: See ℞ **digitoxin.**

C/T/S ⓑ
A preparation of ℞ **clindamycin.**
Formulation: Topical solution.
Availability: Prescription only.
Warnings and side effects: See ℞ **clindamycin.**

Cuprimine ⓑ
A preparation of ℞ **penicillamine.**
Formulation: Oral capsules, available in two strengths.
Availability: Prescription only.
Warnings and side effects: See ℞ **penicillamine.**

Cutar Bath Oil Emulsion ⓑ
A preparation of ℞ **coal tar.**
Formulation: Liquid (to add to bath).
Availability: OTC.
Warnings and side effects: See ℞ **coal tar.**

Cutivate ⓑ
A preparation of ℞ **fluticasone propionate.**
Formulation: Ointment; cream.
Availability: Prescription only.

Warnings and side effects: See ℞ **fluticasone propionate**.

cyanocobalamin ⓖ
(hydroxocobalamin)
Type/Group: **anemia treatment; vitamin**.
Brand(s): Cyanocobalamin: Big Shot B$_{12}$; Crystamine; Crysti 1000; Cyanoject; Cyomin; Nascobal; Rubesol-1000; various generic.
Hydroxocobalamin: Hydro Cobex; Hydro-Crysti-12; LA-12; various generic.
How administered: Injection; orally; intranasal.

Used to treat
Cyanocobalamin and hydroxocobalamin are forms of ⚕ **vitamin B$_{12}$** and are used to treat vitamin B$_{12}$ deficiency, ◑ **pernicious anemia**, and vitamin B$_{12}$ malabsorption syndrome as well as to meet increased vitamin B$_{12}$ requirements in pregnancy and certain diseases. Vitamin B$_{12}$ is readily found in most normal, well-balanced diets (for example, in fish, eggs, liver, and red meat). Vegans, who eat no animal products at all, may eventually suffer from deficiency of this vitamin. A deficiency of vitamin B$_{12}$ eventually causes megaloblastic anemia where large deformed red blood-cells are produced, and this leads to degeneration of nerves in the central and peripheral nervous systems and abnormalities of epithelia (particularly the lining of the mouth and gut). Apart from poor diet, deficiency can also be caused by the lack of an intrinsic factor necessary for absorption in the stomach (pernicious anemia) and by various malabsorption syndromes in the gut (sometimes due to drugs). Hydroxocobalamin is preferred to cyanocobalamin for initial treatment, but either may be used in maintenance treatment. Cyanocobalamin is used to treat nutritional vitamin B$_{12}$ deficiency. Different routes of administration are used for different purposes.

Warnings
• It should not be given to people with known hypersensitivity to these agents, or with optic nerve atrophy. The nasal form should not be used by people with symptoms of nasal congestion, allergic rhinitis, or upper respiratory tract infections until symptoms have subsided.
• At levels above the recommended daily allowance, it should be used during pregnancy only if benefit outweighs potential risk to the fetus.
• It does appear in breast milk. Vitamin B$_{12}$ is a necessary nutrient and needs are increased in pregnancy and when breast-feeding.
• Rarely, intensive vitamin B$_{12}$ treatment may produce life-threatening hypokalemia (low blood potassium levels) in those with severe megaloblastic anemia; monitoring may be required.

Interactions
• ℞ **Aminosalicylates**, ℞ **chloramphenicol**, colchicine, and alcohol may reduce the effects of cyanocobalamin.

Side effects
• There may be skin itching in overdose, also fever, headache, chills, hot flushes, dizziness, allergic reactions, and diarrhea.

Cyanoject ⑧
A preparation of ⚕ **cyanocobalamin**.
Formulation: Injection.
Availability: Prescription only.

Warnings and side effects: See ⚕ **cyanocobalamin**.

cyclizine ⓖ
Type/Group: **antihistamine; antinauseant**.
Brand(s): Marezine.
How administered: Orally.

Used to treat
Cyclizine is used to prevent and treat the nausea, vomiting, and dizziness of ◑ **motion sickness**.

Warnings
• It should not be given to people with known hypersensitivity to this drug (or with known sensitivity to other antihistamines) or with severe heart failure.
• Antihistamines should be given with caution to people with lower respiratory disease or asthma (and never during an attack), heart disease, hypertension, hyperthyroidism, epilepsy, porphyria, increased intraocular pressure (pressure in the eyeball, as in glaucoma), enlarged prostate, urinary retention, or certain obstructive bladder or gastrointestinal conditions.
• Cyclizine should be used during pregnancy only if the potential benefit outweighs the possible risk to the fetus.
• Nursing mothers should discontinue using this drug or discontinue breast-feeding.
• This drug must not be given to infants, and for children under the age of 12 the manufacturer's or medical instructions must be followed closely.
• Because of its sedative side effects, the performance of skilled tasks, such as driving, may be impaired.
• Side effects are more frequent in the elderly.

Interactions
• ℞ **MAOI** antidepressants may prolong and intensify the ℞ **anticholinergic** effects of antihistamines (see Side effects below).
• If used with ℞ **tricyclic** antidepressants, other antihistamines, ℞ **skeletal muscle relaxants**, ℞ **opioids**, ℞ **barbiturates**, ℞ **hypnotics**, ℞ **sedatives**, or ℞ **antianxiety** drugs, there is a risk of intensified side effects.
• Alcohol may intensify side effects such as drowsiness and impaired mental alertness.

Side effects
• These depend on how it is administered. For this type of antihistamine, there is commonly drowsiness, headache, impaired muscular coordination or dizziness, and anticholinergic effects (dry mouth, blurred vision, urinary retention, gastrointestinal disturbances).
• Less frequently, rashes and photosensitivity (abnormal sensitivity to light), palpitations and heart arrhythmias.
• Rarely, there may be stimulation instead of sedation (paradoxical stimulation), especially in children (and convulsions in overdose), hypersensitivity reactions, blood disorders, liver disturbances, depression, sleep disturbances, and hypotension.

cyclobenzaprine ⓖ
Type/Group: **skeletal muscle relaxant**.
Brand(s): Flexeril; various generic.

Key to symbols: ⓓ = Drug type/group   ⓖ = Generic name   ⑧ = Brand name

How administered: Orally.
Used to treat
Cyclobenzaprine is a skeletal muscle relaxant that can be used as an additional treatment along with other measures (such as rest and physical therapy) for the relief of acute muscle pain. It works by an action on the central nervous system.
Warnings
• It should not be used by people with known hypersensitivity to cyclobenzaprine, or who have certain heart conditions, intermittent porphyria or thyroid disease.
• It should be given with caution to people with kidney or liver disease, a history of urinary retention, angle-closure glaucoma, increased ocular pressure, or who are elderly (increased risk of anticholinergic side effects).
• It should be used during pregnancy only if clearly needed.
• Medical judgment is required if breast-feeding is being considered. It is not known whether this drug is excreted in breast milk.
• It should be used for only short period (2 to 3 weeks).
• It may impair the perfomance of skilled tasks, such as driving.
• Alcohol and other CNS depressants should be avoided.
Interactions
• Cyclobenzaprine is similar in structure to ℞ **tricyclic** antidepressants, which can cause serious or fatal reactions if taken with ℞ **MAOI** antidepressants. Because this drug could interact in a similar way, it should not be used, or within 14 days of discontinuing, MAOIs.
• ℞ **tricyclic** antidepressants may increase the risk of side effects and overdosage.
Side effects
• Commonly, drowsiness, dry mouth, and dizziness.
• Rarely, fatigue, tiredness, weakness, blurred vision, headache, nervousness, confusion, gastrointestinal upsets, and disorders of heart rhythm.

Cyclogyl Ⓑ
A preparation of ℞ **cyclopentolate hydrochloride**.
Formulation: Ophthalmic solution.
Availability: Prescription only.
Warnings and side effects: See ℞ **cyclopentolate hydrochloride**.

cyclopentolate hydrochloride Ⓖ
Type/Group: **anticholinergic; cycloplegic; mydriatic**.
Brand(s): Cyclogyl; AK-Pentolate; Pentolair; various generic.
How administered: Topically (eye).
Used to treat
Cyclopentolate is used to dilate the pupil and paralyze the focusing of the eye for ophthalmic examinations.
Warnings
• It should not be given to people with narrow-angle glaucoma.
• It should be given with caution to people over 65, because they are more at risk of increased intraocular pressure (pressure in the eyeball). Also, use with caution in children as this drug has been associated with mental and behavioral disturbances in children.
• Cyclopentolate should be used during pregnancy only when it is clearly needed and when the potential benefits outweigh the risks to the fetus.
• Medical judgment is required if breast-feeding is being considered. It is not known whether this drug appears in breast milk.
• It may cause blurred vision. Any skilled task, such as driving, should be avoided while the pupils are dilated.
Interactions
No significant interactions specific to this drug are known.
Side effects
• Increased intraocular pressure, stinging, burning, irritation of eyes, dry mouth and skin, light sensitivity, speeded heartbeat, central nervous system disturbances, fever, flushing, respiratory depression, abdominal discomfort, and irregular pulse.

cyclophosphamide Ⓖ
Type/Group: **cytotoxic; anticancer; immunosuppressant**.
Brand(s): Cytoxan; Neosar.
How administered: Orally; injection.
Used to treat
Cyclophosphamide is a cytotoxic drug (an alkylating agent) that is used in the treatment of chronic lymphocytic ✪ **leukemia**, ✪ **lymphomas**, and some solid ✪ **tumors**. It works by interfering with DNA and so preventing normal cell replication. Although not stated by the manufacturer for such use, it can also be used as an immunosuppressant for complicated ✪ **rheumatoid arthritis** and other connective tissue diseases.
Warnings
• It should not be given to people with known hypersensitivity to cyclophosphamide, or with suppressed bone marrow function.
• It should be given with caution to people with kidney or liver dysfunction or certain blood disorders, and anyone who has previously had radiation therapy or chemotherapy. This is a specialist drug which will be used following a full evaluation by specialist physicians.
• Cyclophosphamide is not recommended for use during pregnancy unless it is medically judged to be essential, because it may cause birth defects. Becoming pregnant while using this drug must be avoided.
• It should not be used if breast-feeding.
• It causes blood changes that may reduce resistance to infection.
• In common with many anticancer drugs this drug is associated with the development of secondary malignancies (new cancers).
• Heart damage is possible at high doses.
• It may interfere with wound healing.
• Inform your physician if you experience unusual bleeding or bruising, fever, nausea, skin rash, chills, sore throat, shortness or breath, cough or wheezing, amenorrhea, unusual lumps, joint, stomach, flank pain, sores in mouth or yellowing skin or eyes.
• It can impair fertility in men and women (which may be reversible).
Interactions
• ℞ **thiazide** ℞ **diuretics** increase the level of side effects.
• The effects of ℞ **digoxin** and ℞ **quinolones** may be decreased.

Key to symbols: ✪ = Disorder Section ℞ = Drug Section ♣ = Herbal Section ♊ = Supplement Section

• The effects of ℞ **succinylcholine**, ℞ **doxorubicin hydrochloride**, and ℞ **anticoagulants** may be enhanced.
• ℞ **chloramphenicol** and ℞ **phenobarbital** may reduce the levels of cyclophosphamide.

Side effects
• Frequently, nausea, vomiting several hours after administration, and hair loss.
• Occasionally, diarrhea, darkening of the skin or fingernails, mucosal irritation, mouth ulcers, headache, sweating.
• Rarely, severe allergic reaction, colitis with bleeding, pain and redness at injection site, bladder and kidney infections.

cycloplegic ⒟

Generics: **cyclopentolate hydrochloride; homatropine hydrobromide; tropicamide.**

Actions and uses
Cycloplegic drugs paralyze the focusing muscles of the eye, and are used for certain ophthalmic examinations. Those used are ℞ **anticholinergic** (antimuscarinic) drugs, including ℞ **atropine sulfate**, ℞ **homatropine hydrobromide**, ℞ **tropicamide**, and ℞ **cyclopentolate hydrochloride**.

Limitations
These drugs are most commonly used as ℞ **mydriatic** agents, in order to dilate the pupil for ophthalmic examination or to treat certain inflammatory conditions of the eye, but also where the muscles of the pupil need to be paralyzed. The disadvantage of these drugs is that if they have a long duration of action, they may trigger an attack of ✪ **glaucoma** in susceptible people.

cycloserine ⒢

Type/Group: **antibacterial; antituberculosis.**
Brand(s): Seromycin.
How administered: Orally.

Used to treat
Cycloserine is used specifically in the treatment of ✪ **tuberculosis** that is resistant to the powerful drugs ordinarily used first, or in cases where those drugs are not tolerated, and like all antituberculosis drugs it is taken with other effective chemotherapy. It is also used for acute urinary tract infections, especially when more conventional treatments have failed.

Warnings
• It should not be given to people with known hypersensitivity to cycloserine, or with epilepsy, depression, severe anxiety, psychosis, chronic alcoholism, or severe kidney insufficiency.
• Cycloserine should be used during pregnancy only when it is clearly needed.
• Medical judgment is required if breast-feeding is being considered.
• It may cause CNS (central nervous system) toxicity (for example, convulsions, psychosis, somnolence, depression, confusion, headache, tremor). The risk of convulsions is increased in alcoholics.
• Alcohol should be avoided while taking this drug.

Interactions
• ℞ **isoniazid** increases the risk of CNS toxicity.

Side effects
• Headache, dizziness, drowsiness, depression, convulsions, tremor, allergic dermatitis, and effects on blood components and the liver.
• Rarely, seizure and congestive heart failure.

cyclosporine ⒢

(ciclosporin)
Type/Group: **antirheumatic; immunosuppressant.**
Brand(s): Gengraf; Neoral; Sandimmune; SangCya; generic.
How administered: Orally; intravenous infusion.

Used to treat
Cyclosporine is used particularly to limit tissue rejection during and following organ transplant surgery. It can also be used to treat severe, active ✪ **rheumatoid arthritis** and some skin conditions such as severe, resistant atopic ✪ **dermatitis** and (under special supervision) ✪ **psoriasis**. It has very little effect on the blood-cell producing capacity of the bone marrow, but does have kidney toxicity.

Warnings
• It should not be given to people with known hypersensitivity to this drug (or when injected, other ingredients in the injection). When used to treat rheumatoid arthritis, cyclosporine should not be used by anyone with kidney impairment, uncontrolled high blood pressure, or any kind of malignancy (cancer). This is a specialist drug and is used only after a full medical assessment.
• It is thought that cyclosporine may have the potential to harm the fetus, and it should be used in pregnancy only when the potential benefits outweigh the possible risk to the fetus.
• Medical judgment is required if breast-feeding is being considered.
• Cyclosporine is prescribed only by doctors experienced in immunosuppressive therapy and in settings equipped to monitor and manage the effects of therapy. (Close monitoring of kidney function is necessary, as well as periodic checks of blood values and other vital signs.)
• Treatment with cyclosporine inevitably leaves the body vulnerable to infection.
• There may be a higher vulnerability to certain cancers, as well, and people taking cyclosporine should protect themselves from excessive exposure to the sun.

Interactions
• If taken with ℞ **lovastatin** there is the possibility of muscle breakdown (including heart muscle).
• The levels of ℞ **digoxin** and ℞ **etoposide** may be raised, with the possibility of toxic effects.
• ℞ **Aminoglycosides** (for example, ℞ **gentamicin**, ℞ **tobramycin**), ℞ **amiodarone hydrochloride**, ℞ **amphotericin B**, ℞ **androgens**, ℞ **azoles** (antifungals), ℞ **bromocriptine**, ℞ **calcium-channel blockers**, ℞ **cimetidine**, ℞ **colchicine**, ℞ **diclofenac**, ℞ **oral contraceptives**, ℞ **corticosteroids**, ℞ **foscarnet**, ℞ **macrolide** antibiotics, ℞ **melphalan**, ℞ **metoclopramide**, ℞ **naproxen**, protease inhibitors (for example, ℞ **indinavir**, ℞ **ritonavir**, ℞ **saquinavir**), ℞ **ranitidine**, ℞ **sulindac**, ℞ **tacrolimus**, and ℞ **vancomycin** may increase the

levels of cyclosporine or intensify its effects, with a higher potential for toxicity (particularly for kidney damage).

• Potassium-sparing ℞ **diuretics** (for example, ℞ **amiloride**, ℞ **spironolactone**, ℞ **triamterene**) may cause a serious increase of potassium (hyperkalemia). These drugs should not be used with cyclosporine.

• Other ℞ **immunosuppressants** (but not corticosteroids) increase the risk of infections, or lymphoma and other neoplasms (tumors).

• Live ℞ **vaccines** should not be used during treatment with cyclosporine.

• ℞ **Anticonvulsants** (for example, ℞ **carbamazepine**, ℞ **phenobarbital**, ℞ **phenytoin**), ℞ **nafcillin**, ℞ **octreotide**, probucol, ℞ **rifampin**, ℞ **rifabutin**, ℞ **sulfamethoxazole**, ℞ **terbinafine**, ℞ **ticlopidine**, and ℞ **trimethoprim (TMP)** may decrease the levels or effectiveness of cyclosporine.

• Grapefruit juice may increase levels of cyclosporine, with the potential for toxic effects.

Side effects

These depend on the use and how it is administered.

• The most dangerous effects are, kidney effects (nephrotoxicity), and there may also be changes in blood enzymes, disturbances in liver and cardiovascular function, excessive hair growth, gastrointestinal disturbances, lethargy, tremor, gum growth, edema, fatigue and tingling sensations in the hands and feet, among others. Anaphylactic reactions are quite rare.

Cycofed Pediatric Syrup ®

A preparation of ℞ **codeine phosphate**, ℞ **guaifenesin**, and ℞ **pseudoephedrine**.
Formulation: Oral syrup.
Availability: May or may not require a prescription.
Warnings and side effects: See ℞ **codeine phosphate**; ℞ **guaifenesin**; ℞ **pseudoephedrine**.

Cyklokapron ®

A preparation of ℞ **tranexamic acid**.
Formulation: Oral tablets; injection.
Availability: Prescription only.
Warnings and side effects: See ℞ **tranexamic acid**.

cyproheptadine hydrochloride Ⓖ

Type/Group: **antihistamine; antiallergic**.
Brand(s): Periactin Tablets, Syrup; various generic.
How administered: Orally.

Used to treat

Cyproheptadine is used for the symptomatic relief of allergic symptoms such as ✪ **hay fever** (seasonal allergic rhinitis), perennial rhinitis, vasomotor rhinitis, allergic ✪ **conjunctivitis**, and skin manifestations of ✪ **urticaria** and ✪ **angioedema**. It differs from other antihistamines in having additional actions including as an antagonist of serotonin receptors and as a ℞ **calcium-channel blocker**. Although not stated by the manufacturer for such treatments, it is sometimes prescribed for a wider range of conditions, including as an ℞ **appetite stimulant** and as an ℞ **antimigraine** agent for the prevention of attacks and for cluster headache.

Warnings

• It should not be given to people with known hypersensitivity to this drug (or with known sensitivity to other antihistamines).

• Antihistamines should be given with caution to people with lower respiratory disease or asthma (and never during an attack), heart disease, hypertension, hyperthyroidism, epilepsy, porphyria, increased intraocular pressure (pressure in the eyeball, as in glaucoma), enlarged prostate, urinary retention, or certain obstructive bladder or gastrointestinal conditions.

• Cyproheptadine should be used during pregnancy only if it is clearly needed, but not in the third trimester, as newborns or premature infants may have severe reactions, including convulsions, to antihistamines.

• Nursing mothers should discontinue using this drug or discontinue breast-feeding.

• This drug must not be given to infants, and for children under the age of 12 the manufacturer's or medical instructions must be followed closely.

• Because of its sedative side effects, the performance of skilled tasks, such as driving, may be impaired.

• Side effects are more frequent in the elderly.

Interactions

• ℞ **MAOI** antidepressants may prolong and intensify the ℞ **anticholinergic** effects of antihistamines (see Side effects below).

• If used with ℞ **tricyclic** antidepressants, other antihistamines, ℞ **skeletal muscle relaxants**, ℞ **phenothiazines**, ℞ **opioids**, ℞ **barbiturates**, ℞ **hypnotics**, ℞ **sedatives**, or ℞ **antianxiety** drugs, there is a risk of intensified side effects.

• The effects of ℞ **SSRIs** (for example, ℞ **fluoxetine**) may be lessened or reversed by cyproheptadine.

• Alcohol may intensify side effects such as drowsiness and impaired mental alertness.

Side effects

• These depend on how it is administered. For this type of antihistamine, there is commonly drowsiness, headache, impaired muscular coordination or dizziness, anticholinergic effects (dry mouth, blurred vision, urinary retention, gastrointestinal disturbances), occasional rashes and photosensitivity (abnormal sensitivity to light), palpitations and heart arrhythmias.

• Rarely, there may be stimulation instead of sedation (paradoxical stimulation), especially in children (and convulsions in overdose), hypersensitivity reactions, blood disorders, liver disturbances, depression, sleep disturbances, and hypotension. It may cause weight gain.

Cystex ®

A preparation of ℞ **methenamine**, ℞ **sodium salicylate**, and ℞ **benzoic acid**.
Formulation: Oral Tablets.
Availability: OTC.
Warnings and side effects: See ℞ **methenamine**; ℞ **sodium salicylate**; ℞ **benzoic acid**.

Cystospaz; Cystospaz-M ®

A preparation of ℞ **hyoscyamine** sulfate.
Formulation: Timed release capsules.
Availability: Prescription only.
Warnings and side effects: See ℞ hyoscyamine.

Cytadren ®

A preparation of ℞ **aminoglutethimide**.
Formulation: Tablets.
Availability: Prescription only.
Warnings and side effects: See ℞ aminoglutethimide.

cytarabine ©

Type/Group: **anticancer; cytotoxic.**
Brand(s): Tarabine TFS; Cytosar-U; DepoCyt; various generic.
How administered: Intravenous infusion; injection; intrathecal.

Used to treat

Cytarabine is a cytotoxic drug (an antimetabolite) that is used for acute ○ **leukemias.** It works by interfering with pyrimidine synthesis (a chemical needed for cell replication/DNA) and so prevents cell replication.

Warnings

• It should not be given to people with known hypersensitivity to cytarabine.
• It should be given with caution to people with impaired liver or kidney function. This is a specialist drug which will be used following a full evaluation by specialist physicians.
• Cytarabine is not recommended for use during pregnancy unless it is medically judged to be essential, because it may cause birth defects. Becoming pregnant while using this drug must be avoided.
• It should not be used if breast-feeding.
• It can cause bone marrow depression, which may lead to bleeding and a reduced resistance to infection.
• When used in the encapsulated form given directly into the cerebrospinal fluid, chemical arachnitis (a syndrome characterized by nausea, vomiting, headache, and fever) is common and must be treated.
• It may cause adverse CNS (central nervous system) effects. A doctor must be contacted if signs of neurotoxicity (for example, gait disturbances, handwriting difficulties, numbness) develop.
• Some people have had serious allergic reactions to this drug.
• At high doses, severe adverse effects on the CNS, gastrointestinal system, and lungs may occur.

Interactions

• The effects of ℞ **digoxin** and ℞ **gentamicin** may be reduced.

Side effects

• Gastrointestinal problems, oral or anal inflammation, headache, liver dysfunction, fever, rash, blood clots, or bleeding. "Cytarabine syndrome" (fever, pain in bones and/or joints, and occasionally chest pain, rash, eye inflammations, and malaise) may occur 6 to 12 hours after treatment.

Cytomel ®

A preparation of ℞ **liothyronine**.

Formulation: Tablets in several strengths.
Availability: Prescription only.
Warnings and side effects: See ℞ liothyronine.

cytoprotectant ⓓ

Generics: **dexrazoxane; mesna; sucralfate.**

Actions and uses

℞ **Cytoprotectants** have the capacity to protect tissue from damage. The term is most commonly used for drugs with the capacity to protect the gastric mucosa (the lining of the stomach) by forming a cytoprotectant barrier over an ○ **ulcer,** so protecting it from acid, bile salts, and the enzyme pepsin which can cause erosion and pain in ○ **peptic ulcers,** and so allowing it to heal. They may be used as long-term ℞ **ulcer-healing drugs,** as well as providing short-term relief from discomfort and helping relive stress-ulceration. They may also be used to treat esophageal ulceration and inflammation.
Sometimes the term cytoprotectant is used to include drugs (such as ℞ **dexrazoxane,** ℞ **mesna** and ℞ **dexrazoxane**) that are taken along with ℞ **cytotoxic** drugs when used in the treatment of cancer to reduce the incidence and severity of tissue damage toxicity.

Limitations

See the individual drug entries.

Cytosar-U ®

A preparation of ℞ **cytarabine**.
Formulation: Powder or vial for injection.
Availability: Prescription only.
Warnings and side effects: See ℞ cytarabine.

Cytotec ®

A preparation of ℞ **misoprostol**.
Formulation: Oral tablets, available in two strengths.
Availability: Prescription only.
Warnings and side effects: See ℞ misoprostol.

cytotoxic ⓓ

Generics: **altretamine; azathioprine; bleomycin; busulfan; carboplatin; carmustine; chlorambucil; cyclophosphamide; cladribine; cisplatin; cytarabine; cyclosporine; dacarbazine; dactinomycin; daunorubicin; docetaxel; doxorubicin hydrochloride; epirubicin hydrochloride; fludarabine phosphate; fluorouracil; gemcitabine; hydroxyurea; idarubicin hydrochloride; irinotecan hydrochloride; lomustine; mechlorethamine hydrochloride; melphalan; methotrexate; mercaptopurine; mitomycin; mitoxantrone; paclitaxel; pentostatin; procarbazine; rituximab; thiotepa; thioguanine; topotecan; valrubicin; vinblastine sulfate; vincristine sulfate; vindesine sulfate; vinorelbine tartrate.**

Actions and uses

℞ **cytotoxic** drugs are used mainly in the treatment of ○ **cancer** and are the biggest group of ℞ **anticancer** drugs. They have the essential property of preventing cell replication and so inhibiting the growth of cancerous tumors or of excess production of cells in body fluids. There are several mechanisms by which they do this, but in every case they inevitably also affect the growth of normal (non-cancerous) healthy cells and cause toxic side effects.

The most-used cytotoxics are the alkylating agents, which work by interfering with the action of DNA in cell replication (including ℞ **busulfan**, ℞ **carmustine**, ℞ **chlorambucil**, ℞ **cyclophospha-mide**, ℞ **lomustine**, ℞ **melphalan**, ℞ **mechlorethamine hydro-chloride**, and ℞ **thiotepa**).

The ℞ **vinca alkaloid** drugs (for example, ℞ **vinblastine sulfate**, ℞ **vincristine sulfate**, ℞ **vindesine sulfate**, and ℞ **vinorelbine tartrate**) are also effective cytotoxics and work by arresting division (metaphase of miosis) in new-forming cells, however, they have severe side effects, such as damage to peripheral nerves, which limits their use.

A number of cytotoxics chemically are ℞ **antibiotic** in origin (although their ℞ **antimicrobial** properties are not relevant) which work by a direct action on DNA (for example, ℞ **bleomycin**, ℞ **dactinomycin**, ℞ **daunorubicin**, ℞ **doxorubicin hydrochlo-ride**, ℞ **epirubicin**, ℞ **idarubicin hydrochloride**, ℞ **mitomycin**, ℞ **mitoxantrone**, ℞ **pentostatin**). Some other cyctotoxics are referred to as antimetabolites because they combine with cellular components and interfere with the metabolic pathways involved in DNA synthesis and so prevent cellular division (for example, ℞ **cladribine**, ℞ **cytarabine**, ℞ **fludarabine phosphate**, ℞ **gem-citabine**, ℞ **mercaptopurine**, ℞ **methotrexate**, and ℞ **thiogua-nine**). A new development has been the taxane drugs which are based on a chemical found in the yew tree, and these show promise in the treatment of ovarian and breast cancer (for example, ℞ **paclitaxel** and ℞ **docetaxel**). Another new group is the topoi-somerase I inhibitors (for example, ℞ **irinotecan hydrochloride** and ℞ **topotecan**) which act on an enzyme involved in DNA rep-lication.

℞ **rituximab** is one of a relatively new class of drug, a monoclonal antibody, which causes lysis (destruction) of B lymphocytes and so it can be described as a specific cytotoxic agent with defined ℞ **immunosuppressant** actions. It is used to treat chemotherapy-resistant or recurrent follicular non-Hodgkin's lymphoma.

There are some cytotoxics that are not only used in the treatment of cancer, but also as ℞ **immunosuppressant** drugs to limit tissue rejection during and following transplant surgery and in the treat-ment of autoimmune diseases, such as ✪ **rheumatoid arthritis** and lupus erythematosus (see ✪ **lupus**). Of these, some are, in practice, used for both purposes (for example, ℞ **chlorambucil** and ℞ **cyclophosphamide**), and others for immunosuppression alone (℞ **azathiaprine**, ℞ **cyclosporine**, ℞ **methotrexate**).

Limitations

As mentioned, cytotoxic anticancer drugs cause profound changes in cellular metabolism in the body. They inevitably also affect the growth of normal healthy cells and cause many toxic side effects. Normally, myelosuppression (a reduction in blood-cell production of the bone marrow, including leukocytes and so decreased resis-tance to infection) is one of the most serious side effects, but con-versely this is the cytotoxic effect exploited in cytotoxic drug treatment of leukemias. Some of the serious discomfort experi-enced by people undergoing cancer treatment, for instance nau-sea, vomiting and hair loss, can be minimized by careful adjustment

of chemotherapy and radiotherapy regimens. Other side effects can include impaired healing of wounds, depression of growth in children, and damage to the lining (epithelium) of the gastrointes-tinal tract, sterility, kidney damage, and some drugs may even cause cancer themselves, for example, ℞ **altretamine** can cause secondary malignancies (new cancers) and this will monitored. The use of live vaccine immunization while taking cytotoxics is danger-ous.

When taking cytotoxic anticancer drugs, such as alkylators and antimetabolites, contraceptive measures must be taken. Most of these drugs are in the Food and Drug Administration's Pregnancy Category D, that is, they are not recommended for use during pregnancy, unless medically judged to be essential, because they may cause birth defects. Also, breast-feeding should be avoided because of the potential for harming the infant.

See also the individual drug entries.

Cytovene ®

A preparation of ℞ **ganciclovir (DHPG)**.
Formulation: Oral capsules, powder for injection.
Availability: Prescription only.
Warnings and side effects: See ℞ **ganciclovir (DHPG)**.

Cytoxan ®

A preparation of ℞ **cyclophosphamide**.
Formulation: Oral tablets; powder for injection.
Availability: Prescription only.
Warnings and side effects: See ℞ **cyclophosphamide**.

Cytra-2; Cytra-3; Citra-K; Cytra-LC ®

A preparation of ℞ **citrates**.
Formulation: Oral solution.
Availability: Prescription only.
Warnings and side effects: See ℞ **citrates**.

d4T ⑥

see ℞ **stavudine**.

dacarbazine ⑥

Type/Group: **anticancer; cytotoxic**.
Brand(s): DTIC-Dome.
How administered: Injection.

Used to treat

Dacarbazine is used comparatively rarely because of its high toxic-ity. It may be used to treat the skin (mole) cancer ✪ **melanoma** and, in combination with other anticancer drugs, the lymphatic cancer ✪ **Hodgkin's disease**. Although not stated by the manufac-turer for such use, it may also be prescribed, in combination with other drugs, to treat some soft-tissue sarcomas (see ✪ **cancer**).

Warnings

• It should not be given to people with known hypersensitivity dacarbazine. This is a specialist drug which will be used following a full evaluation by specialist physicians.

• Dacarbazine is not recommended for use during pregnancy unless it is medically judged to be essential, because it may cause

Key to symbols: ✪ = Disorder Section ℞ = Drug Section ♣ = Herbal Section ⚗ = Supplement Section

birth defects. Becoming pregnant while using this drug must be avoided.

• It should not be used if breast-feeding.

• It can cause bone marrow depression, which may lead to bleeding and a reduced resistance to infection.

• In common with many anticancer drugs, dacarbazine may cause cancer.

Interactions
No interactions specific to this drug are known.

Side effects
• Frequently, nausea, vomiting, and loss of appetite.

• Occasionally, facial flushing, tingling sensations, hair loss, flu-like syndrome, skin reactions, CNS (central nervous system) symptoms (for example, confusion, blurred vision).

• Rarely, diarrhea, inflammation of mouth mucosa, burning or redness of mouth, gums or tongue, intractable nausea and vomiting, light sensitivity, and severe allergic reaction.

daclizumab
Type/Group: **immunosuppressant**.
Brand(s): Zenapax.
How administered: Intravenous infusion.

Used to treat
Daclizumab is one of a relatively new class of drug, a monoclonal antibody (a form of pure antibody produced by a type of molecular engineering). In this case the cloned antibody is one that prevents proliferation of the white blood cells, T-lymphocytes, which have an important role in immunity and cell rejection. It is used for prophylaxis (prevention) of rejection in kidney transplantation, and is used together with ℞ **cyclosporine** and ℞ **corticosteroids**.

Warnings
• It should not be given to people with known hypersensitivity to this drug or to any product prepared with mouse protein. This is a specialist drug and is used only after a full medical assessment.

• The effects of daclizumab in pregnancy are not known, but adverse effects on the fetus are thought possible. It should be used only if the potential benefit outweighs the possible risk to the fetus. Women of childbearing potential should use effective contraception during treatment and for two months afterwards.

• Medical judgment is required if breast-feeding is being considered.

• Daclizumab is prescribed only by specialists in immunosuppressive therapy and used under qualified supervision.

• It is not known whether this drug has long-term effects on the immune system's response to new antigens (for example, viruses or bacteria that were not previously encountered by the body's defenses).

• Anyone receiving immunosuppressive treatment may have a greater risk of opportunistic infection and lymphoproliferative disorders, although no higher risk is now associated with daclizumab.

Interactions
No drug interactions of significance are known.

Side effects
This drug is still under evaluation and side effects that probably or possibly are associated with it have not been identified. (And since it is used in combination with cyclosporine and corticosteroids, and only in people undergoing major surgery, any immediate side effects it may have are difficult to distinguish.)

dactinomycin
(actinomycin D; ACT)
Type/Group: **anticancer**; **cytotoxic**.
Brand(s): Cosmegen.
How administered: Injection; intrapleural infusion.

Used to treat
Dactinomycin is a cytotoxic (an antibiotic in origin) that is used particularly to treat ✪ **cancer** in children.

Warnings
• It should not be given to people with chicken pox or herpes zoster, because a severe, potentially fatal generalized disease could occur. This is a specialist drug which will be used following a full evaluation by specialist physicians.

• It is not recommended for use during pregnancy unless it is medically judged to be essential, because it may cause birth defects. Becoming pregnant while using this drug must be avoided.

• It should not be used if breast-feeding.

• It is associated with many abnormalities of kidney, liver, and bone marrow function.

• In common with many anticancer drugs, dactinomycin may cause cancer or genetic mutations in cells.

Interactions
• Radiation may worsen adverse side effects, including the incidence of secondary cancers.

Side effects
• Frequently, nausea and vomiting, irritation of skin, mouth, or throat, and rash.

• Occasionally, loss of appetite, loss of hearing, and abdominal distress.

D.A. II Tablets; Chew Tabs ⓑ
A preparation of methscopolamine nitrate, ℞ **chlorpheniramine maleate**, and ℞ **phenylephrine hydrochloride**.
Formulation: Oral tablets.
Availability: Prescription only.
Warnings and side effects: See ℞ **scopolamine hydrobromide**; ℞ **chlorpheniramine maleate**; ℞ **phenylephrine hydrochloride**.

Dakin's ⓑ
A preparation of ℞ **sodium hypochlorite**.
Formulation: Topical solution.
Availability: OTC.
Warnings and side effects: See ℞ **sodium hypochlorite**.

Dalalone; Dalalone DP; Dalalone LA ⓑ
A preparation of ℞ **dexamethasone** acetate (Dalalone DP, Dalalone LA) and dexamethasone sodium phosphate (Dalalone).

Formulation: Injection.
Availability: Prescription only.
Warnings and side effects: See ℞ **dexamethasone**.

Dallergy-D Syrup ⓑ

A preparation of ℞ **phenylephrine hydrochloride** and
℞ **chlorpheniramine maleate**.
Formulation: Oral syrup.
Availability: OTC.
Warnings and side effects: See ℞ **phenylephrine hydrochloride**;
℞ **chlorpheniramine maleate**.

Dallergy-JR Capsules ⓑ

A preparation of ℞ **pseudoephedrine** and ℞ **brompheniramine
maleate**.
Formulation: Oral capsules, sustained release.
Availability: Prescription only.
Warnings and side effects: See ℞ **pseudoephedrine**;
℞ **brompheniramine maleate**.

Dallergy Tablets; Dallergy Syrup ⓑ

A preparation of methscopolamine nitrate, ℞ **chlorpheniramine
maleate**, and ℞ **phenylephrine hydrochloride**.
Formulation: Oral tablets; syrup.
Availability: Prescription only.
Warnings and side effects: See ℞ **scopolamine hydrobromide**;
℞ **chlorpheniramine maleate**; ℞ **phenylephrine hydrochloride**.

Dalmane ⓑ

A preparation of ℞ **flurazepam**.
Formulation: Oral capsules in several strengths.
Availability: Prescription only.
Warnings and side effects: See ℞ **flurazepam**.

dalteparin sodium ⓖ

Type/Group: anticoagulant.
Brand(s): Fragmin.
How administered: Injection (subcutaneous).

Used to treat

Dalteparin sodium is a low molecular weight heparin, an anticoagulant. It can be to prevent ✺ **deep vein thrombosis** after hip
replacement or abdominal surgery (in certain at-risk patients), to
lower the chance of complications from embolism. When administered with ℞ **aspirin**, it may be used to reduce the risk of ischemic
complications in certain acute cardiac conditions.

Warnings

• It should not be given to people with known hypersensitivity to
this drug or to pork products, or where lab testing shows antibodies
to platelets when taking this drug. It will be administered by
experienced personnel after a full medical assessment.
• It should be given with caution to people with an increased risk
of hemorrhage (for example, uncontrolled hypertension, bleeding
disorders, active ulcer, recent stroke, or surgery), and in those who
have experienced a reduction of platelet (thrombocyte) levels after
taking heparin. It also should be used with caution in people with

a tendency to bleed or recent gastrointestinal bleeding, with low
thrombocyte levels or platelet defects, or with severe kidney or liver
impairment.
• It should be used during pregnancy only if it is clearly needed.
• Medical judgment is required if breast-feeding is being
considered. It is not known whether this drug appears in breast
milk.

Interactions

• If taken with other anticoagulants, antiplatelet agents, or
℞ **NSAID**s, there is a higher risk for bleeding (caution is advised).

Side effects

• The most common are hematoma (a trapped accumulation of
blood) at the injection site and post-operative bleeding, which may
occasionally occur at non-surgical sites, particularly in the
gastrointestinal tract.
• Changes in liver function may occur and hyperkalemia (high
blood potassium levels) has been reported. Rarely, allergic
reactions (for example, rash, itching, fever) and very rarely,
anaphylaxis.

Damason-P Tablets ⓑ

A preparation of ℞ **hydrocodone bitartrate** and ℞ **aspirin**.
Formulation: Oral tablets.
Availability: Prescription only.
Warnings and side effects: See ℞ **hydrocodone bitartrate**;
℞ **aspirin**.

danaparoid sodium ⓖ

Type/Group: **anticoagulant**.
Brand(s): Organ.
How administered: Injection (subcutaneous).

Used to treat

Danaparoid is a heparinoid, derived from the same substances as
℞ **heparin**, but excluding certain components. Some people who
are hypersensitive to heparin itself can tolerate this drug. It can be
used to prevent ✺ **deep vein thrombosis** after hip replacement
surgery, to reduce the chance of complications from embolism.

Warnings

• It should not be given to people with known hypersensitivity to
this drug or pork products, or anyone with hemophilia or major
active bleeding site. It will be administered by experienced
personnel after a full medical assessment.
• It should be given with caution to people with an increased risk
of hemorrhage (for example, uncontrolled hypertension, bleeding
disorders, active ulcer, recent stroke, or surgery), or with severe
kidney impairment.
• Danaparoid should be used during pregnancy only if it is clearly
needed.
• Medical judgment is required if breast-feeding is being
considered. It is not known whether this drug appears in breast
milk.
• There is a risk that administration of spinal or epidural anesthesia,
or other spinal puncture procedures, may result in bleeding
(hematoma) and paralysis in people taking danaparoid.

Interactions

• If taken with other anticoagulants, antiplatelet agents, or ℞ **NSAIDs**, there is a higher risk for bleeding (caution is advised).

Side effects

• The most common is post-operative bleeding, which may occasionally occur at non-surgical sites, particularly in the gastrointestinal tract. Other common side effects may include fever, gastrointestinal disturbances (for example, nausea, constipation, vomiting), rash, and itching.

• Less frequently, edema, insomnia, headache, dizziness, urinary tract infection and urine retention, and joint pain. At the site of injection there may be pain, irritation or hematoma (a trapped accumulation of blood). Anemia may occur.

danazol Ⓖ

Type/Group: **androgen; antiestrogen**.
Brand(s): Danocrine.
How administered: Orally.

Used to treat

Danazol has weak androgen effects that inhibits output of the ℞ **gonadotrophins**, FSH and LH, and is used to treat ✿ **endometriosis** (a growth of the lining of the uterus at inappropriate sites) and symptoms of fibrocystic breast disease. It is also used to prevent attacks of hereditary ✿ **angioedema** (characterized by swelling in extremities, abdominal pain, and potentially fatal swelling of the larynx) in males and females. Although not stated by the manufacturer for such use, danazol may be prescribed to treat precocious puberty, male breast growth, and excessive or prolonged menstruation.

Warnings

• It should not be used by people with undiagnosed abnormal genital bleeding, porphyria, or markedly impaired liver, kidney or heart function.

• It should be given with caution to people with breast cancer, epilepsy, migraine, or heart, kidney, or liver dysfunction.

• Danazol must not be used during pregnancy, and pregnancy must be ruled out before beginning treatment. It may cause masculinization of a female fetus.

• It should not be used by nursing mothers.

• Long-term use might lead to toxicity.

• Blood clots, embolisms strokes, and benign intracranial hypertension (elevated blood pressure in the head) have been reported.

• Serious liver disease may develop with prolonged use.

• Use a nonhormonal method of contraception during treatment.

Interactions

• Response to oral ℞ **anticoagulants** (for example, ℞ **warfarin sodium**) may be increased.

• ℞ **insulin** requirements in diabetics may increase.

Side effects

• Female virilization (deepening voice, growth of body hair, acne, clitoral enlargement, irregular periods), pancreatitis, fluid retention, dizziness, increased emotionality, nervousness, sleep disorders, elevated blood pressure, gastrointestinal effects, flushing, sweating, glucose intolerance, weight gain.

Danocrine Ⓑ

A preparation of ℞ **danazol**.
Formulation: Oral capsules in several strengths.
Availability: Prescription only.
Warnings and side effects: See ℞ **danazol**.

Dantrium Ⓑ

A preparation of ℞ **dantrolene sodium**.
Formulation: Oral; injection.
Availability: Prescription only.
Warnings and side effects: See ℞ **dantrolene sodium**.

dantrolene sodium Ⓖ

Type/Group: **skeletal muscle relaxant**.
Brand(s): Dantrium.
How administered: Orally; injection.

Used to treat

Dantrolene sodium acts directly on skeletal muscle and can be used for relieving severe spasticity of muscles in spasm, resulting from upper neuron disorders such as spinal cord injury, cerebral palsy, or multiple sclerosis. It is also used in the treatment of malignant hyperthermia (a rare, but serious complication of anesthesia). Although not stated by the manufacturers for such use, it may be prescribed for exercise-induced muscle pain, neuroleptic malignant syndrome (a potentially life-threatening reaction to antipsychotic drugs), or heatstroke.

Warnings

• It should not be used by people with known hypersensitivity to dantrolene, active liver disease, or those in whom spasticity is helpful for sustaining balance in walking or for increased function, or spasticity that results from rheumatic disorders.

• It should be given with caution to people with a history of liver disease or dysfunction, or with impaired heart, liver, or lung function.

• It should be used during pregnancy only if medically judged that the benefits outweigh the risks to the fetus.

• It should not be used by breast-feeding mothers.

• It may cause liver damage. The risk appears to be greater in women over 35, and in people taking other medication along with dantrolene.

• Alcohol and other CNS depressants should be avoided.

• It may impair the perfomance of skilled tasks, such as driving.

• Exposure to sunlight may cause photosensitivity.

Interactions

• ℞ **clofibrate** and ℞ **warfarin** may reduce the effects of dantrolene.

• Although a link has not definitely been established, liver damage may occur more frequently in women over 35 who are taking ℞ **estrogens** (for example, in the oral contraceptive pill, and HRT).

• If taken with ℞ **verapamil**, there is a possibility of elevated potassium levels and depression of heart muscle function.

Side effects

• Commonly, drowsiness, dizziness, weakness, general malaise, fatigue, and diarrhea (these usually occur only during early treatment).

• Occasionally, confusion, headache, insomnia, constipation, and urinary frequency.

• Rarely, CNS excitement or restlessness, tingling sensation, ringing in ears, slurred speech, tremor, blurred vision, dry mouth, bedwetting, impotence, and potentially serious side effects such as gastrointestinal bleeding, liver damage, and pulmonary edema.

Dapacin Capsules ℞

A preparation of ℞ **acetaminophen**.
Formulation: Oral capsules.
Availability: OTC.
Warnings and side effects: See ℞ **acetaminophen**.

dapsone ⓖ

Type/Group: antibacterial; antimalarial; amebicide and antiprotozoal.
Brand(s): Generic.
How administered: Orally.

Used to treat

Dapsone is a ℞ **sulfone** used in the treatment of ✪ **leprosy**, and also to treat dermatitis herpetiformis (a chronic skin disease). Although not stated by the manufacturer for such use, dapsone may also be prescribed for *Pneumocystis carinii* ✪ **pneumonia** (PCP), to prevent travelers in tropical regions from contracting ✪ **malaria**, and as an immunosuppressive agent (for relapsing polychondritis and systemic lupus erythematosus: see ✪ **lupus**). Dapsone also has been used to treat various serious skin conditions.

Warnings

• It should not be given to people with known hypersensitivity to dapsone.

• It should be given with caution to people with kidney or liver disease, G6PD- or methemoglobin reductase deficiencies (genetic enzyme disorders), or severe cardiopulmonary disease.

• Dapsone should be used during pregnancy only if it is clearly needed.

• It is not recommended for use while nursing. It does appear in breast milk.

• Serious blood disorders have been known to occur.

• It may cause serious allergic skin reactions.

• It can cause kidney or liver damage.

• As dapsone may cause photosensitivity, prolonged exposure to sunlight or sunlamps should be avoided.

Interactions

• ℞ **activated charcoal**, ℞ **didanosine (ddI)**, para-aminobenzoic acid, and ℞ **rifampin** may reduce the effects of dapsone.

• Folic acid antagonists (for example, ℞ **pyrimethamine**) and ℞ **probenecid** may increase the effects, especially blood-related side effects, of dapsone.

• If used with ℞ **trimethoprim (TMP)**, the levels and effects of both drugs may be increased.

Side effects

• Nausea, vomiting, loss of appetite, and photosensitivity (increased sensitivity to sun or ultraviolet light).

• Less frequently, tingling in extremities, drug-induced lupus erythematosus, or nerve disorders.

Darvocet-N ℞

A preparation of propoxyphene napsylate and ℞ **acetaminophen**.
Formulation: Oral tablets; available in two strengths.
Availability: Prescription only.
Warnings and side effects: See ℞ **propoxyphene hydrochloride**; ℞ **acetaminophen**.

Darvon Compound-65 Pulvules ℞

A preparation of ℞ **propoxyphene hydrochloride**, ℞ **aspirin**, and ℞ **caffeine**.
Formulation: Oral capsules.
Availability: Prescription only.
Warnings and side effects: See ℞ **propoxyphene hydrochloride**; ℞ **aspirin**; ℞ **caffeine**.

Darvon-N ℞

A preparation of propoxyphene napsylate.
Formulation: Oral tablets.
Availability: Prescription only.
Warnings and side effects: See ℞ **propoxyphene hydrochloride**.

Darvon Pulvules ℞

A preparation of ℞ **propoxyphene hydrochloride**.
Formulation: Oral capsules.
Availability: Prescription only.
Warnings and side effects: See ℞ **propoxyphene hydrochloride**.

daunorubicin ⓖ

Type/Group: anticancer; cytotoxic.
Brand(s): DaunoXome; various generic.
How administered: Injection; intravenous infusion.

Used to treat

Daunorubicin is a recently introduced drug (an anthracycline antibiotic in origin) with properties similar to ℞ **doxorubicin hydrochloride**. It is used particularly for advanced HIV-related ✪ **Kaposi's sarcoma** (as daunorubicin citrate liposomal) and for acute ✪ **leukemias** (as daunorubicin hydrochloride).

Warnings

• It should not be given to people with known hypersensitivity to daunorubicin or any of its components.

• It should be given with caution to people with kidney or liver dysfunction, who have had previous chemotherapy or radiation, and those with a history of heart disease. This is a specialist drug which will be used following a full evaluation by specialist physicians.

• Daunorubicin is not recommended for use during pregnancy unless it is medically judged to be essential, because it may cause birth defects. Becoming pregnant while using this drug must be avoided.

• It should not be used if breast-feeding.

• Bone marrow depression is a major toxic side effect of this drug, and may lead to infection or hemorrhage.

• Adverse effects on the heart may occur, particularly at high doses. These may appear during treatment or months or years later.

• It can impair fertility in males (which may be reversible).

• In common with many anticancer drugs, it may cause cancer or genetic mutations in cells.

Interactions

• ℞ cyclophosphamide may increase adverse effects on the heart.

• Other agents that suppress bone marrow may increase such effects.

• ℞ methotrexate and other drugs with adverse effects on liver increase the risk of toxicity.

Side effects

• Frequently, hair loss, gastrointestinal disturbances, and fever.

• Occasionally, inflammation in the mouth and discoloration of fingernails and toenails.

• Rarely, chills.

DaunoXome ⑧

A preparation of ℞ daunorubicin.
Formulation: Injection.
Availability: Prescription only.
Warnings and side effects: See ℞ daunorubicin.

Daypro ⑧

A preparation of ℞ oxaprozin.
Formulation: Oral tablets.
Availability: Prescription only.
Warnings and side effects: See ℞ oxaprozin.

Daypro Caplets ⑧

A preparation of ℞ oxaprozin.
Formulation: Oral tablets.
Availability: Prescription only.
Warnings and side effects: See ℞ oxaprozin.

DDAVP ⑧

A preparation of ℞ desmopressin.
Formulation: Oral tablets; nasal solution; injection.
Availability: Prescription only.
Warnings and side effects: See ℞ desmopressin.

Decadron; Decadron LA ⑧

A preparation of ℞ dexamethasone and dexamethasone acetate (Decadron LA).
Formulation: Oral tablets in several strengths; injection (Decadron LA).
Availability: Prescription only.
Warnings and side effects: See ℞ dexamethasone.

Decadron with Xylocaine ⑧

A preparation of ℞ dexamethasone, ℞ sodium phosphate, and ℞ lidocaine.
Formulation: Injection.
Availability: Prescription only.
Warnings and side effects: See ℞ dexamethasone.

Deca-Durabolin ⑧

A preparation of ℞ nandrolone.
Formulation: Injection.
Availability: Prescription only.
Warnings and side effects: See ℞ nandrolone.

Decaject ⑧

A preparation of ℞ dexamethasone sodium phosphate.
Formulation: Injection.
Availability: Prescription only.
Warnings and side effects: See ℞ dexamethasone.

Decaspray ⑧

A preparation of ℞ dexamethasone.
Formulation: Aerosol spray.
Availability: Prescription only.
Warnings and side effects: See ℞ dexamethasone.

Decholin ⑧

A preparation of ℞ dehydrocholic acid.
Formulation: Oral tablets.
Availability: OTC.
Warnings and side effects: See ℞ dehydrocholic acid.

Declomycin ⑧

A preparation of ℞ demeclocycline.
Formulation: Oral capsules; oral tablets in two strengths.
Availability: Prescription only.
Warnings and side effects: See ℞ demeclocycline.

Decofed Syrup ⑧

A preparation of ℞ pseudoephedrine.
Formulation: Oral syrup.
Availability: OTC.
Warnings and side effects: See ℞ pseudoephedrine.

Decohistine DH Liquid ⑧

A preparation of ℞ codeine phosphate, ℞ pseudoephedrine, and ℞ chlorpheniramine maleate.
Formulation: Oral liquid.
Availability: May or may not require a prescription.
Warnings and side effects: See ℞ codeine phosphate; ℞ pseudoephedrine; ℞ chlorpheniramine maleate.

Deconamine CX Liquid ⑧

A preparation of ℞ hydrocodone bitartrate, ℞ pseudoephedrine, and ℞ guaifenesin.
Formulation: Oral syrup.
Availability: Prescription only.
Warnings and side effects: See ℞ hydrocodone bitartrate; ℞ pseudoephedrine; ℞ guaifenesin.

Deconamine SR Capsules; Tablets; Syrup ⑧

A preparation of ℞ pseudoephedrine and ℞ chlorpheniramine maleate.

Formulation: Oral capsules, sustained release; tablets; syrup.
Availability: Prescription only.
Warnings and side effects: See ℞ **pseudoephedrine;**
℞ **chlorpheniramine maleate.**

decongestant Ⓓ

Generics: **antihistamine; beclomethasone dipropionate; brompheniramine maleate; budesonide; dimenhydrinate; ephedrine; epinephrine; flunisolide; fluticasone propionate; ketotifen; mometasone; naphazoline hydrochloride; nedocromil sodium; oxymetazoline hydrochloride; pheniramine maleate; phenylephrine hydrochloride; pseudoephedrine; tetrahydrozoline hydrochloride; thymol.**

Actions and uses

℞ **decongestant** drugs are used to relieve or reduce the symptoms of congestion of the airways and/or nose. Nasal decongestants are generally applied in the form of nosedrops or as a nasal spray, which avoids the tendency of such drugs to have side effects, such as raising blood pressure, although some are taken by mouth and this side effect can be a problem.

Most decongestants are ℞ **sympathomimetic** agents with a ℞ **vasoconstrictor** action (narrow blood vessels) and work by constricting blood vessels in the mucous membranes of the airways and nasal cavity, so reducing the thickness of this nasal lining, improving drainage and possibly decreasing mucus and fluid secretions. Some of these drugs are direct acting ℞ **alpha-adrenergic stimulant** agents (including ℞ **epinephrine,** ℞ **naphazoline hydrochloride,** ℞ **oxymetazoline hydrochloride,** ℞ **phenylephrine hydrochloride**), others are indirect sympathomimetics that act through releasing norepinephrine from sympathetic nerve endings (for instance, ℞ **pseudoephedrine,** ℞ **ephedrine**).

Rhinitis, especially when caused by an allergy (for example, hay fever), is usually dealt with by using ℞ **antihistamine** agents, which inhibit the detrimental and congestive effects of histamine released by an allergic response. These include; ℞ **dimenhydrinate,** ℞ **brompheniramine maleate,** ℞ **ketotifen,** ℞ **pheniramine maleate.** Other ℞ **antiallergic** drugs may help relieve congestion of the nose (and any eye symptoms that may be present) when applied locally to inhibit the allergic response itself and therefore effectively reduce inflammation (for example, ℞ **cromolyn sodium**). Other antiallergics used topically (externally) include ℞ **corticosteroid** preparations, such as ℞ **beclomethasone dipropionate,** ℞ **flunisolide,** ℞ **fluticasone propionate,** ℞ **budesonide,** and ℞ **mometasone.**

Decongestants are often included in ℞ **cold and cough preparation** remedies that contain a number of other constituents, each one treating or relieving a different symptom. These may include aromatics such as ℞ **thymol,** which has weak decongestant properties when used by inhalation.

Limitations

Drugs for nasal decongestion are generally, and most safely, used in the form of nosedrops or as a nasal spray, which avoids the tendency of such drugs to cause side effects like raised blood pressure that occurs when taken by mouth. However, most people are unaware of this, but it is important to realize that the vasoconstric-

tion, speeding of the heart, and hypertension often caused by sympathomimetic drugs are detrimental and potentially dangerous if taken by people who have certain cardiovascular disorders. Further, sympathomimetics can have serious interactions with a number of other drug classes, especially (℞ **MAOI**) ℞ **antidepressant** drugs. It is better to use topical preparations of vasoconstrictor drugs to minimize systemic side effects (important for those with cardiovascular problems). It is also believed that there may be "rebound" congestion phase after treatment with some decongestants. See also the individual drug entries.

Deconsal II Tablets Ⓑ

A preparation of ℞ **pseudoephedrine** and ℞ **guaifenesin.**
Formulation: Oral tablets, sustained release.
Availability: Prescription only.
Warnings and side effects: See ℞ **pseudoephedrine;**
℞ **guaifenesin.**

Deconsal Pediatric Syrup Ⓑ

A preparation of ℞ **codeine phosphate,** ℞ **guaifenesin,** and ℞ **pseudoephedrine.**
Formulation: Oral syrup.
Availability: May or may not require a prescription.
Warnings and side effects: See ℞ **codeine phosphate;**
℞ **guaifenesin;** ℞ **pseudoephedrine.**

Deconsal Sprinkle Capsules Ⓑ

A preparation of ℞ **phenylephrine hydrochloride** and ℞ **guaifenesin.**
Formulation: Oral capsules, sustained release.
Availability: Prescription only.
Warnings and side effects: See ℞ **phenylephrine hydrochloride;**
℞ **guaifenesin.**

Deep-Down Rub Ⓑ

A preparation of ℞ **methyl salicylate,** ℞ **menthol,** and ℞ **camphor.**
Formulation: Topical ointment.
Availability: OTC.
Warnings and side effects: See ℞ **methyl salicylate;** ℞ **menthol;**
℞ **camphor.**

DeFed-60 Tablets Ⓑ

A preparation of ℞ **pseudoephedrine.**
Formulation: Oral tablets.
Availability: OTC.
Warnings and side effects: See ℞ **pseudoephedrine.**

Defen-LA Tablets Ⓑ

A preparation of ℞ **pseudoephedrine** and ℞ **guaifenesin.**
Formulation: Oral tablets, sustained release.
Availability: Prescription only.
Warnings and side effects: See ℞ **pseudoephedrine;**
℞ **guaifenesin.**

Degas ®

A preparation of ℞ **simethicone**.
Formulation: Oral tablets, chewable.
Availability: OTC.
Warnings and side effects: See ℞ **simethicone**.

dehydrocholic acid ©

Type/Group: **laxative; gallstone treatment**.
Brand(s): Cholan-HMB; Decholin; various generic.
How administered: Orally.

Used to treat

Dehydrocholic acid is used for temporary relief of ✪ **constipation**. It also acts on bile, diluting it somewhat with water and causing greater flow. For this reason dehydrocholic acid may be used after biliary surgery to help flush debris from the biliary tract or in other conditions in which increased fluid flow in the bile tract is desirable. (It is not thought effective, however, in dissolving gallstones, nor does it increase the amount of bile produced.)

Warnings

• It should not be given to people with known hypersensitivity to this drug or to bile salts, with any form of intestinal, urinary or biliary obstruction, liver impairment, or children under 12.
• The effects of dehydrocholic acid in pregnancy have not been studied, and so it should be used only if it is clearly needed.
• Medical judgment is required if breast-feeding is being considered. It is not known whether it appears in breast milk.
• Do not use if there is abdominal pain, nausea, or vomiting, unless directed by a doctor.
• As a laxative, it takes 6 to 12 hours to work.
• Chronic use of laxatives may cause fluid and electrolyte imbalances, vitamin and mineral deficiencies, and abnormal bowel function. Generally, they should not be used for more than a week.
• A doctor must be consulted first before taking any other medication (including OTCs, herbal remedies, and supplements), because laxatives may alter the absorption of a wide range of drugs.

Interactions

• No drug interactions of significance are known.
• Laxatives can alter the absorption of a wide range of drugs.

Side effects

• Rarely, there may be allergic symptoms such as itching or inflamed skin.

Deladumone ®

A preparation of ℞ **estradiol** and ℞ **testosterone** enanthate.
Formulation: Injection.
Availability: Prescription only.
Warnings and side effects: See ℞ **estradiol**; ℞ **testosterone**.

Delatestryl ®

A preparation of ℞ **testosterone** ethanate.
Formulation: Injection.
Availability: Prescription only.
Warnings and side effects: See ℞ **testosterone**.

Delcort ®

A preparation of ℞ **hydrocortisone**.
Formulation: Cream in two strengths. Higher strength is prescription.
Availability: OTC or prescription only depending on label.
Warnings and side effects: See ℞ **hydrocortisone**.

Del-Mycin ®

A preparation of ℞ **erythromycin**.
Formulation: Topical solution.
Availability: Prescription only.
Warnings and side effects: See ℞ **erythromycin**.

Delsym ®

A preparation of ℞ **dextromethorphan**.
Formulation: Liquid, sustained action.
Availability: OTC.
Warnings and side effects: See ℞ **dextromethorphan**.

Delta-Cortef ®

A preparation of ℞ **prednisolone**.
Formulation: Oral tablets.
Availability: Prescription only.
Warnings and side effects: See ℞ **prednisolone**.

Deltasone ®

A preparation of ℞ **prednisone**.
Formulation: Oral tablets in several strengths.
Availability: Prescription only.
Warnings and side effects: See ℞ **prednisone**.

Delta-Tritex ®

A preparation of ℞ **triamcinolone**.
Formulation: Ointment; cream.
Availability: Prescription only.
Warnings and side effects: See ℞ **triamcinolone**.

Demadex ®

A preparation of ℞ **torsemide**.
Formulation: Oral tablets (4 strengths); injection.
Availability: Prescription only.
Warnings and side effects: See ℞ **torsemide**.

demeclocycline ©

Type/Group: **tetracycline; antibiotic; antibacterial**.
Brand(s): Declomycin.
How administered: Orally.

Used to treat

Demeclocycline is a broad-spectrum drug used to treat many kinds of infection, but particularly those of the respiratory tract, the gastrointestinal and genitourinary tracts, ✪ **acne**, ✪ **syphilis**, ✪ **urethritis**, chronic ✪ **bronchitis**, ✪ **Rocky Mountain spotted fever**, ✪ **psittacosis**, and a wide variety of soft-tissue infections. Although not represented by the manufacturer for such treatment, it is also prescribed, quite separately from its use as an antibiotic, as a ℞ **hormone antagonist** to treat over-secretion of antidiuretic hormone (ADH) through an action on the kidney.

Warnings

• It should not be given to people with known hypersensitivity to tetracyclines, or to children under 8 years of age.

• It should be given with caution to people with kidney or liver impairment.

• Democlocycline should be avoided in the last half of pregnancy because of the risk of dental staining and inhibiting the skeletal growth of the fetus.

• It should not be used by nursing mothers.

• Superinfections due to the altered bacterial balance caused by antibiotic treatment may occur. A doctor must be contacted if abdominal pain, moderate to severe diarrhea, or any new or unusual symptoms occur.

• It may cause photosensitivity reactions (abnormal sensitivity to sunlight), so exposure to direct sunlight must be minimized.

• It may cause permanent discoloration of teeth and the thin tooth enamel in children from the time of tooth formation, which begins in the uterus and ends at the age of 8. It may also retard bone development during the same period.

• It must not be used after the discard date, as it becomes harmful to the kidneys as it degrades.

• Prolonged treatment with demeclocycline has been associated with reversible kidney disorders.

Interactions

• ℞ **Bismuth subsalicylate**, ℞ **barbiturates**, ♒ **calcium**, ♒ **iron**, ♒ **magnesium**, ℞ **cholestyramine**, ℞ **sodium bicarbonate**, ♒ **zinc**, ℞ **colestipol hydrochloride** may decrease the absorption of tetracyclines.

• The levels of ℞ **digoxin** may be reduced.

• The effects of ℞ **penicillin** are impaired.

• The effectiveness of ℞ **oral contraceptives** may be reduced.

• ℞ **Carbamazepine** and ℞ **phenytoin** may decrease concentrations of demeclocycline.

• There is the potential of enhancing the anticoagulant effect of ℞ **warfarin sodium**.

Side effects

• Frequently, gastrointestinal upsets (take with food to minimize) and difficulty swallowing.

• Rarely, rash, hives, liver toxicity, pancreatitis, blood and skin disorders, and kidney damage.

dementia treatment ⓓ

(Alzheimer's treatment; senile dementia treatment)

Generics: **citalopram; donepezil; ergoloid mesylates; fluphenazine; rivastigmine; selegiline hydrochloride; tacrine hydrochloride**.

Actions and uses

Dementia treatment seeks to restore some of the cognitative brain function agents lost in the group of neurological diseases referred to as ⓞ **dementia**, characterized by a general decline in all areas of mental ability. Causes include brain tumors, cerebrovascular disease such as stroke, syphilis, head injury, ⓞ **Huntington's disease** and ⓞ **Parkinson's disease**, pernicious anaemia, and alcoholism.

Although some of these causes can be treated, the changes are not always reversible. Where the cerebrovascular disease originates from impaired blood supply, some cerebral ℞ **vasodilator** drugs (for example, ℞ **ergoloid mesylates**) may be tried.

ⓞ **Alzheimer's disease** and similar neurodegenerative diseases have long been thought to involve defective function of nerves (cholinergic neurones) in the central nervous system (with impaired release or action of the neurotransmitter, acetylcholine. For this reason ℞ **anticholinesterases**, (for example, ℞ **tacrine hydrochloride**, ℞ **donepezil**, ℞ **rivastigmine**) have been recently introduced for the symptomatic treatment of mild to moderate dementia of Alzheimer's disease, where they may slow the rate of cognitive and non-cognitive deterioration in up to half of people treated (although there is no effect in people with other causes of confusion or dementia).

Other drugs sometimes used in the general treatment of dementias, particularly anxiety states, include the ℞ **SSRI** antidepressant ℞ **citalopram**, the ℞ **antipsychotic** drug ℞ **fluphenazine**, and the ℞ **antiparkinsonism** drug ℞ **selegiline hydrochloride**.

Limitations

Unfortunately, none of the current treatments for dementias are very successful, and in general it seems doubtful that marked degenerative changes in the brain are reversible by drug treatment, although some of the newly trialed or introduced anticholinesterase drugs for Alzheimer's disease show moderate promise in early cases. Future approaches include the development of vaccines that prevent the formation of the amyloid plaque proteins in the brain (which are characteristic of Alzheimer's disease), and of drugs that increase the release of neurotransmitters from cholinergic neurons. Until then, the best hope lies in prevention of neurodegenerative changes in the first place, for instance, by rapid and effective treatment of stroke, or partial prevention with a low dose of aspirin. Lifestyle drugs such as food supplements containing ♒ **antioxidants** that reduce free radicals, and possibly ♒ **vitamin B₁₂**, are worth consideration.

Demerol ®

A preparation of ℞ **meperidine hydrochloride**.

Formulation: Oral tablets; syrup; injection.

Availability: Prescription only.

Warnings and side effects: See ℞ **meperidine hydrochloride**.

Demser ®

A preparation of ℞ **metyrosine**.

Formulation: Oral capsules.

Availability: Prescription only.

Warnings and side effects: See ℞ **metyrosine**.

demulcent ⓓ

Generics: **alginic acid; glycerin**.

Actions and uses

Demulcent agents are preparations that soothe or protect mucous membranes, and help relieve pain and irritation. They work by forming a protective film and are incorporated into ℞ **antacid** preparations for protecting the gastric mucosa (stomach lining), and into mouthwashes and gargles to soothe the membranes of the mouth. The most commonly used demulcent agent is ℞ **alginic acid** (usually in the form of magnesium alginate or sodium alginate). Syrup, honey, and ℞ **glycerin** soothe mucous membranes as well as sweetening medications.

Limitations

See the individual drug entries.

Demulen Ⓑ

A preparation of ℞ **ethinyl estradiol**, ethynodiol diacetate (etynodiol diacetate).

Formulation: Calendar pack of oral tablets.
Availability: Prescription only.
Warnings and side effects: See ℞ **ethinyl estradiol**; ℞ **progestins**.

Denavir Ⓑ

A preparation of ℞ **penciclovir**.
Formulation: Topical cream.
Availability: Prescription only.
Warnings and side effects: See ℞ **penciclovir**.

Denorex; Extra Strength Ⓑ

A preparation of ℞ **coal tar** and ℞ **menthol**.
Formulation: Shampoo.
Availability: OTC.
Warnings and side effects: See ℞ **coal tar**; ℞ **menthol**.

Dentipatch Ⓑ

A preparation of ℞ **lidocaine**.
Formulation: Oral patch in two strengths.
Availability: Prescription only.
Warnings and side effects: See ℞ **lidocaine**.

Depacon Ⓑ

A preparation of ℞ **valproate sodium**.
Formulation: Injection.
Availability: Prescription only.
Warnings and side effects: See ℞ **valproate sodium**.

Depakene Capsules; Syrup Ⓑ

A preparation of ℞ **valproate sodium**.
Formulation: Oral capsules; syrup.
Availability: Prescription only.
Warnings and side effects: See ℞ **valproate sodium**.

Depakote Tablets; Sprinkle Capsules Ⓑ

A preparation of ℞ **divalproex**.
Formulation: Oral capsules (contents may be sprinkled on food); tablets, delayed release, available in 3 strengths.
Availability: Prescription only.
Warnings and side effects: See ℞ **divalproex**.

depAndro Ⓑ

A preparation of ℞ **testosterone** cypionate.

Formulation: Injection in two strengths (100 and 200).
Availability: Prescription only.
Warnings and side effects: See ℞ **testosterone**.

Depen Ⓑ

A preparation of ℞ **penicillamine**.
Formulation: Oral tablets.
Availability: Prescription only.
Warnings and side effects: See ℞ **penicillamine**.

depGynogen Ⓑ

A preparation of ℞ **estradiol**.
Formulation: Injection.
Availability: Prescription only.
Warnings and side effects: See ℞ **estradiol**.

DepoCyt Ⓑ

A preparation of ℞ **cytarabine**.
Formulation: Liposomal injection.
Availability: Prescription only.
Warnings and side effects: See ℞ **cytarabine**.

Depo-Estradiol Ⓑ

A preparation of ℞ **estradiol**.
Formulation: Injection.
Availability: Prescription only.
Warnings and side effects: See ℞ **estradiol**.

DepoGen Ⓑ

A preparation of ℞ **estradiol**.
Formulation: Injection.
Availability: Prescription only.
Warnings and side effects: See ℞ **estradiol**.

Depoject Ⓑ

A preparation of ℞ **methylprednisolone** acetate.
Formulation: Injection.
Availability: Prescription only.
Warnings and side effects: See ℞ **methylprednisolone**.

Depo-Medrol Ⓑ

A preparation of ℞ **methylprednisolone** acetate.
Formulation: Injection.
Availability: Prescription only.
Warnings and side effects: See ℞ **methylprednisolone**.

Deponit Ⓑ

A preparation of ℞ **nitroglycerin**.
Formulation: Transdermal patch, available in two release rates.
Availability: Prescription only.
Warnings and side effects: See ℞ **nitroglycerin**.

Depopred Ⓑ

A preparation of ℞ **methylprednisolone** acetate.
Formulation: Injection.

Key to symbols: ⒟ = **Drug type/group**   ⒢ = **Generic name**   Ⓑ = **Brand name**

Availability: Prescription only.
Warnings and side effects: See ℞ **methylprednisolone**.

Depo-Provera ⑧

A preparation of ℞ **medroxyprogesterone**.
Formulation: Injectable solutions in different strengths for the different uses.
Availability: Prescription only.
Warnings and side effects: See ℞ **medroxyprogesterone**.

Depotest ⑧

A preparation of ℞ **testosterone** cypionate.
Formulation: Injection in two strengths.
Availability: Prescription only.
Warnings and side effects: See ℞ **testosterone**.

Depo-Testadiol ⑧

A preparation of ℞ **estradiol** and ℞ **testosterone** cypionate.
Formulation: Injection.
Availability: Prescription only.
Warnings and side effects: See ℞ **estradiol**; ℞ **testosterone**.

Depotestogen ⑧

A preparation of ℞ **estradiol** cypoinate and ℞ **testosterone** cypionate.
Formulation: Injection.
Availability: Prescription only.
Warnings and side effects: See ℞ **estradiol**; ℞ **testosterone**.

Depo-Testosterone ⑧

A preparation of ℞ **testosterone** cypionate.
Formulation: Injection in two strengths.
Availability: Prescription only.
Warnings and side effects: See ℞ **testosterone**.

Deproist Expectorant with Codeine Liquid ⑧

A preparation of ℞ **codeine phosphate**, ℞ **guaifenesin**, and ℞ **pseudoephedrine**.
Formulation: Oral liquid.
Availability: May or may not require a prescription.
Warnings and side effects: See ℞ **codeine phosphate**; ℞ **guaifenesin**; ℞ **pseudoephedrine**.

Dermacort ⑧

A preparation of ℞ **hydrocortisone**.
Formulation: Lotion; cream.
Availability: Prescription only.
Warnings and side effects: See ℞ **hydrocortisone**.

DermaFlex ⑧

A preparation of ℞ **lidocaine**.
Formulation: Topical gel.
Availability: OTC.
Warnings and side effects: See ℞ **lidocaine**.

Dermal-Rub Balm ⑧

A preparation of ℞ **methyl salicylate**, ℞ **menthol**, and ℞ **camphor**.
Formulation: Topical ointment.
Availability: OTC.
Warnings and side effects: See ℞ **methyl salicylate**; ℞ **menthol**; ℞ **camphor**.

Dermamycin ⑧

A preparation of ℞ **diphenhydramine hydrochloride**.
Formulation: Topical cream, spray.
Availability: OTC.
Warnings and side effects: See ℞ **diphenhydramine hydrochloride**.

Derma-Pax Lotion ⑧

A preparation of ℞ **chlorpheniramine maleate** and ℞ **pyrilamine maleate**.
Formulation: Topical lotion.
Availability: OTC.
Warnings and side effects: See ℞ **chlorpheniramine maleate**; ℞ **pyrilamine maleate**.

Dermarest Plus ⑧

A preparation of ℞ **diphenhydramine hydrochloride**, benzalkonium chloride, ℞ **resorcinol**, and ℞ **menthol**.
Formulation: Topical gel; spray.
Availability: OTC.
Warnings and side effects: See ℞ **diphenhydramine hydrochloride**; benzalkonium chloride; ℞ **resorcinol**; ℞ **menthol**.

Derma-Smoothe/FS ⑧

A preparation of ℞ **fluocinolone acetonide**.
Formulation: Topical oil.
Availability: Prescription only.
Warnings and side effects: See ℞ **fluocinolone acetonide**.

Dermolate ⑧

A preparation of ℞ **hydrocortisone**.
Formulation: Cream.
Availability: OTC.
Warnings and side effects: See ℞ **hydrocortisone**.

Dermol HC ⑧

A preparation of ℞ **hydrocortisone**.
Formulation: Cream in two strengths; ointment.
Availability: Prescription only.
Warnings and side effects: See ℞ **hydrocortisone**.

Dermoplast ⑧

A preparation of ℞ **benzocaine** with ℞ **menthol**, aloe, and emollients.
Formulation: Topical spray.
Availability: OTC.

Warnings and side effects: See ℞ benzocaine; ℞ menthol.

Dermtex HC with Aloe ⑧

A preparation of ℞ **hydrocortisone**.
Formulation: Cream.
Availability: OTC.
Warnings and side effects: See ℞ hydrocortisone.

DES ⑥

see ℞ **diethylstilbestrol**.

Desenex ⑧

A preparation of ℞ **clotrimazole**.
Formulation: Topical powder; topical cream; soap.
Availability: OTC.
Warnings and side effects: See ℞ clotrimazole.

desensitizing products ⑥

Type/Group: **desensitizing vaccine**.
Brand(s): Albay; Pharmalgen; various generic (over 900 different allergens available).
How administered: Injection (usually subcutaneous).

Used to treat

Desensitizing vaccines are preparations of particular allergens (substances to which a person has an allergic reaction) which are given, in progressive doses, to reduce the degree of allergic reaction that exposure causes; a procedure called hyposensitization. For example, preparations of grass pollens are administered for the treatment of ○ **hay fever**, or bee venom or wasp venom to protect against the effects of subsequent stings. The mechanism by which they work is not clear, and the course of therapy may take four to six months or longer. They are also used in very small amounts (just a skin prick) to diagnose which substances might cause allergy in an individual.

Warnings

• They should not be used by people with frequent or acute reactions to this therapy, or where simple avoidance of an allergen is possible.
• They should also be avoided by people with acute asthma or feverish conditions.
• Although no risks are particularly associated with the use of these substances during pregnancy, release of histamine and other inflammatory mediators can induce contractions of the uterus. Desensitizing vaccines are often discontinued or given at reduced dosage during pregnancy.
• There are no known problems when used by breast-feeding mothers.
• Injections should be given under close medical supervision and where emergency facilities for full cardiorespiratory resuscitation are immediately available (in case of anaphylactic reaction), with monitoring for at least an hour after administration.
• A doctor must be notified immediately if symptoms such as fainting, wheezing, hypotension, or slow heart beat develop.

• Although allergens may be used to diagnose allergies to various foods, there is no evidence that using them as desensitizing vaccines is effective.
• Many of these allergens should only be given in the "off season" (for example, for allergy to grasses), because the effects of high environmental exposure and desensitizing agents can enhance the problem.

Interactions

• ℞ **antihistamines** and ℞ **corticosteroids** may suppress the allergic reaction and make diagnosis difficult.

Side effects

• There may be allergic reactions, especially in small children, including such symptoms as pallor, fainting, slow heart beat, hypotension, wheezing, cough, rhinitis, conjunctivitis, angioedema (allergic swelling), hives, and anaphylaxis.

desensitizing vaccine ⓪

Generics: **desensitizing products**.

Actions and uses

Desensitizing vaccines are preparations of particular allergens (substances to which a person has an allergic reaction) which are used, in progressive doses, to reduce the degree of allergic reaction a person suffers when exposed to the allergen following treatment—a procedure called *hyposensitization*. For example, grass pollens are administered for the treatment of ○ **hay fever**, or bee venom or wasp venom to protect against the effects of subsequent stings. They are given by injection (usually subcutaneous). The mechanism by which they work is not clear, and the course of treatment may take four to six months or longer. They are also used in very small amounts (just a skin prick) to diagnose which substances might cause allergy in an individual.

Limitations

They should not be given to people with frequent or acute reactions to this treatment, or where simple avoidance of an allergen is possible, or to anyone with acute asthma or a feverish condition. Although no risks are particularly associated with use of these substance during pregnancy, release of histamine and other inflammatory mediators can induce contractions of the uterus. Desensitizing vaccines are often discontinued or given at reduced dosage during pregnancy. (They come in the Food and Drug Administration's Pregnancy Category C.) No problems are known in use by nursing women.

Injections should be given under close medical supervision and in locations where emergency facilities for full cardiorespiratory resuscitation are immediately available (in case of ○ **anaphylactic reaction**), with monitoring for at least an hour after administration. A doctor must be contacted immediately if symptoms such as fainting, wheezing, hypotension, or slow heartbeat develop.

Although allergens may be used to diagnose allergies to various foods, there is no evidence that using them as desensitizing vaccines is effective. Many of these allergens should only be given in the "off season" (for example, for allergy to grasses), as the effects of high environmental exposure and desensitizing agents can be additive.

There may be allergic reactions, especially in small children, including such symptoms as pallor, fainting, slow heartbeat, hypotension, wheezing, cough, rhinitis, conjunctivitis, angioedema (allergic swelling), hives, and anaphylactic reaction.

Antihistamines and corticosteroids may suppress an allergic reaction and make diagnosis difficult.

Desferal ®

A preparation of ℞ **desferoxamine mesylate**.
Formulation: Oral tablets.
Availability: Prescription only.
Warnings and side effects: See ℞ **desferoxamine mesylate**.

desferoxamine mesylate Ⓖ

Type/Group: antidote; chelating agent.
Brand(s): Desferal.
How administered: Injection.

Used to treat

Desferoxamine mesylate is is used as an antidote to treat iron poisoning or an overload of iron in the tissues (for example, in aplastic anemia due to repeated blood transfusions). It has been investigated, with some success, for the treatment of aluminum overload (for example, in kidney dialysis patients).

Warnings

• Depending on use, it should be not be used by people with kidney impairment or anuria (absence of urine, from whatever cause).
• Desferoxamine mesylate has been associated with birth defects and should not be used during pregnancy, especially in late pregnancy, except where it is medically judged that the potential benefit outweighs potential risk to the fetus.
• Medical judgment is also required for breast-feeding mothers.
• With extended use, desferoxamine may increase the risk of hearing and visual disturbances, including cataracts. Periodic check-ups are necessary.
• Dizziness or visual side effects may impair the performance of skilled tasks such as driving.

Interactions

• Desferoxamine taken with ℞ **prochlorperazine** may lead to a temporary impairment of consciousness.
• Levels of ♒ **vitamin C** fall in iron overload and supplementation may be needed, but this must be done with caution, especially in people with heart disorders as heart problems have occurred with combined desferoxamine and vitamin C therapy.

Side effects

• There may be pain at the site of injection, gastrointestinal disturbances, hypotension, heart rate changes, anaphylaxis, convulsions, dizziness, disturbances in vision and hearing, and skin, heart and liver disorders.
• There is some evidence to suggest that desferoxamine can raise susceptibility to some gastrointestinal infections (with strains of *Yersinia*); its use is discontinued until the infection is resolved.

desipramine hydrochloride Ⓖ

Type/Group: antidepressant; tricyclic.
Brand(s): Norpramin; various generic.

How administered: Orally.

Used to treat

Desipramine hydrochloride can be used to treat ✚ **depression**. Although not stated by the manufacturer for such use, it is sometimes used for the treatment of eating disorders and panic disorder, and to help in cocaine withdrawal. It has fewer ℞ **anticholinergic** side effects than some other tricyclics. As is the case with other antidepressants, this drug is also being evaluated for other uses.

Warnings

• It should not be given to people with known hypersensitivity to this drug, who are just recovering from myocardial infarction (heart attack), or anyone taking or have stopped taking ℞ **MAOI** antidepressants within the previous 14 days.
• It should be given with extreme caution to people with a history of seizures, urinary retention, increased intraocular pressure (pressure in the eyeball), narrow-angle glaucoma, cardiovascular or heart disease, thyroid disease, prostatic hypertrophy, kidney or liver disease, who are receiving electroconvulsive therapy, or are over the age of 65.
• It should be used during pregnancy only if the benefits outweigh the risk to the fetus.
• It should not be used by nursing mothers.
• Other symptoms of a psychiatric illnesses may worsen.
• Episodes of mania or hypomania may occur.
• Exposure to sunlight should be minimized because of possible photosensitization (sensitivity to light).
• Treatment should be stopped gradually by lowering the dose over a period of time.
• It is not generally given to children under the age of 12.
• It may be 4 to 6 weeks before there are any signs of improvement.
• It may impair the performance of skilled tasks such as driving.
• Alcohol, grapefruit juice, and smoking can all affect tricyclics (see Interactions below).

Interactions

• Serious or even fatal reactions can occur if ℞ **MAOI** antidepressants are taken at the same time as tricyclics.
• The effects of ℞ **epinephrine**, ℞ **norepinephrine**, and ℞ **phenylephrine** on blood pressure are intensified.
• Grapefruit juice increases the levels of tricyclics.
• ℞ **clonidine hydrochloride** should not be used with tricyclics, because a dangerous increase in blood pressure and hypertensive crisis is possible.
• The effects of ℞ **guanethidine monosulfate**, ℞ **levodopa**, and ℞ **sympathomimetics** may be reduced by tricyclics.
• The effects of ℞ **anticholinergics**, dicumarol, ℞ **quinolones**, grepafloxacin, and sparfloxacin may be enhanced by tricyclics.
• ℞ **Barbiturates**, ℞ **activated charcoal**, and rifamycin-related antibiotics may reduce the effectiveness of tricyclics.
• ℞ **Cimetidine**, ℞ **SSRIs**, ℞ **haloperidol**, ℞ **bupropion**, ℞ **valproate sodium** (and other valproic acid derivatives), and histamine ℞ **H₂-antagonist** may increase the levels of tricyclics in the blood.
• The levels of ℞ **carbamazepine** may increase, while blood levels of tricyclics decrease.
• Smoking may affect the metabolism of tricyclics.

• The effects of alcohol may be enhanced.

Side effects

• Desipramine has fewer anticholinergic side effects than some other tricyclics. It may cause constipation, dry mouth, dizziness, postural hypotension (lowered blood pressure on standing), blurred vision, and urinary retention.

• Less frequently, anxiety, confusion, fatigue, headache, insomnia, mental changes, tremors, weakness, ECG changes, elevated blood pressure, speeded heartbeat or palpitations, fainting, gastrointestinal disorders, skin sensitivity reactions, and weight gain.

• Older adults may experience extrapyramidal symptoms (uncontrollable movement). Rare but serious side effects include blood cell disorders and abnormal heart rhythm.

Desitin; Desitin Creamy Ⓑ

A preparation of ℞ zinc oxide, ℞ petrolatum; ℞ lanolin, and ℞ cod-liver oil.

Formulation: Topical ointment.

Availability: OTC.

Warnings and side effects: See ℞ zinc oxide; ℞ petrolatum; ℞ lanolin; ℞ cod-liver oil.

desmopressin Ⓖ

Type/Group: **diabetes insipidus treatment;** hemostatic; antidiuretic; **hormone; anterior pituitary hormone.**

Brand(s): DDAVP; Stimate.

How administered: Injection; orally; intranasal.

Used to treat

Desmopressin is a major synthetic analog of antidiuretic hormone (ADH), also called ℞ vasopressin. ADH is released from the posterior pituitary gland and naturally reduces urine production. Desmopressin is used to treat ✪ bed-wetting, neurogenic ✪ diabetes insipidus, temporary increased urination following head trauma or surgery in the pituitary region, and bleeding (by boosting clotting factors; VIII) in certain cases of ✪ hemophilia A and von Willebrand's disease (Type I).

Warnings

• It should not be used by people with known hypersensitivity to this drug. Intranasal formulations should not be used by anyone with nasal scarring, blockage, or other impairment, or with an impaired level of consciousness.

• It should be given with caution to people with coronary artery disease or hypertensive cardiovascular disease, and to children under the age of 6.

• It should be used during pregnancy only if medically judged to be needed.

• Medical judgment is also required if breast-feeding is being considered.

• Infants and young children must have their fluid intake restricted to prevent possible low sodium levels or water intoxication, which can cause serious adverse reactions. Older adults should restrict their fluid intake as well.

• Upper respiratory tract infections, nasal congestion, and allergies may decrease the effectiveness of desmopressin when it is taken intranasally.

Interactions

• ℞ **carbamazepine,** ℞ **chlorpropamide,** and ℞ **clofibrate** may increase the effects of desmopressin.

• ℞ **demeclocycline,** ℞ **lithium,** and ℞ **norepinephrine** may decrease the effects of desmopressin.

Side effects

These depend on the how administered, dose, and use.

• When given by injection, there may occasionally be pain, redness or swelling at the injection site, headache, abdominal cramps, vulva pain, flushed skin, mild elevation of blood pressure, and nausea with high doses.

• Nasal administration occasionally causes a runny or stuffy nose, and slight elevation of blood pressure.

Desogen Ⓑ

A preparation of ℞ ethinyl estradiol and ℞ desogestrel.

Formulation: Calendar pack of oral tablets.

Availability: Prescription only.

Warnings and side effects: See ℞ ethinyl estradiol; ℞ desogestrel.

desogestrel Ⓖ

Type/Group: **progestin; oral contraceptive.**

Brand(s): Desogen; Mircette; Ortho-Cept.

How administered: Orally.

Used to treat

Desogestrel is a progestin which is used as a constituent of the combined oral contraceptives that contain an estrogen and a progestin.

Warnings

• It should not be given to people with clotting disorders, history of deep vein thrombophlebitis or thromboembolic disorders, cerebral vascular or coronary artery disease, known or suspected breast cancer or estrogen-dependent cancer, undiagnosed abnormal genital bleeding, cholestatic jaundice in prior pill use, certain liver disorders, or known or suspected pregnancy.

• Desogestrel should not be used while pregnant because there is a risk to the fetus. A doctor must be contacted if pregnancy occurs while taking this drug.

• It is not recommended for use by nursing mothers.

• The use of oral contraceptives is associated with a risk of serious cardiovascular side effects (for example, embolism, stroke, heart attack), particularly in those over age 35. Cigarette smoking increases the risk. This added risk gets larger with age and with heavy smoking (>15 per day), and is quite marked in women over the age of 35.

• Benign liver tumors, increased risk of gallbladder disease, and elevated blood pressure have been associated with oral contraceptive use.

Interactions

• ℞ Rifampin and ℞ barbiturates reduce the effects of estrogen.

• The steroid effect of ℞ corticosteroids is increased.

• If used with ℞ **phenytoin**, there is a loss of seizure control and levels of estrogen are reduced.
• If used with ℞ **warfarin sodium** and similar anticoagulants, there is a theoretical increase in the risk of thromboembolism.

Side effects
• Nausea and vomiting, breakthrough bleeding, spotting, change in menstrual flow, temporary infertility after discontinuation, edema, breast changes, changes in cervical erosion and secretion, cholestatic jaundice, migraine, rash, mental depression, reduced tolerance to carbohydrates, vaginal candidiasis, steepening in corneal curvature, and intolerance to contact lenses.

desoxymetasone Ⓖ

Type/Group: **corticosteroid; anti-inflammatory.**
Brand(s): Topicort; various generic.
How administered: Topically.

Used to treat
Desoxymetasone is used for the topical (applied externally) treatment of psoriasis, eczema, and contact dermatitis, and for pruritus.

Warnings
• It should not be used by people with known hypersensitivity to corticosteroids, or who have fungal infections.
• It must not be used on the face, groin, or armpits.
• It should be given with caution to anyone with a bacterial or viral infection, and to children, who may be more susceptible to systemic side effects.
• Corticosteroids can cross the placenta. It is unknown whether external application could result in sufficient systemic absorption to create a hazard to the fetus. Desoxymetasone, therefore, should be used during pregnancy only if it is medically judged to be essential.
• Medical judgment is also required if breast-feeding is being considered. When taken internally, corticosteroids are excreted in breast milk and may suppress growth and interfere with the production of natural corticosteroids in the infant. It is unknown whether external application could result in sufficient systemic absorption to produce detectable amounts in breast milk.
• Topical corticosteroids can be absorbed in sufficient amounts to produce systemic effects. Therefore, do not use over large surface areas or for a prolonged period, in order to minimize the risk of systemic absorption.
• Bandages or dressings must not be put over the treated area unless directed by a doctor, as this may increase the risk of adverse skin reactions.
• Weeping, denuded, or infected areas, and the eyes must be avoided.
• A doctor must be notified and use of desoxymetasone stopped if local irritation or fever develops.

Interactions
No significant interactions have been reported.

Side effects
• Occasionally, irritation, and itching.
• Rarely, allergic rash, systemic effects are possible (for example, adrenal insufficiency), reversible liver changes, reduced glucose tolerance, and white blood cell disorders.

Desoxyn; Desoxyn Gradumet Ⓑ

A preparation of ℞ **methamphetamine.**
Formulation: Oral tablets; sustained release capsules (Gradumet).
Availability: Prescription only.
Warnings and side effects: See ℞ **methamphetamine.**

desquamating agent Ⓓ

see ℞ **keratolytic.**

Desquam X Wash; Desquam-E Ⓑ

A preparation of ℞ **benzoyl peroxide.**
Formulation: Topical liquid, topical gel. Available in varying strengths.
Availability: Prescription only.
Warnings and side effects: See ℞ **benzoyl peroxide.**

Desyrel; Desyrel Dividose Ⓑ

A preparation of ℞ **trazodone hydrochloride.**
Formulation: Oral tablets in varying strengths.
Availability: Prescription only.
Warnings and side effects: See ℞ **trazodone hydrochloride.**

Detrol Ⓑ

A preparation of ℞ **tolterodine tartrate.**
Formulation: Oral tablets.
Availability: Prescription only.
Warnings and side effects: See ℞ **tolterodine tartrate.**

Detussin Expectorant Liquid Ⓑ

A preparation of ℞ **hydrocodone bitartrate,** ℞ **pseudoephedrine,** and ℞ **guaifenesin.**
Formulation: Oral syrup.
Availability: Prescription only.
Warnings and side effects: See ℞ **hydrocodone bitartrate;** ℞ **pseudoephedrine;** ℞ **guaifenesin.**

Detussin Liquid Ⓑ

A preparation of ℞ **hydrocodone bitartrate** and ℞ **pseudoephedrine.**
Formulation: Oral liquid.
Availability: Prescription only.
Warnings and side effects: See ℞ **hydrocodone bitartrate;** ℞ **pseudoephedrine.**

Dex4 Glucose Ⓑ

A preparation of ℞ **glucose.**
Formulation: Oral tablets.
Availability: OTC.
Warnings and side effects: See ℞ **glucose.**

Dexacidin Ⓑ

A preparation of ℞ **dexamethasone,** ℞ **neomycin,** and ℞ **polymyxin B sulfate.**
Formulation: Opthalmic solution.
Availability: Prescription only.

Warnings and side effects: See ℞ **dexamethasone**; ℞ **neomycin**; ℞ **polymyxin B sulfate**.

Dexacidin Ophthalmic Solution ⑧

A preparation of benzalkonium chloride, and ℞ **dexamethasone**, ℞ **neomycin**, and ℞ **polymyxin B sulfate**.
Formulation: Ophthalmic solution.
Availability: Prescription only.
Warnings and side effects: See ℞ **dexamethasone**; ℞ **neomycin**; ℞ **polymyxin B sulfate**.

Dexameth ⑧

A preparation of ℞ **dexamethasone**.
Formulation: Oral tablets.
Availability: Prescription only.
Warnings and side effects: See ℞ **dexamethasone**.

dexamethasone ⑥

Type/Group: corticosteroid; anti-inflammatory; immunosuppressant.
Brand(s): AK-Dex; Cortastat; Dalalone; Decadron; Decadron Phosphate; Decaspray; Dexameth; Dexasone; Dexone; Hexadrol; Maxidex; Solurex; various generic. Combinations: With *lidocaine*: Decadron with Xylocaine. With *neomycin*: Neo-Decadron; Ak-Neo-Dex; Neo-Dexameth. With *neomycin and polymyxin B*: Dexacidin; Maxitrol; Ak-Trol. With *tobramycin*: Tobradex.
How administered: Orally; topically; injection.

Used to treat

Dexamethasone is used for the treatment of many kinds of inflammation, especially eye disorders. It has major and varied effects on metabolism, and modifies the operation of the immune system. Therefore, it may be used to treat a range of conditions, including adrenal insufficiency, congenital adrenal hyperplasia, rheumatic disorders, such as ✪ **arthritis** and ✪ **osteoarthritis**, allergic states, collagen diseases, allergic eye disorders, intestinal tract, liver and kidney disorders, skin diseases, respiratory diseases (such as bronchial ✪ **asthma**), edemas, and malignancies.

Warnings

These depend on use.
• It should not be used by people with known hypersensitivity to corticosteroids, or those with systemic fungal infections. It should not be used in the eye if there are certain eye infections.
• It should be given with caution to anyone with low thyroid function, peptic ulcers, hepatitis, cirrhosis, ocular herpes simplex, history of tuberculosis, nonspecific colitis, congestive heart failure, diabetes mellitus, glaucoma, myocardial infarction (heart attack), hypertension, psychosis, or kidney insufficiency. Also, it should be given with caution to anyone 65 and by children. External use by those with marked circulation impairment should be undertaken with care.
• Corticosteroids cross the placenta, and dexamethasone, therefore, should be used during pregnancy only if it is medically judged to be essential.
• It should not be used by breast-feeding mothers. It is excreted in breast milk and could suppress growth and interfere with

production of corticosteroids in the infant. It is not known whether, or under what conditions, enough of the drug is absorbed from topical use to create these risks.
• May mask signs of infection and interfere with the body's ability to keep infection from spreading.
• Live vaccines must not be taken while using this drug.
• It may reactivate latent tuberculosis or amebiasis.
• Prolonged use in children can inhibit skeletal growth, and so growth will be monitored.
• It causes increased excretion of calcium and other minerals, and so supplements may be needed.
• Prolonged use may lead to adrenal insufficiency. A doctor must be notified if there is unusual weight gain, swelling of the legs or feet, muscle weakness, black tarry stools, vomiting of blood, puffing of the face, menstrual irregularities, or prolonged sore throat, fever, cold, or infection.
• Those on long-term steroid therapy should wear a medic-alert bracelet or the equivalent.
• Any other medication (including herbal remedies and supplements) must not be taken without consulting a doctor.
• When used in the eye, ophthalmic checks are recommended.
• Discontinuation of treatment must be gradual and under medical supervision to avoid adverse reactions.
• Dentists and other doctors must be informed of the use of this drug during, and for 12 months after discontinuing, treatment. Supportive drugs may be required in the event of severe illness, surgery, or trauma.
• Topical corticosteroids can be absorbed in sufficient amounts to produce systemic effects. Therefore, do not use over large surface areas, cover with bandages, or for a prolonged period, to minimize risk of systemic absorption.

Interactions

• Dexamethasone taken with ℞ **amphotericin** or ℞ **diuretics** may further reduce potassium levels.
• The effects of ℞ **aspirin**, ℞ **oral hypoglycemics**, ℞ **insulin**, ℞ **diuretics**, and ⚭ **potassium** supplements may be reduced.
• ℞ **Barbiturates**, ℞ **hydantoins**, ℞ **rifampin**, and ℞ **ephedrine** may reduce the effects of dexamethasone.
• ℞ **Ketoconazole**, ℞ **estrogens**, ℞ **oral contraceptives**, and nondepolarizing muscle relaxants may increase the effects of corticosteroids.
• Oral ℞ **anticoagulants** and ℞ **theophylline** may alter the effects of either corticosteroids or the other drug, or both.
• The effectiveness of ℞ **anticholinesterases**, ℞ **isoniazid**, ℞ **salicylates**, and ℞ **somatrem** may be reduced.
• ℞ **Cyclosporine** and digitalis may increase the risk of toxicity.

Side effects

These depend on how administered, dose, duration of treatment, and use.
• Systemic use: Frequently, insomnia, facial swelling, abdominal tightness, indigestion, increased appetite, nervousness, facial flushing, and increased sweating. Occasionally, dizziness, decreased or blurred vision. Rarely, general allergic reaction, psychic changes, false sense of well-being, hallucinations, and depression.

• Topical use: Occasionally, allergic rash, blood-containing blisters, thinning of skin with easy bruising, and raised dark red spots on skin.

• Ophthalmic (topical) use: Frequently, blurred vision. Occasionally, decreased vision, watery eyes, eye pain, nausea, vomiting, burning, stinging, and redness in eyes.

dexamphetamine sulfate ⓖ

see ℞ dextroamphetamine.

Dexaphen-S.A. Tablets ⓑ

A preparation of pseudoephedrine sulfate and dexbromphe-niramine maleate.

Formulation: Oral tablets, sustained release.

Availability: Prescription only.

Warnings and side effects: See ℞ **pseudoephedrine;** ℞ **brompheniramine maleate.**

Dexasone ⓑ

A preparation of ℞ **dexamethasone** sodium phosphate.

Formulation: Injection.

Availability: Prescription only.

Warnings and side effects: See ℞ **dexamethasone.**

Dexedrine ⓑ

A preparation of ℞ **dextroamphetamine.**

Formulation: Oral tablets; sustained release capsules. Contains tartrazine, which may cause an allergic reaction in susceptible individuals. Incidence is low, but it is more frequent in those who are allergic to aspirin.

Availability: Prescription only.

Warnings and side effects: See ℞ **dextroamphetamine.**

DexFerrum ⓑ

A preparation of ℞ **iron dextran.**

Formulation: Injection.

Availability: Prescription only.

Warnings and side effects: See ℞ **iron dextran.**

Dexone; Dexone LA ⓑ

A preparation of ℞ **dexamethasone** and ℞ **dexamethasone** acetate (Dexone LA).

Formulation: Oral tablets in several strengths; injection (Dexone LA).

Availability: Prescription only.

Warnings and side effects: See ℞ **dexamethasone.**

dexrazoxane ⓖ

Type/Group: chelating agent; cytoprotectant.

Brand(s): Zinecard.

How administered: Intravenous infusion.

Used to treat

Dexrazoxane, a synthetic agent (and derivative of EDTA), and is used with ℞ **doxorubicin hydrochloride** in the treatment of

✪ **breast cancer** as a cardioprotectant to reduce the incidence and severity of heart damage.

Warnings

• It is a specialist drug and is used after a full assessment for suitability.

• It may harm the fetus or cause birth defects and so should be used during pregnancy only if the potential benefit outweighs the risk to the fetus.

• Taking dexrazoxane when nursing is not recommended.

• It may somewhat increase adverse blood changes associated with ℞ **anticancer** drugs.

Interactions

No significant interactions specific to this drug are known.

Side effects

• Frequently, hair loss, nausea, vomiting, fatigue, weakness, loss of appetite, stomatitis (mouth sores), fever, infection, and diarrhea.

• Occasionally, pain from injection, neurological effects, phlebitis, and skin reactions.

dextroamphetamine ⓖ

(dexamphetamine sulfate)

Type/Group: **CNS stimulant; sympathomimetic.**

Brand(s): Dexedrine; various generic.

How administered: Orally.

Used to treat

Dextroamphetamine, in adults, works directly on the brain as a stimulant and can be used to treat ✪ **narcolepsy** (irresistible attacks of sleep during the day). It can also be used to treat ✪ **attention deficit disorder** in children. Although not stated by the manufacturer for such use, it may be prescribed as an adjunct (additional treatment to enhance effectiveness) in the short-term treatment of ✪ **obesity.**

Warnings

• It should not be used by people with known hypersensitivity to sympathomimetic amines, advanced arteriosclerosis, symptomatic heart disease, hypertension, hyperthyroidism, glaucoma, agitated states, or a history of drug abuse, or those taking ℞ **MAOI** antidepressants (see Interactions below).

• It is not known whether or not dextroamphetamine can harm the fetus, therefore, it should be used during pregnancy only if medically judged to be needed.

• It should not be used by breast-feeding mothers.

• It may impair the ability to perform skilled tasks requiring alertness, such as driving.

• It has a high abuse potential and should not be used in larger doses or for a longer period than prescribed. Tolerance, extreme psychological dependence, and severe social disability may occur.

• Dextroamphetamine is a Schedule II controlled substance.

• Other medications (including OTC preparations, herbal remedies, and supplements) must not be taken without consulting a doctor.

Interactions

• Dextroamphetamine must not be taken with, or within two weeks of discontinuing, ℞ **MAOI** antidepressants. Severe and even fatal reactions can occur.

• ℞ **selegiline** and ℞ **furazolidone** may cause severe hypertensive reactions.

• ℞ **tricyclic** antidepressants and ℞ **urinary acidifiers** may reduce levels of amphetamines.

• ℞ **sodium bicarbonate** may increase the effects of amphetamines.

Side effects

• Frequently, headache, nervousness, dizziness, hypersalivation, talkativeness, restlessness, nausea diarrhea, dry mouth, depression, anxiety, insomnia, delayed sleep, euphoria, restlessness, and changes in heartbeat.

dextromethorphan ⓓ

Type/Group: **antitussive; opioid**.

Brand(s): Benylin Adult; Benylin DM; Benylin Pediatric; Children's Hold; Creo-Terpin; Delsymn; Diabetes CF; Drixoral Cough Liquid Caps; Pertussin CS, ES; Robitussin Cough Calmers; Robitussin Pediatric; St. Joseph Cough Suppressant; Scot-Tussin DM Cough Chasers; Silphen DM; Sucrets 4-Hour Cough; Sucrets Cough Control; Suppress; Trocal; Vicks 44 Cough Relief; various generic. Combinations: With pseudoephedrine: Children's Sudafed; Robitussin Maximum Strength Cough & Cold Liquid, Pediatric; Vicks 44D Cough & Head Congestion Relief. (Plus) *carbinoxamine maleate*: Carbodec DM Syrup, Drops; Cardec DM Syrup, Drops; Pseudo-Car DM Syrup; Rondamine-DM Drops; Rondec-DM Syrup, Drops; Sildec-DM Syrup, Pediatric Drops; Tussafed Syrup, Drops. (Plus) *brompheniramine maleate*: Bromadine-DM; Bromarest DX Cough Syrup; Bromatane DX Cough Syrup; Bromfed DM Cough Syrup; Bromphen DX Cough Syrup; Dimetane-DX Cough Syrup; Myphetane DX Cough Syrup. (Plus) *chlorpheniramine maleate*: Children's Vicks Nyquil; Rescon-DM Liquid; Rhinosyn-DM Liquid; Triaminic Night Time Maximum Strength. With pseudoephedrine and acetaminophen: Alka-Seltzer Plus Cold & Flu Liqui-Gels; Contac Severe Cold & Flu Non-Drowsy Caplets; Thera-Flu Non-Drowsy Formula Maximum Strength; Robitussin Multi Symptom Honey Flu; Sudfed Severe Cold Formula Caplets, Tablets; Tylenol Flu Maximum Strength Non-Drowsy Gelcaps; Vicks Dayquil. (Plus) *chlorpheniramine maleate*: Alka-Seltzer Plus Cold & Cough LiquiGels; Children's Tylenol Cold Plus Cough Chewable Tablets; Comtrex Maximum Strength Multi-Symptom Cold & Cough Relief Caplets, Tablets; Contac Severe Cold & Flu Caplets; Genacol Tablets; Kolephrin/DM Caplets; Medi-Flu Liquid; Multi-Symptom Tylenol Cold Caplets, Tablets; NightTime TheraFlu Powder; Robitussin Nighttime Honey Flu; Triaminic Severe Cold & Fever; Vicks 44M Cold & Flu Relief. (Plus) *doxylamine succinate*: Alka-Seltzer Plus NightTime Cold Liqui-Gels; Genite Liquid; Nytcold Medicine Liquid; Vicks NyQuil. (Plus) *guaifenesin*: Sudafed Cold & Cough Liquid Caps; Robitussin Cold Multi-Symptom Cold & Flu Liqui-Gels, Caplets; Vicks DayQuil LiquiCaps. (Plus) *pyrilamine maleate*: Robitussin Night Relief Liquid. With pseudoephedrine and guaifenesin: Anatuss DM Tablets, Syrup; Ambenyl-D Liquid; Benylin Multi-Symptom Liquid; Dimacol Caplets; MED-Rx DM Tablets; Novahistine DMX; PamMist-DM Syrup; Primatuss Cough Mixture 4D Liquid; Protuss DM Tablets; Rhinosyn-S Liquid; Robitussin Cold & Congestion Liqui-Gels, Caplets, Infant Drops;

Ru-Tuss Expectorant Liquid; Touro CC; Tussafed-LA. With guaifenesin: Aquatab DM; Benylin Expectorant Liquid; Cheracol D Cough Liquid; Clear Tussin 30 Liquid; Diabetic Tussin DM Syrup; Duratuss DM; Fenesin DM Tablets; Genatuss DM Syrup; Guaifenex DM Tablets; Halotussin-DM Liquid, Sugar Free Liquid; Humibid DM Tablets, Sprinkles; Iobid DM Tablets; Kolephrin GG/DM Liquid; Muco-Fen-DM Tablets; Mytussin DM Liquid; Naldecon Senior DX Liquid; Phanatuss DM Syrup; Phenadex Senior Liquid; Respa-DM Tablets; Rhinosyn DMX Syrup; Robafen DM Syrup; Robitussin-DM Liquid, Infant Drops; Safe Tussin 30 Liquid; Scot-Tussin Senior Clear Liquid; Siltussin DM Syrup; Synacol CF Tablets; Tolu-Sed DM Syrup; Touro-DM Tablets; Tusibron-DM Syrup; Tuss-DM Tablets; Tussin DM Liquid; Uni-tussin DM Syrup; Vicks 44E Liquid; Vicks Pediatric Formula 44E Liquid. With phenylephrine: (Plus) *chlorpheniramine maleate*: Cerose-DM Liquid. (Plus) *chlorpheniramine maleate and guaifenesin*: Donatussin Syrup. (Plus) *pyrilamine maleate*: Codimal DM Syrup. With other constituents: With *chlorpheniramine maleate*: Primatuss Cough Mixture 4 Liquid; Scot-Tussin DM Liquid; Tricodene Sugar Free Liquid. With *promethazine*: Phenameth DM Syrup; Phenergan w/Dextromethorphan Syrup; Pherazine DM Syrup. (Most combinations available as generics.)

How administered: Orally.

Used to treat

Dextromethorphan is used alone or with other drugs to relieve a dry or painful non-productive ✪ **cough**.

Warnings

• It should not be given to people with known hypersensitivity to this drug. It should be used only under medical supervision by anyone with a high fever, rash, persistent headache, nausea or vomiting.

• There are no known risks in pregnancy or nursing.

• It should not be used by anyone taking a ℞ **MAOI** antidepressant, or until two weeks after stopping MAOI treatment.

• Do not use to treat a persistent or chronic cough (as from smoking, asthma, or emphysema), or a cough with heavy secretions.

Interactions

• If used with MAOI antidepressants, ℞ **isocarboxazid** or ℞ **phenelzine**, there is an increased risk of toxicity.

• If used with ℞ **sibutramine**, there is an increased risk of serotonin syndrome.

Side effects

• These are rare, but nausea, slight drowsiness or dizziness may occur.

dextropropoxyphene hydrochloride ⓓ

see ℞ **propoxyphene hydrochloride**.

Dextrostat ⓑ

A preparation of ℞ **dextroamphetamine**.

Formulation: Oral tablets.

Availability: Prescription only.

Warnings and side effects: See ℞ **dextroamphetamine**.

D.H.E. 45 ®

A preparation of ℞ **dihydroergotamine mesylate.**
Formulation: Injection.
Availability: Prescription only.
Warnings and side effects: See ℞ dihydroergotamine mesylate.

DHS Tar ®

A preparation of ℞ **coal tar.**
Formulation: Shampoo.
Availability: OTC.
Warnings and side effects: See ℞ coal tar.

DHT ®

see ℞ **dihydrotachysterol (DHT).**

DiaBeta ®

A preparation of ℞ **glyburide.**
Formulation: Oral tablets in several strengths.
Availability: Prescription only.
Warnings and side effects: See ℞ glyburide.

Diabetes CF ®

A preparation of ℞ **dextromethorphan.**
Formulation: Oral syrup.
Availability: OTC.
Warnings and side effects: See ℞ dextromethorphan. It contains the sweetener aspartame (with phenylalanine), which should be avoided by individuals with phenylketonuria.

diabetes insipidus treatment ⊙

Generics: **benzthiazide; desmopressin; chlorothiazide; chlorpropamide; indapamide; lypressin; vasopressin.**

Actions and uses

Diabetes insipidus treatment involves the use of drugs to counter-act the under-production of, or decrease the kidney response to, antidiuretic hormone (ADH; also called ℞ **vasopressin**), which is secreted by the posterior pituitary gland, and which is a character-istic of ⊙ **diabetes insipidus.**

Where the defect is in release, then either of its two natural forms (℞ **vasopressin** and ℞ **lypressin**) may be used, but must be given by injection (the hormone is a peptide and so is broken down in the gastrointestinal tract). The analog ℞ **desmopressin** (a syn-thetic peptide) can be given in the form of a nasal spray (it is absorbed into the systemic circulation from the nasal mucosa) or by mouth. For nephrogenic diabetes insipidus (where the defect is in the kidney), ℞ **diuretic** drugs of the ℞ **thiazide** class (including ℞ **benzthiazide**, ℞ **chlorothiazide**, and ℞ **indapamide**) have become a major part of treatment.

Unusually for a ℞ **sulfonylurea** drug (a class normally used for ⊙ **diabetes mellitus** treatment), ℞ **chlorpropamide** can also be used as in diabetes insipidus treatment, although only in mild forms caused by pituitary or thalamic malfunction.

Limitations

Diabetes insipidus is a rare disease and has no connection at all with diabetes mellitus, which is also a hormone disorder, but due to the under-production of, or the body's response, to ℞ **insulin** by the pancreas gland. However, in both conditions symptoms include thirst and a production of large quantities of dilute urine. See also the individual drug entries.

Diabetic Tussin DM Syrup ®

A preparation of ℞ **dextromethorphan** and ℞ **guaifenesin.**
Formulation: Oral liquid.
Availability: OTC.
Warnings and side effects: See ℞ dextromethorphan; ℞ guaifenesin.

Diabetic Tussin EX Liquid ®

A preparation of ℞ **guaifenesin.**
Formulation: Oral syrup.
Availability: OTC.
Warnings and side effects: See ℞ guaifenesin.

Diabinese ®

A preparation of ℞ **chlorpropamide.**
Formulation: Oral tablets.
Availability: Prescription only.
Warnings and side effects: See ℞ chlorpropamide.

diagnostic agent ⓪

Generics: **cosyntropin; corticotropin; fluorescein sodium; tropicamide; tuberculin.**

Actions and uses

Diagnostic agents are used for investigational purposes, particu-larly in the diagnosis of disease. There are many drugs that can be used and a few of the more popular ones are described in this entry. A number of ℞ **hormone** drugs are used to investigate endocrine disorders, and sometimes the natural hormone is used, or alterna-tively a synthetic analog. Thus ℞ **corticotropin** (adrenocorti-cotrophic hormone (ACTH)) is used for diagnostic testing of adrenocortical function, and sometimes the synthetic derivative ℞ **cosyntropin** is used instead. ℞ **fluorescein sodium** is a dye used on the surface of the eye in ophthalmic diagnostic procedures, or is injected in ophthalmic angiography. ℞ **tropicamide** is a short-acting ℞ **anticholinergic** drug, which can be used also in oph-thalmic examination to dilate the pupil and paralyze the focusing of the eye. ℞ **tuberculin** (in the form tuberculin purified protein derivative; PPD) is a diagnostic agent prepared from protein parts of the tuberculosis mycobacterium. It is used to test whether or not a person has antibodies to tuberculosis, which may indicate active disease or that there has been contact with someone who does have active infection.

Limitations

See the individual drug entries.

Dialume ®

A preparation of ℞ **aluminum hydroxide.**
Formulation: Oral capsules.
Availability: OTC.
Warnings and side effects: See ℞ aluminum hydroxide.

Diamox Tablets; Capsules ®

A preparation of ℞ **acetazolamide**.
Formulation: Oral tablets, available in two strengths; sustained release capsules; powdered form for injection.
Availability: Prescription only.
Warnings and side effects: See ℞ **acetazolamide**.

Diaparene Diaper Rash ®

A preparation of ℞ **zinc oxide** and ℞ **petrolatum**.
Formulation: Topical ointment.
Availability: OTC.
Warnings and side effects: See ℞ **zinc oxide**; ℞ **petrolatum**.

Diaper Guard ®

A preparation of ℞ **zinc oxide**.
Formulation: Topical ointment.
Availability: OTC.
Warnings and side effects: See ℞ **zinc oxide**.

Diaper Guard Ointment ®

A preparation of dimethicone, ℞ **petrolatum**, cocoa butter, ⚖ **vitamin A** and ⚖ **D**, and ℞ **zinc oxide**.
Formulation: Topical ointment.
Availability: OTC.
Warnings and side effects: See ℞ **simethicone**; ℞ **petrolatum**; ⚖ **vitamin A**; ⚖ **vitamin D**; ℞ **zinc oxide**.

Diapid ®

A preparation of ℞ **lypressin**.
Formulation: Nasal spray.
Availability: Prescription only.
Warnings and side effects: See ℞ **lypressin**.

Diar-Aid Caplets ®

A preparation of ℞ **loperamide hydrochloride**.
Formulation: Oral tablets.
Availability: OTC.
Warnings and side effects: See ℞ **loperamide hydrochloride**.

Diastat; Pediatric ®

A preparation of ℞ **diazepam**.
Formulation: Rectal gel in several strengths (including pediatric).
Availability: Prescription only.
Warnings and side effects: See ℞ **diazepam**.

diazepam ©

Type/Group: antianxiety; sedatives; anticonvulsant; skeletal muscle relaxant; benzodiazepine; antiepileptic.
Brand(s): Diastat; Valium; various generic.
How administered: Orally; injection; suppository.

Used to treat

Diazepam can be used in the short-term treatment of ✪ **anxiety**, for ✪ **insomnia**, as an additional treatment of convulsions due to poisoning, seizure disorders and fever, as a sedative in preoperative medication, and as a skeletal muscle relaxant. It is used also to assist in the treatment of acute alcohol withdrawal symptoms and to control intermittent episodic increased seizure frequency in epilepsy. Although not stated by the manufacturer for such use, it may be given for the control of panic disorder, tremor, tension headaches, or for night terrors and sleepwalking in children.

Warnings

• It should not be given to people with known hypersensitivity to benzodiazepines, with psychosis, or narrow-angle glaucoma.
• It should be given with caution to people with liver or kidney disease, with low blood levels of albumin, who are in a weakened condition (debilitated), over 65, or children.
• Diazepam should almost always be avoided during pregnancy, particularly in the first trimester. A doctor must be contacted if pregnancy occurs while diazepam is being taken.
• It should not normally be used by nursing mothers.
• It may cause drowsiness and so impair the performance of skilled tasks such as driving.
• Avoid alcohol consumption, because side effects may be increased (see Side effects below).
• Avoid other psychotropic medications unless prescribed by a doctor.
• A doctor must be consulted before discontinuing use or increasing dosage, because benzodiazepines may produce psychological and physical dependence and withdrawal symptoms.

Interactions

• ℞ **carbamazepine**, ℞ **phenytoin**, and ℞ **rifampin** markedly reduce the effects of diazepam.
• ℞ **cimetidine**, ℞ **ciprofloxacin**, ℞ **clarithromycin**, delavirdine, ℞ **disulfiram**, ℞ **erythromycin**, ℞ **fluconazole**, ℞ **fluoxetine**, ℞ **fluvoxamine**, ℞ **isoniazid**, ℞ **itraconazole**, ℞ **ketoconazole**, ℞ **metoprolol tartrate**, ℞ **omeprazole**, ℞ **quinolones**, and troleandomycin may increase the effects of diazepam.
• The effects of ℞ **levodopa** may be reduced by diazepam.
• If used with ℞ **clozapine**, respiratory and cardiovascular side effects are increased.
• If used with alcohol, adverse side effects may be increased.

Side effects

• Depending on use, dose, how it is administered, and type, there may be drowsiness and lightheadedness; postural hypotension (lowered blood pressure on standing), and blurred vision.
• Less frequently, confusion, impaired movement and coordination (particularly in older adults), mental changes, memory loss, aggression, vertigo, headache, hypotension, salivation changes, rashes, visual disturbances, changes in libido, urinary retention, liver and blood disorders, jaundice, and gastrointestinal disorders.
• Rare but serious side effects include respiratory depression.

diazoxide ©

Type/Group: antihypertensive; hypotensive; antihypoglycemic.
Brand(s): Hyperstat; Proglycem.
How administered: Orally; injection.

Used to treat

Diazoxide has two separate actions and uses. It is a hyperglycemic drug and can be used by mouth to treat chronic hypoglycemia (abnormally low levels of glucose in the bloodstream), for example, where a pancreatic tumor causes excessive secretion of insulin. A second unrelated use is as a vasodilator that can lower blood pressure rapidly on injection, and can therefore be used to treat acute hypertensive crisis.

Warnings
• It should not be given to people with a history of hypersensitivity to ℞ **thiazide** derivatives (it is chemically similar).
• It should be given with caution to people with impaired kidney function or compromised heart reserve.
• It crosses the placenta and may have adverse effects on the fetus. It should be used during pregnancy only if the potential benefit outweighs the risk to the fetus.
• Medical judgment is required if breast-feeding is being considered, as this drug appears in breast milk and may have adverse effects on the infant.
• An overdose may cause hyperglycemia.

Interactions
• ℞ **carboplatin** and ℞ **cisplatin** increase the risk of kidney damage.
• ℞ **hydralazine hydrochloride** can cause a severe hypotensive reaction.
• ℞ **phenytoin** levels are reduced in children.
• ℞ **thiazide** ℞ **diuretics** cause hyperglycemia.

Side effects
• Frequently, edema.
• Occasionally, speeded heartbeat, altered taste, constipation, loss of appetite, nausea, vomiting, and abdominal pain.
• Rarely, allergic reactions, confusion, tingling or numbness, postural hypotension (dizziness when standing up), angina, heart rhythm changes, and platelet disorders.

Dibent Ⓑ
A preparation of ℞ **dicyclomine hydrochloride**.
Formulation: Injection.
Availability: Prescription only.
Warnings and side effects: See ℞ **dicyclomine hydrochloride**.

Dibenzyline Ⓑ
A preparation of ℞ **phenoxybenzamine**.
Formulation: Oral capsules.
Availability: Prescription only.
Warnings and side effects: See ℞ **phenoxybenzamine**.

dibucaine Ⓖ
(cinchocaine)
Type/Group: **local anesthetic**.
Brand(s): Nupercainil; various generic.
How administered: Topically (external).

Used to treat
Dibucaine is used topically (externally) to treat the pain and itching of skin disorders, sunburn, toothache, rash, minor wounds, and rectal irritation.

Warnings
• It should not be given to people with known hypersensitivity to dibucaine or other amide anesthetics, or to infants under one year.
• It should be given with caution to children under six.
• Dibucaine should be used during pregnancy only if it is clearly needed.
• Medical judgment is required if breast-feeding is being considered.
• It should not be applied to large areas.

Interactions
No significant interactions have been reported.

Side effects
• Irritation, rash, and allergic reaction.

Dicarbosil Ⓑ
A preparation of ℞ **calcium carbonate**.
Formulation: Oral tablets, chewable.
Availability: OTC.
Warnings and side effects: See ℞ **calcium carbonate**.

dichlorphenamide Ⓖ
Type/Group: **glaucoma treatment**.
Brand(s): Daranide.
How administered: Orally.

Used to treat
Dichlorphenamide is a sulfonamide derivative used to treat ✪ **glaucoma**. It is most effective when used in combination with other drugs.

Warnings
• It should not be given to people with known hypersensitivity to this drug, liver insufficiency, kidney failure, adrenocortical insufficiency, hyperchloremic acidosis, hypokalemia (low blood potassium), hyponatremia, or impaired alveolar ventilation.
• It should be given with caution to people with respiratory acidosis or cirrhosis, or who are taking steroids or ACTH.
• It should be used during pregnancy only if the potential benefits outweigh the possible risks to the fetus.
• Medical judgment is required if breast-feeding is being considered.
• It may cause drowsiness.

Interactions
• If used with ℞ **salicylates**, there is an increased risk of CNS (central nervous system) toxicity.
• The levels of ℞ **flecainide**, ℞ **mexiletine**, and ℞ **quinidine** are increased.
• If used with ℞ **methenamine**, the alkalization of urine decreases the antibacterial effects.
• If used with ℞ **phenytoin**, there is an increased risk of osteomalacia (a bone disorder).
• There may be a decrease in the levels of ℞ **primidone**.

Side effects
• Most frequently, fatigue, tingling in hands or feet, weakness, loss of appetite, diarrhea, nausea, taste alteration, vomiting, urinary frequency, and hypokalemia (low potassium levels).

Key to symbols: ✪ = Disorder Section ℞ = Drug Section ♣ = Herbal Section ᪥ = Supplement Section

• Rare but serious effects include seizure, blood disorders, and Stevens-Johnson syndrome (a skin disorder).

diclofenac Ⓖ

Type/Group: **anti-inflammatory; antirheumatic; non-narcotic analgesic; NSAID; antigout.**

Brand(s): Cataflam; Voltaren; Voltaren-XR; various generic. For ophthalmic use: Voltaren Solution. Combinations: With *misoprostol*, Arthrotec.

How administered: Orally; topically (eye).

Used to treat

Diclofenac is used to treat pain and inflammation in rheumatic disease and other ✪ **musculoskeletal disorders** (such as ✪ **rheumatoid arthritis,** ✪ **ankylosing spondylitis,** and ✪ **osteoarthritis**) and to relieve symptoms of menstrual dysfunction. It is also used in some ophthalmic procedures. It is being increasingly used to treat pain immediately after certain surgical procedures (for example, to reduce inflammation of the eye after cataract removal).

Warnings

• It should not be used by people with known hypersensitivity to this drug, or to other NSAIDs (including ℞ **aspirin**), who have chronic kidney disease, porphyria, certain bleeding disorders or conditions (for example, hemophilia, vitamin K deficiency, low blood-platelet levels), or who have a tendency to, or active, peptic ulceration.

• It should be given with caution to people taking certain drugs for gout, with allergic disorders (especially asthma and skin conditions), who are elderly, or with any kind of kidney impairment or certain liver disorders.

• When used topically in the eye (for example, after ophthalmic surgery), soft contact lenses should not be worn because they may cause redness and burning.

• Diclofenac should be used during pregnancy only when medically judged to be clearly needed, but not at all in the third trimester, because of risk to the fetus. (Some preparations contain diclofenac in combination with ℞ **mifepristone**, which is an FDA pregnancy category X drug and should not be used by pregnant or breast-feeding mothers.)

• Breast-feeding mothers should either discontinue this drug or stop breast feeding.

• With regular, long-term use (as in the treatment of osteoarthritis), NSAIDs may cause gastrointestinal bleeding, ulceration, or perforation. Any signs of bleeding (for example, black stools) should be reported to a physician immediately.

• Most NSAIDs have the potential, particularly with regular use, to cause liver damage. This potential is higher with diclofenac, and periodic evaluation of liver function is necessary in long-term therapy (more than two months).

• Side effects are more frequent in the elderly.

• Gastrointestinal upsets may be minimized by taking it with milk or food.

Interactions

• There is generally no added benefit in taking other NSAIDs or other ℞ **salicylates** at the same time, but there is a higher risk of gastrointestinal upsets and bleeding.

• Diclofenac taken with alcohol or ℞ **corticosteroids** increases the risk of bleeding, particularly if there is an existing ulcer.

• ℞ **Anticoagulants** (for example, ℞ **warfarin sodium**) and ℞ **misoprostol** should be used with caution, because they may make bleeding more likely.

• The effects of ℞ **cyclosporine,** ℞ **digoxin,** ℞ **lithium,** and ℞ **methotrexate** may be exaggerated, with potential for serious toxicity.

• Diclofenac taken with ℞ **insulin** or ℞ **oral hypoglycemics** may alter the glucose-lowering effect.

• ℞ **Beta-blockers,** ℞ **diuretics,** and ℞ **hydrochlorothiazide** may lose some of their effectiveness.

• ℞ **colestipol hydrochloride** and ℞ **sucralfate** may lower the absorption or effectiveness of diclofenac.

• Foodstuffs and herbals with ℞ **antiplatelet** properties, such as ♣ **ginger,** ⚘ **garlic,** and various herbal preparations, may add to the antiplatelet effect of NSAIDs.

Side effects

These vary in severity and how often they occur, and also depend on how the drug is administered, use, dose, and duration of treatment.

• Commonly, gastrointestinal upsets, nausea, heartburn, diarrhea, constipation, and flatulence.

• Less frequently, there may be vomiting, dizziness, headache, rash, ringing in the ears, fluid retention, edema, fatigue, and sleep disturbances.

• Prolonged bleeding time (with a resulting risk of ulceration) is possible with high dosage, and other blood changes can occur, including anemia.

• Hypersensitivity reactions may include symptoms such as swelling of eyelids, tongue, lips, or larynx, rash, chest tightness, asthma, or bronchospasm.

• Reversible kidney failure, particularly in renal impairment, has occurred. Liver damage is rare.

• These systemic effects are unlikely (though possible) with topical (ophthalmic) use, however, there may be burning, stinging, itching, or blurred vision when used as eyedrops.

dicloxacillin sodium Ⓖ

Type/Group: **antibiotic; penicillin.**

Brand(s): Dynapen; Pathocil; Dycill; various generics.

How administered: Orally; injection.

Used to treat

Dicloxacillin sodium is a semisynthetic penicillinase-resistant penicillin used to treat ✪ **bacterial infections** of the bone and localized skin and skin structure.

Warnings

• It should not be used by anyone with known hypersensitivity to penicillins.

• It should be given with caution to people with allergies to ℞ **cephalosporins** or ℞ **imipenem**, with asthma, eczema, and mononucleosis (may cause rash).

• Penicillins cross the placenta and should be used in pregnancy only if medically judged to be needed.

• Dicloxacillin should not be used while breast-feeding.

• Serious and occasionally fatal hypersensitivity reactions can occur. A doctor must be contacted if skin rash, itching, hives, severe diarrhea, shortness of breath, black tongue, sore throat, nausea, fever, swollen joints, or any unusual bleeding or bruising occurs.

• Superinfections from the altered bacterial balance created by antibiotic treatment may occur and may result in ⊕ **pseudomembranous colitis**. A doctor must be contacted if there is severe abdominal pain, or moderate to severe diarrhea.

• Take on an empty stomach (one hour before or two hours after eating).

• The full course of treatment prescribed must be completed or infection may return.

Interactions

• ℞ **chloramphenicol**, ℞ **macrolide** antibiotics, and ℞ **tetracyclines** may be reduce the effectiveness of penicillin.

• The effectiveness of ℞ **oral contraceptives** may be reduced.

• The effects of ℞ **warfarin sodium** may be inhibited.

• ℞ **methotrexate** levels may be increased.

Side effects

• Frequently, mild allergic reaction, nausea, gastrointestinal effects.

• Possible but rare serious side effects include kidney and bladder infections, bone marrow depression, seizures, and blood changes.

dicumarol ⓖ

Type/Group: **anticoagulant**.
Brand(s): Generic.
How administered: Orally; injection.

Used to treat

Dicumarol is used to prevent the formation of clots in certain heart disorders or after heart surgery (especially following implantation of prosthetic heart valves), and to treat or prevent venous ⊕ **thrombosis** and ⊕ **pulmonary embolism**, especially after a heart attack.

Warnings

• It should not be given to people with known hypersensitivity to this drug, with active bleeding, a tendency to bleed or blood-forming disorders, pericarditis or bacterial endocarditis, uncontrolled high blood pressure, injury or surgery that is still healing, or recent surgery involving the eye or nervous system. It will be administered by experienced personnel after a full medical assessment.

• It should be given with caution to people with vascular disease or congestive heart failure, indwelling catheters, gastrointestinal infection, high blood pressure, severe diabetes mellitus, serious vitamin C deficiency, polycythemia vera, recent traumatic injury, or liver impairment.

• This drug is not used by women who are or may become pregnant.

• Medical judgment is required if breast-feeding is being considered.

• Dicumarol should not be given to people who may not be able to cope with self-administration (for example, who are senile, alcoholic, psychotic, or uncooperative), nor should it be used where there are no facilities for performing periodic blood testing.

• A doctor should be contacted immediately if any unusual symptoms or bleeding occur, such as pain, swelling or discomfort, prolonged bleeding from a cut, nosebleeds or bleeding gums from brushing, increased menstrual flow, bruising, dark urine, red or tar black stools, headache, dizziness or weakness.

• Notify a doctor of any illness.

• Activities that might cause traumatic injury (for example, sports) should be avoided.

• Diet should be normal and balanced. Significant changes in the amount of vitamin K in the diet (as from eating large amounts of green leafy vegetables) can alter the anticoagulant effect of dicumarol.

• Dicumarol may free tiny bits of plaque that may lodge (usually) in the smaller blood vessels, which may result in abrupt, sharp pain in a leg, foot, the toes, back, or flank. ("Purple toes syndrome" appears as mottled, purplish discoloration of the toes.) More serious obstructions are possible, and may cause kidney insufficiency, pancreatitis, penile gangrene, hypertension, paralysis, or stroke. Use of dicumarol should be stopped if any of these occur.

Interactions

• The following drugs may increase the levels and effects of dicumarol, with an increased risk of bleeding: ℞ **acetaminophen**; ℞ **allopurinol**; ℞ **amiodarone hydrochloride**; ℞ **androgens**; ℞ **beta-blockers**; ℞ **chloral hydrate**; ℞ **chloramphenicol**; ℞ **chlorpropamide**; ℞ **cimetidine**; ℞ **clofibrate**; ℞ **corticosteroids**; ℞ **cyclophosphamide**; ℞ **disulfiram**; ℞ **erythromycin**; ℞ **fluconazole**; ℞ **gemfibrozil**; ℞ **glucagon**; ℞ **hydantoins**; ℞ **ifosfamide**; ℞ **influenza virus vaccine**; ℞ **isoniazid**; ℞ **ketoconazole**; loop ℞ **diuretics**; ℞ **lovastatin**; ℞ **metronidazole**; ℞ **miconazole**; ℞ **moricizine**; ℞ **nalidixic acid**; ℞ **omeprazole**; ℞ **propafenone**; ℞ **propoxyphene**; ℞ **quinidine**; ℞ **quinine**; ℞ **quinolones**; ℞ **streptokinase**; ℞ **sulfinpyrazone**; ℞ **sulfonamides**; ℞ **tamoxifen**; ℞ **thyroid hormones**; ℞ **trimethoprim and sulfamethoxazole**; and ℞ **urokinase**. Use of streptokinase or urokinase with dicumarol may be hazardous.

• ℞ **Aminoglycosides**, ℞ **mineral oil**, ℞ **tetracyclines**, and ♖♖ **vitamin E** interfere with vitamin K and may cause an increased risk of bleeding when taken with dicumarol.

• ℞ **Cephalosporins**, ℞ **diflunisal**, ℞ **NSAIDs**, ℞ **penicillins**, and ℞ **salicylates** may have various effects that make bleeding more likely when used with dicumarol.

• The following drugs may reduce the levels and effects of dicumarol: alcohol; ℞ **aminoglutethimide**; ℞ **barbiturates**; ℞ **carbamazepine**; ℞ **cholestyramine**; ℞ **oral contraceptives**; ℞ **dicloxacillin**; ℞ **estrogens**; etretinate; ℞ **glutethimide**; ℞ **griseofulvin**; ℞ **nafcillin**; ℞ **rifampin**; ℞ **spironolactone**;

℞ **sucralfate**; ℞ **thiazide** diuretics; ℞ **trazodone**; ꙮ **vitamin C** (at high doses); ꙮ **vitamin K.**

Side effects
• The chief complication is hemorrhage, which may occur at virtually any site in the body.
• Infrequent side effects may include allergic reactions, jaundice and liver disorders, gastrointestinal disturbances (for example, abdominal pain, nausea, vomiting, diarrhea), hair loss, and tingling sensations.

dicyclomine hydrochloride Ⓖ
(dicyloverine hydrochloride)
Type/Group: **anticholinergic; antispasmodic.**
Brand(s): Antispas; Bentyl; Byclomine; Dibent; Dilomine; Di-Spaz; Or-Tyl; various generic.
How administered: Orally; injection.

Used to treat
Dicyclomine hydrochloride is used for the symptomatic relief of muscle spasm in the gastrointestinal tract, especially in treating ✪ **irritable bowel syndrome.**

Warnings
• It should not be given to people with known hypersensitivity to anticholinergics, infants under 6 months old, those with myasthenia gravis, narrow-angle glaucoma, urinary obstruction, or with any infection or obstructive condition of the gastrointestinal tract.
• It should be given with caution to people with kidney or liver impairment, enlarged prostate, heart disease or high blood pressure, hyperthyroidism, ulcerative colitis, hiatal hernia, glaucoma, brain damage, or Down's syndrome.
• Dicyclomine should be used during pregnancy only if it is clearly needed.
• It may appear in breast milk and it should be avoided by nursing mothers.
• It has been associated with serious adverse reactions in infants under 6 months of age.
• Anticholinergics in general should not be given to anyone with a febrile (feverish) illness or who must work or live in a hot environment.
• The frequency and severity of side effects is higher in young children and the elderly.
• Because side effects may include drowsiness or visual disturbances, it may impair the performance of skilled tasks, such as driving.

Interactions
• ℞ **amantadine**, some ℞ **antiarrhythmic** agents (for example, ℞ **disopyramide**, ℞ **procainamide**, ℞ **quinidine**), some ℞ **antihistamines** (for example, ℞ **promethazine**, ℞ **carbinoxamine**, ℞ **diphenhydramine hydrochloride**), ℞ **antiparkinsonism** agents, ℞ **glutethimide**, ℞ **meperidine**, ℞ **phenothiazines**, and ℞ **tricyclic** antidepressants all have some anticholinergic effects which may increase when taken with dicyclomine to cause side effects.
• The levels of ℞ **digoxin** may rise if taken in the slow-dissolving form (but not as capsules or elixir).

• Anticholinergics and ꙮ **potassium chloride** (in tablet form) should be used together with caution, because the tablet form of potassium chloride may stay in the intestines longer, and so there is a greater risk of irritation and lesions.
• Dicyclomine should be taken at least an hour before an ℞ **antacid.**
• ℞ **ketoconazole** should be taken least two hours before an anticholinergic.

Side effects
These tend to occur less frequently and are weaker than with other anticholinergics (for example, ℞ **atropine**), but may include:
• Dry mouth, thirst, blurred vision and other visual disturbances, urinary hesitancy, palpitation, dizziness (when injected), and constipation, especially at higher doses;
• Uncommonly, increased intraocular pressure (pressure in the eyeball), headache, unusual or absent taste sensation, nervousness, drowsiness, flushing, and nausea;
• Although rare, hives, other skin eruptions, and anaphylaxis may occur in extreme allergic reactions;
• Injection of dicyclomine may cause irritation at the site of injection.

dicyloverine hydrochloride Ⓖ
see ℞ **dicyclomine hydrochloride.**

didanosine (ddl) Ⓖ
Type/Group: **antiviral.**
Brand(s): Videx.
How administered: Orally.

Used to treat
Didanosine is a reverse transcriptase antiviral, an antiretroviral, which can be used in the treatment of ✪ **HIV** infection. It is mainly given in combination with other antivirals to people who are intolerant to, or have not benefited from, other drugs.

Warnings
• It should not be given to people with known hypersensitivity to didanosine.
• It should be given with caution to people with kidney or liver dysfunction, alcoholism, elevated triglycerides, low T-cell counts, or a history of pancreatitis.
• Didanosine's safety during pregnancy has not been established and its use is not recommended.
• The Centers for Disease Control and Prevention recommend that HIV-infected mothers do not breast-feed.
• It is a specialist drug, and there will be full assessment and patient monitoring throughout treatment.
• It should be taken on an empty stomach.
• Pancreatitis is a major and serious toxicity.
Interactions:
• Food reduces the levels of didanosine.
• ℞ **allopurinol** increases the risk of toxicity in people with kidney impairment.
• The absorption of ℞ **dapsone** may be reduced.
• ℞ **Ganciclovir (DHPG)** may increase levels of didanosine.

• The levels of ℞ **itraconazole**, ℞ **ketoconazole**, and ℞ **quinolones** may be decreased.

Side effects

These include:

• Diarrhea, peripheral neuropathy (for example, loss of feeling in the feet), raised uric acid levels in the blood (monitoring is necessary), nausea, headache, vomiting, confusion, insomnia, fever and headache, dry mouth, effects on the eye, skin rashes, pancreatitis, and blood disorders.

Di-Delamine ®

A preparation of ℞ **diphenhydramine hydrochloride**, and benzalkonium chloride, and tripelennamine.

Formulation: Topical gel; non-aerosol spray.

Availability: OTC.

Warnings and side effects: See ℞ **diphenhydramine hydrochloride; benzalkonium chloride.

Didronel ®

A preparation of ℞ **etidronate disodium.**

Formulation: Oral tablets.

Availability: Prescription only.

Warnings and side effects: See ℞ **etidronate disodium.**

dienestrol ©

(dienoestrol)

Type/Group: **sex hormone; estrogen.**

Brand(s): Ortho Dienestrol.

How administered: Topically.

Used to treat

Dienestrol is a synthetic nonsteroidal estrogen derivative which is used as a topical treatment for atrophy of the vagina and kraurosis vulvae (such as in the treatment of symptoms of the ✪ menopause).

Warnings

• It should not be used by people with breast cancer, active thromboembolic disease, known or suspected estrogen-dependent cancers, or undiagnosed abnormal genital bleeding.

• It should be given with caution to people with hypertension, gallbladder disease, congestive heart failure, diabetes mellitus, bone disease, depression, migraine headache, seizure disorders, liver disease, or kidney disease, or a family history of breast or endometrial cancer.

• Dienestrol must not be use during pregnancy. A doctor must be contacted if pregnancy occurs while using this drug.

• Medical judgment is required if breast-feeding is being considered. It may reduce quality and quantity of breast milk.

• Use of progestins along with estrogen is recommended for menopausal or postmenopausal women with an intact uterus. Taking estrogen increases the risk of endometrial cancer in these women, but adding progestins reduces the risk.

Interactions

• Dienestrol taken with ℞ **cyclosporine** may increase the risk of toxicity.

• The steroid effects of ℞ **corticosteroids** may be increased.

• ℞ **Phenytoin** causes loss of seizure control and decreased estrogen levels.

• With ℞ **warfarin sodium** and similar ℞ **anticoagulants** there is a possible increase in the risk of thromboembolism.

Side effects

• Commonly, nausea.

• Less frequently, depression, dizziness, headache, edema, elevated blood pressure, blood clots, contact lens intolerance, loss of appetite cramps, diarrhea, gallbladder disease, increased appetite and weight, endometrial hyperplasia (an abnormal increase in cell growth), and skin disorders.

• Rare but serious side effects include pancreatitis, stroke, pulmonary embolism, and heart attack.

dienoestrol ©

see ℞ **dienestrol**.

diethylstilbestrol ©

(DES)

Type/Group: **sex hormone; estrogen; anticancer.**

Brand(s): Stilphostrol.

How administered: Injection.

Used to treat

Diethylstilbestrol is a synthetic estrogen that is used to treat inoperable cancer of the prostate in men. Although not represented by the manufacturer for such use, it may be prescribed to treat advanced metastatic breast cancer in men. It is currently not available in the US except in the form of an injection.

Warnings

• It should not be used by women, or people with active thrombophlebitis or thromboembolic (blood-clotting) disorders, a history of such disorders when treated with estrogen, undiagnosed vaginal bleeding, known or suspected estrogen-dependent neoplasms (unless being treated for this), or with hypersensitivity to estrogen.

• It should be given with caution to people with heart, kidney, or liver dysfunction, epilepsy, migraine, metabolic bone disease, or depression.

• Diethylstilbestrol must not be used during pregnancy as it may cause serious harm to the fetus.

• It should not be used by breast-feeding mothers.

• Long-term, continuous administration of estrogens may increase risk of heart attack, stroke, blood-clotting disorders, and certain cancers.

Interactions

• The steroid effects of ℞ **corticosteroids** are increased.

• ℞ **Phenytoin** causes loss of seizure control and decreased estrogen levels.

• With ℞ **warfarin sodium** and similar ℞ **anticoagulants** there is a possible increase in the risk of thromboembolism.

Side effects

• Commonly, nausea and loss of appetite at high doses, breakthrough bleeding, amenorrhea breast tenderness and enlargement.

• With ℞ **warfarin sodium** and similar ℞ **anticoagulants** there is a possible increase in the risk of thromboembolism.

Differin ®

A preparation of ℞ **adapalene**.
Formulation: Topical gel.
Availability: Prescription only.
Warnings and side effects: See ℞ **adapalene**.

Diflucan ®

A preparation of ℞ **fluconazole**.
Formulation: Oral tablets, oral suspension, injection.
Availability: Prescription only.
Warnings and side effects: See ℞ **fluconazole**.

diflunisal ©

Type/Group: **anti-inflammatory; antirheumatic; non-narcotic analgesic; salicylate**.
Brand(s): Dolobid Tablets; various generic.
How administered: Orally.

Used to treat

Diflunisal is derived from ℞ **aspirin**, but is quite powerful and with a longer duration of action. It can be used in the treatment of mild to moderate pain and ✪ **inflammation** (especially in rheumatic disease and other ✪ **musculoskeletal disorders**) and also, although not stated by the manufacturer, for ✪ **dysmenorrhea** (period pain), ✪ **migraine**, and tendonitis.

Warnings

• Diflunisal should not be used by people with known hypersensitivity to this drug or to other ℞ **NSAIDs** (including aspirin), who have chronic kidney disease, certain bleeding disorders or conditions (for example, hemophilia, vitamin K deficiency, low platelet levels), or who have a tendency to, or active, peptic ulceration.

• It should be given with caution to people taking certain drugs for gout or diabetes mellitus, or with allergic disorders (especially asthma and skin conditions), in the elderly, children or teenagers, in those with any kind of kidney impairment, or with certain liver disorders.

• Diflunisal may adversely affect the health both of a pregnant woman and the fetus. It should be used during pregnancy only if potential benefit outweighs potential risk, but not in the third trimester, when risk to the fetus is at its highest.

• Breast-feeding mothers should either discontinue this drug or stop breast-feeding.

• Although no direct association has been shown with diflunisal, there is a link between ℞ **salicylates** and the rare, but serious, condition called ✪ **Reye's syndrome** (which causes inflammation of the brain and liver). Because diflunisal is a salicylate derivative, it is recommended that it is not given to children or teenagers who have, or might have, chickenpox or influenza. As so many infections resemble flu in their initial symptoms, salicylates should not, as a general rule, be used to treat fever, ache, and malaise by anyone in this age group except on the advice of a doctor.

• If dizziness, change in hearing, or ringing in the ears (tinnitus) occurs, stop using this drug. These are usually the first symptoms of overdose.

• Diflunisal can produce the same allergic-like symptoms (including bronchospasm) that may occur after taking NSAIDs, including bronchospasm in "aspirin-sensitive" asthmatics.

Interactions

• There is a greater risk of liver damage if taken with ℞ **acetaminophen**, and so these drugs should not be used together except on medical advice and with careful monitoring.

• There is generally no added benefit in taking other NSAIDs (especially ℞ **indomethacin**) or other salicylates at the same time, but there is a higher risk of gastrointestinal upsets and bleeding.

• If taken with alcohol, there is an increased risk of bleeding, particularly of an existing ulcer.

• ℞ **Anticoagulants** have an additive effect in prolonging bleeding time.

• The effects of ℞ **cyclosporine** and ℞ **methotrexate** may be exaggerated with potentially toxic results.

• ℞ **Hydrochlorothiazide** may lose some of its therapeutic effect.

• ℞ **Antacids** (when used routinely) may lower the absorption or therapeutic effect of diflunisal.

• Foods high in salicylates, such as curry powder, gherkins, licorice, paprika, prunes, raisins, and tea, may increase the risk of side effects.

Side effects

These vary in severity and in the frequency with which they occur.

• The most common are gastrointestinal upsets, nausea, heartburn, diarrhea, headache, and rash. (The gastrointestinal upsets may be minimized by taking the drug with milk or food.)

• Prolonged bleeding time (with consequent risk of ulceration) is possible with high dosage.

• Less frequently there may be vomiting, constipation, flatulence, dizziness, ringing in the ears, fatigue, and sleep disturbances.

• Hypersensitivity reactions may include symptoms such as fever and chills, hives, rash, bronchospasm, edema, blood disorders, and fluid retention.

• Reversible kidney failure, particularly in renal impairment, has occurred. Liver damage is rare.

Di-Gel Advanced Formula Tablets ®

A preparation of ℞ **calcium carbonate**, ℞ **magnesium hydroxide**, and ℞ **simethicone**.
Formulation: Oral tablets, chewable.
Availability: OTC.
Warnings and side effects: See ℞ **calcium carbonate**; ℞ **magnesium hydroxide**; ℞ **simethicone**.

Di-Gel Liquid ®

A preparation of ℞ **aluminum hydroxide** and ℞ **simethicone**.
Formulation: Oral liquid.
Availability: OTC.
Warnings and side effects: See ℞ **aluminum hydroxide**; ℞ **simethicone**.

Digepepsin Tablets Ⓑ

A preparation of ℞ **pancreatin** (amylase, lipase, protease), pepsin, bile salts.

Formulation: Oral tablets.

Availability: Prescription only.

Warnings and side effects: See ℞ pancreatin.

digestive enzyme Ⓓ

Generics: **pancreatin.**

Actions and uses

Digestive enzyme preparations are used to make up a deficiency in the secretion of one of the digestive enzymes, so that a more normal digestion of foods may take place. The only enzyme given by mouth for this purpose is a pancreatic enzyme mixture. ℞ **pancreatin** is the term used to describe extracts of the pancreas that contain the pancreatic enzymes amylase, lipase, and protease. (In a more concentrated form and with a higher percentage of lipase, the extract is called *pancrelipase*.) It can be given by mouth to treat ✪ **digestive system disorders** and deficiencies due to impaired natural secretion by the pancreas, such as in ✪ **cystic fibrosis**, and also following operations involving removal of pancreatic tissue, such as panreatectomy and gastrectomy.

This approach has been tried in the past with various enzymes, but they have tended to erode the upper digestive tract. Also the enzymes that help digest protein, starch, and fat, are inactivated by stomach acid. To circumvent this, in the case of pancreatin, preparations are taken with food or with certain other drugs, such as ℞ **H₂-antagonists**, which reduce acid secretion. Alternatively, pancreatin is available as enteric-coated tablets and capsules, which give it some protection from stomach acid. However, they are destroyed by heat and should, therefore, be mixed with food after its preparation. The majority of pancreatin preparations are of porcine (pig) origin.

Limitations

See the individual drug entries.

Digibind Ⓑ

A preparation of ℞ **digoxin immune Fab.**

Formulation: Injection.

Availability: Prescription only.

Warnings and side effects: See ℞ digoxin immune Fab.

digitoxin Ⓖ

Type/Group: cardiac glycoside; heart failure treatment; cardiac stimulant; antiarrhythmic.

Brand(s): Crystodigin.

How administered: Orally.

Used to treat

Digitoxin is derived from the leaves of *Digitalis* foxgloves. It increases the force of contraction (beneficial in the treatment of ✪ **heart failure**, and can also be used to treat certain heartbeat irregularities (see ✪ **arrhythmia**).

Warnings

• It should not be given to people who have had a previous toxic or allergic response to this drug, or who have beriberi, heart disease, or ventricular tachycardia or fibrillation.

• It should be given with caution to people who have had a recent heart attack, with certain arrhythmias and heart conditions (for example, those caused by episodes of rheumatic fever), hypothyroidism, severe lung disease, who are elderly, or with impaired kidney function.

• It should be used during pregnancy only when it is clearly needed.

• Medical judgment is required if breast-feeding is being considered. No adverse effects in infants have been reported in nursing women taking digitoxin, but its safety has not been established.

• Once an effective digitoxin dose and routine has been established, it should not be stopped without first checking with a doctor. Adverse effects are possible with abrupt discontinuation.

• Because a beneficial digitoxin dose lies within a very narrow range for each person, a large number of other drugs may significantly affect its circulating levels or effects. Other medication (including some OTC antacids, cold, allergy and diet drugs, and herbal remedies) should not be used without first consulting a doctor.

• A doctor must be contacted if there is irregular heartbeat, troubled breathing, nausea, diarrhea, unusual weakness or tiredness, skin rash, or blurred or yellow vision.

• Regular monitoring of blood potassium and other electrolyte levels is usual, as well as periodic monitoring of heart function (ECG).

Interactions

• ℞ **amiodarone hydrochloride**, ℞ **amphotericin B**, ℞ **anticholinergics**, ℞ **benzodiazepines**, ℞ **beta-blockers**, some ℞ **calcium-channel blockers** (for example, ℞ **diltiazem hydrochloride**, ℞ **verapamil**), ☊ **calcium salts**, ℞ **cyclosporine**, ℞ **diphenoxylate**, thiazide and loop ℞ **diuretics**, ℞ **esmolol**, ℞ **felodipine**, ℞ **flecainide**, ℞ **hydroxychloroquine sulfate**, ℞ **ibuprofen**, ℞ **indomethacin**, ℞ **itraconazole**, ℞ **omeprazole**, ℞ **propafenone**, ℞ **propantheline**, ℞ **quinidine**, ℞ **quinine**, nondepolarizing ℞ **skeletal muscle relaxants**, ℞ **succinylcholine**, ℞ **sympathomimetics** (for example, ℞ **ephedrine**, ℞ **epinephrine**, ℞ **isoproterenol**), ℞ **tolbutamide**, and ℞ **triamterene** may increase the levels or effects of digitoxin, with possibly adverse effects.

• Some anti-infectives (for example, ℞ **clarithromycin**, ℞ **erythromycin**, ℞ **tetracycline**) may also increase digitoxin levels (but only in some people).

• ℞ **amiloride**, ℞ **aminoglutethimide**, ℞ **aminosalicylate**, aluminum or magnesium ℞ **antacids**, certain ℞ **anticancer** drugs, kaolin or pectin ℞ **antidiarrheals**, ℞ **antihistamines**, ℞ **barbiturates**, ℞ **cholestyramine**, ℞ **colestipol hydrochloride**, ℞ **hydantoins**, oral ℞ **hypoglycemic** agents, ℞ **metoclopramide**, ℞ **neomycin**, ℞ **penicillamine**, ℞ **rifampin**, ℞ **sucralfate**, ℞ **sulfasalazine**, and ℞ **thyroid hormones** may decrease the levels or effects of digitoxin.

• The effects of oral ℞ **aminoglycosides** and ℞ **spironolactone** on digitoxin are not consistent.

Side effects

• There are serious and common side effects (adverse effects are usually signs of toxicity; the minimization of which depends on finding a suitable dosage schedule for each person and regular monitoring): loss of appetite, nausea and vomiting, with a consequent weight loss, diarrhea and abdominal pain, visual disturbances, fatigue, confusion, delirium and hallucinations.

• Overdosage may lead to arrhythmias or heart block.

digoxin Ⓖ

Type/Group: **cardiac glycoside; heart failure treatment; cardiac stimulant; antiarrhythmic.**

Brand(s): **Lanoxicaps, Lanoxin**; various generic.

How administered: Orally; injection.

Used to treat

Digoxin is derived from the leaves of *Digitalis* foxgloves and is the most-used of the cardiac glycosides. It increases the force of contraction, which is beneficial in the treatment of ✚ **heart failure**, and can be used to treat certain heartbeat irregularities (see ✚ **arrhythmia**).

Warnings

• It should not be given to people who have had a previous toxic or allergic response to this drug, or who have beriberi, heart disease, or ventricular tachycardia or fibrillation.

• It should be given with caution to people who have had a recent heart attack, certain arrhythmias and heart conditions (for example, rheumatic fever), hypothyroidism, severe lung disease, who are elderly, or have impaired kidney function.

• Digoxin should be used during pregnancy only when it is clearly needed.

• Medical judgment is required if breast-feeding is being considered. No adverse effects in infants have been reported, but its safety has not been established.

• Once an effective digoxin dose and routine has been established, it should not be stopped without first checking with a doctor, as adverse effects are possible.

• Because a beneficial digoxin dose lies within a very narrow range for each person, a large number of other drugs may significantly affect its levels and effects. Other medication (including some OTC antacids, cold, allergy and diet drugs, and herbal remedies) must not be taken without first consulting a doctor.

• A doctor must be contacted if irregular heartbeat, troubled breathing, nausea, diarrhea, unusual weakness or tiredness, skin rash, blurred or yellow vision occur.

• Regular monitoring of blood potassium and other electrolyte levels is usual, as well as periodic monitoring of heart function (ECG).

Interactions

• ℞ **amiodarone hydrochloride**, ℞ **amphotericin B**, ℞ **anticholinergics**, ℞ **benzodiazepines**, ℞ **beta-blockers**, some ℞ **calcium-channel blockers** (for example, ℞ **diltiazem hydrochloride**, ℞ **verapamil**), ⚘ **calcium**, ℞ **cyclosporine**, ℞ **diphenoxylate**, thiazide and loop ℞ **diuretics**, ℞ **esmolol**, ℞ **felodipine**, ℞ **flecainide**, ℞ **hydroxychloroquine sulfate**, ℞ **ibuprofen**, ℞ **indomethacin**, ℞ **itraconazole**, ℞ **omeprazole**,

℞ **propafenone**, ℞ **propantheline**, ℞ **quinidine**, ℞ **quinine**, nondepolarizing ℞ **skeletal muscle relaxants**, ℞ **succinylcholine**, ℞ **sympathomimetics** (for example, ℞ **ephedrine**, ℞ **epinephrine**, ℞ **isoproterenol**), ℞ **tolbutamide**, and ℞ **triamterene** may increase the levels or effects of digoxin, with possibly adverse effects.

• Some anti-infectives (for example, ℞ **clarithromycin**, ℞ **erythromycin**, ℞ **tetracycline**) may also increase digoxin levels (but only in some people), and the risk of interaction may be reduced by using digoxin available in liquid-filled capsules (a rapidly absorbed form).

• ℞ **amiloride**, ℞ **aminoglutethimide**, ℞ **aminosalicylate**, aluminum or magnesium ℞ **antacids**, certain ℞ **anticancer** drugs, kaolin or pectin ℞ **antidiarrheals**, ℞ **antihistamines**, ℞ **barbiturates**, ℞ **cholestyramine**, ℞ **colestipol hydrochloride**, ℞ **hydantoins**, oral ℞ **hypoglycemic** agents, ℞ **metoclopramide**, ℞ **neomycin**, ℞ **penicillamine**, ℞ **rifampin**, ℞ **sucralfate**, ℞ **sulfasalazine**, and ℞ **thyroid hormones** may decrease the levels or effects of digoxin.

• The effects of oral ℞ **aminoglycosides** and ℞ **spironolactone** on digoxin are not consistent.

Side effects

• There are serious and common side effects (adverse effects are usually signs of toxicity; the minimization of which depends on finding a suitable dosage schedule for each person and regular monitoring): loss of appetite, nausea and vomiting, with a consequent weight loss, diarrhea and abdominal pain, visual disturbances, fatigue, confusion, delirium and hallucinations.

• Overdosage may lead to arrhythmias or heart block.

digoxin immune Fab Ⓖ

(digoxin-specific antibody fragment)

Type/Group: **antidote.**

Brand(s): **Digibind.**

How administered: Injection.

Used to treat

Digoxin immune Fab is composed of antibody fragments that react with the glycosides and can be used as an antidote to overdosage by ℞ **digoxin** and ℞ **digitoxin**.

Warnings

• There are no absolute contraindications.

• It should be given with caution to people with impaired heart and kidney function, or with allergies to sheep-derived products.

• It should be used during pregnancy only when it is clearly needed and when the potential benefits outweigh the possible risks to the fetus.

• Medical judgment is required if breast-feeding is being considered. It is not known whether this drug appears in breast milk.

• It may cause an allergic reaction.

• It is a specialist drug used under controlled conditions.

Interactions

No significant interactions are known.

Side effects
• Hypokalemia (low blood potassium levels), low cardiac output, and congestive heart failure.

digoxin-specific antibody fragment Ⓖ
see ℞ digoxin immune Fab.

dihydroergotamine mesilate Ⓖ
see ℞ dihydroergotamine mesylate.

dihydroergotamine mesylate Ⓖ
(dihydroergotamine mesilate)
Type/Group: **antimigraine; ergot alkaloid.**
Brand(s): **D.H.E. 45; Migranol.**
How administered: Injection; orally; nasal spray.
Used to treat
Dihydroergotamine mesylate is used to treat vascular headaches, such as ✪ **migraine**, that are not relieved by ordinary painkilling drugs. It is most effective if used during the "aura"—the initial symptoms—of an attack and probably works as a vasoconstrictor (narrows blood vessels) on the cranial arteries. However, although the pain may be relieved, other symptoms, such as the visual disturbances and nausea, may not (but other drugs may be used to treat these symptoms separately). Although it has less vasoconstrictor activity than ℞ **ergotamine**, it acts more rapidly and has effects on venous circulation that are being investigated for the prevention of ✪ **deep vein thrombosis**.
Warnings
• It should not be given to people with known hypersensitivity to any ergot alkaloid, or who have vascular disease (for example, Raynaud's disease), certain kidney or liver disorders, severe hypertension, porphyria, malnutrition, sepsis, or hyperthyroidism.
• Dihydroergotamine must not be used during pregnancy.
• Ergot alkaloids do appear in breast milk and may cause symptoms in infants, such as vomiting or diarrhea.
• This drug should be used only to treat, not to prevent, migraine attacks. For best results, it should be used at the first sign of an attack.
• If there is numbness or tingling in the extremities, treatment must be stopped and a doctor contacted.
Interactions
• ℞ **methysergide** and dihydroergotamine should not be used within 24 hours of one another.
• If used with ℞ **beta-blockers**, circulation to the extremities may be restricted to the point that gangrene occurs.
• If used with ℞ **macrolides** (for example, ℞ **erythromycin**), there is a risk of intensified and serious side effects.
• ℞ **Vasodilators** may cause dangerously high blood pressure.
• ℞ **Naratriptan**, ℞ **rizatriptan**, ℞ **sumatriptan**, and ℞ **zolmitriptan** (antimigraine drugs) may increase effects with dihydroergotamine, with potentially serious circulatory side effects.
Side effects
• Depending on how it is administered, dose, and use, there may be vomiting, nausea, vertigo, abdominal pain and diarrhea,

cramps, chest pain, itching, pain, tingling and numbness in the extremities, and fast or slow heartbeat.
• Repeated high dosage may cause confusion, gangrene, and peritoneal fibrosis.

dihydrotachysterol (DHT) Ⓖ
Type/Group: **vitamin.**
Brand(s): DHT; Hytakerol.
How administered: Orally.
Used to treat
Dihydrotachysterol is a synthetic form of vitamin D (related to D_2 and D_3) which is used to treat postoperative and idiopathic (unknown cause) tetany (a condition involving cramps and convulsions), hypoparathyroidism, and to make up body deficiencies of this vitamin.
Warnings
• It should not be given to people with known hypercalcemia, elevated levels of vitamin D, decreased kidney function, malabsorption syndrome, or abnormal sensitivity to the effects of vitamin D.
• It should be given with caution to people with kidney stones, kidney failure, and heart disease.
• It should be used during pregnancy only if the potential benefit outweighs the possible risk to the fetus. This does not apply to amounts below the RDA.
• Medical judgment is required if breast-feeding is being considered. Calcium levels of the infant should be monitored if pharmacologic doses are taken.
• It may be toxic at high doses. A check should be kept of the amount of vitamin D in the diet and dietary supplements to avoid excess.
Interactions
• If used with magnesium-containing ℞ **antacids**, people on dialysis may develop elevated serum levels of magnesium.
• If used with digitalis glycosides or ℞ **verapamil**, there are adverse cardiac effects from hypercalcemia.
• ℞ **Cholestyramine**, ℞ **ketoconazole**, ℞ **mineral oil**, ℞ **phenytoin**, and ℞ **phenobarbital** may reduce vitamin D synthesis.
• If used with ℞ **thiazide** ℞ **diuretics**, there is an increased risk of hypercalcemia.
Side effects
• Infrequently, weakness, headache, somnolence, gastrointestinal effects, mental changes, weight loss, and urinary changes.

Dilacor XR Ⓑ
A preparation of ℞ **diltiazem hydrochloride.**
Formulation: Oral capsules, sustained release, available in 3 strengths.
Availability: Prescription only.
Warnings and side effects: See ℞ **diltiazem hydrochloride.**

Dilantin Ⓑ
A preparation of ℞ **phenytoin.**

Formulation: Oral tablets; Infatab is chewable; capsules, available in three strengths.
Availability: Prescription only.
Warnings and side effects: See ℞ **phenytoin**.

Dilatrate-SR ⑧

A preparation of ℞ **isosorbide dinitrate**.
Formulation: Oral capsules, sustained release.
Availability: Prescription only.
Warnings and side effects: See ℞ **isosorbide dinitrate**.

Dilaudid ⑧

A preparation of ℞ **hydromorphone hydrochloride**.
Formulation: Oral tablets; liquid; rectal suppositories; injection.
Availability: Prescription only.
Warnings and side effects: See ℞ **hydromorphone hydrochloride**.

Dilocaine ⑧

A preparation of ℞ **lidocaine**.
Formulation: Injection.
Availability: Prescription only.
Warnings and side effects: See ℞ **lidocaine**.

Dilomine ⑧

A preparation of ℞ **dicyclomine hydrochloride**.
Formulation: Injection.
Availability: Prescription only.
Warnings and side effects: See ℞ **dicyclomine hydrochloride**.

Dilor-G Tablets; Liquid ⑧

A preparation of ℞ **guaifenesin** and diphylline.
Formulation: Oral tablets; liquid.
Availability: Prescription only.
Warnings and side effects: See ℞ **guaifenesin**; ℞ **theophylline**.

Diltia XT ⑧

A preparation of ℞ **diltiazem hydrochloride**.
Formulation: Oral capsules, extended release, available in 3 strengths.
Availability: Prescription only.
Warnings and side effects: See ℞ **diltiazem hydrochloride**.

diltiazem hydrochloride ⑥

Type/Group: **calcium-channel blocker; antianginal; antiarrhythmic; antihypertensive**.
Brand(s): Cardizem; Dilacor XR; Diltia XT; Tiamate; Tiazac; various generic.
How administered: Orally; injection.

Used to treat

Diltiazem hydrochloride is used in oral form for the treatment of ✪ **hypertension** and in the management of ✪ **angina pectoris**. When injected, it is used to control conduction disturbances such as atrial flutter or fibrillation (see ✪ **arrhythmia**).

Warnings

• It should not be given to people with known hypersensitivity to this drug, or with certain heart arrhythmias.
• It should be given with caution to people with congestive heart failure, impaired liver or kidney function, or who are elderly.
• It should be used during pregnancy only if the potential benefits outweigh the risk to the fetus.
• Breast-feeding women should either discontinue using this drug or stop breast-feeding.
• If diltiazem is given to replace a ℞ **beta-blocker**, then withdrawal of the beta-blocker should not be abrupt. Calcium-channel blockers, also, should not be discontinued abruptly.

Interactions

• Medical judgment is required if using diltiazem in combination with any drug that affects heart action, as there may be additive effects which are not always consistent or predictable.
• The levels of ℞ **beta-blockers** and ℞ **digoxin** may be increased, although effects are not clear, and so caution is advised.
• ℞ **cimetidine** may increase the levels and effects of diltiazem.
• The levels of ℞ **lithium** may be affected, with various adverse results.
• The levels of ℞ **carbamazepine** and ℞ **cyclosporine** may be increased, with potential for toxic effects, when used with diltiazem taken orally.

Side effects

• Frequently, effects on the heart (for example, slow heart beat), swelling of the extremities, headache, and dizziness.
• Less commonly, gastrointestinal disturbances (for example, constipation, dyspepsia, nausea), feeling of weakness, hypotension, rash, and urinary frequency.
• Changes in liver function and effects on the heart may occur.
• Hypotension occurs more often if the drug is given by injection, and there may be itching or burning at the site of injection.

Dimacol Caplets ⑧

A preparation of ℞ **dextromethorphan**, ℞ **pseudoephedrine**, and ℞ **guaifenesin**.
Formulation: Oral caplets.
Availability: OTC.
Warnings and side effects: See ℞ **dextromethorphan**; ℞ **pseudoephedrine**; ℞ **guaifenesin**.

dimenhydrinate ⑥

Type/Group: **antihistamine; antinauseant**.
Brand(s): Calm-X; Dimetabs; Children's Dramamine; Dramamine Tablets, Chewable Tablets, Liquid; Dinate; Dramanate; Dymenate; Hydrate; TripTone; various generic.
How administered: Orally.

Used to treat

Dimenhydrinate is used particularly for preventing and treating nausea and vomiting associated with ✪ **motion sickness**. It may be prescribed for vertigo caused by disorders of the balance function of the inner ear (for example, ✪ **Ménière's disease**).

Warnings

• It should not be given to people with known hypersensitivity to this drug (or with known sensitivity to other antihistamines), or who have a seizure disorder or porphyria.

• Antihistamines should be given with caution to people with lower respiratory disease or asthma (and never during an attack), heart disease, hypertension, hyperthyroidism, increased intraocular pressure (pressure in the eyeball, as in glaucoma), enlarged prostate, urinary retention, or certain obstructive bladder or gastrointestinal conditions.

• Dimenhydrinate should be used during pregnancy only if it is clearly needed, but not in the third trimester, as newborns or premature infants may have severe reactions, including convulsions, to antihistamines.

• Nursing mothers should discontinue using this drug or discontinue breast-feeding.

• This drug must not be given to infants, and for children under the age of 12 the manufacturer's or medical instructions must be followed closely.

• Because of its sedative side effects, the performance of skilled tasks, such as driving, may be impaired.

• Side effects are more frequent in the elderly.

Interactions

• ℞ **MAOI** antidepressants may prolong and intensify the ℞ **anticholinergic** effects of antihistamines (see Side effects below).

• If used with ℞ **tricyclic** antidepressants, other antihistamines, ℞ **skeletal muscle relaxants**, ℞ **opioids**, ℞ **barbiturates**, ℞ **hypnotics**, ℞ **sedatives**, or ℞ **antianxiety** drugs, there is a risk of intensified side effects.

• Dimenhydrinate can mask the toxic effects (to the ears) that are possible with the use of ℞ **aminoglycoside** antibiotics.

• Alcohol may intensify side effects such as drowsiness and impaired mental alertness.

Side effects

• These depend on how it is administered. For this type of antihistamine, there is commonly drowsiness, headache, impaired muscular coordination or dizziness, anticholinergic effects (dry mouth, blurred vision, urinary retention, gastrointestinal disturbances), occasional rashes and photosensitivity (abnormal sensitivity to light), palpitations and heart arrhythmias.

• Rarely, there may be stimulation instead of sedation (paradoxical stimulation), especially in children (and convulsions in overdose), hypersensitivity reactions, blood disorders, liver disturbances, depression, sleep disturbances, and hypotension. It may cause weight gain.

dimercaprol (BAL) Ⓖ

Type/Group: **antidote; chelating agent**.
Brand(s): BAL in Oil.
How administered: Injection.

Used to treat

Dimercaprol is used as an antidote to poisoning with arsenic, gold, mercury, and (with ℞ **edetate calcium disodium**) lead. It is thought to be of questionable value in treating poisoning with anti-

mony, bismuth, chromium, copper, nickel, tungsten, and zinc, and is not effective against thallium, tellurium, or vanadium.

Warnings

• It should not be used by people with severe liver or kidney impairment, or with hypersensitivity to peanuts (the drug is prepared in solution with peanut oil).

• It should be given with caution to anyone with G6PD deficiency, acidic urine, hypertension, or kidney damage.

• Dimercaprol has been associated with birth defects and should not be used during pregnancy, except in cases of life-threatening poisoning and it is medically judged that the potential benefit outweighs potential risk to the fetus.

• Medical judgment is also required for breast-feeding mothers.

• This drug should never be used as an antidote to poisoning by iron, cadmium, selenium or uranium, as the chemical resultants are more toxic than the metals themselves.

• Urinary alkalinization is recommended with dimercaprol to protect the kidneys.

Interactions

• ♒ **iron** may cause toxic effects.

Side effects

• Hypertension, increase in heart rate, sweating, malaise, nausea and vomiting, excessive tears, constriction of the throat and chest, burning sensation (eyes and mouth), headache, muscle spasms, pain in the abdomen, tingling in extremities, and pain and abscess at injection site.

Dimetabs Ⓑ

A preparation of ℞ **dimenhydrinate**.
Formulation: Oral tablets.
Availability: Prescription only.
Warnings and side effects: See ℞ **dimenhydrinate**.

Dimetane Decongestant Caplets Ⓑ

A preparation of ℞ **phenylephrine hydrochloride** and ℞ **brompheniramine maleate**.
Formulation: Oral tablets.
Availability: OTC.
Warnings and side effects: See ℞ **phenylephrine hydrochloride;** ℞ **brompheniramine maleate**.

Dimetane Decongestant Elixir Ⓑ

A preparation of ℞ **phenylephrine hydrochloride** and ℞ **brompheniramine maleate**.
Formulation: Oral liquid.
Availability: OTC.
Warnings and side effects: See ℞ **phenylephrine hydrochloride;** ℞ **brompheniramine maleate**.

Dimetane-DX Cough Syrup Ⓑ

A preparation of ℞ **dextromethorphan**, ℞ **brompheniramine maleate**, and ℞ **pseudoephedrine**.
Formulation: Oral syrup.
Availability: Prescription only.

Warnings and side effects: See ℞ **dextromethorphan**; ℞ **brompheniramine maleate**; ℞ **pseudoephedrine**.

dimethicone ⒢

see ℞ **simethicone**.

dimeticone ⒢

see ℞ **simethicone**.

Dinate Ⓑ

A preparation of ℞ **dimenhydrinate**.
Formulation: Injection.
Availability: Prescription only.
Warnings and side effects: See ℞ **dimenhydrinate**.

dinoprostone ⒢

(E₂; PGE₂)
Type/Group: prostaglandin; abortifacient; uterine stimulant.
Brand(s): Cervidil; Prepidil Gel, Prostin E₂; various generic.
How administered: Intravaginal; intracervical.

Used to treat

Dinoprostone is the prostaglandin E₂, which has the effect of causing contractions in the muscular walls of the uterus. It is used to ripen the cervix for labor induction, for benign hydatiform mole, and occasionally as an abortifacient.

Warnings

• It should not be given to people with known hypersensitivity to this or other prostaglandins, acute pelvic inflammatory disease, or active heart, kidney, liver or lung disease.
• It should be given with caution to people with cervical or vaginal infections, blood pressure disease, anemia, jaundice, diabetes mellitus, epilepsy, uterine fibroids, previous uterine surgery or heart, kidney, or liver disease.
• Failed attempts at pregnancy termination should be completed by other means.
• This is a specialist drug for hospital use only.

Interactions

• If taken with ℞ **oxytocics**, effects are increased.

Side effects

• Frequently, gastrointestinal symptoms fever, joint swelling, and leg cramps.
• Occasionally, headache, chills, hives, shortness of breath, wheezing, slowed heart rate, and bronchoconstriction.
• Rarely, flushing, ileus, or edema.

Diocto C Syrup Ⓑ

A preparation of casanthranol and ℞ **docusate sodium**.
Formulation: Oral syrup.
Availability: OTC.
Warnings and side effects: See ℞ **cascara sagrada**; ℞ **docusate sodium**.

Diocto Liquid; Syrup Ⓑ

A preparation of ℞ **docusate sodium**.
Formulation: Oral liquid; syrup.

Availability: OTC.
Warnings and side effects: See ℞ **docusate sodium**.

Diovan HCT Ⓑ

A preparation of ℞ **hydrochlorothiazide** and ℞ **valsartan**.
Formulation: Oral tablets, in two (valsartan) strengths.
Availability: Prescription only.
Warnings and side effects: See ℞ **hydrochlorothiazide**; ℞ **valsartan**.

Dipentum Ⓑ

A preparation of ℞ **olsalazine sodium**.
Formulation: Oral capsules.
Availability: Prescription only.
Warnings and side effects: See ℞ **olsalazine sodium**.

Diphen AF Liquid; Cough Syrup Ⓑ

A preparation of ℞ **diphenhydramine hydrochloride**.
Formulation: Oral liquid; syrup.
Availability: OTC.
Warnings and side effects: See ℞ **diphenhydramine hydrochloride**.

Diphenhist Captabs; Solution Ⓑ

A preparation of ℞ **diphenhydramine hydrochloride**.
Formulation: Oral tablets; liquid.
Availability: OTC.
Warnings and side effects: See ℞ **diphenhydramine hydrochloride**.

diphenhydramine hydrochloride ⒢

antihistamine; antiallergic; antinauseant; antiemetic; cold and cough preparation; sleep-aid product.
Brand(s): Benadryl Allergy Ultratabs, Kapseals, Chewables, Allergy Liquid, Dye-Free Allergy Liqui-Gels, Dye-Free Liquid; Banophen Capsules, Caplets; Diphenhist Captabs, Solution; AllerMax Caplets, Allergy & Cough Formula Liquid; Nighttime Sleep Aid; Genahist; Scot-Tussin Allergy DM; Diphen AF, Cough Syrup; Siladryl Elixir; Tusstat Syrup; Hyrexin-50. Combinations: With pseudoephedrine: Actifed Allergy Tablets; Banophen Decongestant Capsules; Benadryl Allergy Decongestant Tablets, Decongestant Liquid. (Plus) *acetaminophen*: Actifed Sinus Daytime/Nighttime Caplets, Tablets; Benadryl Allergy/Cold Tablets; Contac Day & Night Allergy/Sinus Caplets; Tylenol Flu Night Time Maximum Strength Powder (has *phenylalanine*). (Topical preparations): Benadryl Itch Relief Stick, Itch Stopping Cream, Itch Stopping Spray, Itch Stopping Gel; Dermamycin Cream, Spray; Di-Delamine; Dermarest Plus Gel; Ziradryl Lotion. (Most combinations available as generics.)
How administered: Orally; topically (external); injection.

Used to treat

Diphenhydramine can be used for the symptomatic relief of allergic symptoms, such as ✪ **hay fever** (seasonal allergic rhinitis), allergic ✪ **conjunctivitis**, and skin manifestations of ✪ **angioedema** and ✪ **urticaria**. It is also incorporated into a number of preparations for ✪ **colds** and ✪ **coughs**. It is also used to alleviate symptoms of parkinsonism, and to prevent and treat ✪ **motion sickness**. Diphenhydramine has marked sedative properties and can be used for the relief of occasional ✪ **insomnia** in adults.

Warnings

• It should not be given to people with known hypersensitivity to this drug (or with known sensitivity to other antihistamines).

• Antihistamines should be given with caution to people with lower respiratory disease or asthma (and never during an attack), heart disease, hypertension, hyperthyroidism, epilepsy, porphyria, increased intraocular pressure (pressure in the eyeball, as in glaucoma), enlarged prostate, urinary retention, or certain obstructive bladder or gastrointestinal conditions, liver disease.

• Diphenhydramine should be used during pregnancy only if it is clearly needed, but not in the third trimester, as newborns or premature infants may have severe reactions, including convulsions, to antihistamines.

• Nursing mothers should discontinue using this drug or discontinue breast-feeding.

• ℞ **MAOI** antidepressants may prolong and intensify the ℞ **anticholinergic** and sedative effects of antihistamines (see Side effects below).

• This drug must not be given to infants, and for children under the age of 12 the manufacturer's or medical instructions must be followed closely.

• Because of its sedative side effects, the performance of skilled tasks, such as driving, may be impaired.

• Side effects are more frequent in the elderly.

• Topical forms (used externally) of this drug should not be applied with other antihistamine preparations, to large areas of the body (risk of absorbed overdose), or on damaged skin (for example, blistered or oozing).

Interactions

• ℞ **MAOI** antidepressants may prolong and intensify the anticholinergic (see Side effects below) effects of antihistamines.

• If used with ℞ **tricyclic** antidepressants, other antihistamines, ℞ **skeletal muscle relaxants**, ℞ **opioids**, ℞ **barbiturates**, ℞ **hypnotics**, ℞ **sedatives**, or ℞ **antianxiety** drugs, there is a risk of intensified side effects.

• Alcohol may intensify side effects such as drowsiness and impaired mental alertness.

Side effects

• These depend on how it is administered. For this type of antihistamine, there is commonly drowsiness, headache, impaired muscular coordination or dizziness, anticholinergic effects (dry mouth, blurred vision, urinary retention, gastrointestinal disturbances), occasional rashes and photosensitivity (abnormal sensitivity to light), palpitations and heart arrhythmias.

• Rarely, there may be stimulation instead of sedation (paradoxical stimulation), especially in children (and convulsions in overdose), hypersensitivity reactions, blood disorders, liver disturbances, depression, sleep disturbances, and hypotension.

diphenoxylate hydrochloride ⓖ

Type/Group: **antidiarrheal; opioid**.

Brand(s): (All in combination with *atropine*): Logen; Lomenate; Lomotil Liquid, Tablets; Lonox Tablets.

How administered: Orally.

Used to treat

Diphenoxylate hydrochloride is used to treat ✪ **diarrhea**. It is generally available only in combination with ℞ **atropine sulfate**, so some warnings apply to the combination. Note that difenoxine, which is the active metabolite of diphenoxylate hydrochloride in the body, is incorporated into some preparations in the place of the latter.

Warnings

• It should not be given to people with known hypersensitivity to this drug, or who have an intestinal infection, liver or kidney disease or abnormal function. It should not be given to children under the age of 2, as its effects are unpredictable, with occasional serious toxicity.

• Diphenoxylate should be used during pregnancy only if the benefits outweigh the potential risks.

• Medical judgment is required if breast-feeding is being considered. It probably appears in breast milk.

• Drowsiness may affect the performance of skilled tasks such as driving.

• The effects of alcohol may be enhanced (including respiratory depression).

• Prolonged use may lead to impaired gastrointestinal function.

• This is a Schedule IV controlled drug.

Interactions

• If used with ℞ **barbiturates**, ℞ **general anesthetics**, ℞ **opioids**, ℞ **tranquilizers** (for example, ℞ **phenothiazines**), ℞ **sedatives**, ℞ **benzodiazepines** (for example, ℞ **diazepam**, ℞ **lorazepam**), or alcohol increased effects are possible.

Side effects

• Depending on use and dose, there may be nausea and vomiting, drowsiness, loss of appetite, constipation, and commonly sedation.

diphosphonate ⓓ

see ℞ **bisphosphonate**.

diphtheria and tetanus toxoid, adsorbed (DT; Td) ⓖ

Type/Group: **vaccine**.

Brand(s): Various generic.

How administered: Intramuscular injection.

Used to treat

Adsorbed onto a mineral carrier, this combination of ✪ **diphtheria** (toxoid) vaccine and ✪ **tetanus** (toxoid) vaccine is used for the primary immunization of children (in a series of administrations including a booster before nursery school entry) and as an alternative to adsorbed diphtheria, tetanus, and pertussis vaccine (DTwP), for children who can not be given the pertussis vaccine. A similar but different form is used for adolescents and adults. The formulation denoted DT or "Pediatric" is for children under 7; Td or "Adult" is for anyone 7 or older.

Warnings

• It should not be given to people with known hypersensitivity or allergy to the vaccine, or anyone who has a current or recent febrile (feverish) illness or infection.

• It should not be used during pregnancy; but if immunization is necessary, it should preferably occur in the last two trimesters.

• Medical judgment is required if breast-feeding is being considered.

• It should never be used to treat actual diphtheria, tetanus, or pertussis infection.

• If a particularly acute skin inflammation, often progressing to abscess, occurs (Arthus reaction), further tetanus toxoids should not be administered more frequently than 10-year intervals, even in an emergency.

• After administration, people will be required to wait for some time to ensure that there is no serious reaction (such as anaphylaxis).

Interactions

• ℞ **Immunosuppressants** may reduce the effectiveness of the vaccine.

• Caution is required if ℞ **anticoagulants** are being taken.

• ℞ **Tetanus immune globulin (TIG)** may delay immunity, and should not be injected in the same arm.

Side effects

• These range from little or no reactions to severe discomfort, high temperature, and pain.

• Rarely, there may be anaphylactic shock.

diphtheria and tetanus vaccine (DTaP) ⒢

Full name: **diphtheria and tetanus toxoids and acellular pertussis vaccine (DTaP)**

Type/Group: **vaccine**.

How administered: Intramuscular injection.

Brand(s): Acel-Imune; Tripedia; Infanrix; Certiva.

Used to treat

DTaP may be administered as an alternative to DTwP for the fourth and fifth shots in a series for immunization against ⊘ **diphtheria**, ⊘ **tetanus**, and ⊘ **pertussis** (whooping cough). The pertussis component is prepared differently than in DTwP and causes somewhat reduced side effects, such as less pain, swelling, fever, vomiting, and loss of appetite.

Warnings

• It should not be given to people with known hypersensitivity or allergy to the vaccine, or anyone who has a current or recent febrile (feverish) illness or infection.

• It is not recommended for adults or for children 7 years or older.

• It should be avoided during pregnancy, but if immunization is necessary, it should preferably occur in the last two trimesters.

• Medical judgment is required if breast-feeding is being considered.

• It should never be used to treat actual diphtheria, tetanus, or pertussis infection.

• It should not be given to children who have already had (confirmed) pertussis.

• If a particularly acute skin inflammation, often progressing to abscess, occurs (Arthus reaction), further tetanus toxoids should

not be administered more frequently than 10-year intervals, even in an emergency.

• After administration, people will be required to wait for some time to ensure that there is no serious reaction (such as anaphylaxis).

Interactions

• ℞ **Immunosuppressants** may reduce the effectiveness of the vaccine.

• Caution is required if ℞ **anticoagulants** are being taken.

• ℞ **Tetanus immune globulin (TIG)** may delay immunity, and should not be injected in the same arm.

Side effects

• These range from little or no reactions to severe discomfort, high temperature, and pain.

• Rarely, there may be anaphylactic shock.

diphtheria and tetanus vaccine (DTwP) ⒢

Full name: **diphtheria and tetanus toxoids and whole-cell pertussis vaccine, adsorbed (DTwP)**

Type/Group: **vaccine**.

Brand(s): Tri-Immunol; various generic.

How administered: Intramuscular injection.

Used to treat

DTwP is for immunization against ⊘ **diphtheria**, ⊘ **tetanus**, and ⊘ **pertussis** (whooping cough). It consists of diphtheria (toxoid) vaccine, tetanus (toxoid) vaccine and pertussis vaccine adsorbed onto a mineral carrier. This triple vaccine is used for the primary immunization of children (during first year of life), and is administered by injection. Generally, a basic series of three injections is administered, followed by one or two more at longer intervals.

Warnings

• It should not be given to people with known hypersensitivity or allergy to the vaccine, or anyone who has a current or recent febrile (feverish) illness or infection.

• It is not recommended for adults or for children 7 years or older.

• Its use should be avoided during pregnancy, but if immunization is necessary, it should preferably occur in the last two trimesters.

• Medical judgment is required if breast-feeding is being considered.

• It should never be used to treat actual diphtheria, tetanus, or pertussis infection.

• It should not be given to children who have already had (confirmed) pertussis.

• If a particularly acute skin inflammation, often progressing to abscess, occurs (Arthus reaction), further tetanus toxoids should not be administered more frequently than 10-year intervals, even in an emergency.

• After administration, people will be required to wait for some time to ensure that there is no serious reaction, such as anaphylaxis.

Interactions

• ℞ **Immunosuppressants** may reduce the effectiveness of the vaccine.

• Caution is required if ℞ **anticoagulants** are being taken.

• ℞ **Tetanus immune globulin (TIG)** may delay immunity, and should not be injected in the same arm.

Side effects

• These range from little or no reactions to severe discomfort, high temperature, and pain.
• Rarely, there may be anaphylactic shock.

diphtheria and tetanus vaccine (DTwP-Hib) ⓖ

Full name: **diphtheria and tetanus toxoids and acellular pertussis vaccine and** *Haemophilus influenzae* **type b conjugate vaccine (DTwP-Hib)**
Type/Group: **vaccine**.
Brand(s): TriHIBit.
How administered: Intramuscular injection.

Used to treat

DTwP-Hib provides additional immunity, against *Haemophilus influenzae* type b (a bacterium, not the "flu"), within the usual series of vaccinations administered in early childhood against ⊘ **diphtheria**, ⊘ **tetanus**, and ⊘ **pertussis** (whooping cough).

Warnings

• It should not be given to people with known hypersensitivity or allergy to the vaccine, or anyone who has a current or recent febrile (feverish) illness or infection.
• It is not recommended for adults or for children 7 years or older.
• Its use should be avoided during pregnancy, but if immunization is necessary, it should preferably occur in the last two trimesters.
• Medical judgment is required if breast-feeding is being considered.
• It should never be used to treat actual diphtheria, tetanus, pertussis, or *H. influenzae* infection.
• It should not be given to children who have already had (confirmed) pertussis.
• If a particularly acute skin inflammation, often progressing to abscess, occurs (Arthus reaction), further tetanus toxoids should not be administered more frequently than 10-year intervals, even in an emergency.
• After administration, people will be required to wait for some time to ensure that there is no serious reaction (such as anaphylaxis).

Interactions

• ℞ **Immunosuppressants** may reduce the effectiveness of the vaccine.
• Caution is required if ℞ **anticoagulants** are being taken.
• ℞ **Tetanus immune globulin (TIG)** may delay immunity, and should not be injected in the same arm.

Side effects

• These range from little or no reactions to severe discomfort, high temperature, and pain.
• Rarely, there may be anaphylactic shock.

diphtheria antitoxin ⓖ

Type/Group: **antitoxin**.
Brand(s): Generic.
How administered: Injection.

Used to treat

Diphtheria antitoxin is a preparation that neutralizes the toxins produced by ⊘ **diphtheria** bacteria (*Corynebacterium diphtheriae*). It is not used for prevention (most people will have been immunized to diphtheria; see ℞ **immunization**), but only to provide passive immunity to people who have been exposed to suspected outbreaks or contact with patients infected with diphtheria. It is also used in the treatment of the disease. The antitoxin is produced in horses and so hypersensitivity reactions are common.

Warnings

• It should not be given to people with known hypersensitivity to this antitoxin or any serum produced in horses.
• It should be given with extreme caution to people with a history of allergic reaction or asthma.
• It should be used during pregnancy only when it is clearly needed.
• It is not known whether these antitoxins appear in breast milk, and no problems have been documented.
• A sensitivity test (a skin scratch test) should always be performed before administering this antitoxin.
• After administration, people will be required to wait for some time to ensure that there is no serious reaction (such as anaphylaxis).

Interactions

None of significance have been reported.

Side effects

• Commonly, hives, fever, itching, malaise, skin rash, swelling of lymph glands, and aching in the joints.
• Anaphylaxis is not uncommon and is usually characterized by sudden appearance of hives, difficulty breathing, and collapse.

dipivefrine hydrochloride ⓖ

see ℞ **dipivefrin hydrochloride**.

dipivefrin hydrochloride ⓖ

(dipivefrine hydrochloride)
Type/Group: **glaucoma treatment; sympathomimetic**.
Brand(s): Propine; AKPro; various generic.
How administered: Topically (eyes).

Used to treat

Dipivefrin hydrochloride is a derivative of the sympathomimetic ℞ **epinephrine** and is a prodrug that is converted in the body into epinephrine. It is used in treatment of open-angle ⊘ **glaucoma** to reduce intraocular pressure (pressure in the eyeball) and is used instead of epinephrine because it is thought to pass more rapidly through the cornea.

Warnings

• It should not be given to people with known hypersensitivity to dipivefrin, or to anyone with narrow-angle glaucoma.
• It should be given with caution to children.
• Dipivefrin's safety during pregnancy has not been established. It should be used only if it is clearly needed.
• Medical judgment is required if breast-feeding is being considered.
• It may cause reversible macular edema in aphakic individuals (those lacking a lens).

Interactions

• ℞ **tricyclic** antidepressants can reduce the effects of dipivefrin.

Side effects

• Burning and stinging of eyes, light sensitivity, systemic side effects (because it can be absorbed through the eye into the body) such as elevated blood pressure, speeded heart beat and, rarely, dysrhythmias are possible.

Diprolene Ⓑ

A preparation of ℞ **betamethasone** dipropionate.
Formulation: Ointment; cream (Diprolene AF); gel; lotion.
Availability: Prescription only.
Warnings and side effects: See ℞ **betamethasone**.

Diprosone Ⓑ

A preparation of ℞ **betamethasone** dipropionate.
Formulation: Ointment; cream; lotion; aerosol spray.
Availability: Prescription only.
Warnings and side effects: See ℞ **betamethasone**.

dipyridamole Ⓖ

Type/Group: **antiplatelet**.
Brand(s): Persantine; various generic. Combinations: With *aspirin*: Aggrenox.
How administered: Orally; intravenous injection.

Used to treat

Dipyridamole is an antiplatelet drug which is used, together with coumarin ℞ **anticoagulants**, to prevent ✪ **thrombosis**, but does not have an anticoagulant action. It seems to work by stopping platelets sticking to one another or to surgically inserted tubes and valves (particularly artificial heart valves), although its action is not completely understood. In injectable form, dipyridamole is used to improve diagnosis in coronary arteriography (it has ℞ **vasodilator** effects which are useful in this regard).

Warnings

• It should not be given to people with known hypersensitivity to this drug.
• It should be given with caution to people with hypotension, coronary artery disease or conduction disorders, or myasthenia gravis.
• It should be used during pregnancy only if clearly needed.
• Medical judgment is required if breast-feeding is being considered. It appears in breast milk.
• This drug is used in a hospital setting, with monitoring of heart function when given by injection.

Interactions

• If taken with ℞ **adenosine**, there is a risk that the effects of adenosine are increased, with the potential for serious adverse effects.
• There may be additive effects in slowing heart rate when used with ℞ **beta-blockers**.
• ℞ **theophylline** and other xanthines (for example, ℞ **caffeine**) may interfere with the diagnostic use of injectable dipyridamole.

Side effects

• There may be dizziness, gastrointestinal disturbances, headache, or rash.

• When given by injection, additional side effects may include chest pain or angina pectoris, low blood pressure, disturbances of heart rhythm, flushing, and muscle ache.
• Although rare, serious cardiac events and bronchospasm have been reported with the use of injectable dipyridamole.

dirithromycin Ⓖ

Type/Group: **macrolide**; **antibiotic**; **antibacterial**.
Brand(s): Dynabac.
How administered: Orally; injection.

Used to treat

Dirithromycin has activity mainly against Gram-negative organisms and is used to treat ✪ **bacterial infections** as an alternative for people allergic to penicillin, primarily in the treatment of mild to moderate respiratory tract infections.

Warnings

• It should not be given to people with known hypersensitivity to any of the macrolide antibiotics. It must not be used in the treatment of septicemia.
• It should be given with caution to people with kidney or liver dysfunction.
• Dirithromycin should be used during pregnancy only if it is clearly needed and if the potential benefits outweigh the possible risk to the fetus.
• Medical judgment is required if breast-feeding is being considered. It is not known if this drug appears in breast milk.
• Superinfections due to the altered bacterial balance created by the use of antibiotics may occur. A doctor must be contacted if there is severe abdominal pain, moderate to severe diarrhea, or any new or unusual symptoms.
• Rare, serious allergic reactions have occurred.
• Take with food or within an hour of eating to enhance absorption.

Interactions

• The effectiveness of ℞ **penicillins** may be reduced.
• There is a risk of a fatal reaction if macrolides are used with ℞ **pimozide**.
• ℞ **Antacids** and ℞ **H2-antagonists** may increase the effects of dirithromycin.

Side effects

• Frequently, gastrointestinal upsets (nausea, abdominal pain, diarrhea).
• Occasionally, dizziness, nonspecific pain, and weakness.
• Rarely, increased cough, rash, itching, hives, and insomnia.

Disalcid Tablets; Capsules Ⓑ

A preparation of ℞ **salsalate**.
Formulation: Oral capsules; tablets, available in two strengths.
Availability: Prescription only.
Warnings and side effects: See ℞ **salsalate**.

disinfectant Ⓓ

Generics: **chlorhexidine**; **glutaraldehyde**; **phenol**; **sodium hypochlorite**.

Actions and uses

℞ **disinfectants** are used to destroy microorganisms, or inhibit their activity to such an extent that they are less, or no longer, harmful to health. The term can be applied to agents used on inanimate objects (including surgical equipment, catheters, and so on) as well as to preparations used to treat the skin and living tissue (although in the latter case the name ℞ **antiseptic** is often used instead).

Limitations

See the individual drug entries.

Disobrom Tablets ℬ

A preparation of pseudoephedrine sulfate, and dexbrompheniramine maleate.

Formulation: Oral tablets, sustained release.

Availability: Prescription only.

Warnings and side effects: See ℞ **pseudoephedrine**; ℞ **brompheniramine maleate**.

disodium cromoglycate Ⓖ

see ℞ **cromolyn sodium**.

disodium etidronate Ⓖ

see ℞ **etidronate disodium**.

disodium pamidronate Ⓖ

see ℞ **pamidronate disodium**.

Disophrol Chronotabs ℬ

A preparation of ℞ **pseudoephedrine** sulfate and dexbrompheniramine maleate.

Formulation: Oral tablets, sustained release.

Availability: OTC.

Warnings and side effects: See ℞ **pseudoephedrine**; ℞ **brompheniramine maleate**.

Disophrol Tablets ℬ

A preparation of ℞ **pseudoephedrine** and ℞ **brompheniramine maleate**.

Formulation: Oral tablets.

Availability: Prescription only.

Warnings and side effects: See ℞ **pseudoephedrine**; ℞ **brompheniramine maleate**.

disopyramide Ⓖ

Type/Group: **antiarrhythmic**.

Brand(s): Norpace, Norpace CR; various generic.

How administered: Orally.

Used to treat

Disopyramide (also prepared as disopyramide phosphate) is used to regularize the heartbeat, but generally only for life-threatening ✛ **arrhythmias**, especially sustained ventricular tachycardia.

Warnings

• It should not be given to people with known hypersensitivity to this drug, hypotension, certain heart disorders, or uncompensated heart failure.

• It should be given with caution to people with urinary retention, glaucoma, myasthenia gravis, or with liver or kidney impairment. This is a specialist drug and treatment will be carried out by experienced clinicians who are thoroughly familiar with this drug. Periodic monitoring of heart function and blood values is necessary.

• Disopyramide should be used during pregnancy only if the potential benefits outweigh the possible risk to the fetus.

• It is present in breast milk and nursing women should discontinue using this drug or stop breast-feeding.

• It can, occasionally, provoke arrhythmias.

• If there are persistent symptoms such as dry mouth, difficulty in urinating, dizziness, breathing difficulty, constipation or blurred vision, a doctor should be notified, but the drug should not be stopped without instructions from the doctor.

Interactions

• ℞ **Anticholinergics**, other antiarrhythmics, and ℞ **macrolides** (for example, ℞ **erythromycin**) may intensify the effects of disopyramide.

• ℞ **Beta-blockers** may have unpredictable effects.

• The levels of ℞ **quinidine** may fall, while those of disopyramide rise.

• ℞ **Hydantoins** and ℞ **rifampin** may lower the levels and effect of disopyramide.

Side effects

• Frequent side effects include dry mouth, urinary hesitancy or retention, gastrointestinal disturbances (nausea, bloating, constipation), dizziness, blurred vision, dry nose, eyes or throat, fatigue and headache.

• Palpitations, breathlessness, fainting or chest pain may also occur.

• Occasionally, rash and itching, and rarely anaphylactic reactions. The most serious, though not frequent, adverse reactions are hypotension and worsening of congestive heart failure.

disulfiram Ⓖ

Type/Group: **substance-dependence treatment**.

Brand(s): Antabuse.

How administered: Orally.

Used to treat

Disulfiram is used as an additional treatment for chronic alcoholism. It is an enzyme inhibitor that blocks a stage in the break down of alcohol (ethanol) in the body, resulting in a accumulation in a metabolite (acetaldehyde). If even only a very small amount of alcohol is taken, disulfiram causes very unpleasant, reactions, such as flushing, headache, palpitations, nausea and vomiting. Therefore, if an alcoholic takes disulfiram on a regular basis, there is a powerful disincentive to drink alcoholic beverages.

Warnings

• It should not be given to people with known hypersensitivity to this or similar agents, for example, a history of contact dermatitis when skin contacts rubber (since this often contains thiuram derivatives; disulfiram is a thiuram derivative), or with psychoses or cardiovascular disease.

• It should be given with caution to people with low thyroid function, liver disease, diabetes mellitus, seizure disorders, kidney infection, or who have had a stroke.

• It must not be used during pregnancy.

• It should not be used by nursing mothers.

• The effects that disulfiram causes, if even a small amount of alcohol is taken, are potentially very dangerous. Medicines, foods (including vinegars), and even products such as lotions or colognes that contain alcohol must be avoided. Reaction to alcohol may occur up to two weeks after last dose.

• Herbal remedies in the form of tinctures must be avoided (they contain alcohol).

• Disulfiram may impair the performance of skilled tasks such as driving.

Interactions

• The effects of oral ℞ **anticoagulants** may be increased.

• The levels of ℞ **phenytoin** may be increased.

• ℞ **Isoniazid** may increase CNS (central nervous system) effects.

• ℞ **Metronidazole** may increase toxicity.

Side effects

• Frequently, drowsiness and headache.

• Occasionally, nerve damage, inflammation of the optic nerve, mental changes, impotence, bad taste in the mouth, skin rash, and unusual tiredness.

• Rarely, liver damage or seizures.

Dital ®

A preparation of ℞ **phendimetrazine**.
Formulation: Sustained release capsules.
Availability: Prescription only.
Warnings and side effects: See ℞ **phendimetrazine**.

dithranol ©

see ℞ **anthralin**.

Ditropan; Ditropan XL ®

A preparation of ℞ **oxybutynin**.
Formulation: Oral tablets; extended release tablets (XL).
Availability: Prescription only.
Warnings and side effects: See ℞ **oxybutynin**.

Diucardin ®

A preparation of ℞ **hydroflumethiazide**.
Formulation: Oral tablets.
Availability: Prescription only.
Warnings and side effects: See ℞ **hydroflumethiazide**.

Diurese ®

A preparation of ℞ **trichlormethiazide**.
Formulation: Oral tablets.
Availability: Prescription only.
Warnings and side effects: See ℞ **trichlormethiazide**.

diuretic ⑩

Generics: **acetazolamide; amiloride; ammonium chloride; bendroflumethiazide; benzthiazide; benzthiazide; chlorothiazide; chlorthalidone; dichlorphenamide; dorzolamide; hydrochlorothiazide; hydroflumethiazide; indapamide; mannitol; methyclothiazide; metolazone; polythiazide; quinethazone; spironolactone; triamterene; trichlormethiazide; urea**.

Actions and uses

Diuretic drugs used to reduce excess fluid in the body by increasing the excretion of water and mineral salts (sodium) by an action on the kidney, so increasing urine production (hence the term "water tablets") and reversing ✪ **fluid retention**. They have a wide range of uses, because edema due to excess fluid retention in sites such as the lungs, ankles, and eyeball is a symptom of a number of disorders. Reducing edema is, in itself, of benefit in some of these disorders, and diuretics may be used in acute pulmonary (lung) edema, in congestive ℞ **heart failure treatment**, some liver and kidney disorders, ℞ **glaucoma treatment** and in certain electrolyte disturbances, such as hypercalcemia (raised calcium levels) and hyperkalemia (raised potassium levels). Their most common use is as ℞ **antihypertensive** agents, where their action of reducing edema is of value in relieving the load on the heart, which then (over some days or weeks) gives way to a beneficial reduction in blood pressure (see ✪ **hypertension**), which partly may be due to a ℞ **vasodilator** action.

In relation to their specific actions and uses, the diuretics are divided into a number of distinct classes. *Osmotic diuretics* (for example, ℞ **mannitol** and ℞ **urea**) are inert (not chemically active) compounds secreted into the kidney proximal tubules and are not resorbed and therefore carry water and salts with them into the urine. *Loop diuretics* (for example, ℞ **frusemide** and ℞ **bumetanide**) have a very vigorous action on the loop of Henlé (inhibiting resorption of sodium, chloride, and water, and also some potassium) and are used especially in ✪ **heart failure**. *Thiazide* and *thiazide-like* diuretics (for example, ℞ **chlorothiazide** and ℞ **hydrochlorothiazide**) are the most commonly used and have a moderate action in inhibiting sodium reabsorption at the distal tubule of the kidney, allowing their prolonged use as antihypertensives in treating hypertension. But they may cause potassium loss from the blood to the urine, which needs correction (sometimes through using preparations that combine the diuretic and a potassium salt in tablets). *Potassium-sparing* diuretics (for example, ℞ **amiloride**, ℞ **triamterene**, and ℞ **spironolactone**) have a weak action on the distal tubule of the kidney and (as the name suggests) cause retention of potassium, making them suitable for combination with some of the other diuretic classes and for some specific conditions. *Aldosterone antagonists* (also ℞ **spironolactone**) work by blocking the action of the normal mineralocorticoid hormone aldosterone, and this makes them suitable for treating edema associated with aldosteronism, liver failure, and certain heart conditions. *Carbonic anhydrase inhibitors* (for example, ℞ **acetazolamide**) are weak diuretics and are now rarely used to treat systemic edema. However, they have a similar action in the eye and some (℞ **acetazolamide**, ℞ **dorzolamide** and ℞ **dichlo-**

rphenamide) are useful in reducing fluid in the eye which causes ✪ **glaucoma**.

℞ **ammonium chloride** is a mild diuretic and is used in some non-prescription preparations for the relief of premenstrual water retention. In the treatment of hypertension, diuretics are commonly used in combination with other classes of drugs, particularly ℞ **beta-blocker** drugs.

Limitations
See the individual drug entries.

Diurigen ⓑ
A preparation of ℞ **chlorothiazide**.
Formulation: Oral tablets.
Availability: Prescription only.
Warnings and side effects: See ℞ **chlorothiazide**.

Diuril Tablets; Oral Suspension; Injection ⓑ
A preparation of ℞ **chlorothiazide**.
Formulation: Oral tablets (2 strengths); oral liquid; injection.
Availability: Prescription only.
Warnings and side effects: See ℞ **chlorothiazide**.

divalproex sodium ⓖ
Type/Group: **anticonvulsant; antiepileptic**.
Brand(s): Depakote; Depakote Sprinkle.
How administered: Orally.

Used to treat
Divalproex sodium is used to control and prevent seizures in ✪ **epilepsy**, to prevent ✪ **migraine** headache, and to treat mania associated with ✪ **bipolar disorder**. It is very similar in its properties and action to ℞ **valproate sodium** and valproic acid (it is a stable chemical compound comprised of these two).

Warnings
• Avoid its use in people with known hypersensitivity to this drug, or with a history of liver disease or known liver abnormality.
• It should be used with extreme caution in children under two years of age.
• This drug is associated with an increase in frequency of certain birth defects and should not be used during pregnancy. However, because uncontrolled seizures can also threaten fetal health, medical judgment is needed to weigh potential benefits and risks.
• Valproate sodium appears in breast milk, though its effects are not known, and so medical judgment is also required if breast-feeding is being considered.
• Treatment should be stopped immediately if there is vomiting, jaundice, stomach pain, drowsiness, anorexia, or loss of seizure control; rashes; or various signs of liver or blood disorder. Patients or their care providers should be instructed how to recognize signs of blood or liver disorders, and they are advised to seek immediate medical attention if symptoms develop.
• Withdrawal should be gradual otherwise it may precipitate attacks.
• As this drug may cause drowsiness, driving or other hazardous activity should be avoided.

Interactions
• Divalproex sodium taken with ℞ **clonazepam** may induce absence-type seizure in those with a history of this kind of seizure.
• ℞ **chlorpromazine**, ℞ **erythromycin**, felbamate, and ℞ **salicylates** (such as ℞ **aspirin**) may increase levels of divalproex and so a higher risk of side effects.
• ℞ **rifampin** may decrease levels of divalproex.
• The effects of the following drugs may be intensified, while at the same time the therapeutic effect of divalproex is reduced: ℞ **carbamazepine**; ℞ **lamotrigine**; ℞ **phenobarbital** (and other ℞ **barbiturates**); ℞ **phenytoin**.
• Divalproex may increase levels of the following drugs, and so increase the risk of side effects or overdose symptoms: ℞ **amitriptyline** (and ℞ **nortriptyline**); ℞ **benzodiazepines**; ℞ **ethosuximide**; felbamate; ℞ **tolbutamide**; ℞ **warfarin sodium**; ℞ **zidovudine**.

Side effects
Many have been reported and depending on the use, how administered, and dose they include:
• Stomach irritation and nausea, drowsiness, unsteady gait, and muscle tremor;
• Feeling of weakness, weight loss or weight gain, thinning and curling hair;
• Edema and blood changes;
• Divalproex may cause pancreas and potentially serious liver damage;
• At high dosage tremor, hair loss, and blood abnormalities are frequent.

Doak Tar ⓑ
A preparation of ℞ **coal tar**.
Formulation: Shampoo; bath oil; topical liquid; topical lotion.
Availability: OTC.
Warnings and side effects: See ℞ **coal tar**.

Doan's Extra Strength Caplets ⓑ
A preparation of ℞ **magnesium salicylate**.
Formulation: Oral tablets.
Availability: OTC.
Warnings and side effects: See ℞ **magnesium salicylate**.

dobutamine hydrochloride ⓖ
Type/Group: **beta-adrenergic stimulant; sympathomimetic; dopamine-receptor stimulant; cardiac stimulant**.
Brand(s): Dobutrex; various generic.
How administered: Intravenous infusion.

Used to treat
Dobutamine is used to treat serious heart disorders, including cardiogenic shock, septic shock, and during open-heart surgery. It works by increasing the heart's force of contraction.

Warnings
• It should not be given to people with known hypersensitivity to this drug, or with certain forms of aortic stenosis.
• It should be given with caution to people with hypertension, low blood volume, or who have certain heart arrhythmias.

Key to symbols: ✪ = Disorder Section   ℞ = Drug Section   ♣ = Herbal Section   ⏁⏁ = Supplement Section

• Dobutamine should be used during pregnancy only when it is clearly needed.

• Medical judgment is required if breast-feeding is being considered. Its effects in breast-feeding are unknown.

• This is a powerful drug, used only under hospital conditions and with continuous monitoring of heart function, blood pressure, and other vital signs.

Interactions

• Halogenated ℞ **general anesthetics** (for example, halothane) or cyclopropane have the potential for serious adverse effects on heart rhythm, and must be used with extreme caution.

• ℞ **bretylium tosylate**, ℞ **guanethidine monosulfate**, oxytocics (for example, ℞ **oxytocin**, ℞ **ergonovine**), and ℞ **tricyclics** may intensify the various effects of dobutamine, with potential for serious adverse reactions.

• ℞ **Beta-blockers** may reduce or negate the effects of dobutamine.

Side effects

• There may be irregular or fast heartbeat, rapid change in blood pressure (either increase or decrease), chest pain or angina pectoris, headache, nausea or shortness of breath.

• Occasionally, phlebitis may occur at the infusion site, allergic reactions (including rash, fever, bronchospasm) have been reported and are sometimes caused by sulfites used in some commercially available preparations.

Dobutrex ⑧

A preparation of ℞ **dobutamine hydrochloride**.
Formulation: Intravenous infusion.
Availability: Prescription only.
Warnings and side effects: See ℞ **dobutamine hydrochloride**.

docetaxel Ⓖ

Type/Group: **anticancer; cytotoxic**.
Brand(s): Taxotere.
How administered: Intravenous infusion.

Used to treat

Docetaxel is a cytotoxic agent from a new group of drugs termed the taxanes. It is used in the treatment of (anthracycline-resistant) ✪ **breast cancer** and non-small-cell lung ✪ **cancer**.

Warnings

• It should not be given to people with a history of severe hypersensitivity to docetaxel, or other drugs formulated with polysorbate 80, low blood counts, or elevated bilirubin levels.

• It should be given with caution to people with abnormal liver function (or liver function test results) and those receiving higher doses than normal. This is a specialist drug which will be used following a full evaluation by specialist physicians.

• Docetaxel is not recommended for use during pregnancy unless it is medically judged to be essential, because it may cause birth defects. Becoming pregnant while using this drug must be avoided.

• It should not be used if breast-feeding.

• Treatment-related deaths have occurred.

• Severe fluid retention may develop.

• Serious allergic reactions to this drug have occurred.

• Virtually everyone experiences blood-cell changes and monitoring is required.

• Treatable conduction abnormalities (heart disorders) can develop.

• In common with many anticancer drugs, docetaxel can cause genetic mutations in chromosomes.

Interactions

• ℞ **cyclosporine**, ℞ **ketoconazole**, ℞ **erythromycin**, troleandomycin, and other drugs metabolized by the same route may increase the levels of docetaxel.

Side effects

• Frequently, hair loss, weakness, gum or tongue inflammation, gastrointestinal disturbances, fever, nail changes, vomiting, and aches and pains.

• Occasionally, hypotension, redness, rash, swelling, loss of appetite, headache, weight gain, infection, and dizziness.

• Rarely, dry skin, sensory disorders, bone and joint pain, weight loss, conjunctivitis, and blood or protein in urine.

Doctar ⑧

A preparation of ℞ **coal tar**.
Formulation: Shampoo.
Availability: OTC.
Warnings and side effects: See ℞ **coal tar**.

Docu Liquid; Syrup ⑧

A preparation of ℞ **docusate sodium**.
Formulation: Oral liquid; syrup.
Availability: OTC.
Warnings and side effects: See ℞ **docusate sodium**.

docusate sodium Ⓖ

Type/Group: **laxative**.
Brand(s): Colace Capsules, Liquid, Syrup; Diocto Liquid, Syrup; Docu Liquid, Syrup; D.O.S.; D-S-S; ex-lax Stool Softener; Genasoft; Modane Soft; Phillips' Liqui-Gels; Regulax SS; Silace; various generic. Combinations: With *casanthranol*: Diocto C Syrup; DOK-Plus; Doxidan; Peri-Colace; Silace-C Syrup; various generic. With *glycerin*: Therevac-SB. (Plus): *benzocaine*: Therevac-Plus. With *senna*: Senokot-S.

How administered: Orally; topically (rectal enema).

Used to treat

Docusate sodium is a weak, (surfactant) laxative, with both stimulant and stool softener properties. It is used to relieve ✪ **constipation**, often in combination with other laxatives, and also to evacuate the rectum prior to abdominal radiological procedures. It is a constituent of many OTC compound laxatives because it seems to have few adverse side effects. It works like a surfactant, by applying a very thin film of low surface tension (similar to a detergent) over the surface of the intestinal wall. Very similar compounds, docusate calcium and docusate potassium, are also used in many OTC products.

Warnings

• It should not be given to people with certain gastrointestinal disorders such as fecal impaction or obstruction.

• No ill effects in pregnancy have been associated with this drug, but a doctor should always be consulted before taking any drug when pregnant.

• Medical judgment is required if breast-feeding is being considered. It is not known whether this drug appears in breast milk.

• In general, no stool softener should be used together with any oral drug where the difference between therapeutic dose and overdose toxicity is small ("low therapeutic index"). For example, ℞ **antiarrhythmics**, many ℞ **anticancer** drugs, ℞ **digoxin**, ℞ **lithium**, ℞ **theophylline**, and ℞ **warfarin sodium**. Stool softeners may cause higher absorption in the intestines, and so increase levels of drugs in the circulation. A doctor must be consulted first before taking any other medication (including OTCs, herbal remedies, and supplements).

• Do not use if there is abdominal pain, nausea or vomiting, unless directed by a doctor.

• Rectal preparations should not be used by people with hemorrhoids or an anal fissure.

• Chronic use of laxatives may cause fluid and electrolyte imbalances, vitamin and mineral deficiencies, and abnormal bowel function. Generally, they should not be used for more than a week.

Interactions

• The absorption of the laxatives ℞ **mineral oil** and phenolphthalein may be increased, reducing their effectiveness. In the case of mineral oil, higher absorption may cause toxicity, and so docusate sodium and mineral oil should not be used together.

• There may be a higher risk of intestinal irritation or bleeding if taken with ℞ **aspirin**.

Side effects

• Although side effects are rare, throat irritation and nausea may occur and abdominal cramps. Rashes have been reported.

DOK-Plus ⓑ

A preparation of casanthranol and ℞ **docusate sodium**.
Formulation: Oral syrup.
Availability: OTC.
Warnings and side effects: See ℞ **cascara sagrada**; ℞ **docusate sodium**.

Dolacet Capsules ⓑ

A preparation of ℞ **hydrocodone bitartrate** and ℞ **acetaminophen**.
Formulation: Oral capsules.
Availability: Prescription only.
Warnings and side effects: See ℞ **hydrocodone bitartrate**; ℞ **acetaminophen**.

dolasetron mesylate ⓖ

Type/Group: antiemetic; antinauseant.
Brand(s): Anzemet.
How administered: Orally; injection.

Used to treat

Dolasetron mesylate may be used to give relief from nausea and vomiting, especially in people receiving ℞ **cytotoxic** chemotherapy, or for nausea after surgery. It has been used, as well, to relieve nausea following radiotherapy. Dolasetron and its active metabolite hydrodolasetron, act as ℞ **serotonin-receptor antagonists**, blocking the action of the natural neurotransmitter serotonin.

Warnings

• It should not be given to people with known hypersensitivity to this drug.

• It should be given with caution to people with certain heart conduction disorders, who are taking certain ℞ **antiarrhythmic** drugs, and anyone with low potassium (hypokalemia) or magnesium (hypomagnesemia) levels.

• Dolasetron mesylate should be used during pregnancy only if it is clearly needed.

• Medical judgment is required if breast-feeding is being considered. It is not known whether this drug appears in breast milk.

• Some people may experience significant changes in heart conduction and rhythm, although these effects decrease as drug levels in the blood fall.

• ℞ **Diuretics** that may cause electrolyte imbalance (for example, ℞ **thiazides**) should be used with dolasetron mesylate with caution, as electrolyte imbalance increases the potential for effects on the heart.

• The use of this drug should be stopped at the first sign of rash or other allergic responses, and a doctor informed.

Interactions

• ℞ **Atenolol** and ℞ **cimetidine** may increase the levels and effects of dolasetron.

• ℞ **Rifampin** may lower the levels and effects of dolasetron.

Side effects

• The most common are headache, dizziness, diarrhea, constipation, dyspepsia, and hypotension. There may be changes in heart and liver function.

• Less frequent side effects may include rash, sweating, flushing, and abnormalities of taste or vision.

• Serious hypersensitivity reactions are rare, but anaphylaxis, hives, shortness of breath, and facial swelling have been reported.

Dolgic Tablets ⓑ

A preparation of ℞ **acetaminophen** and ℞ **butabarbital**.
Formulation: Oral tablets.
Availability: Prescription only.
Warnings and side effects: See ℞ **acetaminophen**; ℞ **butabarbital**.

Dolobid Tablets ⓑ

A preparation of ℞ **diflunisal**.
Formulation: Oral tablets, available in two strengths.
Availability: Prescription only.
Warnings and side effects: See ℞ **diflunisal**.

Dolophine ®

A preparation of ℞ **methadone hydrochloride.**
Formulation: Oral tablets, syrup; injection.
Availability: Prescription only.
Warnings and side effects: See ℞ **methadone hydrochloride.**

Dolorac ®

A preparation of ℞ **capsaicin.**
Formulation: Topical cream.
Availability: OTC.
Warnings and side effects: See ℞ **capsaicin.**

Dolsed ®

A preparation of ℞ **atropine sulfate,** ℞ **hyoscyamine,** and
℞ **methenamine,** methylene blue, phenyl ℞ **salicylate,** and
℞ **benzoic acid.**
Formulation: Oral tablets.
Availability: Prescription only.
Warnings and side effects: See ℞ **atropine sulfate;**
℞ **hyoscyamine;** ℞ **methenamine;** ℞ **salicylates;** ℞ **benzoic
acid.**

Domebro Powder; Tablets ®

A preparation of aluminum sulfate and calcium acetate.
Formulation: Topical powder; effervescent tablets.
Availability: OTC.
Warnings and side effects: See ℞ **aluminum acetate.**

Dome-Paste ®

A preparation of ℞ **zinc oxide** and ℞ **calamine.**
Formulation: Topical ointment.
Availability: OTC.
Warnings and side effects: See ℞ **zinc oxide;** and ℞ **calamine.**

Donatussin DC Syrup ®

A preparation of ℞ **hydrocodone bitartrate,** ℞ **guaifenesin,** and
℞ **phenylephrine hydrochloride.**
Formulation: Oral syrup.
Availability: Prescription only.
Warnings and side effects: See ℞ **hydrocodone bitartrate;**
℞ **guaifenesin;** ℞ **phenylephrine hydrochloride.**

Donatussin Drops ®

A preparation of ℞ **phenylephrine hydrochloride,**
℞ **guaifenesin,** and ℞ **chlorpheniramine maleate.**
Formulation: Oral liquid.
Availability: Prescription only.
Warnings and side effects: See ℞ **phenylephrine hydrochloride;**
℞ **guaifenesin;** ℞ **chlorpheniramine maleate.**

donepezil ⓖ

Type/Group: dementia treatment; anticholinesterase.
Brand(s): Aricept.
How administered: Orally

Used to treat
Donepezil is for the symptomatic treatment of mild to moderate
dementia of ✪ **Alzheimer's disease.**
Warnings
• It should not be used by people with known hypersensitivity to
donepezil or to piperidine, or who are currently using other
cholinesterase inhibitors.
• It should be given with caution to anyone with chronic
obstructive pulmonary disease (COPD), asthma, seizure disorders,
bradycardia, hyperthyroidism, heart arrythmias, a history of
gastrointestinal ulcers, or a history of bladder outflow obstruction.
• It is not known whether or not donepezil can harm the fetus,
therefore, it should be used during pregnancy only if medically
judged to be essential.
• Medical judgment is also required if breast-feeding is being
considered, as it is not known whether it is excreted in breast milk.
• Overdose can cause a cholinergic crisis, which is characterized by
severe nausea, vomiting, salivation, sweating, bradycardia,
hypotension, collapse, and convulsions.
• Because it acts to increase cholinergic activity, ulcers or other
gastrointestinal symptoms may develop, and heart rate may be
affected.
Interactions
• ℞ **fluvoxamine** levels may be increased if taken with donepezil.
Side effects
• Diarrhea, and muscle cramps.
• Less frequently nausea, vomiting, fatigue, insomnia, dizziness,
effects on the heart and gastrointestinal systems, and psychiatric
disturbances.

Donnamar ®

A preparation of ℞ **hyoscyamine.**
Formulation: Oral tablets.
Availability: Prescription only.
Warnings and side effects: See ℞ **hyoscyamine.**

Donnatal Capsules; Elixir; Extentabs; Tablets ®

A preparation of ℞ **atropine sulfate,** ℞ **hyoscyamine,**
℞ **scopolamine hydrobromide,** and ℞ **phenobarbital.**
Formulation: Oral capsules, tablets, elixir, and extentabs (higher
dose, extended release).
Availability: Prescription only.
Warnings and side effects: See ℞ **atropine sulfate;**
℞ **hyoscyamine;** ℞ **scopolamine hydrobromide;**
℞ **phenobarbital.**

Donnazyme Tablets ®

A preparation of ℞ **pancreatin** (amylase, lipase, protease).
Formulation: Oral tablets.
Availability: Prescription only.
Warnings and side effects: See ℞ **pancreatin.**

dopamine antagonist ⓓ

see ℞ **dopamine-receptor antagonist.**

dopamine hydrochloride ⑥

Type/Group: **dopamine-receptor stimulant; cardiac stimulant.**
Brand(s): Intropin; various generic.
How administered: Intravenous infusion.

Used to treat

Dopamine hydrochloride is the chemical form of naturally occurring dopamine. It is used in heart surgery and in the treatment of shock arising from a number of causes, such as heart attack, trauma, septicemia, kidney failure, or heart-related events. Its effects are somewhat complicated: as well as stimulating the heart, it has some ℞ **vasoconstrictor** actions (especially in the extremities) and some ℞ **vasodilator** (especially in the kidneys) action, depending on dose and parts of the body affected.

Warnings

• It should not be given to people with pheochromocytoma or certain heart arrhythmia.
• It should be given with caution to people with low blood volume or occlusive vascular diseases (for example, arteriosclerosis, Raynaud's disease, Buerger's disease, frostbite, or other obstructive conditions).
• Dopamine should be used during pregnancy only if the potential benefit outweighs the possible risk to the fetus.
• Medical judgment is required if breast-feeding is being considered. Its effects in breast-feeding are unknown.
• This is a powerful drug, used only under hospital conditions and with continuous monitoring of heart function, blood pressure, and other vital signs.
• Because of a significant interaction with ℞ **MAOI** (monoamine-oxidase inhibitor) antidepressants, dopamine should be given with caution and at greatly reduced dose to people who have used MAOIs within two to three weeks of the dopamine dose.

Interactions

• ℞ **MAOIs** may greatly increase the effects of dopamine, with the potential for serious adverse effects.
• Halogenated ℞ **general anesthetics** (for example, halothane) or cyclopropane have the potential for serious adverse effects on heart rhythm, and must be used with extreme caution.
• ℞ **bretylium tosylate**, oxytocics (for example, ℞ **oxytocin**, ℞ **ergonovine**), ℞ **tricyclics**, and ℞ **vasoconstrictors** may intensify the various effects of dopamine, with the potential for serious adverse reactions.
• ℞ **Alpha-adrenergic blockers** and ℞ **beta-blockers** may reduce or negate the effects of dopamine.
• ℞ **Diuretics** may increase effects if used with dopamine (at low dosage), with increased urinary output.
• ℞ **Phenytoin** may cause hypotension and slow heartbeat.
• ℞ **Haloperidol**, ℞ **phenothiazines**, and ℞ **opioids** may reduce dopamine's vasodilator effects (in the kidney and intestinal circulation).

Side effects

• There may be irregular or fast heartbeat, rapid change in blood pressure (either increase or decrease), chest pain or angina, headache, nausea or shortness of breath.
• At high doses or with long-term use, gangrene of the extremities has occurred.

dopamine-receptor agonist ⓪

see ℞ **dopamine-receptor stimulant.**

dopamine-receptor antagonist ⓪

(dopamine antagonist; dopamine-receptor blocker)
Generics: **chlorpromazine; haloperidol; metoclopramide hydrochloride; promazine; trifluoperazine.**

Actions and uses

℞ **dopamine-receptor antagonists** block the actions of dopamine and other ℞ **dopamine-receptor stimulant** agents at receptors that "recognize" the neurotransmitter dopamine, which is a neurotransmitter in the brain and some other sites in the body. It is possible that some psychoses may in part be caused by abnormalities in the metabolism of dopamine, because dopamine-receptor antagonist drugs (especially of the ℞ **phenothiazine** group) that prevent some of its actions can be used as ℞ **antipsychotic** drugs (for example, ℞ **chlorpromazine**, ℞ **promazine**, ℞ **haloperidol**, and ℞ **trifluoperazine**) to relieve some of the symptoms of ✪ **schizophrenia**. Another type of dopamine-receptor antagonist is ℞ **metoclopramide hydrochloride**, which is an effective ℞ **antiemetic** and ℞ **antinauseant** with useful ℞ **motility stimulant** properties.

Limitations

A major disadvantage of dopamine-receptor antagonist drugs used as antipsychotic drugs, is the high incidence of side effects, including extrapyramidal symptoms and, on prolonged administration, tardive dyskinesia (see ℞ **antipsychotic** entry). See also the individual drug entries.

dopamine-receptor blocker ⓪

see ℞ **dopamine-receptor antagonist.**

dopamine-receptor stimulant ⓪

(dopamine-receptor agonist)
Generics: **bromocriptine; cabergoline; dobutamine hydrochloride; dopamine hydrochloride; fenoldopam mesylate; levodopa; pergolide; pramipexole; ropinirole.**

Actions and uses

℞ **dopamine-receptor stimulant** drugs act at the receptors that "recognize" the neurotransmitter dopamine. Dopamine is chemically a monoamine and is both an intermediate product in the biosynthetic pathway in the brain and sympathetic nervous system that manufactures and stores norepinephrine (noradrenaline) and epinephrine (adrenaline), and a neurotransmitter in its own right in relaying nerve messages. Like the sympathetic neurotransmitters, it is particularly concentrated in the brain and adrenal glands. Drugs that act as dopamine-receptor stimulants or that lead to increased dopamine production or concentrations in the brain play an important part in the treatment of parkinsonism and related disorders. Dopamine-receptor stimulant drugs that mimic some aspects of the action of dopamine in the brain (including ℞ **bromocriptine**, ℞ **pergolide**, ℞ **pramipexole**, ℞ **ropinirole**, and ℞ **cabergoline**) can be used both for ℞ **antiparkinsonism** treatment and to relieve a number of hormone disorders. Similarly, drugs that lead to increased levels of dopamine in the brain also lead indirectly to increased dopamine-receptor stimulation, and such antiparkinsonism drugs include ℞ **levodopa** (a synthetic version of dopamine's natural precursor amino acid DOPA), and also enzyme inhibitors that slow down dopamine's breakdown in the body (℞ **carbidopa**, ℞ **entacapone**, ℞ **selegiline hydrochloride**, ℞ **tolcapone**).

Dopamine has other roles in the brain, apart from control of movement. It is thought also to act as a ℞ **hypothalamic hormone**, *prolactin release-inhibiting factor* (PRIF), which has a controlling role on the release of prolactin, the hormone that causes lactation as an end-effect. For this reason, dopamine-receptor stimulants, such as ℞ **bromocriptine** and ℞ **cabergoline**, have alternative uses to inhibit prolactin secretion by the pituitary gland and to reduce or halt lactation (in galactorrhea) or prolactinoma (a tumor of the pituitary gland which leads to excess prolactin secretion).

In the periphery (that is, in the body rather than the brain), dopamine in the form of the synthetic drug ℞ **dopamine hydrochloride** is used in medicine as a ℞ **cardiac stimulant** in heart surgery. Its effects are complicated and as well as stimulating the heart, it has some ℞ **vasoconstrictor** (narrows blood vessels, especially in the extremities) and some ℞ **vasodilator** (widens blood vessels, especially in kidneys) action, depending on dose and parts of the body affected. The related drug ℞ **dobutamine hydrochloride** may be used as a cardiac stimulant in the treatment of cardiogenic shock associated with a ✚ **myocardial infarction** (heart attack) or heart surgery and in the treatment of shock arising from a number of causes, such as heart attack, trauma, septicemia, kidney failure, or heart-related events. Its beneficial effects are thought to result partly through actions as a ℞ **beta-adrenergic stimulant** in the heart and partly at dopamine receptors in blood vessels. Another analog, ℞ **fenoldopam mesylate**, has similar actions and is used, in hospitals, to quickly reduce blood pressure in hypertensive emergencies.

Members of this group of drugs have some important therapeutic uses. A number of these drugs were quite recently introduced, and further drugs with these actions can be expected.

Limitations

See the individual drug entries.

Dopram ⓑ

A preparation of ℞ **doxapram**.
Formulation: Injection.
Availability: Prescription only.
Warnings and side effects: See ℞ **doxapram**.

Doral ⓑ

A preparation of ℞ **quazepam**.
Formulation: Oral tablets in several strengths.
Availability: Prescription only.
Warnings and side effects: See ℞ **quazepam**.

dornase alfa ⓖ

Type/Group: mucolytic; enzyme.
Brand(s): Pulmozyme.
How administered: Inhalation.

Used to treat

Dornase alfa is a version, manufactured by genetic engineering, of a naturally occurring human enzyme which breaks down deoxyribonucleic acid (DNA) in sputum which reduces sputum viscoelasticity. Because of this effect, it is used in ✚ **cystic fibrosis** to improve lung function and reduce respiratory infections (excess secretions exacerbate infections).

Warnings

• It should not be given to people with known hypersensitivity or allergy to this drug. Its safety has not been established for children under the age of 5.

• It should be used in pregnancy only when medically judged to be clearly needed.

• Medical judgment is required if breast-feeding is being considered. It is not known whether this drug is present in breast milk.

• Do not dilute or mix dornase with other drugs, as this could lead to chemical or functional changes in one or more of the drugs.

• It must be kept refrigerated right up to use (between 36–46°F, 2–8°C;) and kept away from strong light.

Interactions

No significant interactions have been reported.

Side effects

• Frequently, sore throat, chest pain or discomfort, and voice changes.

• Occasionally, conjunctivitis, hoarseness, and skin rash.

• Rarely, adverse gastrointestinal or respiratory effects.

Doryx ⓑ

A preparation of ℞ **doxycycline**.
Formulation: Oral capsules with coated pellets.
Availability: Prescription only.
Warnings and side effects: See ℞ **doxycycline**.

dorzolamide ⓖ

Type/Group: **carbonic anhydrase inhibitor; glaucoma treatment.**
Brand(s): Trusopt Ocumeter. Combinations: With *timolol maleate*: Cosopt Ocumeter.
How administered: Topically (eyes).

Used to treat

Dorzolamide is used to treat ✚ **glaucoma**, alone or in combination with ℞ **beta-blockers**, because it reduces the formation of aqueous humor (fluid) in the eye and ocular hypertension.

Warnings

• It should not be given to people with known hypersensitivity to dorzolamide or ℞ **sulfonamides**.

• It should be given with caution to people with severe kidney or liver impairment.

• Dorzolamide's safety during pregnancy has not been established. It should be used only if the potential benefit outweighs the possible risk to the fetus.

• It should not be used by nursing mothers, so avoid if possible.

• Dorzolamide is a sulfonamide and is absorbed systemically (into the body) and so has the potential for producing the adverse reactions seen with other sulfonamides.

• The preservative in dorzolamide solution, benzalkonium chloride, may be absorbed by soft contact lenses, and so it should be used 15 minutes before putting in the lenses.

Interactions
No significant interactions have been reported.

Side effects
• Burning, stinging or discomfort, bitter taste, allergic reaction, transient corneal inflammation, blurred vision, tearing, dryness, and light sensitivity.

• Rarely, systemic side effects such as headache, nausea, and fatigue.

D.O.S. ⑧
A preparation of ℞ **docusate sodium**.
Formulation: Oral gelcaps.
Availability: OTC.
Warnings and side effects: See ℞ **docusate sodium**.

Dostinex ⑧
A preparation of ℞ **cabergoline**.
Formulation: Oral tablets.
Availability: Prescription only.
Warnings and side effects: See ℞ **cabergoline**.

Double Ice ArthriCare Gel ⑧
A preparation of ℞ **camphor** and ℞ **menthol**.
Formulation: Topical gel.
Availability: OTC.
Warnings and side effects: See ℞ **camphor**; ℞ **menthol**.

Dovonex ⑧
A preparation of ℞ **calcipotriene**.
Formulation: Topical cream, ointment, solution.
Availability: Prescription only.
Warnings and side effects: See ℞ **calcipotriene**.

doxapram ⑥
Type/Group: **respiratory stimulant**.
Brand(s): Dopram; various generic.
How administered: Injection.

Used to treat
Doxapram is used to relieve severe respiratory difficulties in people who suffer from ✪ **chronic obstructive pulmonary disease** (COPD), or who undergo respiratory depression following major surgery or drug overdose.

Warnings
Doxapram is a specialist hospital drug, and a full evaluation will be carried out.

• It should not be used by anyone with seizure disorders, severe hypertension, bronchial asthma, certain heart, lung or airway disorders, head injury, or stroke.

• It should be given with caution to anyone with heart rhythm disorders, pheochromocytoma, or hypertension.

• It is not known whether or not doxapram can harm the fetus, therefore, it should be used during pregnancy only if medically judged to be needed.

• Medical judgment is also required if breast-feeding is being considered, as it is not known whether this drug is excreted in breast milk.

• Ttreatment must take place in a hospital.

Interactions
• Doxapram taken with a ℞ **MAOI** antidepressant may enhance the effect on blood pressure.

Side effects
• Muscle weakness, anorexia and weight loss, dizziness, drowsiness, agitation and confusion, insomnia, depression, headache, sweating, feeling of being unwell, and tremor.

• Rarely, angina pectoris, gastrointestinal hemorrhage, fainting, convulsions, and there can also be bladder outflow obstruction.

doxazosin mesylate ⑥
Type/Group: **alpha-adrenergic blocker; antihypertensive**.
Brand(s): Cardura.
How administered: Orally.

Used to treat
Doxazosin is used in the treatment of ✪ **hypertension**, often with other antihypertensives (for example, ℞ **beta-blockers** or ℞ **thiazide** ℞ **diuretics**). It can also be used to treat urinary retention in ✪ **benign prostatic hyperplasia** (BPH).

Warnings
• It should not be given to people with known hypersensitivity to this drug or to any other quinazoline derivative (for example, ℞ **prazosin**, ℞ **terazosin**), or with impaired liver function.

• Doxazosin should be used in pregnancy only if it is clearly needed.

• Medical judgment is required if breast-feeding is being considered. It is not known whether this drug appears in breast milk.

• Postural hypotension (lowered blood pressure on standing, usually causing dizziness) occurs frequently and may result in fainting. Sudden or prolonged standing or exercise should be avoided when taking doxazosin. During initial dosing, it is necessary also for the person to identify situations in which fainting would be dangerous. These hypotensive effects may be aggravated by hot environments.

• Because of possible sedative side effects, caution is advised for potentially hazardous activities, such as driving, that require mental alertness.

• Rarely, priapism (prolonged and painful erection) has been reported with use of this drug. This condition, should it occur, should be treated promptly, or permanent dysfunction may result.

Interactions
• If used with other antihypertensives and diuretics, the effects of these drugs may be increased. This additive effect is sometimes used to advantage in combination treatments for high blood pressure.

Side effects

• These may include postural hypotension, dizziness and vertigo, headache, fatigue, muscle weakness, edema, sleepiness, nausea, and rhinitis.

• Less frequently, abdominal discomfort, diarrhea and vomiting, agitation, muscle tremor, rash and pruritus.

• Rare side effects include blurred vision, nosebleed, slight blood changes, liver problems and jaundice, urinary incontinence, priapism, and impotence.

doxepin Ⓖ

Type/Group: **antidepressant; tricyclic; antihistamine; antipruritic**.

Brand(s): (Antidepressant): Sinequan; Adapin; various generic. (Topical): Zonalon.

How administered: Orally; topically (external).

Used to treat

Doxepin can be used, as doxepin hydrochloride, to treat ✪ **depression** and ✪ **anxiety**, especially in people where sedation would be helpful. It is recommended as a treatment for depression and/or anxiety associated with alcoholism and organic disease, and for psychotic depressive disorders, including ✪ **bipolar disorder** (manic-depressive illness). Although not stated by the manufacturer for such treatment, it is sometimes prescribed together with analgesics for pain associated with peptic ulcer disease and certain skin disorders. It also has ℞ **antihistamine** properties, and is used externally for the treatment of pruritis (itching) associated with certain types of ✪ **eczema**. As is the case with other antidepressants, this drug is also being evaluated for other uses.

Warnings

• It should not be given to people with known hypersensitivity to this drug, or who are just recovering from myocardial infarction (heart attack), or with narrow-angle glaucoma, urinary retention, who are taking or have stopped taking MAOI antidepressants within the previous 14 days.

• It should be given with caution to people with a history of elevated intraocular pressure (pressure in the eyeball), cardiovascular, heart, kidney, liver or thyroid disease, or diabetes mellitus.

• Doxepin should be used during pregnancy only if the benefits outweigh the risk to the fetus.

• It should not be used by nursing mothers.

• Other symptoms of a psychiatric illnesses may worsen.

• Episodes of mania or hypomania may occur.

• Exposure to sunlight should be minimized because of possible photosensitization (sensitivity to light).

• Treatment should be stopped gradually by lowering the dose over a period of time.

• It is not generally given to children under the age of 12.

• It may be 4 to 6 weeks before there are any signs of improvement.

• It may impair the performance of skilled tasks such as driving.

• Alcohol, grapefruit juice, and smoking can all affect tricyclics (see Interactions below).

Interactions

• Serious or even fatal reactions can occur if ℞ **MAOI** antidepressants are taken at the same time as tricyclics.

• The effects of ℞ **epinephrine**, ℞ **norepinephrine**, and ℞ **phenylephrine** on blood pressure are intensified.

• Grapefruit juice increases the levels of tricyclics.

• ℞ **clonidine hydrochloride** should not be used with tricyclics, because a dangerous increase in blood pressure and hypertensive crisis is possible.

• The effects of ℞ **guanethidine monosulfate**, ℞ **levodopa**, and ℞ **sympathomimetics** may be reduced by tricyclics.

• The effects of ℞ **anticholinergics**, dicumarol, ℞ **quinolones**, grepafloxacin, and sparfloxacin may be enhanced by tricyclics.

• ℞ **Barbiturates**, ℞ **activated charcoal**, and rifamycin-related antibiotics may reduce the effectiveness of tricyclics.

• ℞ **Cimetidine**, ℞ **SSRI**s, ℞ **haloperidol**, ℞ **bupropion**, ℞ **valproate sodium** (and other valproic acid derivatives), and histamine ℞ **H$_2$-antagonists** may increase the levels of tricyclics in the blood.

• The levels of ℞ **carbamazepine** may increase, while blood levels of tricyclics decrease.

• Smoking may affect the metabolism of tricyclics.

• The effects of alcohol may be enhanced.

Side effects

These depend on the how it is administered.

• Oral use: It has pronounced ℞ **anticholinergic** side effects, notably drowsiness and difficulty in concentrating, dry mouth, blurred vision, constipation, stoppage of the normal action of the intestine (peristalsis), postural hypotension (lowered blood pressure on standing), and urinary retention. Less frequently, white blood cell disorders, hypertension, and irregular or speeded heartbeat. It may also cause weight gain.

• Topical use: There may be burning, stinging, or skin sensitization, and enough can be absorbed into the body to cause drowsiness.

Doxidan Ⓑ

A preparation of casanthranol, ℞ **cascara sagrada**, and ℞ **docusate sodium**.

Formulation: Oral capsules.

Availability: OTC.

Warnings and side effects: See ℞ **cascara sagrada**; ℞ **docusate sodium**.

Doxil Ⓑ

A preparation of ℞ **doxorubicin hydrochloride**.

Formulation: Liposomal injection.

Availability: Prescription only.

Warnings and side effects: See ℞ **doxorubicin hydrochloride**.

doxorubicin hydrochloride Ⓖ

Type/Group: **anticancer; cytotoxic**.

Brand(s): Adriamycin; Doxil; Rubex; various generic.

How administered: Intravenous injection.

Used to treat

Doxorubicin is a cytotoxic drug (an anthracycline antibiotic in origin) used particularly for acute ⊕ **leukemia**, ⊕ **lymphomas**, some solid ⊕ **tumors**, and ⊕ **Kaposi's sarcoma** (as doxorubicin liposomal) in people with AIDS.

Warnings

• It should not be given to people with known hypersensitivity to doxorubicin, with marked bone marrow depression from previous cancer treatment, or anyone previously treated with complete cumulative doses of this or any of several related drugs.

• It should be given with caution to people with a history of heart disease, hypertension, or liver impairment. The elderly or very young are more at risk of experiencing serious adverse effects on the heart.

• Medical judgment is required if the liposomal form is to be given to people with a history of cardiovascular disease. This is a specialist drug which will be used following a full evaluation by specialist physicians.

• Doxorubicin is not recommended for use during pregnancy unless it is medically judged to be essential, because it may cause birth defects. Becoming pregnant while using this drug must be avoided.

• It should not be used if breast-feeding.

• Bone marrow depression is a major toxic side effect of this drug, and may lead to infection or hemorrhage.

• Mucositis (sores formed in the mucous membrane lining of the gastrointestinal tract) may occur and may lead to serious infection and/or bleeding.

• Adverse effects on the heart may be produced, particularly at high doses, during treatment or even months to years later.

• In common with many anticancer drugs, doxorubicin may cause cancer or genetic mutations in cells.

Interactions

• ℞ **Cyclophosphamide** may increase adverse effects on heart.

• ℞ **Paclitaxel**, ℞ **progesterone**, streptozocin, and ℞ **verapamil** may increase concentrations of doxorubicin.

• The effects of ℞ **actinomycin D**, ℞ **cyclophosphamide**, and ℞ **mercaptopurine** may be increased.

• The levels of ℞ **digoxin** and ℞ **phenytoin** may be reduced.

• The toxicity of radiation therapy is increased.

Side effects

• Frequently, hair loss, gastrointestinal disturbances, inflamed esophagus, and reddish urine.

• Occasionally, darkening of nails, fingers or toes, and skin creases.

• Rarely, fever, chills, and tearing or inflammation of the eyes.

doxycycline ⓖ

Type/Group: **tetracycline; antibiotic; antibacterial; antimalarial**.
Brand(s): Doryx; Monodox; Periostat; Vibra-Tabs; Vibramycin; various generic.
How administered: Orally; injection.

Used to treat

Doxycycline is used to treat many kinds of infection, for example, of the respiratory and genital tracts, ⊕ **trachoma**, ⊕ **acne**, and ⊕ **syphilis**. It can also be used, in combination with other drugs, to treat ⊕ **brucellosis** and ⊕ **pelvic inflammatory disease**, ⊕ **Lyme disease**, ⊕ **Rocky Mountain spotted fever**, Q fever, and ⊕ **psittacosis**. It is also used as an preventive treatment for ⊕ **malaria**.

Warnings

• It should not be given to people with known hypersensitivity to tetracyclines, or to children under 8 years of age.

• It should be given with caution to people with kidney or liver impairment.

• Doxycycline should be avoided in the last half of pregnancy because of a risk of dental staining and inhibiting the skeletal growth of the fetus.

• It should not be used by nursing mothers.

• Superinfections due to the altered bacterial balance caused by antibiotic treatment may occur. A doctor must be contacted if severe abdominal pain, moderate to severe diarrhea, or any new or unusual symptoms occur.

• It may cause photosensitivity reactions (abnormal sensitivity to sunlight).

• It may cause permanent discoloration of teeth and the thin tooth enamel in children from the time of tooth formation, which begins in the uterus and ends at the age of 8. It may also retard bone development during the same period.

• It must not be used after the discard date, as it becomes harmful to the kidneys as it degrades.

• It must not be taken with antacids or iron supplements.

Interactions

• Avoid using ℞ **antacids** within two hours before or after a dose of doxycycline.

• ℞ **Bismuth subsalicylate**, ℞ **barbiturates**, ⚗ **calcium**, ⚗ **iron**, ⚗ **magnesium**, ℞ **cholestyramine**, ℞ **sodium bicarbonate**, ⚗ **zinc**, ℞ **colestipol hydrochloride** may decrease the absorption of tetracyclines.

• The levels of ℞ **digoxin** may be reduced.

• The effects of ℞ **penicillin** are impaired.

• The effectiveness of ℞ **oral contraceptives** may be reduced.

• ℞ **Carbamazepine** and ℞ **phenytoin** may decrease concentrations of doxycycline.

• There is the potential of enhancing the anticoagulant effect of ℞ **warfarin sodium**.

Side effects

• Frequently, gastrointestinal upsets (take with food to minimize) and difficulty swallowing.

• Rarely, rash, hives, liver toxicity, pancreatitis, blood and skin disorders.

doxylamine ⓖ

Type/Group: **antihistamine; cold and cough preparation**.
Brand(s): Unisom Nighttime Sleep Aid; various generic.
Combinations: With *pseudoephedrine, dextromethorphan, and acetaminophen*: Alka-Seltzer Plus NightTime Cold Liqui-Gels; Genite Liquid; Nytcold Medicine Liquid; Vicks NyQuil.
How administered: Orally.

Used to treat

Doxylamine is incorporated into a proprietary ℞ **analgesic** and cold and cough preparations for temporary relief of ✪ **cold** and ✪ **cough** symptoms. It is strongly sedating and is used also as a ℞ **sleep-aid product**.

Warnings

• It should not be given to people with known hypersensitivity to this drug (or with known sensitivity to other antihistamines).

• Antihistamines should be given with caution to people with asthma (and never during an attack) or lower respiratory disease, heart disease, hypertension, hyperthyroidism, epilepsy, porphyria, increased intraocular pressure (pressure in the eyeball, as in glaucoma), enlarged prostate, urinary retention, or certain obstructive bladder or gastrointestinal conditions.

• Doxylamine should be used during pregnancy only if the potential benefit outweighs the possible risk to the fetus.

• Nursing mothers should discontinue using this drug or discontinue breast-feeding.

• This drug must not be given to infants, and for children under the age of 12 the manufacturer's or medical instructions must be followed closely.

• Because of its sedative side effects, the performance of skilled tasks, such as driving, may be impaired.

• Side effects are more frequent in the elderly.

Interactions

• ℞ **MAOI** antidepressants may prolong and intensify the ℞ **anticholinergic** effects of antihistamines (see Side effects below).

• If used with ℞ **tricyclic** antidepressants, other antihistamines, ℞ **phenothiazines**, ℞ **skeletal muscle relaxants**, ℞ **opioids**, ℞ **barbiturates**, ℞ **hypnotics**, ℞ **sedatives**, or ℞ **antianxiety** drugs, there is a risk of intensified side effects.

• Alcohol may intensify side effects such as drowsiness and impaired mental alertness.

Side effects

• These depend on how it is administered. For this type of antihistamine, there is commonly drowsiness, headache, impaired muscular coordination or dizziness, anticholinergic effects (dry mouth, blurred vision, urinary retention, gastrointestinal disturbances), occasional rashes and photosensitivity (abnormal sensitivity to light), palpitations and heart arrhythmias.

• Rarely, there may be stimulation instead of sedation (paradoxical stimulation), especially in children (and convulsions in overdose), hypersensitivity reactions, blood disorders, liver disturbances, depression, sleep disturbances, and hypotension.

Dramamine Less Drowsy Formula ⑧

A preparation of ℞ **meclizine hydrochloride**.
Formulation: Oral tablets.
Availability: OTC.
Warnings and side effects: See ℞ **meclizine hydrochloride**.

Dramamine Tablets; Chewable Tablets; Liquid ⑧

A preparation of ℞ **dimenhydrinate**.

Formulation: Oral tablets; chewable tablets; liquid.
Availability: OTC; Liquid is prescription only.
Warnings and side effects: See ℞ **dimenhydrinate**. The chewable tablets contain the sweetener aspartame (with phenylalanine), which should be avoided by individuals with phenylketonuria they also contain tartrazine (FD&C yellow No 5), a dye that may cause allergic reaction in a few people, but especially those with sensitivity to aspirin.

Dramanate ⑧

A preparation of ℞ **dimenhydrinate**.
Formulation: Injection.
Availability: Prescription only.
Warnings and side effects: See ℞ **dimenhydrinate**.

Drisdol ⑧

A preparation of ℞ **ergocalciferol**.
Formulation: Oral liquid drops; oral capsules.
Availability: Liquid is OTC; capsules are prescription only.
Warnings and side effects: See ℞ **ergocalciferol**.

Dristan 12 Hr Nasal ⑧

A preparation of ℞ **oxymetazoline hydrochloride**.
Formulation: Nasal drops.
Availability: OTC.
Warnings and side effects: See ℞ **oxymetazoline hydrochloride**.

Dristan Cold Caplets ⑧

A preparation of ℞ **pseudoephedrine** and ℞ **acetaminophen**.
Formulation: Oral tablets.
Availability: OTC.
Warnings and side effects: See ℞ **pseudoephedrine**; ℞ **acetaminophen**.

Dristan Cold Multi-Symptom Formula Tablets ⑧

A preparation of ℞ **phenylephrine hydrochloride**, ℞ **acetaminophen**, and ℞ **chlorpheniramine maleate**.
Formulation: Oral tablets.
Availability: OTC.
Warnings and side effects: See ℞ **phenylephrine hydrochloride**; ℞ **acetaminophen**; ℞ **chlorpheniramine maleate**.

Dristan Nasal Spray ⑧ ·

A preparation of ℞ **phenylephrine hydrochloride** and ℞ **pheniramine maleate**.
Formulation: Nasal spray.
Availability: OTC.
Warnings and side effects: See ℞ **phenylephrine hydrochloride**; ℞ **pheniramine maleate**.

Dristan Saline Spray ⑧

A preparation of ℞ **sodium chloride**.
Formulation: Nasal Spray.

Availability: OTC.

Warnings and side effects: See ℞ **sodium chloride**.

Dristan Sinus Caplets Ⓑ

A preparation of ℞ **pseudoephedrine** and ℞ **ibuprofen**.

Formulation: Oral tablets.

Availability: OTC.

Warnings and side effects: See ℞ **pseudoephedrine**;
℞ **ibuprofen**.

Drithocreme; Dritho-Scalp Ⓑ

A preparation of ℞ **anthralin**.

Formulation: Topical cream in two strengths; scalp cream (Dritho-Scalp).

Availability: Prescription only.

Warnings and side effects: See ℞ **anthralin**.

Drixomed Tablets Ⓑ

A preparation of pseudoephedrine sulfate and dexbrompheniramine maleate.

Formulation: Oral tablets.

Availability: Prescription only.

Warnings and side effects: See ℞ **pseudoephedrine**;
℞ **brompheniramine maleate**.

Drixoral Cold & Allergy Tablets Ⓑ

A preparation of ℞ **pseudoephedrine** sulfate and
℞ **brompheniramine maleate**.

Formulation: Oral tablets, sustained release.

Availability: OTC.

Warnings and side effects: See ℞ **pseudoephedrine**;
℞ **brompheniramine maleate**.

Drixoral Cold & Flu Tablets Ⓑ

A preparation of ℞ **pseudoephedrine** sulfate, ℞ **acetaminophen**, and dexbrompheniramine maleate.

Formulation: Oral tablets (extended release).

Availability: OTC.

Warnings and side effects: See ℞ **pseudoephedrine**;
℞ **acetaminophen**; ℞ **brompheniramine maleate**.

Drixoral Cough Liquid Caps Ⓑ

A preparation of ℞ **dextromethorphan**.

Formulation: Oral capsules.

Availability: OTC.

Warnings and side effects: See ℞ **dextromethorphan**.

Drixoral Non-Drowsy Formula Tablets Ⓑ

A preparation of ℞ **pseudoephedrine** sulfate.

Formulation: Oral tablets.

Availability: OTC.

Warnings and side effects: See ℞ **pseudoephedrine**.

Drixoral Syrup Ⓑ

A preparation of ℞ **pseudoephedrine** sulfate and
℞ **brompheniramine maleate**.

Formulation: Oral syrup.

Availability: OTC.

Warnings and side effects: See ℞ **pseudoephedrine**;
℞ **brompheniramine maleate**.

dronabinol Ⓖ

Type/Group: **antiemetic; antinauseant; appetite stimulant**.

Brand(s): Marinol.

How administered: Orally.

Used to treat

Dronabinol is the principal psychoactive constituent of marijuana (*Cannabis sativa*). Although its action is not fully understood, it is known that it acts at specific receptors on the brain and elsewhere. This drug both stimulates appetite and effectively suppresses ✚ **nausea** and ✚ **vomiting**. It is used for the control of such symptoms in people undergoing chemotherapy or radiotherapy for cancer, and to restore appetite in those with AIDS.

Warnings

• It should not be given to people with known hypersensitivity to this drug or to marijuana or sesame oil.

• It should be given with caution to people with heart disease or high blood pressure, or who are manic, depressive, or schizophrenic.

• Dronabinol should be used during pregnancy only if it is clearly needed.

• Its effects while breast-feeding are unknown, and so nursing women should discontinue this drug or discontinue breast-feeding.

• Observation is recommended when first beginning treatment, as unusual responses are possible.

• Psychotropic side effects may be more likely in the elderly.

• It may cause drowsiness or dizziness, and so hazardous or skilled tasks, such as driving, should be avoided.

• It is considered highly abusable and is a Class III controlled substance.

Interactions

• There is a potential for significant additive hypertensive effect and rapid heartbeat if used with ℞ **amphetamines**,
℞ **anticholinergics**, ℞ **antihistamines**, ℞ **cocaine**,
℞ **sympathomimetics**, or ℞ **tricyclic** antidepressants.

• There is a possibility of intensified effects on the central nervous system if used with alcohol, ℞ **hypnotics**, or ℞ **sedatives**.

• ℞ **Disulfiram** and ℞ **fluoxetine** may cause hypomania (elation, restlessness, irritability).

• The levels and effects of ℞ **theophylline** may be decreased.

Side effects

• The most common side effect is euphoria. Others may include dizziness, paranoid reaction, drowsiness, nausea, and vomiting.

• Less frequently there may be palpitations or rapid heartbeat, amnesia, confusion, hallucinations or abnormal thinking, vision problems, speech difficulties, depression, or diarrhea.

Key to symbols: ✚ = Disorder Section ℞ = Drug Section ♣ = Herbal Section ⚕ = Supplement Section

droperidol Ⓖ

Type/Group: **antiemetic; antinauseant; sedatives**.
Brand(s): Inapsine; various generic.
How administered: Injection.

Used to treat

Droperidol belongs to the antipsychotic butyrophenone group, but is used to tranquilize and reduce the incidence of nausea and vomiting in patients about to undergo surgery or diagnostic procedures. It may be combined with a ℞ **narcotic analgesic** to decrease anxiety and pain. It is also used as an additional treatment to maintain general anesthesia during surgical procedures. Although not stated by the manufacturer for such use, it may be prescribed to treat nausea and vomiting caused by chemotherapy.

Warnings

• It should not be given to people with known hypersensitivity to this or similar drugs.
• It should be given with caution to anyone over 65, and to anyone with heart, cardiovascular, liver, kidney, or Parkinson's disease.
• Droperidol should be used during pregnancy only when it is medically judged to be clearly needed. It has been used in Cesarean section deliveries with no apparent harm to the newborn.
• Medical judgment is also required if breast-feeding is being considered, as it is not known whether this drug is excreted in breast milk.
• The doctor must be informed if CNS depressants are being used (such as, ℞ **antidepressants**, ℞ **barbiturates**).

Interactions

• CNS depressants increase the effects of droperidol.

Side effects

• Drowsiness, reduced blood pressure, speeded heart beat, chills, dizziness, and respiratory depression.

Drotic Ⓑ

A preparation of ℞ **hydrocortisone**, ℞ **neomycin**, and ℞ **polymyxin B sulfate**.
Formulation: Ear drops.
Availability: Prescription only.
Warnings and side effects: See ℞ **hydrocortisone**; ℞ **neomycin**; ℞ **polymyxin B sulfate**.

Dr Scholl's Clear Away Disks; One Step Strips Ⓑ

A preparation of ℞ **salicylic acid**.
Formulation: Topical, adhesive medicated strips, disks.
Availability: OTC.
Warnings and side effects: See ℞ **salicylic acid**.

Dr Scholl's Wart Remover Kit; Corn/Callus Remover Ⓑ

A preparation of ℞ **salicylic acid** and various.
Formulation: Topical liquid.
Availability: OTC.
Warnings and side effects: See ℞ **salicylic acid**.

Dry Eyes Ⓑ

A preparation of ℞ **polyvinyl alcohol** and benzalkonium chloride.
Formulation: Ophthalmic solution.
Availability: OTC.
Warnings and side effects: See ℞ **polyvinyl alcohol**.

Dryox 2.5; 5 Ⓑ

A preparation of ℞ **benzoyl peroxide**.
Formulation: Topical gel in two strengths.
Availability: OTC.
Warnings and side effects: See ℞ **benzoyl peroxide**.

Dryox Wash Ⓑ

A preparation of ℞ **benzoyl peroxide**.
Formulation: Topical liquid (wash); topical gel in several strengths.
Availability: OTC.
Warnings and side effects: See ℞ **benzoyl peroxide**.

Drysol Ⓑ

A preparation of ℞ **aluminum chloride**.
Formulation: Topical solution.
Availability: Prescription only.
Warnings and side effects: See ℞ **aluminum chloride**.

Drytex Lotion Ⓑ

A preparation of ℞ **salicylic acid** and various.
Formulation: Topical lotion.
Availability: OTC.
Warnings and side effects: See ℞ **salicylic acid**.

D-S-S Ⓑ

A preparation of ℞ **docusate sodium**.
Formulation: Oral capsules.
Availability: OTC.
Warnings and side effects: See ℞ **docusate sodium**.

DTIC-Dome Ⓑ

A preparation of ℞ **dacarbazine**.
Formulation: Injection.
Availability: Prescription only.
Warnings and side effects: See ℞ **dacarbazine**.

DTwP Ⓖ

see ℞ **diphtheria and tetanus toxoids and whole-cell pertussis vaccine adsorbed (DTwP)**.

DTwP-Hib Ⓖ

see ℞ **diphtheria and tetanus toxoids and acellular pertussis and Haemophilus influenzae type b conjugate vaccine (DTaP-HIB)**.

Dulcolax Tablets; Suppositories Ⓑ

A preparation of ℞ **bisacodyl**.
Formulation: Oral tablets; rectal suppositories.
Availability: OTC.

Warnings and side effects: See ℞ bisacodyl.

Dull-C ®

A preparation of ℞ **ascorbic acid.**
Formulation: Oral powder.
Availability: OTC.
Warnings and side effects: See ℞ ascorbic acid.

Duocet Capsules ®

A preparation of ℞ **hydrocodone bitartrate** and ℞ **acetaminophen.**
Formulation: Oral capsules.
Availability: Prescription only.
Warnings and side effects: See ℞ hydrocodone bitartrate; ℞ acetaminophen.

Duo-Cyp ®

A preparation of ℞ **estradiol** and ℞ **testosterone** cypionate.
Formulation: Injection.
Availability: Prescription only.
Warnings and side effects: See ℞ estradiol; ℞ testosterone.

DuoFilm Liquid; Transdermal Patch ®

A preparation of ℞ **salicylic acid.**
Formulation: Topical liquid; adhesive medicated patch.
Availability: OTC.
Warnings and side effects: See ℞ salicylic acid.

DuoPlant Gel ®

A preparation of ℞ **salicylic acid.**
Formulation: Topical gel.
Availability: OTC.
Warnings and side effects: See ℞ salicylic acid.

Duphalac ®

A preparation of ℞ **lactulose.**
Formulation: Oral liquid.
Availability: Prescription only.
Warnings and side effects: See ℞ lactulose.

Duplex Liquid Face Cleanser ®

A preparation of ℞ **sodium lauryl sulfate.**
Formulation: Topical liquid.
Availability: OTC.
Warnings and side effects: See ℞ sodium lauryl sulfate.

Duplex T ®

A preparation of ℞ **coal tar.**
Formulation: Shampoo.
Availability: OTC.
Warnings and side effects: See ℞ coal tar.

Duracef ®

A preparation of ℞ **cefadroxil.**
Formulation: Tablets; capsule; oral liquid.

Availability: Prescription only.
Warnings and side effects: See ℞ cefadroxil.

Duraclon ®

A preparation of ℞ **clonidine hydrochloride.**
Formulation: Injection (epidural infusion).
Availability: Prescription only.
Warnings and side effects: See ℞ clonidine hydrochloride.

Duragesic-25; -50; -75; -100 ®

A preparation of ℞ **fentanyl.**
Formulation: Skin patch.
Availability: Prescription only.
Warnings and side effects: See ℞ fentanyl; doses larger than Duragesic-25 must be used only by those who are already opioid tolerant.

Duralex Capsules ®

A preparation of ℞ **pseudoephedrine** and ℞ **chlorpheniramine maleate.**
Formulation: Oral capsules, sustained release.
Availability: Prescription only.
Warnings and side effects: See ℞ pseudoephedrine; ℞ chlorpheniramine maleate.

Duralone ®

A preparation of ℞ **methylprednisolone** acetate.
Formulation: Injection.
Availability: Prescription only.
Warnings and side effects: See ℞ methylprednisolone.

Duramist Plus ®

A preparation of ℞ **oxymetazoline hydrochloride.**
Formulation: Nasal spray.
Availability: OTC.
Warnings and side effects: See ℞ oxymetazoline hydrochloride.

Duramorph ®

A preparation of ℞ **morphine sulfate.**
Formulation: Injection, available in two strengths.
Availability: Prescription only.
Warnings and side effects: See ℞ morphine sulfate.

Duranest ®

A preparation of ℞ **etidocaine.**
Formulation: Injection.
Availability: Prescription only.
Warnings and side effects: See ℞ etidocaine.

Duratest ®

A preparation of ℞ **testosterone** cypionate.
Formulation: Injection in two strengths.
Availability: Prescription only.
Warnings and side effects: See ℞ testosterone.

Durathate ®

A preparation of ℞ **testosterone** enanthate.
Formulation: Injection.
Availability: Prescription only.
Warnings and side effects: See ℞ **testosterone**.

Duration ®

A preparation of ℞ **oxymetazoline hydrochloride**.
Formulation: Nasal spray.
Availability: OTC.
Warnings and side effects: See ℞ **oxymetazoline hydrochloride**.

Duratuss DM Syrup ®

A preparation of ℞ **dextromethorphan** and ℞ **guaifenesin**.
Formulation: Oral syrup.
Availability: Prescription only.
Warnings and side effects: See ℞ **dextromethorphan**; ℞ **guaifenesin**.

Duratuss-G Tablets ®

A preparation of ℞ **guaifenesin**.
Formulation: Oral tablets.
Availability: Prescription only.
Warnings and side effects: See ℞ **guaifenesin**.

Duratuss HD Elixir ®

A preparation of ℞ **hydrocodone bitartrate**, ℞ **pseudoephedrine**, and ℞ **guaifenesin**.
Formulation: Oral liquid.
Availability: Prescription only.
Warnings and side effects: See ℞ **hydrocodone bitartrate**; ℞ **pseudoephedrine**; ℞ **guaifenesin**.

Duratuss Tablets ®

A preparation of ℞ **pseudoephedrine** and ℞ **guaifenesin**.
Formulation: Oral tablets, long acting.
Availability: Prescription only.
Warnings and side effects: See ℞ **pseudoephedrine**; ℞ **guaifenesin**.

Dyazide ®

A preparation of ℞ **hydrochlorothiazide** and ℞ **triamterene**.
Formulation: Oral capsules.
Availability: Prescription only.
Warnings and side effects: See ℞ **hydrochlorothiazide**; ℞ **triamterene**.

Dycill ®

A preparation of ℞ **dicloxacillin sodium**.
Formulation: Oral capsules in several strengths.
Availability: Prescription only.
Warnings and side effects: See ℞ **dicloxacillin sodium**.

Dyflex-G Tablets ®

A preparation of ℞ **guaifenesin** and diphylline.
Formulation: Oral tablets.
Availability: Prescription only.
Warnings and side effects: See ℞ **guaifenesin**; ℞ **theophylline**.

Dyline G.G. Tablets; Liquid ®

A preparation of ℞ **guaifenesin** and diphylline.
Formulation: Oral tablets, liquid.
Availability: Prescription only.
Warnings and side effects: See ℞ **guaifenesin**; ℞ **theophylline**.

Dymelor ®

A preparation of ℞ **acetohexamide**.
Formulation: Oral tablets.
Availability: Prescription only.
Warnings and side effects: See ℞ **acetohexamide**.

Dymenate ®

A preparation of ℞ **dimenhydrinate**.
Formulation: Injection.
Availability: Prescription only.
Warnings and side effects: See ℞ **dimenhydrinate**.

Dynacin ®

A preparation of ℞ **minocycline**.
Formulation: Oral capsules in several strengths.
Availability: Prescription only.
Warnings and side effects: See ℞ **minocycline**.

DynaCirc; DynaCirc CR ®

A preparation of ℞ **isradipine**.
Formulation: Oral tablets, controlled release (two strengths); capsules (CR, two strengths).
Availability: Prescription only.
Warnings and side effects: See ℞ **isradipine**.

Dynafed Asthma Relief Tablets ®

A preparation of ℞ **ephedrine** and ℞ **guaifenesin**.
Formulation: Oral tablets.
Availability: OTC.
Warnings and side effects: See ℞ **ephedrine**; ℞ **guaifenesin**.

Dynafed Extra Strength Tablets; Children's Dynafed Jr. ®

A preparation of ℞ **acetaminophen**.
Formulation: Oral tablets; Dynafed Jr. tablets are chewable.
Availability: OTC.
Warnings and side effects: See ℞ **acetaminophen**.

Dynafed Pseudo Tablets ®

A preparation of ℞ **pseudoephedrine**.
Formulation: Oral tablets.
Availability: OTC.
Warnings and side effects: See ℞ **pseudoephedrine**.

Dynapen ⓑ

A preparation of ℞ **dicloxacillin sodium**.
Formulation: Oral capsules in several strengths; oral suspension.
Availability: Prescription only.
Warnings and side effects: See ℞ **dicloxacillin sodium**.

Dyprotex Pads ⓑ

A preparation of ℞ **zinc oxide**, ℞ **petrolatum**, dimethicone, ℞ **cod-liver oil**, and aloe.
Formulation: Topical application pads.
Availability: OTC.
Warnings and side effects: See ℞ **zinc oxide**; ℞ **petrolatum**; ℞ **simethicone**; ℞ **cod-liver oil**.

Dyrenium ⓑ

A preparation of ℞ **triamterene**.
Formulation: Oral capsules, available in two strengths.
Availability: Prescription only.
Warnings and side effects: See ℞ **triamterene**.

Ear-Eze ⓑ

A preparation of ℞ **hydrocortisone**; ℞ **neomycin**, and ℞ **polymyxin B sulfate**.
Formulation: Ear drops.
Availability: Prescription only.
Warnings and side effects: See ℞ **hydrocortisone**; ℞ **neomycin**; ℞ **polymyxin B sulfate**.

E-Base ⓑ

A preparation of ℞ **erythromycin**.
Formulation: Oral tablets.
Availability: Prescription only.
Warnings and side effects: See ℞ **erythromycin**.

echothiopate iodide ⓖ

see ℞ **echothiopate iodide**.

echothiopate iodide ⓖ

(echothiopate iodide)
Type/Group: **glaucoma treatment; anticholinesterase**.
Brand(s): Phospholine Iodide.
How administered: Topically (external).

Used to treat

Echothiopate iodide is a cholinesterase inhibitor used to treat open-angle ⊙ **glaucoma** and for accommodative esotropia (reflex crossing of the eyes) in farsighted children.

Warnings

• It should not be given to people with known active inflammation of the uvea or most of those with angle-closure glaucoma.
• It should be given with caution to people with asthma, bradycardia, parkinsonism, peptic ulcer, myasthenia gravis, spastic gastrointestinal disease, recent heart attack, epilepsy, or a history of uveitis.

• It is not known whether echothiopate iodide crosses the placenta. It should be used during pregnancy only if the potential benefits outweigh the risks to the fetus.
• Medical judgment is required if breast-feeding is being considered.
• Exercise care while driving at night or performing other hazardous tasks in poor light.
• This drug causes lens opacities in half of those using it for over 6 months.
• Systemic side effects are possible.

Interactions

• If used with ℞ **succinylcholine**, neuromuscular blocking effects are prolonged.

Side effects

• Frequently, headache, brow ache, burning, tearing, and visual blurring.
• Less frequently, other eye effects, gastrointestinal effects, urinary incontinence, difficulty breathing, sweating, and fainting.

econazole ⓖ

Type/Group: **antifungal; azole**.
Brand(s): Spectazole.
How administered: Topically (external).

Used to treat

Econazole is a broad-spectrum synthetic azole/imidazole antifungal used to treat ⊙ **fungal infections** of the skin, including jock itch, ⊙ **athlete's foot**, and ringworm.

Warnings

• It should not be given to people with known sensitivity to econazole.
• It should be used during the first trimester of pregnancy only if medically judged to be essential, and used during the second and third trimester only if clearly needed.
• Medical judgment is required if breast-feeding is being considered. It is not known if the drug appears in breast milk.
• Contact with the eyes must be avoided.
• The prescribed treatment time must be completed even if symptoms improve.

Interactions

No significant interactions have been reported when used topically.

Side effects

• Burning, stinging, redness, and itching.

Econopred; Econopred Plus ⓑ

A preparation of ℞ **prednisolone**.
Formulation: Eye drops in two strengths.
Availability: Prescription only.
Warnings and side effects: See ℞ **prednisolone**.

Ecotrin Regular Strength Tablets; Low Strength Tablets; Maxi ⓑ

A preparation of ℞ **aspirin**.
Formulation: Oral tablets, all are enteric coated.
Availability: OTC.

Warnings and side effects: See ℞ **aspirin.** Adult Low Strength contains tartrazine (FD&C yellow No. 5), a dye that may cause allergic reaction in a few people, but especially those with sensitivity to aspirin.

Ed A-Hist Tablets; Liquid ⑧

A preparation of ℞ **phenylephrine hydrochloride** and ℞ **chlorpheniramine maleate.**
Formulation: Oral tablets; liquid.
Availability: Prescription only.
Warnings and side effects: See ℞ **phenylephrine hydrochloride;** ℞ **chlorpheniramine maleate.**

Edecrin Tablets; Injection ⑧

A preparation of ℞ **ethacrynic acid.**
Formulation: Oral tablets (2 strengths); injection.
Availability: Prescription only.
Warnings and side effects: See ℞ **ethacrynic acid.**

edetate calcium disodium ⑥

(calcium EDTA)
Type/Group: **antidote; chelating agent.**
Brand(s): Calcium Disodium Versenate.
How administered: Injection.

Used to treat

Edetate calcium disodium is used to treat poisoning by lead. It acts as a chelating agent by binding to metals to form a compound that can be excreted from the body. It has been investigated as an antidote to poisoning by other metals, including fission products such as plutonium, uranium, and thorium, and non-radioactive heavy metals such as chromium, manganese, nickel and zinc. It is not effective in treating poisoning by mercury, gold, or arsenic.

Warnings

• It should not be used by people with anuria (absence of urine, from whatever cause), or with active kidney disease, or hepatitis.
• It should be given with caution to anyone with impaired kidney function.
• Edetate calcium disodium should be used in pregnancy only if medically judged that it is clearly needed.
• Medical judgment is also required for breast-feeding mothers.
• It can produce toxic side effects that may be fatal, therefore, medical monitoring of kidney, liver, and heart function is necessary.
• A physician must be contacted if urine stops for a period of 12 hours.

Interactions

• Edetate calcium disodium may interfere with ℞ **insulin** absorption from insulin preparations containing zinc.
• ℞ **Corticosteroids** may increase the risk of side effects.

Side effects

There are a number, but edetate calcium disodium is only used under specialist care. Among the more frequent are:
• Hypotension, arrhythmias, urinary and kidney changes, nausea and vomiting, malaise, tremors, headache, numbness, and thirst.

Edex ⑧

A preparation of ℞ **alprostadil.**
Formulation: Injection.
Availability: Prescription only.
Warnings and side effects: See ℞ **alprostadil.**

edrophonium chloride ⑥

Type/Group: **anticholinesterase.**
Brand(s): Enlon; Reversol; Tensilon. Combinations: With *atropine sulfate*: Enlon-Plus.
How administered: Injection.

Used to treat

Edrophonium enhances the effects of the neurotransmitter acetylcholine (and of certain cholinergic drugs). It has a short duration of action and can be used in the diagnosis, evaluation, and treatment of ⊙ **myasthenia gravis**, as well as at the termination of operations to reverse the actions of neuromuscular blocking agents (when it is often administered with atropine sulfate).

Warnings

• It should not be used by people with known hypersensitivity to anticholinesterases, or with mechanical, urinary or intestinal obstruction.
• It should be given with caution to anyone with seizure disorder, asthma, certain heart conditions, hyperthyroidism, peptic ulcer, megacolon or poor gastrointestinal motility, or hypotension.
• It is not known whether this drug can harm the fetus, but it would not be expected to cross the placenta or be excreted into breast milk. In pregnancy, it may cause premature labor if given near term. It should be given with caution to breast-feeding mothers.
• Allergic reactions are possible.

Interactions

• ℞ **Tacrine** may increase cholinergic effects.
• ℞ **aminoglycoside** antibiotics (such as, ℞ **neomycin**, ℞ **streptomycin**) may increase the effects of edrophonium.
• ℞ **Corticosteroids**, ⚕ **magnesium**, and ℞ **local anesthetics** may interfere with the action of edrophonium.

Side effects

• Gastrointestinal upsets, dizziness, drowsiness, headache, incoordination, muscle cramps, rash and potentially serious effects on the cardiovascular and respiratory systems.

ED-TLC Liquid ⑧

A preparation of ℞ **hydrocodone bitartrate,** ℞ **chlorpheniramine maleate,** and ℞ **phenylephrine hydrochloride.**
Formulation: Oral liquid.
Availability: Prescription only.
Warnings and side effects: See ℞ **hydrocodone bitartrate;** ℞ **chlorpheniramine maleate;** ℞ **phenylephrine hydrochloride.**

ED-TLS Liquid ⑧

A preparation of ℞ **hydrocodone bitartrate,** ℞ **chlorpheniramine maleate,** and ℞ **phenylephrine hydrochloride.**
Formulation: Oral liquid.

Availability: Prescription only.
Warnings and side effects: See ℞ hydrocodone bitartrate; ℞ chlorpheniramine maleate; ℞ phenylephrine hydrochloride.

E.E.S. ⑧

A preparation of ℞ **erythromycin**.
Formulation: Oral tablets; oral solution; both in several strengths.
Availability: Prescription only.
Warnings and side effects: See ℞ **erythromycin**.

efavirenz ⑥

Type/Group: **antiviral**.
Brand(s): Sustiva.
How administered: Orally.

Used to treat

Efavirenz is one of the non-nucleoside group of reverse transcriptase inhibitors, and can be used in the treatment of ✚ **HIV** infection, usually in combination with other antiviral drugs.

Warnings

• It should not be given to people with known hypersensitivity or allergy to this drug.
• It should be given with caution to people with liver disease or depressive illness.
• Efavirenz's use during pregnancy should be avoided if possible.
• HIV-infected mothers are advised not to breast-feed.
• A doctor must be contacted before taking any other drug with efavirenz (including OTCs, herbal remedies, and supplements) to avoid potentially serious interactions.
• It is a specialist drug, and there will be full assessment and patient monitoring throughout treatment.

Interactions

• The levels of the following drugs may be increased: astemizole; ℞ fexofenadine; ℞ midazolam; ℞ triazolam; ℞ simvastatin; ℞ nelfinavir; ℞ ethinyl estradiol; ℞ lovastatin, ℞ oral contraceptives; ℞ ergotamine and analogs; ℞ warfarin sodium.
• ℞ amprenavir, ℞ barbiturates, ℞ carbamazepine, ℞ phenytoin, ℞ rifampin, and ℞ saquinavir may reduce the effects of efavirenz.
• The effects of ℞ clarithromycin, ℞ indinavir, and ℞ rifabutin may be reduced.
• The effects of ℞ ritonavir may be increased.

Side effects

• Rash, dizziness, headache, insomnia, sleepiness, disturbing dreams, fatigue, impaired concentration, depression, psychotic state, nausea, raised blood lipids, liver enzyme changes, and diarrhea (pancreatitis has been reported).

Effexor; SR ⑧

A preparation of ℞ **venlafaxine**.
Formulation: Oral tablets in varying strengths; oral capsules, extended release (SR).
Availability: Prescription only.
Warnings and side effects: See ℞ **venlafaxine**.

Efidac/24 Tablets ⑧

A preparation of ℞ **pseudoephedrine**.
Formulation: Oral tablets.
Availability: OTC.
Warnings and side effects: See ℞ **pseudoephedrine**.

ELA-Max ⑧

A preparation of ℞ **lidocaine**.
Formulation: Topical cream.
Availability: OTC.
Warnings and side effects: See ℞ **lidocaine**.

Elase-Chloramycetin ⑧

A preparation of ℞ **chloramphenicol**, desoxyribonuclease.
Formulation: Topical ointment.
Availability: Prescription only.
Warnings and side effects: See ℞ **chloramphenicol**.

Elavil ⑧

A preparation of ℞ **amitriptyline hydrochloride**.
Formulation: Oral tablets in several strengths; vials for injection.
Availability: Prescription only.
Warnings and side effects: See ℞ **amitriptyline hydrochloride**.

Eldecort ⑧

A preparation of ℞ **hydrocortisone**.
Formulation: Cream.
Availability: Prescription only.
Warnings and side effects: See ℞ **hydrocortisone**.

Eldepryl ⑧

A preparation of ℞ **selegiline hydrochloride**.
Formulation: Oral capsules.
Availability: Prescription only.
Warnings and side effects: See ℞ **selegiline hydrochloride**.

Eldisine ⑧

A preparation of ℞ **vindesine sulfate**.
Formulation: Injection (intravenous).
Availability: Prescription only.
Warnings and side effects: See ℞ **vindesine sulfate**.

electrolyte ⑩

(rehydration solution)
Generics: **ammonium chloride; calcium carbonate; citrates; sodium chloride**.

Actions and uses

An electrolyte is, chemically, a compound that when in solution dissociates into ions. Physiologically, the functioning of the body depends on maintaining a proper balance of these essential ions, which are derived from minerals in the diet. The main essential ions are sodium, potassium, and chloride. It is on these ions that all electrical activity in the cells of the body depends, so it is not surprising that in electrolyte upsets, the functioning of muscles, nerves, and the brain is disturbed.

Key to symbols: ✚ = Disorder Section   ℞ = Drug Section   ♣ = Herbal Section   ᐂᐂ = Supplement Section

Many medical conditions are characterized, in part, by electrolyte disturbances, particularly when one or more types of ion are depleted by excess excretion in the urine. Such conditions include ⊙ diarrhea, ⊙ heatstroke, ⊙ dehydration, ⊙ dysentery, ⊙ food poisoning, ⊙ cholera, ⊙ gastroenteritis, ⊙ hyponatremia, ⊙ muscle cramps, and ⊙ alkalosis.

In most of these conditions, the main cause of the electrolyte disturbance is diarrhea. Although ℞ antidiarrheal preparations containing ℞ opioid (℞ opiate) drugs, which work by reducing peristalsis (the rhythmic movement of the intestines) and so slow down the movement of fecal material, are generally available without prescription, the main and most important medical treatment of diarrhea while it lasts is always the replacement of fluids and minerals (particularly sodium) with *rehydration solutions* (and simple rehydration by drinking water). Rehydration solutions are available OTC (over-the-counter) for oral use, but are also used by intravenous infusion in medical emergencies. Rehydration solutions are a combination of various salts made into a dilute solution with water. They usually contain ℞ sodium chloride, potassium chloride, and ℞ citrates of sodium and potassium (which allows adjustment of the pH), and often glucose.

Sometimes other electrolyte solutions are required. For instance, ℞ sodium bicarbonate can be taken to replace lost electrolytes or as an alkalinizing agent to relieve conditions of severe metabolic ⊙ acidosis—when the acid-base equilibrium of the body is badly out of balance—which may occur in kidney failure, cardiac insufficiency, or diabetic coma. ℞ citrates, when taken by mouth, have the effect of making the urine alkaline instead of acid, which is an action that is useful for relieving pain in some infections of the urinary tract or the bladder, in the treatment of gout, and to treat chronic metabolic acidosis such as that caused by renal tubular acidosis. ℞ calcium carbonate may be used as a source of calcium in conditions that deplete calcium levels in the body (for example, hypoparathyroidism, chronic diarrhea, sprue, pregnancy, osteoporosis, pancreatitis, alkalosis, and hyperphosphatemia). ℞ ammonium chloride can cause metabolic acidosis and so can be used to correct metabolic alkalosis. It is used in the therapeutic acidification of urine, which increases the rate of excretion of some drugs and poisons, and is therefore effectively an antidote. It is also used in some OTC preparations for the relief of premenstrual ⊙ fluid retention.

Limitations
See the individual drug entries.

Elimite ℬ
A preparation of ℞ permethrin.
Formulation: Topical cream.
Availability: Prescription only.
Warnings and side effects: See ℞ permethrin.

Elixomin ℬ
A preparation of ℞ theophylline.
Formulation: Oral elixir.
Availability: Prescription only.
Warnings and side effects: See ℞ theophylline.

Elixophyllin ℬ
A preparation of ℞ theophylline.
Formulation: Oral tablets; oral capsules; elixir.
Availability: Prescription only.
Warnings and side effects: See ℞ theophylline.

Elixophyllin GG Liquid ℬ
A preparation of ℞ guaifenesin and ℞ theophylline.
Formulation: Oral liquid.
Availability: Prescription only.
Warnings and side effects: See ℞ guaifenesin; ℞ theophylline.

Ellence ℬ
A preparation of ℞ epirubicin hydrochloride.
Formulation: Injection.
Availability: Prescription only.
Warnings and side effects: See ℞ epirubicin hydrochloride.

Elocon ℬ
A preparation of ℞ mometasone.
Formulation: Topical cream.
Availability: Prescription only.
Warnings and side effects: See ℞ mometasone.

Emadine ℬ
A preparation of ℞ emedastine.
Formulation: Ophthalmic solution.
Availability: Prescription only.
Warnings and side effects: See ℞ emedastine.

Embeline E ℬ
A preparation of ℞ clobetasol propionate.
Formulation: Cream.
Availability: Prescription only.
Warnings and side effects: See ℞ clobetasol propionate.

Emcyt ℬ
A preparation of ℞ estramustine phosphate sodium.
Formulation: Oral capsules.
Availability: Prescription only.
Warnings and side effects: See ℞ estramustine phosphate sodium.

emedastine ℊ
Type/Group: antihistamine; antiallergic.
How administered: Topically (eye).
Brand(s): Emadine.
Used to treat
Emedastine is used for seasonal allergic ⊙ conjunctivitis.
Warnings
• It should not be given to people with known hypersensitivity to this drug.
• It should be given with caution to children.
• Emedastine should be used during pregnancy only if it is clearly needed.

• Medical judgment is required if breast-feeding is being considered.

• Do not use contact lenses if the eyes are red and wait at least 10 minutes after use before inserting soft contact lenses.

Interactions
No significant interactions are known.

Side effects
• Burning or stinging, blurred vision, corneal infiltrates or staining, dry eyes, foreign body sensation, inflammation, itching, nasal or sinus inflammation, and tearing.

emetic Ⓓ
Generics: **ipecac syrup**.

Actions and uses
Emetic agents cause vomiting (emesis). They are used primarily to treat certain types of ✪ **poisoning** by non-corrosive substances when the person is conscious, especially drugs taken in overdose. Some affect the vomiting center in the brain and/or irritate the gastrointestinal tract. The best-known and most-used emetic is ℞ **ipecacuanha** (℞ **ipecac syrup**).

Limitations
A number of drugs cause nausea and vomiting as an undesirable side effect, especially ℞ **narcotic analgesics** and many ℞ **cytotoxic** drugs used in ℞ **anticancer** therapy. See also the ipecac syrup entry.

Eminase Ⓑ
A preparation of ℞ **anistreplase**.
Formulation: Intravenous injection.
Availability: Prescription only.
Warnings and side effects: See ℞ **anistreplase**.

emollient Ⓓ
Generics: **carbomer; glycerin; lanolin; mineral oil; petrolatum**.

Actions and uses
Emollient agents soothe, soften, and moisturize the skin, particularly when it is cracked, dry or scaling. They are usually emulsions of water, fats, waxes, and oils, which may be animal (℞ **lanolin**), plant (℞ **castor oil**), mineral (℞ **mineral oil**, ℞ **petrolatum**, and ℞ **glycerin**) or synthetic (℞ **carbomer**) products. They can be used alone or in combination to help hydrate the skin, sometimes with an added ℞ **hydrating agent** such as ℞ **urea**. They are used to treat various skin conditions such as ✪ **dermatitis**, including ✪ **eczema** and ✪ **psoriasis**. Emollients can be applied as creams, ointments, lotions, or added to bath water. A number of other agents may also be incorporated (see ℞ **skin preparation**).

Limitations
Many of these preparations contain preservatives to which some people may be allergic. This may worsen a condition by causing contact allergic dermatitis. Similarly, some people are allergic to some of the major constituents (particularly ℞ **lanolin**). See also the individual drug entries.

Empirin Ⓑ
A preparation of ℞ **aspirin**.

Formulation: Oral tablets.
Availability: OTC.
Warnings and side effects: See ℞ **aspirin**.

Empirin w/Codeine Ⓑ
A preparation of ℞ **codeine phosphate** and ℞ **aspirin**.
Formulation: Oral tablets, available in two strengths.
Availability: Prescription only.
Warnings and side effects: See ℞ **codeine phosphate**; ℞ **aspirin**.

Emulsoil Ⓑ
A preparation of ℞ **castor oil**.
Formulation: Oral emulsion.
Availability: OTC.
Warnings and side effects: See ℞ **castor oil**.

E-Mycin Ⓑ
A preparation of ℞ **erythromycin**.
Formulation: Oral tablets in several strengths.
Availability: Prescription only.
Warnings and side effects: See ℞ **erythromycin**.

enalapril maleate Ⓖ
Type/Group: **ACE inhibitor; vasodilator; antihypertensive; heart failure treatment**.
Brand(s): Vasotec, Vasotec I.V.; various generic. Combinations: With *felodipine*: Lexxel. With *hydrochlorothiazide*: Vaseretic.
How administered: Orally.

Used to treat
Enalapril is used to reduce blood pressure in ✪ **hypertension**, to treat congestive ✪ **heart failure**, and to prevent ischemia (lack of blood supply) in patients with left ventricular failure. It is often used with other classes of drug, particularly ℞ **thiazide** ℞ **diuretics**.

Warnings
• It should not be given to people with known hypersensitivity to this drug or to any other ACE inhibitor.

• It should be given with caution to people with severe congestive heart failure, or certain other cardiovascular disorders, a history of anaphylaxis, collagen vascular disease (for example, systemic lupus erythematosus; SLE), diabetes mellitus, depressed immune response, or with impaired kidney function or who are on dialysis.

• ACE inhibitors can cause injury to the fetus, even death. The use of these drugs should stop as soon as pregnancy is detected.

• Medical judgment is required if breast-feeding is being considered. Enalapril appears in breast milk.

• Its use should stop and a doctor contacted immediately if signs of angioedema appear (swelling of the face, eyes, lips, tongue, larynx, or extremities; difficulty in breathing or swallowing). Swelling of the larynx, closing off the airway, can be life-threatening.

• Anyone taking an ACE inhibitor should not interrupt or discontinue treatment without first checking with a doctor.

　　Key to symbols: ✪ = Disorder Section ℞ = Drug Section ♣ = Herbal Section ⚕⚕ = Supplement Section

• A doctor must be contacted if any suspected infections (for example, fever, sore throat) develop. ACE inhibitors may cause blood changes which can affect immune response.

• ACE inhibitors generally have less effect on blood pressure in blacks than in non-blacks, and the likelihood of angioedema is higher among blacks, as well.

Interactions

• ACE inhibitors have apparently triggered life-threatening anaphylactoid reactions when used by people also receiving ℞ **desensitizing vaccines**.

• ℞ **Anesthetics** (for example, in surgery), ℞ **phenothiazines**, and ℞ **probenecid** may increase the levels or hypotensive effect of enalapril.

• Levels of ℞ **lithium** may be increased, with the potential for toxic effects.

• If used with potassium-sparing ℞ **diuretics** or other preparations containing potassium (for example, supplements and salt substitutes), levels of potassium may rise.

• ℞ **NSAID**s may increase the risk of kidney damage or (in some cases) reduce the effects of ACE inhibitors.

• ℞ **Antacids** and ℞ **rifampin** may reduce the effects of enalapril. Antacids should not be used for several hours after a dose of an ACE inhibitor (a doctor should be consulted for full instructions and cautions).

• If used with other antihypertensives and diuretics, the effects of these drugs may be increased. This additive effect is sometimes used to advantage in combination treatments for high blood pressure.

Side effects

• The most frequent is low blood pressure (hypotension).

• Occasionally, dizziness, postural hypotension (lowered blood pressure on standing), headache, fainting, fatigue, weakness, tachycardia or rhythm disturbances, rash or gastrointestinal disturbances (for example, diarrhea, nausea and vomiting, indigestion, constipation).

• Infrequently, insomnia, blurred vision, tingling in the extremities, hair loss, or photosensitivity (abnormal sensitivity to light). Although it is uncommon, ACE inhibitors can cause very marked hypotension (especially when beginning treatment) and kidney impairment. They may also cause persistent dry cough.

• Rarely, there may be angioedema, altered liver function, jaundice, hepatitis, pancreatitis, or changes in blood counts.

Enbrel ⓑ

A preparation of ℞ **etanercept**.
Formulation: Subcutaneous injection.
Availability: Prescription only.
Warnings and side effects: See ℞ **etanercept**.

Endafed Capsules ⓑ

A preparation of ℞ **pseudoephedrine** and ℞ **brompheniramine maleate**.
Formulation: Oral capsules, sustained release.
Availability: Prescription only.

Warnings and side effects: See ℞ **pseudoephedrine**; ℞ **brompheniramine maleate**.

Endagen-HD Liquid ⓑ

A preparation of ℞ **hydrocodone bitartrate**; ℞ **chlorpheniramine maleate**; and ℞ **phenylephrine hydrochloride**.
Formulation: Oral liquid.
Availability: Prescription only.
Warnings and side effects: See ℞ **hydrocodone bitartrate**; ℞ **chlorpheniramine maleate**; ℞ **phenylephrine hydrochloride**.

Endal-HD Liquid; Endal Plus Liquid ⓑ

A preparation of ℞ **hydrocodone bitartrate**, ℞ **chlorpheniramine maleate**, and ℞ **phenylephrine hydrochloride**.
Formulation: Oral liquid, in two hydrocodone strengths.
Availability: Prescription only.
Warnings and side effects: See ℞ **hydrocodone bitartrate**; ℞ **chlorpheniramine maleate**; ℞ **phenylephrine hydrochloride**.

Endal Tablets ⓑ

A preparation of ℞ **phenylephrine hydrochloride** and ℞ **guaifenesin**.
Formulation: Oral tablets, time release.
Availability: Prescription only.
Warnings and side effects: See ℞ **phenylephrine hydrochloride**; ℞ **guaifenesin**.

End Lice ⓑ

A preparation of ℞ **pyrethrin**.
Formulation: Topical liquid.
Availability: OTC.
Warnings and side effects: See ℞ **pyrethrin**.

Endocet Tablets ⓑ

A preparation of ℞ **oxycodone** and ℞ **acetaminophen**.
Formulation: Oral tablets.
Availability: Prescription only.
Warnings and side effects: See ℞ **oxycodone**; ℞ **acetaminophen**.

Endocodone ⓑ

A preparation of ℞ **oxycodone**.
Formulation: Oral tablets.
Availability: Prescription only.
Warnings and side effects: See ℞ **oxycodone**.

Enduron ⓑ

A preparation of ℞ **methyclothiazide**.
Formulation: Oral tablets.
Availability: Prescription only.
Warnings and side effects: See ℞ **methyclothiazide**.

Engerix-B ℞

A preparation of ℞ **hepatitis B vaccine**.
Formulation: Intramuscular injection.
Availability: Prescription only.
Warnings and side effects: See ℞ **hepatitis B vaccine**.

Enlon ℞

A preparation of ℞ **edrophonium chloride**.
Formulation: Injection.
Availability: Prescription only.
Warnings and side effects: See ℞ **edrophonium chloride**.

Enlon-Plus ℞

A preparation of ℞ **edrophonium chloride** and ℞ **atropine sulfate**.
Formulation: Injection.
Availability: Prescription only.
Warnings and side effects: See ℞ **edrophonium chloride**;
℞ **atropine sulfate**.

enoxacin Ⓖ

Type/Group: quinolone; antibacterial.
Brand(s): Penetrex.
How administered: Orally.

Used to treat

Enoxacin is used to treat ✪ **gonorrhea** and urinary tract infections
(see ✪ **urinary tract disorders**).

Warnings

• It should not be given to people with known hypersensitivity to
enoxacin or other quinolones, or to children under 18, as there is
a possibility of damage to joints and cartilage in growing children.
• It should be given with caution to people with kidney disease or
any predisposition to seizures.
• It should not be used during pregnancy because it may harm the
mother and the fetus.
• Medical judgment is required if breast-feeding is being
considered.
• Superinfections due to the altered bacterial balance caused by
antibiotic treatment may occur. A doctor must be contacted if
there is severe abdominal pain, or moderate to severe diarrhea.
• Rare, but serious, side effects of quinolones include seizure and
other CNS (central nervous system) effects, and severe allergic
reactions.
• Adequate fluid intake should be maintained.
• There is a risk of photosensitivity (abnormal sensitivity to light)
and so excessive exposure to sunlight should be avoided.
• Doses should be taken one hour before or two hours after meals.
• ♘♘ **calcium**, ♘♘ **iron** preparations, ♘♘ **magnesium**, aluminum,
and ♘♘ **zinc** reduce the effects of enoxacin and so should not be
taken within 4 hours (before or after) of a dose (this includes
supplements).

Interactions

• ℞ **Bismuth subsalicylate** reduces the effects of enoxacin.
• ℞ **Antacids** calcium, iron preparations, magnesium, aluminum,
℞ **sodium bicarbonate**, and zinc reduce the effects of enoxacin

and so should not be taken within 4 hours (before or after) of a
dose.
• ℞ **Didanosine (ddl)** reduce the effects of enoxacin.
• The levels of ℞ **theophylline**, antipyrine, ℞ **caffeine**,
℞ **diazepam**, ℞ **metoprolol**, ℞ **pentoxifylline**, ℞ **phenytoin**,
℞ **propranolol**, ℞ **ranitidine**, ℞ **ropinirole**, ℞ **tacrine**,
℞ **xanthine**, and ℞ **warfarin sodium** may be increased.
• The effects of oral ℞ **anticoagulants** may be increased.
• If used with ℞ **foscarnet**, the risk of seizure is increased.

Side effects

• Frequently, nausea and vomiting.
• Occasionally, abdominal pain, diarrhea, headache, and dizziness.
• Rarely, dry mouth, heartburn, constipation, flatulence, fatigue,
drowsiness, insomnia, anxiety, seizures, and confusion.

enoxaparin sodium Ⓖ

Type/Group: anticoagulant.
Brand(s): Lovenox.
How administered: Injection (subcutaneous).

Used to treat

Enoxaparin sodium is a low molecular weight heparin, an anticoagulant. It can be used (with ℞ **warfarin sodium**) in the treatment
of acute ✪ **deep vein thrombosis**, and after hip or knee replacement or abdominal surgery (in certain at-risk people) to prevent
complications from embolism. When administered with ℞ **aspirin**,
it may be used to reduce the risk of ischemic complications in certain acute cardiac conditions.

Warnings

• It should not be given to people with known hypersensitivity to
this drug or to heparin or pork products, or where lab testing shows
antibodies to platelets when taking this drug. It will be
administered by experienced personnel after a full medical
assessment.
• It should be given with caution to people with an increased risk
of hemorrhage (for example, uncontrolled hypertension, bleeding
disorders, active ulcer, recent stroke, or surgery), and in those who
have experienced a reduction of platelet (thrombocyte) levels after
taking heparin, and in the elderly or in anyone with kidney
impairment.
• Enoxaparin should be used during pregnancy only if it is clearly
needed.
• Medical judgment is required if breast-feeding is being
considered. It is not known whether this drug appears in breast
milk.
• There is a risk that administration of spinal or epidural anesthesia,
or other spinal puncture procedures, may result in bleeding and
paralysis in people taking low molecular weight heparins.

Interactions

• If taken with other anticoagulants, antiplatelet agents, or
℞ **NSAIDs**, there is a higher potential for bleeding (caution is
advised).

Side effects

• The most common is post-operative bleeding, which may
occasionally occur at non-surgical sites, particularly in the
gastrointestinal tract. At the site of injection there may be irritation

Key to symbols: ✪ = Disorder Section ℞ = Drug Section ♣ = Herbal Section ♘♘ = Supplement Section

or hematoma (a trapped accumulation of blood). Anemia and changes in liver function may occur.

• Other side effects may include fever, nausea, edema, and allergic reaction.

entacapone ⑤

Type/Group: **antiparkinsonism.**

Brand(s): Comtan.

How administered: Orally.

Used to treat

Entacapone is a recently introduced drug that is used in antiparkinsonism treatment because it inhibits one of the enzymes that break down the neurotransmitter dopamine in the brain. It is thought that dopamine deficiency in the brain causes ✪ **Parkinson's disease**. It is used in combination with ℞ **levodopa** (which is converted to dopamine in the brain) together with a further enzyme inhibitor, ℞ **carbidopa**, to reduce symptoms of "wearing off" at the end of dose periods.

Warnings

• It should not be used by anyone with known sensitivity to this drug, or who are taking ℞ **MAOI** antidepressants.

• It should be used with caution by anyone with liver or kidney impairment.

• Entacapone's effects in pregnancy are unknown. It should be used only if clearly needed and if the benefits outweigh the possible risk to the fetus.

• Medical judgment is also required if breast-feeding is being considered.

• Treatment with entacapone must be ended gradually and not abruptly.

• It may increase some side effects of levodopa/carbidopa, including hallucinations, postural hypotension (lowered blood pressure on standing) and fainting, diarrhea, dyskinesia (abnormal movement), and discoloration of urine (which is harmless).

Interactions

• The absorption of iron may decrease.

• The metabolism of isoproterenol, ℞ **epinephrine**, ℞ **norepinephrine**, ℞ **dopamine**, ℞ **dobutamine hydrochloride**, isoetherine, and bitolterol may be decreased.

Side effects

• Frequently, nausea, change in the level of involuntary body movements, dizziness, abdominal pain.

• Occasionally, fatigue, anxiety, excessive sleeping, agitation, high fever, abdominal pain, diarrhea, constipation, vomiting, upset stomach, taste disturbance, back pain, shortness of breath, itching, and increased sweating.

Entex PSE Tablets ⑧

A preparation of ℞ **pseudoephedrine** and ℞ **guaifenesin**.

Formulation: Oral tablets, long acting.

Availability: Prescription only.

Warnings and side effects: See ℞ **pseudoephedrine**; ℞ **guaifenesin**.

Entuss-D Tablets; Jr. Liquid ⑧

A preparation of ℞ **hydrocodone bitartrate**, ℞ **pseudoephedrine**, and ℞ **guaifenesin**.

Formulation: Oral tablets; liquid.

Availability: Prescription only.

Warnings and side effects: See ℞ **hydrocodone bitartrate**; ℞ **pseudoephedrine**; ℞ **guaifenesin**.

Entuss Expectorant Tablets ⑧

A preparation of ℞ **hydrocodone bitartrate** and ℞ **guaifenesin**.

Formulation: Oral tablets.

Availability: Prescription only.

Warnings and side effects: See ℞ **hydrocodone bitartrate**; ℞ **guaifenesin**.

Enulose ⑧

A preparation of ℞ **lactulose**.

Formulation: Oral liquid.

Availability: Prescription only.

Warnings and side effects: See ℞ **lactulose**.

Enzone Cream ⑧

A preparation of ℞ **hydrocortisone** and ℞ **pramoxine hydrochloride**.

Formulation: Cream.

Availability: Prescription only.

Warnings and side effects: See ℞ **hydrocortisone**; ℞ **pramoxine hydrochloride**.

enzyme ⑩

Generics: **dornase alfa; hyaluronidase; imiglucerase; pancreatin**.

Actions and uses

Enzymes are proteins that play an essential part in the body's metabolism by acting as catalysts in specific, necessary biochemical reactions. Their physiological functions range from the digestion of food within the digestive tract through to the formation of proteins and other structural elements of the body. Impaired enzyme functioning underlies many diseases (particularly those that run in families), and may cause food intolerances that require special diets (for example, phenylkenonuria and favism). Specialized enzymes are involved in the metabolism and detoxification of chemicals, including drugs, which are foreign to the body. Impaired capacity of these enzymes (which again is often familial) may make persons hypersensitive to these chemicals, and is a prominent cause of adverse drug reactions (for example, ✪ **G6PD-deficiency** and ✪ **porphyria**). Liver enzyme metabolism is often also slower in the young, the elderly, and in people with liver disease (including ✪ **cirrhosis**).

Many drugs have been developed that work selectively, affecting only certain enzymes. These can be used to manipulate the biochemistry of the body (for example, ℞ **MAOI** antidepressants, ℞ **anticholinesterase** agents, and ℞ **phosphodiesterase inhibitor** drugs). In a few instances, the enzymes themselves are used as drugs. However, their chemical nature makes it difficult to deliver them to their targeted site of action. In addition, because they are proteins which, in most cases, are derived from animals there are often serious allergic side effects.

Some fibrinolytic drugs (used in ℞ **thrombolytic** treatment) are enzymes, and are given by injection or infusion in order to dissolve blood clots. They are used in the treatment of life-threatening conditions, such as acute ✪ **myocardial infarction**, venous thrombi, ✪ **pulmonary embolism**, and clots in the eye (the best known of these plasminogen activators is ℞ **streptokinase**).

A number of enzymes are taken by mouth, with food, to supplement deficiencies in the production of proteolytic (protein-digesting) enzymes (see ℞ **digestive enzyme**). This approach, however, is not generally very successful and such agents tend to erode the upper gastrointestinal tract (for example, ℞ **pancreatin**, which is isolated from the pancreas of a cow or pig). Other proteolytic enzymes have diverse uses, for example, dissolving wound debris, by inhalation into the lungs to liquefy viscous sputum (℞ **dornase alfa**).

Enzymes that dissolve connective tissue are used in the treatment of skin extravasation injuries such as burns and inflammatory injuries (to promote reabsorption of excess fluids and blood), to increase the permeability of soft tissues to injected drugs, and in ophthalmic (eye) procedures (for example, ℞ **hyaluronidase**).

℞ **imiglucerase** is an enzyme that is used as a replacement in the specialist treatment of Gaucher's disease, which is a genetically determined enzyme-deficiency disease that affects the spleen, liver, bone marrow, and lymph nodes.

Limitations

There are a number of difficulties in using enzymes in medicine. A major one is that enzymes must normally be given by injection since, because they are proteins, they are broken down by digestive enzymes in the stomach or intestine. Even in the case of ℞ **digestive enzyme** treatment with ℞ **pancreatin**, some of the enzyme activity is lost in the stomach unless it is given together with drugs that decrease acid production. In the case of the ℞ **mucolytic** drug ℞ **dornase alfa** (used, for example, to treat ✪ **cystic fibrosis**) it is given by inhalation because the enzyme has to act on the bronchioles. In the past, the major problem was in isolating enzymes from plant or animal tissues (still the case with ℞ **pancreatin**). However, enzymes can now be made by recombinant DNA technology, which is the case with ℞ **imiglucerase**.

ephedrine ⓖ

Type/Group: **sympathomimetic; bronchodilator; vasoconstrictor; CNS stimulant**.

Brand(s): Kondon's Nasal; Pretz-D; various generic (for injection). Combinations: With theophylline (or derivatives): Marax Tablets; Primatene Dual Action Tablets (has *guaifenesin*). (Plus) *phenobarbital*: Lufyllin-EPG Tablets, Elixir (both have *guaifenesin* and *dyphylline*); Mudrane GG Tablets (has *guaifenesin* and *aminophylline*); Mudrane Tablets (has *potassium iodide* and *aminophylline*); Quadrinal Tablets; Tedrigen Tablets; Theodrine Tablets. (Plus) *hydroxyzine hydrochloride*: Hydrophed Tablets; Marax-DF Syrup; Theomax DF Syrup. With guaifenesin: Broncholate Softgels, Syrup; Bronkaid Dual Action Caplets;

Dynafed Asthma Relief Tablets; Mini Thin Asthma Relief Tablets; Primatene Tablets. (Plus) *chlorpheniramine maleate*: Bronkotuss Expectorant Liquid Other: KIE Syrup (with *potassium iodide*); Norisodrine w/Calcium (with *anhydrous calcium iodide*). (In hemorrhoid preparations): Pazo Hemorrhoid Ointment, Suppositories.

How administered: Orally; nasal spray; injection; topically (external).

Used to treat

Ephedrine is sometimes used as a bronchodilator, for instance in ✪ **asthma**. It is a vasoconstrictor (narrows blood vessels) and is used as a nasal ℞ **decongestant**. Sometimes it is used to raise the blood pressure in emergencies (for example shock) where other methods have not worked. It is incorporated, as ephedrine hydrochloride or ephedrine sulfate, into proprietary hay fever and nasal decongestant preparations. It has weak CNS stimulant properties. Although not stated by the manufacturer for such use, ephedrine is sometimes used for ✪ **bed-wetting** and ✪ **myasthenia gravis**. It is also available in ✪ **hemorrhoid** preparations.

Warnings

• It should not be given to people with narrow-angle glaucoma.

• It should be given with caution to people with certain heart, kidney, cardiovascular and thyroid disorders, diabetes, and hypertension. Care should be taken to avoid interaction with other drugs (especially ℞ **MAOI** antidepressants in case of hypertensive crisis: see Interactions below).

• Ephedrine's effects during pregnancy are not known, and so it should be used with caution and only if there is clear benefit.

• If taken by mouth, this drug should not be used by nursing mothers.

• Ephedrine should not be used together with, or within two weeks of discontinuing, a MAOI antidepressant.

• The last dose should be taken several hours before retiring to bed, as it can cause wakefulness.

• Nasal use should be for no longer than three to five days.

Interactions

• ℞ **MAOI** antidepressants can cause dangerous hypertension (raised blood pressure).

• If used with ℞ **theophylline**, there is a higher incidence of side effects of both drugs.

• ℞ **furazolidone**, ℞ **procarbazine**, and ℞ **selegiline** may increase blood pressure.

• If used with other ℞ **sympathomimetics** or ℞ **ergotamine**, effects are increased, with the potential for toxicity.

• ℞ **General anesthetics** may cause heart arrhythmias.

• ℞ **guanethidine monosulfate** may lose some of its antihypertensive effectiveness when used with ephedrine.

• ℞ **Adrenergic-neuron blockers**, ℞ **methyldopa**, and ℞ **reserpine** lower the effects of ephedrine.

• The effects of ℞ **insulin** and ℞ **hypoglycemics** may be lowered.

Side effects

• These depend on how it is administered, dose, and use. There may be changes in heart rate and blood pressure, anxiety, restlessness, tremor, insomnia, dry mouth, cold fingertips and toes, and changes in the prostate gland.

• When used as a nasal decongestant, it may cause irritation in the nose.

• More serious but rarer side effects include seizures and disorders of heart rhythm.

Epifoam Aerosol Foam ⑧

A preparation of ℞ **hydrocortisone** and ℞ **pramoxine hydrochloride**.

Formulation: Aerosol foam.
Availability: Prescription only.
Warnings and side effects: See ℞ **hydrocortisone**; ℞ **pramoxine hydrochloride**.

Epifrin ⑧

A preparation of ℞ **epinephrine**.
Formulation: Eye drops, available in 3 strengths.
Availability: Prescription only.
Warnings and side effects: See ℞ **epinephrine**.

epileptic treatment ⑩

see ℞ **antiepileptic**.

E-Pilo-1; -2; -4; -6 ⑧

A preparation of ℞ **pilocarpine** and ℞ **epinephrine**.
Formulation: Ophthalmic solution, available in 4 strengths.
Availability: Prescription only.
Warnings and side effects: See ℞ **pilocarpine**; ℞ **epinephrine**.

epinephrine ⑥

(adrenaline)
Type/Group: **alpha-adrenergic stimulant; beta-adrenergic stimulant; sympathomimetic; vasoconstrictor; cardiac stimulant; glaucoma treatment**.
Brand(s): (For ophthalmic use): Epifrin; Glaucon. (As vasoconstrictor or bronchodilator): Ana-Guard; AsthmaHaler Mist; AsthmaNefrin; Epipen, Epipen Jr.; microNefrin; Nephron; Primatene Mist; S-2; Sus-Phrine; various generic (as either epinephrine or adrenaline). Combinations: With *pilocarpine*: E-Pilo-1, -2, -4, -6; P_1E_1, P_2E_1, P_4E_1, P_6E_1.
How administered: Inhalation; topically (intranasal; eye); injection (including specialized methods with local anesthetics).

Used to treat

The main form of epinephrine used clinically is prepared in pure form or as hydrochloride, sulfate, or bitartrate, which alters its strength of action and absorption properties. It has both alpha-adrenergic stimulant and beta-adrenergic stimulant activity, and is not very greatly used therapeutically because its actions are so widespread within the body. In emergencies, however, it may be injected in cardiac arrest, to treat the circulatory collapse and bronchoconstriction of anaphylactic shock (see ⊙ **anaphylactic reaction**), and in ⊙ **angioedema**. More commonly, epinephrine is included in several local anesthetic preparations, because its pronounced vasoconstrictor actions (narrows blood vessels) considerably prolong anesthesia by preventing the local anesthetic from being removed in the bloodstream. Also, it is used in solution in eyedrops to treat certain types of ⊙ **glaucoma**, for the temporary relief of symptoms of certain types of ⊙ **asthma**, and as a decongestant for nasal congestion.

Warnings

• Depending on use, and not when used in emergency, life-saving situations, it is not suitable for people with brain damage or cerebral arteriosclerosis, in cardiovascular shock (but it is used for anaphylactic shock), or with narrow-angle glaucoma.

• It should be given with caution to people with certain heart, cardiovascular, kidney, and thyroid disorders, diabetes, parkinsonism, enlarged prostate, and hypertension. Care must be taken to avoid interaction with other drugs, especially ℞ **MAOI** antidepressants (because of the risk of a hypertensive crisis), and it should not be used with certain ℞ **general anesthetics** or during labor (see Interactions below).

• Epinephrine should be used during pregnancy only if the potential benefit outweighs the possible risks.

• Nursing mothers should discontinue this drug or discontinue breast-feeding.

• This is a powerful drug and there may be severe drug interactions in people already taking a number of other drugs, especially antidepressants and beta-blockers.

• Epinephrine can cause or aggravate psychiatric symptoms, including panic, hallucinations, delusions, and aggressive behavior.

• It may cause severe tissue damage at the site of injection, so continuous monitoring is necessary. It should never be injected in the extremities (fingers, toes, ears, and so on).

• Do not use in the eye when wearing soft contact lenses.

Interactions

• If used with ℞ **beta-blockers**, there is a risk of severe hypertension followed by slowed heart rhythm.

• If used with ℞ **theophylline**, the side effects of both drugs are more likely to occur.

• Epinephrine should not be used with ℞ **MAOI** antidepressants (or within two weeks of stopping MAOI treatment) or other ℞ **sympathomimetics** because this may cause a hypertensive crisis.

• Other sympathomimetics, ℞ **antihistamines**, ℞ **cardiac glycosides**, ℞ **general anesthetics**, MAOIs, ℞ **tricyclic** antidepressants, ℞ **oxytocics** (for example, ℞ **oxytocin**, ℞ **ergonovine**), ℞ **guanethidine monosulfate**, and ℞ **levothyroxine** may intensify the effects of epinephrine, with the potential for serious adverse reactions.

• Epinephrine may lower the effectiveness of ℞ **insulin** and ℞ **hypoglycemics**.

• ℞ **Alpha-adrenergic blockers**, ℞ **phenothiazines**, and ℞ **diuretics** may reverse or decrease the therapeutic effects of epinephrine.

Side effects

• Depending on how it is administered, there may be an increase in heart rate and irregular rhythms, muscle tremor, dry mouth, anxiety or fear, and coldness in the fingertips and toes.

• High dosage may lead to tremor, the accumulation of fluid in the lungs, and cerebral hemorrhage and other effects.

Key to symbols: ⑩ = Drug type/group   ⑥ = Generic name   ⑧ = Brand name

• Epinephrine in eyedrops may cause redness and smarting of the eye and browache.

Epipen; Epipen Jr. ®
A preparation of ℞ **epinephrine**.
Formulation: Injection.
Availability: Prescription only.
Warnings and side effects: See ℞ **epinephrine**.

epirubicin hydrochloride ©
Type/Group: **cytotoxic; anticancer**.
Brand(s): Ellence.
How administered: Intravenous infusion.
Used to treat
Epirubicin (an anthracycline antibiotic in origin) is used in the treatment of ✪ **breast cancer**.
Warnings
• It should not be given to people with certain blood and heart disorders, hypersensitivity to epirubicin or related drugs, severe liver dysfunction, or anyone who has previously been treated with anthracyclines up to the maximum cumulative dose. It is a specialist drug and a full assessment for suitability will be carried out.
• It should be given with caution to people with bone marrow or liver dysfunction and blood disorders.
• It may harm the fetus and should be used during pregnancy only if it is medically warranted. Becoming pregnant while using this drug should be avoided.
• It is not recommended for use while breast-feeding.
• It is a specialist drug which will be administered by specialists in an appropriate facility. Monitoring will be carried out.
Interactions
• If used with ℞ **calcium-channel blockers**, there is a risk of heart failure.
• There is increased toxicity when used with other cytotoxic drugs.
Side effects
• Frequently, nausea, diarrhea, vomiting, stomatitis (mouth sores), hair loss, and myelosuppression.
• Occasionally, loss of appetite, infection, conjunctivitis, rash, and itching. It may cause liver toxicity, damage to heart muscle, metabolic abnormalities, and secondary cancers.

Epitol ®
A preparation of ℞ **carbamazepine**.
Formulation: Oral tablets.
Availability: Prescription only.
Warnings and side effects: See ℞ **carbamazepine**.

Epivir ®
A preparation of ℞ **lamivudine**.
Formulation: Oral tablets; oral solution.
Availability: Prescription only.
Warnings and side effects: See ℞ **lamivudine**.

EPO ®
see ℞ **epoetin alfa**.

epoetin alfa ©
(erythropoietin; EPO)
Type/Group: **hematopoietic**.
Brand(s): Epogen; Procrit.
How administered: Injection or infusion.
Used to treat
Epoetin alfa is a form of human erythropoietin synthesized by recombinant techniques. It is used in the treatment of types of ✪ **anemia** known to be associated with erythropoietin deficiency, as in chronic renal (kidney) failure and in people undergoing some forms of cancer chemotherapy or receiving zidovudine for ✪ **HIV** infection. It may also be used to build up red-cell levels in people about to undergo surgery.
Warnings
• It should not be given to people with known hypersensitivity to this drug or to human albumin, or with uncontrolled hypertension.
• It should be given with caution to people with porphyria, poorly controlled blood pressure, a history of convulsions, heart disease, or a malignant disease. This is a specialist drug and is used only after a full medical assessment.
• Epoetin alfa should be used during pregnancy only when the potential benefit outweighs the possible risk to the fetus.
• Medical judgment is required if breast-feeding is being considered.
• Epoetin alfa is used only under qualified medical supervision and with frequent monitoring of blood values.
• Because of the potential for seizures, mostly during the first 3 months of treatment, potentially hazardous activities, such as driving, should be avoided.
• Iron deficiency often develops, requiring an iron supplement.
Interactions
No interactions of significance are known.
Side effects
• High blood pressure (hypertension) is the most frequent.
• Depending on the underlying cause for treatment, other side effects may include headache, a feverish feeling, joint pain, nausea, vomiting, and seizures.
• Changes in blood clotting may occur and potassium levels may increase. Hypersensitivity reactions (for example, rash or hives) are rare.

epoprostenol sodium ©
Type/Group: **prostaglandin; antihypertensive; antiplatelet; vasodilator**.
Brand(s): Flolan.
How administered: Intravenous infusion.
Used to treat
Epoprostenol (prostacyclin) is present naturally in the walls of blood vessels. It is a powerful dilator of blood vessels and is used to treat pulmonary hypertension. When given by intravenous infusion it also has antiplatelet activity and so inhibits blood coagulation by preventing the aggregation of platelets.

Warnings

• It should not be given to people with known hypersensitivity to this drug, with certain kinds of heart failure, or who develop a buildup of fluid in the lungs during initial dosing with this drug.

• It should be given with caution to elderly people.

• Epoprostenol should be used during pregnancy only if it is clearly needed.

• Medical judgment is required if breast-feeding is being considered. It is not known whether it appears in breast milk.

• Initial dosing with epoprostenol should take place in a medical facility, supervised by a clinician experienced in the treatment of pulmonary hypertension.

• Continued use of this drug is often by self-administration through an indwelling catheter. Thorough instruction from a doctor is necessary for preparing and self-administering epoprostenol.

• Even brief interruptions in dosage can cause hypertensive symptoms to reappear, such as breathlessness, dizziness, and weakness.

Interactions

• Other antihypertensives, ℞ **vasodilators**, and ℞ **diuretics** have increased effects in reducing blood pressure.

• ℞ **anticoagulant** and ℞ **antiplatelet** drugs may increase the risk of bleeding.

• There may be a short-term increase in the levels and effects of ℞ **digoxin**.

Side effects

• When first using the drug and establishing dosage, there may be flushing, headache, nausea and vomiting, hypotension, anxiety, chest pain, dizziness, slowed heart rate, and abdominal pain.

• In continued use, there may be jaw and neck pain, gastrointestinal disturbances (loss of appetite, diarrhea), palpitations or disturbances of heart rhythm, bleeding, sweating, rash or skin ulcer, and mental depression.

eprosartan mesylate Ⓖ

Type/Group: **angiotensin-receptor blocker; antihypertensive; vasodilator**.

Brand(s): Teveten.

How administered: Orally.

Used to treat

Eprosartan is an angiotensin II receptor (AT1 receptors) blocker, and is used, alone or in combination with other drugs, to treat ✪ **hypertension**. Angiotensin II is a circulating hormone that is a powerful vasoconstrictor (narrows blood vessels) and blocking its effects leads to a fall in blood pressure.

Warnings

• It should not be given to people with known hypersensitivity to this drug.

• It should be given with caution to people with severe congestive heart failure, severely impaired liver or kidney function, or renal stenosis. Any fluid- or salt-depleted condition (as from diuretic use) should be corrected before using this drug.

• Risk in pregnancy increases substantially from the first through to the second and third trimesters. Angiotensin-receptor blockers can

cause injury to the fetus. The use of these drugs should be stopped as soon as pregnancy is detected.

• Medical judgment is required if breast-feeding is being considered.

• Blood pressure should be checked regularly.

Interactions

No drug interactions of significance are known.

Side effects

• Angiotensin-receptor blockers in general appear to cause few and infrequent side effects (often indistinguishable from placebo effects). The most common, with eprosartan, may include upper respiratory infection, sore throat, rhinitis, fatigue, dry cough, or joint pain.

• Uncommonly, headache, muscle pain, dizziness, gastrointestinal disturbances, chest pain, or edema. Symptoms such as rash, weakness, and effects on heart rhythm seldom occur. There may be changes in kidney or liver function, and angioedema (an allergic swelling reaction, often of the face) has been reported.

eptifibatide Ⓖ

Type/Group: **antiplatelet**.

Brand(s): Integrelin.

How administered: Intravenous injection or infusion.

Used to treat

Eptifibatide is an antiplatelet drug which is used to prevent ✪ **thrombosis** (blood-clot formation). It works by stopping platelets sticking to one another or to the walls of blood vessels. It can be used (usually together with ℞ **heparin** and ℞ **aspirin**) to prevent thrombosis in acute cardiac conditions in which ✪ **myocardial infarction** (heart attack) has already occurred or is likely to occur.

Warnings

• It should not be given to people with known hypersensitivity to this drug, with active internal bleeding (for example, peptic ulcer) or within 30 days of such active bleeding (including stroke, major surgery, or injury), with a history of intracranial hemorrhage, aneurysm or certain vascular malformations, with active pericarditis, severe high blood pressure, or who are on kidney dialysis. Eptifibatide should not be used together with any drug that has similar antiplatelet action. It will be administered by experienced personnel after a full medical assessment.

• It should be given with caution to people with low platelet count or severe kidney impairment.

• It should be used during pregnancy only if it is clearly needed.

• Medical judgment is required if breast-feeding is being considered. It is not known whether this drug appears in breast milk.

• It is used only in a hospital setting, with periodic monitoring of blood values and close observation for potential bleeding.

Interactions

• If used with ℞ **anticoagulants**, ℞ **clopidogrel**, ℞ **NSAIDs**, ℞ **dipyridamole**, ℞ **thrombolytic** (for example, ℞ **streptokinase**), or ℞ **ticlopidine**, there is a higher potential for bleeding (caution is advised).

Side effects

• The most common is bleeding, although major bleeding is infrequent.

• Other side effects may include hypotension and gastrointestinal disturbances.

Equagesic Tablets Ⓑ

A preparation of ℞ **aspirin** and ℞ **meprobamate**.
Formulation: Oral tablets.
Availability: Prescription only.
Warnings and side effects: See ℞ **aspirin**; ℞ **meprobamate**.

Equanil Ⓑ

A preparation of ℞ **meprobamate**.
Formulation: Oral tablets in several strengths.
Availability: Prescription only.
Warnings and side effects: See ℞ **meprobamate**.

Equilet Ⓑ

A preparation of ℞ **calcium carbonate**.
Formulation: Oral tablets, chewable.
Availability: OTC.
Warnings and side effects: See ℞ **calcium carbonate**.

Ercaf Ⓑ

A preparation of ℞ **ergotamine tartrate**, ℞ **caffeine**, ℞ **belladonna alkaloid**, and pentobarbital.
Formulation: Oral tablets.
Availability: Prescription only.
Warnings and side effects: See ℞ **ergotamine tartrate**; ℞ **caffeine**; ℞ **belladonna alkaloid**.

Ergamisol Ⓑ

A preparation of ℞ **levamisole hydrochloride**.
Formulation: Oral tablets.
Availability: Prescription only.
Warnings and side effects: See ℞ **levamisole hydrochloride**.

ergocalciferol Ⓖ

Type/Group: vitamin; osteoporosis treatment.
Brand(s): Calciferol; Drisdol.
How administered: Orally; injection.

Used to treat

Ergocalciferol (calciferol, vitamin D_2) is one of the natural forms of calciferol (🜂🜂 **vitamin D**), which are formed in plants by the action of sunlight. It is vitamin D_2 but in medicine it is usually referred to as ergocalciferol or simply calciferol, and is used to treat ✪ **osteoporosis**, refractory ✪ **rickets**, familial hypophosphatemia and ✪ **hypoparathyroidism**.

Warnings

• It should not be given to people with known hypercalcemia, malabsorption syndrome, hypervitaminosis D, or those with decreased kidney function.

• It should be given with caution to people with kidney stones, coronary disease, arteriosclerosis, and those over 65.

• It should be used during pregnancy only if the potential benefit outweighs the possible risk to the fetus.

• Medical judgment is required if breast-feeding is being considered. Calcium levels in the infant should be monitored if pharmacologic doses are taken.

• Adequate dietary calcium is necessary for clinical response to treatment. At pharmacological dosages, periodic monitoring may be recommended.

Interactions

• If used with magnesium-containing ℞ **antacids**, people on dialysis may develop elevated serum levels of magnesium.

• If used with digitalis glycosides or ℞ **verapamil**, there are adverse cardiac effects from hypercalcemia.

• ℞ **Cholestyramine**, ℞ **ketoconazole**, ℞ **mineral oil**, ℞ **phenytoin**, and ℞ **phenobarbital** may reduce vitamin D synthesis.

• If used with ℞ **thiazide** diuretics, there is an increased risk of hypercalcemia.

Side effects

• Infrequently, weakness, headache, somnolence, gastrointestinal effects, mental changes, weight loss, and urinary changes (for example, excess urine production).

ergolide Ⓓ

see ℞ **ergot alkaloid**.

ergoloid Ⓓ

see ℞ **ergot alkaloid**.

ergoloid mesylates Ⓖ

(co-dergocrine mesilates)
Type/Group: ergot alkaloid; dementia treatment; alpha-adrenoceptor antagonist.
Brand(s): Gerimal; Hydergine; various generic.
How administered: Orally.

Used to treat

Ergoloid mesylates is a mixture, a combination of ergot alkaloid derivatives, which affects the blood vessels of the brain. Chemically, it consists of dihydroergocornine mesylate, dihydroergocristine mesylate, and alpha- and beta-dihydroergocryptine mesylates, which have alpha-receptor antagonist actions. It has been claimed to be a nootropic agent, that is, it improves brain function, but clinical results of psychological tests during and following treatment have neither proved nor disproved such a claim. It is for the treatment of senile ✪ **dementia** that the drug is most frequently used.

Warnings

• It should not be given to people with known hypersensitivity to these drugs, or who have any kind of acute or chronic psychosis.

• It should be given with caution to people who have a very slow heart rate.

• As this drug mixture is not used by women of childbearing age, it has not been evaluated for effects in pregnancy and breast-feeding.

• Sublingual tablets (placed beneath the tongue) should be allowed to dissolve fully under the tongue and not crushed or chewed.

Interactions
None known.

Side effects
• There may be gastrointestinal disturbances, dizziness, flushing, a blocked nose, headache, rash, postural hypotension (lowered blood pressure on standing) in people with hypertension, nausea, vomiting, and irritation under the tongue (if the sublingual tablets are used).

Ergomar ®
A preparation of ℞ **ergotamine tartrate**.
Formulation: Sublingual tablets.
Availability: Prescription only.
Warnings and side effects: See ℞ **ergotamine tartrate**.

ergometrine maleate ⑥
see ℞ **ergonovine maleate**.

ergonovine maleate ⑥
(ergometrine maleate)
Type/Group: **ergot alkaloid; uterine stimulant; vasoconstrictor**.
Brand(s): Ergotrate Maleate.
How administered: Orally; injection.

Used to treat
Ergonovine is used routinely in obstetrics (an area of medicine to do with pregnancy and childbirth). Ergonovine, or a closely related compound ℞ **methylergonovine**, may be given to prevent excessive postnatal bleeding and also bleeding due to incomplete abortion (when it may be combined with ℞ **oxytocin**). It may be used, as well, to speed up the third stage of labor (the delivery of the placenta), although oxytocin is currently preferred for this purpose. Although not stated by the manufacturer for such use, it is sometimes given for migraine.

Warnings
• It should not be given to people with known hypersensitivity to this drug, or with vascular disease, certain kidney, liver, heart and other cardiovascular or lung disorders, sepsis, calcium deficiency, severe hypertension, or eclampsia. It should not be used during pregnancy, or to induce labor, or when spontaneous abortion seems likely.
• It should be given with caution to people with a very slow heart rate.
• Ergonovine should not be taken during pregnancy.
• Medical judgment is required if breast-feeding is being considered. It may decrease the production of milk.

Interactions
• If used with other vasoconstrictors or ergot alkaloids, there is a possibility of intensified side effects.

Side effects
• Depending on how it is administered, use, and dose, there may be nausea and vomiting, palpitations, breathlessness, slowing of the heartbeat, headache, dizziness, and abdominal and chest pain.

• Rarely, there are cardiovascular complications.

ergot alkaloid ⓓ
(ergolide; ergoloid)
Generics: **bromocriptine; dihydroergotamine mesylate; ergoloid mesylates; ergonovine maleate; ergotamine tartrate; methylergonovine maleate; methysergide; pergolide**.

Actions and uses
Ergot alkaloids are ℞ **alkaloids** derived, directly isolated or semi-synthetically modified, from a mold or fungus called *Claviceps purpurea*, which grows on infected damp rye. These alkaloids are powerful ℞ **vasoconstrictor** substances that narrow the blood vessels in the fingers and toes, in particular, and cause a tingling sensation that progressively develops into pain then gangrene. Ergot poisoning was known as St. Anthony's Fire and was caused by eating bread made from rye contaminated with ergot. In medicine, the dose of individual alkaloids is adjusted carefully to avoid the development of the more serious side effects. ℞ **Ergotamine tartrate** is the main vasoconstrictor used in medicine and is usually given for ✪ **migraine** as an ℞ **antimigraine** treatment; ℞ **ergonovine maleate** is used to contract the uterus in the last stages of labor and to minimize postpartum (after childbirth) bleeding (it is the drug of choice because its effects on blood vessels are less pronounced). Some notable examples of semisynthetic ergot derivatives, which are used for a variety of purposes, include ℞ **methylergonovine maleate**, ℞ **bromocriptine**, ℞ **dihydroergotamine mesylate**, ℞ **ergoloid mesylates**, ℞ **ergotamine tartrate**, ℞ **pergolide**, and ℞ **methysergide**. All the ergot alkaloids are chemically derivatives of lysergide acid, and lysergide (lysergic acid diethylamide) is the medical name for LSD.

Limitations
See individual drug entries.

ergotamine tartrate ⑥
Type/Group: **ergot alkaloid; antimigraine; vasoconstrictor**.
Brand(s): Ergomar. Combinations: With *caffeine* and *belladonna alkaloids*: Cafatine; Cafergot; Cafetrate; Ercaf; Wigraine. With *belladonna alkaloids* and *phenobarbital*: Bel-Phen-Ergot SR; Bellacane SR; Bellergal-S; Folergot-DF; Phenerbel-S.
How administered: Orally; suppository.

Used to treat
Ergotamine is used to treat vascular headaches, such as ✪ **migraine**, that are not relieved by ordinary painkilling drugs. It is most effective if administered during the "aura"—the initial symptoms—of an attack and probably works as a vasoconstrictor (narrows blood vessels) on the cranial arteries. However, although the pain may be relieved, other symptoms, such as the visual disturbances and nausea, may not (but other drugs may be used to treat these symptoms separately).

Warnings
• It should not be given to people with known hypersensitivity to any ergot alkaloid, or anyone with vascular disease (for example, Raynaud's disease), certain kidney or liver disorders, severe hypertension, porphyria, malnutrition, sepsis, or hyperthyroidism.
• Ergotamine must not be used during pregnancy.

• It does appear in breast milk and may cause effects, such as vomiting or diarrhea, in infants.

• If there is numbness or tingling in the extremities, treatment must be stopped and a doctor contacted.

• It should be used only to treat, not to prevent, migraine attacks. For best results, it should be used at the first sign of an attack.

• Regular use may result in withdrawal headaches.

Interactions

• ℞ **ritonavir** must not be used with any form of ergotamine.

• If used with ℞ **beta-blockers**, circulation to the extremities may be restricted to the point that gangrene occurs.

• If used with ℞ **macrolides** (for example, ℞ **erythromycin**), there is a risk of intensified and serious side effects.

• ℞ **Vasodilators** may cause dangerously high blood pressure.

• If the following drugs are used with ergotamine, effects are increased with potentially serious circulatory results: ℞ **naratriptan**; ℞ **rizatriptan**; ℞ **sumatriptan**; ℞ **zolmitriptan** (antimigraine drugs).

Side effects

• These depend on the use, how it is administered, and dose. There may be vomiting, nausea, vertigo, abdominal pain and diarrhea, cramps, chest pain, and a fast or slow heartbeat.

• Repeated high dosage may cause confusion, gangrene, and peritoneal fibrosis.

Ergotrate Maleate ℬ

A preparation of ℞ **ergonovine maleate**.
Formulation: Injection.
Availability: Prescription only.
Warnings and side effects: See ℞ **ergonovine maleate**.

Eryc ℬ

A preparation of ℞ **erythromycin**.
Formulation: Oral capsules, delayed release.
Availability: Prescription only.
Warnings and side effects: See ℞ **erythromycin**.

Eryderm ℬ

A preparation of ℞ **erythromycin**.
Formulation: Topical solution.
Availability: Prescription only.
Warnings and side effects: See ℞ **erythromycin**.

Erymax ℬ

A preparation of ℞ **erythromycin**.
Formulation: Topical solution.
Availability: Prescription only.
Warnings and side effects: See ℞ **erythromycin**.

EryPed ℬ

A preparation of ℞ **erythromycin**.
Formulation: Chewable tablets; oral suspension in several strengths.
Availability: Prescription only.
Warnings and side effects: See ℞ **erythromycin**.

Ery-Tab ℬ

A preparation of ℞ **erythromycin**.
Formulation: Oral tablets in two strengths, both delayed release.
Availability: Prescription only.
Warnings and side effects: See ℞ **erythromycin**.

erythromycin Ⓖ

Type/Group: **macrolide; antibiotic; antibacterial**.
Brand(s): Akne-mycin; A/T/S; Del-Mycin; E-Base; E.E.S.; E-Mycin; Eryc; Eryderm; Erymax; EryPed; Ery-Tab; Ilotycin; PCE Dispertab; Staticin; various generic. Combinations: With *sulfisoxazole*: Eryzole; Pediazole. With *benzoyl peroxide*: Benzamycin.
How administered: Orally; topically (external); topically (eye); injection.

Used to treat

Erythromycin is an original member of the macrolide group and is effective in treating ✪ **bacterial infection** caused by many Gram-positive bacteria, including streptococci (infections of the soft tissue and respiratory tract), mycoplasma (✪ **pneumonia**), Legionella (✪ **Legionnaires' disease**) and chlamydia (✪ **urethritis**). It can also be used in the treatment of ✪ **acne**, ✪ **rosacea**, chronic ✪ **prostatitis**, eye infections, ✪ **diphtheria**, and whooping cough (✪ **pertussis**). It has a similar range of action to penicillin, but acts in a different way (macrolides work by inhibiting microbial protein synthesis). Its principal use is as an alternative to penicillin for people who are allergic to that drug. However, bacterial resistance to erythromycin is quite common.

Warnings

• It should not be given to people with known hypersensitivity to any of the macrolide antibiotics.

• It should be given with caution to people with kidney or liver dysfunction, certain infections, or myasthenia gravis (it may aggravate weakness).

• Erythromycin should be used during pregnancy only if it is clearly needed and if the potential benefits outweigh the possible risk to the fetus.

• Medical judgment is required if breast-feeding is being considered. Although use of this drug is compatible with breast-feeding, it does appear in breast milk and could possibly affect the baby.

• Superinfections due to the altered bacterial balance created by the use of antibiotics may occur. A doctor must be contacted if there is severe abdominal pain, moderate to severe diarrhea, or any new or unusual symptoms.

• Rarely, serious allergic reactions and liver disease have occurred.

Interactions

• Erythromycin must not be used with astemizole, ℞ **fexofenadine**, cisapride, or ℞ **pimozide** because of the risk of serious heartbeat disorders.

• There is the possibility of ergotism if used with ℞ **ergotamine**.

• The effects of ℞ **alfentanil**, ℞ **atorvastatin**, ℞ **bromocriptine**, ℞ **buspirone**, ℞ **carbamazepine**, ℞ **clozapine**, ℞ **colchicine**, ℞ **cyclosporine**, ℞ **diazepam**, ℞ **digoxin**, ℞ **disopyramide**, ℞ **felodipine**, ℞ **itraconazole**, ℞ **lovastatin**, ℞ **methylprednisolone**, ℞ **midazolam**, ℞ **quinidine**,

℞ sildenafil, ℞ simvastatin, ℞ tacrolimus, ℞ theophylline, ℞ triazolam, ℞ valproic acid, ℞ warfarin sodium and zopiclone may be increased.

• The levels of ℞ amprenavir, ℞ indinavir, ℞ nelfinavir, ℞ ritonavir, and ℞ saquinavir, and of clarithromycin, may be increased.

• The effects of ℞ penicillin and ℞ zafirlukast may be decreased.

Side effects

• Systemic use: Frequently, abdominal discomfort and thrombophlebitis when given intravenously. Occasionally, gastrointestinal upsets, rash, and hives. Rarely, heart rhythm disorders.

• Topical use: Frequently, dry skin. Rarely, hives. Ophthalmic use (eyes): Rarely, allergic reaction causing increased eye irritation, and temporary blurring of vision.

erythropoietin ⑥

see ℞ epoetin alfa.

Eryzole ⑧

A preparation of ℞ erythromycin and ℞ sulfisoxazole.
Formulation: Oral suspension.
Availability: Prescription only.
Warnings and side effects: See ℞ erythromycin; ℞ sulfisoxazole.

Esgic Tablets, Capsules; Esgic-Plus Tablets, Capsules ⑧

A preparation of ℞ acetaminophen, ℞ caffeine, and ℞ butabarbital.
Formulation: Oral tablets; capsules.
Availability: Prescription only.
Warnings and side effects: See ℞ acetaminophen; ℞ butabarbital; ℞ caffeine.

Esidrix ⑧

A preparation of ℞ hydrochlorothiazide.
Formulation: Oral tablets, available in two strengths.
Availability: Prescription only.
Warnings and side effects: See ℞ hydrochlorothiazide.

Esimil ⑧

A preparation of ℞ guanethidine monosulfate and ℞ hydrochlorothiazide.
Formulation: Oral tablets.
Availability: Prescription only.
Warnings and side effects: See ℞ guanethidine monosulfate; ℞ hydrochlorothiazide.

Eskalith; Eskalith CR ⑧

A preparation of ℞ lithium.
Formulation: Oral tablets or capsules; oral tablets, extended release (CR).
Availability: Prescription only.
Warnings and side effects: See ℞ lithium.

esmolol hydrochloride ⑥

Type/Group: **beta-blocker; antiarrhythmic; antihypertensive.**
Brand(s): Brevibloc.
How administered: Intravenous infusion.

Used to treat

Esmolol is used to control blood pressure or rapid heart rate during operations and in short-term antiarrhythmic treatment (see ✪ arrhythmia), generally in a medical facility. Beta-blockers are generally not prescribed to people with asthma or other bronchospastic disease (for example, chronic bronchitis or emphysema), but esmolol may be used with medical judgment when other antihypertensive treatments have failed and an injectable agent is required.

Warnings

• It should not be given to people with known hypersensitivity to any beta-blocking drug, who have certain heartbeat irregularities or heart failure. It should not be used in cardiogenic shock.

• It should be given with caution to people with diabetes mellitus or hypoglycemia, hyperthyroidism, myasthenia gravis, congestive heart failure, peripheral vascular disease, or liver or kidney impairment.

• Esmolol should be used during pregnancy only if the potential benefit outweighs the risk to the fetus.

• Medical judgment is required if breast-feeding is being considered. This drug appears in breast milk and may cause adverse effects in nursing infants.

• The use of this drug may mask signs of hyperthyroidism or hypoglycemia.

Interactions

• The effects of ℞ alpha-adrenergic stimulants, ℞ clonidine hydrochloride, ℞ ergot alkaloids, ℞ epinephrine, and ℞ lidocaine may be increased, with the risk of serious adverse effects.

• ℞ Calcium-channel blockers, ℞ guanethidine monosulfate, and ℞ reserpine have the potential for increasing undesirable effects, with exaggerated slowing of heartbeat or hypotension.

• The effects of nondepolarizing ℞ skeletal muscle relaxants may be variable, with the possible risk of significant adverse effects associated with major surgery.

• The effects of ℞ insulin and ℞ sulfonylureas may be reduced by esmolol.

• ℞ Antacids (for example, ℞ aluminum hydroxide, ℞ magnesium hydroxide), ℞ barbiturates, ☍ calcium salts, ℞ cholestyramine, ℞ colestipol hydrochloride, ℞ NSAIDs, ℞ phenytoin, ℞ penicillins, ℞ rifampin, and ℞ salicylates may reduce the levels and effectiveness of esmolol.

• If used with ℞ diuretics and other antihypertensive drugs, there are additive effects which are often used to therapeutic advantage.

Side effects

• Frequently, hypotension, often accompanied by dizziness or headache.

• Less frequently, nausea, cold extremities, or fatigue.

• Uncommonly, mental confusion, slowing of the heart rate, wheezing, vomiting, pallor, dry mouth, and inflammation at the site of infusion.

Estar

A preparation of ℞ **simethicone** and ℞ **coal tar**.
Formulation: Topical gel.
Availability: OTC.
Warnings and side effects: See ℞ **simethicone**; ℞ **coal tar**.

estazolam ⑥

Type/Group: hypnotic; benzodiazepine.
Brand(s): ProSom.
How administered: Orally.

Used to treat

Estazolam is a benzodiazepine (chemically a triazolobenzodiazepine) used for short-term treatment of ✪ **insomnia**.

Warnings

• It should not be given to people with known hypersensitivity to benzodiazepines, narrow-angle glaucoma, or psychosis.
• It should be given with caution to people with kidney or liver impairment, a history of drug abuse, respiratory depression, sleep apnea, or anyone over 65.
• Estazolam should not be used during pregnancy. A doctor must be contacted if pregnancy occurs while taking this drug.
• It should not be used by nursing mothers.
• It must not be used beyond the period prescribed by the doctor, because benzodiazepines may produce psychological and physical dependence and withdrawal symptoms.
• Judgment, thinking, and physical skills may be impaired.
• Avoid alcohol consumption because adverse side effects may be increased (see Side effects below).
• Avoid other psychotropic medications unless prescribed by a doctor.
• A doctor must be consulted before discontinuing use or increasing dosage.
• Sleep may be disturbed for one or two nights after stopping the drug.

Interactions

• ℞ **azole** antifungals (for example, ℞ **ketoconazole**, ℞ **itraconazole**), ℞ **beta-blockers** (for example, ℞ **propranolol**), ℞ **cimetidine**, ℞ **disulfiram**, ℞ **isoniazid**, ℞ **macrolide** antibiotics (for example, ℞ **erythromycin**, ℞ **clarithromycin**, troleandomycin), ℞ **omeprazole**, ℞ **SSRIs**, and ℞ **quinolones** may increase levels of estazolam.
• If used with ℞ **clozapine**, there maybe an increased risk of cardiorespiratory collapse.
• If used with ℞ **antipsychotics**, there is an increased risk of sedation and respiratory depression.
• ℞ **rifampin** may reduce effects of estazolam.
• Alcohol may increase adverse side effects.

Side effects

• Daytime sleepiness, dizziness, impaired coordination, and decreased physical activity.
• Less often, abnormal thinking or emotions, hangover, decreased reflexes, sleep problems, stupor, heart palpitations, fainting, eye, ear or nose pain or inflammation, gastrointestinal effects, shortness of breath, and skin dryness or inflammation.

• Rarely, seizures, irregularities of heart rhythm, and blood cell disorders which can be serious.

esterified estrogens ⑥

Type/Group: sex hormone; estrogen; anticancer.
Brand(s): Estratab; Menest.
How administered: Orally.

Used to treat

These combinations of estrogens are used to treat symptoms of ✪ **menopause**, ✪ **breast cancer**, ✪ **prostate cancer**, ✪ **hypogonadism** (subnormal secretion of sex hormones), female castration, primary ovarian failure, and atrophic vaginitis, as well as to prevent ✪ **osteoporosis**.

Warnings

• It should not be used by people with breast cancer (except when being treated for this), active thromboembolic disease, known or suspected estrogen-dependent cancers, undiagnosed abnormal genital bleeding.
• It should be given with caution to people with hypertension, gallbladder disease, congestive heart failure, diabetes mellitus, depression, migraine headache, seizure disorders, liver disease, family history of breast or endometrial cancer, history of thromboembolic disorders, uterine fibroids, hypertriglyceridemia, or hypercalcemia.
• Not for use during pregnancy. A doctor must be contacted if pregnancy occurs while using this drug.
• Medical judgment is required if breast-feeding is being considered. It may reduce the quality and quantity of breast milk.
• Taking estrogen increases the risk of endometrial cancer. Use of progestins along with estrogen is recommended for menopausal or postmenopausal women with an intact uterus, since progestins reduce the risk.
• Risk of gallbladder disease is increased.
• It may cause increases in blood pressure.
• The risk of thromboembolic disease (blood-clotting disorders) may be increased.
• It may worsen glucose tolerance in diabetics.

Interactions

• The effects of estrogen may be decreased by ℞ **rifampin** and ℞ **barbiturates**.
• The steroid effect of ℞ **corticosteroids** is increased.
• ℞ **Phenytoin** causes loss of seizure control and decreased estrogen levels.
• With ℞ **warfarin sodium** and similar ℞ **anticoagulants** there is a theoretical increase in the risk of thromboembolism.

Side effects

• Nausea and vomiting, breakthrough bleeding, spotting.
• Less frequently, depression, migraine headache, emotional lability, elevated blood pressure, edema, contact lens intolerance, bloating, benign liver tumors, amenorrhea, change in cervical secretions, breast enlargement, breast tenderness, elevated triglyceride or calcium levels, darkening of the skin of the face, changes in libido, and weight gain.

Key to symbols: ✪ = Disorder Section   ℞ = Drug Section   ♣ = Herbal Section   ᨚ = Supplement Section

Estrace ®

A preparation of ℞ estradiol.
Formulation: Oral tablets in several strengths; vaginal cream.
Availability: Prescription only.
Warnings and side effects: See ℞ estradiol.

Estraderm ®

A preparation of ℞ estradiol.
Formulation: Transdermal patch.
Availability: Prescription only.
Warnings and side effects: See ℞ estradiol.

estradiol ⓖ

Type/Group: sex hormone; estrogen; anticancer; hormone replacement.
Brand(s): Climara; Estrace; Estraderm; Estring; Fempatch; Gynodiol; Innofem; Vivelle; Vivelle-Dot; various generic. (As *estradiol cypionate*): Depo-Estradiol; DepoGen; depGynogen; Estro-Cyp. (As *estradiol hemihydrate*): Vagifem. (As *estradiol valerate*): Estra-L; Gynogen L.A.; Valergen. Combinations: With *norethindrone*: Combipatch. With *norgestimate*: Ortho-Prefest. (As *estradiol cypionate*): With *testosterone cypionate*: Depo-Testadiol; Depotestogen; Duo-Cyp. (As *estradiol valerate*):With *testosterone enanthate*: Deladumone; Valertest No.1.
How administered: Orally; injection; transdermal transfer (absorbed through the skin); vaginal insertion.

Used to treat

Estradiol is the main female sex hormone produced and secreted by the ovaries. It is used to treat symptoms associated with ✪ **menopause**, ✪ **breast cancer**, ✪ **prostate cancer**, atrophic ✪ **vaginitis**, ✪ **hypogonadism**, castration, and primary ovarian failure, as well as for the prevention of ✪ **osteoporosis**.

Warnings

• It should not be given to people with breast cancer (except for those being treated for breast cancer with estradiol), active thromboembolic disease, known or suspected estrogen-dependent cancers, or undiagnosed abnormal genital bleeding.
• It should be given with caution to people with hypertension, gallbladder disease, congestive heart failure, diabetes mellitus, depression, migraine headache, seizure disorders, liver disease, a family history of breast or endometrial cancer, a history of thromboembolic disorders, uterine fibroids, hypertriglyceridemia, or hypercalcemia.
• Estradiol should not be used during pregnancy. A doctor must be contacted if pregnancy occurs while using this drug.
• Medical judgment is required if breast-feeding is being considered. It may reduce the quality and quantity of breast milk.
• The use of progestins along with estrogen is recommended for menopausal or postmenopausal women with an intact uterus. Taking estrogen increases the risk of endometrial cancer in these women, but adding progestins reduces the risk.

Interactions

• ℞ Rifampin and ℞ barbiturates may decrease the effects of estradiol.
• The steroid effects of a ℞ corticosteroid may be increased.

• If used with ℞ phenytoin, there may be loss of seizure control and decreased estrogen levels.
• If used with ℞ warfarin sodium and similar anticoagulants, there is a theoretical increase in the risk of thromboembolism.

Side effects

• Nausea and vomiting, breakthrough bleeding, and spotting.
• Less frequently, depression, migraine headache, increased emotionality, elevated blood pressure, venous thrombosis, edema, contact lens intolerance, gallbladder disease, bloating, benign liver tumors, cessation of menses, change in cervical secretions, breast enlargement, breast tenderness, elevated blood glucose, elevated triglyceride or calcium levels, darkening of the skin of the face.
• Rare but serious side effects include arterial thromboembolism, pulmonary embolis.

Estra-L ®

A preparation of ℞ estradiol.
Formulation: Injection.
Availability: Prescription only.
Warnings and side effects: See ℞ estradiol.

estramustine phosphate sodium ⓖ

Type/Group: sex hormone; estrogen; anticancer.
Brand(s): Emcyt.
How administered: Orally.

Used to treat

Estramustine phosphate sodium is used to treat advanced ✪ **prostate cancer**. Chemically, it is formed by a combination of estradiol and the alkylating agent nornitrogen mustard.

Warnings

• It should not be used by people with known hypersensitivity to estradiol or nitrogen mustard, or with active thrombophlebitis or thrombotic disease unless tumor is a cause of the disorder and benefits clearly outweigh risks.
• It should be given with caution to people with a history of clotting disorders, cerebrovascular or coronary artery disease, impaired liver function, or metabolic bone diseases associated with abnormally high levels of calcium in the blood.
• This drug must not be used by pregnant women.
• Long-term administration of estrogen may increase the risk of certain cancers.
• There may be an increase in blood pressure.
• The risk of thromboembolic disease (blood-clotting disorders) may be increased.
• Glucose tolerance in diabetics may worsen.

Interactions

• It must not be taken with milk, milk products, calcium-rich foods, or calcium-containing antacids (impairs the absorption of estramustine phosphate sodium).
• ℞ Rifampin and ℞ barbiturates decrease the effects of estrogen.
• The steroid effects of ℞ corticosteroids are increased.
• ℞ Phenytoin causes loss of seizure control and decreased estrogen levels.
• With ℞ warfarin sodium and similar ℞ anticoagulants there is a theoretical increase in the risk of thromboembolism.

Side effects

• Commonly, swelling of the lower extremities, breast tenderness or enlargement, and gastrointestinal upsets.

• Occasionally, dry skin, easy bruising, flushing, thinning hair, and night sweats.

• Rarely, headache, rash, fatigue, insomnia, and vomiting. The risk of thromboembolic disease (blood-clotting disorders) may be increased.

Estratab ⑧

A preparation of ℞ esterified estrogens.
Formulation: Tablets in several strengths.
Availability: Prescription only.
Warnings and side effects: See ℞ esterified estrogens.

Estring ⑧

A preparation of ℞ estradiol.
Formulation: Vaginal insert.
Availability: Prescription only.
Warnings and side effects: See ℞ estradiol.

Estro-Cyp ⑧

A preparation of ℞ estradiol.
Formulation: Injection.
Availability: Prescription only.
Warnings and side effects: See ℞ estradiol.

estrogen ⑩

(oestrogen)

Generics: **dienestrol; diethylstilbestrol; esterified estrogens; estrogens, conjugated; estrone; estropipate; ethinyl estradiol; mestranol.**

Actions and uses

Estrogen is the name given to the group of (℞ **steroid**) ℞ **sex hormones** that promote the growth and functioning of the female sex organs and the development of female sexual characteristics. In their natural forms, they are produced and secreted mainly by the ovary (and to a small extent the placenta of pregnant women), the adrenal cortex in both sexes and, in men, the testis.

Natural (for example, estriol, estradiol) and synthetic estrogens can be used in medicine, sometimes in combination with progestogens, to treat menstrual problems (for example, absence of menstrual periods in primary amenorrhoria), menopausal problems (℞ **hormone replacement**), or other gynecological problems, and as ℞ **oral contraceptive** agents (normally in combination with ℞ **progestogen** hormones). Some synthetic estrogens are also used to treat certain cancers (for example, ✺ **prostate cancer** and ✺ **breast cancer**). The best-known and most-used estrogens are: ℞ **estradiol**; ℞ **dienestrol**; ℞ **diethylstilbestrol**; ℞ **esterified estrogens**; ℞ **estrogens, conjugated**; ℞ **estrone**; ℞ **estropipate**; ℞ **ethinyl estradiol**; ℞ **mestranol.**

Limitations

There are a number of risks in taking estrogens for any period of time, and the severity of the condition to be treated will be taken into account. In the case of oral contraceptives, a very low dose is taken (generally combined with a progestin) and the risks for most women are considered acceptable in relation to the risk of unwanted pregnancy—although expert counseling may be advisable. For other conditions, estrogens come under the Food and Drug Administration's Pregnancy Category X, that is, they are not for use in pregnancy, and a doctor must be contacted if pregnancy occurs or is suspected while using these drugs.

In ℞ **hormone replacement** during the ✺ **menopause**, the use of progestins along with estrogen is recommended for menopausal or postmenopausal women with an intact uterus, since progestins reduce the risks of adverse cardiovascular effects. The risks are increased (for example, ✺**thromboembolism**, ✺ **stroke**, and heart attack) in particular in those over 35 years old. Cigarette smoking also increases the risks, and this added risk gets larger with age and with heavy smoking or high blood pressure. The risk of blood-clotting disorders may be increased. Glucose tolerance may worsen in diabetics.

See also the individual drug entries.

estrogen antagonist ⑩

see ℞ **antiestrogen.**

estrogens, conjugated ⑥

Type/Group: **sex hormone; estrogen; anticancer; osteoporosis treatment.**
Brand(s): **Premarin, Cenestin.** Combinations: With *medroxyprogesterone*: **Prempro, Premphase.**
How administered: Orally; injection.

Used to treat

Conjugated estrogens are sodium salts of estrogenic compounds. They can be manufactured from pregnant mare's urine, yams, or soy. They are used to treat symptoms of ✺ **menopause**, ✺ **breast cancer**, ✺ **prostate cancer**, dysfunctional uterine bleeding, ✺ **hypogonadism**, female castration, primary ovarian failure, atrophic vaginitis, and to prevent ✺ **osteoporosis**.

Warnings

• They should not be used by people with breast cancer (except for those being treated), active thromboembolic disease, known or suspected estrogen-dependent cancers, undiagnosed abnormal genital bleeding.

• They should be given with caution to people with hypertension, gallbladder disease, congestive heart failure, diabetes mellitus, depression, migraine headache, seizure disorders, liver disease, family history of breast or endometrial cancer, history of thromboembolic disorders, uterine fibroids, hypertriglyceridemia, or hypercalcemia.

• They should not be used during pregnancy. A doctor must be contacted if pregnancy occurs while using this drug.

• Medical judgment is required if breast-feeding is being considered. The quality and quantity of breast milk may be reduced.

• Taking estrogen increases the risk of endometrial cancer. The use of progestins along with estrogen is recommended for menopausal or postmenopausal women with an intact uterus, since progestins reduce the risk.

Key to symbols: ✺ = Disorder Section ℞ = Drug Section ♣ = Herbal Section ◊◊ = Supplement Section

- The risk of gallbladder disease is increased.
- May cause increases in blood pressure.
- The risk of thromboembolic disease (blood-clotting disorders) may be increased.
- Glucose tolerance in diabetics may worsen.

Interactions

- ℞ **Rifampin** and ℞ **barbiturates** may decrease the effects of estrogen.
- The steroid effects of ℞ **corticosteroids** are increased.
- ℞ **Phenytoin** causes loss of seizure control and decreased estrogen levels.
- With ℞ **warfarin sodium** and similar ℞ **anticoagulants** there is a theoretical increase in the risk of thromboembolism.

Side effects

- Nausea and vomiting, breakthrough bleeding, and spotting.
- Less frequently, depression, migraine headache, increased emotionality, elevated blood pressure, edema, contact lens intolerance, bloating, benign liver tumors, amenorrhea, change in cervical secretions, breast enlargement, breast tenderness, elevated triglyceride or calcium levels, darkening of the skin of the face, changes in libido, and weight gain.

estrone ⑥

Type/Group: **estrogen; sex hormone; anticancer**.
Brand(s): Generic only.
How administered: Injection.

Used to treat

Estrone is an estrogen used to treat symptoms of ⊙ **menopause**, ⊙ **prostate cancer**, dysfunctional uterine bleeding, ⊙ **hypogonadism**, and primary ovarian failure.

Warnings

- It should not be used by people with breast cancer, active thromboembolic disease, known or suspected estrogen-dependent cancers, or undiagnosed abnormal genital bleeding.
- It should be given with caution to people with hypertension, gallbladder disease, congestive heart failure, diabetes mellitus, depression, migraine headache, seizure disorders, liver disease, family history of breast or endometrial cancer, history of thromboembolic disorders, hypertriglyceridemia, or hypercalcemia.
- Estrone should not be used during pregnancy. A doctor must be contacted if pregnancy occurs while using this drug.
- Medical judgment is required if breast-feeding is being considered. It may reduce the quality and quantity of breast milk.
- Taking estrogen increases the risk of endometrial cancer. The use of progestins along with estrogen is recommended for menopausal or postmenopausal women with an intact uterus, since progestins reduce the risk.
- The risk of gallbladder disease is increased.
- It may cause increases in blood pressure.
- The risk of thromboembolic disease (blood-clotting disorders) may be increased.
- It may worsen glucose tolerance in diabetics.

Interactions

- ℞ **Rifampin** and ℞ **barbiturates** may decrease the effects of estrone.
- The steroid effects of ℞ **corticosteroids** are increased.
- ℞ **Phenytoin** causes loss of seizure control and decreased estrogen levels.
- With ℞ **warfarin sodium** and similar ℞ **anticoagulants** there is a theoretical increase in the risk of thromboembolism.

Side effects

- Nausea and vomiting, breakthrough bleeding, and spotting.
- Less frequently, depression, migraine headache, increased emotionality, elevated blood pressure, edema, contact lens intolerance, bloating, benign liver tumors, cessation of menses, change in cervical secretions, breast enlargement, breast tenderness, elevated triglyceride or calcium levels, darkening of the skin of the face, changes in libido, and weight gain.

estropipate ⑥

Type/Group: **estrogen; sex hormone**.
Brand(s): Ogen; Ortho-Est.
How administered: Injection.

Used to treat

Estropipate is used in the treatment of symptoms of the ⊙ **menopause**, the prevention of ⊙ **osteoporosis**, and female ⊙ **hypogonadism** (subnormal secretion of sex hormones), female castration, or primary ovarian failure.

Warnings

- It should not be used by people with breast cancer (except for selected individuals being treated for metastatic disease), active thromboembolic disease, known or suspected estrogen-dependent cancers, or undiagnosed abnormal genital bleeding.
- It should be given with caution to people with hypertension, gallbladder disease, congestive heart failure, diabetes mellitus, depression, migraine headache, seizure disorders, liver disease, family history of breast or endometrial cancer, history of thromboembolic disorders, hypertriglyceridemia, or hypercalcemia.
- Estropipate must not be used during pregnancy. A doctor must be contacted if pregnancy occurs while using this drug.
- Medical judgment is required if breast-feeding is being considered. It may reduce the quality and quantity of breast milk.
- Taking estrogen increases the risk of endometrial cancer. The use of progestins along with estrogen is recommended for menopausal or postmenopausal women with an intact uterus, since progestins reduce the risk.
- The risk of gallbladder disease is increased.
- It may cause increases in blood pressure.
- The risk of thromboembolic disease (blood-clotting disorders) may be increased.
- It may worsen glucose tolerance in diabetics.

Interactions

- ℞ **Rifampin** and ℞ **barbiturates** may decrease the effects of estrogen.
- The steroid effects of ℞ **corticosteroids** are increased.

• R Phenytoin causes loss of seizure control and decreased estrogen levels.
• With R **warfarin sodium** and similar R **anticoagulants** there is a theoretical increase in the risk of thromboembolism.

Side effects
• Nausea and vomiting, breakthrough bleeding, and spotting.
• Less frequently, depression, migraine headache, increased emotionality, elevated blood pressure, edema, contact lens intolerance, bloating, benign liver tumors, cessation of menses, change in cervical secretions, breast enlargement, breast tenderness, elevated triglyceride or calcium levels, darkening of the skin of the face, changes in libido, and weight gain.

Estrostep ®
A preparation of R **ethinyl estradiol** and R **norethindrone**.
Formulation: Calendar pack of oral tablets.
Availability: Prescription only.
Warnings and side effects: See R **ethinyl estradiol**; R **norethindrone**.

Estrostep Fe ®
A preparation of R **ethinyl estradiol**, R **norethindrone**, and ♐ **iron** (ferrous fumarate).
Formulation: Calendar pack of oral tablets.
Availability: Prescription only.
Warnings and side effects: See R **ethinyl estradiol**; R **norethindrone**; ♐ **iron**.

etanercept ⑤
Type/Group: **antirheumatic; immunomodulator; immunosuppressant**.
Brand(s): Enbrel.
How administered: Subcutaneous injection.

Used to treat
Etanercept is used to treat moderately to severely active ✪ **rheumatoid arthritis** (RA). It can be used in combination with R **methotrexate**. It is a synthesized molecule that binds to and neutralizes a substance called human tumor necrosis factor (TNF), which has an important association with the inflammatory process in rheumatoid arthritis.

Warnings
• It should not be given to people with known hypersensitivity to this drug or to substances in the injection (benzyl alcohol, mannitol, latex), or to anyone with sepsis.
• It should be given with caution to people with a history of recurring infection or a condition that predisposes to infection, such as poorly controlled diabetes mellitus. This is a specialist drug and is used only after a full medical assessment.
• Studies have not been done on its safety during pregnancy and so it should be used only if it is clearly needed.
• Medical judgment is required if breast-feeding is being considered.
• Treatment should not start when an infection is present, and should be stopped if infection occurs.

• Live R **vaccines** should not be given during a course of treatment.
• The possibility exists of a higher risk of infection or malignancy in treatments that neutralize tumor necrosis factor (TNF), although there is no evidence as yet that etanercept has such an effect.
• Antibodies to "self" (autoantibodies) may be created, but no new autoimmune disease (for example, lupus) has been reported with use of this drug.

Interactions
No interactions of significance are known, but studies have not been carried out.

Side effects
• The most common side effect is upper respiratory infection.
• Other effects include non-respiratory infections, headache, rhinitis, cough, sore throat, indigestion, abdominal pain, rash, and a feeling of weakness.
• There may be redness, pain, and inflammation at the site of injection. Allergic reactions are rare and anaphylaxis has not been reported.

ethacrynic acid ⑤
Type/Group: **diuretic; heart failure treatment**.
Brand(s): Edecrin.
How administered: Orally; injection.

Used to treat
Ethacrynic acid is a powerful diuretic of the loop class. It can be used to treat edema (including edema associated with congestive heart failure, kidney disease, cirrhosis of the liver and fluid build-up in the lungs).

Warnings
• It should not be given to people with known hypersensitivity to this drug, with anuria (no urine), in an electrolyte-depleted state, or who develop severe watery diarrhea when using ethacrynic acid.
• It should be given with caution to people with cirrhosis of the liver, or who have certain kidney disorders, gout, diabetes mellitus, electrolyte depletion, an enlarged prostate gland, chronic obstructive pulmonary disease (COPD), or porphyria.
• Ethacrynic acid should be used in pregnancy only if it is clearly needed.
• Medical judgment is required if breast-feeding is being considered.
• Dehydration may result from too intense a diuretic effect, particularly in elderly people or those on restricted sodium diets.
• Early symptoms of electrolyte imbalance may include muscle weakness or cramps, nausea, or dizziness. A doctor must be contacted if such symptoms appear.
• Loop diuretics may aggravate symptoms of diabetes mellitus or gout, and worsen or activate lupus erythematosus.
• Periodic monitoring of electrolytes, and kidney and liver and other functions will be carried out.
• There may be photosensitivity (abnormal sensitivity to sunlight) and so exposure should be minimized.

Interactions
• The risk of R **lithium** toxicity is increased and generally these two drugs should not be used together.

• The effects of ℞ **aminoglycosides**, other ℞ **antihypertensives**, ℞ **cardiac glycosides**, ℞ **chloral hydrate**, and ℞ **propranolol** may be increased, with the potential for significant side effects or toxicity. An increased effect is sometimes used to advantage in combining loop diuretics with other antihypertensives.

• If taken with ℞ **sulfonylureas**, blood sugar levels may be raised in diabetics with previously stabilized regimens.

• If taken with ℞ **cisplatin**, there is the potential for additive effects and toxicity.

• ℞ **Amphotericin B**, ℞ **corticosteroids**, and ℞ **corticotropin** may increase the diuretic effect of reducing potassium levels, with the possibility of severe depletion.

• The levels of ℞ **warfarin sodium** may rise and a reduction of dose may be necessary.

• The effects of nondepolarizing ℞ **skeletal muscle relaxants** and ℞ **theophylline** become unpredictable.

• ℞ **Activated charcoal**, ℞ **hydantoins**, ℞ **NSAIDs**, and antigout agents (for example, ℞ **probenecid**, ℞ **sulfinpyrazone**) may reduce the effects of ethacrynic acid.

Side effects

• There may be an abnormally low blood pressure (hypotension), gastrointestinal disturbances, raised levels of urea in the blood or gout, raised blood glucose, changes in fats in the blood, headache, dizziness, ringing in the ears and hearing loss. Electrolyte levels in the blood (for example, potassium, sodium, magnesium, and chloride) may be lowered. There may be skin rashes, photosensitivity, effects on bone marrow, blood changes, or pancreatitis. Many of these effects are only seen with high or prolonged dosage. Hearing loss (usually reversible) is associated with rapid injection, high dosage, and using at the same time other drugs that affect hearing.

ethambutol Ⓖ

Type/Group: **antibacterial; antituberculosis**.
Brand(s): Myambutol.
How administered: Orally.

Used to treat

Ethambutol is used in the treatment of ✛ **tuberculosis** that is resistant to other types of drug. It is used in combination (to cover resistance and for maximum effect) with other antituberculosis drugs, such as ℞ **isoniazid**, ℞ **pyrazinamide**, and ℞ **rifampicin**. Although not stated by the manufacturer for such use, it may also be prescribed to treat mycobacterium avium complex (MAC) in people with ✛ **AIDS**.

Warnings

• It should not be given to people with known hypersensitivity to ethambutol or with known inflammation of the optic nerve.

• It should be given with caution to people with kidney liver and blood dysfunction, gout, or certain eye problems.

• Ethambutol should be used during pregnancy only when it is clearly needed.

• It is compatible with breast-feeding.

• It may have adverse, usually reversible, effects on vision. A doctor must be contacted promptly if changes in vision (for example, blurring, red-green color blindness, eye pain) occur.

Interactions

• Aluminum salts may delay or reduce the absorption of ethambutol.

Side effects

• Occasionally, acute gout, confusion, gastrointestinal effects, headache, and visual disturbances.

• Rarely, rash, fever, inflammation of peripheral nerves, blood cell changes, and severe allergic reaction.

Ethamolin Ⓑ

A preparation of ℞ **ethanolamine oleate**.
Formulation: Injection.
Availability: Prescription only.
Warnings and side effects: See ℞ **ethanolamine oleate**.

ethanolamine oleate Ⓖ

(monoethanolamine oleate)
Type/Group: **sclerosing agent**.
Brand(s): Ethamolin.
How administered: Injection.

Used to treat

Ethanolamine is used in sclerotherapy, which is a technique to treat ✛ **varicose veins** by the injection of an irritant solution. It is used specifically in the treatment of varices (enlarged, tortuous knots of blood vessels) in the esophagus that have recently bled.

Warnings

• It should not be given to people with known hypersensitivity to this drug or to oleic acid.

• It should be given with caution to people who are elderly or debilitated, with heart or respiratory disease, or liver or kidney impairment.

• Ethanolamine's safety during pregnancy has not been established and it should be used only if clearly needed.

• Medical judgment is required if breast-feeding is being considered.

• A severe reaction is possible at the site of injection, with death of the surrounding tissue. This drug will only be given by physicians familiar with the appropriate technique.

Interactions

No drug interactions of significance are known, and thorough studies have not been performed.

Side effects

• There may be pleural (the membrane covering the lungs) inflammation, ulcer, or constriction of the esophagus, fever or pain beneath the sternum.

• Aspiration pneumonia and allergic reactions (including anaphylaxis) have been reported.

ethinyl estradiol Ⓖ

Type/Group: **sex hormone; estrogen; contraceptive; anticancer**.
Brand(s): Estinyl. Combinations: With *desogestrel*: Mircett; Desogen; Ortho-Cept. With *ethynodiol diacetate*: Demulen; Zovia. With *levonorgestrel*: Alesse; Levlen; Levlite; Levora; Nordette; Preven; Tri-Leven; Triphasil; Trivora-28. With *norethindrone*

(menopausal symptoms): Femhrt, Activella, CombiPatch. With *norethindrone* (contraception): Brevicon; Estrostep; Estrostep Fe; Jenest-28; Loestrin; Loestrin Fe; Modicon; Necon; Nelova; Norinyl; Ovcon; Ortho-Novum; Tri-Norinyl. With *norgestimate:* Ortho-Cyclen; Ortho-Tri-Cyclen. With *norgestrel:* Ogestrel; LoOvral; Ovral-28; Low-Ogestrel.

How administered: Orally.

Used to treat
Ethinyl estradiol is a synthetic estrogen and is used as a contraceptive in combination with progestins. It is also used to treat symptoms associated with ✪ **menopause**, atrophic vaginitis, ✪ **hypogonadism**, inoperable female ✪ **breast cancer**, and ✪ **prostate cancer**. Although not stated by the manufacturer for such treatment, it may be prescribed for kraurosis vulvae, postpartum breast engorgement, and for the prevention of ✪ **osteoporosis**.

Warnings
• It should not be used by people with breast cancer (except for those being treated with ethinyl estradiol), active thromboembolic disease, known or suspected estrogen-dependent cancers, or undiagnosed abnormal genital bleeding.

• It should be given with caution to people with hypertension, gallbladder disease, congestive heart failure, diabetes mellitus, depression, migraine headache, seizure disorders, liver disease, family history of breast or endometrial cancer, history of thromboembolic disorders, uterine fibroids, hypertriglyceridemia, or hypercalcemia.

• Ethinyl estradiol must not be used during pregnancy. A doctor must be contacted if pregnancy occurs while using this drug.

• Medical judgment is required if breast-feeding is being considered. It may reduce the quality and quantity of breast milk.

• The use of progestins along with estrogen is recommended for menopausal or postmenopausal women with an intact uterus. Taking estrogen increases the risk of endometrial cancer in these women, but adding progestins reduces the risk.

• The use of oral contraceptives including those containing ethinyl estradiol are associated with a risk of serious cardiovascular side effects (for example, embolism, stroke, heart attack), particularly in those over the age of 35. Cigarette smoking increases the risk. This added risk gets larger with age and with heavy smoking (over 15 per day), and is quite marked in women over 35.

Interactions
• ℞ **Rifampin** and ℞ **barbiturates** may decrease the effects of estrogen.

• The steroid effects of ℞ **corticosteroids** are increased.

• ℞ **Phenytoin** causes loss of seizure control and decreased estrogen levels.

• With ℞ **warfarin sodium** and similar ℞ **anticoagulants** there is a theoretical increase in the risk of thromboembolism.

Side effects
• Depending on use, there may be nausea and vomiting, breakthrough bleeding, and spotting.

• Less frequently, depression, migraine headache, increased emotionality, elevated blood pressure, venous thrombosis, edema, contact lens intolerance, gallbladder disease, bloating, benign liver

tumors, cessation of menses, change in cervical secretions, breast enlargement, breast tenderness, elevated blood glucose, elevated triglyceride or calcium levels, darkening of the skin of the face, changes in libido, and weight gain.

• Rarely, endometrial cancer.

• The risk of thromboembolic disease (blood-clotting disorders) may be increased.

Ethmozine ®
A preparation of ℞ **moricizine hydrochloride**.
Formulation: Oral tablets (three strengths).
Availability: Prescription only.
Warnings and side effects: See ℞ **moricizine hydrochloride**.

ethosuximide ©
Type/Group: **anticonvulsant; antiepileptic**.
Brand(s): Zarontin Tablets, Syrup; various generic.
How administered: Orally.

Used to treat
Ethosuximide is used to treat ✪ **epilepsy**, mainly absence seizures (petit mal), and some other types of seizures.

Warnings
• Avoid its use in people with known hypersensitivity to this drug.

• It should be given with caution to people with porphyria, kidney or liver impairment.

• Ethosuximide is associated with an increase in frequency of certain birth defects and should not be used during pregnancy. However, because uncontrolled seizures can also threaten fetal health, medical judgment is needed to weigh potential benefits and risks.

• Medical judgment is also required if breast-feeding is being considred.

• If symptoms such as skin rash, joint pain, blurred vision, sore throat, fever, bruising or mouth ulcers occur, medical help should be sought.

• When used alone to treat mixed forms of epilepsy, ethosuximide may cause an increase in grand mal seizures.

• Withdrawal should be gradual otherwise it may precipitate attacks.

• Ethosuximide may cause drowsiness, and so driving or other hazardous activity should be avoided.

Interactions
• Ethosuximide may raise levels of the drugs ℞ **mephenytoin** and ℞ **phenytoin**.

• When taken with ℞ **valproate sodium** the effects are unpredictable, but levels of ethosuximide may rise or fall.

• The levels of ℞ **primidone** and ℞ **phenobarbital** (and other ℞ **barbiturates**) may be reduced.

Side effects
There are a wide range and include:

• Drowsiness, dizziness, unsteady gait, and gastrointestinal disturbances;

• Itching, confusion, headache, hiccup, and heartburn;

• Lethargy, depression, or mild euphoria, and aggressive behavior;

• Rashes, liver and potentially serious kidney changes, and effects on blood;
• Rarely, psychotic states, suicidal behavior, and auditory hallucinations.

Ethyol ⑧

A preparation of ℞ **amifostine**.
Formulation: Injection (infusion).
Availability: See Prescription only.

etidocaine ⑥

Type/Group: local anesthetic.
Brand(s): Duranest.
How administered: Local injection.
Used to treat
Etidocaine is used for peripheral and central nerve block and infiltration, for anesthesia in intra-abdominal, pelvic, and lower limb surgery, and cesarean section procedures. It is particularly long-acting.
Warnings
• It should not be given to people with known hypersensitivity to etidocaine. It is a specialist drug and there will be a full medical assessment.
• Etodocaine should be used during pregnancy only if it is clearly needed.
• Medical judgment is required if breast-feeding is being considered.
• It can cause cardiac depression, peripheral vasodilatation, or CNS (central nervous system) toxicity.
Interactions
• There may be additive effects if used with ℞ **antiarrhythmics** (for example, ℞ **tocainide**, ℞ **mexiletine**).
Side effects
• Occasionally, pain at injection site, burning, stinging, or tenderness where applied.
• Rarely (generally with a high dose), drowsiness, dizziness, disorientation, lightheadedness, tremors, apprehension, euphoria, sensation of heat, cold, or numbness, blurred or double vision, ringing or roaring in ears, nausea, or allergic reactions.

etidronate disodium ⑥

(disodium etidronate)
Type/Group: bisphosphonate; calcium-metabolism modifier.
Brand(s): Didronel.
How administered: Orally; intravenous infusion.
Used to treat
Etidronate is used to treat ✪ **Paget's disease (of the bone)**, to prevent and treat heterotropic ossification due to spinal cord injury or hip replacement, and to treat hormone-induced disorders of bone metabolism, bone pain in prostate and breast cancer, and ✪ **hypercalcemia** due to malignancy.
Warnings
• It should not be given to people with known hypersensitivity to bisphosphonates, or severe kidney function impairment.

• It should be given with caution to people with enterocolitis, kidney impairment, and those who are unable to maintain adequate intake of vitamin D or calcium.
• It should be used during pregnancy only if clearly needed.
• Medical judgment is required if breast-feeding is being considered. It is not known if it appears in breast milk.
• It should be taken on an empty stomach, two hours before meals.
• Kidney damage is possible with intravenous infusion.
Interactions
• ℞ **Antacids** reduce absorption.
Side effects
• Frequently, nausea, diarrhea, increased, continuing, or more frequent bone pain in people with Paget's disease.
• Occasionally, bone fractures, and altered taste.
• Rarely, allergic skin reaction.

etodolac ⑥

Type/Group: anti-inflammatory; antirheumatic; non-narcotic analgesic; NSAID.
Brand(s): Lodine Tablets, Capsules, Lodine XL; various generic.
How administered: Orally.
Used to treat
Etodolac is used primarily for long-term management of ✪ **arthritis** (for example, osteoarthritis) and ✪ **pain**.
Warnings
• It should not be used by people with known hypersensitivity to this drug or to other NSAIDs (including ℞ **aspirin**), who have chronic kidney disease, certain bleeding disorders or conditions (for example, hemophilia, vitamin K deficiency, low blood-platelet levels), or who have a tendency to, or active, peptic ulceration.
• It should be given with caution to people taking certain drugs for gout, or with allergic disorders (especially asthma and skin conditions), who are elderly, or with any kind of kidney impairment or with certain liver disorders.
• Etodolac should be used during pregnancy only when medically judged to be needed. Its risks to the fetus increase In the third trimester, however, and so should only be used if the benefits outweigh the risks to the fetus, which are higher at this time.
• Breast-feeding mothers should either discontinue this drug or stop breast-feeding.
• With regular, long-term use (as in the treatment of osteoarthritis), NSAIDs may cause gastrointestinal bleeding, ulceration, or perforation. Any signs of bleeding (for example, black stools) should be reported to a physician immediately.
• Most NSAIDs have the potential, particularly with regular use, to cause liver damage. Periodic evaluation of liver function is necessary in long-term therapy (more than two months).
• Side effects are more frequent in the elderly.
• Gastrointestinal upsets may be minimized by taking it with milk or food.
Interactions
• There is generally no added benefit in taking other NSAIDs or other ℞ **salicylates** at the same time, but there is a higher risk of gastrointestinal upsets and bleeding.

• ℞ **Anticoagulants** (for example, ℞ **warfarin sodium**) may prolong bleeding.

• Alcohol increases the risk of bleeding, particularly if there is an existing ulcer.

• The effects of ℞ **cyclosporine**, ℞ **digoxin**, ℞ **lithium**, and ℞ **methotrexate** may be exaggerated, with potential for serious toxicity.

• Etodolac taken with ℞ **insulin** or ℞ **oral hypoglycemic**s may alter the glucose-lowering effect.

• ℞ **Beta-blockers**, ℞ **diuretics**, and ℞ **hydrochlorothiazide** may lose some of their effectiveness.

• ℞ **colestipol hydrochloride** and ℞ **sucralfate** may lower the absorption or effectiveness of etodolac.

• Foodstuffs and herbals with ℞ **antiplatelet** properties, for example ♣ **ginger**, ♒ **garlic**, and various herbal preparations, may enhance the antiplatelet effect of NSAIDs.

Side effects

These vary in severity and how often they occur.

• Commonly, gastrointestinal upsets, nausea, diarrhea, flatulence, dizziness, and malaise.

• Less frequently there may be constipation, vomiting, headache, rash, ringing in the ears, fluid retention, edema, fatigue, and sleep disturbances.

• Prolonged bleeding time (with consequent risk of ulceration) is possible with high dosage, and other blood changes can occur, including anemia.

• Hypersensitivity reactions may include symptoms such as hives, chest tightness, asthma, or bronchospasm.

• Reversible kidney failure, particularly in renal impairment, has occurred. Liver damage is rare.

Etopophos ®

A preparation of ℞ etoposide.
Formulation: Injection.
Availability: Prescription only.
Warnings and side effects: See ℞ etoposide.

etoposide ⑥

(V-16)
Type/Group: **anticancer; cytotoxic.**
Brand(s): Etopophos; Toposar; VePesid; various generic.
How administered: Orally; intravenous injection.

Used to treat

Etoposide is used primarily to treat small cell ✪ **lung cancer**, ✪ **lymphomas**, and sometimes cancer of the testes. It works in much the same way as the ℞ **vinca alkaloids** by disrupting the replication of cancer cells and so preventing further growth.

Warnings

• It should not be given to people with known hypersensitivity to etoposide or any of its components.

• It should be given with caution to people with active infections, certain blood disorders, kidney or liver dysfunction, who have had previous chemotherapy or radiation, and those with a history of herpes infections. This is a specialist drug which will be used following a full evaluation by specialist physicians.

• Etoposide is not recommended for use during pregnancy unless it is medically judged to be essential, because it may cause birth defects. Becoming pregnant while using this drug must be avoided.

• It should not be used if breast-feeding.

• Bone marrow depression is a major toxic side effect of this drug.

• Occasionally, adverse effects on liver may occur.

• It can impair fertility (which may be reversible).

• A physician must be contacted if fever, chills, difficulty breathing, or rapid heartbeat occur.

• In common with many anticancer drugs, this drug may cause cancer.

Interactions

• ℞ **cyclosporine** may increase the effects of etoposide.

• The effects of ℞ **warfarin sodium** may be increased.

Side effects

• Frequently, nausea, vomiting, and loss of hair.

• Occasionally, diarrhea, loss of appetite, inflammation of mouth mucosa.

• Rarely, hypotension and effects on peripheral nerves (for example, burning or tingling sensation).

Etrafon ®

A preparation of ℞ **perphenazine** and ℞ **amitriptyline hydrochloride.**
Formulation: Oral tablets in several strengths.
Availability: Prescription only.
Warnings and side effects: See ℞ **perphenazine**; ℞ **amitriptyline hydrochloride**.

Eucerin Cream ®

A preparation of ℞ **petrolatum** and ℞ **mineral oil**.
Formulation: Topical cream.
Availability: OTC.
Warnings and side effects: See ℞ **petrolatum** and ℞ **mineral oil**.

Eucerin Moisturizing ®

A preparation of ℞ **mineral oil**, ℞ **lanolin**, and ℞ **sorbitol**.
Formulation: Topical lotion.
Availability: OTC.
Warnings and side effects: See ℞ **mineral oil**; ℞ **lanolin**; ℞ **sorbitol**.

Eudal-SR Tablets ®

A preparation of ℞ **pseudoephedrine** and ℞ **guaifenesin**.
Formulation: Oral tablets, sustained release.
Availability: Prescription only.
Warnings and side effects: See ℞ **pseudoephedrine**; ℞ **guaifenesin**.

Eulexin ®

A preparation of ℞ **flutamide**.
Formulation: Oral capsules.
Availability: Prescription only.
Warnings and side effects: See ℞ **flutamide**.

Eurax ®

A preparation of ℞ **crotamiton**.
Formulation: Topical cream; topical lotion.
Availability: Prescription only.
Warnings and side effects: See ℞ **crotamiton**.

Evista ®

A preparation of ℞ **raloxifene**.
Formulation: Oral tablets.
Availability: Prescription only.
Warnings and side effects: See ℞ **raloxifene**.

Evoxac ®

A preparation of ℞ **cevimeline hydrochloride**.
Formulation: Oral capsules.
Availability: Prescription only.
Warnings and side effects: See ℞ **cevimeline hydrochloride**.

Exact ®

A preparation of ℞ **salicylic acid**, ℞ **menthol**, and various.
Formulation: Topical liquid.
Availability: OTC.
Warnings and side effects: See ℞ **salicylic acid**; ℞ **menthol**.

Excedrin Aspirin Free Caplets, Geltabs ®

A preparation of ℞ **acetaminophen** and ℞ **caffeine**.
Formulation: Oral tablets; geltabs.
Availability: OTC.
Warnings and side effects: See ℞ **acetaminophen**; ℞ **caffeine**.

Excedrin Migraine; Extra Strength Caplets; Tablets; Geltabs ®

A preparation of ℞ **acetaminophen**, ℞ **aspirin**, and ℞ **caffeine**.
Formulation: Oral tablets; gel tablets.
Availability: OTC.
Warnings and side effects: See ℞ **acetaminophen**; ℞ **aspirin**; ℞ **caffeine**.

Exelderm ®

A preparation of ℞ **sulconazole nitrate**.
Formulation: Topical cream, topical solution.
Availability: Prescription only.
Warnings and side effects: See ℞ **sulconazole nitrate**.

Exelon ®

A preparation of ℞ **rivastigmine**.
Formulation: Oral capsules; solution.
Availability: Prescription only.
Warnings and side effects: See ℞ **rivastigmine**.

exemestane Ⓖ

Type/Group: **anticancer; hormone antagonist**.
Brand(s): Aromasin.
How administered: Orally.

Used to treat

Exemestane is used to treat advanced ✪ **breast cancer** in post-menopausal women whose disease has progressed following anti-estrogen (for example, tamoxifen) treatment. It is an aromatase inhibitor that works by inhibiting the conversion of androgens (male sex hormones) into estrogens. Although not stated by the manufacturer for such treatment, it may be prescribed to prevent ✪ **prostate cancer**.

Warnings

• It should not be used by people with known hypersensitivity to this drug, or whose disease is not responsive to antiestrogen treatment.
• It should be given with caution to people with impaired liver function.
• Exemestane should not be used during pregnancy. A doctor must be notified if pregnancy occurs while taking this drug.
• Should be used with care by nursing mothers.
• It may cause a decline in lymphocyte levels, although there will probably be no significant increased tendency to viral infections.

Interactions

• Blood levels of the drug may increase markedly after a high-fat meal.

Side effects

• Gastrointestinal effects, nausea, fatigue, hot flashes, pain, depression, insomnia, anxiety, dizziness, headache, edema, sweating, and elevated blood pressure.

Ex-Histine Syrup ®

A preparation of methscopolamine nitrate, ℞ **chlorpheniramine maleate**, and ℞ **phenylephrine hydrochloride**.
Formulation: Oral syrup.
Availability: Prescription only.
Warnings and side effects: See ℞ **scopolamine hydrobromide**; ℞ **chlorpheniramine maleate**; ℞ **phenylephrine hydrochloride**.

ex-lax; ex-lax chocolated ®

A preparation of ℞ **senna**.
Formulation: Oral tablets (and chocolated tablet preparation).
Availability: OTC.
Warnings and side effects: See ℞ **senna**.

Ex-lax Stool Softener ®

A preparation of ℞ **docusate sodium**.
Formulation: Oral tablets.
Availability: OTC.
Warnings and side effects: See ℞ **docusate sodium**.

Exna ®

A preparation of ℞ **benzthiazide**.
Formulation: Oral tablets.
Availability: Prescription only.
Warnings and side effects: See ℞ **benzthiazide**. Tablets contain tartrazine (FD&C yellow No 5), a dye that may cause allergic reaction in a few people, but especially those with sensitivity to aspirin.

Exocaine Medicated Rub; Exocaine Plus Rub ⑧

A preparation of ℞ **methyl salicylate** and various.
Formulation: Topical ointment.
Availability: OTC.
Warnings and side effects: See ℞ **methyl salicylate**.

expectorant ⑩

Generics: ammonium chloride; guaifenesin; ipecac syrup.

Actions and uses

Expectorants are incorporated into medicated liquids intended to change the viscosity of sputum (phlegm), so making it more watery and easier to cough up (an action of ℞ **mucolytic** drugs). In high dosage, some expectorants, for example, ipecacuanha (℞ **ipecac syrup**), can also be used as ℞ **emetic** drugs (to induce vomiting). It is because of this that they are usually thought to act as expectorants by stimulating nerves in the stomach to cause a reflex secretion of fluid by the bronchioles in the lungs (see ⊙ **catarrh**, ⊙ **bronchial congestion**). However, it is not known for sure how expectorants work and, further, there is considerable doubt about their effectiveness. The most commonly used is ℞ **guaifenesin** (guaiphenesin), and it (and ammonium chloride) is incorporated into many ℞ **cold and cough preparation** OTC (over-the-counter) mixtures.

Limitations

See the individual drug entries.

Extendryl Chewable Tablets; Jr. Capsules; Syrup ⑧

A preparation of methscopolamine nitrate, ℞ **chlorpheniramine maleate**, and ℞ **phenylephrine hydrochloride**.
Formulation: Oral tablets; capsules; syrup.
Availability: Prescription only.
Warnings and side effects: See ℞ **scopolamine hydrobromide**; ℞ **chlorpheniramine maleate**; ℞ **phenylephrine hydrochloride**.

Eye-Sed ⑧

A preparation of ℞ **zinc sulfate**.
Formulation: Eyedrops.
Availability: OTC.
Warnings and side effects: See ℞ **zinc sulfate**.

Eyesine ⑧

A preparation of ℞ **tetrahydrozoline hydrochloride**.
Formulation: Eye drops.
Availability: OTC.
Warnings and side effects: See ℞ **tetrahydrozoline hydrochloride**.

eye treatment ⑩

Generics: fluorescein sodium; rose bengal; tropicamide; verteporfin.

Actions and uses

Many different classes of drugs are used in eye treatments. ⊙ **glaucoma** is a common and potentially serious condition, and ℞ **glaucoma treatment** involves the use of drugs to lower the raised intraocular pressure (raised pressure in the eyeball) that usually is a characteristic of this group of eye conditions. Drugs used include ℞ **carbonic anhydrase inhibitor** drugs, ℞ **beta-blocker** drugs, some ℞ **sympathomimetic** drugs, and certain ℞ **parasympathomimetic** cholinergic drugs. Either to treat disease states, or to allow certain ophthalmic investigations, ℞ **miotic** agents (that constrict the pupil), and ℞ **cycloplegic** drugs (that paralyze the focusing muscles of the eye) and ℞ **mydriatic** drugs (that dilate the pupil of the eye) are used. ℞ **artificial tears** are used where there is tear deficiency and dryness of the eyes due to disease, such as Sjögren's syndrome. Where there is infection of the eye and its orbit, (often ℞ **antibiotic**) ℞ **antibacterial** agents and sometimes ℞ **antifungal** or ℞ **antiviral** drugs are used, normally as eyedrops or an eye ointment.

Various other agents are used diagnostically on the eye, including ℞ **fluorescein sodium** and ℞ **rose bengal**, which are dyes used in ophthalmic diagnostic procedures or ophthalmic angiography. The unusual agent ℞ **verteporfin** is used in the treatment of age-related macular degeneration (AMD), and the drug is used for ophthalmic phototherapy where the retina is exposed to non-thermal red laser light.

Limitations

See the individual drug entries.

Ezide ⑧

A preparation of ℞ **hydrochlorothiazide**.
Formulation: Oral tablets.
Availability: Prescription only.
Warnings and side effects: See ℞ **hydrochlorothiazide**.

Factor IX ⑥

(Factor IX complex)
Type/Group: hemostatic.
Brand(s): (Derived from human plasma): With *Factor IX* only: Mononine. With *Factors II, VII, IX, X*: AlphaNine SD; Hemonyne; Konyne 80; Profilnine SD; Proplex T. (Recombinant synthetic; *Factor IX* only): Benefix.
How administered: Intravenous infusion.

Used to treat

Factor IX is a hemostatic and antihemophilic agent used to prevent or control bleeding episodes in persons with a deficiency in Factor IX (Christmas Factor), ⊙ **hemophilia** B (Christmas disease). Some of these substances are prepared from human blood plasma, others are synthesized by recombinant techniques. Several also contain clotting Factors II, VII, and X (and in other plasma-derived forms, these factors may be present in nearly undetectable amounts).

Warnings

• It should not be given to people with known hypersensitivity to mouse protein (applies only to the brand Mononine) or hamster protein (applies only to Benefix). It will be administered by experienced personnel after a full medical assessment.

• It should be given with caution to people with liver disease.

• It should be used during pregnancy only when it is clearly needed.

• Medical judgment is required if breast-feeding is being considered.

• In using those substances that are derived from human blood plasma, there is risk of exposure to viral infection (for example, AIDS and hepatitis A, B, and C). Where possible, vaccination, for instance against hepatitis A and B, is recommended, but infection with hepatitis C is most likely.

• There is some risk of thrombosis when these clotting factors are used. If uncontrolled generalized clotting (disseminated intravascular coagulation; DIC) occurs, the use of Factor IX should stop immediately.

• Hypersensitivity symptoms, such as hives, tightness of the chest or wheezing, should be reported to a doctor—although such reactions have only been reported with use of the brand form Mononine, which contains traces of mouse protein.

• Trace amounts of the proteins that distinguish the blood groups (ABO) may be present. With large or frequent doses the possibility exists for blood-type incompatibility reactions (for example, hemolytic anemia) in persons with type A, B, or AB blood.

Interactions

• ℞ **aminocaproic acid** should not be used with Factor IX.

• The levels of oral ℞ **anticoagulants** (for example, ℞ **warfarin sodium**, ℞ **anisindione**) may be lowered.

Side effects

• Rapid infusion may result in headache, flushing, changes in blood pressure or heart rate, fever, chills, tingling sensations, or nausea.

• High doses have been linked with heart attack, venous thrombosis, and pulmonary embolism.

Factor VIII Ⓖ
see ℞ **antihemophilic factor**.

Factor VIII inhibitor bypassing fraction Ⓖ
see ℞ **anti-inhibitor coagulant complex**.

famciclovir Ⓖ
Type/Group: **antiviral**.
Brand(s): Famvir.
How administered: Orally.

Used to treat
Famciclovir is used to treat acute infections caused by herpes zoster and for recurrent genital herpes (see ✪ **herpes**). It is similar to ℞ **acyclovir**, but can be given less often. It is a prodrug of ℞ **penciclovir**.

Warnings

• It should not be given to people with known hypersensitivity to famciclovir.

• It should be given with caution to people with kidney function impairment.

• Famciclovir's safety during pregnancy has not been established, and it should be used only when the potential benefits outweigh the possible risk to the fetus.

• Medical judgment is required if breast-feeding is being considered.

• Intercourse should be avoided when genital herpes symptoms are active to avoid infecting the partner.

Interactions
No significant interactions have been reported.

Side effects

• Frequently, headache, diarrhea, and nausea.

• Occasionally, dizziness, drowsiness, numbness of feet, gastrointestinal effects, fatigue, fever, sore throat, sinusitis, and itching.

• Rarely, insomnia, back pain, and joint pain.

famotidine Ⓖ
Type/Group: **H_2-antagonist; ulcer-healing drug**.
Brand(s): Pepcid, Pepcid AC.
How administered: Orally; injection; infusion.

Used to treat
Famotidine is used to assist in the treatment of benign ✪ **peptic ulcers** (gastric and duodenal), to relieve heartburn in cases of reflux esophagitis, ✪ **Zollinger-Ellison syndrome**, and a variety of conditions where reduction of acidity is beneficial. It is now also available without prescription (in a limited amount and for short-term uses only) for the relief of heartburn, ✪ **indigestion**, acid indigestion/hyperacidity, and sour stomach. It works by reducing the secretion of gastric acid (by acting as a histamine receptor—H_2-receptor—antagonist), so reducing erosion and bleeding from peptic ulcers and allowing them a chance to heal. However, treatment with famotidine should not begin before a full diagnosis of gastric bleeding or serious pain has been completed, because its action in restricting gastric secretions may possibly mask the presence of stomach cancer.

Warnings

• It should not be given to people with known hypersensitivity to this drug.

• It should be given with caution to people with kidney or liver impairment.

• Famotidine should be used during pregnancy only if it is clearly needed.

• It may appear in breast milk and should not be used by nursing mothers.

• Although rare, confusional states (depression, anxiety, psychosis, hallucinations) have occurred. The risk is highest among those who are severely ill or have existing kidney or liver disease. These conditions clear up within a few days of discontinuing the drug.

• H_2-antagonists, like this one, may mask symptoms of gastric cancer. This possibility must be eliminated with particular care in persons who have reached middle-age.

• The frequency and severity of side effects is higher in the elderly.

Interactions

• Cigarette smoking reverses some of the effects of famotidine, and interferes with ulcer healing.

• ℞ **Anticholinergics** and ℞ **metoclopramide** may decrease the absorption of famotidine, reducing its effect.

Side effects
These are infrequent and may include:

• Headache, dizziness, constipation, or diarrhea.

• Rare side effects may include flushing, ringing in the ears, fever, arthralgia (joint pain), hair loss, hypersensitivity reactions (including bronchospasm, facial swelling, hives, rash, anaphylaxis), blood disorders, seizures, and effects on the heart.

• Confusional states occur predominately in those who are severely ill.

Famvir Ⓑ

A preparation of ℞ **famciclovir**.
Formulation: Oral tablets in several strengths.
Availability: Prescription only.
Warnings and side effects: See ℞ **famciclovir**.

Fansidar Ⓑ

A preparation of ℞ **sulfadoxine** and ℞ **pyrimethamine**.
Formulation: Oral Tablets.
Availability: Prescription only.
Warnings and side effects: See ℞ **sulfadoxine**; ℞ **pyrimethamine**.

Fareston Ⓑ

A preparation of ℞ **toremifene**.
Formulation: Oral tablets.
Availability: Prescription only.
Warnings and side effects: See ℞ **toremifene**.

Fastin Ⓑ

A preparation of ℞ **phentermine**.
Formulation: Oral capsules.
Availability: Prescription only.
Warnings and side effects: See ℞ **phentermine**.

Fedahist Expectorant Syrup Ⓑ

A preparation of ℞ **pseudoephedrine** and ℞ **guaifenesin**.
Formulation: Oral syrup.
Availability: OTC.
Warnings and side effects: See ℞ **pseudoephedrine**; ℞ **guaifenesin**.

Fedahist Tablets; Timecaps; Gyrocaps Ⓑ

A preparation of ℞ **pseudoephedrine** and ℞ **chlorpheniramine maleate**.
Formulation: Oral tablets; capsules, sustained release.
Availability: OTC; Timecaps and Gyrocaps are prescription only.
Warnings and side effects: See ℞ **pseudoephedrine**; ℞ **chlorpheniramine maleate**.

Feen-a-mint Ⓑ

A preparation of ℞ **bisacodyl**.
Formulation: Oral tablets.
Availability: OTC.
Warnings and side effects: See ℞ **bisacodyl**.

Feiba VH Immuno Ⓑ

A preparation of ℞ **anti-inhibitor coagulant complex**.

Formulation: Injection (intravenous).
Availability: Prescription only.
Warnings and side effects: See ℞ **anti-inhibitor coagulant complex**.

Feldene Ⓑ

A preparation of ℞ **piroxicam**.
Formulation: Oral capsules, available in two strengths.
Availability: Prescription only.
Warnings and side effects: See ℞ **piroxicam**.

felodipine Ⓖ

Type/Group: **calcium-channel blocker; antihypertensive**.
Brand(s): Plendil. Combinations: With *enalapril maleate*: Lexxel.
How administered: Orally.

Used to treat

Felodipine is used alone or with other drugs to treat ✚ **hypertension**. Although not stated by the manufacturer, it is sometimes used to treat ✚ **Raynaud's disease**.

Warnings

• It should not be given to people with known hypersensitivity to this drug.

• It should be given with caution to people with congestive heart failure, impaired liver function, or who are elderly.

• It should be used during pregnancy only if the potential benefit outweighs the risk to the fetus.

• Breast-feeding women should either discontinue using this drug or stop breast-feeding.

• Swelling of the gums, usually mild, has been reported. Good dental hygiene may relieve or eliminate this adverse effect.

• Grapefruit juice should be avoided as it can increase the levels of felodipine in blood plasma.

• If felodipine is given to replace a ℞ **beta-blocker**, then withdrawal of the beta-blocker should not be abrupt. Calcium-channel blockers, also, should not be discontinued abruptly.

Interactions

• The levels of beta-blockers (for example, ℞ **metoprolol**) may be increased, although effects are not clear, and so caution is advised.

• ℞ **Cimetidine** may increase the levels and effects of felodipine.

• ℞ **Anticonvulsants** (for example, ℞ **carbamazepine**, ℞ **phenobarbital**, ℞ **phenytoin**) may reduce the levels and effects of felodipine.

Side effects

• These are generally mild and the most frequent are swelling of the extremities, flushing and sensations of warmth, headache, or dizziness.

• Occasionally, significant hypotension and, rarely, fainting.

Fem-1 Tablets Ⓑ

A preparation of ℞ **acetaminophen** and pamabrom.
Formulation: Oral tablets.
Availability: OTC.
Warnings and side effects: See ℞ **acetaminophen**.

Femara ⑧

A preparation of ℞ **letrozole**.
Formulation: Oral tablets.
Availability: Prescription only.
Warnings and side effects: See ℞ **letrozole**.

FemBack Caplets ⑧

A preparation of ℞ **acetaminophen**, ℞ **salicylamide**, and phenyltoloxamine citrate.
Formulation: Oral tablets.
Availability: OTC.
Warnings and side effects: See ℞ **acetaminophen**;
℞ **salicylamide**.

Femhrt ⑧

A preparation of ℞ **ethinyl estradiol** and ℞ **norethindrone**.
Formulation: Oral tablets.
Availability: Prescription only.
Warnings and side effects: See ℞ **ethinyl estradiol**;
℞ **norethindrone**.

Femiron ⑧

A preparation of ℞ **ferrous fumarate**.
Formulation: Oral tablets.
Availability: OTC.
Warnings and side effects: See ℞ **ferrous fumarate**.

Femizol-M ⑧

A preparation of ℞ **miconazole**.
Formulation: Vaginal cream.
Availability: OTC.
Warnings and side effects: See ℞ **miconazole**.

Fempatch ⑧

A preparation of ℞ **estradiol**.
Formulation: Transdermal patch.
Availability: Prescription only.
Warnings and side effects: See ℞ **estradiol**.

Femstat 3 ⑧

A preparation of ℞ **butoconazole**.
Formulation: Vaginal cream.
Availability: OTC.
Warnings and side effects: See ℞ **butoconazole**.

Fenesin ⑧

A preparation of ℞ **dextromethorphan** and ℞ **guaifenesin**.
Formulation: Oral tablets.
Availability: Prescription only.
Warnings and side effects: See ℞ **dextromethorphan**;
℞ **guaifenesin**.

Fenesin Tablets ⑧

A preparation of ℞ **guaifenesin**.
Formulation: Oral tablets, sustained release.

Availability: Prescription only.
Warnings and side effects: See ℞ **guaifenesin**.

fenofibrate ⑤

Type/Group: **lipid-regulating drug; fibrate**.
Brand(s): Tricor.
How administered: Orally.

Used to treat

Fenofibrate is used in ⊙ **hyperlipidemia** to reduce the levels, or change the proportions, of various lipids in the bloodstream. Generally, it is given only to people in whom a strict and regular dietary regime alone is not having the desired effect.

Warnings

• It should not be given to people with active liver or renal disease, or primary biliary cirrhosis.
• It should be given with caution to people with kidney impairment, heart disease, who are over 65, or who are using anticoagulant drugs.
• It should be used during pregnancy only if the potential benefits outweigh the possible risks to the fetus.
• It should not be used while breast-feeding.
• When taking fenofibrate, any unusual muscle pain or tenderness should be reported to a doctor immediately and treatment stopped, because it has the potential to cause destruction of muscle tissue.

Interactions

• ℞ **gemfibrozil**, ℞ **colestipol hydrochloride**, and ℞ **cholestyramine** reduce the effects of fenofibrate.
• If taken with ℞ **lovastatin**, ℞ **atorvastatin**, ℞ **fluvastatin**, ℞ **pravastatin**, or ℞ **cyclosporine** there is an increased risk of kidney damage.
• The effects of ℞ **sulfonylureas** may be reduced.

Side effects

• Gastrointestinal effects, rash, itching, photosensitivity, headache, dizziness, drowsiness, blurred vision, potential for liver disease, jaundice, and kidney failure.

fenoldopam mesylate ⑤

Type/Group: **dopamine-receptor stimulant; antihypertensive; vasodilator**.
Brand(s): Corlopam.
How administered: Intravenous infusion.

Used to treat

Fenoldopam is used, in hospitals, to quickly reduce blood pressure in hypertensive emergencies. Generally, it is not administered for longer than 48 hours.

Warnings

• It is a specialist drug and will be administered only by experienced personnel following full patient evaluation and with monitoring.
• It will be used with caution in people with high intraocular pressure (pressure in the eyeball, for example, glaucoma), or with a history of stroke.
• It should be used during pregnancy only when it is clearly needed.
• Medical judgment is required if breast-feeding is being considered.

• This drug should be used only in an adequately equipped medical facility and with frequent blood pressure monitoring.

• Potassium levels may fall after administration, and electrolytes should be monitored.

Interactions

• There is limited experience of using fenoldopam with other antihypertensives (for example, ℞ **ACE inhibitors**, ℞ **beta-blockers**, ℞ **alpha-adrenergic blockers**, ℞ **calcium-channel blockers**, and ℞ **diuretics**), and so caution is advised.

Side effects

• These include headache, flushing, nausea, or hypotension.

• Less frequently, palpitations and effects on heart function (rapid heartbeat may occur with higher dosage), shortness of breath, or changes in kidney function or blood sugar levels.

fenoprofen ⓖ

Type/Group: **anti-inflammatory; antirheumatic; non-narcotic analgesic; NSAID.**
Brand(s): Nalfon Pulvules; various generic.
How administered: Orally.

Used to treat

Fenoprofen is used for the relief of symptoms of ⊕ **rheumatoid arthritis** and ⊕ **osteoarthritis**, including for flare-ups and long-term management. It is also used for mild to moderate pain.

Warnings

• It should not be used by people with known hypersensitivity to this drug or to other NSAIDs (including ℞ **aspirin**), who have chronic kidney disease, certain bleeding disorders or conditions (for example, hemophilia, vitamin K deficiency, low blood-platelet levels), or who have a tendency to, or active, peptic ulceration.

• It should be given with caution to people taking certain drugs for gout, with peripheral edema or allergic disorders (especially asthma and skin conditions), who are elderly, or with any kind of kidney impairment or with certain liver disorders.

• Fenoprofen should be used during pregnancy only when medically judged to be clearly needed. Its risks to the fetus increase in the third trimester, however, and so should only be used if the benefits outweigh the risks to the fetus, which are higher at this time.

• Breast-feeding mothers should either discontinue this drug or stop breast-feeding.

• With regular, long-term use (as in treatment of osteoarthritis), NSAIDs may cause gastrointestinal bleeding, ulceration, or perforation. Any signs of bleeding (for example black stools) should be reported to a physician immediately.

• Most NSAIDs have the potential, particularly with regular use, to cause liver damage. Periodic evaluation of liver function is necessary in long-term therapy (more than two months).

• Because of its sedative side effects, the performance of skilled tasks, such as driving, may be impaired.

• Side effects are more frequent in the elderly.

• Gastrointestinal upsets may be minimized by taking the drug with milk or food.

Interactions

• There is generally no added benefit in taking other NSAIDs or other ℞ **salicylates** (especially aspirin) at the same time, but there is a higher risk of gastrointestinal upsets and bleeding.

• Alcohol and ℞ **corticosteroids** increase the risk of bleeding, particularly if there is an existing ulcer.

• ℞ **anticoagulant**, ℞ **antiplatelet**, and ℞ **thrombolytic** drugs may increase bleeding time.

• Fenoprofen may reduce the effectiveness of ℞ **diuretics**, ℞ **ACE inhibitors**, and ℞ **beta-blockers**.

• The effects of ℞ **sulfonamides**, ℞ **sulfonylureas**, and ℞ **hydantoin** may be exaggerated, with potential for toxicity.

• ℞ **phenobarbital** may lower the concentration of fenoprofen.

• Foodstuffs and herbals with ℞ **antiplatelet** properties, for example, ♣ **ginger**, ⚭ **garlic**, and various herbal preparations, may add the antiplatelet effect of NSAIDs.

Side effects

These vary in severity and how often they occur.

• Commonly, gastrointestinal upsets, nausea, constipation, swelling of the extremities, drowsiness and ringing in the ears.

• Less frequently, diarrhea, vomiting, headache, dizziness, confusion, sweating, itching, rash, fatigue, and sleep disturbances.

• Prolonged bleeding time (with consequent risk of ulceration) is possible with high dosage, and other blood changes can occur, including anemia.

• Hypersensitivity reactions may include symptoms such as hives, chest tightness, asthma, or bronchospasm.

• Reversible kidney failure, particularly in renal impairment, has occurred. Liver damage is rare.

fentanyl ⓖ

Type/Group: **narcotic analgesic; opioid.**
Brand(s): Actiq; Duragesic; Fentanyl Oralet; Sublimaze; various generic. Combination: With *droperidol*: (generic) fentanyl citrate and droperidol.
How administered: Injection; infusion; orally; transdermal (absorbed through the skin).

Used to treat

Fentanyl is used to treat moderate to severe pain (in operative procedures, but also used transdermally (absorbed through the skin) for chronic pain, such as in cancer), to enhance the effect of ℞ **general anesthetics**, and to depress spontaneous respiration in people having their breathing assisted.

Warnings

• It should not be given to people with known hypersensitivity to this drug. Opioids (even the weaker ones) should not be given to people with asthma, to anyone with seriously depressed breathing disorders, prostatic hypertrophy, convulsive disorders, raised intracranial pressure, or a head injury.

• It should be given with caution to the elderly, or to anyone with hypotension, certain liver, kidney, heart or adrenal disorders, hypothyroidism (under-activity of the thyroid gland), or alcoholism.

• Fentanyl should be used during pregnancy only if the benefits outweigh the potential risks.

• It does appear in breast milk and should not be used by nursing mothers.

• It is a Schedule II controlled substance.

• Prolonged use of narcotics can lead to physical dependence (addiction), although this rarely happens in routine medical use.

• This is a powerful drug and all but the smallest initiating doses can be toxic to those whose bodies are not already opioid-tolerant through prior medication with this or another morphine-like drug.

• In injectable or oral form fentanyl should not be given to children under 2, and transdermally (as a skin patch) to children under 12, although depending on weight and age this may need to be adjusted upward.

• Drowsiness may affect the performance of skilled tasks such as driving.

• The effects of alcohol may be enhanced (including a higher risk of respiratory depression).

Interactions

• If the following drugs are used with fentanyl, then effects may be enhanced with potentially serious results: ℞ **barbiturates**; inhalant ℞ **anesthetics**; ℞ **MAOIs**; ℞ **opioids**; protease inhibitors (for example, ℞ **nelfinavir**, ℞ **ritonavir**, ℞ **saquinavir**); ℞ **antihistamines**; alcohol; ℞ **chlorpromazine**; ℞ **thioridazine**; ℞ **diazepam**; nitrous oxide.

• If used with ℞ **droperidol**, there is a risk of severe hypotension and respiratory depression. Although fentanyl may be used with droperidol, it is given in a hospital under close medical supervision.

Side effects

• Depending on use and dose, there may be drowsiness, nausea and vomiting, constipation, dry mouth, sweating, confusion, pruritis, sleepiness, and loss of energy or weakness.

• There is occasionally euphoria, which may lead to a state of mental detachment or abnormal thinking. Less commonly, there may be nervousness, anxiety, depression, hallucinations, tremor, loss of appetite, headache, or inadequate breathing.

• With overdose, fentanyl may cause rigidity of skeletal muscles, particularly of the trunk. There is also a risk of serious respiratory depression.

Fentanyl Oralet ®

A preparation of ℞ **fentanyl**.
Formulation: Lozenges; 4 strengths, including the lowest, initiating dosage.
Availability: Prescription only.
Warnings and side effects: See ℞ **fentanyl**.

Feosol ®

A preparation of ℞ **ferrous sulfate**.
Formulation: Oral elixir, tablets.
Availability: OTC.
Warnings and side effects: See ℞ **ferrous sulfate**.

Feostat ®

A preparation of ℞ **ferrous fumarate**.
Formulation: Oral tablets, oral suspension, oral drops.
Availability: OTC.

Warnings and side effects: See ℞ **ferrous fumarate**.

Fergon ®

A preparation of ℞ **ferrous gluconate**.
Formulation: Oral tablets.
Availability: OTC.
Warnings and side effects: See ℞ **ferrous gluconate**.

Fer-In-Sol ®

A preparation of ℞ **ferrous sulfate**.
Formulation: Oral syrup; oral drops.
Availability: OTC.
Warnings and side effects: See ℞ **ferrous sulfate**.

ferrous fumarate ⓖ

Type/Group: anemia treatment.
Brand(s): Feostat; Ircon; Femiron; various generic.
How administered: Orally.

Used to treat

Ferrous fumarate is a drug rich in iron which is used in the treatment of iron-deficiency anemia to restore iron to the body or to prevent deficiency.

Warnings

• It should not be given to people with certain blood diseases or known sensitivity to any ingredient in the preparations.

• Ferrous fumarate is safe for use during pregnancy.

• It is compatible with nursing.

• Anyone with a normal iron balance should not take iron supplements regularly.

• It is best absorbed when taken on an empty stomach. Take with food to minimize gastrointestinal upsets.

Interactions

• If used with ℞ **antacids** or ℞ **cimetidine**, the absorption of iron may be reduced.

• If used with ℞ **ascorbic acid** or ℞ **chloramphenicol**, the absorption of iron may be increased.

• The effects of ℞ **levodopa**, ℞ **levothyroxine**, ℞ **methyldopa**, ℞ **penicillamine**, and ℞ **quinolones** may be reduced.

• The absorption of ℞ **tetracyclines** and iron salts may be reduced.

Side effects

• Occasionally, mild, transient nausea.

• Rarely, heartburn, anorexia, constipation, or diarrhea.

ferrous gluconate ⓖ

Type/Group: anemia treatment.
Brand(s): Fergon; various generic.
How administered: Orally.

Used to treat

Ferrous gluconate is a drug rich in iron which is used in the treatment of iron-deficiency anemia to restore iron to the body or to prevent deficiency.

Warnings

• It should not be given to people with certain blood diseases or known sensitivity to any ingredient in the preparations.

• Ferrous gluconate is safe for use during pregnancy.

• It is compatible with nursing.

• Anyone with a normal iron balance should not take iron supplements regularly.

• It is best absorbed when taken on an empty stomach. Take with food to minimize gastrointestinal upsets.

Interactions

• If used with ℞ **antacids** or ℞ **cimetidine**, the absorption of iron may be reduced.

• If used with ℞ **ascorbic acid** or ℞ **chloramphenicol**, the absorption of iron may be increased.

• The effects of ℞ **levodopa**, ℞ **levothyroxine**, ℞ **methyldopa**, ℞ **penicillamine**, and ℞ **quinolones** may be reduced.

• The absorption of ℞ **tetracyclines** and iron salts may be reduced.

Side effects

• Occasionally, mild, transient nausea.

• Rarely, heartburn, anorexia, constipation, or diarrhea.

ferrous sulfate ⓖ

Type/Group: **anemia treatment**.
Brand(s): Fer-In-Sol; Feosol; various generic.
How administered: Orally.

Used to treat

Ferrous sulfate is a drug rich in iron which is used in the treatment of iron-deficiency anemia to restore iron to the body or to prevent deficiency.

Warnings

• It should not be given to people with certain blood diseases or known sensitivity to any ingredient in the preparations.

• Ferrous sulfate is safe for use during pregnancy.

• It is compatible with nursing.

• Anyone with a normal iron balance should not take iron supplements regularly.

• It is best absorbed when taken on an empty stomach. Take with food to minimize gastrointestinal upsets.

Interactions

• If used with ℞ **antacids** or ℞ **cimetidine**, the absorption of iron may be reduced.

• If used with ℞ **ascorbic acid** or ℞ **chloramphenicol**, the absorption of iron may be increased.

• The effects of ℞ **levodopa**, ℞ **levothyroxine**, ℞ **methyldopa**, ℞ **penicillamine**, and ℞ **quinolones** may be reduced.

• The absorption of ℞ **tetracyclines** and iron salts may be reduced.

Side effects

• Occasionally, mild, transient nausea.

• Rarely, heartburn, anorexia, constipation, or diarrhea.

fertility treatment ⓓ

see ℞ infertility treatment.

Fertinex ⓑ

A preparation of ℞ **urofollitropin**.
Formulation: Injection.
Availability: Prescription only.
Warnings and side effects: See ℞ **urofollitropin**.

Feverall Children's Sprinkles; Junior Strength Sprinkles ⓑ

A preparation of ℞ **acetaminophen**.
Formulation: Capsules containing powder for solution.
Availability: OTC.
Warnings and side effects: See ℞ **acetaminophen**.

fexofenadine hydrochloride ⓖ

Type/Group: **antihistamine; antiallergic**.
Brand(s): AllegraTablets; Capsules. Combinations: With *pseudoephedrine hydrochloride*: Allegra-D.
How administered: Orally.

Used to treat

Fexofenadine is a recently developed antihistamine drug with less sedative side effects than some older members of its class. It is the active metabolite of terfenadine (which is no longer available in the US), and can be used for the symptomatic relief of allergic symptoms such as chronic idiopathic ⚙ **urticaria** and ⚙ **hay fever** (seasonal allergic rhinitis).

Warnings

• It should not be given to people with known hypersensitivity to this drug (or with known sensitivity to other antihistamines, and particularly to terfenadine).

• Antihistamines should be given with caution to people with asthma or lower respiratory disease, heart disease, hypertension, hyperthyroidism, epilepsy, porphyria, increased intraocular pressure (pressure in the eyeball, as in glaucoma), enlarged prostate, urinary retention, certain obstructive bladder or gastrointestinal conditions, kidney or liver impairment, and the elderly.

• Fexofenadine should be used during pregnancy only if the potential benefit outweighs the possible risk to the fetus.

• Medical judgment is required if breast-feeding is being considered.

• Although infrequent with fexofenadine, sedative side effects that may affect the performance of skilled tasks, such as driving, are possible.

• Side effects are more frequent in the elderly.

Interactions

• ℞ **macrolide** antibiotics (for example, ℞ **erythromycin**) and ℞ **azoles** (for example, ℞ **ketoconazole**) may increase the levels of fexofenadine.

• ℞ **Antacids** containing aluminum and magnesium may reduce levels of fexofenadine.

• ℞ **MAOI** antidepressants may prolong and intensify the anticholinergic (see Side effects below) effects of antihistamines.

Side effects

• These depend on how it is administered. For this type of antihistamine, there may be drowsiness, headache, cold and flu symptoms, fatigue, indigestion, dizziness, and menstrual disturbances. The incidence of sedation, anticholinergic (dry mouth, blurred vision, urinary retention, gastrointestinal disturbances), and other side effects of antihistamines is low for this type of drug. Other antihistamine side effects include occasional rashes and photosensitivity (abnormal sensitivity to light), palpitations and heart arrhythmias, stimulation instead of sedation (paradoxical stimulation), especially in children (and convulsions in overdose), hypersensitivity reactions, blood disorders, liver disturbances, depression, sleep disturbances, and hypotension.

• It is not yet clear whether fexofenadine shares some of the adverse side effects (hazardous arrhythmias) of terfenadine.

Fiberall Tropical Fruit Flavor; Orange Flavor ®

A preparation of ℞ **psyllium**.
Formulation: Oral powder.
Availability: OTC.
Warnings and side effects: See ℞ **psyllium**. Powders contain the sweetener aspartame, which should be avoided by individuals with phenylketonuria.

fibrate ⑩

Generics: **clofibrate; fenofibrate; gemfibrozil.**

Actions and uses

Fibrate (or fibric acid derivative) drugs are used in ℞ **lipid-regulating drug** (antihyperlipidemia) treatment. These agents are used in ✪ **hyperlipidemia** to reduce the levels, or change the proportions, of various lipids in the bloodstream. These drugs may lower the levels of very low-density lipoprotein fraction rich in triglycerides, decrease serum cholesterol, increase HDL-cholesterol, and sometimes lower LDL-cholesterol.

Current medical opinion suggests that if diet, or drugs, can be used to lower levels of LDL-cholesterol (low-density lipoprotein) while raising HDL-cholesterol (high-density lipoprotein), then there may be a regression of the progress of coronary ✪ **atherosclerosis** (a diseased state of the arteries of the heart where plaques of lipid material narrow blood vessels, which contributes to angina pectoris attacks and the formation of abnormal clots that go on to cause heart attacks and strokes).

Limitations

See the individual drug entries.

fibric acid derivative ⑩

see ℞ **fibrate**.

fibrinolytic ⑩

Generics: **alteplase, recombinant; anistreplase; reteplase, recombinant; streptokinase; urokinase.**

Actions and uses

Fibrinolytic agents are ℞ **enzyme** agents, or activate enzymes, that lead to the dissolution of fibrin, which is a mesh-like protein that is one of the main components of thrombi (blood clots formed in blood vessels), and which traps platelets (thrombocytes). In medicine they are used as ℞ **thrombolytic** drugs to break up and disperse thrombi, when used rapidly in serious conditions, such as life-threatening venous thrombi, pulmonary embolism, particularly to reopen the blocked coronary arteries, for example, in ✪ **myocardial infarction** (heart attack).

Agents with the reverse of the action of fibrinolytic drugs are available, and are called *antifibrinolytic* agents, for example, ℞ **aprotinin** and ℞ **aminocaproic acid**—see ℞ **hemostatic**.

Limitations

See the individual drug entries.

filgrastim ⑥

Type/Group: **hematopoietic.**
Brand(s): Neupogen.
How administered: Injection.

Used to treat

Filgrastim is a name given to "granulocyte-colony stimulating factor (G-CSF)," a natural blood-stimulating substance that is synthesized using DNA engineering techniques. It reduces neutropenia (a shortage of neutrophil white blood cells in the circulation) by stimulating white cell production (mainly neutrophils) when this has been reduced during chemotherapy in cancer treatment, and this may alleviate several adverse effects of chemotherapy and radiotherapy, including liver and kidney damage, and the risk of infection or sepsis. Additionally, it can be used to stimulate white cell production in conditions unrelated to cancer (for example, fevers or infections) that may cause chronic neutropenia. It may be of benefit in the treatment of ✪ **AIDS**, aplastic ✪ **anemia**, hairy-cell ✪ **leukemia**, and certain other blood disorders.

Warnings

• It should not be given to people with known hypersensitivity to this drug or to proteins derived from *E. coli* (intestinal bacteria).

• It should be used with caution by people with certain heart disorders. This is a specialist drug and is used only after a full medical assessment.

• Filgrastim should be used during pregnancy only when it is clearly needed.

• Medical judgment is required if breast-feeding is being considered.

• It is used only under qualified medical supervision and with frequent monitoring of blood values.

Interactions

• ℞ **Corticosteroids**, ℞ **lithium**, and any other drugs that might intensify the potential of filgrastim for stimulating production of white cells should be used with caution.

Side effects

• Mild to moderate bone pain is the most frequent.

• Depending on the underlying disease being treated, other side effects may include nausea, vomiting, hypertension, rash, headache, or enlargement of the spleen. Inflammation at the site of injection may occur.

Finac Lotion ®

A preparation of ℞ **salicylic acid** and various.
Formulation: Topical liquid.
Availability: OTC.
Warnings and side effects: See ℞ **salicylic acid**.

finasteride ⑥

Type/Group: **antiandrogen; hormone antagonist.**

Brand(s): Propecia; Proscar.

How administered: Orally.

Used to treat

Finasteride is an enzyme inhibitor that acts as an indirect sex hormone antagonist and is used to treat ✪ **benign prostatic hyperplasia** and male pattern baldness.

Warnings

• It should not be used by women, or children, or anyone with known hypersensitivity to the drug.

• It should be given with caution to people with impaired liver function or obstructive uropathy.

• It is not to be used by pregnant women. Pregnant women should avoid handling crushed tablets.

• Condoms should be used if there is any chance of becoming pregnant.

• Women who may become pregnant should avoid handling crushed or broken tablets.

• Several months of treatment may be needed to assess whether the drug is effective.

Interactions

None have been noted.

Side effects

• Decreased libido, decreased volume of ejaculate, and impotence.

Fioricet Tablets ⓑ

A preparation of ℞ **acetaminophen**, ℞ **caffeine**, and ℞ **butabarbital**.

Formulation: Oral tablets.

Availability: Prescription only.

Warnings and side effects: See ℞ **acetaminophen**; ℞ **butabarbital**; ℞ **caffeine**.

Fioricet w/Codeine Capsules ⓑ

A preparation of ℞ **codeine phosphate**, ℞ **acetaminophen**, ℞ **caffeine**, and ℞ **butabarbital**.

Formulation: Oral capsules.

Availability: Prescription only.

Warnings and side effects: See ℞ **codeine phosphate**; ℞ **acetaminophen**; ℞ **caffeine**, and ℞ **butabarbital**.

Fiorinal Capsules ⓑ

A preparation of ℞ **aspirin** and ℞ **butabarbital**.

Formulation: Oral capsules.

Availability: Prescription only.

Warnings and side effects: See ℞ **aspirin**; ℞ **butabarbital**.

Fiorinal w/Codeine Capsules ⓑ

A preparation of ℞ **codeine phosphate**, ℞ **aspirin**, ℞ **caffeine**, and ℞ **butabarbital**.

Formulation: Oral capsules.

Availability: Prescription only.

Warnings and side effects: See ℞ **codeine phosphate**; ℞ **aspirin**; ℞ **caffeine**; ℞ **butabarbital**.

Fiortal Capsules ⓑ

A preparation of ℞ **aspirin**, ℞ **butabarbital**, and ℞ **caffeine**.

Formulation: Oral capsules.

Availability: Prescription only.

Warnings and side effects: See ℞ **aspirin**; ℞ **butabarbital**; ℞ **caffeine**.

5-aminosalicylate ⓓ

see ℞ **aminosalicylate**.

5-aminosalicylic acid ⓖ

see ℞ **mesalamine**.

5-ASA ⓖ

see ℞ **mesalamine**.

5-FC ⓖ

see ℞ **flucytosine**.

5-fluorocytosine ⓖ

see ℞ **flucytosine**.

5-HT receptor agonist ⓓ

see ℞ **serotonin-receptor stimulant**.

5-HT receptor antagonist ⓓ

see ℞ **serotonin-receptor antagonist**.

5-lipoxygenase inhibitor ⓓ

see ℞ **lipoxygenase inhibitor**.

Flagyl; Flagyl ER; Flagyl 375; Flagyl IV ⓑ

A preparation of ℞ **metronidazole**.

Formulation: Oral tablets in several strengths, extended release (ER); oral capsules (375), injection (intravenous).

Availability: Prescription only.

Warnings and side effects: See ℞ **metronidazole**.

Flanders Buttocks ⓑ

A preparation of ℞ **zinc oxide** and ℞ **castor oil**.

Formulation: Topical ointment.

Availability: OTC.

Warnings and side effects: See ℞ **zinc oxide**; ℞ **castor oil**.

Flarex ⓑ

A preparation of ℞ **fluorometholone**.

Formulation: Eye drops.

Availability: Prescription only.

Warnings and side effects: See ℞ **fluorometholone**.

Flatulex Drops ⓑ

A preparation of ℞ **simethicone**.

Formulation: Oral drops.

Availability: OTC.

Warnings and side effects: See ℞ **simethicone**.

Key to symbols: ✪ = Disorder Section ℞ = Drug Section ♣ = Herbal Section ᐜ = Supplement Section

Flatulex Tablets ⑧

A preparation of ℞ **activated charcoal** and ℞ **simethicone**.
Formulation: Oral tablets.
Availability: OTC.
Warnings and side effects: See ℞ **activated charcoal**;
℞ **simethicone**.

flavoxate hydrochloride ⑥

Type/Group: **anticholinergic; antispasmodic.**
Brand(s): Urispas.
How administered: Orally.

Used to treat

Flavoxate is used as an antispasmodic to treat urinary frequency and incontinence associated with urinary tract infections (see ✪ **urinary tract disorders**).

Warnings

• It should not be given to people with known gastrointestinal obstructive disease, hemorrhage, ileus, or urinary obstruction.
• It should be given with caution to people with suspected glaucoma.
• Flavoxate should be used during pregnancy only when it is clearly needed.
• Medical judgment is required if breast-feeding is being considered. It is not known whether this drug appears in breast milk.
• It may cause drowsiness or blurred vision. Driving or any hazardous activity must be avoided while the pupils are dilated.

Interactions

No significant interactions specific to this drug are known.

Side effects

• Frequently, dry mouth or throat, and drowsiness.
• Occasionally, constipation, difficult urination, blurred vision, dizziness, headache, increased light sensitivity, nausea, vomiting, and stomach pain.
• Rarely, confusion, allergic reaction, increased intraocular pressure (pressure in the eyeball), and leucopenia.

flecainide acetate ⑥

Type/Group: **antiarrhythmic.**
Brand(s): Tambocor.
How administered: Orally.

Used to treat

Flecamide is used to regularize the heartbeat when certain life-threatening ✪ **arrhythmias** have developed. It has sometimes been used (where no heart disease is present) to treat some other less severe arrhythmias. Treatment is usually begun in a hospital.

Warnings

• It should not be given to people with known hypersensitivity to this drug, with heart block or certain arrhythmias, or who have had a recent heart attack.
• It should be given with caution to people with congestive heart failure, with pacemakers, or significantly impaired liver or kidney function. This is a specialist drug and treatment will be carried out by experienced clinicians who are thoroughly familiar with this drug. Periodic monitoring of heart function and blood values is necessary.
• Flecainide may have the potential to cause fetal harm and should be used during pregnancy only if the potential benefit outweighs the possible risk to the fetus.
• It is present in breast milk and nursing women should discontinue using this drug or stop breast-feeding.
• Flecainide can, occasionally, provoke arrhythmias.

Interactions

• ℞ **amiodarone hydrochloride**, ℞ **cimetidine**, ℞ **disopyramide**, ℞ **propranolol**, ℞ **verapamil**, and ℞ **urinary alkalinizers** (for example, sodium bicarbonate) may raise the levels or intensify the effects of flecainide.
• The levels of and effects of ℞ **digoxin** may be increased.
• Smoking and urinary acidifiers (for example, ℞ **ammonium chloride**) may reduce the effects of flecainide.

Side effects

• The most serious adverse reactions are arrhythmias, which can be provoked by antiarrhythmic drugs.
• More frequent side effects include dizziness, disturbed vision, breathlessness, headache, nausea, fatigue, palpitations, and chest pain.
• Less frequently, gastrointestinal disturbances, tremor, nervousness or other mental changes (for example, memory loss and confusion), malaise, fever or increased sweating.
• Sensitivity reactions such as rash, hives, itching, allergic swelling and bronchospasm have occurred.
• Liver and blood changes are rare.

Fleet; Phospho-soda Solution ⑧

A preparation of ℞ **sodium phosphate**.
Formulation: Oral liquid; enema.
Availability: OTC.
Warnings and side effects: See ℞ **sodium phosphate**.

Fleet Babylax ⑧

A preparation of ℞ **glycerin**.
Formulation: Rectal liquid.
Availability: OTC.
Warnings and side effects: See ℞ **glycerin**.

Fleet Laxative Tablets; Suppositories; Bisacodyl Enema ⑧

A preparation of ℞ **bisacodyl**.
Formulation: Oral tablets; rectal suppositories; enema.
Availability: OTC.
Warnings and side effects: See ℞ **bisacodyl**.

Fleet Mineral Oil ⑧

A preparation of ℞ **mineral oil**.
Formulation: Enema.
Availability: OTC.
Warnings and side effects: See ℞ **mineral oil**.

Fletcher's Castoria ℬ

A preparation of ℞ **senna**.
Formulation: Oral liquid.
Availability: OTC.
Warnings and side effects: See ℞ **senna**.

Flex-all 454 Gel; Maximum Strength Flex-all 454 ℬ

A preparation of ℞ **methyl salicylate**, ℞ **menthol**, and various.
Formulation: Topical gel.
Availability: OTC.
Warnings and side effects: See ℞ **methyl salicylate**; ℞ **menthol**.

Flexall Ultra Plus ℬ

A preparation of ℞ **methyl salicylate**, ℞ **menthol**, ℞ **camphor**, and various.
Formulation: Topical ointment.
Availability: OTC.
Warnings and side effects: See ℞ **methyl salicylate**; ℞ **menthol**; ℞ **camphor**.

Flexaphen ℬ

A preparation of ℞ **chlorzoxazone** and ℞ **acetaminophen**.
Formulation: Oral tablets.
Availability: Prescription only.
Warnings and side effects: See ℞ **chlorzoxazone**; ℞ **acetaminophen**.

Flexiril ℬ

A preparation of ℞ **cyclobenzaprine**.
Formulation: Oral tablets.
Availability: Prescription only.
Warnings and side effects: See ℞ **cyclobenzaprine**.

Flexoject ℬ

A preparation of ℞ **orphenadrine**.
Formulation: Injection.
Availability: Prescription only.
Warnings and side effects: See ℞ **orphenadrine**.

Flexon ℬ

A preparation of ℞ **orphenadrine**.
Formulation: Injection.
Availability: Prescription only.
Warnings and side effects: See ℞ **orphenadrine**.

Flextra-DS Tablets ℬ

A preparation of ℞ **acetaminophen** and phenyltoloxamine citrate.
Formulation: Oral tablets.
Availability: Prescription only.
Warnings and side effects: See ℞ **acetaminophen**.

Flolan ℬ

A preparation of ℞ **epoprostenol sodium**.
Formulation: Intravenous infusion.
Availability: Prescription only.
Warnings and side effects: See ℞ **epoprostenol sodium**.

Flomax ℬ

A preparation of ℞ **tamsulosin hydrochloride**.
Formulation: Oral capsules.
Availability: Prescription only.
Warnings and side effects: See ℞ **tamsulosin hydrochloride**.

Florida Sunburn Relief ℬ

A preparation of ℞ **phenol**, ℞ **camphor**, and ℞ **menthol**.
Formulation: Topical lotion.
Availability: OTC.
Warnings and side effects: See ℞ **phenol**; ℞ **camphor**; ℞ **menthol**.

Florinef ℬ

A preparation of ℞ **fludrocortisone**.
Formulation: Oral tablets.
Availability: Prescription only.
Warnings and side effects: See ℞ **fludrocortisone**.

Flovent; Flovent Rotadisk ℬ

A preparation of ℞ **fluticasone propionate**.
Formulation: Aerosol spray; powder.
Availability: Prescription only.
Warnings and side effects: See ℞ **fluticasone propionate**.

Floxin ℬ

A preparation of ℞ **ofloxacin**.
Formulation: Oral tablets; injection; eardrops.
Availability: Prescription only.
Warnings and side effects: See ℞ **ofloxacin**.

fluconazole Ⓖ

Type/Group: **antifungal; azole**.
Brand(s): Diflucan.
How administered: Orally; injection.

Used to treat

Fluconazole is a triazole/azole antifungal drug used in the treatment of *Candida* ✪ **fungal infections** (candidiasis) of the throat and mouth, vagina, esophagus and urinary tract, peritonitis, systemic candidal infections, and cryptococcal meningitis. It can also be used to prevent fungal infections in immunocompromised patients following chemotherapy or radiotherapy.

Warnings

• It should not be given to people with known hypersensitivity to fluconazole.
• It should be given with caution to people hypersensitive to other azoles or with kidney disease.
• It may harm the fetus and should be used during pregnancy only if the potential benefits outweigh the risks to the fetus.
• Medical judgment is required if breast-feeding is being considered. Fluconazole does appear in breast milk.

• It has been associated with rare cases of serious liver damage, usually reversible. A doctor must be contacted if dark urine, pale stools, fatigue, yellowing skin, fever, or pronounced gastrointestinal upsets occur.

• Alcohol must be avoided.

• Long-term therapy may be needed to clear the infection.

Interactions

• ℞ **Antacids** and ℞ **ulcer-healing drugs** should be taken at least two hours after fluconazole to avoid reducing its effectiveness.

• The effects of ℞ **alprazolam**, ℞ **amprenavir**, atevirdine, ℞ **atorvastatin**, ℞ **buspirone**, ℞ **chlordiazepoxide**, ℞ **cyclosporine**, ℞ **diazepam**, ℞ **felodipine**, ℞ **fluvastatin**, ℞ **indinavir**, ℞ **lovastatin**, ℞ **methadone**, ℞ **methylprednisolone**, ℞ **midazolam**, ℞ **nelfinavir**, ℞ **pravastatin**, ℞ **quinidine**, ℞ **ritonavir**, ℞ **saquinavir**, ℞ **simvastatin**, ℞ **tacrolimus**, ℞ **tolbutamide**, ℞ **triazolam**, and ℞ **warfarin sodium** may be reduced by fluconazole.

• ℞ **Aluminum hydroxide**, ⚕ **calcium**, ℞ **cimetidine**, ℞ **didanosine**, ℞ **famotidine**, ℞ **lansoprazole**, ⚕ **magnesium**, ℞ **nizatidine**, and ℞ **sodium bicarbonate** may reduce the effects of fluconazole.

• If used with ℞ **rifampin** the effects of both drugs are reduced.

Side effects

These depend on how it is administered, dose, and use.

• Occasionally, allergic reaction, dizziness, drowsiness, headache, and gastrointestinal upset.

• Rarely, serious liver, skin, and blood disorders have been reported.

flucytosine ⑤

(5-FC; 5-fluorocytosine)

Type/Group: **antifungal**.
Brand(s): Neutrexin.
How administered: Orally.

Used to treat

Flucytosine is a synthetic antifungal drug that can be used to treat especially serious systemic yeast and ✪ **fungal infections**, such as systemic *Candida* and by *Cryptococcus* infections.

Warnings

• It should not be given to people with known hypersensitivity to flucytosine.

• It should be given with caution to people with kidney function impairment or bone marrow suppression.

• It is unknown whether flucytosine harms the fetus. It should be used during pregnancy only if the potential benefit outweighs the possible risks.

• Because of the possibility of serious reactions in infants, flucytosine should not be used while breast-feeding.

• Close monitoring of blood, kidney, and liver status is essential because of the potential for serious adverse reactions.

• Gastrointestinal reactions can be minimized by spreading the dose out over several minutes rather than taking all at once.

Interactions

• ℞ **Amphotericin B** may increase the effects of flucytosine.

• Cytosine may inactivate the antifungal activity of flucytosine.

Side effects

• Frequently, gastrointestinal upset, rashes, confusion, hallucinations, headaches, dizziness, sedation, blood, liver, kidney and heart problems.

Fludara ⑧

A preparation of ℞ **fludarabine phosphate**.
Formulation: Injection.
Availability: Prescription only.
Warnings and side effects: See ℞ **fludarabine phosphate**.

fludarabine phosphate ⑤

Type/Group: **anticancer; cytotoxic**.
Brand(s): Fludara.
How administered: Intravenous infusion.

Used to treat

Fludarabine is a cytotoxic drug (an antimetabolite) that is used primarily for certain ✪ **leukemias** (B-cell chronic lymphatic leukemia).

Warnings

• It should not be given to people with known hypersensitivity to this drug.

• It should be given with caution to people with impaired kidney function. This is a specialist drug which will be used following a full evaluation by specialist physicians.

• Fludarabine is not recommended for use during pregnancy unless it is medically judged to be essential, because it may cause birth defects. Becoming pregnant while using this drug must be avoided.

• It should not be used if breast-feeding.

• It can cause bone marrow depression, which may lead to bleeding and a reduced resistance to infection.

• High doses may produce severe, even fatal, neurological effects (though these are rare at recommended dose).

• It may impair fertility in males (which may be reversible).

• Breaking up of tumors may lead to "tumor lysis syndrome," which is a complication of treatment involving increased levels of certain minerals in the blood that can have adverse effects on kidney function.

Interactions

No interactions specific to this drug are known.

Side effects

• Fever, chills, infection, gastrointestinal effects, swelling in limbs, dry skin, rash, reddened skin, pain, confusion, chilliness, fatigue, weakness, and sinusitis.

• Rarely, tingling or burning sensations on skin, headaches, hearing loss, visual disturbances, urinary problems, and bleeding.

fludrocortisone ⑤

Type/Group: **corticosteroid; anti-inflammatory**.
How administered: Orally.
Brand(s): Florinef.

Used to treat

Fludrocortisone is used as partial replacement therapy to correct an insufficiency of hormone from the adrenal gland in ✪ **Addison's disease**. It is also used to an adjunctive treatment (additional treatment to enhance effectiveness) of salt-losing forms of congenital adrenogenital syndrome. Although not stated by its manufacturers for such use, it has also been prescribed as a treatment of severe postural hypotension (dizziness, faintness when arising from a sitting or lying position).

Warnings

• It should not be used by people with a known hypersensitivity to fludrocortisone or with systemic fungal infections.

• It should be given with caution to anyone with congestive heart failure, hypertension, or kidney insufficiency.

• It is not known whether this drug crosses the placenta or is excreted in breast milk, but other corticosteroids do. Therefore, it should only be used during pregnancy if medically judged to be essential, and it is also a matter for medical judgment if breast-feeding is being considered.

• Dentists and other doctors must be informed of the use of this drug during, and for 12 months after discontinuing, treatment. Supportive drugs may be required in the event of severe illness, surgery, or trauma.

• Anyone on long-term steroid therapy should wear a medic-alert bracelet or the equivalent. or the equivalent.

• Discontinuation of treatment must be gradual and under medical supervision following prolonged therapy.

• Aspirin or any other medication (including herbal remedies and supplements) must not be taken without consulting a doctor.

• It may cause serious decrease in potassium levels, and so awareness of signs and symptoms (weakness and muscle cramps, numbness or tingling (especially in the legs or feet), nausea and vomiting, and irritability) is essential. A doctor must be contacted if they develop.

Interactions

• Fludrocortisone taken with ℞ **amphotericin** or ℞ **diuretics** may further reduce potassium levels.

• The effects of ℞ **aspirin**, ℞ **oral hypoglycemics**, ℞ **insulin**, ℞ **diuretics**, and ♧♧ **potassium** supplements may be reduced.

• The ulcerogenic (causes or exacerbates peptic ulcers) effect of aspirin is increased.

• ℞ **Barbiturates**, ℞ **hydantoins**, ℞ **rifampin**, and ℞ **ephedrine** reduce the effects of corticosteroids.

• ℞ **Ketoconazole**, ℞ **estrogens**, ℞ **oral contraceptives**, nondepolarizing muscle relaxants, and ℞ **cholestyramine** may increase the effects of fludrocortisone.

• Oral ℞ **anticoagulants** and ℞ **theophylline** may alter the effects of either corticosteroids or the other drug, or both.

• The effectiveness of ℞ **anticholinesterases**, ℞ **isoniazid**, ℞ **salicylates**, and ℞ **somatrem** may be reduced.

• ℞ **Cyclosporine** and digitalis glycosides may increase the risk of toxicity.

Side effects

• Frequently, increased appetite, edema, exaggerated sense of well-being, abdominal distention, weight gain, insomnia, and mood swings.

• Occasionally, headache, dizziness, menstrual difficulty or amenorrhea, and ulcers.

• Rarely, an allergic reaction may occur.

Flumadine ℞

A preparation of ℞ **rimantadine**.
Formulation: Oral tablets; oral syrup.
Availability: Prescription only.
Warnings and side effects: See ℞ **rimantadine**.

flumazenil Ⓖ

Type/Group: **antidote**.
Brand(s): Romazicon.
How administered: Injection.

Used to treat

Flumazenil is a specialized drug, a benzodiazepine antagonist, which can be used to reverse the sedative effects of ℞ **benzodiazepine** drugs on the central nervous system induced during anesthesia, in intensive care, for diagnostic procedures, or from overdose.

Warnings

• It should not be used by people with known hypersensitivity to this or similar drugs, or in cases of serious cyclic antidepressant overdose, or when benzodiazepines have been given to control a life-threatening condition.

• It should be given with caution to anyone with a head injury, impaired kidney or liver function, seizure disorder, active alcoholism, or drug dependence. It is a specialist drug and full patient evaluation and monitoring will be carried out.

• Flumazenil's should be used during pregnancy only when it is medically judged to be clearly needed.

• Medical judgment is also required if breast-feeding is being considered, as it is not known whether this drug is excreted in breast milk.

• Do not engage in activities requiring complete alertness for 18 to 24 hours after taking the drug, and only with your doctor's advice. The effects of benzodiazepine (sedation) may recur even after a period of alertness.

• Do not use alcohol or nonprescription drugs for 18 to 24 hours after taking the drug.

• It may provoke panic attacks in people with a history of panic disorder.

Interactions

• The effects of other drugs that may have been masked by benzodiazepine may appear after flumazenil reverses the benzodiazepine effects.

Side effects

• Anxiety, agitation, dry mouth, shortness of breath, insomnia, palpitations and effects on heart rhythm, tremors, headache, blurred vision, dizziness, unsteadiness and incoordination, nausea, and vomiting.

• Occasionally, fatigue, flushing, hearing disturbances, rash.

• Rarely, hives, itching, and hallucinations.

flunisolide Ⓖ

Type/Group: **corticosteroid; anti-inflammatory**.
Brand(s): AeroBid; Nasalide; Nasarel.
How administered: Inhalation; intranasal.

Used to treat

Flunisolide is prescribed as a respiratory inhalant for treatment and prevention of bronchial ⊙ **asthma**, and as a treatment for nasal inflammation from allergies (such as seasonal allergic rhinitis and perennial allergic rhinitis).

Warnings

• It should not be used by people with known hypersensitivity to corticosteroids, or with systematic fungal infections.

• It should be given with caution to anyone with adrenal insufficiency, untreated infections, and certain nasal conditions (intranasal use).

• Corticosteroids can cross the placenta, and therefore flunisolide should only be used during pregnancy if medically judged to be essential.

• Medical judgment is also required if breast-feeding is required. When taken internally, corticosteroids are excreted in breast milk and may suppress growth and interfere with the production of natural corticosteroids in the infant. It is not known whether, or under what conditions, enough of the drug is absorbed from topical use to create these risks.

• Localized fungal infections (thrush) have occurred in the mouths and throats of people using corticosteroid inhalants.

• Because corticosteroids suppress the immune system, anyone using long-term inhalant therapy is particularly susceptible to infections (for example, chickenpox, measles), and may become sicker than others, so risk of exposure must be minimized.

• Growth in children and adolescents must be monitored because there is evidence that oral corticosteroids may suppress growth when used long term or at high doses.

• Special care and monitoring is required by asthmatics who are transferred from using systemically active to inhaled corticosteroids because serious reactions (even fatal) can occur during times of stress due to adrenal insufficiency. People will be advised of what to do (for example, resume systemic corticosteroids) during times of stress or severe asthma attacks and a medic-alert bracelet/ warning card should be carried explaining this.

Interactions

No significant interactions have been reported.

Side effects

These depend on how administered, dose, duration of treatment, and use.

• Inhalation: Frequently, nausea, vomiting, sore throat, diarrhea, unpleasant taste, upset stomach, cold symptoms, and nasal congestion. Occasionally, dizziness, irritability; nervousness, abdominal pain, heartburn, and edema.

• Intranasal: Occasionally, mild nose or throat irritation, dryness, rebound congestion, asthma, runny nose, loss of sense of taste. There may be systemic effects (see ℞ **corticosteroid**).

fluocinolone acetonide Ⓖ

Type/Group: **corticosteroid; anti-inflammatory**.
Brand(s): Flurosyn; Synalar; FS Shampoo; Fluonid; Derma-Smoothe/FS; various generic.
How administered: Topically.

Used to treat

Fluocinolone is used to treat non-infective inflammation of the skin caused by conditions such as ⊙ **eczema** and ⊙ **psoriasis**, atopic ⊙ **dermatitis**, ⊙ **pruritis**, and contact dermatitis.

Warnings

• It should not be used by people with known hypersensitivity to corticosteroids, or with fungal infections.

• It should be given with caution to anyone with bacterial or viral infections, and to children, who may be more susceptible to systemic side effects.

• It must not be used on the face, groin, or armpits.

• Corticosteroids can cross the placenta. It is unknown whether external application could result in sufficient systemic absorption to create a hazard to the fetus. Therefore, fluocinolone acetonide should only be used during pregnancy if medically judged to be essential.

• Medical judgment is also required if considering breast-feeding. When taken internally, corticosteroids are excreted in breast milk and may suppress growth and interfere with the production of natural corticosteroids in the infant. It is unknown whether external application could result in sufficient systemic absorption to produce detectable amounts in breast milk.

• Topical (applied externally) corticosteroids can be absorbed in sufficient amounts to produce systemic effects. Therefore do not use over large surface areas or for prolonged periods in order to minimize the risk of systemic absorption.

• Bandages or dressings must not be placed over the treated area unless directed by a doctor, as this may increase the risk of adverse skin reactions.

• Weeping, denuded, or infected areas, and the eyes must be avoided.

• A doctor must be notified and use of flucinolone stopped if local irritation or fever develops.

Interactions

No significant interactions have been reported.

Side effects

• Occasionally, irritation, and itching.

• Rarely, allergic rash. Systemic effects are possible (see ℞ **corticosteroid**).

fluocinonide Ⓖ

Type/Group: **corticosteroid; anti-inflammatory**.
Brand(s): Fluonex; Lidex; various generic.
How administered: Topically.

Used to treat

Fluocinonide is used to treat non-infective inflammation of the skin caused by conditions such as ⊙ **eczema**, ⊙ **psoriasis**, ⊙ **pruritis**, contact ⊙ **dermatitis** and atopic dermatitis.

Warnings

• It should not be used by people with known hypersensitivity to corticosteroids, or with fungal infections.

• It should be given with caution to anyone with a bacterial or viral infection, and to children, who may be more susceptible to systemic side effects.

• It must not be used on the face, groin, or armpits.

• Corticosteroids can cross the placenta. It is unknown whether external application could result in sufficient systemic absorption to create a hazard to the fetus. Therefore, fluocinonide should only be used in pregnancy if medically judged to be essential.

• Medical judgment is required if breast-feeding is being considered. When taken internally, corticosteroids are excreted in breast milk and may suppress growth and interfere with the production of natural corticosteroids in the infant. It is unknown whether external application could result in sufficient systemic absorption to produce detectable amounts in breast milk.

• Topical (applied externally) corticosteroids can be absorbed in sufficient amounts to produce systemic effects. Therefore, fluocinonide should not be applied over large surface areas or for a prolonged period to minimize the risk of systemic absorption.

• Bandages or dressings must not be placed over the treated area unless directed by a doctor, as this may increase the risk of adverse skin reactions.

• Weeping, denuded, or infected areas, and the eyes must be avoided.

• A doctor must be notified and use of fluocinide stopped if local irritation or fever develops.

Interactions
No significant interactions have been reported.

Side effects
• Occasionally, irritation, and itching.

• Rarely, allergic rash. There may be systemic effects (see ℞ **corticosteroid**).

Fluogen ⑧
A preparation of ℞ **influenza virus vaccine**.
Formulation: Intramuscular injection.
Availability: Prescription only.
Warnings and side effects: See ℞ **influenza virus vaccine**.

Fluonex ⑧
A preparation of ℞ **fluocinonide**.
Formulation: Cream in several strengths.
Availability: Prescription only.
Warnings and side effects: See ℞ **fluocinonide**.

Fluonid ⑧
A preparation of ℞ **fluocinolone acetonide**.
Formulation: Solution.
Availability: Prescription only.
Warnings and side effects: See ℞ **fluocinolone acetonide**.

fluorescein sodium ⑥
Type/Group: diagnostic agent.
Brand(s): AK-Fluor; Fluorescite; Ful-Glo; Fluorets; various generic.
How administered: Topically (eye); injection.

Used to treat
Fluorescein sodium is a dye that is used on the surface of an eye in ophthalmic diagnostic procedures, or is injected in ophthalmic angiography.

Warnings
• It should not be given to people with known hypersensitivity to fluorescein or any component of the product.

• The injectable form should not be used during the first trimester. Either form should be used during pregnancy only when they are clearly needed.

• Medical judgment is required if breast-feeding is being considered. It is not known whether this drug is found in breast milk.

• It may discolor soft contact lenses.

Interactions
No significant interactions specific to this drug are known.

Side effects
• Strong taste, discoloration of skin and urine. With the injected form: nausea, headache, gastrointestinal distress, vomiting, fainting, and allergic reaction.

Fluorescite ⑧
A preparation of ℞ **fluorescein sodium**.
Formulation: Injection.
Availability: Prescription only.
Warnings and side effects: See ℞ **fluorescein sodium**.

Fluorets ⑧
A preparation of ℞ **fluorescein sodium**.
Formulation: Ophthalmic strips.
Availability: Prescription only.
Warnings and side effects: See ℞ **fluorescein sodium**.

fluorometholone ⑥
Type/Group: **corticosteroid; anti-inflammatory**.
Brand(s): Fluor-Op; FML; Flarex; various generic. Combinations: With *sulfacetamide*: FML-S Liquifilm.
How administered: Topically.

Used to treat
Fluorometholone is used to treat inflammatory conditions of the eye, corneal injury, post-operative inflammation after eye surgery, and graft rejection after cornea replacement surgery.

Warnings
• It should not be used by people with known hypersensitivity to corticosteroids. This drug is not appropriate for use in certain eye disorders.

• It must be given with caution to children.

• Corticosteroids can cross the placenta. It is unknown whether external application could result in sufficient systemic absorption to create a hazard to the fetus. Therefore, fluorometholone should only be used in pregnancy if medically judged to be essential.

• Medical judgment is also required if breast-feeding is being considered. When taken internally, corticosteroids are excreted in breast milk and may suppress growth and interfere with the production of natural corticosteroids in the infant. It is unknown whether external application could result in sufficient systemic absorption to produce detectable amounts in breast milk.

• Prolonged use may result in secondary eye infections. A doctor must be notified if the condition worsens, persists, or if pain, itching, or swelling of the eye occurs.

• A doctor must be contacted if there is no improvement after two days, but treatment must not be stopped without consulting a physician.

Interactions

No significant interactions have been reported.

Side effects

• Occasionally, cataracts, decreased acuity, worsening of glaucoma, stinging or burning, and visual field defects.

• Rarely, optic nerve damage.

• Sytemic effects are possible (see ℞ **corticosteroid**).

Fluor-Op ⑧

A preparation of ℞ **fluorometholone**.
Formulation: Eye drops.
Availability: Prescription only.
Warnings and side effects: See ℞ **fluorometholone**.

fluoroquinolone ⑩

see ℞ **quinolone**.

fluorouracil ⑥

Type/Group: anticancer; cytotoxic.
Brand(s): Adrucil; various generic.
How administered: Intravenous injection; topically (external).

Used to treat

Fluorouracil is a cytotoxic drug (an antimetabolite) that is used primarily in the treatment of solid ✪ **tumors** (for example, of the colon and breast). It works by preventing the cancer cells from replicating and so prevents the growth of the cancer. It is sometimes given with other drugs (in advanced colorectal (large intestine) cancer). It is sometimes given by injection together with floxuridine, which is converted in the body to fluorouracil, but the two drugs in combination can have a greater effect. It is also given topically (externally) to treat superficial basal cell carcinomas and multiple actinic or solar keratosis.

Warnings

• It should not be given to people with known hypersensitivity to this drug, with poor nutritional status, depressed bone marrow function, or potentially serious infections. This is a specialist drug which will be used following a full evaluation by specialist physicians.

• Fluorouracil is not recommended for use during pregnancy unless it is medically judged to be essential, because it may cause birth defects. Becoming pregnant while using this drug must be avoided.

• It should not be used if breast-feeding.

• It can cause bone marrow depression, which may lead to bleeding and a reduced resistance to infection.

• When applied topically, ulcerated or inflamed skin must be avoided.

• When used topically, exposure to UV radiation must be avoided.

• It can impair fertility in men and women (which may be reversible).

• In common with many anticancer drugs, genetic mutations have occurred with its use.

• It may cause adverse effects on the heart.

Interactions

• ℞ **Leucovorin** increases toxicity.

Side effects

• Diarrhea, fever, weakness, other gastrointestinal disturbances, blood changes, and hair loss.

• When used topically, pain, itching, irritation, darkened skin, scarring, burning on site of application, and allergic contact dermatitis.

fluoxetine ⑥

Type/Group: SSRI; antidepressant.
Brand(s): Prozac; Sarefem (for premenstrual symptoms).
How administered: Orally.

Used to treat

Fluoxetine is used to treat ✪ **depression**, premenstrual dysphoric disorder, ✪ **bulimia** nervosa, and ✪ **obsessive-compulsive disorder** (OCD). It has the advantage over some earlier antidepressants because it has relatively less sedative and ℞ **anticholinergic** side effects. It may take some weeks to reach full effect and the decline of its effects after ending treatment is also slow. Although not stated by the manufacturer for such used, it is sometimes used to treat anorexia nervosa, attention-deficit hyperactivity disorder, bipolar disorder (manic-depressive illness), cataplexy and narcolepsy, kleptomania, migraine and other headaches, post-traumatic stress disorder, schizophrenia, trichotillomania, levodopa-induced dyskinesia, recurrent fainting, Tourette's syndrome, and social phobia.

Warnings

• It should not be given to people with known hypersensitivity to this type of drug or to anyone taking a ℞ **MAOI** antidepressant (see Interactions below).

• It should be given with caution to people with liver or severe kidney impairment, heart disorders, a history of seizures, diabetes mellitus, psychosis, bipolar disorder, or anyone receiving electroconvulsive therapy.

• Fluoxetine should be used during pregnancy only if the benefits outweigh the possible risk to the fetus.

• Medical judgment is required if breast-feeding is being considered.

• A doctor must be consulted before taking any other medications, including OTC preparations, herbal remedies (especially ♣ St. John's wort), supplements (for example the ⚯ amino acids tryptophan and tyramine) or any other natural or alternative products.

• Avoid or minimize alcohol consumption.

• Judgment, thinking, and physical skills may be impaired, so use caution when first taking the drug.

• It may cause sensitivity to sunlight.

• Treatment should be stopped gradually, lowering the dose over a period of time.

• It may be 4 to 6 weeks before there are any signs of improvement.

Interactions

• Serious and even fatal reactions have occurred when ℞ **MAOI** antidepressants are taken with other antidepressants. There should be at least a 14-day gap between discontinuing a MAOI and starting to use fluoxetine, and at least 5 weeks between stopping fluoxetine and starting a MAOI.

• Tryptophan (see ⚭ **amino acids**) increases the risk of adverse effects (for example agitation, gastrointestinal effects) due to excessive serotonin.

• The levels of ℞ **antihistamines** (non-sedating), ℞ **imipramine** and other ℞ **tricyclics**, ℞ **benzodiazepines** (for example, ℞ **diazepam**), ℞ **beta-blockers** (for example, ℞ **metoprolol**) ℞ **dextromethorphan**, ℞ **haloperidol**, ℞ **carbamazepine**, statin/HMG-CoA reductase inhibitors (for example, ℞ **lovastatin**), and ℞ **phenytoin** may be increased by fluoxetine.

• If used with ℞ **buspirone**, the effects of both drugs may be reduced, and seizures are possible.

• ℞ **Cyproheptadine** and ℞ **serotonin-receptor antagonist** may reverse the effects of fluoxetine.

• Loop ℞ **diuretics** (for example, ℞ **bumetanide**) may increase the risk of severe low sodium levels.

• If used with ℞ **lithium**, neurotoxicity has been reported.

Side effects

• Gastrointestinal effects (related to dose; including nausea and vomiting, indigestion, and loose stools) and anorexia. Also, anxiety, insomnia, dizziness, headache, drowsiness, tiredness, and tremor.

• Important sensitivity reactions (skin reactions including angioedema and urticaria, muscle pain and other allergic reactions) can occur.

• Less frequently, absence of emotion, sexual dysfunction, mental changes, hot flashes, palpitations, visual disturbance, taste changes, painful menstruation, changes in blood glucose levels, joint or muscle pain, sweating, and fever.

• Rare but serious side effects include seizures.

fluoxymesterone ⑥

Type/Group: **sex hormone; androgen; anticancer**.
Brand(s): Halotestin; various generic.
How administered: Orally.

Used to treat

Fluoxymesterone is a synthetic ℞ **testosterone** derivative used to treat male ⚬ **hypogonadism** (subnormal secretion of sex hormones) and delayed puberty in males. In women it is used as a treatment for advanced metastatic ⚬ **breast cancer**. It is also sometimes used for postpartum breast pain and engorgement.

Warnings

• It should not be used by people with serious heart, liver or kidney disease, or hypersensitivity to androgens; or by men with cancer of the breast or prostate.

• It should be given with caution to people with acute intermittent porphyria, history of myocardial infarction, cardiovascular disease, coronary artery disease, seizure disorder, or benign prostatic

hyperplasia, or diabetes mellitus. It should be given with extreme caution to children and anyone over 65.

• Fluoxymesterone should not be used during pregnancy.

• Medical judgment is required if breast-feeding is being considered.

• It should not be used to enhance athletic performance.

• In males over 65 there is an increased risk of prostatic cancer, and it may markedly increase libido.

• Fluoxymesterone is a Schedule III controlled substance.

Interactions

• The response to oral ℞ **anticoagulants** (for example, ℞ **warfarin sodium**) may be increased.

• Levels of ℞ **cyclosporine** are increased with potential for toxic effects.

Side effects

• In women there is commonly virilization (deepening voice, growth of body hair, acne, clitoral enlargement, irregular periods).

• In men there is commonly breast soreness or enlargement, urinary tract infection, excessive frequency and duration of penile erections.

• Occasionally, impotence and testicular atrophy. Also, edema, nausea, vomiting, mild acne, diarrhea, and stomach pain.

• Rarely, white blood cell disorders. Prolonged use of high doses may cause serious liver disease, and, rarely, cancer in women. In men, reduced sperm count and ejaculatory volume may occur after prolonged or excessive use.

• When given to children, it may speed up bone maturation without producing proportional increase in height, which can affect final adult stature. It may cause reduction of bone calcium in immobilized patients.

fluphenazine ⑥

Type/Group: **antipsychotic; phenothiazine**.
Brand(s): Permitil; Prolixin; various generic.
How administered: Orally; injection.

Used to treat

Fluphenazine is used in the treatment of psychoses (see ⚬ **psychotic disorders**), such as ⚬ **schizophrenia**. Although not stated by the manufacturer for such use, it is sometimes given for ⚬ **Huntington's disease**, control of acute agitation, and ⚬ **dementia**.

Warnings

• It should not be given to people with known hypersensitivity to this drug, liver damage, cerebral arteriosclerosis, coronary artery disease, severe high or low blood pressure, certain blood diseases, coma, subcortical brain damage, or bone marrow depression.

• It should be given with caution to people with depression, acute lung infection, chronic respiratory disorders, cardiovascular disease, glaucoma, seizure disorder (epilepsy), impaired kidney or liver function, to anyone receiving electroconvulsive therapy, who is experiencing alcohol withdrawal, or is over 65.

• Fluphenazine should be used during pregnancy only if the benefits outweigh the possible risk to the fetus.

• Medical judgment is required if breast-feeding is being considered.

• Judgment, thinking, and physical skills may be impaired.

• It may increase susceptibility to heat stroke, exercise caution in hot weather.

• It may cause postural hypotension (lowered blood pressure on standing), so rise slowly from a reclining position. Older people in particular should exercise caution.

• It may cause sensitivity to sunlight (photosensitivity), so minimize exposure (use a sunscreen, sunglasses, and so on).

• If used for a long time, tardive dyskinesia (see ℞ **antipsychotics**) occasionally develops.

• It may color urine reddish-brown or pink.

• Treatment should be stopped gradually.

• Avoid alcohol.

Interactions

• Fluphenazine may inhibit the antiparkinsonian effect of ℞ **levodopa**.

• If used with ℞ **anticholinergics**, the effects of fluphenazine are lowered, while those of the anticholinergics are increased.

• ℞ **Antimalarials** (amodiaquine, chloroquine, sulfadoxine, pyrimethamine) increase the effects of fluphenazine.

• ℞ **Barbiturates** and ℞ **orphenadrine** reduce the effects of fluphenazine.

• If used with a ℞ **beta-blocker** or a ℞ **tricyclic** antidepressant, potentially the effects of both drugs are increased.

• If used with ℞ **bromocriptine**, the effects of both drugs are reduced.

• Fluphenazine reduces the effects of ℞ **guanadrel**.

• Fluphenazine may alter the response to ℞ **epinephrine**.

• If used with ℞ **meperidine**, blood pressure is lowered and there is excessive CNS (central nervous system) depression.

• Rarely, there is severe neurotoxicity (nerve damage) in acutely manic patients when used with ℞ **lithium**.

• If an antipsychotic is taken with alcohol, there may be increased sedative effects.

Side effects

• These depend on how it is administered and can be serious. Fluphenazine is less sedating than some phenothiazines, but there is more of a risk of extrapyramidal side effects (see ℞ **antipsychotics**).

• Also, there may be pseudoparkinsonism (parkinson symptoms) restlessness, abnormal muscle tone, postural hypotension, loss of appetite, constipation, nausea, and vomiting.

• Less frequently, drowsiness, fatigue, headache, vertigo, ECG changes, increases in blood pressure, speeded heartbeat, eye changes, weight gain, urinary disorders, male sexual disorders, priapism (prolonged, painful penile erection), metabolic abnormalities, SIADH (syndrome of inappropriate antidiuretic hormone secretion), bronchial spasm, shortness of breath, spasm of the larynx, rash, and heat intolerance.

• Rare but serious side effects include, seizures, tardive dyskinesia (which usually takes longer to develop), hepatitis, stoppage of peristalsis (normal intestinal motion), serious blood disorders, heart attack, neuroleptic malignant syndrome (a potentially fatal condition characterized by very high fever, muscle rigidity,

changes in mental status, and irregular pulse, blood pressure and/or heart rhythm).

flurandrenolide Ⓖ

(fludroxycortide)

Type/Group: **corticosteroid; anti-inflammatory**.

Brand(s): Cordran; various generic.

How administered: Topically.

Used to treat

Flurandrenolide is used to treat non-infective inflammation of the skin caused by conditions such as contact ✪ **dermatitis**, ✪ **pruritis**, ✪ **eczema**, and ✪ **psoriasis**.

Warnings

• It should not be used by people with known hypersensitivity to corticosteroids, or those with fungal infections.

• It should be given with caution to anyone with a bacterial or viral infection, and children, who may be more susceptible to systemic side effects.

• It must not be used on the face, groin, or armpits.

• Corticosteroids can cross the placenta. It is unknown whether external application could result in sufficient systemic absorption to create a hazard to the fetus. Therefore, fluocinonide should only be used during pregnancy if medically judged to be essential.

• Medical judgment is also required if breast-feeding is being considered. When taken internally, corticosteroids are excreted in breast milk and may suppress growth and interfere with the production of natural corticosteroids in the infant. It is unknown whether external application could result in sufficient systemic absorption to produce detectable amounts in breast milk.

• Topical (applied externally) corticosteroids can be absorbed in sufficient amounts to produce systemic effects. Therefore, do not use over large surface areas or for a prolonged period to minimize the risk of systemic absorption.

• Bandages or dressings must not cover the treated area unless directed by a doctor, as this may increase the risk of adverse skin reactions.

• Avoid weeping, denuded, or infected areas, and the eyes.

• A doctor must be notified and use of flurandrenolide stopped if local irritation or fever develops.

Interactions

No significant interactions have been reported.

Side effects

• Occasionally, irritation, and itching.

• Rarely, allergic rash. Systemic effects are possible (see ℞ **corticosteroid**).

flurazepam Ⓖ

Type/Group: **hypnotic; benzodiazepine**.

Brand(s): Dalmane.

How administered: Orally.

Used to treat

Flurazepam is used for the short-term treatment of ✪ **insomnia** where some sedation during the daytime is acceptable.

Warnings

• It should not be given to people with known hypersensitivity to benzodiazepines.

• It should be given with caution to people with kidney or liver impairment, depression, a history of drug abuse, respiratory depression, sleep apnea, or anyone over 65.

• Flurazepam is not recommended for use during pregnancy. A doctor must be contacted if pregnancy occurs while taking this drug.

• Medical judgment is required if breast-feeding is being considered.

• It may cause drowsiness the next day and so judgment, thinking, and physical skills may be impaired.

• Avoid alcohol consumption because adverse side effects may be increased (see Side effects below).

• Avoid other psychotropic medications unless prescribed by a doctor.

• A doctor must be consulted before discontinuing use or increasing dosage, because benzodiazepines may produce psychological and physical dependence and withdrawal symptoms.

• Sleep may be disturbed for the first or second night after discontinuing the drug.

Interactions

• ℞ **azole** antifungals (for example, ℞ **ketoconazole**, ℞ **itraconazole**), ℞ **beta-blockers** (for example, ℞ **propranolol**), ℞ **cimetidine**, ℞ **disulfiram**, ℞ **isoniazid**, ℞ **macrolide** antibiotics (for example, ℞ **erythromycin**, ℞ **clarithromycin**, troleandomycin), ℞ **omeprazole**, ℞ SSRIs, and ℞ **quinolones** may increase levels of flurazepam.

• If used with ℞ **clozapine**, there maybe an increased risk of cardiorespiratory collapse.

• When used with ℞ **loxapine**, there have been isolated cases of respiratory depression and stupor, although the role of drug interaction has not been established.

• ℞ **rifampin** may reduce effects of flurazepam.

• Alcohol may increase adverse side effects.

Side effects

• Daytime sedation and drowsiness.

• Less frequently, anxiety, confusion, dizziness, headache, irritability, chest pain, heart or pulse changes, gastrointestinal effects, allergic skin reactions, flushing, and sweating.

• Rare but serious side effects include blood cell disorders.

flurbiprofen Ⓖ

Type/Group: **anti-inflammatory; antirheumatic; non-narcotic analgesic; NSAID**.
Brand(s): Ansaid; various generic. (For ophthalmic use): Ocufen Solution; various generic.
How administered: Orally; topically (eye).

Used to treat

Flurbiprofen has similar uses to those of ℞ **aspirin**. It is used particularly in the acute or long-term treatment of ○ **rheumatoid arthritis** and ○ **osteoarthritis**. It can also used in the eye, for example, to reduce inflammation, and also for the pain of conditions such as ○ **dysmenorrhea**.

Warnings

• It should not be used by people with known hypersensitivity to this drug or to other NSAIDs (including aspirin), who have chronic kidney disease, certain bleeding disorders or conditions (for example, hemophilia, vitamin K deficiency, low blood-platelet levels), or who have a tendency to, or active, peptic ulceration.

• It should be given with caution to people taking certain drugs for gout, or with allergic disorders (especially asthma and skin conditions), who are elderly, or with any kind of kidney impairment or with certain liver disorders.

• Flurbiprofen should be used only when medically judged that the benefits outweigh risk to the fetus. However, it should not be used in the third trimester when risk to the fetus is at its highest.

• Breast-feeding mothers should either discontinue this drug or stop breast-feeding.

• With regular, long-term use (as in the treatment of osteoarthritis), NSAIDs may cause gastrointestinal bleeding, ulceration, or perforation. Any signs of bleeding (for example, black stools) should be reported to a physician immediately.

• Most NSAIDs have the potential, particularly with regular use, to cause liver damage. Periodic evaluation of liver function is necessary in long-term therapy (more than two months).

• Side effects are more frequent in the elderly.

• Gastrointestinal upsets, when taken orally, may be minimized by taking the drug with milk or food.

Interactions

• There is generally no added benefit in taking other NSAIDs or other ℞ **salicylates** (especially aspirin) at the same time, but there is a higher risk of gastrointestinal upsets and bleeding.

• Alcohol increases the risk of bleeding, particularly if there is an existing ulcer.

• ℞ **anticoagulant**, ℞ **antiplatelet**, and ℞ **thrombolytic** drugs may increase bleeding time.

• Flurbiprofen may reduce the effectiveness of ℞ **diuretics**, ℞ **ACE inhibitors**, and ℞ **beta-blockers**.

• The effects of ℞ **lithium** and ℞ **methotrexate** may be exaggerated, with potential for serious toxicity.

• Foodstuffs and herbals with ℞ **antiplatelet** properties, for example, ♣ **ginger**, ⚭ **garlic**, and various herbal preparations, may add to the antiplatelet effect of NSAIDs.

Side effects

These depend on how it is administered, dose, duration of treatment, and use, and vary in severity and how often they occur.

• Commonly gastrointestinal upsets, diarrhea, nausea, headache and swelling of the extremities. dizziness, and malaise.

• Less frequently, constipation, flatulence, vomiting, rash, ringing in the ears, blurred vision, dizziness, nervousness, malaise, and depression.

• Prolonged bleeding time (with consequent risk of ulceration) is possible with high dosage, and other blood changes can occur, including anemia.

• Hypersensitivity reactions may include symptoms such as swelling of eyelids, tongue, lips, or larynx, rash, chest tightness, asthma, or bronchospasm.

• Reversible kidney failure, particularly in renal impairment, has occurred. Liver damage is rare.

• There may be burning, stinging, itching, or blurred vision when used as eyedrops.

Flurosyn Ⓑ

A preparation of ℞ **fluocinolone acetonide**.
Formulation: Cream in several strengths; ointment.
Availability: Prescription only.
Warnings and side effects: See ℞ **fluocinolone acetonide**.

FluShield Ⓑ

A preparation of ℞ **influenza virus vaccine**.
Formulation: Intramuscular injection.
Availability: Prescription only.
Warnings and side effects: See ℞ **influenza virus vaccine**.

flutamide Ⓖ

Type/Group: **hormone antagonist; antiandrogen; anticancer**.
Brand(s): Eulexin.
How administered: Orally.

Used to treat

Flutamide is used as an anticancer drug, along with other drugs (for example, leuprolide), for the treatment of ✚ **prostate cancer** (specifically for management of locally confined stage B_2 to C and Stage D_2 metastatic prostate carcinoma).

Warnings

• It should not be used by people with known hypersensitivity to this drug.

• It should be given with caution to people with certain liver disorders (liver function may be monitored).

• Flutamide should not be used by pregnant women.

• Feminization may occur during therapy.

• Treatment must not be stopped without notifying a doctor.

Interactions

• Flutamide may interfere with the effects of ℞ **anticoagulants** (for example, ℞ **warfarin sodium**).

Side effects

• Hot flashes, diarrhea, nausea, vomiting, decreased libido, impotence, growth and tenderness of breasts, and anemia.

• Rare but serious side effects include hepatitis and certain blood-cell disorders.

Flutex Ⓑ

A preparation of ℞ **triamcinolone** acetate.
Formulation: Cream; ointment, both in several strengths.
Availability: Prescription only.
Warnings and side effects: See ℞ **triamcinolone**.

fluticasone propionate Ⓖ

Type/Group: **corticosteroid; anti-inflammatory**.
Brand(s): Cutivate; Flovent; various generic.

How administered: Topically; inhalant.

Used to treat

Fluticasone propionate is used to treat non-infective inflammation of the skin caused by conditions such as ✚ **eczema** and ✚ **psoriasis**. It can be used as a respiratory inhalant for prevention of bronchial ✚ **asthma** and seasonal allergic rhinitis, perennial allergic rhinitis, and non-allergic rhinitis.

Warnings

• It should not be used by people with known hypersensitivity to corticosteroids, or with fungal infections.

• It should be given with caution to anyone with a bacterial or viral infection, and to children, who may be more susceptible to systemic side effects.

• It is not used for the relief of acute bronchospasm.

• Corticosteroids can cross the placenta, and therefore fluocinonide should only be used during pregnancy if medically judged to be essential.

• Medical judgment is also required if breast-feeding is being considered. When taken internally, corticosteroids are excreted in breast milk and may suppress growth and interfere with the production of natural corticosteroids in the infant. It is unknown whether external application could result in sufficient systemic absorption to produce detectable amounts in breast milk.

• Topical (applied externally) corticosteroids can be absorbed in sufficient amounts to produce systemic effects. Therefore, do not use over large surface areas or for a prolonged period to minimize the risk of systemic absorption.

• Bandages or dressings must not cover the treated area unless directed by a doctor, as this may increase the risk of adverse skin reactions.

• Avoid weeping, denuded, or infected areas.

• Localized fungal infections (thrush) have occurred in the mouths and throats of people using corticosteroid inhalants.

• Because corticosteroids suppress the immune system, anyone using long-term inhalant therapy is particularly susceptible to infections (for example, chickenpox, measles), and may become sicker than others, so risk of exposure must be minimized.

• Growth in children and adolescents must be monitored because there is evidence that oral corticosteroids may suppress growth with long-term or high doses of use.

• Special care and monitoring is required by asthmatics who are transferred from using systemically active to inhaled corticosteroids because serious reactions (even fatal) can occur during times of stress due to adrenal insufficiency. People will be advised of what to do (for example, resume systemic corticosteroids) during times of stress or severe asthma attacks and a medic-alert bracelet/warning card should be carried explaining this.

Interactions

• ℞ **ketoconazole** may increase the concentration of fluticasone, but there is no significant clinical effect.

Side effects

These depend on how administered, dose, duration of treatment, and use.

• Topical use: Occasionally, irritation, and itching. Rarely, allergic rash.

• Inhalation: Frequently, headache, upper respiratory infections, sore throat, and nasal congestion. Occasionally, gastrointestinal effects, fever. Rarely, allergic reactions. Systemic effects may occur (see ℞ **corticosteroid**).

fluvastatin ⑥

Type/Group: **lipid-regulating drug; statin.**
Brand(s): Lescol.
How administered: Orally.

Used to treat

Fluvastatin is a (statin/HMG-CoA reductase inhibitor) lipid-regulating drug that can be used in ⚙ **hyperlipidemia** to reduce the levels, or change the proportions, of various lipids in the bloodstream. It is usually given only to people in whom a strict and regular dietary regime alone is not having the desired effect. It is also used to help prevent heart attacks.

Warnings

• It should not be given to people with active liver disease.
• It should be given with caution to people with a history of liver disease, kidney insufficiency, conditions predisposing to kidney failure, severe endocrine, metabolic, or electrolyte disorders, or heavy users of alcohol.
• Fluvastatin is considered quite hazardous to the fetus. It is given to women of childbearing age only when they are thought highly unlikely to conceive and have been informed of the risks.
• It should not be used while breast-feeding.
• When taking fluvastatin, any unusual muscle pain or tenderness should be reported to a doctor immediately and treatment stopped, because it has the potential to cause destruction of muscle tissue.
• Potentially harmful changes in liver function may occur, so periodic tests may be necessary to check the drug's effect.

Interactions

• ℞ **Azoles** (antifungals such as ℞ **itraconazole,** ℞ **ketoconazole**), ℞ **danazol,** ℞ **cimetidine,** ℞ **ranitidine,** ℞ **omeprazole,** mibefradil, ℞ **erythromycin,** ℞ **clarithromycin,** ℞ **nefazodone,** ℞ **cyclosporine,** ℞ **gemfibrozil,** ℞ **niacin,** and (℞ **nicotinic acid,** a B vitamin) increase the levels of fluvastatin and the risk of adverse effects.
• ℞ **Cholestyramine,** ℞ **colestipol hydrochloride,** and ℞ **rifampin** interfere with the effects of fluvastatin.
• The effects of ℞ **warfarin sodium** may be increased.
• Alcohol may increase levels of fluvastatin.

Side effects

• Headache, gastrointestinal effects, muscle pain or inflammation, insomnia, destruction of muscle tissue, and kidney or liver damage.

fluvoxamine ⑥

Type/Group: **antidepressant; SSRI.**
Brand(s): Luvox.
How administered: Orally.

Used to treat

Fluvoxamine is used for ⚙ **obsessive-compulsive disorder** (OCD) and also, although not stated by the manufacturer for such treat-

ment, for ⚙ **depression.** As is the case with other drugs of this type, it is being investigated for use in other disorders.

Warnings

• It should not be given to people with known hypersensitivity to this type of drug or to anyone taking a ℞ **MAOI** antidepressant (see Interactions below).
• It should be given with caution to people with liver or severe kidney impairment, heart disorders, a history of seizures, diabetes mellitus, psychosis, bipolar disorder (manic depression), or anyone receiving electroconvulsive therapy.
• Fluvoxamine should be used during pregnancy only if the benefits outweigh the possible risk to the fetus.
• Medical judgment is required if breast-feeding is being considered.
• A doctor must be consulted before taking any other medications, including OTC preparations, herbal remedies (especially ♣ **St. John's wort**), supplements (for example the ⚬⚬ **amino acids** tryptophan and tyramine) or other natural or alternative products.
• Avoid or minimize alcohol consumption.
• Judgment, thinking, and physical skills may be impaired, so use caution when first taking the drug.
• It may cause sensitivity to sunlight.
• Treatment should be stopped gradually, lowering the dose over a period of time.
• It may be more than a week before there are any signs of improvement.

Interactions

• Serious and even fatal reactions have occurred when ℞ **MAOIs** are taken with other antidepressants. There should be at least a 14-day gap between discontinuing a MAOI and starting another type.
• Cisapride and ℞ **pimozide** should not normally be taken at the same time as fluvoxamine.
• The risk of toxicity from non-sedating ℞ **antihistamines** (such as astemizole and ℞ **fexofenadine**), ℞ **phenytoin,** and ℞ **theophylline** is increased.
• The metabolism of ℞ **clozapine,** ℞ **tricyclic,** antidepressants, ℞ **trazodone,** ℞ **benzodiazepines,** ℞ **carbamazepine,** ℞ **beta-blockers,** and HMG-CoA reductase inhibitors (℞ **atorvastatin,** ℞ **lovastatin**), and ℞ **theophylline** may be inhibited.
• The effects of ℞ **warfarin sodium** may be increased.
• If used with ℞ **lithium,** a serious adverse reaction is possible.

Side effects

• Headache, insomnia, sleepiness, diarrhea, dry mouth, nausea, indigestion, and effects on the heart.
• Less frequently, postural hypotension (lowered blood pressure on standing), confusion and hallucinations, unsteady gait, abnormal liver function, hypersensitivity reactions (rash, itching, muscle pain), sexual disorders (abnormal ejaculation, sexual dysfunction) and urinary frequency.

Fluzone ⑧

A preparation of ℞ **influenza virus vaccine.**
Formulation: Intramuscular injection.
Availability: Prescription only.
Warnings and side effects: See ℞ **influenza virus vaccine.**

FML; FML Forte; FML S.O.P. ®

A preparation of ℞ **fluorometholone**.
Formulation: Eye drops in two strengths (Forte is higher strength); ointment (S.O.P.).
Availability: Prescription only.
Warnings and side effects: See ℞ **fluorometholone**.

Foamicon ®

A preparation of ℞ **aluminum hydroxide**, ℞ **magnesium trisilicate**, and ℞ **sodium bicarbonate**.
Formulation: Oral tablets, chewable.
Availability: OTC.
Warnings and side effects: See ℞ **aluminum hydroxide**; ℞ **magnesium trisilicate**; ℞ **sodium bicarbonate**.

Foille; Foille Plus ®

A preparation of ℞ **benzocaine** and ℞ **chloroxylenol**.
Formulation: Topical aerosol; topical spray.
Availability: OTC.
Warnings and side effects: See ℞ **benzocaine** ℞ **chloroxylenol**.

Folergot-DF ®

A preparation of ℞ **ergotamine tartrate**, ℞ **belladonna alkaloid**, and ℞ **phenobarbital**.
Formulation: Oral tablets.
Availability: Prescription only.
Warnings and side effects: See ℞ **ergotamine tartrate**; ℞ **belladonna alkaloid**; ℞ **phenobarbital**.

folic acid ⑥

Type/Group: anemia treatment; vitamin.
Brand(s): Folvite; various generic (prescription or over-the-counter depending upon strength).
How administered: Orally; injection.

Used to treat

Folic acid, also known as pteroylglutamic acid, is a vitamin of the B complex and is used to treat certain forms of ✪ **anemia** (for example, megaloblastic anemia). It has an important role in the synthesis of nucleic acids (DNA and RNA). Good food sources of folic acid include liver and vegetables and its consumption is particularly necessary during the first few months of pregnancy. Folic acid supplements are recommended before and during pregnancy to help prevent neural tube defects. See also ℞ **folic acid** in the Supplements part.

Warnings

• It should not be given to people with known allergy to folic acid preparations or with anemias in which vitamin B_{12} is deficient (it will not be effective).
• It is safe for use during pregnancy, but avoid high total levels of folic acid consumption except on a doctor's advice.
• It is compatible with breast-feeding, but very high doses should be avoided.
• It must be used under medical supervision.

• There is a potential danger that folic acid taken by people with undiagnosed ✪ **pernicious anemia** will mask manifestations of the disease and allow neurologic complications to progress.

Interactions

• ℞ **Aminosalicylates**, ℞ **oral contraceptives**, ℞ **methotrexate** and related agents, ℞ **sulfasalazine**, and ℞ **phenytoin** may reduce the effects of folic acid.
• The effects of ℞ **hydantoins** may be reduced.

Side effects

• Folic acid is relatively non-toxic, but at high doses it has been associated with altered sleep patterns, difficulty in concentrating, irritability, excitement, confusion, and gastrointestinal effects.

folinic acid ⑥

see ℞ **leucovorin calcium**.

Follistim ®

A preparation of ℞ **follitropin alfa/follitropin beta**.
Formulation: Injection.
Availability: Prescription only.
Warnings and side effects: See ℞ follitropin alfa/follitropin beta.

follitropin alfa/follitropin beta ⑥

Type/Group: gonadotropin; sex hormone; fertility treatment; anterior pituitary hormone.
Brand(s): Gonal-F; Follistim.
How administered: Injection.

Used to treat

Follitropin alfa and follitropin beta (which are considered therapeutically interchangeable) are used as an infertility treatment in women whose infertility is due to abnormal pituitary gland function, or who do not respond to the commonly used fertility drug ℞ **clomiphene citrate**. They are also used in superovulation treatment for assisted conception, such as in *in vitro* fertilization. In addition, they may be prescribed to treat infertility in men by stimulating sperm production. These follitropin are synthetic forms of the sex hormone, follicle-stimulating hormone (FSH), which is secreted by the anterior pituitary gland and the chorionic tissue of the placenta. In women (in conjunction with luteinizing hormone (LH), it causes the monthly ripening in one ovary of a follicle and stimulates ovulation. In men, it stimulates the production of sperm in the testes.

Warnings

• Not to be used in people with known sensitivity to this drug, uncontrolled thyroid or adrenal dysfunction, sex hormone dependent tumors of the reproductive tract and accessory organs, hypothalamus or pituitary gland.
• In women, it should not be used if there is heavy or irregular vaginal bleeding of undetermined origin or ovarian cyst enlargement of undetermined origin.
• Not for use during pregnancy.
• Not to be used by breast-feeding mothers.
• The risk of multiple births is markedly increased.

Key to symbols: ⑩ = Drug type/group   ⑥ = Generic name   ® = Brand name

• Overstimulation of the ovary may occur. If there is significant ovarian enlargement after ovulation, intercourse must be avoided because of the danger of ruptured ovarian cyst.

• In some cases ovarian hyperstimulation syndrome, a serious medical event, may occur. Early warning signs are severe nausea and vomiting and weight gain; a doctor must be contacted if these develop.

Interactions
Drug interactions for follitropin alfa/beta have not been documented.

Side effects
• Serious lung and circulatory conditions may develop.

• There may be ovarian cysts, gastrointestinal symptoms, pain or irritation at the site of injection, breast tenderness, headache, and skin reactions.

Folvite ®
A preparation of ℞ **folic acid**.
Formulation: Injection.
Availability: Prescription only.
Warnings and side effects: See ℞ **folic acid**.

fomepizole ©
Type/Group: **antidote**.
Brand(s): Antizol.
How administered: Injection.

Used to treat
Fomepizole is used as an antidote to poisoning by ethylene glycol (antifreeze).

Warnings
• It should not be given to people with known severe hypersensitivity to this drug or other pyrazoles.

• It should be given with caution to people over 65.

• Its use should be avoided during the first trimester, and it should be used during pregnancy at any other time only when it is clearly needed.

• Medical judgment is required if breast-feeding is being considered. It is not known whether this drug appears in breast milk.

• It may impair fertility in men.

Interactions
• If used with alcohol, there is a reduced elimination of both drugs.

Side effects
• Abdominal pain, vomiting, hypotension, headache, dizziness, rash, blood changes, seizures, and pain at injection site.

formaldehyde ©
Type/Group: **keratolytic**.
Brand(s): Formaldehyde-10; Lazer formaldehyde.
How administered: Topically (external).

Used to treat
Formaldehyde is a powerful keratolytic agent, which is used, in mild solution to dissolve away layers of toughened or warty skin, especially in the treatment of ✪ **verrucas** (plantar warts) on the soles of the feet.

Warnings
None significant.
Interactions
None significant.
Side effects
None significant.

Formaldehyde-10 ®
A preparation of ℞ **formaldehyde**.
Formulation: Topical spray.
Availability: Prescription only.
Warnings and side effects: See ℞ **formaldehyde**.

Fortaz ®
A preparation of ℞ **ceftazidime**.
Formulation: Injection.
Availability: Prescription only.
Warnings and side effects: See ℞ **ceftazidime**.

Fortovase ®
A preparation of ℞ **saquinavir**.
Formulation: Oral capsules.
Availability: Prescription only.
Warnings and side effects: See ℞ **saquinavir**.

Fosamax ®
A preparation of ℞ **alendronate sodium**.
Formulation: Oral tablets.
Availability: Prescription only.
Warnings and side effects: See ℞ **alendronate sodium**.

foscarnet sodium ©
Type/Group: **antiviral**.
Brand(s): Foscavir.
How administered: Intravenous infusion.

Used to treat
Foscarnet is used to treat cytomegaloviral (CMV) retinitis in patients with ✪ **AIDS** and also resistant herpes simplex and herpes zoster infections (see ✪ **herpes**).

Warnings
• It should not be given to people with known hypersensitivity to foscarnet.

• It should be given with caution to people with neurologic or heart abnormalities, a history of kidney impairment, or altered calcium or other electrolyte levels.

• Foscarnet's safety during pregnancy has not been established, and it should be used only when the potential benefits outweigh the possible risks to the fetus.

• Medical judgment is required if breast-feeding is being considered.

• It often causes kidney impairment.

• Seizures and mineral-electrolyte imbalances may be life-threatening. Any tingling or numbness in the extremities and mouth must be reported to a doctor.

• It does not cure CMV retinitis and relapse may occur.

• It is a specialist drug, and there will be full assessment and patient monitoring throughout treatment.

Interactions
• ℞ **Quinolones** increase the risk of seizure.

Side effects
These can be many and include:
• Frequently, fever and gastrointestinal effects;
• Occasionally, loss of appetite, pain and inflammation at injection site, malaise, change in blood pressure, headache, tingling and numbness, dizziness, rash, and increased sweating;
• Rarely, back or chest pain, edema, flushing, itching constipation, and dry mouth;
• Potentially serious side effects include blood disorders, seizures, and kidney dysfunction.

Foscavir ⑧
A preparation of ℞ **foscarnet sodium**.
Formulation: Intravenous infusion.
Availability: Prescription only.
Warnings and side effects: See ℞ **foscarnet sodium**.

fosfomycin ⑥
Type/Group: **antibiotic; antibacterial.**
Brand(s): Monurol.
How administered: Orally.

Used to treat
Fosfomycin is a broad-spectrum antibiotic used to treat uncomplicated urinary tract bacterial infections (such as ✪ **cystitis**) in women. It is generally used for women for whom the usual treatments are inappropriate.

Warnings
• It should not be given to people with known hypersensitivity to fosfomycin.
• It should be given with caution to people with kidney function impairment.
• Its effects in pregnancy are unknown, and it should be used only if clearly needed.
• Medical judgment is required if breast-feeding is being considered. It is not known whether fosfomycin appears in breast milk.
• It must be mixed with water before taking.

Interactions
• ℞ **Metoclopramide** decreases the levels of fosfomycin.

Side effects
• Frequently, diarrhea, nausea, skin rash, and itching.
• Occasionally, headache, taste alteration, temporary tongue discoloration, yeast and fungal infections.
• Rarely, low blood-platelet count, increased blood pressure, irregular heartbeat or palpitations.

fosinopril sodium ⑥
Type/Group: **ACE inhibitor; antihypertensive; heart failure treatment; vasodilator.**
Brand(s): Monopril.
How administered: Orally.

Used to treat
Fosinopril is used to reduce blood pressure in ✪ **hypertension** and in the treatment of congestive ✪ **heart failure**. It is often used with other classes of drug, particularly ℞ **thiazide** ℞ **diuretics**.

Warnings
• It should not be given to people with known hypersensitivity to this drug or to any other ACE inhibitor.
• It should be given with caution to people with severe congestive heart failure, or certain other cardiovascular disorders, a history of anaphylaxis, collagen vascular disease (for example, systemic lupus erythematosus; SLE), diabetes, depressed immune response, or with impaired liver or kidney function or on dialysis.
• Risk in pregnancy increases substantially from the first through to the second and third trimesters. ACE inhibitors can cause injury to the fetus, even death. The use of these drugs should stop as soon as pregnancy is detected.
• Medical judgment is required if breast-feeding is being considered.
• Its use should be stopped and a doctor contacted immediately if signs of angioedema appear (swelling of the face, eyes, lips, tongue, larynx, or extremities; difficulty in breathing or swallowing). Swelling of the larynx, closing off the airway, can be life-threatening.
• Anyone taking an ACE inhibitor should not interrupt or discontinue treatment without first checking with a doctor.
• If any suspected infections (for example, fever, sore throat) occur, a doctor must be contacted at once. ACE inhibitors may cause blood changes which can affect immune response.
• ACE inhibitors generally have less effect on blood pressure in blacks than in non-blacks, and the likelihood of angioedema is higher among blacks, as well.

Interactions
• ACE inhibitors have apparently triggered life-threatening anaphylactoid reactions when used by people also receiving ℞ **desensitizing vaccines**.
• ℞ **Anesthetics** (for example, in surgery), ℞ **phenothiazines**, and ℞ **probenecid** may increase the levels or hypotensive effect of fosinopril.
• Levels of ℞ **lithium** may be increased, with the potential for toxic effects.
• If used with potassium-sparing ℞ **diuretics** or other preparations containing potassium (for example, supplements and salt substitutes), levels of potassium may rise.
• ℞ **NSAIDs** may increase the risk of kidney damage or (in some cases) reduce the effects of ACE inhibitors.
• ℞ **Antacids** and ℞ **rifampin** may reduce the effects of fosinopril. Antacids should not be used for several hours after a dose of an ACE inhibitor (a doctor should be consulted for full instructions and cautions).
• If used with other antihypertensives and diuretics, the effects of these drugs may be increased. This additive effect is sometimes used to advantage in combination treatments for high blood pressure.

Side effects
• The most common are dizziness and dry cough.

• Occasionally, headache, fatigue, insomnia, or gastrointestinal disturbances (for example, nausea and vomiting, diarrhea, constipation).

• Infrequently, chest and muscle pains, tingling in the extremities, tachycardia or photosensitivity (abnormal sensitivity to light). Although it is uncommon, ACE inhibitors can cause very marked hypotension (especially when beginning treatment) and kidney impairment.

• Rarely, there may be angioedema, altered liver function, jaundice, hepatitis, pancreatitis, or changes in blood counts.

fosphenytoin ⓖ

Type/Group: **anticonvulsant; antiepileptic.**
Brand(s): Cerebyx.
How administered: Injection.

Used to treat

Fosphenytoin is a recently introduced drug, one of the chemical goup of hydantoins used to treat ✪ **epilepsy**. It is is a pro-drug of ℞ **phenytoin**, and has the advantage over the older drug in that it can be given more rapidly and when given intravenously causes fewer reactions at the injection site. (However, there are interactions (see below) for phenytoin—the form present in the body.) It can be used in the emergency treatment of status epilepticus and convulsive seizures during neurosurgical operations or head injury.

Warnings

• Avoid its use in people with known hypersensitivity to this drug, phenytoin, or other hydantoins, or with certain heart conduction disorders, or porphyria.

• Fosphenytoin should be used with caution by anyone with hypotension or liver impairment. This is a specialist drug and full patient evaluation will be carried out.

• Fosphenytoin is associated with an increase in frequency of certain birth defects and should not be used during pregnancy. However, because uncontrolled seizures can also threaten fetal health, medical judgment is needed to weigh potential benefits and risks.

• Breast-feeding mothers should either discontinue using this drug or stop breast-feeding.

• It use should be discontinued if a skin rash appears.

• Fosphenytoin may raise blood glucose levels, and so medical judgment is advised for diabetics.

• A relationship has been suggested between phenytoin (this drug's active form) and some disorders of the lymphatic system, therefore, any lymphatic symptoms (tenderness or swelling) should be investigated.

Interactions

• Fosphenytoin and ℞ **tricyclic** antidepressants may precipitate seizures.

• The following drugs may intensify the effect of phenytoin, and so increase the risk of side effects: ℞ **amiodarone hydrochloride;** ℞ **chloramphenicol;** ℞ **chlordiazepoxide;** ℞ **diazepam;** ℞ **dicumarol;** ℞ **disulfiram;** ℞ **estrogens;** ℞ **fluoxetine;** ℞ H_2-antagonists; halothane; ℞ **isoniazid;** ℞ **methylphenidate;** ℞ **phenothiazines;** phenylbutazone; ℞ **salicylates;** succinimides

(for example, ethosuximide, methsuximide); ℞ **sulfonamides;** ℞ **tolbutamide;** ℞ **trazodone.**

• Fosphenytoin may increase the effects of ℞ **lithium** and ℞ **primidone,** with potential for toxicity.

• The effects if taken with ℞ **clonazepam,** ℞ **phenobarbital,** ℞ **sodium valproate,** or ℞ **valproic acid** are unpredictable.

• Alcohol, depending on drinking habits, may either raise or lower levels of phenytoin.

• The therapeutic effect of the following drugs may be reduced: ℞ **acetaminophen;** ℞ **corticosteroids;** coumarin ℞ **anticoagulants;** ℞ **digitoxin;** ℞ **dopamine;** ℞ **doxycycline;** ℞ **estrogens;** ℞ **furosemide;** oral ℞ **contraceptives;** ℞ **quinidine;** ℞ **rifampin;** ℞ **theophylline;** ⚗ **vitamin D.**

• ℞ **carbamazepine,** ℞ **reserpine,** and ℞ **sucralfate** lower levels of phenytoin.

Side effects

• Eye-flicker, itching, dizziness, drowsiness, nausea, confusion, slurred speech, nervousness, headache, insomnia, and strange taste sensations;

• Rarely, movement disorders, peripheral nerve disorders, rashes, acne, enlargement of the gums, growth of excess hair, and blood disorders;

• Hypersensitivity reactions (swollen lymph glands, fever, aches, rash) have occurred.

Fostex 10% Wash; Fostex ⓑ

A preparation of ℞ **benzoyl peroxide.**
Formulation: Topical lotion; topical bar.
Availability: OTC.
Warnings and side effects: See ℞ **benzoyl peroxide.**

Fostex Acne Cleansing Cream ⓑ

A preparation of ℞ **salicylic acid** and various.
Formulation: Topical cream.
Availability: OTC.
Warnings and side effects: See ℞ **salicylic acid.**

Fostex Acne Medication Cleansing Bar ⓑ

A preparation of ℞ **salicylic acid.**
Formulation: Bar soap.
Availability: OTC.
Warnings and side effects: See ℞ **salicylic acid.**

Fostex Cream ⓑ

A preparation of ℞ **salicylic acid.**
Formulation: Topical cream.
Availability: OTC.
Warnings and side effects: See ℞ **salicylic acid.**

Fototar ⓑ

A preparation of ℞ **coal tar.**
Formulation: Topical cream.
Availability: OTC.
Warnings and side effects: See ℞ **coal tar.**

4-quinolone Ⓓ

see ℞ quinolone.

4-Way Long Lasting Nasal; Spray Ⓑ

A preparation of ℞ oxymetazoline hydrochloride.
Formulation: Nasal; spray.
Availability: OTC.
Warnings and side effects: See ℞ oxymetazoline hydrochloride.

Fragmin Ⓑ

A preparation of ℞ dalteparin sodium.
Formulation: Subcutaneous injection.
Availability: Prescription only.
Warnings and side effects: See ℞ dalteparin sodium.

Freezone Ⓑ

A preparation of ℞ salicylic acid.
Formulation: Topical liquid.
Availability: OTC.
Warnings and side effects: See ℞ salicylic acid.

frusemide Ⓖ

see ℞ furosemide.

FS Shampoo Ⓑ

A preparation of ℞ fluocinolone acetonide.
Formulation: Shampoo.
Availability: Prescription only.
Warnings and side effects: See ℞ fluocinolone acetonide.

Ful-Glo Ⓑ

A preparation of ℞ fluorescein sodium.
Formulation: Ophthalmic strips.
Availability: Prescription only.
Warnings and side effects: See ℞ fluorescein sodium.

Fulvicin U/F; Fulvicin P/G Ⓑ

A preparation of ℞ griseofulvin.
Formulation: Oral tablets in several strengths.
Availability: Prescription only.
Warnings and side effects: See ℞ griseofulvin.

Fungizone Ⓑ

A preparation of ℞ amphotericin B.
Formulation: Injection (intravenous); topical cream; topical ointment; topical lotion.
Availability: Prescription only.
Warnings and side effects: See ℞ amphotericin B.

Fungoid; Fungoid Tincture; Fungoid Creme Ⓑ

A preparation of ℞ triacetin.
Formulation: Topical solution, topical cream.
Availability: Prescription only.
Warnings and side effects: See ℞ triacetin.

Fungoid AF Ⓑ

A preparation of ℞ undecylenic acid.
Formulation: Topical solution.
Availability: OTC.
Warnings and side effects: See ℞ undecylenic acid.

Furadantin Ⓑ

A preparation of ℞ nitrofurantoin.
Formulation: Oral suspension.
Availability: Prescription only.
Warnings and side effects: See ℞ nitrofurantoin.

furazolidone Ⓖ

Type/Group: antibacterial; amebicide and antiprotozoal.
Brand(s): Furoxone.
How administered: Orally.

Used to treat

Furazolidone is used primarily to treat ☉ **diarrhea** and ☉ **enteritis.** It inhibits the enzyme monoamine oxidase (MAO).

Warnings

• It should not be given to people with known hypersensitivity to furazolidone.
• It should be given with caution to people with hypertension, diabetes mellitus, or G6PD deficiency (a genetic enzyme disorder).
• Its effects during pregnancy are unknown, and it should be used only if clearly needed and if the potential benefits outweigh the risks to the fetus.
• Medical judgment is required if breast-feeding is being considered. It is not known whether furazolidone appears in breast milk.
• Avoid drinking alcohol while using this drug and for 4 days after therapy, otherwise an unpleasant adverse reaction characterized by flushing, fever, and fainting may be experienced.
• Avoid tyramine-containing foods, herbal remedies, or supplements, particularly if taking the drug for more than 5 days. Marked elevation in blood pressure, hypertensive crisis or hemorrhagic stroke could occur.
• It may color urine brown.

Interactions

• ℞ Amphetamines, ℞ ephedrine, and ℞ MAOI antidepressants increase the risk of hypertensive crisis.

Side effects

• Headache, malaise, nausea, postural hypotension (lowered blood pressure on standing), hypoglycemia, and gastrointestinal disturbances.

furosemide Ⓖ

(frusemide)
Type/Group: diuretic; antihypertensive.
Brand(s): Lasix; various generic.
How administered: Orally; injection.

Key to symbols: Ⓓ = Drug type/group   Ⓖ = Generic name   Ⓑ = Brand name

Used to treat

Furosemide is a powerful loop diuretic which can be used to treat edema (including fluid build-up in the lungs), low urine production (oliguria) due to kidney failure, and also, alone or with other drugs, ✪ **hypertension**.

Warnings

• It should not be given to people with known hypersensitivity to this drug (or to ℞ **sulfonamide**-derived drugs), with anuria (no urine), or in an electrolyte-depleted state.

• It should be given with caution to people with cirrhosis of the liver, certain kidney disorders, gout, diabetes mellitus, an enlarged prostate gland, or porphyria.

• It should be used during pregnancy only if the potential benefit outweighs the possible risk to the fetus.

• Medical judgment is required if breast-feeding is being considered.

• Dehydration may result from too intense a diuretic effect, particularly in elderly people or anyone with a restricted sodium intake.

• Early symptoms of electrolyte imbalance may include muscle weakness or cramps, nausea, vomiting, restlessness or lethargy, dry mouth, excessive thirst, fast pulse, or dizziness. A doctor must be contacted if such symptoms occur.

• Loop diuretics may aggravate symptoms of diabetes or gout, and worsen or activate lupus erythematosus.

• Periodic monitoring of electrolytes, and kidney and liver function is needed.

• Photosensitivity may develop and so precautions such as protective clothing or sunscreens should be used.

• It may cause postural hypotension (lowered blood pressure on standing up), so get up slowly.

Interactions

• There is a risk of ℞ **lithium** toxicity, and so generally these two drugs should not be used together.

• The effects of ℞ **aminoglycosides**, ℞ **anticoagulants**, other antihypertensives, ℞ **cardiac glycosides**, ℞ **chloral hydrate**, and ℞ **propranolol** may be increased, with the potential of significant side effects or toxicity. An additive effect is sometimes used to advantage in combining loop diuretics with other antihypertensives.

• ℞ **Sulfonylureas** may raise blood sugar levels in diabetics with previously stabilized regimens.

• If taken with ℞ **cisplatin**, there is a potential for increased effects and toxicity.

• ℞ **Amphotericin B**, ℞ **corticosteroids**, and ℞ **corticotropin** may increase the effect of reducing potassium levels, with the possibility of severe depletion.

• ℞ **clofibrate** may intensify the diuretic effect of furosemide.

• The effects of nondepolarizing ℞ **skeletal muscle relaxants** and ℞ **theophylline** are unpredictable.

• ℞ **Activated charcoal**, ℞ **hydantoins**, ℞ **NSAIDs**, and antigout agents (for example, ℞ **probenecid**, ℞ **sulfinpyrazone**) may reduce the effects of furosemide.

Side effects

• There may be abnormally low blood pressure (hypotension), gastrointestinal disturbances, raised levels of urea in the blood or gout, raised blood glucose, changes in fats in the blood, headache, dizziness, ringing in the ears and hearing loss. Electrolyte levels in the blood (for example, potassium, sodium, magnesium, and chloride) may be lowered. There may be skin rashes, photosensitivity, effects on bone marrow, blood changes, or pancreatitis. Many of these effects are only seen with high or prolonged dosage. Hearing loss (usually reversible) is associated with rapid injection, high dosage, and the use of other drugs that affect hearing.

Furoxone   ®

A preparation of ℞ **furazolidone**.
Formulation: Oral tablets; oral liquid.
Availability: Prescription only.
Warnings and side effects: See ℞ **furazolidone**.

gabapentin   Ⓖ

Type/Group: **anticonvulsant; antiepileptic**.
Brand(s): Neurontin.
How administered: Orally.

Used to treat

Gabapentin is used in the treatment of ✪ **epilepsy** as an adjunct (an additional treatment) to assist in the control of partial seizures that have not responded to other antiepileptic drugs.

Warnings

• Avoid its use in people with known hypersensitivity to this drug.

• It should be given with caution to anyone with certain kidney disorders.

• Gabapentin may have the potential to cause birth defects. However, because uncontrolled seizures can also threaten fetal health, medical judgment is needed to weigh potential benefits and risks.

• It appears in breast milk, though its effects are not known, and so it should be used by breast-feeding mothers only if the potential benefit outweighs risk to the infant.

• Withdrawal should be gradual otherwise it may precipitate attacks.

• As this drug may cause drowsiness, driving or other hazardous activity should be avoided.

Interactions

• ℞ **Antacids** may reduce the availability and effectiveness of gabapentin.

• ℞ **Cimetidine** may raise gabapentin levels slightly.

• The levels of oral ℞ **contraceptives** may be slightly increased.

Side effects

• Fatigue, sleepiness, dizziness, unsteady gait, eye-flicker, and double vision;

• Headache, tremor, nausea, and vomiting;

• Rhinitis, weight gain, convulsions, and indigestion;

• Cough, aches, pains, and tingling.

Gabatril Flimtabs ⑧

A preparation of ℞ **tiagabine**.
Formulation: Oral tablets, available in 4 strengths.
Availability: Prescription only.
Warnings and side effects: See ℞ **tiagabine**.

Gabitril Filmtabs ⑧

A preparation of ℞ **tiagabine**.
Formulation: Oral tablets, available in 4 strengths.
Availability: Prescription only.
Warnings and side effects: See ℞ **tiagabine**.

gallstone treatment ⑩

Generics: **dehydrocholic acid; monoctanoin; ursodiol**.
Actions and uses
℞ **Gallstone treatments** are used to treat gallstone (✪ **calculus**) disorders. The most common class of drug used is the *choliolythics*, which help dissolve stones in the gallbladder or bile duct so that they may be dislodged. ℞ **Ursodiol**, which is made from a naturally occurring bile acid, is the main drug used and, over a period, it helps to decrease the cholesterol content of bile and gallstones by reducing hepatic cholesterol secretion, and the reabsorption of cholesterol by the intestine. Another bile acid, ℞ **dehydrocholic acid**, does not significantly dissolve stones, but it dilutes bile, causing greater flow. For this reason it may be used after biliary surgery to help flush debris from the biliary tract or in other conditions in which increased fluid flow in the bile tract is desirable. It also is a ℞ **laxative**. ℞ **Monoctanoin** is a drug that can be used to dissolve some gallstones (only those made up of cholesterol) *in situ*, when other methods have failed or cannot be used.

Limitations
Treatment is only necessary if the stones cause symptoms. This may be by breaking up the stones using ultrasound therapy, or by surgical removal of the stones or gallbladder. Choliolythic drug treatment with ℞ **ursodiol** is not suitable for acute cases because it may take months to have any effect, the reoccurrence of stones is common, and treatment does not work for all types of stones. See also the individual drug entries.

Gamimune N ⑧

A preparation of ℞ **immune globulin, human (IG)**.
Formulation: Intravenous infusion, available in two concentrations.
Availability: Prescription only.
Warnings and side effects: See ℞ **immune globulin, human (IG)**.

gamma benzene hexachloride ⑤

see ℞ **lindane**.

Gammar-P I.V. ⑧

A preparation of ℞ **immune globulin, human (IG)**.
Formulation: Intravenous infusion, supplied as a powder.
Availability: Prescription only.

Warnings and side effects: See ℞ **immune globulin, human (IG)**.

ganciclovir (DHPG) ⑤

Type/Group: **antiviral**.
Brand(s): Cytovene.
How administered: Orally; injection.
Used to treat
Ganciclovir is related to ℞ **acyclovir**, and although it is more active against certain ✪ **viral infections** (cytomegalovirus) it is more toxic. Its use is, therefore, restricted to the treatment of life-threatening or sight-threatening cytomegalovirus (CMV) infections in immunocompromised patients, and the prevention of cytomegalovirus disease in transplant patients and people with ✪ **AIDS**.
Warnings
• It should not be given to people with known hypersensitivity to ganciclovir.
• It should be given with caution to people with pre-existing cytopenia, kidney function impairment, low platelet counts, who are over 65, or infants under 6 months of age.
• Ganciclovir's safety during pregnancy has not been established and its use is not recommended.
• It is not recommended for use while breast-feeding.
• Because of major blood toxicity risk, laboratory monitoring is essential.
• It is a specialist drug, and there will be full assessment and patient monitoring throughout treatment.
Interactions
• ℞ **Didanosine (ddI)** and ℞ **zidovudine** increase blood toxicity.
Side effects
These are many and include:
• Various blood-cell deficiencies, headache, sore throat and swelling of the face, fever and rash, effects on liver function, gastrointestinal disturbances, and a number of other reactions.

ganglion-blocker ⑩

Generics: **mecamylamine hydrochloride; trimetaphan camsilate**.
Actions and uses
Ganglion-blockers form a class of drugs that block nerve transmission in the peripheral autonomic nervous system at the nervous junction, called the ganglia. These drugs work by preventing the actions of acetylcholine—the neurotransmitter at these junctions—and so, in effect, ganglion-blockers are a type of ℞ **anticholinergic** drug. The cholinergic receptors at which ganglion-blockers act are called nicotinic receptors (since ℞ **nicotine** is a strong stimulant at such receptors) and these are similar, but not identical, to the cholinergic receptors of the same name, which are found at the skeletal neuromuscular junction.

℞ **trimetaphan camsilate** lowers blood pressure by reducing vascular (blood vessel) tone, which is normally induced by the sympathetic nervous system. It is short-acting, which makes it a useful ℞ **hypotensive** for controlling blood pressure during surgery, or to quickly reduce blood pressure in hypertensive emergencies. ℞ **Mecamylamine** hydrochloride is a potent ganglion-blocker, which can be used to treat moderately severe to severe hypertension.

Limitations
The ganglion-blockers were introduced as ℞ **antihypertensive** drugs—and are very effective as such—but their actions and side effects are so widespread that they are now rarely used in medicine because safer and more selective alternatives are available.

Gani-Tuss NR ⑧
A preparation of ℞ **codeine phosphate** and ℞ **guaifenesin**.
Formulation: Oral liquid.
Availability: May or may not require a prescription.
Warnings and side effects: See ℞ **codeine phosphate**; ℞ **guaifenesin**.

Gantanol ⑧
A preparation of ℞ **sulfamethoxazole**.
Formulation: Oral tablets.
Availability: Prescription only.
Warnings and side effects: See ℞ **sulfamethoxazole**.

Gantrisin Ophthalmic ⑧
A preparation of ℞ **sulfisoxazole** diolamine.
Formulation: Eye drops.
Availability: Prescription only.
Warnings and side effects: See ℞ **sulfisoxazole**.

Gantrisin Pediatric ⑧
A preparation of ℞ **sulfisoxazole**.
Formulation: Oral suspension.
Availability: Prescription only.
Warnings and side effects: See ℞ **sulfisoxazole**.

Garamycin ⑧
A preparation of ℞ **gentamicin**.
Formulation: Injection; topical ointment; topical cream; eye drops; ophthalmic ointment.
Availability: Prescription only.
Warnings and side effects: See ℞ **gentamicin**.

Gas Ban ⑧
A preparation of ℞ **calcium carbonate** and ℞ **simethicone**.
Formulation: Oral tablets.
Availability: OTC.
Warnings and side effects: See ℞ **calcium carbonate**; ℞ **simethicone**.

Gas Ban DS Liquid ⑧
A preparation of ℞ **aluminum hydroxide**, ℞ **magnesium hydroxide**, and ℞ **simethicone**.
Formulation: Oral liquid.
Availability: OTC.
Warnings and side effects: See ℞ **aluminum hydroxide**; ℞ **magnesium hydroxide**; ℞ **simethicone**.

Gastrocrom ⑧
A preparation of ℞ **cromolyn sodium**.
Formulation: Oral concentrate.
Availability: Prescription only.
Warnings and side effects: See ℞ **cromolyn sodium**.

gastrointestinal anti-inflammatory agent ⑩
see ℞ **aminosalicylate**.

Gastrosed Tablets ⑧
A preparation of ℞ **hyoscyamine**.
Formulation: Oral tablets.
Availability: Prescription only.
Warnings and side effects: See ℞ **hyoscyamine**.

Gas-X Tablets; Extra Strength Capsules ⑧
A preparation of ℞ **simethicone**.
Formulation: Oral tablets, chewable; capsules.
Availability: OTC.
Warnings and side effects: See ℞ **simethicone**.

gatifloxacin ⑥
Type/Group: **quinolone; antibacterial**.
Brand(s): Tenquin.
How administered: Orally; injection.

Used to treat
Gatifloxacin is a recently introduced synthetic quinolone that can be used to treat ✚ **bacterial infections**, including respiratory infections such as bacteria-caused worsening of chronic ✚ **bronchitis**, community-acquired (caught from the environment) ✚ **pneumonia**, and acute ✚ **sinusitis**, as well as urinary tract, prostate, and kidney infections, gonorrhea, and rectal infections in women.

Warnings
• It should not be given to people with known hypersensitivity to gatifloxacin or other quinolones. It should not be given to children under 18, because there is a possibility of damage to joints and cartilage in growing children.

• It should be given with caution to people with liver or kidney disease, diabetes mellitus, certain heart conditions, a history of photosensitivity reactions (abnormal sensitivity to light), or any predisposition to seizures.

• Gatifloxacin should not be used during pregnancy or while breast-feeding unless the potential benefit outweighs the possible risk to the fetus or infant.

• Superinfections due to the altered bacterial balance caused by antibiotic treatment may occur. A doctor must be contacted if there is severe abdominal pain, or moderate to severe diarrhea.

• Rare, but serious, side effects of quinolones include seizure and other CNS (central nervous system) effects, and severe, allergic reactions.

• Adequate fluid intake must be maintained.

• Photosensitivity reactions may occur when using quinolones and so excessive exposure to sunlight should be avoided.

• Do not take products such as supplements containing ⚭ **calcium**, ⚭ **magnesium**, aluminum, ⚭ **iron**, or ⚭ **zinc** less than four hours before or two hours after taking gatifloxacin, because they may reduce its effects.

Interactions

• ℞ **Antacids**, ℞ **didanosine (ddI)**, and iron sucralfate may reduce the effects of gatifloxacin.

• The levels of ℞ **theophylline**, antipyrine, ℞ **caffeine**, ℞ **diazepam**, ℞ **metoprolol**, ℞ **pentoxifylline**, ℞ **phenytoin**, ℞ **propranolol**, ℞ **ropinirole**, ℞ **xanthine**, and ℞ **warfarin sodium** may be increased.

• The effects of oral ℞ **anticoagulants** may be increased.

• If used with ℞ **foscarnet**, the risk of seizure is increased.

Side effects

• Frequently, nausea.

• Occasionally, diarrhea, headache, dizziness, and vaginitis.

Gaviscon Extra Strength Relief Formula Tablets ®

A preparation of ℞ **aluminum hydroxide**, ℞ **magnesium carbonate**, and ℞ **sodium bicarbonate**.

Formulation: Oral tablets, chewable.

Availability: OTC.

Warnings and side effects: See ℞ **aluminum hydroxide**; ℞ **magnesium carbonate**; ℞ **sodium bicarbonate**.

Gaviscon Liquid; Extra Strength Relief Formula Liquid ®

A preparation of ℞ **aluminum hydroxide**, ℞ **magnesium carbonate**, and sodium alginate.

Formulation: Oral liquid. (Extra Strength also contains ℞ **simethicone**.)

Availability: OTC.

Warnings and side effects: See ℞ **aluminum hydroxide**; ℞ **magnesium carbonate**; ℞ **alginic acid**; ℞ **simethicone**.

Gaviscon Tablets; Gaviscon-2 Double Strength Tablets ®

A preparation of ℞ **aluminum hydroxide**, ℞ **magnesium trisilicate**, ℞ **sodium bicarbonate**, and ℞ **alginic acid**.

Formulation: Oral tablets, chewable.

Availability: OTC.

Warnings and side effects: See ℞ **aluminum hydroxide**; ℞ **magnesium trisilicate**; ℞ **sodium bicarbonate**; ℞ **alginic acid**.

Gelhist Pediatric Suspension ®

A preparation of phenylephrine tannate, chlorpheniramine tannate, and pyrilamine tannate.

Formulation: Oral liquid.

Availability: Prescription only.

Warnings and side effects: See ℞ **phenylephrine hydrochloride**; ℞ **chlorpheniramine maleate**; ℞ **pyrilamine maleate**.

Gelusil Tablets ®

A preparation of ℞ **aluminum hydroxide**, ℞ **magnesium hydroxide**, and ℞ **simethicone**.

Formulation: Oral tablets, chewable.

Availability: OTC.

Warnings and side effects: See ℞ **aluminum hydroxide**; ℞ **magnesium hydroxide**; ℞ **simethicone**.

gemcitabine ⓖ

Type/Group: anticancer; cytotoxic.

Brand(s): Adrucil; various generic.

How administered: Intravenous injection.

Used to treat

Gemcitabine is a cytotoxic (an antimetabolite) that is used for locally advanced or metastatic non-small cell ✪ **lung cancer** and pancreatic cancer.

Warnings

• It should not be given to people with known hypersensitivity to this drug.

• It should be given with caution to people with impaired kidney function or liver insufficiency. This is a specialist drug which will be used following a full evaluation by specialist physicians.

• Gemcitabine is not recommended for use during pregnancy unless it is medically judged to be essential, because it may cause birth defects. Becoming pregnant while using this drug must be avoided.

• It should not be used if breast-feeding.

• It can cause bone marrow depression, which may lead to bleeding and a reduced resistance to infection.

• Many people may experience fever and flu-like symptoms even in the absence of infection.

Interactions

• ℞ **Leucovorin** increases toxicity.

Side effects

• Frequently, nausea and vomiting, pain, fever, and rash.

• Occasionally, breathing problems, other gastrointestinal symptoms, bleeding, infection, hearing loss, sleepiness, tingling or burning sensations.

gemfibrozil ⓖ

Type/Group: lipid-regulating drug; fibrate.

Brand(s): Lopid.

How administered: Orally.

Used to treat

Gemfibrozil is used in the treatment of ✪ **hyperlipidemia** to reduce the levels, or change the proportions, of various lipids (for example, to lower triglycerides and lower LDL-cholesterol and raise LDL-cholesterol) in the bloodstream and to reduce the risk of heart disease. Generally, it is given only to people in whom a strict and regular dietary regime alone is not having the desired effect.

Warnings

• It should not be given to people with known hypersensitivity to gemfibrozil, liver dysfunction, severe kidney dysfunction, primary biliary cirrhosis, or pre-existing gallbladder disease.

• It should be given with caution to people with hypothyroidism or diabetes mellitus, or to anyone taking ℞ **estrogen** or ℞ **anticoagulants**.

• Gemfibrozil's safety in pregnancy has not been established, but the drug is not absorbed systemically. It may, however, interfere with maternal absorption of fat-soluble vitamins. It should be used only if the potential benefits outweigh the possible risks to the fetus.

• It should not be used while breast-feeding.

• It may impair the performance of skilled tasks, for example, driving should be avoided if dizziness occurs.

• Any other kind of medication (including OTCs, herbal remedies, and supplements) must not be taken without consulting a doctor.

Interactions

• Binding resins reduce the effects of gemfibrozil.

• Glyburide increases the risk of hypoglycemia.

• ℞ **lovastatin**, ℞ **simvastatin**, ℞ **atorvastatin**, and ℞ **pravastatin** increase the likelihood of drug-induced muscle damage.

• ℞ **warfarin sodium** increases anticoagulant effects.

Side effects

• Frequently, upset stomach; abdominal pain, diarrhea, and dyspepsia.

• Occasionally, gastrointestinal effects, effects on the heart, and fatigue.

• Rarely, acute appendicitis, dizziness, headache, rash, altered taste, pancreatitis, and blood disorders.

Genacol Tablets ℞

A preparation of ℞ **dextromethorphan**, ℞ **acetaminophen**, ℞ **chlorpheniramine maleate**, and ℞ **pseudoephedrine**.
Formulation: Oral tablets.
Availability: OTC.
Warnings and side effects: See ℞ **dextromethorphan**; ℞ **acetaminophen**; ℞ **chlorpheniramine maleate**; ℞ **pseudoephedrine**.

Genac Tablets ℞

A preparation of ℞ **pseudoephedrine** and ℞ **triprolidine hydrochloride**.
Formulation: Oral tablets.
Availability: OTC.
Warnings and side effects: See ℞ **pseudoephedrine**; ℞ **triprolidine hydrochloride**.

Genahist ℞

A preparation of ℞ **diphenhydramine hydrochloride**.
Formulation: Oral liquid.
Availability: OTC.
Warnings and side effects: See ℞ **diphenhydramine hydrochloride**.

Genapap Tablets ℞

Also: **Extra Strength Tablets, Caplets; Children's Infants' Drops**
A preparation of ℞ **acetaminophen**.
Formulation: Oral tablets; chewable tablets; liquid, drops.

Availability: OTC.
Warnings and side effects: See ℞ **acetaminophen**.

Genaphed Tablets ℞

A preparation of ℞ **pseudoephedrine**.
Formulation: Oral tablets.
Availability: OTC.
Warnings and side effects: See ℞ **pseudoephedrine**.

Genasal ℞

A preparation of ℞ **oxymetazoline hydrochloride**.
Formulation: Nasal drops.
Availability: OTC.
Warnings and side effects: See ℞ **oxymetazoline hydrochloride**.

Genasoft ℞

A preparation of ℞ **docusate sodium**.
Formulation: Oral gelcaps.
Availability: OTC.
Warnings and side effects: See ℞ **docusate sodium**.

Genasoft Plus Softgels ℞

A preparation of ℞ **docusate sodium**, casanthranol, and ℞ **sorbitol**.
Formulation: Oral gelcaps.
Availability: OTC.
Warnings and side effects: See ℞ **docusate sodium**; ℞ **sorbitol**.

Genasyme Tablets; Drops ℞

A preparation of ℞ **simethicone**.
Formulation: Oral tablets, chewable; drops.
Availability: OTC.
Warnings and side effects: See ℞ **simethicone**.

Genaton Extra Strength Tablets ℞

A preparation of ℞ **aluminum hydroxide**, ℞ **magnesium carbonate**, ℞ **alginic acid**, and ℞ **sodium bicarbonate**.
Formulation: Oral tablets, chewable.
Availability: OTC.
Warnings and side effects: See ℞ **aluminum hydroxide**; ℞ **magnesium carbonate**; ℞ **alginic acid**; ℞ **sodium bicarbonate**.

Genaton Liquid ℞

A preparation of ℞ **aluminum hydroxide**, sodium alginate, ℞ **sorbitol**, and ℞ **magnesium carbonate**.
Formulation: Oral liquid.
Availability: OTC.
Warnings and side effects: See ℞ **aluminum hydroxide**; ℞ **magnesium carbonate**; ℞ **alginic acid**; ℞ **sorbitol**.

Genaton Tablets ℞

A preparation of ℞ **aluminum hydroxide**, ℞ **magnesium trisilicate**, ℞ **alginic acid**, and ℞ **sodium bicarbonate**.

Key to symbols: ✚ = Disorder Section ℞ = Drug Section ♣ = Herbal Section ⚖ = Supplement Section

Formulation: Oral tablets, chewable.
Availability: OTC.
Warnings and side effects: See ℞ **aluminum hydroxide;** ℞ **magnesium trisilicate;** ℞ **alginic acid;** ℞ **sodium bicarbonate.**

Genatuss DM Syrup Ⓑ

A preparation of ℞ **dextromethorphan** and ℞ **guaifenesin.**
Formulation: Oral syrup.
Availability: OTC.
Warnings and side effects: See ℞ **dextromethorphan;** ℞ **guaifenesin.**

Genatuss Syrup Ⓑ

A preparation of ℞ **guaifenesin.**
Formulation: Oral syrup.
Availability: OTC.
Warnings and side effects: See ℞ **guaifenesin.**

Gendecon Tablets Ⓑ

A preparation of ℞ **phenylephrine hydrochloride,** ℞ **acetaminophen,** and ℞ **chlorpheniramine maleate.**
Formulation: Oral tablets.
Availability: OTC.
Warnings and side effects: See ℞ **phenylephrine hydrochloride;** ℞ **acetaminophen;** ℞ **chlorpheniramine maleate.**

Genebs Tablets; Extra Strength Tablets, Caplets Ⓑ

A preparation of ℞ **acetaminophen.**
Formulation: Oral tablets.
Availability: OTC.
Warnings and side effects: See ℞ **acetaminophen.**

general anesthetic Ⓓ

Actions and uses

General anesthetics are drugs that reduce sensation in the whole body with a loss of consciousness. They are used for surgical procedures. ℞ **Local anesthetics,** in contrast, affect sensation in a specific, local area without the loss of consciousness. The general anesthetic that is used to bring about (induce) anesthesia is often different from the drug, or drugs, used to maintain the anesthesia. For induction, short-acting general anesthetics that can be injected are convenient (for example, thiopental sodium, etomidate, propofol), but for maintenance during long operations, inhalation anesthetics are commonly used (for example, halothane, desflurane, diethyl ether, isoflurane, and enflurane). In order to minimize the depth of anesthesia necessary for a surgical procedure, premedication with, or concurrent use of, other drugs is usually necessary. A range of ancillary drugs are also valuable, including ℞ **tranquilizer** or ℞ **sedative** agents (especially ℞ **benzodiazepine** drugs), ℞ **narcotic analgesic** drugs, ℞ **skeletal muscle relaxant** drugs, and using local anesthetics at the same time.

Limtiations

The use of general anesthetics is a specialized hospital procedure, so details of individual agents are not given in this book.

Geneye Ⓑ

A preparation of ℞ **tetrahydrozoline hydrochloride.**
Formulation: Eye drops.
Availability: OTC.
Warnings and side effects: See ℞ **tetrahydrozoline hydrochloride.**

Genfiber; Genfiber Orange Flavor Ⓑ

A preparation of ℞ **psyllium.**
Formulation: Oral powder.
Availability: OTC.
Warnings and side effects: See ℞ **psyllium.**

Gengraf Ⓑ

A preparation of ℞ **cyclosporine.**
Formulation: Oral capsules.
Availability: Prescription only.

Genite Liquid Ⓑ

A preparation of ℞ **dextromethorphan,** ℞ **acetaminophen,** ℞ **pseudoephedrine,** and ℞ **doxylamine.**
Formulation: Oral liquid.
Availability: OTC.
Warnings and side effects: See ℞ **dextromethorphan;** ℞ **acetaminophen;** ℞ **pseudoephedrine;** ℞ **doxylamine.**

Genoptic; Genoptic S.O.P. Ⓑ

A preparation of ℞ **gentamicin.**
Formulation: Eye drops: ophthalmic ointment (S.O.P.).
Availability: Prescription only.
Warnings and side effects: See ℞ **gentamicin.**

Genotropin Ⓑ

A preparation of ℞ **somatropin.**
Formulation: Injection in several strengths.
Availability: Prescription only.
Warnings and side effects: See ℞ **somatropin.**

Genpril Ⓑ

A preparation of ℞ **ibuprofen.**
Formulation: Oral tablets.
Availability: OTC.
Warnings and side effects: See ℞ **ibuprofen.**

Gentak Ⓑ

A preparation of ℞ **gentamicin.**
Formulation: Eye drops: ophthalmic ointment.
Availability: Prescription only.
Warnings and side effects: See ℞ **gentamicin.**

gentamicin Ⓖ

Type/Group: **aminoglycoside; antibiotic; antibacterial.**
Brand(s): **Systemic:** Garamycin. Ophthalmic: Garamycin; Genoptic; Genoptic S.O.P. **Topical:** Garamycin; Gentak; G-myticin. Combinations: With *prednisolone*: Pred-G.

How administered: Injection; intravenous infusion; topically (eye, skin).

Used to treat

Gentamicin is used primarily against serious ○ **bacterial infections** caused by Gram-negative bacteria, although it does have activity against Gram-positive bacteria. It is the most widely used of the aminoglycoside family. It is given for the treatment of, for example, ○ **septicemia**, ○ **meningitis**, infections of the heart (sometimes in conjunction with penicillin), the biliary and urinary tracts, the eyes and skin, and ○ **pneumonia** in hospital patients.

Warnings

• It should not be given to people with known hypersensitivity to gentamicin or other aminoglycosides, or with severe kidney disease.

• It should be given with caution to people with mild kidney disease, hearing deficits or vertigo, dehydration, with muscular disorders, such as myasthenia gravis or parkinsonism, and those over 65.

• Medical judgment is required when giving to very young infants.

• Gentamicin should be used during pregnancy if medically judged to be clearly needed and if the potential benefits outweigh the risks to the fetus (it crosses the placenta and could cause damage to ears or kidneys).

• Medical judgment is required if breast-feeding is being considered.

• Aminoglycosides are associated with nephrotoxicity (damage to the kidneys) and ototoxicity (damage in the ears). Irreversible vestibular impairment can occur, resulting in vertigo and difficulty maintaining balance. Permanent hearing loss in one or both ears can also occur. The risk is greatest in those with pre-existing impairments, with high doses, and with prolonged use.

• A doctor must be contacted if there are problems with hearing, vision, balance, urination, or headaches, even after the course of treatment is completed.

• When used in the eye, a doctor must be notified if redness, swelling, decreased vision, or pain persists, or stinging, burning, or itching becomes pronounced.

• The use of antibiotics may result in superinfection due to bacterial imbalance.

Interactions

• ℞ **Atracurium**, ℞ **succinylcholine**, ℞ **vecuronium**, or neuromuscular blocking agents taken with gentamicin increases respiratory depression.

• ℞ **ethacrynic acid** and ℞ **carboplatin** increase the risk of ear damage.

• ℞ **Amphotericin B**, ℞ **cephalosporins**, ℞ **cyclosporine**, methoxyflurane, and ℞ **NSAID**s may increase the risk of kidney damage.

• ℞ **carboplatin**, ℞ **cisplatin**, and ℞ **vancomycin** increase the risk of ear or kidney damage.

• ℞ **carbenicillin**, ℞ **penicillins**, ℞ **piperacillin**, and ℞ **ticarcillin** could inactivate gentamicin in people with kidney failure.

• ℞ **Diuretics** should not be taken at the same time as aminoglycosides.

Side effects

• Frequently, gastrointestinal upsets.

• Occasionally, rash, fever, hives, and itching.

• Rarely, hair loss, elevated blood pressure, and weakness.

• Additional serious effects include neurotoxicity (nerve damage), blood changes, ototoxicity, deafness, and kidney damage. When used in the eye there may be temporary blurring of vision.

gentian violet ⓖ

(crystal violet; methylrosaniline chloride)
Type/Group: **antiseptic; astringent**.
Brand(s): Generic only.
How administered: Topically (external).

Used to treat

Gentian violet is a dye with astringent and oxidizing properties. It is used as an antiseptic and occasionally to treat ○ **fungal infections** of the skin, or abrasions and minor wounds.

Warnings

• It should not be given to people with known hypersensitivity to gentian violet.

• It is not recommended for use during pregnancy.

• Medical judgment is required if breast-feeding is being considered.

• Wounds must not be covered.

• Will stain skin and clothing.

Interactions

No significant interactions have been reported when used topically (externally).

Side effects

None significant when used topically.

Gen-Xene ⓑ

A preparation of ℞ **clorazepate dipotassium**.
Formulation: Oral tablets.
Availability: Prescription only.
Warnings and side effects: See ℞ **clorazepate dipotassium**.

Geocillin ⓑ

A preparation of ℞ **carbenicillin**.
Formulation: Oral tablets.
Availability: Prescription only.
Warnings and side effects: See ℞ **carbenicillin**.

Geref ⓑ

A preparation of ℞ **sermorelin**.
Formulation: Injection.
Availability: Prescription only.
Warnings and side effects: See ℞ **sermorelin**.

Gerimal ⓑ

A preparation of ℞ **ergoloid mesylates**.
Formulation: Oral and sublingual tablets.
Availability: Prescription only.
Warnings and side effects: See ℞ **ergoloid mesylates**.

Glandosane ⑧

A preparation of ℞ **carboxymethylcellulose sodium** and various.
Formulation: Topical solution.
Availability: OTC.
Warnings and side effects: See ℞ **carboxymethylcellulose sodium**.

glatiramer acetate ⑥

Type/Group: **immunosuppressant**.
Brand(s): Copaxone.
How administered: Subcutaneous injection.

Used to treat

Glatiramer acetate is used to reduce the frequency of relapses in people with the relapsing form of ✪ **multiple sclerosis** (MS). Although its action is not well understood, it is thought to act by modifying immune response to the important (nerve-insulating) substance myelin.

Warnings

• It should not be given to people with known hypersensitivity to this drug or to mannitol.
• Thorough studies have not been done and it should be used during pregnancy only if it is clearly needed.
• Medical judgment is required if breast-feeding is being considered.
• Photosensitivity may develop and so precautions such as protective clothing or sunscreens should be used.
• As with any drug that suppresses some part of immune function, there may be unwanted effects, although none have been associated so far with this drug.
• Immediately after injection there may be flushing, chest pain, palpitations, shortness of breath, throat constriction, or hives. This kind of reaction, which has not required special treatment, occurs several months after starting to this drug.

Interactions

No interactions of significance are known, but a full study has not been carried out.

Side effects

• These include itching and rash, nausea, swollen lymph glands, facial swelling, joint pain, dry eyes, neck pain, peripheral edema, weight gain, and vaginal moniliasis.
• In addition to the syndrome of flushing and chest pain associated with later injections, there is often pain, redness, and inflammation at the site of injection.

glaucoma treatment ⑩

Generics: acetazolamide; apraclonidine; betaxolol hydrochloride; brimonidine tartrate; carbachol; carteolol; dichlorphenamide; dipivefrine hydrochloride; dorzolamide; epinephrine; latanoprost; levobunolol; metipranolol; pilocarpine; timolol maleate.

Actions and uses

Glaucoma treatment involves the use of drugs to lower the raised intraocular pressure (pressure in the eyeball) that usually is a characteristic of the group of eye conditions called ✪ **glaucoma**, in which the optic nerve, and so vision, is damaged within the eye. A number of types of drug help reduce this pressure (which has nothing directly to do with blood pressure). It is usually caused by a reduced outflow of fluid (aqueous humor) from the eye, so drugs often work by increasing this outflow. The drug used depends on what sort of glaucoma is being treated (for example, open-angle or closed-angle).

℞ **beta-blocker** drugs are effective in most cases, for example, in chronic simple glaucoma (for example, ℞ **betaxolol hydrochloride**, ℞ **carteolol**, ℞ **timolol maleate**, ℞ **metipranolol**, and ℞ **levobunolol**). Some ℞ **sympathomimetic** drugs are used, including ℞ **epinephrine** and ℞ **dipivefrin hydrochloride** (which is converted into epinephrine in the body), and the unusual drugs ℞ **apraclonidine** and ℞ **brimonidine tartrate** (which are selective for the alpha$_2$-subtype of adrenergic receptor). ℞ **parasympathomimetic** cholinergic agents may also be given, such as ℞ **carbachol** and ℞ **pilocarpine** (these act as ℞ **miotic** agents; that is, they constrict the pupil). Certain ℞ **carbonic anhydrase inhibitor** drugs, including ℞ **acetazolamide**, ℞ **dorzolamide**, and ℞ **dichlorphenamide**, may be prescribed because they reduce the formation of aqueous humor in the eye. A novel treatment is the ℞ **prostaglandin** analog, latanoprost, which is now used to treat open-angle glaucoma and ocular hypertension when other drugs are inappropriate (it increases the outflow of aqueous humor).

Limitations

It is important to note that certain classes of drugs, such as the ℞ **corticosteroid** drugs and ℞ **anticholinergic** drugs (for example, atropine sulfate), cause a rise in intraocular pressure and if given to people predisposed to glaucoma, they may cause an acute attack.

Glaucon ⑧

A preparation of ℞ **epinephrine**.
Formulation: Eye drops, available in two strengths.
Availability: Prescription only.
Warnings and side effects: See ℞ **epinephrine**.

Gliadel ⑧

A preparation of ℞ **carmustine**.
Formulation: Wafer for surgical emplacement.
Availability: Prescription only.
Warnings and side effects: See ℞ **carmustine**.

glibenclamide ⑥

see ℞ **glyburide**.

glimepiride ⑥

Type/Group: **antidiabetic; oral hypoglycemic; sulfonylurea**.
Brand(s): Amaryl.
How administered: Orally.

Used to treat

Glimepiride is used in the treatment of type 2 ✪ **diabetes mellitus** (non-insulin-dependent diabetes mellitus; NIDDM). It works by augmenting what remains of insulin production in the pancreas.

Warnings

• It should not be given to people with type 1 diabetes mellitus or ketoacidosis.

• It should be given with caution to people with heart, thyroid, kidney, or liver disease, severe hypoglycemic reactions, adrenal or pituitary insufficiency, who are over 65, or severely debilitated.

• It is inappropriate for use during pregnancy (insulin is the drug of choice).

• Medical judgment is required if breast-feeding is being considered. It is not known whether it is appears in breast milk.

• Alcohol should be avoided while using this drug, as it can cause unpleasant symptoms and interfere with blood sugar control.

• There are potentially multiple drug interactions with glimepiride. A doctor should be consulted before taking any other medication (including OTCs, herbal remedies, and supplements).

Interactions

• ℞ NSAIDs, ℞ salicylates, ℞ sulfonamides, ℞ chloramphenicol, coumarins, ℞ probenecid, ℞ MAOIs, and ℞ beta-blockers may enhance the hypoglycemic effect of sulfonylureas.

• ℞ Thiazide and other ℞ diuretics, ℞ corticosteroids, ℞ phenothiazines, ℞ thyroid hormones, ℞ estrogens, ℞ oral contraceptives, ℞ phenytoin, ℞ niacin, ℞ sympathomimetics, and ℞ isoniazid may lead to the loss of control of sugar levels.

• Oral ℞ miconazole, ℞ diclofenac, ℞ ibuprofen, ℞ naproxen, and ℞ mefenamic acid have the potential for severe hypoglycemia.

Side effects

• Frequently, altered taste sensation, dizziness, weight gain, gastrointestinal effects, and headache.

• Occasionally, photosensitivity, peeling skin, itching, and rash.

• Rarely, hypoglycemia, gastrointestinal bleeding, liver disorders, and blood changes.

glipizide ⓖ

Type/Group: **antidiabetic; oral hypoglycemic; sulfonylurea.**
Brand(s): Glucotrol; various generic.
How administered: Orally.

Used to treat

Glipizide is used to treat type 2 ✪ **diabetes mellitus** (non-insulin-dependent diabetes mellitus; NIDDM). It works by augmenting what remains of insulin production in the pancreas.

Warnings

• It should not be given to people with type 1 diabetes mellitus or ketoacidosis.

• It should be given with caution to people with heart, thyroid, kidney, or liver disease, severe hypoglycemic reactions, adrenal or pituitary insufficiency, who are over 65, or severely debilitated.

• It is inappropriate for use during pregnancy (insulin is the drug of choice).

• Medical judgment is required if breast-feeding is being considered, as this drug appears in breast milk.

• Alcohol should be avoided while using this drug, as it can cause unpleasant symptoms and interfere with blood sugar control.

• There are multiple drug interactions with glipizide. Consult a doctor before taking any other medication (including OTCs, herbal remedies, and supplements).

Interactions

• ℞ NSAIDs, ℞ salicylates, ℞ sulfonamides, ℞ chloramphenicol, coumarins, ℞ probenecid, ℞ MAOIs, and ℞ beta-blockers may enhance the hypoglycemic effect of sulfonylureas.

• ℞ Thiazide and other ℞ diuretics, ℞ corticosteroids, ℞ phenothiazines, ℞ thyroid hormones, ℞ estrogens, ℞ oral contraceptives, ℞ phenytoin, ℞ niacin, ℞ sympathomimetics, and ℞ isoniazid may lead to the loss of control of sugar levels.

• Oral ℞ miconazole, ℞ diclofenac, ℞ ibuprofen, ℞ naproxen, and ℞ mefenamic acid have the potential for severe hypoglycemia.

Side effects

• Frequently, altered taste sensation, dizziness, weight gain, gastrointestinal effects, and headache.

• Occasionally, photosensitivity, peeling skin, itching, and rash.

• Rarely, hypoglycemia, gastrointestinal bleeding, liver disorders, and blood changes.

glucagon ⓖ

Type/Group: **hormone; antihypoglycemic; diagnostic agent.**
Brand(s): Glucagon Emergency Kit.
How administered: Injection.

Used to treat

Glucagon is a hormone produced and secreted by the pancreas in order to cause an increase in blood sugar levels; that is, it is a hyperglycemic agent. It is normally part of a balancing mechanism with insulin, which has the opposite effect (see ℞ **hypoglycemics**). Therapeutically, glucagon can be given to people with low blood sugar levels (hypoglycemia) in an emergency, but it is mainly used for diagnostic purposes.

Warnings

• It should not be given to people with known sensitivity to glucagon, or with pheochromocytoma (it may cause a sudden increase in blood pressure).

• It should be given with caution to people with a history of insulinoma or pheochromocytoma.

• Its safety in pregnancy is not established. It should be used only if medically judged to be clearly needed.

• Medical judgment is required if breast-feeding is being considered. It is not known whether this drug appears in breast milk.

• People should become familiar with techniques for administering glucagon before an emergency arises.

Interactions

• The effects of ℞ anticoagulants may be increased.

Side effects

• Nausea, vomiting, generalized allergic reaction, hives, respiratory distress, and hypotension.

Glucagon Emergency Kit Ⓑ

A preparation of ℞ **glucagon.**

Formulation: Injection.
Availability: Prescription only.
Warnings and side effects: See ℞ **glucagon**.

Glucophage ⑧

A preparation of ℞ **metformin**.
Formulation: Oral tablets.
Availability: Prescription only.
Warnings and side effects: See ℞ **metformin**.

glucose ⑥

Type/Group: **antihypoglycemic**.
Brand(s): B-D Glucose; Dex4 Glucose; Glucose-40; Glutose; Insta-Glucose; various generic.
How administered: Orally; intravenous infusion; topically (eye).

Used to treat

Glucose, or dextrose, is a simple sugar and is an important source of energy for the body (it is the main source of energy for the brain). Once digested, it is stored in tissues, including the liver and muscles, in the form of glycogen and is broken down in the muscles back into glucose produces energy. The level of glucose in the blood is critical and harmful symptoms can occur if the level is too high or too low. Therapeutically, it may be administered as a dietary supplement in conditions of low blood sugar level, to treat abnormally high acidity of body fluids (acidosis), or to increase glucose levels in the liver following liver damage. Diabetics on certain hypoglycemic drugs need to carry glucose as an antihypoglycemic agent to take by mouth to deal with possible hypotensive crises. It may also be prescribed for topical (external) treatment of corneal edema.

Interactions

None significant.

Side effects

• Applied externally, it may cause irritation.

Glucose-40 ⑧

A preparation of ℞ **glucose**.
Formulation: Ophthalmic solution.
Availability: Prescription only.
Warnings and side effects: See ℞ **glucose**.

Glucotrol; Glucotrol XL ⑧

A preparation of ℞ **glipizide**.
Formulation: Oral tablets, extended release tablets, each in two strengths.
Availability: Prescription only.
Warnings and side effects: See ℞ **glipizide**.

glutaraldehyde ⑥

Type/Group: **disinfectant; antiseptic**.
Brand(s): Cidex.

Used to treat

Glutaraldehyde is similar to ℞ **formaldehyde**, but is stronger and faster-acting. It is mostly used to sterilize medical and surgical equipment.

glutethimide ⑥

Type/Group: **hypnotic**.
Brand(s): Generic only.
How administered: Orally.

Used to treat

Glutethimide is used as a short-term treatment for ⊙ **insomnia**. It produces effects similar to those of ℞ **barbiturates** and it has generally been replaced with other drugs considered to be safer.

Warnings

• It should not be given to people with known hypersensitivity to glutethimide or with porphyria.
• It should be given with caution to people with a history of drug abuse or to anyone over 65.
• Glutethimide should be used during pregnancy only if it is clearly needed.
• It should not be used by nursing mothers.
• Physical and psychological dependence (addiction) may occur, and should not be used for more than one week at a time.
• Avoid driving or other activities requiring alertness.
• Do not drink alcohol.
• Treatment must not be stopped abruptly.
• This drug is a Schedule II controlled substance.

Interactions

• There is a decreased response to oral ℞ **anticoagulants** (for example, ℞ **warfarin sodium**).
• ℞ **Activated charcoal** reduces the effects of glutethimide.
• Alcohol increases the effects of glutethimide.

Side effects

• Skin rash, nausea, hangover, dizziness, and drowsiness.
• Less frequently, vertigo, headache, depression, unsteadiness and incoordination, confusion, edema, indigestion, lightheadedness, vomiting, dry mouth, euphoria, impaired memory, slurred speech, and ringing in the ears.
• Rarely, paradoxical excitation, blurred vision, acute hypersensitivity, porphyria, and blood abnormalities.

Glutose ⑧

A preparation of ℞ **glucose**.
Formulation: Oral gel.
Availability: OTC.
Warnings and side effects: See ℞ **glucose**.

Glyate Syrup ⑧

A preparation of ℞ **guaifenesin**.
Formulation: Oral syrup.
Availability: OTC.
Warnings and side effects: See ℞ **guaifenesin**.

glyburide ⑥

(glibenclamide)
Type/Group: **antidiabetic; oral hypoglycemic; sulfonylurea**.
Brand(s): Diabeta; Glynase Prestab; Micronase; various generic.
How administered: Orally.

Used to treat

Glyburide is used in the treatment of type 2 ✛ **diabetes mellitus** (non-insulin-dependent diabetes mellitus; NIDDM). It works by augmenting what remains of insulin production in the pancreas.

Warnings

• It should not be given to people with juvenile diabetes or ketoacidosis.

• It should be given with caution to people with heart, thyroid, kidney, or liver disease, severe hypoglycemic reactions, adrenal or pituitary insufficiency, who are over 65, or severely debilitated.

• It is inappropriate for use during pregnancy (insulin is the drug of choice).

• Medical judgment is required if breast-feeding is being considered because this drug appears in breast milk.

• Alcohol should be avoided while using this drug, as it can cause unpleasant symptoms and interfere with blood sugar control.

• There are potentially multiple drug interactions with glyburide. A doctor should be consulted before taking any other medication (including OTCs, herbal remedies, and supplements).

Interactions

• ℞ **NSAIDs**, ℞ **salicylates**, ℞ **sulfonamides**, ℞ **chloramphenicol**, coumarins, ℞ **probenecid**, ℞ **MAOI**s, and ℞ **beta-blockers** may enhance the hypoglycemic effect of sulfonylureas.

• ℞ **Thiazide** and other ℞ **diuretics**, ℞ **corticosteroids**, ℞ **phenothiazines**, ℞ **thyroid hormones**, ℞ **estrogens**, ℞ **oral contraceptives**, ℞ **phenytoin**, ℞ **niacin**, ℞ **sympathomimetics**, and ℞ **isoniazid** may lead to the loss of control of sugar levels.

• Oral ℞ **miconazole**, ℞ **diclofenac**, ℞ **ibuprofen**, ℞ **naproxen**, and ℞ **mefenamic acid** have the potential for severe hypoglycemia.

Side effects

• Frequently, altered taste sensation, dizziness, weight gain, gastrointestinal effects, and headache.

• Occasionally, photosensitivity, peeling skin, itching, and rash.

• Rarely, hypoglycemia, gastrointestinal bleeding, liver disorders, and blood changes.

glycerin ⓖ

(glycerol; glycerine)

Type/Group: **emollient; laxative; eye treatment; anorectal preparation; demulcent.**

Brand(s): (Rectal application): Colace Suppositories; Fleets Babylax; Sani-Supp; various generic. (Ophthalmic, oral): Osmoglyn. (Ophthalmic, topical): Ophthalgan. Combinations: With *docusate sodium*: Therevac-SB. (Plus): *benzocaine*: Therevac-Plus.

How administered: Orally; topically (rectal suppositories); topically (eyes).

Used to treat

Glycerin is a colorless, sweet viscous liquid that is chemically an alcohol. It is used in many emollient skin preparations, as a sweetening agent for medications, and as a laxative in the form of rectal suppositories. Applied to the eye, as an ointment, it rapidly clears corneal haze or puffiness, aiding in diagnosis of certain eye disorders. It may also be given internally, as an oral liquid, to interrupt acute attacks in ✛ **glaucoma**, or to reduce intraocular pressure (pressure in the eyeball) before or after eye surgery.

Warnings

• Depending on use, it should be used with caution in people with diabetes mellitus, who require a low galactose diet, with certain lung, kidney or heart conditions (oral use), with any form of intestinal obstruction, or certain other gastrointestinal disorders (as laxative).

• The effects of glycerin in pregnancy have not been studied, and it should be used only if it is clearly needed.

• Medical judgment is required if breast-feeding is being considered. It is not known whether this drug appears in breast milk.

• Do not use as a laxative if there is abdominal pain, nausea, or vomiting, unless directed by a doctor.

• Chronic use of laxatives may cause fluid and electrolyte imbalances, vitamin and mineral deficiencies, and abnormal bowel function. Generally, they should not be used for more than a week.

• A doctor must be consulted first before taking any other medication (including OTCs, herbal remedies, and supplements), because laxatives may alter the absorption of a wide range of drugs.

Interactions

No significant drug interactions are known.

Side effects

• As a rectal suppository it may cause local irritation, dizziness, abdominal pain, flatulence, and bloating.

• With oral and rectal use, there may be effects on the heart.

• With oral use alone, there may be vomiting, confusion, and headache.

• When applied to the eye, it may cause irritation or pain.

glycerine ⓖ

see ℞ **glycerin**.

glycerol ⓖ

see ℞ **glycerin**.

Glyceryl-T Capsules; Liquid ⓡ

A preparation of ℞ **guaifenesin** and ℞ **theophylline**.

Formulation: Oral capsules; liquid.

Availability: Prescription only.

Warnings and side effects: See ℞ **guaifenesin**; ℞ **theophylline**.

glyceryl trinitrate ⓖ

see ℞ **nitroglycerin**.

glycopyrrolate ⓖ

(glycopyrronium bromide)

Type/Group: **anticholinergic; antispasmodic.**

Brand(s): Rubinul; various generic.

How administered: Injection; orally.

Used to treat

Glycopyrrolate is used in preoperative medication for drying up saliva and other secretions, and postoperatively to reverse neuro-

Key to symbols: ✛ = Disorder Section ℞ = Drug Section ♣ = Herbal Section ৯ = Supplement Section

muscular blockade. It may also be prescribed as an additional treatment for ⊙ peptic ulcer.

Warnings

• It should not be given to people with known severe hypersensitivity to this drug or similar agents, or those with narrow-angle glaucoma, obstructive urinary tract or gastrointestinal tract disorders, acute hemorrhage, severe ulcerative colitis, toxic megacolon, or myasthenia gravis.

• It should be given with caution to people with glaucoma, prostatic hypertrophy, kidney disease, congestive heart failure, lung disease, myasthenia gravis, hyperthyroidism, coronary artery disease, or hypertension. Its safety as an ulcer treatment in children under 12 has not been established.

• Glycopyrrolate's safety during pregnancy has not been established and it should be used only when it is clearly needed.

• Medical judgment is required if breast-feeding is being considered. It is not known whether this drug appears in breast milk.

• In hot weather heat prostration is more likely in those who are taking any anticholinergic drug, such as this one.

Interactions

No significant interactions specific to this drug are known.

Side effects

• Frequently, constipation and dry mouth.

• Less frequently, mental changes, drowsiness, sedation, weakness, heartbeat changes, postural hypotension (lowered blood pressure on standing), visual changes, nasal congestion, difficulty swallowing, gastrointestinal difficulties, urinary hesitancy or retention, impotence, allergic skin reactions, and decreased sweating.

glycopyrronium bromide Ⓖ

see ℞ glycopyrrolate.

Glycotuss Tablets Ⓑ

A preparation of ℞ guaifenesin.
Formulation: Oral tablets.
Availability: OTC.
Warnings and side effects: See ℞ guaifenesin.

Glynase Prestab Ⓑ

A preparation of ℞ glyburide.
Formulation: Oral tablets in several strengths.
Availability: Prescription only.
Warnings and side effects: See ℞ glyburide.

Gly-Oxide Liquid Ⓑ

A preparation of ℞ carbamide peroxide.
Formulation: Topical solution.
Availability: OTC.
Warnings and side effects: See ℞ carbamide peroxide.

Glyset Ⓑ

A preparation of ℞ miglitol.
Formulation: Oral tablets in several strengths.

Availability: Prescription only.
Warnings and side effects: See ℞ miglitol.

Glytuss Tablets Ⓑ

A preparation of ℞ guaifenesin.
Formulation: Oral tablets.
Availability: OTC.
Warnings and side effects: See ℞ guaifenesin.

G-myticin Ⓑ

A preparation of ℞ gentamicin.
Formulation: Topical ointment; topical cream.
Availability: Prescription only.
Warnings and side effects: See ℞ gentamicin.

Gold Bond Medicated Baby Powder Ⓑ

Also: Gold Bond Cornstarch Plus Medicated Baby Powder
A preparation of ℞ zinc oxide.
Formulation: Topical powder.
Availability: OTC.
Warnings and side effects: See ℞ zinc oxide.

gold compound Ⓓ

Generics: auranofin; aurothioglucose.
Actions and uses

Gold compounds are used in ℞ antirheumatic treatment to help in the management of severe, progressive ⊙ rheumatoid arthritis (and juvenile ⊙ arthritis), when ℞ NSAID treatment alone is not adequate. The main drugs used are organic compounds of gold—including ℞ aurothioglucose (gold sodium thiomalate) and ℞ auranofin and are 50 percent and 29 percent gold, respectively. They have an ℞ anti-inflammatory action through a mechanism that is not fully understood.

℞ aurothioglucose is also used to treat psoriatic arthritis, Felty's syndrome, and ⊙ Sjögren's syndrome.

Limitations

Gold compounds work extremely slowly and take several months to have any beneficial effect. These drugs should be discontinued if at all possible when pregnancy is discovered. If a pregnancy is planned, gold therapy should be stopped before pregnancy, because gold is cleared from the body's tissues only slowly. Nursing mothers should either discontinue this type of drug or discontinue breast feeding. See also the individual drug entries.

gonadorelin Ⓖ

Type/Group: hormone; sex hormone; diagnostic agent; infertility treatment; hypothalamic hormone.
Brand(s): Factrel (gonadorelin hydrochloride); Lutrepulse (gonadorelin acetate).
How administered: Injection.

Used to treat

Gonadorelin is a synthetic version of ℞ gonadotropin-releasing hormone (GnRH; LH-RH) and is used to evaluate pituitary function (as gonadorelin hydrochloride) and to induce ovulation in women with primary hypothalamic amenorrhea (as gonadorelin acetate).

It works by acting on the pituitary gland to release the gonadotropins (luteinizing hormone: LH, and follicle-stimulating hormone; FSH). Although not stated by the manufacturer for such treatment, it may be prescribed to inhibit ovulation or to treat precocious puberty.

Warnings
• It should not be used by people with known hypersensitivity to gonadorelin.
• Gonadorelin should not be used by women who must avoid pregnancy, have ovarian cysts, or conditions that would be worsened by reproductive hormones, such as hormone-dependent tumors (because treatment leads to production of reproductive hormones), or whose failure to ovulate is other than hypothalamic in origin.
• It should be used during pregnancy only if clearly needed.
• Medical judgment is required if breast-feeding is being considered.
• Rarely, severe allergic reactions may occur. Any signs of rash, urticaria, difficulty in swallowing or breathing, or rapid heart beat must be reported to a doctor immediately.
• Treatment will be carried out by specialists.

Interactions
No significant interactions have been reported.

Side effects
• Gonadorelin acetate: Occasionally, multiple pregnancy, inflammation, infection, and mild phlebitis. Rarely, ovarian hyperstimulation.
• Gonadorelin hydrochloride: Rarely, headache, nausea, lightheadedness, and abdominal discomfort.

gonadotrophin ✪
see ℞ **gonadotropin**.

gonadotropin ✪
(gonadotrophin)
Generics: **follitropin alfa/follitropin beta; menotropins; urofollitropin**.

Actions and uses
Gonadotropins (so called because of their actions on gonadal (sex) cells) are a group of hormones that are ℞ **anterior pituitary hormone** agents secreted by the anterior pituitary gland when stimulated in a pulsitile manner by a ℞ **hypothalamic hormone** called gonadotropin-releasing hormone. In pregnancy, large amounts are produced by the placenta.
Gonadotropins act on the ovary in women and the testes in men to promote the production in turn of ℞ **sex hormones** and of ova (eggs) or sperm, respectively. The major gonadotropins are follicle-stimulating hormone (FSH) and luteinizing hormone (LH; in men this is also called interstitial cell stimulating hormone, ICSH). There are very similar hormones released by the chorionic tissue of the placenta in pregnancy, which are called ℞ **chorionic gonadotropin**, and evidence in the urine for the presence of this is the basis of many pregnancy tests. These hormones are used mainly as drugs in ℞ **infertility treatment** where infertility is due to lack of ovulation (release of an ovum, egg, in women) but gonadotropins may also be prescribed to treat infertility in men by stimulating sperm production.
Preparations available include ℞ **urofollitropin** (a highly purified preparation of FSH extracted from the urine of menopausal women), ℞ **menotropins** (a collective name for hormone preparations consisting of combinations of the gonadotropin hormones), and ℞ **follitropin alfa/follitropin beta** (two synthetic forms considered therapeutically interchangeable).

Limitations
These hormone preparations are complex peptides that must be taken by injection over a period of 7–10 days for the induction of ovulation and pregnancy in carefully assessed individuals for whom infertility is not caused by primary ovarian failure. They are also used in assisted conception (such as in *in vitro* fertilization; IVF). Often the more common drug ℞ **clomiphene citrate** may be tried first. Although the procedure in women is often successful, there may be overstimulation of the ovary, increasing the risk of multiple births. There may be allergic reactions to the peptide drugs. See also the individual drug entries.

Gonal-F ℞
A preparation of ℞ **follitropin alfa/follitropin beta**.
Formulation: Injection.
Availability: Prescription only.
Warnings and side effects: See ℞ **follitropin alfa/follitropin beta**.

Goody's Body Pain Powder ℞
A preparation of ℞ **acetaminophen** and ℞ **aspirin**.
Formulation: Soluble powder (oral).
Availability: OTC.
Warnings and side effects: See ℞ **acetaminophen**; ℞ **aspirin**.

Goody's Extra Strength Headache Powder ℞
A preparation of ℞ **acetaminophen**, ℞ **aspirin**, and ℞ **caffeine**.
Formulation: Soluble powder (oral).
Availability: OTC.
Warnings and side effects: See ℞ **acetaminophen**; ℞ **aspirin**; ℞ **caffeine**.

Gordofilm ℞
A preparation of ℞ **salicylic acid**.
Formulation: Topical liquid.
Availability: OTC.
Warnings and side effects: See ℞ **salicylic acid**.

Gordogesic Creme ℞
A preparation of ℞ **methyl salicylate**, ℞ **mineral oil**, and various.
Formulation: Topical cream.
Availability: OTC.
Warnings and side effects: See ℞ **methyl salicylate**; ℞ **mineral oil**.

goserelin Ⓖ

Type/Group: **hypothalamic hormone**; sex hormone; **anticancer**.
Brand(s): Zoladex.
How administered: Subdermal implant.

Used to treat

Goserelin is a synthetic analog of gonadotropin-releasing hormone (GNRH) used to treat ✪ **prostate cancer**, ✪ **endometriosis**, and advanced ✪ **breast cancer** in premenopausal women. It is also prescribed as an endometrial thinning agent in cases of dysfunctional uterine bleeding.

Warnings

• It should not be used by people with known hypersensitivity, or with undiagnosed uterine bleeding.
• It should be given with caution to people at major risk of osteoporosis (such as alcoholics, heavy smokers, and those taking corticosteroids for prolonged periods).
• Goserelin should not be used during pregnancy. A doctor must be notified if pregnancy occurs while taking this drug.
• It should not be used by breast-feeding mothers.
• Pain and urinary difficulties associated with prostatic cancer may increase at the beginning of treatment.
• Gonadotropin and sex steroids rise above baseline initially; side effects are greatest during the first week of treatment, and signs and symptoms may increase before decreasing.
• Becoming pregnant must be avoided while using this drug, and only nonhormonal contraception used.
• Effective doses should stop menstruation. A doctor must be notified if it continues.
• There is a loss in bone mineral density. It may increase the risk of osteoporosis in those who are most susceptible.

Interactions

None have been noted.

Side effects

• In women, hot flashes, headache, vaginal dryness, changes in breast size, edema, headache, sweating, increased emotionality, depression, acne, vaginitis, and changes in libido.
• In men, hot flashes, sexual dysfunction, pain, lethargy, gastrointestinal symptoms, respiratory infection, edema, sweating, rash, and heart disease.
• It may increase cholesterol levels.

gramicidin Ⓖ

Type/Group: **antibiotic; antibacterial; eye treatment**.
Brand(s): Neosporin Ophthalmic; generic.

Used to treat

Gramicidin is incorporated into eye preparations along with ℞ **neomycin** and ℞ **polymyxin B sulfate**.

Warnings

It is too toxic to be used systemically so is only ever used topically in combination with other antibacterials for local infections.

Interactions

See Warnings.

Side effects

See Warnings.

granisetron Ⓖ

Type/Group: **serotonin-receptor antagonist; antiemetic; antinauseant**.
Brand(s): Kytril.
How administered: Orally; injection.

Used to treat

Granisetron may be used to give relief from nausea and vomiting, especially in patients receiving ℞ **cytotoxic** radiotherapy or chemotherapy. It has been used, as well, for relieving nausea after surgery. It acts as a serotonin receptor antagonist, blocking the action of the natural neurotransmitter serotonin.

Warnings

• It should not be given to people with known hypersensitivity to this drug.
• It should be used in pregnancy only if it is clearly needed.
• Medical judgment is required if breast-feeding is being considered. It is not known whether it appears in breast milk.
• It should be discontinued at the first sign of rash or other allergic response, and a doctor informed.

Interactions

No interactions of significance are known.

Side effects

• The most common are headache, feeling of weakness, constipation, and diarrhea.
• There may be changes in liver function. Hypersensitivity reactions are rare, but anaphylaxis, hives, shortness of breath and fall in blood pressure have been reported.

Grifulvin V Ⓑ

A preparation of ℞ **Griseofulvin**.
Formulation: Oral tablets in several strengths; oral suspension.
Availability: Prescription only.
Warnings and side effects: ℞ **Griseofulvin**

Grisactin; Grisactin Ultra Ⓑ

A preparation of ℞ **Griseofulvin**.
Formulation: Oral tablets in several strengths; oral capsules.
Availability: Prescription only.
Warnings and side effects: ℞ **Griseofulvin**

Griseofulvin Ⓑ

A preparation of ℞ **griseofulvin**.
Formulation: Oral tablets in several strengths.
Availability: Prescription only.
Warnings and side effects: See ℞ **griseofulvin**.

griseofulvin Ⓖ

Type/Group: **antifungal; antibiotic**.
Brand(s): Fulvicin; Grifulvin V; Grisactin; Gris-PEG; various generic.
How administered: Orally.

Used to treat

Griseofulvin is a powerful antifungal drug of antibiotic origin. It is used to treat ringworm infections of the skin, hair and nails, and also other ✪ **fungal infections** such as athlete's foot, and barber's itch.

Warnings

• It should not be given to people with known hypersensitivity to griseofulvin, with porphyria, or certain liver disorders.

• It should be given with caution to people with penicillin allergy (because they may be allergic to griseofulvin as well) or lupus erythematosus (because this drug sometimes causes a lupus-like reaction, or worsens symptoms of lupus).

• It is unknown whether this drug harms the fetus. It should be used during pregnancy only if medically judged to be essential.

• Medical judgment is required if breast-feeding is being considered. It is not known if it appears in breast milk.

• It may cause photosensitivity reactions (abnormal sensitivity to light), and so excessive exposure to sunlight or ultra-violet light must be avoided.

• A doctor must be contacted if a sore throat or skin rash develops.

Interactions

• The effects of ℞ **aspirin**, ℞ **cyclosporine**, ℞ **tacrolimus**, and ℞ **warfarin sodium** may be reduced.

• ℞ **Oral contraceptives** taken with griseofulvin may cause menstrual irregularities and increase the risk of pregnancy.

• ℞ **Phenobarbital** may reduce the effects of griseofulvin.

Side effects

• Occasionally, allergic reaction (such as rash, itching, hives), headache, nausea, diarrhea, excessive thirst, flatulence, oral thrush, dizziness, and insomnia.

• Rarely, tingling in hands and feet, protein excretion in urine. Also, serious reactions may occur, usually due to high dosages, or taking for long periods of time, or both. These include gastrointestinal bleeding, alteration in blood constituents, liver damage, and lupus-like syndrome.

Gris-PEG ®

A preparation of ℞ **Griseofulvin**.
Formulation: Oral tablets in several strengths.
Availability: Prescription only.
Warnings and side effects: ℞ **Griseofulvin**

growth factor Ⓓ

Generics: **becaplermin; filgrastim; interferons; sargramostim**.

Actions and uses

Growth factors are natural mediator chemicals within the body which control, modulate, or promote cell division and differentiation. They are protein or peptide molecules and often of some considerable chemical complexity. They are elaborated and released in tiny quantities by one cell type in the body, to act nearby (*paracrine*) or on the original cell (*autocrine*), and so serve as *local hormones*.

Many mediators can be regarded as growth factors, some of which are known as cytokines. Well-known member growth factors include platelet-derived growth factor (PDGF), epidermal growth factor (RGF), nerve growth factor (NGF), fibroblast growth factor, vascular endothelial growth factor, and insulin-like growth factor. Others are specifically involved in blood cell division and differentiation, and these are grouped together in the colony-stimulating factor family.

Of the main growth factors, human platelet-derived growth factor, which is manufactured by recombinant technology (DNA technology) in a form known as ℞ **becaplermin**, has recently been introduced as a ℞ **wound-healing agent** in the treatment of neuropathic diabetic ulcers.

Members of the colony-stimulating factor family are ℞ **hematopoietic** substances and some are now manufactured to be used to stimulate the production of blood cells. These include granulocyte-colony stimulating factor (G-CSF), which is now available (in a form synthesized using DNA engineering techniques) as ℞ **filgrastim**. This is used to reverse neutropenia (decrease in the number of neutrophils) by stimulating white cell production (mainly neutrophils) when this has been reduced during chemotherapy in ℞ **anticancer** treatment. Also, granulocyte macrophage-colony stimulating factor (GM-CSF), in its synthesized form ℞ **sargramostim**, also reduces neutropenia by stimulating white cell production (all granulocytes and monocytes) also when reduced during chemotherapy in the treatment of cancer.

The cytokine superfamily of mediators includes interleukins, chemokines, interferons, tumor necrosis factor, and transforming growth factor, as well as the growth factors and colony-stimulating factors discussed above. Of the remainder, a number (especially ℞ **interferons**) are involved in inflammatory processes in the body, and some aspects of this are discussed in the ℞ **immunomodulator** entry.

Limitations

There is evidently a huge potential for these agents in medicine, but progress has been delayed for two main reasons.

First, basic research has only recently acquired the experimental tools—largely those of molecular biology—to make any substantial inroads into identifying the agents involved (well over 50 are now characterized) and their corresponding actions. The amounts of protein molecule made, and released, by cells are quite tiny, so alternative approaches often have to be used. When, eventually, receptor antagonists to these agents are discovered, it will be easier to dissect the workings of cytokines on cells, in health or disease.

Second, these proteins turn out to be of great chemical complexity, and in the past have been impossible to synthesize or manufacture. Recently, however, it has become possible to harness the techniques of molecular biology to manufacture these proteins by recombinant technology. However, they are very expensive to make, and the cost factor is likely to limit their application to mainstream medicine for some time to come. Since they are proteins that would be digested in the gut, all have to be injected. Even so, most do not last long in the body, and agents that are eventually widely used will most likely be chemical variants of the natural molecules, which prolong their duration in the body.

See also the individual drug entries.

Guaifed Capsules; PD Capsules ®

A preparation of ℞ **pseudoephedrine** and ℞ **guaifenesin**.
Formulation: Oral capsules, timed release; PD capsules, long acting.
Availability: Prescription only.

Warnings and side effects: See ℞ **pseudoephedrine**; ℞ **guaifenesin**.

guaifenesin ⑥

(guaiphenesin)

Type/Group: expectorant.

Brand(s): Anti-Tuss Syrup; Breonesin Capsules; Diabetic Tussin EX Liquid; Duratuss-G Tablets; Fenesin Tablets; Genatuss Syrup; Glyate Syrup; Glycotuss Tablets; Glytuss Tablets; Humibid Sprinkle Capsules, L.A. Tablets; Hytuss 2X Capsules, Tablets; Liquibid Tablets; Muco-Fen-LA Tablets; Mytussin Syrup; Naldecon Senior EX Liquid; Organidin NR Liquid, NR Tablets; Respa-GF Tablets; Robitussin Syrup; Scot-Tussin Expectorant Syrup; Siltussin Syrup; Sinumist-SR Capsulets; Touro EX Tablets; Tusibron Syrup; Uni-tussin Syrup. Combinations: With codeine: Brontex; Cheracol Cough Syrup; Gani-Tuss NR; Guiatussin w/Codeine Expectorant Liquid; Halotussin AC; Mytussin AC Cough Syrup; Robitussin A-C Syrup; Romilar AC; Tussi-Organidin-S NR Liquid. With codeine and pseudoephedrine: Cycofed Pediatric Syrup; Deconsal Pediatric Syrup; Deproist Expectorant with with Codeine Liquid; Guiatussin DAC Syrup; Isoclor Expectorant Liquid; Mytussin DAC Liquid; Novagest Expectorant Liquid; Nucofed Expectorant Syrup; Nucofed Pediatric Expectorant Syrup; Nucotuss Expectorant Codeine Liquid; Nucotuss Pediatric Expectorant Syrup; Phenhist Expectorant Liquid; Robafen DAC Syrup; Robitussin-DAC Syrup; Ryna-CX Liquid. With dextromethorphan: Aquatab DM; Benylin Expectorant Liquid; Cheracol D Cough Liquid; Clear Tussin 30 Liquid; Diabetic Tussin DM Syrup; Duratuss DM; Fenesin DM Tablets; Genatuss DM Syrup; Guaifenex DM Tablets; Halotussin-DM Liquid, Sugar Free Liquid; Humibid DM Tablets, Sprinkles; Iobid DM Tablets; Kolephrin GG/DM Liquid; Muco-Fen-DM Tablets; Mytussin DM Liquid; Naldecon Senior DX Liquid; Phanatuss DM Syrup; Phenadex Senior Liquid; Respa-DM Tablets; Rhinosyn DMX Syrup; Robafen DM Syrup; Robitussin-DM Liquid, Infant Drops; Safe Tussin 30 Liquid; Scot-Tussin Senior Clear Liquid; Siltussin DM Syrup; Synacol CF Tablets; Tolu-Sed DM Syrup; Touro-DM Tablets; Tusibron-DM Syrup; Tuss-DM Tablets; Tussin DM Liquid; Uni-tussin DM Syrup; Vicks 44E Liquid; Vicks Pediatric Formula 44E Liquid. With dextromethorphan and pseudoephedrine: Anatuss DM Tablets, Syrup; Ambenyl-D Liquid; Benylin Multi-Symptom Liquid; Dimacol Caplets; MED-Rx DM Tablets; Novahistine DMX; PamMist-DM Syrup; Primatuss Cough Mixture 4D Liquid; Protuss DM Tablets; Rhinosyn-S Liquid; Robitussin Cold & Congestion Liqui-Gels, Caplets, Infant Drops; Ru-Tuss Expectorant Liquid; Touro CC; Tussafed-LA. With dextromethorphan, pseudoephedrine and acetaminophen: Sudafed Cold & Cough Liquid Caps; Robitussin Cold Multi-Symptom Cold & Flu Liqui-Gels, Caplets; Vicks DayQuil LiquiCaps. With ephedrine: Broncholate Softgels, Syrup; Bronkaid Dual Action Caplets; Dynafed Asthma Relief Tablets; Mini Thin Asthma Relief Tablets; Primatene Tablets. (Plus) *chlorpheniramine maleate*: Bronkotuss Expectorant Liquid. With ephedrine and theophylline (or derivatives): Primatene Dual Action Tablets. (Plus) *phenobarbital*: Lufyllin-EPG Tablets, Elixir (both have *diphylline*); Mudrane GG Tablets (has *aminophylline*). With hydrocodone: Atuss EX Syrup; Codiclear DH Syrup; Co-Tuss Liquid; Entuss Expectorant Tablets; HycoClear Tuss Syrup; Hycosin; Hycotuss Expectorant Syrup; Kwelcof Liquid; Pneumotussin Tablets, HC Syrup; Vicodin Tuss Syrup. (Plus) *phenylephrine*: Atuss-G Syrup; Donatussin DC Syrup; P-V-Tussin Tablets; Tussafed HC Syrup. (Plus) *pseudoephedrine*: Cophene XP Liquid; Deconamine CX Liquid; Detussin Expectorant Liquid; Duratuss HD Elixir; Entuss-D Tablets, Entuss Jr. Liquid; Pancof XP Liquid; SRC Expectorant Liquid; SUTUSS Elixir; Tussafin Expectorant Liquid; Vanex Expectorant Liquid. With phenylephrine: Deconsal Sprinkle Capsules; Endal Tablets; Liquibid-D Tablets; Rescon-GG Liquid; Sinupan Capsules. (Plus) *chlorpheniramine*: Donatussin Drops; Donatussin Syrup (has *dextromethorphan*). With pseudoephedrine: Anatuss LA Tablets; Congess SR Capsules, JR. Capsules; Congestac Caplets; Deconsal II Tablets; Defen-LA Tablets; Duratuss Tablets; Entex PSE Tablets; Eudal-SR Tablets; Fedahist Expectorant Syrup; Guaifed Capsules, PD Capsules; Guaifenex PSE 120 Tablets, PSE 60 Tablets, Rx Tablets, Rx AM Tablets, Rx DM Tablets; Guaimax-D Tablets; Guaitab Tablets; Guaivent/PSE Tablets, Capsules, PD Capsules; GuiaCough PE Liquid; Guiatex PSE Tablets; Guiatuss PE Syrup; Histalet X Tablets, Syrup; Iosal II Tablets; MED-Rx Tablets; Nasabid SR Tablets, Capsules; Nasatab LA Tablets; PanMist LA, JR Tablets, Syrup; Polaramine Expectorant Liquid (has *dexchlorpheniramine maleate*); Refenesan Plus Tablets; Respaire 120 Capsules, 60 Capsules; Robitussin PE Syrup, Severe Congestion Liqui-Gels; Ru-tuss DE Tablets; Rymed Capsules, Liquid; Sinufed Timecelles; Sinutab Non-Drying Capsules; Stamoist E Tablets; Sudal 120/600 Tablets, 60/500 Tablets; Syn-Rx Tablets; Touro LA Caplets; Tuss-LA Tablets; Tussin PE; V-Dec-M Tablets; Versacaps Capsules; Zephrex LA Tablets, Tablets. With theophylline (or derivatives): Elixophyllin GG Liquid; Glyceryl-T Capsules, Liquid; Quibron Capsules, -300 Capsules; Mudrane GG-2 Tablets; Slo-Phyllin GG Capsules, Syrup; Synophylate-GG Syrup. (*With diphylline*): Dilor-G Tablets, Liquid; Dyflex-G Tablets; Dyline G.G. Tablets, Liquid; Lufyllin-GG Tablets, Elixir; Panfil G Tablets, Liquid. (Most combinations available as generics.)

How administered: Orally.

Used to treat

Guaifenesin is used in a number of brands for ✪ **coughs** and ✪ **colds** (particularly for dry non-productive coughs). Although not stated by the manufacturers for such us, it is also used for ✪ **sinusitis**. However, strong evidence of its benefits is lacking.

Warnings

• It should not be given to people with known hypersensitivity to this drug.

• Guaifenesin should be used during pregnancy only if it is clearly needed.

• Nursing mothers should discontinue this drug or discontinue breast-feeding.

• It is regarded as safe in normal use. However, some authorities believe that it should be avoided by people with certain respiratory problems.

• If a cough persists for more than a week, a doctor should be consulted.

Interactions

In ordinary use guaifenesin has no significant interactions with other drugs.

Side effects

• There are no significant side effects if it is used in recommended doses.

• In high doses it may cause nausea and vomiting, dizziness, drowsiness, skin rash, and headache.

Guaifenex DM Tablets ®

A preparation of ℞ **dextromethorphan** and ℞ **guaifenesin**.

Formulation: Oral tablets, extended release.

Availability: Prescription only.

Warnings and side effects: See ℞ **dextromethorphan**; ℞ **guaifenesin**.

Guaifenex PSE 120 Tablets; PSE 60 Tablets; Rx Tablets; Rx AM ®

A preparation of ℞ **pseudoephedrine** and ℞ **guaifenesin**.

Formulation: Oral tablet, extended release.

Availability: Prescription only.

Warnings and side effects: See ℞ **pseudoephedrine**; ℞ **guaifenesin**.

Guaimax-D Tablets ®

A preparation of ℞ **pseudoephedrine** and ℞ **guaifenesin**.

Formulation: Oral tablets, extended release.

Availability: Prescription only.

Warnings and side effects: See ℞ **pseudoephedrine**; ℞ **guaifenesin**.

Guaitab Tablets ®

A preparation of ℞ **pseudoephedrine** and ℞ **guaifenesin**.

Formulation: Oral tablets.

Availability: OTC.

Warnings and side effects: See ℞ **pseudoephedrine**; ℞ **guaifenesin**.

Guaivent/PSE Tablets; Capsule; PD Capsules ®

A preparation of ℞ **pseudoephedrine** and ℞ **guaifenesin**.

Formulation: Oral capsules, long acting; PSE tablets, sustained release.

Availability: Prescription only.

Warnings and side effects: See ℞ **pseudoephedrine**; ℞ **guaifenesin**.

guanabenz acetate ©

Type/Group: alpha-adrenergic stimulant; antisympathetic; antihypertensive.

Brand(s): Wytensin; various generic.

How administered: Orally.

Used to treat

Guanabenz prevents the release of norepinephrine from sympathetic nerves. It can be used to reduce high blood pressure in ✪ **hypertension**, alone or with a ℞ **thiazide** ℞ **diuretic**.

Warnings

• It should not be given to people with known hypersensitivity to this drug.

• It should be given with caution to people with severe coronary insufficiency, recent heart attack, cerebrovascular disease, or impaired liver or kidney function.

• Guanabenz should be used during pregnancy only if the potential benefit outweighs the possible risk to the fetus.

• Medical judgment is required if breast-feeding is being considered. It is not known whether this drug appears in breast milk.

• Abruptly discontinuing using this drug or missing regular doses may cause a "rebound" rise in blood pressure.

• Because of possible sedative side effects, caution is advised for potentially hazardous activities, such as driving, that require mental alertness.

• A doctor must be consulted before taking any other medication (including OTCs, herbal remedies, supplements, or alternative remedies of any kind).

Interactions

• If taken with alcohol, ℞ **anesthetics**, ℞ **barbiturates**, ℞ **benzodiazepines**, ℞ **opioids**, ℞ **phenothiazines**, or ℞ **sedatives**, there is a general potential for increased or intensified effects.

• ℞ **MAOIs** or ℞ **tricyclic** antidepressants may reduce the antihypertensive effect of guanabenz.

• If used with other antihypertensives and diuretics, the effects of these drugs may be increased. This additive effect is sometimes used to advantage in combination treatments for high blood pressure.

Side effects

• Except for rebound hypertension that can occur with abrupt withdrawal, side effects are generally mild. Dry mouth, drowsiness or sedation are fairly common, as well as dizziness, weakness or gastrointestinal disturbances (for example, nausea, abdominal pain, diarrhea, vomiting).

• Less frequently, chest pain, edema, mental changes (for example, anxiety, depression or sleep disturbances), urinary frequency, rashes, palpitations or arrhythmias, or aches in the extremities.

guanadrel ©

Type/Group: antihypertensive; adrenergic-neuron blocker; antisympathetic.

Brand(s): Hylorel.

How administered: Orally.

Used to treat

Guanadrel prevents release of ℞ **norepinephrine** (also called noradrenaline) from sympathetic nerves, and can be used alone or with other drugs to reduce high blood pressure, including ✪ **hypertension** arising from certain kidney diseases.

Key to symbols: ✪ = Disorder Section   ℞ = Drug Section   ♣ = Herbal Section   ⧖ = Supplement Section

Warnings

• It should not be given to people with known hypersensitivity to this drug, with pheochromocytoma, congestive heart failure, or anyone taking an ℞ **MAOI** antidepressant.

• It should be given with caution to the elderly, to anyone with bronchial asthma, peptic ulcer, coronary or cerebral arteriosclerosis, or impaired kidney function.

• Guanadrel's safety during pregnancy has not been established and it should be used only if the potential benefit outweighs the risk to the fetus.

• Nursing women should either discontinue this drug or discontinue breast-feeding.

• Postural hypotension (lowered blood pressure on standing) occurs frequently and fainting may result. Sudden or prolonged standing or exercise should be avoided. These hypotensive effects may be aggravated by hot environments. Sit or lie down immediately if you experience weakness or dizziness.

• Because of possible sedative side effects, caution is advised for potentially hazardous and skilled activities, such as driving.

• A doctor must be consulted before taking any other medication, including OTCs, herbal remedies (especially for colds, allergy, or asthma), or supplements.

Interactions

• ℞ **MAOI** antidepressants should not be used with guanadrel or within one week of discontinuing an MAOI.

• ℞ **Beta-blockers** and ℞ **vasodilators** may cause exaggerated hypotension or slowing of the heart rate.

• The effects of direct-acting ℞ **sympathomimetics**, such as ℞ **vasoconstrictors** (for example, ℞ **metaraminol**, ℞ **norepinephrine**, ℞ **phenylephrine**) and nasal ℞ **decongestants** may be intensified or prolonged by guanadrel.

• Guanadrel treatment should be stopped two or three days before any surgery because of possible interactions with anesthetics.

• Alcohol may increase the risk and severity of hypotensive effects.

• ℞ **amphetamines**, ℞ **ephedrine**, ℞ **phenothiazines**, and ℞ **tricyclic** antidepressants may reduce or antagonize the antihypertensive effect of guanadrel.

• If taken with another antihypertensive or a ℞ **diuretic**, the effects of both drugs may be increased, which is sometimes used to advantage in combination treatments for high blood pressure.

Side effects

• The most frequent are postural hypotension, diarrhea, drowsiness, failure to ejaculate, and slowing of heart rate.

• There may also be gastrointestinal disturbances (for exampe, loss of appetite, nausea, vomiting), chest pain, cough, palpitations, urinary retention, edema, or shortness of breath.

• Dry mouth, nasal stuffiness, disturbances of vision, muscle pain, tingling sensations, confusion, or mental depression may also occur.

guanethidine monosulfate Ⓖ

(guanethidine monosulphate)
Type/Group: **adrenergic-neuron blocker; antisympathetic; antihypertensive**.

Brand(s): Ismelin; various generic. Combinations: With *hydrochlorothiazide*: Esimil.
How administered: Orally.

Used to treat

Guanethidine monosulfate prevents the release of ℞ **norepinephrine** (also called noradrenaline) from sympathetic nerves. It can be used alone or with other drugs to reduce high blood pressure, including ◗ **hypertension** arising from certain kidney diseases.

Warnings

• It should not be given to people with known hypersensitivity to this drug, with pheochromocytoma, congestive heart failure, or by anyone taking an ℞ **MAOI** antidepressant.

• It should be given with caution to elderly people and to anyone with bronchial asthma, peptic ulcer, coronary or cerebral arteriosclerosis, or impaired kidney function.

• Guanethidine's safety during pregnancy has not been established and it should be used only if the potential benefit outweighs the possible risk to the fetus.

• Medical judgment is required if breast-feeding is being considered.

• Postural hypotension (lowered blood on standing) occurs frequently and fainting may result. Sudden or prolonged standing or exercise should be avoided. These hypotensive effects may be aggravated by hot environments.

• Because of possible sedative side effects, caution is advised for potentially hazardous activities, such as driving, that require mental alertness.

• A doctor must be consulted before taking any other medication (including OTCs, herbal remedies, supplements, or any other kind of alternative remedy).

• A doctor must be contacted if severe diarrhea, frequent dizziness, or fainting occur.

Interactions

• Guanethidine should not be taken with a ℞ **MAOI** antidepressant, or within one week of discontinuing MAOI treatment.

• ℞ **Cardiac glycosides** may cause a significant slowing of the heart rate.

• The effects of direct-acting ℞ **sympathomimetics** such as ℞ **vasoconstrictors** (for example, ℞ **metaraminol**, ℞ **norepinephrine**, ℞ **phenylephrine**) and nasal ℞ **decongestants** may be intensified or prolonged.

• It is recommended that guanethidine treatment should stop at least two weeks before any planned surgery due to possble interactions with ℞ **anesthetics**.

• There is a risk of increased hypotensive effects if taken with alcohol, ℞ **levodopa**, or ℞ **methotrimeprazine** (particularly for postural hypotension with methotrimeprazine).

• ℞ **amphetamine**, diethylpropion, ℞ **ephedrine**, ℞ **haloperidol**, mephentermine, ℞ **methylphenidate**, ℞ **oral contraceptives**, some ℞ **phenothiazines**, ℞ **thiothixene**, and ℞ **tricyclic** antidepressants may reduce or block the antihypertensive effect of guanethidine.

• If used with other antihypertensives and diuretics, the effects of these drugs may be increased. This additive effect is sometimes used to advantage in combination treatments for high blood pressure.

Side effects

• Frequently, postural hypotension (which may cause dizziness, weakness, lassitude or fainting), diarrhea, nasal congestion, failure to ejaculate, drowsiness, and slowing of the heart rate.

• Less commonly, gastrointestinal disturbances (for example, loss of appetite, nausea, vomiting), urinary retention, edema, or shortness of breath. Dry mouth or tender salivary glands, drooping eyelids, blurred vision, muscle pain, mental depression, and angina pectoris have also been reported.

guanethidine monosulphate Ⓖ

see ℞ guanethidine monosulfate.

guanfacine hydrochloride Ⓖ

Type/Group: **alpha-adrenergic stimulant; antisympathetic; antihypertensive**.
Brand(s): Tenex.
How administered: Orally.

Used to treat

Guanfacine is an antisympathetic drug which decreases neurotransmitter release from sympathetic nerves (it is thought to act as an alpha-adrenergic stimulant (alpha$_2$-receptor subtype) in the brain). It can be used to reduce high blood pressure in ✪ **hypertension** in combination with a ℞ **thiazide** ℞ **diuretic**.

Warnings

• It should not be given to people with known hypersensitivity to this drug.

• It should be given with caution to people with severe coronary insufficiency, recent heart attack, cerebrovascular disease, or impaired liver or kidney function.

• Guanfacine should be used during pregnancy only if it is clearly needed.

• Medical judgment is required if breast-feeding is being considered. It is not known whether it appears in breast milk.

• Abruptly discontinuing using this drug or missing regular doses may cause a "rebound" rise in blood pressure.

• Because of possible sedative side effects, caution is advised for potentially hazardous activities, such as driving, that require mental alertness.

• A doctor must be consulted beore taking any other medication (including OTCs, herbal remedies, supplements, or any other kind of alternative remedy).

Interactions

• If taken with alcohol, ℞ **anesthetics**, ℞ **barbiturates**, ℞ **benzodiazepines**, ℞ **opioids**, ℞ **phenothiazines**, or ℞ **sedatives**, there is a general potential for increased or intensified effects.

• ℞ **Phenytoin** may reduce the levels and effects of guanfacine.

• There may be some reduction of the antihypertensive effect of guanfacine if taken with ℞ **MAOI** or ℞ **tricyclic** antidepressants.

• If used with other antihypertensives and diuretics, the effects of these drugs may be increased. This additive effect is sometimes used to advantage in combination treatments for high blood pressure.

Side effects

• Except for rebound hypertension that can occur with abrupt withdrawal, these are generally mild. Dry mouth, drowsiness, dizziness, and constipation are fairly common. Other effects may include weakness or gastrointestinal disturbances (for example, abdominal pain, diarrhea, indigestion).

• Less frequently, chest pain, edema, mental changes (for example, anxiety, depression, or sleep disturbances), urinary frequency, blurred vision, palpitations or arrhythmias, impotence, leg cramps, tingling in the extremities, or rash. There may be changes in liver function.

guanidine hydrochloride Ⓖ

Type/Group: **parasympathomimetic**.
Brand(s): Generic only.
How administered: Orally.

Used to treat

Guanidine enhances the release of the neurotransmitter acetylcholine after a nerve impulse. It is used to treat Eaton-Lambert syndrome, which is a condition that resembles ✪ **myasthenia gravis**, but not for myasthenia gravis itself.

Warnings

• It should not be used by anyone with known hypersensitivity to guanidine.

• It is not known whether guanidine can harm the fetus, therefore, it should be used during pregnancy only if medically judged to be needed.

• It should not be used by breast-feeding mothers.

• Fatal bone-marrow suppression can occur. Blood cell count should be monitored.

• Kidney function may be affected in some people.

• It should not be used any longer than necessary.

Interactions

No interactions have been reported.

Side effects

• Dry mouth, loss of appetite, nausea, diarrhea, tingling sensation, cold sensations, nervousness, elevated liver enzymes, palpitations, changes in heart rate, hypotension, fever, and sore throat.

GuiaCough PE Liquid Ⓑ

A preparation of ℞ **pseudoephedrine** and ℞ **guaifenesin**.
Formulation: Oral liquid.
Availability: OTC.
Warnings and side effects: See ℞ **pseudoephedrine**; ℞ **guaifenesin**.

Guiatussin DAC Syrup Ⓑ

A preparation of ℞ **codeine phosphate**, ℞ **guaifenesin**, and ℞ **pseudoephedrine**.
Formulation: Oral syrup.
Availability: May or may not require a prescription.

　　　Key to symbols:　✪ = Disorder Section　℞ = Drug Section　♣ = Herbal Section　◬ = Supplement Section

Warnings and side effects: See ℞ codeine phosphate; ℞ guaifenesin; ℞ pseudoephedrine.

Guiatussin w/Codeine Expectorant Liquid ⓑ

A preparation of ℞ codeine phosphate and ℞ guaifenesin.
Formulation: Oral liquid.
Availability: May or may not require a prescription.
Warnings and side effects: See ℞ codeine phosphate; ℞ guaifenesin.

Guiatuss PE Syrup ⓑ

A preparation of ℞ pseudoephedrine and ℞ guaifenesin.
Formulation: Oral syrup.
Availability: OTC.
Warnings and side effects: See ℞ pseudoephedrine; ℞ guaifenesin.

Gynazole ⓑ

A preparation of ℞ butoconazole.
Formulation: Vaginal cream.
Availability: Prescription only.
Warnings and side effects: See ℞ butoconazole.

Gynecort Female Creme ⓑ

A preparation of ℞ hydrocortisone.
Formulation: Cream.
Availability: OTC.
Warnings and side effects: See ℞ hydrocortisone.

Gyne Sulf ⓑ

A preparation of ℞ triple sulfa cream.
Formulation: Topical cream.
Availability: Prescription only.
Warnings and side effects: See ℞ triple sulfa cream.

Gynodiol ⓑ

A preparation of ℞ estradiol.
Formulation: Oral tablets in several strengths; vaginal cream.
Availability: Prescription only.
Warnings and side effects: See ℞ estradiol.

Gynogen L.A. ⓑ

A preparation of ℞ estradiol.
Formulation: Injection.
Availability: Prescription only.
Warnings and side effects: See ℞ estradiol.

H_2-antagonist ⓓ

(H_2-histamine receptor antagonist; histamine H_2-receptor antagonist)
Generics: **cimetidine; famotidine; nizatidine; ranitidine hydrochloride.**

Actions and uses

H_2-antagonist drugs act to block the actions of histamine at a class of histamine receptor called H_2, which is found in the gastric mucosa (stomach lining) and promotes secretion of gastric acid (peptic acid, hydrochloric acid). The overproduction of gastric acid may be involved in ulceration of the gastric (stomach) and duodenal (first part of small intestine) linings, or be the cause of pain in reflux esophagitis (regurgitation of acid and enzymes into the esophagus). Technically, these drugs are ℞ antihistamine drugs, but somewhat confusingly this term is not applied to them because it is reserved for the much earlier class of drugs that act at H_1-receptors and which have quite different actions.

H_2-antagonists (for example, ℞ cimetidine, ℞ ranitidine hydrochloride, ℞ famotidine and ℞ nizatidine) are commonly used in the treatment of ulcers (see ℞ ulcer-healing drug) and for a wide variety of ⊙ indigestion (dyspepsia) and other peptic acid complaints. They promote healing of ⊙ peptic ulcers, so are used in the treatment of benign peptic (gastric and duodenal) ulcers, ℞ NSAID-induced ulceration, and as a preventive to relieve heartburn in cases of reflux esophagitis, Zollinger-Ellison syndrome, and a variety of conditions where reduction of acidity is beneficial.

Limitations

H_2-antagonist drugs are generally well tolerated with few serious side effects. However, treatment with these drugs should not start before a full diagnosis of gastric bleeding or serious pain has been made, because their action in restricting gastric secretions may possibly mask the presence of stomach cancer. Nevertheless H_2-antagonists are available OTC (over-the-counter), though at low doses, for heartburn, acid indigestion, and sour stomach due to overindulgence. Cigarette smoking reverses some of the effects of these drugs and so will delay ulcer healing.
See also the individual entries.

H_2-histamine receptor antagonist ⓓ

see ℞ H_2-antagonist.

Habitrol ⓑ

A preparation of ℞ nicotine.
Formulation: Transdermal patch.
Availability: Prescription only.
Warnings and side effects: See ℞ nicotine.

haematopoietic ⓓ

see ℞ hematopoietic.

Haemophilus b conjugate vaccine ⓖ

Type/Group: vaccine.
Brand(s): ActHIB; HibTITER; OmniHIB; PedvaxHIB; ProHIBit.
How administered: Intramuscular injection.

Used to treat

Haemophilus b conjugate vaccine is a vaccine for immunizing young children, usually 6 years or under, against *Haemophilus influenzae* type b, which is a bacterium that may cause serious illness, such as ⊙ meningitis and ⊙ pneumonia, chiefly in children.

Warnings

• It should not be given to people with known hypersensitivity or allergy to the vaccine, or anyone who has a current or recent febrile (feverish) illness or infection.

• The effectiveness of this vaccine has not been evaluated in adults and older children.

• Its use is not recommended during pregnancy.

• Medical judgment is required if breast-feeding is being considered.

• After vaccination, people will be required to wait for some time to ensure that there is no serious reaction (such as anaphylaxis).

Interactions

• Caution is required if ℞ **anticoagulants** are being taken.

• ℞ **Tetanus immune globulin (TIG)** may delay immunity, and should not be injected in the same arm.

Side effects

• These range from little or no reactions to fever, diarrhea, vomiting, irritability, sleepiness, and loss of appetite.

• Rarely, there may be anaphylactic shock.

haemorrhoid/hemorrhoid preparation ⓪

see ℞ **anorectal preparation**.

haemostatic ⓪

see ℞ **hemostatic**.

hair-growth promoter ⓪

Generics: **minoxidil**.

Actions and uses

Hair-growth promoter agents are for treating balding (✪ **alopecia**). However, few such drugs have ever been shown to be effective. Recently, ℞ **minoxidil** (normally used systemically as a ℞ **vasodilator** to treat high blood pressure) has become available for use in external application to treat alopecia—hair loss that occurs as "male pattern baldness" in men, and as hair thinning around the forehead and temples in women. Signs of new hair growth generally take four months or more to appear.

Limitations

See the individual drug entry.

halazepam ⓖ

Type/Group: **antianxiety; benzodiazepine**.
Brand(s): Paxipam.
How administered: Orally.

Used to treat

Halazepam is used to treat ✪ **anxiety**.

Warnings

• It should not be given to people with known hypersensitivity to benzodiazepines, narrow-angle glaucoma, or psychosis.

• It should be given with caution to people with kidney or liver impairment, a history of drug abuse, respiratory depression, sleep apnea, or anyone over 65.

• Halazepam is not recommended for use during pregnancy. A doctor must be consulted if pregnancy occurs while taking this drug.

• It should not be used by nursing mothers.

• Judgment, thinking, and physical skills may be impaired.

• Avoid alcohol because adverse side effects may be increased (see Side effects below).

• Avoid other psychotropic medications unless prescribed by a doctor.

• A doctor must be consulted before discontinuing use or increasing dosage, because benzodiazepines may produce psychological and physical dependence and withdrawal symptoms.

Interactions

• ℞ **azole** antifungals (for example, ℞ **fluconazole**, ℞ **ketoconazole**, ℞ **itraconazole**), ℞ **beta-blockers** (for example, ℞ **propranolol**, ℞ **metoprolol**), ℞ **cimetidine**, ℞ **ciprofloxacin**, delavirdine, ℞ **disulfiram**, ℞ **isoniazid**, ℞ **macrolide** antibiotics (for example, ℞ **erythromycin**, ℞ **clarithromycin**, troleandomycin), ℞ **omeprazole**, ℞ SSRIs, and ℞ **quinolones** may increase levels of halazepam.

• ℞ **carbamazepine**, ℞ **phenytoin**, and ℞ **rifampin** may reduce the effects of halazepam.

• ℞ **clozapine** may have additive effects on respiratory and cardiovascular depression.

• Alcohol may increase adverse side effects.

Side effects

• Abnormal sleepiness, weakness, and decrease in physical activity.

• Less frequently, abnormal thinking and emotions, decreased reflexes, joint pain, seizure, sleep disorder, stupor, irregular heartbeat, fainting, eye, ear, nose or throat pain and inflammation, gastrointestinal effects, urinary problems, menstrual cramps, vaginal discharge, back or leg pain, asthma, shortness of breath, skin inflammation, dry skin, and blood cell disorders that can be serious.

halcinonide ⓖ

Type/Group: **corticosteroid; anti-inflammatory**.
Brand(s): Halog; various generic.
How administered: Topically.

Used to treat

Halcinonide is used to treat non-infective inflammation of the skin caused by conditions such as ✪ **eczema**, ✪ **psoriasis**, contact ✪ **dermatitis**, and ✪ **pruritus**.

Warnings

• It should not be used by people with known hypersensitivity to corticosteroids, or with fungal infections.

• It should be given with caution to anyone with a bacterial or viral infection, and to children, who may be more susceptible to systemic side effects.

• It must not be used on the groin, face, or armpits.

• Corticosteroids can cross the placenta. It is unknown whether external application could result in sufficient systemic absorption to create a hazard to the fetus. Therefore, halcinonide should only be used in pregnancy if medically judged to be essential.

• Medical judgment is also required if breast-feeding is being considered. When taken internally, corticosteroids are excreted in breast milk and may suppress growth and interfere with the

Key to symbols: ✪ = Disorder Section ℞ = Drug Section ♣ = Herbal Section ⚯ = Supplement Section

production of natural corticosteroids in the infant. It is unknown whether external application could result in sufficient systemic absorption to produce detectable amounts in breast milk.

• Topical (applied externally) corticosteroids can be absorbed in sufficient amounts to produce systemic effects (see ℞ **corticosteroids**). Therefore, do not use over large surface areas or for a prolonged period to minimize the risk of systemic absorption.

• Bandages or dressings must not cover the treated area unless directed by a doctor, as this may increase the risk of adverse skin reactions.

• Avoid weeping, denuded, or infected areas, and the eyes.

• A doctor must be notified and use of halcinonide stopped if local irritation or fever develops.

Interactions
• No significant interactions have been reported.

Side effects
• Occasionally, irritation, and itching.
• Rarely, allergic rash. There may be systemic effects.

Halcion ℬ

A preparation of ℞ **triazolam**.
Formulation: Oral tablets in several strengths.
Availability: Prescription only.
Warnings and side effects: See ℞ triazolam.

Haldol; decanoate ℬ

A preparation of ℞ **haloperidol**.
Formulation: Oral tablets in several strengths; oral concentrate; injectable solutions, regular and Decanoate, which has a longer duration of action.
Availability: Prescription only.
Warnings and side effects: See ℞ haloperidol.

Halenol Children's Liquid ℬ

A preparation of ℞ **acetaminophen**.
Formulation: Oral liquid.
Availability: OTC.
Warnings and side effects: See ℞ acetaminophen.

Haley's M-O ℬ

A preparation of ℞ **magnesium hydroxide** and ℞ **mineral oil**.
Formulation: Oral liquid.
Availability: OTC.
Warnings and side effects: See ℞ magnesium hydroxide; ℞ **mineral oil**.

Halfprin 81; 1/2 Halfprin ℬ

A preparation of ℞ **aspirin**.
Formulation: Oral tablets; all are enteric coated.
Availability: OTC.
Warnings and side effects: ℞ aspirin.

Hall's; Plus Maximum Strength; Sugar Free Mentholyptus ℬ

A preparation of ℞ **menthol**.
Formulation: Tablets, lozenges.
Availability: OTC.
Warnings and side effects: See ℞ menthol.

halofantrine hydrochloride ⑥

Type/Group: **antimalarial; amebicide and antiprotozoal**.
Brand(s): Halfan.
How administered: Orally.

Used to treat
Halofantrine is used to treat infection by uncomplicated, chloroquine-resistant *Plasmodium falciparum* species ✪ **malaria**, or chloroquine-resistant *Plasmodium vivax* species of malaria.

Warnings
• It should not be given to people with known hypersensitivity to halofantrine or related compounds.
• It should be given with caution to people with certain heart disorders, unexplained syncope (fainting), or thiamine deficiency.
• This is a specialist drug that is only prescribed by physicians who have experience in the treatment of malaria.
• Halofantrine must not be used during pregnancy.
• It is not recommended for use while nursing.
• ℞ **mefloquine** should not be used along with or following halofantrine, because potentially fatal changes in heart rhythm may occur.

Interactions
• Mefloquine, and other drugs known to prolong QTc interval, may cause serious changes in heart rhythm.

Side effects
• Abdominal pain, diarrhea, nausea/vomiting, heart rhythm changes, hypersensitivity reaction.

Halofed Tablets ℬ

A preparation of ℞ **pseudoephedrine**.
Formulation: Oral tablets.
Availability: OTC.
Warnings and side effects: See ℞ pseudoephedrine.

Halog; Halog-E ℬ

A preparation of ℞ **halcinonide**.
Formulation: Cream in several strengths; ointment (Halog-E).
Availability: Prescription only.
Warnings and side effects: See ℞ halcinonide.

haloperidol ⑥

Type/Group: **antipsychotic**.
Brand(s): Haldol.
How administered: Orally, injection.

Used to treat
Haloperidol is used to treat and tranquilize patients with psychotic disorders (such as ✪ **schizophrenia**, and in manic episodes: see also ✪ **psychotic disorders**) and as an ℞ **antianxiety** drug for

other behavioral disturbance, especially for emergency control. It can also be used in the short-term treatment of hyperactive children. Quite separately from the previous uses, it can be administered to treat Tourette's syndrome. Although not stated by the manufacturer for such use, it is sometimes given in small doses as an ℞ **antinauseant** and ℞ **antiemetic** to treat nausea and vomiting.

Warnings

• It should not be given to people with known hypersensitivity to this drug, a history of allergic reactions to drugs, with severe toxic CNS (central nervous system) depression, in a comatose state from any cause, or with Parkinson's disease.

• It should be given with caution to people over 65, or with severe cardiovascular disorders, seizure disorder, liver dysfunction, glaucoma, chronic obstructive pulmonary disease (COPD), or to anyone undergoing alcohol withdrawal, or receiving electroconvulsive therapy.

• Haloperidol should be used during pregnancy only if the benefits outweigh the risk to the fetus.

• It should not be used by nursing mothers.

• It may cause postural hypotension (lowered blood pressure on standing), so rise slowly from a reclining position. Older people in particular should exercise caution.

• It may impair physical and mental abilities.

• Avoid alcohol.

• It may cause sensitivity to sunlight (photosensitivity), so exposure must be minimized (use a sunscreen, sunglasses, and so on).

• If used for a long time, tardive dyskinesia (see ℞ **antipsychotics**) occasionally develops.

• The dose should be reduced gradually when discontinuing treatment.

• Take special precautions to stay cool in hot weather.

• It is not generally used in children less than 3 years of age.

Interactions

• Haloperidol may inhibit the ℞ **antiparkinsonian** effect of ℞ **levodopa**.

• ℞ **Anticholinergics**, ℞ **barbiturates**, ℞ **narcotic analgesics**, and ℞ **orphenadrine** lower the levels of ℞ **antipsychotic** and/or increase the occurrence of anticholinergic and/or CNS (central nervous system) effects.

• If used with ℞ **bromocriptine**, the levels of both drugs may be decreased.

• ℞ **guanethidine monosulfate**'s effects on blood pressure may be reduced.

• If used with ℞ **lithium**, rarely, neurotoxicity (nerve damage) may occur.

• ℞ **Quinidine** increases the concentrations of haloperidol.

• If an antipsychotic is taken with alcohol, there may be increased sedative effects.

Side effects

• These depend on the how it is administered and the use, but there may be drowsiness, extrapyramidal symptoms (see ℞ **antipsychotics**), headache, loss of appetite and weight loss, constipation, dry mouth, and nausea.

• Less frequently, anxiety, catatonic-like behavioral states, confusion, depression, euphoria, worsening of psychotic symptoms, restlessness, vertigo, ECG changes, changes in hormone function (irregular menstruation, growth of breasts, abnormal milk production, impotence, increased libido), changes in blood pressure, speeded heartbeat, blurred vision, eye changes, vomiting, priapism (prolonged, painful penile erection), urinary retention, spasmodic constriction of the bronchi or larynx, respiratory depression, increased sweating, loss of hair, and skin reactions.

• Rarely, seizure, blood cell disorders, neuroleptic malignant syndrome (a potentially fatal condition characterized by very high fever, muscle rigidity, changes in mental status, and irregular pulse, blood pressure and/or heart rhythm).

haloprogin ⓖ

Type/Group: **antifungal**.
Brand(s): Halotex.
How administered: Topically (external).

Used to treat

Haloprogin is a synthetic antifungal used to treat athlete's foot, jock itch, ringworm, and other ✪ **fungal infections**.

Warnings

• It should not be given to people with known hypersensitivity to haloprogin.

• It is not known whether haloprogin harms the fetus. It should be used during pregnancy only if clearly needed.

• Medical judgment is required if breast-feeding is being considered.

• A doctor must be contacted if the condition worsens or if irritation, redness, swelling, stinging, or burning persists.

Interactions

No significant interactions when used topically (externally).

Side effects

• Local irritation, burning, redness, scaling, and itching.

Halotestin ⓑ

A preparation of ℞ **fluoxymesterone**.
Formulation: Oral tablets in several strengths.
Availability: Prescription only.
Warnings and side effects: See ℞ **fluoxymesterone**.

Halotussin AC ⓑ

A preparation of ℞ **codeine phosphate** and ℞ **guaifenesin**.
Formulation: Oral liquid.
Availability: May or may not require a prescription.
Warnings and side effects: See ℞ **codeine phosphate**; ℞ **guaifenesin**.

Halotussin-DM Liquid; Sugar Free Liquid ⓑ

A preparation of ℞ **dextromethorphan** and ℞ **guaifenesin**.
Formulation: Oral liquid.
Availability: OTC.
Warnings and side effects: See ℞ **dextromethorphan**; ℞ **guaifenesin**.

Havrix ®

A preparation of ℞ **hepatitis A vaccine, inactivated.**
Formulation: Intramuscular injection.
Availability: Prescription only.
Warnings and side effects: See ℞ **hepatitis A vaccine, inactivated.**

Hawaiian Tropic Baby Faces Sunblock ®

A preparation of ℞ **cinnamates** and ℞ **titanium dioxide.**
Formulation: Topical lotion.
Availability: OTC.
Warnings and side effects: See ℞ **cinnamates;** ℞ **titanium dioxide.**

Hayfebrol Liquid ®

A preparation of ℞ **pseudoephedrine,** ℞ **menthol,** and ℞ **chlorpheniramine maleate.**
Formulation: Oral liquid.
Availability: OTC.
Warnings and side effects: See ℞ **pseudoephedrine;** ℞ **menthol;** ℞ **chlorpheniramine maleate.**

HBIG ©

see ℞ **hepatitis B immune globulin (HBIG).**

H-BIG ®

A preparation of ℞ **hepatitis B immune globulin (HBIG).**
Formulation: Intramuscular injection.
Availability: Prescription only.
Warnings and side effects: See ℞ **hepatitis B immune globulin (HBIG).**

HC Derma-Pax Liquid ®

A preparation of ℞ **chlorpheniramine maleate,** and ℞ **pyrilamine maleate,** and ℞ **hydrocortisone.**
Formulation: Topical liquid.
Availability: OTC.
Warnings and side effects: See ℞ **chlorpheniramine maleate;** ℞ **pyrilamine maleate;** ℞ **hydrocortisone.**

HCG ©

see ℞ **chorionic gonadotropin.**

Head and Shoulders Intensive Treatment Dandruff Shampoo ®

A preparation of ℞ **selenium sulfide.**
Formulation: Topical lotion/shampoo.
Availability: OTC.
Warnings and side effects: See ℞ **selenium sulfide.**

heart failure treatment ⓓ

amiloride; benazepril hydrochloride; captopril; carvedilol; digitoxin; digoxin; enalapril maleate; fosinopril sodium; hydralazine hydrochloride; inamrinone lactate; isosorbide dinitrate; isosorbide mononitrate; lisinopril; milrinone; nitroglycerin; quinapril hydrochloride; ramipril; sodium nitroprusside; spironolactone; trandolapril; triamterene.

Actions and uses

The aim of heart failure treatment is to rectify the functioning of a failing heart. It can involve the use of a number of different drug types. ✪ **heart failure** is a term used for the condition in which the amount of blood pumped by the heart is not sufficient to meet the oxygen and metabolic needs of the body either during work or at rest. The causes of heart failure include disease within the heart (mainly ischemia—an inadequate supply of blood to the muscle that can also cause ✪ **angina pectoris** pain) or an excessive load imposed on the heart by arterial and other forms of ✪ **hypertension.**

Drugs of the ℞ **cardiac glycoside** group (℞ **digoxin,** ℞ **digitoxin**) increase the force of contraction of the heart and have been widely used in heart failure treatment, although today they are usually used in with other drugs. Drugs that cause blood vessels to dilate and therefore reduce the workload of the heart may be valuable and are widely used as ℞ **antihypertensive** agents. These particularly include the ℞ **ACE inhibitor** drugs (including ℞ **captopril,** ℞ **enalapril maleate,** ℞ **lisinopril,** ℞ **quinapril hydrochloride,** ℞ **ramipril,** ℞ **trandolapril,** ℞ **benazepril hydrochloride,** and ℞ **fosinopril sodium**). Alternatively, direct-acting ℞ **vasodilator** drugs can be used, such as the ℞ **nitrate** agents (for example, ℞ **sodium nitroprusside,** ℞ **nitroglycerin,** ℞ **isosorbide dinitrate,** ℞ **isosorbide mononitrate**). ℞ **carvedilol** (a combined ℞ **beta-blocker** and ℞ **alpha-adrenergic blocker**) is another vasodilator and can be used, alone or in combination with other drugs, to reduce high blood pressure, and to treat congestive heart failure.

Some of the ℞ **diuretic** agents (including ℞ **amiloride,** ℞ **spironolactone,** ℞ **triamterene**) are useful because heart failure can lead to fluid retention (edema; especially of the lungs, legs, ankles, and feet), and diuretics may be used in treating this. There is an increasing use of ℞ **phosphodiesterase inhibitor** agents relatively specific for the form of this enzyme in the heart (type III), since drugs of this type (℞ **milrinone** and ℞ **inamrinone lactate**), have a stimulatory action on heart muscle (myocardium), and can be used in severe congestive heart failure. In practice, many different drug types may be used simultaneously to maintain people with congestive heart failure. A major part of treatment is likely to be a diuretic drug combined with antihypertensive therapy, possibly with added vasodilators.

Limitations

See the individual drug entries.

Heartline ®

A preparation of ℞ **aspirin.**
Formulation: Oral tablets, enteric coated.
Availability: OTC.
Warnings and side effects: See ℞ **aspirin.**

Helicobacter pylori eradication regime ⓓ

Generics: amoxicillin; bismuth subsalicylate; clarithromycin; lansoprazole; metronidazole; omeprazole; pantoprazole sodium; ranitidine bismuth citrate; ranitidine hydrochloride; tetracycline hydrochloride.

Actions and uses

Helicobacter pylori eradication regime is a combination treatment for ✪ **peptic ulcer** where there is an infection by an unusual sort of bacteria, *Helicobacter pylori*, which has now been strongly linked with the development of these ulcers. Three main drug classes are used in the treatment, with a drug from two or all three groups being used at the same time.

First, an agent that reduces acid secretion is used, which may be an ℞ **H₂-antagonist** (for instance, ℞ **ranitidine hydrochloride**) or a ℞ **proton-pump inhibitor** (for instance, ℞ **omeprazole**, ℞ **pantoprazole**, or ℞ **lansoprazole**). Second, an ℞ **antibacterial** drug is used that is effective against this atypical organism, for example, the ℞ **antibiotic** agents ℞ **clarithromycin**, ℞ **amoxicillin**, and ℞ **tetracycline hydrochloride**, or the synthetic drug ℞ **metronidazole** (sometimes two are used at the same time). Third, some compound containing bismuth is sometimes included, for example, ℞ **bismuth subsalicylate**, or the compound of ranitidine and bismuth called ℞ **ranitidine bismuth citrate**.

Most eradication regimes are used for a period between two and four weeks. Normally, a test is made before and after treatment for the presence of the *Helicobacter pylori* organism to confirm eradication.

Limitations

See the individual drug entries.

Helidac ℞

A preparation of ℞ **bismuth subsalicylate**, ℞ **metronidazole**, and ℞ **tetracycline**.
Formulation: Capsules and tablets.
Availability: Prescription only.
Warnings and side effects: See ℞ **bismuth subsalicylate**; ℞ **metronidazole**; ℞ **tetracycline**.

Helixate ℞

A preparation of ℞ **antihemophilic factor** (recombinant).
Formulation: Intravenous infusion.
Availability: Prescription only.
Warnings and side effects: See ℞ **antihemophilic factor**.

Hemabate ℞

A preparation of ℞ **carboprost**.
Formulation: Injection.
Availability: Prescription only.
Warnings and side effects: See ℞ **carboprost**.

hematopoietic ⓓ

(colony-stimulating factor; haematopoietic; hematopoietic growth factors)
Generics: epoetin alfa; filgrastim; sargramostim; oprelvekin.

Actions and uses

Hematopoietic agents stimulate hematopoiesis, which is the formation and development of blood elements in the bone marrow. Physiologically, a number of hematopoietic factors—specialized

℞ **growth factor** mediators—promote the proliferation of blood cells. These include erythropoietin, colony-stimulating factors, and interleukin. Some are now available in forms synthesized by recombinant techniques (DNA technology).

℞ **epoetin alfa** is a synthesized (recombinant) version of one form of *human* erythropoietin. It is used to treat types of ✪ **anemia** known to be associated with erythropoietin deficiency, as in chronic renal failure and in people undergoing certain forms of ✪ **cancer** chemotherapy, or ✪ **HIV** treatment. It is also used to build up red-cell levels in people about to have surgery.

℞ **filgrastim** is a name given to *granulocyte-colony stimulating factor* (G-CSF), which is a natural blood-stimulating substance that is synthesized using DNA engineering techniques. It reduces neutropenia (a shortage of neutrophil white blood-cells in the circulation) by stimulating the production of white cells (mainly neutrophils). Similarly, ℞ **sargramostim** is a name given to *granulocyte macrophage-colony stimulating factor* (GM-CSF), another natural blood-stimulating substance that reduces neutropenia by stimulating white cell production (all granulocytes and monocytes), when this has been reduced during chemotherapy in anticancer treatment. This may alleviate several adverse effects of chemotherapy and radiotherapy, including liver and kidney damage, and the risk of infection or sepsis.

Certain cytokines (the *interleukins*) stimulate the production of blood platelets (thrombocytes), which are critical to blood clotting. A synthetic version of interleukin 11 (IL-11) (℞ **oprelvekin**) is used to help restore platelet levels when these have been suppressed during chemotherapy in anticancer treatment, and so reducing the need for platelet transfusions.

Limitations

These agents are all complex protein-like chemicals that have only recently become available. This is due to the harnessing of the techniques of molecular biology to manufacture them by recombinant technology. However, they are generally very expensive to make in pure form, and this is likely to limit their application in mainstream medicine for some time to come. Being proteins—and therefore digested in the gut—all have to be injected. Even so, most do not last long in the body, and it is to be expected that those agents that are eventually widely used will be chemical variations on the natural molecules, which prolong their duration in the body.

These drugs are given by experienced personnel following a full medical assessment. They have significant contraindications and side effects, and are not generally used during pregnancy. See the individual drug entries.

hematopoietic growth factors ⓓ

see ℞ **hematopoietic**.

Hemofil M ℞

A preparation of ℞ **antihemophilic factor** (human).
Formulation: Intravenous infusion.
Availability: Prescription only.
Warnings and side effects: See ℞ **antihemophilic factor**.

Hemonyne ⑧

A preparation of ℞ **Factor IX complex** (human; also contains Factors II, VII, X).
Formulation: Intravenous infusion.
Availability: Prescription only.
Warnings and side effects: See ℞ **Factor IX complex**.

Hemorid For Women Cream; Suppositories ⑧

A preparation of ℞ **phenylephrine hydrochloride** with ℞ **pramoxine hydrochloride** (cream) or ℞ **zinc oxide** (suppositories).
Formulation: Topical cream; rectal suppositories.
Availability: OTC.
Warnings and side effects: See ℞ **phenylephrine hydrochloride**; ℞ **pramoxine hydrochloride**; ℞ **zinc oxide**.

Hemorrhoidal HC ⑧

A preparation of ℞ **hydrocortisone**.
Formulation: Rectal suppository.
Availability: Prescription only.
Warnings and side effects: See ℞ **hydrocortisone**.

hemostatic ⑩

(haemostatic)
Generics: **antihemophilic factor; anti-inhibitor coagulant complex; coagulation Factor VIIa recombinant; rFVIIa; desmopressin; Factor IX; vasopressin.**

Actions and uses

Hemostatic agents include a wide range of drugs that enhance the process of hemostasis in the body; that is, they act to slow or prevent bleeding (hemorrhage). They are used mostly to treat disorders in which bleeding is prolonged and potentially dangerous. For treating certain types of ✪ **hemophilia**, the specific deficient factor can be replaced, for instance ℞ **Factor IX** (Christmas Factor, hemophilia B), ℞ **antihemophilic factor** (for classical hemophilia (hemophilia A), in which there is a deficiency of the clotting factor, Factor VIII). Some antihemophilic factors are prepared from human blood plasma, some from a porcine (pig) source, and some is synthesized by recombinant techniques. Several of these blood preparations also contain clotting Factors II, VII and X (and in other plasma-derived forms, these factors may be present at low levels). To treat hemophilia A or B with inhibitors to Factor VIII or Factor IX, ℞ **coagulation Factor VIIa** (synthesized by recombinant techniques, utilizing no human serum or proteins) may be taken for bleeding episodes. Similarly, in persons with inhibitors to Factor VIII, ℞ **anti-inhibitor coagulant complex** which is prepared from human blood plasma and contains various clotting factors, may be used in bleeding episodes or before surgery.

Agents with the opposite action of ℞ **fibrinolytic** drugs are available. ℞ **aprotinin** is a natural enzyme inhibitor obtained from bovine lung which has antifibrinolytic activity—it inhibits the proteolytic enzymes that normally dissolve blood clots. In medicine, it can be used to reduce blood loss in people having repeated heart bypass surgery and in selected cases of a first bypass operation.

Similarly ℞ **aminocaproic acid** and ℞ **tranexamic acid** are synthetic drugs that inhibit the activation of plasminogen, which is an enzyme in the blood that dissolves blood clots. Therefore, aminocaproic acid is antifibrinolytic. It is used to control excessive bleeding, particularly in life-threatening situations, sometimes "off-label" use for the prevention or recurrence of subarachnoid hemorrhage, the management of certain bleeding disorders, bleeding that results from certain surgical procedures (heart bypass, tonsillectomy, or prostate surgery), reduction of bleeding after stomach or intestinal hemorrhage, in cancer, and for recurrent nosebleeds and in other short-term bleeding.

The natural coagulation vitamin necessary for the production of a number of clotting factors is vitamin K (Koagulation in German). This is used in the form of ℞ **phytonadione** (vitamin K_1) to treat vitamin-K deficiency; but not deficiency caused by malabsorption states (in such cases vitamin K_1 or menadiol sodium phosphate, the synthetic form of vitamin K_3, must be used). It is given as a single intramuscular injection, or by mouth to prevent vitamin-K deficiency bleeding in newborn babies, and to treat hypothrombinemia by promoting production of prothrombin in the liver.

Some forms of acute emergency hemorrhage are treated with ℞ **vasoconstrictors**, which work directly by constricting small blood vessels and so can reduce bleeding. For example, for bleeding from varices in the esophagus, ℞ **desmopressin** or ℞ **vasopressin** may be used, and these two forms of ℞ **posterior pituitary hormone** can also act to boost clotting factors.

Limitations

Most of these drugs will be prescribed by specialists following a full medical assessment. There is a danger of causing too much or too little blood coagulation activity, and careful laboratory monitoring of various blood levels is required. See also the individual drug entries.

Hem-Prep Ointment; Suppositories ⑧

A preparation of ℞ **phenylephrine hydrochloride**, ℞ **zinc oxide**, and ℞ **petrolatum** (ointment only).
Formulation: Topical ointment; rectal suppositories.
Availability: OTC.
Warnings and side effects: See ℞ **phenylephrine hydrochloride**; ℞ **zinc oxide**; ℞ **petrolatum**.

Hemril-HC Uniserts ⑧

A preparation of ℞ **hydrocortisone**.
Formulation: Rectal suppository.
Availability: Prescription only.
Warnings and side effects: See ℞ **hydrocortisone**.

heparin ⑥

Type/Group: **anticoagulant**.
Brand(s): Various generic.
How administered: Injection (subcutaneous or intravenous) or intravenous infusion.

Used to treat

Heparin is a natural anticoagulant in the body. It is produced by the liver, leukocytes (white blood cells), and is found in some other sites, including mast cells. It inhibits the action of the enzyme thrombin, which is needed for the final stages of blood coagulation. For therapeutic use, it is purified after extraction from bovine lungs and porcine intestinal mucosa. It is available in several forms, including low molecular-weight forms ℞ **dalteparin sodium** and ℞ **enoxaparin sodium**. Also, there are heparinoid forms (℞ **danaparoid sodium**). Heparin is widely used for preventing or treating venous ✪ **thrombosis**, especially ✪ **deep vein thrombosis** after surgery, prevention of clotting in arterial or cardiac surgery, and prevention of embolism (including that which may be associated with atrial fibrillation). It is also used as an anticoagulant in blood transfusions, dialysis, and blood samples.

Warnings

• It should not be given to people with known hypersensitivity to this drug, with severely reduced levels of platelets (thrombocytes) or active, uncontrollable bleeding. It will be administered by experienced personnel after a full medical assessment.

• It should be given with extreme caution to people with indwelling catheters or who have an increased risk of hemorrhage (for example, uncontrolled hypertension, bleeding disorders, active ulcer, menstruation, recent stroke or surgery—especially to the eye or nervous system) or severe liver, kidney, or biliary disease. Also, use with caution in women over 60.

• Heparin should be used during pregnancy only if it is clearly needed.

• It does not appear in breast milk and is considered safe for use by nursing women.

• It is necessary to perform repeated tests of clotting time when heparin is being administered.

• Should hemorrhage occur, it may be difficult to stop the bleeding for a time—although, because heparin is so short-acting, merely discontinuing treatment is usually effective fairly quickly.

• Bleeding may occur at virtually any site. Shortness of breath, pain (for example, head, chest abdomen, joints), unexplained swelling or shock, or paralysis may arise from undetected hemorrhage.

• A paradoxic "white clot syndrome" has occurred with heparin use and is associated with markedly reduced numbers of platelets (thrombocytes). Heparin should be discontinued if platelet (thrombocyte) count falls below a certain level.

Interactions

• If used with other anticoagulants, ℞ **antiplatelet** agents, ℞ **hydroxychloroquine sulfate**, or ℞ **NSAIDs**, there is a higher potential for bleeding (caution is advised).

• ℞ **Antihistamines**, dextran, ℞ **digoxin**, ℞ **nicotine**, ℞ **streptokinase**, and ℞ **tetracyclines** may partially counteract the effects of heparin.

Side effects

• The chief complication is hemorrhage, which is more frequent with high doses. Some decline in platelet (thrombocyte) count and changes in liver function are not uncommon.

• In longer-term use, there are rare reports of osteoporosis, suppressed kidney function, hair loss, and priapism (abnormal, prolonged penile erection).

• Allergic reactions are rare, and may include chills, fever, hives, asthma, rhinitis, nausea, itching and burning (especially of the soles of the feet), or shock.

hepatitis A vaccine, inactivated ©

Type/Group: **vaccine**.
Brand(s): Havrix; Vaqta.
How administered: Intramuscular injection.

Used to treat

Hepatitis A vaccine, inactivated consists of a vaccine used for immunization that is prepared from biosynthetic inactivated hepatitis A virus (HAV). It is an alternative to human normal immunoglobulin and may be administered to those with known exposure to ✪ **hepatitis** A, chronic liver disease, or who are in a high-risk population (for example, Native Americans, users of illicit injectable drugs), to frequent travelers in moderate-to-high risk areas, and to high-risk laboratory staff, including those who work with the virus.

Warnings

• It should not be given to people with known hypersensitivity to this vaccine.

• It should be used during pregnancy only when it is clearly needed.

• Medical judgment is required if breast-feeding is being considered.

• This vaccine confers no immunity to other forms of viral hepatitis (types B, C, or E) and may not prevent hepatitis A infection when the disease (unrecognized) is already present.

• After administration, people will be required to wait for some time to ensure that there is no serious reaction (such as anaphylaxis).

Interactions

• ℞ **Immunosuppressants** may reduce the effectiveness of the vaccine and additional does may be needed.

• Caution is required if ℞ **anticoagulants** are being taken.

Side effects

• Most of the side effects are mild, though anaphylactoid reactions have occurred.

• There may be swelling, irritation or tenderness at the site of vaccination, and headache, nausea, fever, or malaise.

• Infrequently, skin rash, hives, itching, swelling of lymph glands, and achy joints.

hepatitis B immune globulin (HBIG) ©

Type/Group: **immune globulin**.
Brand(s): Bay-Hep B; H-BIG; HyperHep; Nabi-HB.
How administered: Intramuscular injection.

Used to treat

Hepatitis B immune globulin is a specific immune globulin that is used for ℞ **immunization** to give immediate passive immunity against infection by the ✪ **hepatitis** B virus. It may be used, for example, to immunize people in medical laboratories and hospitals after an accidental "needle stick" or other accident, to treat babies of mothers infected by the virus during pregnancy, or to confer immunity more quickly in those being vaccinated with hepatitis B vaccine.

Warnings
• It should not be given to people with known hypersensitivity to this globulin.
• It should be given with caution to people with a known deficiency of the naturally occurring IgA immunoglobulin.
• It should be given to pregnant women only if medically judged to be clearly needed.
• Medical judgment is required if breast-feeding is being considered.
• This immune globulin confers no immunity to other forms of viral hepatitis (types A, C or E) and may not prevent hepatitis B infection when the disease (unrecognized) is already present.
• In those who are immunosuppressed, either through existing disease or drug therapy, additional or larger doses of the vaccine may be needed.
• After administration, people will be required to wait for some time to ensure that there is no serious reaction (such as anaphylaxis).
• Because this immune globulin is extracted from human blood, the possibility exists that it might contain virus or other disease agents; however, multiple screenings and filters (chemical and physical) are used in its preparation, and its potential to transmit infection is considered nearly nonexistent.

Interactions
• Immune response to live virus vaccines (for example, ℞ **MMR vaccine**) may not be satisfactory. A delay of three months is recommended after administering HBIG.
• Caution is required if ℞ **anticoagulants** are being taken.

Side effects
• Most of the side effects are mild. There may be swelling, irritation or tenderness at the site of vaccination, and headache, nausea, fever, or malaise.
• Infrequently, skin rash, hives, itching, swelling of lymph glands, and achy joints.
• Although rare, anaphylactic shock has been reported.

hepatitis B vaccine Ⓖ
Type/Group: **vaccine**.
Brand(s): Comvax; Engerix-B; Recombivax HB.
How administered: Intramuscular injection.

Used to treat
Hepatitis B vaccine consists of a vaccine, used for immunization, that is prepared from noninfectious subunits of the virus (prepared by recombinant DNA technology using yeast cells, and not involving human blood products), specifically from the ⊙ **hepatitis** B virus surface antigen (HBsAg). It is recommended for everyone, but especially for those with a higher risk of infection from the hepatitis B virus (for example, those from an area where the disease is endemic, with chronic liver disease, intravenous-injecting drug users or their sex partners, and healthcare workers who handle blood samples). Because hepatitis D only infects people who have hepatitis B, this vaccine also protects against hepatitis D.

Warnings
• It should not be given to people with known hypersensitivity to this vaccine (or to yeast).

• It should be given to pregnant women only when medically judged to be clearly needed.
• Medical judgment is required if breast-feeding is being considered.
• This vaccine confers no immunity to other forms of viral hepatitis (types A, C, or E) and may not prevent hepatitis B infection when the disease (unrecognized) is already present.
• There may be an association between this vaccine and flare-ups of symptoms of multiple sclerosis (MS). For people with MS the benefits of the vaccine must be weighed against potential risk of worsening the existing disease.
• In those who are immunosuppressed, either through existing disease or drug therapy, additional or larger doses of the vaccine may be needed.
• After administration, people will be required to wait for some time to ensure that there is no serious reaction (such as anaphylaxis).

Interactions
• ℞ **Immunosuppressants** may reduce the effectiveness of the vaccine and additional does may be needed.
• Caution is required if ℞ **anticoagulants** are being taken.
• Response to ℞ **yellow fever vaccine** may be inadequate when given within a month of hepatitis B vaccine.
• Interleukin-2 may aid response to hepatitis B vaccine in those who are immunocompromised, but had no additional effect in otherwise healthy people.

Side effects
• There may be swelling, irritation, or tenderness at the site of vaccination, and fatigue, headache, or dizziness.
• Infrequently, skin rash, hives, itching, swelling of lymph glands, malaise, flu-like symptoms, and achiness.
• Hypersensitivity reactions may include facial swelling, arthritis, fever, or anaphylaxis.

Herplex Ⓑ
A preparation of ℞ **idoxuridine**.
Formulation: Eye drops.
Availability: Prescription only.
Warnings and side effects: See ℞ **idoxuridine**.

hexachlorophene Ⓖ
(hexochlorophane)
Type/Group: **antiseptic**.
Brand(s): pHisoHex.
How administered: Topically (external).

Used to treat
Hexachlorophene is used on the skin as a surgical scrub and cleanser.

Warnings
• It should not be given to people with known hypersensitivity to this drug or any component or with primary sensitivity to halogenated phenol derivatives.
• Hexachlorophene should be used during pregnancy only if it is clearly needed. It crosses the placenta.
• Medical judgment is required if breast-feeding is being considered. It is not known whether it appears in breast milk.

• It should not be used routinely for bathing infants, as it can have systemic effects.
• Avoid burned or denuded skin or routine bathing, as a wet pack, on burns or any mucous membrane, or on serious generalized dermatological conditions. Toxic systemic effects are possible.

Interactions
No significant interactions are known when used in this way.

Side effects
• People with highly sensitive skin may develop redness, mild scaling, or dryness.
• Rarely, there may be allergic skin reactions.

Hexadrol; Hexadrol Phosphate ®
A preparation of ℞ **dexamethasone** and dexamethasone sodium phosphate (Hexadrol Phosphate).
Formulation: Oral tablets; injection; each in several strengths.
Availability: Prescription only.
Warnings and side effects: See ℞ **dexamethasone**.

Hexalen ®
A preparation of ℞ **altretamine**.
Formulation: Oral capsules.
Availability: Prescription only.
Warnings and side effects: See ℞ **altretamine**.

hexamethylmelamine ⑥
see ℞ **altretamine**.

hexochlorophane ⑥
see ℞ **hexachlorophene**.

hexylresorcinol ⑥
Type/Group: **antiseptic**.
Brand(s): Sucrets Sore Throat.
How administered: Topically (external).

Used to treat
Hexylresorcinol is used for topical oral care.

Warnings
None significant.

Interactions
None significant.

Side effects
None significant.

HibTITER ®
A preparation of ℞ **Haemophilus b conjugate vaccine**.
Formulation: Injection.
Availability: Prescription only.
Warnings and side effects: See ℞ **Haemophilus b conjugate vaccine**.

Hi-Cor ®
A preparation of ℞ **hydrocortisone**.
Formulation: Cream.
Availability: Prescription only.

Warnings and side effects: See ℞ **hydrocortisone**.

High Potency Tar ®
A preparation of ℞ **coal tar**.
Formulation: Shampoo, gel.
Availability: OTC.
Warnings and side effects: See ℞ **coal tar**.

Hiprex ®
A preparation of ℞ **methenamine**.
Formulation: Oral Tablets. Contains tartrazine. Some individuals are allergic to tartrazine, particularly those who are allergic to aspirin.
Availability: Prescription only.
Warnings and side effects: See ℞ **methenamine**.

Histagesic Modified Tablets ®
A preparation of ℞ **phenylephrine hydrochloride**, ℞ **acetaminophen**, and ℞ **chlorpheniramine maleate**.
Formulation: Oral tablets.
Availability: OTC.
Warnings and side effects: See ℞ **phenylephrine hydrochloride**; ℞ **acetaminophen**; ℞ **chlorpheniramine maleate**.

Histalet Syrup ®
A preparation of ℞ **pseudoephedrine** and ℞ **chlorpheniramine maleate**.
Formulation: Oral syrup.
Availability: Prescription only.
Warnings and side effects: See ℞ **pseudoephedrine**; ℞ **chlorpheniramine maleate**.

Histalet X Tablets ®
A preparation of ℞ **pseudoephedrine** and ℞ **guaifenesin**.
Formulation: Oral tablets.
Availability: Prescription only.
Warnings and side effects: See ℞ **pseudoephedrine**; ℞ **guaifenesin**.

histamine H2-receptor antagonist ⑩
see ℞ **H₂-antagonist**.

Histatab Plus Tablets ®
A preparation of ℞ **phenylephrine hydrochloride** and ℞ **chlorpheniramine maleate**.
Formulation: Oral tablets.
Availability: OTC.
Warnings and side effects: See ℞ **phenylephrine hydrochloride**; ℞ **chlorpheniramine maleate**.

Histerone ®
A preparation of ℞ **testosterone**.
Formulation: Injection.
Availability: Prescription only.
Warnings and side effects: See ℞ **testosterone**.

Histex HC ⓑ

A preparation of ℞ hydrocodone bitartrate;
℞ pseudoephedrine; and ℞ carbinoxamine maleate.
Formulation: Oral syrup.
Availability: Prescription only.
Warnings and side effects: See ℞ hydrocodone bitartrate;
℞ pseudoephedrine; ℞ carbinoxamine maleate.

Histex PD Liquid ⓑ

A preparation of ℞ carbinoxamine maleate.
Formulation: Oral liquid.
Availability: Prescription only.
Warnings and side effects: See ℞ carbinoxamine maleate.

Histex SR ⓑ

A preparation of ℞ phenylephrine hydrochloride,
℞ acetaminophen, and ℞ chlorpheniramine maleate.
Formulation: Oral tablets, sustained release.
Availability: Prescription only.
Warnings and side effects: See ℞ phenylephrine hydrochloride;
℞ acetaminophen; ℞ chlorpheniramine maleate.

Histinex D ⓑ

A preparation of ℞ hydrocodone bitartrate and
℞ pseudoephedrine.
Formulation: Oral liquid.
Availability: Prescription only.
Warnings and side effects: See ℞ hydrocodone bitartrate;
℞ pseudoephedrine.

Histinex PV Syrup ⓑ

A preparation of ℞ hydrocodone bitartrate,
℞ pseudoephedrine, and ℞ chlorpheniramine maleate.
Formulation: Oral syrup.
Availability: Prescription only.
Warnings and side effects: See ℞ hydrocodone bitartrate;
℞ pseudoephedrine; ℞ chlorpheniramine maleate.

Histor-D Syrup ⓑ

A preparation of ℞ phenylephrine hydrochloride and
℞ chlorpheniramine maleate.
Formulation: Oral syrup.
Availability: Prescription only.
Warnings and side effects: See ℞ phenylephrine hydrochloride;
℞ chlorpheniramine maleate.

Histussin D ⓑ

A preparation of ℞ hydrocodone bitartrate and
℞ pseudoephedrine.
Formulation: Oral liquid.
Availability: Prescription only.
Warnings and side effects: See ℞ hydrocodone bitartrate;
℞ pseudoephedrine.

Histussin HC Syrup ⓑ

A preparation of ℞ hydrocodone bitartrate,
℞ chlorpheniramine maleate, and ℞ phenylephrine hydrochloride.
Formulation: Oral syrup.
Availability: Prescription only.
Warnings and side effects: See ℞ hydrocodone bitartrate;
℞ chlorpheniramine maleate; ℞ phenylephrine hydrochloride.

Hi-Vegi-Lip Tablets ⓑ

A preparation of ℞ pancreatin (amylase, lipase, protease).
Formulation: Oral tablets.
Availability: OTC.
Warnings and side effects: See ℞ pancreatin.

Hivid ⓑ

A preparation of ℞ zalcitabine.
Formulation: Oral tablets in two strengths.
Availability: Prescription only.
Warnings and side effects: See ℞ zalcitabine.

homatropine hydrobromide ⓖ

Type/Group: **belladonna alkaloid; anticholinergic; eye treatment; mydriatic; cycloplegic.**
Brand(s): Isopto Homatropine; various generic.
How administered: Topically (eye).

Used to treat

Homatropine hydrobromide can be used to dilate the pupil and paralyze the focusing of the eye for ophthalmic examination, and to treat ✪ uveitis.

Warnings

• It should not be given to people with known severe hypersensitivity to this or similar agents, or those with adhesions between the iris and lens, primary glaucoma, or narrow anterior chamber angle.
• It should be given with caution to people over 65 and young children.
• Its safety during pregnancy has not been established and it should be used only when it is clearly needed.
• It is compatible with breast-feeding.
• It may cause blurred vision, so driving and other skilled activities should be avoided while the pupils are dilated.
• It may cause light sensitivity and so the eyes should be protected from bright light.

Interactions

No interactions specific to this drug are known.

Side effects

• Increased intraocular pressure (pressure in the eyeball), blurred vision, photophobia, edema, and irritation of the eye.
• Also, systemic effects if absorbed into the body, including, infrequently, mental changes, fever, headache, speeded heartbeat, vasodilatation, decreased gastrointestinal motility, dry mouth, urinary retention, dry skin, and rash.

hormone ⓓ

Actions and uses

Hormone mediators are substances produced and secreted by glands. These are endocrine hormones, that is, hormones liberated from a gland to act at a distance, and normally carried in the bloodstream to the organs on which they have their effect. Hormones can be divided into families on the basis of the glands that secrete them and their functions. Few hormones act independently—mainly they are under the control of other hormones, the brain, or the levels of the hormone that they secrete, which influences release by a feedback process.

The brain has a considerable (unconscious) effect on hormone balance. In the base of the brain, an area called the hypothalamus secretes a number of ℞ **hypothalamic hormone** mediators or factors. These act on the anterior part of the nearby pituitary gland to initiate or inhibit the release into the bloodstream of a number of ℞ **anterior pituitary hormone** substances. The anterior part of the nearby pituitary gland also releases ℞ **posterior pituitary hormone** mediators, which act directly on target tissues in the body. The anterior pituitary hormones tend not to have direct actions on body tissues, but instead stimulate further glands; the thyroid glands in the neck to release ℞ **thyroid hormone** substances; the cortex (outer part) of the adrenal glands near the kidneys to release ℞ **corticosteroid** hormones; and the sex glands to release ℞ **sex hormone** mediators (see ℞ **gonadotropin**).

Other endocrine glands include the parathyroid glands at the base of the neck; the adrenal medulla (the inner part of the adrenal gland), which secretes mainly ℞ **epinephrine**; and the glucose-regulatory hormones that are produced by the pancreas (for example, glucagon and insulin).

The above discussion deals mainly with endocrine hormones. There are also various types of mediators that do not act at a distance, but instead act on adjacent tissues, cells, or even the same cells that release them—these agents are sometimes called local hormones (for example, histamine and the ℞ **prostaglandin** mediators). A number of hormones act—at different sites—both as hormones and neurotransmitters (released from nerves and act on an immediately adjacent nerve or other cell type). However, in all cases the underlying mechanism is similar; a stimulus causes the release of a highly specific chemical mediator, which travels to a target site to specifically activate a special receptor that "recognizes" it and responds in a physiologically appropriate manner.

In nearly all cases, synthetic forms and chemical analogs of these hormones have been developed for use as drugs. They act on the natural receptors that physiologically recognize the hormone. In most cases these are given to make up a deficiency in the body of a hormone, which has been caused by developmental failures, disease, or age (see ℞ **hormone replacement**; ℞ **antidiabetic**; ℞ **thyroid hormone**). Changing the balance or cycle of hormone action may also influence normal body physiology, for example, to prevent ⓓ **pregnancy** (see ℞ **oral contraceptive**). Also, synthetic ℞ **hormone antagonist** drugs have been developed either to reduce the release of hormones (for example, in ⓓ **cancer** therapy of endocrine glands) or, with sex hormones, to reduce normal release or the effects of normal levels of hormone, for example, where this inhibition benefits cancers of certain organs such as the prostate gland, the endometrium of the uterus, or the breast.

Limitations

See the type/group and individual drug entries.

hormone antagonist ⓓ

Generics: **bicalutamide; demeclocycline; flutamide; gonadorelin; goserelin; leuprolide acetate; nafarelin acetate; nilutamide; octreotide; phenoxybenzamine; prazosin hydrochloride; propranolol hydrochloride; tamoxifen; toremifene.**

Actions and uses

Hormone antagonist drugs are used to prevent specific actions of natural ℞ **hormone** agents, which are their synthetic drug counterparts and chemical analogs.

The first type of such antagonist drugs act directly at hormone receptors (special recognition sites on cells, which "recognize" the individual hormones) where they compete for the binding, and prevent the activation of these sites by the natural hormone. Drugs working this way include certain ℞ **antiestrogen** drugs, which bind to estrogen receptors (for example, ℞ **tamoxifen** and ℞ **toremifene**); ℞ **antiandrogen** drugs working at androgen (testosterone) receptors (℞ **bicalutamide**, ℞ **flutamide**, and ℞ **nilutamide**); and ℞ **demeclocycline** when used to treat oversecretion of antidiuretic hormone (ADH) by directly blocking the action of the hormone on the kidney tubules. Further, when epinephrine and norepinephrine are released from the adrenal medulla (or ⓓ **pheochromocytoma** tumors) into the bloodstream they act as endocrine hormones (rather than their other role in the body as neurotransmitters when they are released from nerve endings), and here many receptor antagonists are available that can be used to limit their actions (for example, on blood pressure in ⓓ **hypertension**). These include both ℞ **alpha-adrenergic blocker** (for example, ℞ **phenoxybenzamine**, ℞ **prazosin hydrochloride**) and ℞ **beta-blocker** (for example, ℞ **propranolol hydrochloride**) drugs.

A second type of drug often referred to as hormone antagonists, work more indirectly—for instance, by interfering with the production or release of the hormone. For example, drugs called aromatase inhibitors work by inhibiting the conversion of ℞ **androgen** hormones (predominantly male sex hormones) into female ℞ **estrogen** steroid hormones. These drugs are used to treat advanced ⓓ **breast cancer** in postmenopausal women whose disease has progressed after a period of treatment with tamoxifen.

A third group of drugs, also referred to as hormone antagonists, work even more indirectly. For instance, the ℞ **hypothalamic hormone** called gonadotropin-releasing hormone (LH-RH), used in its synthetic drug form, ℞ **gonadorelin**, or as synthetic chemical analogs (for example, ℞ **goserelin**, ℞ **nafarelin acetate**, and ℞ **leuprolide acetate**) is used in the treatment of cancer and sex hormone disorders to suppress the formation, or inhibit the release, of sex hormones, including both estrogens and androgens. They do this through their initial action on the anterior pituitary gland which, in turn, affects the sex glands that release these sex hormones.

The fourth type of hormone antagonist is the very useful drug ℞ **octreotide**. This is a stable analog of the hypothalamic hormone somatostatin, which is not selective in that it does not act on just one gland or site, but has widespread inhibitory or blocking effects. As such, it can be used to "damp-down" the release of a number of types of hormone from several types of cancerous endocrine or paracrine cells around the body.

Limitations

Drugs that are used to modify the actions or release of hormones tend to have widespread side effects, and these are generally regarded as acceptable if the condition being treated warrants them. The majority of the drugs used are for the purpose of modifying sex hormone activity in the body. This can be involved in a number of serious disorders that require intervention. Some of these are disorders of sexual development or fertility, but probably most are used in ℞ **anticancer** therapy to help treat hormone-dependent tumors of the breast, uterus, or prostate.

Future development toward more acceptable hormone antagonists may be expected to feature receptor antagonists, since such drugs are generally relatively specific in their actions and effects. For example, ℞ **tamoxifen** is sufficiently well tolerated that it is being taken by some relatively young, "at-risk" women (for example, where there is a family history of breast cancer), who have not yet developed the condition, but are using the drug as a preventive measure against its early development.

hormone (posterior pituitary) Ⓓ

see ℞ **posterior pituitary hormone**.

hormone replacement Ⓓ

(hormone replacement therapy; HRT; menopausal hormone therapy)

Generics: **dienestrol; esterified estrogens; estrogens, conjugated; estrone; estropipate; ethinyl estradiol; hydroxyprogesterone caproate; insulin; medroxyprogesterone; methyltestosterone; somatrem; vasopressin.**

Actions and uses

Hormone replacement is a term that can be applied to drug treatment for menopausal women (see Ⓞ **menopause**) to supplement the reduced production of ℞ **estrogen** hormones (a major type of ℞ **sex hormone**) by the body during the menopause (whether natural, due to illness, or surgery):

Replacement therapy is essentially estrogen replacement therapy, and consists of the administration of small doses of natural or synthetic estrogens (for example, ℞ **estradiol**; ℞ **dienestrol**, ℞ **esterified estrogens**, ℞ **estrogens, conjugated**, ℞ **estrone**, ℞ **estropipate**, ℞ **ethinyl estradiol**), sometimes (for women who have an intact uterus) in combination with ℞ **progestin** female hormone (℞ **hydroxyprogesterone caproate**, ℞ **medroxyprogesterone**), and occasionally ℞ **androgen** (for example, ℞ **methyltestosterone**). The object is to alleviate symptoms of the Ⓞ **menopause** such as vasomotor symptoms (for example, flushing), night sweats, thinning and drying of the vagina, palpitations, tingling, possibly mood changes, and other symptoms in women

whose lives are inconvenienced by these conditions. Additionally, there is good evidence that such therapy will reduce postmenopausal Ⓞ **osteoporosis** (brittle bones).

It should be noted that, in a more general sense, the term hormone replacement therapy is also used to refer to the use of any synthetic or natural hormone that supplements a deficiency in the body, for example, ℞ **thyroid hormone**, ℞ **corticosteroid** hormones, growth hormone (℞ **somatrem**) antidiuretic hormone (℞ **vasopressin**), and ℞ **insulin**.

Limitations

While there is good evidence that vasomotor symptoms and vaginal symptoms are generally improved, and that there is a decreased incidence of osteoporosis, there is less good evidence that hormone replacement may be beneficial in reducing the risk of Ⓞ **atherosclerosis**, Ⓞ **myocardial infarction** (heart attack), and Ⓞ **stroke**, and these will not normally be a reason for prescribing the therapy. Whether or not this treatment as any affect on the development of Ⓞ **Alzheimer's disease** is unresolved.

Prior to treatment, a number of risk factors need to be taken into account (in particular a possible increase in blood clotting) according to the person's medical background (including previous drug treatments, familial and genetic traits, history of stroke or hypertension, smoking habits, exercise and body weight, and likelihood of breast cancer) and so expert counseling is necessary. In those at risk of osteoporosis, treatment may be advised to start prior to the menopause. In women who have had a hysterectomy, long-term treatment with estrogen alone may be used, but otherwise a ℞ **progestin** may also be prescribed (to reduce the risk of endometrial cystic hyperplasia and possible cancer of the uterus). Administration of the drugs, often cyclically, can be oral as tablets, by injection, or by topical (external) application (for example, vaginal cream, skin gels, or skin patches). Possible side effects are given under the individual drug entries.

hormone replacement therapy Ⓓ

see ℞ **hormone replacement**.

HRT Ⓓ

see ℞ **hormone replacement**.

H-Tuss-D Ⓑ

A preparation of ℞ **hydrocodone bitartrate** and ℞ **pseudoephedrine**.

Formulation: Oral liquid.

Availability: Prescription only.

Warnings and side effects: See ℞ **hydrocodone bitartrate**; ℞ **pseudoephedrine**.

Humalog Ⓑ

A preparation of ℞ **insulin analog (lispro)**.

Formulation: Vials and cartridges for injection.

Availability: Prescription only.

Warnings and side effects: See ℞ **insulin analog (lispro)**.

Humalog Mix75/25 ⓑ

A preparation of ℞ insulin lispro and insulin lispro protamine.
Formulation: Cartridges for injection.
Availability: Prescription only.
Warnings and side effects: See ℞ insulin lispro and insulin lispro protamine.

human chorionic gonadotropin ⓖ

see ℞ chorionic gonadotropin.

human normal immunoglobulin (HNIG) ⓖ

see ℞ immune globulin, human (IG).

Humatrope ⓑ

A preparation of ℞ somatropin.
Formulation: Injection.
Availability: Prescription only.
Warnings and side effects: See ℞ somatropin.

Humegon ⓑ

A preparation of ℞ menotropins.
Formulation: Injection.
Availability: Prescription only.
Warnings and side effects: See ℞ menotropins.

Humibid DM Tablets ⓑ

A preparation of ℞ dextromethorphan and ℞ guaifenesin.
Formulation: Oral tablets, sustained release.
Availability: Prescription only.
Warnings and side effects: See ℞ dextromethorphan; ℞ guaifenesin.

Humibid Sprinkle Capsules; L.A. Tablets ⓑ

A preparation of ℞ guaifenesin.
Formulation: Oral capsules; tablets; both forms are sustained release.
Availability: Prescription only.
Warnings and side effects: See ℞ guaifenesin.

Humulin 50/50 ⓑ

A preparation of ℞ insulin, regular and isophane mixture.
Formulation: Bottles and cartridges for injection.
Availability: OTC.
Warnings and side effects: See ℞ insulin, regular and isophane mixture.

Humulin 70/30 ⓑ

A preparation of ℞ insulin, regular and isophane mixture.
Formulation: Bottles and cartridges for injection.
Availability: OTC.
Warnings and side effects: See ℞ insulin, regular and isophane mixture.

Humulin L ⓑ

A preparation of ℞ insulin zinc suspension (lente).

Formulation: Bottles for injection.
Availability: OTC.
Warnings and side effects: See ℞ insulin zinc suspension (lente).

Humulin N ⓑ

A preparation of ℞ insulin, isophane suspension (insulin, NPH).
Formulation: Bottles and cartridges for injection.
Availability: OTC.
Warnings and side effects: See ℞ insulin, isophane suspension (insulin, NPH).

Humulin-R ⓑ

A preparation of ℞ insulin, regular.
Formulation: Bottles and cartridges for injection.
Availability: OTC.
Warnings and side effects: See ℞ insulin, regular.

Humulin U Ultralente ⓑ

A preparation of ℞ insulin zinc suspension (lente).
Formulation: Bottles for injection.
Availability: OTC.
Warnings and side effects: See ℞ insulin zinc suspension (lente).

hyaluronidase ⓖ

Type/Group: enzyme.
Brand(s): Wydase.
How administered: Topically (external).

Used to treat
Hyaluronidase is an enzyme that can be used to increase the permeability of soft tissues to injected drugs, and to help reabsorption of excess blood and fluids.

Warnings
• It should not be given to people with known hypersensitivity to this drug.
• Its safety during pregnancy has not been established and it should be used only when it is clearly needed.
• Medical judgment is required if breast-feeding is being considered. It is not known if it appears in breast milk.
• Allergic reaction to hyaluronidase may occur.

Interactions
• It may shorten the duration of action of local ℞ anesthetics and increase systemic effects.

Side effects
• Itching, rash, and hives.

Hybolin Decanoate ⓑ

A preparation of ℞ nandrolone.
Formulation: Injection.
Availability: Prescription only.
Warnings and side effects: See ℞ nandrolone.

Hycamtin ⓑ

A preparation of ℞ topotecan.

Key to symbols: ✪ = Disorder Section ℞ = Drug Section ♣ = Herbal Section ⚖ = Supplement Section

Formulation: Powder for injection.
Availability: Prescription only.
Warnings and side effects: See ℞ **topotecan**.

HycoClear Tuss Syrup ⓑ

A preparation of ℞ **hydrocodone bitartrate** and ℞ **guaifenesin**.
Formulation: Oral syrup.
Availability: Prescription only.
Warnings and side effects: See ℞ **hydrocodone bitartrate**;
℞ **guaifenesin**.

Hycodan Syrup; Tablets ⓑ

A preparation of ℞ **hydrocodone bitartrate** and ℞ **homatropine hydrobromide**.
Formulation: Oral syrup; tablets.
Availability: Prescription only.
Warnings and side effects: See ℞ **hydrocodone bitartrate**;
℞ **homatropine hydrobromide**.

Hycomine Compound Tablets ⓑ

A preparation of ℞ **hydrocodone bitartrate**,
℞ **chlorpheniramine maleate**, ℞ **phenylephrine hydrochloride**,
℞ **acetaminophen**, and ℞ **caffeine**.
Formulation: Oral tablets.
Availability: Prescription only.
Warnings and side effects: See ℞ **hydrocodone bitartrate**;
℞ **chlorpheniramine maleate**; ℞ **phenylephrine hydrochloride**;
℞ **acetaminophen**; ℞ **caffeine**.

Hycort ⓑ

A preparation of ℞ **hydrocortisone**.
Formulation: Ointment.
Availability: Prescription only.
Warnings and side effects: See ℞ **hydrocortisone**.

Hycosin ⓑ

A preparation of ℞ **hydrocodone bitartrate** and ℞ **guaifenesin**.
Formulation: Oral liquid.
Availability: Prescription only.
Warnings and side effects: See ℞ **hydrocodone bitartrate**;
℞ **guaifenesin**.

Hycotuss Expectorant Syrup ⓑ

A preparation of ℞ **hydrocodone bitartrate** and ℞ **guaifenesin**.
Formulation: Oral syrup.
Availability: Prescription only.
Warnings and side effects: See ℞ **hydrocodone bitartrate**;
℞ **guaifenesin**.

hydantoin ⓓ

see ℞ **antiepileptic**.

Hydeltrasol ⓑ

A preparation of ℞ **prednisolone** sodium phosphate.
Formulation: Injection in several strengths.

Availability: Prescription only.
Warnings and side effects: See ℞ **prednisolone**.

Hydergine ⓑ

A preparation of ℞ **ergoloid mesylates**.
Formulation: Oral and sublingual tablets; liquid capsules; liquid.
Availability: Prescription only.
Warnings and side effects: See ℞ **ergoloid mesylates**.

hydralazine hydrochloride ⓖ

Type/Group: vasodilator; antihypertensive; heart failure treatment.
Brand(s): Apresoline; various generic. Combinations: With *hydrochlorothiazide*: Apresazide. With *hydrochlorothiazide and reserpine*: Hydrap-ES; Marpres; Ser-Ap-Es; Tri-Hydroserpine. (Combinations available as generic.)
How administered: Orally; injection.

Used to treat

Hydralazine is used for the long-term control of ⊕ **hypertension**) and is often given with other drugs. It may be used in the treatment of ⊕ **heart failure**, certain heart valve defects, and short-term support after heart valve surgery (but such uses are still being studied and evaluated).

Warnings

• It should not be given to people with known hypersensitivity to this drug, with coronary artery disease, or certain kinds of damage from rheumatic heart disease.
• It should be given with caution to people who have a history of stroke or with significantly impaired kidney function.
• Hydralazine's safety during pregnancy has not been established, and it should be used only if the potential benefit outweighs the possible risk to the fetus.
• Medical judgment is required if breast-feeding is being considered.
• This drug may cause an immune response with symptoms resembling those of systemic lupus erythematosus (SLE: see ⊕ **lupus**). Periodic blood counts are performed to detect changes or presence of antibodies associated with SLE. Symptoms such as joint or chest pain, fever or malaise should be reported to a doctor. If signs of SLE are confirmed, or other significant blood changes occur, the use of hydralazine is generally stopped.
• Because this drug may cause dizziness or weakness, caution is advised for potentially hazardous activities, such as driving, that require mental alertness.
• Stools may turn black.
• A doctor must be consulted beore taking any other medication (including OTCs, herbal remedies, supplements, or any other kind of alternative remedy).

Interactions

• If taken with ℞ **MAOI** antidepressnts, the combined effect may cause marked hypotension (lowered blood pressure).
• The effect of ℞ **epinephrine** may be reduced by hydralazine.
• If used with other antihypertensives and ℞ **diuretics**, the effects of these drugs may be increased. This additive effect is sometimes

used to advantage in combination treatments for high blood pressure.

Side effects

• Frequently, headache, palpitations, or rapid heartbeat. Other effects may include gastrointestinal disturbances (for example, loss of appetite, nausea, vomiting, diarrhea), nasal congestion, flushing, edema, muscle cramps, or weakness.

• Uncommonly, rash, hives, shortness of breath, numbness or tingling of the extremities, dizziness, postural hypotension (lowered blood pressure on standing, usually causing dizziness), tremors and difficulty in urination. Blood changes or lupus-like illness (with fever, joint pain, enlarged spleen and lymph glands, weakness, and characteristic facial rash) may also occur.

Hydrap-ES ®

A preparation of ℞ **hydralazine hydrochloride,** ℞ **hydrochlorothiazide,** and ℞ **reserpine**.
Formulation: Oral tablets.
Availability: Prescription only.
Warnings and side effects: See ℞ **hydralazine hydrochloride;** ℞ **hydrochlorothiazide;** ℞ **reserpine.**

Hydrate ®

A preparation of ℞ **dimenhydrinate**.
Formulation: Injection.
Availability: Prescription only.
Warnings and side effects: See ℞ **dimenhydrinate.**

hydrating agent ⑩

Generics: **urea**.

Actions and uses

A hydrating agent is a substance that is used to help in the treatment of conditions where the skin is dry or flaky. Hydrating agents such as ℞ **urea** are often used in preparations where they are combined with ℞ **emollient** agents, which soothe, soften, and moisturize the skin, and are given to treat various sorts of ✪ **dermatitis,** including ✪ **eczema** and ✪ **psoriasis.**

Hydrea ®

A preparation of ℞ **hydroxyurea.**
Formulation: Oral capsules.
Availability: Prescription only.
Warnings and side effects: See ℞ **hydroxyurea.**

Hydrisinol ®

A preparation of ℞ **castor oil.**
Formulation: Topical cream, lotion.
Availability: OTC.
Warnings and side effects: See ℞ **castor oil.**

Hydrocet Capsules ®

A preparation of ℞ **hydrocodone bitartrate** and ℞ **acetaminophen.**
Formulation: Oral capsules.
Availability: Prescription only.

Warnings and side effects: See ℞ **hydrocodone bitartrate;** ℞ **acetaminophen.**

hydrochlorothiazide Ⓖ

Type/Group: **diuretic; thiazide; antihypertensive; diabetes insipidus treatment.**
Brand(s): Esidrix; Ezide; HydroDIURIL; Hydro-Par; Microzide Capsules; Oretic; various generic. Combinations: With *amiloride*: Moduretic. With *benazepril*: Lotensin HCT. With *bisoprolol fumarate*: Ziac Tablets. With *captopril*: Capozide. With *enalapril maleate*: Vaseretic. With *guanethidine monosulfate*: Esimil. With *hydralazine*: Apresazide. With *hydralazine and reserpine*: Hydrap-ES; Marpres; Ser-Ap-Es; Tri-Hydroserpine. With *irbesartan*: Avalide. With *lisinopril*: Prinzide; Zestoretic. With *losartan potassium*: Hyzaar. With *metoprolol tartrate*: Lopressor HCT. With *methyldopa*: Aldoril. With *moexipril*: Uniretic. With *propranolol*: Inderide, Inderide LA. With *quinapril*: Accuretic. With *reserpine*: Hydro-Serp; Hydroserpine. With *spironolactone*: Aldactazide. With *timolol maleate*: Timolide. With *triamterene*: Dyazide; Maxide. With *valsartan*: Diovan HCT. (Many combinations available as generic.)
How administered: Orally.

Used to treat

Hydrochlorothiazide is used in the treatment of ✪ **hypertension,** either alone or with other types of diuretic or other drugs (for example, ℞ **beta-blockers**). It can also be used in the treatment of edema. Thiazide diuretics have also become a major part of the treatment for nephrogenic ✪ **diabetes insipidus.**

Warnings

• It should not be given to people with known hypersensitivity to thiazides (or to ℞ **sulfonamide**-derived drugs), or severe kidney or liver disorders.

• It should be given with caution to elderly people, or anyone with high cholesterol or triglyceride levels, or liver or kidney impairment.

• It should be used in pregnancy only when the potential benefit outweighs the possible risk to the fetus.

• Medical judgment is required if breast-feeding is being considered.

• Early symptoms of electrolyte imbalance may include muscle weakness or cramps, nausea, vomiting, restlessness or lethargy, dry mouth, excessive thirst, fast pulse, or dizziness. A doctor must be consulted if such symptoms occur.

• Thiazides may aggravate symptoms of diabetes or gout, and worsen or activate lupus erythematosus.

• Periodic monitoring of electrolytes (particularly potassium, sodium, chloride, and bicarbonate) is needed.

• Photosensitivity may develop and so precautions such as protective clothing or sunscreens should be used.

• Thiazides interact with a number of drugs, including some over-the-counter preparations. A doctor must be consulted before taking any other medications (including OTCs, herbal remedies, and supplements).

Interactions

• There is a higher risk of a hypersensitivity reaction to ℞ **allopurinol.**

• The effects of ℞ **anesthetics**, ℞ **anticancer** drugs, other antihypertensives, ℞ **diazoxide**, ⚖ **calcium** salts, ℞ **cardiac glycosides**, ℞ **lithium**, loop diuretics, ℞ **methyldopa**, nondepolarizing ℞ **skeletal muscle relaxants**, and ⚖ **vitamin D** may be increased, with the potential for significant adverse effects or toxicity. An additive effect is sometimes used to advantage in combining thiazides with other antihypertensives.
• The effects of ℞ **anticoagulants** and antigout agents (for example, ℞ **probenecid**, ℞ **sulfinpyrazone**) may be lowered by thiazides.
• The doses of ℞ **insulin** and ℞ **sulfonylureas** may need to be adjusted, as thiazides may increase blood sugar levels.
• ℞ **Amphotericin B**, ℞ **anticholinergics**, ℞ **corticosteroids**, ℞ **corticotropin**, and ℞ **MAOIs** may increase the effects of thiazides, with the possibility of significant electrolyte loss, especially potassium.
• ℞ **cholestyramine**, ℞ **colestipol hydrochloride**, ℞ **methenamine**, and ℞ **NSAIDs** (especially ℞ **indomethacin**) may reduce the effectiveness of thiazide diuretics.
• There is an increased possibility of postural hypotension (lowered blood pressure on standing) if taken with alcohol, ℞ **barbiturates**, or ℞ **opioids**.

Side effects

• There may be dizziness, headache, muscle cramps, mild gastrointestinal upsets, postural hypotension, reversible impotence, low blood potassium, sodium, magnesium and chloride, raised blood urea, glucose and lipids, and gout.
• Rarely, photosensitivity, blood disorders, skin reactions, and pancreatitis.

Hydrocil Instant Ⓑ

A preparation of ℞ **psyllium**.
Formulation: Oral powder.
Availability: OTC.
Warnings and side effects: See ℞ **psyllium**.

Hydro Cobex Ⓑ

A preparation of ℞ **hydroxocobalamin**.
Formulation: Injection.
Availability: Prescription only.
Warnings and side effects: See ℞ **hydroxocobalamin**.

hydrocodone bitartrate Ⓖ

Type/Group: **narcotic analgesic**; **opioid**; **antitussive**.
Brand(s): (All are combinations): With acetaminophen: Anexia Tablets; Bancap HC Capsules; Ceta-Plus Capsules; Co-Gesic Tablets; Dolacet Capsules; Duocet Capsules; Hydrocet Capsules; Hydrogesic; Hy-Phen Tablets; Lorcet-HD Capsules, Lorcet Plus, Lorcet 10/500 Tablets; Lortab Elixir, Tablets; Margesic H Capsules; Norco Tablets; Oncet Capsules; Panacet Tablets; Stagesic Capsules; T-Gesic Capsules; Vicodin Tablets, ES, HP, Vicoprofen Tablets; Zydone Tablets. With aspirin: Alor Tablets; Damason-P Tablets; Lortab ASA Tablets; Panasal Tablets. With chlorpheniramine maleate: S-T Forte Liquid. (Plus) *phenylephrine*: Atuss MS, HD, HD Syrup, DM Syrup; ED-TLC Liquid; ED Tuss HC Liquid; Endagen-HD Liquid; Endal-HD Liquid, Plus Liquid; Hitussin HC Syrup; Histinex HC Syrup; Iodal HD; Iotussin HC Syrup; Tussanil DH Syrup; Vanex-HD Liquid. (Plus) *phenylephrine, acetaminophen, caffeine*: Hycomine Compound Tablets. With guaifenesin: Atuss EX Syrup; Codiclear DH Syrup; Co-Tuss Liquid; Entuss Expectorant Tablets; HycoClear Tuss Syrup; Hycosin; Hycotuss Expectorant Syrup; Kwelcof Liquid; Pneumotussin Tablets, HC Syrup; Vicodin Tuss Syrup. (Plus) *phenylephrine*: Atuss-G Syrup; Donatussin DC Syrup; P-V-Tussin Tablets; Tussafed HC Syrup. With homatropine: Hydromet Syrup; Hycodan Syrup, Tablets; Tussigon Tablets. With pseudoephedrine: Detussin Liquid; Entuss-D Liquid; Histinex D; Histussin D, HC; H-Tuss D. (Plus) *carbinoxamine*: Histex HC. (Plus) *brompheniramine maleate*: Anaplex HD Syrup: (Plus) *chlorpheniramine maleate*: Histinex PV Syrup; Hyphed; Pancof-HC Liquid; P-V-Tussin Syrup. (Plus) *guaifenesin*: Cophene XP Liquid; Deconamine CX Liquid; Detussin Expectorant Liquid; Duratuss HD Elixir; Entuss-D Tablets, Entuss Jr. Liquid; Pancof XP Liquid; SRC Expectorant Liquid; SUTUSS Elixir; Tussafin Expectorant Liquid; Vanex Expectorant Liquid. (Most combinations available as generic.)
How administered: Orally; topically (external); injection.

Used to treat

Hydrocodone bitartrate is used to treat moderate to moderately severe pain and, as an antitussive, it is included in many cough linctuses or syrups (in preference to stronger opioids of the narcotic analgesic type) for non-productive ✪ **coughs**.

Warnings

• It should not be given to people with known hypersensitivity to this drug. Opioids (even the weaker ones) should not be given to people with asthma, with seriously depressed breathing disorders, prostatic hypertrophy, convulsive disorders, raised intracranial pressure, or a head injury.
• Depending on use and dose, they should be given with caution to the elderly, or to anyone with hypotension, urethral stricture, acute abdominal conditions, porphyria, certain liver, kidney, or adrenal disorders, hypothyroidism (under-activity of the thyroid gland), alcoholism, or a history of drug abuse.
• Withdrawal symptoms have been observed in newborns and it should be used during pregnancy only if the benefits outweigh the potential risks.
• Medical judgment is required if breast-feeding is being considered. It is not known whether this drug appears in breast milk, but similar drugs do.
• Hydrocodone is a Schedule III controlled substance.
• Prolonged use of narcotics can lead to physical dependence (addiction), although this rarely happens in routine medical use.
• Drowsiness may affect the performance of skilled tasks such as driving.
• The effects of alcohol may be enhanced (including respiratory depression).

Interactions

If the following drugs are used with hydrocodone, then effects may be enhanced with potentially serious results: ℞ **barbiturates**; ℞ **general anesthetics**; ℞ **MAOI** antidepressants; ℞ **opioids**; ℞ **tranquilizers** (for example, ℞ **phenothiazines**); ℞ **sedatives**,

℞ **antihistamines**; ℞ **tricyclic** antidepressants; ℞ **benzodiaz-epines** (for example, ℞ **diazepam**, ℞ **lorazepam**); alcohol.

Side effects

• These are infrequent with hydrocodone and depend on the dose, how it is administered, and use, but there may be sedation, drowsiness, dizziness, and vomiting and nausea.

• Less commonly, lethargy, anxiety, mental clouding, postural hypotension (lowered blood pressure on standing), mood changes, loss of appetite, constipation, urinary retention, and rashes.

• Rare, but serious, side effects include respiratory depression.

Hydrocort ®

A preparation of ℞ **hydrocortisone**.
Formulation: Cream.
Availability: Prescription only.
Warnings and side effects: See ℞ **hydrocortisone**.

hydrocortisone ©

Type/Group: **corticosteroid; anti-inflammatory; immunosuppressant.**

How administered: Orally; rectal; topically; injection.

Brand(s): Acticort 100; Ala-Cort; Ala-Scalp; Anucort-HC; Anumed HC; Anusol-HC; Bactine Hydrocortisone; Cetacort; Cortaid; Cort-Dome High Potency; Cortenema; Cortifoam; Cortizone; Cortizone for Kids; Delcort; Dermacort; Dermol HC; Dermolate; Dermtex HC with Aloe; Eldecort; Hemril Uniserts; Hemorrhoidal HC;. Hi-Cor; Hycort; Hydrocort; Hydrotex; Hytone; Keri-Cort 10 Maximum Strength; LactiCare-HC; Nutracort; 1% HC; Penecort; Procort; Proctocort; Proctocream HC; Scalpicin; S-T Cort; Synacort; Tegrin-HC; Texacort; T/Scalp; various generic (prescription or OTC depending on label) As *hydrocortisone acetate*: Caldecort Maximum Strength; Cortaid with Aloe; Cortaid Maximum Strength; Cortef Feminine Itch; Corticaine; Gynecort Female Crème; Hydrocortone Acetate; Lanacort; various generic (OTC or prescription, depending on label). As *hydrocortisone buteprate*: Pandel. As *hydrocortisone butyrate*: Locoid. As *hydrocortisone cypionate*: Cortef. As *hydrocortisone sodium phosphate*: Hydrocortone Phosphate. As *hydrocortisone sodium succinate*: A-Hydrocort; Solu-Cortef. As *hydrocortisone valerate*: Westcort; various generic. With *pramoxine hydrochloride*: Analpram-HC; Enzone Cream; Epifoam Aerosol Foam; Pramasome; Proctofoam-HC; Pramoxine HC. With *clioquinol*: Ala-Quin; Corque; Hysone; Pedi-Cort V; Zone-A-Forte. With *clioquinol and pramoxine*: 1 + 1-F Crème. With *urea*; Anusol-HC-1; Carmol HC Cream; Massingill Medicated Towelettes. With *iodoquinol;* Vytone Cream. With *lidocaine*: Lida-Mantle-HC Cream. With *benzoyl peroxide*: Vanoxide-HC Lotion. With *polymyxin B*: Cortisporin Cream; Otobiotic Otic. With *bacitracin zinc, neomycin,* and *polymyxin B*: Cortisporin; Neotricin-HC. With *oxytetracycline*: Terra-Cortil. With *neomycin and polymyxin B*: AK-Spore H.C; AntibiOtic; Cortatrigen Modified; Corticosporin Otic; Drotic; Ear-Eze; Lazer-Sporin-C; Octicair; Otic-Care; Otocort; Otomycin-HPN; With *ciprofloxacin*: Cipro HC. With *chloramphenicol*: Chloromycetin-HC Ophthalmic Solution;

Ophthocort. With *pyrilamine maleate* and *chlorpheniramine*: HC Derma-Pax.

Used to treat

Hydrocortisone is used for the treatment of many kinds of ✪ **inflammation**. It has major and varied effects on metabolism, and modifies the operation of the immune system; therefore, it may be used to treat a range of conditions, including adrenal insuffi-ciency, congenital adrenal hyperplasia, rheumatic disorders (such as ✪ **arthritis** and ✪ **osteoarthritis**), allergic states, collagen dis-eases, allergic and inflammatory eye disorders, intestinal tract, liver, and kidney disorders, skin diseases, respiratory diseases (such as bronchial ✪ **asthma**), edemas, and malignancies.

Warnings

Depending on route of administration, dose, and use:

• It should not be given to anyone with known hypersensitivity to corticosteroids, or with systemic fungal infections.

• It should be given with caution to anyone with low thyroid function, a peptic ulcer, hepatitis, cirrhosis, ocular herpes simplex, history of tuberculosis, nonspecific colitis, congestive heart failure, myocardial infarction (heart attack), diabetes mellitus, hypertension, psychosis, or kidney insufficiency. Also, anyone over 65 and children. External use by people with marked circulation impairment should be undertaken with care.

• Corticosteroids cross the placenta, and therefore hydrocortisone should only be used during pregnancy if medically judged to be essential.

• It should not be used by breast-feeding mothers. It is excreted in breast milk and could suppress growth and interfere with the production of corticosteroids in the infant. It is not known whether, or under what conditions, enough of the drug is absorbed from topical use to create these risks.

• It may mask signs of infection and interfere with the body's ability to keep infection from spreading.

• Live vaccines must not be taken while using this drug.

• It may reactivate latent tuberculosis or amebiasis.

• It increases the excretion of calcium and other minerals, and supplements may be needed.

• Prolonged use may lead to adrenal insufficiency. A doctor must be notified if there is unusual weight gain, swelling of the legs or feet, muscle weakness, black tarry stools, vomiting of blood, puffing of the face, menstrual irregularities, or prolonged sore throat, fever, cold, or infection (signs/symptoms of adrenal insufficiency).

• Anyone on long-term steroid therapy should wear medic-alert bracelet or the equivalent.

• Other medication (including OTC, herbal remedies, and supplements) must not be taken without consulting a doctor.

• Dentists and other doctors must be informed of the use of this drug during, and for 12 months after discontinuing, treatment. Supportive drugs may be required in the event of severe illness, surgery, or trauma.

• The contraceptive effect of IUDs (intrauterine device) may be decreased.

• Discontinuation of treatment must be gradual and under medical supervision in order to avoid adverse reactions.

• When using topically, do not use over large surface areas, for a prolonged period, or cover with bandages to minimize the risk of systemic absorption and accompanying side effects.

Interactions

• Hydrocortisone taken with ℞ **amphotericin** or ℞ **diuretics** may further reduce potassium levels.
• The effects of ℞ **aspirin**, ℞ **oral hypoglycemics**, ℞ **insulin**, ℞ **diuretics**, and ⚖ **potassium** supplements may be reduced.
• ℞ **aspirin** and ℞ **NSAIDs** increase the risk of gastric ulceration.
• ℞ **Barbiturates**, ℞ **hydantoins**, ℞ **rifampin**, and ℞ **ephedrine** may reduce the effects of corticosteroids.
• ℞ **Ketoconazole**, ℞ **estrogens**, ℞ **oral contraceptives**, nondepolarizing muscle relaxants, and ℞ **cholestyramine** may increase the effects of hydrocortisone.
• Oral ℞ **anticoagulants** and ℞ **theophylline** may alter the effects of either corticosteroids or the other drug, or both.
• The effectiveness of ℞ **anticholinesterases**, ℞ **isoniazid**, ℞ **salicylates**, and ℞ **somatrem** may be reduced.
• ℞ **Cyclosporine** and digitalis glycosides may increase the risk of toxicity.

Side effects

These depend on how administered, dose, duration of treatment, and use.
• Systemically: Frequently, insomnia, heartburn, nervousness, abdominal tightness, increased sweating, acne, mood swings, increased appetite, facial flushing, delayed wound healing, increased susceptibility to infection, and diarrhea or constipation. Occasionally, edema, headache, change in skin color, frequent urination. Rarely, speeded heartbeat, allergic skin reaction, psychological changes and potentially serious side effects such as gastrointestinal hemorrhage and pancreatitis.
• Topically: Occasionally, irritation, and itching. Rarely, allergic rash. Systemic side effects (see above) are possible if absorbed.

Hydrocortone Acetate Ⓑ

A preparation of ℞ **hydrocortisone**.
Formulation: Injection in two strengths.
Availability: Prescription only.
Warnings and side effects: See ℞ **hydrocortisone**.

Hydrocortone Phosphate Ⓑ

A preparation of ℞ **hydrocortisone** sodium phosphate.
Formulation: Injection.
Availability: Prescription only.
Warnings and side effects: See ℞ **hydrocortisone**.

Hydro-Crysti-12 Ⓑ

A preparation of ℞ **hydroxocobalamin**.
Formulation: Injection.
Availability: Prescription only.
Warnings and side effects: See ℞ **hydroxocobalamin**.

HydroDIURIL Ⓑ

A preparation of ℞ **hydrochlorothiazide**.
Formulation: Oral tablets, available in 3 strengths.
Availability: Prescription only.
Warnings and side effects: See ℞ **hydrochlorothiazide**.

hydroflumethiazide Ⓖ

Type/Group: **diuretic**; **thiazide**; **antihypertensive**; **diabetes insipidus treatment**.
Brand(s): Diucardin; various generic. Combinations: With *reserpine*: Salutensin, Salutensin-Demi.
How administered: Orally.

Used to treat

Hydroflumethiazide is used in the treatment of ✪ **hypertension**, either alone or with other types of diuretic or other drugs (for example, ℞ **beta-blockers**). It can also be used in the treatment of edema. Thiazide diuretics have also become a major part of the treatment for nephrogenic ✪ **diabetes insipidus**.

Warnings

• It should not be given to people with known hypersensitivity to thiazides (or to ℞ **sulfonamide**-derived drugs), or severe kidney or liver disorders.
• It should be given with caution to elderly people, or anyone with high cholesterol or triglyceride levels, or with liver or kidney impairment.
• Hydroflumethiazide should be used in pregnancy only when the potential benefit outweighs the possible risk to the fetus.
• Medical judgment is required if breast-feeding is being considered.
• Early symptoms of electrolyte imbalance may include muscle weakness or cramps, nausea, vomiting, restlessness or lethargy, dry mouth, excessive thirst, fast pulse, or dizziness. A doctor must be contacted if such symptoms occur.
• Thiazides may aggravate symptoms of diabetes or gout, and worsen or activate lupus erythematosus.
• Periodic monitoring of electrolytes (particularly potassium, sodium, chloride, and bicarbonate) is needed.
• Photosensitivity may develop and so precautions such as protective clothing or sunscreens should be used.
• Thiazides interact with a number of drugs, including some over-the-counter preparations. A doctor must be consulted before taking any other medications (including OTCs, herbal remedies, and supplements).

Interactions

• There is a higher risk of a hypersensitivity reaction to ℞ **allopurinol**.
• The effects of ℞ **anesthetics**, ℞ **anticancer** drugs, other antihypertensives, ℞ **diazoxide**, ⚖ **calcium** salts, ℞ **cardiac glycosides**, ℞ **lithium**, loop diuretics, ℞ **methyldopa**, nondepolarizing ℞ **skeletal muscle relaxants**, and ⚖ **vitamin D** may be increased, with the potential for significant adverse effects or toxicity. An additive effect is sometimes used to advantage in combining thiazides with other antihypertensives.
• The effects of ℞ **anticoagulants** and antigout agents (for example, ℞ **probenecid**, ℞ **sulfinpyrazone**) may be lowered by thiazides.
• The doses of ℞ **insulin** and ℞ **sulfonylureas** may need to be adjusted, as thiazides may increase blood sugar levels.

• ℞ **Amphotericin B**, ℞ **anticholinergics**, ℞ **corticosteroids**, ℞ **corticotropin**, and ℞ **MAOIs** may increase the effects of thiazides, with the possibility of significant electrolyte loss, especially potassium.
• ℞ **cholestyramine**, ℞ **colestipol hydrochloride**, ℞ **methenamine**, and ℞ **NSAIDs** (especially ℞ **indomethacin**) may reduce the effectiveness of thiazide diuretics.
• There is an increased possibility of postural hypotension (lowered blood pressure on standing) if taken with alcohol, ℞ **barbiturates**, or ℞ **opioids**.

Side effects
• There may be dizziness, headache, muscle cramps, mild gastrointestinal upsets, postural hypotension, reversible impotence, low blood potassium, sodium, magnesium and chloride, raised blood urea, glucose and lipids, and gout.
• Rarely, photosensitivity, blood disorders, skin reactions, and pancreatitis.

hydrogen peroxide Ⓖ
Type/Group: **antiseptic**.
Brand(s): Peroxil; various generic.
How administered: Topically (external).
Used to treat
Hydrogen peroxide can be used to cleanse and deodorize wounds and ulcers and treat irritations of the mouth.
Warnings
• It should not be given to infants, unless directed by a doctor.
• A doctor should be consulted before using during pregnancy or while breast-feeding.
• Do not use for a longer period of time or in higher doses than recommended.
• If used as a gargle or mouthwash, avoid swallowing.
• If used as a bleach on teeth, it can seriously damage tooth enamel.
Interactions
• Hydrogen peroxide may increase the effects of other substances in the mouth (for example, the carcinogenic [cancer causing] potential of smoking residue).
Side effects
• Strong solutions can be highly irritating to skin, and may result in ulceration and a secondary infection.

Hydrogesic Capsules Ⓑ
A preparation of ℞ **hydrocodone bitartrate** and ℞ **acetaminophen**.
Formulation: Oral capsules.
Availability: Prescription only.
Warnings and side effects: See ℞ **hydrocodone bitartrate**; ℞ **acetaminophen**.

Hydromet Syrup Ⓑ
A preparation of ℞ **hydrocodone bitartrate** and ℞ **homatropine hydrobromide**.
Formulation: Oral syrup.
Availability: Prescription only.

Warnings and side effects: See ℞ **hydrocodone bitartrate**; ℞ **homatropine hydrobromide**.

hydromorphone hydrochloride Ⓖ
Type/Group: **antitussive**; **narcotic analgesic**; **opioid**.
Brand(s): Dilaudid; various generic.
How administered: Orally; rectal suppositories; injection.
Used to treat
Hydromorphone hydrochloride can be used in the treatment of moderate to severe ✚ **pain**, such as in cancer, and to suppress dry, nonproductive cough. Its use quickly tends to tolerance and then dependence (addiction).
Warnings
• It should not be used by anyone with known hypersensitivity to any opioid, or with paralytic ileus (cessation of the normal rhythmic muscle contractions of the intestines). Opioids (even the weaker ones) should not be given to asthmatics, to anyone with seriously depressed breathing disorders, or with prostatic hypertrophy, convulsive disorders, raised intracranial pressure, or a head injury.
• Depending on use and dose, they should be given with caution to the elderly, or to those with hypotension, certain liver, kidney, or adrenal disorders, hypothyroidism (underactivity of the thyroid gland), or alcoholism or a history of drug abuse.
• Hydromorphone should be used during pregnancy only if the benefits outweigh potential risks.
• Because of its potential to cause withdrawal symptoms in breast-fed infants, mothers should either discontinue using this drug or stop breast-feeding.
• Hydromorphone hydrochloride is a Schedule II controlled substance.
• In overdose narcotic analgesics produce serious respiratory depression (decreased breathing), which is occasionally fatal.
• Tolerance occurs extremely readily and dependence (addiction) may follow.
• Drowsiness may affect the performance of skilled tasks, such as driving.
• The effects of alcohol may be enhanced and the likelihood of respiratory depression increased.
Interactions
• Alcohol, ℞ **barbiturates**, ℞ **general anesthetics**, ℞ **MAOIs**, ℞ **opioids**, ℞ **sedatives**, ℞ **hypnotics**, ℞ **tranquilizers**, ℞ **tricyclic** antidepressants, ℞ **phenothiazines**, ℞ **antihistamines**, and ℞ **cimetidine** can enahnce or increase the effects possible with hydromorphone, which can cause potentially serious side effects, especially respiratory depression.
• The effects of ℞ **diuretics** may be decreased in people with congestive heart failure.
Side effects
These depend on how administered, dose and use. The most frequent side-effects include:
• Sedation, euphoria, constipation, dizziness, sweating, nausea and vomiting, loss of appetite, and mood change.
• Less often there may be dry mouth, flushing of the face, headache, palpitations, changes in heart rate, postural hypotension (a lowering of blood pressure on standing, causing

    Key to symbols: ✚ = Disorder Section   ℞ = Drug Section   ♣ = Herbal Section   ⚯ = Supplement Section

dizziness), rashes, miosis (pupil constriction), confusion, and hallucinations. There may also be itching and a rash.

Hydromox ®

A preparation of ℞ **quinethazone**.
Formulation: Oral tablets.
Availability: Prescription only.
Warnings and side effects: See ℞ **quinethazone**.

Hydro-Par ®

A preparation of ℞ **hydrochlorothiazide**.
Formulation: Oral tablets, available in two strengths.
Availability: Prescription only.
Warnings and side effects: See ℞ **hydrochlorothiazide**.

Hydrophed Tablets ®

A preparation of ℞ **ephedrine**, ℞ **theophylline**, and ℞ **hydroxyzine**.
Formulation: Oral tablets.
Availability: Prescription only.
Warnings and side effects: See ℞ **ephedrine**; ℞ **theophylline**; ℞ **hydroxyzine**.

Hydro-Serp ®

A preparation of ℞ **hydrochlorothiazide** and ℞ **reserpine**.
Formulation: Oral tablets.
Availability: Prescription only.
Warnings and side effects: See ℞ **hydrochlorothiazide**; ℞ **reserpine**.

Hydroserpine #1; #2 ®

A preparation of ℞ **hydrochlorothiazide** and ℞ **reserpine**.
Formulation: Oral tablets, two (hydrochlorothiazide) strengths.
Availability: Prescription only.
Warnings and side effects: See ℞ **hydrochlorothiazide**; ℞ **reserpine**.

HydroTex ®

A preparation of ℞ **hydrocortisone**.
Formulation: Cream.
Availability: OTC.
Warnings and side effects: See ℞ **hydrocortisone**.

hydroxocobalamin ⑥

see ☍ **cyanocobalamin**.

hydroxycarbamide ⑥

see ℞ **hydroxyurea**.

hydroxychloroquine sulfate ⑥

Type/Group: antimalarial; antirheumatic.
Brand(s): Plaquenil; various generic.
How administered: Orally.

Used to treat

Hydroxychloroquine is a (4-aminoquinoline) drug used for acute attacks and suppression of ✪ **malaria**, and also to treat ✪ **rheumatoid arthritis** (including juvenile arthritis) and systemic and discoid lupus erythematosus (see ✪ **lupus**). It is usually used when other, more common treatments (for example, ℞ **NSAIDs**) are unsuccessful. Its effects may not be seen for 4 to 6 months.

Warnings

• It should not be used by people with known hypersensitivity to any 4-aminoquinoline drug, or with retinal damage from taking such a drug, or those who have psoriasis or porphyria (although cases may arise where potential benefit outweighs potential risk).
• Children should not receive this drug in long-term therapy.
• Medical judgment is required for people with G6PD deficiency, alcoholism, or who have impaired of kidney or liver function.
• Hydroxychloroquine sulfate should not be used during pregnancy, except where the benefits outweigh the potential risk to the fetus. Birth defects have been reported in cases where a closely related drug, ℞ **chloroquine**, was used for lupus erythematosus (although not where it was used for prevention of malaria). Study and evaluation is incomplete.
• Breast-feeding mothers should either discontinue using this drug or stop breast-feeding.
• Hydroxychloroquine is very toxic in overdose, and in acute cases, seizures and death may occur within two hours.
• In long-term use, eye examinations, medical monitoring of liver function, and blood cell counts are necessary.

Interactions

• Circulating levels of ℞ **digoxin** may be elevated by hydroxychloroquine.
• Hydroxychloroquine should not be taken with ℞ **amiodarone hydrochloride** or levacetylmethadol because of the risk of heart rhythm disorders.

Side effects

• Damage to the retina and other parts of the eye is of great concern in long-term use.
• Other side effects include nausea and vomiting, headache, and gastrointestinal disturbance, and occasionally, itching and rash.
• Susceptible people may suffer psychotic episodes, blood disorders, and effects (such as bleaching) to the hair.

hydroxyethylcellulose ⑥

Type/Group: artificial tears; artificial saliva.
How administered: Topically (external).
Brand(s): Adsorbonac; Comfort Tears; Optimoist; TearGuard.

Used to treat

Hydroxyethylcellulose is a constituent of preparations used to relieve corneal edema, and as artificial tears and is given to people with dry eyes (tear deficiency) and/or dry mouth due to disease (for example, Sjögren's syndrome).

Warnings

• It should not be given to people with known hypersensitivity to this drug.
• A doctor must be consulted before using during pregnancy or while breast-feeding.

• It may cause mild stinging or temporary blurred vision.

Interactions
No significant interactions are known.

Side effects
No significant side effects are known.

hydroxyprogesterone caproate ⓖ
Type/Group: **sex hormone; progestin; anticancer**.
Brand(s): Hylutin; Prodrox; generic.
How administered: Injection.

Used to treat
Hydroxyprogesterone caproate is used for dysfunctional uterine bleeding and amenorrhea, and also for endometrial cancer. Although not stated by the manufacturer for such treatment, it may be prescribed in combination with ℞ **estrogen** for symptoms of the ✺ **menopause**, and for obesity-hypoventilation syndrome, obstructive sleep apnea, hirsutism, or homozygous sickle-cell disease.

Warnings
• It should not be used by people with known hypersensitivity to this drug, or with impaired liver function or disease, breast cancer, undiagnosed vaginal bleeding, missed abortion, thrombophlebitis, or a history of thromboembolic disease or stroke.
• It should be given with caution to people with epilepsy, migraine, asthma, heart or kidney dysfunction, depression, or diabetes mellitus.
• It should not be used during pregnancy because there is evidence of risk to the fetus. A doctor must be contacted if pregnancy occurs while taking this drug.
• Medical judgment is required if breast-feeding is being considered.
• Diabetics must monitor blood glucose levels during treatment.
• Ultraviolet light, including sunlight, must be avoided.

Interactions
• ℞ **aminoglutethimide** may reduce the levels of hydroxyprogesterone.

Side effects
• Dizziness, headache, insomnia, fatigue, nausea, cholestatic jaundice, increased weight, nausea, appetite changes, amenorrhea, breakthrough bleeding.
• Less frequently, depression, edema, breast changes, decreased libido, hot flashes, decreased bone density, acne, hair loss, body hair growth, acne, oily skin, photosensitivity, rash, and darkening of skin on face.

hydroxypropyl methylcellulose ⓖ
(hypromellose)
Type/Group: **artificial tears**.
Brand(s): OcuCoat; Tears Naturale; Ultra Tears.
How administered: Topically (external).

Used to treat
Hydroxypropyl methylcellulose is a constituent of preparations used as artificial tears and is used by people with dry eyes due to certain disorders.

Warnings
• It should not be given to people with known hypersensitivity to this drug.
• A doctor must be consulted before using during pregnancy or while breast-feeding.
• It may cause mild stinging or temporary blurred vision.

Interactions
No significant interactions are known.

Side effects
No significant side effects are known.

hydroxyurea ⓖ
(hydroxycarbamide)
Type/Group: **anticancer; cytotoxic**.
Brand(s): Hydrea; generic.
How administered: Orally.

Used to treat
Hydroxyurea is a cytotoxic drug used in the treatment of squamous cell carcinoma and chronic myelocytic ✺ **leukemia**, and ovarian cancer (see ✺ **cancer**).

Warnings
• It should not be given to people with marked bone marrow depression or severe anemia.
• It should be given with caution to people with marked kidney impairment. This is a specialist drug which will be used following a full evaluation by specialist physicians.
• Hydroxyurea is not recommended for use during pregnancy unless it is medically judged to be essential, because it may cause birth defects. Becoming pregnant while using this drug must be avoided.
• It should not be used if breast-feeding.
• It can cause bone marrow depression, resulting in blood-cell changes and abnormalities.
• It may temporarily impair kidney function.
• A doctor must be contacted if fever, chills, sore throat, signs of local infection, unusual bleeding, or bruising occur.

Interactions
• Radiation may worsen skin reactions.

Side effects
• Gastrointestinal effects, mild reversible rash, facial flushing, itching, fever, chills, malaise, hair loss, headache, drowsiness, dizziness, and disorientation.

hydroxyzine ⓖ
Type/Group: **antihistamine; antiallergic; antianxiety; antipruritic**.
Brand(s): Atarax Tablets, Syrup; Vistaril Capsules, Oral Suspension, Injection; various generic. Combinations: With *ephedrine and theophylline*: Hydrophed Tablets; Marax-DF Syrup; Theomax DF Syrup.
How administered: Orally; injection.

Used to treat
Hydroxyzine is an antihistamine with some additional antianxiety properties. It can be used for the relief of allergic symptoms, such as pruritus due to ✺ **urticaria** and dermatoses (✺ **skin conditions**),

or for the short-term treatment of ☉ **anxiety**, and as a sedative as premedication and after general anesthesia. Two forms are used in drug preparations, hydroxyzine hydrochloride and hydroxyzine pamoate.

Warnings

• It should not be given to people with known hypersensitivity to this drug (or with known sensitivity to other antihistamines).

• Antihistamines should be given with caution to people with lower respiratory disease or asthma (and never during an attack), heart disease, hypertension, hyperthyroidism, epilepsy, porphyria, increased intraocular pressure (pressure in the eyeball, as in glaucoma), enlarged prostate, urinary retention, or certain obstructive bladder or gastrointestinal conditions.

• Hydroxyzine should be used during pregnancy only if the potential benefit outweighs the potential risk to the fetus.

• Nursing mothers should discontinue using this drug or discontinue breast-feeding.

• In injected form, this drug may cause severe irritation at the site of injection.

• Hydroxyzine must not be given to infants, and for children under the age of 12 the manufacturer's or medical instructions must be followed closely.

• Because of its sedative side effects, the performance of skilled tasks, such as driving, may be impaired.

• Side effects are more frequent in the elderly.

Interactions

• ℞ MAOI antidepressants may prolong and intensify the ℞ **anticholinergic** effects of antihistamines.

• If used with ℞ **tricyclic** antidepressants, other antihistamines, ℞ **phenothiazines**, ℞ **skeletal muscle relaxants**, ℞ **opioids**, ℞ **barbiturates**, ℞ **hypnotics**, ℞ **sedatives**, or ℞ **antianxiety** drugs, there is a risk of intensified side effects.

• Alcohol may intensify side effects such as drowsiness and impaired mental alertness.

Side effects

• These depend on how it is administered. For this type of antihistamine, there is commonly drowsiness, headache, impaired muscular coordination or dizziness, and anticholinergic effects (dry mouth, blurred vision, urinary retention, gastrointestinal disturbances).

• Less frequently, rashes and photosensitivity (abnormal sensitivity to light), palpitations and heart arrhythmias.

• Rarely, there may be stimulation instead of sedation (paradoxical stimulation), especially in children (and convulsions in overdose), hypersensitivity reactions, blood disorders, liver disturbances, depression, sleep disturbances, and hypotension.

Hygroton ⓑ

A preparation of ℞ **chlorthalidone**.
Formulation: Oral tablets.
Availability: Prescription only.
Warnings and side effects: See ℞ **chlorthalidone**.

Hylutin ⓑ

A preparation of ℞ **hydroxyprogesterone caproate**.

Formulation: Injection.
Availability: Prescription only.
Warnings and side effects: See ℞ **hydroxyprogesterone caproate**.

hyoscine hydrobromide ⓖ

see ℞ **scopolamine hydrobromide**.

hyoscyamine ⓖ

Type/Group: belladonna alkaloid; anticholinergic; antispasmodic.
Brand(s): Anaspaz; A-Spas S/L; Cystospaz, Cystospaz-M; Donnamar; Gastrosed; Levsin Tablets, Levsin S/L; Levbid; Levsinex Timecaps; various generic. Combinations: With *phenobarbital*: Bellacane Tablets. With *phenobarbital, atropine* and *scopolamine*: Barbidonna Tablets; Donnatal Capsules, Elixir, Extentabs, Tablets; Hyosophen Elixir, Tablets. With *digestive enzymes, atropine* and *phenobarbital*: Arco-Lase Plus Tablets. With *methenamine* and *multiple analgesic/antibacterial agents*: Atrosept; Dolsed; Prosed/DS; Trac Tabs 2X; Urimar-T; Urised Tablets; Urisedamine; Urogesic Blue. With *phenazopyridine* and *butabarbital*: Pyridium Plus.
How administered: Orally; injection.

Used to treat

Hyoscyamine is similar to ℞ **atropine** (chemically it is the *(S)-* form of atropine, and has many of the same properties) and they are often used together. Hyoscyamine relieves spasm and overactivity of the digestive tract, lessens respiratory secretions, and symptomatically relieves ☉ **inflammation** of the bladder and urinary tract.

Warnings

• It should not be given to people with known hypersensitivity to belladonna alkaloids. Depending on how it is given and dose, it should not be given to anyone with closed-angle glaucoma, myasthenia gravis, prostate gland enlargement, and certain gastrointestinal disorders.

• It should be given with caution to people with urinary retention, ulcerative colitis, pyloric stenosis, liver, cardiovascular and kidney disorders, chronic obstructive pulmonary disease (COPD), thyrotoxicosis, or Down's syndrome. It may worsen gastroesophageal reflux and certain cardiovascular disorders. Additionally, the anticholinergic effects of hyoscyamine may worsen and prolong any intestinal infection.

• Hyoscyamine should be used during pregnancy only if it is clearly needed.

• Medical judgment is required if breast-feeding is being considered. It appears in breast milk and as a general rule nursing mothers should not use this drug.

• Long-term use in children is not recommended, as this is a powerful drug with potentially serious side effects that develop more quickly in children.

• In hot weather heat prostration (fever and heat stroke due to decreased sweating) is more likely to affect anyone taking an anticholinergic drug, such as hyoscyamine.

Interactions

• ℞ **amantadine**, ℞ **tricyclic** antidepressants, and ℞ MAOIs may increase side effects.

• The effects of ℞ **atenolol** and ℞ **digoxin** may be intensified by hyoscyamine.

• Hyoscyamine may lessen the antipsychotic effects of ℞ **phenothiazines**.

• ℞ **Antacids** may affect the absorption of hyoscyamine.

Side effects

• Depending on how it is administered and dose, there may be dry mouth, difficulty in swallowing and thirst, dry skin with flushing, slowing then speeding of the heart, urgency then difficulty in urination, constipation, palpitations and heart arrhythmias, confusion, and stimulation (especially in the elderly).

• Rarely, there may be high temperature accompanied by delirium or hallucinations.

Hyosophen Tablets; Elixir ℗

A preparation of ℞ **atropine sulfate**, ℞ **hyoscyamine**, ℞ **scopolamine hydrobromide**, and ℞ **phenobarbital**.

Formulation: Oral tablets; elixir.

Availability: Prescription only.

Warnings and side effects: See ℞ **atropine sulfate**; ℞ **hyoscyamine**; ℞ **scopolamine hydrobromide**; ℞ **phenobarbital**.

Hyperab ℗

A preparation of ℞ **rabies immune globulin, human (RIG)**.

Formulation: Injection.

Availability: Prescription only.

Warnings and side effects: See ℞ **rabies immune globulin, human (RIG)**.

HyperHep ℗

A preparation of ℞ **hepatitis B immune globulin (HBIG)**.

Formulation: Intramuscular injection.

Availability: Prescription only.

Warnings and side effects: See ℞ **hepatitis B immune globulin (HBIG)**.

Hyperstat ℗

A preparation of ℞ **diazoxide**.

Formulation: Injection.

Availability: Prescription only.

Warnings and side effects: See ℞ **diazoxide**.

Hyper-Tet ℗

A preparation of ℞ **tetanus immune globulin**.

Formulation: Intramuscular injection.

Availability: Prescription only.

Warnings and side effects: See ℞ **tetanus immune globulin**.

Hyphed ℗

A preparation of ℞ **hydrocodone bitartrate**, ℞ **pseudoephedrine**, and ℞ **chlorpheniramine maleate**.

Formulation: Oral syrup.

Availability: Prescription only.

Warnings and side effects: See ℞ **hydrocodone bitartrate**; ℞ **pseudoephedrine**; ℞ **chlorpheniramine maleate**.

Hy-Phen Tablets ℗

A preparation of ℞ **hydrocodone bitartrate** and ℞ **acetaminophen**.

Formulation: Oral capsules.

Availability: Prescription only.

Warnings and side effects: See ℞ **hydrocodone bitartrate**; ℞ **acetaminophen**.

hypnotic ⓓ

Generics: **butabarbital**; **chloral hydrate**; **chlorpheniramine maleate**; **diphenhydramine hydrochloride**; **flurazepam**; **glutethimide**; **lorazepam**; **paraldehyde**; **phenobarbital**; **promethazine hydrochloride**; **quazepam**; **secobarbital sodium**; **temazepam**; **triazolam**; **zolpidem**.

Actions and uses

Hypnotic drugs ("sleeping pills") induce sleep. They act on neurons in the brain to depress electrical activity and the release of neurotransmitters in areas controlling wakefulness. Older drugs like the ℞ **barbiturate** group, depress most areas of the brain—they are ℞ **general anesthetic** agents in larger doses—and have only a small margin of safety because they also depress parts of the brain controlling respiration and blood pressure. Newer drugs, including the ℞ **benzodiazepine** group, depress mainly brain areas affecting wakefulness and awareness, and a person can be easily roused after taking a normal dose. The benzodiazepines act on specific receptors in certain brain areas only, and work by increasing the actions of the inhibitory neurotransmitter GABA.

Hypnotics are mainly used to treat ✪ **insomnia**, and sometimes to heavily sedate patients who are mentally ill or in some disease states. They can be used for the short-term treatment of insomnia due to jetlag, shiftwork, emotional problems, or serious illness. The benzodiazepines also have useful ℞ **antianxiety** actions which may be of benefit for some sleep disorders, and they are prescribed at lower doses and are taken during the day for treating anxiety.

Benzodiazepines that are used as hypnotics have virtually replaced earlier drugs, such as the ℞ **barbiturate** drugs (℞ **secobarbital sodium**, ℞ **butabarbital**, ℞ **phenobarbital**) and ℞ **chloral hydrate**, because they are just as effective but much safer in overdose. Those used include some with a long duration of action, such as ℞ **flurazepam** and ℞ **lorazepam**, and so should be used only if some degree of sedation the next day is acceptable (or valuable, if the insomnia is associated with anxiety states). Alternatively, there are some short-acting agents that are eliminated rapidly from the system compared to other benzodiazepines, but may cause withdrawal problems the day after use (and are only prescribed for very short courses), and these include ℞ **quazepam**, ℞ **temazepam**, and ℞ **triazolam**.

℞ **zolpidem** is a hypnotic that is not chemically a benzodiazepine, but which works on the same receptors in the brain as the benzodiazepines. Other types of hypnotics used in the short term in special circumstances include ℞ **glutethimide** and ℞ **paraldehyde**, but they are potentially more hazardous than the benzodiazepines in overdose. Some older ℞ **antihistamine** drugs (℞ **diphenhydramine hydrochloride**, ℞ **chlorpheniramine maleate**, ℞ **promethazine hydrochloride**) are used as ℞ **sleep-aid products** because they have quite marked sedative actions, and some brands are available OTC (over-the-counter).

Limitations

In the event of benzodiazepine overdosage, benzodiazepine receptor antagonist, ℞ **flumazenil**, is available. See also the individual drug entries.

hypoglycemic ⓓ

see ℞ **oral hypoglycemic**.

Hypo Tears ⓑ

A preparation of ℞ **polyvinyl alcohol**.
Formulation: Ophthalmic solution.
Availability: OTC.
Warnings and side effects: See ℞ **polyvinyl alcohol**.

hypotensive ⓓ

Generics: **sodium nitroprusside; trimethaphan camsylate; diazoxide.**

Actions and uses

Hypotensive drugs lower blood pressure and there are many drugs that have such an action. Some drugs do so on acute (short-term) administration as a deliberate part of their medical use. Few drugs are actually used for this purpose, but some direct-acting ℞ **vasodilator** drugs are suitable for controlling severe hypertensive crises, and as a hypotensive for controlled low blood pressure in surgery, including ℞ **sodium nitroprusside** and ℞ **diazoxide**. A ℞ **ganglion-blocker** agent, ℞ **trimethaphan camsylate**, is short-acting and is used as a hypotensive for controlled blood pressure during surgery or to quickly reduce blood pressure in hypertensive emergencies. These drugs may be given by intravenous infusion in emergency treatment.

Although the term hypotensive can be applied to drugs that cause marked falls in blood pressure on an acute basis, the term ℞ **antihypertensive** is, by convention, usually used to describe drugs that are used to lower an abnormally high blood pressure (see ⊙ **hypertension**) on a long-term basis. Such antihypertensive drugs do not necessarily lower blood pressure in people with normal blood pressure, but hypotensive drugs do.

Limitations

See the individual drug entries.

hypothalamic hormone ⓓ

Generics: **cetrorelix; dopamine hydrochloride; goserelin; leuprolide acetate; nafarelin acetate; octreotide; gonadorelin; protirelin; sermorelin.**

Actions and uses

Hypothalamic hormones, sometimes called hypothalamic factors, travel through a specialized system of portal blood vessels the short distance from the hypothalamus (a brain area in the base of the brain) to the pituitary gland to control the release of ℞ **anterior pituitary hormone**, which in turn controls various other glands.

These hypothalamic hormone factors include corticotropin-releasing hormone (CRH; or corticotropin-releasing factor, CRF); gonadotropin-releasing hormone, (gonadotrophin-releasing hormone) GnRH; or gonadotropin-releasing factor, GRF, LH-RH, synthetic drug form ℞ **gonadorelin**); growth hormone-releasing hormone (GHRH, or growth hormone-releasing factor, GHRF); growth hormone release-inhibiting hormone (GH-RIH; or growth hormone release-inhibiting factor, GH-RIF, somatostatin); thyrotropin-releasing hormone; TRH; protirelin); prolactin release-inhibiting factor (PRIF); prolactin-releasing factor and others.

Some of these hormones, or chemical analogs, are used in therapeutics, mainly as ℞ **diagnostic agents**. ℞ **protirelin**, a synthetic version of thyrotropin-releasing hormone is used as a diagnostic agent to assess thyroid function. ℞ **sermorelin**, a synthetic analog of growth hormone-releasing hormone, is used diagnostically in a test to assess the secretion of growth hormone.

Gonadorelin is a synthetic version of gonadotropin-releasing hormone and is used as a diagnostic agent for pituitary function, to induce ovulation in women with primary hypothalamic amenorrhea, or to treat precocious puberty. A number of synthetic analogs of gonadorelin (including ℞ **leuprolide**, ℞ **goserelin**, ℞ **nafarelin acetate**) are used for various purposes, including to treat prostate cancer, breast cancer endometriosis, precocious puberty and for assisted fertility (see ⊙ **infertility**).

Octreotide, a long-lasting analog of somatostatin, reduces the release of a number of hormones from the pituitary gland and other sites, and is used to treat symptoms caused by the release of hormones from cancerous and noncancerous tumors (and for other purposes).

Limitations

Since most hypothalamic hormones are chemically peptides, they cannot be given by mouth because they would be digested, and instead have to be injected. This limits their use (although this does not matter when they are used as diagnostic agents). However, it is possible to develop synthetic analogs that are more stable, and octreotide is a good example of a drug that, although it still has to be injected, can be used for long-term treatment. Also, the various synthetic analogs of gonadorelin are relatively stable and very useful in medicines.

PRIF is probably identical to the neurotransmitter dopamine, and because PRIF controls the release of prolactin, the hormone that causes lactation as an end-effect, this is thought to be the reason why ℞ **dopamine-receptor antagonist** drugs sometimes cause lactation.

HypRho-D, Mini-Dose ⓑ

A preparation of ℞ $Rh_0(D)$ immune globulin (human).
Formulation: Intramuscular injection.
Availability: Prescription only.
Warnings and side effects: See ℞ $Rh_0(D)$ immune globulin (human).

Hyprogest ⓑ

A preparation of ℞ **hydroxyprogesterone caproate**.
Formulation: Injection.

Availability: Prescription only.

Warnings and side effects: See ℞ **hydroxyprogesterone caproate.**

hypromellose Ⓖ

see ℞ **hydroxypropyl methylcellulose.**

Hyrexin-50 Ⓑ

A preparation of ℞ **diphenhydramine hydrochloride.**

Formulation: Injection.

Availability: Prescription only.

Warnings and side effects: See ℞ **diphenhydramine hydrochloride.**

Hysone Ⓑ

A preparation of ℞ **hydrocortisone** and ℞ **clioquinol.**

Formulation: Cream.

Availability: Prescription only.

Warnings and side effects: See ℞ **hydrocortisone;** ℞ **clioquinol.**

Hytakerol Ⓑ

A preparation of ℞ **dihydrotachysterol (DHT).**

Formulation: Oral capsules.

Availability: Prescription only.

Warnings and side effects: See ℞ **dihydrotachysterol (DHT).**

Hytone Ⓑ

A preparation of ℞ **hydrocortisone.**

Formulation: Ointment in several strengths; cream in two strengths; lotion in two strengths.

Availability: Prescription only.

Warnings and side effects: See ℞ **hydrocortisone.**

Hytrin Ⓑ

A preparation of ℞ **terazosin.**

Formulation: Oral capsules, available in 4 strengths.

Availability: Prescription only.

Warnings and side effects: See ℞ **terazosin.**

Hytuss 2X Capsules; Tablets Ⓑ

A preparation of ℞ **guaifenesin.**

Formulation: Oral capsules; tablets.

Availability: OTC; tablets are prescription only.

Warnings and side effects: See ℞ **guaifenesin.**

Hyzaar Ⓑ

A preparation of ℞ **hydrochlorothiazide** and ℞ **losartan potassium.**

Formulation: Oral tablets, in two strengths.

Availability: Prescription only.

Warnings and side effects: See ℞ **hydrochlorothiazide;** ℞ **losartan potassium.**

ibuprofen Ⓖ

Type/Group: anti-inflammatory; antirheumatic; non-narcotic analgesic; NSAID; cold and cough preparation.

Brand(s): Advil Tablets, Caplets, Gel Caplets, Liqui-Gels, Junior Strength Tablets, Junior Strength Chewable Tablets, Children's Oral Suspension, Infants' Drops; Genpril; Motrin Tablets, Motrin IB Tablets, Caplets, Gelcaps, Children's Chewable Tablets, Children's Oral Suspension, Infants' Concentrated Drops; Nuprin Tablets, Caplets; Pediacare Fever Suspension, Oral Drops. Combinations: With *pseudoephedrine hydrochloride*: Advil Cold & Sinus Caplets; Dristan Sinus Caplets; Motrin IB Sinus Caplets; Sine-Aid IB Caplets.

How administered: Orally; topically.

Used to treat

Ibuprofen is used primarily to treat ✛ **rheumatoid arthritis,** ✛ **osteoarthritis,** and other ✛ **musculoskeletal disorders,** and also moderate pain of inflammatory origin and postoperative pain. Accordingly, it was the first and only modern NSAID for oral use approved for non-prescription, over-the-counter sale. It has extensive use both in its own right and as the major active constituent in compound analgesic preparations for the treatment of minor or moderate pain, including headache, migraine, dysmenorrhea (period pain), toothache, and muscle ache. Its ℞ **antipyretic** action helps symptomatic relief of the fever associated with colds and influenza. It is also available for use in babies (for example, to reduce fever in babies over 6 months) and children (including juvenile arthritis).

Warnings

• It should not be used by people with known hypersensitivity to this drug or to other NSAIDs (including ℞ **aspirin**), who have chronic kidney disease, certain bleeding disorders or conditions (for example, hemophilia, vitamin K deficiency, low blood-platelet levels), or who have a tendency to, or active, peptic ulceration.

• It should be given with caution to people taking certain drugs for diabetes mellitus, or with allergic disorders (especially asthma and skin conditions), who are elderly, or with any kind of kidney impairment or with certain liver disorders.

• Ibuprofen should be used when pregnant only if medically judged to be clearly needed. It should not be used in the third trimester, however, because this is when risk to the fetus is highest.

• Breast-feeding mothers should either discontinue this drug or stop breast-feeding.

• With regular, long-term use (as in the treatment of osteoarthritis), NSAIDs may cause gastrointestinal bleeding, ulceration, or perforation. Any signs of bleeding (for example, black stools) should be reported to a physician immediately.

• Most NSAIDs have the potential, particularly with regular use, to cause liver damage. Periodic evaluation of liver function is necessary in long-term therapy (more than two months).

• Side effects are more frequent in the elderly.

• Gastrointestinal upsets may be minimized by taking it with milk or food.

• If blurred or reduced vision is experienced, a doctor or ophthalmologist must be contacted and use of the drug stopped.

Key to symbols: ✛ = Disorder Section   ℞ = Drug Section   ♣ = Herbal Section   ᔆᔆ = Supplement Section

Interactions

• There is generally no added benefit in taking other NSAIDs or other ℞ **salicylates** (especially aspirin) at the same time, but there is a higher risk of gastrointestinal upsets and bleeding.
• Alcohol and ℞ **corticosteroids** increase the risk of bleeding, particularly if there is an existing ulcer.
• ℞ **anticoagulant**, ℞ **antiplatelet**, and ℞ **thrombolytic** drugs may increase bleeding time.
• Ibuprofen may reduce the effectiveness of ℞ **diuretics**, ℞ **ACE inhibitors**, and ℞ **beta-blockers**.
• The effects of ℞ **lithium** and ℞ **methotrexate** may be exaggerated, with potential for serious toxicity.
• Foodstuffs and herbals with ℞ **antiplatelet** properties, for example, ♣ **ginger**, ♧ **garlic**, and various herbal preparations, may add to the antiplatelet effect of NSAIDs.

Side effects

These depend on how it is administered, dose, duration of treatment, and use. Ibuprofen is better tolerated and causes less gastrointestinal disturbances than the majority of its class, but severe reactions and side effects are still possible, especially with long-term use.
• Commonly heartburn, gastrointestinal upsets, nausea, diarrhea, constipation, flatulence, swelling of the extremities, itching, rash, dizziness, and headache.
• Prolonged bleeding time (with consequent risk of ulceration) is possible with high dosage, and other blood changes can occur, including anemia.
• Less frequently, vomiting, dizziness, mood swings, ringing in the ears, edema, fatigue, or blurred vision.
• Hypersensitivity reactions may include symptoms such as fever, chills, chest tightness, asthma, or bronchospasm.
• Reversible kidney failure, particularly in renal impairment, has occurred. Liver damage is rare.

ichthammol ⒢

Type/Group: **keratolytic; anti-infective; antifungal**.
Brand(s): Boyol Salve.
How administered: Topically (external).

Used to treat

Ichthammol is a thick, dark brown liquid derived from bituminous oils. It is used in ointments or in glycerol solution for the topical treatment of ulcers and inflammation of the skin. It is milder than coal tar and is useful in treating the less-severe forms of ✪ **eczema**.

Warnings

None significant.

Interactions

No significant interactions are known.

Side effects

No significant side effects are known.

Icy Hot Balm; Stick Ⓑ

A preparation of ℞ **methyl salicylate**, ℞ **menthol**, and various.
Formulation: Topical ointment; cream; solid.
Availability: OTC.
Warnings and side effects: See ℞ methyl salicylate; ℞ menthol.

Icy Hot Cream Ⓑ

A preparation of ℞ **methyl salicylate**, ℞ **menthol**, ℞ **camphor**, and ℞ **carbomer**.
Formulation: Topical Cream.
Availability: OTC.
Warnings and side effects: See ℞ methyl salicylate; ℞ menthol; ℞ camphor; ℞ carbomer.

Idamycin Ⓑ

A preparation of ℞ **idarubicin hydrochloride**.
Formulation: Injection.
Availability: Prescription only.
Warnings and side effects: ℞ idarubicin hydrochloride

idarubicin hydrochloride ⒢

Type/Group: **anticancer; cytotoxic**.
Brand(s): Idamycin.
How administered: Intravenous infusion.

Used to treat

Idarubicin is a cytotoxic drug (an anthracycline antibiotic in origin) with properties similar to ℞ **doxorubicin hydrochloride** and is used for acute myeloid ✪ **leukemia**.

Warnings

• It should not be given to people with known hypersensitivity to idarubicin or related drugs.
• It should be given with caution to people with pre-existing bone marrow suppression, a history of heart disease, who have had a previous course of treatment with anthracyclines or other cardiotoxic agents, or with kidney or liver impairment. This is a specialist drug which will be used following a full evaluation by specialist physicians.
• Idarubicin is not recommended for use during pregnancy unless it is medically judged to be essential, because it may cause birth defects. Becoming pregnant while using this drug must be avoided.
• It should not be used if breast-feeding.
• It can cause bone marrow depression, which may lead to bleeding and a reduced resistance to infection.
• This drug may be associated with the development of myelogenous leukemia.
• Adverse effects on the heart, leading to congestive heart failure, may occur.
• In common with many anticancer drugs, idarubicin may impair fertility, induce genetic mutations in cells, or cause cancer.

Interactions

No interactions specific to this drug are known.

Side effects

• Infection, hair loss, nausea and vomiting, abdominal pain, diarrhea, esophageal inflammation, loss of appetite, darkening of nail beds or skin, fever, chills, eye inflammation and tearing.

idoxuridine ⒢

(IDU)
Type/Group: **antiviral**.
Brand(s): Herplex.

How administered: Topically (eye).

Used to treat

Idoxuridine is used in ophthalmic solution to treat eye infections caused by a herpes simplex virus (see ✪ herpes). It has rather weak and variable results. It works by stopping the virus multiplying by interfering with DNA synthesis.

Warnings

• It should not be given to people with known hypersensitivity to iodine.

• Idoxuridine's safety during pregnancy has not been established.

• Medical judgment is required if breast-feeding is being considered.

• It is an investigational drug and this status will be reviewed.

• Sunglasses should be worn to decrease sensitivity to bright light.

Interactions

• A precipitate can form if taken with ⚗ **boric acid**.

Side effects

• Initial irritation and stinging on administration.

IDU ⓖ

see ℞ **idoxuridine**.

Ifex ⑧

A preparation of ℞ **ifosfamide**.
Formulation: Powder for injection.
Availability: Prescription only.
Warnings and side effects: ℞ **ifosfamide**

ifosfamide ⓖ

Type/Group: **anticancer; cytotoxic**.
Brand(s): Ifex.
How administered: Intravenous injection.

Used to treat

Ifosfamide is an alkylating agent used particularly in the treatment of testicular ✪ **cancer**, which is its only labeled use. It works by interfering with cellular DNA and so inhibits cell replication. It is often given simultaneously with ℞ **mesna**, in order to reduce the toxic side effects.

Warnings

• It should not be given to people with known hypersensitivity to ifosfamide or severe bone marrow depression.

• It should be given with caution to people with impaired kidney or liver function, or compromised bone marrow function. This is a specialist drug which will be used following a full evaluation by specialist physicians.

• Ifosfamide is not recommended for use during pregnancy unless it is medically judged to be essential, because it may cause birth defects. Becoming pregnant while using this drug must be avoided.

• It should not be used if breast-feeding.

• Urotoxicities (harm to the urinary tract), as will as CNS (central nervous system) toxicity, such as confusion and coma, have been associated with this drug.

• It can cause severe bone marrow suppression, which may lead to bleeding and a reduced resistance to infection.

• In common with many anticancer drugs, it may cause cancer.

Interactions

No interactions specific to this drug are known.

Side effects

• Frequently, nausea, vomiting, blood in urine, loss of hair, bladder infection, decreased urination, or urinary frequency.

• Occasionally, confusion, sleepiness, psychosis, hallucinations, and infection.

• Rarely, dizziness, seizures, disorientation, fever, malaise, inflammation of mouth mucosa.

IL-11 ⓖ

see ℞ **oprelvekin**.

Ilotycin; Ilotycin Gluceptate ⑧

A preparation of ℞ **erythromycin**.
Formulation: Ophthalmic ointment; injection (Gluceptate).
Availability: Prescription only.
Warnings and side effects: ℞ **erythromycin**

Imdur ⑧

A preparation of ℞ **isosorbide mononitrate**.
Formulation: Oral tablets, extended release, available in 3 strengths.
Availability: Prescription only.
Warnings and side effects: ℞ **isosorbide mononitrate**

imiglucerase ⓖ

Type/Group: **enzyme; metabolic disorder treatment**.
Brand(s): Cerezyme.
How administered: Intravenous infusion.

Used to treat

Imiglucerase is an enzyme made by recombinant DNA technology, which is used as a replacement in the specialist treatment of Type 1 Gaucher's disease (a genetically determined enzyme deficiency disease affecting the spleen, liver, bone marrow, and lymph nodes).

Warnings

• It should not be given to people with known with hypersensitivity to this drug.

• Imiglucerase's safety during pregnancy has not been established. It should be used only if the potential benefit justifies the possible risk.

• Medical judgment is required if breast-feeding is being considered. It is not known whether it appears in breast milk.

• This is a specialist drug and a full assessment for suitability will be carried out.

Interactions

No interactions specific to this drug are known. Full studies have not been completed.

Side effects

• Itching, pain, swelling or abscess at injection site, hypersensitivity reactions, nausea and vomiting, diarrhea and abdominal pain, fatigue, headache, dizziness, rash, and fever.

Key to symbols: ✪ = Disorder Section ℞ = Drug Section ♣ = Herbal Section ⚗ = Supplement Section

imipramine-cilastatin Ⓖ

Type/Group: **beta-lactam; antibiotic.**
Brand(s): Primaxin.
How administered: Injection.

Used to treat

Imipenem-cilastatin is a drug pair, with the two drugs always used together. It is prescribed for respiratory tract, skin and skin structure, gynecologic, bone, joint, intra-abdominal, and urinary tract infections. It can also used in cases of ✪ **endocarditis**, ✪ **septicemia**, and other mild to moderately severe infections. Imipenem is a new sort of beta-lactam with a broad spectrum of activity against many Gram-positive and Gram-negative bacteria. However, it is partly degraded by an enzyme in the kidney and is therefore combined with cilastatin, which is an enzyme inhibitor.

Warnings

• It should not be given to people with known hypersensitivity to imipenem-cilastatin or other beta-lactams.
• It should be given with caution to people with allergies to penicillins, cephalosporins, or other allergens, or to anyone with impaired kidney function and CNS (central nervous system) disorders.
• It crosses the placenta and should be used in pregnancy only if the benefits outweigh the possible risk to the fetus.
• Medical judgment is required if breast-feeding is being considered. It does appear in breast milk.
• Superinfections due to the altered bacterial balance caused by antibiotic treatment may occur. A doctor must be contacted if there is severe abdominal pain or moderate to severe diarrhea.
• There is a possibility of severe allergic reaction.
• Rarely, seizures or other adverse CNS events may occur in susceptible people (for example, anyone with brain lesions or impaired kidney function).

Interactions

• If used with ℞ **cyclosporine** or ℞ **tacrolimus**, there is a risk of CNS toxicity.
• ℞ **theophylline** increases the risk of seizure.

Side effects

• Occasionally, diarrhea, nausea, and vomiting.
• Rarely, rash and blood disorders.

imipramine Ⓖ

Type/Group: **antidepressant; tricyclic.**
Brand(s): Tofranil; various generic.
How administered: Orally; injection.

Used to treat

Imipramine can be used to treat ✪ **depression**. It can also be used as part of the treatment for childhood enuresis including ✪ **bed-wetting** (nocturnal enuresis) and in the management of unstable bladder conditions. Because it has a less sedative effect than many other tricyclics, it is more suited for the treatment of withdrawn and apathetic patients than those who are agitated and restless. Although not stated by the manufacturer for such use, it may be prescribed for headaches. As is the case with other antidepressants, this drug is also being evaluated for other uses.

Warnings

• It should not be given to people with known hypersensitivity to this drug, or who are just recovering from myocardial infarction (heart attack), with convulsive disorders or prostatic hypertrophy, who are taking or have stopped taking MAOIs antidepressants within the previous 14 days.
• It should be given with caution to people with severe depression, increased intraocular pressure (pressure in the eyeball), narrow-angle glaucoma, urinary retention, or heart, cardiovascular, liver or thyroid disease, or if they are receiving electroshock therapy, or they are over 65.
• Imipramine should be used during pregnancy only if the benefits outweigh the possible risk to the fetus.
• It should not be used by nursing mothers.
• Other symptoms of a psychiatric illnesses may worsen.
• Episodes of mania or hypomania may occur, especially in those with affective bipolar disorder (manic depression).
• Exposure to sunlight should be minimized because of possible photosensitization (sensitivity to light).
• Treatment should be stopped gradually by lowering the dose over a period of time.
• It is not generally given to children under the age of 6.
• It may be one to three weeks before there are any signs of improvement.
• It may impair the performance of skilled tasks such as driving.
• Alcohol, grapefruit juice, and smoking can all affect tricyclics (see Interactions below).

Interactions

• Serious or even fatal reactions can occur if ℞ **MAOI** antidepressants are taken at the same time as tricyclics.
• The effects of ℞ **epinephrine**, ℞ **norepinephrine**, and ℞ **phenylephrine** on blood pressure are intensified.
• Grapefruit juice increases the levels of tricyclics.
• ℞ **clonidine hydrochloride** should not be used with tricyclics, because a dangerous increase in blood pressure and hypertensive crisis is possible.
• The effects of ℞ **guanethidine monosulfate**, ℞ **levodopa**, and ℞ **sympathomimetics** may be reduced by tricyclics.
• The effects of ℞ **anticholinergics**, dicumarol, ℞ **quinolones**, grepafloxacin, and sparfloxacin may be enhanced by tricyclics.
• ℞ **Barbiturates**, ℞ **activated charcoal**, and rifamycin-related antibiotics may reduce the effectiveness of tricyclics.
• ℞ **Cimetidine**, ℞ **SSRIs**, ℞ **haloperidol**, ℞ **bupropion**, ℞ **valproate sodium** (and other valproic acid derivatives), and histamine ℞ **H₂-antagonists** may increase the levels of tricyclics in the blood.
• The levels of ℞ **carbamazepine** may increase, while blood levels of tricyclics decrease.
• Smoking may affect the metabolism of tricyclics.
• The effects of alcohol may be enhanced.

Side effects

• Along with other members of this class, it has ℞ **anticholinergic** side effects, notably drowsiness and difficulty in concentrating, dry mouth, blurred vision, constipation, postural hypotension (lowered blood pressure on standing), urinary retention, ECG changes, speeded heartbeat, gastrointestinal distress, and skin sensitivity reactions.

• Older adults may experience extrapyramidal symptoms (uncontrollable movement). Rarely, acute renal failure or bone marrow depression may occur.

• When used in children for enuresis, the most common side effects are nervousness, sleep disorders, and gastrointestinal disturbances.

• There may be allergic reactions when used by injection.

imiquimod Ⓖ

Type/Group: **keratolytic; antiviral; immunomodulator.**
Brand(s): Aldara.
How administered: Topically (external).

Used to treat

Imiquimod can be used to treat and dissolve ✪ **warts** of the external genital and perianal areas. It is not clear how it works but may locally release cytokines such as the interferons.

Warnings

• It should not be given to people with known hypersensitivity to imiquimod.

• There have been no well-controlled studies in pregnant women. It should be used only if the potential benefits outweigh the possible risks to the fetus.

• Medical judgment is required if breast-feeding is being considered. It is not known whether it appears in breast milk.

• Severe skin reactions can occur. The cream must be washed off and a doctor contacted if they do.

• Do not bandage or wrap affected area.

• Sexual contact should be avoided while the cream is on the skin.

• It may weaken condoms and vaginal diaphragms.

Interactions

No significant interactions are known.

Side effects

• Commonly, reddening, erosion, peeling, flaking, and swelling at application site.

Imitrex Ⓡ

A preparation of ℞ **sumatriptan succinate.**
Formulation: Oral tablets, available in two strengths; nasal spray; injection (subcutaneous).
Availability: Prescription only.
Warnings and side effects: See ℞ **sumatriptan succinate.**

immune globulin, human (IG) Ⓖ

(human normal immunoglobulin (HNIG))
Type/Group: **immune globulin.**
Brand(s): BayGam; Gamimune N; Gammar-P I.V.; Iveegam EN IGIV; Polygam S/D; Sandoglobulin; Venoglobulin-S.
How administered: Intramuscular injection; intravenous infusion.

Used to treat

Immune globulin, human (also known as gamma globulin or normal immunoglobulin) is used to give passive immunity by the injection of immune globulin (antibody) prepared from the pooled blood plasma donated by individuals with antibodies to viruses prevalent in the general population, including ✪ **hepatitis** A virus,

✪ **measles**, and ✪ **rubella** (German measles). It is commonly given to people at risk, such as infants who cannot tolerate vaccines that incorporate live (though weakened) viruses (active immunity), for rubella in pregnancy, and hepatitis A short-term protection for travelers in areas were the disease is endemic. Administration is normally by intramuscular injection, but there are also special forms for replacement therapy given by intravenous infusion, including formulations for patients undergoing a bone-marrow transplant, or patients with certain congenital blood component deficiencies, for example, agammaglobulinemia, hypogammaglobulinemia, idiopathic thrombocytopenic purpura, and Kawasaki syndrome. It is sometimes used in the treatment of Guillain-Barré syndrome.

Warnings

• It should not be given to people with known hypersensitivity to immune globulins.

• It should be given with caution to people with a known deficiency of the naturally occurring IgA immunoglobulin.

• Its effects in pregnancy have not been fully studied, but immune globulin is generally considered safe enough to be used when clearly needed.

• Medical judgment is required if breast-feeding is being considered (antibodies do appear in breast milk).

• When given in intravenous (IV) form, immune globulin occasionally causes a sharp fall in blood pressure with flushing, chills, tightness in the chest, or nausea 30 minutes to an hour after commencing an infusion. (This reaction is thought to be related to the rate of infusion, which must be discontinued and, after symptoms have been controlled, readjusted.) Close medical monitoring during an infusion is necessary.

• Because this immune globulin is extracted from human blood, the possibility exists that it might contain virus or other disease agents. However, multiple screenings and filters (chemical and physical) are used in its preparation, and its potential to transmit infection is considered nearly nonexistent.

• After administration, people will be required to wait for some time to ensure that there is no serious reaction (such as anaphylaxis).

Interactions

• The immune response to live virus vaccines (for example, ℞ **MMR vaccine**) may not be satisfactory. A delay of at least three months (more for some vaccines, or their specific uses) is recommended after administering immune globulin. This does not apply, however, to the live vaccines for polio (oral form), typhoid (oral form), or yellow fever, which may given at the same time as immune globulin.

• Caution is required if ℞ **anticoagulants** are being taken.

Side effects

• Most of the side effects are mild, and depend somewhat on whether given intravenously or intramuscularly.

• There may be swelling, irritation or tenderness at the site of injection, and headache, nausea, fever, or malaise.

• Infrequently, skin rash, hives, itching, swelling of lymph glands, and achy joints.

• Although rare, anaphylactic shock has been reported.

immune globulin ⒟
(immunoglobulin)

Generics: **hepatitis B immune globulin (HBIG); immune globulin, human (IG); rabies immune globulin, human (RIG); Rh$_0$(D) immune globulin (human); tetanus immune globulin TIG.**

Actions and uses
Immune globulin (immunoglobulin) is a term used to describe any of approximately five classes of proteins in the immune system that naturally act as antibodies in the bloodstream. They are created in response to the presence of a specific antigen (any substance the body regards as foreign or dangerous) and circulate within the blood. Immunoglobulin deficiencies are often associated with an increased risk of infection. These antibodies can be given by injection or infusion for immediate immunity, commonly known as passive immunity, against certain ✪ **infections** (see ℞ **immunization**). To minimize the risk of allergic reactions, immunoglobulins are normally of human origin rather than from an animal (when they are usually referred to as antiserum or antisera). Different types of human immunoglobulins are used to protect people either suffering from infection or exposed to infection. Standard immune globulin—℞ **immune globulin, human (IG)** or gamma globulin—is prepared from the pooled serum of a large sample of donors who have antibodies to viruses prevalent in a normal population. Specific immune globulins are prepared in a similar way, except that the pooled blood plasma used to obtain the immunoglobulins is from hyperimmunized donors with high levels of the particular antibody that is required. See ℞ **antitoxin**; ℞ **immunization**.

Limitations
Because immune globulin is extracted from human blood, the possibility exists that it might contain a virus or other disease agents. However, multiple screenings and filters (chemical and physical) are used in its preparation, and its potential to transmit infection is considered nearly nonexistent.

Local or systemic (throughout the body) allergic hypersensitivity reactions to immune globulin can occur. Where the immune globulin has been prepared in an animal species (for example, horse for ℞ **diphtheria antitoxin**), it is referred to as an ℞ **antitoxin** (or antiserum), and the risk of an allergic reaction is very much higher.

Where the immune globulin is raised in an animal species to be used as an ℞ **antidote** to neutralize the poison in a snakebite, a scorpion's sting or a bite from any other poisonous creature (such as a spider), it is called an ℞ **antivenin** (or antivenom), and here again there is considerable risk of an allergic reaction.

immunization ⒟

Actions and uses
Immunization agents are used in the immunization procedure, which can be used either to prevent someone from contracting specific ✪ **infections**, or help treat an existing infection. This is achieved by using one of two methods, active or passive immunity. Active immunity is conferred by vaccination (that is, by administering a ℞ **vaccine**), which involves the injection or administration of bacterial or viral agents that are live (but weakened, "attenuated"), dead, or toxoids (chemically-modified microbial toxins; also called

detoxified exotoxins). These agents act as antigens to trigger the body's own defense mechanisms to manufacture antibodies. This method gives long-lasting, but not necessarily permanent, protection.

Passive immunity is conferred by the injection of a quantity of prepared blood serum already containing mixed antibodies (standard immune globulin—also called gamma globulin) or of selected antibodies, and so helps to prevent the person contracting the infection or helps to treat an already existing infection. This method gives immediate protection but only lasts several weeks.

An injection of ℞ **antitoxin** (an agent that neutralizes the toxins that are produced by the disease-causing organism) is another way of imparting passive immunity.

Vaccination in advance of possible infection is generally the preferred and safer option. This method gives long-lasting protection, but this is not necessarily permanent, either because the infective organism tends to change (for example, the influenza virus) or because immunization "wears-off."

Limitations
See ℞ **antitoxin**; ℞ **antivenin**; ℞ **immune globulin**; ℞ **vaccine**.

immunomodulator ⒟
Generics: **aldesleukin; etanercept; imiquimod; infliximab; interferons; levamisole hydrochloride.**

Actions and uses
Immunomodulator agents (biological response modifiers or immune response modifiers) are used to modify the activity of the body's immune system, normally improving defense against infection and possibly malignant growths. These terms are not used in an exact sense, and some very different types of drug are commonly referred to as biological response modifiers. In practice, the meaning somewhat overlaps the terms ℞ **immunostimulant** and ℞ **immunosuppressant**.

The biggest group of natural agents generally termed ℞ **immunomodulator**, are certain *cytokine* proteins or peptide molecules. These are often of some considerable chemical complexity and are produced in tiny quantities by cells, and act as natural mediator chemicals within the body. Some act as ℞ **growth factor**  agents to control, modulate, or promote cell division and differentiation, others are more concerned with inflammatory processes. When manufactured using the techniques of molecular biology, these agents become (very expensive) drugs that can be given by injection.

℞ **interferons** are a group of inducible proteins synthesized in response to viruses (and also some mammalian cells). They can modify the host response by inducing the production of enzymes, for instance, that inhibit translocation of viral mRNA into viral protein, and so prevent virus reproduction. However, they have been less effective against viruses than was hoped, and have so many different actions that they can be difficult to use. There are several kinds currently in use (all are copies of complete, naturally occurring human interferons, except alfacon-1, which is a "designer" construction of protein elements common to the alfa type of interferon). These include: interferon alfa-2a, interferon alfa-2b, interferon alfacon-1, interferon beta-1a, interferon beta-1b, interferon gamma-1b. Their uses include for certain forms of ✪ **leukemia** and AIDS-related ✪ **Kaposi's sarcoma**, investigation of over 20 forms of cancer, for hairy-cell leukemia, malignant melanoma, condyloma (certain warts), chronic ✪ **hepatitis** B and C infections, for relapsing ✪ **multiple sclerosis** (MS), for chronic granulomatous disease (CGD), and to delay progression of severe ✪ **osteoporosis** (see ℞ **osteoporosis treatment**; these are detailed in the ℞ **interferon** article).

℞ **aldesleukin** (recombinant interleukin-2) is another of the cytokine inflammatory mediators, an interleukin, produced naturally by cells of the immune system in response to infection or antigenic challenge (a foreign body). Synthetic (recombinant; DNA technology) versions can be used as an ℞ **anticancer** drug, licensed for use to treat metastatic renal cell carcinoma. It is being investigated, with beneficial reports, in the treatment of melanoma, colorectal cancer, and non-Hodgkin's lymphoma, and also for use in Kaposi's sarcoma.

Both ℞ **etanercept** and ℞ **infliximab** bind with, and inhibit the action of, a particular mediator substance—tumor necrosis factor alpha. This is a ℞ **growth factor** found in unusually high levels at inflamed sites in ✪ **rheumatoid arthritis** and ✪ **Crohn's disease**. ℞ **etanercept** and ℞ **infliximab** can be regarded as ℞ **immunosuppressant** or ℞ **immunomodulator** agents.

The ℞ **anticancer** drug ℞ **levamisole**, which is used as an additional treatment with an *antimetabolite* anticancer drug after surgery in certain people with colon cancer, is regarded as a biological response modifier because it restores depressed immune function and enhances T-lymphocyte responses (T-lymphocytes are white blood cells involved in cell immunity).

℞ **imiquimod** is a new sort of ℞ **keratolytic** agent which can be used to treat and dissolve warts of the external genital and perianal areas. It is regarded as an immune response modifier because it induces cytokines in the skin.

Limitations

These are specialist drugs and are used only after a full medical assessment. The ℞ **interferons** should be used during pregnancy only if the potential benefits outweigh the possible risk to the fetus. Medical judgment is required if breast-feeding is being considered. Regular blood counts are essential during treatment, particularly to check the levels of white blood cells. Of particular concern are blood changes (which may include anemia and white-cell suppression) and mental depression.

℞ **aldesleukin** is a very toxic drug, which causes tumor shrinkage in a small number of patients. Toxicity is universal and often severe. A common acute problem is the development of a capillary leak syndrome causing pulmonary edema and hypotension. It is used in specialist units only.

See also the individual drug entries.

immunostimulant ⑩

Generics: **BCG intravesical; pegademase bovine.**

Actions and uses

Immunostimulant agents are used to boost the efficiency of the body's immune system, and so improve defense against ✪ **infections** and possibly malignant growths (✪ **cancer**).

Vaccination uses ℞ **vaccine** preparations for systemic long-term immunostimulation against specific bacterial or viral organisms, through the use of live but weakened (attenuated) organisms, dead but immunogenic organisms, or live, non-pathogenic organisms closely related to the invading microbe. Many vaccines are administered with immunoadjuvant drugs (for example, aluminum phosphate) to enhance their immunostimulant actions. ℞ **interferons** and interleukins are discussed in the ℞ **immunomodulator** entry.

℞ **pegademase bovine** is an ℞ **enzyme** which acts as a replacement enzyme for one that is lacking in a rare inherited disorder that causes a form of severe combined immunodeficiency disease (SCID). Infants born with this enzyme deficiency are unable to maintain adequate levels of white blood cells, and hence have little immunity even to common infections. This condition is often fatal. The drug can be termed an immunostimulant because it boosts immunity under these conditions.

℞ **BCG intravesical** is a drug used in the treatment of bladder cancer *in situ*. BCG vaccine was originally developed as an antituberculosis vaccine produced from a live attenuated strain of the tuberculosis bacillus, but can be used for this unrelated indication. It is not known exactly how it works, but it appears to stimulate T-lymphocytes and so can be regarded as an immunostimulant.

Limitations

In the past, many preparations of inactivated bacteria (other than specific ones used as vaccines) and other potential antigen proteins have been injected in the hope of stimulating the natural immune system, including in ℞ **anticancer** therapy. This particular approach has not proved very successful and has largely been discontinued, although a number of similar agents are currently being evaluated or are licensed in other countries (some for use against certain forms of cancer). Pegademase bovine is prescribed only by specialists and used only under expert supervision.

immunosuppressant ⑩

(immunosuppressive)

Generics: **azathiaprine; basiliximab; betamethasone; cortisone; cyclophosphamide; cyclosporine; daclizumab; dexamethasone; etanercept; glatiramer acetate; hydrocortisone; infliximab; leflunomide; methotrexate; methylprednisolone; muromonab-CD3; mycophenolate mofetil; prednisolone; rituximab; sirolimus; tacrolimus.**

Actions and uses

Immunosuppressants are used to prevent tissue rejection following donor grafting or transplant surgery (although this carries the risk of unopposed infection). They impair the immunologic defensive responses of the body, which are activated against anything the body considers to be foreign (for example, infective agents or foreign bodies). They are also commonly used to treat autoimmune diseases (where the immune system is triggered into inappropriately acting against part of the body itself, because the body incorrectly considers a part of itself to be a "foreign body"). In this way, immunosuppressant drugs can be used to treat chronic inflammatory diseases, such as ✪ **rheumatoid arthritis**, ✪ **lupus** erythematosus, and collagen disorders (some of which may have an autoimmune component).

The best-known and most-used immunosuppressants are the ℞ **corticosteroid** drugs (for example, ℞ **betamethasone**, ℞ **cortisone**, ℞ **dexamethasone**, ℞ **hydrocortisone**, ℞ **methylprednisolone**, and ℞ **prednisolone**), which also have potent ℞ **anti-inflammatory** activity and are used for the treatment of many kinds of diseases. Of the non-steroid agents, ℞ **cyclosporine** is used as an immunosuppressant, particularly to limit tissue rejection during and following organ transplant surgery. It can also be used to treat severe, active ✪ **rheumatoid arthritis** and some skin conditions, such as severe, resistant atopic ✪ **dermatitis** and (under special supervision) ✪ **psoriasis**. Similarly ℞ **cyclophosphamide** has many actions, but can be prescribed ("off-label") as an immunosuppressant in the treatment of complicated rheumatoid arthritis and other connective tissue diseases. ℞ **tacrolimus** is a drug that chemically is antibiotic in nature, but is used particularly as an immunosuppressant to limit tissue rejection during and following organ transplant surgery (especially of the liver). A similar agent is ℞ **mycophenolate mofetil**, which is used mainly as an immunosuppressant to reduce tissue rejection in heart or kidney transplants. Generally it is used in combination with ℞ **corticosteroid** drugs and ℞ **cyclosporine**. Another drug of this type is ℞ **sirolimus**, which is also used to prevent organ rejection.

℞ **methotrexate** has many actions (including as a ℞ **cytotoxic** agent in ℞ **anticancer** treatment), and is probably working mainly as an immunosuppressant when used as a disease-modifying ℞ **antirheumatic** agent to treat rheumatoid arthritis—and also resistant psoriasis (when these conditions are severe and disabling and other treatments have proven inadequate). A similar drug is ℞ **leflunomide**, which has been recently introduced as a disease-modifying ℞ **antirheumatic** to treat active episodes of rheumatic arthritis. The beneficial effect does not develop until after several weeks and takes a long time to wear off.

℞ **Azathiaprine** is a powerful cytotoxic and immunosuppressant. It is mainly used to reduce tissue rejection in transplant patients, but it can also be used to treat rheumatoid arthritis. It has been investigated—with varied success—in the treatment of ✪ **ulcerative colitis**, ✪ **myasthenia gravis**, ✪ **Crohn's disease**, and ✪ **Behçet's syndrome** (especially any eye symptoms). Another drug ℞ **glatiramer acetate** is used to reduce the frequency of relapses in persons with the relapsing form of ✪ **multiple sclerosis** (MS). Although its action is not well understood, it is thought to modify the immune response to the important (nerve-insulating) substance myelin.

There is a group of recently introduced agents with immunosuppressant properties which are quite different in the way they have been designed. They are *monoclonal antibodies*, a form of pure antibody produced by molecular engineering, and are designed to react with a specific protein structure in the body to alter cellular functioning. ℞ **basiliximab** is an antibody that prevents proliferation of the white blood cells—T-lymphocytes—which have an important role in immunity and cell rejection. It is used for prophylaxis (prevention) of rejection in kidney transplantation, and is used with ℞ **cyclosporine** and ℞ **corticosteroid** drugs. The monoclonal antibody ℞ **daclizumab** has the same properties and is used for the same purpose. ℞ **rituximab** is a monoclonal antibody which causes lysis (destruction) of B lymphocytes, so effectively it can be regarded as a specific ℞ **cytotoxic** agent with defined immunosuppressant actions, and can be used to treat chemotherapy-resistant or recurrent follicular non-Hodgkin's lymphoma. ℞ **infliximab** is a monoclonal antibody that binds with, and inhibits the action of, a particular mediator substance (tumor necrosis factor alpha; TNF-alpha), which is found in unusually high levels at inflamed sites in ✪ **rheumatoid arthritis** and ✪ **Crohn's disease**. ℞ **etanercept** works in the same way and is used for the same purpose. The mouse monoclonal antibody that makes up ℞ **muromonab-CD3** is targeted to react with a specific region within T-lymphocytes, and can be used to reverse rejection following organ transplants.

Limitations
Most of these drugs are prescribed only by doctors experienced in immunosuppressive treatment and in settings equipped to monitor and manage their effects. See also the individual drug entries.

immunosuppressive Ⓓ
see ℞ immunosuppressant.

Imodium A-D Caplets; Liquid Ⓑ
A preparation of ℞ **loperamide hydrochloride**.
Formulation: Oral tablets; liquid.
Availability: OTC.
Warnings and side effects: ℞ **loperamide hydrochloride**

Imovax Rabies I.D. vaccine Ⓑ
A preparation of ℞ **rabies vaccine** (human diploid cell).
Formulation: Injection, intramuscular only; single-dose syringe.
Availability: Prescription only.
Warnings and side effects: See ℞ **rabies vaccine**.

Imovax Rabies Vaccine Ⓑ
A preparation of ℞ **rabies vaccine** (human diploid cell).
Formulation: Injection, intramuscular only.
Availability: Prescription only.
Warnings and side effects: See ℞ **rabies vaccine**.

impotence treatment Ⓓ
Generics: alprostadil; papaverine; sildenafil.
Actions and uses
Impotence treatment drugs are given to men to treat erectile dysfunction. They are ℞ **vasodilator** drugs that act on intracavernosal vessels in the penis to cause engorgement with blood, and consequently erection. The agents used formerly were given by direct intracavernosal injection into the penis or by urethral application. Such drugs include ℞ **alprostadil**, a ℞ **prostaglandin** (PGE₁), and ℞ **papaverine** (on an investigative basis). However, the recently introduced drug ℞ **sildenafil** (Viagra), a ℞ **phosphodiesterase inhibitor**, is much more convenient since it is taken by mouth.
Limitations
The injected agents are liable to cause local scaring and pain at the injection site. They are not suitable for those with anatomical deformations of the penis (for example, Peyronie's disease). Sildenafil has

marked vasodilator and ℞ **cardiac stimulant** properties. It should not be used while undergoing treatment with nitrates (for example, for heart failure or angina pectoris) because a fatal heart attack is possible. It is not suitable for those with kidney or liver function impairment, malformation of the penis, predisposition to prolonged erection (for example, in sickle-cell anemia, leukemia, multiple myeloma), serious heart disease, bleeding disorders, peptic ulcer and a number of other conditions. Careful medical counseling is necessary before use. See also the individual drug entries.

Imuran ®

A preparation of ℞ **azathiaprine**.
Formulation: Oral tablets; injection (infusion).
Availability: Prescription only.
Warnings and side effects: See ℞ **azathiaprine**.

inamrinone lactate ©

Type/Group: phosphodiesterase inhibitor; heart failure treatment; cardiac stimulant.
Brand(s): Generic.
How administered: Intravenous infusion.

Used to treat

Inamrinone lactate is used in short-term treatment of congestive ✪ **heart failure** where other drugs (for example, ℞ **digoxin**, ℞ **diuretics**, or ℞ **vasodilators**) have been unsuccessful.

Warnings

• It should not be given to people with known hypersensitivity to this drug (or to bisulfite), or who have had a recent heart attack, or certain kinds of heart valve disease.
• Inamrinone should be used during pregnancy only if the potential benefit outweighs the possible risk to the fetus.
• Medical judgment is required if breast-feeding is being considered. It is not known whether this drug appears in breast milk.
• This drug is only used in a medical facility, with close monitoring of electrolytes, fluids, and heart and kidney function. Serious arrhythmias are possible.

Interactions

No interactions of significance are known, but experience with this drug is still limited.

Side effects

• There may be irregular heartbeat, hypotension, nausea, vomiting, fever, loss of appetite or abdominal pain, and reduction in blood platelets.
• Marked changes in liver enzymes may mean stopping treatment.

Inapsine ®

A preparation of ℞ **droperidol**.
Formulation: Injection.
Availability: Prescription only.
Warnings and side effects: See ℞ **droperidol**.

indapamide ©

Type/Group: diuretic; thiazide; antihypertensive.
Brand(s): Lozol.

How administered: Orally.

Used to treat

Indapamide is used in the treatment of ✪ **hypertension**, either alone or with other types of diuretic or other drugs (for example, ℞ **beta-blockers**). It can also be used in the treatment of edema. Thiazide diuretics have also become a major part of treatment for nephrogenic ✪ **diabetes insipidus**.

Warnings

• It should not be given to people with known hypersensitivity to thiazides (or to ℞ **sulfonamide**-derived drugs), or severe kidney or liver disorders.
• It should be given with caution to elderly people, or anyone with liver or kidney impairment.
• Indapamide should be used during pregnancy only when the potential benefit outweighs the possible risk to the fetus.
• Medical judgment is required if breast-feeding is being considered.
• Early symptoms of electrolyte imbalance may include muscle weakness or cramps, nausea, vomiting, restlessness or lethargy, dry mouth, excessive thirst, fast pulse, or dizziness. A doctor must be contacted if such symptoms occur.
• Thiazides may aggravate symptoms of diabetes or gout, and worsen or activate lupus erythematosus.
• Periodic monitoring of electrolytes (particularly potassium, sodium, chloride and bicarbonate) is needed.
• Photosensitivity may develop and so precautions such as protective clothing or sunscreens should be used.
• Thiazides interact with a number of drugs, including some over-the-counter preparations. A doctor must be consulted before taking any other medications (including OTCs, herbal remedies, and supplements).

Interactions

• There is a higher risk of a hypersensitivity reaction to ℞ **allopurinol**.
• The effects of ℞ **anesthetics**, ℞ **anticancer** drugs, other antihypertensives, ℞ **diazoxide**, ⚖ **calcium** salts, ℞ **cardiac glycosides**, ℞ **lithium**, loop diuretics, ℞ **methyldopa**, nondepolarizing ℞ **skeletal muscle relaxants**, and ⚖ **vitamin D** may be increased, with the potential for significant adverse effects or toxicity. An additive effect is sometimes used to advantage in combining thiazides with other antihypertensives.
• The effects of ℞ **anticoagulants** and antigout agents (for example, ℞ **probenecid**, ℞ **sulfinpyrazone**) may be lowered by thiazides.
• The doses of ℞ **insulin** and ℞ **sulfonylureas** may need to be adjusted, as thiazides may increase blood sugar levels.
• ℞ **Amphotericin B**, ℞ **anticholinergics**, ℞ **corticosteroids**, ℞ **corticotropin**, and ℞ **MAOIs** may increase the effects of thiazides, with the possibility of significant electrolyte loss, especially potassium.
• ℞ **cholestyramine**, ℞ **colestipol hydrochloride**, ℞ **methenamine**, and ℞ **NSAIDs** (especially ℞ **indomethacin**) may reduce the effectiveness of thiazide diuretics.

• There is an increased possibility of postural hypotension (lowered blood pressure on standing) if taken with alcohol, ℞ **barbiturates**, or ℞ **opioids**.

Side effects

• There may be dizziness, headache, muscle cramps, mild gastrointestinal upsets, postural hypotension, reversible impotence, low blood potassium, sodium, magnesium and chloride, raised blood urea and glucose, and gout.

• Rarely, photosensitivity, blood disorders, skin reactions, and pancreatitis.

Inderal Tablets; Inderal LA; Injection ⑧

A preparation of ℞ **propranolol hydrochloride**.

Formulation: Oral tablets (5 strengths); sustained-release capsules (LA); injection.

Availability: Prescription only.

Warnings and side effects: See ℞ **propranolol hydrochloride**.

Inderide 40/25, 80/25 Tablets; Inderide LA 80/50, 120/50 ⑧

A preparation of ℞ **hydrochlorothiazide** and ℞ **propranolol hydrochloride**.

Formulation: Oral tablets, in two (propranolol/ hydrochlorothiazide) strengths; long-acting capsules in three strengths.

Availability: Prescription only.

Warnings and side effects: See ℞ **hydrochlorothiazide**; ℞ **propranolol hydrochloride**.

indinavir ⑥

Type/Group: **antiviral**.

Brand(s): Crixivan.

How administered: Orally.

Used to treat

Indinavir is a protease inhibitor antiviral used as an antiretroviral drug often together with reverse transcriptase antivirals in the treatment of ✺ **HIV** infection.

Warnings

• It should not be given to people with known hypersensitivity to indinavir.

• It should be given with caution to people with kidney and liver function impairment, who are dehydrated, or children.

• Indinavir's safety during pregnancy has not been established, and it should be used only when the potential benefits clearly outweigh the possible risks to the fetus.

• HIV-infected mothers are advised not to breast-feed.

• Kidney disease may occur.

• It is a specialist drug, and there will be full assessment and patient monitoring throughout treatment.

• Grapefruit juice and meals high in fat can reduce the absorption of indinavir.

Interactions

• ℞ **rifampin** must not be used with indinavir, because it reduces the effects of indinavir.

• The effects of ℞ **barbiturates**, ℞ **carbamazepine**, ℞ **phenytoin**, and ℞ **rifabutin** are increased while the effects of indinavir are decreased.

• The effects and levels of ℞ **clarithromycin**, ℞ **ergot alkaloids**, ℞ **lovastatin**, ℞ **midazolam**, ℞ **ritonavir**, ℞ **saquinavir**, ℞ **simvastatin**, and ℞ **triazolam** may be increased.

• Delavirdine, ℞ **ketoconazole**, and ℞ **nelfinavir** may increase the levels of indinavir.

• If taken with ℞ **erythromycin**, the effects of both drugs may be reduced.

• If taken with ℞ **nevirapine**, the levels of indinavir may be reduced.

Side effects

• Frequently, gastrointestinal effects (especially nausea) and headache.

• Occasionally, muscle pain, fatigue, insomnia, and accumulation of fat on the waist, abdomen, or back of the neck.

• Rarely, abnormal taste sensation, heartburn, urinary tract disease, and transient kidney dysfunction.

Indocin; Indocin SR; Oral Suspension; Suppositories ⑧

A preparation of ℞ **indomethacin**.

Formulation: Oral liquid; capsules (two strengths); SR is sustained release capsule; rectal suppositories.

Availability: Prescription only.

Warnings and side effects: See ℞ **indomethacin**.

indometacin ⑥

see ℞ **indomethacin**.

indomethacin ⑥

(indometacin)

Type/Group: **anti-inflammatory; antirheumatic; non-narcotic analgesic; NSAID**.

Brand(s): Indocin, Indocin SR, Oral Suspension, Suppositories; various generic.

How administered: Orally; topically (rectal suppositories); injection.

Used to treat

Indomethacin is used to treat ✺ **osteoarthritis**, acute gouty ✺ **arthritis**, ✺ **ankylosing spondylitis**, ✺ **rheumatoid arthritis**, ✺ **bursitis**, and tendonitis. Most of its proprietary preparations are not normally given to children, but one form is used (under specialist supervision with extensive monitoring) in premature babies who have patent ductus arteriosus (failure of this connecting vessel between the pulmonary artery and aorta to close after birth). Although not stated by the manufacturer, it is sometimes used for many other inflammatory and painful disorders.

Warnings

• It should not be used by anyone with known hypersensitivity to this drug or to other NSAIDs (including ℞ **aspirin**), who have epilepsy, chronic kidney disease, certain bleeding disorders or conditions (for example, hemophilia, vitamin K deficiency, low blood-platelet levels), or who have a tendency to, or active, peptic ulceration.

• It should be given with caution to people taking certain drugs for diabetes mellitus, with epilepsy, parkinsonism, psychiatric disturbances, or with allergic disorders (especially asthma and skin conditions), who are elderly, or with any kind of kidney impairment or with certain liver disorders.

• Indomethacin should not be used during pregnancy, and especially not during the third trimester.

• Breast-feeding mothers should either discontinue this drug or stop breast-feeding.

• With regular, long-term use (as in the treatment of osteoarthritis), NSAIDs may cause gastrointestinal bleeding, ulceration, or perforation. Any signs of bleeding (for example, black stools) should be reported to a physician immediately.

• Most NSAIDs have the potential, particularly with regular use, to cause liver damage. Periodic evaluation of liver function is necessary in long-term therapy (more than two months).

• Side effects are more frequent in the elderly.

• Gastrointestinal upsets may be minimized by taking it with milk or food.

Interactions

• There is generally no added benefit in taking other NSAIDs (especially ℞ **diflunisal**) or other ℞ **salicylates** (especially aspirin) at the same time, but there is a higher risk of gastrointestinal upsets and bleeding.

• Alcohol and ℞ **corticosteroids** increase the risk of bleeding, particularly if there is an existing ulcer.

• ℞ **anticoagulant**, ℞ **antiplatelet**, and ℞ **thrombolytic** drugs may increase bleeding time.

• Indomethacin may reduce the effectiveness of ℞ **diuretics** (for example, ℞ **furosemide**), ℞ **ACE inhibitors**, and ℞ **beta-blockers**.

• It should not be taken with ℞ **triamterene** because there is a risk of kidney failure.

• The effects of ℞ **cyclosporine**, ℞ **digoxin**, ℞ **lithium**, ℞ **methotrexate**, and penicillamine may be exaggerated, with potential for toxicity.

• Indomethacin should be started at a low dose when used with ℞ **probenecid** for treating gout, because probenecid increases its concentration and effect.

• Foodstuffs and herbals with ℞ **antiplatelet** properties, for example, ♣ **ginger**, ⚕ **garlic**, and various herbal preparations, may add to the antiplatelet effect of NSAIDs.

Side effects

These depend on how administered, dose, duration of treatment, and use.

• Commonly, headache, dizziness, gastrointestinal upsets, flatulence, or nausea.

• Less frequently there may be vomiting, diarrhea, constipation, mood swings, malaise, ringing in the ears, edema, fatigue, blurred vision, or changes in blood pressure.

• Prolonged bleeding time (with consequent risk of ulceration) is possible with high dosage, and other blood changes can occur, including anemia.

• Hypersensitivity reactions may include symptoms such as hives, chest tightness, asthma, or bronchospasm.

• Reversible kidney failure, particularly in renal impairment, has occurred. Liver damage is rare.

Infanrix ℞

A preparation of ℞ **diphtheria and tetanus toxoids and acellular pertussis vaccine (DTaP)**.

Formulation: Injection.

Availability: Prescription only.

Warnings and side effects: See ℞ **diphtheria and tetanus toxoids and acellular pertussis vaccine (DTaP)**.

InFeD ℞

A preparation of ℞ **iron dextran**.

Formulation: Injection.

Availability: Prescription only.

Warnings and side effects: ℞ **iron dextran**

Infergen ℞

A preparation of ℞ **interferon** alfacon-1.

Formulation: Injection.

Availability: Prescription only.

Warnings and side effects: See ℞ **interferons**.

infertility treatment ⓓ

Generics: chorionic gonadotropin; clomiphene citrate; follitropin alfa/follitropin beta; gonadorelin; menotropins; progesterone; urofollitropin.

Actions and uses

Drugs for infertility are used to treat couples who are unable to conceive. Infertility can result from defects in hormonal release or action, and functional and organic disorders in the man or the woman. Drugs are used in a variety of ways depending on the reason for infertility. Some forms of ℞ **gonadotropin** hormones (℞ **urofollitropin**, ℞ **menotropins**, ℞ **follitropin alfa/follitropin beta**, and ℞ **chorionic gonadotropin**) are administered for 7–10 days to correct a lack of ovulation which is of pituitary origin, whether as part of assisted conception (such as in *in vitro* fertilization, IVF, or assisted reproductive technology therapy, ART) or natural fertilization. Usually ℞ **clomiphene** is tried first or used with gonadotropins. Gonadotropins can also be taken by subfertile men to stimulate sperm production.

℞ **clomiphene citrate** is a sex ℞ **hormone antagonist** (an ℞ **antiestrogen**) which is used as a fertility treatment in women whose condition is linked to the persistent presence of estrogens and a consequent failure to ovulate (characterized by sparse or infrequent periods). It prevents the action of estrogens and this increases the secretion of gonadotrophins, which cause ovulation. It is also sometimes used by infertile men.

Gonadotropin-releasing hormone (LH-RH), in its synthetic drug form ℞ **gonadorelin** (or sometimes as synthetic chemical analogs), when initially given by injection causes the pituitary gland to release the gonadotropins, but with continued use suppresses their production. Both uses may form part of diagnosis or treatment of infertility in women, including as part of ART.

This natural ℞ **progestin** ℞ **progesterone** is sometimes used to treat luteal phase deficiency (inadequate production of progesterone during the luteal phase of menstruation) in women undergoing (ART).

Limitations

Most of these hormone preparations are complex peptides that cannot be given by mouth and must normally be given by injection over a period (although some synthetic analogs can now be taken by nasal spray, which allows absorption into the circulation from the nasal mucosa). The induction of ovulation and pregnancy is only carried out in carefully assessed people, in whom infertility is not caused by primary ovarian failure, and also in assisted conception (such as in *in vitro* fertilization; IVF). Although the procedure is often successful, there may be overstimulation of the ovary and the risk of multiple births is markedly increased. There may also be allergic reactions. See also the individual drug entries and ℞ **impotence treatment**.

Inflamase Mild; Inflamase Forte ⓑ

A preparation of ℞ **prednisolone**.
Formulation: Eye drops in two strengths (Forte is stronger).
Availability: Prescription only.
Warnings and side effects: See ℞ **prednisolone**.

infliximab ⓖ

Type/Group: **anti-inflammatory; antirheumatic**.
Brand(s): Remicade.
How administered: Injection.

Used to treat

Infliximab is used, usually in combination with ℞ **methotrexate**, in the treatment of ⊙ **rheumatoid arthritis** and (in very limited dosage) ⊙ **Crohn's disease**. Infliximab belongs to a relatively new class of drug, those copied directly—or cloned—from substances occurring naturally in the body. It is a monoclonal antibody: a biologically engineered version of an antibody with a specific human region (as well as a mouse sequence). This antibody binds with and inhibits the action of a particular mediator substance (tumor necrosis factor alpha; TNF-alpha) which is found in unusually high levels at inflamed sites in rheumatoid arthritis and Crohn's disease.

Warnings

• It should not be given to people with known hypersensitivity to this drug or to any product prepared with mouse protein. It should not be given to anyone with a significant, active infection.

• It should be given with caution to people with a history of chronic infection.

• The effects of infliximab in pregnancy are not known and it should be used only if clearly necessary.

• Medical judgment is required if breast-feeding is being considered.

• This is a specialist drug, a full assessment for suitability and monitoring will be carried out.

• Autoantibodies (antibodies to "self") may form with use of infliximab; this drug should be discontinued if any lupus-like symptoms are observed.

• Antibodies to infliximab may also form; which may make an "infusion reaction" more likely with subsequent doses. (But persons already taking immunosuppressant drugs may experience fewer adverse reactions.)

• Risk of infections, some potentially serious, may be higher with use of infliximab.

Interactions

• Live ℞ **vaccines** must not be given during treatment with infliximab.

Side effects

• More frequent side effects may include headache, rash, abdominal pain, or fatigue.

• Within a few hours of taking infliximab there may be an infusion reaction, with symptoms such as fever, chills, hypotension, breathlessness, chest pain, itching or hives.

• Upper respiratory infections, with symptoms such as coughing, sinusitis and sore throat, may become more frequent.

influenza virus vaccine ⓖ

Type/Group: **vaccine**.
Brand(s): Fluogen; FluShield; Fluzone.
How administered: Intramuscular injection.

Used to treat

Influenza virus vaccine is used for ℞ **immunization** to help protect people from catching ⊙ **influenza**. It is recommended for anyone wishing to reduce the chances of coming down with the flu, but particularly for people at risk of complications from flu infection, such as the elderly, asthmatics, diabetics, those with chronic heart or kidney disease, or women who will be in the second or third trimester of pregnancy during the flu season. It is also recommended for health professionals, who might expose a more vulnerable population to infection. The immunity conferred by this vaccine is highly variable: unlike some viruses, the influenza viruses A and B are constantly changing in physical form and antibodies manufactured in the body to deal with one strain at one time will not necessarily be effective on the same strain at another time. For this reason, influenza vaccine is reformulated each year to be effective against the virus strains thought most likely to cause infection.

Warnings

• Because this vaccine is prepared from virus strains grown in chicken embryos, it should not be given to people with known sensitivity to eggs. It should not be administered to those with ⊙ **Guillain-Barré syndrome** (GBS) unless potential benefit (to someone at high risk of flu complications) outweighs potential risk. If possible, its use should be postponed for someone with an existing moderate-to-severe febrile illness.

• It should be used during pregnancy only when medically judged to be clearly needed.

• Medical judgment is required if breast-feeding is being considered.

• Fewer side effects, especially in children, have been reported in the use of vaccines prepared from virus parts ("split-virus") rather than from whole virus.

• After administration, people will be required to wait for some time to ensure that there is no serious reaction (such as anaphylaxis).

Interactions

• ℞ **Immunosuppressants** may reduce the effectiveness of the vaccine and additional does may be needed.

• Caution is required if ℞ **anticoagulants** are being taken.

Side effects

• Most of the side effects are mild, the most severe reactions generally occurring in those with an undetected allergy to chicken eggs.

• There may be swelling, irritation or tenderness at the site of vaccination, and headache, nausea, fever, or malaise.

• Infrequently, skin rash, hives, itching, swelling of lymph glands, and achy joints.

Infumorph ℞

A preparation of ℞ **morphine sulfate**.
Formulation: Injection, available in two strengths.
Availability: Prescription only.
Warnings and side effects: ℞ **morphine sulfate**

InnoGel Plus ℞

A preparation of ℞ **pyrethrin**.
Formulation: Topical gel.
Availability: OTC.
Warnings and side effects: See ℞ pyrethrin.

Insta-Glucose ℞

A preparation of ℞ **glucose**.
Formulation: Oral gel.
Availability: OTC.
Warnings and side effects: See ℞ glucose.

insulin, human regular and human NPH mixture ⓖ

see ℞ insulin, regular and isophane mixture.

insulin, isophane suspension (insulin, NPH) ⓖ

(NPH: isophane protamine insulin; isophane insulin suspension (NPH: isophane protamine insulin))
Type/Group: **antidiabetic; insulin analog**.
Brand(s): NPH Iletin I; NPH-N; NPH Iletin II; Humulin N; Novolin N; Novolin N PenFill; Novolin N Prefilled.
How administered: Injection.

Used to treat

It is used to maintain people with ⊙ **diabetes mellitus**. It is a form of highly purified bovine, porcine or human insulin, prepared as a sterile complex with protamine. Its effects last for an intermediate length of time.

Warnings

• It should not be given to people who have previously been using another form of insulin, without medical supervision. Any changes in insulin must be made with caution.

• It should be given with caution to people with kidney impairment.

• It should be used during pregnancy only if it is clearly needed.

• Medical judgment is required if breast-feeding is being considered (dose adjustment may be required).

• Expert counseling and training, and blood-glucose monitoring is required because individuals must maintain a stable blood-glucose level over long periods. The choice of suitable preparations, or combinations of preparations, may take some time to establish.

• Excessive alcohol use may cause hypoglycemia (low glucose levels in the blood).

• Cigarette smoking and marijuana may increase glucose levels.

Interactions

• ℞ **Beta-blockers** may mask the signs and symptoms of hypoglycemia.

• ℞ **Anabolic steroids** have variable effects on blood glucose levels.

• The following drugs may increase blood glucose levels or mask symptoms of hypoglycemia: ℞ **calcium-channel blockers**; ℞ **corticosteroids**; ℞ **isoniazid**; ℞ **oral contraceptives**; ℞ **estrogens**; ℞ **phenothiazines**; ℞ **thyroid hormone**, ℞ **sympathomimetics** (for example, ℞ **epinephrine**); ℞ **thiazide** ℞ **diuretics**; ℞ **furosemide**; ℞ **ethacrynic acid**; ℞ **lipid-regulating drugs** (for example, ℞ **niacin**).

• Other antidiabetic drugs, ℞ **sulfonamides**, ℞ **salicylates**, ℞ **ACE inhibitors**, ℞ **MAOI** antidepressants, ℞ **octreotide**, ℞ **tetracyclines**, and ℞ **guanethidine monosulfate** decrease blood glucose levels.

Side effects

• Hypoglycemia, and there may also be allergic reactions.

insulin, regular ⓖ

Type/Group: **antidiabetic; insulin analog**.
Brand(s): Regular Iletin I; Regular Iletin II; Regular Purified Pork Insulin; Novolin R; Velosulin Human BR; Novolin R PenFill; Novolin R Prefilled; Humulin-R.
How administered: Injection.

Used to treat

Insulin, regular is used to maintain people with ⊙ **diabetes mellitus**. It is a form of highly purified bovine, porcine or human insulin injection, prepared as a sterile complex with zinc salts. It takes effect relatively rapidly and lasts for a relatively short length of time.

Warnings

• It should not be given to people who have previously been using another form of insulin, without medical supervision. Any changes in insulin must be made with caution.

• It should be given with caution to people with kidney impairment.

• It should be used during pregnancy only if it is clearly needed.

• Medical judgment is required if breast-feeding is being considered (dose adjustment may be required).

Key to symbols: ⊙ = Disorder Section ℞ = Drug Section ♣ = Herbal Section ⟐ = Supplement Section

• Expert counseling and training, and blood-glucose monitoring is required because patients must maintain a stable blood-glucose level over long periods. The choice of suitable preparations, or combinations of preparations, may take some time to establish.

• Excessive alcohol use may cause hypoglycemia (low glucose levels in the blood).

• Cigarette smoking and marijuana may increase glucose levels.

Interactions

• ℞ **Beta-blockers** may mask the signs and symptoms of hypoglycemia.

• ℞ **Anabolic steroids** have variable effects on blood glucose levels.

• The following drugs may increase blood glucose levels or mask symptoms of hypoglycemia: ℞ **calcium-channel blockers**; ℞ **corticosteroids**; ℞ **isoniazid**; ℞ **oral contraceptives**; ℞ **estrogens**; ℞ **phenothiazines**; ℞ **thyroid hormone**, ℞ **sympathomimetics** (for example, ℞ **epinephrine**); ℞ **thiazide** ℞ **diuretics**; ℞ **furosemide**; ℞ **ethacrynic acid**; ℞ **lipid-regulating drugs** (for example, ℞ **niacin**).

• Other antidiabetic drugs, ℞ **sulfonamides**, ℞ **salicylates**, ℞ **ACE inhibitors**, ℞ **MAOI** antidepressants, ℞ **octreotide**, ℞ **tetracyclines**, and ℞ **guanethidine monosulfate** decrease blood glucose levels.

Side effects

Hypoglycemia (too little glucose in the blood). There may also be allergic reactions.

insulin, regular and isophane mixture ⓖ

(insulin, human regular and human NPH mixture; insulin mixture (isophane insulin suspension and insulin regular))

Type/Group: **antidiabetic; insulin analog.**

Brand(s): Humulin 70/30; Novolin 70/30; Novolin 70/30 PenFill; Novolin 70/30 Prefilled; Humulin 50/50.

How administered: Injection.

Used to treat

Insulin, regular and isophane mixture is used to maintain people with ⊙ **diabetes mellitus**. It is a form of purified insulin which is prepared as a sterile buffered suspension of porcine insulin complexed with protamine in a solution of porcine insulin, or human insulin complex in a solution of human insulin. Its effects last for an intermediate length of time.

Warnings

• It should not be given to people who have previously been using another form of insulin, without medical supervision. Any changes in insulin must be made with caution.

• It should be given with caution to people with kidney impairment.

• It should be used during pregnancy only if it is clearly needed.

• Medical judgment is required if breast-feeding is being considered (dose adjustment may be required).

• Expert counseling and training, and blood-glucose monitoring is required because patients must maintain a stable blood-glucose level over long periods. The choice of suitable preparations, or combinations of preparations, may take some time to establish.

• Excessive alcohol use may cause hypoglycemia (low glucose levels in the blood).

• Cigarette smoking and marijuana may increase glucose levels.

Interactions

• ℞ **Beta-blockers** may mask the signs and symptoms of hypoglycemia.

• ℞ **Anabolic steroids** have variable effects on blood glucose levels.

• The following drugs may increase blood glucose levels or mask symptoms of hypoglycemia: ℞ **calcium-channel blockers**; ℞ **corticosteroids**; ℞ **isoniazid**; ℞ **oral contraceptives**; ℞ **estrogens**; ℞ **phenothiazines**; ℞ **thyroid hormone**, ℞ **sympathomimetics** (for example, ℞ **epinephrine**); ℞ **thiazide** ℞ **diuretics**; ℞ **furosemide**; ℞ **ethacrynic acid**; ℞ **lipid-regulating drugs** (for example, ℞ **niacin**).

• Other antidiabetic drugs, ℞ **sulfonamides**, ℞ **salicylates**, ℞ **ACE inhibitors**, ℞ **MAOI** antidepressants, ℞ **octreotide**, ℞ **tetracyclines**, and ℞ **guanethidine monosulfate** decrease blood glucose levels.

Side effects

• Hypoglycemia, and there may also be allergic reactions.

insulin ⓓ

Insulin is a hormone with an important role in regulating glucose in the body. It is secreted into the bloodstream in pulses every 15 to 30 minutes by the B-cells of the islets of Langerhans in the pancreas gland. Because it is released into the bloodstream it acts on target cells throughout the body. Insulin causes uptake of glucose into cells, which is then stored in another form, such as glycogen. This process lowers blood glucose in the short-term, but maintains it at safe levels in the long-term.

Good control of blood-glucose levels is achieved with the aid of two other pancreatic hormones: amylin (also secreted by the B-cells); and ℞ **glucagon** (secreted by the A-cells of the pancreas). These two hormones oppose the action of insulin, that is, they tend to increase blood glucose by stimulating the breakdown of glycogen and by other means.

In a normal healthy person, very fine control of blood glucose is normally achieved because the pancreas is sensitive to levels of glucose in the blood. However, in ⊙ **diabetes mellitus**, glucose is not stored efficiently and so is wasted, and is removed in the urine with water with it (which causes the characteristic frequent urination, body wastage, weight loss and other symptoms of diabetes). This disease is due either to the secretion of insulin being decreased (type 1 "juvenile-onset" diabetes mellitus) or by the tissues becoming unresponsive to insulin (type 2 "adult-onset" diabetes mellitus). Type 1 diabetes mellitus is treated with diet and by injections of a variety of forms of insulin (see the ℞ **insulin analog** entry). Type 2 diabetes mellitus is treated with diet and ℞ **oral hypoglycemic drugs**.

insulin analog ⓓ

Generics: **insulin, regular; insulin analog (lispro); insulin aspart recombinant; insulin lispro and insulin lispro protamine; insulin, regular and isophane mixture; insulin, isophane** suspension (insulin, NPH); insulin glargine; insulin zinc suspension (lente).

Actions and uses

Insulin analog drugs are used in ℞ **antidiabetic** (✪ **diabetes mellitus**) treatment. Mainly in the control of blood glucose (sugar) levels in type 1 ✪ **diabetes mellitus** (insulin-dependent diabetes mellitus; IDDM; juvenile-onset diabetes), or type 2 diabetes mellitus when ℞ **oral hypoglycemic** agents are no longer adequate.

There are numerous preparations of insulin available, all of which have to be injected, and these can be grouped in various ways. In origin, some are from bovine or porcine sources, and newer ones of human form are now available. The effects of human insulin tends to be quicker in onset (that is, it quickly starts working) and it generally has a shorter duration of action. The most important property when choosing an insulin preparation is its duration of action. Those with a longer duration require less frequent injection. The rate of onset of action is more important when insulin needs to be injected to quickly control raised blood glucose levels. Often the individual advantages of two different insulins can be combined by mixing them, and preparations of mixed insulins are available. Some are packaged in vials, some in preloaded syringes. The properties of the main types of insulin available at the time of writing, are summarized as follows, and some of these are only recently available, displacing others.

Rapid acting and/or short duration versions are: ℞ **insulin, regular** is a highly purified bovine, porcine or human insulin, prepared as a complex with zinc salts, and it takes effect relatively rapidly (0.5–1 hour) and has a relatively short duration of action (8–12 hours); ℞ **insulin analog (lispro)** is a recombinant (DNA technology) human insulin analog with a rapid onset of action; ℞ **insulin aspart recombinant** is a human insulin analog that has a rapid onset and a short duration of action.

Intermediate acting: ℞ **insulin lispro and insulin lispro protamine** is a recombinant human insulin analog (lispro). It is a biphasic form (containing mixed insulin analog lispro and insulin analog lispro protamine, which have different rates of onset and offset of action) and has an intermediate duration of action; ℞ **insulin, regular and isophane mixture** is a form of purified porcine insulin complexed with protamine in a solution of porcine insulin, or human insulin complex in a solution of human insulin. It has an intermediate duration of action; ℞ **insulin, isophane suspension (insulin, NPH)** is a form of highly purified bovine, porcine or human insulin, prepared as a complex with protamine. It has an intermediate duration of action (up to 24 hours).

Long acting: ℞ **insulin glargine** is a recombinant human insulin analog that has a intermediate to long duration of action; ℞ **insulin zinc suspension (lente)** is a form of highly purified bovine and/or porcine insulin or human insulin, prepared as a sterile neutral complex with zinc salts. It has a long duration of action (up to 24 hours). A similar form is *extended insulin zinc suspension,* a preparation of human insulin zinc suspension with an even longer duration of action (more than 36 hours).

Limitations

Nearly two million people in the US suffer from insulin-dependent diabetes mellitus, and considerable efforts are being made to develop insulin preparations that are more effective, more convenient to use, and safe to use. The material from bovine or porcine sources that traditionally has been used is being replaced or augmented with recombinant human form insulin (insulin, a protein is made up of amino acids and actually some recombinant forms do differ chemically but only in one amino acid) due to progress in the techniques of molecular biology for the manufacture of proteins. An advantage of the human form is that it is less likely to cause the production of antibodies compared to those forms of animal origin which the body may treat as foreign bodies—although it is not yet clear to what extent it is better. This is important because it is this antibody development with chronic usage of insulin that is thought to lie behind sensitivity reactions and the development of insulin resistance.

Insulin preparations have to be injected because insulin is a protein that would be digested in the same way as dietary protein if taken by mouth. Advances have been made in producing preparations of insulin that last longer (by complexing it with zinc or protamine, using microcrystals and so forth), or are more convenient to inject (preloaded syringes). Efforts are being made to develop a system that can inject insulin rapidly into the skin as a powder, or forms that can be absorbed from a nasal or buccal spray (where it is absorbed between the cheek and teeth or gums).

See also the individual drug entries.

insulin analog (lispro)   Ⓖ

Type/Group: **antidiabetic; insulin analog.**
Brand(s): Humalog.
How administered: Injection.

Used to treat

Insulin analog (lispro) is used to maintain people with ✪ **diabetes mellitus**. It is a recombinant (DNA technology) human insulin analog, which takes effect rapidly and lasts for a relatively short length of time.

Warnings

• It should not be given to people who have previously been using another form of insulin, without medical supervision.

• It should be given with caution to people with kidney impairment. Any changes in insulin must be made with caution.

• Insulin analog (lispro) should be used during pregnancy only if it is clearly needed.

• Medical judgment is required if breast-feeding (dose adjustment may be required).

• Expert counseling, initial training, and blood-glucose monitoring is required, because the person must maintain a stable blood-glucose level over long periods. The choice of suitable preparations, or combinations of preparations, may take some time to establish.

• Excessive alcohol use may cause hypoglycemia (low glucose levels in the blood).

• Cigarette smoking and marijuana may increase glucose levels.

Interactions

• ℞ **Beta-blockers** may mask the signs and symptoms of hypoglycemia.

• ℞ **Anabolic steroids** have variable effects on blood glucose levels.

• The following drugs may increase blood glucose levels or mask symptoms of hypoglycemia: ℞ **calcium-channel blockers;** ℞ **corticosteroids;** ℞ **isoniazid;** ℞ **oral contraceptives;** ℞ **estrogens;** ℞ **phenothiazines;** ℞ **thyroid hormone,** ℞ **sympathomimetics** (for example, ℞ **epinephrine**); ℞ **thiazide** ℞ **diuretics;** ℞ **furosemide;** ℞ **ethacrynic acid;** ℞ **lipid-regulating drugs** (for example, ℞ **niacin**).

• Other antidiabetic drugs, ℞ **sulfonamides,** ℞ **salicylates,** ℞ **ACE inhibitors,** ℞ **MAOI** antidepressants, ℞ **octreotide,** ℞ **tetracyclines,** and ℞ **guanethidine monosulfate** decrease blood glucose levels.

Side effects
• Hypoglycemia, and there may also be allergic reactions.

insulin analog lispro and insulin analog protamine ⓖ
see ℞ insulin lispro and insulin lispro protamine.

insulin analog lispro mixture ⓖ
see ℞ insulin lispro and insulin lispro protamine.

insulin aspart recombinant ⓖ
Type/Group: **antidiabetic; insulin analog.**
Brand(s): NovoLog.
How administered: Injection.

Used to treat
It is used to maintain people with ⊙ **diabetes mellitus** by controlling hyperglycemia (too much glucose in the blood). Insulin aspart is a human insulin analog which takes effect rapidly and has a short duration of action.

Warnings
• It should not be given to people with known hypersensitivity to insulin aspart or any of its constituents, or anyone experiencing an episode of hypoglycemia. Anyone who has previously been using another form of insulin should not use without medical supervision. Any changes in insulin must be made with caution.

• It should be given with caution to people with kidney or liver impairment.

• It should be used during pregnancy only if it is clearly needed.

• Medical judgment is required if breast-feeding is being considered (dose adjustment may be required).

• Because it takes effect so rapidly, the injection of insulin aspart should immediately be followed by a meal.

• Because of the short duration of action, people with type 1 diabetes also require a longer-acting insulin to maintain adequate glucose control.

• Expert counseling and training, and blood-glucose monitoring is required because patients must maintain a stable blood-glucose level over long periods. The choice of suitable preparations, or combinations of preparations, may take some time to establish.

• Excessive alcohol use may cause hypoglycemia (low levels of glucose in the blood).

Interactions
• ℞ **Beta-blockers** may mask the signs and symptoms of hypoglycemia.

• ℞ **Anabolic steroids** have variable effects on blood glucose levels.

• The following drugs may increase blood glucose levels or mask symptoms of hypoglycemia: ℞ **calcium-channel blockers;** ℞ **corticosteroids;** ℞ **isoniazid;** ℞ **oral contraceptives;** ℞ **estrogens;** ℞ **phenothiazines;** ℞ **thyroid hormone,** ℞ **sympathomimetics** (for example, ℞ **epinephrine**); ℞ **thiazide** ℞ **diuretics;** ℞ **furosemide;** ℞ **ethacrynic acid;** ℞ **lipid-regulating drugs** (for example, ℞ **niacin**).

• Other antidiabetic drugs, ℞ **sulfonamides,** ℞ **salicylates,** ℞ **ACE inhibitors,** ℞ **MAOI** antidepressants, ℞ **octreotide,** ℞ **tetracyclines,** and ℞ **guanethidine monosulfate** decrease blood glucose levels.

Side effects
• Hypoglycemia, and there may also be allergic reactions.

insulin glargine ⓖ
Type/Group: **antidiabetic; insulin analog.**
Brand(s): Lantus.
How administered: Injection.

Used to treat
It is used to maintain people with ⊙ **diabetes mellitus** by controlling hyperglycemia (too much glucose in the blood). Insulin glargine is a recombinant (DNA technology) human insulin analog. Its effects last for up to 24 hours.

Warnings
• It should not be given to people who have previously been using another form of insulin, without medical supervision. Any changes in insulin must be made with caution.

• It should be given with caution to people with kidney impairment.

• It should be used during pregnancy only if it is clearly needed.

• Medical judgment is required if breast-feeding is being considered (dose adjustment may be required).

• Expert counseling and training, and blood-glucose monitoring is required because patients must maintain a stable blood-glucose level over long periods. The choice of suitable preparations, or combinations of preparations, may take some time to establish.

• Excessive alcohol use may cause hypoglycemia (low levels of glucose in the blood).

• Do not mix with another insulin solution.

Interactions
• ℞ **Beta-blockers** may mask the signs and symptoms of hypoglycemia.

• ℞ **Anabolic steroids** have variable effects on blood glucose levels.

• The following drugs may increase blood glucose levels or mask symptoms of hypoglycemia: ℞ **calcium-channel blockers;** ℞ **corticosteroids;** ℞ **isoniazid;** ℞ **oral contraceptives;** ℞ **estrogens;** ℞ **phenothiazines;** ℞ **thyroid hormone,** ℞ **sympathomimetics** (for example, ℞ **epinephrine**); ℞ **thiazide** ℞ **diuretics;** ℞ **furosemide;** ℞ **ethacrynic acid;** ℞ **lipid-regulating drugs** (for example, ℞ **niacin**).

• Other antidiabetic drugs, ℞ **sulfonamides,** ℞ **salicylates,** ℞ **ACE inhibitors,** ℞ **MAOI** antidepressants, ℞ **octreotide,**

℞ tetracyclines, and ℞ **guanethidine monosulfate** decrease blood glucose levels.

Side effects

• Hypoglycemia, and there may also be allergic reactions.

insulin lispro and insulin lispro protamine Ⓖ

(insulin analog (lispro) mixture; insulin analog (lispro) and insulin (analog) protamine)

Type/Group: **antidiabetic; insulin analog**.

Brand(s): Humalog Mix 75/25.

How administered: Injection.

Used to treat

Insulin lispro and insulin lispro protamine is used to maintain people with ❂ **diabetes mellitus**. It is a recombinant (DNA technology) human insulin analog (lispro). It is a biphasic form (containing mixed insulin analog lispro and insulin analog lispro protamine, which have different rates of onset and offset of action) and its effects last for an intermediate length of time.

Warnings

• It should not be given to people who have been using another form of insulin, without medical supervision. Any changes in insulin must be made with caution.

• It should be used with caution by anyone with kidney impairment.

• It should be used during pregnancy only if it is clearly needed.

• Medical judgment is required if breast-feeding is being considered (dose adjustment may be required).

• Expert counseling and training, and blood-glucose monitoring is required because people must maintain a stable blood-glucose level over long periods. The choice of suitable preparations, or combinations of preparations, may take some time to establish.

• Excessive alcohol use may cause hypoglycemia (low glucose levels in the blood).

• Cigarette smoking and marijuana may increase glucose levels.

Interactions

• ℞ **Beta-blockers** may mask the signs and symptoms of hypoglycemia.

• ℞ **Anabolic steroids** have variable effects on blood glucose levels.

• The following drugs may increase blood glucose levels or mask symptoms of hypoglycemia: ℞ **calcium-channel blockers**; ℞ **corticosteroids**; ℞ **isoniazid**; ℞ **oral contraceptives**; ℞ **estrogens**; ℞ **phenothiazines**; ℞ **thyroid hormone**, ℞ **sympathomimetics** (for example, ℞ **epinephrine**); ℞ **thiazide diuretics**; ℞ **furosemide**; ℞ **ethacrynic acid**; ℞ **lipid-regulating drugs** (for example, ℞ **niacin**).

• Other antidiabetic drugs, ℞ **sulfonamides**, ℞ **salicylates**, ℞ **ACE inhibitors**, ℞ **MAOI** antidepressants, ℞ **octreotide**, ℞ **tetracyclines**, and ℞ **guanethidine monosulfate** decrease blood glucose levels.

Side effects

• Hypoglycemia, and there may also be allergic reactions.

insulin mixture isophane Ⓖ

Full name: **insulin mixture isophane insulin suspension and insulin regular**

see ℞ **insulin, regular and isophane mixture**.

Insulin Reaction Ⓑ

A preparation of ℞ **glucose**.

Formulation: Oral gel.

Availability: OTC.

Warnings and side effects: See ℞ **glucose**.

insulin zinc suspension (lente) Ⓖ

Type/Group: **antidiabetic; insulin analog**.

How administered: Injection.

Brand(s): Lente Iletin II; Lente L; Humulin L; Humulin U Ultralente; Novolin L.

Used to treat

It is used to maintain people with ❂ **diabetes mellitus**. It is a form of highly purified bovine and/or porcine insulin or human insulin, prepared as a sterile neutral complex with zinc salts. Its effects last a long time. A further form is extended insulin zinc suspension (Ultralente), a preparation of human insulin zinc suspension with an even longer duration of action.

Warnings

• It should not be given to people who have previously been using another form of insulin, without medical supervision. Any changes in insulin must be made with caution.

• It should be given with caution to people with kidney impairment.

• It should be used during pregnancy only if it is clearly needed.

• Medical judgment is required if breast-feeding is being considered (dose adjustment may be required).

• Expert counseling and training, and blood-glucose monitoring is required because patients must maintain a stable blood-glucose level over long periods. The choice of suitable preparations, or combinations of preparations, may take some time to establish.

• Excessive alcohol use may cause hypoglycemia (low glucose levels in the blood).

• Cigarette smoking and marijuana may increase glucose levels.

Interactions

• ℞ **Beta-blockers** may mask the signs and symptoms of hypoglycemia.

• ℞ **Anabolic steroids** have variable effects on blood glucose levels.

• The following drugs may increase blood glucose levels or mask symptoms of hypoglycemia: ℞ **calcium-channel blockers**; ℞ **corticosteroids**; ℞ **isoniazid**; ℞ **oral contraceptives**; ℞ **estrogens**; ℞ **phenothiazines**; ℞ **thyroid hormone**, ℞ **sympathomimetics** (for example, ℞ **epinephrine**); ℞ **thiazide diuretics**; ℞ **furosemide**; ℞ **ethacrynic acid**; ℞ **lipid-regulating drugs** (for example, ℞ **niacin**).

• Other antidiabetic drugs, ℞ **sulfonamides**, ℞ **salicylates**, ℞ **ACE inhibitors**, ℞ **MAOI** antidepressants, ℞ **octreotide**, ℞ **tetracyclines**, and ℞ **guanethidine monosulfate** decrease blood glucose levels.

Side effects
• Hypoglycemia, and there may also be allergic reactions.

Intal ®

A preparation of ℞ **cromolyn sodium**.
Formulation: Aerosol spray; solution for nebulizer.
Availability: Prescription only.
Warnings and side effects: See ℞ **cromolyn sodium**.

Integrilin ®

A preparation of ℞ **eptifibatide**.
Formulation: Intravenous injection or infusion.
Availability: Prescription only.
Warnings and side effects: See ℞ **eptifibatide**.

interferons ⑥

Type/Group: immunomodulator; anticancer; antiviral.
Brand(s): (*Alfa-2a*): Roferon-A. (*Alfa-2b*): Intron A. (*Alfa-2b with ribavirin*): Rebetron. (*Alfacon-1*): Infergen. (*Beta-1a*): Avonex. (*Beta-1b*): Betaseron. (*Gamma-1b*): Actimmune.
How administered: Injection.

Used to treat
Interferons are proteins produced in tiny quantities by cells infected by a virus and which have the ability to inhibit further growth of the virus. Genetic engineering, including the use of bacteria as host cells has enabled interferons to be mass-produced (though at great expense), but they have been less effective against viruses than was hoped. Because they are immunomodulators (biological response modifiers), they also have complex effects on cells, cell function, and immunity, which has limited their use. There are several kinds currently in use (all are copies of complete, naturally occurring human interferons, except alfacon-1, which is a "designer" construction of protein elements common to the alfa types of interferon):
Interferon alfa-2a; [rIFN-A; IFLrA]: for some forms of leukemia and AIDS-related ✪ **Kaposi's sarcoma**. It is being investigated for treatment of many forms of ✪ **cancer**.
Interferon alfa-2b; [IFN-alpha 2; rIFN-(2; (-2-interferon)] for hairy-cell ✪ **leukemia**, malignant ✪ **melanoma**, condyloma (certain warts), AIDS-related Kaposi's sarcoma, and chronic ✪ **hepatitis** B and C infections. It is being investigated for treatment of over 20 forms of cancer. In combination with ℞ **ribavirin**, it is used to treat hepatitis C infection;
Interferon alfacon-1: for chronic hepatitis C infection; it may be effective against hairy-cell leukemia.
Interferon beta (includes types *beta-1a; beta-1b*): for relapsing ✪ **multiple sclerosis** (MS); and being investigated for treatment of various cancers and viral hepatitis infection.
Interferon gamma-1b: for chronic granulomatous disease (CGD) and to delay progression of severe ✪ **osteoporosis**.

Warnings
• It should not be given to people with known hypersensitivity to this drug.
• It should be given with caution to people with severe kidney or liver impairment, heart disease, seizure or neurological disorder, or bone marrow suppression. These are specialist drugs and are used only after a full medical assessment.
• They should be used during pregnancy only if the potential benefits outweigh the possible risk to the fetus.
• Medical judgment is required if breast-feeding is being considered.
• Depression (including suicidal behavior) is associated with use of these drugs.
• Regular blood counts are essential during treatment, particularly to check the levels of white blood cells. Other tests (for example, of liver and kidney function) are also performed periodically.

Interactions
• Interleukin-2 taken with *alfa-2a* creates a potential risk of kidney failure.
• The effects of aminophylline and ℞ **theophylline** may be increased.
• If ℞ **zidovudine** is taken with *alfa-2b*, there is the possiblity of additive effects in reducing certain white-cell counts.
• Myelosuppressive drugs (that is, drugs that cause bone marrow suppression) increase the risk of serious blood effects.
• If taken with CNS (central nervous system) drugs (for example, ℞ **antipsychotics**, ℞ **sedatives**, ℞ **hypnotics**, ℞ **anticonvulsants**), there may be an increase in the risk of adverse effects.

Side effects
• Commonly, all the interferons may cause fatigue, headache, and severe flu-like symptoms. Also frequent are loss of appetite, nausea and vomiting, dizziness, various muscle and joint pains, rashes and other skin and hair changes.
• Of particular concern are blood changes (which may include anemia and white-cell suppression) and mental depression.
• There may also be high or low blood pressure, heartbeat irregularities, liver or kidney toxicity, mental confusion, and serious hypersensitivity reactions.
• Thyroid abnormalities and high triglyceride levels have been reported with the alfa interferons.

interleukin 11 ⑥
see ℞ **oprelvekin**.

Intron A ®

A preparation of ℞ **interferon** alfa-2b.
Formulation: Injection.
Availability: Prescription only.
Warnings and side effects: See ℞ **interferons**.

Inversine ®

A preparation of ℞ **mecamylamine hydrochloride**.
Formulation: Oral tablets.
Availability: Prescription only.
Warnings and side effects: See ℞ **mecamylamine hydrochloride**.

Invirase ®

A preparation of ℞ **saquinavir**.

Formulation: Oral capsules.
Availability: Prescription only.
Warnings and side effects: See ℞ **saquinavir**.

Iobid DM Tablets ⑧

A preparation of ℞ **dextromethorphan** and ℞ **guaifenesin**.
Formulation: Oral tablets, sustained release.
Availability: Prescription only.
Warnings and side effects: See ℞ **dextromethorphan**;
℞ **guaifenesin**.

Iocon ⑧

A preparation of ℞ **coal tar**.
Formulation: Shampoo, gel.
Availability: OTC.
Warnings and side effects: See ℞ **coal tar**.

Iodal HD ⑧

A preparation of ℞ **hydrocodone bitartrate** and
℞ **chlorpheniramine maleate** and ℞ **phenylephrine hydrochloride**.
Formulation: Oral liquid.
Availability: Prescription only.
Warnings and side effects: See ℞ **hydrocodone bitartrate**;
℞ **chlorpheniramine maleate**; ℞ **phenylephrine hydrochloride**.

iodine; povidone-iodine ⓖ

Type/Group: antiseptic.
Brand(s): Operand; Polydine; Betadine; various generic (both iodine and povidone iodine).
How administered: Topically (external).

Used to treat

Iodine is a non-metallic element that is used in solution as an antiseptic. Iodine is accumulated by the body in the thyroid gland (situated at the base of the neck) and is used by the cells of this gland to synthesize the thyroid hormones thyroxine and triiodothyronine, which control a number of normal metabolic processes and growth. Povidone iodine is a complex of iodine on an organic carrier that is also used as an antiseptic. It is topically applied to the skin, especially in sensitive areas (such as the vulva). It works by slowly releasing the iodine it contains.

Warnings

• It should not be used in low birth-weight infants, as systemic effects are possible.
• Medical judgment is required if it is used during pregnancy or if breast-feeding is being considered.
• Do not use for a longer period or at higher doses than recommended.
• Avoid severe burns or large wounds.
• Bandages must not be used with iodine, but they can with povidone iodine.
• It may stain skin and clothing.
• The eyes and mucous membranes must be avoided.
• It is highly toxic if ingested.

Interactions

No significant interactions are known.
Side effects
• Rarely, it may cause irritation or inflammation.

iodochlorhydroxyquin ⓖ

see ℞ **clioquinol**.

Iofed Capsules; PD Capsules ⑧

A preparation of ℞ **pseudoephedrine** and ℞ **brompheniramine maleate**.
Formulation: Oral capsules, sustained release.
Availability: Prescription only.
Warnings and side effects: See ℞ **pseudoephedrine**;
℞ **brompheniramine maleate**.

Ionax Astringent Cleanser ⑧

A preparation of ℞ **salicylic acid** and various.
Formulation: Topical liquid.
Availability: OTC.
Warnings and side effects: See ℞ **salicylic acid**.

Ionil Plus ⑧

A preparation of ℞ **salicylic acid**.
Formulation: Shampoo.
Availability: OTC.
Warnings and side effects: See ℞ **salicylic acid**.

Ionil T ⑧

A preparation of ℞ **salicylic acid** and ℞ **coal tar**.
Formulation: Shampoo.
Availability: OTC.
Warnings and side effects: See ℞ **salicylic acid**; ℞ **coal tar**.

Ionil T Plus ⑧

A preparation of ℞ **coal tar**.
Formulation: Shampoo.
Availability: OTC.
Warnings and side effects: See ℞ **coal tar**.

Iopidine ⑧

A preparation of ℞ **apraclonidine**.
Formulation: Eye drops in two strengths.
Availability: Prescription only.
Warnings and side effects: See ℞ **apraclonidine**.

Iosal II Tablets ⑧

A preparation of ℞ **pseudoephedrine** and ℞ **guaifenesin**.
Formulation: Oral tablets, extended release.
Availability: Prescription only.
Warnings and side effects: See ℞ **pseudoephedrine**;
℞ **guaifenesin**.

Iosopan Liquid ⑧

A preparation of ℞ **magaldrate**.

Formulation: Oral liquid.
Availability: OTC.
Warnings and side effects: See ℞ **magaldrate**.

Iosopan Plus Liquid ⑧

A preparation of ℞ **magaldrate** and ℞ **simethicone**.
Formulation: Oral liquid.
Availability: OTC.
Warnings and side effects: See ℞ **magaldrate**; ℞ **simethicone**.

Iotussin HC Syrup ⑧

A preparation of ℞ **hydrocodone bitartrate**,
℞ **chlorpheniramine maleate**, and ℞ **phenylephrine hydrochloride**.
Formulation: Oral syrup.
Availability: Prescription only.
Warnings and side effects: See ℞ **hydrocodone bitartrate**; ℞ **chlorpheniramine maleate**; ℞ **phenylephrine hydrochloride**.

ipecac syrup ⑥

(ipecacuanha)
Type/Group: emetic.
Brand(s): Various generic.
How administered: Orally.

Used to treat

Ipecac syrup is an extract from the ipecac plant. It contains two alkaloids (emetine and cephaeline) that have an irritant action on the gastrointestinal tract and is therefore a powerful emetic. It can be used to clear the stomach in certain cases of non-corrosive poisoning when the patient is conscious (particularly in children). Emetine (and certain derivatives) has been used as an amebicidal (see ℞ **amebicide and antiprotozoal** drugs).

Warnings

• It should not be given to people who are unconscious or semiconscious, or to anyone who has ingested corrosives (such as alkalis or strong acids), petroleum distillates, or strychnine.
• Ipecac syrup should be used during pregnancy only if the potential benefit outweighs the possible risks.
• Medical judgment is required if breast-feeding is being considered. It is not known whether this drug appears in breast milk.
• If not vomited, and allowed to be absorbed, ipecac may cause serious heart disturbances.
• Ipecac has been abused by persons with eating disorders (bulimia and anorexia nervosa) with occasionally serious, even fatal, results.
• It should be used with water and *not* with milk or carbonated beverages.

Interactions

• Ipecac should be used before ℞ **activated charcoal** after vomiting has occurred.

Side effects

• Depending on use, there may be excessive vomiting, effects on the heart and blood pressure (if absorbed) and damage to the epithelium (surface tissues) of the gastrointestinal tract.
• High doses can cause severe gastric upset.

ipecacuanha ⑥

see ℞ **ipecac syrup**.

IPOL ⑧

A preparation of poliovirus vaccine, inactivated (IPV).
Formulation: Injection.
Availability: Prescription only.
Warnings and side effects: See ℞ **poliovirus vaccine**.

ipratropium bromide ⑥

Type/Group: antiasthmatic; bronchodilator; anticholinergic.
Brand(s): Atrovent; various generic. Combinations: with *albuterol*: Combivent.
How administered: Inhalation; topically (nasal spray).

Used to treat

Ipratropium bromide is mainly used for maintenance treatment of bronchospasm in chronic obstructive pulmonary disease (COPD), including ✪ **bronchitis** and ✪ **emphysema**, as well as for symptomatic relief of rhinorrhea (blocked nose) associated with colds and allergies (perennial rhinitis).

Warnings

• It should not be given to people with known hypersensitivity to ℞ **atropine** (it is chemically related to atropine) or similar agents.
• It should be given with caution to people with angle-closure glaucoma, prostatic hypertrophy, bladder neck obstruction, or urinary retention.
• It should be used during pregnancy only if medically judged to be clearly needed.
• Medical judgment is required if breast-feeding is being considered. It is not known if it appears in breast milk.
• Avoid getting the drug into the eyes, particularly people with glaucoma.

Interactions

No significant interactions have been reported.

Side effects

• Nausea, cough, worsening of symptoms, anxiety, dizziness, headache, nervousness, palpitations, blurred vision, dry mouth, metallic taste, stomach pain, cramps, vomiting, rash, and allergic reaction.

irbesartan ⑥

Type/Group: angiotensin-receptor blocker; antihypertensive; vasodilator.
Brand(s): Avapro. Combinations: With *hydrochlorothiazide*: Avalide.
How administered: Orally.

Used to treat

Irbesartan is an angiotensin II receptor (AT1 receptors) blocker. Angiotensin II is a circulating hormone that is a powerful vasoconstrictor (narrows blood vessels) and blocking its effects leads to a fall in blood pressure. Irbesartan can be used, alone or with other drugs, to treat ✪ **hypertension**.

Warnings

• It should not be given to people with known hypersensitivity to this drug.

• It should be given with caution to people with severe congestive heart failure, with severely impaired liver or kidney function, or renal stenosis. Any fluid- or salt-depleted condition (as from diuretic use) should be corrected before using this drug.

• Risk in pregnancy increases substantially from the first through to the second and third trimesters. Angiotensin-receptor blockers can cause injury to the fetus. The use of these drugs should be stopped as soon as pregnancy is detected.

• Medical judgment is required if breast-feeding is being considered.

• Blood pressure should be checked regularly.

Interactions

No drug interactions of significance are known.

Side effects

• Angiotensin-receptor blockers in general appear to cause few and infrequent side effects (often indistinguishable from placebo effects). The most common, with irbesartan, may include upper respiratory infection, fatigue, and gastrointestinal disturbances (for example, diarrhea, indigestion, heartburn).

• Uncommon side effects include headache, joint pain, dizziness, dry cough, chest pain, or edema. Rash, weakness, and effects on heart rhythm occasionally occur. There may be changes in kidney function and angioedema (an allergic swelling reaction, often of the face) has been reported.

Ircon ®

A preparation of ℞ **ferrous fumarate**.
Formulation: Oral tablets.
Availability: OTC.
Warnings and side effects: See ℞ **ferrous fumarate**.

irinotecan hydrochloride ⑥

Type/Group: **anticancer; cytotoxic**.
Brand(s): Camptosar.
How administered: Injection.

Used to treat

Irinotecan is one of a new group of drugs termed topoisomerase I inhibitors. It is used in the treatment of colon or rectal ✪ **cancer**.

Warnings

• It should not be given to people with known hypersensitivity to irinotecan.

• It should be given with caution to people who have previously received pelvic or abdominal irradiation, or who are over 65, as there is an increased risk of bone marrow suppression. This is a specialist drug which will be used following a full evaluation by specialist physicians.

• Irinotecan is not recommended for use during pregnancy unless it is medically judged to be essential, because it may cause birth defects. Becoming pregnant while using this drug must be avoided.

• It should not be used if breast-feeding.

• It can cause severe bone marrow suppression, which may lead to bleeding and a reduced resistance to infection.

• Diarrhea appearing more than 24 hours after administration may be serious and should be treated promptly with ℞ **loperamide**.

• This drug may rarely produce severe allergic reactions.

• A doctor must be contacted if vomiting, fever, or evidence of infection, fainting, lightheadedness, or dizziness is noted (for example, at home) following treatment.

Interactions

No interactions specific to this drug are known.

Side effects

• Commonly, diarrhea, nausea, and weakness.

• Frequently, vomiting, loss of appetite, fever, abdominal pain and cramps, and hair loss.

• Occasionally, constipation, flatulence, inflammation of mouth mucosa, headache, back pain, swelling, decreased body weight, dehydration, rash, sweating, shortness of breath, increased cough, nasal irritation, insomnia, and dizziness.

iron dextran ⑥

Type/Group: **anemia treatment**.
Brand(s): InFeD; DexFerrum.
How administered: Injection.

Used to treat

Iron dextran is a complex of ferric hydroxide with dextran, a derivative of dextrose. It is rich in iron and is used in the treatment of iron-deficiency ✪ **anemia** to restore iron to the body when treatment by mouth is unsatisfactory or impossible.

Warnings

• It should not be given to people with known hypersensitivity to the product or anyone in the acute phase of infectious kidney disease. Those with serious liver function impairment use with extreme caution.

• Iron dextran should be used during pregnancy only if the potential benefits outweigh the possible risk to the fetus.

• Medical judgment is required if breast-feeding is being considered.

• Injection of iron-carbohydrate complexes such as iron dextran has resulted in serious, even fatal, allergic reactions. Injections will be carried out by experienced personnel under controlled conditions.

• Intramuscular injection of iron-carbohydrate complexes such as iron dextran may create a risk of cancer.

Interactions

• If used with ℞ **chloramphenicol**, iron levels may be increased.

Side effects

• Bone and muscle aches, chills, dizziness, fever, headache, malaise, nausea, and vomiting.

Ismelin ®

A preparation of ℞ **guanethidine monosulfate**.
Formulation: Oral tablets, available in two strengths.
Availability: Prescription only.
Warnings and side effects: See ℞ **guanethidine monosulfate**.

ISMO ®

A preparation of ℞ **isosorbide mononitrate**.
Formulation: Oral tablets.
Availability: Prescription only.

Key to symbols: ✪ = Disorder Section ℞ = Drug Section ♣ = Herbal Section ⬧⬧ = Supplement Section

Warnings and side effects: See ℞ **isosorbide mononitrate.**

Isocaine ⑧

A preparation of ℞ **mepivacaine hydrochloride.**
Formulation: Injection.
Availability: Prescription only.
Warnings and side effects: See ℞ **mepivacaine hydrochloride.**

isocarboxazid ⑥

Type/Group: antidepressant; MAOI.
Brand(s): Marplan.
How administered: Orally.

Used to treat

Isocarboxazid is used to treat ✪ **depression** that has proven resistant to other forms of treatment.

Warnings

• It should not be given to people with known hypersensitivity to MAOI antidepressants, or to people with pheochromocytoma, cardiovascular or cerebrovascular disease, hypertension, congestive heart failure, known or suspected liver disease, severe kidney impairment or heart disease, or a history of frequent or severe headache.

• It should be given with caution to people over the age of 60, to anyone with low blood pressure, bipolar disorder (manic-depressive illness), schizophrenia, hyperactivity, diabetes mellitus, seizure disorder, angina pectoris, blood disorders, porphyria, or thyroid disease.

• Isocarboxazid should be used during pregnancy only if it is clearly needed.

• It should not be used by nursing mothers.

• Foods with a high tyramine, dopamine, or tryptophan content should be avoided (see Interactions below).

• Do not drink alcoholic beverages.

• A doctor must be consulted before taking any other medication, including OTC drugs, herbal remedies, supplements, or any other alternative preparation (especially cold, hay fever, or weight-reduction products).

• Minimize caffeine intake.

• A doctor must be contacted at once if headache, palpitations, nausea, neck stiffness, sweating, photophobia, or other unusual symptoms develop. They can indicate a potentially serious reaction.

• It is not generally given to children under the age of 16.

• It may aggravate anxiety and agitation.

• Treatment should be stopped gradually, lowering the dose over a period of time, after long-term use.

• It may impair the performance of skilled tasks requiring mental alertness or physical skills, such as driving.

Interactions

• Foods containing tyramine, such as cheeses, sour cream, yogurt, liver, fermented sausages (for example, salami, bologna), smoked, spoiled dried or pickled fish, meat tenderizer, game meats, beer, red wine, sherry, spirits, tofu, bananas, raspberries (other fruits especially if dried or overripe), sauerkraut, yeast extracts, broad beans, chocolate, and ginseng, may cause dangerously high blood pressure.

• Herbal remedies, such as ginseng or caffeine, and others, that contain amines may cause dangerously high blood pressure.

• Supplements containing tryptophan and tyramine (see ⚖ **amino acids**) may cause dangerously high blood pressure.

• Serious and even fatal reactions have occurred when MAOI antidepressants are taken with other antidepressants (such as SSRIs or tricyclics). At least 14 days should elapse between discontinuing one and starting the other, and 21 days for some including clomipramine or imipramine.

• If used with ℞ **dextromethorphan**, agitation or seizure are possible.

• If used with ℞ **ephedrine**, ℞ **amphetamine**, ℞ **phenylephrine**, or ℞ **pseudoephedrine**, severe high blood pressure is possible.

• Sensitivity to ℞ **barbiturates**, ℞ **antidiabetics**, and ℞ **beta-blockers** may be increased.

• If used with ℞ **methylphenidate**, ℞ **carbamazepine**, ℞ **cyclobenzaprine**, or ℞ **levodopa**, raised blood pressure, sometimes to dangerous levels, may occur.

• ℞ **guanethidine monosulfate**'s effects on blood pressure may be inhibited by MAOIs.

• Toxic reactions are possible with ℞ **meperidine**, ℞ **sulfonamide**, or ℞ **sumatriptan**.

• Adverse reactions may occur with ℞ **methyldopa**, Rauwolfia ℞ **alkaloids**, ℞ **sympathomimetics**, ℞ **thiazide** ℞ **diuretics**, or *l*-tryptophan.

Side effects

• These include dizziness, drowsiness, and loss of appetite.

• Less frequently, blurred vision, mental changes, headache, sleep disturbance, gastrointestinal disturbances, weight gain, change in sexual interest, anemia, flushing, jaundice, increased sweating, and rash.

• Rare but serious side effects include changes in heart rhythm and dangerously high blood pressure.

Isoclor Expectorant Liquid ⑧

A preparation of ℞ **codeine phosphate**, ℞ **guaifenesin**, and ℞ **pseudoephedrine**.
Formulation: Oral liquid.
Availability: May or may not require a prescription.
Warnings and side effects: See ℞ **codeine phosphate**; ℞ **guaifenesin**; ℞ **pseudoephedrine**.

isoetharine ⑥

Type/Group: antiasthmatic; sympathomimetic; beta-adrenergic stimulant.
Brand(s): Generic.
How administered: Inhalant.

Used to treat

Isoethrine is used for bronchial ✪ **asthma** and reversible bronchospasm that occurs with ✪ **bronchitis** and ✪ **emphysema**.

Warnings

• It should not be given to people with a known history of allergy to sympathomimetics.

• It should be given with caution to people with hypertension, heart disease, hyperthyroidism, or diabetes mellitus.

• It should be used during pregnancy only if medically judged to be clearly needed.

• Medical judgment is required if breast-feeding is being considered. It is not known if it appears in breast milk.

• Rarely, it may have adverse effects on heart and blood pressure, or may lead to paradoxical bronchoconstriction.

Interactions

• ℞ **Beta-blockers** decrease the effects of isoetharine.

• If used with ℞ **furosemide**, there is a risk of enhancing furosemide's potassium-lowering effect.

• ℞ **Digoxin** may increase the risk of arrhythmias.

Side effects

• Occasionally, anxiety, tremor, nausea, nervousness, palpitations, speeded heartbeat, peripheral vasodilatation, dry mouth or throat, dizziness, vomiting, insomnia, headache, and increased blood pressure.

isometheptene mucate ⓖ

Brand(s): **Midrin**.

How administered: Orally.

Type/Group: sympathomimetic; beta-adrenergic stimulant.

Used to treat

Isometheptene mucate is used as an ℞ **antimigraine** treatment for acute attacks. It is available only in combination with dichloral-phenazone, a mild sedative, and ℞ **acetaminophen**.

Warnings

• It should not be given to people with glaucoma, severe kidney disease, severe liver disease, or organic heart disease.

• It should be given with caution to people with hypertension, peripheral vascular disease, and those who have had a recent cerebrovascular accident.

• Consult a doctor before using this drug during pregnancy or while breast-feeding. Data specific to this combination is not available.

• Side effects and warnings applicable to acetaminophen apply to the combination product.

Interactions

• If used with ℞ **bromocriptine**, there is potential for adverse effects on heart.

Side effects

• Transient dizziness and skin rash.

isoniazid ⓖ

Type/Group: **antibacterial; antituberculosis**.

Brand(s): Laniazid; Nydrazid; various generic. Combinations: With *rifampin*: Rifamate. With *pyrazinamide* and *rifampin*: Rifater.

How administered: Orally; injection.

Used to treat

Isoniazid is used, in combination with other drugs, in the treatment of ⊙ **tuberculosis**. It can also be used to prevent the contraction of tuberculosis.

Warnings

• It should not be given to people with known hypersensitivity to isoniazid, acute liver disease, or a history of liver damage with previous use of isoniazid.

• It should be given with caution to people with chronic liver disease, alcoholism, malnutrition, slow alkylators, diabetes, or severe kidney impairment.

• Isoniazid should be used during pregnancy only when it is clearly needed. Preventive treatment may be postponed until after delivery.

• It is compatible with breast-feeding, but the infant must be periodically examined.

• Severe and sometimes fatal hepatitis may develop, which is more likely if alcohol is drunk everyday.

• Serious allergic reaction may occur.

• A doctor must be contacted if weakness, loss of appetite, fatigue, nausea, yellowing skin or eyes, darkened urine, or tingling or numbness in feet or hands occur.

• Foods, histamine or tyramine may cause adverse effects.

Interactions

• ℞ **Antacids**, aluminum salts, and ℞ **corticosteroids** may reduce the absorption of isoniazid taken by mouth.

• The toxicity of ℞ **carbamazepine** and ℞ **phenytoin** may be increased.

• The levels of ℞ **ketoconazole** may be decreased.

• ℞ **Disulfiram**, ℞ **meperidine**, and ℞ **cycloserine** may increase CNS (central nervous system) effects.

• ℞ **rifampin**, enflurane, halothane, and acetaminophen may increase the risk of liver toxicity.

• The effects of ℞ **benzodiazepines**, oral ℞ **anticoagulants**, ℞ **theophylline**, and ℞ **valproic acid** may be increased.

Side effects

• Frequently, gastrointestinal effects.

• Occasionally, pain at injection site and inflammation of optic nerve.

• Rarely, nerve damage, liver damage, hepatitis, blood disorders, and skin disorders.

isophane insulin suspension NPH: isophane protamine insulin ⓖ

see ℞ **insulin, isophane suspension** (insulin, NPH).

isoprenaline ⓖ

see ℞ **isoproterenol**.

isoproterenol ⓖ

(isoprenaline)

Type/Group: **sympathomimetic; cardiac stimulant**.

Brand(s): Isuprel; various generic.

How administered: Injection, infusion.

Used to treat

Isoproterenol is similar to ℞ **epinephrine**, which stimulates the heart, and so it can produce an increased rate and force of contraction. It is used to treat mild episodes of heart block (see ⊙ **cardiovascular disorders**), to treat shock (along with other drugs), and in an emergency to reverse cardiac arrest. It is also used for bronchospasm, for example, during anesthesia.

Warnings

• It should not be given to people with existing arrhythmias other than those treated by this drug, or angina pectoris.

• It should be given with caution to people who are elderly or who have heart or coronary artery disease, hyperthyroidism, diabetes mellitus, kidney impairment, or low blood volume.

• Isoproterenol should be used during pregnancy only if the potential benefit outweighs the possible risk to the fetus.

• Medical judgment is required if breast-feeding is being considered.

• This is a powerful drug, used only under hospital conditions and with continuous monitoring of heart function, blood pressure, and other vital signs.

Interactions

• Halogenated ℞ **general anesthetics** (for example, halothane) or cyclopropane have the potential for serious adverse effects on heart rhythm. Generally, they should not be used together with isoproterenol.

• There is a risk of arrhythmias if taken with ℞ **digoxin**.

• ℞ **bretylium tosylate**, ℞ **ergot alkaloids** (for example, ℞ **ergonovine**, ℞ **ergotamine**), ℞ **guanethidine monosulfate**, ℞ **oxytocin**, other ℞ **sympathomimetics**, and ℞ **tricyclics** may intensify the effects of isoproterenol, with the potential for serious adverse reactions. Other sympathomimetics and isoproterenol should not be administered within 4 hours of one another.

• ℞ **Beta-blockers** may decrease the therapeutic action of isoproterenol.

Side effects

• There may be irregular or fast heartbeat, rapid change in blood pressure (either increase or decrease), flushing, sweating, nervousness, headache, dizziness, chest pain, or nausea.

• Allergic reactions (including rash, wheezing, bronchospasm) have been caused by sulfites used in some commercially available preparations.

Isoptin Tablets; SR Tablets; Injection Ⓑ

A preparation of ℞ **verapamil hydrochloride**.
Formulation: Oral tablets (3 strengths); sustained release tablets (SR, 3 strengths).
Availability: Prescription only.
Warnings and side effects: See ℞ **verapamil hydrochloride**. Isoptin SR is used only for control of high blood pressure.

Isopto Atropine Ⓑ

A preparation of ℞ **atropine sulfate**.
Formulation: Eyedrop solution.
Availability: Prescription only.
Warnings and side effects: See ℞ **atropine sulfate**.

Isopto Carbachol Ⓑ

A preparation of ℞ **carbachol**.
Formulation: Eye drops.
Availability: Prescription only.

Warnings and side effects: See ℞ **carbachol**.

Isopto Carpine Ⓑ

A preparation of ℞ **pilocarpine**.
Formulation: Ophthalmic solution in several strengths.
Availability: Prescription only.
Warnings and side effects: See ℞ **pilocarpine**.

Isopto Cetapred Ⓑ

A preparation of ℞ **prednisolone**, ℞ **sodium phosphate**, and sodium sulfacemide.
Formulation: Eye drops.
Availability: Prescription only.
Warnings and side effects: See ℞ **prednisolone**; sodium sulfacemide.

Isopto Homatropine Ⓑ

A preparation of ℞ **homatropine hydrobromide**.
Formulation: Ophthalmic solution.
Availability: Prescription only.
Warnings and side effects: See ℞ **homatropine hydrobromide**.

Isopto Hyoscine Ⓑ

A preparation of ℞ **scopolamine hydrobromide**.
Formulation: Eyedrops.
Availability: Prescription only.
Warnings and side effects: See ℞ **scopolamine hydrobromide**.

Isordil Sublingual Tablets Ⓑ

A preparation of ℞ **isosorbide dinitrate**.
Formulation: Sublingual tablets, available in 3 strengths.
Availability: Prescription only.
Warnings and side effects: See ℞ **isosorbide dinitrate**.

Isordil Titradose Tablets; Tembids Ⓑ

A preparation of ℞ **isosorbide dinitrate**.
Formulation: Oral tablets (5 strengths); sustained release tablets or capsules (Tembids).
Availability: Prescription only.
Warnings and side effects: See ℞ **isosorbide dinitrate**.

isosorbide dinitrate Ⓖ

Type/Group: nitrate; vasodilator; antianginal; heart failure treatment.
Brand(s): Dilatrate-SR; Isordil Titradose, Tembids; Sorbitrate; various generic.
How administered: Orally.

Used to treat

Isosorbide dinitrate is used to prevent attacks of ✪ **angina pectoris**, for instance when taken before exercise, and for symptomatic relief during an acute attack. It has been used, as well, to lighten heart exertion in congestive ✪ **heart failure** or after a heart attack. It works by dilating the veins returning blood to the heart and so reducing the heart's workload. It is short-acting when absorbed rapidly, but its effect can be extended through the use of modified-release sublingual tablets (which dissolve under the tongue) or oral sustained-release tablets.

Warnings

• It should not be given to people with known hypersensitivity to nitrates, or who have postural hypotension (lowered blood pressure on standing), marked anemia, head injury or brain hemorrhage, or closed-angle glaucoma.

• It should be given with caution to people who have only very recently had a heart attack, with certain cardiovascular disorders, glaucoma, or kidney, liver or thyroid impairment. Extended-release forms should be given to people with intestinal malabsorption and hypermotility disorders.

• Isosorbide's safety during pregnancy has not been established, and it should be used only when it is clearly needed.

• Medical judgment is required if breast-feeding is being considered.

• Alcohol should be avoided because severe hypotension or circulatory collapse is possible.

• Postural hypotension may occur, even with small doses, and measures such as deep breathing or lowering the head may be needed to overcome dizziness or prevent fainting. Sublingual tablets should be taken in a sitting position.

• When using sublingual tablets, if pain is not relieved by 3 tablets taken one after another at 5-minute intervals, a doctor must be contacted immediately or go to an emergency room.

• A doctor should be notified of symptoms such as blurred vision, dry mouth, or persistent headache.

• There can be some variation in effect among different brands, and it is important not to switch brands without first checking with a pharmacist or doctor.

Interactions

• Alcohol, other ℞ **antihypertensive** drugs, ℞ **calcium-channel blockers**, ℞ **beta-adrenergic blockers**, ℞ **phenothiazines**, and ℞ **sildenafil** have the potential for increasing effects, with marked or severe hypotension. Dosages may need adjustment.

• ℞ **Dihydroergotamine** may have antagonistic, unpredictable effects.

Side effects

• These include throbbing headache, flushing, or dizziness. Some people experience an increase in heart rate and postural hypotension.

• Less frequently, gastrointestinal disturbances, arthralgia (joint pain), pallor, and perspiration or cold sweat.

isosorbide mononitrate Ⓖ

Type/Group: **nitrate; antianginal; heart failure treatment**.
Brand(s): Monoket; Imdur; ISMO; Isotrate ER; various generic.
How administered: Orally.

Used to treat

Isosorbide mononitrate is a ℞ **vasodilator** used to prevent attacks of ✚ **angina pectoris**, for instance when taken before exercise (but not during an attack). It has been used, as well, to lighten heart exertion in congestive ✚ **heart failure** or after a heart attack. It works by dilating the veins returning blood to the heart and so reducing the heart's workload.

Warnings

• It should not be given to people with known hypersensitivity to nitrates, or who have postural hypotension (lowered blood pressure on standing), marked anemia, head injury or brain hemorrhage, or closed-angle glaucoma.

• It should be given with caution to people who have only very recently had a heart attack, with certain cardiovascular disorders, glaucoma, or kidney, liver or thyroid impairment. Extended-release forms should not be given to people with intestinal malabsorption and hypermotility disorders.

• Isosorbide's safety during pregnancy has not been established, and so it should only be used when clearly needed.

• Medical judgment is required if breast-feeding is being considered.

• Alcohol should be avoided, as severe hypotension or circulatory collapse is possible.

• Postural hypotension may occur, even with small doses, and measures such as deep breathing or lowering the head may be needed to overcome dizziness or prevent fainting.

• A doctor should be notified of symptoms such as blurred vision, dry mouth, or persistent headache.

• There can be some variation in effect among different brands, and it is important not to switch brands without first checking with a pharmacist or doctor.

Interactions

• Alcohol, other ℞ **antihypertensive** drugs, ℞ **calcium-channel blockers**, ℞ **beta-adrenergic blockers**, ℞ **phenothiazines**, and ℞ **sildenafil** have the potential for additive effects, with marked or severe hypotension. Dosages may need adjustment.

• ℞ **Dihydroergotamine** may have antagonistic, unpredictable effects.

Side effects

• These include throbbing headache, flushing, or dizziness. Some people experience an increase in heart rate and postural hypotension.

• Less frequently, gastrointestinal disturbances, arthralgia (joint pain), pallor, and perspiration or cold sweat.

Isotrate ER Ⓡ

A preparation of ℞ **isosorbide mononitrate**.
Formulation: Oral tablets, extended release.
Availability: Prescription only.
Warnings and side effects: See ℞ **isosorbide mononitrate**.

isotretinoin Ⓖ

Type/Group: **acne treatment; retinoid**.
Brand(s): Accutane.
How administered: Orally.

Used to treat

Isotretinoin is chemically a retinoid (a derivative of retinol, or ♻ **vitamin A**) and has a marked effect on the cells that make up the skin epithelium (surface tissues). Actually, it is a chemical form of ℞ **tretinoin** (an isomer). It can be used for the long-term, systemic treatment of severe ✚ **acne** (severe recalcitrant cystic acne).

Warnings

• It should not be given to people with known hypersensitivity to this drug.

• It should be given with caution to people with diabetes mellitus, obesity, a family history of elevated triglyceride levels, inflammatory bowel disease, or wearers of contact lenses.

• Isotretinoin must not be used while pregnant, and becoming pregnant must be avoided while using this drug. There is a very high risk of birth defects from taking this drug, even in small amounts and for short periods. It will be prescribed only after obtaining a report of a negative pregnancy test and once the woman concerned has started her menstrual period. Women of childbearing potential are given special counseling before isotretinoin is prescribed.

• It is not known whether this drug appears in breast milk, but, because of the potential for severe adverse effects, it should not be used while nursing.

• It can cause raised blood pressure around the brain. A doctor must be contacted if headache, visual disturbances, or swelling of the eyes occur.

• Rarely, it may be linked with inflammatory bowel disease, in which case treatment should stop.

• It may temporarily raise cholesterol levels, particularly in people who drink alcohol.

• It may reduce night vision (which can happen suddenly), so use caution when driving at night.

• It may be linked with damage to the liver.

• Ultraviolet light should be avoided and exposure to sunlight minimized.

• Blood must not be donated for 30 days following use of this drug because of its potential for causing birth defects.

Interactions

• The absorption of isotretinoin is increased when taken with food.

• Vitamin A supplements must not be taken otherwise there will be additive effects.

• If taken with ℞ **tetracycline** or ℞ **minocycline**, there is a risk of adverse side effects.

• The levels of ℞ **carbamazepine** are reduced.

Side effects

• Frequently, inflammation around the lips and cracking lips (cheilitis), dryness of the skin, mucous membranes, eyes, nose, and mouth, itching, nosebleeds, gastrointestinal effects, conjunctivitis, bone or joint pain, and muscle aches.

• Rarely, decreased night vision or depression.

isradipine ⑥

Type/Group: **calcium-channel blocker; antihypertensive.**
Brand(s): Dynacirc.
How administered: Orally.

Used to treat

Isradipine is used to treat ✪ **hypertension**, either alone or with thiazide ℞ **diuretics.**

Warnings

• It should not be given to people with known hypersensitivity to this drug, or who have marked hypotension or porphyria.

• It should be given with caution to people with congestive heart failure, impaired liver or kidney function, or who are elderly.

• It should be used during pregnancy only if the potential benefits outweigh the risk to the fetus.

• Breast-feeding women should either discontinue using this drug or stop breast-feeding.

• Regular monitoring of blood pressure is necessary to establish a safe, effective dosage.

• If isradipine is given to replace a ℞ **beta-blocker**, then withdrawal of the beta-blocker should not be abrupt. Calcium-channel blockers, also, should not be discontinued abruptly.

• Grapefruit juice should be avoided as it can increase the levels of isradipine in blood plasma.

Interactions

• Beta-blockers (for example, ℞ **propranolol**) occasionally cause adverse reactions, though the effects are unclear, so caution is advised.

• ℞ **Anticonvulsants** (for example, ℞ **phenytoin**) may produce anticonvulsant toxic effects over time.

• There may be a risk of severe hypotension if taken with ℞ **fentanyl**, so caution is advised.

• Other hypotensive agents (for example, ℞ **captopril**, ℞ **hydralazine hydrochloride**, ℞ **methyldopa**) may have additive effects, and severe hypotension is possible.

• Alcohol, ℞ **cimetidine** and grapefruit juice may increase the levels and effects of isradipine.

• The levels of ℞ **digoxin** may be increased by isradipine.

• The levels of ℞ **quinidine** may fall when isradipine treatment is begun, and rise when it is stopped.

Side effects

• Frequently, headache, dizziness, swelling of the extremities, nausea or abdominal pain, flushing and sensations of warmth, or palpitations.

• Less commonly, rash and itching, urinary frequency, breathlessness, chest pain, or rapid heartbeat.

• Occasionally, it may cause significant hypotension and, rarely, fainting.

Isuprel ⑧

A preparation of ℞ **isoproterenol**.
Formulation: Injection; infusion.
Availability: Prescription only.
Warnings and side effects: See ℞ **isoproterenol**. This drug contains sodium metabisulfite, which may cause serious allergic reaction (for example, hives, wheezing, anaphylaxis) in susceptible individuals.

Itch-X ⑧

A preparation of ℞ **pramoxine hydrochloride**.
Formulation: Topical cream.
Availability: OTC.
Warnings and side effects: See ℞ **pramoxine hydrochloride**.

itraconazole ⑥

Type/Group: **antifungal; azole.**

Brand(s): Sporanox.

How administered: Orally; injection.

Used to treat

Itraconazole can be used to treat ✪ **fungal infections** in and outside the lungs, infections of the fingernails, ringworm, and athlete's foot. In oral solution, it is used for esophageal candidiasis (thrush). Although not stated by the manufacturer for such use, it may also be prescribed to treat other superficial and systemic fungal infections, including infections of the mucous membranes and vaginal ✪ **candidiasis**.

Warnings

• It should not be given to people with known hypersensitivity to itraconazole.

• It should be given with caution to people sensitive to other azoles or with liver function impairment.

• It is not known if itraconazole harms the fetus. It should be used during pregnancy only if the benefits outweigh the potential risk.

• Medical judgment is required if breast-feeding is being considered. It does appear in breast milk.

• It must not be taken with ℞ **pimozide** or ℞ **quinidine**. Life-threatening heart arrhythmias have occurred in people using these drugs together.

• Rarely, hepatitis and liver injury, usually reversible, have been associated with itraconazole. A doctor must be contacted if dark urine, pale stools, fatigue, yellowing skin, fever, or pronounced gastrointestinal upsets develop.

• A doctor must be contacted before adding or changing medications (including OTCs, herbal remedies, and supplements), because itraconazole interacts with many drugs.

• Some minerals, including magnesium and calcium, can reduce the effects of itraconazole. Supplements containing these must be avoided.

Interactions

These are many and include:

• ℞ **Antacids** and ℞ **ulcer-healing drugs** should be taken at least two hours after itraconazole to avoid reducing its effectiveness.

• The effects of ℞ **alprazolam**, ℞ **amprenavir**, atevirdine, ℞ **atorvastatin**, ℞ **buspirone**, ℞ **chlordiazepoxide**, ℞ **cyclosporine**, ℞ **diazepam**, ℞ **felodipine**, ℞ **fluvastatin**, ℞ **indinavir**, ℞ **lovastatin**, ℞ **methadone**, ℞ **methylprednisolone**, ℞ **midazolam**, ℞ **nelfinavir**, ℞ **pravastatin**, ℞ **quinidine**, ℞ **ritonavir**, ℞ **saquinavir**, ℞ **simvastatin**, ℞ **tacrolimus**, ℞ **tolbutamide**, ℞ **triazolam**, and ℞ **warfarin sodium** may be reduced by itraconazole.

• Astemizole, cisapride, ℞ **pimozide**, ℞ **quinidine**, and ℞ **fexofenadine** can cause potentially serious (even life-threatening) arrhythmias.

• ℞ **Aluminum hydroxide**, ⚖ **calcium**, ℞ **cimetidine**, ℞ **didanosine**, ℞ **famotidine**, ℞ **lansoprazole**, ⚖ **magnesium**, ℞ **nizatidine**, and ℞ **sodium bicarbonate** may reduce the effects of itraconazole.

• ℞ **Rifampin** - the effects of both drugs may be reduced.

Side effects

• Frequently, nausea, rash, constipation, and headache.

• Occasionally, vomiting, diarrhea, elevated blood pressure, swelling in legs or ankles, and fatigue.

• Rarely, abdominal pain, loss of appetite, itching, fever, loss of libido and impotence, sleepiness, and rash.

Ivarest Ⓑ

A preparation of ℞ **calamine**.

Formulation: Topical cream, topical lotion.

Availability: OTC.

Warnings and side effects: See ℞ **calamine**.

Iveegam EN IGIV Ⓑ

A preparation of ℞ **immune globulin, human (IG)**.

Formulation: Intravenous infusion, supplied as a powder.

Availability: Prescription only.

Warnings and side effects: See ℞ **immune globulin, human (IG)**.

ivermectin Ⓖ

Type/Group: **anthelmintic**.

Brand(s): Stromectol.

How administered: Orally.

Used to treat

Ivermectin is a a synthetic anthelmintic drug that is very effective in the treatment of the tropical disease onchocerciasis (infestation by the nematode parasite *Onchocerca volvulus*) and also for strongyloidiasis (nematode *Strongyloides* infection) (see ✪ **worms**). It is now the drug of choice because a single treatment produces a large reduction in the level of parasites, although more than one course of treatment may be necessary to eradicate the infestation.

Warnings

• It should not be given to people with known hypersensitivity to this drug.

• It should not be used during pregnancy, because its safety has not been established.

• Medical judgment is required if breast-feeding is being considered. The drug is found in breast milk.

• Rapid killing of microfilariae may cause systemic or ocular inflammatory responses, characterized by itching rash, enlarged lymph nodes, and fever (the Mazzotti reaction).

Interactions

No significant interactions have been reported.

Side effects

• Dizziness, sleepiness, tremor, gastrointestinal effects, changes in liver enzymes and blood, itching, rash, and hives.

Jenest-28 Ⓑ

A preparation of ℞ **ethinyl estradiol** and ℞ **norethindrone**.

Formulation: Calendar pack of oral tablets.

Availability: Prescription only.

Warnings and side effects: See ℞ **ethinyl estradiol**; ℞ **norethindrone**.

Kabolin Ⓑ

A preparation of ℞ **nandrolone**.

Formulation: Injection.
Availability: Prescription only.
Warnings and side effects: See ℞ **nandrolone**.

Kadian ⑧

A preparation of ℞ **morphine sulfate**.
Formulation: Oral capsules, sustained release, available in 3 strengths.
Availability: Prescription only.
Warnings and side effects: See ℞ **morphine sulfate**.

kanamycin ⑥

Type/Group: **aminoglycoside; antibiotic; antibacterial**.
Brand(s): Kantrex.
How administered: Orally; injection.

Used to treat

Kanamycin is used primarily to reduce the levels of bacteria in the colon prior to intestinal surgery or examination, or in liver failure, but it is also used for some serious ✪ **bacterial infections**, for example, of the central nervous system, urinary, and respiratory tracts.

Warnings

• It should not be given to people with known hypersensitivity to kanamycin or other aminoglycosides, or with severe kidney disease.
• It should be given with caution to people with mild kidney disease, dehydration, hearing deficits or vertigo, muscular disorders, such as myasthenia gravis or parkinsonism, and those over 65.
• Medical judgment is required when giving to very young infants.
• Kanamycin should only be used during pregnancy if medically judged to be clearly needed and if the potential benefits outweigh the risks to the fetus (it crosses the placenta and could cause damage to ears or kidneys).
• Medical judgment is required if breast-feeding is being considered. This drug appears in breast milk.
• Aminoglycosides are associated with nephrotoxicity (damage to the kidneys) and ototoxicity (damage in the ears). Irreversible vestibular impairment can occur, resulting in vertigo and difficulty maintaining balance. Permanent hearing loss in one or both ears can also occur. The risk is greatest in those with pre-existing impairments, with high doses, and with prolonged use.
• A doctor must be contacted if there are problems with hearing, vision, balance, urination, or headaches, even after the course of treatment is completed.
• The use of antibiotics may result in superinfection due to bacterial imbalance.

Interactions

• ℞ **Atracurium**, ℞ **succinylcholine**, ℞ **vecuronium**, or neuromuscular blocking agents taken with kanamycin increases respiratory depression.
• ℞ **ethacrynic acid** and ℞ **carboplatin** increase the risk of ear damage.
• ℞ **Amphotericin B**, ℞ **cephalosporins**, ℞ **cyclosporine**, methoxyflurane, and ℞ **NSAIDs** may increase the risk of kidney damage.

• ℞ **carboplatin**, ℞ **cisplatin**, and ℞ **vancomycin** increase the risk of ear or kidney damage.
• ℞ **carbenicillin**, ℞ **penicillins**, ℞ **piperacillin**, and ℞ **ticarcillin** could inactivate kanamycin in people with kidney failure.

Side effects

• Frequently, gastrointestinal upsets when taken orally.
• Occasionally, rash, fever, hives, and itching.
• Rarely, headache, and potentially serious effects including ototoxicity and deafness, kidney damage, and muscular paralysis.

Kank-A ⑧

A preparation of ℞ **benzocaine**, benzyl alcohol, and ℞ **castor oil**.
Formulation: Topical liquid film.
Availability: OTC.
Warnings and side effects: See ℞ **benzocaine**; benzyl alcohol; ℞ **castor oil**.

Kantrex ⑧

A preparation of ℞ **kanamycin**.
Formulation: Oral capsules; injection.
Availability: Prescription only.
Warnings and side effects: See ℞ **kanamycin**.

Kaodene Non-Narcotic Liquid ⑧

A preparation of ℞ **bismuth subsalicylate**, ℞ **kaolin**, and pectin.
Formulation: Oral liquid.
Availability: OTC.
Warnings and side effects: See ℞ **bismuth subsalicylate**; ℞ **kaolin**.

kaolin ⑥

Type/Group: **antidiarrheal; adsorbent**.
Brand(s): (in combination with pectin): Kao-Spen; various generic.
How administered: Orally.

Used to treat

Kaolin is a purified and sometimes powdered white clay (china clay) that is available in combination with pectin as a treatment for ✪ **diarrhea**. It is also used as an adsorbent in other antidiarrheal preparations (with or without ℞ **opioids**, such as ℞ **codeine phosphate** or ℞ **morphine sulfate**).

Warnings

None significant.

Interactions

No significant interactions are known.

Side effects

No significant side effects are known.

Kaopectate II Caplets ⑧

A preparation of ℞ **loperamide hydrochloride**.
Formulation: Oral tablets.
Availability: OTC.
Warnings and side effects: See ℞ **loperamide hydrochloride**.

Kao-Spen ⑧

A preparation of ℞ **kaolin** and pectin.

Formulation: Oral suspension.
Availability: OTC.
Warnings and side effects: See ℞ **kaolin**.

karaya ⓖ
(sterculia gum)
Type/Group: **laxative**.
Brand(s): Various generic.
How administered: Orally.

Used to treat
Karaya is a vegetable gum that can absorb large amounts of water and is traditionally used as a (bulking-agent) laxative. It works by increasing the overall mass of stool and so stimulating bowel movement, although the full effect may not be achieved for several hours. It is a useful in relieving a range of bowel conditions, including ✪ **diverticular disease** and ✪ **irritable bowel syndrome**. It has been used (controversially) as an appetite suppressant to treat serious ✪ **obesity** with the intention that small amounts of food ingested may be bulked up internally, so achieving a feeling of fullness.

Warnings
• It should not be given to people with gastrointestinal obstruction, esophageal obstruction, or who have difficulty swallowing.
• No ill effects in pregnancy or breast-feeding have been associated with karaya, but a doctor should always be consulted before taking any drug when pregnant.
• Adequate fluid intake must be maintained, and a glass of liquid must be drunk when taking this bulking agent. (It swells up, becoming bulkier. Obstruction can form in the esophagus if the substance is not carried all the way down, or in the bowel if insufficient liquid is present.) It should not be taken just before bed.
• Do not use if there is abdominal pain, nausea, or vomiting, unless directed by a doctor.
• A doctor must be consulted first before taking any other medication (including OTCs, herbal remedies, and supplements), because laxatives may alter the absorption of a wide range of drugs.

Interactions
No drug interactions of significance are known.

Side effects
• There may be flatulence and abdominal distension, intestinal obstruction.

Kayexalate ⓡ
A preparation of ℞ **sodium polystyrene sulfonate**.
Formulation: Powder for suspension, to be administered orally, rectally, or by nasogastric tube.
Availability: Prescription only.
Warnings and side effects: See ℞ **sodium polystyrene sulfonate**.

Keflex ⓡ
A preparation of ℞ **cephalexin**.
Formulation: Capsules; oral suspension.
Availability: Prescription only.
Warnings and side effects: See ℞ **cephalexin**.

Keftab ⓡ
A preparation of ℞ **cephalexin**.
Formulation: Tablets.
Availability: Prescription only.
Warnings and side effects: See ℞ **cephalexin**.

Kefurox ⓡ
A preparation of ℞ **cefuroxime**.
Formulation: Injection.
Availability: Prescription only.
Warnings and side effects: See ℞ **cefuroxime**.

Kefzol ⓡ
A preparation of ℞ **cefazolin sodium**.
Formulation: Injection in several strengths.
Availability: Prescription only.
Warnings and side effects: See ℞ **cefazolin sodium**.

Kenacort ⓡ
A preparation of ℞ **triamcinolone**.
Formulation: Oral tablets in two strengths; syrup. Yellow tablets contain tartrazine. Some individuals are allergic to tartrazine, particularly those who are allergic to aspirin.
Availability: Prescription only.
Warnings and side effects: See ℞ **triamcinolone**.

Kenaject ⓡ
A preparation of ℞ **triamcinolone** acetate.
Formulation: Suspension for injection.
Availability: Prescription only.
Warnings and side effects: See ℞ **triamcinolone**.

Kenalog Suspension ⓡ
A preparation of ℞ **triamcinolone** acetate.
Formulation: Suspension for injection in several strengths.
Availability: Prescription only.
Warnings and side effects: See ℞ **triamcinolone**.

Keppra ⓡ
A preparation of ℞ **levetiracetam**.
Formulation: Oral tablets, available in 3 strengths.
Availability: Prescription only.
Warnings and side effects: See ℞ **levetiracetam**.

Keralyt ⓡ
A preparation of ℞ **salicylic acid**.
Formulation: Topical gel.
Availability: OTC.
Warnings and side effects: See ℞ **salicylic acid**.

keratolytic ⓓ
Generics: **azelaic acid; benzoic acid; benzoyl peroxide; coal tar; formaldehyde; ichthammol; imiquimod; podofilox; resorcinol; salicylic acid**.

Key to symbols: ✪ = Disorder Section ℞ = Drug Section ♣ = Herbal Section ⚕ = Supplement Section

Actions and uses

Keratolytic agents (desquamating agents) are used to clear the skin of hyperkeratoses (thickened and horny patches), which are the scaly areas that occur in some forms of ✪ **eczema**, ichthyosis, and ✪ **psoriasis**, and also in ℞ **acne treatment** to help clear the plugs of keratin that develop in the pores and form pimples. The standard keratolytic is ℞ **salicylic acid**, but there are others such as ℞ **benzoyl peroxide**, ℞ **benzoic acid**, ℞ **resorcinol**, ℞ **azelaic acid**, ℞ **coal tar**, and ℞ **ichthammol** (several of which can usefully be applied in the form of a paste inside an impregnated bandage). Stronger keratolytics form the basis of various ✪ **wart** and ✪ **verruca** treatments (including ℞ **formaldehyde**, ℞ **imiquimod**, ℞ **podofilox** and more concentrated ℞ **salicylic acid**).

Limitations

All of these drug solutions are caustic and can cause skin reactions. Some can cause reddening, erosion, peeling, flaking, and swelling at the application site. A trial application should be made, particularly when preparations for genital warts are to be used. See also the individual drug entries.

Keri ®

A preparation of ℞ **lanolin**.
Formulation: Lotion.
Availability: OTC.
Warnings and side effects: See ℞ **lanolin**.

KeriCort-10 Maximum Strength ®

A preparation of ℞ **hydrocortisone**.
Formulation: Cream.
Availability: OTC.
Warnings and side effects: See ℞ **hydrocortisone**.

Kerlone ®

A preparation of ℞ **betaxolol hydrochloride**.
Formulation: Oral tablets.
Availability: Prescription only.
Warnings and side effects: See ℞ **betaxolol hydrochloride**.

ketoconazole Ⓖ

Type/Group: **antifungal; azole**.
Brand(s): Nizoral; Nizoral A-D; various generic.
How administered: Orally; Topically (external).

Used to treat

Ketoconazole is a synthetic imidazole/azole antifungal drug that can be used to treat deep-seated, serious ✪ **fungal infections** (mycoses). In particular, it is used to treat resistant ✪ **candidiasis** (thrush), gastrointestinal infections, and other infections including seborrheic ✪ **dermatitis** and pityriasis versicolor. Although not stated by the manufacturer for such use, it may also be prescribed to treat ringworm, vaginal candidiasis, advanced ✪ **prostate cancer**, and ✪ **Cushing's syndrome**.

Warnings

• It should not be given to people with known hypersensitivity to ketoconazole, or taking oral ℞ **triazolam**.
• It should be given with caution to people with liver disease.

• It is not known if ketoconazole can harm the fetus. It should be used during pregnancy only if the benefits outweigh the risks.
• Medical judgment is required if breast-feeding is being considered. It is not known if it appears in breast milk.
• Liver injury, usually reversible, has been associated with ketoconazole. A doctor must be contacted if dark urine, pale stools, fatigue, yellowing skin, fever, or pronounced gastrointestinal upsets occur.
• Alcohol must be avoided.
• A doctor must be consulted before adding or changing medications (including OTCs, herbal remedies, and supplements), as ketoconazole interacts with many drugs.
• Some minerals, including magnesium and calcium, can reduce the effects of ketoconazole, and so supplements containing these should be avoided.

Interactions

These are many and include:
• ℞ **Antacids** and ℞ **ulcer-healing drugs** should be taken at least two hours after ketoconazole to avoid reducing its effectiveness.
• The effects of ℞ **alprazolam**, ℞ **amprenavir**, atevirdine, ℞ **atorvastatin**, ℞ **buspirone**, ℞ **chlordiazepoxide**, ℞ **cyclosporine**, ℞ **diazepam**, ℞ **felodipine**, ℞ **fluvastatin**, ℞ **indinavir**, ℞ **lovastatin**, ℞ **methadone**, ℞ **methylprednisolone**, ℞ **midazolam**, ℞ **nelfinavir**, ℞ **pravastatin**, ℞ **quinidine**, ℞ **ritonavir**, ℞ **saquinavir**, ℞ **simvastatin**, ℞ **tacrolimus**, ℞ **tolbutamide**, ℞ **triazolam**, and ℞ **warfarin sodium** may be reduced by ketoconazole.
• Astemizole, cisapride, ℞ **pimozide**, ℞ **quinidine**, and ℞ **fexofenadine** can cause potentially serious (even life-threatening) arrhythmias.
• ℞ **Aluminum**, ⚖ **calcium**, ℞ **cimetidine**, ℞ **didanosine**, ℞ **famotidine**, ℞ **lansoprazole**, ⚖ **magnesium**, ℞ **nizatidine**, and ℞ **sodium bicarbonate** may reduce the effects of ketoconazole.
• ℞ **Rifampin** - the effects of both drugs may be reduced.

Side effects

These depend on how it is administered.
• Occasionally, nausea, and vomiting.
• Rarely, abdominal pain diarrhea, headache, dizziness, itching, blood disorders, liver disorders, impotence, and breast enlargement in men.

ketoprofen Ⓖ

Type/Group: **anti-inflammatory; antirheumatic; non-narcotic analgesic; NSAID**.
Brand(s): Orudis Capsules; Orudis KT Tablets; Oruvail Capsules; various generic.
How administered: Orally.

Used to treat

Ketoprofen is used to treat the signs and symptoms of ✪ **osteoarthritis** and ✪ **rheumatoid arthritis**, mild to moderate pain of rheumatic or muscular inflammation, or after surgery, to alleviate the discomfort of toothache, backache, and dysmenorrhea (period pain), and as an ℞ **antipyretic** to reduce fever.

Warnings

• It should not be used by people with known hypersensitivity to this drug or to other NSAIDs (including ℞ **aspirin**), who have epilepsy, chronic kidney disease, certain bleeding disorders or conditions (for example, hemophilia, vitamin K deficiency, low blood-platelet levels), or who have a tendency to, or active, peptic ulceration.

• It should be given with caution to people with allergic disorders (especially asthma and skin conditions), who are elderly, or with any kind of kidney impairment or with certain liver disorders.

• Ketoprofen should be used during pregnancy only when medically judged to be needed. In the third trimester, however, its risk to the fetus increase, and so it should only be used if the benefits outweigh the risks, which are at their highest during this time.

• Breast-feeding mothers should either discontinue this drug or stop breast-feeding.

• With regular, long-term use (as in the treatment of osteoarthritis), NSAIDs may cause gastrointestinal bleeding, ulceration, or perforation. Any signs of bleeding (for example, black stools) should be reported to a physician immediately.

• Most NSAIDs have the potential, particularly with regular use, to cause liver damage. Periodic evaluation of liver function is necessary in long-term therapy (more than two months).

• Side effects are more frequent in the elderly.

• Gastrointestinal upsets may be minimized by taking it with milk or food.

Interactions

• There is generally no added benefit in taking other NSAIDs or other ℞ **salicylates** (especially aspirin) at the same time, but there is a higher risk of gastrointestinal upsets and bleeding.

• Alcohol and ℞ **corticosteroids** increase the risk of bleeding, particularly if there is an existing ulcer.

• ℞ **anticoagulant**, ℞ **antiplatelet**, and ℞ **thrombolytic** drugs may increase bleeding time.

• The effectiveness of ℞ **ACE inhibitors** and ℞ **beta-blockers** may be reduced.

• There is a risk of damaging kidney function if taken with ℞ **diuretics** (for example, ℞ **furosemide**).

• It should not be taken with ℞ **triamterene** because there is a risk of kidney failure.

• The effects of ℞ **cyclosporine**, ℞ **lithium**, and ℞ **methotrexate** may be exaggerated, with potential for toxicity.

• Ketoprofen should not be used with ℞ **probenecid**.

• Foodstuffs and herbals with ℞ **antiplatelet** properties, for example, ♣ **ginger**, ◊◊ **garlic**, and various herbal preparations, may add to the antiplatelet effect of NSAIDs.

Side effects

• Commonly, gastrointestinal upsets, flatulence, nausea, diarrhea, constipation, headache, and edema.

• Less frequently, vomiting, mood swings, malaise, dizziness, ringing in the ears, fatigue, blurred vision, or changes in blood pressure.

• Prolonged bleeding time (with consequent risk of ulceration) is possible with high dosage, and other blood changes can occur, including anemia.

• Hypersensitivity reactions may include symptoms such as hives, chest tightness, asthma, or bronchospasm.

• Reversible kidney failure, particularly in renal impairment, has occurred. Liver damage is rare.

ketorolac trometamol ⑤

see ℞ **ketorolac tromethamine**.

ketorolac tromethamine ⑤

(ketorolac trometamol)

Type/Group: **anti-inflammatory; antirheumatic; non-narcotic analgesic; NSAID**.

Brand(s): Toradol Tablets, Injection; various generic. (For ophthalmic use): Acular.

How administered: Orally; topically; injection.

Used to treat

Ketorolac tromethamine is used in the short-term management of moderate to severe acute postoperative pain, and to prevent and reduce inflammation following eye surgery (for example, cataract extraction). It is also used for the relief of itchy eyes due to seasonal allergic rhinitis.

Warnings

• It should not be used by people with known hypersensitivity to this drug or to other NSAIDs (including ℞ **aspirin**), who have epilepsy, chronic kidney disease, certain bleeding disorders or conditions (for example, hemophilia, vitamin K deficiency, low blood-platelet levels), or who have a tendency to, or active, peptic ulceration.

• It should be given with caution to people taking certain drugs for gout or epilepsy, or with allergic disorders (especially asthma and skin conditions), who are elderly, or with any kind of kidney impairment or with certain liver disorders.

• Ketorolac should be used when pregnant only if medically judged that the benefits outweigh the risk to the fetus. It should not be used during the third trimester, however, when risk to the fetus is highest.

• Breast-feeding mothers should either discontinue this drug or stop breast-feeding.

• It should not be taken for more than five days (at recommended doses) because the risk of adverse effects increases greatly.

• It should not be used with aspirin or other ℞ **NSAIDs**, as serious side effects are more likely.

• Side effects are more frequent in the elderly.

• Gastrointestinal upsets may be minimized by taking the drug with milk or food.

• Do not wear soft-contact lenses when using the ophthalmic solution.

• It is not for long-term use.

Interactions

• There is generally no added benefit in taking other NSAIDs or other ℞ **salicylates** (especially aspirin) at the same time, but there is a higher risk of gastrointestinal upsets and bleeding.

• Alcohol and ℞ **corticosteroids** increase the risk of bleeding, particularly if there is an existing ulcer.

• ℞ **anticoagulant**, ℞ **antiplatelet**, and ℞ **thrombolytic** drugs may increase bleeding time.

• The effectiveness of ℞ **ACE inhibitors**, ℞ **beta-blockers**, and ℞ **diuretics** (for example, ℞ **furosemide**) may be reduced.

• ℞ **antiepileptics** may increase the risk of seizure.

• There is a possibility of respiratory depression if taken with ℞ **skeletal muscle relaxants**.

• The effects of ℞ **cyclosporine**, ℞ **lithium**, and ℞ **methotrexate** may be exaggerated, with potential for toxicity.

• ketorolac should not be used with ℞ **probenecid**.

• Foodstuffs and herbals with ℞ **antiplatelet** properties, for example, ♣ **ginger**, ⚭ **garlic**, and various herbal preparations, may add to the antiplatelet effect of NSAIDs.

Side effects

These depend on how administered, dose, duration of treatment, and use.

• Commonly, gastrointestinal upsets, flatulence, nausea, diarrhea, constipation, headache, drowsiness, dizziness, and edema.

• Less frequently, vomiting, nervousness, euphoria, hallucinations, incoordination, tremor, or changes in blood pressure.

• Prolonged bleeding time (with consequent risk of ulceration) is possible with high dosage, and other blood changes can occur, including anemia. Other kinds of blood disorder may arise, though infrequently.

• Hypersensitivity reactions may include symptoms such as hives, swelling of the tongue or larynx, chest tightness, asthma, or bronchospasm.

• Reversible kidney failure, particularly in renal impairment, has occurred. Liver damage is rare.

• There may be pain at the site of injection, or irritation with suppositories.

• When used as eyedrops, there may be burning, stinging, itching, or blurred vision.

ketotifen ⒢

Type/Group: **antihistamine; antiallergic; decongestant.**
Brand(s): Zaditor.
How administered: Topically (eyedrops).

Used to treat

Ketotifen has anti-allergic properties similar to those of ℞ **cromolyn sodium**, and can be used to prevent itching of the eye due to allergic ✷ **conjunctivitis**.

Warnings

• It should not be given to people with known hypersensitivity to this drug (or with known sensitivity to other antihistamines). When used topically in the eye, it should not be used when contact lenses are worn.

• Ketotifen should be used during pregnancy only if the potential benefit outweighs the potential risk to the fetus.

• Medical judgment is required if breast-feeding is being considered.

• This drug is currently for topical (eye) use only.

Interactions

When used topically at recommended doses, no significant interactions are known.

Side effects

• There may be reactions such as stinging, burning or itching of the eye, eye pain or painful sensitivity to light (photophobia). Allergic reactions such as rash, irritated throat and flu-like feeling may also occur.

Key-Pred (acetate) Ⓑ

A preparation of ℞ **prednisolone** acetate.
Formulation: Injection in several strengths.
Availability: Prescription only.
Warnings and side effects: See ℞ **prednisolone**.

Key-Pred (sodium phosphate) Ⓑ

A preparation of ℞ **prednisolone** sodium phosphate.
Formulation: Injection in several strengths.
Availability: Prescription only.
Warnings and side effects: See ℞ **prednisolone**.

KIE Syrup Ⓑ

A preparation of ℞ **ephedrine** and potassium iodide.
Formulation: Oral syrup.
Availability: Prescription only.
Warnings and side effects: See ℞ **ephedrine**.

Klerist-D Capsules; Tablets Ⓑ

A preparation of ℞ **pseudoephedrine** and ℞ **chlorpheniramine maleate**.
Formulation: Oral capsules, sustained release; tablets.
Availability: Prescription only.
Warnings and side effects: See ℞ **pseudoephedrine**; ℞ **chlorpheniramine maleate**.

Klonopin Ⓑ

A preparation of ℞ **clonazepam**.
Formulation: Oral tablets in several strengths.
Availability: Prescription only.
Warnings and side effects: See ℞ **clonazepam**.

Koate-HP Ⓑ

A preparation of ℞ **antihemophilic factor** (human).
Formulation: Intravenous infusion.
Availability: Prescription only.
Warnings and side effects: See ℞ **antihemophilic factor**.
Contains a small amount of ℞ **heparin**.

Kof-Eze Ⓑ

A preparation of ℞ **menthol**.
Formulation: Lozenges.
Availability: OTC.
Warnings and side effects: See ℞ **menthol**.

Kogenate; Kogenate FS Ⓑ

A preparation of ℞ **antihemophilic factor** (recombinant).
Formulation: Intravenous infusion.
Availability: Prescription only.

Warnings and side effects: See ℞ antihemophilic factor.
Kogenate FS contains no albumin (human).

Kolephrin Caplets ℬ

A preparation of ℞ **pseudoephedrine**, ℞ **acetaminophen**, and ℞ **chlorpheniramine maleate**.
Formulation: Oral tablets.
Availability: OTC.
Warnings and side effects: See ℞ pseudoephedrine; ℞ acetaminophen; ℞ chlorpheniramine maleate.

Kolephrin/DM Caplets ℬ

A preparation of ℞ **dextromethorphan**, ℞ **acetaminophen**, ℞ **chlorpheniramine maleate**, and ℞ **pseudoephedrine**.
Formulation: Oral caplets.
Availability: OTC.
Warnings and side effects: See ℞ dextromethorphan; ℞ acetaminophen; ℞ chlorpheniramine maleate; ℞ pseudoephedrine.

Kolephrin GG/DM Liquid ℬ

A preparation of ℞ **dextromethorphan** and ℞ **guaifenesin**.
Formulation: Oral liquid.
Availability: OTC.
Warnings and side effects: See ℞ dextromethorphan; ℞ guaifenesin.

Kondon's Nasal ℬ

A preparation of ℞ **ephedrine**.
Formulation: Jelly.
Availability: OTC.
Warnings and side effects: See ℞ ephedrine.

Kondremul Plain ℬ

A preparation of ℞ **mineral oil**.
Formulation: Oral emulsion.
Availability: OTC.
Warnings and side effects: See ℞ mineral oil.

Konsyl; Konsyl-D; Konsyl-Orange; Easy Mix Formula ℬ

A preparation of ℞ **psyllium**.
Formulation: Oral powder.
Availability: OTC.
Warnings and side effects: See ℞ psyllium.

Konyne 80 ℬ

A preparation of ℞ **Factor IX complex** (human; also contains Factors II, VII, X).
Formulation: Intravenous infusion.
Availability: Prescription only.
Warnings and side effects: See ℞ Factor IX complex.

Kronofed-A Capsules; Jr. Capsules ℬ

A preparation of ℞ **pseudoephedrine** and ℞ **chlorpheniramine maleate**.
Formulation: Oral capsules, sustained release.
Availability: Prescription only.
Warnings and side effects: See ℞ pseudoephedrine; ℞ chlorpheniramine maleate.

Kudrox Double Strength Suspension ℬ

A preparation of ℞ **aluminum hydroxide**, ℞ **magnesium hydroxide**, and ℞ **simethicone**.
Formulation: Oral liquid.
Availability: OTC.
Warnings and side effects: See ℞ aluminum hydroxide; ℞ magnesium hydroxide; ℞ simethicone.

Ku-Zyme HP Capsules ℬ

A preparation of ℞ **pancreatin** (amylase, lipase, protease).
Formulation: Oral capsules.
Availability: Prescription only.
Warnings and side effects: See ℞ pancreatin.

Kwelcof Liquid ℬ

A preparation of ℞ **hydrocodone bitartrate** and ℞ **guaifenesin**.
Formulation: Oral liquid.
Availability: Prescription only.
Warnings and side effects: See ℞ hydrocodone bitartrate; ℞ guaifenesin.

Kytril ℬ

A preparation of ℞ **granisetron**.
Formulation: Oral tablets; injection.
Availability: Prescription only.
Warnings and side effects: See ℞ granisetron.

LA-12 ℬ

A preparation of ℞ **hydroxocobalamin**.
Formulation: Injection.
Availability: Prescription only.
Warnings and side effects: See ℞ hydroxocobalamin.

labetalol hydrochloride Ⓖ

Type/Group: **beta-blocker; alpha-adrenergic blocker; vasodilator; antihypertensive**.
Brand(s): Normodyne; Trandate; various generic.
How administered: Orally; injection.

Used to treat

Labetalol is an unusual drug that combines both beta-blocker and alpha-adrenergic blocker properties. It can be used, alone or in combination with other drugs, to reduce high blood pressure (see ✪ **hypertension**). Because it has less effect on the heart than other beta-blockers, labetalol is often used in hypertensive "emergencies," where it is necessary to reduce blood pressure quickly (for example, some brain injuries, aneurysm, eclampsia, heart attack). It is sometimes used for ✪ **pheochromocytoma**.

Warnings

• It should not be given to people with known hypersensitivity to any beta-blocking drug, who have certain heartbeat irregularities or heart failure, severe hypotension, or bronchial asthma. It should not be used in cardiogenic shock.

• It should be given with caution to people with diabetes mellitus or hypoglycemia, hyperthyroidism, myasthenia gravis, congestive heart failure, peripheral vascular disease, or liver impairment. Beta-blockers are generally not given to anyone with a chronic obstructive pulmonary disease, including asthma.

• Labetalol should be used during pregnancy only if the potential benefit outweighs the possible risk to the fetus.

• Medical judgment is required if breast-feeding is being considered. This drug appears in breast milk.

• Labetalol, in rare instances, has caused liver damage. Any early symptoms, such as dark urine, jaundice, right upper quadrant tenderness (over the liver), an unexplained "flu-like" feeling, or persistent loss of appetite should be reported to a doctor. Periodic monitoring of liver function is required.

• Abruptly stopping using a beta-blocker may have adverse effects, including on the heart.

• The use of this drug may mask signs of hyperthyroidism or hypoglycemia.

• Other medications (including OTCs, herbal remedies, and supplements) must not be taken without consulting a doctor. Some ℞ **nasal decongestants**, commonly available over the counter, contain ℞ **alpha-adrenergic stimulants** (for example, ℞ **phenylephrine**) that may cause a severe hypertensive reaction if taken with beta-blockers.

Interactions

• A serious blood pressure increase may occur after withdrawal from ℞ **clonidine hydrochloride** or both drugs at the same time.

• Other ℞ **antiarrhythmics** (for example, ℞ **amiodarone**, ℞ **disopyramide**, ℞ **quinidine**, ℞ **procainamide**) and ℞ **tricyclics** have the potential for significant adverse effects on heart rhythm. Tricyclics used together with labetalol are associated with development of tremor in some individuals.

• The effects of ℞ **alpha-adrenergic stimulants**, ℞ **ergot alkaloids**, ℞ **epinephrine**, ℞ **hydralazine hydrochloride**, ℞ **lidocaine**, and ℞ **theophylline** may be increased, with the risk of serious adverse effects.

• ℞ **Calcium-channel blockers** (particularly ℞ **diltiazem hydrochloride** and ℞ **verapamil**), ℞ **guanethidine monosulfate**, ℞ **MAOIs**, and ℞ **reserpine** have the potential for increasing undesirable effects, with exaggerated slowing of heartbeat or hypotension.

• The effects of nondepolarizing ℞ **skeletal muscle relaxants** may be variable, with the possible risk of significant adverse effects associated with major surgery.

• The effects of ℞ **beta-adrenergic stimulant** (for example, ℞ **albuterol**, ℞ **terbutaline**), ℞ **insulin**, ℞ **nitroglycerin**, and ℞ **sulfonylureas** may be reduced.

• ℞ **Cimetidine** may increase the effect of labetalol.

• ℞ **Antacids** (for example, ℞ **aluminum hydroxide**, ℞ **magnesium hydroxide**), ℞ **barbiturates**, ⚗ **calcium** salts,

℞ **cholestyramine**, ℞ **colestipol hydrochloride**, ℞ **NSAIDs**, ℞ **phenytoin**, ℞ **penicillins**, ℞ **rifampin**, and ℞ **salicylates** may reduce the levels and effectiveness of beta-blockers. Antacids should not be taken within two hours of beta-blockers.

• If used with ℞ **diuretics** and other antihypertensive drugs, there are additive effects which are often used to therapeutic advantage.

Side effects

These are infrequent and may include:

• Dizziness, fatigue, nausea, shortness of breath, nasal stuffiness, sexual dysfunction, postural hypotension (low blood pressure when standing up), loss of appetite, headache or tingling of the scalp, and bronchospasm;

• Heart failure, should it develop, generally requires withdrawal (gradually, if possible) of this drug.

• Unusual antibodies may develop, though lupus-like symptoms (fever, myalgia, pleurisy, various inflammations) seldom occur;

• Postural hypotension occurs frequently after intravenous administration of labetalol.

LactiCare-HC ®

A preparation of ℞ **hydrocortisone**.
Formulation: Lotion.
Availability: Prescription only.
Warnings and side effects: See ℞ **hydrocortisone**.

lactulose Ⓖ

Type/Group: **laxative**.
Brand(s): Cephulac; Cholac; Chronulac; Constulose; Duphalac; Enulose; various generic.
How administered: Orally; topically (rectal).

Used to treat

Lactulose is an osmotic laxative and is a sugar-like compound. It relieves ✪ **constipation** by retaining fluid in the intestine and may take up to 48 hours to have full effect. It can also be used to treat hepatic (portal system) encephalopathy.

Warnings

• It should not be given to people with any form of intestinal obstruction, or who require a low galactose diet.

• It should be given with caution to people with diabetes mellitus.

• The effects of lactulose in pregnancy have not been studied, and it should be used only if it is clearly needed.

• Medical judgment is required if breast-feeding is being considered. It is not known whether this drug appears in breast milk.

• It should not be used with other laxatives.

• Do not use if there is abdominal pain, nausea, or vomiting, unless directed by a doctor.

• Chronic use of laxatives may cause fluid and electrolyte imbalances, vitamin and mineral deficiencies, and abnormal bowel function. Generally, they should not be used for more than a week.

• A doctor must be consulted first before taking any other medication (including OTCs, herbal remedies, and supplements), because laxatives may alter the absorption of a wide range of drugs.

Interactions
• Nonabsorbable ℞ **antacids** may interfere with the action of lactulose.

Side effects
• There may be flatulence, intestinal cramps or abdominal discomfort, belching, and nausea.

Lamictal Tablets; Chewable Dispersible Tablets ⓑ
A preparation of ℞ **lamotrigine**.
Formulation: Oral tablets, available in 4 strengths; chewable tablets.
Availability: Prescription only.
Warnings and side effects: See ℞ **lamotrigine**.

Lamisil ⓑ
A preparation of ℞ **terbinafine**.
Formulation: Oral tablets; topical gel; topical cream.
Availability: Oral formulation is prescription only; topical cream is OTC.
Warnings and side effects: See ℞ **terbinafine**.

lamivudine ⓖ
(3TC)
Type/Group: **antiviral**.
Brand(s): Epivir. Combinations: with *zidovudine*: Combivir. With *zidovudine* and *abacavir*: Trizivir.
How administered: Orally.

Used to treat
Lamivudine is a reverse transcriptase antiviral drug that can be used in antiretroviral treatment of ✚ **HIV** infection, normally in combination with other antiviral drugs. It can also be used for chronic ✚ **hepatitis** B infection.

Warnings
• It should not be given to people with known hypersensitivity to lamivudine.
• It should be given with caution to people with peripheral neuropathy or a history of peripheral neuropathy, impaired kidney function, or children with a history of pancreatitis.
• Lamivudine's safety during pregnancy has not been established, and it should be used only when the potential benefits outweigh the possible risk to the fetus.
• Medical judgment is required if breast-feeding is being considered. HIV-infected mothers are advised not to breast-feed.
• Pancreatitis may occur in a significant number of children.
• It is a specialist drug, and there will be full assessment and patient monitoring throughout treatment.

Interactions
• ℞ **trimethoprim and sulfamethoxazole** (Bactrim) increases lamivudine concentration.

Side effects
• Frequently, gastrointestinal effects, headache, cough, malaise, insomnia, muscular pain, nasal symptoms, and peripheral neuropathy.
• Occasionally, depression, muscle pain, and abdominal cramps.

• Rarely, pancreatitis, blood disturbances, and changes in liver enzymes.

lamotrigine ⓖ
Type/Group: **anticonvulsant; antiepileptic**.
Brand(s): Lamictal Tablets, Chewable Dispersible Tablets.
How administered: Orally.

Used to treat
This is a recently introduced anticonvulsant and antiepileptic drug, which is used to treat ✚ **epilepsy**, including partial and tonic-clonic seizures.

Warnings
• Avoid its use in people with known hypersensitivity to this drug, or with liver impairment.
• Lamotrigine should be given with caution to children and anyone with certain kidney disorders or heart impairment.
• It should be used in pregnancy only when potential benefit outweighs risk to the fetus.
• Breast-feeding mothers should either discontinue using this drug or stop breast-feeding.
• A doctor must be notified if a skin rash appears. Although they are rare, serious, and even life-threatening rashes have been associated with this drug, particularly when used together with valproic acid.
• Withdrawal should be gradual otherwise it may precipitate attacks.
• As this drug may cause drowsiness, driving or other hazardous activity should be avoided.
• Avoid prolonged exposure to direct sunlight.

Interactions
• Valproic acid (for example, ℞ **valproate sodium**, ℞ **divalproex sodium**) may markedly raise concentrations of lamotrigine, while the levels of valproic acid fall.
• ℞ **carbamazepine** may cause levels of lamotrigine to fall, and carbamazepine levels to rise.
• ℞ **acetaminophen**, ℞ **phenobarbital**, ℞ **phenytoin**, and ℞ **primidone** may lower levels of lamotrigine and so decrease its therapeutic effect.
• Lamotrigine interferes with the metabolism of folate (℞ **folic acid**).

Side effects
These are many and may include:
• Dizziness, rashes, headache, visual disturbances, gastrointestinal upsets, nausea, and vomiting;
• Fever, malaise, flu-like symptoms, and drowsiness;
• Dizziness, headache, unsteady gait, and drowsiness are more frequent at high doses;
• Rarely, liver dysfunction, blood changes, movement and mood changes;
• Potentially serious side effects include certain skin reactions and a worsening of seizures.

Lanabiotic ⓑ
A preparation of ℞ **neomycin**, ℞ **polymyxin B sulfate**, ℞ **bacitracin**, and ℞ **lidocaine**.

Formulation: Topical ointment.
Availability: OTC.
Warnings and side effects: See ℞ neomycin; ℞ polymyxin B sulfate; ℞ bacitracin; ℞ lidocaine.

Lanacane Cream; Lanacane Spray ⑧

A preparation of ℞ benzocaine.
Formulation: Topical cream.
Availability: OTC.
Warnings and side effects: See ℞ benzocaine.

Lanacort-5; Lanacort 10 ⑧

A preparation of ℞ hydrocortisone.
Formulation: Cream in two strengths; ointment.
Availability: OTC.
Warnings and side effects: See ℞ hydrocortisone.

Laniazid; Laniazid CT ⑧

A preparation of ℞ isoniazid.
Formulation: Oral tablets in two strengths; oral syrup.
Availability: Prescription only.
Warnings and side effects: See ℞ isoniazid.

lanolin ⑥

Type/Group: **emollient**.
Brand(s): Desitin; Bottom Better; Keri; Lubritears; Nivea Moisturizing; Preparation H.
How administered: Topically (external).
Used to treat
Lanolin is a fatty substance obtained from sheep's wool that is incorporated into several emollient preparations. It can be used on cracked, dry or scaling skin, where it encourages hydration and is commonly combined with ℞ **mineral oil**.
Warnings
• It should not be given to people with known hypersensitivity to lanolin.
• A doctor must be consulted before using during pregnancy or while breast-feeding.
• Some people are allergic to lanolin, in which case a skin rash develops.
Interactions
No significant interactions are known.
Side effects
Lanolin is considered safe in normal topical use.

Lanophyllin ⑧

A preparation of ℞ theophylline.
Formulation: Oral elixir.
Availability: Prescription only.
Warnings and side effects: See ℞ theophylline.

Lanoxicaps; Lanoxin Tablets, Pediatric Elixir, Injection ⑧

A preparation of ℞ digoxin.
Formulation: Oral tablets; capsules (Lanoxicaps); liquid; injection.

Availability: Prescription only.
Warnings and side effects: See ℞ digoxin.

lansoprazole ⑥

Type/Group: **proton-pump inhibitor; ulcer-healing drug**.
Brand(s): Prevacid. Combinations: With *amoxicillin, clarithromycin*: Prevpac.
How administered: Orally.
Used to treat
Lansoprazole works as an inhibitor of gastric acid secretion in the parietal (acid-producing) cells of the stomach lining by acting as a proton-pump inhibitor. It is used for the treatment of benign gastric and duodenal ulcers (see ◐ **peptic ulcer**) (including those complicating ℞ **NSAID** therapy), ◐ **indigestion**, ◐ **Zollinger-Ellison syndrome**, and reflux esophagitis. It can also be used with antibiotics to treat gastric *Helicobacter pylori* infection.
Warnings
• It should not be given to people with known hypersensitivity to this drug, or to any substituted benzimidazoles (that is, other proton-pump inhibitors, such as ℞ **omeprazole**, ℞ **rabeprazole**, ℞ **pantoprazole**).
• It should be given with caution to people with severe liver impairment.
• Lansoprazole should be used during pregnancy only if the potential benefit outweighs the possible risk to the fetus.
• Medical judgment is required if breast-feeding is being considered. It is not known whether this drug appears in breast milk, but there is reason to believe its effects would be harmful.
• Before treatment, it should be confirmed that there is no gastric cancer or other disease.
• Drug levels may vary depending whether ethnic origin is Asian or Caucasian. (But this difference is not as significant as it is with ℞ **omeprazole**.)
• Food reduces the absorption of lansoprazole, and so the drug should be taken before eating.
Interactions
• The levels and effects of ℞ **theophylline** may be decreased.
• Proton-pump inhibitors, like lansoprazole, should be taken at least 30 minutes before ℞ **sucralfate** or they may not be absorbed efficiently.
• The levels and effects of ℞ **digoxin**, ferrous salts (◊◊ **iron supplements**), ℞ **ketoconazole**, and ℞ **ampicillin** may be decreased when taken with lansoprazole.
• It is thought possible that deficiency of ◊◊ **vitamin B$_{12}$** can occur with long-term use of lansoprazole.
Side effects
• These are uncommon with lansoprazole, consisting mainly of diarrhea and abdominal pain, but proton-pump inhibitors may also cause headache, rashes and itching, dizziness, nausea and vomiting, constipation, and flatulence. These drugs also decrease gastric acidity and so may increase the risk of gastrointestinal infections.
• Rarer side effects may include hives, other allergic reactions, fever, malaise, nosebleed, muscle and joint pain, kidney problems, pancreatitis, sleepiness, insomnia, temporary mental disturbances,

hair loss, peripheral edema, effects on the liver and the heart, and various blood changes. (When used together with ℞ **clarithromycin** and ℞ **amoxicillin** the commonest side effects are diarrhea, headache and strange taste sensation; with amoxicillin alone there may be diarrhea and headache.)

• Very rare but occasionally reported are menstrual problems, growth of breasts in men, and impotence.

Lantus ®

A preparation of ℞ **insulin glargine**.
Formulation: Injection.
Availability: Prescription only.
Warnings and side effects: See ℞ **insulin glargine**.

Larodopa ®

A preparation of ℞ **levodopa**.
Formulation: Oral tablets in several strengths.
Availability: Prescription only.
Warnings and side effects: See ℞ **levodopa**.

Lasix ®

A preparation of ℞ **furosemide**.
Formulation: Oral tablets, available in 3 strengths.
Availability: Prescription only.
Warnings and side effects: See ℞ **furosemide**.

latanoprost ©

Type/Group: glaucoma treatment; prostaglandin.
Brand(s): Xalatan.
How administered: Topically (eyes).

Used to treat

Latanoprost is used as a novel treatment of open-angle ✪ **glaucoma** and ocular hypertension in people for whom other drugs are not suitable. It increases the outflow of aqueous humor (fluid in the eye).

Warnings

• It should not be given to people with known hypersensitivity to this drug or with corneal disease.

• Latanoprost's safety during pregnancy has not been established. It should be used only if the potential benefit outweighs the possible risk to the fetus.

• Medical judgment is required if breast-feeding is being considered.

• It can cause an increase in brown pigment in the iris and change the color of the eyes (which may not be noticeable for months).

• It must not be administered while wearing contact lenses.

• The preservative in latanoprost solution, benzalkonium chloride, may be absorbed by soft contact lenses, and so it should be used 15 minutes before putting in the lenses.

Interactions

No significant interactions have been reported.

Side effects

• Blurred vision, burning and stinging, increased blood flow to conjunctiva, foreign body sensation, and itching.

• Systemic side effects (because it can be absorbed into the body through the eye) such as respiratory tract infections, back and joint pain, and rash.

laxative Ⓞ

Generics: bisacodyl; cascara sagrada; castor oil; dehydrocholic acid; docusate sodium; glycerin; karaya; lactulose; magnesium carbonate; magnesium hydroxide; magnesium sulfate; methylcellulose; mineral oil; psyllium; senna; sodium phosphate.

Actions and uses

Laxative and other purgatives are preparations that promote defecation and so relieve ✪ **constipation**. They can be divided into several different types. The *fecal softener* laxatives (for example, ℞ **mineral oil**) soften the feces for easier evacuation. The *bulking-agent* laxatives increase the overall volume of the feces, which then stimulates bowel movement. Bulking agents are usually some form of fiber, for example, ℞ **psyllium**, ℞ **methylcellulose**, or ℞ **karaya** (sterculia gum). The *stimulant* laxatives act on the intestinal muscles to increase motility (movement). Many traditional remedies for constipation are stimulants, such as ℞ **cascara sagrada**, ℞ **castor oil**, ℞ **senna**, and elixir of figs. However, there are modern variants with less of a stimulant action and which also have other properties, for example, ℞ **bisacodyl** and ℞ **docusate sodium**. Finally, the *osmotic* laxatives which are chemical salts that work by retaining water in the intestine, so increasing overall liquidity, for example, ℞ **lactulose**, ℞ **magnesium hydroxide**, ℞ **magnesium carbonate**, and ℞ **magnesium sulfate** (note that magnesium salts are also used as ℞ **antacid** drugs). Suppositories and enemas (for instance, containing ℞ **sodium phosphate** or ℞ **glycerin**) also aid in promoting defecation. ℞ **dehydrocholic acid**, a bile salt derivative is sometimes used as a mild laxative.

Laxatives are also used to treat constipation which results as a side effect of another drug, to clear the alimentary tract before radiological or surgical procedures, and to help expel parasites after ℞ **anthelmintic** treatment.

Limitations

Chronic use of laxatives may cause fluid and electrolyte imbalances, vitamin and mineral deficiencies, and abnormal bowel function. Generally, they should not be used for more than a week.

In general, no stool softener should be used together with any oral drug whose margin between therapeutic dose and overdose toxicity is narrow ("low therapeutic index"). Examples are ℞ **antiarrhythmic** drugs, many ℞ **anticancer** drugs, also ℞ **digoxin**, ℞ **lithium**, ℞ **theophylline**, and ℞ **warfarin sodium**. Stool softeners may allow for a higher absorption in the intestines and so higher levels of drugs in circulation. A doctor should always be consulted in such cases. Anyone taking any medication, including OTC (over-the-counter) brands, herbal remedies, supplements, or any kind of alternative renedy, should consult a doctor before deciding to self-administer a laxative.

Lazer Formaldehyde ®

A preparation of ℞ **formaldehyde**.
Formulation: Topical solution.

Availability: Prescription only.
Warnings and side effects: See ℞ **formaldehyde**.

LazerSporine-C ⑧
A preparation of ℞ **hydrocortisone**, ℞ **neomycin**, and ℞ **polymyxin B sulfate**.
Formulation: Ear drops.
Availability: Prescription only.
Warnings and side effects: See ℞ **hydrocortisone**; ℞ **neomycin**; ℞ **polymyxin B sulfate**.

leflunomide ⑤
Type/Group: **antirheumatic; immunosuppressant**.
Brand(s): Arava.
How administered: Orally.

Used to treat
Leflunomide is a recently introduced drug used to treat active episodes of ✪ **rheumatoid arthritis**. The beneficial effect does not develop until after several weeks and takes a long time to wear off.

Warnings
• It should not be used by people with known hypersensitivity to this drug. As its effects have not yet been fully studied, it is not recommended for use in those with kidney or liver impairment, conditions that might impair the immune system (for example, bone marrow suppresion, uncontrolled infection), or within a short time of vaccination with any live ℞ **vaccine**. This is a specialist drug, and full patient evaluation will be carried out.
• Leflunomide should not be used during pregnancy or when the possibility of becoming pregnant exists (women with childbearing potential should use reliable contraception).
• Breast-feeding mothers should either discontinue using this drug or stop breast-feeding.
• Use of this drug may increase the risk of malignancy, particularly of a lymphatic kind.
• During treatment with leflunomide, change in liver function is common and usually reversible, but regular medical monitoring is necessary.

Interactions
• Live ℞ **vaccines** should not be administered until leflunomide has cleared the body (it is removed only slowly).
• Leflunomide taken with ℞ **methotrexate** or other drugs that impair liver function (hepatotoxic) may increase the risk of damage to the liver.
• ℞ **rifampin** may raise leflunomide concentration.
• ℞ **cholestyramine** and ℞ **activated charcoal** lower concentrations of leflunomide.

Side effects
This is a new drug and possible side effects and warnings are extensive. It is only used under specialist supervision. There may be:
• Diarrhea, abnormal liver function, hair loss, rash, and itchiness;
• Less frequently, effects such as fever, malaise, palpitations, constipation, flatulence, anemia, bone pain, ache, herpes skin manifestations, blurred vision, and odd taste sensations. Other than anemia, blood changes are rare.
• Anaphylactic reaction is extremely rare.

Lente Iletin II ⑧
A preparation of ℞ **insulin zinc suspension (lente)**.
Formulation: Bottles for injection.
Availability: OTC.
Warnings and side effects: See ℞ **insulin zinc suspension (lente)**.

Lente L ⑧
A preparation of ℞ **insulin zinc suspension (lente)**.
Formulation: Vials for injection.
Availability: OTC.
Warnings and side effects: See ℞ **insulin zinc suspension (lente)**.

lepirudin ⑤
Type/Group: **anticoagulant**.
Brand(s): Refludan.
How administered: Intravenous infusion or injection.

Used to treat
Lepirudin is an anticoagulant, a synthetic (recombinant process) version of natural hirudin from the salivary glands of the medicinal leech. It is a parenteral anticoagulant (not active by mouth, and must be injected), and can be used for anticoagulation where antithrombotic treatment is needed, but there is adverse reaction to ℞ **heparin** (for example, thrombocytopenia).

Warnings
• It should not be given to people with known hypersensitivity to this drug. It will be administered by experienced personnel after a full medical assessment.
• It should be given with extreme caution to people with an increased risk of hemorrhage (for example, uncontrolled hypertension, bleeding disorders, active ulcer, bacterial endocarditis, recent stroke or surgery—especially to the eye or nervous system) or with severe kidney or liver impairment. Also, use with caution in people with kidney insufficiency.
• Lepirudin should be used during pregnancy only if it is clearly needed.
• Medical judgment is required if breast-feeding is being considered. It is not known whether this drug appears in breast milk.
• Lepirudin used with ℞ **streptokinase** or similar ℞ **thrombolytic** may cause life-threatening intracranial bleeding.
• Regular blood testing is required to check the effect of doses and to adjust dose levels. Antibodies to this substance often form and may alter the levels and effect of lepirudin.

Interactions
• If used with other anticoagulants, ℞ **antiplatelet** agents, ℞ **aspirin**, or thrombolytics (for example, streptokinase), there is a higher potential for bleeding (caution is advised).

Side effects
• The most common is bleeding, which may occur at virtually any site (for example, a puncture or wound, gastrointestinal tract, respiratory tract, other organs), although intracranial bleeding has not been reported, except when lepirudin has been used with certain thrombolytic drugs.

• Other side effects may include a change in liver or kidney function, heart failure or effects on other organs. Some allergic reactions are common with lepirudin (for example, cough, bronchospasm, shortness of breath). Rash, hives, chills, fever and anaphylactoid responses occur less frequently.
• Allergic swelling of face, tongue, or larynx is rare.

Lescol ℞

A preparation of ℞ **fluvastatin**.
Formulation: Oral capsules.
Availability: Prescription only.
Warnings and side effects: See ℞ **fluvastatin**.

letrozole Ⓖ

Type/Group: **anticancer; hormone antagonist**.
Brand(s): Femara.
How administered: Orally.

Used to treat

Letrozole is used to treat advanced breast cancer in postmeno-pausal women whose disease has progressed following antiestro-gen treatment. It is an aromatase inhibitor that works by inhibiting the conversion of androgens (male sex hormones) into estrogens.

Warnings

• It should not be used by people with known hypersensitivity to this drug, or whose disease is not responsive to antiestrogen therapy.
• It should be given with caution to people with impaired liver function.
• Letrozole must not be used during pregnancy. A doctor must be notified if pregnancy occurs while taking this drug.
• Medical judgment is required if breast-feeding is being considered.
• It may be associated with the impairment of liver function. elevated blood pressure, rash.

Interactions

None have been noted.

Side effects

• Achiness, gastrointestinal effects, hot flashes, fatigue, edema, headache, coughing, and shortness of breath.

leucovorin calcium Ⓖ

(calcium folinate; folinic acid)
Type/Group: **anemia treatment; antidote**.
Brand(s): Wellcovorin; various generic.
How administered: Intravenous infusion; orally.

Used to treat

Leucovorin calcium is the usual form in which folinic acid (a deriv-ative of ℞ **folic acid**, which is a vitamin of the vitamin-B complex) is given as a supplement to people who are susceptible to some of the toxic effects caused by the folate-antagonist activity of certain ℞ **anticancer** drugs, especially ℞ **methotrexate**. It is also used, along with the anticancer drug ℞ **fluorouracil**, to treat colorectal (large intestine) ✚ **cancer**. In addition, it can be used to treat meg-aloblastic ✚ **anemias** when oral treatment is not feasible.

Warnings

• It should not be given to people with known anemias secondary to vitamin B_{12} deficiency.
• Its safety during pregnancy has not been established, and should be used only if it is clearly needed.
• Medical judgment is required if breast-feeding is being considered.
• Rarely, severe allergic reactions may occur.

Interactions

• The effects of ℞ **anticonvulsants** may be reduced.
• The toxicity of ℞ **fluorouracil** may be enhanced.
• At high doses, leucovorin may interfere with the therapeutic effects of ℞ **methotrexate**.

Side effects

• Hives, skin irritation, and rarely anaphylactic reactions. No other adverse reactions have been attributed to leucovorin alone.

Leukeran ℞

A preparation of ℞ **chlorambucil**.
Formulation: Oral tablets.
Availability: Prescription only.
Warnings and side effects: See ℞ **chlorambucil**.

Leukine ℞

A preparation of ℞ **sargramostim**.
Formulation: Injection or infusion.
Availability: Prescription only.

leukotriene antagonist Ⓓ

see ℞ **leukotriene receptor antagonist**.

leukotriene receptor antagonist Ⓓ

(leukotriene antagonist)
Generics: **montelukast sodium; zafirlukast**.

Actions and uses

Leukotriene receptor antagonists are a recently introduced class of drugs which work as ℞ **antiallergic** agents by blocking the actions of leukotrienes. These are natural inflammatory mediators released in most tissues and organs including the lungs. ℞ **montelukast sodium** is used in ℞ **antiasthmatic** treatment as a form of add-on therapy for people not adequately controlled by inhaled ℞ **corticosteroid** therapy and short-acting ℞ **beta-adrenergic stimulant** drugs. It helps to prevent mild-to-moderate ✚ **asthma** attacks (including exercise-induced bronchospasm), but not to treat acute attacks. A further example is ℞ **zafirlukast**.

Limitations

These drugs are relatively well tolerated, although there are some common side effects. It is too early to say how important this group will be in overall antiasthma therapy. See the individual drug entries.

leuprolide acetate Ⓖ

(leuprorelin acetate)
Type/Group: **hypothalamic hormone; anticancer**.
Brand(s): Lupron.

Key to symbols: ✚ = Disorder Section ℞ = Drug Section ♣ = Herbal Section ⚌ = Supplement Section

How administered: Injection.

Used to treat

Leuprolide is a synthetic analog of the hypothalamic hormone ℞ **gonadotropin**-releasing hormone (GnRH) and is used to treat advanced ○ **prostate cancer**, ○ **endometriosis**, and precocious puberty. It is also used, along with iron therapy, as a preoperative treatment for anemia caused by fibroid tumors of the uterus. After an initial surge, on prolonged administration, it reduces secretion of GnRH by the pituitary gland, which results in reduced secretion of ℞ **sex hormones** by the ovaries or testes.

Warnings

• It should not be given to people with known hypersensitivity to this drug or with undiagnosed uterine bleeding.

• It should not be used during pregnancy. A doctor must be contacted if pregnancy occurs while taking this drug.

• It should not be used by nursing mothers.

• Pain and urinary difficulties associated with prostatic cancer may increase at the beginning of treatment.

• Side effects are greatest during the first week of treatment, and signs and symptoms may increase before decreasing.

• Continuous treatment is vital for treatment of precocious puberty.

• Effective doses should stop menstruation. A doctor must be contacted if it continues.

• A loss of bone mineral density occurs with treatment. It may increase the risk of osteoporosis in those with major risk factors.

Interactions

None noted.

Side effects

• Depending on use, there may be hot flashes, edema, ECG changes, elevated blood pressure, breast changes, androgen-like effects, decreased libido, decreased testicular size, impotence, dizziness, and shortness of breath.

• Possible serious side effects include stroke and heart irregularities.

leuprorelin acetate ⑥

see ℞ **leuprolide acetate**.

Leustatin ⑧

A preparation of ℞ **cladribine**.
Formulation: Injection.
Availability: Prescription only.
Warnings and side effects: See ℞ **cladribine**.

levalbuterol hydrochloride ⑥

((*R*)-albuterol hydrochloride)
Type/Group: **beta-adrenergic stimulant; antiasthmatic; sympathomimetic**.
Brand(s): Xopenex.
How administered: Inhalant.

Used to treat

Levalbuterol is used to treat and prevent bronchospasm in individuals with reversible obstructive airway disease (○ **asthma**). It is also available in another chemical form, ℞ **albuterol**, of which it is one of the isomers.

Warnings

• It should not be given to people with known hypersensitivity to levalbuterol, heart arrhythmias, or severe heart disease.

• It should be given with caution to people with certain heart diseases, hyperthyroidism, diabetes mellitus, hypertension, or prostatic hypertrophy.

• Levalbuterol may cross the placenta, and inhibit uterine contractions, and so should be used in pregnancy only if clearly needed.

• Medical judgment is required if breast-feeding is being considered. It is not known if it appears in breast milk.

• Rarely, it may have adverse effects on heart and blood pressure, or may lead to paradoxical bronchoconstriction.

Interactions

• ℞ **Beta-blockers** decrease the effects of levalbuterol.

• ℞ **Digoxin** increases the risk of ECG changes or elevated potassium levels.

• ℞ **MAOIs** and ℞ **tricyclic** antidepressants may increase the effects of levalbuterol. The recommendation is to wait two weeks after treatment with an antidepressant is stopped before taking levalbuterol.

Side effects

• Frequently, nervousness, tremor, nasal inflammation, and viral infection.

• Occasionally, generalized pain, speeded heart rate, increased blood glucose levels, flu syndrome, upset stomach, leg cramps, and migraine.

levamisole hydrochloride ⑥

Type/Group: **immunomodulator; anticancer**.
Brand(s): Ergamisol.
How administered: Orally.

Used to treat

Levamisole is used as an additional treatment with ℞ **fluorouracil** after surgery in certain patients with colon cancer.

Warnings

• It should not be given to people with known hypersensitivity to the drug or any of its components. This is a specialist drug and a full assessment for suitability will be carried out before treatment.

• It should be used during pregnancy only if the potential benefits outweigh the possible risks.

• It is not recommended for use while nursing.

• A doctor must be contacted if flu-like symptoms or malaise occur.

• Avoid alcohol (see Interactions).

• Rarely, this drug has been associated with an acute neurologic syndrome with varied symptoms including coma, confusion, lethargy, and memory loss.

• Blood disorders may occur days to weeks after treatment. Blood monitoring will be required.

Interactions

• It may interfere with alcohol metabolism and cause unpleasant reactions.

• The levels of ℞ **phenytoin** are increased.

• The anticoagulants effects of ℞ **warfarin sodium** and similar agents are increased.

Side effects

• Frequently, diarrhea, nausea, and metallic taste.

• Occasionally, muscle or joint pain, anxiety, dizziness, headache, insomnia, unusual tiredness, skin rash and itching, vomiting, hair loss, and stomatitis (mouth sores).

• Rarely, numbness in the hands, face, and feet, blurred vision, confusion, seizures, tardive dyskinesia, tremors, and liver toxicity.

Levatol ⓑ

A preparation of ℞ **penbutolol sulfate**.
Formulation: Oral tablets.
Availability: Prescription only.
Warnings and side effects: See ℞ **penbutolol sulfate**.

Levbid ⓑ

A preparation of ℞ **hyoscyamine**.
Formulation: Extended release tablets.
Availability: Prescription only.
Warnings and side effects: See ℞ **hyoscyamine**.

levetiracetam ⓖ

Type/Group: anticonvulsant; antiepileptic.
Brand(s): Keppra.
How administered: Orally.

Used to treat

Levetiracetam is a recently introduced drug which may be used in the treatment of ⚙ **epilepsy** to assist in the control of partial seizures.

Warnings

• Avoid its use in people with known hypersensitivity to this drug.

• It should be given with caution to anyone with kidney impairment, neuropsychiatric conditions, or blood and liver disorders.

• Studies suggest adverse developmental effects on the fetus, therefore this drug should be used in pregnancy only when potential benefit outweighs potential risk to the fetus.

• It is not known whether this drug appears in breast milk, and so medical judgment is required if considering breast-feeding.

• Withdrawal should be gradual otherwise it may precipitate attacks.

• As this drug may cause drowsiness, driving or other hazardous activity should be avoided.

Interactions

No significant drug interactions have been documented.

Side effects

These include:

• Drowsiness, feelings of weakness, sleepiness, mood swings, sore throat, dizziness, and uncoordinated movements, though these symptoms tend to decline after several weeks of use;

• There are a range of side effects which occur less frequently to rarely, including visual or hearing disturbances, aches and pains, gastrointestinal upsets, rash, confusion, abnormal thinking, and tremor.

Levite ⓑ

A preparation of ℞ **ethinyl estradiol** and ℞ **levonorgestrel**.
Formulation: Calendar pack of oral tablets.
Availability: Prescription only.
Warnings and side effects: See ℞ **ethinyl estradiol**; ℞ **levonorgestrel**.

Levlen ⓑ

A preparation of ℞ **ethinyl estradiol** and ℞ **levonorgestrel**.
Formulation: Calendar pack of oral tablets.
Availability: Prescription only.
Warnings and side effects: See ℞ **ethinyl estradiol**; ℞ **levonorgestrel**.

levobunolol ⓖ

Type/Group: beta-blocker; glaucoma treatment.
Brand(s): AKBeta; Betagan Liquifilm; various generic.
How administered: Topically (eyes).

Used to treat

Levobunolol is used to treat chronic simple ⚙ **glaucoma**. It is thought to work by slowing the rate of production of aqueous humor (fluid) in the eye.

Warnings

• It should not be given to people with known hypersensitivity to levobunolol, or with certain heart disorders.

• It should be given with caution to people undergoing major surgery, who have diabetes mellitus, kidney disease, thyroid disease, chronic obstructive pulmonary disease (COPD), asthma, heart failure, or peripheral vascular disease. It can be absorbed systemically (into the body).

• Levobunolol's safety during pregnancy has not been established. It should be used only if the potential benefit outweighs the possible risk to the fetus.

• Medical judgment is required if breast-feeding is being considered. It is not known whether it appears in breast milk.

Interactions

• Oral ℞ **beta-blockers** can increase systemic effects.

• The effects of ℞ **verapamil** and ℞ **quinidine** are increased.

Side effects

• Frequently, eye irritation, transient burning or stinging, and visual disturbances.

• Occasionally, increased light sensitivity, and watering of the eyes.

• Rarely, dry eye, conjunctivitis, and eye pain. Because it can be absorbed through the eye, systemic side effects are possible, particularly on the cardiovascular and respiratory systems.

levobupivacaine ⓖ

Type/Group: local anesthetic.
Brand(s): Chirocaine.
How administered: Local injection.

Used to treat

Levobupivacaine is a recently introduced local anesthetic of the amide group which is long-lasting. It is used for spinal anesthesia, including epidural injection (especially during labor), for nerve block, and by local infiltration.

   Key to symbols: ⚙ = Disorder Section   ℞ = Drug Section   ♣ = Herbal Section   ◔◑ = Supplement Section

Warnings

• It should not be given to people with known hypersensitivity to local anesthetics or para-aminobenzoic acid. It is a specialist drug and there will be a full medical assessment.

• Its safety in pregnancy has not been established and it should be used only if it is clearly needed.

• Medical judgment is required if breast-feeding is being considered. It is unknown whether this drug appears in breast milk.

• Its use during labor may prolong delivery.

• It can cause cardiac depression, peripheral vasodilatation, or CNS (central nervous system) toxicity.

Interactions

• ℞ **Metoprolol**, ℞ **nadolol**, ℞ **propranolol**, and ℞ **cimetidine** increase the levels of bupivacaine.

Side effects

• Hypotension, nausea, anemia, post-operative pain, vomiting, back pain, fever, and dizziness.

levocabastine hydrochloride Ⓖ

Type/Group: **antiallergic; antihistamine**.
Brand(s): Livostin.
How administered: Topically (eyedrops).

Used to treat

Levocabastine can be used topically for the relief of seasonal allergic ✪ **conjunctivitis**.

Warnings

• It should not be given to people with known hypersensitivity to this drug.

• Levocabastine should be used during pregnancy only when the potential benefit outweighs the possible risk to the fetus.

• It appears in breast milk in small amounts. Nursing women should discontinue this drug or discontinue breast-feeding.

• It should not be applied while wearing contact lenses.

Interactions

No interactions are known when used topically as directed.

Side effects

• There may be brief stinging and burning or headache.

• Less frequently, vision disturbances, dry mouth, eye pain or redness, swollen eyelids, rash, nausea, or shortness of breath.

levocarnitine Ⓖ

(L-carnitine)
Type/Group: **metabolic disorder treatment**.
Brand(s): Carnitor; various generic.
How administered: Orally.

Used to treat

Levocarnitine is an amino acid used to treat deficiency of the naturally occurring amino acid carnitine, either where there is a primary deficiency due to an inborn error of metabolism, or where there is a secondary deficiency in hemodialysis patients.

Warnings

• It should not be given to people with known hypersensitivity to this drug or any of its constituents.

• It should be given with caution to people with kidney impairment.

• Levocarnitine should be used during pregnancy only if it is clearly needed.

• Medical judgment is required if breast-feeding is being considered. It is not known whether this drug appears in breast milk.

• Levels of carnitine in blood and urine may be monitored.

• A doctor must be consulted before taking any supplements; dl-carnitine (sold as vitamin B_T in health-food stores) inhibits the action of this drug and can cause a deficiency.

• There is a risk of mild myasthenia in uremic patients.

Interactions

• Vitamin B_T (DL-carnitine) inhibits the action of this drug and can cause a deficiency.

Side effects

• Gastrointestinal complaints (nausea, vomiting, diarrhea, abdominal cramps) and body odor.

levodopa Ⓖ

Type/Group: **antiparkinsonism; dopamine-receptor stimulant**.
Brand(s): Larodopa. Combination: With *carbidopa*: Sinemet; various generic.
How administered: Orally.

Used to treat

Levodopa is used to treat parkinsonism, but not the symptoms of parkinsonism induced by drugs. It is also used to treat postencephalitic parkinsonism and parkinsonism associated with cerebral arteriosclerosis, or following injury to the CNS (central nervous system) by carbon monoxide or manganese intoxication. Levodopa is converted into the neurotransmitter ℞ **dopamine** within the brain and works by replenishing dopamine levels in the part of the brain (striatum) where there is depletion in ✪ **Parkinson's disease**. It is effective in reducing the slowness of movement and rigidity associated with parkinsonism, but is not as successful in controlling the tremor. It is most often combined with the enzyme inhibitor ℞ **carbidopa**, which inhibits the conversion of levodopa to dopamine outside the brain, therefore enabling as much levodopa as possible to reach the brain before it is converted; and sometimes additionally with the enzyme inhibitor ℞ **entacapone**. This means a lower dose can be used, with a consequent reduction in side effects. Although not stated by the manufacturer, levodopa is sometimes used in the treatment of herpes zoster and restless leg syndrome.

Warnings

• It should not be used by people with known hypersensitivity to this drug, narrow-angle glaucoma, or who have a history of melanoma or suspicious undiagnosed skin lesions (can activate malignant melanoma).

• It should be given with caution to anyone with severe heart or lung disease, bronchial asthma, certain circulatory disorders, kidney, liver, or endocrine disease, depression, mania, or major psychoses, heart dysrhythmias, a history of peptic ulcer, or wide-angle glaucoma.

• Levodopa should be used during pregnancy only if clearly needed and if the benefits outweigh the potential risk to the fetus.

• This drug is excreted in breast milk and should not be used by breast-feeding mothers.

• It must not be used while taking, or within two weeks after having discontinued, an ℞ **MAOI** antidepressant, because serious interactive effects are possible.

• It may affect the performance of skilled tasks, such as driving.

• Diabetics should check with a doctor before making dosage adjustments based on abnormal urine tests for sugar or ketones, because levodopa may interfere with such tests.

• It may cause darkening of the urine or sweat, which is not harmful.

Interactions

• Food high in protein and/or ⚖ **iron** may inhibit the effectiveness of levodopa. Tell your clinician of any supplements you are taking.

• Levodopa taken with ℞ **benzodiazepines** may possibly worsen parkinsonism.

• ℞ **Antipsychotics**, ℞ **methionine**, ℞ **phenytoin**, ⚖ **pyridoxine**, spiramycin, and ℞ **tacrine** may inhibit the effectiveness of levodopa.

• Moclobemide increases the risk of side effects.

• ℞ **MAOI** antidepressants may cause an abnormal rise in blood pressure.

Side effects

• Very frequently, uncontrolled body movements (including face, tongue, arms, upper body), nausea and vomiting, dry mouth, gastrointestinal disturbances, and loss of appetite.

• Occasionally, depression, anxiety, confusion, nervousness, mental changes, difficulty urinating, irregular heartbeats, dizziness, lightheadedness, blurred vision, constipation, dry mouth, flushed skin, headache, insomnia, diarrhea, unusual tiredness.

• Rarely, hypertension, ulcer, hemolytic anemia.

levofloxacin ⓖ

Type/Group: **quinolone; antibacterial**.
Brand(s): Levaquin.
How administered: Orally; injection.

Used to treat

Levofloxacin is a synthetic antibiotic-like antibacterial that is active against both Gram-positive and Gram-negative organisms. It can be used to treat respiratory infections, including worsening of chronic ⊕ **bronchitis** caused by bacteria, community-acquired (caught from the environment) ⊕ **pneumonia**, and acute ⊕ **sinusitis**, as well as infections of the urinary tract, kidneys, and skin and soft tissues.

Warnings

• It should not be given to people with known hypersensitivity to levofloxacin or other quinolones, a history of photosensitivity (abnormal sensitivity to light) reactions, or certain heart conditions. It should not be given to children under 18, because there is a possibility of damage to joints and cartilage in growing children.

• It should be given with caution to people with liver or kidney disease, diabetes mellitus, or with any predisposition to seizures.

• Levofloxacin should not be used during pregnancy or while breast-feeding unless the potential benefit outweighs the possible risk to the fetus or infant.

• Superinfections due to the altered bacterial balance caused by antibiotic treatment may occur. A doctor must be contacted if there is severe abdominal pain, or moderate to severe diarrhea.

• Rare, but serious side effects of quinolones include seizure and other CNS (central nervous system) effects, and severe allergic reactions.

• Adequate fluid intake should be maintained.

• Photosensitivity reactions can occur and so excessive exposure to sunlight should be avoided.

• Do not take products such as supplements containing ⚖ **calcium**, ⚖ **magnesium**, aluminum, ⚖ **iron**, or ⚖ **zinc** less than two hours before or two hours after taking levofloxacin because they reduce its effects.

Interactions

• ℞ **Antacids**, ℞ **didanosine (ddI)**, and ℞ **sodium bicarbonate** may reduce the effects of levofloxacin.

• The levels of ℞ **theophylline**, antipyrine, ℞ **caffeine**, ℞ **diazepam**, ℞ **metoprolol**, ℞ **pentoxifylline**, ℞ **phenytoin**, ℞ **propranolol**, ℞ **ropinirole**, ℞ **xanthine**. The effect of oral anticoagulants such as ℞ **warfarin** may be increased.

• The effects oral ℞ **anticoagulants** may be increased.

• If used with ℞ **foscarnet**, the risk of seizure is increased.

Side effects

• Frequently, dizziness, lightheadedness, insomnia, drowsiness, and gastrointestinal effects.

• Occasionally, seizure.

levonorgestrel ⓖ

Type/Group: **sex hormone; progestin; contraceptive**.
Brand(s): Norplant System; Plan B. Combinations: With *ethinyl estradiol*: Alesse; Levlen; Levlite; Levora; Nordette; Preven; Tri-Leven; Triphasil; Trivora-28.
How administered: Orally; subdermal implant.

Used to treat

Levonorgestrel is a synthetic progestin used as a contraceptive implant under the skin, orally as an emergency contraceptive following unprotected intercourse, and, in combination with ℞ **estrogen**, as an oral contraceptive for regular use.

Warnings

• It should not be used by people with known hypersensitivity to this drug, or with active thrombophlebitis or thromboembolic disorders, undiagnosed abnormal genital bleeding, who are pregnant, with acute liver disease, liver tumors, or breast cancer.

• It should be given with caution to people with diabetes mellitus, impaired liver function, conditions aggravated by fluid retention, history of depression, or who wear contact lens.

• Levonorgestrel must not be used during pregnancy. A doctor must be contacted if pregnancy occurs while using this drug.

• Medical judgment is required if breast-feeding is being considered.

• The menstrual cycle may be disrupted and irregular and unpredictable bleeding or spotting may result.

• Implants can be removed at any time for any reason or at the end of 5 years. Removal is harder than insertion.

• The effectiveness of emergency contraception is better if taken as soon as possible after unprotected intercourse.

Interactions

• ℞ **Carbamazepine**, ℞ **phenobarbital**, and ℞ **phenytoin** may decrease the effectiveness of levonorgestrel.

Side effects

These depend on use, dose, duration of use, and how administered.

• When used as an emergency contraceptive, the most common side effect is nausea.

• Other side effects include dizziness, headache, nervousness, edema, weight gain, change of appetite, ovarian cysts, cessation of menses, vaginal infection, breast changes, altered glucose tolerance, musculoskeletal pain, acne, skin inflammation, changes in hair growth, infection, and pain or itching at implantation site.

Levophed ℞

A preparation of ℞ **norepinephrine bitartrate**.
Formulation: Injection; infusion.
Availability: Prescription only.
Warnings and side effects: See ℞ **norepinephrine bitartrate**.

Levoprome ℞

A preparation of ℞ **methotrimeprazine**.
Formulation: Injection.
Availability: Prescription only.
Warnings and side effects: See ℞ **methotrimeprazine**.

Levoquin ℞

A preparation of ℞ **levofloxacin**.
Formulation: Oral tablets; injection.
Availability: Prescription only.
Warnings and side effects: See ℞ **levofloxacin**.

Levora ℞

A preparation of ℞ **ethinyl estradiol** and ℞ **levonorgestrel**.
Formulation: Calendar pack of oral tablets.
Availability: Prescription only.
Warnings and side effects: See ℞ **ethinyl estradiol**; ℞ **levonorgestrel**.

levothyroxine sodium Ⓖ

Type/Group: **thyroid hormone; diagnostic agent**.
How administered: Orally; injection.
Brand(s): Eltroxin; Levothroid; Levoxyl; Synthroid; various generic. Combinations: liotrix (a uniform mixture of synthetic T_4 and T_3 in a 4 to 1 ratio): Thyrolar.

Used to treat

Levothyroxine sodium is a synthetic form of the naturally occurring thyroid hormone, thyroxine (T_4; L-thyroxine; *levo*-thyroxine (denoting *levo*-isomer)). It is chemically identical to that produced in the human thyroid gland. It is used to treat thyroid deficiency, including congenital ⊙ **hypothyroidism**, myxedema (severe

hypothyroidism), and non-toxic goiter. It is also prescribed to treat conditions involving pituitary TSH suppression, including thyroid nodules, Hashimoto's disease (an autoimmune thyroid disease), multinodular goiter, and thyrotoxicosis (in conjunction with antithyroid drugs), as well as to manage thyroid cancer. It may also be used in a diagnostic test of thyroid function.

Warnings

• It should not be used by people with apparent hypersensitivity, thyrotoxicosis (a disease caused by excessive thyroid hormones; except in conjunction with antithyroid drugs), or myocardial infarction.

• It should be given with caution to people over 65, and those with cardiovascular disease, diabetes mellitus, diabetes insipidus, Addison's disease, or myxedema.

• It does not cross the placenta and no adverse effects when taken during pregnancy have been observed.

• Medical judgment is required if breast-feeding is being considered.

• Excessive doses may produce the signs and symptoms of hyperthyroidism. A doctor must be contacted if headache, nervousness, diarrhea, excessive sweating, heat intolerance, chest pain, increased pulse rate, or any unusual events occur.

• Children may have partial hair loss during the first few months of treatment, but hair growth usually resumes.

• Long-term treatment has been associated with decreased bone density in women. Bone density should therefore be monitored regularly.

• One brand of this drug should not be changed to another without consulting a doctor first. Different brands may not have the same effects.

• It may take a few weeks for levothyroxine sodium to start working.

• Treatment should not be stopped without consulting a doctor.

Interactions

• The effects of oral ℞ **anticoagulants** may be increased.

• ℞ **cholestyramine**, ℞ **colestipol hydrochloride**, and ℞ **estrogens** may decrease the absorption of levothyroxine sodium.

• ℞ **Sympathomimetics** may increase the effects of levothyroxine sodium, possibly leading to heart failure.

Side effects

• Insomnia, tremors, palpitations, and fast heart rate.

• Rarely, dry skin, upset stomach, skin reactions, severe headache, menstrual irregularities, fever, heat intolerance, and seizures.

Levsinex Timecaps ℞

A preparation of ℞ **hyoscyamine**.
Formulation: Timed release capsules.
Availability: Prescription only.
Warnings and side effects: See ℞ **hyoscyamine**.

Levsin Tablets; Elixir; Injection; Levsin S/L ℞

A preparation of ℞ **hyoscyamine**.
Formulation: Oral tablets; elixir; injection; S/L are sublingual tablets.

Availability: Prescription only.
Warnings and side effects: See ℞ **hyoscyamine**.

Lexxel 5-2.5; 5-5 Ⓑ

A preparation of ℞ **enalapril maleate** and ℞ **felodipine**.
Formulation: Oral tablets, available in two (felodipine) strengths.
Availability: Prescription only.
Warnings and side effects: See ℞ **enalapril maleate**;
℞ **felodipine**.

Librax Ⓑ

A preparation of clidinium and ℞ **chlordiazepoxide**.
Formulation: Oral capsules.
Availability: Prescription only.
Warnings and side effects: See ℞ **chlordiazepoxide**.

Librium Ⓑ

A preparation of ℞ **chlordiazepoxide**.
Formulation: Oral tablets in several strengths; injectable solution.
Availability: Prescription only.
Warnings and side effects: See ℞ **chlordiazepoxide**.

Lida-Mantle-HC Ⓑ

A preparation of ℞ **hydrocortisone** and ℞ **lidocaine**.
Formulation: Cream.
Availability: Prescription only.
Warnings and side effects: See ℞ **hydrocortisone**; ℞ **lidocaine**.

Lidex; Lidex E Ⓑ

A preparation of ℞ **fluocinonide**.
Formulation: Cream; ointment (Lidex E); solution; gel.
Availability: Prescription only.
Warnings and side effects: See ℞ **fluocinonide**.

lidocaine Ⓖ

(lignocaine hydrochloride)
Type/Group: antiarrhythmic; local anesthetic.
Brand(s): Anestacon; Burn-O-Jel; Dentipatch; DermaFlex; Dilocaine; ELA-Max; Lidoject; Nervocaine; Numby Stuff; Solarcaine; Xylocaine; Zilactin-L; various generic. Combinations: With *dexamethasone*: Decadron. With *hydrocortisone*: Lida-Mantle-HC.
How administered: Local injection; systemic; topically (external).

Used to treat

Lidocaine is the most commonly used of all the local anesthetics. It can be given by a number of routes and always close to its site of action. When administered by injection or infiltration, it can be used for dental and minor surgery (such as sutures). By epidural injection (into a space surrounding the nerves of the spinal cord), it can be used in childbirth or major surgery (sometimes in combination with a general anesthetic). When injected into a vascular region, it is co-injected with epinephrine, which acts as a vasoconstrictor and so limits the rate at which the lidocaine is washed away. When applied topically, it is well absorbed from mucous membranes and abraded skin and can be used to treat discomfort at many sites. Additionally, lidocaine (as hydrochloride) is used as an ℞ antiarrhythmic (particularly in the emergency treatment of ✪ **arrhythmias** and fibrillation following heart attack), when it is administered by intravenous injection.

Warnings

• It should not be given to people with known hypersensitivity to amide-type anesthetics. It is a specialist drug and there will be a full medical assessment.
• Its safety during pregnancy has not been established and it should be used only if it is clearly needed.
• It is compatible with breast-feeding.
• Severe adverse reactions to lidocaine are uncommon, but high dosage by any route may have effects on the heart.

Interactions

• If used with ℞ **disopyramide**, heart dysrhythmia or heart failure may occur in predisposed people.
• ℞ **Metoclopramide**, ℞ **nadolol**, ℞ **propranolol**, and ℞ **cimetidine** increase the levels of lidocaine.
• There is a risk of additive toxicity with ℞ **antiarrhythmics** (for example, ℞ **tocainide**, ℞ **mexiletine**).

Side effects

• Occasionally, pain at injection site, burning, stinging, or tenderness where applied.
• Rarely (generally with high dose), drowsiness, dizziness, disorientation, lightheadedness, tremors, apprehension, euphoria, sensation of heat, cold, or numbness, blurred or double vision, ringing or roaring in ears, and nausea.

Lidoject Ⓑ

A preparation of ℞ **lidocaine**.
Formulation: Injection.
Availability: Prescription only.
Warnings and side effects: See ℞ **lidocaine**.

lignocaine hydrochloride Ⓖ

see ℞ **lidocaine**.

Limbitrol Ⓑ

A preparation of ℞ **chlordiazepoxide** and ℞ **amitriptyline hydrochloride**.
Formulation: Oral tablets, regular and double strength.
Availability: Prescription only.
Warnings and side effects: See ℞ **chlordiazepoxide**; ℞ **amitriptyline hydrochloride**.

lindane Ⓖ

(gamma benzene hexachloride)
Type/Group: scabicide and pediculicide.
Brand(s): Generics.
How administered: Topically (lotion and shampoo).

Used to treat

Lindane is used to treat infestation by head lice, crab lice (see ✪ **lice and mite infestations**), and ✪ **scabies** when other treatments have not worked or are inappropriate.

Warnings

• It should not be given to people with Norwegian (crusted) scabies, seizure disorders, or known hypersensitivity to this drug or any component of the product. Premature infants should not be treated with lindane because the drug may be more easily absorbed through their skin, and their livers may not be sufficiently developed to metabolize it adequately. Anyone over 65 may require a reduced dose because of the potential for increased absorption.

• There are no adequate and well-controlled studies in pregnant women. The recommended dosage should not be exceeded, and it should not be used more than twice during pregnancy.

• Medical judgment is required if breast-feeding is being considered. It is found in breast milk, although at levels that are probably insignificant.

• Lindane penetrates the skin and has the potential for causing toxic CNS (central nervous system) effects (dizziness, seizures), particularly if not used according to the instructions. (Such reactions are extremely rare when the drug is properly used.)

• Oils may enhance absorption, so use of creams, ointments, or oils at the same time as lindane should be avoided. Oil-based hair products, such as conditioners after applying lindane shampoo, should be avoided.

• Do not apply to the face, broken skin, or the eyes.

Interactions

No significant drug interactions are known.

Side effects

• Irritation and eczema.

linezolid Ⓖ

Type/Group: **antibacterial**.

Brand(s): Zyvox.

How administered: Orally; infusion; injection.

Used to treat

Linezolid is a recently introduced synthetic antibacterial of the oxalolidinone class that is used to treat Gram-positive infections, ✪ pneumonia, skin and skin structure infections, and certain ℞ vancomycin-resistant infections. It is also a nonselective monoamine-oxidase inhibitor (MAOI).

Warnings

• It should not be given to people with known hypersensitivity to linezolid.

• It should be given with caution to people with thrombocytopenia (low blood platelet count).

• Its effects during pregnancy are unknown, and so it should be used only if clearly needed and if the potential benefits outweigh the risks to the fetus.

• Medical judgment is required if breast-feeding is being considered. It is not known whether linezolid appears in breast milk.

• Superinfections from the altered bacterial balance created by antibiotics may occur. A doctor must be contacted if there is severe abdominal pain, moderate to severe diarrhea, or any new or unusual symptoms.

• Avoid large quantities of tyramine-containing foods (for example, aged cheeses; aged, smoked, pickled, or processed meat and fish; red wine: see a doctor for a complete list).

• Avoid caffeine and alcohol while taking this drug.

• Do not take any other medication, including herbal remedies, decongestants, weight-reducing products, or those used for hay fever, or colds without consulting a doctor. Ingredients in such products may interact with linezolid and cause serious reactions.

Interactions

• Other ℞ MAOIs (for example, ℞ isocarboxazid, ℞ phenelzine, ℞ tranylcypromine, ℞ selegiline) or drugs that possess MAOI-like activity (for example, ℞ furazolidone, ℞ procarbazine) must not be taken with, or within two weeks before or after taking, linezolid, otherwise a severe reaction could occur.

• ℞ Brimonidine, ℞ bupropion, ℞ levodopa, tramadol, ⚕ tryptophan, ⚕ tyrosine, ℞ naratriptan, ℞ sumatriptan, ℞ rizatriptan, and ℞ zolmitriptan should not be taken with, or within two weeks of taking, linezolid if possible.

• ℞ Dopamine, ℞ dobutamine hydrochloride, ℞ epinephrine, ℞ guanadrel, ℞ guanethidine monosulfate, and ℞ reserpine may raise blood pressure.

• ℞ dextromethorphan and other ℞ antidepressants could create an excess of serotonin, which causes serious adverse reactions.

Side effects

• Frequently, diarrhea, nausea, skin rash, and itching.

• Occasionally, headache, taste alteration, temporary tongue discoloration, yeast and fungal infections.

• Rarely, low blood-platelet count, increased blood pressure, and irregular heartbeat or palpitations.

Lioresal Ⓑ

A preparation of ℞ baclofen.

Formulation: Oral tablets; implanted pump for continuous infusion.

Availability: Prescription only.

Warnings and side effects: See ℞ cisatracurium.

liothyronine Ⓖ

Type/Group: **thyroid hormone; diagnostic agent**.

Brand(s): Cytomel; Triostat; various generic. Combinations: *lotrix* (a uniform mixture of synthetic T_4 and T_3 in a 4 to 1 ratio): Thyrolar.

How administered: Orally; injection.

Used to treat

Liothyronine is a synthetic form of the naturally occurring thyroid hormone, triiodothyronine (T_3), and is used to treat thyroid deficiency, including congenital hypothyroidism, myxedema (severe hypothyroidism), and non-toxic goiter. It is also prescribed to treat conditions involving pituitary TSH suppression, including thyroid nodules, Hashimoto's disease (an autoimmune thyroid disease), multinodular goiter, and thyroid cancer. It may also be used in a diagnostic test of thyroid function. Liothyronine has a more rapid onset of action and shorter half-life than other similar drugs.

Warnings

- It should not be used by people with known hypersensitivity to this drug, with thyrotoxicosis, or myocardial infarction uncomplicated by hypothyroidism.
- It should be given with caution to people over 65, or anyone with cardiovascular disease, diabetes mellitus, or diabetes insipidus.
- It does not cross the placenta and no adverse effects from its use during pregnancy have been observed.
- Medical judgment is required if breast-feeding is being considered.
- Excessive doses may produce the signs and symptoms of hyperthyroidism. A doctor must be contacted if headache, nervousness, diarrhea, excessive sweating, heat intolerance, chest pain, increased pulse rate (symptoms of hyperthyroidism), or any unusual events occur.
- Children may have partial hair loss during the first few months of therapy, but hair growth usually resumes.
- Long-term treatment has been associated with decreased bone density in women. Bone density should therefore be monitored regularly.
- Treatment should not be stopped without consulting a doctor.

Interactions

- The effects of oral ℞ **anticoagulants** may be increased.
- ℞ **cholestyramine**, ℞ **colestipol hydrochloride**, and ℞ **estrogens** may decrease the absorption of liothyronine.
- ℞ **Sympathomimetics** may increase the effects of liothyronine, possibly leading to heart failure.

Side effects

- Insomnia, tremors, palpitations, and fast heart rate.
- Rarely, dry skin, upset stomach, skin reactions, severe headache, menstrual irregularities, fever, heat intolerance, and arrhythmias.

lipid-lowering drug ⓓ

see ℞ lipid-regulating drug.

lipid-regulating drug ⓓ

Generics: **atorvastatin; cerivastatin sodium; cholestyramine; clofibrate; colesevelam; fenofibrate; gemfibrozil; lovastatin; niacin; pravastatin sodium; simvastatin.**

Actions and uses

Lipid-regulating drug (lipid-lowering; antihyperlipidemia) treatment is used in clinical conditions of ⓞ **hyperlipidemia**, where the blood plasma contains very high levels of certain of the lipids of cholesterol and/or triglycerides (natural fats of the body). Because these drugs lower some lipid levels while raising others, this group are now referred to as *lipid-regulating* rather than *lipid-lowering* drugs. Lipid-regulating drugs are used where there is a family history of hyperlipidemia, or clinical signs (for example, cardiovascular disorders, or those with the highest plasma concentrations of cholesterol) indicating the need for intervention. In most people, however, an appropriate low-fat diet can adequately do what is required.

Lipid-lowering drugs work in a number of ways. ℞ **statin** drugs (technically called HMG-CoA reductase inhibitors) work by competitively inhibiting an enzyme called *HMG-CoA reductase*, which is an early rate-limiting step in the production of cholesterol. These drugs may moderately lower levels of triglycerides, dramatically reduce both overall serum and LDL-cholesterol, and moderately raise HDL-cholesterol. They include ℞ **atorvastatin**, ℞ **cerivastatin**, ℞ **lovastatin**, ℞ **pravastatin** and ℞ **simvastatin**. ℞ **fibrate** (or fibric acid derivative) drugs lower the levels of very low-density lipoprotein fraction rich in triglycerides, decrease serum cholesterol, increase HDL-cholesterol, and sometimes lower LDL-cholesterol. They include ℞ **gemfibrozil**, ℞ **fenofibrate**, and ℞ **clofibrate**. *Bile acid sequestrants* (℞ **cholestyramine** and ℞ **colesevelam**) are resins that bind bile acids in the gut, and so reduce absorption of bile salts from the gut, resulting in changed cholesterol metabolism in the liver. They can be used as a lipid-regulating drugs in hyperlipidemia to reduce the levels, or change the proportions, of various lipids in the bloodstream. Usually, there is a decrease in overall serum cholesterol, a fall in LDL-cholesterol, and sometimes a small rise in HDL-cholesterol and triglycerides. The *nicotinic acid derivatives* (see ℞ **niacin**) can lower total cholesterol, LDL-cholesterol and triglyceride levels by an action on enzymes in the liver.

Current medical opinion suggests that if diet, or drugs, can be used to lower levels of LDL-cholesterol (low-density lipoprotein) while raising HDL-cholesterol (high-density lipoprotein), then there may be a regression of the progress of coronary ⓞ **atherosclerosis** (a diseased state of the arteries of the heart where plaques of lipid material narrow blood vessels, which contributes to angina pectoris attacks and the formation of abnormal clots that go on to cause heart attacks and strokes). They can be used in ℞ **antianginal** and ℞ **heart failure treatment** through reduction of atheromatous disease.

There are a number of types of hyperlipidemia (classified into groups I to V), and some drug groups are better suited to particular purposes. Patient evaluation is best done by specialists, and drug treatment will involve regular blood lipid measurement.

Limitations

These drugs are not without side effects, especially gastrointestinal effects. A rare adverse effect with some drugs of the statin group is the destruction of muscle tissue (rhabdomyolysis) with resulting damage to the kidneys and even kidney failure (any muscle pain should be reported to a doctor). Bile acid sequestrants may interfere with absorption of fat-soluble vitamins. See also the individual drug entries.

Lip Medex ®

A preparation of ℞ **camphor** and ℞ **phenol**.
Formulation: Topical ointment.
Availability: OTC.
Warnings and side effects: See ℞ camphor; ℞ phenol.

Lipo-Nicin ®

A preparation of ℞ **niacin** and ℞ **niacinamide**.
Formulation: Oral tablets in two strengths.
Availability: Prescription only.
Warnings and side effects: See ℞ niacin; ℞ niacinamide.

lipoxygenase inhibitor ⒟

Generics: zileuton.

Actions and uses

Lipoxygenase inhibitors are a new class of drug, which are also called *5-lipoxygenase inhibitors*. They work as ℞ **antiallergic** drugs by blocking the production of leukotrienes, which are natural inflammatory mediators released, for example, in the lungs. The first such drug in use, ℞ **zileuton**, is taken by mouth in the chronic treatment and prevention of ✪ **asthma**.

Limitations

It is too early to say how important this group will be in overall ℞ **antiasthmatic** treatment.

Liver changes may occur, and periodic monitoring is required. A doctor should be contacted if there is pain in the right upper quadrant of the abdomen, nausea, fatigue, lethargy, itching, jaundice, or flu-like symptoms (these are signs and symptoms of liver disease). The drug is only used in pregnancy if the potential benefits clearly justify the possible risk to the fetus. See also the individual drug entry.

Lipram; Lipram-UL20 Ⓑ

A preparation of ℞ **pancreatin** (amylase, lipase, protease).
Formulation: Oral capsules, 6 strengths.
Availability: Prescription only.
Warnings and side effects: See ℞ **pancreatin**.

Liquibid-D Tablets Ⓑ

A preparation of ℞ **phenylephrine hydrochloride** and ℞ **guaifenesin**.
Formulation: Oral tablets.
Availability: Prescription only.
Warnings and side effects: See ℞ **phenylephrine hydrochloride**; ℞ **guaifenesin**.

Liquibid Tablets Ⓑ

A preparation of ℞ **guaifenesin**.
Formulation: Oral tablets, sustained release.
Availability: Prescription only.
Warnings and side effects: See ℞ **guaifenesin**.

Liqui-Char Ⓑ

A preparation of ℞ **activated charcoal**.
Formulation: Liquid.
Availability: OTC.
Warnings and side effects: See ℞ **activated charcoal**.

Liqui-Doss Ⓑ

A preparation of ℞ **mineral oil**.
Formulation: Oral emulsion.
Availability: OTC.
Warnings and side effects: See ℞ **mineral oil**.

liquid paraffin ⒢

see ℞ **mineral oil**.

Liquid Pred Ⓑ

A preparation of ℞ **prednisone**.
Formulation: Oral syrup.
Availability: Prescription only.
Warnings and side effects: See ℞ **prednisone**.

Liquifilm tears Ⓑ

A preparation of ℞ **polyvinyl alcohol**.
Formulation: Ophthalmic solution.
Availability: OTC.
Warnings and side effects: See ℞ **polyvinyl alcohol**.

Liquiprin Drops for Children Ⓑ

A preparation of ℞ **acetaminophen**.
Formulation: Oral liquid.
Availability: OTC.
Warnings and side effects: See ℞ **acetaminophen**.

lisinopril ⒢

Type/Group: ACE inhibitor; antihypertensive; heart failure treatment.
Brand(s): Prinivil; Zestril. Combinations: With *hydrochlorothiazide*: Prinzide; Zestoretic.
How administered: Orally.

Used to treat

Lisinopril can be used in the treatment of ✪ **hypertension** and congestive ✪ **heart failure**. Additionally, it can be used following ✪ **myocardial infarction** (damage to heart muscle, usually after a heart attack). It is often used with other classes of drug, particularly ℞ **thiazide** ℞ **diuretics**.

Warnings

• It should not be given to people with known hypersensitivity to this drug or to any other ACE inhibitor.

• It should be given with caution to people with severe congestive heart failure, or certain other cardiovascular disorders, a history of anaphylaxis, collagen vascular disease (for example, systemic lupus erythematosus; SLE), diabetes, depressed immune response, or with impaired kidney function or on dialysis.

• Risk in pregnancy increases substantially from the first through to the second and third trimesters. ACE inhibitors can cause injury to the fetus, even death. The use of these drugs should be stopped as soon as pregnancy is detected.

• Medical judgment is required if breast-feeding is being considered.

• Use of this drug should be stopped and a doctor contacted immediately if signs of angioedema appear (swelling of the face, eyes, lips, tongue, larynx, or extremities; difficulty in breathing or swallowing). Swelling of the larynx, closing off the airway, can be life-threatening.

• Anyone taking an ACE inhibitor should not interrupt or discontinue treatment without first checking with a doctor.

• Any suspected infections (for example, fever, sore throat) should be reported to a doctor, because ACE inhibitors may cause blood changes which can affect immune response.

• ACE inhibitors generally have less effect on blood pressure in blacks than in non-blacks, and the likelihood of angioedema is higher among blacks, as well.

Interactions

• ACE inhibitors have apparently triggered life-threatening anaphylactoid reactions when used by people also receiving ℞ **desensitizing vaccines**.

• ℞ **Anesthetics** (for example, in surgery), ℞ **phenothiazines**, and ℞ **probenecid** may increase the levels or hypotensive effect of lisinopril.

• ℞ **Antacids** and ℞ **rifampin** may reduce the effects of lisinopril. Antacids should not be used for several hours after a dose of an ACE inhibitor (a doctor should be consulted for full instructions and cautions).

• If used with other antihypertensives and diuretics, the effects of these drugs may be increased. This additive effect is sometimes used to advantage in combination treatments for high blood pressure.

Side effects

• Commonly, dizziness, dry cough, and headache.

• Occasionally, fatigue, postural hypotension (lowered blood pressure on standing), muscle cramps, tingling in the extremities, upper respiratory infection or nasal congestion, sexual dysfunction, rash, weakness or gastrointestinal disturbances (for example, diarrhea, nausea and vomiting, constipation).

• Infrequently, chest and muscle pains, tachycardia, insomnia, confusion and mood changes, or photosensitivity (abnormal sensitivity to light). Although it is uncommon, ACE inhibitors can cause very marked hypotension (especially when beginning treatment) and kidney impairment.

• Rarely, there may be angioedema, altered liver function, jaundice, hepatitis, pancreatitis, or changes in blood counts.

Listerine ℬ

A preparation of ℞ **thymol**, eucalyptol, ℞ **methyl salicylate**, and alcohol.

Formulation: Topical liquid.

Availability: OTC.

Warnings and side effects: See ℞ thymol; ℞ methyl salicylate.

Listermint Arctic Mint ℬ

A preparation of poloxamer 335, ℞ **glycerin**, ℞ **sodium lauryl sulfate**; and ℞ **benzoic acid**.

Formulation: Topical liquid.

Availability: OTC.

Warnings and side effects: See ℞ glycerin; ℞ sodium lauryl sulfate; ℞ benzoic acid.

lithium Ⓖ

Type/Group: antimania.

Brand(s): Eskalith; Eskalith CR; Lithotabs; Lithobid; Lithonate; Cibalith-S.

How administered: Orally.

Used to treat

Lithium, as carbonate or citrate, is singularly effective as an antimania drug to control or prevent the hyperactive manic episodes in bipolar affective disorder (see ○ **bipolar disorder**). It may also reduce the frequency and severity of depressive episodes. How it works remains imperfectly understood, but its use is so successful that the side effects (caused by its toxicity) are deemed to be justified. Although not stated by the manufacturer for such use, it may be prescribed to prevent ○ **depression** in recurrent depressive illness and other behavioral problems, and to treat ○ **premenstrual syndrome** (PMS), ○ **bulimia**, alcoholism, tardive dyskinesia, overactive thyroid, postpartum affective psychosis, and to prevent cluster headache. It may also be prescribed to treat SIADH (syndrome of inappropriate antidiuretic hormone release).

Warnings

• It should not be given to people with certain heart or kidney disorders, or imperfect sodium balance in the bloodstream.

• It should be given with caution to people taking diuretics, or with myasthenia gravis, thyroid disease, tartrazine sensitivity, diabetes mellitus, to children, or anyone over 65.

• Lithium should be avoided during pregnancy if possible, especially during the first trimester. A doctor must be contacted if pregnancy occurs while taking this drug.

• Medical judgment is required if breast-feeding is being considered. It should not normally be used by nursing mothers.

• Lithium is prescribed after a full medical assessment, and people are monitored regularly.

• Take with meals to avoid stomach upset.

• Drink 8 to 12 glasses of water or other liquid every day.

• Do not restrict sodium in the diet, because too high or too low levels of sodium may alter the effects of lithium.

• Visual disturbances, worsening gastric problems, vomiting, muscle weakness, twitching, tremor and lack of coordination (and eventually convulsions and coma) indicate lithium intoxication. Stop taking the medication and contact a doctor if these symptoms occur.

• Prolonged treatment may cause serious kidney damage and thyroid gland dysfunction. Prolonged overdosage eventually causes serious effects on the brain.

• Caution must be exercised when performing tasks that require alertness, such as driving.

Interactions

• If used with ℞ **MAOI**s, a dangerously high fever may occur.

• ℞ **ACE inhibitors**, ℞ **methyldopa**, ℞ **NSAID**s, ℞ **phenytoin**, and ℞ **thiazide** diuretics may increase the effects of lithium.

• ℞ **diltiazem hydrochloride**, ℞ **verapamil**, ℞ **amitriptyline**, ℞ **carbamazepine**, ℞ **fluoxetine**, and ℞ **fluvoxamine** may cause neurotoxicity (damage to nerves), including seizures.

• There is a reduced response to ℞ **antipsychotics**, and severe neurotoxicity is possible in acute manic patients.

• If used with ℞ **potassium iodide**, there is an increased risk of decline in thyroid function.

• ℞ **sodium bicarbonate** and ℞ **theophylline** decrease the effects of lithium.

Side effects

• Nausea, thirst, excessive urination, gastrointestinal disturbance, including vomiting and diarrhea, weakness and tremor, dizziness, drowsiness, headache, lowered blood pressure, loss of appetite, and dry mouth.

• There may be fluid retention and consequent weight gain.

• Rare but serious side effects include circulatory collapse, seizures, abnormal heart rhythm, and angioedema.

Lithobid ⑧

A preparation of ℞ **lithium**.
Formulation: Oral extended release tablets.
Availability: Prescription only.
Warnings and side effects: See ℞ **lithium**.

Lithonate ⑧

A preparation of ℞ **lithium**.
Formulation: Oral capsules.
Availability: Prescription only.
Warnings and side effects: See ℞ **lithium**.

Lithostat ⑧

A preparation of ℞ **acetohydroxamic acid (AHA)**.
Formulation: Oral tablets.
Availability: Prescription only.
Warnings and side effects: See ℞ **acetohydroxamic acid (AHA)**.

Lithotabs ⑧

A preparation of ℞ **lithium**.
Formulation: Oral tablets.
Availability: Prescription only.
Warnings and side effects: See ℞ **lithium**.

Lobac ⑧

A preparation of ℞ **acetaminophen**, ℞ **salicylamide**, and phenyltoloxamine citrate.
Formulation: Oral capsules.
Availability: Prescription only.
Warnings and side effects: See ℞ **acetaminophen**; ℞ **salicylamide**.

Lobana Body Shampoo ⑧

A preparation of ℞ **chloroxylenol**.
Formulation: Topical liquid.
Availability: OTC.
Warnings and side effects: See ℞ **chloroxylenol**.

local anesthetic ⑩

Generics: benzocaine; bupivacaine; chloroprocaine hydrochloride; cocaine; dibucaine; etidocaine; prilocaine hydrochloride; levobupivacaine; lidocaine; mepivacaine hydrochloride; pramoxine hydrochloride; procainamide hydrochloride; procaine; proparacaine; ropivacaine hydrochloride; tetracaine; tocainide hydrochloride.

Actions and uses

Local anesthetic drugs are used to reduce sensation (especially pain) in a specific, local area of the body and without loss of consciousness. In contrast, ℞ **general anesthetics** decrease sensation only because of a loss of consciousness. Local anesthetics work by reversibly blocking the transmission of impulses in nerves.

They can be administered by a number of routes and always close to their site of action. By local injection or infiltration, they can be used for dental and minor surgery (such as sutures) and vasectomy. A more extensive loss of sensation with nerve block (for example, injected near to the nerve supplying a limb) or with spinal anesthesia (for example, epidural injection in childbirth) or intrathecal block (for extensive procedures) produces a loss of sensation in whole areas of the body sufficient to allow major surgery (though with some, quickly reversible paralysis). Local anesthetics are particularly valuable where the use of a general anesthetic carries a high risk, or when the cooperation of the patient is required. When administered into a vascular region, ℞ **epinephrine** is co-injected and acts as a ℞ **vasoconstrictor** to limit the rate at which the anesthetic is washed away in the blood. When applied topically, certain local anesthetics are well absorbed from mucous membranes and abraded skin and can be used to treat discomfort at many sites such as teething in babies, hemorrhoids.

Limitations

Local anesthetics should only be administered by those with special training depending on the route of administration, including training for emergency resuscitation procedures (including dental use).

There can be hypersensitivity reactions, adverse effects on the heart, and respiratory depression. coma and death in overdose.

Some local anesthetics are only used for their ℞ **antiarrhythmic** effects on the heart (including ℞ **tocainide hydrochloride** and ℞ **procainamide**).

Locoid ⑧

A preparation of ℞ **hydrocortisone**.
Formulation: Cream.
Availability: Prescription only.
Warnings and side effects: See ℞ **hydrocortisone**.

Lodine Tablets, Capsules; Lodine XL ⑧

A preparation of ℞ **etodolac**.
Formulation: Oral tablets (two strengths); capsules (two strengths); XL tablets are extended release.
Availability: Prescription only.
Warnings and side effects: See ℞ **etodolac**.

lodoxamide tromethamine ⑥

Type/Group: anti-inflammatory.
How administered: Topically (eye).
Brand(s): Alomide.

Used to treat

Lodoxamide tromethamine is an anti-inflammatory drug (a mast-cell stabilizer) used for seasonal allergic ✪ **conjunctivitis**.

Warnings

• It should not be given to people with known hypersensitivity to any component of the product.
• It should be used during pregnancy only if it is clearly needed.
• Medical judgment is required if breast-feeding is being considered.
• Soft contact lenses should not be worn during treatment (a component of the currently available formulation can damage them).

Interactions

No significant interactions are known.

Side effects

• Short-lived mild burning and stinging, itching and excess tear formation. Also, flushing and dizziness.

Lodrane LD Capsules ®

A preparation of ℞ **pseudoephedrine** and ℞ **brompheniramine maleate**.
Formulation: Oral capsules, sustained release.
Availability: Prescription only.
Warnings and side effects: See ℞ **pseudoephedrine**; ℞ **brompheniramine maleate**.

Loestrin ®

A preparation of ℞ **ethinyl estradiol** and ℞ **norethindrone**.
Formulation: Calendar pack of oral tablets. Available in two strengths.
Availability: Prescription only.
Warnings and side effects: See ℞ **ethinyl estradiol**; ℞ **norethindrone**.

Loestrin Fe ®

A preparation of ℞ **ethinyl estradiol**, ℞ **norethindrone**, and ⚶ **iron** (ferrous fumarate).
Formulation: Calendar pack of oral tablets. Available in two strengths.
Availability: Prescription only.
Warnings and side effects: See ℞ **ethinyl estradiol**; ℞ **norethindrone**; ⚶ **iron**.

Logen ®

A preparation of ℞ **atropine sulfate** and ℞ **diphenoxylate hydrochloride**.
Formulation: Oral tablets.
Availability: Prescription only.
Warnings and side effects: See ℞ **atropine sulfate**; ℞ **diphenoxylate hydrochloride**.

lomefloxacin Ⓖ

Type/Group: **quinolone; antibacterial**.
Brand(s): Maxaquin.
How administered: Orally.

Used to treat

Lomefloxacin is a recently introduced synthetic broad-spectrum quinolone, an antibiotic-like antibacterial, which can be used to treat ✚ **bacterial infections**, including lower respiratory tract infections, urinary tract infections, and to prevent preoperative and postoperative urinary tract infections connected with certain surgical procedures.

Warnings

• It should not be given to people with known hypersensitivity to lomefloxacin or other quinolones, with kidney disease, or any predisposition to seizures. It should not be given to children under 18, because there is a possibility of damage to joints and cartilage in growing children.
• Lomefloxacin should not be used during pregnancy or while breast-feeding if possible. There is a risk of joint damage to the fetus or infant.
• Superinfections due to the altered bacterial balance caused by antibiotic therapy may occur. A doctor must be contacted if there is severe abdominal pain, or moderate to severe diarrhea.
• Rare, but serious, side effects of quinolones include seizure and other CNS (central nervous system) effects, and severe allergic reactions.
• Adequate fluid intake should be maintained.
• The absorption of lomefloxacin is delayed by food.
• Products, such as supplements, containing these ingredients must not be taken less than four hours before or two hours after taking lomefloxacin.
• Photosensitivity reactions (abnormal sensitivity to light) can occur, and so excessive exposure to sunlight should be avoided.

Interactions

• Food delays and reduces the absorption of lomefloxacin.
• ℞ **Antacids**, ⚶ **calcium**, ℞ **didanosine (ddI)**, ⚶ **iron** preparations, ⚶ **magnesium**, ℞ **sodium bicarbonate**, ⚶ **zinc** reduce the effects of levofloxacin. Do not take products containing these ingredients less than four hours before or two hours after taking lomefloxacin.
• The levels of ℞ **theophylline**, antipyrine, ℞ **caffeine**, ℞ **diazepam**, ℞ **metoprolol**, ℞ **pentoxifylline**, ℞ **phenytoin**, ℞ **propranolol**, ℞ **ropinirole**, ℞ **xanthine**, and ℞ **warfarin sodium** may be increased.
• The effects of oral ℞ **anticoagulants** may be increased.
• If used with ℞ **foscarnet**, the risk of seizure is increased.

Side effects

• Frequently, nausea, also diarrhea, headache, dizziness, visual disturbances, and rash.

Lomenate ®

A preparation of ℞ **atropine sulfate** and ℞ **diphenoxylate hydrochloride**.
Formulation: Oral liquid.
Availability: Prescription only.
Warnings and side effects: See ℞ **atropine sulfate**; ℞ **diphenoxylate hydrochloride**.

Lomotil Liquid; Tablets ®

A preparation of ℞ **atropine sulfate** and ℞ **diphenoxylate hydrochloride**.
Formulation: Oral tablets.

Availability: Prescription only.
Warnings and side effects: See ℞ atropine sulfate;
℞ diphenoxylate hydrochloride.

lomustine Ⓖ

(CCNU)
Type/Group: **anticancer; cytotoxic**.
Brand(s): CeeNu.
How administered: Orally.

Used to treat
Lomustine is an alkylating agent that is used particularly for
✪ **Hodgkin's disease** and brain ✪ **tumors**. It works by disrupting
cellular DNA and so inhibiting cell replication.

Warnings
• It should not be given to people with known hypersensitivity to
lomustine.
• It should be given with caution to people with certain blood
disorders. This is a specialist drug which will be used following a
full evaluation by specialist physicians.
• Lomustine is not recommended for use during pregnancy unless
it is medically judged to be essential, because it may cause birth
defects. Becoming pregnant while using this drug must be
avoided.
• It should not be used if breast-feeding.
• It can cause severe bone marrow suppression, which may lead to
bleeding and a reduced resistance to infection.
• In common with many anticancer drugs, this drug is associated
with development of secondary malignancies (new cancers).
• It can impair fertility in men and women (which may be
reversible).
• It may have adverse effects on the kidneys, liver, or lungs.

Interactions
No interactions specific to this drug are known.

Side effects
• Nausea, vomiting, and loss of appetite.
• Occasionally, nerve disorders, inflammation of mouth mucosa,
darkening of the skin, diarrhea, skin rash, itching, and hair loss.

Loniten Ⓑ

A preparation of ℞ **minoxidil**.
Formulation: Oral tablets, available in two strengths.
Availability: Prescription only.
Warnings and side effects: See ℞ **minoxidil**.

Lonox Tablets Ⓑ

A preparation of ℞ **atropine sulfate** and ℞ **diphenoxylate hydro-
chloride**.
Formulation: Oral tablets.
Availability: Prescription only.
Warnings and side effects: See ℞ atropine sulfate;
℞ diphenoxylate hydrochloride.

loperamide hydrochloride Ⓖ

Type/Group: **antidiarrheal; opioid**.

Brand(s): Diar-Aid Caplets; Imodium A-D; Kaopectate; Maalox
Anti-Diarrheal; Neo-Diaral; Pepto Diarrhea Control; various
generic. Combinations: With *simethicone*: Imodium Advanced.
How administered: Orally.

Used to treat
Loperamide acts on the nerves of the intestine to inhibit peristalsis
(the waves of muscular activity that move along the contents of the
intestines), so reducing motility (movement), and also decreases
fluid secretion in the intestines. It is used for ✪ **diarrhea**, including
traveler's diarrhea and chronic diarrhea in inflammatory bowel
disease.

Warnings
• It should not be given to people with known hypersensitivity to
this drug, with a fever, or who must for medical reasons avoid
constipation or where diarrhea is caused by invasive organisms
such as *E. coli, Salmonella* or *Shigella*, or pseudomembranous colitis.
• It should be given with caution to people with liver disease, severe
ulcerative colitis, or dehydration. It should also be given with
caution to children.
• Loperamide should be used during pregnancy only when it is
clearly needed and when the benefits outweigh the potential risks.
• Medical judgment is required if breast-feeding is being
considered. This drug has not been evaluated for safety in nursing
mothers.
• Drowsiness may affect the performance of skilled tasks such as
driving.
• It should not be used after 48 hours if there is no improvement.
• A doctor must be contacted if fever or swelling of the abdomen
occur.

Interactions
None of significance.

Side effects
• Usually minor, but may include abdominal pain or discomfort,
constipation, dry mouth, nausea, vomiting, fatigue, dizziness, and
drowsiness.
• Rarely, toxic megacolon (a serious condition affecting the colon).

Lopid Ⓑ

A preparation of ℞ **gemfibrozil**.
Formulation: Oral tablets.
Availability: Prescription only.
Warnings and side effects: See ℞ **gemfibrozil**.

Lopressor Ⓑ

A preparation of ℞ **metoprolol tartrate**.
Formulation: Oral tablets (two strengths); injection.
Availability: Prescription only.
Warnings and side effects: See ℞ **metoprolol tartrate**.

Lopressor HCT 50/25; 100/25; 100/50 Ⓑ

A preparation of ℞ **hydrochlorothiazide** and ℞ **metoprolol tartrate**.
Formulation: Oral tablets, in three (metoprolol/
hydrochlorothiazide) strengths.
Availability: Prescription only.

Warnings and side effects: See ℞ **hydrochlorothiazide**; ℞ **metoprolol tartrate**.

loratadine ⓖ

Type/Group: **antihistamine; antiallergic**.
Brand(s): Claritin Tablets, Reditabs, Syrup. Combinations: With *pseudoephedrine hydrochloride*: Claritin-D, 24-hour Tablets.
How administered: Orally.

Used to treat
Loratadine is a recently developed antihistamine which has less sedative side effects than some older members of its class and can be used for the symptomatic relief of allergic symptoms, such as ⊕ **hay fever** (seasonal allergic rhinitis) and ⊕ **urticaria**.

Warnings
• It should not be given to people with known hypersensitivity to this drug (or with known sensitivity to other antihistamines).
• Antihistamines should be given with caution to people with liver or kidney impairment, asthma or lower respiratory disease, heart disease, hypertension, hyperthyroidism, epilepsy, porphyria, increased intraocular pressure (pressure in the eyeball, as in glaucoma), enlarged prostate, urinary retention, or certain obstructive bladder or gastrointestinal conditions.
• Loratadine should be used during pregnancy only if it is clearly needed.
• Nursing mothers should discontinue using this drug or discontinue breast-feeding.
• Although infrequent with loratadine, possible sedative side effects may affect the performance of skilled tasks, such as driving.
• Side effects are more frequent in the elderly.

Interactions
• ℞ **macrolide** antibiotics (for example, ℞ **erythromycin**), ℞ **azoles** (for example, ℞ **ketoconazole**), and ℞ **cimetidine** may increase levels of loratadine.

Side effects
• These depend on how it is administered. For this type of antihistamine, there is occasionally drowsiness, headache, impaired muscular coordination or dizziness, and anticholinergic effects (dry mouth, blurred vision, urinary retention, gastrointestinal disturbances) (although the occurrence of sedation and anticholinergic side effects is low).
• Rarely, there may be occasional rashes and photosensitivity (abnormal sensitivity to light), palpitations and heart arrhythmias, stimulation instead of sedation (paradoxical stimulation), especially in children (and convulsions in overdose), hypersensitivity reactions, blood disorders, liver disturbances, depression, sleep disturbances, and hypotension.

lorazepam ⓖ

Type/Group: **antianxiety; sedatives; hypnotic; antiepileptic; benzodiazepine; antiemetic**.
Brand(s): Ativan.
How administered: Orally, injection.

Used to treat
Lorazepam is used in the short-term treatment of ⊕ **anxiety**, as an antiepileptic in status epilepticus, and as a sedative in preoperative medication, because its ability to cause amnesia means that the patient forgets the unpleasant procedure. Although not stated by the manufacturer for such use, it may be prescribed for ⊕ **insomnia**, for acute alcohol withdrawal symptoms, as an additional, supportive treatment in endoscopic procedures, and for chemotherapy-induced nausea and vomiting.

Warnings
• It should not be given to people with known hypersensitivity to benzodiazepines, with narrow-angle glaucoma, or psychosis.
• It should be used with caution by those with liver or kidney disease, chronic obstructive pulmonary disease (COPD), in a weakened condition (debilitated), with a history of drug abuse, or anyone over 65.
• Lorazepam is not recommended for use during pregnancy. Its use in the first trimester should almost always be avoided. A doctor must be contacted if pregnancy occurs while this drug is being taken.
• Medical judgment is required if breast-feeding is being considered.
• It may cause drowsiness and so judgment, thinking, and the performance of skilled tasks may be impaired, such as driving.
• Avoid alcohol because adverse side effects may be increased (see Side effects below).
• Avoid other psychotropic medications unless prescribed by a doctor.
• A doctor must be consulted before discontinuing use or increasing dosage, because benzodiazepines may produce psychological and physical dependence and withdrawal symptoms.

Interactions
• ℞ **fluconazole** and ℞ **itraconazole** may increase levels of lorazepam.
• If used with CNS (central nervous system) depressants (for example, ℞ **narcotic analgesics**), effects may be increased.
• Alcohol may increase some adverse effects.

Side effects
• Depending on how it is administered, dose, and use, there may be dizziness, drowsiness, postural hypotension (lowered blood pressure on standing), and blurred vision.
• Less frequently, anxiety, confusion, depression, fatigue, hallucinations, headache, insomnia, stimulation, tremors, unsteadiness, ECG changes, speeded heartbeat, ringing in the ears (tinnitus), gastrointestinal symptoms, and skin sensitivity reactions.

Lorcet-HD Capsule; Plus Tablets; 10/650 Tablets ®

A preparation of ℞ **hydrocodone bitartrate** and ℞ **acetaminophen**.

Formulation: Oral tablets; capsules.

Availability: Prescription only.

Warnings and side effects: See ℞ **hydrocodone bitartrate**; ℞ **acetaminophen**.

Lortab Elixir, Tablets ⓑ

A preparation of ℞ **hydrocodone bitartrate** and
℞ **acetaminophen**.
Formulation: Oral liquid; tablets, available in 3 strengths.
Availability: Prescription only.
Warnings and side effects: See ℞ **hydrocodone bitartrate**;
℞ **acetaminophen**.

Lortab ASA Tablets ⓑ

A preparation of ℞ **hydrocodone bitartrate** and ℞ **aspirin**.
Formulation: Oral tablets.
Availability: Prescription only.
Warnings and side effects: See ℞ **hydrocodone bitartrate**;
℞ **aspirin**.

losartan potassium ⓖ

**Type/Group: angiotensin-receptor blocker; antihypertensive;
vasodilator**.
Brand(s): Cozaar. Combinations: With *hydrochlorothiazide*: Hyzaar.
How administered: Orally.

Used to treat

Losartan potassium is an angiotensin II receptor (AT1 receptors)
blocker. Angiotensin II is a circulating hormone that is a powerful
vasoconstrictor (narrows blood vessels) and blocking its effects
leads to a fall in blood pressure. Losartan was the first drug introduced in this class. It can be used, alone or with other drugs, in the
treatment of ✪ **hypertension**.

Warnings

• It should not be given to people with known hypersensitivity to
this drug.
• It should be given with caution to people with severe congestive
heart failure, with impaired liver function, severe kidney
insufficiency, or renal stenosis. Any fluid- or salt-depleted condition
(as from diuretic use) should be corrected before using this drug.
• Risk in pregnancy increases substantially from the first through
to the second and third trimesters. Angiotensin-receptor blockers
can cause injury to the fetus. The use of these drugs should stop as
soon as pregnancy is detected.
• Medical judgment is required if breast-feeding is being
considered.
• Blood pressure should be checked regularly.
• Losartan may have less effect on blood pressure in blacks than in
non-blacks.

Interactions

No drug interactions of significance are known.

Side effects

• Angiotensin-receptor blockers in general appear to cause few and
infrequent side effects (often indistinguishable from placebo
effects). The most common, with losartan, include dizziness,
muscle cramps, back and leg pain, and upper respiratory
symptoms or infection.
• Uncommonly, insomnia, headache, gastrointestinal
disturbances, chest pain or edema; symptoms such as fatigue, rash,
weakness and effects on heart rhythm seldom occur. There may be

changes in kidney function; angioedema (an allergic swelling
reaction, often of the face) has been reported.

Lotensin ⓑ

A preparation of ℞ **benazepril hydrochloride**.
Formulation: Oral tablets, available in 4 strengths.
Availability: Prescription only.
Warnings and side effects: See ℞ **benazepril hydrochloride**.

Lotensin HCT 5/6.25; 10/12.5; 20/12.5; 20/25 ⓑ

A preparation of ℞ **benazepril hydrochloride** and
℞ **hydrochlorothiazide**.
Formulation: Oral tablets, in four (benazepril/
hydrochlorothiazide) strengths.
Availability: Prescription only.
Warnings and side effects: See ℞ **benazepril hydrochloride**;
℞ **hydrochlorothiazide**.

Lotrel ⓑ

A preparation of ℞ **amlodipine besylate** and ℞ **benazepril
hydrochloride**.
Formulation: Oral capsules, available in 3 strengths.
Availability: Prescription only.
Warnings and side effects: See ℞ **amlodipine besylate**;
℞ **benazepril hydrochloride**.

Lotrimin ⓑ

A preparation of ℞ **clotrimazole**.
Formulation: Topical cream; topical lotion; topical solution.
Availability: Prescription only.
Warnings and side effects: See ℞ **clotrimazole**.

Lotrimin-AF ⓑ

A preparation of ℞ **clotrimazole**.
Formulation: Topical powder; topical spray powder; topical liquid
spray.
Availability: OTC.
Warnings and side effects: See ℞ **clotrimazole**.

Lotrisone ⓑ

A preparation of ℞ **betamethasone** dipropionate and
℞ **clotrimazole**.
Formulation: Cream.
Availability: Prescription only.
Warnings and side effects: See ℞ **betamethasone**;
℞ **clotrimazole**.

lovastatin ⓖ

Type/Group: lipid-regulating drug; statin.
Brand(s): Mevacor.
How administered: Orally.

Used to treat

Lovastatin is a (statin/HMG-CoA reductase inhibitor) lipid-regulating drug used in ✪ **hyperlipidemia** to reduce the levels, or change

the proportions, of various lipids in the bloodstream. It is usually given only to people in whom a strict and regular dietary regime alone is not having the desired effect, or who have high total blood cholesterol levels and coronary heart disease.

Warnings

• It should not be given to people with liver disease or a history of heavy alcohol consumption.

• It should be given with caution to people with past liver disease, severe metabolic, or electrolyte disorders.

• Lovastatin is considered quite hazardous to the fetus and must not be used during pregnancy. It is given to women of childbearing age only when they are thought highly unlikely to conceive and have been informed of the risks.

• It is not known whether lovastatin appears in breast milk, but because of the potential for serious harm to an infant, mothers should not breast-feed.

• This drug can cause destruction of muscle tissue with resulting damage to the kidneys and even kidney failure. When taking lovastatin, any unusual muscle pain or tenderness should be reported to a doctor immediately and treatment stopped.

• Potentially harmful changes in liver function may occur, so periodic tests are necessary to check the drug's effect.

Interactions

• ℞ Azoles (antifungals such as ℞ itraconazole, ℞ ketoconazole), mibefradil, ℞ erythromycin, ℞ clarithromycin, ℞ nefazodone, ℞ cyclosporine, ℞ gemfibrozil, and ℞ niacin (nicotinic acid, a B vitamin) may increase levels of atorvastatin.

• ℞ warfarin sodium may increase anticoagulant effects.

Side effects

• Constipation, abdominal pain, muscle cramps, rash, and insomnia.

Lovenox ®

A preparation of ℞ **enoxaparin sodium**.
Formulation: Injection.
Availability: Prescription only.
Warnings and side effects: See ℞ **enoxaparin sodium**.

Low-ogestrel ®

A preparation of ℞ **ethinyl estradiol** and ℞ **norgestrel**.
Formulation: Calendar pack of oral tablets.
Availability: Prescription only.
Warnings and side effects: See ℞ **ethinyl estradiol**; ℞ **norgestrel**.

Lowsium Plus Suspension ®

A preparation of ℞ **magaldrate** and ℞ **simethicone**.
Formulation: Oral liquid.
Availability: OTC.
Warnings and side effects: See ℞ **magaldrate**; ℞ **simethicone**.

loxapine ©

Type/Group: antipsychotic; dopamine-receptor antagonist.

Used to treat

Loxapine is used to treat acute and chronic ✪ **psychotic disorders**.
Brand(s): Loxitane.
How administered: Orally; injection.

Warnings

• It should not be given to people with severe drug-induced depressive states or coma.

• It should be given with caution to people with seizure disorders, porphyria, liver disease, heart disease, prostatic hypertrophy, glaucoma, or chronic obstructive pulmonary disease. It should also be used with caution in children.

• Loxapine should be used during pregnancy only when it is clearly needed.

• Medical judgment is required if breast-feeding is being considered. It is not known whether this drug appears in breast milk.

• It may cause postural hypotension (lowered blood pressure on standing), so rise slowly from a reclining position. Older people should use particular caution.

• It may impair physical and mental abilities.

• Avoid alcohol.

• It may cause sensitivity to sunlight, so minimize exposure and use a sunscreen and sunglasses.

• With prolonged use, tardive dyskinesia (see ℞ **antipsychotics**) occasionally develops.

• The dosage must be reduced gradually when stopping treatment.

• Take special precautions to stay cool in hot weather.

Interactions

• ℞ **Anticholinergics** reduce the effect of loxapine.

• Loxapine reduces the effects of ℞ **bromocriptine**.

• If used with ℞ **lithium**, there is increased neurotoxicity.

• If used with ℞ **lorazepam**, there is a potential for serious adverse reaction.

Side effects

• Frequently, blurred vision, confusion, drowsiness, dry mouth, dizziness, and lightheadedness.

• Occasionally, allergic reaction, decreased urination, constipation, decreased sexual ability, enlarged breasts in men, headache, increased sensitivity of skin to sunlight, nausea, vomiting, insomnia, and weight gain.

• Rarely, extrapyramidal symptoms (see ℞ **antipsychotics**) seizure, blood cell disorders, and neuroleptic malignant syndrome (a potentially fatal condition characterized by very high fever, muscle rigidity, changes in mental status, and irregular pulse, blood pressure and/or heart rhythm).

Loxitane ®

A preparation of ℞ **loxapine**.
Formulation: Oral capsules; oral liquid; injection.
Availability: Prescription only.
Warnings and side effects: See ℞ **loxapine**.

Lozol ®

A preparation of ℞ **indapamide**.
Formulation: Oral tablets, available in two strengths.

Availability: Prescription only.
Warnings and side effects: See ℞ **indapamide**.

LubriTears Ⓑ

A preparation of ℞ **petrolatum**, ℞ **mineral oil**, and ℞ **lanolin**.
Formulation: Ophthalmic ointment.
Availability: OTC.
Warnings and side effects: See ℞ **petrolatum**; ℞ **mineral oil**; ℞ **lanolin**.

Ludiomil Ⓑ

A preparation of ℞ **maprotiline hydrochloride**.
Formulation: Oral tablets in several strengths.
Availability: Prescription only.
Warnings and side effects: See ℞ **maprotiline hydrochloride**.

Lufyllin-EPG Tablets; Elixir Ⓑ

A preparation of ℞ **ephedrine**, diphylline, ℞ **guaifenesin**, and ℞ **phenobarbital**.
Formulation: Oral tablets; liquid.
Availability: Prescription only.
Warnings and side effects: See ℞ **ephedrine**; ℞ **theophylline**; ℞ **guaifenesin**; ℞ **phenobarbital**.

Lufyllin-GG Tablets; Elixir Ⓑ

A preparation of ℞ **guaifenesin** and diphylline.
Formulation: Oral tablets, liquid.
Availability: Prescription only.
Warnings and side effects: See ℞ **guaifenesin**; ℞ **theophylline**.

Luminal Ⓑ

A preparation of ℞ **phenobarbital**.
Formulation: Injection.
Availability: Prescription only.
Warnings and side effects: See ℞ **phenobarbital**.

Lupron; Lupron Depots Ⓑ

A preparation of ℞ **leuprolide acetate**.
Formulation: Injection in several strengths; depots are microspheres for extended release; they come with several durations of action.
Availability: Prescription only.
Warnings and side effects: See ℞ **leuprolide acetate**.

Luvox Ⓑ

A preparation of ℞ **fluvoxamine**.
Formulation: Oral tablets in varying strengths.
Availability: Prescription only.
Warnings and side effects: See ℞ **fluvoxamine**.

Luxiq Ⓑ

A preparation of ℞ **betamethasone** valerate.
Formulation: Topical (foam).
Availability: Prescription only.
Warnings and side effects: See ℞ **betamethasone**.

Lyme disease vaccine (recombinant OspA) Ⓖ

Type/Group: **vaccine**.
Brand(s): LYMErix.
How administered: Intramuscular injection.

Used to treat

Lyme disease vaccine is a recently developed vaccine, which provides active immunization against the tick-borne bacterium *Borrelia burgdorferi*. The vaccine is prepared using modern biotechnological methods to synthesize an outer surface protein of the bacterium, a protein which stimulates production of effective antibodies when introduced into humans. This method of manufacture makes it possible to eliminate use of any substances of animal origin in the vaccine. Because previous infection does not necessarily result in immunity, this vaccine may be useful even for those who have already had ❍ **Lyme disease**, although the protective effect of the vaccine is not total (estimated between approx. 50 percent and 75 percent). It is indicated particularly for people at risk such as those who work or live or plan to travel in *B. burgdorferi*-infected tick-infested grassy or wooded areas.

Warnings

• It should not be given to people with known hypersensitivity to this vaccine.
• It should not be used to treat the active disease.
• Its use should be postponed in anyone with respiratory infections or any acute febrile (feverish) illness.
• Its effects in pregnancy have not been studied, and so should be used only when medically judged to be clearly needed.
• Medical judgment is required if breast-feeding is being considered.
• This vaccine should not be administered less than two weeks prior to starting a course of treatment with any kind of immunosuppressant drug.
• Lyme disease vaccine should only be used in persons 15 to 70 years of age.
• A rare complication of the disease, Lyme arthritis, is associated with significant reactions to the vaccine; it should not be given to people who have experienced this complication.
• After administration, people will be required to wait for some time to ensure that there is no serious reaction (such as anaphylaxis).

Interactions

• ℞ **Immunosuppressants** (for example, ℞ **corticosteroids**, ℞ **cytotoxics**, and radiation therapy) may reduce the effectiveness of the vaccine in conferring immunity. It is recommended that vaccination is postponded until three months after ending immunosuppressive treatment.
• Caution is required if ℞ **anticoagulants** are being taken.

Side effects

• Swelling or tenderness at the site of vaccination is common, but other side effects are infrequent and mild, notably muscle or joint aches.
• Side effects, including fatigue, rash and fever, as well as muscle and joint pain, are more likely to occur in people who have already had Lyme disease.

LYMErix ®

A preparation of ℞ **Lyme disease vaccine (recombinant OspA)**.
Formulation: Intramuscular injection.
Availability: Prescription only.
Warnings and side effects: See ℞ **Lyme disease vaccine (recombinant OspA)**.

lypressin ©

Type/Group: diabetes insipidus treatment; antidiuretic; hormone; anterior pituitary hormone.
Brand(s): Diapid.
How administered: Intranasal.

Used to treat

Lypressin (8-Lysine vasopressin) is a synthetic version of one of the two forms of antidiuretic hormone (ADH), also called ℞ **vasopressin**, found in nature. It is used to treat pituitary-originated ✪ **diabetes insipidus**.

Warnings

• It should not be used by people with known hypersensitivity to this drug or chronic kidney infection.
• It should be given with extreme caution to people with coronary artery disease or other circulatory disease.
• It should be used during pregnancy only if medically judged to be needed.
• Medical jusgment is also required if breast-feeding is being considered.
• Rarely, allergic reactions can occur.
• Upper respiratory tract infections, nasal congestion, and allergies may decrease effectiveness of lypressin, because it is administered as a nasal spray (for absorption from the nasal mucosa into the bloodstream).

Interactions

• ℞ **carbamazepine**, ℞ **chlorpropamide**, and ℞ **clofibrate** may increase the effects of lypressin.
• ℞ **demeclocycline**, ℞ **lithium**, and ℞ **norepinephrine** may decrease the effects of lypressin.

Side effects

• Infrequently, nasal congestion or irritation, conjunctivitis, abdominal cramps, heartburn, and nausea.

Maalox Antacid Caplets ®

A preparation of ℞ **calcium carbonate**.
Formulation: Oral tablets.
Availability: OTC.
Warnings and side effects: See ℞ **calcium carbonate**.

Maalox Anti-Diarrheal Caplets ®

A preparation of ℞ **loperamide hydrochloride**.
Formulation: Oral tablets.
Availability: OTC.
Warnings and side effects: See ℞ **loperamide hydrochloride**.

Maalox Anti-Gas ®

A preparation of ℞ **simethicone**.
Formulation: Oral tablets, chewable.
Availability: OTC.
Warnings and side effects: See ℞ **simethicone**.

Maalox Extra Strength Suspension ®

A preparation of ℞ **aluminum hydroxide**, ℞ **magnesium hydroxide**, and ℞ **simethicone**.
Formulation: Oral liquid.
Availability: OTC.
Warnings and side effects: See ℞ **aluminum hydroxide**; ℞ **magnesium hydroxide**; ℞ **simethicone**.

Maalox Suspension; Therapeutic Concentrate Suspension ®

A preparation of ℞ **aluminum hydroxide** and ℞ **magnesium hydroxide**.
Formulation: Oral liquid.
Availability: OTC.
Warnings and side effects: See ℞ **aluminum hydroxide**; ℞ **magnesium hydroxide**.

Macrobid ®

A preparation of ℞ **nitrofurantoin**.
Formulation: Oral capsules.
Availability: Prescription only.
Warnings and side effects: See ℞ **nitrofurantoin**.

Macrodantin ®

A preparation of ℞ **nitrofurantoin**.
Formulation: Oral capsules in several strengths.
Availability: Prescription only.
Warnings and side effects: See ℞ **nitrofurantoin**.

macrolide ⓓ

Actions and uses

Macrolide agents are a chemical class of ℞ **antibiotic** drugs which are used for their ℞ **antibacterial** action. They have a similar spectrum of action to the ℞ **penicillin** class, but they work in a different way by inhibiting microbial protein synthesis—they are bacteriostatic. The original and best-known, member of the group is ℞ **erythromycin**, which is effective against many Gram-positive bacteria, including streptococci (which can cause soft tissue and respiratory tract infections), *Legionella* (✪ **Legionnaires' disease**), and *Chlamydia* (✪ **urethritis**), and is also used in the treatment of ✪ **acne**, chronic ✪ **prostatitis**, ✪ **diphtheria**, and ✪ **pertussis** (whooping cough.) The macrolides are relatively non-toxic and although they do have side effects, serious side effects are rare. Derivatives with similar properties include ℞ **azithromycin**, ℞ **dirithromycin** and ℞ **clarithromycin** (the last-named being additionally used in ℞ **Helicobacter pylori eradication regimes**, and for mycobacterial infections in advanced HIV).

Limitations

The principal use of the macrolides is as an alternative antibiotic in people who are allergic to penicillin. However, they are far from free from all side effects, which frequently include gastrointestinal upsets (diarrhea, nausea, dyspepsia, abdominal discomfort) and occasionally superinfections due to the altered bacterial balance caused by antibiotic treatment may occur. A doctor must be contacted if severe abdominal pain, moderate to severe diarrhea, or any new or unusual symptoms develop.

Interactions with a wide variety of other drugs (including ℞ **fexofenadine** (an ℞ **antihistamine**) and ℞ **pimozide**) can be a problem, including the provoking of serious heart rate disorders. See also the individual drug entries.

mafenide Ⓖ

Type/Group: **sulfonamide; antibacterial.**
Brand(s): Sulfamylon.
How administered: Topically (external).

Used to treat
Mafenide is used in the treatment of ✪ **burns** to reduce the bacterial population.

Warnings
• It should not be given to people with known hypersensitivity to this drug.
• It should be given with caution to people with acute kidney impairment, lung function, G6PD deficiency (a genetic enzyme disorder), and blood dyscrasias (abnormal condition).
• Mafenide's safety during pregnancy has not been established. It is not recommended for use unless the burn area us more than 20 percent of the body surface. Do not use near term.
• Medical judgment is required if breast-feeding is being considered. Sulfonamides are found in breast milk.
• If used over extensive areas of the body, or areas in which skin is seriously compromised, enough of the drug may be absorbed to create the potential for rare adverse reactions associated with systemic use of sulfonamides: serious or even fatal allergic reactions, liver failure, and serious blood disorders. A doctor must be contacted if any adverse reactions, particularly a rash, occur.
• The use of antibiotics may result in a superinfection from non-susceptible organisms.

Interactions
No significant interactions have been reported.

Side effects
• Frequently, burning or pain.
• Occasionally, allergic reaction, metabolic acidosis, and hyperventilation.

magaldrate Ⓖ

Type/Group: **antacid.**
Brand(s): Iosopan; Riopan; various generic. Combinations: With *simethicone*: Iosopan Plus Liquid; Lowsium Plus Suspension; Riopan Plus Tablets, Suspension, Double Strength Tablets, Suspension; various generic.
How administered: Orally.

Used to treat
Magaldrate comprises a chemical mixture of basic salts of aluminum and magnesium (actually it is aluminum magnesium hydroxide sulfate). It is incorporated into preparations for the relief of hyperacidity and ✪ **indigestion**. Since magnesium-containing antacids tend to be laxative whereas aluminum-containing antacids

may be constipating, a mixture of the two is considered sometimes to be an advantage.

Warnings
• It should not be used by people with hypophosphatemia (low blood phosphates) or kidney disease.
• It should be used with caution by people with impaired kidney function, heart disorders, sodium-restricted diets, gastrointestinal disorders, cirrhosis, porphyria, or who are taking certain drugs.
• No ill-effects during pregnancy have been associated with magaldrate, but a doctor should always be consulted before taking any drug during pregnancy.
• Medical judgment is required if breast-feeding is being considered.
• Overusing antacids may cause "acid rebound," which is an increase in stomach acid secretion. Magaldrate, therefore, should not be used for more than 2 weeks continuously.
• Do not use when there is abdominal pain, nausea, or vomiting, unless directed by a doctor.
• Anyone taking any medication, including OTCs, herbal remedies, or supplements, should consult a doctor before using an antacid, as antacids may alter the absorption of a wide range of drugs.

Interactions
• ℞ **Sodium polystyrene sulfonate** resins must not be taken with magnesium or aluminum antacids, because there is potential for systemic ✪ **alkalosis.**
• Buffered ℞ **aspirin**/antacid combinations should not be used in any long-term treatment, for example, for rheumatic inflammation.
• The following drugs may have their absorption and actions impaired: ℞ **ACE inhibitors** (for example, ℞ **captopril**); ℞ **allopurinol**; ℞ **atenolol**; ℞ **chloroquine**; ℞ **corticosteroids** (for example, ℞ **dexamethasone**), ℞ **diflunisal**, ℞ **digoxin**; ℞ **ethambutol**; ℞ **H2-antagonists** (for example, ℞ **cimetidine**; ℞ **ranitidine**); iron salts, ℞ **indomethacin**, ℞ **isoniazid**; ℞ **ketoconazole**; ℞ **nitrofurantoin**; ℞ **penicillamine**; ℞ **phenothiazines**; ℞ **quinolones**; ℞ **tetracyclines**; ℞ **thyroid hormones**; and ℞ **ticlopidine**. Doses of these drugs should be taken several hours apart from doses of the antacid (a doctor should be consulted for full instructions and cautions).
• ℞ **Benzodiazepines**, ℞ **dicumarol**, ℞ **levodopa**, ℞ **quinidine**, ℞ **sulfonylureas**, and ℞ **valproate sodium** may have their absorption increased and so there is a higher potential for adverse effects.

Side effects
• Magaldrate may occasionally cause the chief side effects of its two constituents, aluminum (constipation) and magnesium (diarrhea); nausea and vomiting may also occur.

Magan Tablets Ⓑ

A preparation of ℞ **magnesium salicylate.**
Formulation: Oral tablets.
Availability: Prescription only.
Warnings and side effects: See ℞ **magnesium salicylate.**

Magnalox Liquid ®

A preparation of ℞ **aluminum hydroxide** and ℞ **magnesium hydroxide**.

Formulation: Oral liquid.

Availability: OTC.

Warnings and side effects: See ℞ **aluminum hydroxide**; ℞ **magnesium hydroxide**.

Magnaprin Tablets; Arthritis Strength Captabs ®

A preparation of ℞ **aspirin**, ℞ **aluminum hydroxide**, ℞ **magnesium hydroxide**, ℞ **calcium carbonate**.

Formulation: Oral tablets.

Availability: OTC.

Warnings and side effects: See ℞ **aspirin**; ℞ **aluminum hydroxide**; ℞ **magnesium hydroxide**; ℞ **calcium carbonate**.

magnesium carbonate ©

Type/Group: **antacid**; **laxative**.

Brand(s): Various generic. Combinations: With *calcium carbonate*: Marblen Tablets, Liquid; Mi-Acid Gelcaps; Mylagen Gelcaps; Mylanta Gelcaps. With *aluminum hydroxide*: Alenic Alka Liquid, Extra Strength Tablets; Gaviscon Liquid, Extra Strength Relief Formula Liquid (also has *simethicone*); Genaton Liquid. (Plus): *sodium bicarbonate*: Gaviscon Extra Strength Relief Formula Tablets; Genaton Extra Strength Tablets.

How administered: Orally.

Used to treat

Magnesium carbonate is an antacid that also has laxative properties. It is a mild antacid but fairly long-acting and is a constituent of many over-the-counter preparations used to relieve hyperacidity, ♦ **dyspepsia**, and the symptoms of ♦ **peptic ulcer**.

Warnings

• It should be used with caution by people with impaired kidney function, low phosphate levels, or who are taking certain drugs.

• No ill effects during pregnancy have been associated with magnesium carbonate, but a doctor should always be consulted before taking any drug during pregnancy.

• Medical judgment is required if breast-feeding is being considered.

• Overusing antacids may cause "acid rebound," which is an increase in stomach acid secretion. Magnesium carbonate, therefore, should not be used for more than two weeks continuously.

• Do not use when there is abdominal pain, nausea, or vomiting, unless directed by a doctor.

• Antacids containing magnesium, with prolonged use, may cause kidney damage or symptoms of magnesium toxicity.

• Anyone taking any medication, including OTCs, herbal remedies, or supplements, should consult a doctor before taking an antacid or laxative, as they may alter the absorption of a wide range of drugs.

Interactions

• ℞ **Sodium polystyrene sulfonate** resins must not be taken with magnesium or aluminum antacids, because there is potential for systemic ♦ **alkalosis**.

• Buffered ℞ **aspirin**/antacid combinations should not be used in any long-term treatment, for example, for rheumatic inflammation.

• The following drugs may have their absorption and actions impaired: ℞ **ACE inhibitors** (for example, ℞ **captopril**); ℞ **benzodiazepines**; ℞ **chloroquine**; ℞ **corticosteroids** (for example, ℞ **dexamethasone**); ℞ **digoxin**; ℞ **H₂-antagonists**, (for example, ℞ **cimetidine**, ℞ **ranitidine hydrochloride**); ℞ **hydantoins**; ℞ **indomethacin**; iron salts; ℞ **isoniazid**; ℞ **nitrofurantoin**; ℞ **penicillamine**; ℞ **phenothiazines**; ℞ **quinolones**; ℞ **tetracyclines**; and ℞ **ticlopidine**. Doses of these drugs should be taken several hours apart from doses of the antacid (a doctor should be consulted for full instructions and cautions).

• The absorption of ℞ **dicumarol**, ℞ **quinidine**, ℞ **sulfonylureas**, and ℞ **valproate sodium** may be increased, with a higher potential for adverse effects.

Side effects

• There may be belching due to the internal liberation of carbon dioxide, and diarrhea.

magnesium hydroxide ©

Type/Group: **antacid**; **laxative**.

Brand(s): Phillips' Chewable Tablets; Phillips' Milk of Magnesia; various generic. Combinations: With *aluminum hydroxide*: Almag Suspension; Maalox Suspension, Therapeutic Concentrate; Magnalox Liquid; Magnox Suspension; Mintox Tablets, Suspenion; Rulox Tablets, Suspension. (Plus): *simethicone*: Almag Plus Suspension; Almacone Tablets, Almacone II; Aludrox; Gas Ban DS Liquid; Gelusil; Kudrox Double Strength; Maalox Extra Strength Suspension; Mi-Acid II; Mintox Plus, Extra Strength; Mygel II; Mylagen II; Mylanta Tablets, Double Strength Tablets, Liquid; Rulox Plus Tablets, Suspension; Simaal Gel 2 Liquid; Tempo Tablets (also has *calcium carbonate*). With *calcium carbonate*: Mylanta Supreme; Rolaids Calcium Rich Tablets. (Plus): *simethicone*: Di-Gel Advanced Formula. With *mineral oil*: Haley's M-O.

How administered: Orally.

Used to treat

Magnesium hydroxide, or hydrated magnesium oxide (magnesia), is an antacid that also has laxative properties. As an antacid it is comparatively weak but fairly long-acting and is a constituent of many OTC preparations used for hyperacidity, ♦ **indigestion**, and symptomatic relief of ♦ **peptic ulcer**. It can also be used to treat ♦ **constipation**.

Warnings

• It should be used with caution by people with impaired kidney function, gastrointestinal disease or impairment, or who are taking certain drugs.

• No ill effects during pregnancy have been associated with magnesium hydroxide, but a doctor should always be consulted before taking any drug during pregnancy.

• Medical judgment is required if breast-feeding is being considered.

• Overusing antacids may cause "acid rebound," which is an increase in stomach acid secretion. Magnesium hydroxide, therefore, should not be used for more than one week continuously.

• Do not use when there is abdominal pain, nausea, or vomiting, unless directed by a doctor.

• Prolonged use of antacids containing magnesium may cause kidney damage or symptoms of magnesium toxicity.

• Anyone taking any medication, including OTCs, herbal remedies, or supplements, should consult a doctor before taking an antacid or laxative, as they may alter the absorption of a wide range of drugs.

Interactions

• ℞ **Sodium polystyrene sulfonate** resins must not be taken with magnesium or aluminum antacids, because there is potential for systemic ✪ **alkalosis**.

• Buffered ℞ **aspirin**/antacid combinations should not be used in any long-term treatment, for example, for rheumatic inflammation.

• The following drugs may have their absorption and actions impaired: ℞ **ACE inhibitors** (for example, ℞ **captopril**); ℞ **benzodiazepines**; ℞ **chloroquine**; ℞ **corticosteroids** (for example, ℞ **dexamethasone**); ℞ **digoxin**; ℞ **H₂-antagonist** (for example, ℞ **cimetidine**, ℞ **ranitidine**); ℞ **hydantoins**; ℞ **indomethacin**; iron salts; ℞ **isoniazid**; ℞ **nitrofurantoin**; ℞ **penicillamine**; ℞ **phenothiazines**; ℞ **quinolones**; ℞ **tetracyclines**; and ℞ **ticlopidine**. Doses of these drugs should be taken several hours apart from doses of the antacid (a doctor should be consulted for full instructions and cautions).

• The absorption of ℞ **dicumarol**, ℞ **quinidine**, ℞ **sulfonylureas**, and ℞ **valproate sodium** may be increased, with a higher potential for adverse effects.

Side effects

• There may be diarrhea.

• Less commonly, abdominal pain, nausea, vomiting, and dehydration.

magnesium salicylate ⑥

Type/Group: **antipyretic; anti-inflammatory; antirheumatic; non-narcotic analgesic.**

Brand(s): **Doan's Extra Strength Caplets; Magan Tablets; Mobidin Tablets; Momentum Muscular Backache Formula Caplets; Nuprin Backache Caplets.** Combinations: With *choline salicylate*: **Tricosal Tablets; Trilisate Tablets, Liquid**; various generic. With *phenyltoloxamine citrate*: **Magsal Tablets; Mobigesic Tablets.** How administered: Orally.

Used to treat

Magnesium salicylate has similar effects to ℞ **aspirin**, although usually with less marked gastrointestinal side effects. It is used to relieve mild to moderate pain, and in the treatment of ✪ **rheumatoid arthritis**, ✪ **osteoarthritis**, and related rheumatic disorders. This and other ℞ **salicylates** do not possess aspirin's degree of ℞ **antiplatelet** activity, and so should not be used as an aspirin sub-

stitute when aspirin's preventive ℞ **antithrombotic** effects are required.

Warnings

• It should not be used by people with known hypersensitivity to this drug or to other salicylates (including aspirin), who have chronic kidney disease, certain bleeding disorders or conditions (for example, hemophilia, vitamin K deficiency, low platelet levels), or who have a tendency to, or active, peptic ulceration.

• It should be used with care by people taking certain drugs for gout or diabetes mellitus, or with allergic disorders (especially asthma and skin conditions), in the elderly, children or teenagers, in anyone with any kind of kidney impairment, or with certain liver disorders.

• Salicylates can adversely affect the health both of a pregnant woman and the fetus. They should not be used during pregnancy, and especially not in the third trimester, when risk to the fetus is at its highest.

• Breast-feeding mothers should either discontinue this drug or stop breast-feeding.

• Because of a link between salicylates and the rare, but serious, condition called ✪ **Reye's syndrome** (which causes inflammation of the brain and liver), salicylates should not be given to children or teenagers who have, or might have, chickenpox or influenza. As so many infections resemble flu in their initial symptoms, salicylates should not, as a general rule, be used to treat fever, ache, and malaise by anyone in this age group except on advice of a doctor.

• Excessive use in babies for teething upsets has resulted in poisoning.

• If dizziness, change in hearing, or ringing in the ears (tinnitus) occurs, stop using this drug. These are usually the first symptoms of overdose.

• Salicylates can produce the same allergic-like symptoms (including bronchospasm) that may occur after taking NSAIDs, including bronchospasm in "aspirin-sensitive" asthmatics.

Interactions

• ℞ **Anticoagulants** have an additive effect in prolonging bleeding time.

• There is generally no added benefit in taking other NSAIDs or other salicylates at the same time, but there is a higher risk of gastrointestinal upsets and bleeding.

• If taken with alcohol, there is an increased risk of bleeding, particularly of an existing ulcer.

• ℞ **Antacids**, ℞ **corticosteroids**, ℞ **urinary alkalinizers**, and ℞ **activated charcoal** may lower the absorption or therapeutic effect of salicylates.

• ℞ **Carbonic-anhydrase inhibitors** (for example, ℞ **acetazolamide**) increase the risk of overdose symptoms for both salicylates and these drugs.

• The effects of the following drugs may be exaggerated: ℞ **phenytoin**; ℞ **nitroglycerin**; ℞ **valproate sodium** (and other valproic acid derivatives); ℞ **methotrexate**.

• Magnesium salicylate taken with ℞ **insulin** or ℞ **sulfonylureas** may cause a greater glucose-lowering effect.

• The therapeutic effects of ℞ **angiotensin-receptor blockers**, ℞ **beta-blockers**, loop ℞ **diuretics**, and ℞ **spironolactone** may be reduced by salicylates.

• ℞ **Uricosuric** agents (used in the treatment of gout, for example, phenylbutazone, ℞ **probenecid**, and ℞ **sulfinpyrazone**) may lose their effectiveness.

• There is a risk of accidental overdose and toxic effects if taken with OTC medications containing salicylates in some form (for example, some ℞ **antacids**).

• Foods high in salicylates, such as curry powder, gherkins, licorice, paprika, prunes, raisins, and tea, may increase the risk of side effects.

Side effects

These vary in severity and in the frequency with which they occur.

• The most common are gastrointestinal upsets, nausea, heartburn, diarrhea, and prolonged bleeding time (with consequent risk of ulceration). (The gastrointestinal upsets may be minimized by taking the drug with milk or food.)

• There may be hypersensitivity reactions, including hives, rash, bronchospasm, edema, headache, blood disorders, ringing in the ears, dizziness, and fluid retention.

• Reversible kidney failure, particularly in renal impairment, has occurred. Liver damage is rare.

magnesium sulfate Ⓖ

Type/Group: **anticonvulsant; antiepileptic; laxative; antiarrhythmic**.

Brand(s): As an oral laxative: various generic, usually known as Epsom salts. Injected form: various generic.

How administered: Orally; topically; injection.

Used to treat

Magnesium sulfate (also known as Epsom salts) is an osmotic laxative. It works by preventing the reabsorption of water within the intestines and can be used to facilitate rapid bowel evacuation. In its injected form, its uses are quite different: in emergency treatment of heart ✚ **arrhythmias** and for people thought to have suffered ✚ **myocardial infarction** (heart attack); to control or prevent seizures or convulsions that may occur in ✚ **eclampsia**, glomerulonephritis, ✚ **epilepsy**, and ✚ **hypothyroidism**; and as a supplement in magnesium deficiency that may arise from such conditions as alcoholism, cirrhosis of the liver, acute pancreatitis, and malabsorption disorders. It may also be used in counteracting the effects of barium poisoning.

Warnings

• Use with caution in anyone with kidney impairment.

• As a laxative medication, magnesium sulfate is considered safe when used as recommended. When injected there is generally little risk to the fetus, unless high dosages are delivered by slow infusion (particularly in the hours before delivery); use only when clearly needed.

• Magnesium sulfate should not be given by injection in the two hours before delivery.

• Medical judgment is required if an injection is being considered for breast-feeding mothers.

• Extra fluid intake may be necessary to keep up normal urinary function.

Interactions

• Magnesium sulfate may intensify the effects of neuromuscular blockers (for example, ℞ **succinylcholine**, tubocurarine, ℞ **vecuronium**).

Side effects

• When taken orally, there may be colic and diarrhea.

• After excess doses (orally or by injection) there may be nausea, vomiting, thirst, flushing, effects on heart and blood pressure, depression, confusion, drowsiness, and other effects.

magnesium trisilicate Ⓖ

Type/Group: **antacid**.

Brand(s): Various generic. Combinations: With *aluminum hydroxide, sodium bicarbonate*: Foamicon; Gaviscon Tablets, Gaviscon-2 Double Strength Tablets; Genaton Tablets.

How administered: Orally.

Used to treat

Magnesium trisilicate has a long duration of action. It is a constituent of many over-the-counter preparations that are used to relieve hyperacidity and ✚ **indigestion**, and also for the symptomatic relief of a ✚ **peptic ulcer**.

Warnings

• It should be used with caution by people with impaired kidney function, with gastrointestinal disease or impairment, or who are taking certain drugs.

• No ill effects during pregnancy have been associated with magnesium trisilicate, but a doctor should always be consulted before taking any drug during pregnancy.

• Medical judgment is required if breast-feeding is being considered.

• Overusing antacids may cause "acid rebound," which is an increase in stomach acid secretion. Magnesium trisilicate, therefore, should not be used for more than 2 weeks continuously.

• Do not use if there is abdominal pain, nausea, or vomiting, unless directed by a doctor.

• Antacids containing magnesium, with prolonged use, may cause kidney damage or symptoms of magnesium toxicity.

• Anyone taking any medication, including OTCs, herbal remedies, or supplements, should consult a doctor before taking an antacid, as it may alter the absorption of a wide range of drugs.

Interactions

• ℞ **Sodium polystyrene sulfonate** resins must not be taken with magnesium or aluminum antacids, because there is potential for systemic ✚ **alkalosis**.

• Buffered ℞ **aspirin**/antacid combinations should not be used in any long-term treatment, for example, for rheumatic inflammation.

• The following drugs may have their absorption and actions impaired: ℞ **ACE inhibitors** (for example, ℞ **captopril**); ℞ **benzodiazepines**; ℞ **chloroquine**; ℞ **corticosteroids** (for example, ℞ **dexamethasone**); ℞ **digoxin**; ℞ **H₂-antagonist** (for example, ℞ **cimetidine**, ℞ **ranitidine**); ℞ **hydantoins**; ℞ **indomethacin**; iron salts; ℞ **isoniazid**; ℞ **nitrofurantoin**;

℞ penicillamine; ℞ phenothiazines; ℞ quinolones; ℞ tetracyclines; and ℞ ticlopidine. Doses of these drugs should be taken several hours apart from doses of the antacid (a doctor should be consulted for full instructions and cautions).

• The absorption of ℞ dicumarol, ℞ quinidine, ℞ sulfonylureas, and ℞ valproate sodium may be increased, with a higher potential for adverse effects.

Side effects
• There may be diarrhea.
• Less commonly, abdominal pain, nausea, vomiting, and dehydration.

Magnox Suspension ⓑ
A preparation of ℞ aluminum hydroxide and ℞ magnesium hydroxide.
Formulation: Oral liquid.
Availability: OTC.
Warnings and side effects: See ℞ aluminum hydroxide; ℞ magnesium hydroxide.

Magsal Tablets ⓑ
A preparation of ℞ magnesium salicylate and phenyltoloxamine citrate.
Formulation: Oral tablets.
Availability: Prescription only.
Warnings and side effects: See ℞ magnesium salicylate.

major tranquilizer ⓓ
see ℞ antipsychotic.

malaria treatment ⓓ
see ℞ antimalarial.

malathion ⓖ
Type/Group: scabicide and pediculicide.
Brand(s): Ovide.
How administered: Topically (external).

Used to treat
Malathion is an insecticidal drug used as a pediculicidal to treat infestations by head lice and their eggs (see ✪ lice and mite infestation).

Warnings
• It should not be given to people with known hypersensitivity to this drug or any components of the product. Its safety and effectiveness in children under 2 years of age have not been established.
• It should be given with caution to people with asthma or eczema (especially preparations containing alcohol).
• Malathion should be used during pregnancy only if it is clearly needed.
• Medical judgment is required if breast-feeding is being considered. It is not known whether it appears in breast milk.
• It must not be applied around the eyes.
• It is toxic if taken internally.

• Exposure to insecticides or pesticides must be avoided during treatment.

Interactions
• ℞ Aminoglycosides (when injected) increase the risk of respiratory depression.
• Local ℞ anesthetics increase the risk of systemic toxicity.
• ℞ edrophonium chloride increases the risk of adverse effects in people with myasthenia gravis.
• If taken with cholinesterase inhibitors (including ophthalmic agents), there is increased toxicity.
• The effects of ℞ succinylcholine may be increased.

Side effects
• Scalp irritation.

male sex hormone ⓓ
see ℞ androgen.

Mallamint ⓑ
A preparation of ℞ calcium carbonate.
Formulation: Oral tablets, chewable.
Availability: OTC.
Warnings and side effects: See ℞ calcium carbonate.

Mandol ⓑ
A preparation of ℞ cefamandole.
Formulation: Injection.
Availability: Prescription only.
Warnings and side effects: See ℞ cefamandole.

manic-depressive treatment ⓓ
see ℞ antimanic.

mannitol ⓖ
Type/Group: diuretic; glaucoma treatment.
Brand(s): Osmitrol; various generic.
How administered: Intravenous infusion.

Used to treat
Mannitol is one of the osmotic class of diuretics, and the most widely used of this class. It consists of substances secreted into the kidney proximal tubules, which are not resorbed and so carry water and mineral salts into the urine, therefore increasing the volume produced. It is used primarily to treat edema, particularly cerebral (brain) edema, low urinary output (oliguria) in acute kidney failure, and to accelerate urinary excretion of some toxic substances (for example, in the overdose of ℞ aspirin or ℞ barbiturates). It may also be used in the treatment of ✪ glaucoma to decrease pressure within the eyeball in acute attacks, when other agents have not worked satisfactorily.

Warnings
• It should not be given to people with severe degrees of kidney disease, lung congestion, heart failure or dehydration, where the use of mannitol causes or worsens such conditions, or when there is active bleeding within the brain.
• It should be given with caution to people with less severe degrees of all the above disorders.

• Mannitol should be used in pregnancy only if it is clearly needed.

• Medical judgment is required if breast-feeding is being considered.

• An escape of mannitol into the tissues from the site of infusion (vein) can cause inflammation and death of the surrounding skin tissue.

• Fluids, electrolytes (especially potassium and sodium), and kidney function are monitored during treatment, because significant depletion is possible.

Interactions

• Mannitol increases the clearance of ℞ **lithium** from the body (most diuretics have an opposite effect) and so the effects of lithium may be decreased.

Side effects

• Commonly, fluid and electrolyte imbalance. Other side effects may include dry mouth, thirst, urinary retention, headache, blurred vision, nausea and vomiting, chills, dizziness, and hypotension.

MAOI ⑩

(monoamine-oxidase inhibitor)

Generics: **phenelzine; tranylcypromine; isocarboxazid.**

Actions and uses

MAOI is a class ℞ **antidepressant** drugs—technically referred to as monoamine-oxidase inhibitors—which are used to relieve the symptoms of the affective disorder ✪ **depression**.

All types of antidepressants may be used to elevate mood, help resume normal functioning, and reduce the frequency of depressive episodes in chronic depressive states. There are several different groups of antidepressants, but they all work by changing the levels of monoamine neurotransmitters (mainly serotonin and norepinephrine) in areas of the brain that regulate mood. The MAOI group work by blocking the metabolic breakdown of the monoamine neurotransmitters by inhibiting specific monoamine-oxidase enzymes.

Limitations

All antidepressant drugs have significant side effects, although these do generally become less troublesome with time. The MAOI group has a serious limitation in that strict dietary restrictions must be followed. Because the enzyme monoamine-oxidase also detoxifies the amine tyramine in the body, when certain foodstuffs that contain this amine are eaten (for example, ripe cheese, fermented soya bean products, meat or yeast extracts, and some alcoholic beverages) or medicines that contain ℞ **sympathomimetic** amines are taken (for example, cough and cold remedies that contain ℞ **ephedrine** or ℞ **pseudoephedrine**) the outcome may be a hypertensive crisis. Drugs of the ℞ **amphetamine** class also have serious, potentially fatal, hypertensive interactions with MAOIs. In the search for the best treatment, switching between different groups is not easy because each needs a quite long wash-out period before the next type can be tried. A doctor must always be consulted before taking any other medications, including herbal remedies and supplements, if you are taking MAOIs.

Mapap Regular Strength Tablets; Extra Strength Tablets ⑧

A preparation of ℞ **acetaminophen**.
Formulation: Oral tablets; chewable tablets; liquid.
Availability: OTC.
Warnings and side effects: See ℞ **acetaminophen**.

maprotiline hydrochloride ⑥

Type/Group: **antidepressant; tricyclic.**
Brand(s): Ludiomil; various generic.
How administered: Orally.

Used to treat

Maprotiline hydrochloride can be used to treat ✪ **depression**. It differs in structure from the tricyclic compounds, but its effects are similar. Although not stated by the manufacturer for such treatment, it is sometimes used for ✪ **anxiety**.

Warnings

• It should not be given to people with known hypersensitivity to this drug, or anyone just recovering from myocardial infarction (heart attack), or who are taking or have stopped taking MAOI antidepressants within the previous 14 days. There is a danger of convulsions and precipitated epileptic episodes, and so it is not recommended for epileptics.

• It should be given with caution to people with a history of urinary retention, elevated intraocular pressure (pressure in the eyeball), narrow-angle glaucoma, cardiovascular, heart or thyroid disease, diabetes mellitus, angle-closure glaucoma, or kidney or liver disease.

• Maprotiline should be used during pregnancy only if the benefits outweigh the possible risk to the fetus.

• Medical judgment is required if breast-feeding is being considered.

• The effects of alcohol may be enhanced.

• Treatment should be stopped gradually by lowering the dose over a period of time.

• It is not generally given to children.

• It may be two to three weeks before there are any signs of improvement.

• It may impair the performance of skilled tasks such as driving.

Interactions

• Serious or even fatal reactions can occur if ℞ **MAOI** antidepressants are taken at the same time as tricyclics.

• The effects of ℞ **epinephrine**, ℞ **norepinephrine**, and ℞ **phenylephrine** on blood pressure are intensified.

• ℞ **clonidine hydrochloride** should not be used with tricyclics, because a dangerous increase in blood pressure and hypertensive crisis is possible.

• The ℞ **antihypertensive** effects of ℞ **guanethidine monosulfate**, are reduced.

• The effects of ℞ **anticholinergics** and ℞ **sympathomimetics** may be enhanced.

• ℞ **Barbiturates**, alcohol, and hepatic enzyme inducers may reduce the effectiveness of maprotiline.

• ℞ **Cimetidine** hepatic enzyme inhibitors may increase the levels of maprotiline in the blood.

• ℞ **Benzodiazepines,** ℞ **phenothiazines,** and ℞ **thyroid hormones** may increase the risk of seizure or heart problems.

Side effects

• Although it has fewer ℞ **anticholinergic** side effects than some other tricyclics, it can cause drowsiness and difficulty in concentrating, dry mouth, blurred vision, constipation, postural hypotension (lowered blood pressure on standing), and urinary retention. Rashes are common. Irregular heartbeat or gastric or intestinal distress may also occur.

• Although rare, seizures, white cell blood and platelet disorders, and stoppage of normal intestinal action (peristalsis) can occur.

Marax-DF Syrup Ⓑ

A preparation of ℞ **ephedrine,** ℞ **theophylline,** and ℞ **hydroxyzine.**
Formulation: Oral syrup.
Availability: Prescription only.
Warnings and side effects: See ℞ **ephedrine;** ℞ **theophylline;** ℞ **hydroxyzine.**

Marax Tablets Ⓑ

A preparation of ℞ **ephedrine,** ℞ **theophylline** and ℞ **hydroxyzine.**
Formulation: Oral tablets.
Availability: Prescription only.
Warnings and side effects: See ℞ **ephedrine;** ℞ **theophylline;** ℞ **hydroxyzine.**

Marblen Tablets; Liquid Ⓑ

A preparation of ℞ **calcium carbonate** and ℞ **magnesium carbonate.**
Formulation: Oral tablets; liquid.
Availability: OTC.
Warnings and side effects: See ℞ **calcium carbonate;** ℞ **magnesium carbonate.**

Marcaine Ⓑ

A preparation of ℞ **bupivacaine.**
Formulation: Injection.
Availability: Prescription only.
Warnings and side effects: See ℞ **bupivacaine.**

Marcillin Ⓑ

A preparation of ℞ **ampicillin.**
Formulation: Oral capsules.
Availability: Prescription only.
Warnings and side effects: See ℞ **ampicillin.**

Marezine Ⓑ

A preparation of ℞ **cyclizine.**
Formulation: Oral tablets.
Availability: Prescription only.
Warnings and side effects: See ℞ **cyclizine.**

Margesic Capsules Ⓑ

A preparation of ℞ **acetaminophen,** ℞ **caffeine,** and ℞ **butabarbital.**
Formulation: Oral capsules.
Availability: Prescription only.
Warnings and side effects: See ℞ **acetaminophen;** ℞ **butabarbital;** ℞ **caffeine.**

Margesic H Capsules Ⓑ

A preparation of ℞ **hydrocodone bitartrate** and ℞ **acetaminophen.**
Formulation: Oral capsules.
Availability: Prescription only.
Warnings and side effects: See ℞ **hydrocodone bitartrate;** ℞ **acetaminophen.**

Marplan Ⓑ

A preparation of ℞ **isocarboxazid.**
Formulation: Oral tablets.
Availability: Prescription only.
Warnings and side effects: See ℞ **isocarboxazid.**

Marpres Ⓑ

A preparation of ℞ **hydralazine hydrochloride,** ℞ **hydrochlorothiazide,** and ℞ **reserpine.**
Formulation: Oral tablets.
Availability: Prescription only.
Warnings and side effects: See ℞ **hydralazine hydrochloride;** ℞ **hydrochlorothiazide;** ℞ **reserpine.**

Marten-Tab Ⓑ

A preparation of ℞ **acetaminophen** and ℞ **butabarbital.**
Formulation: Oral tablets.
Availability: Prescription only.
Warnings and side effects: See ℞ **acetaminophen;** ℞ **butabarbital.**

Marthritic Tablets Ⓑ

A preparation of ℞ **salsalate.**
Formulation: Oral tablets.
Availability: Prescription only.
Warnings and side effects: See ℞ **salsalate.**

Massengil Medicated Towelettes Ⓑ

A preparation of ℞ **hydrocortisone,** diazolidinyl urea and propylene glycol.
Formulation: Saturated wipe.
Availability: OTC.
Warnings and side effects: See ℞ **hydrocortisone.**

Matulane Ⓑ

A preparation of ℞ **procarbazine.**
Formulation: Oral capsules.
Availability: Prescription only.
Warnings and side effects: See ℞ **procarbazine.**

Mavik ®

A preparation of ℞ **trandolapril**.
Formulation: Oral tablets, available in 3 strengths.
Availability: Prescription only.
Warnings and side effects: See ℞ **trandolapril**.

Maxair Inhaler; Maxair Autohaler ®

A preparation of ℞ **pirbuterol**.
Formulation: Aerosol inhalers.
Availability: Prescription only.
Warnings and side effects: See ℞ **pirbuterol**.

Maxalt; Maxalt-MLT ®

A preparation of ℞ **rizatriptan benzoate**.
Formulation: Oral tablets; MLT are orally disintegrating tablets; both are available in two strengths.
Availability: Prescription only.
Warnings and side effects: See ℞ **rizatriptan benzoate**. MLT tablets contain the sweetener aspartame, which should be avoided by individuals with phenylketonuria.

Maxaquin ®

A preparation of ℞ **lomefloxacin**.
Formulation: Oral tablets.
Availability: Prescription only.
Warnings and side effects: See ℞ **lomefloxacin**.

Maxidex ®

A preparation of ℞ **dexamethasone**.
Formulation: Eye drops.
Availability: Prescription only.
Warnings and side effects: See ℞ **dexamethasone**.

Maximum Strength Sudafed Sinus Tablets, Caplets ®

A preparation of ℞ **pseudoephedrine** and ℞ **acetaminophen**.
Formulation: Oral tablets.
Availability: OTC.
Warnings and side effects: See ℞ **pseudoephedrine**; ℞ **acetaminophen**.

Maximum Strength Dristan Cold Caplets ®

A preparation of ℞ **pseudoephedrine**, ℞ **acetaminophen**, and ℞ **brompheniramine maleate**.
Formulation: Oral tablets.
Availability: OTC.
Warnings and side effects: See ℞ **pseudoephedrine**; ℞ **acetaminophen**; ℞ **brompheniramine maleate**.

Maximum Strength Dynafed Tablets ®

A preparation of ℞ **pseudoephedrine** and ℞ **acetaminophen**.
Formulation: Oral tablets.
Availability: OTC.
Warnings and side effects: See ℞ **pseudoephedrine**; ℞ **acetaminophen**.

Maximum Strength Meted ®

A preparation of ℞ **salicylic acid** and ℞ **sulfur**.
Formulation: Shampoo.
Availability: OTC.
Warnings and side effects: See ℞ **salicylic acid**; ℞ **sulfur**.

Maximum Strength Sine-Aid Tablets; Caplets; Gelcaps ®

A preparation of ℞ **pseudoephedrine** and ℞ **acetaminophen**.
Formulation: Oral tablets; capsules.
Availability: OTC.
Warnings and side effects: See ℞ **pseudoephedrine**; ℞ **acetaminophen**.

Maximum Strength Tylenol Allergy Sinus Caplets; Gelcaps ®

A preparation of ℞ **pseudoephedrine**, ℞ **acetaminophen**, and ℞ **chlorpheniramine maleate**.
Formulation: Oral tablets; capsules.
Availability: OTC.
Warnings and side effects: See ℞ **pseudoephedrine**; ℞ **acetaminophen**; ℞ **chlorpheniramine maleate**.

Maximum Strength Tylenol Sinus Tablets ®

Also: **Caplets; Gelcaps; Geltabs**
A preparation of ℞ **pseudoephedrine** and ℞ **acetaminophen**.
Formulation: Oral tablets; capsules.
Availability: OTC.
Warnings and side effects: See ℞ **pseudoephedrine**; ℞ **acetaminophen**.

Maxipime ®

A preparation of ℞ **cefepime**.
Formulation: Injection.
Availability: Prescription only.
Warnings and side effects: See ℞ **cefepime**.

Maxitrol ®

A preparation of ℞ **dexamethasone**, ℞ **neomycin**, and ℞ **polymyxin B sulfate**.
Formulation: Opthalmic ointment.
Availability: Prescription only.
Warnings and side effects: See ℞ **dexamethasone**; ℞ **neomycin**; ℞ **polymyxin B sulfate**.

Maxitrol Ophthalmic Solution ®

A preparation of ℞ **neomycin**, ℞ **dexamethasone**, and benzalkonium hydrochloride.
Formulation: Eye drops.
Availability: Prescription only.
Warnings and side effects: See ℞ **neomycin**; ℞ **dexamethasone**.

Maxivate ⑧

A preparation of ℞ **betamethasone** dipropionate.
Formulation: Topical (ointment; cream; lotion).
Availability: Prescription only.
Warnings and side effects: See ℞ **betamethasone**.

Maxolon ⑧

A preparation of ℞ **metoclopramide hydrochloride**.
Formulation: Oral tablets.
Availability: Prescription only.
Warnings and side effects: See ℞ **metoclopramide hydrochloride**.

M-Caps ⑧

A preparation of ℞ **methionine**.
Formulation: Oral capsules.
Availability: Prescription only.
Warnings and side effects: See ℞ **methionine**.

measles-mumps-rubella virus vaccine, live ⑥

see ℞ **MMR vaccine**.

Mebaral ⑧

A preparation of mephenobarbital (see ℞ **phenobarbital**).
Formulation: Oral tablets; oral capsules.
Availability: Prescription only.
Warnings and side effects: See ℞ **phenobarbital**.

mebendazole ⑥

Type/Group: anthelmintic; azole.
Brand(s): Vermox; various generic.
How administered: Orally.

Used to treat

Mebendazole is a a synthetic azole anthelmintic drug that can be used in the treatment of infestation by roundworm, pinworm, whipworm, and hookworm (common and American) (see ✚ **worms**).

Warnings

• It should not be given to people with known hypersensitivity or allergy to this drug.
• It is not generally recommended for use in pregnancy.
• Medical judgment is required if breast-feeding is being considered.
• The tablets should be chewed or crushed, and taken with food.
• It may take 3 days for the parasite to be killed and removed from the digestive tract. A doctor should be contacted if the condition is not cured within 3 weeks.

Interactions

• ℞ **carbamazepine** and ℞ **phenytoin** decrease levels of mebendazole.

Side effects

• Dizziness, fever, diarrhea, and transient abdominal pain.

mecamylamine hydrochloride ⑥

Type/Group: ganglion-blocker; vasodilator; antihypertensive.
Brand(s): Inversine.
How administered: Orally.

Used to treat

Mecamylamine is used to treat moderately severe to severe ✚ **hypertension**.

Warnings

• It should not be given to people with known hypersensitivity to this drug, with coronary insufficiency or recent heart attack, uremia, glaucoma, certain kidney disorders, or with less severe degrees of hypertension.
• It should be given with caution to people with cerebral or kidney insufficiency, or with any bladder or urethral obstruction (including benign prostate hypertrophy; BPH).
• Mecamylamine should be used during pregnancy only if the potential benefit outweighs the possible risk to the fetus.
• Medical judgment is required if breast-feeding is being considered.
• Treatment should be stopped gradually and with the appropriate substitution of other antihypertensives. A sudden withdrawal may cause serious hypertensive effects.
• Postural hypotension (lowered blood pressure on standing) occurs frequently and fainting may result. Sudden or prolonged standing should be avoided when taking this drug. These hypotensive effects may be intensified by a number of factors, including fever, infection, vigorous exercise, excessive heat, pregnancy, surgery, alcohol consumption, or salt depletion (as from diarrhea, excessive sweating, or diuretics).
• Mecamylamine has effects in the brain and, although rare, symptoms such as tremor, abnormal movements, mental aberrations, and convulsions have occurred (but usually at high doses or in people with cerebral or kidney insufficiency).
• Because of the possible sedative side effects, caution is advised for potentially hazardous activities, such as driving, that require mental alertness.
• Complete inaction of the bowels (ileus) is a concern, and use of this drug should be stopped at the first signs of this (often swollen abdomen and absence of any intestinal sounds).

Interactions

• ℞ **acetazolamide**, ℞ **sodium bicarbonate**, and other drugs that increase urinary pH may increase the effects of mecamylamine, with the potential for toxicity.
• ℞ **Antibiotics** and ℞ **sulfonamides** should not be used with mecamylamine.
• Alcohol, ℞ **anesthetics**, and ℞ **bethanechol** may intensify the effects of mecamylamine.
• If used with other antihypertensives and ℞ **diuretics**, the effects of these drugs may be increased. This additive effect is sometimes used to advantage in combination treatments for high blood pressure.

Side effects

• There may be postural hypotension and dizziness (and sometimes fainting), weakness, fatigue, headache, drowsiness, and gastrointestinal disturbances (for example, loss of appetite, nausea and vomiting, diarrhea, constipation).

• Other side effects may include dry mouth, dilated pupils, blurred vision, impotence, and urinary retention.

mechlorethamine hydrochloride Ⓖ

(chlormethine hydrochloride)

Type/Group: **anticancer; cytotoxic**.

Brand(s): Mustargen.

How administered: Injection. Also intrapleural, intraperitonial, intracardiac injection.

Used to treat

Mechlorethamine hydrochloride is an alkylating agent which is used in the treatment of ✚ **Hodgkin's disease** and certain metastatic ✚ **cancers**.

Warnings

• It should not be given to people with known severe hypersensitivity to mechlorethamine, or anyone with an infectious disease.

• It should be given with caution to people with chronic lymphatic leukemia, amyloidosis, or herpes zoster. This is a specialist drug which will be used following a full evaluation by specialist physicians.

• Mechlorethamine is not recommended for use during pregnancy unless it is medically judged to be essential, because it may cause birth defects. Becoming pregnant while using this drug must be avoided.

• It should not be used if breast-feeding.

• It can cause severe bone marrow depression, which may lead to bleeding and a reduced resistance to infection.

• It can impair fertility in men (which may be reversible).

• In common with many anticancer drugs, this drug may be associated with the development of secondary malignancies (new cancers).

Interactions

No interactions specific to this drug are known.

Side effects

• Frequently, nausea, vomiting, reduced white blood-cell count, loss of appetite, diarrhea, and dehydration (caused by vomiting).

• Occasionally, weakness, headache, drowsiness, lightheadedness, and rash.

• Rarely, hair loss, ringing ears, fever, seizures, and tingling sensations.

Meclan Ⓑ

A preparation of ℞ **meclocycline sulfosalicylate**.

Formulation: Ointment.

Availability: Prescription only.

Warnings and side effects: See ℞ **meclocycline sulfosalicylate**.

meclizine hydrochloride Ⓖ

(meclozine hydrochloride)

Type/Group: **antihistamine; antinauseant**.

Brand(s): Antivert, Antivert/25, Antivert/50; Antrizine Tablets; Dramamine Less Drowsy Formula; Bonine Chewable Tablets; Meni-D Capsules; Vergon Capsules.

How administered: Orally.

Used to treat

Meclizine is used primarily as an antinauseant in the treatment or prevention of ✚ **motion sickness** and vomiting. It is thought that it may be effective for the control of vertigo caused by disorders of the balance function of the inner ear.

Warnings

• It should not be given to people with known hypersensitivity to this drug (or with known sensitivity to other antihistamines).

• Antihistamines should be given with caution to people with lower respiratory disease or asthma (and never during an attack), heart disease, hypertension, hyperthyroidism, epilepsy, porphyria, increased intraocular pressure (pressure in the eyeball, as in glaucoma), enlarged prostate, urinary retention, or certain obstructive bladder or gastrointestinal conditions.

• Meclizine should be used during pregnancy only if clearly needed.

• As the safety of this drug has not been established in breast-feeding, nursing mothers should discontinue using this drug or discontinue breast-feeding.

• Meclizine must not be given to infants, and for children under the age of 12 the manufacturer's or medical instructions must be followed closely.

• Because of its sedative side effects, the performance of skilled tasks, such as driving, may be impaired.

• Side effects are more frequent in the elderly.

Interactions

• If used with ℞ **tricyclic** antidepressants, other antihistamines, ℞ **skeletal muscle relaxants**, ℞ **opioids**, ℞ **barbiturates**, ℞ **hypnotics**, ℞ **sedatives**, or ℞ **antianxiety** drugs, there is a risk of intensified side effects.

• Alcohol may intensify side effects such as drowsiness and impaired mental alertness.

Side effects

• These depend on how it is administered. For this type of antihistamine, there is commonly drowsiness, headache, impaired muscular coordination or dizziness, and anticholinergic effects (dry mouth, blurred vision, urinary retention, gastrointestinal disturbances).

• Less frequently, rashes and photosensitivity (abnormal sensitivity to light), palpitations and heart arrhythmias.

• Rarely, there may be stimulation instead of sedation (paradoxical stimulation), especially in children (and convulsions in overdose), hypersensitivity reactions, blood disorders, liver disturbances, depression, sleep disturbances, and hypotension.

meclocycline sulfosalicylate Ⓖ

Type/Group: **tetracycline; antibiotic; antibacterial; acne treatment**.

Brand(s): Meclan.

How administered: Topically (external).

Used to treat

Meclocycline is used to treat ✪ **acne**.

Warnings

• It should not be given to people with known hypersensitivity to tetracyclines or any component of the product.

• It should be given with caution to people with kidney or liver function impairment, because significant absorption through the skin may result from prolonged use.

• It should be used during pregnancy only if it is clearly needed and if the benefits outweigh the potential harm to the fetus.

• Medical judgment is required if breast-feeding is being considered.

• It may temporarily stain hair.

Interactions

No significant interactions have been reported.

Side effects

• Rarely, skin irritation and rash. Systemic effects are unlikely.

meclofenamamic acid ⓖ

see ℞ **meclofenamate sodium**.

meclofenamate sodium ⓖ

(meclofenamamic acid)

Type/Group: **anti-inflammatory; antirheumatic; non-narcotic analgesic; NSAID.**

Brand(s): **Various generic.**

How administered: Orally.

Used to treat

Meclofenamate sodium is used to treat mild to moderate pain and inflammation in ✪ **rheumatoid arthritis**, ✪ **osteoarthritis**, and other ✪ **musculoskeletal disorders**. It is also used to treat ✪ **dysmenorrhea** (period pain) and ✪ **menorrhagia** (heavy bleeding).

Warnings

• It should not be used by people with known hypersensitivity to this drug or to other NSAIDs (including ℞ **aspirin**), who have chronic kidney disease, certain bleeding disorders or conditions (for example, hemophilia, vitamin K deficiency, low blood-platelet levels), or who have a tendency to, or active, peptic ulceration.

• It should be given with caution to people with diabetes mellitus, porphyria, SLE (systemic lupus erythematosus), peripheral edema, or allergic disorders (especially asthma and skin conditions), who are elderly, or with any kind of kidney impairment or with certain liver disorders.

• Meclofenamate should be used during pregnancy only when medically judged that it is needed. In the third trimester, its risk to the fetus increases, and so it should only be used if the benefits outweigh the risks to the fetus, which are higher at this time.

• Breast-feeding mothers should either discontinue this drug or stop breast-feeding.

• With regular, long-term use (as in the treatment of osteoarthritis), NSAIDs may cause gastrointestinal bleeding, ulceration, or perforation. Any signs of bleeding (for example, black stools) should be reported to a physician immediately.

• Most NSAIDs have the potential, particularly with regular use, to cause liver damage. Periodic evaluation of liver function is necessary in long-term therapy (more than two months).

• If a rash appears during treatment, its use should be stopped and a physician consulted.

• Its side effects (such as dizziness) may impair the performance of skilled tasks, such as driving.

• Side effects are more frequent in the elderly.

• Gastrointestinal upsets may be minimized by taking the drug with milk or food.

Interactions

• There is generally no added benefit in taking other NSAIDs or other ℞ **salicylates** (especially aspirin) at the same time, but there is a higher risk of gastrointestinal upsets and bleeding.

• Alcohol and ℞ **corticosteroids** increase the risk of bleeding, particularly if there is an existing ulcer.

• ℞ **anticoagulant**, ℞ **antiplatelet**, and ℞ **thrombolytic** drugs may increase bleeding time.

• The effectiveness of ℞ **ACE inhibitors**, ℞ **beta-blockers**, and ℞ **diuretics** may be reduced.

• The effects of ℞ **cyclosporine**, ℞ **digoxin**, ℞ **lithium**, and ℞ **methotrexate** may be exaggerated, with potential for toxicity.

• Foodstuffs and herbals with ℞ **antiplatelet** properties, for example, ♣ **ginger**, ⚭ **garlic**, and various herbal preparations, may add to the antiplatelet effect of NSAIDs.

Side effects

• Among the drugs in this class, meclofenamate has the highest incidence of diarrhea, sometimes severe enough to require discontinuing its use.

• Commonly, diarrhea, nausea, gastrointestinal upsets, vomiting, dizziness, and headache.

• Less frequently, constipation, flatulence, swelling of the extremities, malaise, blurred vision, ringing in the ears, nervousness, fatigue, and sleep disturbances.

• Prolonged bleeding time (with consequent risk of ulceration) is possible with high dosage, and other blood changes can occur, including anemia.

• Hypersensitivity reactions may include symptoms such as hives, rash, chest tightness, asthma, or bronchospasm.

• Reversible kidney failure, particularly in renal impairment, has occurred. Liver damage is rare.

meclozine hydrochloride ⓖ

see ℞ **meclizine hydrochloride**.

Medacote Lotion ⓑ

A preparation of ℞ **pyrilamine maleate**, ℞ **camphor**, ℞ **menthol**, ℞ **zinc oxide**, and dimethyl polysiloxane.

Formulation: Topical lotion.

Availability: OTC.

Warnings and side effects: See ℞ **pyrilamine maleate**; ℞ **camphor**; ℞ **menthol**; ℞ **zinc oxide**.

Medi-Flu Liquid ℞

A preparation of ℞ **dextromethorphan**, ℞ **acetaminophen**, ℞ **chlorpheniramine maleate**, and ℞ **pseudoephedrine**.
Formulation: Oral liquid.
Availability: OTC.
Warnings and side effects: See ℞ **dextromethorphan**; ℞ **acetaminophen**; ℞ **chlorpheniramine maleate**; ℞ **pseudoephedrine**.

Medigesic Capsules ℞

A preparation of ℞ **acetaminophen**, ℞ **caffeine**, and ℞ **butabarbital**.
Formulation: Oral capsules.
Availability: Prescription only.
Warnings and side effects: See ℞ **acetaminophen**; ℞ **caffeine**; ℞ **butabarbital**.

Mediplast ℞

A preparation of ℞ **salicylic acid**.
Formulation: Topical plaster (patches).
Availability: OTC.
Warnings and side effects: See ℞ **salicylic acid**.

Medi-Quick Ointment ℞

A preparation of ℞ **neomycin**, ℞ **polymyxin B sulfate**, and ℞ **bacitracin**.
Formulation: Topical ointment.
Availability: OTC.
Warnings and side effects: See ℞ **neomycin**; ℞ **polymyxin B sulfate**; ℞ **bacitracin**.

Medotar ℞

A preparation of ℞ **coal tar**.
Formulation: Topical ointment.
Availability: OTC.
Warnings and side effects: See ℞ **coal tar**.

Medralone ℞

A preparation of ℞ **methylprednisolone** acetate.
Formulation: Injection.
Availability: Prescription only.
Warnings and side effects: See ℞ **methylprednisolone**.

Medrol ℞

A preparation of ℞ **methylprednisolone**.
Formulation: Oral tablets in several strengths.
Availability: Prescription only.
Warnings and side effects: See ℞ **methylprednisolone**. Yellow tablet contains tartrazine. Some individuals are allergic to tartrazine, particularly those who are allergic to aspirin.

medroxyprogesterone ⓖ

Type/Group: **sex hormone; progestin; anticancer; contraceptive**.

Brand(s): Amen; Depo-Provera; Provera; various generic.
Combinations: With *conjugated estrogens*: Prempro; Premphase.
How administered: Orally, injection.

Used to treat

Medroxyprogesterone acetate is used for dysfunctional uterine bleeding, amenorrhea, and for contraception. It is also used as an anticancer treatment for endometrial, breast, and kidney cancer. Although not stated by the manufacturer for such treatment, it may be prescribed in combination with ℞ **estrogen** for symptoms of menopause, and for obesity-hypoventilation syndrome, obstructive sleep apnea, hirsutism, or homozygous sickle-cell disease.

Warnings

• It should not be used by people with known hypersensitivity to this drug, impaired liver function or disease, breast cancer, undiagnosed vaginal bleeding, missed abortion, thrombophlebitis, or a history of thromboembolic disease or stroke.
• It should be given with caution to people with epilepsy, migraine, asthma, heart or kidney dysfunction, depression, or diabetes mellitus.
• Medroxyprogesterone must not be used during pregnancy, because there is evidence of risk to the fetus. A doctor must be contacted if pregnancy occurs while taking this drug.
• It may be used by breast-feeding mothers.
• Take with food to avoid upset stomach.
• When used as a contraceptive, the menstrual cycle may be disrupted and become irregular, and may cease entirely as treatment continues.
• Diabetic patients must monitor blood glucose levels during treatment.
• Avoid exposure to ultraviolet light, including sunlight.

Interactions

• ℞ **aminoglutethimide** may reduce levels of medroxyprogesterone.

Side effects

These depend on use, duration of use, how administered, and dose.
• Commonly, dizziness, headache, insomnia, fatigue, cholestatic jaundice, increased weight, nausea, appetite changes, amenorrhea, and breakthrough bleeding.
• Less frequently, depression, edema, breast changes, decreased libido, delayed return to fertility, hot flashes, decreased bone density, acne, hair loss, body hair growth, oily skin, photosensitivity, rash, and darkening of skin on face.

MED-Rx DM Tablets ℞

A preparation of ℞ **dextromethorphan**, ℞ **pseudoephedrine**, and ℞ **guaifenesin**.
Formulation: Oral tablets.
Availability: Prescription only.
Warnings and side effects: See ℞ **dextromethorphan**; ℞ **pseudoephedrine**; ℞ **guaifenesin**.

MED-Rx Tablets ℞

A preparation of ℞ **pseudoephedrine** and ℞ **guaifenesin**.
Formulation: Oral tablets.

Key to symbols: ✚ = Disorder Section ℞ = Drug Section ♣ = Herbal Section ⌗⌗ = Supplement Section

Availability: Prescription only.
Warnings and side effects: See ℞ **pseudoephedrine**; ℞ **guaifenesin**.

mefenamic acid ⓖ

Type/Group: **anti-inflammatory; antirheumatic; non-narcotic analgesic; NSAID.**
Brand(s): Ponstel.
How administered: Orally.

Used to treat

Mefenamic acid is used primarily as a short-term (one week or less) treatment of mild to moderate pain, such as lower back pain. It is also used to treat ✪ **dysmenorrhea** (period pain) and, although not stated by the manufacturer, it is sometimes used to treat ✪ **menorrhagia** (heavy bleeding).

Warnings

• It should not be used by people with known hypersensitivity to this drug or to other NSAIDs (including ℞ **aspirin**), who have chronic kidney disease, certain bleeding disorders or conditions (for example, hemophilia, vitamin K deficiency, low blood-platelet levels), or who have a tendency to, or active, peptic ulceration.
• It should be given with caution to people taking certain drugs for gout, with porphyria, with allergic disorders (especially asthma and skin conditions), who are elderly, or with any kind of kidney impairment or with certain liver disorders.
• Mefenamic acid should be used during pregnancy only when medically judged to be needed. In the third trimester, its risk to the fetus rises, and so it should only be used if the benefits outweigh the risks, which are higher at this time.
• Breast-feeding mothers should either discontinue this drug or stop breast-feeding.
• NSAIDs may cause gastrointestinal bleeding, ulceration, or perforation. Any signs of bleeding (for example, black stools) should be reported to a physician immediately.
• If a rash appears, discontinue its use and consult a physician.
• Its side effects (such as dizziness and visual disturbances) may impair the performance of skilled tasks, such as driving.
• Side effects are more frequent in the elderly.
• Gastrointestinal upsets may be minimized by taking the drug with milk or food.
• It is for short-term use only.

Interactions

• There is generally no added benefit in taking other NSAIDs or other ℞ **salicylates** (especially aspirin) at the same time, but there is a higher risk of gastrointestinal upsets and bleeding.
• Alcohol and ℞ **corticosteroids** increase the risk of bleeding, particularly if there is an existing ulcer.
• ℞ **Anticoagulant,** ℞ **antiplatelet,** and ℞ **thrombolytic** drugs may increase bleeding time.
• The effectiveness of ℞ **ACE inhibitors** and ℞ **beta-blockers** may be reduced.
• There is a risk of damaging kidney function if taken with ℞ **diuretics** (for example, ℞ **furosemide**).
• The effects of ℞ **cyclosporine,** ℞ **lithium,** and ℞ **methotrexate** may be exaggerated, with potential for toxicity.

• It should not be used with ℞ **probenecid**.
• Foodstuffs and herbals with ℞ **antiplatelet** properties, for example, ♣ **ginger,** ⚘ **garlic,** and various herbal preparations, may add to the antiplatelet effect of NSAIDs.

Side effects

• Mefenamic acid has weaker anti-inflammatory properties than most drugs of this class and a higher incidence of diarrhea.
• Commonly, diarrhea, gastrointestinal upsets, nausea, vomiting, drowsiness, and dizziness.
• Less frequently, constipation, flatulence, headache, blurred vision, nervousness, fatigue, and sleep disturbances.
• Prolonged bleeding time (with consequent risk of ulceration) is possible with high dosage, and other blood changes can occur, including anemia.
• Hypersensitivity reactions may include symptoms such as facial swelling, hives, rash, chest tightness, asthma, or bronchospasm.
• Reversible kidney failure, particularly in renal impairment, has occurred. Liver damage is rare.

mefloquine ⓖ

Type/Group: **antimalarial; amebicide and antiprotozoal.**
Brand(s): Lariam.
How administered: Orally.

Used to treat

Mefloquine is a (*4-aminoquinoline*) drug used to prevent and treat ✪ **malaria** infection, including uncomplicated falciparum malaria (caused by *Plasmodium falciparum*) and chloroquine-resistant vivax malaria (caused by *Plasmodium vivax*).

Warnings

• It should not be given to people with known hypersensitivity to mefloquine or related compounds.
• It should be given with caution to people with heart rhythm disorders, psychiatric disorders, and myasthenia gravis or other neurological disorders.
• Mefloquine should be used with extreme caution during the first trimester of pregnancy, and after that only if the potential benefits outweigh the possible risk to the fetus.
• It does appear in breast milk and is not recommended for use while nursing.
• Exercise caution when driving or performing other skills requiring alertness, because this drug may cause dizziness.
• It has caused eye damage in animals when given at high doses over an extended period.
• It has been associated with emotional disturbances (confusion, disorientation, hallucinations).
• Halofantrine must not be used along with or following mefloquine, because potentially fatal changes in heart rhythm may occur.

Interactions

• ℞ **Beta-blockers** and ℞ **chloroquine** increase the risk of heart and neurologic side effects.
• ℞ **Anticonvulsants** may reduce the effects of these medications.
• If used with halofantrine, potentially fatal changes in heart rhythm may occur.

• If used with ℞ **quinine** or ℞ **quinidine**, there is an increased risk of severe heart and neurologic side effects.

Side effects

• Frequently, gastrointestinal effects, dizziness, loss of balance, headache, drowsiness, and sleep disorders.
• Occasionally, heart rate changes, ringing in the ears, aches, itching, and rash.
• Rare, but serious effects include blood disorders and seizures.

Mefoxin ®

A preparation of ℞ **cefoxitin**.
Formulation: Injection.
Availability: Prescription only.
Warnings and side effects: See ℞ **cefoxitin**.

Megace ®

A preparation of ℞ **megestrol acetate**.
Formulation: Oral tablets in two strengths; oral suspension (for appetite enhancement).
Availability: Prescription only.
Warnings and side effects: See ℞ **megestrol acetate**.

megestrol acetate ⑥

Type/Group: **sex hormone; progestin; anticancer**.
Brand(s): Megace; generic.
How administered: Orally.

Used to treat

Megestrol acetate can be used for cancer of the uterus (endometrium) and breast. It is also used as a treatment for loss of appetite, emaciation, or unexplained serious weight loss in AIDS patients.

Warnings

• It should not be used by people with known hypersensitivity to this drug.
• It should be given with caution to people with diabetes mellitus or a history of thrombophlebitis.
• Megestrol acetate must not be used during pregnancy, because there is evidence of risk to the fetus. A doctor must be contacted if pregnancy occurs while taking this drug.
• It should not be used by breast-feeding mothers.
• Contraceptive measures are recommended during therapy.
• Diabetic patients should monitor blood glucose carefully.

Interactions

• ℞ **insulin** requirements may be increased in diabetic patients.

Side effects

• Commonly, weight gain due to increased appetite.
• Less frequently, nausea, breakthrough bleeding, backache, headache, breast tenderness, and carpal tunnel syndrome.

Mellaril ®

A preparation of ℞ **thioridazine**.
Formulation: Oral concentrate; tablets; suspension.
Availability: Prescription only.
Warnings and side effects: See ℞ **thioridazine**.

meloxicam ⑥

Type/Group: **anti-inflammatory; antirheumatic; non-narcotic analgesic; NSAID**.
Brand(s): Mobic; various generic.
How administered: Orally.

Used to treat

Meloxicam is used to treat pain and inflammation in ✪ osteoarthritis.

Warnings

• It should not be used by people with known hypersensitivity to this drug or to other NSAIDs (including ℞ **aspirin**), who have chronic kidney disease, certain bleeding disorders or conditions (for example, hemophilia, vitamin K deficiency, low blood-platelet levels), or who have a tendency to, or active, peptic ulceration.
• It should be given with caution to people with peripheral edema, or allergic disorders (especially asthma and skin conditions), who are elderly, or with any kind of kidney impairment, with certain liver disorders, or who are dehydrated.
• Meloxicam should be used when pregnant only if medically judged to be needed. In the third trimester, its risks to the fetus rise, and so it should only be used if the benefits outweigh the risks, which are higher at this time.
• Breast-feeding mothers should either discontinue this drug or stop breast-feeding.
• With regular, long-term use (as in the treatment of osteoarthritis), NSAIDs may cause gastrointestinal bleeding, ulceration, or perforation. Any signs of bleeding (for example, black stools) should be reported to a physician immediately.
• Most NSAIDs have the potential, particularly with regular use, to cause liver damage. Periodic evaluation of liver function is necessary in long-term therapy (more than two months).
• Side effects are more frequent in the elderly.
• Gastrointestinal upsets may be minimized by taking the drug with milk or food.

Interactions

• There is generally no added benefit in taking other NSAIDs (especially ℞ **diflunisal**) or other ℞ **salicylates** (especially aspirin) at the same time, but there is a higher risk of gastrointestinal upsets and bleeding.
• Alcohol and ℞ **corticosteroids** increase the risk of bleeding, particularly if there is an existing ulcer.
• ℞ **Anticoagulants** (for example, ℞ **warfarin sodium**) may increase bleeding time.
• The effectiveness of ℞ **ACE inhibitor** and ℞ **diuretics** may be reduced.
• ℞ **Cholestyramine** may reduce the levels of meloxicam.
• The effects of ℞ **cyclosporine**, ℞ **lithium**, and ℞ **methotrexate** may be exaggerated, with potential for toxicity.

Side effects

These vary in severity and how often they occur, although there is a relatively higher risk of gastric bleeding associated with meloxicam in long-term use at high dosage.
• Commonly, diarrhea, nausea, gastrointestinal upsets, and dehydration.

• Less frequently, vomiting, constipation, flatulence, swelling of the extremities, dizziness, headache, malaise, ringing in the ears, nervousness, fatigue, and insomnia.
• Prolonged bleeding time (with consequent risk of ulceration) is possible with high dosage, and other blood changes can occur, including anemia.
• Hypersensitivity reactions may include symptoms such as facial swelling, hives, rash, chest tightness, asthma, or bronchospasm.
• Reversible kidney failure, particularly in renal impairment, has occurred. Liver damage is rare.

melphalan Ⓖ

Type/Group: **anticancer; cytotoxic**.
Brand(s): Alkeran.
How administered: Injection.

Used to treat

Melphalan is used in the treatment of multiple myeloma and certain ovarian ✪ **cancers**.

Warnings

• It should not be given to people with known hypersensitivity to melphalan, or whose cancer has proven resistant to melphalan.
• It should be given with caution to people with kidney impairment. This is a specialist drug which will be used following a full evaluation by specialist physicians.
• Melphalan is not recommended for use during pregnancy unless it is medically judged to be essential, because it may cause birth defects. Becoming pregnant while using this drug must be avoided.
• It should not be used if breast-feeding.
• It can cause severe bone marrow depression, which may lead to bleeding and a reduced resistance to infection.
• It can impair fertility in men and women (which may be reversible).
• In common with many anticancer drugs, it is associated with the development of secondary malignancies (new cancers).
• A doctor must be contacted if fever, sore throat, signs of local infections, easy bruising, unusual bleeding, excessive tiredness or weakness, blood in urine or stools, or flank pain occur.

Interactions

• ℞ **Cisplatin** and ℞ **nalidixic acid** increase the risk of adverse side effects.
• ℞ **Interferon** alfa may reduce the effects of melphalan.
• The levels of ℞ **carmustine** and ℞ **cyclosporine** may be increased.

Side effects

• Frequently, nausea and vomiting.
• Occasionally, other gastrointestinal effects, rash, itching, and hair loss.

Menest Ⓑ

A preparation of ℞ **estrogens, conjugated**.
Formulation: Injection.
Availability: Prescription only.
Warnings and side effects: See ℞ **estrogens, conjugated**.

Meni-D Capsules Ⓑ

A preparation of ℞ **meclizine hydrochloride**.
Formulation: Oral capsules.
Availability: Prescription only.
Warnings and side effects: See ℞ **meclizine hydrochloride**.

meningococcal polysaccharide vaccine Ⓖ

Type/Group: **vaccine**.
Brand(s): Menomune-A/C/Y/W-135.
How administered: Subcutaneous injection.

Used to treat

Meningococcal polysaccharide vaccine is used for ℞ **immunization** against (but not for treatment of) infection from the organism meningococcus (*Neisseria meningitidis*), which can cause serious illness, such as ✪ **meningitis**. It may be given to those intending to travel "rough" through parts of the world where the risk of meningococcal infection is much higher than in the US (for example, parts of India and much of Africa), or to those groups at higher risk (certain blood or spleen disorders, occupational exposure, or during outbreaks of infection).

Warnings

• It should not be given to people with known hypersensitivity to this vaccine, to thimerosal (contained in the vaccine), or those with acute illness.
• It should be used in pregnancy only when medically judged to be clearly needed.
• Medical judgment is required if breast-feeding is being considered.
• This is a polyvalent vaccine, conferring immune response to meningococci of Groups A, C Y, and W-135, but immunity to Groups A and C decreases more rapidly than to the others. It should not be assumed that immunity lasts for more than three years from the time of vaccination.
• After administration, people will be required to wait for some time to ensure that there is no serious reaction (such as anaphylaxis).

Interactions

• Whole-cell pertussis (in DTWP) or ℞ **typhoid vaccine** may not be well tolerated.
• ℞ **Immunosuppressants** may reduce the effectiveness of the vaccine in conferring immunity. It is recommended to delay vaccination until 3 months after ending immunosuppressant treatment.
• Caution is required if ℞ **anticoagulants** are being taken.

Side effects

• Most of the side effects are mild. There may be swelling, irritation or tenderness at the site of vaccination, and headache, fatigue, malaise, or slight fever.
• Infrequently, skin rash or gastrointestinal disturbances.

Menomune-A/C/Y/W-135 Ⓑ

A preparation of ℞ **meningococcal polysaccharide vaccine**.
Formulation: Subcutaneous injection.
Availability: Prescription only.
Warnings and side effects: See ℞ **meningococcal polysaccharide vaccine**.

Key to symbols: Ⓓ = Drug type/group   Ⓖ = Generic name   Ⓑ = Brand name

menopausal hormone therapy Ⓓ
see ℞ hormone replacement.

menotropins Ⓖ
Type/Group: **sex hormone; gonadotropin; fertility treatment**.
Brand(s): Humegon; Pergonal; Repronex.
How administered: Injection.

Used to treat
"Menotropins" is a collective name for hormone preparations consisting of combinations of the gonadotrophin hormones follicle-stimulating hormone (FSH), and luteinizing hormone (LH) in a ratio of 1:1. In conjunction with human chorionic gonadotropin (HCG), it is used as an infertility treatment in both women and men whose infertility is due to abnormal pituitary gland function. In women, it stimulates ovulation, and in men, it stimulates sperm production. In addition, it is used in superovulation treatment for assisted conception, such as *in vitro* fertilization.

Warnings
• It should not be used by women with primary ovarian failure, abnormal bleeding, thyroid or adrenal dysfunction, organic intracranial lesion, ovarian cysts, or who are pregnant.
• It should not be used by men with primary testicular failure, normal pituitary function, or an infertility disorder other than hypogonadotropic hypogonadism.
• Menotropin should not be used during pregnancy.
• Medical judgment is required if breast-feeding is being considered.
• The risk of multiple births is markedly increased.
• Overstimulation of the ovary may occur. If there is significant ovarian enlargement after ovulation, intercourse must be avoided because of the danger of ruptured ovarian cyst.
• In some cases ovarian hyperstimulation syndrome, a serious medical event, may occur. Early warning signs are severe nausea and vomiting and weight gain. A doctor must be contacted if these develop.

Interactions
No significant interactions have been reported.

Side effects
• Commonly, in women, abdominal pain, bloating, and nausea. Occasionally, shortness of breath, irregular heartbeat, dizziness, loss of appetite, headache, and fainting.
• In men, breast growth.

menthol Ⓖ
Type/Group: **terpene; counter-irritant; local anesthetic**.
Brand(s): Florida Sunburn Relief; Hall's Mentholyptus; Halls-Plus Maximum Strength; Hall's Mentholyptus Sugar Free; Kof-Eze; Robitussin Cough Drops; Robitussion Honey Cough; Robitussin Liquid Center Cough Drops; Nice n Clear; N'Ice Throat Spray; Vicks Cherry Cough Drops; Vicks Extra Strength Cough Drops.
How administered: Topically (external); inhalation.

Used to treat
Menthol is a white, crystalline substance derived from peppermint oil (an essential oil extracted from a plant of the mint family) and is chemically a terpene. It is available in several specific chemical forms, of which levomenthol is one of the preferred isomers. It is commonly used, with or without the volatile substance eucalyptus oil, in inhalations intended to clear the nasal or catarrhal congestion associated with colds, rhinitis (inflammation of the nasal mucous membrane), or sinusitis. It has mild local anesthetic actions, and is included in some counter-irritant, or rubefacient, preparations that are rubbed into the skin to relieve muscle or joint pain.

Warnings
• It should not be given to children under six years as an inhalant, or under two years when used topically.
• A doctor must be consulted before using during pregnancy or while breast-feeding.
• Avoid using on cuts or abraded skin.

Interactions
No significant interactions are known.

Side effects
• Rarely, skin reactions such as itching, rashes, and inflammation.

MenthoRub Ointment Ⓑ
A preparation of ℞ camphor, ℞ menthol, and ℞ thymol.
Formulation: Topical gel.
Availability: OTC.
Warnings and side effects: See ℞ camphor; ℞ menthol; ℞ thymol.

mepenzolate bromide Ⓖ
Type/Group: **anticholinergic; antispasmodic**.
Brand(s): Cantil.
How administered: Orally.

Used to treat
Mepenzolate has been used in combination with other drugs (for example, ℞ phenobarbital) in the treatment of ✪ peptic ulcer. It is not now considered to be nearly as effective as more recent treatments (against *H. pylori* bacteria).

Warnings
• It should not be given to people with known hypersensitivity to anticholinergics, with myasthenia gravis, narrow-angle glaucoma, urinary obstruction, or with any infection or obstructive condition of the gastrointestinal tract.
• It should be given with caution to people with kidney or liver impairment, enlarged prostate, heart disease or high blood pressure, hyperthyroidism, ulcerative colitis, hiatal hernia, glaucoma, brain damage, or Down's syndrome.
• Mepenzolate should be used during pregnancy only when the potential benefit outweighs the possible risk to the fetus.
• It may appear in breast milk and should be avoided by nursing mothers.
• Anticholinergic in general should not be given to anyone with a febrile (feverish) illness or who must work or live in a hot environment.
• The safety of this drug has not been established for children and infants.
• The frequency and severity of side effects is higher in the elderly.
• Because side effects may include drowsiness or visual disturbances, caution is advised in driving and other tasks requiring

alertness or good vision. A doctor must be contacted if any eye pain develops.

Interactions

• The following drugs have some anticholinergic properties and may interact with mepenzolate to increase side effects: ℞ **amantadine**; some ℞ **antiarrhythmic** drugs (for example, ℞ **disopyramide**, ℞ **procainamide**, ℞ **quinidine**); some ℞ **antihistamines** (for example, ℞ **promethazine**, ℞ **carbinoxamine**, ℞ **diphenhydramine hydrochloride**); ℞ **antiparkinsonism** drugs; ℞ **glutethimide**; ℞ **meperidine**; ℞ **phenothiazines**; ℞ **tricyclic** antidepressants.

• The levels of ℞ **digoxin** may rise if taken in its slow-dissolving form, but not as capsules or elixir.

• Anticholinergics and ⚕ **potassium chloride** (in tablet form) should be used together with caution, because the tablet form of potassium chloride may stay in the intestines longer, and so there is a greater risk of irritation and lesions.

• Mepenzolate should be taken at least one hour before an ℞ **antacid**.

• ℞ **Ketoconazole** should be taken at least two hours before an anticholinergic such as mepenzolate.

Side effects

• These may include dry mouth, thirst, blurred vision and other visual disturbances, urinary hesitancy, palpitations, and constipation.

• Uncommon effects may include increased intraocular pressure (pressure in the eyeball), headache, unusual or absent taste sensation, nervousness, drowsiness, flushing, and nausea.

• Although rare, hives, other skin eruptions, and anaphylaxis may occur in extreme allergic reactions.

Mepergan ℬ

A preparation of ℞ **meperidine hydrochloride** and ℞ **promethazine hydrochloride**.

Formulation: Oral capsules; injection.

Availability: Prescription only.

Warnings and side effects: See ℞ **meperidine hydrochloride**; ℞ **promethazine hydrochloride**.

meperidine hydrochloride ⑥

(pethidine hydrochloride)

Type/Group: narcotic analgesic; opioid.

Brand(s): Demerol; various generic. Combinations: With *promethazine hydrochloride*: Mepergan. With *atropine sulfate*: various generic.

How administered: Orally; injection.

Used to treat

Meperidine is used primarily for the relief of moderate to severe ✪ **pain**, especially during labor and operations. It is less effective than ℞ **morphine** and not suitable for relieving severe, chronic pain. Its effect is rapid and short-lasting, so its sedative properties are made use of only as a premedication prior to surgery, or to enhance the effects of anesthetic drugs during or following surgery.

Warnings

• It should not be taken by people with known hypersensitivity to this drug, or at the same time as or within 14 days of ℞ **MAOI** antidepressants. Opioids (even the weaker ones) should not be taken by people with asthma, anyone with seriously depressed breathing disorders, prostatic hypertrophy, convulsive disorders, raised intracranial pressure, a head injury, or with severe kidney damage.

• Depending on use and dose, they should be taken with caution by the elderly, or anyone with hypotension, porphyria, certain liver, kidney or adrenal disorders, urethral stricture, hypothyroidism (under-activity of the thyroid gland), alcoholism, or a history of drug abuse.

• Meperidine should be used during pregnancy (except during labor and delivery) only if the potential benefits outweigh the possible risks. Withdrawal symptoms and respiratory depression have been observed in newborns.

• Medical judgment is required if breast-feeding is being considered. It appears in high concentrations in breast milk.

• ℞ **MAOI** antidepressants have caused severe, even fatal reactions. Meperidine should not be administered within 14 days after discontinuing MAOI treatment.

• Meperidine is a Schedule II controlled substance.

• Prolonged use of narcotics can lead to physical dependence (addiction), although this rarely happens in routine medical use.

• Drowsiness may affect the performance of skilled tasks such as driving.

• The effects of alcohol may be enhanced (including a higher risk of respiratory depression).

Interactions

• Most protease inhibitors (for example, ℞ **nelfinavir**, ℞ **saquinavir**) should be used with caution with meperidine, except ℞ **ritonavir**, which must never be used at the same time.

• If used with ℞ **furazolidone**, ℞ **chlorpromazine**, or ℞ **thioridazine**, there is a far greater risk of significant side effects.

• If the following drugs are used with meperidine, then effects may be increased: ℞ **barbiturates**; ℞ **general anesthetics**; ℞ **MAOIs**; ℞ **opioids**; ℞ **tranquilizers** (for example, ℞ **phenothiazines**); ℞ **sedatives**; ℞ **benzodiazepines** (for example, ℞ **diazepam**, ℞ **lorazepam**); ℞ **tricyclic** antidepressants; alcohol.

• ℞ **hydantoin** analogs (for example, ℞ **phenytoin**, ℞ **mephenytoin**) decrease the effects of meperidine.

Side effects

• These depend on the dose, use, and how it is administered. Compared to many opioids, it is less likely to cause constipation and there is less depression of respiration in the newborn when used to relieve pain during labor. Overdose can cause convulsions. There may be sedation, dizziness, vomiting, nausea, and sweating. There is occasionally euphoria, which may lead to a state of mental detachment or confusion. Also, there may be headache, palpitations, changes in heart rate, postural hypotension (a lowering of blood pressure on standing, causing dizziness), constipation, urinary retention, rashes, miosis (pupil constriction), dry mouth, flushing of the face, loss of appetite, mood change, and hallucinations.

mephenytoin ⓖ

Type/Group: **anticonvulsant; antiepileptic.**
Brand(s): Mesantoin.
How administered: Orally.

Used to treat

Mephenytoin is one of the chemical group of hydantoins used to treat most forms of ✪ epilepsy (except absence seizures), but its use is generally confined to conditions that are not successfully managed with less toxic anticonvulsants (such as ℞ phenobarbital, ℞ phenytoin, and ℞ primidone).

Warnings

• Avoid its use in people with known hypersensitivity to this drug.
• Avoid its use in anyone with porphyria.
• Medical judgment is required if someone has liver impairment.
• This drug is associated with an increase in frequency of certain birth defects and should not be used during pregnancy. However, because uncontrolled seizures can also threaten fetal health, medical judgment is needed to weigh potential benefits and risks.
• Breast-feeding mothers should either discontinue using this drug or stop breast-feeding.
• Discontinue using and seek medical advice if a skin rash appears.
• Mephenytoin may raise blood glucose levels, and so caution is advised for diabetics.
• Withdrawal should be gradual otherwise it may precipitate attacks.

Interactions

• ℞ tricyclic antidepressants may precipitate seizures.
• The following drugs may intensify the effects of mephenytoin, and so there is a higher risk of side effects: ℞ **amiodarone hydrochloride**; ℞ **chloramphenicol**; ℞ **chlordiazepoxide**; ℞ **diazepam**; ℞ **dicumarol**; disulfiram; ℞ **estrogens**; ℞ **fluoxetine**; ℞ **H₂-antagonists**; halothane; ℞ **isoniazid**; ℞ **methylphenidate**; ℞ **phenothiazines**, phenylbutazone, ℞ **salicylates**, succinimides (for example, ℞ **ethosuximide**, ℞ **methsuximide**), ℞ **sulfonamides**; ℞ **tolbutamide**; ℞ **trazodone**.
• Mephenytoin may increase the effects of ℞ **lithium** and ℞ **primidone**, with potentially toxic results.
• If taken with ℞ **clonazepam**, ℞ **phenobarbital**, ℞ **sodium valproate**, or ℞ **valproic acid**, the effects are unpredictable.
• Alcohol may either raise or lower levels of mephenytoin, depending on a person's drinking habits.
• The therapeutic effect of the following drugs may be reduced: ℞ **acetaminophen**; ℞ **corticosteroids**; coumarin ℞ **anticoagulants**; ℞ **digitoxin**; ℞ **dopamine**; ℞ **doxycycline**; ℞ **estrogens**; ℞ **furosemide**; oral ℞ **contraceptives**; ℞ **quinidine**; ℞ **rifampin**; ℞ **theophylline**; ℞ **calcitriol** (vitamin D).
• ℞ **Carbamazepine**, ℞ **reserpine**, and ℞ **sucralfate** lower levels of mephenytoin.

Side effects

These vary widely and tend to occur frequently. They include:
• Drowsiness, eye-flicker, and movement disorders;
• Slurred speech, confusion, headache, fatigue, depression, and tremor;
• Rarely, peripheral nerve disorders, rashes, acne, enlargement of the gums, growth of excess hair and blood disorders;
• Nausea, vomiting, nervousness, dizziness, and insomnia may occur when first taking the drug, but tend to disappear;
• Hypersensitivity reactions (swollen lymph glands, fever, aches, rash) and systemic lupus erythematosus have occurred;
• Although mephenytoin may cause less gastrointestinal disturbance, gum inflammation or movement abnormality than phenytoin, frequency of serious blood effects is higher.

mephobarbital ⓖ

Type/Group: **sedatives; anticonvulsant; antiepileptic; barbiturate; antianxiety.**
Brand(s): Mebaral.
How administered: Orally; injection.

Used to treat

Mephobarbital is used for the relief of ✪ anxiety, tension, and apprehension, and also as an anticonvulsant in the treatment of ✪ epilepsy.

Warnings

• It should not be given to people with known hypersensitivity to barbiturates, with respiratory depression, severe liver impairment, or porphyria.
• It should be given with caution to people with anemia, addiction to barbiturates, liver disease, myasthenia gravis, chronic obstructive pulmonary disease (COPD), emphysema, thyroid conditions, kidney disease, high blood pressure, acute or chronic pain, mental depression, a history of drug abuse, or anyone over 65.
• Mephobarbital should not be used during pregnancy if possible. A doctor must be consulted if pregnancy occurs while using this drug.
• Medical judgment is required if breast-feeding is being considered.
• There is a high risk of dependence (addiction) and abuse.
• It loses some of effectiveness for treating insomnia after about two weeks.
• Avoid driving or other activities requiring alertness.
• Do not drink alcohol.
• Treatment must not be stopped abruptly after long-term use.
• It is very dangerous in overdose and tests will regularly be carried out.
• A doctor must be consulted if fever, sore throat, bruising, or mouth sores develop.

Interactions

• The response to oral ℞ **anticoagulants** (for example ℞ **warfarin sodium**) is decreased.
• If used with ℞ **acetaminophen**, there is an increased risk of toxic effects on the liver.
• The levels and therapeutic effects of the following drugs may be reduced: ℞ **antidepressants**; ℞ **beta-blockers**; ℞ **calcium-channel blockers**; ℞ **corticosteroids**; ℞ **cyclosporine**; ℞ **digitoxin**; ℞ **disopyramide**; ℞ **doxycycline**; ℞ **estrogens**; ℞ **griseofulvin**; ℞ **oral contraceptives**; ℞ **propafenone**; ℞ **quinidine**; ℞ **tacrolimus**; ℞ **theophylline**.

• ℞ **MAOI** antidepressants prolong the effects of barbiturates.

• If used with an ℞ **antipsychotic**, the effects of both drugs are reduced.

• If used with ℞ **chloramphenicol**, barbiturate levels are increased, while the levels of chloramphenicol are reduced.

• If used with methoxyflurane, adverse effects on the kidneys are increased.

• The effects of ℞ **narcotic analgesics** may be altered, with increased central nervous system (CNS) depression.

• ℞ **Valproic acid** increases levels of barbiturates.

• If used with alcohol, there can be excessive central nervous system (CNS) depression.

Side effects

• Depending on how it is administered, dose, and use, there may be hangover with drowsiness, lack of energy, or rash.

• Less frequently, central nervous system depression, dizziness, headache, lightheadedness, mental depression, physical dependence, slurred speech, excitement in children and those over 65, vertigo, slowed heartbeat, lowered blood pressure, gastrointestinal upset, and hives.

• Rare but serious side effects include blood cell disorders, breathing stoppages, respiratory depression, spasms of the bronchi or larynx, Stevens-Johnson syndrome (a severe skin disorder), and angioedema.

Mephyton ®

A preparation of ℞ **phytonadione**.

Formulation: Oral tablets.

Availability: Prescription only.

Warnings and side effects: See ℞ **phytonadione**.

mepivacaine hydrochloride ©

Type/Group: **local anesthetic**.

Brand(s): Carbocaine; Isocaine; Polocaine; various generic.

How administered: Local injection.

Used to treat

Mepivacaine is used particularly for nerve block and infiltration during labor and delivery, and in dental procedures.

Warnings

• It should not be given to people with known hypersensitivity to mepivacaine, or those rare patients with methemoglobinemia (a serious blood disorder). It is a specialist drug and there will be a full medical assessment.

• It should be used during pregnancy only when it is clearly needed.

• Medical judgment is required if breast-feeding is being considered.

• It can cause cardiac depression, peripheral vasodilatation, or CNS (central nervous system) toxicity.

Interactions

• There is a risk of additive toxicity with ℞ **antiarrhythmics** (for example, ℞ **tocainide**, ℞ **mexiletine**).

• ℞ **Sedatives** may cause increased CNS effects.

Side effects

• Occasionally, pain at injection site, burning, stinging, or tenderness where applied.

• Rarely (generally with high dose), drowsiness, dizziness, disorientation, lightheadedness, tremors, apprehension, euphoria, sensation of heat, cold, or numbness, blurred or double vision, ringing or roaring in ears, nausea, or allergic reactions.

meprobamate ©

Type/Group: **antianxiety; hypnotic; antianxiety**.

Brand(s): Equanil; Miltown; Neuramate; various generic.

How administered: Orally.

Used to treat

Meprobamate is sometimes used in the short-term treatment of ✪ **anxiety**. It is potentially more hazardous than the ℞ **benzodiazepines** in overdose.

Warnings

• It should not be given to people with known hypersensitivity to the drug, with porphyria, or certain lung and breathing disorders.

• It should be given with caution to people with respiratory difficulties, epilepsy, impaired liver or kidney function, a history drug or alcohol abuse, or anyone over 65.

• Meprobamate should almost always not be used during pregnancy. A doctor must be contacted if pregnancy occurs while taking this drug.

• It should not be used by nursing mothers.

• Physical and psychological dependence may occur.

• It may impair the performance of skilled tasks such as driving.

• Avoid alcohol.

• Treatment must not be stopped abruptly after long-term use.

Interactions

• If used with CNS (central nervous system) depressants (for example, ℞ **barbiturates**, ℞ **narcotic analgesics**, alcohol), increased effects will occur.

Side effects

Drowsiness, dizziness, slurred speech, gastrointestinal disturbances, changes in heart rhythm, low blood pressure, tingling in the extremities, weakness, headache, and disturbances of vision. Rare but serious side effects include seizures, irregular heart rhythm, cessation of urination, blood disorders, spasm of the bronchi, and severe skin and blood cell disorders.

mercaptopurine ©

Type/Group: **anticancer; cytotoxic**.

Brand(s): Purinethol.

How administered: Orally.

Used to treat

Mercaptopurine is a cytotoxic drug (an antimetabolite) that is used as a treatment of acute ✪ **leukemias**. It works by preventing cell replication.

Warnings

• It should not be given to people with known hypersensitivity or resistance to this drug.

• It should be given with caution to people with impaired kidney function. This is a specialist drug which will be used following a full evaluation by specialist physicians.

• Mercaptopurine is not recommended for use during pregnancy unless it is medically judged to be essential, because it may cause birth defects. Becoming pregnant while using this drug must be avoided.

• It should not be used if breast-feeding.

• It can cause bone marrow depression, which may lead to bleeding and a reduced resistance to infection.

• It may have toxic effects on the liver.

• In common with many anticancer drugs, this drug causes chromosomal changes and may cause cancer.

• A doctor must be contacted if symptoms of infection or bleeding, yellow discoloration of skin or eyes, abdominal, flank or joint pain, swelling of the feet or legs, or excessive tiredness or weakness occur.

Interactions

• Ṟ **Allopurinol**, Ṟ **trimethoprim (TMP)**, and Ṟ **sulfamethoxazole** may increase the likelihood of severe adverse effects.

Side effects

• Gastrointestinal disturbances, darkening of the skin, diarrhea, headache, skin rash, itching, weakness, and decreased appetite.

Meridia ®

A preparation of Ṟ **sibutramine**.
Formulation: Oral capsules.
Availability: Prescription only.
Warnings and side effects: See Ṟ **sibutramine**.

meropenem ⓖ

Type/Group: antibacterial; beta-lactam; antibiotic.
Brand(s): Merrem IV.
How administered: Injection.

Used to treat

Meropenem is a new sort of beta-lactam (a carbapenem) with a broad-spectrum of activity against many Gram-positive and Gram-negative bacteria. Unlike the earlier similar drug Ṟ **imipenem**, it is not degraded by an enzyme in the kidney. It can be used to treat ⊙ **bacterial infections**, including ⊙ **peritonitis**, appendicitis, ⊙ **meningitis**, and intra-abdominal infections.

Warnings

• It should not be given to people with known hypersensitivity to meropenem or other beta-lactams.

• It should be given with caution to people with allergies to penicillins, cephalosporins, or other substances, and those with kidney function impairment or CNS (central nervous system) disorders.

• Meropenem's safety in pregnancy has not been established. It should be used only if the benefits outweigh the possible risk to the fetus.

• Medical judgment is required if breast-feeding is being considered. It is unknown whether it appears in breast milk.

• Rarely, seizures may occur in susceptible people (for example, those with brain lesions or impaired kidney function).

• Superinfections due to the altered bacterial balance caused by antibiotic treatment may occur. A doctor must be contacted if severe abdominal pain, or moderate to severe diarrhea occur.

Interactions

• Ṟ **Probenecid** inhibits the metabolism of meropenem and the two should not be used at the same time.

Side effects

• Frequently, diarrhea, nausea, vomiting, headache, and inflammation at injection site.

• Occasionally, oral thrush, rash, and itching.

• Rarely, constipation or sore tongue.

Merrem IV ®

A preparation of Ṟ **meropenem**.
Formulation: Injection.
Availability: Prescription only.
Warnings and side effects: See Ṟ **meropenem**.

Meruvax II ®

A preparation of Ṟ **rubella vaccine, live**.
Formulation: Subcutaneous injection.
Availability: Prescription only.
Warnings and side effects: See Ṟ **rubella vaccine, live**.

mesalamine ⓖ

(mesalazine; 5-aminosalicylic acid; 5-ASA)
Type/Group: **aminosalicylate; anti-inflammatory**.
Brand(s): Asacol; Pentasa; Rowasa.
How administered: Orally; topically (rectal suppository or suspension).

Used to treat

Mesalamine can be used in the treatment of chronic inflammatory bowel disease (such as ⊙ **ulcerative colitis**), also proctitis and proctosigmoiditis, as an alternative to Ṟ **sulfasalazine**. It is formed in the body when sulfasalazine is taken orally (it is split into mesalamine and sulfapyridine), but some people have an adverse hypersensitivity to sulfapyridine (which as a member of the Ṟ **sulfonamide** group).

Warnings

• It should not be given to people with known hypersensitivity to mesalamine or to any Ṟ **salicylate** (especially sulfasalazine).

• It should be given with caution to people with kidney impairment.

• Mesalamine should not be used during pregnancy.

• Medical judgment is required if breast-feeding is being considered. It is known that this drug appears in breast milk and its effects have not been studied.

• A doctor must be contacted if unexplained bruising, bleeding, sore throat, fever or malaise occur, as these could be symptoms of blood changes that would require treatment to be stopped.

• Kidney function should be monitored.

• Although rare, serious complications such as pericarditis and acute pancreatitis have been associated with mesalamine.

Interactions

• The levels of Ṟ **digoxin** and Ṟ **folic acid** may be reduced.

Side effects

These vary somewhat depending on how it is administered:

• Commonly, gastrointestinal disturbances (abdominal discomfort, belching, nausea, and so on) headache, fever, malaise, and dizziness.

• Less frequently, flu-like feeling, rash, joint pain, hair loss and blood, liver and kidney abnormalities.

• Occasionally, mesalamine has made colitis worse, apparently in those with hypersensitivity to the drug. Acute abdominal pain, cramping, and bloody diarrhea are signs the drug should be immediately discontinued.

mesalazine ⑥

see ℞ **mesalamine**.

Mesantoin ⑧

A preparation of ℞ **mephenytoin**.
Formulation: Oral tablets.
Availability: Prescription only.
Warnings and side effects: See ℞ **mephenytoin**.

Mescolor Tablets ⑧

A preparation of methscopolamine nitrate, ℞ **chlorpheniramine maleate**, and ℞ **pseudoephedrine**.
Formulation: Oral tablets.
Availability: Prescription only.
Warnings and side effects: See ℞ **scopolamine hydrobromide**; ℞ **chlorpheniramine maleate**; ℞ **pseudoephedrine**.

mesna ⑥

Type/Group: **cytoprotectant**.
Brand(s): Mesnex.
How administered: Intravenous injection.

Used to treat

Mesna is a synthetic drug which combats hemorrhagic ⊙ **cystitis** that is a toxic complication caused by ℞ **cytotoxic** drugs (for example, ℞ **ifosfamide**). It works by reacting with a toxic metabolite (a breakdown product called acrolein) produced by the cytotoxic drugs and which is the cause of the hemorrhagic cystitis. Mesna is therefore used as an adjunct in the treatment of certain forms of cancer.

Warnings

• It should not be given to people with known hypersensitivity to this drug (or to thiol compounds), or who are hypotensive or dehydrated.

• The effects of mesna in pregnancy are not known and so it should be used only if the potential benefit outweighs the possible risk to the fetus.

• Medical judgment is required if breast-feeding is being considered.

• Pretreatment with an ℞ **antihistamine** or ℞ **corticosteroid**, or both, is advised for persons with autoimmune disorders, as they experience hypersensitivity (which may include anaphylactic reactions) to mesna more frequently.

Interactions

No interactions of significance are known.

Side effects

• These may include a bad taste in the mouth (very frequent), soft stools or diarrhea, limb pain, headache, fatigue, nausea, hypotension and allergic reactions (for example, itching, hives, facial swelling).

Mesnex ⑧

A preparation of ℞ **mesna**.
Formulation: Injection.
Availability: Prescription only.
Warnings and side effects: See ℞ **mesna**.

mesoridazine ⑥

Type/Group: **antipsychotic; phenothiazine**.
Brand(s): Serentil.
How administered: Orally; injection.

Used to treat

Mesoridazine is a member of the phenothiazines and has more of a sedative effect, which makes it a useful treatment for ⊙ **schizophrenia** and behavioral problems associated with mental deficiency and chronic brain syndrome. It can also be used as an additional treatment for ⊙ **alcoholism**, also for personality disorders, and for ⊙ **anxiety** and tension associated with neuroses.

Warnings

• It should not be given to people with known hypersensitivity to this drug or with severe CNS (central nervous system) depression or coma.

• It should be given with caution to people with severe cardiovascular disorders, epilepsy, liver or kidney disease, glaucoma, prostatic hypertrophy, low calcium levels, chronic obstructive pulmonary disease (COPD), or anyone over 65.

• Mesoridazine should be used during pregnancy only if the benefits outweigh the possible risks to the fetus.

• Medical judgment is required if breast-feeding is being considered.

• It may cause drowsiness and so the performance of skilled tasks, such as driving, may be impaired.

• It may cause postural hypotension (lowered blood pressure on standing), so rise slowly from a reclining position. Older individuals in particular should exercise caution.

• Avoid alcohol consumption.

• It may cause sensitivity to sunlight (photosensitivity), so minimize exposure (use a sunscreen, sunglasses and so on).

• Treatment should be stopped gradually.

• If used for a long time, tardive dyskinesia (see ℞ **antipsychotics**) occasionally develops.

Interactions

• Mesoridazine may inhibit the ℞ **antiparkinsonism** effect of ℞ **levodopa**.

• The levels of some ℞ **antidepressants** may be increased.

• ℞ **Antimalarials** may cause the levels of antipsychotics to increase.

• If used with ℞ **bromocriptine** or ℞ **lithium**, the effects of both drugs are reduced.

• ℞ **Anticholinergics**, ℞ **barbiturates**, ℞ **narcotic analgesics**, and ℞ **orphenadrine** lower the levels of antipsychotics and/or increase the occurrence of anticholinergic and/or CNS (central nervous system) effects.

• Mesoridazine may interfere with response to ℞ **clonidine hydrochloride**, ℞ **guanadrel**, and ℞ **guanethidine monosulfate**.

• Antipsychotics may change the response to ℞ **epinephrine**.

• If an antipsychotic is taken with alcohol, there may be increased sedative effects.

Side effects

• These depend on how it is administered and use. There may be drowsiness, headache, loss of appetite, constipation, dry mouth, and nausea.

• Less frequently, extrapyramidal symptoms (see ℞ **antipsychotics**), anxiety, agitation, confusion, euphoria, worsening of psychotic symptoms, heat or cold intolerance, insomnia, lethargy, restlessness, ECG changes, blood pressure changes, speeded heart rate, eye changes, indigestion, increased saliva, priapism (prolonged, painful penile erection), sexual dysfunction, urinary retention, breast changes, anemia, changes in blood sugar levels, high cholesterol, low blood sodium levels, impotence, increased libido, menstrual irregularities, respiratory depression, spasm of the larynx, increased sweating loss of hair, and skin reactions.

• Rare but serious side effects include white blood cell disorders, spasm of the bronchi, neuroleptic malignant syndrome (a potentially fatal condition characterized by very high fever, muscle rigidity, changes in mental status, and irregular pulse, blood pressure and/or heart rhythm), and seizure.

Mestinon ®

A preparation of ℞ **pyridostigmine bromide**.
Formulation: Oral tablets, sustained release tablets, syrup.
Availability: Prescription only.
Warnings and side effects: See ℞ **pyridostigmine bromide**.

mestranol ©

Type/Group: **estrogen; oral contraceptive**.
Brand(s): Combinations: With *norethindrone*: Necon 1/50; Nelova 1/50M; Norcept-E; Norethin; Norinyl 1 + 50; Ortho-Novum 1/50.
How administered: Orally.

Used to treat

Mestranol is a synthetic estrogen that is a constituent in several combined oral contraceptives and is also used in ℞ **hormone replacement**.

Warnings

• It should not be given to people with breast cancer, active thromboembolic disease, known or suspected estrogen-dependent cancers, or undiagnosed abnormal genital bleeding.

• It should be given with caution to people with hypertension, gallbladder disease, congestive heart failure, diabetes mellitus, depression, migraine headache, seizure disorders, liver disease, a family history of breast or endometrial cancer, a history of

thromboembolic disorders, uterine fibroids, hypertriglyceridemia, or hypercalcemia.

• It should not be used during pregnancy. A doctor must be contacted if pregnancy occurs while using this drug.

• Medical judgment is required if breast-feeding is being considered. It may reduce the quality and quantity of breast milk.

• The use of oral contraceptives is associated with a risk of serious cardiovascular side effects (for example, embolism, stroke, heart attack), particularly in those over age 35. Cigarette smoking increases the risk. This added risk gets larger with age and with heavy smoking (>15 per day), and is quite marked in women over 35.

• Benign liver tumors, increased risk of gallbladder disease, and elevated blood pressure have been associated with oral contraceptive use.

Interactions

• ℞ **Rifampin** and ℞ **barbiturates** reduce the effects of estrogen.

• The steroid effect of ℞ **corticosteroids** is increased.

• If used with ℞ **phenytoin**, there is a loss of seizure control and levels of estrogen are reduced.

• If used with ℞ **warfarin sodium** and similar anticoagulants, there is a theoretical increase in the risk of thromboembolism.

Side effects

• Nausea and vomiting, breakthrough bleeding, and spotting.

• Less frequently, depression, migraine headache, increased emotionality, elevated blood pressure, venous thrombosis, edema, contact lens intolerance, gallbladder disease, bloating, benign liver tumors, cessation of menses, change in cervical secretions, breast enlargement, breast tenderness, elevated blood glucose, elevated triglyceride or calcium levels, darkening of the skin of the face, changes in libido, and weight gain.

• Rarely, endometrial cancer.

metabolic disorder treatment ⓓ

Generics: **imiglucerase; levocarnitine; penicillamine**.

Used to treat

Metabolic disorder treatment drugs or dietary supplements are used to correct defects in the body's metabolism, some of them due to inborn errors of metabolism which are caused by an inherited defective enzyme. Some of these drugs are ℞ **chelating agent** chemicals that work by chemically binding to certain metallic ions and other substances, making them less toxic and allowing their excretion (for example, of copper in ❂ **Wilson's disease**, for which ℞ **penicillamine** is used).

In many of the known cases of inborn errors of metabolism, such enzyme deficiencies may lead to a shortage in the body of an amino acid (for example, carnitine deficiency; treated with a dietary supplement of carnitine as ℞ **levocarnitine**), or of high levels of a precursor, for example, ❂ **phenylketonuria** where failure of conversion of phenylalanine into tyrosine leads to a build up of excess of the former which causes the disorder; treated by a special diet containing low levels of phenylalanine.

Commonly, an error of metabolism leads to production of an enzyme which functions abnormally. ℞ **Sodium phenylbutyrate** is a soluble salt of the amino acid phenylbutyric acid, and is used as a treatment for urea cycle disturbances due to specific enzyme deficiencies that cause a buildup of ammonia in the body. Ideally, a replacement form of a deficient enzyme is required, and ℞ **imiglucerase** is an ℞ **enzyme** drug made by recombinant DNA technology which is used as a replacement in the specialist treatment of Type 1 Gaucher's disease (a genetically determined enzyme deficiency disease affecting the spleen, liver, bone marrow, and lymph nodes).

Limitations

Our increasing knowledge of the human genome, and the production of proteins that it controls, is beginning to highlight just how many diseases are due to a fault, often genetic in origin, in the enzyme proteins. Ideally, these deficiencies would be rectified by administration of the missing ℞ **enzyme** as a drug, and in the future by correcting the deficient gene. However, there are a number of difficulties in using enzymes in medicine. A major one is that enzymes must normally be given by injection because they are proteins and so are broken down by digestive enzymes in the stomach or intestine. Another difficulty in the past was in isolating an enzyme from plant or animal tissues, but now enzymes can be made by recombinant DNA technology, which is the case with imiglucerase. However, the cost of such drugs is likely to be great. See also the individual drug entries.

Metahydrin ℞

A preparation of ℞ **trichlormethiazide**.
Formulation: Oral tablets.
Availability: Prescription only.
Warnings and side effects: See ℞ **trichlormethiazide**. Contains tartrazine (FD&C yellow No. 5), a dye that may cause allergic reaction in a few people, but especially those with sensitivity to aspirin.

Metamucil Original; Orange; Sugar Free; Wafers ℞

A preparation of ℞ **psyllium**.
Formulation: Oral powder (available as original or smooth texture); oral wafers.
Availability: OTC.
Warnings and side effects: See ℞ **psyllium**. Sugar Free powders contain the sweetener aspartame, which should be avoided by individuals with phenylketonuria.

metaproterenol ℗

(orciprenaline sulfate)
Type/Group: **beta-adrenergic stimulant; sympathomimetic; bronchodilator; antiasthmatic**.
Brand(s): Alupent; Metaprel; various generic.
How administered: Orally; inhalant.

Used to treat

Metaproterenol has some beta$_2$-receptor selectivity (though is less selective than ℞ **albuterol** and because of this is therefore more likely to cause side effects). It is mainly used to treat bronchial ✪ **asthma** and reversible bronchospasm associated with ✪ **bronchitis** and ✪ **emphysema**.

Warnings

• It should not be taken by people with known hypersensitivity to this drug, or who have pre-existing heart dysrhythmias associated with speeded heartbeat.
• It should be taken with caution by people with ischemic heart disease, other heart dysrhythmias, hypertension, hyperthyroidism, and diabetes mellitus.
• It should be used during pregnancy only if medically judged to be clearly needed.
• Medical judgment is required if breast-feeding is being considered. It is not known if it appears in breast milk.
• Rarely, it may have adverse effects on heart and blood pressure, or may lead to paradoxical bronchoconstriction.

Interactions

• ℞ **Beta-blockers** decrease the effects of metaproterenol.
• If used with ℞ **furosemide**, there is a risk of enhancing furosemide's potassium-lowering effect.

Side effects

• Frequently, tremors, speeded heartbeat, shakiness, nervousness, nausea, vomiting, and dry mouth.
• Occasionally, palpitations, dizziness, weakness, headache, gastrointestinal distress, cough, and dry throat.
• Rarely, changes in blood pressure, drowsiness, and unusual taste.

metaraminol ℗

Type/Group: **alpha-adrenergic stimulant; sympathomimetic; vasoconstrictor**.
Brand(s): Aramine.
How administered: Injection, infusion.

Used to treat

Metaraminol is used primarily to treat cases of acute ✪ **hypotension**, particularly in emergency situations (for example, bleeding, allergic drug reactions, brain injury, surgical complications), and during the administration of spinal anesthetics.

Warnings

• It should not be given to people with known hypersensitivity to this drug (or to sulfites, present in this preparation).
• It should be given with caution to people with heart or artery disease, hyperthyroidism, diabetes mellitus, cirrhosis of the liver, or low blood volume. It is a specialist hospital drug, and a full assessment for suitability will be carried out.
• Metaraminol should be used during pregnancy only if it is clearly needed.
• Medical judgment is required if breast-feeding is being considered.
• This is a powerful drug and is used only under hospital conditions, with continuous monitoring of heart function, blood pressure, and other vital signs.

Interactions

• Halogenated ℞ **general anesthetics** (for example, halothane) or cyclopropane have the potential for serious adverse effects on heart rhythm. Generally they should not be used together with metaraminol.
• There is a risk of arrhythmias if taken with ℞ **digoxin**.

• ℞ **Ergot alkaloids** (for example, ℞ **ergonovine**, ℞ **ergotamine**), ℞ **guanethidine monosulfate**, ℞ **MAOIs**, ℞ **oxytocin**, other sympathomimetics, and ℞ **tricyclics** may intensify the effects of metaraminol, with the potential for serious adverse reactions.

• The effects of ℞ **reserpine** may be unpredictable.

• ℞ **Alpha-adrenergic blockers**, ℞ **beta-blockers**, and ℞ **diuretics** may decrease the therapeutic effects of metaraminol.

• ℞ **Atropine sulfate** enhances some effects of metaraminol, while blocking its tendency to produce slowed heartbeat. This is a usually beneficial interaction.

Side effects

• There may be excessive rise in blood pressure, palpitations, nervousness, dizziness, sweating, pallor, breathlessness, headache (often severe), nausea or vomiting.

• Rarely, abscess or tissue death may occur at the site of injection.

metformin Ⓖ

Type/Group: **antidiabetic; oral hypoglycemic; biguanide**.
Brand(s): Glucophage.
How administered: Orally.

Used to treat

Metformin hydrochloride is a non-sulfonylurea (it is a biguanide) used in the treatment of type 2 ✪ **diabetes mellitus** (non-insulin-dependent diabetes mellitus; NIDDM). It is thought to involve an effect on glucose uptake by skeletal muscle, glucose absorption, and production.

Warnings

• It should not be given to people with a history of lactic acidosis, conditions associated with hypoxemia, hypersensitivity to metformin, kidney disease or dysfunction, abnormal creatinine clearance, or acute or chronic metabolic acidosis, including diabetic ketoacidosis.

• It should be given with caution to people with uncontrolled thyroid disease, heart disease, liver impairment, decreased kidney function, congestive heart failure, chronic respiratory difficulty, who are over 65, taking drugs that affect kidney function, and children.

• Its safety in pregnancy is not established. It should be used only if clearly needed.

• It is not recommended for use while breast-feeding.

• Lactic acidosis occurs rarely, but is a serious, often fatal complication. A doctor must be contacted and use of the drug stopped if unexplained hyperventilation, muscle aches, extreme tiredness, or unusual sleepiness develop.

• Avoid excess alcohol.

Interactions

• ℞ **cimetidine** increases levels of metformin.

• ℞ **MAOIs** increase the possibility of hypoglycemia.

Side effects

• Frequently, gastrointestinal disturbances (which usually disappear).

• Occasionally, unpleasant taste, skin irritation, rash, and impaired vitamin B_{12} absorption.

methadone hydrochloride

Type/Group: **narcotic analgesic; opioid**.
Brand(s): Dolophine; various generic.
How administered: Orally; injection.

Used to treat

Methadone is used primarily for the relief of severe ✪ **pain**. It is less effective and less sedative than ℞ **morphine** but acts for a longer time. It is used in an oral preparation as a substitute for more powerful addictive opioids (for example, heroin) in detoxification therapy.

Warnings

• It should not be taken by people with known hypersensitivity to this drug. Opioids (even the weaker ones) should not be taken by people with asthma, anyone with seriously depressed breathing disorders, prostatic hypertrophy, convulsive disorders, raised intracranial pressure, or a head injury.

• Depending on use and dose, it should be taken with caution by the elderly, or anyone with hypotension, porphyria, certain liver, kidney or adrenal disorders, urethral stricture, hypothyroidism (under-activity of the thyroid gland), or alcoholism.

• It should be used during pregnancy only if the benefits outweigh the potential risks. Withdrawal symptoms have been observed in newborns.

• Methadone appears in high concentration in breast milk, with an addictive effect in newborns.

• Methadone is a Schedule II controlled substance.

• Use of methadone in detoxification or maintenance is regulated by US law.

• Withdrawal effects of methadone may persist for six to seven weeks.

• Drowsiness may affect the performance of skilled tasks such as driving.

• The effects of alcohol may be enhanced (including a higher risk of respiratory depression).

Interactions

• If the following drugs are used with methadone, then effects may be increased: ℞ **barbiturates**; ℞ **general anesthetics**; ℞ **opioids**; ℞ **tranquilizers** (for example, ℞ **phenothiazines**); protease inhibitors (for example, ℞ **nelfinavir**, ℞ **ritonavir**, ℞ **saquinavir**); ℞ **sedatives**; ℞ **benzodiazepines** (for example, ℞ **diazepam**, ℞ **lorazepam**); alcohol; ℞ **cimetidine**; ℞ **fluvoxamine**.

• ℞ **hydantoin** analogs (for example, ℞ **phenytoin**, ℞ **mephenytoin**) ℞ **rifampin** decrease the effect of methadone.

• The levels of ℞ **desipramine** may increase when taken with methadone.

Side effects

• These depend on use, dose, and how it is administered. There may be sedation, dizziness, vomiting, nausea, loss of appetite, excessive sweating, and constipation. There is occasionally euphoria, which may lead to a state of mental detachment or confusion. Also, there may be sweating, headache, palpitations, changes in heart rate, postural hypotension (a lowering of blood pressure on standing, causing dizziness), rashes, miosis (pupil constriction), dry mouth, flushing of the face, mood change, and hallucinations.

Methagual ⑧

A preparation of ℞ **methyl salicylate**, guaiacol, and various.
Formulation: Topical ointment.
Availability: OTC.
Warnings and side effects: See ℞ **methyl salicylate**.

Methalgen Cream ⑧

A preparation of ℞ **methyl salicylate**, ℞ **camphor**, ℞ **menthol**, and various.
Formulation: Topical cream.
Availability: OTC.
Warnings and side effects: See ℞ **methyl salicylate**; ℞ **camphor**; ℞ **menthol**.

methamphetamine ⑤

Type/Group: CNS stimulant; sympathomimetic; appetite suppressant; obesity treatment.
Brand(s): Desoxyn.
How administered: Orally.

Used to treat

Methamphetamine, in adults, works directly on the brain as a stimulant and can be used as an adjunct (additional treatment to enhance effectiveness) in the short-term treatment of ✪ **obesity**. It can also be used in the treatment of ✪ **attention deficit disorder** with hyperactivity in children.

Warnings

• It should not be used by people with known hypersensitivity to sympathomimetic amines, advanced arteriosclerosis, symptomatic cardiovascular disease, hypertension, hyperthyroidism, glaucoma, agitated states, a history of drug abuse, or when taking ℞ **MAOI** antidepressants (see Interactions below).
• It should be given with caution to anyone with Tourette's syndrome.
• It is not known whether or not methamphetamine can harm the fetus, therefore, it should be used during pregnancy only if medically judged to be needed.
• It should not be used by breast-feeding mothers.
• It may impair the ability to perform skilled tasks requiring alertness, such as driving.
• It has a high abuse potential, and should not be taken in higher doses or for a longer period than prescribed. Tolerance, extreme psychological dependence, and severe social disability may occur.
• The sustained-release form must not be crushed or chewed.
• Methamphetamine is a Schedule II controlled substance.
• Other medications (including OTC preparations, herbal remedies, and supplements) must not be taken without consulting a doctor.

Interactions

• Methamphetamine must not be taken with, or within two weeks of discontinuing, ℞ **MAOI** antidepressants. Severe and even fatal reactions can occur.
• ℞ **selegiline** and ℞ **furazolidone** may cause severe hypertensive reactions.
• ℞ **tricyclic** antidepressants and ℞ **urinary acidifiers** may reduce levels of amphetamines.

• ℞ **Sodium bicarbonate** may increase the effects of amphetamines.

Side effects

• Frequently, headache, nervousness, dizziness, hypersalivation, nausea, diarrhea, hyperactivity, dry mouth, depression, anxiety, insomnia, delayed sleep, euphoria, restlessness and, at high doses, potentially serious effects on heart rhythm.

methantheline bromide ⑤

Type/Group: **anticholinergic; antispasmodic**.
Brand(s): Banthine.
How administered: Orally.

Used to treat

Methantheline has been used in combination with other drugs (for example, ℞ **phenobarbital**) in the treatment of ✪ **peptic ulcer**. It is not now considered to be nearly as effective as more recent treatments (against *H. pylori* bacteria). It may also be used to treat a type of ✪ **incontinence** that arises from nerve damage in the control of bladder function.

Warnings

• It should not be given to people with known hypersensitivity to anticholinergics, with myasthenia gravis, narrow-angle glaucoma, urinary obstruction, or with any infection or obstructive condition of the gastrointestinal tract.
• It should be given with caution to people with kidney or liver impairment, enlarged prostate, heart disease or high blood pressure, hyperthyroidism, ulcerative colitis, hiatal hernia, glaucoma, brain damage, or Down's syndrome.
• Methantheline should be used during pregnancy only when the potential benefit outweighs the possible risk to the fetus.
• Medical judgment is required if breast-feeding is being considered. It may appear in breast milk.
• Anticholinergics in general should not be given to anyone with a febrile (feverish) illness or who must work or live in a hot environment.
• The safety of this drug has not been established for children and infants.
• The frequency and severity of side effects is higher in the elderly.
• Because side effects may include drowsiness or visual disturbances, caution is advised in driving and other tasks requiring alertness or good vision. A doctor must be contacted if any eye pain develops.

Interactions

• The following drugs have some anticholinergic properties and may interact with methantheline to increase side effects:
℞ **amantadine**; some ℞ **antiarrhythmic** drugs (for example, ℞ **disopyramide**, ℞ **procainamide**, ℞ **quinidine**); some ℞ **antihistamines** (for example, ℞ **promethazine**, ℞ **carbinoxamine**, ℞ **diphenhydramine hydrochloride**); ℞ **antiparkinsonism** drugs; ℞ **glutethimide**; ℞ **meperidine**; ℞ **phenothiazines**; ℞ **tricyclic** antidepressants.
• The levels of ℞ **digoxin** may rise if taken in its slow-dissolving form, but not as capsules or elixir.
• Anticholinergics and ⚖ **potassium chloride** (in tablet form) should be used together with caution, because the tablet form of

potassium chloride may stay in the intestines longer, and so there is a greater risk of irritation and lesions.

• Methantheline should be taken at least one hour before an ℞ **antacid**.

• ℞ **Ketoconazole** should be taken at least two hours before an anticholinergic.

Side effects

• These may include dry mouth, thirst, blurred vision and other visual disturbances, urinary hesitancy, palpitations, and constipation.

• Uncommonly, intraocular pressure (pressure in the eyeball), headache, unusual or absent taste sensation, nervousness, drowsiness, flushing, and nausea.

• Although rare, hives, other skin eruptions, and anaphylaxis may occur in extreme allergic reactions.

methazolamide Ⓖ

Type/Group: **carbonic anhydrase inhibitor; glaucoma treatment**.

Brand(s): Neptazine.

How administered: Orally.

Used to treat

Methazolamide is a sulfonamide derivative that acts as a carbonic anhydrase inhibitor that reduces the rate of formation of fluid in the eye, and is used to treat open-angle ✪ **glaucoma** and to lower intraocular pressure (pressure in the eyeball) in acute angle-closure glaucoma when surgery is delayed. It may also be prescribed to treat acute mountain sickness.

Warnings

• It should not be given to people with kidney disease, severe liver disease, electrolyte imbalance, adrenocortical insufficiency, or cirrhosis.

• It should be given with caution to people with a severe loss of respiratory capacity, diabetes mellitus, hypercalciuria (abnormal levels of calcium in the urine), or gout, and also to children.

• Methazolamide should be used during pregnancy only if the potential benefits outweigh the possible risks.

• Medical judgment is required if breast-feeding is being considered.

• Take with food to avoid gastrointestinal upsets.

Interactions

• If used with ℞ **salicylates**, there is an increased risk of central nervous system toxicity.

• The levels of ℞ **amphetamines**, ℞ **ephedrine**, ℞ **flecainide**, ℞ **mexiletine**, and ℞ **quinidine** are increased.

• The alkalization of urine decreases the antibacterial effects of ℞ **methenamine**.

• If used with ℞ **phenytoin**, there is an increased risk of osteomalacia.

Side effects

• Most frequently, nausea, vomiting, loss of appetite, tingling in hands or feet, and urinary frequency.

• Rare but serious effects include seizure, blood disorders, and severe skin disorders.

methenamine Ⓖ

Type/Group: **antibacterial**.

Brand(s): As *hippurate*: Hiprex; Urex. As *mandelate*: various generic. Combinations: With *hyoscyamine sulfate* and *multiple analgesic/ antibacterial agents*: Atrosept; Dolsed; Prosed/DS; Trac Tabs 2X; Urimar-T; Urised Tablets; Urisedamine; Urogesic Blue. With *sodium salicylate* and *benzoic acid*: Cystex. With *sodium acid phosphate*: Uroquid-Acid No. 2.

How administered: Orally.

Used to treat

Methenamine, as hippurate and mandelate, is a synthetic antibacterial used to treat recurrent ✪ **bacterial infections** of the urinary tract.

Warnings

• It should not be given to people with known hypersensitivity to methenamine, with kidney insufficiency, severe liver impairment (this applies to methenamine hippurate), or severe dehydration (also methenamine hippurate).

• Its safety in pregnancy has not been established, but methenamine has been used in the last trimester without apparent ill effects. It should be used only if clearly needed and if the potential benefits outweigh the risks to the fetus.

• This drug appears in breast milk, but no adverse effects have been reported.

• Plenty of fluids must be drunk to ensure adequate urine flow.

• Urine must be kept acidic, and it may be necessary to acidify it by, for example, drinking cranberry juice or taking ascorbic acid.

Interactions

• ℞ **Sulfonamides** taken with methenamine may cause formation of hard crystals in the urine.

• ℞ **Acetazolamide** and ℞ **antacids** interfere with methenamine's antibacterial activity.

Side effects

• Frequently, gastrointestinal upsets and appetite loss.

• Occasionally, itching, hives, bladder irritation, urinary frequency or urgency, and headache.

• Rarely, generalized edema, cessation of urination, blood in urine, muscle cramps, and transient changes in liver function.

Methergine Ⓡ

A preparation of ℞ **methylergonovine maleate**.

Formulation: Injection; oral tablets.

Availability: Prescription only.

Warnings and side effects: See ℞ **methylergonovine maleate**.

methimazole Ⓖ

Type/Group: **antithyroid; hormone antagonist**.

Brand(s): Tapazole.

How administered: Orally

Used to treat

Methimazole acts as an indirect hormone antagonist by inhibiting the thyroid gland's production of ℞ **thyroid hormones**, thereby preventing an excess of thyroid hormone entering the blood and so is useful in the treatment of the symptoms that excess thyroid hormones cause (thyrotoxicosis). It is also used to lessen hyperthyroidism in preparation for surgery or radiation therapy.

Warnings

• It should not be used by people with known hypersensitivity to this drug.

• It should be given with caution to people with infections, bone marrow depression, liver disease, and to children, as liver toxicity has been reported.

It should be used during pregnancy only if medically judged to be needed and benefit outweighs risk to the fetus.

It should not be used by breast-feeding mothers.

• It may cause agranulocytosis (a serious blood disease resulting in increased susceptibility to infection). A doctor must be contacted if hay fever, sore throat, skin eruptions, fever, headache, or general malaise (symptoms of agranulocytosis) develop. The risk is increased in people over the age of 40.

Interactions

• The effects of oral ℞ **anticoagulants** may be altered.

• Drugs containing ◌◌ **iodine** (for example, potassium iodide) may decrease the response to methimazole.

• The levels of ℞ **digoxin** may be increased.

• The risk of agranulocytosis is increased if other drugs that can also cause this condition (for example, ℞ **tricyclic** antidepressants) are taken with methimazole.

Side effects

• Frequently, hives, rash, itching, nausea and vomiting, darkening of skin, hair loss, headache, and tingling sensation.

• Occasionally, drowsiness, enlarged lymph nodes, dizziness. Rarely, drug fever, lupus-like syndrome, hepatitis, and potentially serious blood and skin disorders.

methionine ⓖ

Type/Group: **skin preparation**

Brand(s): M-Caps; Pedameth; Uracid; various generic.

How administered: Orally.

Used to treat

Methionine is a natural amino acid that is used for diaper rash in infants and for the control of odor and irritation caused by urine in incontinent adults (see ◑ **incontinence**). The acid-producing effect of methionine creates ammonia-free urine. Methioine is also taken orally as a dietary supplement (see ◌◌ **amino acid**).

Warnings

• It should not be given to people with a history of liver disease, as large doses may exaggerate the adverse effects of liver disease.

• A doctor must be consulted before using during pregnancy or if breast-feeding.

• Excessive use in infants may result in less than normal weight gain.

• It should be taken with food or liquid.

Interactions

No significant interactions are known.

Side effects

It is considered safe in normal use.

methocarbamol ⓖ

Type/Group: **skeletal muscle relaxant.**

Brand(s): Robaxin; various generic. Combination: With *aspirin*: Robaxisal.

How administered: Orally; injection.

Used to treat

Methocarbamol is used as an additional along with other measures (such as rest and physical therapy) for the relief of acute muscle pain. It may also be prescribed to control the neuromuscular manifestations of tetanus. It works by an action on the central nervous system (CNS).

Warnings

• It should not be used by people with known hypersensitivity to methocarbamol. The injectable form should not be used by anyone with known or suspected kidney disorders.

• It should be given with caution to epileptics.

• It should be used during pregnancy only if medically judged that the benefits outweigh the risks to the fetus.

• Medical judgment is also required if breast-feeding is being considered.

• It may impair the perfomance of skilled tasks, such as driving.

• Alcohol and other CNS depressants should be avoided.

• It may darken urine.

Interactions

None of significance have been reported.

Side effects

• Commonly, dizziness, drowsiness, and lightheadedness.

• Rarely, fainting, allergic skin reactions, blurred or double vision, gastrointestinal upset, muscular incoordination, blood disorders, and seizures.

methotrexate ⓖ

Type/Group: **cytotoxic; antirheumatic; immunosuppressant.**

Brand(s): Rhumatrex; various generic.

How administered: Orally; injection.

Used to treat

Methotrexate is an (antimetabolite) ℞ **cytotoxic** drug which is used primarily as an ℞ **anticancer** treatment of childhood acute lymphoblastic ◑ **leukemia**, and also to treat non-Hodgkin's lymphomas, choriocarcinoma, and some solid tumors. It is sometimes used for many types of cancer and other disorders, although not stated by the manufacturer for all these uses. It works by inhibiting the activity of an enzyme essential to the DNA metabolism in cells. It is also used as an immunosuppressant to treat ◑ **rheumatoid arthritis** and resistant ◑ **psoriasis**, but only when these conditions are severe and disabling, and other treatments have proven inadequate. This drug is administered only by physicians familiar with its risks, and close medical monitoring for toxic effects is necessary.

Warnings

• It should not be used by people with known hypersensitivity to this drug, with existing liver disease, alcoholism, severe kidney impairment, porphyria, or certain blood abnormalities. Use with extreme caution where there is kidney impairment, peptic ulcer, colitis, or general physical debility. This is a specialist drug administered by experts who will make a full patient assessment pior to treatment.

• Methotrexate should not be used during pregnancy, nor by either partner when the possibility of becoming pregnant exists (women with childbearing potential should use reliable contraception). Pregnancy should be avoided by women for at least one ovulatory cycle after discontinuing methotrexate, and for 3 months if the man has been taking the drug.

• Breast-feeding mothers should either discontinue using this drug or stop breast feeding.

• The appearance of the following symptoms means that use must be discontinued, at least for a medical evaluation: lung symptoms (especially dry, nonproductive cough), diarrhea, and bleeding mouth sores (ulcerative stomatitis).

• When it is to be self-administered, and before it is prescribed people taking this drug must be absolutely certain of correct dosage and schedule; overdose has led to fatalities.

• There will be continual medical monitoring throughout treatment.

Interactions

• ℞ **Penicillins**, ℞ **salicylates**, ℞ **sulfonamides**, ℞ **sulfonylureas**, etretinate, phenylbutazone, ℞ **phenytoin**, and ℞ **probenecid** may increase the risk of methotrexate toxicity.

• Methotrexate taken with any nephrotoxic drug (for example, ℞ **cisplatin**) will increase the risk of toxic effects.

• Medical judgment is required if using ℞ **NSAIDs** or ℞ **theophylline**.

• Live ℞ **vaccines** should not be administered until methotrexate has cleared the body.

• ℞ **Folic acid** may decrease the response to methotrexate. Similarly, an existing folate deficiency may increase potential for toxicity.

• Oral ℞ **antibiotics** (such as, ℞ **tetracycline**, ℞ **chloramphenicol**) may lower the absorption of methotrexate.

Side effects

The treatment of cancer is very complex and is carried out by specialists (oncologists). Counselling and explanations of what side effects are to be expected, and what to look out for, will be provided. Many of these side effects also apply to people using methotrexate for other disorders (such as, rheumatoid arthritis).

• Some of the serious discomfort, for instance nausea, vomiting, and hair loss, can be minimized by careful adjustment of therapy regimens.

• The more common side effects include nausea, vomiting, impaired liver function, mouth sores, blood abnormalities, rash, itchiness, diarrhea, hair loss, and dizziness.

• In common with cytotoxic drugs as a group, methotrexate may cause impaired wound healing, depression of growth in children, and damage to the lining (epithelium) of the gastrointestinal tract, sterility, and kidney damage.

methotrimeprazine Ⓖ

Type/Group: **non-narcotic analgesic; anxiolytic; sedatives**.
Brand(s): Levoprome.
How administered: Injection.

Used to treat

Methotrimeprazine is used to treat moderate to severe pain in bed-ridden patients, to provide preoperative sedation, and to provide analgesia and sedation during labor. It is a ℞ **phenothiazine** derivative.

Warnings

• It should not be used by anyone with hypersensitivity to methotrimeprazine or sulfites, or by those with severe kidney, heart or liver disease, seizure disorders, who are in a coma, or with clinically significant hypotension.

• It should be given with caution to anyone who is unable to get out of bed, because it can cause substantial postural hypotension (a lowering of blood pressure on standing, causing dizziness), anyone over 65, and children.

• It is not known whether methotrimeprazine can harm the fetus. It does not affect the force, duration, and frequency of uterine contractions during labor.

• Medical judgment is required if breast-feeding is being considered.

• It should not be used for longer than 30 days. Adverse effects on liver and red blood cells can occur.

Interactions

• CNS (central nervous system) depressants may enhance effects.

• ℞ **Atropine**, ℞ **scopolamine**, or ℞ **succinylcholine** taken with methotrimeprazine can cause speeded heartbeat, decreased blood pressure, effects on the central nervous system, and extrapyramidal symptoms (involuntary movement).

Side effects

• Frequently, postural hypotension.

• Occasionally, amnesia, disorientation, excessive sedation, seizures, changes in heart rate, abdominal symptoms, urinary disorders, and potentially serious side-effects such as blood cell disorders, liver toxicity, seizures, and respiratory depression.

methoxamine hydrochloride Ⓖ

Type/Group: **alpha-adrenergic stimulant; sympathomimetic; vasoconstrictor**.
Brand(s): Vasoxyl.
How administered: Injection, infusion.

Used to treat

Methoxamine hydrochloride is used primarily to maintain or restore blood pressure (for example, when falling blood pressure is caused by anesthesia), or to treat atrial tachycardia by raising blood pressure (see Ⓞ **arrhythmia**).

Warnings

• It should not be given to people with known hypersensitivity to this drug, or with severe hypertension.

• It should be given with caution to people with heart or artery disease, hyperthyroidism, or low blood volume. It is a specialist hospital drug, and a full assessment of suitability will be carried out.

• It is thought that methoxamine may harm the fetus and so it should be used during pregnancy only if the potential benefit outweighs the possible risk.

• Medical judgment is required if breast-feeding is being considered.

• This is a powerful drug, used only under hospital conditions, and with continuous monitoring of heart function, blood pressure, and other vital signs.

Interactions

• There is a risk of significant hypertension if taken with ℞ **beta-blockers**.

• ℞ **Bretylium tosylate**, ℞ **ergot alkaloids** (for example, ℞ **ergonovine**, ℞ **ergotamine**), ℞ **MAOI**s, ℞ **oxytocin**, other sympathomimetics, and ℞ **tricyclics** may intensify the effects of methoxamine, with the potential for serious adverse reactions.

• ℞ **Alpha-adrenergic blockers**, ℞ **diuretics**, and ℞ **phenothiazines** may reverse or decrease the therapeutic effects of methoxamine.

• ℞ **Atropine sulfate** enhances some effects of methoxamine, while blocking its tendency to produce slowed heartbeat. This is a usually beneficial interaction.

Side effects

• There may be an excessive rise in blood pressure, palpitations, nervousness, dizziness, sweating, pallor, breathlessness, headache (often severe), nausea or vomiting.

methsuximide ⑥

Type/Group: **anticonvulsant; antiepileptic**.
Brand(s): Celontin Kapseals.
How administered: Orally.

Used to treat

Methsuximide is used in the treatment of ⊘ **epilepsy**, mainly to treat refractory absence (petit mal).

Warnings

• Avoid its use in people with known hypersensitivity to this drug.

• Medical judgment is required for people with porphyria, kidney or liver impairment.

• Methsuximide is associated with an increase in frequency of certain birth defects and should not be used during pregnancy. However, because uncontrolled seizures can also threaten fetal health, medical judgment is needed to weigh potential benefits and risks.

• Medical judgment is also required for breast-feeding mothers.

• If symptoms such as skin rash, joint pain, blurred vision, sore throat, fever, bruising, or mouth ulcers occur, medical help should be sought.

• When used alone to treat mixed forms of epilepsy, methsuximide may cause an increase in grand mal seizures.

• Withdrawal should be gradual otherwise it may precipitate attacks.

• As this drug may cause drowsiness, driving or other hazardous activity should be avoided.

Interactions

• Methsuximide may raise the levels of ℞ **mephenytoin** and ℞ **phenytoin**.

• The effects if taken with ℞ **valproate sodium** are unpredictable, and levels of methsuximide may rise or fall.

• The levels of ℞ **primidone** and ℞ **phenobarbital** (and other ℞ **barbiturates**) may be reduced.

Side effects

These are a wide ranging, and include:

• Drowsiness, dizziness, unsteady gait, gastrointestinal disturbances, vomiting, nausea, and loss of appetite;

• Itching, confusion, headache, hiccup, depression or mild euphoria, and aggressive behavior;

• Rashes, liver and kidney changes, and effects on blood;

• Rarely, psychotic states, suicidal behavior, and auditory hallucinations;

• Potentially serious side effects include blood-cell disorders and skin disorders.

methyclothiazide ⑥

Type/Group: **diuretic; thiazide; antihypertensive**.
Brand(s): Aquatensen; Enduron; various generic.
How administered: Orally.

Used to treat

Methyclothiazide is used in the treatment of ⊘ **hypertension**, either alone or with other types of diuretic or other drugs (for example, ℞ **beta-blockers**). It can also be used in the treatment of edema. Thiazide diuretics have also become a major part of treatment for nephrogenic ⊘ **diabetes insipidus**.

Warnings

• It should not be given to people with known hypersensitivity to thiazides (or to ℞ **sulfonamide**-derived drugs), or severe kidney or liver disorders.

• It should be given with caution to elderly people, or anyone with high cholesterol or triglyceride levels, or with liver or kidney impairment.

• Methyclothiazide should be used during pregnancy only when the potential benefit outweighs the possible risk to the fetus.

• Medical judgment is required if breast-feeding is being considered.

• Early symptoms of electrolyte imbalance may include muscle weakness or cramps, nausea, vomiting, restlessness or lethargy, dry mouth, excessive thirst, fast pulse, or dizziness. A doctor must be contacted if such symptoms occur.

• Thiazides may aggravate symptoms of diabetes or gout, and worsen or activate lupus erythematosus.

• Periodic monitoring of electrolytes (particularly potassium, sodium, chloride, and bicarbonate) will be carried out.

• There may be photosensitivity (abnormal sensitivity to sunlight) and so exposure should be minimized.

• Thiazides interact with a number of drugs, including some over-the-counter preparations. A doctor must be consulted if any other medications are being taken (including OTCs, herbal remedies, and supplements).

Interactions

• There is a higher risk of a hypersensitivity reaction to ℞ **allopurinol**.

• The effects of ℞ **anesthetics**, ℞ **anticancer** drugs, other antihypertensives, ℞ **diazoxide**, ☊ **calcium** salts, ℞ **cardiac glycosides**, ℞ **lithium**, loop diuretics, ℞ **methyldopa**, nondepolarizing ℞ **skeletal muscle relaxants**, and ☊ **vitamin D** may be increased, with the potential for significant side effects or toxicity. An increased effect is sometimes used to advantage in combining loop diuretics with other antihypertensives.

• The effects of ℞ **anticoagulants**, antigout agents (for example, ℞ **probenecid**, ℞ **sulfinpyrazone**) may be lowered by thiazides.

• The dosage of ℞ **insulin** and ℞ **sulfonylureas** may need to be adjusted, as thiazides may increase blood sugar levels.

• ℞ **Amphotericin B**, ℞ **anticholinergics**, ℞ **corticosteroids**, ℞ **corticotropin**, and ℞ **MAOIs** may increase the diuretic effect of thiazides with the possibility of significant electrolyte loss, especially of potassium.

• ℞ **Cholestyramine**, ℞ **colestipol hydrochloride**, ℞ **methenamine**, and ℞ **NSAIDs** (especially ℞ **indomethacin**) may reduce the effectiveness of thiazide diuretics.

• If taken with alcohol, ℞ **barbiturates**, or ℞ **opioids**, there is an increased possibility of postural hypotension (lowered blood pressure on standing).

Side effects

• There may be dizziness, headache, muscle cramps, mild gastrointestinal upsets, postural hypotension, reversible impotence, low blood potassium, sodium, magnesium and chloride, raised blood urea, glucose and lipids, and gout.

• Rarely, photosensitivity, blood disorders, skin reactions, or pancreatitis.

methylcellulose ⑥

Type/Group: **laxative. obesity treatment**.
Brand(s): Citrucel.
How administered: Orally.

Used to treat

Methylcellulose is a bulking-agent laxative which works by increasing the overall mass of stool while at the same time retaining a lot of water and so stimulating bowel movement. However, the full effect may not be achieved for many hours. It may be used when treating a range of bowel conditions, including diverticular disease and irritable bowel syndrome. Separately, it may be used as part of the treatment for ⊙ **obesity** to reduce food intake, since it may act as an appetite suppressant through giving a feeling of fullness. A very similar compound, carboxymethylcellulose, is also used in OTC laxative preparations.

Warnings

• It should not be given to people with gastrointestinal obstruction, esophageal obstruction, or who have difficulty swallowing.

• No ill effects in pregnancy or breast-feeding have been associated with methylcellulose, but a doctor should always be consulted before taking any drug during pregnancy.

• Adequate fluid intake must be maintained, and at least a glass of liquid must be drunk when taking this bulking agent. (It swells up, becoming bulkier. Obstruction can form in the esophagus if the substance is not carried all the way down, or in the bowel if insufficient liquid is present.) It should not be taken just before bed.

• Do not use if there is abdominal pain, nausea, or vomiting, unless directed by a doctor.

• A doctor must be consulted first before taking any other medication (including OTCs, herbal remedies, and supplements), because laxatives may alter the absorption of a wide range drugs.

Often it is recommended that a bulk-forming laxative dose be separated by at least 3 hours from doses of medications that might be affected (for example, digitalis, ℞ **nitrofurantoin**, ℞ **salicylates**).

Interactions

Laxatives can affect the absorption of a wide range of drugs. No specific drug interactions of significance are known.

Side effects

• There may be flatulence and abdominal distension, and intestinal obstruction.

methyldopa ⑥

Type/Group: **alpha-adrenergic stimulant; antisympathetic; antihypertensive**.
Brand(s): Aldomet; various generic. Combinations: With *chlorothiazide*: Aldoclor-150, 250 Tablets. With *hydrochlorothiazide*: Aldoril.
How administered: Orally; injection.

Used to treat

Methyldopa is an antisympathetic drug which decreases neurotransmitter release from sympathetic nerves (it is thought to act as an alpha-adrenergic stimulant (alpha$_2$-receptor subtype) in the brain). It can be used (commonly in combination with other drugs) to treat moderate to severe ⊙ **hypertension** and in hypertensive crisis. The form used in injectable preparations is methyldopate hydrochloride.

Warnings

• It should not be given to people with known hypersensitivity to this drug, with active liver disease or previous liver problems associated with the use of methyldopa, or to anyone taking a ℞ **MAOI** antidepressant. It is not recommended for those with pheochromocytoma.

• It should be given with caution to elderly people and to anyone with impaired liver or kidney function.

• Risk in pregnancy increases with the injectable form. Methyldopa should be used during pregnancy only if it is clearly needed.

• Medical judgment is required if breast-feeding is being considered.

• Tests to monitor liver function and possible blood changes are generally required.

• Because of possible sedative side effects, caution is advised for potentially hazardous activities, such as driving, that require mental alertness.

• A doctor must be contacted if unusual, prolonged tiredness, fever, or jaundice occur.

• This drug is removed by dialysis, which may cause blood pressure to rise.

• A doctor must be consulted beore taking any other medication (including OTCs, herbal remedies, supplements, or any other kind of alternative remedy).

Interactions

• ℞ **MAOI** antidepressants should not be used with methyldopa.

• The effects of ℞ **norepinephrine** may be intensified or prolonged.

• If used with ℞ **general anesthetics** or ℞ **methotrimeprazine**, there is a risk of increased hypotensive effects.

• If used with ℞ **lithium**, it may cause symptoms of lithium toxicity.

• There is the possibility of an additive hypotensive effect and mental effects, such as psychosis, with ℞ **levodopa**.

• ℞ **amphetamines**, ℞ **haloperidol**, ⚕ **iron** preparations (for example, ferrous sulfate, ferrous gluconate), ℞ **phenothiazines**, and ℞ **tricyclic** antidepressants may reduce the levels or antihypertensive effect of methyldopa. In addition, the effects of haloperidol may be exaggerated, with slowed movements, memory impairment, or difficulty concentrating.

• If used with other antihypertensives and ℞ **diuretics**, the effects of these drugs may be increased. This additive effect is sometimes used to advantage in combination treatments for high blood pressure.

Side effects

• These are many and may include drowsiness or sedation, dry mouth, nasal stuffiness, gastrointestinal disturbances, and fluid retention.

• Less commonly, sleep disturbances, depression, headache, dizziness, slowing of heart rate, fever, aches and pains, tingling in the extremities, disturbances of sexual function (and breast enlargement), fainting, impaired liver function, skin and blood disorders, and parkinsonian symptoms.

• Rarely, darkening of urine. Sensitivity reactions including rash, hives, sores on the soles of the feet, and lupus-like symptoms have occurred.

methylergonovine maleate Ⓖ

Type/Group: **ergot alkaloid; uterine stimulant; vasoconstrictor**.
Brand(s): Methergine.
How administered: Orally; injection.

Used to treat

Methylergonovine is used routinely in obstetrics (an area of medicine to do with pregnancy and childbirth). Methylergonovine, or a closely related compound ℞ **ergonovine**, may be given to prevent excessive postnatal bleeding and also bleeding due to incomplete abortion (when it may be combined with ℞ **oxytocin**). It may be used, as well, to speed up the third stage of labor (the delivery of the placenta), although oxytocin is currently preferred for this purpose.

Warnings

• It should not be given to people with known hypersensitivity to this drug, or with vascular disease, certain kidney, liver, heart and other cardiovascular or lung disorders, sepsis, calcium deficiency, severe hypertension, or eclampsia. It should not be used during pregnancy, or to induce labor, or when spontaneous abortion seems likely.

• It should be given with caution to people who have a very slow heart rate.

• Methylergonovine should not be taken during pregnancy.

• Medical judgment is required if breast-feeding is being considered. It may decrease the production of milk.

Interactions

• If used with other vasoconstrictors or ergot alkaloids, there is a possibility of intensified side effects.

Side effects

• Depending on how it is administered, use, and dose, there may be nausea and vomiting, palpitations, breathlessness, slowing of the heartbeat, headache, dizziness, and abdominal and chest pain.

• Rarely, there are cardiovascular complications.

Methylin Ⓑ

A preparation of ℞ **methylphenidate**.
Formulation: Oral tablets, sustained release tablets, both in several strengths.
Availability: Prescription only.
Warnings and side effects: See ℞ **methylphenidate**.

methylphenidate Ⓖ

Type/Group: **CNS stimulant; obesity treatment**.
Brand(s): Ritalin; Methylin; various generic.
How administered: Orally.

Used to treat

Methylphenidate is an amphetamine derivative. In adults it works directly on the brain as a stimulant and can be used to treat ✪ **narcolepsy** (irresistible attacks of sleep during the day). It can also be used to treat ✪ **attention deficit disorder** with hyperactivity in children. Although not stated by the manufacturer for such use, it can be prescribed for depression in people with cancer, or who have suffered a stroke, and in those over 65.

Warnings

• It should not be used by people with known hypersensitivity to sympathomimetic amines, glaucoma, or a history of Tourette's syndrome or motor tics. It should also be avoided by anyone experiencing marked anxiety, tension, and agitation.

• It should be given with caution to anyone with severe depression, seizure disorders, hypertension, or a history of drug abuse.

• It is not known whether or not methylphenidate can harm the fetus, therefore, it should be used during pregnancy only if medically judged to be needed.

• Medical judgment is also required if breast-feeding is being considered.

• It may impair the ability to perform skilled tasks requiring alertness, such as driving.

• It has a high abuse potential and should not be taken in higher doses or for a longer period than prescribed. Tolerance, extreme psychological dependence, and severe social disability may occur.

• The sustained-release form must not be crushed or chewed.

• The effects of long-term use in children are not established. Prolonged use may produce a temporary suppression of normal growth in weight and/or height.

• Methylphenidate is a Schedule II controlled substance.

Interactions

• Methylphenidate must not be taken with, or within two weeks of discontinuing, ℞ **MAOI** antidepressants. Severe and even fatal reactions can occur.

• The effects of ℞ **guanethidine monosulfate** may be reduced.

• ℞ **tricyclic** antidepressants may reduce the levels of amphetamines.

Side effects
• Frequently, nervousness, insomnia, loss of appetite.
• Occasionally, dizziness, drowsiness, headache, nausea, stomach pain, fever, rash, and joint pain.
• Rarely, blurred vision, Tourette's syndrome, seizure (more likely in those with a history of such disorders), changes in rate of heartbeat, angina, blood, and skin disorders.

methylprednisolone ⑥
Type/Group: **corticosteroid; anti-inflammatory; immunosuppressant.**
Brand(s): Medrol; various generic. As *methylprednisolone acetate*: Adlone; Depo-Medrol; Depoject; Depopred; Duralone; M-Prednisol; Medralone; various generic. As *methylprednisolone succinate*: A-Methapred; Solu-Medrol; various generic.
Combinations: With *neomycin*: Neo-Medrol.
How administered: Orally; injection.

Used to treat
Methylprednisolone is used for the treatment of acute and chronic adrenal insufficiency, congenital adrenal hyperplasia, and adrenal insufficiency secondary to pituitary insufficiency. In addition it can also used for arthritis, rheumatic heart disease, allergic, collagen, intestinal tract, liver, ocular, kidney, and skin diseases, bronchial asthma, cerebral edema (fluid retention in the brain), and some cancers.

Warnings
• It should not be used by anyone with known hypersensitivity to corticosteroids, or with systemic fungal infections.
• It should be given with caution to anyone with low thyroid function, peptic ulcers, hepatitis, cirrhosis, ocular herpes simplex, diabetes mellitus, history of tuberculosis, ulcerative colitis, congestive heart failure, myocardial infarction (heart attack), hypertension, psychosis, or kidney insufficiency, or anyone over 65 and children.
• Corticosteroids can cross the placenta, and therefore methylprednisolone should only be used during pregnancy if medically judged to be essential.
• It should not be used by breast-feeding mothers. It is excreted in breast milk and could suppress growth and interfere with production of corticosteroids in the infant.
• It may mask the signs of infection and interfere with the body's ability to keep infection from spreading.
• Live vaccines must not be taken while using this drug.
• Prolonged use in children can inhibit skeletal growth, and so growth must be monitored.
• The contraceptive effect of IUDs (intrauterine device) may be decreased.
• It may reactivate latent tuberculosis or amebiasis.
• It causes increased excretion of calcium and other minerals, and so supplements may be needed.
• Prolonged use may lead to adrenal insufficiency. Notify a doctor if there is unusual weight gain, swelling of the legs or feet, muscle weakness, black tarry stools, vomiting of blood, puffing of the face,

menstrual irregularities, or prolonged sore throat, fever, cold, or infection.
• Anyone on long-term steroid therapy should wear a medic-alert bracelet or the equivalent.
• No other medication (including OTC, herbal remedies and supplements) should be taken without consulting a doctor.
• Discontinuation of this drug must be gradual and under medical supervision to avoid adverse reactions.
• Dentists and other doctors must be informed of the use of this drug during, and for 12 months after discontinuing, treatment. Supportive drugs may be required in the event of severe illness, surgery, or trauma.

Interactions
• Methylprednisolone taken with amphotericin or diuretics may further reduce potassium levels.
• The effects of ℞ **aspirin**, ℞ **oral hypoglycemics**, ℞ **insulin**, diuretics, and ⚵ **potassium** supplements may be reduced.
• ℞ **Barbiturates**, ℞ **hydantoins**, ℞ **rifampin**, and ℞ **ephedrine** may reduce the effects of methylprednisolone.
• ℞ **Ketoconazole**, ℞ **estrogens**, ℞ **oral contraceptives**, and nondepolarizing muscle relaxants may increase the effects of corticosteroids.
• ℞ **Aspirin** and ℞ **NSAID**s increase the risk of gastric ulceration.
• Oral ℞ **anticoagulants** and ℞ **theophylline** may alter the effects of either corticosteroids or the other drug, or both.
• The effectiveness of ℞ **anticholinesterases**, ℞ **isoniazid**, ℞ **salicylates**, and ℞ **somatrem** may be reduced.
• ℞ **Cyclosporine** and digitalis glycosides may increase the risk of toxicity.

Side effects
These depend on how administered, dose, duration of treatment, and use.
• Frequently, insomnia, heartburn, nervousness, abdominal tightness, increased sweating, acne, mood swings, increased appetite, facial flushing, gastrointestinal distress, delayed wound healing, diarrhea, and constipation.
• Occasionally, headache, edema, speeded heartbeat, change in skin color, frequent urination, and depression.
• Rarely, psychosis, increased blood coagulability, and hallucinations. Potentially serious side effects include pancreatitis, seizures, and gastrointestinal hemorrhage.

methylrosaniline chloride ⑥
see ℞ **gentian violet**.

methyl salicylate ⑥
Type/Group: **NSAID; counter-irritant.**
Brand(s): Argesic Cream; ArthriCare Triple-Medicated Gel; Ben-Gay Regular Strength Cream, Ultra Strength Cream, Ben-Gay Original Ointment, Arthritis Formula Cream; Deep-Down Rub; Dermal-Rub Balm; Exocaine Medicated Rub, Exocaine Plus Rub; Flexall Ultra Plus, Flexall 454 Gel, Maximum Strength 454 Gel; Gordogesic Creme; Icy Hot Balm, Cream, Stick; Methagual; Methalgen Cream; Minit-Rub; Musterole Deep Strength Rub;

Panalgesic Cream; Soltice Quick-Rub; Thera-Gesic Cream; Ziks Cream.
How administered: Topically (external).

Used to treat

Methyl salicylate can be applied to the skin for symptomatic relief of pain in muscles and underlying organs, for instance in rheumatic and other ✪ **musculoskeletal disorders**. It is administered topically to the skin, and is available as a liniment, ointment, cream, or balsam.

Warnings

• Methyl salicylate should not be used by people with known hypersensitivity to this drug or to other ℞ **salicylates** (including ℞ **aspirin**).

• If used topically as directed, there are no effects in pregnancy or breast-feeding.

• Do not use a topical salicylate with heat (for example, a heating pad or hot water bottle), as absorption may be greatly increased, causing damage to underlying skin, muscle, or organs.

• Topical salicylates should not be used for longer than a week at a time.

• If signs of over-sensitivity occur (redness of the skin, rash, or blisters), discontinue use of this drug.

• Avoid contact with the eyes, mucous membranes, or broken skin.

Interactions

• ℞ **Anticoagulants** have an additive effect in prolonging bleeding time.

Side effects

Normally, little is absorbed into the circulation and local side effects are limited to mild irritation.

• It can cause sensitivity to bright sunlight.

• Systemic effects (including blood disorders, liver, and kidney damage) may occur with prolonged or excessive use.

methyltestosterone Ⓖ

Type/Group: **sex hormone; androgen**.
Brand(s): Android; Oreton Methyl; Virilon; Testred; various generic.
How administered: Orally.

Used to treat

Methyltestosterone is a synthetic ℞ **testosterone** derivative used to treat male primary and secondary ✪ **hypogonadism** (subnormal secretion of sex hormones) and delayed puberty in men. In women, it is used for advanced metastatic ✪ **breast cancer**, and, in conjunction with estrogens, to treat symptoms of ✪ **menopause**. Although not stated by the manufacturers for such use, it may also be prescribed for postpartum breast pain and engorgement.

Warnings

• It should not be used by people with serious heart, liver, or kidney disease, or hypersensitivity to androgens, or by men with cancer of the breast or prostate.

• It should be given with caution to people with acute intermittent porphyria, history of myocardial infarction, coronary artery disease, seizure disorder, or benign prostatic hyperplasia, and with extreme caution to children and those over 65.

• Methyltestosterone must not be used during pregnancy.

• Medical judgment is required if breast-feeding is being considered.

• It should not be used to enhance athletic performance.

• In males over 65, there is an increased risk of prostatic cancer, and it may markedly increase libido.

• When taking buccal tablets, do not eat, drink, or smoke, and do allow them to dissolve between the cheek and gums.

• Methyltestosterone is a Schedule III controlled substance.

Interactions

• The response to oral ℞ **anticoagulants** (for example, ℞ **warfarin sodium**) may be increased.

• The levels of ℞ **cyclosporine** are increased.

Side effects

• In women, virilization (deepening voice, growth of body hair, clitoral enlargement, irregular periods).

• In men, breast enlargement, excessive frequency and duration of penile erections.

• Other side effects include anxiety, depression, tingling or burning sensations, acne, retention of water and minerals, blood changes, nausea, allergic skin reactions, and elevated cholesterol levels.

• Reduced sperm count and ejaculatory volume may occur after prolonged or excessive use.

• Prolonged use of high doses may cause serious liver disease, and, rarely, cancer in women.

• When given to children, it may speed up bone maturation without producing proportional increase in height. This can affect final adult stature.

• It may cause reduction of bone calcium in immobilized patients.

methysergide Ⓖ

Type/Group: **ergot alkaloid; antimigraine**.
Brand(s): Sansert.
How administered: Orally.

Used to treat

Methysergide is a potentially dangerous drug that is used, under strict medical supervision in a hospital, to treat ✪ **migraine** to prevent severe recurrent attacks and similar headaches in people for whom other forms of treatment have failed. Although not stated by the manufacturer for such use, it is also sometimes used in carcinoid syndrome to control diarrhea.

Warnings

• It should not be given to people with certain kidney, lung, liver or cardiovascular disorders, severe hypertension, urinary tract disorders, serious infections, collagen disease, or cellulitis.

• It should be given with caution to people with peptic ulcer.

• Methysergide should not be used during pregnancy or by nursing mothers. Ergot derivatives, like this drug, do appear in breast milk and may cause symptoms in infants, such as vomiting or diarrhea.

• Because it may cause drowsiness, the performance of skilled tasks, such as driving, may be impaired.

• If there is numbness or tingling in the extremities, chest pain, or shortness of breath, stop treatment and contact a doctor.

Interactions

• If used with ℞ **beta-blockers**, circulation may be restricted to the extremities to the point that gangrene occurs.

Side effects

• This is a specialist drug used under supervised conditions. There are many side effects, some of which are serious, including nausea, vomiting, abdominal discomfort, heartburn, insomnia, weight gain, rashes, mental disturbances, hair loss, cramps, effects on the cardiovascular system, edema, drowsiness, and dizziness.

Meticorten ®

A preparation of ℞ **prednisone**.
Formulation: Oral tablets.
Availability: Prescription only.
Warnings and side effects: See ℞ prednisone.

Metimyd ®

A preparation of ℞ **prednisolone** acetate phosphate and sodium ℞ **sulfacetamide**.
Formulation: Eye drops; ophthalmic ointment.
Availability: Prescription only.
Warnings and side effects: See ℞ prednisolone; ℞ sulfacetamide.

metipranolol ©

Type/Group: **beta-blocker; glaucoma treatment**.
Brand(s): Optipranolol.
How administered: Topically (eyes).

Used to treat

Metipranolol is used to treat chronic simple ✪ **glaucoma**. It is thought to work by slowing the rate of production of the aqueous humor (fluid) in the eye.

Warnings

• It should not be given to people with known hypersensitivity to metipranolol, or with certain heart disorders.
• It should be given with caution to people undergoing major surgery, and anyone with diabetes mellitus, kidney disease, thyroid disease, chronic obstructive pulmonary disease (COPD), asthma, heart failure, or peripheral vascular disease. It can be absorbed systemically (into the body).
• Metipranolol's safety during pregnancy has not been established. It should be used only if the potential benefit outweighs the possible risk to the fetus.
• Medical judgment is required if breast-feeding is being considered. It is not known if it appears in breast milk.
• Anaphylactic reactions (acute allergic reactions) may be more severe, and not as responsive to the usual doses of epinephrine used to treat them.

Interactions

• Oral ℞ **beta-blockers** can increase systemic effects.
• The effects of ℞ **verapamil** and ℞ **quinidine** are increased.

Side effects

• Frequently, eye irritation, transient local discomfort, and visual disturbances.
• Occasionally, increased light sensitivity and watering of the eyes.
• Rarely, dry eye, conjunctivitis, and eye pain. Because it can be absorbed through the eye, systemic side effects are possible, particularly headache, allergic reactions, weakness, and effects on the cardiovascular and respiratory systems.

metirosine ©

see ℞ **metyrosine**.

metoclopramide hydrochloride ©

Type/Group: **dopamine-receptor antagonist; antiemetic; antinauseant; motility stimulant**.
Brand(s): Clopra; Maxolon; Octamide Tablets, Octamide PFS; Reclomide; Reglan; various generic.
How administered: Orally; injection.

Used to treat

Metoclopramide can be used to prevent ✪ **vomiting** caused by gastrointestinal disorders, chemotherapy, or radiotherapy (in the treatment of cancer). It works both by a direct action on the vomiting center of the brain and by actions within the intestine. It enhances the strength of esophageal sphincter contraction (preventing the passage of stomach contents up into the gullet), stimulates emptying of the stomach, and increases the rate at which food is moved along the intestine. These last actions lead to its use in non-ulcer indigestion, for gastric stasis, and to prevent reflux esophagitis. It is also used during intestine examination to speed up the movement of barium through the intestine following a barium meal.

Warnings

• It should not be given to people with known hypersensitivity to this drug (or to ℞ **procainamide**), who have pheochromocytoma, obstruction of the gastrointestinal tract, a history of seizures, or are taking drugs that might make seizures or other neurological effects more likely (for example, ℞ **antipsychotic** drugs such as phenothiazines or butyrophenones).
• It should be given with extreme caution to people with depression, suicidal tendencies, or parkinsonism. Care is advised in its use by those with porphyria, hypertension, congestive heart failure, or liver or kidney impairment. Because it is a dopamine antagonist, metoclopramide promotes secretion of the hormone prolactin, which is generally undesirable in breast cancer. This drug should be given with caution to anyone with previously detected breast cancer.
• Metoclopramide should be used during pregnancy only when it is clearly needed.
• Medical judgment is required if breast-feeding is being considered. It appears in breast milk.
• This drug has been associated with depression in people with or without a prior history of depression.
• Extrapyramidal symptoms (uncoordinated or involuntary movements) and Parkinson-like symptoms (such as tremor, rigidity, slow movement) may occur. Although most of these symptoms are reversible or disappear, some may be irreversible (particularly if part of a syndrome called tardive dyskinesia).
• It may cause drowsiness or dizziness, and the performance of skilled tasks, such as driving, may be impaired.
• The sedative effects of alcohol may be increased.

Interactions
• ℞ **Antipsychotics** or ℞ **levodopa** should not be used with metoclopramide.
• The effects of ℞ **cyclosporine**, ℞ **MAOIs**, and ℞ **succinylcholine** may be intensified, with the potential for significant adverse effects.
• Depending on the drug preparation (tablet, capsule, elixir), the absorption and effects of ℞ **digoxin** may be reduced.
• ℞ **Anticholinergics** and ℞ **narcotic analgesics** have an opposing effect to that of metoclopramide.
• The effect of ℞ **cimetidine** may be reduced.

Side effects
• There may be extrapyramidal effects (especially facial, such as grimace or protrusion of the tongue), particularly in the young and elderly. Other common side effects are restlessness, drowsiness, headache, fatigue, diarrhea, nausea, and dizziness.
• Less frequently there may be headache, insomnia, depression, confusion, urinary frequency, blood disorders, and visual disturbances.
• It can cause secretion of milk, growth of breasts, in males as well, and impotence. Allergic symptoms (such as rash, hives, bronchospasm) are uncommon. When given in high intravenous doses or when administered with drugs known to cause liver damage, severe reactions have occurred.

metolazone ⓖ
Type/Group: **diuretic; thiazide; antihypertensive.**
Brand(s): Mykrox; Zaroxolyn.
How administered: Orally.

Used to treat
Metolazone is used in the treatment of ⊙ **hypertension**, either alone or with other types of diuretic or other drugs (for example, ℞ **beta-blockers**). It can also be used in the treatment of edema (but not the rapidly acting preparation, Mykrox). Thiazide diuretics have also become a major part of the treatment for nephrogenic ⊙ **diabetes insipidus**.

Warnings
• It should not be given to people with known hypersensitivity to thiazides (or to ℞ **sulfonamide**-derived drugs), or severe kidney or liver disorders.
• It should be given with caution to elderly people, anyone with high cholesterol or triglyceride levels, or with liver or kidney impairment.
• Metolazone should be used in pregnancy only when the potential benefit outweighs the possible risk to the fetus.
• Medical judgment is required if breast-feeding is being considered.
• Early symptoms of electrolyte imbalance may include muscle weakness or cramps, nausea, vomiting, restlessness or lethargy, dry mouth, excessive thirst, fast pulse, or dizziness. A doctor must be contacted if such symptoms occur.
• Thiazides may aggravate symptoms of diabetes or gout, and worsen or activate lupus erythematosus.
• Periodic monitoring of electrolytes (particularly potassium, sodium, chloride, and bicarbonate) is needed.

• Photosensitivity may develop and so precautions such as protective clothing or sunscreens should be used.
• Thiazides interact with a number of drugs, including some over-the-counter preparations. A doctor must be contacted before taking any other medications (including OTCs, herbal remedies, and supplements).

Interactions
• There is a higher risk of a hypersensitivity reaction to ℞ **allopurinol**.
• The effects of ℞ **anesthetics**, ℞ **anticancer** drugs, other antihypertensives, ℞ **diazoxide**, ⚷ **calcium** salts, ℞ **cardiac glycosides**, ℞ **lithium**, loop diuretics, ℞ **methyldopa**, nondepolarizing ℞ **skeletal muscle relaxants**, and ⚷ **vitamin D** may be increased, with the potential for significant adverse effects or toxicity. An additive effect is sometimes used to advantage in combining thiazides with other antihypertensives.
• The effects of ℞ **anticoagulants** and antigout agents (for example, ℞ **probenecid**, ℞ **sulfinpyrazone**) may be lowered by thiazides.
• The doses of ℞ **insulin** and ℞ **sulfonylureas** may need to be adjusted, as thiazides may increase blood sugar levels.
• ℞ **Amphotericin B**, ℞ **anticholinergics**, ℞ **corticosteroids**, ℞ **corticotropin**, and ℞ **MAOIs** may increase the effects of thiazides, with the possibility of significant electrolyte loss, especially potassium.
• ℞ **Cholestyramine**, ℞ **colestipol hydrochloride**, ℞ **methenamine**, and ℞ **NSAIDs** (especially ℞ **indomethacin**) may reduce the effectiveness of thiazide diuretics.
• There is an increased possibility of postural hypotension (lowered blood pressure on standing) if taken with alcohol, ℞ **barbiturates**, or ℞ **opioids**.

Side effects
• There may be dizziness, headache, muscle cramps, mild gastrointestinal upsets, postural hypotension, reversible impotence, low blood potassium, sodium, magnesium and chloride, raised blood urea, glucose and lipids, and gout.
• Rarely, photosensitivity, blood disorders, skin reactions, and pancreatitis. There can be marked diuresis (urine production) when given with furosemide.

metoprolol tartrate ⓖ
Type/Group: **beta-blocker; antianginal; antihypertensive.**
Brand(s): Lopressor; Toprol-XL; generic. Combinations: With *hydrochlorothiazide*: Lopressor HCT.
How administered: Orally; injection.

Used to treat
Metoprolol tartrate is used to lower blood pressure (see ⊙ **hypertension**) and to relieve the symptoms of and improve exercise tolerance in ⊙ **angina pectoris**. It is also used after heart attack to enhance recovery. Extended-release tablets contain an equivalent form, metoprolol succinate. Beta-blockers are generally not prescribed for persons with asthma or other bronchospastic disease (for example, chronic bronchitis or emphysema), but metoprolol may be used with medical judgment when other antihypertensive treatments have failed.

Warnings

• It should not be given to people with known hypersensitivity to any beta-blocking drug, who have certain heartbeat irregularities or heart failure. It should not be used in cardiogenic shock.

• It should be given with caution to people with diabetes mellitus or hypoglycemia, hyperthyroidism, myasthenia gravis, congestive heart failure, peripheral vascular disease, or liver or kidney impairment.

• Metoprolol should be used during pregnancy only if clearly needed.

• It appears in breast milk, and so nursing women should discontinue using this drug or stop breast-feeding.

• Abruptly stopping using a beta-blocker may have adverse effects such as on the heart.

• The use of this drug may mask signs of hyperthyroidism or hypoglycemia.

• Other medications (including OTCs, herbal remedies, and supplements) must not be taken without consulting a doctor. Some ℞ **nasal decongestants**, commonly available over the counter, contain ℞ **alpha-adrenergic stimulants** (for example, ℞ **phenylephrine**) that may cause a severe hypertensive reaction if taken with beta-blockers.

Interactions

• A serious blood pressure increase may occur after withdrawal from ℞ **clonidine hydrochloride** or both drugs at the same time.

• The effects of ℞ **alpha-adrenergic stimulants**, ℞ **ergot alkaloids**, ℞ **epinephrine**, and ℞ **lidocaine** may be increased, with the risk of serious adverse effects.

• ℞ **Calcium-channel blockers** (particularly ℞ **diltiazem hydrochloride** and ℞ **verapamil**), ℞ **guanethidine monosulfate**, and ℞ **reserpine** have the potential for increasing undesirable effects, with exaggerated slowing of heartbeat or hypotension. Verapamil and metoprolol should not be used together.

• The effects of nondepolarizing ℞ **skeletal muscle relaxants** may be variable, with the possible risk of significant adverse effects associated with major surgery.

• The effects of ℞ **insulin** and ℞ **sulfonylureas** may be reduced.

• ℞ **Cimetidine** may increase the effect of metoprolol.

• ℞ **Antacids** (for example, ℞ **aluminum hydroxide**, ℞ **magnesium hydroxide**), ℞ **barbiturates**, ♉ **calcium** salts, ℞ **cholestyramine**, ℞ **colestipol hydrochloride**, ℞ NSAIDs, ℞ **penicillins**, ℞ **rifampin**, and ℞ **salicylates** may reduce the levels and effectiveness of beta-blockers.

• If used with ℞ **diuretics** and other antihypertensive drugs, there are additive effects which are often used to therapeutic advantage.

Side effects

These are usually mild and may include:

• Dizziness, fatigue, insomnia, gastrointestinal disturbances (for example, diarrhea, nausea, abdominal pain, constipation), slowing of the heart rate and shortness of breath;

• Less frequently, headache, cold extremities, hypotension, dry mouth, peripheral edema, or mental depression. At higher doses asthma-like symptoms and wheezing may occur;

• Heart failure, should it develop, generally requires withdrawal (gradually, if possible) of this drug.

Metric 21 ⑧

A preparation of ℞ **metronidazole**.
Formulation: Oral tablets.
Availability: Prescription only.
Warnings and side effects: See ℞ **metronidazole**.

MetroGel; MetroLotion ⑧

A preparation of ℞ **metronidazole**.
Formulation: Topical gel; topical lotion.
Availability: Prescription only.
Warnings and side effects: See ℞ **metronidazole**.

MetroGel-Vaginal ⑧

A preparation of ℞ **metronidazole**.
Formulation: Vaginal gel.
Availability: Prescription only.
Warnings and side effects: See ℞ **metronidazole**.

metronidazole ⑥

Type/Group: antimicrobial; antibacterial; amebicide and antiprotozoal; Helicobacter pylori eradication regime; azole; candidiasis treatment.
Brand(s): Flagyl; Metric 21; MetroGel; Metro-Gel-Vaginal; MetroLotion; Noritate; Protostat; various generic.
How administered: Orally; intravenous infusion; topically (external); intravaginal.

Used to treat

Metronidazole is an ℞ **azole** antibacterial used to treat ✪ **bacterial infections**, notably vaginal infections caused by *Gardnerella vaginalis* and is incorporated in *Helicobacter pylori* elimination regimes to eliminate the ulcer-causing organism *Helicobacter pylori*. It is also used for intra-abdominal, skin and skin structure, and lower respiratory tract infections. It acts by interfering with bacterial DNA replication. As an antiprotozoal it is specifically active against the protozoa *Entamoeba histolytica*, which causes ✪ **dysentery**, *Giardia lamblia*, which causes an infection (✪ **giardiasis**) of the small intestine, and *Trichomonas vaginalis*, which causes ✪ **vaginitis**. It may also be used to prevent infections during colorectal surgery. Topically, it is prescribed to treat ✪ **acne**. Although not stated by the manufacturer for such use, it is also prescribed to treat antibiotic-induced ✪ **colitis** and ✪ **Crohn's disease**. (When used externally or intravaginally, some warnings and side effects do not apply.)

Warnings

• It should not be given to people with known hypersensitivity to metronidazole or other nitromidazole derivatives.

• It should be given with caution to people with blood disorders, severe liver dysfunction, CNS (central nervous system) disease, severe kidney failure, or over the age of 65.

• It crosses the placenta. The effects on the fetus are unknown. It should not be used to treat trichomoniasis in the first trimester.

• Medical judgment is required if breast-feeding is being considered. If single-dose therapy is used, discontinue breast-feeding for 12 to 24 hours to allow excretion of the drug.

• This drug is carcinogenic in rodents, and so unnecessary use should be avoided.

• Seizure and other neurological side effects (mainly numbness or tingling of arms or legs, dizziness and incoordination, weakness, or insomnia) may occur, particularly when used at high doses for long periods.

• The use of antibacterials can lead to overgrowth of nonsusceptible organisms, leading to a secondary infection.

• Alcohol must not be drunk while using this drug, or for 24 hours after the last dose. A very unpleasant adverse reaction, including irregular heartbeat, nausea, vomiting, and headache, can occur.

• During treatment for trichomoniasis, intercourse must be avoided or condoms used to prevent reinfection.

Interactions

• ℞ **Barbiturates** may stop metronidazole from being effective.

• ℞ **Cimetidine** may increase levels of metronidazole.

• The effects of ℞ **anticoagulants**, ℞ **hydantoins**, and ℞ **lithium** may be increased.

• ℞ **Disulfiram** taken with metronidazole may cause acute psychosis or a confused state.

• Alcohol may cause unpleasant adverse reactions.

Side effects

These depend on how it is administered.

• Frequently, loss of appetite, nausea, dry mouth, and metallic taste.

• Occasionally, gastrointestinal upsets, dizziness, rash, hives, and discolored urine.

• Rarely, with intravenous use, mild transient changes in blood-cell ratios. With vaginal use, irritation, swelling, abdominal cramps, and uterine pain. With topical use, occasional transient redness, dryness, and irritation.

metyrosine Ⓖ

(metirosine)

Type/Group: **antisympathetic; antihypertensive.**

Brand(s): Demser.

How administered: Orally.

Used to treat

Metyrosine inhibits one of the enzymes (tyrosine hydroxylase) that produce norepinephrine (noradrenaline) and is used in the preoperative treatment of ✪ **pheochromocytoma** (sometimes with an ℞ **alpha-adrenergic blocker**) or to manage the condition when surgery is not possible.

Warnings

• It should not be given to people with known hypersensitivity to this drug.

• It should be given with caution to people with kidney or liver impairment.

• The safety of metyrosine for use during pregnancy has not been established, and it should be used only when clearly needed.

• Medical judgment is required if breast-feeding is being considered.

• Increased fluid intake during treatment is essential. Regular checks on overall blood volume may be carried out.

• Because of possible sedative side effects, caution is advised for potentially hazardous activities, such as driving, that require mental alertness.

• Alcohol should be avoided.

Interactions

• The effects of ℞ **haloperidol** and ℞ **phenothiazines** may be exaggerated.

• If used with alcohol, ℞ **hypnotics**, ℞ **sedatives**, or ℞ **tranquilizers**, increased effects are possible.

Side effects

• The most common are drowsiness and sedation (and there may be insomnia after the drug is discontinued).

• Other side effects may include diarrhea (sometimes severe) and extrapyramidal symptoms (for example, drooling, speech difficulty, tremor).

• Infrequently, swelling of the breasts, nasal stuffiness, dry mouth, headache, gastrointestinal disturbances (for example, nausea, vomiting, abdominal pain), and male sexual dysfunction. Blood or liver changes and hypersensitivity reactions (including hives and swelling in the throat) are rare. Crystals may form in the urine, particularly if fluid intake is insufficient.

Mevacor Ⓑ

A preparation of ℞ **lovastatin**.

Formulation: Oral tablets.

Availability: Prescription only.

Warnings and side effects: See ℞ **lovastatin**.

mexiletine hydrochloride Ⓖ

Type/Group: **antiarrhythmic.**

Brand(s): Mexitil.

How administered: Orally.

Used to treat

Mexiletine hydrochloride is used to regularize the heartbeat, but generally only for life-threatening ✪ **arrhythmias**, especially sustained ventricular tachycardia.

Warnings

• It should not be given to people with known hypersensitivity to this drug, or with certain heart disorders.

• It should be given with caution to people with congestive heart failure or certain heart conduction abnormalities, hypotension, impaired liver function, or a history of seizures. This is a specialist drug and treatment will be carried out by experienced clinicians who are thoroughly familiar with this drug. Periodic monitoring of heart function and blood values is necessary.

• Mexiletine crosses the placenta and so it should be used during pregnancy only if the potential benefit outweighs the possible risk to the fetus.

• It is present in breast milk and nursing women should discontinue using this drug or stop breast-feeding.

• Mexiletine can, occasionally, provoke arrhythmias.

• A doctor must be contacted if such symptoms as general tiredness, jaundice, fever or sore throat (can indicate liver damage) occur.

• Changes in diet that could drastically alter the acidity or alkalinity of the urine must be avoided.

Interactions

• ℞ **Metoclopramide** and ℞ **urinary alkalinizers** (for example, ℞ **sodium bicarbonate**) may raise the levels or intensify the effects of mexiletine.

• The effects and levels of mexiletine are unpredictable when taken with ℞ **cimetidine**.

• ℞ **Atropine**, ℞ **hydantoins**, ℞ **opioids**, ℞ **phenobarbital**, ℞ **rifampin**, urinary acidifiers (for example, ℞ **ammonium chloride**) may reduce the effects of mexiletine.

• The levels of ℞ **caffeine** and ℞ **theophylline** may be increased.

Side effects

• The most serious adverse reactions are arrhythmias, which can be provoked by antiarrhythmic drugs.

• Frequently, gastrointestinal disturbances (for example, nausea, vomiting, heartburn, diarrhea), tremor, dizziness, nervousness, sleep disturbances, incoordination, and palpitations.

• Other effects include headache, blurred vision, tingling or numbness, rash, breathlessness, or mental difficulty (for example, speech problems, confusion, short-term memory loss, depression).

• There may be effects on blood pressure. Liver damage has been reported, though it is rare.

Mexitil ℬ

A preparation of ℞ **mexiletine hydrochloride**.
Formulation: Oral capsules (3 strengths).
Availability: Prescription only.
Warnings and side effects: See ℞ **mexiletine hydrochloride**.

Mexsana Medicated ℬ

A preparation of ℞ **zinc oxide**, ℞ **camphor**, and ℞ **kaolin**.
Formulation: Topical powder.
Availability: OTC.
Warnings and side effects: See ℞ **zinc oxide**; ℞ **camphor**; ℞ **kaolin**.

Mezlin ℬ

A preparation of ℞ **mezlocillin**.
Formulation: Injection; intravenous infusion.
Availability: Prescription only.
Warnings and side effects: See ℞ **mezlocillin**.

mezlocillin Ⓖ

Type/Group: **antibiotic; penicillin; antibacterial**.
Brand(s): Mezlin.
How administered: Injection; intravenous infusion.

Used to treat

Mezlocillin is a synthetic penicillin used to treat ✪ **bacterial infections**. It is active against a number of important Gram-negative bacteria, including *Pseudomonas aeruginosa*. It can be used to treat ✪ **septicemia**, ✪ **peritonitis**, infections of the respiratory and urinary tracts, gynecological infections, and for preventing infection during surgical procedures.

Warnings

• It should not be used by people with known hypersensitivity to penicillins.

• It should be given with caution to people with allergies to ℞ **cephalosporins** or ℞ **imipenem**, impaired kidney function, or those who must restrict their sodium intake.

• Penicillins cross the placenta and should be used in pregnancy only if medically judged to be needed.

• Medical judgment is also required for breast-feeding mothers.

• Serious and occasionally fatal hypersensitivity reactions can occur.

• There will be monitoring (for example, blood, kidney, liver) during prolonged treatment.

• Superinfections from the altered bacterial balance created by antibiotic treatment may occur and may result in ✪ **pseudomembranous colitis**. A doctor must be contacted if there is severe abdominal pain, or moderate to severe diarrhea.

Interactions

• The effects of ℞ **aminoglycosides** may be reduced.

• ℞ **Chloramphenicol**, ℞ **macrolide** antibiotics, and ℞ **tetracyclines** may reduce the effectiveness of penicillin.

• Large doses of penicillin may increase levels of ℞ **methotrexate**.

Side effects

• Frequently, rash, hives, pain at injection site, thrombophlebitis when given by intravenous infusion.

• Occasionally, nausea, vomiting, diarrhea, elevated sodium levels. Rarely, bleeding with high intravenous dosage, depressed potassium levels, headache, fatigue, and dizziness.

• Rare but serious effects include kidney infection and seizure.

MG 217 Medicated Tar ℬ

A preparation of ℞ **coal tar**.
Formulation: Shampoo; ointment.
Availability: OTC.
Warnings and side effects: See ℞ **coal tar**.

MG217 Medicated Tar-Free Shampoo; MG400 ℬ

A preparation of ℞ **salicylic acid** and ℞ **sulfur**.
Formulation: Shampoo.
Availability: OTC.
Warnings and side effects: See ℞ **salicylic acid**; ℞ **sulfur**.

MG217 Sal-Acid Ointment ℬ

A preparation of ℞ **salicylic acid** and ⚕ **vitamin E**.
Formulation: Topical ointment.
Availability: OTC.
Warnings and side effects: See ℞ **salicylic acid**; ⚕ **vitamin E**.

Miacalcin ℬ

A preparation of ℞ **calcitonin-salmon**.
Formulation: Injection; nasal spray.
Availability: Prescription only.
Warnings and side effects: See ℞ **calcitonin-salmon**.

Mi-Acid Gelcaps ℬ

A preparation of ℞ **calcium carbonate** and ℞ **magnesium carbonate**.

Formulation: Oral gelcaps.
Availability: OTC.
Warnings and side effects: See ℞ **calcium carbonate**; ℞ **magnesium carbonate.**

Mi-Acid II Liquid ⑧

A preparation of ℞ **aluminum hydroxide,** ℞ **magnesium hydroxide,** and ℞ **simethicone.**
Formulation: Oral liquid.
Availability: OTC.
Warnings and side effects: See ℞ **aluminum hydroxide;** ℞ **magnesium hydroxide;** ℞ **simethicone.**

Mi-Acid Liquid ⑧

A preparation of ℞ **aluminum hydroxide,** ℞ **magnesium hydroxide,** and ℞ **simethicone.**
Formulation: Oral liquid.
Availability: OTC.
Warnings and side effects: See ℞ **aluminum hydroxide;** ℞ **magnesium hydroxide;** ℞ **simethicone.**

Micanol ⑧

A preparation of ℞ **anthralin.**
Formulation: Topical cream.
Availability: Prescription only.
Warnings and side effects: See ℞ **anthralin.**

Micatin ⑧

A preparation of ℞ **miconazole.**
Formulation: Topical powder; topical spray powder; topical liquid spray.
Availability: OTC.
Warnings and side effects: See ℞ **miconazole.**

miconazole ⑥

Type/Group: **antifungal; azole.**
Brand(s): **Femizole; Micatin; Monistat.**
How administered: Topically (external).

Used to treat
Miconazole is a synthetic imidazole/azole antifungal drug used to treat vaginal ⊙ **candidiasis** infections and skin infections, including ringworm (see ⊙ **fungal infections**).

Warnings
• It should not be given to people with known hypersensitivity to miconazole.
• No adverse effects from use during pregnancy have been reported. It should, however, be used during pregnancy only if the benefits outweigh the risk to the fetus.
• Medical judgment is required if breast-feeding is being considered. It is not known if this drug appears in breast milk.
• The vaginal suppository must not be used with contraceptive diaphragms or condoms, as it may damage latex.

Interactions
None significant have been reported when used topically (externally).

Side effects
• Burning, irritation, itching, rash, and pelvic cramps.

Micronase ⑧

A preparation of ℞ **glyburide.**
Formulation: Oral tablets in several strengths.
Availability: Prescription only.
Warnings and side effects: See ℞ **glyburide.**

microNefrin ⑧

A preparation of racepinephrine.
Formulation: Solution for inhalation.
Availability: OTC.
Warnings and side effects: See ℞ **epinephrine.**

Micronor ⑧

A preparation of ℞ **norethindrone.**
Formulation: Oral tablets.
Availability: Prescription only.
Warnings and side effects: See ℞ **norethindrone.**

Microzide Capsules ⑧

A preparation of ℞ **hydrochlorothiazide.**
Formulation: Oral capsules.
Availability: Prescription only.
Warnings and side effects: See ℞ **hydrochlorothiazide.**

Midamor ⑧

A preparation of ℞ **amiloride.**
Formulation: Oral tablets.
Availability: Prescription only.
Warnings and side effects: See ℞ **amiloride.**

midazolam ⑥

Type/Group: **sedatives; benzodiazepine.**
Brand(s): **Versed.**
How administered: Orally, injection.

Used to treat
Midazolam can be used as a sedative in preoperative medication, because its ability to cause amnesia means that any unpleasant procedures are forgotten. It is also used in the induction of general anesthesia and as a sedative for diagnostic procedures such as endoscopy. Because it has been associated with respiratory depression and arrest, it is used only in a hospital or medical facility.

Warnings
• It should not be given to people with known hypersensitivity to benzodiazepines, anyone in shock, coma, intoxicated with alcohol, or with acute narrow-angle glaucoma.
• It should be given with caution to people with chronic obstructive pulmonary disease (COPD), congestive heart failure, chronic kidney failure, liver disease, myasthenia gravis and related diseases, in a weakened condition, or over 65.
• Midazolam is not recommended for use during pregnancy. Its use in the first trimester should almost always be avoided. A doctor

must be contacted if pregnancy occurs while this drug is being taken.

• Medical judgment is required if breast-feeding is being considered.

• It has an additive effect with other CNS (central nervous system) depressants, such as alcohol. The doctor must be told if such substances have been used near the time of administration.

• It is a specialist drug and will be used under controlled conditions.

Interactions

• R Calcium-channel blockers, R erythromycin, R ketoconazole, and R itraconazole increase the levels of midazolam, sedation, and respiratory depression.

• Intensified effects will occur if used with CNS (central nervous system) depressants (for example, R **barbiturates**, R **narcotic analgesics**, alcohol).

Side effects

• Depending on the use, how it is administered, and dose, there may be anxiety, confusion, euphoria, headache, insomnia, slurred speech, tremors, weakness, tingling or burning sensation, heartbeat changes, blocked ears and loss of balance, eye changes, hiccups, increased salivation, nausea, vomiting, breathing irregularities, skin reaction at injection site, and hives.

• Rare but serious effects include respiratory depression and spasm of the bronchi or larynx.

midodrine hydrochloride Ⓖ

Type/Group: **vasoconstrictor; alpha-adrenergic stimulant; sympathomimetic.**

Brand(s): ProAmatine.

How administered: Orally.

Used to treat

Midodrine is used primarily to treat postural hypotension (orthostatic hypotension; lowered blood pressure on standing) that is serious enough to impair quality of life and which cannot be managed in other ways (for example, support hose or lifestyle changes). Midodrine is itself a prodrug—there is little or no therapeutic effect until it is broken down in the body to its more active metabolite, desglymidodrine, which is an alpha-adrenergic stimulant.

Warnings

• It should not be given to people with known hypersensitivity to this drug, or with severe heart or kidney disease, urinary retention, pheochromocytoma, thyrotoxicosis, or excessively high blood pressure when lying down.

• It should be given with caution to people with diabetes mellitus, visual problems, or liver or kidney impairment.

• Midodrine should be used during pregnancy only if the potential benefit outweighs the possible risk to the fetus.

• Medical judgment is required if breast-feeding is being considered.

• Liver and kidney function will be checked before beginning treatment and at appropriate intervals afterwards.

Interactions

• There is a potential for adverse effects on heart rhythm (sometimes serious) if taken with other alpha adrenergic stimulants (for example, R **phenylephrine**, R **ephedrine**), R **beta-blockers**,

R **cardiac glycosides**, R **corticosteroids** (for example, R **fludrocortisone**), R **ergot alkaloids** (for example, R **ergonovine**, R **ergotamine**), R **MAOIs**, and R **tricyclics**.

• R **Alpha-adrenergic blockers** (for example, R **doxazosin**, R **prazosin**) may reverse or reduce the therapeutic effects of midodrine.

• Variable interactions are possible with R **flecainide**, R H$_2$-antagonists (for example, R **cimetidine**, R **ranitidine**), R **metformin**, R **procainamide**, R **quinidine**, and R **triamterene** (these drugs are broken down in similar ways in the body).

Side effects

• The most common are tingling sensations, goosebumps, urinary problems, itching, increased blood pressure when lying down, chills, various pains, and rash.

• Less frequently, there may be headache, a feeling of fullness in the head, facial flushing, confusion or anxiety, and dry mouth.

• Rarely, visual disturbances, sleep problems, weakness, and gastrointestinal distress have been reported.

Midol Maximum Strength Menstrual Caplets, Geltabs Ⓑ

A preparation of R **acetaminophen**, R **caffeine**, and R **pyrilamine maleate**.

Formulation: Oral tablets; geltabs.

Availability: OTC.

Warnings and side effects: See R **acetaminophen**; R **pyrilamine maleate**; R **caffeine**.

Midol Maximum Strength PMS Caplets, Geltabs Ⓑ

A preparation of R **acetaminophen**, pamabrom, and R **pyrilamine maleate**.

Formulation: Oral tablets; geltabs.

Availability: OTC.

Warnings and side effects: See R **acetaminophen**; R **pyrilamine maleate**.

Midrin Ⓑ

A preparation of R **isometheptene mucate**, R **acetaminophen**, and dichloralphenazone.

Formulation: Oral capsules.

Availability: Prescription only.

Warnings and side effects: See R **isometheptene mucate**; R **acetaminophen**.

Mifeprex Ⓑ

A preparation of R **mifepristone**.

Formulation: Oral tablets.

Availability: Prescription only.

Warnings and side effects: See R **mifepristone**.

mifepristone Ⓖ

(RU 486)

Type/Group: **abortifacient.**

Key to symbols: ✪ = Disorder Section   R = Drug Section   ♣ = Herbal Section   ⌀⌀ = Supplement Section

Brand(s): Mifeprex.
How administered: Orally.

Used to treat
Mifepristone is used as an abortifacient for termination of uterine pregnancy. It is taken by mouth under medical supervision and often with another method of termination, a synthetic ℞ **prostaglandin**, ℞ **misoprostol**.

Warnings
• It should not be given to people with a history of allergy to mifepristone, with confirmed or suspected ectopic pregnancy, undiagnosed mass on uterine appendage, an IUD (intrauterine device) in place, chronic adrenal failure, hemorrhagic disorder, inherited porphyria, or those undergoing anticoagulant or long-term corticosteroid therapy. It is a specialist drug and a full assessment of patient suitability with counseling will be made.
• It should be given with caution to people with heart, hypertensive, liver, respiratory or kidney disease, diabetes mellitus, severe anemia, or heavy smokers.
• Mifepristone should not be used during pregnancy except when used as an abortifacient.
• Medical judgment is required if breast-feeding is being considered.
• Administration of the drug must be in a location with access to appropriate emergency medical care.
• The treatment schedule, including follow-up doctor's visit, must be kept to.
• Vaginal bleeding and uterine cramping probably will occur.
• If the treatment fails, surgical termination will be needed.
• If treatment fails, there is a risk of fetal malformation.
• Contraception must be used as soon as termination has been confirmed.

Interactions
• ℞ **Ketoconazole**, ℞ **itraconazole**, ℞ **erythromycin**, and grapefruit juice: may increase blood levels of mifepristone.
• ℞ **Rifampin**, ℞ **dexamethasone**, ♣ **St. John's wort**, and certain ℞ **anticonvulsants** (for example, ℞ **phenytoin**, ℞ **phenobarbital**) may lower blood levels of mifepristone.
• Avoid using ℞ **NSAIDs** for 8 to 12 days after mifepristone.

Side effects
• Uterine pain, nausea and vomiting, faintness, rash, and infections of the uterus and urinary tract.

miglitol Ⓖ
Type/Group: **antidiabetic; oral hypoglycemic**.
Brand(s): Glyset.
How administered: Orally.

Used to treat
Miglitol is a non-sulfonylurea (it is an alpha-glucosidase inhibitor) used to treat type 2 ☉ **diabetes mellitus**, alone or in with a ℞ **sulfonylurea**.

Warnings
• It should not be given to people with ketoacidosis, certain bowel diseases, or hypersensitivity to the drug in any of its forms.
• It should be given with caution to people with kidney function impairment.

• Its safety in pregnancy is not established. It should be used only if clearly needed.
• It is not recommended for use while breast-feeding.
• It does not cause hypoglycemia, but has the potential for increasing hypoglycemic response induced by sulfonylureas when the two are used in combination.

Interactions
• The effects of ℞ **digoxin**, ℞ **glyburide**, ℞ **metformin**, ℞ **propranolol**, and ℞ **ranitidine** may be reduced by miglitol.
• ℞ **Digestive enzymes** and intestinal adsorbents may reduce the effects of miglitol.

Side effects
• Transient skin rash, flatulence, diarrhea, and abdominal pain. Gastrointestinal effects tend to diminish with continued treatment.

migraine treatment Ⓓ
see ℞ **antimigraine**.

Migranol Ⓑ
A preparation of ℞ **dihydroergotamine mesylate**.
Formulation: Nasal spray.
Availability: Prescription only.
Warnings and side effects: See ℞ **dihydroergotamine mesylate**.

Milkinol Ⓑ
A preparation of ℞ **mineral oil**.
Formulation: Oral emulsion.
Availability: OTC.
Warnings and side effects: See ℞ **mineral oil**.

Milophene Ⓑ
A preparation of ℞ **clomiphene citrate**.
Formulation: Oral tablets.
Availability: Prescription only.
Warnings and side effects: See ℞ **clomiphene citrate**.

milrinone Ⓖ
Type/Group: **phosphodiesterase inhibitor; heart failure treatment; cardiac stimulant**.
Brand(s): Primacor.
How administered: Intravenous infusion.

Used to treat
Milrinone is used in the short-term (48 hours or less) treatment of congestive ☉ **heart failure** (especially where other drugs have been unsuccessful).

Warnings
• It should not be given to people with known hypersensitivity to this drug, or who have had a recent heart attack, or with certain kinds of heart valve disease.
• It should be given with special caution to people with arrhythmias not controlled by ℞ **digoxin**, or when previous ℞ **diuretic** treatment may have failed.
• Milrinone should be used during pregnancy only if the potential benefit outweighs the possible risk to the fetus.

• Medical judgment is required if breast-feeding is being considered. It is not known whether this drug appears in breast milk.

• It is only used in a medical facility, with close monitoring of heart function and electrolytes. Serious arrhythmias are possible.

Interactions

No interactions of significance are known, but experience with this drug is still limited.

Side effects

• There may be irregular heartbeats, hypotension, headache, or chest pain.

Miltown ®

A preparation of ℞ **meprobamate.**
Formulation: Oral tablets in several strengths.
Availability: Prescription only.
Warnings and side effects: See ℞ **meprobamate.**

mineral oil ©

(liquid paraffin)

Type/Group: **emollient; laxative.**

Brand(s): Fleet Mineral Oil; Kondremul Plain; Liqui-Doss; Milkinol; various generic. Combinations: With *aluminum hydroxide*: Nephrox Liquid. With *magnesium hydroxide*: Haley's M-O.

How administered: Orally; topically.

Used to treat

Mineral oil is a traditional (stool-softener) laxative which can be used to relieve ✪ **constipation**. It is also used in many skin treatment preparations as an emollient.

Warnings

When taken orally:

• It should not be given to people with gastrointestinal disorders such as gastrointestinal obstruction.

• In general, mineral oil taken orally should be avoided during pregnancy, except on advice of a doctor.

• Medical judgment is required if breast-feeding is being considered.

• A doctor must be consulted first before taking any other medication (including OTCs, herbal remedies, and supplements), because laxatives may alter the absorption of a wide range drugs.

• It is not a good idea to take mineral oil in a reclining position, because if taken into the lungs it may cause an inflammation (particularly among young children, the elderly, or debilitated).

• Do not use if there is abdominal pain, nausea, or vomiting, unless directed by a doctor.

• It should not be used by people with hemorrhoids or an anal fissures.

• Chronic use of laxatives may cause fluid and electrolyte imbalances, vitamin and mineral deficiencies, and abnormal bowel function. Generally, they should not be used for more than a week.

Interactions

When taken orally:

• If used with other stool softeners (for example, ℞ **docusate sodium**), there may be increased absorption of mineral oil, with adverse effects. docusate sodium and mineral oil should not be used together.

• Mineral oil may interfere with the antibacterial effects of nonabsorbable ℞ **sulfonamides.**

• The absorption of ℞ **oral contraceptives** and ℞ **warfarin sodium** may be lower, reducing their effectiveness.

• Prolonged use of mineral oil may cause a deficiency of carotene and fat-soluble vitamins (♋ **vitamin A**, ♋ **vitamin D**, ♋ **vitamin E**, and ♋ **vitamin K**).

Side effects

• Because only a little of the mineral oil is absorbed in the intestines, seepage may occur from the rectum, causing local irritation, itching, hemorrhoids, and soiling of clothes.

• Used externally, in emollient preparations, no significant side effects are known.

Minipress ®

A preparation of ℞ **prazosin hydrochloride.**
Formulation: Oral capsules, available in 3 strengths.
Availability: Prescription only.
Warnings and side effects: See ℞ **prazosin hydrochloride.**

Mini Thin Asthma Relief Tablets ®

A preparation of ℞ **ephedrine** and ℞ **guaifenesin.**
Formulation: Oral tablets.
Availability: OTC.
Warnings and side effects: See ℞ **ephedrine**; ℞ **guaifenesin.**

Mini Thin Pseudo Tablets ®

A preparation of ℞ **pseudoephedrine.**
Formulation: Oral tablets.
Availability: OTC.
Warnings and side effects: See ℞ **pseudoephedrine.**

Minitran ®

A preparation of ℞ **nitroglycerin.**
Formulation: Transdermal patch, available in 4 release rates.
Availability: Prescription only.
Warnings and side effects: See ℞ **nitroglycerin.**

Minit-Rub ®

A preparation of ℞ **methyl salicylate**, ℞ **camphor**, ℞ **menthol**, and various.
Formulation: Topical ointment.
Availability: OTC.
Warnings and side effects: See ℞ **methyl salicylate**; ℞ **camphor**; ℞ **menthol.**

Minocin ®

A preparation of ℞ **minocycline.**
Formulation: Oral capsules in several strengths; oral suspension; injection.
Availability: Prescription only.
Warnings and side effects: See ℞ **minocycline.**

Key to symbols: ✪ = Disorder Section ℞ = Drug Section ♣ = Herbal Section ♋ = Supplement Section

minocycline Ⓖ

Type/Group: **tetracycline; antibiotic**.
Brand(s): Dynacin; Minocin; Vectrin; various generic.
How administered: Orally; injection.

Used to treat

Minocycline has a wider range of action than most other tetracyclines, and is used to treat many infections including ✚ **syphilis**, ✚ **conjunctivitis**, ✚ **trachoma**, ✚ **acne**, and rickettsial infections such as ✚ **Rocky Mountain spotted fever**. It is also effective in treating certain forms of ✚ **meningitis** (caused by *Neisseria meningitidis*).

Warnings

• It should not be given to people with known hypersensitivity to tetracyclines, or to children under 8 years of age.

• It should be given with caution to people with kidney or liver impairment.

• Minocycline should be avoided in the last half of pregnancy, because of the risk of dental staining and inhibiting the skeletal growth of the fetus.

• It should be avoided by nursing mothers.

• It may cause dizziness and so impair the performance of skilled tasks such as driving.

• Superinfections due to the altered bacterial balance caused by antibiotic treatment may occur. A doctor must be contacted if severe abdominal pain, moderate to severe diarrhea, or any new or unusual symptoms occur.

• It may cause photosensitivity reactions (abnormal sensitivity to sunlight), so exposure to sunlight must be minimized.

• It may cause permanent discoloration of teeth and the thin tooth enamel in children from the time of tooth formation, which begins in the uterus and ends at the age of 8. It may also retard bone development during the same period.

• It must not be used after the discard date, as it becomes harmful to the kidneys as it degrades.

Interactions

• ℞ **Antacids**, ℞ **barbiturates**, ℞ **bismuth subsalicylate**, ⚕ **iron**, ℞ **cholestyramine**, and ℞ **colestipol hydrochloride** may decrease the absorption of tetracyclines.

• The levels of ℞ **digoxin** may be reduced.

• The effects of ℞ **penicillin** are impaired.

• The effectiveness of ℞ **oral contraceptives** may be reduced.

• ℞ **Carbamazepine** and ℞ **phenytoin** may decrease concentrations of minocycline.

• If taken with methoxyflurane, there is a risk of kidney damage.

Side effects

• Frequently, dizziness, lightheadedness, and gastrointestinal effects (diarrhea, nausea, vomiting).

• Occasionally, darkening of the skin, itching, and sore mouth or tongue.

• Rarely, serious blood and skin disorders.

minor tranquilizer Ⓓ

see ℞ antianxiety.

minoxidil Ⓖ

Type/Group: **antihypertensive; vasodilator; hair-growth promoter**.
Brand(s): (Oral use): Loniten; various generic. (Topical use): Rogaine; Minoxidil for Men.
How administered: Orally; topically (external).

Used to treat

Minoxidil is used to treat severe ✚ **hypertension** that cannot be controlled by a combination of other drugs, and it is always given with other drugs In topical application it is used to treat ✚ **alopecia**—hair loss that occurs as "male pattern baldness" in men and as hair thinning around the forehead and temples in women. Signs of new hair growth generally take 4 months or more to appear.

Warnings

These depend on the route of adminsitration and use.

• It should not be given to people with known hypersensitivity to this drug, with pheochromocytoma or who have had a recent heart attack.

• It should be given with caution to people with congestive heart failure, coronary artery disease, or significant kidney impairment. Topical use is not ruled out by such conditions unless evidence of systemic effects appears (for example, rapid heart rate, fluid retention).

• Minoxidil's safety during pregnancy has not been established when used orally, and it should be used only if the potential benefit outweighs the possible risk to the fetus. If used topically, it should not be used during pregnancy.

• Medical judgment is required if breast-feeding is being considered (for oral and topical use).

• A doctor must be contacted if the pulse rate increases by 20 or more beats per minute above normal, if breathing becomes difficult (especially when lying down), or symptoms such as dizziness, fainting, edema or angina pectoris occur (when used for hypertension).

• This is a powerful drug with potential effects on heart muscle, heart conduction, and fluid and electrolyte balance. Appropriate monitoring is necessary when used for hypertension.

• Minoxidil may cause enhanced growth, thickening, and darkening of fine body hair.

• It should not be applied to broken or inflamed skin (for example, psoriasis or sunburn), and contact with the eyes or mucous membranes should be avoided. It should not be used with agents that might enhance absorption through the skin (for example, corticosteroids, retinoids, or petrolatum).

Interactions

These apply to oral use only, as there are no known interactions when used topically.

• ℞ **guanethidine monosulfate** should not be used with minoxidil, because profound postural hypotension (lowered blood pressure on standing) is possible.

• If used with other antihypertensives and ℞ **diuretics**, the effects of these drugs may be increased. This additive effect is sometimes used to advantage in combination treatments for high blood pressure.

Side effects
• Oral use: Fluid retention, rapid heartbeat, growth, and darkening of body hair. Rarely, breast tenderness or growth (in males), changes in skin pigmentation, menstrual disorders, headache, nausea, vomiting, or rash. Serious adverse effects involving heart muscle or conduction and fluid build-up may occur.
• Topical use: Skin reactions and irritation, and allergy (for example, hives, facial swelling).

Mintezol ®
A preparation of ℞ **thiabendazole**.
Formulation: Chewable tablets; oral suspension.
Availability: Prescription only.
Warnings and side effects: See ℞ **thiabendazole**.

Mintox Plus Tablets; Mintox Plus Extra Strength Liquid ®
A preparation of ℞ **aluminum hydroxide**, ℞ **magnesium hydroxide**, and ℞ **simethicone**.
Formulation: Oral tablets; liquid.
Availability: OTC.
Warnings and side effects: See ℞ **aluminum hydroxide**; ℞ **magnesium hydroxide**; ℞ **simethicone**.

Mintox Tablets; Suspension ®
A preparation of ℞ **aluminum hydroxide** and ℞ **magnesium hydroxide**.
Formulation: Oral tablets, chewable; liquid.
Availability: OTC.
Warnings and side effects: See ℞ **aluminum hydroxide**; ℞ **magnesium hydroxide**.

Miochol-E ®
A preparation of ℞ **acetylcholine chloride**.
Formulation: Solution for injection.
Availability: Prescription only.
Warnings and side effects: See ℞ **acetylcholine chloride**.

Miostat ®
A preparation of ℞ **carbachol**.
Formulation: Ophthalmic solution.
Availability: Prescription only.
Warnings and side effects: See ℞ **carbachol**.

miotic ⑩
Generics: **carbachol; pilocarpine**.
Actions and uses
Miotic drugs constrict the pupil of the eye and are used mainly in ℞ **glaucoma treatment**. The only ones used regularly (as eye-drops) are the ℞ **parasympathomimetic** drugs ℞ **carbachol** and ℞ **pilocarpine**, and the ℞ **anticholinesterase** drug ℞ **echothiophate iodide**. They lower intraocular pressure (pressure in the eyeball) by opening up inefficient drainage channels in the trabecular meshwork in the front chamber of the eye, which are caused

by contraction or spasm of the ciliary muscle, and a small pupil is an unfortunate side effect.
Limitations
The small pupil may cause problems with dark adaptation, so care should be taken while driving at night or performing tasks in poor light. Also, there may be browache and headache, which may get worse in the weeks following treatment. See also the individual drug entries.
A number of other types of drug may cause miosis as an undesirable side effect, notably (℞ **opioid**) ℞ **narcotic analgesic** drugs.

Miradon ®
A preparation of ℞ **anisindione**.
Formulation: Oral tablets.
Availability: Prescription only.
Warnings and side effects: See ℞ **anisindione**.

Mirapex ®
A preparation of ℞ **pramipexole**.
Formulation: Oral tablets in several strengths.
Availability: Prescription only.
Warnings and side effects: See ℞ **pramipexole**.

Mircette ®
A preparation of ℞ **ethinyl estradiol**, and desogestrel (℞ **progestin**).
Formulation: Calendar pack of oral tablets.
Availability: Prescription only.
Warnings and side effects: See ℞ **ethinyl estradiol**; ℞ **progestin**.

mirtazapine hydrochloride ⑥
Type/Group: **antidepressant**.
Brand(s): Remeron.
How administered: Orally.
Used to treat
Mirtazapine hydrochloride can be used to treat depressive illness (see ✪ **depression**). It is an "atypical" antidepressant that works by increasing brain neurotransmission of noradrenaline and serotonin (5-HT). It causes sedation during initial treatment. Although not stated by the manufacturer for such treatment, it is sometimes used for preoperative insomnia. As is the case with other antidepressants, this drug is also being evaluated for other uses.
Warnings
• It should not be given to people with known hypersensitivity to this drug, or to anyone who is taking or has stopped taking a ℞ **MAOI** antidepressant in the previous 14 days.
• It should be given with caution to people with kidney or liver impairment, epilepsy, heart disorders, or low blood pressure, a history of seizures, stroke, urinary retention, glaucoma, diabetes mellitus, psychosis, or bipolar disorder (manic depression), and to anyone over the age of 65.
• Mirtazapine should be used during pregnancy only if the benefits outweigh the possible risk to the fetus.
• Medical judgment is required if breast-feeding is being considered.

Key to symbols: ✪ = Disorder Section ℞ = Drug Section ♣ = Herbal Section ⬭⬭ = Supplement Section

• A doctor must be contacted if signs of infection, such as fever, chills or sore throat, develop during treatment.

• A doctor should be consulted before taking any other medications, including OTC preparations, herbal remedies, supplements, or other natural or alternative products.

• Do not drink alcohol.

• Because of its sedative effects it may impair the performance of skilled tasks requiring mental alertness or physical skills, such as driving.

• Treatment should be stopped gradually, lowering the dose over a period of time.

Interactions

• Serious or even fatal reactions can occur if ℞ **MAOI** antidepressants are taken at the same time, or within a period of a few weeks after the use of, other antidepressants.

• If used with ℞ **diazepam** and similar drugs, motor skills may be impaired.

• Alcohol can add to the impairment of motor and cognitive effects caused by mirtazapine.

Side effects

• Sedation, drowsiness, dizziness, increased appetite and weight gain, and dry mouth.

• Less commonly, changed liver enzymes or jaundice (treatment should be stopped).

• Rarely, edema, white blood cell disorders, seizures, and postural hypotension (lowered blood pressure on standing).

misoprostol ⓖ

Type/Group: **prostaglandin; ulcer-healing drug.**
Brand(s): Cytotec.
How administered: Orally.

Used to treat

Misoprostol is a synthetic analog of the ℞ **prostaglandin** E_1 (℞ **alprostadil**). It can be used as a peptic ✪ **ulcer**-healing drug, because it inhibits acid secretion and promotes protective blood flow to the mucosal layer of the intestine. It cannot be used to treat indigestion, but it can be very useful in protecting against stomach ulcers caused by ℞ **NSAIDs** and for this reason it is now available in combination with some (NSAID) ℞ **non-narcotic analgesic** and ℞ **antirheumatic** drugs (for example, ℞ **Arthrotec**) used in the treatment of rheumatic disease where stomach ulcers may result from treatment.

Warnings

• It should not be given to people with known hypersensitivity to this drug, or to any prostaglandin.

• Misoprostol may cause miscarriage. It should not be used during pregnancy and should be prescribed to women with child-bearing ability only when effective contraception is used.

• It is not known whether this drug appears in breast milk, but there is reason to believe its effects would be harmful.

• It does not prevent duodenal ulcers that may be caused by NSAIDs (only effective in the prevention of stomach ulcers).

• It is not effective against the gastrointestinal pain or discomfort associated with NSAIDs.

Interactions

• The concentration of misoprostol is reduced when taken together with food or ℞ **antacids**.

Side effects

• Diarrhea (which may be severe), nausea, flatulence and vomiting, abdominal pain, indigestion, headache, menstrual irregularities, dizziness, and rashes.

mitomycin ⓖ

Type/Group: **anticancer; cytotoxic.**
Brand(s): Mutamycin.
How administered: Injection.

Used to treat

Mitomycin is used to treat ✪ **cancers** of the upper intestinal tract, and, although not stated by the manufacturer for such use, it may be prescribed for bladder and other cancers.

Warnings

• It should not be given to people with known hypersensitivity to mitomycin, certain blood disorders, coagulation disorders, or increased bleeding tendencies from other causes.

• It should be given with caution to people with impaired kidney function, or lung disorders or infections. This is a specialist drug which will be used following a full evaluation by specialist physicians.

• Mitomycin is not recommended for use during pregnancy unless it is medically judged to be essential, because it may cause birth defects. Becoming pregnant while using this drug must be avoided.

• It should not be used if breast-feeding.

• It can cause marked bone marrow depression, which may lead to bleeding and a reduced resistance to infection.

• It is is associated with impairment of kidney function.

• In common with many anticancer drugs, it may cause cancer or genetic mutations in cells.

• Hemolytic uremic syndrome (a serious complication of chemotherapy) has occurred with this drug.

Interactions

• ℞ **Vinca alkaloids** may cause acute respiratory distress.

Side effects

• Frequently, fever, anorexia, nausea, and vomiting.

• Occasionally, inflammation of mouth mucosa, numbness of fingers or toes, purple bands on nails, skin rash, loss of hair, and unusual tiredness.

• Rarely, bloody vomiting and lung disorders.

mitoxantrone ⓖ

Type/Group: **anticancer; cytotoxic.**
Brand(s): Novantrone.
How administered: Intravenous infusion.

Used to treat

Mitoxantrone is a cytotoxic (an anthracycline antibiotic in origin) that is chemically related to ℞ **doxorubicin hydrochloride**. It is used to treat ✪ **leukemia**, and, although not stated by the manufacturer for such use, it is also prescribed for other cancers, for example, ✪ **breast cancer**.

Warnings

• It should not be given to people with a history of allergy to mitoxantrone.

• It should be given with caution to people with pre-existing bone marrow depression. This is a specialist drug which will be used following a full evaluation by specialist physicians.

• Mitoxantrone is not recommended for use during pregnancy unless it is medically judged to be essential, because it may cause birth defects. Becoming pregnant while using this drug must be avoided.

• It should not be used if breast-feeding.

• It can produce severely depressed bone marrow function. A doctor must be contacted if signs or symptoms of bleeding or infection occur.

• It may cause adverse changes in heart function, including congestive heart failure.

• It may cause cancer or genetic mutations in cells.

• Urine or the whites of the eyes may be discolored.

Interactions

No interactions specific to this drug are known.

Side effects

• Frequently, nausea and vomiting, fever, hair loss, other gastrointestinal effects, bleeding, CNS (central nervous system) effects, inflammation of mouth mucosa or stomach lining, cough, shortness of breath, easy bruising, and fungal infection.

Mivacron ®

A preparation of ℞ **mivacurium**.
Formulation: Injection.
Availability: Prescription only.
Warnings and side effects: See ℞ **mivacurium**.

mivacurium ©

Type/Group: **skeletal muscle relaxant**.
Brand(s): Mivacron.
How administered: Injection.

Used to treat

Mivacurium is a non-depolarizing neuromuscular blocking agent used as a skeletal muscle relaxant to induce muscle paralysis during surgery or mechanical ventilation.

Warnings

• It should not be given to people with known hypersensitivity to the drug.

• It should be given with caution to people with certain heart and neuromuscular diseases, electrolyte imbalances, dehydration, kidney, liver, or lung disorders, or other conditions where histamine release is contraindicated.

• Mivacurium should be used during pregnancy only if the benefits outweigh the risk to the fetus.

• Medical judgment is required if breast-feeding is being considered.

• It must be given by trained personnel in hospitals only.

Interactions

• ℞ **Cholinesterase inhibitors** (for example, ℞ **neostigmine**), ℞ **antibiotics**, ℞ **local anesthetics**, cardiovascular drugs,

℞ **calcium-channel blockers**, ℞ **corticosteroids**, and ℞ **thiazide** diuretics may enhance neuromuscular blocking.

• ℞ **Carbamazepine** and ℞ **phenytoin** may reduce the effects of mivacurium.

Side effects

• Flushing, rash, hives, allergic reaction, spasm of the bronchi or larynx, wheezing, speeded heart beat, and arrhythmias.

• Rarely, malignant hyperthermia (a metabolic disorder).

M-M-R II ®

A preparation of ℞ **MMR vaccine**.
Formulation: Subcutaneous injection.
Availability: Prescription only.
Warnings and side effects: See ℞ **MMR vaccine**.

MMR vaccine ©

(measles-mumps-rubella virus vaccine, live)
Type/Group: **vaccine**.
Brand(s): M-M-R II.
How administered: Subcutaneous injection.

Used to treat

MMR is a combined (polyvalent) vaccine used for active immunization, which uses live but weakened (attenuated) strains of the viruses. It was introduced with the objective of eliminating ⊕ **rubella** (German measles), ⊕ **mumps**, and ⊕ **measles** through universal vaccination of children before they began school. The first dose is given to children at 12 to 15 months, with a booster at four to six years. It is also given in the control of outbreaks of measles, and to susceptible children within three days of exposure to infection (measles only). Although vaccines are available to immunize individually against these infections, the combined form is preferred.

Warnings

• It should not be given to people with known hypersensitivity to any component of this vaccine (including gelatin) or who have exhibited immediate, anaphylactoid reaction to eggs (hives, swelling of mouth and throat, difficulty in breathing, shock), or who are sensitive to neomycin (used in virus preparation).

• It should be given with caution to people with a history of febrile (feverish) seizure or cerebral injury, or to those with impaired immune response.

• This vaccine should not be administered during pregnancy. Women should be advised to avoid pregnancy within the three months following vaccination.

• Medical judgment is required if breast-feeding is being considered. The vaccine virus appears in breast milk, although there are no reports of significant effects in newborns.

• It is recommended that children with a history of reaction to eggs be given a sensitivity test before administration of the MMR vaccine.

• After administration, people will be required to wait for some time to ensure that there is no serious reaction (such as anaphylaxis).

Interactions

• The immune response to ℞ **meningococcal polysaccharide vaccine** may be decreased by MMR.

• ℞ **Immune globulins**, ℞ **immunosuppressants** (for example, ℞ **corticosteroids**), and ℞ **interferon** may reduce the effectiveness of the vaccine in conferring immunity. It is recommended to delay vaccination until three months after ending treatment with immune agents.

• Caution is required if ℞ **anticoagulants** are being taken.

• The response to a ℞ **tuberculin** skin test may be depressed or inaccurate.

Side effects

• Most of the side effects are mild. Moderate fever may occur during the month following vaccination. There may be swelling, irritation or tenderness at the site of vaccination, and headache, sore throat, rash, fatigue, malaise, or achiness.

• Rarely, a swelling of the parotid gland (salivary gland in the jaw) after two to three weeks. Arthritic side effects are more common in adults receiving this vaccination. Anaphylactoid reactions have occurred.

Moban ⑧

A preparation of ℞ **molindone**.
Formulation: Oral tablets; oral concentrate.
Availability: Prescription only.
Warnings and side effects: See ℞ **molindone**.

Mobic ⑧

A preparation of ℞ **meloxicam**.
Formulation: Oral tablets.
Availability: Prescription only.
Warnings and side effects: See ℞ **meloxicam**.

Mobidin Tablets ⑧

A preparation of ℞ **magnesium salicylate**.
Formulation: Oral tablets.
Availability: Prescription only.
Warnings and side effects: See ℞ **magnesium salicylate**.

Mobigesic Tablets ⑧

A preparation of ℞ **magnesium salicylate** and phenyltoloxamine citrate.
Formulation: Oral tablets.
Availability: OTC.
Warnings and side effects: See ℞ **magnesium salicylate**.

Moctanin ⑧

A preparation of and ℞ **monoctanoin**.
Formulation: Perfusion (biliary).
Availability: Prescription only.
Warnings and side effects: See ℞ **monoctanoin**

modafinil ⑥

Type/Group: **CNS stimulant**.
Brand(s): Provigil.
How administered: Orally.

Used to treat

Modafinil is used to treat ✪ **narcolepsy** (irresistible attacks of sleep during the day), and, although not stated by the manufacturer, it is sometimes used for other sleep disorders.

Warnings

• It should not be used by people with known hypersensitivity to modafinil.

• It should be given with caution to anyone with hypertension, certain heart or airway disorders, head injury, or stroke, and other cardiovascular disease, a history of emotional instability, drug abuse, psychosis, hypertension, severe liver disease, or severe kidney impairment, and to anyone over 65.

• It is not known whether or not modafinil can harm the fetus, therefore, it should be used during pregnancy only if medically judged to be needed.

• Medical judgment is also required if breast-feeding is being considered, as it is not known if it is excreted in breast milk.

• There is a risk of pregnancy if taken with oral contraceptives.

Interactions

• ℞ **carbamazepine**, ℞ **phenobarbital**, ℞ **rifampin**, ℞ **ketoconazole**, and ℞ **itraconazole** may alter the levels of modafinil.

• ℞ **MAOI** antidepressants may have interactive effects.

• Modafinil may increase the levels of ℞ **tricyclic** antidepressants and ℞ **warfarin sodium**.

• ℞ **methylphenidate** may reduce the effects of modafinil.

Side effects

• Frequently, headache, nervousness, dizziness, hypersalivation, nausea, diarrhea, and dry mouth.

• Occasionally, depression, anxiety, insomnia, delayed sleep, euphoria, and restlessness.

Modane ⑧

A preparation of ℞ **bisacodyl**.
Formulation: Oral tablets.
Availability: OTC.
Warnings and side effects: See ℞ **bisacodyl**.

Modane Bulk ⑧

A preparation of ℞ **psyllium**.
Formulation: Oral powder.
Availability: OTC.
Warnings and side effects: See ℞ **psyllium**.

Modane Soft ⑧

A preparation of ℞ **docusate sodium**.
Formulation: Oral capsules.
Availability: OTC.
Warnings and side effects: See ℞ **docusate sodium**.

Modicon ⑧

A preparation of ℞ **ethinyl estradiol** and ℞ **norethindrone**.
Formulation: Calendar pack of oral tablets.
Availability: Prescription only.

Key to symbols: ⑩ = Drug type/group   ⑥ = Generic name   ⑧ = Brand name

Warnings and side effects: See ℞ ethinyl estradiol; ℞ norethindrone.

Moduretic ⑧

A preparation of ℞ **amiloride** and ℞ **hydrochlorothiazide**.
Formulation: Oral tablets.
Availability: Prescription only.
Warnings and side effects: See ℞ amiloride; ℞ hydrochlorothiazide.

moexipril hydrochloride ⑥

Type/Group: **ACE inhibitor; vasodilator; antihypertensive.**
Brand(s): Univasc. Combinations: With *hydrochlorothiazide*: Uniretic.
How administered: Orally.

Used to treat

Moexipril is used to reduce high blood pressure in ⊕ **hypertension**. It is often used with other classes of drug, particularly ℞ **thiazide** ℞ **diuretics**.

Warnings

• It should not be given to people with known hypersensitivity to this drug or to any other ACE inhibitor.

• It should be given with caution to people with severe congestive heart failure, or certain other cardiovascular disorders, a history of anaphylaxis, collagen vascular disease (for example, systemic lupus erythematosus; SLE), diabetes mellitus, depressed immune response, or with impaired kidney function or on dialysis.

• Risk in pregnancy increases substantially from the first through to the second and third trimesters. ACE inhibitors can cause injury to the fetus, even death. The use of these drugs should be stopped as soon as pregnancy is detected.

• Medical judgment is required if breast-feeding is being considered. It is not known whether moexipril appears in breast milk.

• Use of this drug should be stopped and a doctor contacted immediately if signs of angioedema appear (swelling of the face, eyes, lips, tongue, larynx, or extremities; difficulty in breathing or swallowing). Swelling of the larynx, closing off the airway, can be life-threatening.

• Anyone taking an ACE inhibitor should not interrupt or discontinue treatment without first checking with a doctor.

• Any suspected infections (for example, fever, sore throat) should be reported to a doctor, because ACE inhibitors may cause blood changes which can affect immune response.

• ACE inhibitors generally have less effect on blood pressure in blacks than in non-blacks, and the likelihood of angioedema is higher among blacks, as well.

Interactions

• ACE inhibitors have apparently triggered life-threatening anaphylactoid reactions when used by people also receiving ℞ desensitizing vaccines.

• ℞ Anesthetics (for example, in surgery), ℞ phenothiazines, and ℞ probenecid may increase the levels or hypotensive effect of moexipril.

• Levels of ℞ **lithium** may be increased, with the potential for toxic effects.

• If used with potassium-sparing ℞ **diuretics** or other preparations containing potassium (for example, supplements and salt substitutes), levels of potassium may rise.

• ℞ **NSAIDs** may increase the risk of kidney damage or (in some cases) reduce the effects of ACE inhibitors.

• ℞ **Antacids** and ℞ **rifampin** may reduce the effects of moexipril. Antacids should not be used for several hours after a dose of an ACE inhibitor (a doctor should be consulted for full instructions and cautions).

• If used with other antihypertensives and diuretics, the effects of these drugs may be increased. This additive effect is sometimes used to advantage in combination treatments for high blood pressure.

Side effects

• Commonly, dry cough, dizziness, and a flu-like feeling.

• Occasionally, flushing, fatigue, sore throat, rash, muscle pain, or gastrointestinal disturbances (for example, diarrhea, vomiting, abdominal pain).

• Infrequently, headache, upper respiratory infection, swelling of the extremities, chest pain, urinary frequency, insomnia, fainting, or photosensitivity (abnormal sensitivity to light). Although it is uncommon, ACE inhibitors can cause very marked hypotension (especially when beginning treatment) and kidney impairment.

• Rarely, there may be angioedema, altered liver function, jaundice, hepatitis, pancreatitis, or changes in blood counts.

Moi-stir ⑧

A preparation of ℞ **carboxymethylcellulose sodium**.
Formulation: Topical solution.
Availability: OTC.
Warnings and side effects: See ℞ carboxymethylcellulose sodium.

Moisture Drops ⑧

A preparation of ℞ **hydroxypropyl methylcellulose** and ℞ **povidone**.
Formulation: Ophthalmic solution.
Availability: OTC.
Warnings and side effects: See ℞ hydroxypropyl methylcellulose; ℞ povidone.

molindone ⑥

Type/Group: **antipsychotic.**
Brand(s): Moban.
How administered: Orally.

Used to treat

Molindone is used in the treatment of ⊕ **psychotic disorders**. It is chemically different from other antipsychotics.

Warnings

• It should not be given to people with known hypersensitivity to this drug, severe CNS (central nervous system) depression, or in a coma.

• It should be given with caution to people with high blood pressure, liver disease, heart disease, respiratory disease, brain tumor, glaucoma, urinary retention, diabetes mellitus, prostatic hypertrophy, or anyone over 65.

• Molindone should be used during pregnancy only if the benefits outweigh the risk to the fetus.

• Medical judgment is required if breast-feeding is being considered.

• It may cause drowsiness, and so the performance of skilled tasks, such as driving, may be impaired.

• It may cause increased activity, and so caution must be exercised where increased activity may be harmful.

• It may cause postural hypotension (lowered blood pressure on standing), so rise slowly from a reclining position. Older people in particular should exercise caution.

• Avoid alcohol consumption.

• Treatment should be stopped gradually.

• If used for a long time, tardive dyskinesia (see ℞ **antipsychotics**) occasionally develops.

Interactions

• Molindone may inhibit the ℞ **antiparkinsonism** effect of ℞ **levodopa**.

• ℞ **Barbiturates**, ℞ **benztropine**, ℞ **carbamazepine**, ℞ **orphenadrine**, and ℞ **trihexyphenidyl** may reduce the effects of molindone.

• ℞ **Fluoxetine**, ℞ **paroxetine**, and ℞ **quinidine** may increase the effects of molindone.

• The effects of ℞ **guanethidine monosulfate** and ℞ **lithium** may be reduced.

• If used with ℞ **bromocriptine**, the effects of both drugs may be reduced.

• ℞ **indomethacin** may increase the risk of CNS (central nervous system) side effects.

• If an antipsychotic is taken with alcohol, there may be increased sedative effects.

Side effects

• Molindone has a low level of some side effects, including sedation, compared to other antipsychotics, although a relatively high occurrence of extrapyramidal side effects (see ℞ **antipsychotics**).

• Side effects include loss of appetite, constipation, dry mouth, nausea, and vomiting.

• Less frequently, extrapyramidal symptoms, drowsiness, ECG changes, high blood pressure, speeded heart rate, blurred vision, glaucoma, diarrhea, jaundice, weight gain, anemia, white blood cell disorders, changes in hormone function (irregular menstruation, growth of breasts, abnormal milk production, impotence), urinary frequency or retention, shortness of breath, spasm of the bronchi or larynx, respiratory depression, skin reactions, and decreased sweating.

• Rarely, cardiac arrest, neuroleptic malignant syndrome (a potentially fatal condition characterized by very high fever, muscle rigidity, changes in mental status, and irregular pulse, blood pressure and/or heart rhythm), and seizures.

Momentum Muscular Backache Formula Caplets ⑧

A preparation of ℞ **magnesium salicylate**.

Formulation: Oral tablets.

Availability: OTC.

Warnings and side effects: See ℞ **magnesium salicylate**.

mometasone ⑥

Type/Group: corticosteroid; anti-inflammatory.

Brand(s): Elocon; Nasonex

How administered: Topically; intranasal.

Used to treat

Mometasone is used for the prevention and treatment of nasal symptoms of allergic rhinitis, and as a topical (external) application for skin ⊙ **inflammation** and ⊙ **pruritis**.

Warnings

• It should not be used by people with known hypersensitivity to corticosteroids, or with systematic fungal infections.

• It should be taken with caution by anyone with adrenal insufficiency, children, and seniors.

• Corticosteroids can cross the placenta, and therefore mometasone should only be used during pregnancy if medically judged to be essential.

• Medical judgment is also required if breast-feeding is being considered. When taken internally, corticosteroids are excreted in breast milk and may suppress growth and interfere with the production of natural corticosteroids in the infant.

• A nose spray must be used with caution if recent nasal surgery or trauma has left a wound in the nose, as corticosteroids can slow healing.

• Prolonged use in children can inhibit skeletal growth, and so growth must be monitored.

• Topical (applied externally) corticosteroids can be absorbed in sufficient amounts to produce systemic effects, so do not use over large surface areas or for a prolonged period, to minimize this risk.

• Bandages or dressings must not cover the treated area unless directed by a doctor, as this may increase the risk of adverse skin reactions.

• Avoid weeping, denuded, or infected areas.

• A doctor must be notified and the use of mometasone stopped if local irritation or fever develops.

Interactions

No significant interactions have been reported.

Side effects

These depend on how administered, dose, duration of treatment, and use.

• Topical use: Occasionally, acne-like eruptions, irritation, itching, rash, hair loss, and darkening of the skin. Rarely, allergic rash.

• Intranasal: Occasionally, mild nose or throat irritation, dryness, rebound congestion, asthma, runny nose, and loss of sense of taste. Systemic effects are possible if absorbed.

Monistat 7 ⑧

A preparation of ℞ **miconazole**.

Formulation: Vaginal cream; vaginal suppositories.

Availability: OTC.
Warnings and side effects: See ℞ miconazole.

Monistat-Derm ⑧

A preparation of ℞ **miconazole**.
Formulation: Topical cream.
Availability: Prescription only.
Warnings and side effects: See ℞ miconazole.

monoamine-oxidase inhibitor ⑩

see ℞ MAOI.

Monoclate-P ⑧

A preparation of ℞ **antihemophilic factor**.
Formulation: Intravenous infusion.
Availability: Prescription only.
Warnings and side effects: See ℞ antihemophilic factor.

monoctanoin ⑥

Type/Group: **gallstone treatment**.
Brand(s): Moctanin.
How administered: Infusion (nasobiliary tube).

Used to treat

Monoctanoin can be used to dissolve some ✪ **gallstones** (only those made up of cholesterol) *in situ*, when other methods have failed or cannot be used.

Warnings

• It should not be given to people with significant biliary tract infection, acute pancreatitis, recent duodenal ulcer, jejunitis, impaired liver function (including any abnormal circulatory bypassing of the liver), or any life-threatening problem that might be worsened by perfusing this drug into the biliary tract.
• It should be given with caution to people with jaundice that has been caused by gallstones.
• Monoctanoin's effects in pregnancy are unknown, and it should be used only when the potential benefit outweighs the possible risk to the fetus.
• Medical judgment is required if breast-feeding is being considered. It is not known whether this drug appears in breast milk.
• Liver function should be monitored.
• Treatment should stop if there are symptoms such as fever, loss of appetite, chills, low white-cell count, increasing jaundice, or severe pain in the right upper quadrant of the abdomen.

Interactions

• Side effects may be lessened if perfusion is discontinued during meals.

Side effects

• There is commonly abdominal pain, nausea, vomiting, diarrhea, or fever.
• Other side effects may include loss of appetite, indigestion, itching, fatigue, chills, headache, and allergic reaction.
• Low potassium levels, blood and liver changes, ulcerations in the duodenum (which heal after discontinuation) and bile shock may also occur.

Monodox ⑧

A preparation of ℞ **doxycycline**.
Formulation: Oral capsules in several strengths.
Availability: Prescription only.
Warnings and side effects: See ℞ doxycycline.

monoethanolamine oleate ⑥

see ℞ ethanolamine oleate.

Mono-Gesic Tablets ⑧

A preparation of ℞ **salsalate**.
Formulation: Oral tablets.
Availability: Prescription only.
Warnings and side effects: See ℞ salsalate.

Monoket ⑧

A preparation of ℞ **isosorbide mononitrate**.
Formulation: Oral tablets, available in two strengths.
Availability: Prescription only.
Warnings and side effects: See ℞ isosorbide mononitrate.

Mononine ⑧

A preparation of ℞ **Factor IX** (human).
Formulation: Intravenous infusion.
Availability: Prescription only.
Warnings and side effects: See ℞ Factor IX.

Monopril ⑧

A preparation of ℞ **fosinopril sodium**.
Formulation: Oral tablets, available in 3 strengths.
Availability: Prescription only.
Warnings and side effects: See ℞ fosinopril sodium.

montelukast sodium ⑥

Type/Group: **antiasthmatic; leukotriene receptor antagonist; antiallergic**.
Brand(s): Singulair.
How administered: Orally.

Used to treat

Montelukast is a recently introduced drug that can be used as an add-on therapy for individuals not adequately controlled by inhaled ℞ **corticosteroids** and short-acting ℞ **beta-adrenergic stimulants** to prevent mild to moderate ✪ **asthma** attacks (including, along with other drugs, exercise-induced bronchospasm), but not to treat acute attacks. It represents a new class of drugs called leukotriene receptor antagonists that work as antiallergic agents by blocking the actions of leukotrienes, which are natural inflammatory mediators released in the lungs.

Warnings

• It should not be given to people with known hypersensitivity to montelukast.
• Chewable tablets contain phenylalanine and should be given with caution (if at all) to people with phenylketonuria. Medical judgment is also required for patients with liver disease.

Key to symbols: ✪ = Disorder Section ℞ = Drug Section ♣ = Herbal Section ⚕ = Supplement Section

• The safety and efficacy of this drug in children under two years of age has not been established.

• There have been no adequate or controlled trials in pregnant women and safe use during pregnancy has not been established. It should be used, therefore, only if clearly needed.

• Medical judgment is required if breast-feeding is being considered. Manufacturers of similar agents have recommended against breast-feeding while taking these medications.

• Although a causal relationship has not been established, in rare cases, reduction in oral corticosteroid dose in people taking montelukast has resulted in Churg-Strauss syndrome (a systemic blood disorder). Symptoms may include eosinophilia (abnormal increase in eosinophil blood cells), rash, worsening pulmonary symptoms, heart complications, and/or nerve disorders.

• It is not used to treat acute attacks.

Interactions

• ℞ Carbamazepine, ℞ fosphenytoin, ℞ phenobarbital, ℞ phenytoin, ℞ rifabutin, and ℞ rifampin may decrease the response to montelukast.

• ℞ Ketoconazole, ℞ erythromycin, ℞ amiodarone hydrochloride, ℞ cimetidine, ℞ fluoxetine, and ℞ omeprazole may increase the levels of montelukast.

• Anyone with sensitivity to ℞ aspirin should avoid taking aspirin or other ℞ NSAIDs when taking montelukast.

Side effects

• Frequently, headache.

• Occasionally, influenza.

• Rarely, abdominal pain, cough, upset stomach, dizziness, fatigue, and dental pain. In children 6 to 14, diarrhea, laryngitis, sore throat, nausea, earache, sinusitis, and viral infection.

Monurol Ⓑ

A preparation of ℞ fosfomycin.

Formulation: Granules to mix with water.

Availability: Prescription only.

Warnings and side effects: See ℞ fosfomycin.

moricizine hydrochloride Ⓖ

Type/Group: **antiarrhythmic.**

Brand(s): Ethmozine.

How administered: Orally.

Used to treat

Moricizine hydrochloride is used to regularize the heartbeat, but generally only for life-threatening ⊙ **arrhythmias**, especially sustained ventricular tachycardia.

Warnings

• It should not be given to people with known hypersensitivity to this drug, or with certain heart conduction conditions.

• It should be given with caution to people with congestive heart failure, pacemakers, certain arrhythmias, or significantly impaired liver or kidney function. This is a specialist drug and treatment will be carried out by experienced clinicians who are thoroughly familiar with this drug. Periodic monitoring of heart function and blood values is necessary.

• Moricizine should be used during pregnancy only if it is clearly needed.

• It is present in breast milk and nursing women should discontinue using this drug or stop breast-feeding.

• Moricizine can, occasionally, provoke arrhythmias.

• A doctor must be contacted immediately if there is chest pain or discomfort, pounding in the chest (palpitations), irregular heartbeat, or fever.

Interactions

• ℞ amiodarone hydrochloride, ℞ cimetidine, ℞ disopyramide, ℞ propranolol, ℞ verapamil, and ℞ urinary alkalinizers (for example, ℞ sodium bicarbonate) may raise the levels or intensify the effects of moricizine.

• The levels and effects of ℞ digoxin may be increased.

• Smoking and urinary acidifiers (for example, ℞ ammonium chloride) may reduce the effects of moricizine.

Side effects

• Frequent side effects include dizziness, gastrointestinal disturbances (for example, nausea, abdominal pain, dyspepsia, vomiting, diarrhea), headache, fatigue, palpitations, or breathlessness.

• Other effects may include sweating, muscle pain, dry mouth, blurred vision, tingling sensations, nervousness, or sleep disorders.

• Mental changes (for example, memory loss, confusion, incoordination) and tremor occur infrequently.

• Sensitivity reactions such as rash, hives, itching, fever or swelling of lips and tongue have occurred occasionally. Blood changes are rare.

morphine sulfate Ⓖ

(morphine sulphate)

Type/Group: **narcotic analgesic; opioid.**

Brand(s): Astramorph PF; Duramorph; Infumorph; Kadian; MSIR; MS Contin; OMS Concentrate; Oramorph SR; RMS; Roxanol; various generic.

How administered: Orally; rectal suppository; injection; infusion.

Used to treat

Morphine is the principal ℞ **alkaloid** of opium. It is widely used to treat severe ⊙ **pain** and to relieve associated stress and anxiety, because it induces a state of mental detachment and euphoria. It is used during operations as an analgesic (painkiller) and to enhance the actions of ℞ **general anesthetics**. Although not stated by the manufacturer, it is sometimes used to relieve cough in the terminally ill as an ℞ **antitussive** (it may cause nausea and vomiting), in acute pulmonary edema, and for reducing secretion and peristalsis in the intestine (it has a powerful ℞ **antidiarrheal** and antimotility action and is used in some antidiarrheal mixtures).

Warnings

• It should not be taken by people with known hypersensitivity to any opioid, or who have respiratory depression, hemorrhage, acute asthma attack, or paralytic ileus (cessation of the normal rhythmic muscle contractions of the intestines). Opioids (even the weaker ones) should not be taken by people with asthma, or anyone with seriously depressed breathing disorders, prostatic hypertrophy, convulsive disorders, raised intracranial pressure, or a head injury.

• Depending on use and dose, it should be taken with caution by the elderly, or anyone with hypotension, certain liver, kidney, gastrointestinal or adrenal disorders, hypothyroidism (under-activity of the thyroid gland), or alcoholism.

• Morphine should be used during pregnancy only if the benefits outweigh the potential risks.

• Because of its potential to cause withdrawal symptoms in nursing infants, it is not recommended for use if breast-feeding.

• Morphine is a Schedule II controlled substance.

• In overdose narcotic analgesics produce serious respiratory depression (decreased breathing), which is occasionally fatal.

• Tolerance occurs extremely readily and dependence (addiction) may follow.

• Drowsiness may affect the performance of skilled tasks such as driving.

• The effects of alcohol may be enhanced and the likelihood of respiratory depression increases.

Interactions

• If the following drugs are used with morphine, then effects are increased with potentially serious results: ℞ **barbiturates**; ℞ **general anesthetics**; ℞ **MAOIs**; ℞ **opioids**; protease inhibitors (for example, ℞ **nelfinavir**, ℞ **ritonavir**, ℞ **saquinavir**); ℞ **antihistamines**; alcohol; ℞ **chlorpromazine**; ℞ **thioridazine**; ℞ **chloral hydrate**; ℞ **glutethimide**; ℞ **methocarbamol**; ℞ **amitriptyline**; ℞ **clomipramine**; ℞ **nortriptyline**.

• The anticoagulant effect of ℞ **anticoagulants** (for example, ℞ **warfarin sodium**) is intensified, with the potential for bleeding.

Side effects

• These depend on the how it is administered, dose, and use. The most frequent side effects include sedation, euphoria, constipation, dizziness, drowsiness, sweating, nausea and vomiting, loss of appetite, and mood change.

• Less often there may be dry mouth, flushing of the face, headache, palpitations, changes in heart rate, postural hypotension (a lowering of blood pressure on standing, causing dizziness), miosis (pupil constriction), confusion and hallucinations, and potentially serious respiratory depression. It may also cause itching and a rash.

morphine sulphate Ⓖ

see ℞ morphine sulfate.

Mosco Liquid Ⓑ

A preparation of ℞ **salicylic acid**.
Formulation: Topical liquid.
Availability: OTC.
Warnings and side effects: See ℞ salicylic acid.

motility stimulant Ⓓ

Actions and uses

Motility stimulants (prokinetic agents) increase gut motility (intestinal movement), that is, they stimulate stomach emptying and the rate of passage of food along the intestine. ℞ **metoclopramide hydrochloride** is a drug with useful motility stimulant properties and also effective ℞ **antiemetic** and ℞ **antinauseant** activity. It can be used to prevent vomiting caused by gastrointestinal disorders, chemotherapy, or radiotherapy (in the treatment of cancer). It works both by a direct action on the vomiting center of the brain (where it is an ℞ **dopamine-receptor antagonist**) and by actions within the intestine. It enhances the strength of esophageal sphincter contraction (preventing the passage of stomach contents up into the gullet), stimulates emptying of the stomach, and increases the rate at which food is moved along the intestine. These last actions lead to its use in non-ulcer dyspepsia (Ⓞ **indigestion**), for gastric stasis and to prevent Ⓞ **gastroesophageal reflux**. It is also used during examination of the intestine to speed up the movement of barium through the intestine following a barium meal.

Limitations

A number of drugs of this class have been used in the past, (including cisapride which can be used in certain circumstances), but the only example in common use is ℞ **metoclopramide hydrochloride**. Because of its actions on dopaminergic nerve pathways in the brain, this drug is not normally used by people already taking dopamine-receptor antagonists (for example, ℞ **antipsychotic** drugs such as phenothiazines or butyrophenones), or in who have extreme depression, suicidal tendencies, or parkinsonism or pheochromocytoma. Also, because it is a dopamine antagonist, metoclopramide promotes secretion of the hormone prolactin, which is generally undesirable as it can cause side effects. It should not be used where there is obstruction of the gastrointestinal tract, or where stimulation of the gut might be dangerous. See also the metoclopramide hydrochloride entry.

Motofen Tablets Ⓑ

A preparation of ℞ **atropine sulfate** and difenoxin.
Formulation: Oral tablets.
Availability: Prescription only.
Warnings and side effects: See ℞ atropine sulfate; ℞ diphenoxylate hydrochloride.

Motrin; Children's; Infants' Ⓑ

A preparation of ℞ **ibuprofen**.
Formulation: Oral liquid; tablets, chewable and contain the sweetener aspartame, which should be avoided by individuals with phenylketonuria.
Availability: OTC.
Warnings and side effects: See ℞ ibuprofen.

Motrin IB Sinus Caplets Ⓑ

A preparation of ℞ **pseudoephedrine** and ℞ **ibuprofen**.
Formulation: Oral tablets.
Availability: OTC.
Warnings and side effects: See ℞ pseudoephedrine; ℞ ibuprofen.

Motrin IB Tablets; Caplets; Gelcaps Ⓑ

A preparation of ℞ **ibuprofen**.
Formulation: Oral tablets; gelcaps.
Availability: OTC.
Warnings and side effects: See ℞ ibuprofen.

Motrin Tablets ®

A preparation of ℞ ibuprofen.
Formulation: Oral tablets, available in two strengths.
Availability: Prescription only.
Warnings and side effects: See ℞ ibuprofen.

moxifloxacin ⑥

Type/Group: **quinolone; antibacterial.**
Brand(s): Avelox.
How administered: Orally.

Used to treat

Moxifloxacin is used to treat ✪ **bacterial infections**, especially respiratory infections, including bacteria-caused worsening of chronic ✪ **bronchitis**, community-acquired (caught from the environment) ✪ **pneumonia**, and acute ✪ **sinusitis**, as well as urinary tract infections, kidney infections, and skin and soft tissue infections.

Warnings

• It should not be given to people with known hypersensitivity to moxifloxacin or other quinolones, or to children under 18, as there is a possibility of damage to joints and cartilage in growing children.

• It should be given with caution to people with liver or kidney disease, diabetes mellitus, certain heart conditions, any predisposition to seizures or a history of photosensitivity reactions (abnormal sensitivity to light).

• Moxifloxacin should not be used during pregnancy or while breast-feeding unless the potential benefit justifies the possible risk of joint damage or other harm to the fetus or infant.

• Superinfections due to the altered bacterial balance caused by antibiotic therapy may occur. A doctor must be contacted if severe abdominal pain, or moderate to severe diarrhea occur.

• Rare, but serious, side effects of quinolones include seizure and other CNS (central nervous system) effects, and severe allergic reactions.

• Adequate fluid intake should be maintained.

• ⚶ **calcium**, ⚶ **iron** preparations, ⚶ **magnesium**, and ⚶ **zinc** may reduce the effects of moxifloxacin. Products such as supplements that contain these ingredients must not be taken less than four hours before or four hours after taking moxifloxacin.

• Photosensitivity reactions can occur and so excessive exposure to sunlight should be avoided.

Interactions

• ℞ **Antacids**, ⚶ **calcium**, ℞ **Didanosine (ddl)**, ⚶ **iron** preparations, ⚶ **magnesium**, ℞ **sodium bicarbonate**, and ⚶ **zinc** reduce the effects of moxifloxacin. Do not take products containing these ingredients less than four hours before or two hours after taking moxifloxacin.

• The levels of ℞ **theophylline**, antipyrine, ℞ **caffeine**, ℞ **diazepam**, ℞ **metoprolol**, ℞ **pentoxifylline**, ℞ **phenytoin**, ℞ **propranolol**, ℞ **ropinirole**, ℞ **xanthine**, and ℞ **warfarin sodium** may be increased.

• The effects of oral ℞ **anticoagulants** may be increased.

• If used with ℞ **foscarnet**, the risk of seizure is increased.

Side effects

• Frequently, dizziness, lightheadedness, insomnia, drowsiness, and gastrointestinal effects.

M-Prednisol; ®

A preparation of ℞ **methylprednisolone** acetate.
Formulation: Injection.
Availability: Prescription only.
Warnings and side effects: See ℞ **methylprednisolone**.

MS Contin ®

A preparation of ℞ **morphine sulfate**.
Formulation: Oral tablets, controlled releases, available in four strengths.
Availability: Prescription only.
Warnings and side effects: See ℞ **morphine sulfate**.

MSIR ®

A preparation of ℞ **morphine sulfate**.
Formulation: Oral capsules; tablets; liquid.
Availability: Prescription only.
Warnings and side effects: See ℞ **morphine sulfate**.

Muco-Fen-DM Tablets ®

A preparation of ℞ **dextromethorphan** and ℞ **guaifenesin**.
Formulation: Oral tablets, timed release.
Availability: Prescription only.
Warnings and side effects: See ℞ **dextromethorphan**; ℞ **guaifenesin**.

Muco-Fen-LA Tablets ®

A preparation of ℞ **guaifenesin**.
Formulation: Oral tablets, sustained release.
Availability: Prescription only.
Warnings and side effects: See ℞ **guaifenesin**.

mucolytic ⑩

Generics: **acetylcysteine; dornase alfa.**

Actions and uses

℞ **mucolytic** drugs dissolve, or help break down, mucus. They are generally used in an effort to reduce the viscosity of sputum in the upper airways and so aid expectoration (coughing up sputum). They may also be termed ℞ **expectorant** drugs.

It is believed that ℞ **acetylcysteine** has a mucolytic effect by weakening the chemical (disulfide) bonds between molecules in the mucoprotein of the mucus so that it becomes less viscous. It is used to relieve obstruction in such conditions as ✪ **pneumonia**, chronic bronchopulmonary disease (✪ **emphysema**, ✪ **bronchitis**, tracheobronchitis), ✪ **cystic fibrosis**, and ✪ **tuberculosis**.

℞ **dornase alfa** is a genetically engineered version of a naturally occurring human ℞ **enzyme**, which breaks down deoxyribonucleic acid (DNA) in sputum and so reduces sputum viscoelasticity. It is used in cystic fibrosis to improve lung function and reduce respiratory infections (excess secretions can worsen and encourage infections).

Limitations
Dornase alfa, being an enzyme, is chemically unstable. It needs to be kept refrigerated and then inhaled via a nebulizer system. It is well tolerated with chronic use and should be used as part of a treatment that includes physiotherapy. See also the individual drug entries.

Mucomyst ℞
A preparation of ℞ **acetylcysteine**.
Formulation: Solution.
Availability: Prescription only.
Warnings and side effects: See ℞ **acetylcysteine**.

Mucosil-10; Mucosil-20 ℞
A preparation of ℞ **acetylcysteine**.
Formulation: Solution.
Availability: Prescription only.
Warnings and side effects: See ℞ **acetylcysteine**.

Mudrane GG-2 Tablets ℞
A preparation of ℞ **guaifenesin** and ℞ **theophylline**.
Formulation: Oral tablets.
Availability: Prescription only.
Warnings and side effects: See ℞ **guaifenesin**; ℞ **theophylline**.

Mudrane GG Tablets ℞
A preparation of ℞ **ephedrine**, ℞ **theophylline**, aminophylline, ℞ **guaifenesin**, and ℞ **phenobarbital**.
Formulation: Oral tablets.
Availability: Prescription only.
Warnings and side effects: See ℞ **ephedrine**; ℞ **theophylline**; ℞ **guaifenesin**; ℞ **phenobarbital**.

Mudrane Tablets ℞
A preparation of ℞ **ephedrine**, ℞ **theophylline**, aminophylline (anhydrous), potassium iodide, and ℞ **phenobarbital**.
Formulation: Oral tablets.
Availability: Prescription only.
Warnings and side effects: See ℞ **ephedrine**; ℞ **theophylline**; ℞ **phenobarbital**.

Multi-Symptom Tylenol Cold Caplets; Tablets ℞
A preparation of ℞ **dextromethorphan**, ℞ **acetaminophen**, ℞ **chlorpheniramine maleate**, and ℞ **pseudoephedrine**.
Formulation: Oral caplets; tablets.
Availability: OTC.
Warnings and side effects: See ℞ **dextromethorphan**; ℞ **acetaminophen**; ℞ **chlorpheniramine maleate**; ℞ **pseudoephedrine**.

mupirocin ⓖ
Type/Group: **antibiotic; antibacterial**.
Brand(s): Bactroban.
How administered: Topically (external).

Used to treat
Mupirocin, which is unrelated to any other antibiotic (it is a pseudomonic acid derivative), is used to treat ⊙ **impetigo** and infected skin wounds. It is of value in treating infections caused by bacteria resistant to other antibacterials, for instance methoxycillin-resistant *Staphylococcus aureus*, which is present in the nose.

Warnings
• It should not be given to people with known hypersensitivity to mupirocin.
• It should be given with caution to people with impaired kidney function. The safety of nasal preparations in children has not been established.
• It should be used during pregnancy only if clearly needed and if the potential benefits outweigh the risks to the fetus.
• It is unknown whether this drug appears in breast milk, and is not recommended for use while breast-feeding.
• Superinfections due to the altered bacterial balance created by antibiotic treatment may occur, especially with prolonged or repeated use.

Interactions
No significant interactions have been reported.

Side effects
• Frequently, with nasal use, headache, inflammation, upper respiratory congestion, sore throat, and altered taste.
• Occasionally, with nasal use, burning, stinging, and cough.
• Occasionally, with topical use, stinging on application. Rarely, itching, gastrointestinal upsets, dry skin or dry mouth, and rash.

Murine ℞
A preparation of ℞ **polyvinyl alcohol**.
Formulation: Ophthalmic solution.
Availability: OTC.
Warnings and side effects: See ℞ **polyvinyl alcohol**.

Murine Plus ℞
A preparation of ℞ **tetrahydrozoline hydrochloride**.
Formulation: Eye drops.
Availability: OTC.
Warnings and side effects: See ℞ **tetrahydrozoline hydrochloride**.

Muro 128 ℞
A preparation of ℞ **sodium chloride**.
Formulation: Ophthalmic solution.
Availability: OTC.
Warnings and side effects: See ℞ **sodium chloride**.

muromonab-CD3 ⓖ
Type/Group: **immunosuppressant**.
Brand(s): Orthoclone OKT3.
How administered: Intravenous infusion.

Used to treat
Muromonab-CD3 is used to treat rejection following organ transplants. It is a form of an antibody found in mice.

Key to symbols: ⊙ = Disorder Section ℞ = Drug Section ♣ = Herbal Section ⚕ = Supplement Section

Warnings

• It should not be given to people with known hypersensitivity to this or other agents of mouse origin, including mouse antibodies, with uncompensated heart failure, seizure disorders, or fluid overload. This is a specialist drug and it will used only after a full medical assessment.

• It should be given with caution to people with certain heart, lung or circulatory diseases, or septic shock.

• Muromonab-CD3 should be used during pregnancy only if the potential benefits justify the the possible risk to the fetus.

• Women taking this drug should not breast-feed.

• Some people experience cytokine-release syndrome, which ranges from a "flu-like" illness to a life-threatening shock-like syndrome. A doctor must be contacted immediately if symptoms such as a skin rash, rapid heartbeat, difficulty breathing or swallowing develop. It is most likely to occur after the first few doses.

• Neuropsychiatric events including seizures, encephalopathy, cerebral edema, meningitis, and headaches have occurred.

• Immunosuppression may increase the risk of infection.

• Serious and occasionally fatal allergic reactions have occurred.

• Immunosuppression may increase the risk of developing lymphomas or other cancers.

Interactions

• Other immunosuppressants (for example, ℞ **azathiaprine**, ℞ **corticosteroids**, ℞ **cyclosporine**) increase the risk of side effects.

• If used with ℞ **indomethacin**, there is an increased risk of encephalopathy and other CNS (central nervous system) effects.

• ℞ **Vaccines** are less effective when given with immunosuppressants such as muromonab-CD3.

Side effects

• These can be many and include potentially serious cytokine-release syndrome, commonly chills, headache, fever, abdominal pain, diarrhea, nausea, vomiting, chest pain, breathing problems and wheezing, generalized weakness, muscle and joint aches, and pain.

• Also, potentially serious, pulmonary edema, seizures, headache, and allergic reactions.

Muroptic-5   ⑧

A preparation of ℞ **sodium chloride**.
Formulation: Ophthalmic solution.
Availability: OTC.
Warnings and side effects: See ℞ **sodium chloride**.

muscle relaxant   ⑩

see ℞ skeletal muscle relaxant.

Muse   ⑧

A preparation of ℞ **alprostadil**.
Formulation: Pellets administered via applicator.
Availability: Prescription only.
Warnings and side effects: See ℞ **alprostadil**.

Mustargen   ⑧

A preparation of ℞ **mechlorethamine hydrochloride**.
Formulation: Powder for injection.
Availability: Prescription only.
Warnings and side effects: See ℞ **mechlorethamine hydrochloride**.

Musterole Deep Strength Rub   ⑧

A preparation of ℞ **methyl salicylate**, ℞ **menthol**, and methyl nicotinate.
Formulation: Topical ointment.
Availability: OTC.
Warnings and side effects: See ℞ **methyl salicylate**; ℞ **menthol**.

Mutamycin   ⑧

A preparation of ℞ **mitomycin**.
Formulation: Powder for injection.
Availability: Prescription only.
Warnings and side effects: See ℞ **mitomycin**.

Myambutol   ⑧

A preparation of ℞ **ethambutol**.
Formulation: Oral tablets.
Availability: Prescription only.
Warnings and side effects: See ℞ **ethambutol**.

Mycelex   ⑧

A preparation of ℞ **clotrimazole**.
Formulation: Topical cream in two strengths; vaginal cream in two strengths; oral lozengess.
Availability: Prescription or OTC (creams); Prescription only (lozenges).
Warnings and side effects: See ℞ **clotrimazole**.

Mycifradin   ⑧

A preparation of ℞ **neomycin**.
Formulation: Oral solution.
Availability: Prescription only.
Warnings and side effects: See ℞ **neomycin**.

Myciguent   ⑧

A preparation of ℞ **neomycin**.
Formulation: Ointment; Cream.
Availability: OTC.
Warnings and side effects: See ℞ **neomycin**.

Myci-Spray   ⑧

A preparation of phenylephrine tannate and ℞ **pyrilamine maleate**.
Formulation: Nasal Spray.
Availability: OTC.
Warnings and side effects: See ℞ **phenylephrine hydrochloride**; ℞ **pyrilamine maleate**.

Mycitracin Maximum Strength Triple Antibiotic Ointment ℞

A preparation of ℞ **neomycin**, ℞ **polymyxin B sulfate**, and ℞ **bacitracin**.
Formulation: Topical ointment.
Availability: OTC.
Warnings and side effects: See ℞ **neomycin**, ℞ **polymyxin B sulfate**, ℞ **bacitracin**.

Mycitracin Plus Ointment ℞

A preparation of ℞ **neomycin**, ℞ **polymyxin B sulfate**, ℞ **bacitracin**, and ℞ **lidocaine**.
Formulation: Topical ointment.
Availability: OTC.
Warnings and side effects: See ℞ **neomycin**; ℞ **polymyxin B sulfate**; ℞ **bacitracin**; ℞ **lidocaine**.

Mycobutin ℞

A preparation of ℞ **rifabutin**.
Formulation: Oral capsules.
Availability: Prescription only.
Warnings and side effects: See ℞ **rifabutin**.

mycophenolate mofetil ⑥

Type/Group: **immunosuppressant**.
Brand(s): CellCept.
How administered: Orally; intravenous infusion.
Used to treat
Mycophenolate mofetil is a (℞ **cytotoxic**) immunosuppressant drug used, mainly, to reduce tissue rejection in heart or kidney transplants. Generally, it is used with ℞ **corticosteroids** and ℞ **cyclosporine**.
Warnings
• It should not be given to people with known hypersensitivity to this drug.
• It should be given with caution to people with severe kidney impairment, or gastrointestinal disease or inflammation. This is a specialist drug and is used only after a full medical assessment.
• Mycophenolate may have the potential for harming the fetus and it should not be used during pregnancy. Effective contraception should be used before, during, and for six weeks after treatment has ended.
• Medical judgment is required if breast-feeding is being considered.
• Mycophenolate is prescribed only by physicians experienced in immunosuppressive therapy and in settings adequately equipped to monitor and manage the treatment. Periodic monitoring of blood values is necessary.
• Treatment with mycophenolate inevitably leaves the body vulnerable to infection.
• There may be a higher vulnerability to certain cancers (including lymphoma and skin cancers), and persons taking mycophenolate should protect themselves from excessive exposure to the sun.
• Gastrointestinal bleeding is a particular concern.

Interactions
• The levels of ℞ **acyclovir** and ℞ **ganciclovir (DHPG)** and mycophenolate may increase when used together, especially if there is existing kidney impairment.
• ℞ **Probenecid** and ℞ **salicylates** may raise mycophenolate levels or increase its effects.
• The effectiveness of ℞ **oral contraceptives** may be reduced and other contraceptives or combined methods are recommended.
• Mycophenolate and ℞ **azathiaprine** should not be used together, as the effects have not been studied.
• Live ℞ **vaccines** should not be given during treatment.
• ℞ **Cholestyramine** may lower the levels or effects of mycophenolate, and these drugs should not be used together.
• The levels of ℞ **phenytoin** and ℞ **theophylline** may be increased.
• ℞ **Antacids** (those containing ℞ **aluminum** or ℞ **magnesium hydroxide**) and food may sharply reduce the levels of mycophenolate and should not be taken within a few hours before or after this drug.
Side effects
These are many and may include:
• Nausea and vomiting, diarrhea or constipation, abdominal pain, hypertension, edema, chest pain, shortness of breath, cough, insomnia, headache, dizziness and tremor, susceptibility to a range of infections, various blood effects, or hyperglycemia.

Mycostatin; Mycostatin Pastilles ℞

A preparation of ℞ **nystatin**.
Formulation: Oral tablets; troche (Pastilles); oral suspension; topical cream; topical ointment; topical powder; vaginal tablets.
Availability: Prescription only.
Warnings and side effects: See ℞ **nystatin**.

Mydfrin 2.5% ℞

A preparation of ℞ **phenylephrine hydrochloride**.
Formulation: Eye drops, available in two strengths.
Availability: Prescription only.
Warnings and side effects: See ℞ **phenylephrine hydrochloride**.

Mydriacyl ℞

A preparation of ℞ **tropicamide**.
Formulation: Ophthalmic solution in several strengths.
Availability: Prescription only.
Warnings and side effects: See ℞ **tropicamide**.

mydriatic Ⓓ

Generics: atropine sulfate; cyclopentolate hydrochloride; homatropine hydrobromide; phenylephrine hydrochloride; tropicamide.
Actions and uses
Mydriatic drugs dilate the pupil of the eye (mydriasis), and are used during ophthalmic examinations. The drugs used are either ℞ **sympathomimetic** (℞ **alpha-adrenergic stimulant**) drugs, such as ℞ **phenylephrine hydrochloride**, or ℞ **anticholinergic** drugs, including ℞ **cyclopentolate hydrochloride**, ℞ **tropicam-**

ide, ℞ **homatropine hydrobromide**, and sometimes ℞ **atropine sulfate**.

Limitations

Generally, agents that have an effect for only a short period are used for this purpose (tropicamide, cyclopentolate hydrochloride) but if a longer duration is required, then homatropine hydrobromide, or for very prolonged action, atropine sulfate, may be used. Anticholinergic drugs also paralyze the focusing muscles of the eye (see ℞ **cycloplegic**), which is generally a disadvantage. However, they are sometimes used for this purpose in ophthalmic examinations. A number of drugs may cause mydriasis as an unwanted side effect when given systemically for other purposes, notably most anticholinergics and sympathomimetics. See also the individual drug entries.

Mygel II Suspenion ⓑ

A preparation of ℞ **aluminum hydroxide** and ℞ **magnesium hydroxide** and ℞ **simethicone**.
Formulation: Oral liquid.
Availability: OTC.
Warnings and side effects: See ℞ **aluminum hydroxide**; ℞ **magnesium hydroxide**; ℞ **simethicone**.

Mygel Suspension ⓑ

A preparation of ℞ **aluminum hydroxide** and ℞ **simethicone**.
Formulation: Oral liquid.
Availability: OTC.
Warnings and side effects: See ℞ **aluminum hydroxide**; ℞ **simethicone**.

Mykrox ⓑ

A preparation of ℞ **metolazone**.
Formulation: Oral tablets, rapidly-acting tablets.
Availability: Prescription only.
Warnings and side effects: See ℞ **metolazone**.

Mylagen Gelcaps ⓑ

A preparation of ℞ **calcium carbonate** and ℞ **magnesium carbonate**.
Formulation: Oral gelcaps.
Availability: OTC.
Warnings and side effects: See ℞ **calcium carbonate**; ℞ **magnesium carbonate**.

Mylagen II Liquid ⓑ

A preparation of ℞ **aluminum hydroxide** and ℞ **magnesium hydroxide** and ℞ **simethicone**.
Formulation: Oral liquid.
Availability: OTC.
Warnings and side effects: See ℞ **aluminum hydroxide**; ℞ **magnesium hydroxide**; ℞ **simethicone**.

Mylagen Liquid ⓑ

A preparation of ℞ **aluminum hydroxide** and ℞ **simethicone**.
Formulation: Oral liquid.

Availability: OTC.
Warnings and side effects: See ℞ **aluminum hydroxide**; ℞ **simethicone**.

Mylanta Gas ⓑ

A preparation of ℞ **simethicone**.
Formulation: Oral tablets, chewable (2 strengths).
Availability: OTC.
Warnings and side effects: See ℞ **simethicone**.

Mylanta Gelcaps ⓑ

A preparation of ℞ **calcium carbonate** and ℞ **magnesium carbonate**.
Formulation: Oral gelcaps.
Availability: OTC.
Warnings and side effects: See ℞ **calcium carbonate**; ℞ **magnesium carbonate**.

Mylanta Liquid ⓑ

A preparation of ℞ **aluminum hydroxide** and ℞ **simethicone**.
Formulation: Oral liquid.
Availability: OTC.
Warnings and side effects: See ℞ **aluminum hydroxide**; ℞ **simethicone**.

Mylanta Supreme ⓑ

A preparation of ℞ **calcium carbonate** and ℞ **magnesium hydroxide**.
Formulation: Oral liquid.
Availability: OTC.
Warnings and side effects: See ℞ **calcium carbonate**; ℞ **magnesium hydroxide**.

Mylanta Tablets; Double Strength Liquid ⓑ

A preparation of ℞ **aluminum hydroxide** and ℞ **magnesium hydroxide** and ℞ **simethicone**.
Formulation: Oral tablets, chewable; liquid.
Availability: OTC.
Warnings and side effects: See ℞ **aluminum hydroxide**; ℞ **magnesium hydroxide**; ℞ **simethicone**.

Myleran ⓑ

A preparation of ℞ **busulfan**.
Formulation: Oral tablets.
Availability: Prescription only.
Warnings and side effects: See ℞ **busulfan**.

Mylicon Drops ⓑ

A preparation of ℞ **simethicone**.
Formulation: Oral drops.
Availability: OTC.
Warnings and side effects: See ℞ **simethicone**.

Key to symbols: ⓓ = Drug type/group   ⓖ = Generic name   ⓑ = Brand name

Myochrysine ®

A preparation of gold sodium thiomalate (℞ **aurothioglucose**).
Formulation: Oral tablets.
Availability: Prescription only.
Warnings and side effects: See ℞ **aurothioglucose**.

Myotonachol ®

A preparation of ℞ **bethanechol chloride**.
Formulation: Oral tablets.
Availability: Prescription only.
Warnings and side effects: See ℞ **bethanechol chloride**.

Myphetane DX Cough Syrup ®

A preparation of ℞ **dextromethorphan**, ℞ **brompheniramine maleate**, and ℞ **pseudoephedrine**.
Formulation: Oral syrup.
Availability: Prescription only.
Warnings and side effects: See ℞ **dextromethorphan**; ℞ **brompheniramine maleate**; ℞ **pseudoephedrine**.

Mysoline; Mysoline Suspension ®

A preparation of ℞ **primidone**.
Formulation: Oral liquid; tablets, available in two strengths.
Availability: Prescription only.
Warnings and side effects: See ℞ **primidone**.

Mytelase ®

A preparation of ℞ **ambenonium chloride**.
Formulation: Oral tablets.
Availability: Prescription only.
Warnings and side effects: See ℞ **ambenonium chloride**.

Mytussin AC Cough Syrup ®

A preparation of ℞ **codeine phosphate** and ℞ **guaifenesin**.
Formulation: Oral syrup.
Availability: May or may not require a prescription.
Warnings and side effects: See ℞ **codeine phosphate**; ℞ **guaifenesin**.

Mytussin DAC Liquid ®

A preparation of ℞ **codeine phosphate**, ℞ **guaifenesin**, and ℞ **pseudoephedrine**.
Formulation: Oral liquid.
Availability: May or may not require a prescription.
Warnings and side effects: See ℞ **codeine phosphate**; ℞ **guaifenesin**; ℞ **pseudoephedrine**.

Mytussin DM Liquid ®

A preparation of ℞ **dextromethorphan** and ℞ **guaifenesin**.
Formulation: Oral liquid.
Availability: OTC.
Warnings and side effects: See ℞ **dextromethorphan**; ℞ **guaifenesin**.

Mytussin Syrup ®

A preparation of ℞ **guaifenesin**.
Formulation: Oral syrup.
Availability: OTC.
Warnings and side effects: See ℞ **guaifenesin**.

Nabi-HB ®

A preparation of ℞ **hepatitis B immune globulin (HBIG)**.
Formulation: Intramuscular injection.
Availability: Prescription only.
Warnings and side effects: See ℞ **hepatitis B immune globulin (HBIG)**.

nabumetone Ⓖ

Type/Group: anti-inflammatory; antirheumatic; non-narcotic analgesic; NSAID.
Brand(s): Relafen.
How administered: Orally.

Used to treat

Nabumetone is used primarily to relieve pain and inflammation, particularly in ✛ **osteoarthritis** and ✛ **rheumatoid arthritis**.

Warnings

• It should not be used by people with known hypersensitivity to this drug or to other NSAIDs (including ℞ **aspirin**), who have chronic kidney disease, certain bleeding disorders or conditions (for example, hemophilia, vitamin K deficiency, low blood-platelet levels), or who have a tendency to, or active, peptic ulceration.
• It should be given with caution to people with diabetes mellitus, SLE (systemic lupus erythematosus), peripheral edema, or allergic disorders (especially asthma and skin conditions), who are elderly, or with any kind of kidney impairment or certain liver disorders.
• Nabumetone should be used during pregnancy only if medically judged that it is needed. In the third trimester, its risks to the fetus rise, and so it should only be used if the benefits outweigh the risks, which are higher at this time.
• Breast-feeding mothers should either discontinue this drug or stop breast-feeding.
• With regular, long-term use (as in treatment of osteoarthritis), NSAIDs may cause gastrointestinal bleeding, ulceration, or perforation. Any signs of bleeding should be reported to a physician immediately.
• Most NSAIDs have the potential, particularly with regular use, to cause liver damage. Periodic evaluation of liver function is necessary in long-term therapy (more than two months).
• Side effects are more frequent in the elderly.
• Gastrointestinal upsets may be minimized by taking the drug with milk or food.

Interactions

• There is generally no added benefit in taking other NSAIDs or other ℞ **salicylates** (especially aspirin) at the same time, but there is a higher risk of gastrointestinal upsets and bleeding.
• Alcohol and ℞ **corticosteroids** increase the risk of bleeding, particularly if there is an existing ulcer.
• ℞ **Anticoagulant**, ℞ **antiplatelet**, and ℞ **thrombolytic** drugs may increase bleeding time.

Key to symbols: ✛ = Disorder Section ℞ = Drug Section ♣ = Herbal Section ⚬⚬ = Supplement Section

• The effectiveness of Ŗ **ACE inhibitors**, Ŗ **beta-blockers**, and Ŗ **diuretics** may be reduced.

• The effects of Ŗ **cyclosporine**, Ŗ **digoxin**, Ŗ **lithium**, and Ŗ **methotrexate** may be exaggerated, with potential for toxicity.

• Foodstuffs and herbals with Ŗ **antiplatelet** properties, for example, ♣ **ginger**, ⚯ **garlic**, and various herbal preparations, may add to the antiplatelet effect of NSAIDs.

Side effects

These vary in severity and how often they occur.

• Commonly, diarrhea, gastrointestinal upsets, nausea, constipation, flatulence, swelling of the extremities, dizziness, headache, ringing in the ears, itching, and rash.

• Less frequently, vomiting, sweating, nervousness, fatigue, insomnia, and photosensitivity of the skin.

• Prolonged bleeding time (with consequent risk of ulceration) is possible with high dosage, and other blood changes can occur, including anemia.

• Hypersensitivity reactions may include symptoms such as facial swelling, hives, rash, chest tightness, asthma, or bronchospasm.

• Reversible kidney failure, particularly in renal impairment, has occurred. Liver damage is rare.

nadolol ⒢

Type/Group: **beta-blocker; antianginal; antihypertensive; antimigraine; antianxiety**.
Brand(s): Corgard; various generic. Combinations: With *bendroflumethiazide*: Corzide.
How administered: Orally.

Used to treat

Nadolol can be used as an antihypertensive to lower blood pressure (see ⚙ **hypertension**) and in the treatment of ⚙ **angina pectoris** to relieve symptoms and improve exercise tolerance. Although not stated by the manufacturer, it is also sometimes used in the short-term treatment of thyrotoxicosis, for ⚙ **migraine** to prevent attacks, and ⚙ **anxiety**.

Warnings

• It should not be given to people with known hypersensitivity to any beta-blocking drug, who have certain heartbeat irregularities or heart failure, or bronchial asthma. It should not be used in cardiogenic shock.

• It should be given with caution to people with diabetes mellitus or hypoglycemia, hyperthyroidism, myasthenia gravis, congestive heart failure, peripheral vascular disease, bronchospastic disease (for example, chronic bronchitis or emphysema), or liver or kidney impairment.

• Nadolol should be used during pregnancy only if the potential benefit outweighs the possible risk to the fetus.

• It appears in breast milk, and so nursing women should discontinue using this drug or stop breast-feeding.

• Abruptly stopping using a beta-blocker may have adverse effects such as on the heart.

• The use of this drug may mask signs of hyperthyroidism or hypoglycemia.

• Other medications (including OTCs, herbal remedies, and supplements) must not be taken without consulting a doctor.

Some Ŗ **nasal decongestants**, commonly available over the counter, contain Ŗ **alpha-adrenergic stimulants** (for example, Ŗ **phenylephrine**) that may cause a severe hypertensive reaction if taken with beta-blockers.

Interactions

• A serious blood pressure increase may occur after withdrawal from Ŗ **clonidine hydrochloride** or both drugs at the same time.

• Other Ŗ **antiarrhythmics** (for example, Ŗ **amiodarone**, Ŗ **disopyramide**, Ŗ **procainamide**, Ŗ **quinidine**) and Ŗ **tricyclics** have the potential for significant adverse effects on heart rhythm.

• The effects of Ŗ **alpha-adrenergic stimulants**, Ŗ **ergot alkaloids**, Ŗ **epinephrine**, Ŗ **lidocaine**, and Ŗ **theophylline** may be increased, with the risk of serious adverse effects.

• Ŗ **Calcium-channel blockers** (particularly Ŗ **diltiazem hydrochloride** and Ŗ **verapamil**), Ŗ **MAOIs**, and Ŗ **reserpine** have the potential for increasing undesirable effects, with exaggerated slowing of heartbeat or hypotension. Verapamil and nadolol should not be used together.

• The effects of nondepolarizing Ŗ **skeletal muscle relaxants** may be variable, with the possible risk of significant adverse effects associated with major surgery.

• The effects of Ŗ **beta-adrenergic stimulants** (for example, Ŗ **albuterol**, Ŗ **terbutaline**), Ŗ **insulin**, and Ŗ **sulfonylureas** may be reduced by nadolol.

• Ŗ **Antacids** (for example, Ŗ **aluminum hydroxide**, Ŗ **magnesium hydroxide**), Ŗ **barbiturates**, ⚯ **calcium** salts, Ŗ **cholestyramine**, Ŗ **colestipol hydrochloride**, Ŗ NSAIDs, Ŗ **phenytoin**, Ŗ **penicillins**, Ŗ **rifampin**, and Ŗ **salicylates** may reduce the levels and effectiveness of beta-blockers.

• If used with Ŗ **diuretics** and other antihypertensive drugs, there are additive effects which are often used to therapeutic advantage.

Side effects

These are infrequent and may include:

• Dizziness, cold extremities, fatigue, lethargy, and slowing of the heart rate;

• Occasionally, gastrointestinal disturbances, rash or itching, dry mouth or eyes, or tingling sensations;

• Rarely, bronchospasm has been reported. Heart failure, should it develop, generally requires withdrawal (gradually, if possible) of this drug.

nafarelin acetate ⒢

Type/Group: **sex hormone; antiandrogen; antiestrogen; hormone antagonist**.
Brand(s): Synarel.
How administered: Nasal solution.

Used to treat

Nafarelin is a synthetic gonadotropin-releasing hormone (GnRH) analog used to treat ⚙ **endometriosis** (a growth of the lining of the uterus at inappropriate sites) and gonadotropin-dependent precocious puberty in both sexes. It reduces the secretion of gonadotropin by the pituitary gland, which results in the reduced secretion of sex hormones.

Warnings

• It should not be used by people with known hypersensitivity to gonadotropin-releasing hormones or their analogs, or with undiagnosed abnormal vaginal bleeding.
• Nafarelin acetate should not be used during pregnancy.
• It should not be used by breast-feeding mothers.
• If colds or nasal congestion develops, a doctor must be consulted about using a topical decongestant (nosedrops or spray). Do not use until at least two hours after nafarelin.
• Sneezing during or immediately after dosing must be avoided, as absorption of the drug may be impaired.
• Those taking the drug for endometriosis should notify a doctor if regular menstruation persists. Periods should stop with effective doses. Breakthrough bleeding or ovulation may occur if more than one dose is missed. A nonhormonal method of contraception must be used during treatment.
• Regular and complete daily dosing is very important when the drug is taken for precocious puberty.

Interactions

None have been noted.

Side effects

• In adult women, bone density loss, ovarian cysts, hot flashes, libido decrease, increased emotionality, vaginal dryness, acne, skin disturbances, and weight gain.
• In children, acne, transient breast enlargement, vaginal bleeding, increased emotionality, transient increase in pubic hair and body odor.

Nafazair ®

A preparation of ℞ **naphazoline hydrochloride**.
Formulation: Eye drops.
Availability: Prescription only.
Warnings and side effects: See ℞ **naphazoline hydrochloride**.

nafcillin ©

Type/Group: antibiotic; penicillin; antibacterial.
Brand(s): Nallpen; Unipen.
How administered: Orally; injection.

Used to treat

Nafcillin is a semisynthetic penicillinase-resistant penicillin used for penicillin-resistant staphylococcal ✪ **bacterial infections**.

Warnings

• It should not be used by people with known hypersensitivity to penicillins.
• It should be given with caution to people with allergies to ℞ **cephalosporins** or ℞ **imipenem**, or with impaired kidney or liver function.
• Penicillins cross the placenta and should be used in pregnancy only if medically judged to be needed.
• Nafcillin should not be used while breast-feeding.
• Serious and occasionally fatal hypersensitivity reactions can occur. A doctor must be contacted if skin rash, itching, hives, severe diarrhea, shortness of breath, black tongue, sore throat, nausea, fever, swollen joints, or any unusual bleeding or bruising occurs.

• Superinfections from the altered bacterial balance created by antibiotic treatment may occur and may result in ✪ **pseudomembranous colitis**. A doctor must be contacted if there is severe abdominal pain, or moderate to severe diarrhea.
• Take on an empty stomach (one hour before or two hours after eating).
• The full course of treatment prescribed must be completed or infection may return.

Interactions

• ℞ **Chloramphenicol**, ℞ **macrolide** antibiotics, and ℞ **tetracyclines** may reduce the effectiveness of penicillin.
• The effectiveness of ℞ **oral contraceptives** may be reduced.
• The levels of ℞ **cyclosporine** and ℞ **tacrolimus** may be reduced.
• The effects of ℞ **warfarin sodium** may be inhibited.

Side effects

• Frequently, mild allergic reaction, gastrointestinal effects (diarrhea, nausea, vomiting), vaginitis.
• Occasionally, depressed potassium levels with high intravenous doses, thrombophlebitis.
• Rarely, blood changes, and seizure.

naftifine ©

Type/Group: antifungal.
Brand(s): Naftin.
How administered: Topically (external).

Used to treat

Naftifine is a synthetic antifungal drug used to treat ✪ **fungal infections**, including athlete's foot, jock itch, and ringworm.

Warnings

• It should not be given to people with known hypersensitivity to naftifine.
• It should be used during pregnancy only if the benefits outweigh the risks to the fetus.
• Medical judgment is required if breast-feeding is being considered. It is not known if this drug appears in breast milk.
• Affected areas must not be covered with a bandage unless directed by a doctor.

Interactions

None significant have been reported when used topically (externally).

Side effects

• Burning, stinging, dryness, itching, redness, and local tenderness or irritation.

Naftin ®

A preparation of ℞ **naftifine**.
Formulation: Topical cream; topical gel.
Availability: Prescription only.
Warnings and side effects: See ℞ **naftifine**.

nalbuphine hydrochloride ©

Type/Group: narcotic analgesic; opioid.
Brand(s): Nubain; various generic.
How administered: Injection.

Used to treat

Nalbuphine is very similar to ℞ **morphine** in relieving pain, but with fewer side effects. Like morphine, it is used primarily to relieve moderate to severe ✪ **pain**, especially during or after surgery, and in childbirth.

Warnings

• It should not be given to people with known hypersensitivity to this drug. Opioids (even the weaker ones) should not be given to people with asthma, to anyone with seriously depressed breathing disorders, prostatic hypertrophy, convulsive disorders, raised intracranial pressure, or a head injury.

• Depending on use and dose, they should be given with caution to the elderly, or to anyone with hypotension, porphyria, certain liver, kidney or adrenal disorders, hypothyroidism (under-activity of the thyroid gland), or alcoholism.

• Except for during childbirth, nalbuphine should be used during pregnancy only if the benefits outweigh the possible risks, and with caution in premature delivery.

• Medical judgment is required if breast-feeding is being considered.

• Prolonged use of narcotics can lead to physical dependence (addiction), although this rarely happens in routine medical use.

• Drowsiness may affect the performance of skilled tasks such as driving.

• The effects of alcohol may be enhanced (including a higher risk of respiratory depression).

Interactions

• If the following drugs are used with nalbuphine, then effects are increased: ℞ **barbiturates**; ℞ **general anesthetics**; ℞ **tranquilizers** (for example, ℞ **phenothiazines**); ℞ **sedatives**; ℞ **benzodiazepines** (for example, ℞ **diazepam**, ℞ **lorazepam**); alcohol.

• ℞ **Rifampin** may precipitate withdrawal because it reduces nalbuphine levels.

Side effects

• These depend on dose and use. There is commonly sedation, less frequently sweating, vomiting, vertigo, nausea, dizziness, dry mouth, headache, loss of appetite, and constipation.

• There is occasionally euphoria, which may lead to a state of mental detachment or confusion. Also, there may be palpitations, changes in heart rate, postural hypotension (a lowering of blood pressure on standing, causing dizziness), rashes, miosis (pupil constriction), flushing of the face, mood change, crying, hallucinations, and potentially serious respiratory depression. It is reported to cause less nausea and vomiting than morphine.

Naldecon Senior DX Liquid Ⓑ

A preparation of ℞ **dextromethorphan** and ℞ **guaifenesin**.
Formulation: Oral liquid.
Availability: OTC.
Warnings and side effects: See ℞ **dextromethorphan**; ℞ **guaifenesin**.

Naldecon Senior EX Liquid Ⓑ

A preparation of ℞ **guaifenesin**.

Formulation: Oral liquid.
Availability: OTC.
Warnings and side effects: See ℞ **guaifenesin**.

Nalfon Pulvules Ⓑ

A preparation of ℞ **fenoprofen**.
Formulation: Oral capsules, available in two strengths.
Availability: Prescription only.
Warnings and side effects: See ℞ **fenoprofen**.

nalidixic acid Ⓖ

Type/Group: quinolone; antibacterial.
Brand(s): NegGram.
How administered: Orally.

Used to treat

Nalidixic acid is used primarily to treat ✪ **bacterial infections** of the urinary tract.

Warnings

• It should not be given to people with known hypersensitivity to nalidixic acid or a history of convulsive disorders.

• It should be given with caution to people over 65 and those with kidney disease, liver disease, or severe cerebral arteriosclerosis.

• Nalidixic acid's safety in the first trimester of pregnancy has not been established. It has been used in the second and third trimesters without apparent ill-effect, but it should be used only if the benefits outweigh the possible risk to the fetus.

• Medical judgment is required if breast-feeding is being considered.

• Seizure and other CNS (central nervous system) effects have occurred, usually from overdosage or individual susceptibility to such effects.

• Resistance to this drug may develop during treatment.

• It may cause drowsiness, dizziness, or blurred vision. Exercise care when driving or performing tasks requiring alertness.

Interactions

• The anticoagulant effect of ℞ **warfarin** is increased.

Side effects

• Frequently, dizziness, headache, and gastrointestinal effects (abdominal pain, nausea, vomiting, diarrhea).

• Occasionally, drowsiness, increased intracranial pressure, blurred vision, light sensitivity, rash, itching, and hives.

Nallpen Ⓑ

A preparation of ℞ **nafcillin**.
Formulation: Oral capsules, injection.
Availability: Prescription only.
Warnings and side effects: See ℞ **nafcillin**.

naloxone hydrochloride Ⓖ

Type/Group: **opioid antagonist; antidote.**
Brand(s): Narcan; various generic. Combinations: With *pentazocine*: Talwin NX; various generic.
How administered: Injection; intravenous infusion.

Used to treat

Naloxone is used primarily as an antidote to an overdose of opioid ℞ **narcotic analgesics**. It is quick but short-acting and effectively reverses or prevents the respiratory depression, coma, or convulsions that can follow overdosage of opioids. Administration is by intramuscular or intravenous injection and may be repeated at short intervals until there is some response. It is also used at the end of operations to reverse respiratory depression caused by opioid narcotic analgesics, and in newborn babies where mothers have been administered large amounts of opioid (such as ℞ **meperidine**) for pain-relief during labor. Although not stated by the manufacturer for such treatments, it has been investigated for use in reversing alcohol-induced coma, to treat serious shock, schizophrenia, and dementia in Alzheimer's disease.

Warnings

• It should not be given to people with known hypersensitivity to this drug.

• It should be given with caution to people with heart disease.

• Naloxone should be used during pregnancy only when it is clearly needed.

• Medical judgment is required if breast-feeding is being considered. It is not known whether this drug appears in breast milk.

• It should not be given to patients who are physically dependent on narcotics, except when necessary to reverse overdose symptoms.

• It is a specialist drug and is used in controlled conditions.

Interactions

• Naloxone has no significant interactions when used as a quick-acting and rapidly clearing antidote, other than with the opioids whose action it reverses. It is available in a combination with ℞ **pentazocine**, which is thought to reduce the potential for opioid dependence.

Side effects

• Reversal of opioid effects may cause nausea, vomiting, sweating, rapid heartbeat, and nervousness.

• When used postoperatively, there may be pain (from loss of analgesia).

• There may be changes in blood pressure, disturbance in heart rhythm, pulmonary edema, and, rarely, seizures.

naltrexone hydrochloride ⓖ

Type/Group: **opioid antagonist; substance-dependence treatment**.

Brand(s): ReVia; various generic.

How administered: Orally.

Used to treat

Naltrexone is used in detoxification treatment for formerly opioid-dependent people to help prevent relapse, and to treat recovering alcoholics. Since it is an antagonist of dependence-causing opioids (such as heroin), it will cause withdrawal symptoms in those already taking opioids. During naltrexone treatment, the euphoric effects of habit-forming opioids are blocked, so helping to prevent re-addiction. Treatment is started in specialist clinics. (For overdose with opioids, the related drug ℞ **naloxone** is normally used.)

Although not stated by the manufacturer for such treatments, it is sometimes used for eating disorders, postconcussional syndrome, and as an aid in alcohol withdrawal in alcoholics.

Warnings

• It should not be given to people with known hypersensitivity to this drug, who have acute liver disease, or who are currently taking any opioid drug.

• It should be given with caution to people with certain kidney or liver disorders.

• Naltrexone should be used during pregnancy only if the benefits outweigh the possible risks.

• Medical judgment is required if breast-feeding is being considered. It is not known whether this drug appears in breast milk.

• Opioid-dependent patients should not try to overcome the effects of naltrexone (by taking more opioid) as this can cause dangerous intoxication.

• A doctor must be contacted and use of the drug stopped if symptoms such as abdominal pain lasting several days, yellowing of the eyes, dark urine, or white stools occur.

Interactions

• The effects of ℞ **opioid**-containing products (including certain over-the-counter cough and analgesic preparations) are counteracted by naltrexone, and withdrawal symptoms may appear in people already opioid-tolerant.

• If used with ℞ **thioridazine**, it may cause drowsiness and lethargy.

Side effects

• There may be nausea, vomiting, abdominal pain, anxiety, nervousness, difficulty in sleeping, headache, and pain in the joints and muscles. There may also be diarrhea or constipation, thirst, sweating, dizziness, chills, tearfulness, irritability, depression, rash, lethargy, and decreased sexual potency.

• There have been reports of liver toxicity (that can be serious) and blood abnormalities.

nandrolone ⓖ

Type/Group: **anabolic steroid; sex hormone; anemia treatment**.

Brand(s): DecaDurabolin; Hybolin Decanoate; Kabolin; various generic.

How administered: Injection.

Used to treat

Nandrolone is an anabolic steroid that has similar actions to the male sex hormone ℞ **testosterone** (although it has far fewer masculinizing effects). It is used to treat ✪ **anemia** caused by kidney insufficiency.

Warnings

• It should not be given to people with certain kidney disorders, women with breast cancer with hypercalcemia, or men with breast or prostate cancer.

• It should be given with caution to people over 65, children, anyone with heart disease or risk factors for heart disease, porphyria, kidney or liver disease, seizure disorder, migraine headache, or diabetes mellitus.

• Nandrolone should not be used during pregnancy.

Key to symbols: ✪ = Disorder Section ℞ = Drug Section ♣ = Herbal Section ⚬⚬ = Supplement Section

• Medical judgment is required if breast-feeding is being considered.

• There is a risk of serious liver damage.

• It may cause masculinization in women and premature cessation of growth in children.

• It should not be used to enhance athletic performance. This is a Schedule III controlled substance.

Interactions

• If used with ℞ **antidiabetic** drugs, there are enhanced hypoglycemic effects.

• The levels of ℞ **cyclosporine**, oral ℞ **anticoagulants**, and ℞ **tacrolimus** are increased.

• If used with HMG-CoA reductase inhibitors (for example, ℞ **lovastatin**, ℞ **pravastatin**), the risk of myositis (inflammation of muscle tissue) is increased.

Side effects

• Acne, hair loss, flushing, growth of body hair, rash, sweating, mental changes, rapid, jerky movements, insomnia, edema, deepening of voice, hoarseness, cholestatic jaundice, diarrhea, nausea, amenorrhea, clitoral hypertrophy, decreased breast size, decreased libido, testicular atrophy, vaginitis, decreased glucose tolerance, changes in cholesterol levels, retention of sodium chloride, water, potassium, phosphates or calcium, and hair loss.

naphazoline hydrochloride ⑥

Type/Group: **alpha-adrenergic stimulant; sympathomimetic; vasoconstrictor; decongestant.**

Brand(s): (For ophthalmic use): AK-Con; Albalon; Allerest Eye Drops; Allergy Drops, Maximum Strength; Clear Eyes, ACR; Comfort Eye Drops; Nafazair; Naphcon, Naphcon Forte; 20/20 Eye Drops; VasoClear; Vasocon Regular; various generic. (For nasal decongestion): Privine.

How administered: Nasal; ophthalmic (eye).

Used to treat

Naphazoline is generally used for its vasoconstrictor properties (narrows blood vessels), as a nasal decongestant, and for the symptomatic relief of redness and irritation in the eye.

Warnings

• It should not be given to people with known hypersensitivity to this or any other adrenergic drug, with angle-closure glaucoma, or severe high blood pressure or coronary artery disease.

• It should be given with caution to people taking ℞ **MAOI** antidepressants, or who have high blood pressure, heart disease, hyperthyroidism, diabetes mellitus, enlarged prostate, or increased intraocular pressure (pressure in the eyeball, including glaucoma).

• Naphazoline's effects during pregnancy are not known, it should be used with caution and only if there is clear benefit.

• Medical judgment is required if breast-feeding is being considered.

• In ophthalmic combinations with antazoline, eyedrops should not be used while soft contact lenses are being worn.

• Overuse may cause symptoms such as nervousness and insomnia, and actually make congestion worse, which is an effect called "rebound congestion." No nasal decongestant should be used for longer than three to four days.

• It should be used with caution by the elderly, as they are more likely to suffer side effects.

• The manufacturer's recommendations must be followed carefully when giving to children under 12.

Interactions

• When used topically (externally, to the nose or eyes) at recommended doses, the interactions common to ℞ **sympathomimetics** do not usually apply. However, in overdose there may be interactions similar to ℞ **ephedrine**.

• Naphazoline should not be used with ℞ **MAOI** antidepressants, or within two weeks of stopping MAOI treatment, because this may cause a hypertensive crisis.

Side effects

• These depend on how it is administered. As eyedrops it may cause blurred vision or stinging. When used as a nasal decongestant, it may cause irritation in the nose.

• In nasal or ophthalmic (eye) application systemic side effects are infrequent, and usually occur only with overdose (especially in children) and consist of the usual symptoms associated with sympathomimetics, including changes in heart rate and blood pressure, anxiety, restlessness, tremor, insomnia, dry mouth, cold fingertips and toes, and changes in the prostate gland.

Naphcon; Naphcon Forte ⑧

A preparation of ℞ **naphazoline hydrochloride**.

Formulation: Eye drops.

Availability: OTC; Forte is prescription only.

Warnings and side effects: See ℞ **naphazoline hydrochloride**.

Naphcon A Eye Drops ⑧

A preparation of ℞ **pheniramine maleate**.

Formulation: Eye drops.

Availability: OTC.

Warnings and side effects: See ℞ **pheniramine maleate**.

Naphcon A Solution ⑧

A preparation of ℞ **pheniramine maleate** and ℞ **naphazoline hydrochloride**.

Formulation: Eye drops.

Availability: OTC.

Warnings and side effects: See ℞ **pheniramine maleate**; ℞ **naphazoline hydrochloride**.

Naprelan ⑧

A preparation of ℞ **naproxen**.

Formulation: Oral tablets, controlled release, available in two strengths.

Availability: Prescription only.

Warnings and side effects: See ℞ **naproxen**.

Naprosyn; EC-Naprosyn; Naprosyn Suspension ⑧

A preparation of ℞ **naproxen**.

Formulation: Oral liquid; tablets; EC tablets are delayed release.

Availability: Prescription only.

Warnings and side effects: See ℞ **naproxen.**

naproxen Ⓖ
(naproxen sodium)

Type/Group: anti-inflammatory; antirheumatic; non-narcotic analgesic; NSAID; antigout.

Brand(s): Aleve Tablets, Capsules, Gelcaps; Anaprox, Anaprox DS; Naprelan; Naprosyn, EC-Naprosyn, Naprosyn Suspension; various generic.

How administered: Orally.

Used to treat
Naproxen is used to relieve mild to moderate pain and inflammation, particularly of ✪ **bursitis**, tendonitis, ✪ **osteoarthritis**, ✪ **rheumatoid arthritis**, ✪ **ankylosing spondylitis**, acute ✪ **gout**, juvenile arthritis, and other ✪ **musculoskeletal disorders**; and also mild to moderate pain such as headache and period pain, and as an ℞ **antipyretic** to relieve fever.

Warnings
• It should not be used by people with known hypersensitivity to this drug or to other NSAIDs (including ℞ **aspirin**), who have chronic kidney disease, certain bleeding disorders or conditions (for example, hemophilia, vitamin K deficiency, low blood-platelet levels), or who have a tendency to, or active, peptic ulceration.

• It should be given with caution to people who are taking certain drugs for gout, who have diabetes mellitus, SLE (systemic lupus erythematosus), or allergic disorders (especially asthma and skin conditions), who are elderly, or with any kind of kidney impairment or certain liver disorders.

• Naproxen should be used when pregnant only if medically judged to be needed. However, it must not be used in the third trimester, because this is when risk to the fetus is at irs highest.

• Breast-feeding mothers should either discontinue this drug or stop breast-feeding.

• The two forms of this drug (naproxen and naproxen sodium) should not be used together, because this may cause overdose symptoms and side effects.

• With regular use (as in the treatment of osteoarthritis), NSAIDs may cause gastrointestinal bleeding, ulceration, or perforation. Any signs of bleeding (for example, black stools) should be reported to a physician immediately.

• Most NSAIDs have the potential, particularly with regular use, to cause liver damage. Periodic evaluation of liver function is necessary in long-term therapy (more than two months).

• Its side effects (such as drowsiness and dizziness) may impair the performance of skilled tasks, such as driving.

• Side effects are more frequent in the elderly.

• Gastrointestinal upsets may be minimized by taking the drug with milk or food.

Interactions
• There is generally no added benefit in taking other NSAIDs or other ℞ **salicylates** (especially aspirin) at the same time, but there is a higher risk of gastrointestinal upsets and bleeding.

• Alcohol and ℞ **corticosteroids** increase the risk of bleeding, particularly if there is an existing ulcer.

• ℞ **Anticoagulant**, ℞ **antiplatelet**, and ℞ **thrombolytic** drugs may increase bleeding time.

• The effectiveness of ℞ **ACE inhibitors**, ℞ **beta-blockers**, and ℞ **diuretics** may be reduced.

• Naproxen should not be taken with triamterene, because there is a risk of kidney failure.

• The effects of ℞ **cyclosporine**, ℞ **digoxin**, ℞ **lithium**, and ℞ **methotrexate** may be exaggerated, with potential for toxicity.

• Naproxen should be started at a low dose when used with ℞ **probenecid** for treating gout, because probenecid increases its concentration and effect.

• Foodstuffs and herbals with ℞ **antiplatelet** properties, for example, ♣ **ginger**, ⚬⚬ **garlic**, and various herbal preparations, may add to the antiplatelet effect of NSAIDs.

Side effects
These vary in severity and how often they occur.

• The risk of gastrointestinal side effects is intermediate for its class of drugs.

• Commonly, constipation, gastrointestinal upsets, heartburn, nausea, swelling of the extremities, drowsiness, dizziness, headache, ringing in the ears, itching, and rash.

• Less frequently, diarrhea, vomiting, sweating, mouth sores, blurred vision, depression, malaise, and insomnia.

• Prolonged bleeding time (with consequent risk of ulceration) is possible with high dosage, and other blood changes can occur, including anemia.

• Hypersensitivity reactions may include symptoms such as hives, rash, chest tightness, asthma, or bronchospasm.

• Reversible kidney failure, particularly in renal impairment, has occurred. Liver damage is rare.

naproxen sodium Ⓖ
see ℞ **naproxen.**

Naqua Ⓡ
A preparation of ℞ **trichlormethiazide**.

Formulation: Oral tablets, available in two strengths.

Availability: Prescription only.

Warnings and side effects: See ℞ **trichlormethiazide.**

naratriptan Ⓖ
Type/Group: serotonin-receptor stimulant; vasoconstrictor; antimigraine.

Brand(s): Amerge.

How administered: Orally.

Used to treat
Naratriptan is a recently introduced drug which is used to treat acute ✪ **migraine** attacks (but not to prevent attacks). It works as a ℞ **vasoconstrictor** (through acting as a serotonin receptor stimulant selective for serotonin 5-HT$_1$ receptors), producing a rapid narrowing of blood vessels surrounding the brain.

Warnings
• Avoid its use in people with known hypersensitivity to this drug, or who have certain cardiovascular disorders including peripheral vascular disease, pre-existing heart diseases, including ischemic

heart disease, previous myocardial infarction (heart attack), coronary vasospasm, including some types of angina, or with uncontrolled hypertension; severe kidney or liver impairment.

• Naratriptan should not be used when the headache takes an unusual form, especially migraine in which one half of the body experiences some degree of paralysis during the migraine attack.

• Drugs of this class (that is, those stimulating serotonin 5-HT$_1$ receptors) are used only with great caution where risk factors are present that predispose a person to coronary artery disease. They should be used with care in anyone with impaired liver or kidney function.

• It is recommended that first-time administration of naratriptan to anyone with significant risk factors for coronary artery disease takes place at a physician's office or other medical facility.

• Naratriptan should be used in pregnancy only if the potential benefits outweigh the potential risks to the fetus.

• Medical judgment is also required if it is to be used by a breast-feeding mother.

• If sudden or severe abdominal pain occurs after taking this drug, a doctor must be contacted immediately.

• This drug should not be used at the same time, or shortly after, using ℞ **ergotamine** or other migraine therapies. Ergotamine-like antimigraine drugs should not be taken until 6 hours after this type of antimigraine drug. Also, this type of antimigraine drug should not be taken until at least 24 hours after an ergotamine-like antimigraine drug.

• The dose should not usually be repeated during the same migraine attack.

• Drowsiness may interfere with performance of skilled tasks such as driving.

Interactions

• There is a risk of additive effect, with potentially serious consequences, if taken with ℞ **ergotamine**-containing drugs (such as ℞ **dihydroergotamine** and ℞ **methysergide**).

• Oral ℞ **contraceptives** and ℞ **cimetidine** may increase concentrations of naratriptan.

• ℞ **SSRI** antidepressants (for example, ℞ **fluoxetine**, ℞ **fluvoxamine**, ℞ **paroxetine**, ℞ **sertraline**) may increase the possibility of some less-frequent side effects, such as weakness and incoordination, occurring, and so caution is recommended.

• ♣ **St. John's wort** should not be used at the same time, as there is an increased risk of adverse effects.

Side effects

• Chest pain and tightness in parts of the body, including the chest, jaw, or throat, which may indicate constriction of the blood vessels of the heart (or of anaphylaxis). If the pain is intense, use of naratriptan should stop;

• The most common side effects are sensations of warmth or cold, vertigo, dry mouth, vomiting, tingling, and sensitivity to light (photophobia);

• Less frequently there may be diarrhea, nervousness, confusion, insomnia, palpitations, increased blood pressure, dehydration, thirst, a feeling of weakness, fainting, muscle cramps or pain, blurred vision, drowsiness, and chills or fever;

• Rarely, allergy-like symptoms such as facial swelling, including the eyes, itching, rash, and hives.

Narcan ℞

A preparation of ℞ **naloxone hydrochloride**.
Formulation: Injection.
Availability: Prescription only.
Warnings and side effects: See ℞ **naloxone hydrochloride**.

narcotic analgesic Ⓓ

((opioid) narcotic analgesic)
alfentanil; buprenorphine hydrochloride; codeine phosphate; dextromethorphan; fentanyl; hydrocodone bitartrate; meperidine hydrochloride; methadone hydrochloride; morphine sulfate; nalbuphine hydrochloride; oxycodone; pentazocine; propoxyphene hydrochloride; remifentanil; tramadol hydrochloride.

Actions and uses

Narcotic analgesics are morphine-like drugs which have powerful actions on the central nervous system (CNS) and alter the perception of ✪ **pain**. Many are ℞ **opiate** drugs, that is, they are chemically related to ℞ **morphine** and similar ℞ **alkaloid** agents derived from the opium poppy (*Papaver somniferum*). They are all opioid agents, that is, they work by mimicking the actions of natural opioid neurotransmitters (enkephalins, endorphins, dynorphins) in the brain by activating at their receptors.

Because of the numerous possible side effects, the most important of which is drug dependence (habituation or addiction), this class is usually used under strict medical supervision and preparations are normally available only on prescription. Narcotic analgesics are used for different types and severities of pain, but where there is severe pain (for example, postoperative, post-injury, or terminal cancer) there is little choice but to use this class of agent.

Other notable side effects include depression of breathing, nausea and vomiting, sometimes hypotension (lowered blood pressure), constipation (therefore they can be used as ℞ **antidiarrheal** drugs), inhibition of coughing (so can be used as ℞ **antitussive** drugs to treat troublesome coughing), and constriction of the pupils (miosis).

In practice, care is normally taken to chose a narcotic analgesic no stronger than is needed for the symptoms. Weaker members of the class (for example, ℞ **codeine phosphate**) are used for minor pain, or are combined with ℞ **non-narcotic analgesics**. Somewhat stronger members (for example, ℞ **meperidine hydrochloride**) can be used for preoperative and postoperative medication, and obstetric analgesia (during labor). For treatment of moderate to severe pain, longer-lasting and more powerful agents such as morphine can be used.

Limitations

The side effects of narcotic analgesics can limit their usefulness, and much research effort has been put into developing synthetic drugs with no risk of addiction and less side effects such as respiratory depression. Some small progress has been made, mainly by exploring opioid receptor subtype selective agents, but much remains to be achieved. The analgesic ℞ **tramadol hydrochloride** is one new development where narcotic (opioid) analgesic properties are combined with a second (adrenergic) analgesic action.

In the event of opioid overdose, or in newborn babies after obstetric analgesia, most effects of the opioid narcotic analgesics (the most serious of which is respiratory depression) may be reversed with an ℞ **opioid antagonist** (for example, naloxone hydrochloride). See also the individual drug entries and ℞ **non-narcotic analgesics**.

narcotic antagonist (opioid) Ⓓ

see ℞ opioid antagonist.

Nardil Ⓑ

A preparation of ℞ **phenelzine**.
Formulation: Oral tablets.
Availability: Prescription only.
Warnings and side effects: See ℞ phenelzine.

Naropin Ⓑ

A preparation of ℞ **ropivacaine hydrochloride**.
Formulation: Injection in several strengths.
Availability: Prescription only.
Warnings and side effects: See ℞ ropivacaine hydrochloride.

Nasabid SR Tablets; Capsules Ⓑ

A preparation of ℞ **pseudoephedrine** and ℞ **guaifenesin**.
Formulation: Oral tablets; capsules; both long acting.
Availability: Prescription only.
Warnings and side effects: See ℞ pseudoephedrine; ℞ guaifenesin.

Nasacort; Nasacort AQ Ⓑ

A preparation of ℞ **triamcinolone** propionate.
Formulation: Inhaler; nasal spray (AQ is spray).
Availability: Prescription only.
Warnings and side effects: See ℞ triamcinolone.

Nasalcrom Ⓑ

A preparation of ℞ **cromolyn sodium**.
Formulation: Nasal spray.
Availability: OTC.
Warnings and side effects: See ℞ cromolyn sodium.

nasal decongestant Ⓓ

see ℞ decongestant.

Nasatab LA Tablets Ⓑ

A preparation of ℞ **pseudoephedrine** and ℞ **guaifenesin**.
Formulation: Oral tablets, long acting.
Availability: Prescription only.
Warnings and side effects: See ℞ pseudoephedrine; ℞ guaifenesin.

Nascobal Ⓑ

A preparation of ♧ **cyanocobalamin**.

Formulation: Intranasal gel.
Availability: Prescription only.
Warnings and side effects: See ♧ **cyanocobalamin**.

Nasonex Ⓑ

A preparation of ℞ **mometasone**.
Formulation: Nasal spray.
Availability: Prescription only.
Warnings and side effects: See ℞ mometasone.

Nature's Remedy Tablets Ⓑ

A preparation of aloe and ℞ **cascara sagrada**.
Formulation: Oral tablets.
Availability: OTC.
Warnings and side effects: See ℞ cascara sagrada.

Naturetin Ⓑ

A preparation of ℞ **bendroflumethiazide**.
Formulation: Oral tablets, available in two strengths.
Availability: Prescription only.
Warnings and side effects: See ℞ bendroflumethiazide.

Navane Ⓑ

A preparation of ℞ **thiothixene**.
Formulation: Oral tablets in several strengths; oral concentrate.
Availability: Prescription only.
Warnings and side effects: See ℞ thiothixene.

Navelbine Ⓑ

A preparation of ℞ **vinorelbine tartrate**.
Formulation: Injection (intravenous only).
Availability: Prescription only.
Warnings and side effects: See ℞ vinorelbine tartrate.

ND Clear Capsules Ⓑ

A preparation of ℞ **pseudoephedrine** and ℞ **chlorpheniramine maleate**.
Formulation: Oral capsules, sustained release.
Availability: Prescription only.
Warnings and side effects: See ℞ pseudoephedrine; ℞ chlorpheniramine maleate.

ND-Gesic Tablets Ⓑ

A preparation of ℞ **phenylephrine hydrochloride**, ℞ **acetaminophen**, ℞ **chlorpheniramine maleate**, and ℞ **pyrilamine maleate**.
Formulation: Oral tablets.
Availability: OTC.
Warnings and side effects: See ℞ phenylephrine hydrochloride; ℞ acetaminophen; ℞ chlorpheniramine maleate; ℞ pyrilamine maleate.

Necon 1/50 Ⓑ

A preparation of ℞ **mestranol** and ℞ **norethindrone**.
Formulation: Calendar pack of oral tablets.

　Key to symbols: ✿ = Disorder Section　℞ = Drug Section　♣ = Herbal Section　♧ = Supplement Section

Availability: Prescription only.
Warnings and side effects: See ℞ mestranol; ℞ norethindrone.

nedocromil sodium ⑥

Type/Group: **antiasthmatic; antiallergic**.
Brand(s): Tilade.
How administered: Inhalation.

Used to treat

Nedocromil sodium is used in the maintenance treatment of mild to moderate ✪ **asthma**.

Warnings

• It should not be given to people with known hypersensitivity to this drug.
• It should be used during pregnancy only when it is clearly needed.
• Medical judgment is required if breast-feeding is being considered. It is not known whether this drug is present in breast milk.
• It is not a ℞ **bronchodilator** and is not effective against acute asthma attacks.
• It must be used regularly (even if no symptoms occur) and it may take up to four weeks for its beneficial effects to be felt.

Interactions

No significant interactions have been reported.

Side effects

• Frequently, cough, throat irritation, bronchospasm, headache, and unpleasant taste.
• Occasionally, nasal inflammation, upper respiratory tract infection, abdominal pain, and fatigue.
• Rarely, diarrhea and dizziness.

nefazodone hydrochloride ⑥

Type/Group: **antidepressant**.
Brand(s): Serzone.
How administered: Orally.

Used to treat

Nefazodone hydrochloride is a treatment for ✪ **depression**. It is chemically dissimilar to members of the main antidepressant groups, but like the ℞ **SSRI** and ℞ **tricyclic** groups it inhibits re-uptake of 5-HT. It also blocks 5-HT receptors. It has an advantage over the tricyclics in that it has relatively less sedative and ℞ **anticholinergic** side effects. As is the case with other antidepressants, this drug is also being evaluated for other uses.

Warnings

• It should not be given to people with known hypersensitivity to this drug, or who are taking ℞ **fexofenadine**, astemizole, ℞ **nefazodone**, cisapride, ℞ **pimozide**, ℞ **triazolam**, or ℞ **alprazolam**. It should not be taken by anyone who is taking or has stopped taking a ℞ **MAOI** antidepressant in the previous 14 days.
• It should be given with caution to people with liver or kidney impairment, cardiovascular disease, cerebrovascular disease, dehydration, low blood volume, a history of mania, or seizure disorder.
• Nefazodone should be used during pregnancy only if the benefits outweigh the possible risk to the fetus.

• Medical judgment is required if breast-feeding is being considered.
• Because there have been reports of liver damage, a doctor must be contacted if nausea, vomiting, abdominal pain, fatigue, anorexia, dark urine, jaundice, or other signs or symptoms of liver problems occur.
• A doctor should be consulted before taking any other medications, including OTC preparations, herbal remedies (especially ♣ **St. John's wort**), supplements, or other natural or alternative products.
• Do not drink alcohol.
• It may impair the performance of skilled tasks requiring mental alertness or physical skills, such as driving.
• Treatment should be stopped gradually, lowering the dose over a period of time.
• It may take several weeks before there are any signs of improvement.

Interactions

• Serious or even fatal reactions can occur if ℞ **MAOI** antidepressants are taken at the same time, or within a period of a few weeks after the use of, other antidepressants.
• ℞ **buspirone** and ℞ **sibutramine** may increase the effects of nefazodone.
• The effects of ℞ **benzodiazepines**, ℞ **buspirone**, ℞ **carbamazepine**, cisapride, ℞ **digoxin**, ℞ **pimozide**, ♣ **St. John's wort**, ℞ **trazodone**, ℞ **haloperidol**, hmg-coA reductase inhibitors (for example, ℞ **atorvastatin**, ℞ **fluvastatin**, ℞ **lovastatin**, ℞ **simvastatin**) may be increased.
• The effects of ℞ **propranolol** may be reduced, while the effects of nefazodone may be increased.

Side effects

• Gastrointestinal effects (constipation, diarrhea, dry mouth, increased appetite, nausea), muscle weakness, sleepiness, dizziness, confusion, and headache.
• Less frequently, chills, fever, postural hypotension (lowered blood pressure on standing, and, rarely, fainting), sensitivity reactions, impotence, urinary frequency or retention, vaginitis, lightheadedness, tingling in the extremities, confusion, unsteady gait, and minor visual disturbances.

NeGram ⑧

A preparation of ℞ **nalidixic acid**.
Formulation: Oral caplets; oral suspension.
Availability: Prescription only.
Warnings and side effects: See ℞ nalidixic acid.

nelfinavir ⑥

Type/Group: **antiviral**.
Brand(s): Viracept.
How administered: Orally.

Used to treat

Nelfinavir is a protease inhibitor antiviral drug that is often used together with reverse transcriptase antivirals in antiretroviral treatment of progressive or advanced ✪ **HIV** infection.

Warnings
• It should not be given to people with known hypersensitivity to nelfinavir.
• It should be given with caution to people with phenylketonuria, liver insufficiency, or hemophilia.
• Nelfinavir's safety during pregnancy has not been established, and it should be used only when the potential benefits clearly outweigh the possible risks to the fetus.
• Medical judgment is required if breast-feeding is being considered. HIV-infected mothers are advised not to breast-feed.
• It may cause increased bleeding in hemophiliacs.
• It is a specialist drug, and there will be full assessment and patient monitoring throughout treatment.

Interactions
These are many and include:
• The levels of ℞ **barbiturates**, ℞ **carbamazepine**, ℞ **phenytoin**, and ℞ **rifabutin** are increased while the levels of nelfinavir are decreased;
• The effects of ℞ **ergot alkaloids**, ℞ **lovastatin**, ℞ **midazolam**, ℞ **simvastatin**, and ℞ **triazolam** may be increased;
• If taken with ℞ **erythromycin**, the effects of both drugs are increased;
• The effectiveness of ℞ **oral contraceptives** may be reduced;
• ℞ **Rifampin** reduces the levels of nelfinavir;
• The levels of ℞ **fexofenadine**, astemizole, and cisapride are increased.

Side effects
These can be many and include:
• Nausea, diarrhea and flatulence, rash, hepatitis, changes in blood counts and enzymes, weakness, sexual dysfunction, and others.

Nelova ®
A preparation of ℞ **ethinyl estradiol** and ℞ **norethindrone**.
Formulation: Calendar pack of oral tablets; monophasic form available in two strengths.
Availability: Prescription only.
Warnings and side effects: See ℞ **ethinyl estradiol**; ℞ **norethindrone**.

Nelova 1/50M ®
A preparation of ℞ **mestranol** and ℞ **norethindrone**.
Formulation: Calendar pack of oral tablets.
Availability: Prescription only.
Warnings and side effects: See ℞ **mestranol**; ℞ **norethindrone**.

NeoDecadron Solution ®
A preparation of ℞ **dexamethasone** and ℞ **neomycin**.
Formulation: Opthalmic solution.
Availability: Prescription only.
Warnings and side effects: See ℞ **dexamethasone**; ℞ **neomycin**.

Neo-Dexameth ®
A preparation of ℞ **neomycin** and ℞ **dexamethasone**.
Formulation: Opthalmic solution.

Availability: Prescription only.
Warnings and side effects: See ℞ **neomycin**; ℞ **dexamethasone**.

Neo-Diaral ®
A preparation of ℞ **loperamide hydrochloride**.
Formulation: Oral capsules.
Availability: OTC.
Warnings and side effects: See ℞ **loperamide hydrochloride**.

Neo-fradin ®
A preparation of ℞ **neomycin**.
Formulation: Oral solution.
Availability: Prescription only.
Warnings and side effects: See ℞ **neomycin**.

Neomixin Ointment ®
A preparation of ℞ **neomycin**, ℞ **polymyxin B sulfate**, and ℞ **bacitracin**.
Formulation: Topical Ointment.
Availability: OTC.
Warnings and side effects: See ℞ **neomycin**; ℞ **polymyxin B sulfate**; ℞ **bacitracin**.

neomycin Ⓖ
Type/Group: **aminoglycoside; antibiotic; antibacterial**.
How administered: Orally; topically; eye; ear.
Brand(s): Systemic: Mycifradin; Neo-fradin; various generic. Topical: Myciguent; various generic. Combinations: With *polymyxin B*: Neosporin Cream. With *polymyxin B* and *bacitracin*: Neosporin Maximum Strength; Medi-Quick Ointment; Neomixin Ointment; Neosporin Ointment; Septa Ointment; Mycitracin Maximum; Triple Antibiotic Ointment; Mycitracin Plus; AK-Spore Ophthalmic ointment; Triple Antibiotic Ophthalmic; various generic. With *polymyxin B*, bacitracin, and *lidocaine*: Neosporin Plus; Lanabiotic; Mycitracin; Tribiotic Plus; Clomycin; Campho-Phenique Antibiotic Plus Pain Reliever; Spectrocin Plus. With *polymyxin B, bacitracin, diperodon*: Bactine First Aid Antibiotic Plus Anesthetic Ointment. With *polymyxin B* and *gramicidin*: AK-Spore Solution (eye drops); Neosporin Solution (eye drops); various generic. With *hydrocortisone*: Cortisporin. With *hydrocortisone* and *polymyxin B*: Cortisporin Ophthalmic; AK-Spore H.C. Ophthalmic; Cortisporin Suspension Otic; AntibiOtic; Cortatrigen Modified Ear Drops; Drotic; Ear-Eze; LaserSporin-C Otic; Otic-Care; Octicair; Otocort; Otomycin-HPN. With *hydrocortisone* and *bacitracin*: Cortisporin; Neotricin-HC. With *hydrocortisone* and *bacitracin* and *polymyxin B*: Neotricin HC Ophthalmic. With *triamcinolone*: Mycobiotic II. With *dexamethasone*: NeoDecadron; Neo-Dexamith; AK-Neo-Dex Solution. With *dexamethasone* and *benzalkonium chloride*: Dexacidin Ophthalmic Solution; AK-Trol Ophthalmic solution; Maxitrol Ophthalmic Solution. With *dexamethasone* and *polymyxin B*: Dexacidin Ophthalmic Ointment; AK-Trol Ophthalmic Ointment; Maxitrol Ophthalmic Ointment. With *methylprednisolone*: Neo-Medrol.

Used to treat

Neomycin is an original member of the aminoglycoside family. It is effective in treating some superficial ✪ **bacterial infections** and has quite a widespread use when used topically (in the eyes, ears, or on the skin). However, it is too toxic to be administered by intravenous or intramuscular injection. It is occasionally taken by mouth to reduce the levels of bacteria in the colon prior to intestinal surgery or examination, or in liver failure. When administered orally it is not absorbed from the gastrointestinal tract.

Warnings

• It should not be given to people with known hypersensitivity to neomycin or other aminoglycosides, or with severe kidney disease.

• It should be given with caution to people with mild kidney or liver disease, hearing deficits or vertigo, dehydration, neuromuscular disorders (for example, parkinsonism, myasthenia gravis), and those over 65.

• Medical judgment is required when giving to very young infants and depending on use. It should not be used if there is gastrointestinal disease or intestinal obstruction.

• Neomycin should be used during pregnancy only if medically judged to be clearly needed and if the potential benefits outweigh the risks to the fetus (other aminoglycosides cross the placenta and can cause damage to ears or kidneys).

• Medical judgment is required if breast-feeding is being considered.

• Although only small amounts of neomycin are absorbed when taken orally, or when used topically for short-term therapy not involving extensive areas of skin, aminoglycosides are associated with nephrotoxicity (damage to the kidneys) and ototoxicity (damage in the ears). Irreversible vestibular impairment can occur, resulting in vertigo and difficulty maintaining balance. Permanent hearing loss in one or both ears can also occur.

• A doctor must be contacted if there are problems with hearing, vision, balance, urination, or headaches, even after the course of treatment is completed.

• The use of antibiotics may result in superinfection due to bacterial imbalance.

Interactions

• ℞ **Atracurium**, ℞ **succinylcholine**, ℞ **vecuronium**, or neuromuscular blocking agents taken with neomycin increases respiratory depression.

• ℞ **ethacrynic acid** and ℞ **carboplatin** increase the risk of ear damage.

• ℞ **Amphotericin B**, ℞ **cephalosporins**, ℞ **cyclosporine**, methoxyflurane, and ℞ **NSAIDs** may increase the risk of kidney damage.

• ℞ **Carboplatin**, ℞ **cisplatin**, and ℞ **vancomycin** increase the risk of ear or kidney damage.

• ℞ **Carbenicillin**, ℞ **penicillins**, ℞ **piperacillin**, and ℞ **ticarcillin** could inactivate neomycin in people with kidney failure.

Side effects

• Systemic use: Frequently, gastrointestinal upsets (diarrhea, nausea, vomiting). Rarely, malabsorption syndrome, neuromuscular blockade.

• Topical use: Itching, redness, swelling, and allergic reactions.

Neopap Suppositories ℬ

A preparation of ℞ **acetaminophen**.
Formulation: Rectal suppository.
Availability: OTC.
Warnings and side effects: See ℞ **acetaminophen**.

Neoral ℬ

A preparation of ℞ **cyclosporine**.
Formulation: Oral gelcaps; liquid.
Availability: Prescription only.

Neosar ℬ

A preparation of ℞ **cyclophosphamide**.
Formulation: Powder for injection.
Availability: Prescription only.
Warnings and side effects: See ℞ **cyclophosphamide**.

Neosporin Cream; Neosporin Ointment ℬ

A preparation of ℞ **neomycin** and ℞ **polymyxin B sulfate**.
Formulation: Topical cream.
Availability: OTC.
Warnings and side effects: See ℞ **neomycin**; ℞ **polymyxin B sulfate**.

Neosporin Ointment ℬ

A preparation of ℞ **neomycin**, ℞ **polymyxin B sulfate**, ℞ **bacitracin**, and ℞ **lidocaine**.
Formulation: Topical cream, topical ointment.
Availability: OTC.
Warnings and side effects: See ℞ **neomycin**; ℞ **polymyxin B sulfate**; ℞ **bacitracin**; ℞ **lidocaine**.

Neosporin Ophthalmic Ointment ℬ

A preparation of ℞ **neomycin**, ℞ **polymyxin B sulfate**, and ℞ **bacitracin**.
Formulation: Ophthalmic solution.
Availability: Prescription only.
Warnings and side effects: See ℞ **neomycin**; ℞ **polymyxin B sulfate**; ℞ **bacitracin**.

Neosporin Ophthalmic Solution ℬ

A preparation of ℞ **neomycin**, ℞ **polymyxin B sulfate**, ℞ **gramicidin**.
Formulation: Eye drops.
Availability: Prescription only.
Warnings and side effects: See ℞ **neomycin**; ℞ **polymyxin B sulfate**; ℞ **gramicidin**.

neostigmine methylsulfate ℊ

Type/Group: anticholinesterase.
Brand(s): Prostigmin; various generic.
How administered: Injection.

Used to treat

Neostigmine enhances the effects of the neurotransmitter ℞ **acetylcholine**, and is used to treat ✪ **myasthenia gravis**, to reverse the effects of neuromuscular blocking agents after surgery, and to prevent and treat postoperative urinary distension and retention after a blockage has been removed.

Warnings

• It should not be used by people with known hypersensitivity to anticholinesterases, or with urinary or intestinal obstruction, and peritonitis.

• It should be given with caution to anyone with seizure disorder, asthma, certain heart conditions, hyperthyroidism, peptic ulcer, or hypotension.

• It is not known whether this drug can harm the fetus, but it would not be expected to cross the placenta or be excreted into breast milk. It may cause premature labor if given near term, and transient muscle weakness in newborns. It should be given with caution to breast-feeding mothers.

• It must not be used with any other cholinergic medication except under a doctor's supervision.

• A doctor must be notified promptly of side effects (see below).

Interactions

• ℞ **Tacrine** may increase the cholinergic effects.

• ℞ **aminoglycoside** antibiotics (such as, ℞ **neomycin**, ℞ **streptomycin**) may increase the effects of neostigmine.

• ℞ **Corticosteroids**, ⚖ **magnesium**, and ℞ **local anesthetics** may interfere with the action of neostigmine.

• ℞ **Quinidine** and ℞ **procainamide** may interfere with neostigmine.

Side effects

Report to a doctor any of the following:

• Nausea, vomiting, diarrhea, sweating, increased salivation, irregular heartbeat, muscle weakness, severe abdominal pain, and difficulty in breathing;

• Other possible effects include urinary urgency, frequency, or incontinence, abdominal cramps, increased bronchial secretions, changes in vision, and potentially serious effects on the cardiovascular and respiratory systems.

neostigmine metisulfate ⓖ

see ℞ neostigmine methylsulfate.

Neo-Synephrine ⓑ

A preparation of ℞ **phenylephrine hydrochloride**.
Formulation: Available in many forms: injection (vasoconstrictor); eye drops; nasal drops, spray.
Availability: OTC for nasal use; prescription only for injection and ophthalmic use.
Warnings and side effects: See ℞ **phenylephrine hydrochloride**.

Neotricin HC ⓑ

A preparation of ℞ **neomycin**, ℞ **hydrocortisone**, ℞ **bacitracin** zinc, and ℞ **polymyxin B sulfate**.
Formulation: Ointment; cream.
Availability: Prescription only.
Warnings and side effects: See ℞ **neomycin**; ℞ **hydrocortisone**; ℞ **bacitracin** zinc; ℞ **polymyxin B sulfate**.

Nephron ⓑ

A preparation of racepinephrine.
Formulation: Solution for inhalation.
Availability: OTC.
Warnings and side effects: See ℞ **epinephrine**.

Nephrox Liquid ⓑ

A preparation of ℞ **aluminum hydroxide** and ℞ **mineral oil**.
Formulation: Oral liquid.
Availability: OTC.
Warnings and side effects: See ℞ **aluminum hydroxide**; ℞ **mineral oil**.

Neptazane ⓑ

A preparation of ℞ **methazolamide**.
Formulation: Oral tablets.
Availability: Prescription only.
Warnings and side effects: See ℞ **methazolamide**.

Nervocaine ⓑ

A preparation of ℞ **lidocaine**.
Formulation: Injection.
Availability: Prescription only.
Warnings and side effects: See ℞ **lidocaine**.

Nesacaine ⓑ

A preparation of ℞ **chloroprocaine hydrochloride**.
Formulation: Injection.
Availability: Prescription only.
Warnings and side effects: See ℞ **chloroprocaine hydrochloride**.

netilmicin ⓖ

Type/Group: **aminoglycoside; antibiotic; antibacterial**.
Brand(s): Netromycin.
How administered: Injection; intravenous infusion.

Used to treat

Netilmicin can be used, alone or in combination with other antibiotics, to treat serious ✪ **bacterial infections** caused by Gram-negative bacteria.

Warnings

• It should not be given to people with known hypersensitivity to netilmicin or other aminoglycosides, or with severe kidney disease.

• It should be given with caution to people with mild kidney disease, hearing deficits or vertigo, dehydration, with muscular disorders, such as myasthenia gravis or parkinsonism, and those over 65.

• Medical judgment is required when giving to very young infants.

• Netilmicin should be used during pregnancy only if medically judged to be clearly needed and if the potential benefits outweigh the risks to the fetus (it crosses the placenta and could cause damage to ears or kidneys).

• Medical judgment is required if breast-feeding is being considered. This drug is appears in breast milk, although it is poorly absorbed orally.

• Aminoglycosides are associated with nephrotoxicity (damage to the kidneys) and ototoxicity (damage in the ears). Irreversible vestibular impairment can occur, resulting in vertigo and difficulty maintaining balance. Permanent hearing loss in one or both ears can also occur. The risk is greatest in those with pre-existing impairments, with high doses, and with prolonged use.

• A doctor must be contacted if there are problems with hearing, vision, balance, urination, or headaches, even after the course of treatment is completed.

• The use of antibiotics may result in superinfection due to bacterial imbalance.

Interactions

• ℞ **Atracurium**, ℞ **succinylcholine**, ℞ **vecuronium**, or neuromuscular blocking agents taken with netilmicin increase respiratory depression.

• ℞ **ethacrynic acid** and ℞ **carboplatin** increase the risk of ear damage.

• ℞ **Amphotericin B**, ℞ **cephalosporins**, ℞ **cyclosporine**, methoxyflurane, and ℞ **NSAID**s may increase the risk of kidney damage.

• ℞ **Carboplatin**, ℞ **cisplatin**, and ℞ **vancomycin** increase the risk of ear or kidney damage.

• ℞ **Carbenicillin**, ℞ **penicillins**, ℞ **piperacillin**, and ℞ **ticarcillin** could inactivate netilmicin in people with kidney failure.

Side effects

• Frequently, gastrointestinal upsets.

• Occasionally, rash, fever, hives, and itching.

• Rarely, hair loss, elevated blood pressure, and weakness. Additional serious effects include neurotoxicity (nerve damage), ototoxicity and deafness, kidney damage, blood disorders.

Netromycin ℬ
A preparation of ℞ **netilmicin**.
Formulation: Injection.
Availability: Prescription only.
Warnings and side effects: See ℞ **netilmicin**.

Neumega ℬ
A preparation of ℞ **oprelvekin**.
Formulation: Injection (subcutaneous).
Availability: Prescription only.
Warnings and side effects: See ℞ **oprelvekin**.

Neupogen ℬ
A preparation of ℞ **filgrastim**.
Formulation: Injection.
Availability: Prescription only.
Warnings and side effects: See ℞ **filgrastim**.

Neuramate ℬ
A preparation of ℞ **meprobamate**.
Formulation: Oral tablets.
Availability: Prescription only.
Warnings and side effects: See ℞ **meprobamate**.

neuroleptic Ⓓ
see ℞ **antipsychotic**.

Neurontin ℬ
A preparation of ℞ **gabapentin**.
Formulation: Oral capsules, available in 3 strengths.
Availability: Prescription only.
Warnings and side effects: See ℞ **gabapentin**.

Neutrexin ℬ
A preparation of ℞ **trimetrexate glucuronate**.
Formulation: Injection.
Availability: Prescription only.
Warnings and side effects: See ℞ **trimetrexate glucuronate**.

Neutrogena Chemical-Free Sunblocker ℬ
A preparation of ℞ **titanium dioxide**.
Formulation: Topical lotion.
Availability: OTC.
Warnings and side effects: See ℞ **titanium dioxide**.

Neutrogena Oil-free Acne Wash ℬ
A preparation of ℞ **salicylic acid** and various.
Formulation: Topical liquid.
Availability: OTC.
Warnings and side effects: See ℞ **salicylic acid**.

Neutrogena Sunblock Stick ℬ
A preparation of ℞ **cinnamates**, and other ingredients.
Formulation: Topical stick.
Availability: OTC.
Warnings and side effects: See ℞ **cinnamates**.

Neutrogena T/Gel; Neutrogena T/Derm ℬ
A preparation of ℞ **coal tar**.
Formulation: Shampoo; topical oil.
Availability: OTC.
Warnings and side effects: See ℞ **coal tar**.

Neutrogena T/Sal ℬ
A preparation of ℞ **salicylic acid** and ℞ **coal tar**.
Formulation: Shampoo.
Availability: OTC.
Warnings and side effects: See ℞ **salicylic acid**; ℞ **coal tar**.

nevirapine Ⓖ
Type/Group: **antiviral**.
Brand(s): Viramune.
How administered: Orally.

Used to treat
Nevirapine is a non-nucleoside group reverse transcriptase inhibitor antiviral drug that can be used with other antiretrovirals in the treatment of ⊙ **HIV** infection.

Warnings

• It should not be given to people with known hypersensitivity to nevirapine.

• It should be given with caution to people with Stevens-Johnson syndrome (a skin disorder), liver disease, or central nervous system (CNS) disorders.

• Nevirapine's safety during pregnancy has not been established, and it should be used only when the potential benefits clearly outweigh the possible risks to the fetus.

• HIV-infected mothers are advised not to breast-feed.

• It is a specialist drug, and there will be full assessment and patient monitoring throughout treatment.

• It may cause allergic reactions. A doctor must be contacted if severe rash, or rash with other symptoms, develops.

Interactions

• The levels of ℞ **clarithromycin** are decreased while the levels of nevirapine are increased.

• ℞ **erythromycin**, ℞ **nelfinavir**, and troleandomycin increase levels of nevirapine.

• ℞ **indinavir**, ℞ **rifabutin**, and ℞ **rifampin** may reduce levels of nevirapine.

• The levels of ℞ **ketoconazole** are reduced while the levels of nevirapine are increased.

• ℞ **Methadone** and ℞ **saquinavir** levels are reduced by nevirapine.

Side effects

These can be many and include:

• Fatigue, sedation, skin disorders, jaundice and liver toxicity (which can be serious), nausea and vomiting, diarrhea and abdominal pain, headache, drowsiness and fever, muscle pains, and others.

Nia-Bid ®

A preparation of ℞ **niacin**.
Formulation: Oral capsules, timed release.
Availability: OTC.
Warnings and side effects: See ℞ **niacin**.

Niacels ®

A preparation of ℞ **niacin**.
Formulation: Oral capsules, timed release.
Availability: OTC.
Warnings and side effects: See ℞ **niacin**.

niacin ⓖ

(nicotinic acid; vitamin B$_3$)
Type/Group: lipid-regulating drug; vitamin.
Brand(s): Nia-Bid; Niacels; Niacor; Niaspan; Nico-400; Nicolar; Nicotinex; Slo-Niacin; various generic.
How administered: Orally.

Used to treat

Niacin is a B-complex vitamin. It is a derivative of pyridine and is required in the diet, but is also synthesized in the body to a small degree from the amino acid tryptophan. Dietary deficiency results in the disease ✪ **pellagra**, but deficiency is rare. Niacin can be used to treat pellagra and niacin deficiency. Good food sources include meat, cereals, and yeast extract. It is used as a lipid-regulating drug because it beneficially modifies blood levels of various lipids (HDL and LDL) by inhibiting the synthesis and secretion of lipids in the liver.

Warnings

• It should not be given to people with severe kidney or liver disease, active peptic ulcer, severe hypotension, or hemorrhage.

• It should be given with caution to people with unstable coronary artery disease, gallbladder disease, history of jaundice, liver disease, peptic ulcer, arterial bleeding, gout, or diabetes mellitus.

• Niacin is safe for use during pregnancy at recommended daily intakes (18 to 20 mg). It moves into pregnancy category C in higher doses, and should be used only if the potential benefits outweigh possible risks to the fetus.

• It can be taken while breast-feeding at the 18 to 20 mg daily dosage.

• Alcohol and hot beverages should be avoided to minimize flushing.

• Rarely, hepatitis or severe, life-threatening rash may occur.

Interactions

• Taken with ℞ **lovastatin** there is possibly an increased risk of adverse effects.

Side effects

• Frequently, flushing, gastrointestinal upsets, and itching.

• Occasionally, dizziness, hypotension, headache, blurred vision, and burning or tingling of skin.

• Rarely, hyperglycemia, rash, hyperpigmentation, and dry skin.

niacinamide ⓖ

(nicotinamide)
Type/Group: vitamin; vasodilator.
Brand(s): Generic only.

Warnings

• It can cause liver dysfunction at high doses.

Niacor ®

A preparation of ℞ **niacin**.
Formulation: Oral tablets.
Availability: Prescription only.
Warnings and side effects: See ℞ **niacin**.

nicardipine hydrochloride ⓖ

Type/Group: calcium-channel blocker; antianginal; antihypertensive.
Brand(s): Cardene; generic.
How administered: Orally; injection.

Used to treat

Nicardipine is used to treat ✪ **hypertension** and also in the management of ✪ **angina pectoris**, where it may be used alone or in combination with ℞ **beta-blockers**. The injectable form is used only for short-term treatment, for example, in hypertensive crisis.

Warnings

• It should not be given to people with known hypersensitivity to this drug, or with advanced aortic stenosis.

• It should be given with caution to people with congestive heart failure, impaired liver or kidney function, pheochromocytoma (injectable form), or who are elderly.

• It should be used during pregnancy only if the potential benefits outweigh the risk to the fetus.

• Breast-feeding women should either discontinue using this drug or stop breast-feeding.

• Regular monitoring of blood pressure is necessary to establish a safe, effective dosage. Intravenous use of this drug should be begun in a medical facility equipped to monitor results and to supply resuscitation if needed.

• Grapefruit juice should be avoided as it can increase the levels of nicardipine in blood plasma.

• If nicardipine is given to replace a beta-blocker, then withdrawal of the beta-blocker should not be abrupt. Calcium-channel blockers, also, should not be discontinued abruptly.

Interactions

• ℞ **Beta-blockers** (for example, ℞ **propranolol**) occasionally cause adverse reactions, although the effects are unclear, and so caution is advised.

• ℞ **Anticonvulsants** (for example, ℞ **phenytoin**) may produce anticonvulsant toxic effects over time.

• There may be a risk of severe hypotension if taken with ℞ **fentanyl**, so caution is advised.

• Other hypotensive agents (for example, ℞ **captopril**, ℞ **hydralazine hydrochloride**, ℞ **methyldopa**) may have additive effects, and severe hypotension is possible.

• Alcohol, ℞ **cimetidine** and grapefruit juice may increase the levels and effects of nicardipine.

• The levels of ℞ **digoxin** and ℞ **cyclosporine** may be increased by nicardipine.

• The levels of ℞ **quinidine** may fall when nicardipine treatment is begun, and rise when it is stopped.

Side effects

• Frequently, swollen feet or legs, flushing and sensations of warmth, headache, dizziness, nausea, or palpitations.

• Less commonly, gastrointestinal disturbances, increased salivation, rashes, frequent urination, tingling in the extremities, ringing in the ears, shortness of breath, and impotence.

• Occasionally, significant hypotension and, rarely, fainting. Headache and hypotension are more frequent after intravenous infusion.

N'Ice ℬ

A preparation of ℞ **menthol** and ℞ **glycerin**.
Formulation: Throat spray.
Availability: OTC.
Warnings and side effects: See ℞ **menthol**; ℞ **glycerin**.

N'Ice n' Clear ℬ

A preparation of ℞ **menthol**.
Formulation: Lozenges.
Availability: OTC.
Warnings and side effects: See ℞ **menthol**.

Nico-400 ℬ

A preparation of ℞ **niacin**.
Formulation: Oral capsules, timed release.
Availability: OTC.
Warnings and side effects: See ℞ **niacin**.

Nicoderm CQ ℬ

A preparation of ℞ **nicotine**.
Formulation: Transdermal patch.
Availability: OTC.
Warnings and side effects: See ℞ **nicotine**.

Nicolor ℬ

A preparation of ℞ **niacin**.
Formulation: Oral tablets. Contains tartrazine. Some individuals are allergic to tartrazine, particularly those who are allergic to aspirin.
Availability: Prescription only.
Warnings and side effects: See ℞ **niacin**.

Nicorette; Nicorette DS ℬ

A preparation of ℞ **nicotine**.
Formulation: Chewing gum; two strengths.
Availability: Prescription only.
Warnings and side effects: See ℞ **nicotine**.

nicotinamide ⒢

see ℞ **niacinamide**.

nicotine ⒢

Type/Group: CNS stimulant; substance-dependence treatment.
Brand(s): Habitrol; Nicoderm; Nicorette, Nicorette DS; Nicotrol; Nicotrol NS; Nicotrol Inhaler; ProStep.
How administered: Orally (chewing gum); transdermal (absorbed through the skin); inhalation; nasal spray.

Used to treat

Nicotine is an ℞ **alkaloid** found in tobacco products and is absorbed into the body whether the tobacco is smoked or chewed. It causes a predominantly ℞ **sympathomimetic** effect on the cardiovascular system with a rise in blood pressure and heart rate, and stimulation of the central nervous system (CNS). Like many habituating drugs there is tolerance to its action, so bigger doses are required on continued usage and there is a marked psychological and physical withdrawal syndrome if anyone abruptly stops using it, in other words drug-dependence becomes established. It is available in various replacement forms to help those trying to give up smoking, including as chewing gum (it is absorbed into the circulation from the lining of the mouth) and skin patches for transdermal delivery (absorbed through the skin).

Warnings

• It should not be given to people with known hypersensitivity to this drug.

• Depending on how it is administered, it should be given with caution to people with cardiovascular disease, hypertension, hyperthyroidism, type 1 diabetes mellitus, liver or kidney impairment, pheochromocytoma, gastric ulcers, or skin disorders (with patches).

• Nicotine should be used during pregnancy only if the potential benefit clearly outweighs the possible risks.

• Nicotine appears in breast milk. Nursing mothers should use nicotine in one of the forms used to help quit smoking, if at all.

• People should not smoke or use other nicotine products while receiving treatment of this kind.

• Treatment should last for 10 to 12 weeks.

• Coffee and cola can reduce the absorption of nicotine from the gum form.

Interactions

• Changing from a smoker to a non-smoker may alter a person's dose requirements of certain drugs, particularly any that are ℞ **sympathomimetic** or ℞ **adrenergic-neuron blocking**.

Side effects

• Cold and flu-like symptoms, with headache, nausea, dizziness, insomnia, dreaming, muscle ache, swelling of tongue, sinusitis, dysmenorrhea, constipation or diarrhea, back pain, pruritis, palpitations and changes in heart rhythm, seizures, anxiety, acid stomach, skin reaction (with patches), and others.

Nicotinex Elixir ℞

A preparation of ℞ **niacin**.
Formulation: Oral elixir.
Availability: OTC.
Warnings and side effects: See ℞ **niacin**.

nicotinic acid Ⓖ

see ℞ **niacin**.

Nicotrol ℞

A preparation of ℞ **nicotine**.
Formulation: Transdermal patch.
Availability: OTC.
Warnings and side effects: See ℞ **nicotine**.

Nicotrol Inhaler ℞

A preparation of ℞ **nicotine**.
Formulation: Inhaler.
Availability: Prescription only.
Warnings and side effects: See ℞ **nicotine**.

Nicotrol NS ℞

A preparation of ℞ **nicotine**.
Formulation: Chewing gum.
Availability: Prescription only.
Warnings and side effects: See ℞ **nicotine**.

nifedipine Ⓖ

Type/Group: calcium-channel blocker; antianginal; antihypertensive.
Brand(s): **Adalat; Procardia;** various generic.
How administered: Orally.

Used to treat

Nifedipine is used to prevent attacks of ✪ **angina pectoris** and in the treatment of ✪ **hypertension**. Although not stated by the manufacturer for such use, it has also been widely used to treat ✪ **Raynaud's disease** and sometimes ✪ **migraine**.

Warnings

• It should not be given to people with known hypersensitivity to this drug, or who have marked hypotension or porphyria.

• It should be given with caution to people with congestive heart failure, impaired liver or kidney function, or who are elderly.

• It should be used during pregnancy only if the potential benefits outweigh the risk to the fetus.

• Breast-feeding women should either discontinue using this drug or stop breast-feeding.

• Regular monitoring of blood pressure is necessary to establish a safe, effective dosage.

• The capsules used in the immediate-release preparation are not digested or altered in passing through the intestines, and medical judgment is required for people with significant gastrointestinal obstruction.

• Grapefruit juice should be avoided as it can increase the levels of nifedipine in blood plasma.

• If nifedipine is given to replace a ℞ **beta-blocker**, then withdrawal of the beta-blocker should not be abrupt. Calcium-channel blockers, also, should not be discontinued abruptly.

Interactions

• ℞ **Beta-blockers** (for example, ℞ **propranolol**) occasionally cause adverse reactions, though the effects are unclear, and caution is advised.

• ℞ **Anticonvulsants** (for example, ℞ **phenytoin**) may produce toxic effects over time.

• There is a risk of severe hypotension if taken with ℞ **fentanyl**, and nifedipine should be discontinued at least 36 hours before giving fentanyl.

• Other hypotensive agents (for example, ℞ **captopril**, ℞ **hydralazine hydrochloride**, ℞ **methyldopa**) may have additive effects, and severe hypotension is possible.

• Alcohol, ℞ **cimetidine** and grapefruit juice may increase the levels and effects of nifedipine.

• The levels of ℞ **digoxin** may be increased by nifedipine.

• The levels of ℞ **quinidine** may fall when nifedipine treatment is begun, and rise when it is stopped.

Side effects

• Frequently, flushing and sensations of warmth, dizziness, swelling of the extremities, muscle cramps, nausea or heartburn, headache, or palpitations.

• Occasionally, significant hypotension and, rarely, fainting.

• Side effects are less likely with the extended-release preparations.

Nighttime Sleep Aid ℞

A preparation of ℞ **diphenhydramine hydrochloride**.
Formulation: Oral tablets.
Availability: OTC.
Warnings and side effects: See ℞ **diphenhydramine hydrochloride**.

NightTime Thera-Flu Powder Ⓑ

A preparation of ℞ **dextromethorphan**, ℞ **acetaminophen**, ℞ **chlorpheniramine maleate**, and ℞ **pseudoephedrine**.
Formulation: Powder.
Availability: OTC.
Warnings and side effects: See ℞ **dextromethorphan**; ℞ **acetaminophen**; ℞ **chlorpheniramine maleate**; ℞ **pseudoephedrine**.

Nilandron Ⓑ

A preparation of ℞ **nilutamide**.
Formulation: Oral tablets.
Availability: Prescription only.
Warnings and side effects: See ℞ **nilutamide**.

Nilstat Ⓑ

A preparation of ℞ **nystatin**.
Formulation: Topical cream; topical ointment; oral suspension.
Availability: Prescription only.
Warnings and side effects: See ℞ **nystatin**.

nilutamide Ⓖ

Type/Group: **antiandrogen; anticancer**.
Brand(s): Nilandron.
How administered: Orally.

Used to treat

Nilutamide is a hormone antagonist (an antiandrogen) used for the treatment of ⊙ **prostate cancer**.

Warnings

• It should not be used by people with known hypersensitivity to this drug, or by women, particularly women who are or may become pregnant.
• It should be given with caution to people with certain liver disorders.
• It should not be used during pregnancy unless it is medically judged to be needed.
• It should not be used by breast-feeding mothers.
• Nilutamide has been associated with a risk of pneumonia. Use of the drug must be stopped and a doctor contacted if shortness of breath or other respiratory tract symptoms develop.
• It may cause a delay in visual adaptation to the dark when passing from a lighted to a darker area. Use caution driving at night or through tunnels; tinted glasses should be worn if this problem develops.

Interactions

• Nilutamide may interfere with the effects of ℞ **anticoagulants** (for example, ℞ **warfarin sodium**).
• The effects of ℞ **phenytoin** and ℞ **theophylline** may be increased.

Side effects

• Hot flashes, nausea, constipation, loss of appetite, vomiting, decreased libido, reduced touch perception, breathing problems, sweating, hair loss, dry skin; rash, visual abnormalities, and anemia, reduced tolerance for alcohol.

• Rare but serious side effects include hepatitis and certain blood-cell disorders.

Nimbex Ⓑ

A preparation of ℞ **cisatracurium**.
Formulation: Injection.
Availability: Prescription only.
Warnings and side effects: See ℞ **cisatracurium**.

nimodipine Ⓖ

Type/Group: **calcium-channel blocker; antihypertensive; vasodilator**.
Brand(s): Nimotop.
How administered: Orally.

Used to treat

Nimodipine is used to treat and prevent further brain damage (from new bleeding) following subarachnoid hemorrhage (a relatively rare form of ⊙ **stroke**), by reducing the risk of cerebrovascular vasospasm (spasm in a blood vessel). The course of this preventive treatment is usually three weeks.

Warnings

• It should not be given to people with known hypersensitivity to this drug.
• It should be given with caution to people with impaired liver or kidney function.
• It should be used during pregnancy only if the potential benefits outweigh the risk to the fetus.
• Breast-feeding women should either discontinue using this drug or stop breast-feeding.
• Regular monitoring of blood pressure is necessary.
• If nimodipine is given to replace a ℞ **beta-blocker**, then withdrawal of the beta-blocker should not be abrupt. Calcium-channel blockers, also, should not be discontinued abruptly.
• Grapefruit juice should be avoided as it can increase the levels of nimodipine in blood plasma.

Interactions

• Beta-blockers (for example, ℞ **propranolol**) occasionally cause adverse reactions, although the effects are unclear, and caution is advised.
• ℞ **Anticonvulsants** (for example, ℞ **phenytoin**) may produce anticonvulsant toxic effects over time.
• There is a risk of severe hypotension if taken with ℞ **fentanyl**, so caution is advised.
• Other calcium-channel blockers and hypotensive agents (for example, ℞ **captopril**, ℞ **hydralazine hydrochloride**, ℞ **methyldopa**) may have additive effects, with severe hypotension possible.
• Alcohol, ℞ **cimetidine**, and grapefruit juice may increase the levels and effects of nimodipine.

Side effects

• Frequently, hypotension, headache, swollen feet or legs, or flushing and sensations of warmth.
• Less commonly, dizziness, nausea, palpitations or slow heartbeat, gastrointestinal disturbances (for example, diarrhea, abdominal pain, nausea), rash, breathlessness, or muscle cramps.

Nimotop ®

A preparation of ℞ **nimodipine**.
Formulation: Oral capsules.
Availability: Prescription only.
Warnings and side effects: See ℞ nimodipine.

Nipent ®

A preparation of ℞ **mitoxantrone**.
Formulation: Powder for injection.
Availability: Prescription only.
Warnings and side effects: See ℞ mitoxantrone.

nisoldipine ⓖ

Type/Group: **calcium-channel blocker; antihypertensive.**
Brand(s): Sular.
How administered: Orally.

Used to treat

Nisoldipine is used alone or in combination with other drugs to treat ⊙ **hypertension**.

Warnings

• It should not be given to people with known hypersensitivity to this drug (or to similar calcium-channel blockers).
• It should be given with caution to people with congestive heart failure, severe coronary artery disease, significantly impaired liver or kidney function, or who are elderly.
• It should be used during pregnancy only if the potential benefits outweigh the risk to the fetus.
• Breast-feeding women should either discontinue using this drug or stop breast-feeding.
• Regular monitoring of blood pressure is necessary to establish a safe, effective dosage.
• If nisoldipine is given to replace a ℞ **beta-blocker**, then withdrawal of the beta-blocker should not be abrupt. Calcium-channel blockers, also, should not be discontinued abruptly.
• Grapefruit juice should be avoided as it can increase the levels of nisoldipine in blood plasma.

Interactions

• ℞ **Beta-blockers** (for example, ℞ **propranolol**) occasionally cause adverse reactions, though the effects are unclear, and so caution is advised.
• ℞ **Anticonvulsants** (for example, ℞ **phenytoin**) may produce toxic effects over time.
• There is a risk of severe hypotension if taken with ℞ **fentanyl**, so caution is advised.
• Other calcium-channel blockers and hypotensive agents (for example, ℞ **captopril**, ℞ **hydralazine hydrochloride**, ℞ **methyldopa**) may have additive effects, with severe hypotension possible.
• Alcohol, ℞ **cimetidine**, and grapefruit juice may increase the levels and effects of nisoldipine.
• The levels of ℞ **quinidine** may fall when nisoldipine is first used, and rise when it is stopped.

Side effects

• Frequently, swollen feet or legs, headache, dizziness, flushing and sensations of warmth, nausea, or palpitations.

• Less commonly, chest pain, gastrointestinal disturbances, rash, breathlessness, muscle pain, or cramps.

nitrate ⓓ

Generics: **isosorbide dinitrate; isosorbide mononitrate; nitroglycerin; sodium nitroprusside.**

Actions and uses

℞ **nitrate**s are powerful ℞ **smooth muscle relaxant** agents. They are mainly used for their ℞ **vasodilator** (widens blood vessels) activity to relax the walls of blood vessels in the treatment or prevention of ⊙ **angina pectoris** (see ℞ **antianginal**) and for ⊙ **heart failure**. The best-known and most-used nitrates include ℞ **nitroglycerin**, ℞ **isosorbide dinitrate**, and ℞ **isosorbide mononitrate**. Although ℞ **sodium nitroprusside** is not technically a nitrate, it works on cells in the same way as the nitrates.
How the drug is given is important when it is intended for the relief of an anginal attack. It can be taken as tablets to be held under the tongue (sublingual) until dissolved, buccal tablets (placed between the upper lip and gum), or in aerosol sprays (directed into the mouth). There are various other means of administration, including transdermal patches placed on the skin (the drug is absorbed through the skin).
Nitrates have been in use for a very long time and have proved quite successful in treating acute angina pectoris. Given in a suitable form to prolong their activity, they are also increasingly used to treat the symptoms of congestive heart failure.

Limitations

See the individual drug entries.

Nitrek ®

A preparation of ℞ **nitroglycerin**.
Formulation: Transdermal patch, available in three release rates.
Availability: Prescription only.
Warnings and side effects: See ℞ nitroglycerin.

Nitro-Bid ®

A preparation of ℞ **nitroglycerin**.
Formulation: Topical ointment (applied to chest or back).
Availability: Prescription only.
Warnings and side effects: See ℞ nitroglycerin.

Nitro-Bid IV ®

A preparation of ℞ **nitroglycerin**.
Formulation: Intravenous infusion.
Availability: Prescription only.
Warnings and side effects: See ℞ nitroglycerin.

Nitrodisc ®

A preparation of ℞ **nitroglycerin**.
Formulation: Transdermal patch, available in 3 release rates.
Availability: Prescription only.
Warnings and side effects: See ℞ nitroglycerin.

Nitro-Dur ®

A preparation of ℞ **nitroglycerin**.

Formulation: Transdermal patch, available in 6 release rates.
Availability: Prescription only.
Warnings and side effects: See ℞ **nitroglycerin**.

nitrofurantoin ⓖ

Type/Group: **antibiotic; antibacterial.**
Brand(s): Furadantin; Macrodantin; Macrobid; various generic.
How administered: Orally.

Used to treat
Nitrofurantoin is used to treat ✪ **bacterial infections** of the urinary tract.

Warnings
• It should not be given to people with known hypersensitivity to nitrofurantoin, substantial kidney impairment or reduced urine output.
• It should be given with caution to people with G6PD deficiency (a genetic enzyme disorder), kidney impairment, anemia, diabetes mellitus, electrolyte imbalance, vitamin-B deficiency, or those who are weakened from disease.
• Its safety for use in pregnancy has not been established. It should be used only if clearly needed and if the potential benefits outweigh the risks to the fetus. Do not use at term because of possible adverse effects on newborns.
• Do not nurse infants less than one month old while taking this drug; it is excreted in human breast milk. Medical judgment is required with older infants. Its safety for use by breast-feeding mothers has not been established.
• An adverse reaction affecting the lungs can occur, leading to permanent impairment.
• It may cause liver damage or peripheral nerve damage.
• It may discolor urine.

Interactions
• ℞ **Anticholinergics** and ℞ **probenecid** may increase levels of nitrofurantoin.
• Magnesium salts (such as in supplements) may delay or decrease absorption, so avoid taking at the same time.

Side effects
• Frequently, loss of appetite, nausea and vomiting.
• Occasionally, diarrhea, abdominal pain, rash, itching, hives, hypertension, headache, drowsiness, and dizziness.
• Rarely, photosensitivity (abnormal sensitivity to light), temporary hair loss, asthma, severe allergic reaction, serious skin disorders, liver, nerve, and lung disorders.

Nitrogard ⓑ

A preparation of ℞ **nitroglycerin**.
Formulation: Transmucosal, buccal tablets.
Availability: Prescription only.
Warnings and side effects: See ℞ **nitroglycerin**.

nitroglycerin ⓖ

(glyceryl trinitrate)
Type/Group: **nitrate; vasodilator; antianginal; heart failure treatment.**

Brand(s): (Aerosol, translingual): Nitrolingual. (Injection, IV): Nitro-Bid IV; Tridil; various generic. (Sublingual): NitroQuick; Nitrostat. (Sustained release): Nitro-Time; Nitroglyn; Nitrong; various generic. (Topical ointment): Nitro-Bid; Nitrol; various generic. (Transdermal, patch): Deponit; Minitran; Nitrek; Nitrodisc; Nitro-Dur; Transderm-Nitro; various generic. (Transmucosal, buccal): Nitrogard.
How administered: Orally; transdermal (absorbed through the skin); injection.

Used to treat
Nitroglycerin is used to prevent attacks of ✪ **angina pectoris**, for instance when taken before exercise, and for symptomatic relief during an acute attack. It has been used also to lighten heart exertion in congestive ✪ **heart failure** or after a heart attack. It works by dilating the blood vessels returning blood to the heart and so reducing the workload of the heart. It is short-acting, but its effect can be extended through the use of modified-release sublingual tablets (kept under the tongue) and buccal tablets (kept behind the upper lip). It is also administered by aerosol spray (which is sprayed under the tongue, where it is absorbed into the systemic circulation), by intravenous injection or in skin patches placed on the surface of the chest so that it can be absorbed through the skin. It is also used to control blood pressure, for example, during surgical procedures.

Warnings
• It should not be given to people with known hypersensitivity to nitrates, or who have postural hypotension (lowered blood pressure on standing up), marked anemia, head injury or brain hemorrhage, or closed-angle glaucoma.
• It should be given with caution to people who have recently had a heart attack, with certain cardiovascular disorders, glaucoma, or kidney, liver, or thyroid impairment. Intravenous nitroglycerin should not be given to people with hypotension, low blood volume, or constrictive pericardial conditions. Extended-release forms (sublingual, transdermal) should be avoided by people with intestinal malabsorption and hypermotility disorders.
• Its safety during pregnancy has not been established and so it should be used only when it is clearly needed.
• Medical judgment is required if breast-feeding is being considered. Its safety in breast-feeding has not been established.
• Alcohol should be avoided, as severe hypotension or circulatory collapse is possible.
• Postural hypotension may occur, even with small doses and measures such as deep breathing or lowering the head may be needed to overcome dizziness or prevent fainting. Sublingual nitroglycerin should be taken in a sitting position.
• When using sublingual tablets, if the pain is not relieved by three tablets taken one after another at five-minute intervals, a doctor must be contacted immediately or go to an emergency room.
• A doctor should be notified of symptoms such as blurred vision, dry mouth, or persistent headache.
• There can be some variation in effect among different brands, and it is important not to switch brands without first consulting a pharmacist or doctor.

• Discarded transdermal patches contain enough nitroglycerin to be hazardous to children and pets, and should be disposed of with care.

Interactions

• Alcohol, other antihypertensive drugs, ℞ **calcium-channel blockers**, ℞ **beta-adrenergic blockers**, ℞ **phenothiazines**, and ℞ **sildenafil** have the potential for additive effects, with marked or severe hypotension. Dosages may need adjustment.

• ℞ **dihydroergotamine** may have unpredictable effects.

• The effects of ℞ **heparin** may be reduced.

Side effects

• These include throbbing headache, flushing, or dizziness. Some people experience an increase in heart rate and postural hypotension.

• Less frequently, gastrointestinal disturbances, arthralgia (joint pain), pallor, perspiration or cold sweat.

• Ointments and patches may cause allergic reactions (rash, itching, sores) on the skin, and rarely anaphylactic symptoms.

Nitroglyn ⑧

A preparation of ℞ **nitroglycerin**.
Formulation: Oral capsules, sustained release, available in 3 strengths.
Availability: Prescription only.
Warnings and side effects: See ℞ **nitroglycerin**.

Nitrol ⑧

A preparation of ℞ **nitroglycerin**.
Formulation: Topical ointment (applied to chest or back).
Availability: Prescription only.
Warnings and side effects: See ℞ **nitroglycerin**.

Nitrolingual ⑧

A preparation of ℞ **nitroglycerin**.
Formulation: Aerosol spray, translingual.
Availability: Prescription only.
Warnings and side effects: See ℞ **nitroglycerin**.

Nitrong ⑧

A preparation of ℞ **nitroglycerin**.
Formulation: Oral tablets, sustained release, available in 3 strengths.
Availability: Prescription only.
Warnings and side effects: See ℞ **nitroglycerin**.

Nitropress ⑧

A preparation of ℞ **sodium nitroprusside**.
Formulation: Intravenous infusion.
Availability: Prescription only.
Warnings and side effects: See ℞ **sodium nitroprusside**.

Nitroquick ⑧

A preparation of ℞ **nitroglycerin**.
Formulation: Oral tablets, sublingual, available in three strengths.
Availability: Prescription only.

Warnings and side effects: See ℞ **nitroglycerin**.

Nitrostat ⑧

A preparation of ℞ **nitroglycerin**.
Formulation: Oral tablets, sublingual, available in 3 strengths.
Availability: Prescription only.
Warnings and side effects: See ℞ **nitroglycerin**.

Nitro-Time ⑧

A preparation of ℞ **nitroglycerin**.
Formulation: Oral capsules, sustained release, available in 3 strengths.
Availability: Prescription only.
Warnings and side effects: See ℞ **nitroglycerin**.

Nivea After Tan ⑧

A preparation of ℞ **mineral oil**, ℞ **castor oil**, ℞ **lanolin**, and ℞ **carbomer**.
Formulation: Lotion.
Availability: OTC.
Warnings and side effects: See ℞ **mineral oil**; ℞ **castor oil**; ℞ **lanolin**; ℞ **carbomer**.

Nivea Moisturizing ⑧

A preparation of ℞ **lanolin**, ℞ **mineral oil**, and ℞ **glycerin**.
Formulation: Lotion; topical oil.
Availability: OTC.
Warnings and side effects: See ℞ **lanolin**; ℞ **mineral oil**; ℞ **glycerin**.

Nix ⑧

A preparation of ℞ **permethrin**.
Formulation: Liquid (topical creme rinse).
Availability: OTC.
Warnings and side effects: See ℞ **permethrin**.

nizatidine ⑥

Type/Group: H_2-antagonist; ulcer-healing drug.
Brand(s): Axid; various generic.
How administered: Orally; injection; infusion.
Used to treat
Nizatidine is used to assist in the treatment of benign ✪ **peptic ulcers** (gastric and duodenal), to relieve heartburn in cases of reflux esophagitis (caused by regurgitation of acid and enzymes into the esophagus), and a variety of conditions where reduction of acidity is beneficial. It works by reducing the secretion of gastric acid (by acting as a histamine receptor—H_2-receptor—antagonist), so reducing erosion and bleeding from peptic ulcers and allowing them a chance to heal. However, nizatidine should not be used until a full diagnosis of gastric bleeding or serious pain has been made, because its action in restricting gastric secretions may possibly mask the presence of stomach cancer. Nevertheless it is available OTC (though at lower dosage) for heartburn, acid indigestion, and sour stomach due to overindulgence.

Key to symbols: ✪ = Disorder Section ℞ = Drug Section ♣ = Herbal Section ⬙⬙ = Supplement Section

Warnings

• It should not be given to people with known hypersensitivity to this drug or other H_2-antagonists.

• It should be given with caution to people with kidney or liver impairment.

• Nizatidine should be used during pregnancy only if it is clearly needed.

• It may appear in breast milk and should be avoided by nursing mothers.

• H_2-antagonists, like this one, may mask symptoms of gastric cancer, and this possibility must be eliminated with particular care in persons who have reached middle-age.

• Frequency and severity of side effects are higher in the elderly.

• Doses of nizatidine and antacids must be staggered.

Interactions

• ℞ **Salicylates** (for example, ℞ **aspirin**): In high-dose aspirin therapy, its concentration may be increased when taken with nizatidine.

• Cigarette smoking reverses some of the effects of nizatidine, interfering with ulcer healing.

• ℞ **Anticholinergics** and ℞ **metoclopramide** may decrease the absorption and effect of nizatidine.

Side effects

• These are infrequent and may include drowsiness, headache, dizziness or diarrhea.

• Rarely, sweating, hair loss, blood disorders (including anemia), hypersensitivity reactions (including fever, hives, bronchospasm, swelling of the larynx, anaphylaxis, and inflammation of blood vessels, with associated skin changes), other skin symptoms, temporary mental confusion, raised uric acid levels in the blood, and effects on the liver and the heart.

• There have been occasional reports of impotence and the growth of breasts in men.

Nizoral ⓑ

A preparation of ℞ **ketoconazole**.
Formulation: Oral tablets; topical cream; shampoo.
Availability: Prescription only.
Warnings and side effects: See ℞ **ketoconazole**.

Nizoral A-D ⓑ

A preparation of ℞ **ketoconazole**.
Formulation: Shampoo.
Availability: OTC.
Warnings and side effects: See ℞ **ketoconazole**.

Noctec ⓑ

A preparation of ℞ **chloral hydrate**.
Formulation: Capsules.
Availability: Prescription only.
Warnings and side effects: See ℞ **chloral hydrate**.

No-Drowsiness Allerest Tablets ⓑ

A preparation of ℞ **pseudoephedrine** and ℞ **acetaminophen**.
Formulation: Oral tablets.

Availability: OTC.
Warnings and side effects: See ℞ **pseudoephedrine**; ℞ **acetaminophen**.

no more germies ⓑ

A preparation of ℞ **triclosan**.
Formulation: Soap.
Availability: OTC.
Warnings and side effects: See ℞ **triclosan**.

non-narcotic analgesic ⓓ

(weak analgesic)

Generics: **acetaminophen; aspirin; celecoxib; choline salicylate; diclofenac; diflunisal; etodolac; fenoprofen; flurbiprofen; ibuprofen; indomethacin; ketoprofen; ketorolac tromethamine; magnesium salicylate; meclofenamate sodium; mefenamic acid; meloxicam; methyl salicylate; nabumetone; naproxen; oxaprozin; piroxicam; rofecoxib; salicylamide; salsalate; sodium salicylate; sodium thiosalicylate; sulindac; tolmetin sodium.**

Actions and uses

Non-narcotic analgesics are certain drugs used to treat ⊙ **pain**. The term non-narcotic distinguishes them from the ℞ **narcotic analgesic** class, which includes drugs such as ℞ **morphine**. Non-narcotic analgesics have no tendency to produce dependence (addiction), although they do still have other side effects. Most non-narcotic analgesics are of the type referred to in medical circles as non-steroidal anti-inflammatory drugs or ℞ **NSAIDs**, which refers to the valuable ℞ **anti-inflammatory** action of some members of the class.

Although ℞ **acetaminophen** (paracetamol) shares some of the properties of the NSAID group, it is has little anti-inflammatory potency, and so it is often not classified with them. Acetaminophen, along with all the NSAID drugs, has valuable ℞ **antipyretic** activity, which is the ability to lower body temperature when it is raised in ⊙ **fever**.

Some drugs of this group (for example, ℞ **aspirin**, acetaminophen, and ℞ **ibuprofen**) are available OTC (over-the-counter) in forms to be taken by mouth for the relief of pain of many types (for example, ⊙ **headache**, ⊙ **migraine**, ⊙ **dysmenorrhea** (period pain), toothache, and muscle and joint ache). Drugs in this class are used in combination with other analgesics (including narcotic analgesics such as ℞ **codeine phosphate**) or with drugs of other classes (for example, the ℞ **CNS stimulant** ℞ **caffeine**). They may be incorporated into ℞ **cold and cough preparation** remedies along with ℞ **decongestant**, ℞ **expectorant**, and ℞ **antitussive** drugs.

Some are applied topically (externally) as creams and similar (for example, methyl salicylate) to treat muscle and joint aches and sprains, although whether they work via an NSAID action after absorption into the affected site, or by a separate mechanism as a ℞ **counter-irritant** or rubefacient, is not certain.

Aspirin has an additional ℞ **antiplatelet** action not directly related to its analgesic action, and other NSAIDs are not nearly so powerful in this respect and cannot be substituted (it is due to inhibition of the COX-2 subtype of a cyclo-oxygenase enzyme—rather than inhibition of the COX-1 subtype responsible for its anti-inflammatory action).

Limitations

Although non-narcotic analgesics have no tendency to produce habituation, many do have some very significant side effects. Most of these are gastrointestinal upsets ranging from indigestion to serious bleeding. People with a tendency to dyspepsia or peptic ulcer, should avoid NSAID drugs and use acetaminophen wherever possible. Also, aspirin is now no longer recommended for children because of a perceived risk of causing the rare, but serious, condition of ✪ Reye's syndrome. In general, where an anti-inflammatory analgesic and antipyretic is required for adults or children, ibuprofen is usually considered safe. See also the individual drug entries.

No Pain-HP Ⓑ

A preparation of ℞ **capsaicin**.
Formulation: Topical roll-on.
Availability: OTC.
Warnings and side effects: See ℞ capsaicin.

noradrenaline acid tartrate Ⓖ

see ℞ **norepinephrine bitartrate**.

Norco Tablets Ⓑ

A preparation of ℞ **hydrocodone bitartrate** and ℞ **acetaminophen**.
Formulation: Oral tablets.
Availability: Prescription only.
Warnings and side effects: See ℞ hydrocodone bitartrate; ℞ acetaminophen.

Norcuron Ⓑ

A preparation of ℞ **vecuronium bromide**.
Formulation: Injection.
Availability: Prescription only.
Warnings and side effects: See ℞ vecuronium bromide.

Nordette Ⓑ

A preparation of ℞ **ethinyl estradiol** and ℞ **levonorgestrel**.
Formulation: Calendar pack of oral tablets.
Availability: Prescription only.
Warnings and side effects: See ℞ ethinyl estradiol; ℞ levonorgestrel.

Norditropin Ⓑ

A preparation of ℞ **somatropin**.
Formulation: Injection in several strengths.
Availability: Prescription only.
Warnings and side effects: See ℞ somatropin.

norepinephrine bitartrate Ⓖ

(noradrenaline acid tartrate)
Type/Group: **alpha-adrenergic stimulant; beta-adrenergic stimulant; vasoconstrictor; cardiac stimulant**.

Brand(s): Levophed.
How administered: Intravenous injection, infusion.

Used to treat

Norepinephrine bitartrate is the chemical form of the naturally occurring norepinephrine used in medicine. It has both alpha-adrenergic stimulant and beta-adrenergic stimulant properties, and is not widely used because its actions are so widespread within the body. But in emergencies it may be used as a vasoconstrictor (narrows blood vessels) in acute hypotension (low blood pressure) and, with other drugs, as a cardiac stimulant in cardiac arrest (when it is given by injection).

Warnings

• It should not be given to people with certain thrombotic conditions, or with low blood volume, as from bleeding (except in emergency, life-saving situations).
• It should be given with caution to the elderly, to people with certain cardiovascular (for example, atherosclerosis, arteriosclerosis), heart, kidney, and thyroid disorders, diabetes mellitus, and hypertension. Care must be taken to avoid interaction with other drugs, especially ℞ **MAOI** antidepressants (in case of hypertensive crisis).
• Risk in pregnancy changes depending on circumstances. It should be used during pregnancy only when it is clearly needed.
• Medical judgment is required if breast-feeding is being considered.
• This is a powerful drug, used only in hospitals, and there may be severe drug interactions in people already taking a number of other drugs, especially antidepressants and beta-blockers (see Interactions below).
• Norepinephrine may cause severe tissue damage at the site of injection, so that continuous monitoring is necessary. It should never be injected in the extremities (fingers, toes, ears, and so on).

Interactions

• If used with ℞ **beta-blockers**, there is a risk of severe hypertension followed by slowed heart rhythm.
• Norepinephrine bitartrate should not be used with ℞ **MAOI** antidepressants, or within two weeks of stopping MAOI treatment, because this may cause a hypertensive crisis.
• Other sympathomimetics, ℞ **antihistamines**, ℞ **cardiac glycosides**, halogenated ℞ **general anesthetics**, MAOIs, ℞ **tricyclic** antidepressants, ℞ **oxytocics** (for example, ℞ **oxytocin**, ℞ **ergonovine**), ℞ **bretylium**, ℞ **guanethidine monosulfate**, ℞ **levothyroxine**, and ℞ **methyldopa** may intensify the effects of norepinephrine, with the potential for serious adverse reactions.
• ℞ **alpha-adrenergic blockers**, ℞ **phenothiazines**, and ℞ **diuretics** may reverse or decrease the therapeutic effect of norepinephrine.
• Norepinephrine should not be used with certain ℞ **general anesthetics**.

Side effects

• These depend on how it is administered. There may be palpitation of the heart with slowed and irregular heartbeat, peripheral ischemia (poor circulation in the extremities), breathing difficulty, hypertension, headache, and anxiety.

Norethin ®

A preparation of ℞ **ethinyl estradiol** and ℞ **norethindrone**.
Formulation: Calendar pack of oral tablets.
Availability: Prescription only.
Warnings and side effects: See ℞ ethinyl estradiol;
℞ norethindrone.

norethindrone ©

Type/Group: sex hormone; progestin; contraceptive; oral contraceptive.
Brand(s): Aygestin; Micronor; Nor-Q.D. Combinations: With *ethinyl estradiol* (menopausal symptoms): Femhrt, Activella, Combipatch. With *ethinyl estradiol* (contraception): Brevicon; Estrostep; Estrostep Fe; Gencept; Jenest-28; Loestrin; Loestrin Fe; Modicon; Necon; Nelova; Norinyl; Ovcon; Ortho-Novum; Tri-Norinyl. With *estradiol*: CombiPatch. With *mestranol*: Necon 1/50; Nelova 1/50M; Norcept-E; Norethin; Norinyl 1 + 50; Ortho-Novum 1/50.
How administered: Orally

Used to treat

Norethindrone is used in contraception (alone as "progestin-only pill" or in combination with ℞ **estrogen** as "combined pill"), for secondary amenorrhea, abnormal uterine bleeding, ✪ **endometriosis** (a growth of the lining of the uterus at inappropriate sites), and for the prevention of endometrial hyperplasia (abnormal growth of cells) during postmenopausal estrogen treatment.

Warnings

• It should not be used by people with known hypersensitivity to this drug, or with impaired liver function or disease, breast cancer, undiagnosed vaginal bleeding, thrombophlebitis, or a history of thromboembolic disease or stroke.
• It should be used with caution by people with asthma, heart or kidney dysfunction, depression, diabetes mellitus, epilepsy, or migraine.
• It should not be used during pregnancy. A doctor must be contacted if pregnancy occurs while using this drug.
• It may be used by breast-feeding mothers.
• When used as a contraceptive, the menstrual cycle may be disrupted and irregular and unpredictable bleeding or spotting may result.

Interactions

• ℞ **rifampin** may decrease the effects of norethindrone.

Side effects

• Most commonly, nausea.
• Less frequently, depression, dizziness, fatigue, headache, edema, loss of appetite, cramps, increased weight, vomiting, cessation of menses, breast changes, painful periods, endometriosis (a growth of the lining of the uterus at inappropriate sites), elevated blood glucose levels, acne, hair changes, and darkening of skin on face, rash.
• A rare but serious side effect is cholestatic jaundice.

Norflex ®

A preparation of ℞ **orphenadrine**.

Formulation: Sustained release tablets; injection.
Availability: Prescription only.
Warnings and side effects: See ℞ orphenadrine.

norfloxacin ©

Type/Group: quinolone; antibacterial.
Brand(s): Noroxin; Chilbroxin.
How administered: Orally; injection; topically (ophthalmic solution).

Used to treat

Norfloxacin is used primarily to treat ✪ **bacterial infections** of the urinary tract. It is also prescribed for ✪ **gonorrhea** and ✪ **prostatitis**, traveler's ✪ **diarrhea**, and also for eye infections.

Warnings

• It should not be given to people with known hypersensitivity to norfloxacin or other quinolones or a history of convulsive disorders, or to children under 18, as there is a possibility of damage to joints and cartilage in growing children.
• It should be given with caution to people with kidney disease or any predisposition to seizures.
• Norfloxacin should not be used during pregnancy or while breast-feeding unless the potential benefit outweighs the possible risk of joint damage or other harm to the fetus or infant.
• Superinfections due to the altered bacterial balance caused by antibiotic treatment may occur. A doctor must be contacted if severe abdominal pain, or moderate to severe diarrhea occur.
• Rare, but serious, side effects of quinolones include seizure and other CNS (central nervous system) effects, and severe allergic reactions.
• Adequate fluid intake should be maintained.
• Photosensitivity reactions (abnormal sensitivity to light) can occur, and so excessive exposure to sunlight should be avoided.
• Take one hour before or two hours after meals.
• ᐁ **Calcium**, ᐁ **iron** preparations, ᐁ **magnesium**, and ᐁ **zinc** may reduce the effects of norfloxacin. Products such as supplements that contain these ingredients must not be taken less than four hours before or four hours after taking norfloxacin.

Interactions

• ℞ **Antacids**, ᐁ **calcium**, ℞ **didanosine (ddI)**, ᐁ **iron** preparations, ᐁ **magnesium**, ℞ **sodium bicarbonate**, ᐁ **zinc** reduce the effects of moxifloxacin. Do not take products containing these ingredients less than four hours before or four hours after taking norfloxacin.
• The levels of ℞ **theophylline**, antipyrine, ℞ **caffeine**, ℞ **diazepam**, ℞ **metoprolol**, ℞ **pentoxifylline**, ℞ **phenytoin**, ℞ **propranolol**, ℞ **ropinirole**, ℞ **xanthine**, and ℞ **warfarin sodium** may be increased.
• The effects of oral ℞ **anticoagulants** may be increased.
• If used with ℞ **foscarnet**, the risk of seizure is increased.

Side effects

• Systemic use: Nausea, headache, and dizziness. Rarely, vomiting, diarrhea, dry mouth, bitter taste, nervousness, drowsiness, insomnia, ringing in the ears, crystalluria (hard crystals in urine), and rash fever.

• Ophthalmic (eye) use: Frequently, bad taste in the mouth. Occasionally, temporary blurring of vision and irritation.

Norgesic; Norgesic Forte ®

A preparation of R orphenadrine, R aspirin, and R caffeine.
Formulation: Oral tablets in two strengths.
Availability: Prescription only.
Warnings and side effects: See R orphenadrine; R aspirin; R caffeine.

norgestrel ©

Type/Group: **sex hormone; progestin; contraceptive; oral contraceptive**.
Brand(s): Orvette. Combinations: With *ethinyl estradiol*: Ogestrel; LoOvral; Ovral-28; Low-Ogestrel.
How administered: Orally.

Used to treat

Norgestrel is a progestin which is used in oral contraceptives, alone, and in combination with estrogen.

Warnings

• It should not be given to people with known hypersensitivity to norgestrel, active thromboembolic disease, known or suspected breast cancer, or undiagnosed abnormal genital bleeding.
• It should be given with caution to people with hypertension, gallbladder disease, congestive heart failure, diabetes mellitus, depression, migraine headache, seizure disorders, liver disease, a family history of breast or endometrial cancer, a history of thromboembolic disorders, uterine fibroids, hypertriglyceridemia, or hypercalcemia.
• It should not be used during pregnancy. A doctor must be contacted if pregnancy occurs while using this drug.
• Medical judgment is required if breast-feeding is being considered.
• The use of oral contraceptives is associated with a risk of serious cardiovascular side effects (for example, embolism, stroke, heart attack), particularly in those over age 35. Cigarette smoking increases the risk. This added risk gets larger with age and with heavy smoking (>15 per day), and is quite marked in women over 35.

Side effects

• Nausea and vomiting, breakthrough bleeding, and spotting.
• Less frequently, depression, migraine headache, increased emotionality, elevated blood pressure, venous thrombosis, edema, contact lens intolerance, gallbladder disease, bloating, benign liver tumors, cessation of menses, change in cervical secretions, breast enlargement, breast tenderness, elevated blood glucose, elevated triglyceride or calcium levels, darkening of the skin of the face, changes in libido, and weight gain.

Norinyl 1 + 35 ®

A preparation of R ethinyl estradiol and R norethindrone.
Formulation: Calendar pack of oral tablets.
Availability: Prescription only.
Warnings and side effects: See R ethinyl estradiol; R norethindrone.

Norinyl 1 + 50 ®

A preparation of R mestranol and R norethindrone.
Formulation: Calendar pack of oral tablets.
Availability: Prescription only.
Warnings and side effects: See R mestranol; R norethindrone.

Norisodrine w/Calcium Iodide Syrup ®

A preparation of R isoproterenol sulfate and anhydrous calcium iodide.
Formulation: Oral syrup.
Availability: Prescription only.
Warnings and side effects: See R isoproterenol.

Noritate ®

A preparation of R metronidazole.
Formulation: Topical cream.
Availability: Prescription only.
Warnings and side effects: See R metronidazole.

Normiflo ®

A preparation of R ardeparin sodium.
Formulation: Injection (subcutaneous).
Availability: Prescription only.
Warnings and side effects: See R ardeparin sodium. Contains sodium metabisulfite, methyparaben and propylparaben, which may cause hypersensitivity reaction in a few individuals.

Normodyne Tablets; Injection ®

A preparation of R labetalol hydrochloride.
Formulation: Oral tablets (3 strengths); injection.
Availability: Prescription only.
Warnings and side effects: See R labetalol hydrochloride.

Noroxin ®

A preparation of R norfloxacin.
Formulation: Oral tablets.
Availability: Prescription only.
Warnings and side effects: See R norfloxacin.

Norpace; Norpace CR ®

A preparation of R disopyramide.
Formulation: Oral capsules (two strengths); extended-release capsules (Norpace CR), available in two strengths.
Availability: Prescription only.
Warnings and side effects: See R disopyramide.

Norplant System ®

A preparation of R levonorgestrel.
Formulation: Subdermal implant.
Availability: Prescription only.
Warnings and side effects: See R levonorgestrel.

Norpramin ®

A preparation of R desipramine hydrochloride.
Formulation: Oral tablets.

Key to symbols: ✛ = Disorder Section   R = Drug Section   ♣ = Herbal Section   ⟐ = Supplement Section

Availability: Prescription only.
Warnings and side effects: See ℞ **desipramine hydrochloride.** Also contains tartrazine (FD and C yellow No.5), which may cause adverse reactions, including asthma, in some individuals. Although rare, such reactions are more frequent in those sensitive to aspirin.

Nor Q.-D. ⑧

A preparation of ℞ **norethindrone.**
Formulation: Oral tablets.
Availability: Prescription only.
Warnings and side effects: See ℞ **norethindrone.**

nortriptyline hydrochloride ⑥

Type/Group: antidepressant; tricyclic.
Brand(s): Aventyl; Pamelor; various generic.
How administered: Orally.

Used to treat

Nortriptyline hydrochloride is used in the treatment of ✪ **depression,** and is less sedating than some of the tricyclics. Although not stated by the manufacturer for such treatments, it is sometimes used for panic disorder, premenstrual depression, certain skin disorders, and bed-wetting (nocturnal enuresis). As is the case with other antidepressants, this drug is also being evaluated for other uses.

Warnings

• It should not be given to people with known hypersensitivity to this drug, or who are just recovering from myocardial infarction (heart attack), who are taking or have stopped taking ℞ **MAOI** antidepressants within the previous 14 days.
• It should be given with caution to people with a history of seizures, urinary retention, or elevated intraocular pressure (pressure in the eyeball), narrow-angle glaucoma, liver, cardiovascular, heart, or thyroid disease, diabetes mellitus, epilepsy, or angle-closure glaucoma.
• Nortriptyline should be used during pregnancy only if the benefits outweigh the possible risk to the fetus.
• It should not be used by nursing mothers.
• Other symptoms of psychiatric illnesses may worsen.
• Episodes of mania or hypomania may occur, especially in those with affective bipolar disorder (manic depression).
• Exposure to sunlight should be minimized because of possible photosensitization (sensitivity to light).
• Treatment should be stopped gradually by lowering the dose over a period of time.
• It is not generally given to children under the age of 12.
• It may be two to three weeks before there are any signs of improvement.
• It may impair the performance of skilled tasks such as driving.
• Alcohol, grapefruit juice, and smoking can all affect tricyclics (see Interactions below).

Interactions

• Serious or even fatal reactions can occur if ℞ **MAOI** antidepressants are taken at the same time as tricyclics.
• The effects of ℞ **epinephrine,** ℞ **norepinephrine,** and ℞ **phenylephrine** on blood pressure are intensified.

• Grapefruit juice increases the levels of tricyclics.
• ℞ **clonidine hydrochloride** should not be used with tricyclics, because a dangerous increase in blood pressure and hypertensive crisis is possible.
• The effects of ℞ **guanethidine monosulfate,** ℞ **levodopa,** and ℞ **sympathomimetics** may be reduced by tricyclics.
• The effects of ℞ **anticholinergics,** ℞ **clonidine hydrochloride,** dicumarol, ℞ **quinolones,** grepafloxacin, and sparfloxacin may be enhanced by tricyclics.
• ℞ **Barbiturates,** ℞ **activated charcoal,** and rifamycin-related antibiotics may reduce the effectiveness of tricyclics.
• ℞ **Cimetidine,** ℞ **SSRIs,** ℞ **haloperidol,** ℞ **bupropion,** ℞ **valproate sodium** (and other valproic acid derivatives), and histamine ℞ **H$_2$-antagonists** may increase the levels of tricyclics in the blood.
• The levels of ℞ **carbamazepine** may increase, while blood levels of tricyclics decrease.
• Smoking may affect the metabolism of tricyclics.
• The effects of alcohol may be enhanced.

Side effects

• Along with other members of this class, it has pronounced ℞ **anticholinergic** side effects, including drowsiness and difficulty in concentrating, and also dizziness, dry mouth, blurred vision, constipation, postural hypotension (lowered blood pressure on standing), and urinary retention.
• Less frequently, there may be anxiety, confusion, extrapyramidal symptoms in older adults (uncontrollable movement), mental changes, tremors, weakness, ECG changes, raised blood pressure, heart palpitations, fainting, eye changes, nasal congestion, ringing in the ears (tinnitus), gastrointestinal disorders, hepatitis, jaundice, skin sensitivity reactions, and sweating.
• Rarely, serious side effects including seizures, heart rhythm abnormalities, and blood cell disorders may occur.

Norvasc ⑧

A preparation of ℞ **amlodipine besylate.**
Formulation: Oral tablets, available in 3 strengths.
Availability: Prescription only.
Warnings and side effects: See ℞ **amlodipine besylate.**

Norvir ⑧

A preparation of ℞ **ritonavir.**
Formulation: Oral capsules; oral solution.
Availability: Prescription only.
Warnings and side effects: See ℞ **ritonavir.**

Norwich Extra-Strength ⑧

A preparation of ℞ **aspirin.**
Formulation: Oral tablets.
Availability: OTC.
Warnings and side effects: See ℞ **aspirin.**

Nostrilla ⑧

A preparation of ℞ **oxymetazoline hydrochloride.**
Formulation: Nasal spray.

Availability: OTC.
Warnings and side effects: See ℞ oxymetazoline hydrochloride.

Novacet ℬ

A preparation of (sodium) ℞ **sulfacetamide**.
Formulation: Topical lotion.
Availability: OTC.
Warnings and side effects: See ℞ **sulfacetamide**.

Novafed A Capsules ℬ

A preparation of ℞ **pseudoephedrine** and ℞ **chlorpheniramine maleate**.
Formulation: Oral capsules, sustained release.
Availability: Prescription only.
Warnings and side effects: See ℞ **pseudoephedrine**; ℞ **chlorpheniramine maleate**.

Novagest Expectorant with Codeine Liquid ℬ

A preparation of ℞ **codeine phosphate**, ℞ **guaifenesin**, and ℞ **pseudoephedrine**.
Formulation: Oral liquid.
Availability: May or may not require a prescription.
Warnings and side effects: See ℞ **codeine phosphate**; ℞ **guaifenesin**; ℞ **pseudoephedrine**.

Novahistine DMX ℬ

A preparation of ℞ **dextromethorphan**, ℞ **pseudoephedrine**, and ℞ **guaifenesin**.
Formulation: Oral liquid.
Availability: OTC.
Warnings and side effects: See ℞ **dextromethorphan**; ℞ **pseudoephedrine**; ℞ **guaifenesin**.

Novarel ℬ

A preparation of ℞ **chorionic gonadotropin**.
Formulation: Injection.
Availability: Prescription only.
Warnings and side effects: See ℞ **chorionic gonadotropin**.

Novocain ℬ

A preparation of ℞ **procaine**.
Formulation: Injection.
Availability: Prescription only.
Warnings and side effects: See ℞ **procaine**.

Novolin 70/30 ℬ

A preparation of ℞ **insulin, regular and isophane mixture**.
Formulation: Vials for injection.
Availability: OTC.
Warnings and side effects: See ℞ **insulin, regular and isophane mixture**.

Novolin 70/30 PenFill ℬ

A preparation of ℞ **insulin, regular**.
Formulation: Cartridges for injection.
Availability: OTC.
Warnings and side effects: See ℞ **insulin, regular**.

Novolin 70/30 Prefilled ℬ

A preparation of ℞ **insulin, regular and isophane mixture**.
Formulation: Cartridges for injection.
Availability: OTC.
Warnings and side effects: See ℞ **insulin, regular and isophane mixture**.

Novolin L ℬ

A preparation of ℞ **insulin zinc suspension (lente)**.
Formulation: Bottles for injection.
Availability: OTC.
Warnings and side effects: See ℞ **insulin zinc suspension (lente)**.

Novolin N ℬ

A preparation of ℞ **insulin, isophane suspension (insulin, NPH)**.
Formulation: Bottles for injection.
Availability: OTC.
Warnings and side effects: See ℞ **insulin, isophane suspension (insulin, NPH)**.

Novolin N PenFill ℬ

A preparation of ℞ **insulin, isophane suspension (insulin, NPH)**.
Formulation: Cartridges for injection.
Availability: OTC.
Warnings and side effects: See ℞ **insulin, isophane suspension (insulin, NPH)**.

Novolin N Prefilled ℬ

A preparation of ℞ **insulin, isophane suspension (insulin, NPH)**.
Formulation: Cartridges for injection.
Availability: OTC.
Warnings and side effects: See ℞ **insulin, isophane suspension (insulin, NPH)**.

Novolin R ℬ

A preparation of ℞ **insulin, regular**.
Formulation: Bottles for injection.
Availability: OTC.
Warnings and side effects: See ℞ **insulin, regular**.

Novolin R PenFill ℬ

A preparation of ℞ **insulin, regular**.
Formulation: Cartridges for injection.
Availability: OTC.
Warnings and side effects: See ℞ **insulin, regular**.

Novolin R Prefilled ℬ

A preparation of ℞ **insulin, regular**.

Formulation: Prefilled syringes for injection.

Availability: OTC.

Warnings and side effects: See ℞ insulin, regular.

NovoSeven Ⓑ

A preparation of ℞ coagulation Factor VIIa recombinant; rFVIIa.

Formulation: Intravenous injection.

Availability: Prescription only.

Warnings and side effects: See ℞ coagulation Factor VIIa recombinant; rFVIIa.

NPH: isophane protamine insulin ⒼG

see ℞ insulin, isophane suspension (insulin, NPH).

NPH Iletin I ⒷB

A preparation of ℞ insulin, isophane suspension (insulin, NPH).

Formulation: Bottles for injection.

Availability: OTC.

Warnings and side effects: See ℞ insulin, isophane suspension (insulin, NPH).

NPH Iletin II ⒷB

A preparation of ℞ insulin, isophane suspension (insulin, NPH).

Formulation: Bottle for injection.

Availability: OTC.

Warnings and side effects: See ℞ insulin, isophane suspension (insulin, NPH).

NPH-N ⒷB

A preparation of ℞ insulin, isophane suspension (insulin, NPH).

Formulation: Vial for injection.

Availability: OTC.

Warnings and side effects: See ℞ insulin, isophane suspension (insulin, NPH).

NSAID ⒟D

aspirin; celecoxib; choline salicylate; diclofenac; diflunisal; etodolac; fenoprofen; flurbiprofen; ibuprofen; indomethacin; ketoprofen; ketorolac tromethamine; magnesium salicylate; meclofenamate sodium; mefenamic acid; meloxicam; methyl salicylate; nabumetone; naproxen; oxaprozin; piroxicam; rofecoxib; salsalate; salicylic acid; sodium salicylate; sodium thiosalicylate; sulindac; tolmetin sodium; (acetaminophen).

Actions and uses

NSAID is an abbreviation for non-steroidal anti-inflammatory drug, which is a term used to describe a large group of drugs, of which ℞ aspirin is an original member. Although they are all acidic compounds of different chemical structures, they have several important actions in common. They can be used as ℞ anti-inflammatory drugs (to the extent that some may be used as ℞ antirheumatic treatments), as ℞ non-narcotic analgesic drugs (particularly when the ⊙ pain is associated with inflammation) and as ℞ antipyretic drugs (they lower body temperature only when it is raised in ⊙ fever).

All these actions are thought to be due to the ability of NSAIDs to act as enzyme inhibitors (acting on the cyclo-oxygenase system; COX) to change the synthesis and metabolism of the natural ℞ prostaglandin thromboxane and related inflammatory local hormones. Although ℞ acetaminophen shares some of the properties of the NSAID group, it is a very weak cyclo-oxygenase inhibitor and has little anti-inflammatory activity, and so is often not classified with them. See also ℞ analgesic.

Some NSAIDs are applied topically (externally) as rubbing creams and similar (for example, methyl salicylate) to treat muscle and joint aches and sprains, although whether they work via an NSAID action after absorption into the affected site, or by a separate mechanism as a ℞ counter-irritant or rubefacient is not certain.

Aspirin has an additional ℞ antiplatelet action not directly related to its analgesic action, and other NSAIDs are not nearly so powerful is this respect and cannot be substituted (it is due to inhibition of the COX-2 subtype of a cyclo-oxygenase enzyme—rather than inhibition of the COX-1 subtype responsible for its anti-inflammatory action).

Limitations

In practice, the side effects of NSAIDs are so extensive that the use of individual members depends on the ability of individuals to tolerate their side effects. This toleration is especially important when used for ⊙ rheumatoid arthritis where generally high doses are used for a long period of time. Some with the least side effects are regarded as safe enough for non-prescription, over-the-counter (OTC) sale, such as aspirin and ℞ ibuprofen. Others, such as ℞ ketorolac tromethamine, are used only in exceptional circumstances or only for short periods. Also, aspirin is now no longer recommended for children because of a perceived risk of causing the rare, but serious, condition called ⊙ Reye's syndrome. See the individual drug entries for details.

NTZ Long Acting Nasal Drops; Spray ⒷB

A preparation of ℞ oxymetazoline hydrochloride.

Formulation: Nasal drops; spray.

Availability: OTC.

Warnings and side effects: See ℞ oxymetazoline hydrochloride.

Nubain ⒷB

A preparation of ℞ nalbuphine hydrochloride.

Formulation: Injection.

Availability: Prescription only.

Warnings and side effects: See ℞ nalbuphine hydrochloride.

Nucofed ⒷB

A preparation of ℞ codeine phosphate and ℞ pseudoephedrine.

Formulation: Oral capsules; syrup.

Availability: Prescription only.

Warnings and side effects: See ℞ codeine phosphate; ℞ pseudoephedrine.

Nucofed Expectorant Syrup Ⓑ

A preparation of ℞ **codeine phosphate**, ℞ **guaifenesin**, and ℞ **pseudoephedrine**.
Formulation: Oral syrup.
Availability: Prescription only.
Warnings and side effects: See ℞ **codeine phosphate**; ℞ **guaifenesin**; ℞ **pseudoephedrine**.

Nucofed Pediatric Expectorant Syrup Ⓑ

A preparation of ℞ **codeine phosphate**, ℞ **guaifenesin**, and ℞ **pseudoephedrine**.
Formulation: Oral syrup.
Availability: May or may not require a prescription.
Warnings and side effects: See ℞ **codeine phosphate**; ℞ **guaifenesin**; ℞ **pseudoephedrine**.

Nucotuss Expectorant Syrup Ⓑ

A preparation of ℞ **codeine phosphate**, ℞ **guaifenesin**, and ℞ **pseudoephedrine**.
Formulation: Oral syrup.
Availability: Prescription only.
Warnings and side effects: See ℞ **codeine phosphate**; ℞ **guaifenesin**; ℞ **pseudoephedrine**.

Nucotuss Pediatric Expectorant Syrup Ⓑ

A preparation of ℞ **codeine phosphate**, ℞ **guaifenesin**, and ℞ **pseudoephedrine**.
Formulation: Oral syrup.
Availability: May or may not require a prescription.
Warnings and side effects: See ℞ **codeine phosphate**; ℞ **guaifenesin**; ℞ **pseudoephedrine**.

Numby Stuff Ⓑ

A preparation of ℞ **lidocaine** and ℞ **epinephrine**.
Formulation: Topical solution.
Availability: Prescription only.
Warnings and side effects: See ℞ **lidocaine**; ℞ **epinephrine**.

Numorphan Suppositories; Injection Ⓑ

A preparation of ℞ **oxymorphone hydrochloride**.
Formulation: Rectal suppositories; injection.
Availability: Prescription only.
Warnings and side effects: See ℞ **oxymorphone hydrochloride**.

Numzit Teething Ⓑ

A preparation of ℞ **benzocaine** and ℞ **peppermint oil**.
Formulation: Topical Gel.
Availability: OTC.
Warnings and side effects: See ℞ **benzocaine**; ℞ **peppermint oil**.

Nupercainal Ⓑ

A preparation of ℞ **dibucaine**.
Formulation: Topical cream; topical ointment.
Availability: OTC.

Warnings and side effects: See ℞ **dibucaine**.

Nuprin Backache Caplets Ⓑ

A preparation of ℞ **magnesium salicylate**.
Formulation: Oral tablets.
Availability: OTC.
Warnings and side effects: See ℞ **magnesium salicylate**.

Nuprin Tablets; Caplets Ⓑ

A preparation of ℞ **ibuprofen**.
Formulation: Oral tablets.
Availability: OTC.
Warnings and side effects: See ℞ **ibuprofen**.

Nutracort Ⓑ

A preparation of ℞ **hydrocortisone**.
Formulation: Cream.
Availability: Prescription only.
Warnings and side effects: See ℞ **hydrocortisone**.

Nutropin; Nutropin Depot; Nutropin AQ Ⓑ

A preparation of ℞ **somatropin**.
Formulation: Injection in several strengths; Depot is an extended release form.
Availability: Prescription only.
Warnings and side effects: See ℞ **somatropin**.

Nydrazid Ⓑ

A preparation of ℞ **isoniazid**.
Formulation: Injection.
Availability: Prescription only.
Warnings and side effects: See ℞ **isoniazid**.

nystatin Ⓖ

Type/Group: antifungal; antibiotic; candidiasis treatment.
Brand(s): Mycostatin; Nilstat, Nystex; various generic.
Combinations: With *triamcinolone*: Mycogen II Mycolog-II; Myconel; Mycotriacetate; N.G.T.
How administered: Orally; Topically (external).

Used to treat

Nystatin is a polyene antibiotic with antifungal properties. It is primarily used to treat the yeast infection ✪ **candidiasis** (thrush) of the skin and mucous membranes, including vaginal, intestinal tract, and oral infections. It is effective when administered topically (externally) or orally. When taken orally, it is not absorbed into the blood and its antifungal action is restricted to the mouth and gastrointestinal tract.

Warnings

• It should not be given to people with known hypersensitivity to nystatin.
• The topical forms are safe for use during pregnancy. It is not known if the oral forms can harm the fetus. It should be used during pregnancy only if the benefits outweigh the risks.
• Medical judgment is required if breast-feeding is being considered. It is not known if it appears breast milk.

• Treatment must be continued for at least two days after symptoms have gone.

Interactions

No significant interactions have been reported.

Side effects

• Occasionally, skin or vaginal irritation with topical use.

• Rarely, nausea, vomiting, and diarrhea with oral use.

Nystex Ⓑ

A preparation of ℞ **nystatin**.

Formulation: Oral suspension.

Availability: Prescription only.

Warnings and side effects: See ℞ **nystatin**.

Nytcold Medicine Liquid Ⓑ

A preparation of ℞ **dextromethorphan**, ℞ **acetaminophen**, ℞ **pseudoephedrine**, and ℞ **doxylamine**.

Formulation: Oral liquid.

Availability: OTC.

Warnings and side effects: See ℞ **dextromethorphan**; ℞ **acetaminophen**; ℞ **pseudoephedrine**; ℞ **doxylamine**.

obesity treatment Ⓓ

Generics: karaya; methamphetamine; methylcellulose; orlistat; phendimetrazine; phentermine; psyllium; sibutramine; sterculia gum.

Actions and uses

The treatment of ✪ **obesity** involves dietary and lifestyle changes (for example, more exercise) as well as drug therapy, to reduce body weight where this is a medical risk. Most drugs used in obesity treatment work as ℞ **appetite suppressant**, either acting directly on the brain as ℞ **CNS stimulant** agents (for example, ℞ **phentermine** and ℞ **phendimetrazine**) or as ℞ **bulk-forming agents** which increase the bulk in the intestine which may lead to a feeling of being full (for example, methylcellulose, psyllium, and sterculia). A recently introduced drug, ℞ **orlistat**, works instead by reducing the absorption from the intestine of dietary fat.

Limitations

These drugs are intended to assist in the medical treatment of obesity, where the primary method for reducing weight is an appropriate diet and exercise. They are not for weight loss in non-obese people. See the individual drug entries.

Occlusal-HP Ⓑ

A preparation of ℞ **salicylic acid**.

Formulation: Topical liquid.

Availability: OTC.

Warnings and side effects: See ℞ **salicylic acid**.

Octamide Tablets; PFS Ⓑ

A preparation of ℞ **metoclopramide hydrochloride**.

Formulation: Oral tablets; injection.

Availability: Prescription only.

Warnings and side effects: See ℞ **metoclopramide hydrochloride**.

Octicair Ⓑ

A preparation of ℞ **hydrocortisone**, ℞ **neomycin**, and ℞ **polymyxin B sulfate**.

Formulation: Ear drops.

Availability: Prescription only.

Warnings and side effects: See ℞ **hydrocortisone**; ℞ **neomycin**; ℞ **polymyxin B sulfate**.

octreotide Ⓖ

Type/Group: anticancer; hormone; hypothalamic hormone.

Brand(s): Sandostatin.

How administered: Injection.

Used to treat

Octreotide, a long-lasting analog of the hypothalamic hormone somatostatin (hypothalamic release-inhibiting hormone; GH-RIH or SRIF), reduces the release of a number of hormones from the pituitary gland and other sites. It is used to treat symptoms caused by the release of hormones from cancerous and noncancerous tumors of the endocrine system (neurocarcinomas such as VIPoma), such as severe diarrhea and flushing episodes associated with metastatic carcinoid tumors, as well as for acromegaly (caused by excessive growth hormone). Although not stated by the manufacturer for such uses, it is sometimes used for certain other diarrheal states and to control bleeding from esophageal varices.

Warnings

• It should not be used by people with known hypersensitivity to this drug.

• It should be given with caution to people with insulin-dependent diabetes mellitus, gallbladder disease, or severe kidney dysfunction.

• It should be used during pregnancy only if medically judged to be needed.

• Medical judgment is also required if breast-feeding is being considered.

• It may affect the gallbladder and inhibit bile secretion. There is a risk of gallstones.

• Thyroid function may be reduced by prolonged, high-dosage therapy.

Interactions

• ℞ **insulin**, ℞ **oral hypoglycemics**, ℞ **glucagon**, and growth hormone may alter blood glucose levels.

Side effects

• Frequently, diarrhea, nausea, slow heart rate, constipation, abdominal discomfort, and increased blood glucose levels.

• Occasionally, other gastrointestinal effects, headache, loss of hair, flushing, dizziness, fatigue, changes in heart rhythm, and blurred vision.

• Rarely, there may be depression, decreased libido, heart palpitations, leg cramps, and shortness of breath.

• Rare but serious side effects include hepatitis, pancreatitis gastrointestinal bleeding, and seizures.

• There may be pain at the injection site.

OcuClear Ⓑ

A preparation of ℞ **oxymetazoline hydrochloride**.

Formulation: Eye drops.
Availability: OTC.
Warnings and side effects: See ℞ **oxymetazoline hydrochloride**.

OcuCoat Ⓑ

A preparation of ℞ **hydroxypropyl methylcellulose**.
Formulation: Ophthalmic solution.
Availability: OTC.
Warnings and side effects: See ℞ **hydroxypropyl methylcellulose**.

Ocufen Solution Ⓑ

A preparation of ℞ **flurbiprofen**.
Formulation: Ophthalmic solution.
Availability: Prescription only.
Warnings and side effects: See ℞ **flurbiprofen**.

Ocuflox Ⓑ

A preparation of ℞ **ofloxacin**.
Formulation: Eye drops.
Availability: Prescription only.
Warnings and side effects: See ℞ **ofloxacin**.

Ocupress Ⓑ

A preparation of ℞ **carteolol**.
Formulation: Eye drops.
Availability: Prescription only.
Warnings and side effects: See ℞ **carteolol**.

Ocusert Pilo-20; Pilo-40 Ⓑ

A preparation of ℞ **pilocarpine**.
Formulation: Eye-insert system, continuous 7-day release.
Availability: Prescription only.
Warnings and side effects: See ℞ **pilocarpine**.

Ocusulf-10 Ⓑ

A preparation of ℞ **sulfacetamide**.
Formulation: Eye drops.
Availability: Prescription only.
Warnings and side effects: See ℞ **sulfacetamide**.

oestrogen Ⓓ

see ℞ **estrogen**.

oestrogen antagonist Ⓓ

see ℞ **antiestrogen**.

Off-Ezy Wart Remover Kit Ⓑ

A preparation of ℞ **salicylic acid**.
Formulation: Topical liquid.
Availability: OTC.
Warnings and side effects: See ℞ **salicylic acid**.

ofloxacin Ⓖ

Type/Group: **quinolone; antibacterial**.
Brand(s): Floxin; Ocuflox.
How administered: Orally; injection; ophthalmic (eye).
Used to treat
Ofloxacin can be used to treat ⊙ **bacterial infections** of the genito-urinary tract, including both ⊙ **gonorrhea** and non-gonorrheal infections, some respiratory and eye infections, skin and skin structure infections, and ⊙ **prostatitis**.
Warnings
• It should not be given to people with known hypersensitivity to ofloxacin or other quinolones, or to children under 18, as there is a possibility of damage to joints and cartilage in growing children.
• It should be given with caution to people with kidney disease or any predisposition to seizures.
• Ofloxacin should not be used during pregnancy or while breast-feeding unless the potential benefit outweighs the risk of joint damage or other harm to the fetus or infant.
• Superinfections due to the altered bacterial balance caused by antibiotic treatment may occur. A doctor must be contacted if severe abdominal pain, or moderate to severe diarrhea occur.
• Rare, but serious, side effects of quinolones include seizure and other CNS (central nervous system) effects, and severe allergic reactions.
• Adequate fluid intake should be maintained.
• Photosensitivity reactions (abnormal sensitivity to light) can occur, so excessive exposure to sunlight must be avoided.
• ⚕ **Calcium**, ⚕ **iron** preparations, ⚕ **magnesium**, aluminum, and ⚕ **zinc** reduce the effects of ofloxacin. Any products containing these substances, such as supplements, must not be taken less than four hours before or two hours after using ofloxacin.
• Take on an empty stomach and not with meals.
Interactions
• ℞ Antacids, ⚕ **calcium**, ℞ **didanosine (ddI)**, ⚕ **iron** preparations, ⚕ **magnesium**, ℞ **sodium bicarbonate**, and ⚕ **zinc** reduce the effects of ofloxacin. Do not take products containing these ingredients less than four hours before or two hours after taking ofloxacin.
• The levels of ℞ **theophylline**, antipyrine, ℞ **caffeine**, ℞ **diazepam**, ℞ **metoprolol**, ℞ **pentoxifylline**, ℞ **phenytoin**, ℞ **propranolol**, ℞ **ropinirole**, ℞ **xanthine**, and ℞ **warfarin sodium** may be increased.
• The effects of oral ℞ **anticoagulants** may be increased.
• If used with ℞ **foscarnet**, the risk of seizure is increased.
Side effects
• Systemic use: Nausea, headache, and dizziness. Rarely, vomiting, diarrhea, dry mouth, bitter taste, nervousness, drowsiness, insomnia, ringing in the ears, crystalluria (hard crystals in urine), rash, fever, and seizures.
• Ophthalmic use: Frequently, bad taste in the mouth. Occasionally, temporary blurring of vision and irritation.

Ogen Ⓑ

A preparation of ℞ **estropipate**.
Formulation: Oral tablets in several strengths.

Key to symbols: ⊙ = Disorder Section ℞ = Drug Section ♣ = Herbal Section ⚕ = Supplement Section

Availability: Prescription only.
Warnings and side effects: See ℞ estropipate.

olanzapine ⓖ

Type/Group: **antipsychotic**.
Brand(s): Zyprexa.
How administered: Orally.

Used to treat

Olanzapine is a recently introduced antipsychotic drug (one of a group sometimes termed "atypical" antipsychotics), which can be used to tranquilize patients suffering from ✪ **psychotic disorders**, such as ✪ **schizophrenia**.

Warnings

• It should not be given to people with known hypersensitivity to this drug.
• It should be given with caution to people with liver impairment, a history of certain cardiovascular, kidney and heart diseases, cerebrovascular disease, seizure disorders (epilepsy), prostatic hypertrophy, narrow-angle glaucoma, a history of fecal impaction or paralytic ileus, or anyone at risk for aspiration pneumonia.
• Olanzapine should be used during pregnancy only if the benefits outweigh the risk to the fetus.
• It should not be used by nursing mothers.
• It may cause postural hypotension (lowered blood pressure on standing), so rise slowly from a reclining position. Older people in particular should exercise caution.
• It may impair physical and mental abilities.
• Avoid alcohol.
• Smoking may reduce the effects of the drug.
• Treatment should be stopped gradually.
• Avoid exposure to extreme heat, and take care to avoid dehydration.
• If used for a long time, tardive dyskinesia (see ℞ **antipsychotics**) occasionally develops.

Interactions

• ℞ **Carbamazepine** reduces the effects of clozapine.
• The ℞ **antiparkinsonism** effects of ℞ **levodopa** may be reduced.
• If an antipsychotic is taken with alcohol, there may be increased sedative effects.

Side effects

• Agitation, anxiety, dizziness, headache, hostility, insomnia, nervousness, sleepiness, nasal congestion, constipation, dry mouth, extrapyramidal symptoms (usually mild and transient; see ℞ **antipsychotics**).
• Less frequently, amnesia, articulation impairment, chest pain, edema, low blood pressure, speeded heart rate, eye changes, abdominal pain, increased appetite and weight gain, premenstrual syndrome, back or joint pain, rash, fever, and changes in liver function.
• Rarely, neuroleptic malignant syndrome (a potentially fatal condition characterized by very high fever, muscle rigidity, changes in mental status, and irregular pulse, blood pressure and/or heart rhythm).

olsalazine sodium ⓖ

Type/Group: **aminosalicylate; anti-inflammatory**.
Brand(s): Dipentum.
How administered: Orally.

Used to treat

Olsalazine is used primarily to induce and maintain remission of the symptoms of ✪ **ulcerative colitis**; often in people who are sensitive to the more commonly prescribed ℞ **sulfasalazine**.

Warnings

• It should not be given to people with known hypersensitivity to olsalazine or to any ℞ **salicylate** (especially sulfasalazine).
• It should be given with caution to people with kidney impairment.
• Olsalazine may be harmful to the fetus, and so it should be used only if the potential benefit outweighs the possible risk to the fetus.
• Medical judgment is required if breast-feeding is being considered. It is not known whether this drug appears in breast milk.
• A doctor must be contacted if there is unexplained bruising, bleeding, sore throat, fever or malaise, which could be symptoms of blood changes that would mean stopping treatment.

Interactions

• ℞ **digoxin** and ℞ **folic acid** levels may be reduced.

Side effects

• Commonly, diarrhea and other gastrointestinal disturbances (abdominal discomfort, cramping and pain, nausea).
• Less frequently, headache, fever, dizziness, flu-like feeling, rash, joint pain, photosensitivity, dry mouth, hair loss and blood, liver and kidney abnormalities.
• Occasionally, olsalazine has made colitis worse, apparently in those with hypersensitivity to the drug; acute abdominal pain, cramping and bloody diarrhea are signs that treatment should be stopped.

omeprazole ⓖ

Type/Group: **proton-pump inhibitor; ulcer-healing drug**.
Brand(s): Prilosec.
How administered: Orally.

Used to treat

Omeprazole works by acting as a proton-pump inhibitor and so interferes with the secretion of gastric acid from the parietal (acid-producing) cells of the stomach lining. It is used for the treatment of benign gastric and duodenal ulcers (see ✪ **peptic ulcer**) (including those that complicate ℞ **NSAID** therapy), acid-related indigestion, ✪ **Zollinger-Ellison syndrome**, and reflux esophagitis (inflammation of the esophagus caused by regurgitation of acid and enzymes), and acid reflux disease. It can also be used with antibiotics to treat gastric *Helicobacter pylori* infection. Omeprazole may be useful in cases where there has been a poor response to conventional treatments, especially with ℞ **H₂-antagonists**.

Warnings

• It should not be given to people with known hypersensitivity to this drug, or to any substituted benzimidazoles (that is, other proton-pump inhibitors, such as ℞ **lansoprazole**, ℞ **rabeprazole**, ℞ **pantoprazole**).

• It should be given with caution to people with liver impairment.

• Omeprazole should be used during pregnancy only if the potential benefit outweighs the possible risk to the fetus.

• Medical judgment is required if breast-feeding is being considered. It is not known whether this drug appears in breast milk, but there is reason to believe its effects would be harmful.

• Before treatment, it should be confirmed that there is no gastric cancer or other disease.

• Dose adjustment may be necessary if ethnic origin is Asian. (Concentrations may be four times higher among Asians.)

• It should be taken before eating.

Interactions

• The levels of R **diazepam**, R **phenytoin**, and R **warfarin sodium** may be increased, requiring adjustment of the dose. This effect may occur, to some extent, for a range of drugs that are broken down in the same way by the liver (for example, R **cyclosporine**, R **disulfiram**, R **benzodiazepines**).

• The levels and effects of R **digoxin**, ferrous salts (⚖ **iron** supplements), R **ketoconazole**, and R **ampicillin** may be decreased.

• Proton-pump inhibitors, like this one, should be taken at least 30 minutes before R **sucralfate** or they may not be absorbed efficiently.

• It is thought possible that deficiency of ⚖ **vitamin B$_{12}$** can occur with long-term use of omeprazole.

Side effects

• Proton-pump inhibitors may cause headache, diarrhea, rashes and itching, dizziness, nausea and vomiting, constipation, flatulence, and abdominal pain. These drugs decrease gastric acidity and so may increase the risk of gastrointestinal infections.

• Uncommon side effects may include hives, other allergic reactions, fever, malaise, nosebleed, muscle and joint pain, kidney problems, pancreatitis, sleepiness, insomnia, temporary mental disturbances, effects on the liver and the heart, and various blood changes. (When used with R **clarithromycin**, commonly there is a strange taste sensation and discoloration of the tongue.)

OMS Concentrate ⑧

A preparation of R **morphine sulfate**.
Formulation: Oral liquid (drops).
Availability: Prescription only.
Warnings and side effects: See R **morphine sulfate**.

Oncet Capsules ⑧

A preparation of R **hydrocodone bitartrate** and R **acetaminophen**.
Formulation: Oral capsules.
Availability: Prescription only.
Warnings and side effects: See R **hydrocodone bitartrate**; R **acetaminophen**.

Oncovin ⑧

A preparation of R **vincristine sulfate**.
Formulation: Injection (intravenous only).
Availability: Prescription only.

Warnings and side effects: See R **vincristine sulfate**.

ondansetron ⑥

Type/Group: **serotonin-receptor antagonist; antiemetic; antinauseant**.
Brand(s): Zofran, Zofran ODT.
How administered: Orally; injection.

Used to treat

Ondansetron gives relief from nausea and vomiting, especially in people receiving chemotherapy and where other drugs are ineffective. It has been used, as well, to prevent nausea and vomiting following surgery in which it is important to avoid these complications.

Warnings

• It should not be given to people with known hypersensitivity to this drug.

• It should be given with caution to people with liver impairment.

• Ondansetron should be used during pregnancy only if it is clearly needed.

• Medical judgment is required if breast-feeding is being considered. It is not known whether this drug appears in breast milk.

• Treatment should stop at the first sign of rash or other allergic response, and a doctor contacted.

Interactions

• R **rifampin** may reduce the levels and effect of ondansetron.

Side effects

These vary with how it is administered, but the most common are:

• Headache, malaise, constipation, diarrhea, dizziness, abdominal pain, dry mouth or feeling of weakness;

• At higher doses, sensations of warmth or flushing, hypoxia (low oxygen level in the blood), urinary retention, and itching may occur. There may be changes in liver function;

• Hypersensitivity reactions are rare, but anaphylaxis and bronchospasm have been reported.

1% HC ⑧

A preparation of R **hydrocortisone**.
Formulation: Ointment.
Availability: Prescription only.
Warnings and side effects: See R **hydrocortisone**.

1 + 1-F Creme ⑧

A preparation of R **hydrocortisone**, R **clioquinol**, and R **Pramoxine HC**.
Formulation: Cream.
Availability: Prescription only.
Warnings and side effects: See R **hydrocortisone**; R **clioquinol**; R **Pramoxine HC**.

Operand ⑧

A preparation of R **iodine; povidone-iodine**.
Formulation: Topical aerosol; foam skin cleanser; ointment; perineal wash; prep solution, prep pads; swab sticks; surgical scrub.
Availability: OTC.

Warnings and side effects: See ℞ **iodine; povidone-iodine.**

Ophthalgan ⑧

A preparation of ℞ **glycerin.**
Formulation: Topical ointment (ophthalmic).
Availability: Prescription only.
Warnings and side effects: See ℞ **glycerin.**

ophthalmic treatment ⑩

See ℞ **eye treatment.**

Ophthocort ⑧

A preparation of ℞ **hydrocortisone,** ℞ **chloramphenicol,** and ℞ **polymyxin B sulfate.**
Formulation: Eye drops.
Availability: Prescription only.
Warnings and side effects: See ℞ **hydrocortisone;** ℞ **chloramphenicol;** ℞ **polymyxin B sulfate.**

opiate ⑩

Generics: **codeine phosphate; hydrocodone bitartrate; morphine sulfate; oxycodone.**

Actions and uses

Opiates are members of a group of drugs that are chemically ℞ **alkaloid** agents, and are closely related to one of the groups of natural constituents (for example, ℞ **morphine** and ℞ **codeine phosphate**) of opium extracted from the opium poppy (*Papaver somniferum*). They powerfully influence certain functions of the central nervous system (CNS), and because of this property they can be used as ℞ **narcotic analgesic** drugs to relieve ✪ **pain.** They also have two other actions: first, as ℞ **antitussive** drugs to reduce ✪ **cough;** second, because of an antimotility action (motility is the movement of the intestines), as ℞ **antidiarrheal** drugs to relieve ✪ **diarrhea.** Therapeutically, the natural opiates, used in the form of salts since naturally they are relatively insoluble bases, are ℞ **morphine sulfate** and ℞ **codeine phosphate.** All opiates are potentially habituating (addictive), especially the semisynthetic derivative diamorphine (heroin)—used as an analgesic in some countries but mainly known as a drug of abuse in the US. Other semisynthetic opiates used in medicine include ℞ **hydrocodone bitartrate** and ℞ **oxycodone.**

Today, the term ℞ **opioid** is increasingly used to embrace all drugs acting in this way, irrespective of chemical structure, as well as naturally occurring peptide neurotransmitters, since all share a common pharmacology because of their working at the same receptors (natural recognition sites).

Limitations

See the individual drug entries.

opioid ⑩

Generics: **alfentanil; buprenorphine hydrochloride; codeine phosphate; dextromethorphan; fentanyl; hydrocodone bitartrate; meperidine hydrochloride; methadone hydrochloride; morphine sulfate; nalbuphine hydrochloride; oxycodone; pentazocine; propoxyphene hydrochloride; remifentanil; tramadol hydrochloride.**

Actions and uses

Opioid is a term that in medical circles is used instead of ℞ **opiate,** to include all agents similar in structure and pharmacology to morphine (opiates) as well as agents with peptide or other structures that have similar pharmacological actions and work in the same way. Opioids influence the central nervous system (CNS) and other body systems and may, for instance, be used as ℞ **narcotic analgesic** drugs to relieve ✪ **pain.** They can also be used for their ℞ **antitussive** and ℞ **antidiarrheal** properties (see ✪ **cough;** ✪ **diarrhea**).

It is now recognized that the typical actions of opioids are due to their ability to mimic certain natural neurotransmitters (enkephalins, endorphins, dynorphins) and because of this the term opioid is used for any chemical (synthetic or natural) that acts on opioid receptors to activate them.

Opioid drugs tend to have similar pharmacological actions and potential side effects. However, there are now recognized subtypes of opioid receptors and this allows some variation in the pharmacology of drugs acting on them. The extent of these pharmacologic effects, and the potency of their analgesic (painkilling) and other actions, varies with individual drugs, the dose, and how the drug is taken.

Limitations

In the event of overdose, or the need to terminate or block opioid action, ℞ **opioid antagonist** drugs (for example, naloxone hydrochloride, naltrexone hydrochloride) are now available. See also the individual drug entries.

opioid antagonist ⑩

Generics: **naloxone hydrochloride; naltrexone hydrochloride.**

Actions and uses

Opioid antagonists oppose the actions of ℞ **opioid** drugs. These are used for a number of purposes, especially as ℞ **narcotic analgesic** agents for pain relief, as ℞ **antitussive** drugs to relieve cough, and as ℞ **antidiarrheal** treatments (see ✪ **diarrhea**). Opioids achieve their effects by mimicking the actions of naturally occurring peptide neurotransmitters (enkephalins, endorphins, and dynorphins) through the stimulation of their receptors. The term opioid, therefore, is used to describe any chemical, synthetic or natural, including opiates, that acts by activating opioid receptors.

Opioid antagonists occupy these receptors without stimulating them, and so can reverse the actions of a wide range of opioid drugs. This is a potentially beneficial action, because an opioid antagonist, such as ℞ **naloxone hydrochloride,** can effectively reverse the respiratory depression, coma, or convulsions that result from an overdose of opioids. Administration of naloxone hydrochloride is by intramuscular or intravenous injection and may be repeated at short intervals until there is some response. It is also used at the end of operations to reverse respiratory depression caused by narcotic analgesics, and in newborn babies where mothers have been given large amounts of opioid (such as meperidine hydrochloride) for pain relief during labor. It is also very effective in reviving individuals who have overdosed on diamorphine (heroin) or any other opiate of abuse.

Similarly, the opioid antagonist ℞ **naltrexone hydrochloride** is used in ℞ **substance-dependence treatment** (detoxification therapy) to help prevent relapse of formerly opioid-dependent people. It is able to do this because as an antagonist of dependence-forming opioids (such as heroin), it will largely prevent the euphoric actions of opiates should the person under treatment relapse.

Limitations
See the individual drug entries.

(opioid) narcotic analgesic ⓓ

see ℞ **narcotic analgesic**.

oprelvekin ⓖ

(interleukin 11; IL-11)
Type/Group: **hematopoietic**.
Brand(s): Neumega.
How administered: Injection (subcutaneous).

Used to treat
Oprelvekin is a natural mediator substance, one of the interleukins, that is synthesized using DNA engineering (recombinant) techniques. Among other activities, it stimulates production of thrombocytes (blood platelets), which are critical to blood clotting. It is used medically to help restore thrombocyte levels when these have been suppressed during chemotherapy in ℞ **anticancer** treatment, so reducing the need for such measures as platelet transfusions.

Warnings
• It should not be given to people with known hypersensitivity to this drug. It will be administered by experienced personnel after a full medical assessment.
• It should be given with caution to people with congestive heart failure or certain arrhythmias, conditions that have caused fluid accumulation (for example, pleural effusion, ascites), or who have swelling of the optic disk—which often indicates raised intracranial pressure.
• It is thought oprelvekin may have adverse effects on fetal development. It should be used in pregnancy only when the potential benefit outweighs the possible risk to the fetus.
• Medical judgment is required if breast-feeding is being considered.
• Fluid and electrolyte levels should be closely monitored.
℞ **Diuretics** are often used with oprelvekin (because it may cause fluid retention), and potassium levels may fall dangerously low.

Interactions
No drug interactions of significance are known.

Side effects
• Edema is frequent, also disturbances of heart rhythm, shortness of breath, rhinitis, sore throat and cough, nausea and diarrhea, dizziness, insomnia, oral moniliasis, pleural fluid accumulation, fever, rash, headache and red, swollen conjunctiva (inner side of eyelid).
• Blurred vision, tingling sensations, dehydration, skin discoloration, and bleeding from the eye have also occurred.

Opticron ⓑ
A preparation of ℞ **cromolyn sodium**.
Formulation: Ophthalmic solution.
Availability: Prescription only.
Warnings and side effects: See ℞ **cromolyn sodium**.

Opticyl ⓑ
A preparation of ℞ **tropicamide**.
Formulation: Ophthalmic solution in several strengths.
Availability: Prescription only.
Warnings and side effects: See ℞ **tropicamide**.

Optigene-3 ⓑ
A preparation of ℞ **tetrahydrozoline hydrochloride**.
Formulation: Eye drops.
Availability: OTC.
Warnings and side effects: See ℞ **tetrahydrozoline hydrochloride**.

Optimine ⓑ
A preparation of ℞ **azatadine maleate**.
Formulation: Oral tablets.
Availability: Prescription only.
Warnings and side effects: See ℞ **azatadine maleate**.

Optimoist ⓑ
A preparation of ℞ **hydroxyethylcellulose**.
Formulation: Topical solution.
Availability: OTC.
Warnings and side effects: See ℞ **hydroxyethylcellulose**.

Optipranolol ⓑ
A preparation of ℞ **metipranolol**.
Formulation: Eye drops.
Availability: Prescription only.
Warnings and side effects: See ℞ **metipranolol**.

Orabase Gel ⓑ
A preparation of ℞ **benzocaine**.
Formulation: Gel.
Availability: OTC.
Warnings and side effects: See ℞ **benzocaine**.

Oracit ⓑ
A preparation of ℞ **citrates**.
Formulation: Oral solution.
Availability: Prescription only.
Warnings and side effects: See ℞ **citrates**.

Orajel Mouth-Aid ⓑ
A preparation of ℞ **benzocaine** and ℞ **cetylpyridinium chloride**.
Formulation: Lozenges.
Availability: OTC.
Warnings and side effects: See ℞ **benzocaine**; ℞ **cetylpyridinium chloride**.

Orajel Perioseptic ®

A preparation of ℞ **carbamide peroxide**.
Formulation: Topical liquid.
Availability: OTC.
Warnings and side effects: See ℞ **carbamide peroxide**.

oral contraceptive ⑩

(The "Pill")

desogestrel; ethinyl estradiol; levonorgestrel; medroxyprogesterone; mestranol; norgestrel; norethindrone; progesterone.

Actions and uses

Oral contraceptive preparations are ℞ **sex hormone** drugs which
are taken by women to prevent conception—and are commonly
referred to as the Pill. The majority of oral contraceptives contain
both an ℞ **estrogen** (such as ℞ **ethinyl estradiol** and
℞ **mestranol**) and a ℞ **progestin** (including the natural hormone
℞ **progesterone** and synthetic substances with similar actions;
℞ **desogestrel**, ℞ **norgestrel**, ℞ **levonorgestrel**, ℞ **medroxyprogesterone**, ℞ **norethindrone**, and norethisterone).

Estrogen inhibits the release of the ℞ **gonadotropin** hormone follicle-stimulating hormone (FSH) so preventing egg development.
Progestin inhibits the release of luteinizing hormone (LH), so preventing ovulation, and makes the cervical mucus unsuitable for
sperm. Their combined action is to alter the uterine lining
(endometrium) and prevent any fertilized eggs from implanting.
This type of preparation is known as the "combined pill." Another
type of pill is the "progestin-only pill" (where the progestins used
include norethisterone and ℞ **norgestrel**). This is thought to work
by making the cervical mucus inhospitable to sperm and by preventing implantation. An alternative to the progestin-only pill is to
take the progestin not by mouth, but as an injection or implant
(which is renewed every three months). Post-coital contraception
is also available in an emergency and involves the use of a high-
dose preparation containing ℞ **levonorgestrel** (with or without
℞ **ethinyl estradiol**) taken shortly after sexual intercourse has
occurred.

Limitations

All the oral contraceptive preparations produce some side effects
and a form that is suited to each woman requires expert advice.
Various oral contraceptives are also used in the treatment of certain
menstrual problems. There are a number of risks in taking estrogens
for any period of time. The severity of the condition needs to be
taken into account. In the case of oral contraceptive agents, a very
low dose is taken (generally combined with a progestin) and the
risks for most women are considered acceptable in relation to the
risk of unwanted pregnancy—although expert counseling may be
advisable. See also the individual drug entries.

oral hypoglycemic ⑩

Generics: acarbose; acetohexamide; chlorpropamide;
glimepiride; glipizide; glyburide; metformin; miglitol;
pioglitazone; repaglinide; rosiglitazone maleate; tolazamide;
tolbutamide.

Actions and uses

℞ **oral hypoglycemic** drugs, usually synthetic agents, are taken by
mouth to reduce the levels of glucose (sugar) in the bloodstream.
They are primarily used to treat ☢ **diabetes mellitus**, specifically
type 2 diabetes (non-insulin-dependent diabetes mellitus; NIDDM;
maturity-onset diabetes). The ℞ **sulfonylurea** group (℞ **chlorpropamide**, ℞ **glimepiride**, ℞ **tolazamide**, ℞ **tolbutamide**, ℞ **acetohexamide**, ℞ **glipizide**, ℞ **glimepiride**, and ℞ **glyburide**) are
the most extensively used. The ℞ **biguanide** drug ℞ **metformin**
is used in certain cases. In contrast, ℞ **insulin analog** drugs are
mainly used in type 1 diabetes mellitus (insulin-dependent diabetes
mellitus; IDDM; juvenile-onset diabetes), and cannot be taken by
mouth because they are destroyed by enzymes in the gastrointestinal tract.

Other oral hypoglycemic drugs include ℞ **rosiglitazone** and
℞ **pioglitazone**, which are recently introduced non-sulfonylurea
agents (they are thiazolidinedione compounds) that reduce what
is known as peripheral insulin resistance, and are used in combination with other drugs (particularly ℞ **metformin**) to improve blood
sugar control in type 2 diabetes mellitus. ℞ **repaglinide**, also a
non-sulfonylurea (it is a meglitinide), works by stimulating insulin
release from the pancreas, and can be used together with
℞ **metformin** in diabetic treatment of type 2 diabetes mellitus,
particularly in people who are not totally dependent on additional
supplies of insulin and when diabetes mellitus is not controlled by
diet and exercise. Another non-sulfonylurea is ℞ **miglitol** (it works
as an alpha-glucosidase inhibitor) which is used to treat type 2 diabetes mellitus, alone or in combination with a sulfonylurea. Further
drugs that may be used include ℞ **acarbose**, which delays the conversion in the intestine of starch and sucrose (sugar) to glucose, and
subsequent absorption. It may be of value in people where other
drugs, or diet control, have not been successful, and so is useful in
obese patients.

Oral hypoglycemic drugs are effective in controlling type 2 diabetes mellitus by boosting what remains of insulin production in the
pancreas, and are only used in conjunction with appropriate
dietary changes, exercise, and loss of weight where there is obesity.
Short-term use of these drugs may be sufficient while lifestyle
changes are being made.

The actions of these groups of drugs are discussed in detail at
℞ **sulfonylurea**, ℞ **biguanide**, and ℞ **insulin analog**.

Limitations

See the individual drug entries.

Oramorph SR ®

A preparation of ℞ **morphine sulfate**.
Formulation: Oral tablets, controlled release, available in 4
strengths.
Availability: Prescription only.
Warnings and side effects: See ℞ **morphine sulfate**.

Orap ®

A preparation of ℞ **pimozide**.
Formulation: Oral tablets.
Availability: Prescription only.

Warnings and side effects: See ℞ **pimozide**.

Orasone ⓑ
A preparation of ℞ **prednisone**.
Formulation: Oral tablets in several strengths.
Availability: Prescription only.
Warnings and side effects: See ℞ **prednisone**.

orciprenaline sulfate ⓖ
see ℞ **metaproterenol**.

Oretic ⓑ
A preparation of ℞ **hydrochlorothiazide**.
Formulation: Oral tablets, available in two strengths.
Availability: Prescription only.
Warnings and side effects: See ℞ **hydrochlorothiazide**.

Oreton Methyl ⓑ
A preparation of ℞ **methyltestosterone**.
Formulation: Oral tablets; buccal tablets. The buccal tablets are to be dissolved between cheek and gum.
Availability: Prescription only.
Warnings and side effects: See ℞ **methyltestosterone**.

Organidin NR Tablets; NR Liquid ⓑ
A preparation of ℞ **guaifenesin**.
Formulation: Oral tablets; liquid.
Availability: Prescription only.
Warnings and side effects: See ℞ **guaifenesin**.

Orgaran ⓑ
A preparation of ℞ **danaparoid sodium**.
Formulation: Subcutaneous injection.
Availability: Prescription only.
Warnings and side effects: See ℞ **danaparoid sodium**. The injection contains sodium sulfite, which may cause allergic reactions, including anaphylaxis, in a few people (those with asthma may be more susceptible).

Original Eclipse Sunscreen ⓑ
A preparation of ℞ **aminobenzoic acid (PABA)** (as glyceryl para-aminobenzoic acid) and padimate O.
Formulation: Topical lotion.
Availability: OTC.
Warnings and side effects: See ℞ **aminobenzoic acid (PABA)**.

Orimune ⓑ
A preparation of poliovirus vaccine, live, oral (OPV).
Formulation: Oral liquid.
Availability: Prescription only.
Warnings and side effects: See ℞ **poliovirus vaccine**.

Orinase ⓑ
A preparation of ℞ **tolbutamide**.
Formulation: Oral tablets.

Availability: Prescription only.
Warnings and side effects: See ℞ **tolbutamide**.

orlistat ⓖ
Type/Group: obesity treatment.
Brand(s): Xenical.
How administered: Orally.

Used to treat
Orlistat is used as an additional treatment for ✪ **obesity** (along with a calorie-controlled diet), but unlike other drugs used for this purpose, it is not an appetite suppressant. It is an enzyme inhibitor that blocks the normal action of the enzyme pancreatic lipase in the intestine, so less dietary fat is absorbed into the body, allowing the rest to be excreted.

Warnings
• It should not be given to people with known hypersensitivity to this drug, or who have chronic malabsorption syndrome or cholestasis (impaired bile flow).
• It should be given with caution to people with a history of kidney stones.
• It is not recommended for use during pregnancy.
• Medical judgment is required if breast-feeding is being considered. It is not known whether this drug appears in breast milk.
• Disorders that may cause obesity, such as hypothyroidism, should be ruled out before use of orlistat is considered.
• Diabetic persons using this drug may find that doses of insulin or hypoglycemic drugs (for example, sulfonylureas, metformin) should be reduced.
• Vitamin supplements (fat-soluble vitamins) may be needed.
• If a meal is missed or contains no fat, the dose should not be taken.

Interactions
• The absorption of fat-soluble vitamins (♊ **vitamin A**, ♊ **vitamin D**, ♊ **vitamin E**, and ♊ **vitamin K**) may be sharply reduced. Vitamin K malabsorption may affect stabilized dose regimes for those taking ℞ **warfarin sodium**.
• Changes in dietary intake may influence ℞ **cyclosporine** absorption, and so caution is advised in using orlistat with this drug.
• ℞ **Pravastatin** has an additive effect in lowering lipids.

Side effects
• There may be fatty, oily stool, flatulence, fecal urgency, or incontinence.
• Less frequently, abdominal or rectal pain, headache, menstrual irregularities, fatigue, or anxiety.
• Gastrointestinal effects can be minimized by a reduced-fat diet.

Ornex Caplets; Max Strength Ornex Caplets ⓑ
A preparation of ℞ **pseudoephedrine** and ℞ **acetaminophen**.
Formulation: Oral tablets.
Availability: OTC.
Warnings and side effects: See ℞ **pseudoephedrine**; ℞ **acetaminophen**.

Key to symbols: ✪ = Disorder Section ℞ = Drug Section ♣ = Herbal Section ♊ = Supplement Section

orphenadrine Ⓖ

Type/Group: **skeletal muscle relaxant**.
Brand(s): Norflex; Banflex; Flexoject; Flexon. Combinations: With *aspirin* and *caffeine*: Norgesic; Orphengesic.
How administered: Orally; injection.

Used to treat

Orphenadrine is used as an additional treatment to other measures (such as rest and physical therapy) for the relief of acute muscle pain. It works within the central nervous system (CNS), probably at spinal cord level.

Warnings

• It should not be used by people with known hypersensitivity to orphenadrine, or with glaucoma, intestinal obstruction, prostatic hypertrophy, bladder neck obstruction, or myasthenia gravis.
• It should be given with caution to people with heart disease or sensitivity to sulfites (some products contain sulfites; check product information).
• It is not usually given to children.
• The effects on the fetus are unknown, and so it should be used during pregnancy only if the benefits outweigh the risks to the fetus.
• Medical judgment is required if breast-feeding is being considered.
• It may cause transient lightheadedness, dizziness or fainting, and so it may impair the performance of skilled tasks such as driving.
• Alcohol and other CNS depressants should be avoided.

Interactions

• Orphenadrine may interfere with the effects of ℞ **antipsychotics**, and the CNS side effects will be increased.

Side effects

• Dry mouth, dizziness, drowsiness, difficult urination, constipation, headache, gastrointestinal upset, and skin reactions.
• Rarely, rapid heart rate, palpitations, and mental confusion.

Ortho-Cept Ⓑ

A preparation of ℞ **ethinyl estradiol** and ℞ **desogestrel**.
Formulation: Calendar pack of oral tablets.
Availability: Prescription only.
Warnings and side effects: See ℞ **ethinyl estradiol**; ℞ **desogestrel**.

Orthoclone OKT 3 Ⓑ

A preparation of ℞ **muromonab-CD3**.
Formulation: Injection.
Availability: Prescription only.
Warnings and side effects: See ℞ **muromonab-CD3**.

Ortho-Cyclen Ⓑ

A preparation of ℞ **ethinyl estradiol** and norgestimate.
Formulation: Calendar pack of oral tablets.
Availability: Prescription only.
Warnings and side effects: See ℞ **ethinyl estradiol**; ℞ **progestin**.

Ortho Dienestrol Ⓑ

A preparation of ℞ **dienestrol**.

Formulation: Vaginal cream.
Availability: Prescription only.
Warnings and side effects: See ℞ **dienestrol**.

Ortho-Est Ⓑ

A preparation of esterified ℞ **estropipate**.
Formulation: Oral tablets in several strengths.
Availability: Prescription only.
Warnings and side effects: See esterified ℞ **estropipate**.

Ortho-Novum Ⓑ

A preparation of ℞ **ethinyl estradiol** and ℞ **norethindrone**.
Formulation: Calendar pack of oral tablets, monophasic, biphasic, and triphasic.
Availability: Prescription only.
Warnings and side effects: See ℞ **ethinyl estradiol**; ℞ **norethindrone**.

Ortho-Novum 1/50 Ⓑ

A preparation of ℞ **mestranol** and ℞ **norethindrone**.
Formulation: Calendar pack of oral tablets.
Availability: Prescription only.
Warnings and side effects: See ℞ **mestranol**; ℞ **norethindrone**.

Ortho-Prefest Ⓑ

A preparation of ℞ **estradiol** and norgestimate.
Formulation: Tablets (pink is estradiol only, white is estradiol and norgestimate.
Availability: Prescription only.
Warnings and side effects: See ℞ **estradiol**; ℞ **progestin**s.

Ortho Tri-Cyclen Ⓑ

A preparation of ℞ **ethinyl estradiol** and norgestimate.
Formulation: Calendar pack of oral tablets.
Availability: Prescription only.
Warnings and side effects: See ℞ **ethinyl estradiol**; ℞ **progestin**.

Or-Tyl Ⓑ

A preparation of ℞ **dicyclomine hydrochloride**.
Formulation: Injection.
Availability: Prescription only.
Warnings and side effects: See ℞ **dicyclomine hydrochloride**.

Orudis Capsules Ⓑ

A preparation of ℞ **ketoprofen**.
Formulation: Oral capsules (3 strengths).
Availability: Prescription only.
Warnings and side effects: See ℞ **ketoprofen**.

Orudis KT Tablets Ⓑ

A preparation of ℞ **ketoprofen**.
Formulation: Oral tablets; they contain tartrazine (FD&C yellow No. 5), a dye that may cause allergic reaction in a few people, but especially those with sensitivity to aspirin.
Availability: OTC.

Warnings and side effects: See ℞ **ketoprofen**.

Oruvail Capsules ⑧

A preparation of ℞ **ketoprofen**.
Formulation: Oral capsules (2 strengths), extended release.
Availability: Prescription only.
Warnings and side effects: See ℞ **ketoprofen**.

Osmitrol ⑧

A preparation of ℞ **mannitol**.
Formulation: Intravenous infusion.
Availability: Prescription only.
Warnings and side effects: See ℞ **mannitol**.

Osmoglyn ⑧

A preparation of ℞ **glycerin**.
Formulation: Oral liquid.
Availability: Prescription only.
Warnings and side effects: See ℞ **glycerin**.

osteoporosis treatment ⑩

Generics: alendronate sodium; calcitonin-salmon; calcitriol; calcium carbonate; dihydrotachysterol (DHT); ergocalciferol; estrogens, conjugated; etidronate disodium; pamidronate disodium; tiludronate sodium; raloxifene.

Actions and uses

Osteoporosis treatment seeks to prevent or reverse the loss of ♒ **calcium** (and associated phosphate) from the bone ("thinning of the bones") that tends to occur in women after the menopause. The most effective preventive treatment is to use ℞ **hormone replacement** treatment, using ℞ **estrogen** hormones (for instance, in ℞ **estrogens, conjugated** of natural origin) and sometimes combined with ℞ **progestin** hormones. Where this is not effective or not possible, there are various ℞ **calcium-metabolism modifier** drugs which alter the metabolism and therefore the levels of calcium in the body. Of these the ℞ **bisphosphonate** drugs can be effective. Apart from these invasive drug treatments, vitamin D supplements (as ℞ **ergocalciferol**, ℞ **calcitriol**, or ℞ **dihydrotachysterol**), combined with calcium supplements (for instance, ℞ **calcium carbonate**) may well be effective in protecting against osteoporosis.

Limitations

See the individual drug entries.

Otic-Care ⑧

A preparation of ℞ **hydrocortisone**, ℞ **neomycin**, and ℞ **polymyxin B sulfate**.
Formulation: Ear drops.
Availability: Prescription only.
Warnings and side effects: See ℞ **hydrocortisone**; ℞ **neomycin**; ℞ **polymyxin B sulfate**.

Otocort ⑧

A preparation of ℞ **hydrocortisone**, ℞ **neomycin**, and ℞ **polymyxin B sulfate**.

Formulation: Ear drops.
Availability: Prescription only.
Warnings and side effects: See ℞ **hydrocortisone**; ℞ **neomycin**; ℞ **polymyxin B sulfate**.

Otomycin-HPN Otic ⑧

A preparation of ℞ **hydrocortisone**, ℞ **neomycin**, and ℞ **polymyxin B sulfate**.
Formulation: Ear drops.
Availability: Prescription only.
Warnings and side effects: See ℞ **hydrocortisone**; ℞ **neomycin**; ℞ **polymyxin B sulfate**.

Otrivin; Otrivin Pediatric Nasal Drops ⑧

A preparation of ℞ **xylometazoline hydrochloride**.
Formulation: Nasal drops; spray.
Availability: OTC.
Warnings and side effects: See ℞ **xylometazoline hydrochloride**.

Ovcon-35; Ovcon-50 ⑧

A preparation of ℞ **ethinyl estradiol** and ℞ **norethindrone**.
Formulation: Calendar pack of oral tablets. Available in two strengths.
Availability: Prescription only.
Warnings and side effects: See ℞ **ethinyl estradiol**; ℞ **norethindrone**.

Ovide ⑧

A preparation of ℞ **malathion**.
Formulation: Topical lotion.
Availability: Prescription only.
Warnings and side effects: See ℞ **malathion**.

Ovral-28 ⑧

A preparation of ℞ **ethinyl estradiol** and norgestrel.
Formulation: Calendar pack of oral tablets.
Availability: Prescription only.
Warnings and side effects: See ℞ **ethinyl estradiol**; ℞ **progestin**.

Ovrette ⑧

A preparation of norgestrel.
Formulation: Calendar pack of oral tablets.
Availability: Prescription only.
Warnings and side effects: See ℞ **progestin**.

oxacillin sodium ⑥

Type/Group: **antibiotic; penicillin; antibacterial**.
Brand(s): Bactrocill; various generics.
How administered: Orally; injection.

Used to treat

Oxacillin sodium is a semisynthetic penicillinase-resistant penicillin used to treat ⊙ **bacterial infections** of the upper and lower respiratory tract, skin and skin structures, bones and joints, and also

✪ **meningitis**, ✪ **septicemia**, and ✪ **endocarditis** caused by penicillinase-resistant staphylococci.

Warnings

• It should not be used by people with known hypersensitivity to penicillins.

• It should be given with caution to people with allergies to ℞ **cephalosporins** or ℞ **imipenem**, or impaired kidney function; medical judgment is also required for its use in newborn babies.

• Penicillins cross the placenta and should be used in pregnancy only if medically judged to be needed.

• Oxacillin should not be used while breast-feeding.

• Serious and occasionally fatal hypersensitivity reactions can occur. A doctor must be contacted if skin rash, itching, hives, severe diarrhea, shortness of breath, black tongue, sore throat, nausea, fever, swollen joints, or any unusual bleeding or bruising occurs.

• Superinfections from the altered bacterial balance created by antibiotic treatment may occur and may result in ✪ **pseudomembranous colitis**. A doctor must be contacted if there is severe abdominal pain, or moderate to severe diarrhea.

• Take on an empty stomach (one hour before or two hours after eating).

• The full course of treatment prescribed must be completed or infection may return.

Interactions

• ℞ **Chloramphenicol** and ℞ **tetracyclines** may reduce the effectiveness of penicillin.

• The levels of ℞ **methotrexate** may be increased.

Side effects

• Frequently, mild allergic reaction, gastrointestinal effect.

• Occasionally, thrombophlebitis or phlebitis, liver damage with high intravenous doses, kidney damage and blood changes.

oxamniquine ⓖ

Type/Group: **anthelmintic**.
Brand(s): Vansil.
How administered: Orally.

Used to treat

Oxamniquine is used to treat infection by schistosomes (*Schistosoma mansoni*), which are the worms that can colonize the veins of a human host and cause ✪ **schistosomiasis** (bilharziasis).

Warnings

• It should not be given to people with known hypersensitivity to this drug.

• It should be given with caution to people with seizure disorder.

• There are no adequate and well-controlled studies in pregnant women.

• Medical judgment is required if breast-feeding is being considered.

• It may cause orange-red discoloration of urine.

• Rarely, it may cause seizure.

Interactions

No significant drug interactions are known.

Side effects

• Frequently, dizziness and drowsiness.

• Less frequently, headache, gastrointestinal effects, liver enzyme elevations, and hives.

oxaprozin ⓖ

Type/Group: **anti-inflammatory; antirheumatic; non-narcotic analgesic; NSAID**.
Brand(s): Daypro Caplets.
How administered: Orally.

Used to treat

Oxaprozin is used for the long-term management of ✪ **osteoarthritis** and ✪ **rheumatoid arthritis**, and for mild to moderate pain.

Warnings

• It should not be given to people with known hypersensitivity to this drug or to other NSAIDs (including ℞ **aspirin**), who have chronic kidney disease, certain bleeding disorders or conditions (for example, hemophilia, vitamin K deficiency, low blood-platelet levels), or who have a tendency to, or active, peptic ulceration.

• It should be given with caution to people who are taking certain drugs for gout, with allergic disorders (especially asthma and skin conditions), who are elderly, or with any kind of kidney impairment or certain liver disorders.

• Oxaprozin should be used when pregnant only if medically judged to be needed. In the third trimester, its risks to the fetus rise, and so it should only be used if the benefits outweigh the risks, which are at their highest at this time.

• Breast-feeding mothers should either discontinue this drug or stop breast-feeding.

• With regular use (as in treatment of osteoarthritis), NSAIDs may cause gastrointestinal bleeding, ulceration, or perforation. Any signs of bleeding (for example, black stools) should be reported to a physician immediately.

• Most NSAIDs have the potential, particularly with regular use, to cause liver damage. Periodic evaluation of liver function is necessary in long-term therapy (more than two months).

• Side effects are more frequent in the elderly.

• Gastrointestinal upsets may be minimized by taking the drug with milk or food.

Interactions

• There is generally no added benefit in taking other NSAIDs or other ℞ **salicylates** (especially aspirin) at the same time, but there is a higher risk of gastrointestinal upsets and bleeding.

• Alcohol and ℞ **corticosteroids** increase the risk of bleeding, particularly if there is an existing ulcer.

• ℞ **Anticoagulant**, ℞ **antiplatelet**, and ℞ **thrombolytic** drugs may increase bleeding time.

• The effectiveness of ℞ **ACE inhibitors**, ℞ **beta-blockers**, and ℞ **diuretics** may be reduced.

• The effects of ℞ **digoxin**, ℞ **lithium**, and ℞ **methotrexate** may be exaggerated, with potential for toxicity.

• ℞ **Probenecid** may increase the concentration of oxaprozin, and so the risk of side effects is greater.

• Foodstuffs and herbals with ℞ **antiplatelet** properties, for example, ♣ **ginger**, ⚘ **garlic**, and various herbal preparations, may add to the antiplatelet effect of NSAIDs.

Side effects

These vary in severity and how often they occur.

• Oxaprozin's risk of gastrointestinal side effects is intermediate for its class (NSAID).

• Commonly, gastrointestinal upsets, nausea, constipation, diarrhea, rash, swelling of the extremities, drowsiness, and rash.

• Less frequently, vomiting, flatulence, blurred vision, ringing in the ears, depression, malaise, and sleep disturbances.

• Prolonged bleeding time (with consequent risk of ulceration) is possible with high dosage, and other blood changes can occur, including anemia.

• Hypersensitivity reactions may include symptoms such as hives, rash, chest tightness, asthma, or bronchospasm.

• Reversible kidney failure, particularly in renal impairment, has occurred. Liver damage is rare.

oxazepam Ⓖ

Type/Group: **antianxiety; benzodiazepine**.
Brand(s): Serax; various generic.
How administered: Orally, injectable solution.

Used to treat

Oxazepam is used to treat ✪ **anxiety** disorders, and for the management of anxiety, tension, agitation, and irritability in older patients. It is also used to treat alcohol withdrawal. Although not stated by the manufacturer for such use, it may be prescribed for ✪ **irritable bowel syndrome**.

Warnings

• It should not be given to people with known hypersensitivity to benzodiazepines, narrow-angle glaucoma, or psychosis.

• It should be given with caution to people with liver or kidney disease, a history of drug abuse, in a weakened condition (debilitated), with respiratory depression, or over 65.

• Oxazepam is not recommended for use during pregnancy. Its use in the first trimester should almost always be avoided. A doctor must be contacted if pregnancy occurs while this drug is being taken.

• It should not normally be used by nursing mothers.

• It may cause drowsiness and so the performance of skilled tasks, such as driving, may be impaired.

• Avoid alcohol because adverse side effects may be increased (see Side effects below).

• Avoid other psychotropic medications unless prescribed by a doctor.

• A doctor must be consulted before discontinuing use or increasing dosage, because benzodiazepines may produce psychological and physical dependence and withdrawal symptoms.

Interactions

• The effects of ℞ **cimetidine**, ℞ **disulfiram**, ℞ **fluconazole**, ℞ **itraconazole**, and ℞ **ketoconazole** may be increased.

• If used with ℞ **levodopa**, Parkinsonian symptoms could be increased.

• Alcohol increases some of oxazepam's adverse effects (see Side effects below).

Side effects

• Depending on use, how it is administered, and dose, there may be weakness, reduction in motor activity, and abnormal sleepiness.

• Less frequently, cognitive and emotional changes, impaired movement and coordination, headache, stupor, eye, ear, nose or throat inflammation, gastrointestinal effects, changes in appetite, urinary and vaginal disorders, back or leg pain, and skin reactions.

• Rare but serious side effects include abnormal heart rhythm and blood cell disorders.

oxcarbazepine Ⓖ

Type/Group: **anticonvulsant; antiepileptic**.
Brand(s): Trileptal
How administered: Orally.

Used to treat

Oxcarbazepine can be used, alone or with other drugs, in the treatment of ✪ **epilepsy**. It is used to treat partial seizures in adults, and in combination with other drugs to treat children from age 4 to 16. Although not stated by the manufacturer for such use, it may be prescribed for some cases of panic disorder.

Warnings

• It should not be given to people with known hypersensitivity to this drug.

• It should be given with caution to people with impaired kidney function.

• Oxcarbazepine should be used during pregnancy only if the potential benefit outweighs the possible risk to the fetus.

• Nursing mothers should either discontinue this drug or discontinue breast feeding.

• People with hypersensitivity to ℞ **carbamazepine**, another anticonvulsant drug, often have hypersensitivity reactions to oxcarbazepine.

• Oral contraceptives may not be as effective if being used at the same time as with oxcarbazepine. It is recommended that a non-hormonal contraceptive method is used as well.

• Oxcarbazepine may cause low sodium levels (hyponatremia), and so periodic monitoring is suggested for long-term treatment. Symptoms such as nausea, malaise, headache, lethargy, and confusion or obtundation (a general slowness or cloudiness of consciousness) may be caused by low sodium.

• Because of its sedative side effects, the performance of skilled tasks, such as driving, may be impaired.

Interactions

• Hormonal contraceptives may not be as effective and reliable.

• If taken with ℞ **carbamazepine**, ℞ **phenobarbital**, ℞ **phenytoin**, ℞ **valproate sodium**, and ℞ **verapamil**, levels of oxcarbazepine may be lowered. Also, the levels of phenytoin and phenobarbital may be increased.

• Oxcarbazepine may decrease the levels of ℞ **felodipine**.

• The levels of drugs that are broken down by the body in a certain way (such as diazepam, omeprazole, pentamidine, propranolol) may increase.

Side effects

These are many and varied:

Key to symbols: ✪ = Disorder Section ℞ = Drug Section ♣ = Herbal Section ⚖ = Supplement Section

• The most frequent may be abnormal vision or eye movements, dizziness, drowsiness, incoordination, unusual gait, gastrointestinal disturbances (for example, nausea, vomiting, abdominal pain), tremor, and fatigue;

• Other side effects may include low sodium levels, loss of appetite, muscle weakness, nervousness, abnormal thinking, unusual taste sensations, acne, changes in heart rhythm or blood pressure, and upper respiratory infection;

• Hypersensitivity reactions, including allergic swelling, itching, rash, contact dermatitis, fever, and swollen lymph glands, have been reported.

oxiconazole Ⓖ

Type/Group: **antifungal; azole.**
Brand(s): Oxistat.
How administered: Topically (external).

Used to treat
Oxiconazole is a synthetic imidazole/azole antifungal drug that can be used to treat athlete's foot, jock itch, and ringworm infections (see ✪ **fungal infections**).

Warnings
• It should not be given to people with known hypersensitivity to naftifine.
• It should be used during pregnancy only if the benefits outweigh the risk to the fetus.
• Medical judgment is required if breast-feeding is being considered. It is not known if this drug is distributed in breast milk.
• The affected area must not be covered with a bandage unless directed by a doctor.

Interactions
No significant interactions have been reported when used topically (externally).

Side effects
• Itching, burning, stinging, and irritation.

Oxipor VHC Ⓑ

A preparation of ℞ **coal tar.**
Formulation: Topical (lotion).
Availability: OTC.
Warnings and side effects: See ℞ **coal tar.**

Oxistat Ⓑ

A preparation of ℞ **oxiconazole.**
Formulation: Topical cream; topical lotion.
Availability: Prescription only.
Warnings and side effects: See ℞ **oxiconazole.**

oxpentifylline Ⓖ

see ℞ pentoxifylline.

Oxy 5 Tinted; Oxy 10 Wash Ⓑ

A preparation of ℞ **benzoyl peroxide.**
Formulation: Topical liquid, topical gel. Available in varying strengths.
Availability: OTC.

Warnings and side effects: See ℞ benzoyl peroxide.

oxybutynin Ⓖ

Type/Group: **anticholinergic; antispasmodic.**
Brand(s): Ditropan; various generic.
How administered: Orally.

Used to treat
Oxybutynin is used as an antispasmodic to treat urinary frequency, incontinence, bed-wetting, and bladder spasms.

Warnings
• It should not be given to people with known hypersensitivity to this drug, or those with angle-closure glaucoma and certain other eye conditions, gastrointestinal dysfunction, myasthenia gravis, obstructive urinary tract disease, or with unstable cardiovascular status, or acute hemorrhage.
• It should be given with caution to people over 65 and those with autonomic neuropathy, kidney or liver disease.
• Oxybutynin should be used during pregnancy only when it is clearly needed and when the potential benefits outweigh the possible risks to the fetus.
• Medical judgment is required if breast-feeding is being considered. It is not known whether this drug appears in breast milk.
• It may aggravate certain heart and gastrointestinal diseases.
• Caution must be exercised while driving or performing other skilled tasks.
• Avoid prolonged exposure to hot environments as heat prostration may result.

Interactions
• ℞ **acetaminophen** may delay absorption.
• The effects of ℞ **atenolol**, ℞ **digoxin**, and ℞ **nitrofurantoin** may be increased.
• The effects of ℞ **haloperidol** and ℞ **levodopa** may be reduced.
• The side effects of ℞ **phenothiazines** may be increased and their levels altered.
• The anticholinergic side effects (dry mouth, increased heart rate, and so on) of ℞ **amantadine** may be increased.

Side effects
• Dry mouth, blurred vision, constipation, nausea, abdominal discomfort, difficulty in urination, flushing of the face, headache, dizziness, diarrhea, dry skin, and heart irregularities.

oxycodone Ⓖ

Type/Group: **narcotic analgesic; opioid.**
Brand(s): Percolone; Endocodone; Oxycontin; OxyIR; OxyFAST; Roxicodone; Roxicodone Intensol. Combinations: With _acetaminophen_: Endocet Tablets; Percocet Tablets, Roxicet Tablets, 5/500 Caplets, Oral Solution; Tylox Capsules. With _aspirin_: Percodan Tablets; Roxiprin Tablets. (Most combinations available as generic.)
How administered: Orally.

Used to treat
Oxycodone can be used in the treatment of moderate to moderately severe ✪ **pain**, such as in cancer or postoperative pain.

Warnings

• It should not be given to people with known hypersensitivity to any opioid, acute bronchial asthma or upper airways obstruction, or with paralytic ileus (cessation of the normal rhythmic muscle contractions of the intestines). Opioids (even the weaker ones) should not be given to people with asthma, to anyone with seriously depressed breathing disorders, prostatic hypertrophy, convulsive disorders, raised intracranial pressure, or a head injury.

• Depending on use and dose, they should be given with caution to the elderly, or to anyone with hypotension, certain liver, kidney or adrenal disorders, hypothyroidism (under-activity of the thyroid gland), urethral stricture, alcoholism, or a history of drug abuse.

• Oxycodone should be used during pregnancy only if the benefits outweigh the potential risks.

• Because of its potential to cause withdrawal symptoms in nursing infants, it should not be used if breast-feeding.

• Oxycodone is a Schedule II controlled substance.

• Prolonged use of narcotics can lead to physical dependence (addiction), although this rarely happens in routine medical use.

• Drowsiness may affect the performance of skilled tasks such as driving.

• The effects of alcohol may be enhanced (including a higher risk of respiratory depression).

Interactions

• If the following drugs are used with oxycodone, then effects are increased with potentially serious results: ℞ **barbiturates**, ℞ **anesthetics**, ℞ **MAOIs**; ℞ **opioids**; protease inhibitors (for example, ℞ **nelfinavir**, ℞ **ritonavir**, ℞ **saquinavir**); alcohol; ℞ **chlorpromazine**; ℞ **thioridazine**.

Side effects

• Commonly, sedation.

• Less frequently dizziness, nausea and vomiting, loss of appetite, and constipation. There is occasionally euphoria, which may lead to a state of mental detachment or confusion, dry mouth, flushing of the face, sweating, headache, palpitations, changes in heart rate, postural hypotension (a lowering of blood pressure on standing, causing dizziness), rashes, miosis (pupil constriction), mood change, and hallucinations.

Oxycontin ℗

A preparation of ℞ **oxycodone**.
Formulation: Oral tablets, 5 strengths, controlled release.
Availability: Prescription only.
Warnings and side effects: See ℞ **oxycodone**.

OxyFAST ℗

A preparation of ℞ **oxycodone**.
Formulation: Oral liquid (drops).
Availability: Prescription only.
Warnings and side effects: See ℞ **oxycodone**.

OxyIR ℗

A preparation of ℞ **oxycodone**.
Formulation: Oral capsules.
Availability: Prescription only.
Warnings and side effects: See ℞ **oxycodone**.

Oxy Medicated Cleanser and Pads ℗

A preparation of ℞ **salicylic acid** and various.
Formulation: Medicated pads.
Availability: OTC.
Warnings and side effects: See ℞ **salicylic acid**.

oxymetazoline hydrochloride ⑥

Type/Group: **alpha-adrenergic stimulant**; **sympathomimetic**; **decongestant**; **vasoconstrictor**.

Brand(s): (For ophthalmic use): OcuClear; Visine L.R. (For nasal decongestion): Afrin, Afrin Children's Nose Drops, Afrin Sinus; Allerest 12 Hour Nasal; Cheracol Nasal; Chlorphed-LA; Dristan 12 Hr Nasal; Duramist Plus; Duration; 4-Way Long Lasting Nasal Drops, Spray; Genasal; Nostrilla; NTZ Long Acting Nasal; Sinarest 12 Hour; Vicks Sinex 12-Hour; Twice-A-Day; various generic.

How administered: Nasal; ophthalmic (eye).

Used to treat

Oxymetazoline is generally used for its vasoconstrictor properties (narrows blood vessels) which make it an effective nasal decongestant. It is applied topically (externally) to the nasal passages where it constricts the blood vessels of the nose, reducing congestion in the nasal mucous membranes and possibly also reducing secretions. It may also be used for symptomatic relief of redness due to irritation in the eye.

Warnings

• It should not be given to people with known hypersensitivity to this or any other adrenergic drug, with angle-closure glaucoma, or who have severe high blood pressure or coronary artery disease.

• It should be given with caution, on the advice of a doctor, to people who are taking ℞ **MAOI** antidepressants, or who have high blood pressure, heart disease, hyperthyroidism, diabetes mellitus, enlarged prostate, or increased intraocular pressure (pressure in the eyeball, including glaucoma).

• Oxymetazoline's effects during pregnancy are not known and it should be used only if there is a clear benefit over potential risk to the fetus.

• Medical judgment is required if breast-feeding is being considered.

• Overuse may cause symptoms such as nervousness and insomnia, and may make the congestion worse, which is an effect called "rebound congestion." No nasal decongestant should be used for longer than three to four days.

• It should be used with caution by the elderly, as they are more likely to suffer side effects.

• The manufacturer's recommendations must be followed carefully when giving this drug to children under 12.

Interactions

• When used topically (to the nose or eyes) at recommended doses, the interactions common to ℞ **sympathomimetics** do not usually apply. However, in overdose, there may be interactions and side effects similar to ℞ **ephedrine**.

Key to symbols: ✚ = Disorder Section ℞ = Drug Section ♣ = Herbal Section ⚌ = Supplement Section

• Oxymetazoline should not be used with ℞ **MAOI** antidepressants, or within two weeks of stopping MAOI treatment, because this may cause a hypertensive crisis.

Side effects

• These depend on how it is administered. As eyedrops it may cause blurred vision or stinging. When used as a nasal decongestant, it may cause irritation in the nose, anosmia (impairment of sense of smell), nasal mucosal ulceration, and sneezing.

• In nasal or eye application systemic side effects are infrequent, occurring only with overdose (especially in children) and consist of the usual sympathomimetic symptoms: changes in heart rate and blood pressure, anxiety, restlessness, tremor, insomnia, dry mouth, cold fingertips and toes, and changes in the prostate gland.

oxymorphone hydrochloride Ⓖ

Type/Group: **antitussive; narcotic analgesic; opioid.**
Brand(s): Numorphan.
How administered: Injection; rectal suppositories.

Used to treat

Oxymorphone is used in the treatment of moderate to severe ✪ **pain** (such as in cancer) and before surgery or during labor and delivery. Its use quickly tends to tolerance and then dependence (addiction).

Warnings

• It should not be taken by people with known hypersensitivity to any opioid, or with paralytic ileus (cessation of the normal rhythmic muscle contractions of the intestines). Opioids (even the weaker ones) should not be administered to asthmatics, to anyone with seriously depressed breathing disorders, or with prostatic hypertrophy, convulsive disorders, raised intracranial pressure, or a head injury.

• Depending on use and dose, it should be taken with caution by the elderly, or anyone with hypotension, certain liver, kidney or adrenal disorders, hypothyroidism (under-activity of the thyroid gland), or alcoholism.

• Oxymorphone should be used during pregnancy only if the potential benefit outweighs the possible risk to the fetus. (It is used, however, during delivery—with caution if there is abnormal fetal heart rhythm.)

• Medical judgment is required if breast-feeding is being considered.

• Oxymorphone is a Schedule II controlled substance.

• In overdose narcotic analgesics produce serious respiratory depression (decreased breathing), which is occasionally fatal.

• Tolerance occurs extremely readily and dependence (addiction) may follow.

• Drowsiness may affect the performance of skilled tasks such as driving.

• The effects of alcohol may be enhanced and the likelihood of respiratory depression increased.

Interactions

• Alcohol, ℞ **barbiturates**, ℞ **general anesthetics**, ℞ **MAOI**s, ℞ **opioids**, ℞ **sedatives**, ℞ **hypnotics**, ℞ **tranquilizers**, ℞ **tricyclic** antidepressants, ℞ **phenothiazines**, ℞ **antihistamines**, and ℞ **cimetidine** may increase or intensify the effects of oxymorphone, which can cause potentially serious side effects, especially respiratory depression.

• The effects of ℞ **diuretics** may be decreased in people with congestive heart failure.

Side effects

• The most frequent side effects include sedation, euphoria, constipation, dizziness, sweating, nausea and vomiting, loss of appetite, and mood change.

• Less frequently, dry mouth, flushing of the face, headache, palpitations, changes in heart rate, postural hypotension (lowering of blood pressure on standing, causing dizziness), rashes, miosis (pupil constriction), confusion, and hallucinations. It may also cause itching and a rash.

Oxy Night Watch Maximum Strength Lotion Ⓑ

Also: **Sensitive Skin Lotion**
A preparation of ℞ **salicylic acid** and various.
Formulation: Topical liquid.
Availability: OTC.
Warnings and side effects: See ℞ **salicylic acid**.

Oxy ResiDon't Ⓑ

A preparation of ℞ **triclosan**.
Formulation: Topical liquid.
Availability: OTC.
Warnings and side effects: See ℞ **triclosan**.

oxytetracycline Ⓖ

Type/Group: **tetracycline; antibiotic; antibacterial.**
Brand(s): Uri-Tet; Terramycin; various generic.
How administered: Orally; injection.

Used to treat

Oxytetracycline can be used to treat many serious infections, particularly infections of the urogenital (for example, ✪ **gonorrhea**, ✪ **syphilis**), the respiratory tracts, and of the skin (for example, ✪ **acne**).

Warnings

• It should not be given to people with known hypersensitivity to tetracyclines, or to children under eight years of age.

• It should be given with caution to people with kidney or liver impairment.

• Oxytetracycline should be avoided in the last half of pregnancy, because of the risk of dental staining and inhibiting the skeletal growth of the fetus.

• It should be avoided by nursing mothers.

• Superinfections due to the altered bacterial balance caused by antibiotic treatment may occur. A doctor must be contacted if severe abdominal pain, moderate to severe diarrhea, or any new or unusual symptoms occur.

• It may cause photosensitivity reactions (abnormal sensitivity to sunlight), so exposure to sunlight should be minimized.

• It may produce permanent discoloration of teeth and the thin tooth enamel in children from the time of tooth formation, which begins in the uterus and ends at age eight. It may also retard bone development during the same period.

• It must not be used after the discard date, as it becomes harmful to the kidneys as it degrades.

Interactions

• ℞ **Antacids**, ⚭ **calcium**, ⚭ **magnesium**, and ⚭ **zinc** may decrease the absorption of oxytetracycline and so they should be avoided.

• Milk products may also decrease absorption and should be avoided.

• If taken with methoxyflurane, there is a risk of kidney damage.

• The effectiveness of ℞ **oral contraceptives** may be reduced.

Side effects

• Frequently, gastrointestinal effects.

• Occasionally, darkening of the skin, itching, and sore mouth or tongue.

• Rarely, serious blood, liver, and skin disorders.

oxytocic Ⓓ

see ℞ uterine stimulant.

oxytocin Ⓖ

Type/Group: **hormone; posterior pituitary hormone; uterine stimulant.**
Brand(s): Pitocin; Syntocinon; various generic.
How administered: Injection; intranasal.

Used to treat

Oxytocin is a natural pituitary hormone produced and secreted by the posterior pituitary gland. It is an oxytocic, and increases the contractions of the uterus during normal labor. It also stimulates milk production. It can be given by intravenous injection or infusion to induce or assist labor (or abortion), to speed up the third stage of labor (delivery of the placenta), and with other drugs to help stop bleeding following childbirth and in abortion to control uterine bleeding. It may also be prescribed to promote the flow of breast milk, when it is used as a nasal spray.

Warnings

• It should not be given to people with known hypersensitivity to oxytocin, or who have certain gynecological conditions (injected form).

• It should not harm the fetus when used as indicated. It appears in breast milk and if oxytocin is given after childbirth, breast-feeding should be delayed.

• If used as a nasal spray to stimulate lactation, it should never be continued beyond the first week after childbirth.

• Rarely, adverse fetal effects have been associated with the use of ℞ oxytocics.

• It is a specialist drug and is used under controlled hospital conditions.

Interactions

• When used with ℞ **sympathomimetics**, the pressor effect (causing a rise in blood pressure) is increased.

• If taken with other ℞ **oxytocics**, effects are increased.

Side effects

• Occasionally, speeded heartbeat, hypotension, nausea, and vomiting.

• Rarely, with nasal use, tearing, nasal irritation, runny nose, unexpected uterine bleeding or contractions, or serious water intoxication.

P₁E₁ Ⓑ

Also: P_2E_1; P_4E_1; P_6E_1
A preparation of ℞ **pilocarpine** and ℞ **epinephrine.**
Formulation: Ophthalmic solution, available in four strengths.
Availability: Prescription only.
Warnings and side effects: See ℞ **pilocarpine**; ℞ **epinephrine.**

P-A-C Analgesic Tablets Ⓑ

A preparation of ℞ **aspirin** and ℞ **caffeine.**
Formulation: Oral tablets.
Availability: OTC.
Warnings and side effects: See ℞ **aspirin**; ℞ **caffeine.**

Pacerone Ⓑ

A preparation of ℞ **amiodarone hydrochloride.**
Formulation: Oral tablets.
Availability: Prescription only.
Warnings and side effects: See ℞ **amiodarone hydrochloride.**

Pacis Ⓑ

A preparation of ℞ **BCG intravesical.**
Formulation: Powder for suspension.
Availability: Prescription only.
Warnings and side effects: See ℞ **BCG intravesical.**

paclitaxel Ⓖ

Type/Group: **anticancer; cytotoxic.**
Brand(s): Taxol.
How administered: Intravenous infusion.

Used to treat

Paclitaxel is a cytotoxic drug, the first of a group of drugs termed the taxanes. It is used in the treatment of ovarian and ✪ **breast cancer**, also non-small cell ✪ **lung cancer**, and as a second-line treatment for AIDS-related ✪ **Kaposi's sarcoma.**

Warnings

• It should not be given to people with known hypersensitivity or resistance to paclitaxel or related drugs or, depending on use, in people with very low blood neutrophil levels.

• It should be given with caution to people with a history of certain heart conditions or with liver function impairment. This is a specialist drug which will be used following a full evaluation by specialist physicians.

• Paclitaxel is not recommended for use during pregnancy unless it is medically judged to be essential, because it may cause birth defects. Becoming pregnant while using this drug must be avoided.

• It should not be used if breast-feeding.

• It can cause bone marrow suppression, which may lead to bleeding and a reduced resistance to infection.
• Severe allergic reactions to this drug have occurred.
• Treatable conduction abnormalities (heart disorders) can develop.
• In common with many anticancer drugs, it may cause genetic mutations in cells.

Interactions
• ℞ **cisplatin** may increase the effects of paclitaxel.
• The levels of ℞ **doxorubicin hydrochloride** may be increased.

Side effects
• Frequently, hair loss, pain in joints or muscles, gastrointestinal disturbances, peripheral neuropathy (tingling or numbness in hands or feet), hypotension, abnormal ECG, pain and redness at injection site, inflamed mucosa, and speeded heart rate.

Pain Doctor ⑧
A preparation of ℞ **capsaicin**, ℞ **methyl salicylate**, and ℞ **menthol**.
Formulation: Topical cream.
Availability: OTC.
Warnings and side effects: See ℞ capsaicin; ℞ methyl salicylate; ℞ menthol.

painkiller ⑩
see ℞ **analgesic**.

Pain-X ⑧
A preparation of ℞ **capsaicin**, ℞ **menthol**, and ℞ **camphor**.
Formulation: Topical gel.
Availability: OTC.
Warnings and side effects: See ℞ capsaicin; ℞ menthol; ℞ camphor.

Palgic DS Syrup ⑧
A preparation of ℞ **pseudoephedrine** and ℞ **carbinoxamine maleate**.
Formulation: Oral syrup.
Availability: Prescription only.
Warnings and side effects: See ℞ pseudoephedrine; ℞ carbinoxamine maleate.

Palgic-D Tablets Extended Release ⑧
A preparation of ℞ **pseudoephedrine** and ℞ **carbinoxamine maleate**.
Formulation: Oral tablets, sustained release.
Availability: Prescription only.
Warnings and side effects: See ℞ pseudoephedrine; ℞ carbinoxamine maleate.

palivizumab ⑥
Type/Group: antiviral.
Brand(s): Synagis.
How administered: Intramuscular injection.

Used to treat
Palivizumab is one of a relatively new class of drug, a monoclonal antibody (a form of pure antibody produced by a type of molecular engineering). In this case the cloned antibody is one that neutralizes the respiratory syncytial virus (RSV), which is sometimes responsible for serious lower respiratory disease in infants.

Warnings
• It should not be given to people with known hypersensitivity to this drug or to any product prepared with mouse protein.
• This drug is not used in adults.
• Palivizumab is used to prevent infection and its value in treating active infection has not been established.

Interactions
No drug interactions of significance are known, but full studies have not been completed.

Side effects
• Rhinitis, rash, sore throat, upper respiratory tract infection, pain, reactions at the injection site, or changes in liver function.

Pamelor ⑧
A preparation of ℞ **nortriptyline hydrochloride**.
Formulation: Oral capsules in several strengths, oral solution.
Availability: Prescription only.
Warnings and side effects: See ℞ nortriptyline hydrochloride.

pamidronate disodium ⑥
(disodium pamidronate)
Type/Group: bisphosphonate; calcium-metabolism modifier.
Brand(s): Aredia.
How administered: Intravenous infusion.

Used to treat
Pamidronate (formerly called aminohydroxypropylidenediphosphonate disodium (APD)) is used to treat high blood calcium levels (⊙ **hypercalcemia**) induced by malignant tumors, Paget's disease of the bone and pain due to bone metastases secondary to cancers including breast cancer.

Warnings
• It should not be given to people with known hypersensitivity to bisphosphonates.
• It should be given with caution to people with kidney dysfunction.
• It should be used during pregnancy only if clearly needed.
• Medical judgment is required if breast-feeding is being considered. It is not known if it appears in breast milk.

Interactions
• Calcium-containing medications and vitamin D may reduce the effects of pamidronate sodium.

Side effects
• Frequently, rise in temperature 24 to 28 hours after administration, drug-related redness, swelling, pain at injection site, loss of appetite, nausea, fatigue, and electrolyte changes.
• Occasionally, constipation, gastrointestinal hemorrhage, nasal inflammation, rales, anemia, hypertension, speeded heartbeat, atrial fibrillation, drowsiness, seizure, and bone pain.

Pamprin Multi-Symptom Maximum Strength Caplets, Tablets ℞

A preparation of ℞ **acetaminophen**, pamabrom, and ℞ **pyrilamine maleate**.
Formulation: Oral tablets.
Availability: OTC.
Warnings and side effects: See ℞ **acetaminophen**; ℞ **pyrilamine maleate**.

Panacet 5/500 Tablets ℞

A preparation of ℞ **hydrocodone bitartrate** and ℞ **acetaminophen**.
Formulation: Oral tablets.
Availability: Prescription only.
Warnings and side effects: See ℞ **hydrocodone bitartrate**; ℞ **acetaminophen**.

Panalgesic Cream ℞

A preparation of ℞ **methyl salicylate** and ℞ **menthol**.
Formulation: Topical cream.
Availability: OTC.
Warnings and side effects: See ℞ **methyl salicylate**; ℞ **menthol**.

Panasal 5/500 Tablets ℞

A preparation of ℞ **hydrocodone bitartrate** and ℞ **aspirin**.
Formulation: Oral tablets.
Availability: Prescription only.
Warnings and side effects: See ℞ **hydrocodone bitartrate**; ℞ **aspirin**.

Pancof-HC Liquid ℞

A preparation of ℞ **hydrocodone bitartrate**, ℞ **pseudoephedrine**, and ℞ **chlorpheniramine maleate**.
Formulation: Oral liquid.
Availability: Prescription only.
Warnings and side effects: See ℞ **hydrocodone bitartrate**; ℞ **pseudoephedrine**; ℞ **chlorpheniramine maleate**.

Pancof XP Liquid ℞

A preparation of ℞ **hydrocodone bitartrate**, ℞ **pseudoephedrine**, and ℞ **guaifenesin**.
Formulation: Oral liquid.
Availability: Prescription only.
Warnings and side effects: See ℞ **hydrocodone bitartrate**; ℞ **pseudoephedrine**; ℞ **guaifenesin**.

Pancrease MT 4, MT 10, MT 16, MT 20, MT 25 Capsules ℞

A preparation of ℞ **pancrelipase** (amylase, lipase, protease).
Formulation: Oral capsules (5 strengths).
Availability: Prescription only.
Warnings and side effects: See ℞ **pancreatin**.

pancreatin Ⓖ

(pancrelipase)

Type/Group: **digestive enzyme**.
Brand(s): (As *pancreatin*): Digepepsin Tablets; Donnazyme Tablets; Hi-Vegi-Lip Tablets; Pancrezyme 4X Tablets; various generic. (As *pancrelipase*): Cotazyme, Cotazyme-S; Creon 5, 10, 20; Ku-Zyme HP; Lipram, UL20; Pancrease MT; Ultrase MT; Viokase Tablets, Powder; Zymase; various generic.
How administered: Orally.

Used to treat

Pancreatin is the term used to describe extracts of the pancreas that contain the pancreatic enzymes amylase, lipase, and protease. (In a more concentrated form and with a higher percentage of lipase, the extract is called pancrelipase.) It can be given by mouth to treat digestive disorders and deficiencies due to impaired natural secretion by the pancreas, such as in ⊕ **cystic fibrosis**, and also following operations involving removal of pancreatic tissue, such as pancreatectomy and gastrectomy. The enzymes which help digest protein, starch, and fat, are inactivated by the acid in the stomach and so preparations should be taken with food or with certain other drugs, such as ℞ **H_2-antagonists**, that reduce acid secretion. Alternatively, pancreatin is available as enteric-coated tablets and capsules, which overcome some of these problems, but are destroyed by heat and should be mixed with food after its preparation. The majority of pancreatin preparations are of porcine (pig) origin.

Warnings

• It should not be given to people with known hypersensitivity to pork protein or enzymes, or with pancreatic disease.
• The effects of pancreatin in pregnancy have not been studied and it should be used only if it is clearly needed.
• Medical judgment is required if breast-feeding is being considered. It is not known whether this substance appears in breast milk.
• Contact with pancreatin (in granular or powder form) can cause irritation to skin and mucous membranes, and sensitivity reactions in people with allergy to pork-derived substances. It should be handled with care.
• Tablets must be swallowed quickly and not chewed to reduce the possibility of mouth irritation.
• There are particular problems (fibrotic structures in the bowel) that seem to be associated with high-dose preparations and so these are only to be taken with specialist advice.

Interactions

• ℞ **calcium carbonate** and ℞ **magnesium hydroxide** may decrease or neutralize the beneficial effects of pancreatin.
• The absorption of dietary iron supplements may be reduced.

Side effects

• Irritation of the skin around the mouth and anus, and skin rash. There may be gastrointestinal upsets, including nausea, vomiting and abdominal discomfort; and at high dose there may be raised uric acid levels in the blood and urine.

pancrelipase Ⓖ

see ℞ **pancreatin**.

Pancrezyme 4X Tablets ℞

A preparation of ℞ **pancreatin** (amylase, lipase, protease).

Key to symbols: ⊕ = Disorder Section ℞ = Drug Section ♣ = Herbal Section ⟐ = Supplement Section

Formulation: Oral tablets.
Availability: OTC.
Warnings and side effects: See ℞ **pancreatin**.

pancuronium bromide Ⓖ

Type/Group: skeletal muscle relaxant.
Brand(s): Nimbex.
How administered: Injection.

Used to treat
Pancuronium is a non-depolarizing neuromuscular blocking agent used as a skeletal muscle relaxant to induce muscle paralysis during surgery, or as an aid to mechanical ventilation (breathing) or intubation.

Warnings
• It should not be used by people with known hypersensitivity to this drug.
• It should be taken with caution by people with certain heart and neuromuscular diseases, or with kidney, liver, or lung disorders.
• It is for administration only by trained personnel in hospitals, and individuals will be fully assessed for suitability prior to use.
• It should be used during pregnancy only if the benefits outweigh the risks to the fetus.
• Medical judgment is required if breast-feeding is being considered.

Interactions
This drug is for administration only by trained personnel in hospitals, and an individual's current and future therapy regimes will be fully assessed in order to avoid potential drug interactions.

Side effects
• Hypotension, bradycardia, flushing, and spasm of the bronchi.

Pandel Ⓑ

A preparation of ℞ **hydrocortisone** buteprate.
Formulation: Cream.
Availability: Prescription only.
Warnings and side effects: See ℞ **hydrocortisone**.

P&S Ⓑ

A preparation of ℞ **salicylic acid**.
Formulation: Shampoo.
Availability: OTC.
Warnings and side effects: See ℞ **salicylic acid**.

P & S Plus Ⓑ

A preparation of ℞ **coal tar** and ℞ **salicylic acid**.
Formulation: Topical Gel.
Availability: OTC.
Warnings and side effects: See ℞ **coal tar**; ℞ **salicylic acid**.

Panfil G Tablets; Liquid Ⓑ

A preparation of ℞ **guaifenesin** and diphylline.
Formulation: Oral tablets, liquid.
Availability: Prescription only.
Warnings and side effects: See ℞ **guaifenesin**; ℞ **theophylline**.

PanMist LA; JR Tablets; Syrup Ⓑ

A preparation of ℞ **pseudoephedrine** and ℞ **guaifenesin**.
Formulation: Oral tablets, long acting; syrup.
Availability: Prescription only.
Warnings and side effects: See ℞ **pseudoephedrine**;
℞ **guaifenesin**.

Panmycin Ⓑ

A preparation of ℞ **tetracycline hydrochloride**.
Formulation: Oral capsules.
Availability: Prescription only.
Warnings and side effects: See ℞ **tetracycline hydrochloride**.

PanOxyl Ⓑ

A preparation of ℞ **benzoyl peroxide**.
Formulation: Topical bar; topical gel in several bases.
Availability: OTC (bar); Prescription only (gel).
Warnings and side effects: See ℞ **benzoyl peroxide**.

Panscol Lotion; Ointment Ⓑ

A preparation of ℞ **salicylic acid**.
Formulation: Topical lotion; ointment.
Availability: OTC.
Warnings and side effects: See ℞ **salicylic acid**.

pantoprazole sodium Ⓖ

Type/Group: proton-pump inhibitor; ulcer-healing drug.
Brand(s): Protonix.
How administered: Orally.

Used to treat
Pantoprazole works as an inhibitor of gastric acid secretion in the parietal (acid-producing) cells of the stomach lining by acting as a proton-pump inhibitor. It is administered for the treatment of benign gastric and duodenal ulcers (see ◉ **peptic ulcer**), and also for reflux esophagitis. Additionally, it can be used with antibiotics to treat gastric *Helicobacter pylori* infection.

Warnings
• It should not be given to people with known hypersensitivity to this drug, or to any substituted benzimidazoles (that is, other proton-pump inhibitors, such as ℞ **omeprazole**, ℞ **lansoprazole**, ℞ **rabeprazole**).
• It should be given with caution to people with severe liver impairment.
• Pantoprazole should be used during pregnancy only if the potential benefit outweighs the possible risk to the fetus.
• Medical judgment is required if breast-feeding is being considered. It is not known whether this drug appears in breast milk, but there is reason to believe its effects would be harmful.
• Before treatment, it should be confirmed that there is no gastric cancer or other disease.

Interactions
• Proton-pump inhibitors, like this one, should be taken at least 30 minutes before ℞ **sucralfate** or they may not be absorbed properly.

• The levels and effects of ℞ **digoxin** and ferrous salts (♧ **iron** supplements), ℞ **ketoconazole**, and ℞ **ampicillin** may be reduced.

• It is thought possible that deficiency of ♧ **vitamin B$_{12}$** can occur with long-term use of pantoprazole.

Side effects

• These are uncommon with pantoprazole, consisting mainly of headache, but proton-pump inhibitors in general may also cause diarrhea, abdominal pain, rashes and itching, dizziness, nausea and vomiting, constipation, and flatulence. They decrease gastric acidity and so may increase the risk of gastrointestinal infections.

• Rarer side effects of proton-pump inhibitors may include flu-like syndrome, blood lipid changes, muscle and joint pain, cough, rhinitis, sinusitis, mouth ulcers, kidney problems, pancreatitis, sleepiness, insomnia, temporary mental disturbances, hair loss, hives, other allergic reactions (including anaphylaxis), peripheral edema, effects on the liver and the heart, and various blood changes. Also rare, but occasionally reported, are menstrual problems and impotence.

papaverine ⓖ

Type/Group: **vasodilator; alkaloid; impotence treatment**.
Brand(s): Pavagen TD; various generic.
How administered: Orally; injection.

Used to treat

Papaverine is a constituent of opium but is chemically different from ℞ **morphine** (it is not an opiate or opioid) and is without significant painkilling properties (and no potential for addiction). It is used to relieve arterial spasms that cause restricted circulation and ischemic pain. For the most part, its use in such common vasoconstriction disorders as ⊕ **angina pectoris** and ⊕ **Raynaud's disease** has been superseded by other drugs. There have been some recent trials of its use for impotence treatment by direct injection into the corpus cavernosum.

Warnings

• It should not be given to people with certain heart conduction disorders.

• It should be given with caution to people with glaucoma, liver or cardiovascular disease.

• Papaverine should be used during pregnancy only if the benefits outweigh the possible risks.

• Medical judgment is required if breast-feeding is being considered. It may appear in breast milk and so there is a risk of significant side effects.

• Drowsiness may affect the performance of skilled tasks such as driving.

• The effects of alcohol may be enhanced.

Interactions

• Papaverine may block the action of ℞ **levodopa** and reduce its effects.

Paraflex ⓑ

A preparation of ℞ **chlorzoxazone**.
Formulation: Caplets.
Availability: Prescription only.
Warnings and side effects: See ℞ **chlorzoxazone**.

Parafon Forte DSC ⓑ

A preparation of ℞ **chlorzoxazone**.
Formulation: Caplets.
Availability: Prescription only.
Warnings and side effects: See ℞ **chlorzoxazone**.

Paral ⓑ

A preparation of ℞ **paraldehyde**.
Formulation: Oral liquid; rectal liquid.
Availability: Prescription only.
Warnings and side effects: See ℞ **paraldehyde**.

paraldehyde ⓖ

Type/Group: **anticonvulsant; antiepileptic; hypnotic; sedatives**.
Brand(s): Paral; various generic.
How administered: Orally; rectal.

Used to treat

Paraldehyde is used mainly to treat ⊕ **epilepsy**, in the treatment of status epilepticus (severe and continuous epileptic seizures), and to control seizures that arise from other causes, such as tetanus, eclampsia, or poisoning. It has been widely used to prevent or lessen the effects of alcohol withdrawal (especially delirium tremens) and to reduce anxiety in withdrawal from other drugs, such as opiates or barbiturates.

Warnings

• Avoid its use in people with severe respiratory disease, asthma, or severe liver impairment.

• Medical judgment is required for anyone with any liver impairment, or with gastroenteritis, especially if an ulcer is present.

• It is not known whether paraldehyde causes harm to the fetus, therefore it should be used only when the potential benefit outweighs potential risk. (When used during labor, babies have shown significantly depressed breathing.)

• No problems are known when used by breast-feeding mothers, but medical judgment is required to assess the risks and benefits.

• Alcohol and paraldehyde together may cause extreme respiratory depression, and death.

• Long-term use can lead to dependence, with symptoms of delirium tremens when discontinued abruptly, so withdrawal should be gradual.

• Paraldehyde is irritating to mucous membranes and may cause bleeding in the gastrointestinal tract (including the esophagus when taken orally, and rectum when given rectally). Doses should be taken with beverages or food.

• There is likely to be a strong, unpleasant breath odor.

• As this drug may cause drowsiness, driving or other hazardous activity should be avoided.

Interactions

• There may be potentially serious additive effects if taken with one of the following drugs: alcohol; ℞ **barbiturates**; CNS depressants (such as ℞ **benzodiazepines**, ℞ **opioids**, ℞ **skeletal muscle relaxants**, ℞ **hypnotics**, ℞ **sedatives**, and ℞ **tranquilizers**).

• ℞ **Disulfiram** may cause higher concentrations of paraldehyde, with increased risk of side effects, and so these drugs should not be used together.

Side effects
• Rash and gastrointestinal irritation.
• Impaired liver function, causing yellowing of the eyes or skin (jaundice), with prolonged use.

Paraplatin ⑧

A preparation of ℞ **carboplatin**.
Formulation: Powder for injection.
Availability: Prescription only.
Warnings and side effects: See ℞ **carboplatin**.

parasympathomimetic ⑩

Generics: **acetylcholine chloride; ambenonium chloride; bethanechol chloride; carbachol; cevimeline hydrochloride; donepezil; edrophonium chloride; neostigmine methylsulfate; pilocarpine; pyridostigmine bromide; rivastigmine; tacrine hydrochloride.**

Actions and uses
Parasympathomimetic drugs have effects similar to those of the parasympathetic nervous system. They work by mimicking the actions of the natural neurotransmitter acetylcholine. Direct-acting parasympathomimetics act at (so-called "muscarinic") cholinergic receptors which normally "recognize" acetylcholine. Important parasympathomimetic actions include slowing of the heart, vasodilatation (widening of blood vessels), constriction of the bronchioles of the lung, stimulation of the muscles of the intestine and bladder (and so can be used to treat urinary retention: for example, ℞ **bethanechol chloride**), constriction of the pupil (℞ **miotic** drugs, also used in ℞ **glaucoma treatment**: for example, ℞ **acetylcholine chloride**, ℞ **carbachol**, and ℞ **pilocarpine**), and stimulation of secretions including saliva (℞ **cevimeline hydrochloride** is used for disease states characterized by a dry mouth.
The ℞ **anticholinesterase** drugs act as indirect parasympathomimetics because they prolong the duration of action of the naturally released acetylcholine, and so have some actions in common with the direct-acting parasympathomimetics. Examples include ℞ **edrophonium chloride**, ℞ **pyridostigmine bromide**, ℞ **ambenonium chloride**, and ℞ **neostigmine methylsulfate**. Most of these are, in fact, used for their actions at sites where acetylcholine exerts "nicotinic" actions. Recently, anticholinesterases (for example, ℞ **donepezil**, ℞ **rivastigmine**, and ℞ **tacrine hydrochloride**) have been introduced in ℞ **dementia treatment** for the treatment of dementia of impaired mental cognition.

Limitations
In the event of the actions of a parasympathomimetic drug being too long-acting, as in poisoning or the use of anticholinesterases in warfare, ℞ **anticholinergic** (antimuscarinic) drugs may be used because they oppose some of these actions.

paregoric ⑥

Type/Group: **opioid; antidiarrheal.**
Brand(s): Various generic.

How administered: Orally.
Used to treat
Paregoric (actually a tincture of opium) acts on the nerves of the intestine to inhibit peristalsis (the waves of muscular activity that move along the contents of the intestines), so reducing motility, and also decreases fluid secretion in the intestines.

Warnings
• It should not be given to people with known hypersensitivity to this drug, with a fever, or who must for medical reasons avoid constipation.
• It should be given with caution to people with respiratory disorders, liver disease, or severe prostate enlargement.
• Paregoric should be used during pregnancy only when it is clearly needed and when the benefits outweigh potential risks to the fetus.
• Medical judgment is required if breast-feeding is being considered.
• Drowsiness may affect the performance of skilled tasks, such as driving.
• Discontinue use after 48 hours if there is no improvement.
• A doctor must be contacted if fever or swelling of the abdomen occur.
• This is a Schedule III controlled substance.

Interactions
• ℞ **cimetidine** decreases the metabolism of paregoric.
• ℞ **rifampin** and ℞ **barbiturates** increase the metabolism of paregoric.

Side effects
• Usually minor, but they may include abdominal pain or discomfort, constipation, dry mouth, nausea, vomiting, fatigue, dizziness, and drowsiness.

Parkinson's disease treatment ⑩

see ℞ **antiparkinsonism**.

Parlodel ⑧

A preparation of ℞ **bromocriptine**.
Formulation: Tablets, capsules, snaptabs (break neatly into smaller doses).
Availability: Prescription only.
Warnings and side effects: See ℞ **bromocriptine**.

Parnate ⑧

A preparation of ℞ **tranylcypromine** sulfate.
Formulation: Oral tablets.
Availability: Prescription only.
Warnings and side effects: See ℞ **tranylcypromine**.

paroxetine ⑥

Type/Group: **SSRI; antidepressant.**
Brand(s): Paxil.
How administered: Orally.
Used to treat
Paroxetine can be used to treat ✪ **depression**, ✪ **obsessive-compulsive disorder** (OCD), panic disorder, and social ✪ **anxiety** disorder. It is somewhat more sedating than other SSRIs. As is the case

with other antidepressants, this drug is also being evaluated for other uses.

Warnings
• It should not be given to people with known hypersensitivity to this type of drug, or to anyone taking a ℞ **MAOI** antidepressant (see Interactions below).
• It should be given with caution to people with liver or severe kidney impairment, heart disorders, a history of seizures, diabetes mellitus, psychosis, bipolar disorder (manic depression), or who are receiving electroconvulsive therapy.
• Paroxetine should be used during pregnancy only if the benefits outweigh the possible risk to the fetus.
• Medical judgment is required if breast-feeding is being considered.
• A doctor must be consulted before taking any other medications, including OTC preparations, herbal remedies (especially ♣ **St. John's wort**), supplements (for example the ◌◌ **amino acids** tryptophan and tyramine) or other natural or alternative products.
• Avoid or minimize alcohol consumption.
• Judgment, thinking, and physical skills may be impaired, so use caution when first taking the drug.
• It may cause sensitivity to sunlight.
• Treatment should be stopped gradually, lowering the dose over a period of time.
• It may be four weeks before there are any signs of improvement.

Interactions
• Serious and even fatal reactions have occurred when ℞ **MAOIs** are taken with other antidepressants. There should be at least a 14-day gap between discontinuing a MAOI and starting another type.
• *l*-tryptophan, ℞ **amphetamines** or other psychostimulants, other antidepressants, ℞ **buspirone**, certain ℞ **antiparkinsonism** drugs, ℞ **cimetidine**, ℞ **lithium**, and certain ℞ **antibiotics** may increase or change the effects of SSRIs.
• ℞ **Barbiturates**, ℞ **cyproheptadine**, and smoking may reduce the effects of SSRIs.
• The effects of non-sedating ℞ **antihistamines**, ℞ **benzodiazepines**, ℞ **beta-blockers**, ℞ **buspirone**, ℞ **carbamazepine**, ℞ **clozapine**, ℞ **cyclosporine**, ℞ **diltiazem hydrochloride**, ℞ **digoxin**, ℞ **haloperidol**, ℞ **lithium**, ℞ **methadone**, ℞ **phenothiazines**, ℞ **phenytoin**, ℞ **pimozide**, ℞ **procyclidine**, ♣ **St. John's wort**, ℞ **sumatriptan**, ℞ **sympathomimetics**, tacrine, ℞ **theophylline**, ℞ **tolbutamide**, and ℞ **warfarin sodium** may be altered by SSRIs.

Side effects
• Anxiety, loss of appetite, and nausea.
• Less frequently, sleepiness, dry mouth, sexual problems (particularly males), weakness and loss of energy, sweating, constipation, diarrhea, and tremor.

Pathocil ⑱
A preparation of ℞ **dicloxacillin sodium**.
Formulation: Oral capsules in several strengths; oral suspension.
Availability: Prescription only.
Warnings and side effects: See ℞ **dicloxacillin sodium**.

Pavagen T.D. ⑱
A preparation of ℞ **papaverine**.
Formulation: Oral capsules, timed release.
Availability: Prescription only.
Warnings and side effects: See ℞ **papaverine**.

Paxil ⑱
A preparation of ℞ **paroxetine**.
Formulation: Oral tablets in varying strengths; oral suspension.
Availability: Prescription only.
Warnings and side effects: See ℞ **paroxetine**.

Paxipam ⑱
A preparation of ℞ **halazepam**.
Formulation: Oral tablets in several strengths.
Availability: Prescription only.
Warnings and side effects: See ℞ **halazepam**.

Pazo Hemorrhoid Ointment ⑱
A preparation of ℞ **ephedrine**. Ointment contains ℞ **camphor** and ℞ **zinc oxide**.
Formulation: Topical ointment; rectal suppositories.
Availability: OTC.
Warnings and side effects: See ℞ **ephedrine**; ℞ **camphor**; ℞ **zinc oxide**.

PCE Dispertab ⑱
A preparation of ℞ **erythromycin**.
Formulation: Oral tablets.
Availability: Prescription only.
Warnings and side effects: See ℞ **erythromycin**.

PDE-inhibitor ⑪
see ℞ **phosphodiesterase inhibitor**.

Pedameth ⑱
A preparation of ℞ **methionine**.
Formulation: Oral capsules; oral liquid.
Availability: Prescription only.
Warnings and side effects: See ℞ **methionine**.

Pediacare Fever Suspension; Oral Drops ⑱
A preparation of ℞ **ibuprofen**.
Formulation: Oral liquid.
Availability: OTC.
Warnings and side effects: See ℞ **ibuprofen**.

Pediacare Infants' Decongestant Drops ⑱
A preparation of ℞ **pseudoephedrine**.
Formulation: Oral drops.
Availability: OTC.
Warnings and side effects: See ℞ **pseudoephedrine**.

Key to symbols: ✿ = Disorder Section   ℞ = Drug Section   ♣ = Herbal Section   ◌◌ = Supplement Section

Pediacof Syrup Ⓑ

A preparation of ℞ **codeine phosphate**, ℞ **chlorpheniramine maleate**, ℞ **phenylephrine hydrochloride**, and ℞ **potassium iodide**.
Formulation: Oral syrup.
Availability: May or may not require a prescription.
Warnings and side effects: See ℞ **codeine phosphate**; ℞ **chlorpheniramine maleate**; ℞ **phenylephrine hydrochloride**; ℞ **potassium iodide**.

Pediapred Ⓑ

A preparation of ℞ **prednisolone** sodium phosphate.
Formulation: Oral liquid.
Availability: Prescription only.
Warnings and side effects: See ℞ **prednisolone**.

Pediatric Vicks 44d Dry Hacking Cough and Head Congestion Ⓑ

A preparation of ℞ **dextromethorphan**.
Formulation: Oral syrup.
Availability: OTC.
Warnings and side effects: See ℞ **dextromethorphan**.

Pediazole Ⓑ

A preparation of ℞ **erythromycin** and ℞ **sulfamethoxazole**.
Formulation: Topical solution.
Availability: Prescription only.
Warnings and side effects: See ℞ **erythromycin**; ℞ **trimethoprim and sulfamethoxazole** [℞ **co-trimoxazole**].

Pedi-Boro Soak Paks Ⓑ

A preparation of ℞ **aluminum acetate**.
Formulation: Topical powder packets.
Availability: OTC.
Warnings and side effects: See ℞ **aluminum acetate**.

Pedi-Cort V Creme Ⓑ

A preparation of ℞ **hydrocortisone** and ℞ **clioquinol**.
Formulation: Cream.
Availability: Prescription only.
Warnings and side effects: See ℞ **hydrocortisone**; ℞ **clioquinol**.

pediculicidal Ⓓ

see ℞ **scabicide and pediculicide**.

pediculicide Ⓓ

see ℞ **scabicide and pediculicide**.

Pedituss Cough Syrup Ⓑ

A preparation of ℞ **codeine phosphate**, ℞ **chlorpheniramine maleate**, potassium iodide, and ℞ **phenylephrine hydrochloride**.
Formulation: Oral syrup.
Availability: May or may not require a prescription.
Warnings and side effects: See ℞ **codeine phosphate**; ℞ **chlorpheniramine maleate**; ℞ **phenylephrine hydrochloride**.

PedvaxHIB Ⓑ

A preparation of ℞ **Haemophilus b conjugate vaccine**.
Formulation: Injection.
Availability: Prescription only.
Warnings and side effects: See ℞ **Haemophilus b conjugate vaccine**.

pegademase bovine Ⓖ

Type/Group: enzyme; immunostimulant; metabolic disorder treatment.
Brand(s): Adagen.
How administered: Intramuscular injection.
Used to treat
Pegademase bovine is a replacement enzyme for one that is lacking in a rare inherited disorder that causes a form of severe combined immunodeficiency disease (SCID). Infants born with this enzyme deficiency are unable to maintain adequate levels of white blood cells, and hence have little immunity even to common infections. This condition is often fatal. Although it may be permanently relieved by a bone marrow transplant, this procedure may need to be postponed, or fail, or be ill-advised for some, and so pegademase is recommended for infants from birth or for children of any age when the diagnosis has been made.
Warnings
• It should not be used as a routine support therapy for bone marrow transplantation, as studies fail to find benefit in the practice. This is a specialist drug and is used only after a full medical assessment.
• Its effects in pregnancy are unknown and so it should be used only when it is clearly needed.
• Medical judgment is required if breast-feeding is being considered.
• Improvement in the immune system may take from a few weeks to six months after beginning treatment. Appropriate care, to guard against infection, should be maintained until monitoring shows an improvement in immunity.
• Pegademase bovine is prescribed only by specialists and used only under qualified supervision.
• As with any injection, caution must be exercised with people with thrombocytopenia (difficulty in blood clotting).
Interactions
• If taken with vidarabine or ℞ **pentostatin**, an interaction is possible that reduces the effects of pegademase.
Side effects
Few side effects have been reported, but experience with the drug is limited.

penbutolol sulfate Ⓖ

Type/Group: beta-blocker; antihypertensive.
Brand(s): Levatol; generic.
How administered: Orally.

Used to treat
Penbutolol is used to lower blood pressure (see ✪ **hypertension**).

Warnings
• It should not be given to people with known hypersensitivity to any beta-blocking drug, who have certain heartbeat irregularities or heart failure, or bronchial asthma, allergic bronchospasm or severe chronic obstructive pulmonary disease (COPD). It should not be used in cardiogenic shock.

• It should be given with caution to people with diabetes mellitus or hypoglycemia, hyperthyroidism, myasthenia gravis, congestive heart failure, peripheral vascular disease, moderate bronchospastic disease (for example, chronic bronchitis, emphysema), or liver or kidney impairment.

• Penbutolol's safety during pregnancy has not been established and it should be used only if the potential benefit outweighs the possible risk to the fetus.

• Medical judgment is required if breast-feeding is being considered. It is not known whether this drug appears in breast milk.

• Abruptly discontinuing beta-blocker treatment may have adverse effects on the heart.

• The use of this drug may mask signs of hyperthyroidism or hypoglycemia.

• Beta-blockers may intensify allergic responses to a variety of allergens in people with a history of severe anaphylactic reaction, and the response to the usual dose of epinephrine, to treat anaphylaxis, may be reduced in such people.

• Some nasal ℞ **decongestants**, commonly available over the counter, contain ℞ **alpha-adrenergic stimulants** (for example, ℞ **phenylephrine**) that may cause a severe hypertensive reaction if taken with a beta-blocker. A doctor must be consulted before taking any other medication (including OTCs, herbal remedies, and supplements).

Interactions
• A serious blood pressure increase may occur after withdrawal from ℞ **clonidine**, or both drugs at the same time.

• If taken with ℞ **antiarrhythmics** (for example, ℞ **amiodarone hydrochloride**, ℞ **disopyramide**, ℞ **procainamide**, ℞ **quinidine**) and ℞ **tricyclic** antidepressants, there is the potential for significant adverse effects on heart rhythm.

• The effects of ℞ **alpha-adrenergic stimulants**, ℞ **ergot alkaloids**, ℞ **epinephrine**, ℞ **lidocaine**, and ℞ **theophylline** may be increased, with the risk of serious adverse effects.

• If taken with ℞ **calcium-channel blockers** (especially ℞ **diltiazem hydrochloride**, ℞ **verapamil**), ℞ **guanethidine monosulfate**, or ℞ **reserpine**, there is the potential for undesirable additive effects, with exaggerated slowing of the heartbeat or hypotension.

• The effects of nondepolarizing ℞ **skeletal muscle relaxants** are variable, with a possible risk of significant adverse effects associated with major surgery.

• The effects of ℞ **insulin** and ℞ **sulfonylureas** may be reduced by penbutolol.

• ℞ **Antacids** (for example, ℞ **aluminum hydroxide**, ℞ **magnesium hydroxide**), ℞ **barbiturates**, ᵂ **calcium** salts,

℞ **cholestyramine**, ℞ **colestipol hydrochloride**, ℞ NSAIDs, ℞ **phenytoin**, ℞ **penicillins**, ℞ **rifampin**, and ℞ **salicylates** may reduce the levels and effects of beta-blockers. Antacids should not be taken within two hours of beta-blockers.

• If taken with ℞ **diuretics** or other antihypertensive drugs, there are increased effects which are often used to therapeutic advantage.

Side effects
• These may include dizziness, nausea, headache, fatigue, constipation, or diarrhea.

• Occasionally, insomnia, flatulence, urinary frequency, impotence, or decreased libido.

• Rarely, rash, arrhythmias, joint and muscle pain, confusion, or strange taste sensations.

penciclovir Ⓖ
Type/Group: **antiviral**.
Brand(s): Denavir.
How administered: Topically.

Used to treat
Penciclovir is an antiviral drug that is similar to ℞ **acyclovir**. It is used to treat recurrent labial herpes simplex infection (✪ **cold sores**).

Warnings
• It should not be given to people with known hypersensitivity to penciclovir.

• It should be given with caution to people who are immunocompromised.

• Penciclovir's safety during pregnancy has not been established, and it should be used only when the potential benefits clearly outweigh the possible risks to the fetus.

• Medical judgment is required if breast-feeding is being considered.

• Exposure of cold sores to direct sunlight should be avoided.

Interactions
No significant interactions have been reported with topical (external) use.

Side effects
• Frequently, headache and redness.

• Occasionally, a reaction at the site of application.

• Rarely, altered taste and rash.

Penecort Ⓑ
A preparation of ℞ **hydrocortisone**.
Formulation: Cream; solution.
Availability: Prescription only.
Warnings and side effects: See ℞ **hydrocortisone**.

Penetrex Ⓑ
A preparation of ℞ **enoxacin**.
Formulation: Oral tablets.
Availability: Prescription only.
Warnings and side effects: See ℞ **enoxacin**.

Key to symbols: ✪ = Disorder Section ℞ = Drug Section ♣ = Herbal Section ᵂ = Supplement Section

penicillamine ⓖ

Type/Group: **antirheumatic; chelating agent.**
Brand(s): Cuprimine; Depen.
How administered: Orally.

Used to treat

Penicillamine is a derivative of ℞ **penicillin** and is an extremely effective chelating agent. It binds various metal ions within the body, so facilitating their excretion (elimination from the body). It can be used as an antidote to various types of metallic poisoning (for example, copper and lead) and as a ✪ **metabolic disorder** treatment to reduce copper levels in ✪ **Wilson's disease**; sometimes in autoimmune hepatitis and cystinuria, as well. It is used in the long-term treatment of severe ✪ **rheumatoid arthritis** or juvenile chronic arthritis, where it has ℞ **anti-inflammatory** and antirheumatic actions.

Warnings

• It should not be used by people with known hypersensitivity to this drug or to any of the penicillins, or who have a history of kidney insufficiency. It should be given with caution to anyone with lupus erythematosus. It may take several weeks before improvements are experienced.

• Penicillamine may have the potential to cause birth defects and should not be used during pregnancy except when, in the treatment of Wilson's disease, it is medically judged that the potential benefit outweighs the risk to the fetus.

• Breast-feeding mothers should either discontinue using this drug or stop breast-feeding.

• This drug may cause a wide range of blood abnormalities, including anemia, lowered counts of white blood cells and clotting components, and bone marrow depression. In addition, liver and kidney damage may occur. Therefore, close medical monitoring of blood, liver, and kidney function is necessary.

• Symptoms such sore throat, infection, fever, unexplained bruising, bleeding or purple patches, mouth ulcers, rashes, or non-specific illness should be reported immediately to a physician.

• Taking iron supplements can reduce the absorption of penicillamine and thus its therapeutic effect.

• Urine may turn red.

• Take on an empty stomach.

Interactions

• Gold salts (for example, ℞ **aurothioglucose**), ℞ **antimalarials**, and ℞ **cytotoxics** (for example, ℞ **methotrexate**) may increase the risk of significant adverse effects on the blood and kidneys.

• ℞ **Antacids**, and iron salts (for example, ℞ **ferrous sulfate**) lower the absorption of penicillamine.

• Penicillamine may reduce ℞ **digoxin** levels.

Side effects

• Nausea, loss of appetite, fever, rashes, taste impairment, blood and kidney disturbances diarrhea, and abdominal cramping;

• A lupus-like syndrome, myasthenia (muscle weakness), and pemphigus (a severe inflammatory disease of the skin) have all occurred during penicillamine therapy;

• There may be potentially serious blood or kidney disorders.

penicillin ⓓ

Generics: amoxicillin; ampicillin; carbenicillin; cloxacillin sodium; dicloxacillin sodium; mezlocillin; nafcillin; oxacillin sodium; penicillin G; penicillin V; piperacillin; ticarcillin.

Actions and uses

Penicillins are ℞ **antibacterial** and ℞ **antibiotic** drugs which are used to treat ✪ **bacterial infections** by interfering with the synthesis of bacterial cell walls. The early penicillins were mainly effective against Gram-positive bacteria, although they could be used against the Gram-negative organisms that caused gonorrhoea and meningitis, as well as the organism causing syphilis. Later penicillins (for example, ℞ **ampicillin** and ℞ **piperacillin**) were able to treat a greater range of Gram-negative organisms. They are absorbed rapidly by most (but not all) body tissues and fluids and are removed in the urine. A problem with many of the penicillins is that certain penicillin-resistant bacteria make an enzyme that breaks down some of the penicillin class, effectively rendering them useless. Some later penicillins are penicillinase-resistant, but for some of those that are not, an inhibitor of the bacterial enzyme may be administered at the same time as the antibiotic (see ℞ **penicillinase inhibitor**).

Limitations

One great disadvantage of penicillins is that many people are allergic to them—allergy to one, means allergy to them all—and may have reactions that range from a minor rash right up to anaphylactic shock, which occasionally can be fatal (see ✪ **anaphylactic reaction**). Otherwise they are remarkably non-toxic. Rarely, very high dosage may cause convulsions, hemolytic (destruction of red blood cells) anemia, or abnormally high levels of sodium or potassium with consequent symptoms. Penicillins taken by mouth tend to cause diarrhea and there is also a risk with broad-spectrum penicillins of allowing a ✪ **superinfection** to develop by disturbing the natural bacterial balance within the body.

penicillinase inhibitor ⓓ

(beta-lactamase inhibitor)
Generics: **clavulanic acid; tazobactam.**

Actions and uses

Penicillinase inhibitors are drugs used to inhibit enzymes that are produced by certain (penicillin-resistant) bacteria, which break down some of the ℞ **penicillin** class of ℞ **antibiotic** and ℞ **antibacterial** drugs, effectively making them useless. For example, staphylococci bacteria are commonly resistant to ℞ **benzylpenicillin** through developing an ability to produce penicillinase enzyme. Consequently, treatment of ✪ **bacterial infections** caused by such bacteria has normally necessitated the administration of either penicillinase-resistant penicillins, such as flucloxacillin, or entirely different classes of antibiotic. However, some antibiotic preparations combine a penicillinase-sensitive drug with an inhibitor of the penicillinase enzyme, which then artificially gives that antibiotic penicillinase-resistance (for example, ℞ **clavulanic acid** and ℞ **tazobactam** are inhibitors of penicillinase (beta-lactamase).

Limitations

See the individual drug entries.

penicillin G Ⓖ

(benzylpenicillin)

Type/Group: **antibiotic; penicillin; antibacterial.**
Brand(s): Bicillin; Pfizerpen; Wycillin.
How administered: Injection.

Used to treat

Penicillin G is the drug of choice for many severe ✪ **bacterial infections**, including those caused by sensitive strains of meningococcus (for example, meningitis) and streptococcus (for example, bacterial sore throat, scarlet fever, and septicemia), in serious conditions when the micro-organism causing the disease has not been identified for certain (for example, ✪ **endocarditis**). It has a long-acting form, procaine penicillin, and a very long-acting form, benzathine penicillin, which has an important role in treating syphilis. It is the first of the penicillins to be isolated and used as an antibiotic.

Warnings

• It should not be used by people with known hypersensitivity to penicillins.
• It should be taken with caution by people with allergies to Ŗ **cephalosporins** or Ŗ **imipenem**, or who have impaired kidney function.
• Penicillins cross the placenta and should be used in pregnancy only if medically judged to be needed.
• Penicillin G should not be used while breast-feeding.
• Serious and occasionally fatal hypersensitivity reactions can occur (including hives, fever, joint pains, rashes, anaphylaxis, serum sickness-like reactions, hemolytic anemia, and kidney problems).
• Superinfections from the altered bacterial balance created by antibiotic treatment may occur and may result in ✪ **pseudomembranous colitis**. A doctor must be contacted if there is severe abdominal pain, or moderate to severe diarrhea.

Interactions

• Ŗ **Chloramphenicol**, Ŗ **macrolide** antibiotics, and Ŗ **tetracyclines** may reduce the effectiveness of penicillin.
• Large doses of penicillin may increase levels of Ŗ **methotrexate**.
• Occasionally, the effectiveness of Ŗ **oral contraceptives** is impaired.
• Ŗ **Aspirin**, phenylbutazone, Ŗ **sulfonamides**, Ŗ **indomethacin**, thiazide Ŗ **diuretics**, Ŗ **furosemide**, and ethacrynic acid may interfere with the excretion of penicillin G.
• The effectiveness of Ŗ **anticoagulants** may be reduced.
• Ŗ **Heparin** may increase the risk of bleeding.

Side effects

• Frequently, gastrointestinal effects (diarrhea, nausea, vomiting).
• Occasionally, pain at injection site, electrolyte imbalance.
• Rarely, bleeding. Rare but serious effects include kidney damage, when the procaine form is used, a toxic reaction characterized by confusion, combativeness, and mood changes, and also seizures.

penicillin V Ⓖ

(phenoxymethyl penicillin)

Type/Group: **antibiotic; penicillin; antibacterial.**
Brand(s): Beepen-VK; Pen-Vee K; Veetids.
How administered: Orally.

Used to treat

Penicillin V is particularly effective in treating ✪ **bacterial infections** such as ✪ **tonsillitis**, ✪ **scarlet fever**, infection of the middle ear, and certain skin infections. It is also used to prevent recurrent ✪ **rheumatic fever** or chorea. Although not stated by the manufacturer for such use, it may also be prescribed to treat ✪ **Lyme disease** and for the prevention of ✪ **pneumonia** in children with sickle-cell anemia.

Warnings

• It should not be used by people with known hypersensitivity to penicillins.
• It should be given with caution to people with allergies to Ŗ **cephalosporins** or Ŗ **imipenem**, or with impaired kidney function.
• Penicillins cross the placenta and should be used in pregnancy only if medically judged to be needed.
• Penicillin V should not be used while breast-feeding.
• Serious and occasionally fatal hypersensitivity reactions can occur. A doctor must be contacted if skin rash, itching, hives, severe diarrhea, shortness of breath, black tongue, sore throat, nausea, fever, swollen joints, or any unusual bleeding or bruising occurs.
• Superinfections from the altered bacterial balance created by antibiotic treatment may occur and may result in ✪ **pseudomembranous colitis**. A doctor should be contacted if there is severe abdominal pain, or moderate to severe diarrhea.
• The full course of treatment prescribed must be completed or infection may return.

Interactions

• Ŗ **Chloramphenicol**, Ŗ **macrolide** antibiotics, and Ŗ **tetracyclines** may reduce the effectiveness of penicillin.
• The effectiveness of Ŗ **oral contraceptives** may be reduced.

Side effects

• Frequently, mild allergic reaction, and gastrointestinal effects (diarrhea, nausea, vomiting).
• Rarely, bleeding, and kidney damage.

pentamidine isethionate Ⓖ

(pentamidine isetionate)

Type/Group: **amebicide and antiprotozoal.**
Brand(s): Pentam-300; NebuPent.
How administered: Injection; inhalant.

Used to treat

Pentamidine isethionate is used to treat ✪ **pneumonia** caused by the protozoan microorganism *Pneumocystis carinii* (PCP) in people whose immune system has been suppressed (either following transplant surgery or because of a condition such as ✪ **HIV** infection), and to prevent PCP in high-risk HIV-infected individuals. Although not stated by the manufacturer for such use, it has also been used as an antiprotozoal to treat forms of visceral ✪ **leishmaniasis** and trypanosomiasis.

Warnings

• It should not be given to people with a history of severe allergic reaction to pentamidine isethionate, when given as an inhalant.
• It should be given with caution to people with blood pressure disorders, blood glucose disorders, certain blood disorders, kidney

or liver dysfunction, ventricular tachycardia, pancreatitis, and certain serious skin disorders.
• Pentamidine isethionate should be used during pregnancy only if the potential benefits outweigh the possible risks to the fetus.
• Medical judgment is required if breast-feeding is being considered. It is not known if it appears in breast milk.
• Severe, life-threatening hypotension, blood disorders or heart arrhythmias may develop.
• It may cause kidney damage or liver failure.
• Hypoglycemia and insulin-dependent diabetes mellitus may occur.
• The use of the inhalant may induce bronchospasm or cough, particularly in people with a history of smoking or with asthma.

Interactions
• ℞ **Didanosine (ddl)** may increase the risk of pancreatitis.
• ℞ **foscarnet sodium** may increase adverse reactions.

Side effects
• Frequently, abscess or pain at injection site, nausea, and decreased appetite. If inhaled, fatigue, metallic taste, shortness of breath, gastrointestinal effects, dizziness, rash, and cough.
• Occasionally, when injected, fever, rash, bad taste, and confusion. When inhaled, diarrhea, headache, anemia, muscle pain, serious skin disorder, and pancreatitis.

pentamidine isetionate ⓖ

see ℞ pentamidine isethionate.

Pentasa ⑬

A preparation of ℞ **mesalamine**.
Formulation: Oral capsules, controlled release.
Availability: Prescription only.
Warnings and side effects: See ℞ **mesalamine**.

pentazocine ⓖ

Type/Group: **narcotic analgesic; opioid.**
Brand(s): Talwin. Combinations: With *acetaminophen*: Talacen. With *aspirin*: Talwin Compound. With *naloxone*: Talwin NX; various generic.
How administered: Orally; injection.

Used to treat
Pentazocine can be used to treat moderate to severe ✪ **pain**. It is like ℞ **morphine sulfate** in its effect and action, but is less likely to cause dependence. However, it can precipitate withdrawal symptoms if used in patients dependent on opioids.

Warnings
• It should not be given to people with known hypersensitivity to this drug, or with certain cardiovascular complications. Opioids (even the weaker ones) should not be given to people with asthma, to anyone with seriously depressed breathing disorders, prostatic hypertrophy, convulsive disorders, raised intracranial pressure, or a head injury.
• Depending on use and dose, it should be given with caution to the elderly, or to anyone with hypotension, porphyria, cyanosis, certain liver, kidney or adrenal disorders, hypothyroidism (under-activity of the thyroid gland), alcoholism, or a history of drug abuse.

• Pentazocine should be used during pregnancy only if the benefits outweigh the possible risks. Withdrawal symptoms have been observed in newborns.
• Medical judgment is required if breast-feeding is being considered. Its safety in nursing has not been established.
• The proprietary forms of pentazocine are Schedule IV controlled substances.
• Prolonged use of narcotics can lead to physical dependence (addiction), although this rarely happens in routine medical use.
• Treatment by injection may cause pain and tissue damage at the site of the injection.
• Drowsiness may affect the performance of skilled tasks such as driving.
• The effects of alcohol may be enhanced (with a higher risk of respiratory depression).

Interactions
• If the following drugs are used with pentazocine, then effects are increased: ℞ **barbiturates**; ℞ **general anesthetics**; ℞ **opioids**; ℞ **tranquilizers** (for example, ℞ **phenothiazines**); ℞ **sedatives**; ℞ **benzodiazepines** (for example, ℞ **diazepam**, ℞ **lorazepam**); alcohol.
• If used with ℞ **fluoxetine**, there are exaggerated side effects, including tremor, flushing, and ataxia (incoordinated movement).

Side effects
• There may be sedation, dizziness, vomiting, nausea, and constipation.
• There is occasionally euphoria, which may lead to a state of mental detachment or confusion.
• Less frequently, sweating, headache, palpitations, changes in heart rate, postural hypotension (a lowering of blood pressure on standing, causing dizziness), rashes, miosis (pupil constriction), dry mouth, flushing of the face, mood change, and hallucinations.
• Rarely, serious blood cell disorders, shock, and respiratory depression.

Pentolair ⑬

A preparation of ℞ **cyclopentolate hydrochloride**.
Formulation: Ophthalmic solution.
Availability: Prescription only.
Warnings and side effects: See ℞ **cyclopentolate hydrochloride**.

pentostatin ⓖ

Type/Group: **anticancer; cytotoxic.**
Brand(s): Nipent.
How administered: Injection.

Used to treat
Pentostatin is a cytotoxic drug (an antimetabolite, and an antibiotic in origin) which is used for hairy cell ✪ **leukemia**.

Warnings
• It should not be given to people with known hypersensitivity or resistance to this drug.
• It should be given with caution to people with impaired kidney function, pre-existing bone marrow depression, infections, heart

disease, or impaired liver function. This is a specialist drug which will be used following a full evaluation by specialist physicians.
• Pentostatin is not recommended for use during pregnancy unless it is medically judged to be essential, because it may cause birth defects. Becoming pregnant while using this drug must be avoided.
• It should not be used if breast-feeding.
• It can cause bone marrow depression, which may lead to bleeding and a reduced resistance to infection.
• Higher than recommended doses (overdose) may produce severe kidney, liver, lung, or CNS (central nervous system) toxicity.
• Rashes are common and occasionally severe, and may worsen with treatment.
• It may have toxic effects on kidneys.

Interactions
• ℞ **Fludarabine** should not be used with pentostatin because of the risk of severe adverse effects on lungs.
• Vidarabine increases the adverse reactions of both drugs.

Side effects
• Frequently, nausea, vomiting, fatigue, cough, upper respiratory infection, loss of appetite, and diarrhea (also see Warnings above).
• Occasionally, urinary problems, headache, sore throat, sinusitis, bone and joint pain, swelling of extremities, loss of appetite, blurred vision, conjunctivitis, skin discoloration, sweating, easy bruising, anxiety, depression, dizziness, and confusion.

pentoxifylline Ⓖ
(oxpentifylline)
Type/Group: **vasodilator**.
Brand(s): Trental; various generic.
How administered: Orally.

Used to treat
Pentoxifylline dilates the blood vessels of the extremities and can be used to treat peripheral vascular disease (for example, ✪ **Raynaud's disease**) or intermittent claudication (cramp-like pains in the calves).

Warnings
• It should not be given to people with known hypersensitivity to this drug or to methylxanthines (for example, ℞ **caffeine**, ℞ **theophylline**, theobromine), or with recent cerebral or retinal hemorrhage.
• It should be given with caution to people with any condition or disorder that might make bleeding more likely (for example, recent surgery, peptic ulcer), or with impaired kidney function.
• Pentoxifylline should be used during pregnancy only when it is clearly needed.
• Medical judgment is required if breast-feeding is being considered.
• Anyone with any additional risk factors for bleeding should have periodic examination, including blood counts.

Interactions
• If used with ℞ **warfarin sodium**, there may be an increased risk of bleeding.
• The levels and effects of ℞ **theophylline** may be increased, with potential for toxicity.

• If used with ℞ **antihypertensives**, a slight increase in blood pressure may occur.

Side effects
Most side effects occur much less frequently when pentoxifylline is taken in extended-release form.
• The most common are gastrointestinal disturbances (for example, nausea, vomiting, belching, gas, bloating), dizziness, and headache.
• Uncommon side effects may include anxiety, tremor, nosebleed, flu-like symptoms, blurred vision, brittle fingernails, edema, and hypotension.
• Hypersensitivity reactions (for example, itching, rash, hives, allergic swelling) are also uncommon.
• Anaphylactoid reactions are rare. Liver function and blood changes have been reported.

Pentrax; Pentrax Gold Ⓡ
A preparation of ℞ **coal tar**.
Formulation: Shampoo.
Availability: OTC.
Warnings and side effects: See ℞ **coal tar**.

Pen-Vee K Ⓡ
A preparation of ℞ **penicillin V**.
Formulation: Oral tablets in different strengths; Oral solution.
Availability: Prescription only.
Warnings and side effects: See ℞ **penicillin V**.

Pepcid AC Ⓡ
A preparation of ℞ **famotidine**.
Formulation: Oral tablets; chewable tablets; gelcaps.
Availability: OTC.
Warnings and side effects: See ℞ **famotidine**. Chewable tablets contain the sweetener aspartame, which should be avoided by individuals with phenylketonuria.

Pepcid Tablets; RPD Tablets; Powder for Solution; Injection Ⓡ
A preparation of ℞ **famotidine**.
Formulation: Oral tablets; rapid-disintegration tablets; powder; injection.
Availability: Prescription only.
Warnings and side effects: See ℞ **famotidine**. RPD tablets contain the sweetener aspartame, which should be avoided by individuals with phenylketonuria.

peppermint oil Ⓖ
Type/Group: **antispasmodic**.
Brand(s): Numzit Teething.
How administered: Orally; topically (external).

Used to treat
Peppermint oil is incorporated into preparations of topical ℞ **analgesics**, and may also be used to relieve ✪ **colic** and symptoms of ✪ **irritable bowel syndrome**. See also ♣ **peppermint**.

Warnings

When used topically, the eye and other sensitive areas should be avoided since there may be reactions and irritation.

Interactions

No significant interactions are known.

Side effects

See Warnings above.

Pepto-Bismol; Maximum Strength Ⓑ

A preparation of ℞ bismuth subsalicylate.
Formulation: Oral liquid; caplets; tablets, chewable.
Availability: OTC.
Warnings and side effects: See ℞ bismuth subsalicylate.

Pepto Diarrhea Control Ⓑ

A preparation of ℞ loperamide hydrochloride.
Formulation: Oral liquid.
Availability: OTC.
Warnings and side effects: See ℞ loperamide hydrochloride.

Percocet Tablets Ⓑ

A preparation of ℞ oxycodone and ℞ acetaminophen.
Formulation: Oral tablets.
Availability: Prescription only.
Warnings and side effects: See ℞ oxycodone;
℞ acetaminophen.

Percodan Tablets; Percodan-Demi Ⓑ

A preparation of ℞ oxycodone and ℞ aspirin.
Formulation: Oral tablets.
Availability: Prescription only.
Warnings and side effects: See ℞ oxycodone; ℞ aspirin.

Percolone Ⓑ

A preparation of ℞ oxycodone.
Formulation: Oral tablets.
Availability: Prescription only.
Warnings and side effects: See ℞ oxycodone.

Perdiem Fiber Therapy Ⓑ

A preparation of ℞ psyllium.
Formulation: Oral granules.
Availability: OTC.
Warnings and side effects: See ℞ psyllium.

Perdiem Overnight Relief Ⓑ

A preparation of ℞ psyllium and ℞ senna.
Formulation: Oral granules.
Availability: OTC.
Warnings and side effects: See ℞ psyllium; ℞ senna.

pergolide Ⓖ

Type/Group: antiparkinsonism; ergot alkaloid; dopamine-receptor stimulant.
Brand(s): Permax.

How administered: Orally.

Used to treat

Pergolide is a recently introduced antiparkinsonism drug which is an ℞ **ergot alkaloid** derivative used to treat ⊙ **Parkinson's disease.** It works by stimulating the dopamine receptors in the brain. It is similar to ℞ **bromocriptine** in that it is useful in reducing "off" periods in the disease, and is usually given with ℞ **levodopa** and ℞ **carbidopa.**

Warnings

• It should not be given to people with known hypersensitivity to this or any other ergot derivative.

• It should be given with caution to people with certain heart disorders, dyskinesias (incoordinate movement), a history of confusion or hallucinations, or porphyria.

• Pergolide should be used during pregnancy only if it is clearly needed.

• Because of its potential to cause serious reactions in nursing infants, mothers should either discontinue the drug or discontinue breast-feeding.

• At high doses pergolide may impair fertility in men and women.

Interactions

• ℞ **Dopamine antagonists** (for example, most ℞ **antipsychotics**) and ℞ **metoclopramide** have an opposite action from pergolide and may diminish its effect.

• It should be used with caution with any other drug known to affect protein binding in the blood.

Side effects

• These include hallucinations, confusion, impaired muscle movements, somnolence or insomnia, nausea and abdominal pain, indigestion, double vision, rhinitis, labored breathing, constipation or diarrhea, hypotension and changes in heart rate or rhythm, effects on the lungs, and others.

Pergonal Ⓑ

A preparation of ℞ **menotropins.**
Formulation: Injection.
Availability: Prescription only.
Warnings and side effects: See ℞ menotropins.

Periactin Tablets, Syrup Ⓑ

A preparation of ℞ **cyproheptadine hydrochloride.**
Formulation: Oral tablets; syrup.
Availability: Prescription only.
Warnings and side effects: See ℞ cyproheptadine hydrochloride.

Peri-Colace Ⓑ

A preparation of casanthranol and ℞ **docusate sodium.**
Formulation: Oral syrup.
Availability: OTC.
Warnings and side effects: See ℞ cascara sagrada; ℞ docusate sodium.

Peri-Colace Capsules; Peri-Colace Softgels ®

A preparation of ℞ **docusate sodium**, casanthranol, and ℞ **sorbitol**.
Formulation: Oral capsules; oral gelcaps.
Availability: OTC.
Warnings and side effects: See ℞ docusate sodium; ℞ sorbitol.

perindopril erbumine ©

Type/Group: **ACE inhibitor; vasodilator; antihypertensive.**
Brand(s): Aceon.
How administered: Orally.

Used to treat

Perindopril is used to treat high blood pressure in ✪ **hypertension**, often with other classes of drug, particularly ℞ **thiazide** ℞ **diuretics**.

Warnings

• It should not be given to people with known hypersensitivity to this drug or to any other ACE inhibitor.
• It should be given with caution to people with severe congestive heart failure, or certain other cardiovascular disorders, a history of anaphylaxis, collagen vascular disease (for example, systemic lupus erythematosus; SLE), diabetes, depressed immune response, or with impaired liver or kidney function or on dialysis.
• ACE inhibitors can cause injury to the fetus, even death. The use of these drugs should be stopped as soon as pregnancy is detected.
• Medical judgment is required if breast-feeding is being considered. It is not known whether it appears in breast milk.
• Use of this drug should be stopped and a doctor contacted immediately if signs of angioedema appear (swelling of the face, eyes, lips, tongue, larynx, or extremities; difficulty in breathing or swallowing). Swelling of the larynx, closing off the airway, can be life-threatening.
• Anyone taking an ACE inhibitor should not interrupt or discontinue treatment without first checking with a doctor.
• Any suspected infections (for example, fever, sore throat) should be reported to a doctor, because ACE inhibitors may cause blood changes which can affect immune response.
• ACE inhibitors generally have less effect on blood pressure in blacks than in non-blacks, and likelihood of angioedema is higher among blacks, as well.

Interactions

• ACE inhibitors have apparently triggered life-threatening anaphylactoid reactions when used by people also receiving ℞ **desensitizing vaccines**.
• ℞ **Anesthetics** (for example, in surgery), ℞ **phenothiazines**, and ℞ **probenecid** may increase the levels or hypotensive effect of perindopril.
• Levels of ℞ **lithium** may be increased, with the potential for toxic effects.
• If used with potassium-sparing ℞ **diuretics** or other preparations containing potassium (for example, supplements and salt substitutes), levels of potassium may rise.
• ℞ **NSAIDs** may increase the risk of kidney damage or (in some cases) reduce the effects of ACE inhibitors.

• Caution is advised when using ℞ **gentamicin** with perindopril.
• ℞ **Antacids** and ℞ **rifampin** may reduce the effects of perindopril. Antacids should not be used for several hours after a dose of an ACE inhibitor (a doctor should be consulted for full instructions and cautions).
• If used with other antihypertensives and diuretics, the effects of these drugs may be increased. This additive effect is sometimes used to advantage in combination treatments for high blood pressure.

Side effects

• Commonly, dry cough.
• Occasionally, dizziness, headache, upper respiratory infection or symptoms (for example, rhinitis, sore throat), pain in the extremities or back, weakness, gastrointestinal disturbances (for example, diarrhea, abdominal pain, nausea and vomiting), palpitations or heart rhythm disturbances.
• Infrequently, insomnia, tingling in the extremities, rash, sexual dysfunction, nervousness, fever or sweating. Although it is uncommon, ACE inhibitors can cause very marked hypotension (especially when beginning treatment) and kidney impairment.
• Rarely, there may be angioedema, altered liver function, jaundice, hepatitis, pancreatitis, or changes in blood counts.

Permax ®

A preparation of ℞ **pergolide**.
Formulation: Oral tablets.
Availability: Prescription only.
Warnings and side effects: See ℞ pergolide.

permethrin ©

Type/Group: **scabicide and pediculicide.**
Brand(s): Acticin; Elimite; Nix.
How administered: Topically (external).

Used to treat

Permethrin, a pyrethroid, can be used as a pediculicidal to treat infestations by lice, and as a scabicidal to treat skin infestation by mites (see ✪ **lice and mite infestations**; ✪ **scabies**).

Warnings

• It should not be given to people with known hypersensitivity to this or related drugs, to members of the chrysanthemum family (from which permethrin and other pyrethroids originate), or to any components of the preparations.
• Permethrin should be used during pregnancy only if it is clearly needed.
• It is not known whether it appears in breast milk, but because of the potential for adverse effects its use while nursing is not recommended.
• Contact with eyes or mucous membranes must be avoided.

Interactions

No interactions specific to this drug are known.

Side effects

• Itching, redness, or swelling of the scalp.

Permitil ®

A preparation of ℞ **fluphenazine**.

Formulation: Oral tablets; oral concentrate.
Availability: Prescription only.
Warnings and side effects: See ℞ **fluphenazine.**

Pernox Scrub for Oily Skin ⑧

A preparation of ℞ **salicylic acid** and ℞ **sulfur.**
Formulation: Cleanser.
Availability: OTC.
Warnings and side effects: See ℞ **salicylic acid;** ℞ **sulfur.**

Peroxyl ⑧

A preparation of ℞ **hydrogen peroxide.**
Formulation: Topical solution; topical gel.
Availability: OTC.
Warnings and side effects: See ℞ **hydrogen peroxide.**

perphenazine ⓖ

Type/Group: **antipsychotic; phenothiazine.**
Brand(s): Trilafon. Combinations: With amitriptyline
hydrochloride: Triavil, Etrafon.
How administered: Orally; injection.

Used to treat

Perphenazine is used to treat ✪ **schizophrenia** and other severe
psychoses (see ✪ **psychotic disorders**). Although not stated by the
manufacturer for such use, it is sometimes prescribed as an
℞ **antinauseant** and ℞ **antiemetic** to relieve nausea and vomiting, to treat intractable hiccups, neuromuscular disorder hemibal-
lismus, aggressive behavior, ℞ **tricyclic-**induced tremor, and
organic mental syndromes.

Warnings

• It should not be given to people with known hypersensitivity to
this drug, with severe toxic CNS (central nervous system)
depression, in a coma, with subcortical brain damage, or bone
marrow depression.
• It should be given with caution to people over 65, or with
epilepsy, kidney or liver disease, severe cardiovascular disease,
glaucoma, prostatic hypertrophy, severe asthma, emphysema,
hypocalcemia (low calcium), or chronic obstructive pulmonary
disease (COPD).
• Perphenazine should be used during pregnancy only if the
benefits outweigh the risk to the fetus.
• Medical judgment is required if breast-feeding is being
considered.
• It may cause postural hypotension (lowered blood pressure on
standing), so rise slowly from a reclining position. Older people in
particular should exercise caution.
• It may cause drowsiness, and so the performance of skilled tasks,
such as driving, may be impaired.
• It may cause sensitivity to sunlight (photosensitivity), so minimize
exposure (use a sunscreen, sunglasses, and so on).
• If used for a long time, tardive dyskinesia (see ℞ **antipsychotics**)
occasionally develops.
• Treatment should be stopped gradually.
• Avoid alcohol.

Interactions

• The ℞ **antiparkinsonism** effects of ℞ **levodopa** may be reduced.
• If used with an ℞ **antidepressant** or ℞ **propranolol**, the levels
of both drugs may be increased.
• If used with ℞ **lithium**, the levels of both drugs may be decreased.
• ℞ **Antimalarials** (amodiaquine, chloroquine, sulfadoxine,
pyrimethamine) may increase the levels of perphenazine.
• ℞ **Anticholinergics**, ℞ **barbiturates**, ℞ **narcotic analgesics**,
and ℞ **orphenadrine** lower the levels of an antipsychotic in the
blood, and/or increase the occurrence of anticholinergic and/or
CNS (central nervous system) effects.
• If used with ℞ **clonidine hydrochloride**, ℞ **guanadrel**, or
℞ **guanethidine monosulfate**, a severe lowering of blood
pressure possible.
• If an antipsychotic is taken with alcohol, there may be increased
sedative effects.

Side effects

• Perphenazine is less sedating than some other phenothiazines.
Side effects include extrapyramidal symptoms, especially dystonia
(see ℞ **antipsychotics**), headache, loss of appetite, constipation,
dry mouth, and nausea.
• Less frequently, agitation, anxiety, catatonic-like behavioral
states, confusion, depression, euphoria, worsening of psychotic
symptoms, heat or cold intolerance, insomnia, lethargy,
restlessness, vertigo, ECG changes, changes in blood pressure,
speeded heartbeat, anemia, blood abnormalities, blurred vision,
eye changes, indigestion, increased salivation, vomiting, priapism
(prolonged, painful penile erection), urinary retention, changes in
hormone function (irregular menstruation, growth of breasts,
abnormal milk production, impotence, increased libido), changes
in blood sugar levels, sensitivity reactions, rashes, spasmodic
constriction of the bronchi or larynx, increased sweating, and loss
of hair.
• Rare but serious side effects include neuroleptic malignant
syndrome (a potentially fatal condition characterized by very high
fever, muscle rigidity, changes in mental status, and irregular pulse,
blood pressure and/or heart rhythm) and seizure.

Persa-Gel ⑧

A preparation of ℞ **benzoyl peroxide.**
Formulation: Topical gel in several strengths.
Availability: Prescription only.
Warnings and side effects: See ℞ **benzoyl peroxide.**

Persantine ⑧

A preparation of ℞ **dipyridamole.**
Formulation: Oral tablets, available in 3 strengths.
Availability: Prescription only.
Warnings and side effects: See ℞ **dipyridamole.**

Pertussin CS; ES ⑧

A preparation of ℞ **dextromethorphan.**
Formulation: Oral liquid; ES is higher strength.
Availability: OTC.
Warnings and side effects: See ℞ **dextromethorphan.**

pethidine hydrochloride Ⓖ

see ℞ meperidine hydrochloride.

petrolatum Ⓖ

(yellow soft paraffin; white soft paraffin)

Type/Group: **emollient; barrier cream; artificial tears**.

Brand(s): Borofax Skin Protectant; Bottom Better; Eucerin Cream; Lubritears; Wondra.

How administered: Topically (external).

Used to treat

Petrolatum, also known as petroleum jelly, is a hydrocarbon derived from petroleum that is used as a base for ointments, such as those for hemorrhoids, diaper rash, and dry skin, and as well as other products, such as artificial tears. White petrolatum is petrolatum from which the natural yellowish tinge has been removed so the product will be clearer.

Warnings

• It should not be given to people with a history of skin irritation from white petrolatum (white petrolatum only).

• A doctor should be consulted before using during pregnancy or while breast-feeding, but it is generally regarded as safe.

• Petrolatum may impair the natural healing process when used on superficial burns by blocking exposure to oxygen. A doctor should be consulted before using petrolatum products on burns.

Interactions

No significant interactions are known.

Side effects

No significant side effects are known.

Pfizerpen Ⓑ

A preparation of ℞ penicillin G.

Formulation: Injection.

Availability: Prescription only.

Warnings and side effects: See ℞ penicillin G.

Phanatuss DM Syrup Ⓑ

A preparation of ℞ dextromethorphan and ℞ guaifenesin.

Formulation: Oral syrup.

Availability: OTC.

Warnings and side effects: See ℞ dextromethorphan; ℞ guaifenesin.

Phazyme Tablets; Phazyme 95; 125 Ⓑ

A preparation of ℞ simethicone.

Formulation: Oral tablets; capsules (Phazyme 125).

Availability: OTC.

Warnings and side effects: See ℞ simethicone.

Phenadex Senior Liquid Ⓑ

A preparation of ℞ dextromethorphan and ℞ guaifenesin.

Formulation: Oral liquid.

Availability: OTC.

Warnings and side effects: See ℞ dextromethorphan; ℞ guaifenesin.

Phenameth DM Syrup Ⓑ

A preparation of ℞ dextromethorphan and ℞ promethazine hydrochloride.

Formulation: Oral syrup.

Availability: Prescription only.

Warnings and side effects: See ℞ dextromethorphan; ℞ promethazine hydrochloride.

Phenaphen w/Codeine Capsules Ⓑ

A preparation of ℞ codeine phosphate and ℞ acetaminophen.

Formulation: Oral capsules, available in two strengths.

Availability: Prescription only.

Warnings and side effects: See ℞ codeine phosphate; ℞ acetaminophen.

phendimetrazine Ⓖ

Type/Group: **appetite suppressant; obesity treatment; CNS stimulant**.

Brand(s): Adipost; Bontril PDM; Dital; Plegine; various generic.

How administered: Orally.

Used to treat

Phendimetrazine is used, under medical supervision and on a short-term basis, to aid weight loss in severe ✪ obesity. It is potentially subject to abuse and so its proprietary preparations are on the controlled substances list. There is growing doubt among experts over the medical value of such treatment (for instance, there may be a weight relapse once that treatment has finished).

Warnings

• It should not be used by people with known hypersensitivity to sympathomimetic amines, glaucoma, or a history of drug abuse, cardiovascular disease, advanced arteriosclerosis, hyperthyroidism, or moderate to severe hypertension, those taking ℞ MAOI antidepressants (see Interactions below).

• It should be given with caution to anyone with diabetes mellitus, seizure disorders, or mild hypertension.

• It is not known whether or not phendimetrazine can harm the fetus, therefore, it should be used during pregnancy only if medically judged to be needed.

• Medical judgment is also required if breast-feeding is being considered.

• Treatment must not be ended abruptly.

• It may impair the ability to perform skilled tasks requiring alertness, such as driving.

• Phendimetrazine is related to the ℞ amphetamines and has abuse potential; it is a Schedule III controlled substance.

Interactions

• Phendimetrazine must not be taken with, or within two weeks of discontinuing, ℞ MAOI antidepressants. Severe and even fatal reactions can occur.

• ℞ furazolidone if taken with phendimetrazine may cause a serious hypertensive reaction.

• The effects of ℞ guanethidine monosulfate may be reduced.

• ℞ tricyclic antidepressants may reduce levels of phendimetrazine.

Side effects

• Frequently, nervousness, insomnia, dizziness, over-stimulation, and restlessness.

• Occasionally, headache, gastrointestinal upsets, impotence, testicular pain, and urinary hesitancy.

• Rarely, changes in rate of heart beat, and chest pain.

phenelzine Ⓖ

Type/Group: **antidepressant; MAOI.**
Brand(s): Nardil.
How administered: Orally.

Used to treat

Phenelzine can be used to treat ✪ depression. It is used particularly when treatment with ℞ **tricyclic** antidepressants (for example, ℞ **amitriptyline hydrochloride** or ℞ **imipramine**) has failed. It is one of the safer, less-stimulant MAOIs.

Warnings

• It should not be given to people with known hypersensitivity to MAOI antidepressants, or with pheochromocytoma, cardiovascular or cerebrovascular disease, high blood pressure, congestive heart failure, known or suspected liver disease, severe kidney impairment, or a history of frequent or severe headache.

• It should be given with caution to people over the age of 60, to anyone with low blood pressure, bipolar disorder (manic depression), schizophrenia, hyperactivity, diabetes mellitus, seizure disorder, angina, or thyroid disease.

• Phenelzine should be used during pregnancy only if it is clearly needed.

• It should not be used by nursing mothers.

• Foods with high tyramine, dopamine, or tryptophan content must be avoided (see Interactions below).

• Do not drink alcoholic beverages.

• A doctor must be consulted before taking any other medication, including OTC drugs, herbal remedies, supplements, or any other alternative preparation (especially cold, hay fever, or weight-reduction products).

• Minimize caffeine intake.

• A doctor must be contacted at once if headache, palpitations, nausea, neck stiffness, sweating, photophobia, or other unusual symptoms develop. They can indicate a potentially serious reaction.

• It is not generally given to children under the age of 16.

• It may impair the performance of skilled tasks requiring mental alertness or physical skills, such as driving.

Interactions

• Foods containing tyramine, such as cheeses, sour cream, yogurt, liver, fermented sausages (for example, salami, bologna), smoked, spoiled, dried or pickled fish, meat tenderizer, game meats, beer, red wine, sherry, spirits, tofu, bananas, raspberries (other fruits especially if dried or overripe), sauerkraut, yeast extracts, broad beans, chocolate, may cause dangerously high blood pressure.

• Herbal remedies, such as ginseng or caffeine, and others that contain amines may cause dangerously high blood pressure.

• Supplements containing tryptophan and tyramine (see ✦✦ **amino acids**) may cause dangerously high blood pressure.

• Serious and even fatal reactions have occurred when MAOI antidepressants are taken with other antidepressants (such as SSRIs or tricyclics). At least 14 days should elapse between discontinuing one and starting the other, and 21 days for some including clomipramine or imipramine.

• If used with ℞ **dextromethorphan**, agitation or seizure are possible.

• If used with ℞ **ephedrine**, ℞ **amphetamine**, ℞ **phenylephrine**, or ℞ **pseudoephedrine**, severe high blood pressure is possible.

• Sensitivity to ℞ **barbiturates**, ℞ **antidiabetics**, and ℞ **beta-blockers** may be increased.

• If used with ℞ **dextromethorphan**, ℞ **methylphenidate**, ℞ **carbamazepine**, ℞ **cyclobenzaprine**, ℞ **amphetamine**, ℞ **metaraminol**, ℞ **phenylephrine**, ℞ **pseudoephedrine**, ℞ **ephedrine**, or ℞ **levodopa**, raised blood pressure, sometimes to dangerous levels, may occur.

• ℞ **guanethidine monosulfate**'s and guanadrel's effects on blood pressure may be inhibited by MAOIs.

• Toxic reactions are possible with ℞ **meperidine**, ℞ **sulfonamide**, or ℞ **sumatriptan**.

• Adverse reactions may occur with ℞ **methyldopa**, Rauwolfia ℞ **alkaloids**, ℞ **sympathomimetics**, ℞ **thiazide** ℞ **diuretics**, or *l*-tryptophan.

Side effects

• Drowsiness, dizziness, and postural hypotension (lowered blood pressure on standing).

• Less frequently, fainting, heart palpitations, fainting, headache, confusion, memory impairment, sleep disturbance, gastrointestinal disturbances, dry mouth, weight gain, sexual disturbances, chills, and urinary retention.

• Rare but serious side effects include seizures, raised blood pressure, abnormal heart rhythm, and blood cell disorders.

Phenerbel-S Ⓑ

A preparation of ℞ **ergotamine tartrate**, ℞ **belladonna alkaloid**, and ℞ **phenobarbital**.
Formulation: Oral tablets.
Availability: Prescription only.
Warnings and side effects: See ℞ **ergotamine tartrate**; ℞ **belladonna alkaloid**; ℞ **phenobarbital**.

Phenergan Tablets; Syrup; Suppositories; Injection Ⓑ

A preparation of ℞ **promethazine hydrochloride**.
Formulation: Oral tablets; syrup; rectal suppositories; injection, intramuscular only.
Availability: Prescription only.
Warnings and side effects: See ℞ **promethazine hydrochloride**.

Phenergan VC Syrup Ⓑ

A preparation of ℞ **phenylephrine hydrochloride** and ℞ **promethazine hydrochloride**.
Formulation: Oral syrup.
Availability: Prescription only.

Warnings and side effects: See ℞ phenylephrine hydrochloride; ℞ promethazine hydrochloride.

Phenergan VC with Codeine Syrup ®

A preparation of ℞ **codeine phosphate**, ℞ **phenylephrine hydrochloride**, and ℞ **promethazine hydrochloride**.
Formulation: Oral syrup.
Availability: May or may not require a prescription.
Warnings and side effects: See ℞ **codeine phosphate**; ℞ **phenylephrine hydrochloride**; ℞ **promethazine hydrochloride**.

Phenergan w/Dextromethorphan Syrup ®

A preparation of ℞ **dextromethorphan** and ℞ **promethazine hydrochloride**.
Formulation: Oral syrup.
Availability: Prescription only.
Warnings and side effects: See ℞ **dextromethorphan**; ℞ **promethazine hydrochloride**.

Phenergan with Codeine Syrup ®

A preparation of ℞ **codeine phosphate** and ℞ **promethazine hydrochloride**.
Formulation: Oral syrup.
Availability: May or may not require a prescription.
Warnings and side effects: See ℞ **codeine phosphate**; ℞ **promethazine hydrochloride**.

Phenhist DH w/Codeine Liquid ®

A preparation of ℞ **codeine phosphate**, ℞ **pseudoephedrine**, and ℞ **chlorpheniramine maleate**.
Formulation: Oral liquid.
Availability: May or may not require a prescription.
Warnings and side effects: See ℞ **codeine phosphate**; ℞ **pseudoephedrine**; ℞ **chlorpheniramine maleate**.

Phenhist Expectorant Liquid ®

A preparation of ℞ **codeine phosphate**, ℞ **guaifenesin**, and ℞ **pseudoephedrine**.
Formulation: Oral liquid.
Availability: May or may not require a prescription.
Warnings and side effects: See ℞ **codeine phosphate**; ℞ **guaifenesin**; ℞ **pseudoephedrine**.

pheniramine maleate ©

Type/Group: antihistamine; antiallergic; cold and cough preparation.
Brand(s): Naphcon A Eye Drops. Combinations: With *phenylephrine*: Dristan Nasal Spray; Scot-Tussin Original 5-Action Liquid, Syrup. With *phenyltoloxamine and pyrilamine*: Poly-Histine-D Elixir, Capsules, Ped Caps.
How administered: Orally; ophthalmic (eyedrops).

Used to treat

Pheniramine can be used for the symptomatic relief of allergic symptoms, such as ✪ hay fever (seasonal allergic rhinitis),

✪ **urticaria**, and allergic itchiness and irritation of the eyes. It is also used in several preparations for ✪ **coughs** and ✪ **colds**.

Warnings

• It should not be given to people with known hypersensitivity to this drug (or with known sensitivity to other antihistamines).
• Antihistamines should be given with caution to people with lower respiratory disease or asthma (and never during an attack), heart disease, hypertension, hyperthyroidism, epilepsy, porphyria, increased intraocular pressure (pressure in the eyeball, as in glaucoma), enlarged prostate, urinary retention, or certain obstructive bladder or gastrointestinal conditions.
• It should not be used in the eyes when contact lenses are worn.
• Pheniramine should be used during pregnancy only if it is clearly needed, but not in the third trimester, as newborns or premature infants may have severe reactions, including convulsions, to antihistamines.
• Nursing mothers should discontinue using this drug or discontinue breast-feeding.
• ℞ MAOI antidepressants may prolong and intensify the anticholinergic and sedative effects of antihistamines (see Side effects below).
• Pheniramine must not be given to infants, and for children under the age of 12 the manufacturer's or medical instructions must be followed closely.
• Because of its sedative side effects, the performance of skilled tasks, such as driving, may be impaired.
• Side effects are more frequent in the elderly.

Interactions

• ℞ MAOI antidepressants may prolong and intensify the anticholinergic (see Side effects below) effects of antihistamines.
• If used with ℞ tricyclic antidepressants, other antihistamines, ℞ skeletal muscle relaxants, ℞ opioids, ℞ barbiturates, ℞ hypnotics, ℞ sedatives, or ℞ tranquilizers there is a risk of intensified side effects.
• Pheniramine maleate can mask the toxic effects (to the ears) of ℞ aminoglycoside antibiotics.
• Alcohol may intensify side effects such as drowsiness and impaired mental alertness.

Side effects

• These depend on how it is administered. For this type of antihistamine, there is commonly drowsiness, headache, impaired muscular coordination or dizziness, anticholinergic effects (dry mouth, blurred vision, urinary retention, gastrointestinal disturbances), occasional rashes and photosensitivity (abnormal sensitivity to light), palpitations and heart arrhythmias.
• Rarely, there may be stimulation instead of sedation (paradoxical stimulation), especially in children (and convulsions in overdose), hypersensitivity reactions, blood disorders, liver disturbances, depression, sleep disturbances, and hypotension.
• Applied as eyedrops, there may be stinging, burning or itching of the eye, eye pain or painful sensitivity to light (photophobia).

phenobarbital ©

(phenobarbital sodium)

Type/Group: **anticonvulsant; antiepileptic; barbiturate; hypnotic; sedatives.**
Brand(s): Solfoton; Luminol; various generic.
How administered: Orally; injection.

Used to treat
Phenobarbital is used in the prevention of most types of recurrent seizures in ✪ **epilepsy** and for status epilepticus. It is also used as a sedative and as a hypnotic to treat severe and intractable ✪ **insomnia** and for sedation before operations.

Warnings
• It should not be used by people with known hypersensitivity to barbiturates, respiratory depression, severe liver impairment, or porphyria.
• It should be given with caution to people with anemia, addiction to barbiturates, liver disease, chronic obstructive pulmonary disease (COPD), emphysema, high blood pressure, acute or chronic pain, mental depression, myasthenia gravis, diabetes mellitus, a history of drug abuse, or who are over 65 years of age.
• Phenobarbital should not be used during pregnancy if possible. A physician must be contacted if pregnancy occurs while using this drug.
• Medical judgment is required if breast-feeding is being considered.
• Phenobarbital is a Schedule IV controlled substance.
• It has a high potential for dependence (addiction) and abuse.
• It loses its effectiveness for treating insomnia after about two weeks.
• It impairs the performance of skilled tasks, such as driving, and so these should be avoided.
• Alcohol must be avoided.
• Treatment must not be ended abruptly after long-term use.
• It is very dangerous in overdose.

Interactions
• Phenobarbital decreases the response to oral ℞ **anticoagulants** (for example, ℞ **warfarin sodium**).
• ℞ **Acetaminophen** increases the risk of toxic effects on the liver.
• The concentrations and therapeutic effects of the following drugs may be reduced: ℞ **antidepressants**; ℞ **beta-blockers**; ℞ **calcium-channel blockers**; ℞ **corticosteroids**; ℞ **cyclosporine**; ℞ **digitoxin**; ℞ **disopyramide**; ℞ **doxycycline**; ℞ **estrogens**; ℞ **griseofulvin**; ℞ **oral contraceptives**; ℞ **propafenone**; ℞ **quinidine**; ℞ **tacrolimus**; ℞ **theophylline**.
• ℞ **MAOI** antidepressents prolong the effects of barbiturates.
• Phenobarbital taken with an ℞ **antipsychotic** reduces the effects of both drugs.
• ℞ **Chloramphenicol** increases barbiturate concentrations, but reduces concentrations of itself.
• Methoxyflurane increases the adverse effects on the kidneys.
• The effects of ℞ **narcotic analgesics** may be altered, with increased CNS (central nervous system) depression.
• ℞ **Valproic acid** increases concentration of phenobarbital.

Side effects
Depending on how administered, dose, and use, there may be:
• Hangover with drowsiness, lack of energy, and rash.

• Less frequently, CNS (central nervous system) depression, dizziness, headache, lightheadedness, mental depression, physical dependence, slurred speech, excitement in children and people over 65, vertigo, slowed heartbeat, lowered blood pressure, gastrointestinal upset, and hives.
• Rare but serious side effects include blood cell disorders, breathing stoppages, respiratory depression, spasms of the bronchi or larynx, and Stevens-Johnson syndrome (a severe skin disorder).

phenol ⓖ
(carbolic acid)
Type/Group: **disinfectant; antiseptic.**
Brand(s): Blistex; Campho-Phenique; Cepastat Cherry; Chap Stix; Cheracol Sore Throat; Florida Sun Burn Relief; Phenolated Calamine; Vicks Chloraseptic; Children's Vick's Chloraseptic.
How administered: Topically (external).

Used to treat
Phenol is used for cleaning and relieving pain of minor burns, insect bites, or inflammation, and also for mouth and throat hygiene.

Warnings
• It should not be taken by people with known hypersensitivity to any component of these products.
• A doctor should be consulted before using while pregnant or breast-feeding. It is, however, generally regarded as safe.
• Do not swallow (especially concentrated form).
• Overuse may cause tissue damage and toxicity.

Interactions
No significant interactions are known.

Side effects
• Skin irritation.

Phenolated Calamine ⓑ
A preparation of ℞ **calamine**, ℞ **phenol**, and ℞ **zinc oxide**.
Formulation: Topical lotion.
Availability: OTC.
Warnings and side effects: See ℞ **calamine**; ℞ **phenol**; ℞ **zinc oxide.**

Phenoptic ⓑ
A preparation of ℞ **phenylephrine hydrochloride**.
Formulation: Eye drops, available in two strengths.
Availability: Prescription only.
Warnings and side effects: See ℞ **phenylephrine hydrochloride.**

phenothiazine ⓓ
Generics: **chlorpromazine; haloperidol; loxapine; molindone; perphenazine; piperazine; prochlorperazine; promazine; promethazine hydrochloride; thiethylperazine maleate; thioridazine; mesoridazine; thiothixene; trifluoperazine.**

Actions and uses
℞ **phenothiazine** drugs are a group that all have a similar chemical structure. Many of them are used as ℞ **antipsychotic** drugs (for example, ℞ **chlorpromazine**, ℞ **promazine**, ℞ **perphenazine**, ℞ **prochlorperazine**, ℞ **trifluoperazine**, ℞ **thioridazine** and ℞ **mesoridazine**) and it is thought that their ℞ **dopamine-recep-**

tor blocker activity in the brain is the reason for their usefulness in treating psychoses (see ✚ **psychotic disorder**). Some other drugs resemble the phenothiazines in action and are sometimes grouped with them, including thioxanthenes (℞ **thiothixene**), diphenylbutylpiperidines/butyrophenones (℞ **haloperidol**), and indolones (℞ **molindone**). A number of phenothiazines have powerful ℞ **antinauseant** or ℞ **antiemetic** actions (℞ **chlorpromazine**, ℞ **prochlorperazine**, ℞ **thiethylperazine**, ℞ **prochlorperazine**, ℞ **promethazine**) and can relieve nausea and vomiting, and another (℞ **piperazine**) can be used as an ℞ **anthelmintic** agent to kill worm infestations.

Limitations

See the individual drug entries.

phenoxybenzamine Ⓖ

Type/Group: **alpha-adrenergic blocker; antihypertensive**.
Brand(s): Dibenzyline.
How administered: Orally.

Used to treat

Phenoxybenzamine is used to lower blood pressure quickly in hypertensive crises in ✚ **pheochromocytoma**. It has been investigated and used in other conditions as well, including for urinary obstruction or retention problems.

Warnings

• It should not be given to people where a fall in blood pressure is not desirable.
• It should be given with caution to people with congestive heart failure, significant cerebral or coronary arteriosclerosis, or with respiratory infection.
• Phenoxybenzamine should be used during pregnancy only when it is clearly needed.
• Medical judgment is required if breast-feeding is being considered.
• Tachycardia and other arrhythmias may occur, and so it is often used with a ℞ **beta-blocker**.
• Alcohol should be avoided.

Interactions

• If taken with non-selective adrenergic stimulants (for example, ℞ **ephedrine**, ℞ **epinephrine**, ℞ **metaraminol**), there is a risk of rapid heartbeat and marked hypotension (lowered blood pressure).

Side effects

• These may include postural hypotension (lowered blood pressure on standing), rapid heartbeat, gastrointestinal disturbances, drowsiness, fatigue, inhibition of ejaculation, nasal congestion, and constriction of the pupils.

phenoxymethyl penicillin Ⓖ

see ℞ **penicillin V**.

phentermine Ⓖ

Type/Group: **appetite suppressant; obesity treatment; CNS stimulant**.
Brand(s): Ionamin; Fastin; Zantryl; Adipex-P; various generic.
How administered: Orally.

Used to treat

Phentermine is used, under medical supervision and on a short-term basis, to aid weight loss in severe ✚ **obesity**. It is potentially subject to abuse and so its proprietary preparations are on the controlled substances list. There is growing doubt among experts over the medical value of such treatment (for instance, there may be a weight relapse once that treatment has finished).

Warnings

• It should not be used by people with known hypersensitivity to sympathomimetic amines, glaucoma, or a history of drug abuse, cardiovascular disease, or moderate to severe hypertension.
• It should be given with caution to anyone with diabetes mellitus, seizure disorders, mild hypertension, or who are taking ℞ **MAOI** antidepressants (see Interactions below).
• It is not known whether or not phentermine can harm the fetus, therefore, it should be used during pregnancy only if medically judged to be needed.
• Medical judgment is also required if breast-feeding is being considered.
• Tolerance to the appetite suppressant effects may develop with a few weeks. If this happens, the dosage must not be increased and use of the drug must stop.
• It may impair the ability to perform skilled tasks requiring alertness, such as driving.
• Phentermine is related to the ℞ **amphetamines** and has abuse potential; it is a Schedule IV controlled substance.

Interactions

• Phentermine must not be taken with, or within two weeks of discontinuing, ℞ **MAOI** antidepressants. Severe and even fatal reactions can occur.
• ℞ **furazolidone** may cause a serious hypertensive reaction.
• The effects of ℞ **guanethidine monosulfate** may be reduced.
• ℞ **tricyclic** antidepressants may reduce the levels of phentermine.

Side effects

• Frequently, nervousness, insomnia, dizziness, over-stimulation, and restlessness.
• Occasionally, headache, gastrointestinal upsets, impotence, testicular pain, and urinary hesitancy.
• Rarely, changes in rate of heart beat, and chest pain.

phentolamine mesilate Ⓖ

see ℞ **phentolamine mesylate**.

phentolamine mesylate Ⓖ

(phentolamine mesilate)
Type/Group: **alpha-adrenergic blocker; antihypertensive**.
Brand(s): Regetine.
How administered: Injection.

Used to treat

Phentolamine mesylate is used to lower blood pressure quickly in hypertensive crises in ✚ **pheochromocytoma** (it is also used in the diagnosis of this condition). It is also used to prevent skin necrosis and sloughing that may occur at the site of ℞ **norepinephrine** or ℞ **dopamine** injection. Phentolamine has been investigated and used in other conditions, as well, including hypertensive crises that arise from ℞ **MAOI** food or drug interactions, and for impotence (erectile dysfunction).

Warnings

• It is a specialist drug used under controlled conditions.

• It should not be given to people with known hypersensitivity to phentolamine, or with a history of heart attack or coronary artery disease, or symptoms suggesting it (for example, angina pectoris).

• It should be given with caution to people with gastritis or peptic ulcer.

• The safety of phentolamine for use during pregnancy or while breast-feeding has not been established. It should be used only when the potential benefit outweighs the risk risk to the fetus.

• Heart attack (myocardial infarction) and stroke have occurred with use of this drug, usually after an injection has caused marked hypotension and a shock-like state.

• Tachycardia and other arrhythmias may occur. Administration of cardiac glycosides should be delayed until rhythm has returned to normal.

Interactions

• The effects of ℞ **ephedrine** and ℞ **epinephrine** are reduced (these are vasoconstrictors and work in opposition to phentolamine).

• If taken with other antihypertensive drugs, ℞ **opioids**, or ℞ **sedatives**, they may make a false-positive reaction more likely in diagnostic use of phentolamine for pheochromocytoma. Use of these drugs should be discontinued at least a day before such a test.

Side effects

• These may include weakness, dizziness, flushing, postural hypotension (fall in blood pressure on standing); dry mouth and nasal congestion, chest pains and heart irregularities, and gastrointestinal disturbances (abdominal pain, nausea, vomiting, diarrhea).

phenylephrine hydrochloride Ⓖ

Type/Group: **alpha-adrenergic stimulant; sympathomimetic; decongestant; vasoconstrictor; cold and cough preparation; mydriatic.**

Brand(s): (As vasoconstrictor/nasal decongestant): AH-Chew D Tablets; Alconefrin; Children's Nostril; Neo-Synephrine; Rhinall; Sinex. (For ophthalmic use): AK-Dilate; AK-Nefrin; Mydfrin 2.5%; Neo-Synephrine; Phenoptic; Prefrin Liquifilm; Relief.
Combinations: With acetaminophen: (Plus) *brompheniramine maleate*: Dimetane Decongestant Tablets. (Plus) *chlorpheniramine maleate*: Aclophen Tablets; Covangesic Tablets (has *pyrilamine maleate*); Dristan Cold Multi-Symptom Formula Tablets; Gendecon Tablets; Histagesic Modified Tablets; Histex SR; ND-Gesic Tablets (has *pyrilamine maleate*). With brompheniramine maleate: Dimetane Decongestant Elixir. With chlorpheniramine maleate: Comhist Tablets, LA Capsules (have *phenyltoloxamine citrate*); Dallergy-D Syrup; ED A-Hist Tablets, Liquid; Histatab Plus Tablets; Histor-D Syrup; Rolatuss Plain Liquid; Ru-Tuss Liquid. (Plus) *pyrilamine tannate*: Atrohist Pediatric Suspension; Gelhist Pediatric Suspension; Rhinatate Tablets; R-Tannamine Tablets, Pediatric Suspension; R-Tannate Tablets, Pediatric Suspension; Rynatan

Pediatric Suspension; Triotann Tablets; Tri-Tannate Tablets, Pediatric Suspension. With codeine phosphate: (Plus) *chlorpheniramine and potassium iodide*: Pediacof Syrup; Pedituss Cough Syrup. (Plus) *promethazine*: Phenergan VC with Codeine Syrup; Pherazine VC w/Codeine Syrup; Promethist with Codeine Syrup. (Plus) *pyrilamine*: Codimal PH Syrup. With dextromethorphan: (Plus) *chlorpheniramine maleate*: Cerose-DM Liquid. (Plus) *chlorpheneramine maleate and guaifenesin*: Donatussin Syrup. (Plus) *pyrilamine maleate*: Codimal DM Syrup. With guaifenesin: Deconsal Sprinkle Capsules; Donatussin Drops (has *chlorpheniramine maleate*); Endal Tablets; Liquibid-D Tablets; Rescon-GG Liquid; Sinupan Capsules. With hydrocodone: (Plus) *chlorpheniramine maleate*: Atuss MS, HD, HD Syrup, DM Syrup; ED-TLC Liquid; ED Tuss HC Liquid; Endagen-HD Liquid; Endal-HD Liquid, Plus Liquid; Histinex HC Syrup; Hituss HC Syrup; Hycomine Compound Tablets (has *acetaminophen, caffeine*); Iodal HD; Iotussin HC Syrup; Tussanil DH Syrup; Vanex-HD Liquid. (Plus) *guaifenesin*: Atuss-G Syrup; Donatussin DC Syrup; Tussafed HC Syrup. With pheniramine maleate: Dristan Nasal Spray; Scot-Tussin Original 5-Action Liquid, Syrup. With promethazine: Phenergan VC Syrup; Promethazine VC Plain Syrup. With pyrilamine: Myci-Spray; Ryna-12 S Liquid. (In hemorrhoid preparations): Preparation H Cooling Gel, Ointment, Suppositories; Hem-Prep Ointment, Suppositories; Medicone Suppositories; Hemorid For Women Cream, Suppositories. (Most combinations available as generics.)
How administered: Orally; nasal; ophthalmic (eye); topically (external); injection.

Used to treat

Phenylephrine is used in a number of cold cures and hemorrhoid brands. It is also used as a nasal decongestant (both by mouth and by nasal spray) and as a mydriatic to dilate the pupil for ophthalmic examination. In emergency situations, it can be given by intravenous injection or infusion to increase blood pressure.

Warnings

• It should not be given to people with known hypersensitivity to this or any other adrenergic drug, with angle-closure glaucoma, who are taking ℞ **MAOI** antidepressants, who have severe high blood pressure, or coronary artery disease.

• It should be given with caution to people with certain heart and other cardiovascular disorders, hyperthyroidism, diabetes mellitus, enlarged prostate, or increased intraocular pressure (pressure in the eyeball, including glaucoma).

• Phenylephrine's effects in pregnancy are not known, and it should be used only if there is a clear benefit.

• Medical judgment is required if breast-feeding is being considered.

• Eyedrops should not be used while soft contact lenses are being worn.

• Overuse may cause symptoms such as nervousness and insomnia, and may make congestion worse, which is an effect called "rebound congestion."

• It should be used with caution by the elderly, as they are more likely to suffer side effects.

• The manufacturer's recommendations must be followed carefully when giving this drug to children under 12.

Interactions

These apply to oral and injected doses. When used topically (nose or eyes), at recommended doses, these interactions are less frequent (except in cases of overdose).

• Phenylephrine should not be used with ℞ **MAOI** antidepressants, or within three weeks of stopping MAOI treatment, because this may cause a hypertensive crisis.

• If used with ℞ **theophylline**, there may be unpredictable effects, sometimes with toxicity.

• ℞ **Antacids** taken in high doses slow the removal from the body of phenylephrine, increasing the risk of side effects.

• If used with ℞ **tricyclic** antidepressants, ℞ **guanethidine monosulfate**, and ℞ **methyldopa**, there is a possibility of increased blood pressure.

Side effects

• These depend on how it is administered. As eyedrops it may cause blurred vision, stinging, pain in the eye, and photophobia. When used as a nasal decongestant, it may cause irritation in the nose.

• Although more common with oral or injected doses, all forms of phenylephrine may cause hypertension and headache, changes in heart rate, vomiting, tingling and coolness of the skin, anxiety, dizziness, insomnia, and tremor.

phenytoin ⓖ

Type/Group: **antiarrhythmic; anticonvulsant; antiepileptic.**
Brand(s): **Dilantin Infatab, Dilantin-125, Kapseals;** various generic.
How administered: Orally; injection.

Used to treat

Phenytoin is used to treat most forms of ✪ **epilepsy** (except absence seizures) and to prevent or treat seizures during or following head trauma or in ✪ **Reye's syndrome** or neurosurgery. It has been investigated for treatment of trigeminal (facial) neuralgia, certain arrhythmias, diabetic neuropathy pain, and migraine.

Warnings

• Avoid its use in people with known hypersensitivity to this drug, or with porphyria.

• In its injected form it should not be given to anyone with certain heart conduction disorders.

• Medical judgment is required if there is liver or kidney impairment, or diabetes mellitus.

• Phenytoin is associated with an increase in frequency of certain birth defects and should not be used during pregnancy. However, because uncontrolled seizures can also threaten fetal health, medical judgment is needed to weigh potential benefits and risks.

• Breast-feeding mothers should either discontinue using this drug or stop breast-feeding.

• Medical advice must be sought if a skin rash appears.

• Phenytoin may raise blood glucose levels and so medical judgment is necessary to assess benefits and risks for diabetics.

• Withdrawal should be gradual otherwise it may precipitate attacks.

• A relationship has been suggested between phenytoin and some disorders of the lymph system, therefore, any lymphatic symptoms (tenderness, pain, or swelling) should be brought to the doctor's attention.

Interactions

• ℞ **tricyclic** antidepressants may precipitate seizures.

• The following drugs may increase phenytoin's effects and so increase the risk of side effects: ℞ **amiodarone hydrochloride**; ℞ **chloramphenicol**; ℞ **chlordiazepoxide**; ℞ **diazepam**; ℞ **dicumarol**; ℞ **disulfiram**; ℞ **estrogens**; ℞ **fluoxetine**; ℞ **H₂-antagonists**; halothane; ℞ **isoniazid**; ℞ **methylphenidate**; ℞ **phenothiazines**; phenylbutazone; ℞ **salicylates**; succinimides (for example, ℞ **ethosuximide**, ℞ **methsuximide**), ℞ **sulfonamides**; ℞ **tolbutamide**; ℞ **trazodone**.

• ℞ **Lithium** and ℞ **primidone** may increase phenytoin's effects, with potential for toxicity.

• The effects if taken with ℞ **clonazepam**, ℞ **phenobarbital**, ℞ **sodium valproate**, or ℞ **valproic acid** are unpredictable.

• Alcohol may either raise or lower levels of phenytoin, depending on drinking habits.

• The therapeutic effects of the following drugs may be reduced: ℞ **acetaminophen**; ℞ **corticosteroids**; coumarin ℞ **anticoagulants**; ℞ **digitoxin**; ℞ **dopamine**; ℞ **doxycycline**; ℞ **estrogens**; ℞ **furosemide**; oral ℞ **contraceptives**; ℞ **quinidine**; ℞ **rifampin**; ℞ **theophylline**; ♒ **vitamin D**.

• ℞ **Carbamazepine**, ℞ **reserpine**, and ℞ **sucralfate** lower levels of phenytoin.

Side effects

These depend on dose, use, and how administered. They tend to be frequent and include:

• Nausea, vomiting, confusion, slurred speech, headache, dizziness, nervousness, insomnia;

• Rarely, movement disorders, peripheral nerve disorders, eye-flicker and blurred vision, rashes, acne, enlargement of the gums, growth of excess hair, and blood disorders;

• Hypersensitivity reactions (swollen lymph glands, fever, aches, rash), systemic lupus erythematosus, and hepatitis have occurred;

• Potentially serious side effects include effects on the heart and cardiovascular system, liver, skin, and blood cells.

Pherazine DM Syrup ⓑ

A preparation of ℞ **dextromethorphan** and ℞ **promethazine hydrochloride**.

Formulation: Oral syrup.

Availability: Prescription only.

Warnings and side effects: See ℞ **dextromethorphan**; ℞ **promethazine hydrochloride**.

Pherazine VC with Codeine Syrup ⓑ

A preparation of ℞ **codeine phosphate**, ℞ **phenylephrine hydrochloride**, and ℞ **promethazine hydrochloride**.

Formulation: Oral syrup.

Availability: May or may not require a prescription.

Warnings and side effects: See ℞ **codeine phosphate**; ℞ **phenylephrine hydrochloride**; ℞ **promethazine hydrochloride**.

Pherazine w/Codeine Syrup Ⓜ

A preparation of ℞ **codeine phosphate** and ℞ **promethazine hydrochloride**.
Formulation: Oral syrup.
Availability: May or may not require a prescription.
Warnings and side effects: See ℞ **codeine phosphate**; ℞ **promethazine hydrochloride**.

Phillips' Chewable Tablets Ⓜ

A preparation of ℞ **magnesium hydroxide**.
Formulation: Oral tablets, chewable.
Availability: OTC.
Warnings and side effects: See ℞ **magnesium hydroxide**.

Phillips' Liqui-Gels Ⓜ

A preparation of ℞ **docusate sodium**.
Formulation: Oral gelcaps.
Availability: OTC.
Warnings and side effects: See ℞ **docusate sodium**.

Phillips' Milk of Magnesia Ⓜ

A preparation of ℞ **magnesium hydroxide**.
Formulation: Oral liquid.
Availability: OTC.
Warnings and side effects: See ℞ **magnesium hydroxide**.

pHisoHex Ⓜ

A preparation of ℞ **hexachlorophene**.
Formulation: Liquid.
Availability: Prescription only.
Warnings and side effects: See ℞ **hexachlorophene**.

phosphodiesterase inhibitor Ⓓ

(PDE-inhibitor)
Generics: **milrinone; sildenafil**.

Actions and uses

℞ **phosphodiesterase inhibitor** drugs work by inhibiting certain enzymes called phosphodiesterases that occur in a number of different forms in the body, and have important roles in cell metabolism (the biochemical functioning of cells). Some of the phosphodiesterase inhibitors work relatively selectively at a form of the enzyme (type III) found in the heart and vascular smooth muscle. Agents of this type affect the heart muscle (myocardium) and blood vessels in ways that are very similar to ℞ **beta-adrenergic stimulant** drugs, and act as ℞ **cardiac stimulant** and ℞ **vasodilator** drugs. They have so far mainly been used as short-term cardiac stimulant agents and in short-term severe congestive ℞ **heart failure treatment**, especially where other drugs have been unsuccessful. The group includes ℞ **PDE-inhibitors** (such as ℞ **milrinone**). Also, the vasodilator action (widens blood vessels) is used by ℞ **sildenafil** (Viagra) in ℞ **impotence treatment** for men.

Limitations

This is a relatively new class of drugs and so the potential side effects are not yet fully investigated or known. Those drugs used to treat acute severe congestive heart failure are only used in a hospital environment. See also the individual drug entries.

Phrenilin Forte Ⓜ

A preparation of ℞ **acetaminophen**, and butalbital.
Formulation: Oral capsules.
Availability: Prescription only.
Warnings and side effects: See ℞ **acetaminophen**; ℞ **butabarbital**.

phytonadione Ⓐ

(phytomenadione)
Type/Group: **vitamin; hemostatic**.
Brand(s): AquaMEPHYTON; Mephyton.
How administered: Orally; injection.

Used to treat

Phytonadione (vitamin K_1) is a natural form of vitamin K and is normally obtained from vegetables and dairy products. Phytonadione can be used to treat vitamin K deficiency, but not a deficiency caused by malabsorption states (in such cases vitamin K_1 or menadiol sodium phosphate, the synthetic form of vitamin K_3, must be used). It is given as a single intramuscular injection, or by mouth to prevent vitamin K deficiency bleeding in newborn babies and to treat hypothrombinemia (it promotes production of prothrombin in the liver).

Warnings

• It should not be given to people with known hypersensitivity to any component of the products or severe liver disease.
• It should be given with caution to people with G6PD deficiency.
• Vitamin K crosses the placenta and it should be used during pregnancy only if it is clearly needed.
• Medical judgment is required if breast-feeding is being considered.
• Severe allergic-like reactions have occurred during intravenous infusion.
• Vitamin K does not counteract the anticoagulant action of heparin.

Interactions

• The effects of ℞ **anticoagulants** may be reduced.
• ℞ **Mineral oil** may reduce the absorption of vitamin K.

Side effects

• Headache, flushing sensation, rash, and hives.
• Rarely hyperbilirubinemia in newborns.

Pilocar Ⓜ

A preparation of ℞ **pilocarpine**.
Formulation: Ophthalmic solution in several strengths.
Availability: Prescription only.
Warnings and side effects: See ℞ **pilocarpine**.

pilocarpine Ⓐ

(pilocarpine hydrochloride; pilocarpine nitrate)
Type/Group: **alkaloid; parasympathomimetic**.
Brand(s): Adsorbocarpine; Akarpine; Isopto Carpine; Ocusert Pilo; Pilocar; Piloptic; Pilostat; Pilopine; HS Salagen; various generic.

How administered: Orally; topically (eye).
Used to treat
Pilocarpine is a plant alkaloid drug and can be applied to the eye to treat ✪ **glaucoma** by improving drainage of aqueous fluid from the eye, and to constrict the pupil of the eye after it has been dilated for ophthalmic examination. It can be used to alleviate the symptoms of salivary gland hypofunction with dry mouth following irradiation for head and neck cancer.
Warnings
• It should not be given to people with known hypersensitivity to the drug, with uncontrolled asthma, or those in whom acute contraction of the eye pupil is undesirable.
• It should be given with caution to people with asthma, hypertension, bradycardia, hyperthyroidism, cardiovascular disease, renal colic, biliary disease, epilepsy, or parkinsonism.
• Pilocarpine should be used during pregnancy only if the potential benefits outweigh the possible risk to the fetus.
• Medical judgment is required if breast-feeding is being considered. It is not known whether this drug appears in breast milk and there is a potential for serious adverse reactions.
• It can cause visual disturbances, especially at night, and may impair the ability to drive.
Interactions
• The effects of ℞ **anticholinergics** may be reduced.
• If used with ℞ **beta-blockers**, there may be conduction (nerve impulse) disturbances.
Side effects
• When taken orally, there may be sweating, chills, diarrhea or constipation, nausea and vomiting, abdominal pain, hypertension, tears, dizziness, rhinitis, weakness, increased urinary frequency, headache, upset stomach, vasodilatation, and flushing.
• Other possible side effects include effects on the heart and breathing, confusion, and tremors.

Pilopine HS ℞
A preparation of ℞ **pilocarpine**.
Formulation: Ophthalmic gel.
Availability: Prescription only.
Warnings and side effects: See ℞ **pilocarpine**.

Piloptic 1; 2; 3; 4; 6 ℞
A preparation of ℞ **pilocarpine**.
Formulation: Ophthalmic solution in several strengths.
Availability: Prescription only.
Warnings and side effects: See ℞ **pilocarpine**.

Pilostat ℞
A preparation of ℞ **pilocarpine**.
Formulation: Ophthalmic solution in several strengths.
Availability: Prescription only.
Warnings and side effects: See ℞ **pilocarpine**.

Pima Syrup ℞
A preparation of ℞ **potassium iodide**.
Formulation: Oral syrup.

Availability: Prescription only.
Warnings and side effects: See ℞ **potassium iodide**.

pimozide ℞
Type/Group: **antipsychotic; brain-motor disorder treatment**.
Brand(s): Orap; various generic.
How administered: Orally.
Used to treat
Pimozide is one of the diphenylbutylpiperidines chemical group of antipsychotic drugs. It is sometimes used to treat ✪ **schizophrenia** in certain cases, but is mainly used to treat people who have ✪ **brain-motor disorder** Tourette syndrome who are nonresponsive to other treatments.
Warnings
• It should not be given to people with known hypersensitivity to pimozide, or with certain blood cell disorders, severe CNS (central nervous system) depression, heart arrhythmias, or tics other than those due to Tourette's.
• It should be given with caution to people with breast cancer, kidney or liver disease, heart disease, narrow-angle glaucoma, intestinal blockage, urinary tract blockage or difficult urination, hypokalemia (low blood potassium levels), a history of seizures, or known sensivity to other antipsychotic drugs. It should also be given with caution to anyone over 65 and children.
• Pimozide should be used during pregnancy only if it is clearly needed.
• Although it not known whether it appears in breast milk, its use by nursing mothers is not recommended.
• It has been linked with abnormalities of heart rhythm at high doses.
• Sudden unexpected deaths have occurred in experimental studies not involving use for Tourette's syndrome, which may have been due to adverse effects on the heart. For this reason, monitoring with periodic electrocardiograms is recommended.
• There is a risk of developing a potentially life-threatening blood disorder. A doctor must be contacted immediately if any symptoms of infection, such as lethargy, weakness, fever, or sore throat, develop.
• It causes drowsiness and so the performance of skilled tasks, such as driving, may be impaired.
• Dosage must be reduced gradually when stopping treatment.
• If used for a long time, tardive dyskinesia (see ℞ **antipsychotic**) occasionally develops.
Interactions
• Avoid grapefruit juice because it increases the risk of problems with heart rhythm.
• The following drugs increases the risk of heart arrhythmias and should not be taken with pimozide: ℞ **macrolide** antibiotics (℞ **clarithromycin**, ℞ **erythromycin**, ℞ **azithromycin**, ℞ **dirithromycin**); ℞ **azole** ℞ **antifungals** (℞ **itraconazole** ℞ **ketoconazole**); ℞ **antiviral** protease inhibitors (℞ **ritonavir**, ℞ **saquinavir**, ℞ **indinavir**, ℞ **nelfinavir**, ℞ **nefazodone**); ℞ **tricyclic** antidepressants (for example, ℞ **amitriptyline**, ℞ **desipramine**); ℞ **zileuton**; ℞ **quinidine**.

Key to symbols: ✪ = Disorder Section ℞ = Drug Section ♣ = Herbal Section ◊◊ = Supplement Section

• ℞ Fluoxetine, ℞ paroxetine, and ℞ tacrine increase the risk of extrapyramidal symptoms.

• The antiparkinsonism effects of ℞ levodopa are reduced.

• If used with ℞ clonidine hydrochloride or ℞ meperidine, there is an increased risk of hypotension.

• If used with ℞ lithium the effects of both drugs are reduced.

• ℞ Anticholinergics (for example, ℞ benztropine), ℞ bromocriptine, ℞ carbamazepine, and ℞ phenobarbital reduce the effects of pimozide.

• ℞ amphetamines, ℞ methylphenidate, and pemoline may cause tics, but pimozide is not used to treat tics caused by other medicines. Therefore, these drugs should be discontinued before starting pimozide to make sure that they did not cause the symptoms.

Side effects

• Akathisia (restlessness and urge to keep moving), drowsiness, constipation, dry mouth, extrapyramidal symptoms (see ℞ antipsychotic), and constipation.

• Less frequently, photosensitivity (abnormal sensitivity to light), rash, confusion (especially in older adults), difficulty urinating, blurred vision, decreased sweating, sexual dysfunction, worsening of glaucoma, loss of appetite, and breast changes.

• Rarely, seizure, blood cell disorders, neuroleptic malignant syndrome (a potentially fatal condition characterized by very high fever, muscle rigidity, changes in mental status, and irregular pulse, blood pressure and/or heart rhythm).

pindolol Ⓖ

Type/Group: **beta-blocker; antihypertensive.**
Brand(s): Visken; various generic.
How administered: Orally.

Used to treat

Pindolol is used to lower blood pressure in Ⓞ **hypertension.**

Warnings

• It should not be given to people with known hypersensitivity to any beta-blocking drug, who have certain heartbeat irregularities or heart failure, or bronchial asthma. It should not be used in cardiogenic shock.

• It should be given with caution to people with diabetes mellitus or hypoglycemia, hyperthyroidism, myasthenia gravis, congestive heart failure, peripheral vascular disease, bronchospastic disease (for example, chronic bronchitis or emphysema), or liver impairment.

• Pindolol should be used during pregnancy only if the potential benefit outweighs the possible risk to the fetus.

• It appears in breast milk, and so nursing women should discontinue using this drug or stop breast-feeding.

• Abruptly stopping using a beta-blocker may have adverse effects on the heart.

• The use of this drug may mask signs of hyperthyroidism or hypoglycemia.

• Other medications (including OTCs, herbal remedies, and supplements) must not be taken without consulting a doctor. Some ℞ nasal decongestants, commonly available over the counter, contain ℞ alpha-adrenergic stimulants (for example,

℞ phenylephrine) that may cause a severe hypertensive reaction if taken with beta-blockers.

Interactions

• A serious blood pressure increase may occur after withdrawal from ℞ clonidine hydrochloride or both drugs at the same time.

• The effects of ℞ alpha-adrenergic stimulants, ℞ ergot alkaloids, ℞ epinephrine, and ℞ lidocaine may be increased, with the risk of serious adverse effects.

• ℞ Calcium-channel blockers (particularly ℞ diltiazem hydrochloride and ℞ verapamil), ℞ guanethidine monosulfate, and ℞ reserpine have the potential for increasing undesirable effects, with exaggerated slowing of heartbeat or hypotension. Verapamil and pindolol should not be used together.

• The effects of nondepolarizing ℞ skeletal muscle relaxants may be variable, with the possible risk of significant adverse effects associated with major surgery.

• The effects of ℞ beta-adrenergic stimulants (for example, ℞ albuterol, ℞ terbutaline), ℞ insulin, and ℞ sulfonylureas may be reduced by pindolol.

• ℞ Antacids (for example, ℞ aluminum hydroxide, ℞ magnesium hydroxide), ℞ barbiturates, ⚷ calcium salts, ℞ cholestyramine, ℞ colestipol hydrochloride, ℞ NSAIDs, ℞ penicillins, and ℞ rifampin may reduce the levels and effectiveness of beta-blockers.

• If used with ℞ diuretics and other antihypertensive drugs, there are additive effects which are often used to therapeutic advantage.

Side effects

These are infrequent and may include:

• Dizziness, fatigue, swelling of the extremities, muscle pain or cramps, insomnia, gastrointestinal disturbances (for example, nausea, discomfort, diarrhea), visual disturbances, shortness of breath, and slowing of the heart rate;

• Occasionally, chest pain, cold extremities, wheezing, rash or itching, or abnormal dreams. Changes in liver function may occur;

• Heart failure, should it develop, generally requires withdrawal (gradually, if possible) of this drug.

Pin-Rid Ⓑ

A preparation of ℞ **pyrantel.**
Formulation: Oral capsules; oral liquid.
Availability: OTC.
Warnings and side effects: See ℞ pyrantel.

Pin-X Ⓑ

A preparation of ℞ **pyrantel.**
Formulation: Oral liquid.
Availability: OTC.
Warnings and side effects: See ℞ pyrantel.

pioglitazone Ⓖ

Type/Group: **antidiabetic; oral hypoglycemic.**
Brand(s): Actos.
How administered: Orally.

Used to treat

Pioglitazone, a thiazolidinedione, is used in combination with other drugs to improve blood sugar control in type 2 ✪ **diabetes mellitus**.

Warnings

• It should not be given to people with known sensitivity to pioglitazone.

• Its safety in pregnancy is not established. It should be used only if clearly needed.

• It is not recommended for use while breast-feeding.

• Premenopausal women who have not been ovulating (for example, those with polycystic ovary disease, or taking the contraceptive pill) may resume ovulation and be at risk for pregnancy.

• There is a possibility that this drug may cause liver damage (monitoring of liver function will be carried out). Symptoms such as nausea, abdominal pain, fatigue, appetite loss, dark urine, or jaundice must be reported to a doctor.

• A doctor must be consulted before taking any other medication, including OTCs, herbal remedies, and supplements, as there is a potential for interaction with pioglitazone.

Interactions

• ℞ **ketoconazole** may increase the effects of pioglitazone.

• The effects of ℞ **estrogens** and ℞ **oral contraceptives** are reduced.

• Levels of ℞ **cyclosporine** may be reduced.

Side effects

• Headache, upper respiratory tract infection, and muscle aches.

piperacillin ⓖ

Type/Group: **antibiotic; penicillin; antibacterial**.
Brand(s): Pipracil. Combinations: With *tazobactam*: Zosyn.
How administered: Injection; intravenous infusion.

Used to treat

Piperacillin is a synthetic penicillin used against a number of important Gram-negative bacteria, including *Pseudomonas aeruginosa* as well as some Gram-positive bacteria. It can be used to treat ✪ **bacterial infections** that cause ✪ **septicemia**, ✪ **peritonitis**, infections of the respiratory and urinary tracts, and gynecological, bone, and skin infections. In combination with the beta-lactamase inhibitor tazobactam (which inhibits resistance to penicillin) it may also be used to treat resistant bacterial strains.

Warnings

• It should not be used by people with known hypersensitivity to penicillins, ℞ **cephalosporins**, or ℞ **imipenem**.

• It should be given with caution to people with congestive heart failure and children under 12 years of age.

• Penicillins cross the placenta and should be used in pregnancy only if medically judged to be needed.

• Medical judgment is also needed for breast-feeding mothers.

• Serious and occasionally fatal hypersensitivity reactions can occur.

• Superinfections from the altered bacterial balance created by antibiotic treatment may occur and may result in

✪ **pseudomembranous colitis**. A doctor must be contacted if there is severe abdominal pain, or moderate to severe diarrhea.

Interactions

• The effectiveness of ℞ **aminoglycosides** may be reduced.

• ℞ **Chloramphenicol**, ℞ **macrolide** antibiotics, and ℞ **tetracyclines** may reduce the effectiveness of penicillins.

• Large doses of penicillin may increase the levels of ℞ **methotrexate**.

• The effectiveness of ℞ **oral contraceptives** may be impaired.

Side effects

• Frequently, diarrhea, other gastrointestinal effects, and headache.

• Occasionally, urinary abnormalities, vaginal infection, anemia, increased bleeding time, increased sodium concentration, and reduced potassium levels.

• Rare but serious effects include bone marrow depression, and kidney infections.

piperazine ⓖ

Type/Group: **anthelmintic**.
Brand(s): Generic only.
How administered: Orally.

Used to treat

Piperazine is a synthetic anthelmintic drug (a ℞ **phenothiazine**) used to treat infestation by roundworms and pinworms (see ✪ **worms**).

Warnings

• It should not be given to people with known hypersensitivity to this drug.

• It should be given with caution to people with kidney or liver impairment, neurological or seizure disorders, and children.

• Its safety in pregnancy and breast-feeding has not been studied. Discuss with doctor before using.

• A doctor must be contacted if blurring of vision, clumsiness, crawling or tingling feeling of the skin, fever, irregular, twisting movement (especially of the face, arms, and legs), joint pain, skin rash, or itching occur.

• When used to treat pinworms, infestation may recur.

Interactions

• ℞ **Phenothiazines** increase the risk of seizure.

• If taken with ℞ **pyrantel**, the effects of both drugs are reduced.

Side effects

• Nausea/vomiting, abdominal cramps, headache, dizziness, vertigo, ataxia, seizures, and cataracts.

Pipracil ⓡ

A preparation of ℞ **piperacillin**.
Formulation: Injection; intravenous infusion.
Availability: Prescription only.
Warnings and side effects: See ℞ **piperacillin**.

pirbuterol ⓖ

Type/Group: **beta-adrenergic stimulant; antiasthmatic; sympathomimetic**.
Brand(s): Maxair.

How administered: Inhalation.

Used to treat

Pirbuterol is used to prevent and treat bronchospasm, including in those with ✪ **asthma**.

Warnings

• It should not be given to people with known hypersensitivity to pirbuterol or similar agents.

• It should be given with caution to people with certain heart diseases, diabetes mellitus, prostatic hypertrophy, or hypertension.

• It should be used during pregnancy only if clearly needed, as it may cross the placenta and inhibit uterine contractions.

• Medical judgment is required if breast-feeding is being considered. It is not known if it appears in breast milk.

• Rarely, it may have adverse effects on heart and blood pressure, or lead to paradoxical bronchoconstriction.

Interactions

• ℞ **Beta-blockers** may decrease the effects of pirbuterol.

• If used with ℞ **furosemide**, there is a risk of enhancing furosemide's potassium-lowering effect.

Side effects

• Frequently, tremors, speeded heartbeat, shakiness, nervousness, nausea, vomiting, and dry mouth.

• Occasionally, palpitations, dizziness, weakness, headache, gastrointestinal distress, cough, and dry throat.

• Rarely, changes in blood pressure, drowsiness, unusual taste, and bronchospasm.

piroxicam Ⓖ

Type/Group: **anti-inflammatory; antirheumatic; non-narcotic analgesic; NSAID.**
Brand(s): Feldene; various generic.
How administered: Orally.

Used to treat

Piroxicam has a long duration of action, and is used to treat pain and inflammation in ✪ **musculoskeletal disorders** such as ✪ **osteoarthritis** and ✪ **rheumatoid arthritis.**

Warnings

• It should not be used by people with known hypersensitivity to this drug or to other NSAIDs (including ℞ **aspirin**), who have chronic kidney disease, certain bleeding disorders or conditions (for example, hemophilia, vitamin K deficiency, low blood-platelet levels), or who have a tendency to, or active, peptic ulceration.

• It should be given with caution to people with diabetes, SLE (systemic lupus erythematosus), porphyria, or allergic disorders (especially asthma and skin conditions), who are elderly, or with any kind of kidney impairment or certain liver disorders.

• Piroxicam should be used during pregnancy only if medically judged to be needed. In the third trimester, its risks to the fetus rise, and so it should only be used if the benefits clearly outweigh the risks to the fetus.

• Breast-feeding mothers should either discontinue this drug or stop breast-feeding.

• With regular, long-term use (as in the treatment of osteoarthritis), NSAIDs may cause gastrointestinal bleeding, ulceration, or perforation. Any signs of bleeding (for example, black stools) should be reported to a physician immediately.

• Most NSAIDs have the potential, particularly with regular use, to cause liver damage. Periodic evaluation of liver function is necessary in long-term therapy (more than two months).

• Side effects are more frequent in the elderly.

• Gastrointestinal upsets may be minimized by taking the drug with milk or food.

Interactions

• There is generally no added benefit in taking other NSAIDs or other ℞ **salicylates** (especially aspirin) at the same time, but there is a higher risk of gastrointestinal upsets and bleeding.

• Alcohol, ℞ **corticosteroids**, and ℞ **cholestyramine** increase the risk of bleeding, particularly if there is an existing ulcer.

• ℞ **Anticoagulant**, ℞ **antiplatelet**, and ℞ **thrombolytic** drugs may increase bleeding time.

• The effectiveness of ℞ **ACE inhibitors**, ℞ **beta-blockers**, and ℞ **diuretics** may be reduced.

• ℞ **Ritonavir** and piroxicam must not be taken together.

• The effects of ℞ **digoxin**, ℞ **lithium**, and ℞ **methotrexate** may be exaggerated, with potential for toxicity.

• Foodstuffs and herbals with ℞ **antiplatelet** properties, for example, ♣ **ginger**, ⚘ **garlic**, and various herbal preparations, may add to the antiplatelet effect of NSAIDs.

Side effects

These vary in severity and how often they occur. For its class, piroxicam has a slightly higher risk of gastric bleeding.

• Commonly, gastrointestinal upsets, heartburn, nausea, swelling of the extremities, dizziness and headache.

• Less frequently, constipation, diarrhea, vomiting, blurred vision, ringing in the ears, itching, rash, drowsiness, depression, malaise, and insomnia.

• Prolonged bleeding time (with consequent risk of ulceration) is possible with high dosage, and other blood changes can occur, including anemia.

• Hypersensitivity reactions may include symptoms such as hives, rash, chest tightness, asthma, or bronchospasm.

• Reversible kidney failure, particularly in renal impairment, has occurred. Liver damage is rare.

Pitocin Ⓑ

A preparation of ℞ **oxytocin.**
Formulation: Injection.
Availability: Prescription only.
Warnings and side effects: See ℞ **oxytocin.**

Pitressin Synthetic Ⓑ

A preparation of ℞ **vasopressin.**
Formulation: Injection.
Availability: Prescription only.
Warnings and side effects: See ℞ **vasopressin.**

pituitary hormone (anterior) Ⓓ

see ℞ anterior pituitary hormone.

pituitary hormone (posterior) Ⓓ

see ℞ posterior pituitary hormone.

Plan B Ⓑ

A preparation of ℞ levonorgestrel.
Formulation: Oral tablets.
Availability: Prescription only.
Warnings and side effects: See ℞ levonorgestrel.

Plaquenil Sulfate Ⓑ

A preparation of ℞ hydroxychloroquine sulfate.
Formulation: Oral tablets.
Availability: Prescription only.
Warnings and side effects: See ℞ hydroxychloroquine sulfate.

Platinol-AQ Ⓑ

A preparation of ℞ cisplatin.
Formulation: Powder for injection.
Availability: Prescription only.
Warnings and side effects: See ℞ cisplatin.

Plavix Ⓑ

A preparation of ℞ clopidogrel.
Formulation: Oral tablets.
Availability: Prescription only.
Warnings and side effects: See ℞ clopidogrel.

Plegine Ⓑ

A preparation of ℞ phendimetrazine.
Formulation: Oral tablets.
Availability: Prescription only.
Warnings and side effects: See ℞ phendimetrazine.

Plendil Ⓑ

A preparation of ℞ felodipine.
Formulation: Oral tablets, extended release, available in 3 strengths.
Availability: Prescription only.
Warnings and side effects: See ℞ felodipine.

Pletal Ⓑ

A preparation of ℞ cilostazol.
Formulation: Oral tablets, available in two strengths.
Availability: Prescription only.
Warnings and side effects: See ℞ cilostazol.

PMB Ⓑ

A preparation of ℞ estrogens, conjugated and ℞ meprobamate.
Formulation: Oral tablets.
Availability: Prescription only.
Warnings and side effects: See ℞ estrogens, conjugated; ℞ meprobamate.

pneumococcal vaccine Ⓖ

Type/Group: **vaccine.**

Brand(s): Pneumovax 23; Pnu-Immune 23; Prevnar.
How administered: Injection.

Used to treat

Pneumococcal vaccines are used for ℞ immunization against ✚ pneumonia caused by strains of the bacterium *Streptococcus pneumoniae*. Two types are available: *pneumococcal vaccine, polyvalent* (for adults and children over two) and the recently approved *pneumococcal 7-valent conjugate vaccine* (for infants and toddlers), which confers a narrower range of immunity than the polyvalent vaccine. The adult vaccine is intended only for those people at particular risk from a pneumococcal infection prevalent within a community (such as people with chronic lung, liver, kidney, or heart disease, or with diabetes or HIV); the infant vaccine may be used whenever immunization is thought desirable. The duration of protection is considered to be about five years.

Warnings

• It should not be given to people with known hypersensitivity to this vaccine or, in the case of 7-valent conjugate vaccine, to diphtheria toxoid (which is bound to pneumococcal antigens in this version).
• Its use should be postponed for people with respiratory infections or any acute febrile (feverish) illness.
• It is not recommended for use in pregnancy, though it may be given when medically judged to be clearly needed.
• Medical judgment is required if breast-feeding is being considered.
• This vaccine should not be administered less than two weeks prior to starting a course of treatment with any kind of ℞ immunosuppressant agent.
• After administration, people will be required to wait for some time to ensure that there is no serious reaction (such as anaphylaxis).

Interactions

• Immunosuppressants (for example, ℞ corticosteroids, ℞ cytotoxics, radiation therapy) may reduce the effectiveness of the vaccine in conferring immunity.
• Caution is required if ℞ anticoagulants are being taken.

Side effects

• There may be swelling, irritation or tenderness at the site of vaccination, and low grade fever, mild achiness, or headache.
• Infrequently, skin rash, hives, arthralgia, and acute fever.
• Rarely, anaphylaxis has been reported.

Pneumotussin Tablets; HC Syrup Ⓑ

A preparation of ℞ hydrocodone bitartrate and ℞ guaifenesin.
Formulation: Oral tablets; syrup.
Availability: Prescription only.
Warnings and side effects: See ℞ hydrocodone bitartrate; ℞ guaifenesin.

Pneumovax 23 Ⓑ

A preparation of pneumococcal vaccine, polyvalent.
Formulation: Injection.
Availability: Prescription only.
Warnings and side effects: See ℞ pneumococcal vaccine.

Pnu-Immune 23 ®
A preparation of pneumococcal vaccine, polyvalent.
Formulation: Injection.
Availability: Prescription only.
Warnings and side effects: See ℞ **pneumococcal vaccine**.

Podocon-25 ®
A preparation of ℞ **podofilox**.
Formulation: Topical liquid.
Availability: Prescription only.
Warnings and side effects: See ℞ **podofilox**.

podofilox ⑥
Type/Group: **keratolytic**.
Brand(s): Condylox; Podocon-25; Podofin.
How administered: Topically (external).

Used to treat
Podofilox is a keratolytic and caustic agent that can be used to treat and dissolve venereal ✪ **warts**. Another form, *podophyllum resin*, is used only under medical supervision.

Warnings
• It should not be given to people with known hypersensitivity to this drug or any components of the formulation. Podophyllum resin should not be used by anyone with diabetes, using steroids, or with poor blood circulation.
• Podofilox's safety during pregnancy has not been established. It should be used only if the benefits outweigh the possible risk to the fetus. *Podophyllum resin* should not be used in pregnancy, as it has been associated with birth defects and stillbirths.
• Neither form is not recommended for use while breast-feeding.
• Contact with the eyes and broken or irritated skin must be avoided.

Interactions
No significant interactions are known.

Side effects
• Burning, pain, inflammation, erosion of skin, and itching.

Podofin ®
A preparation of podofyllium resin.
Formulation: Topical liquid.
Availability: Prescription only.
Warnings and side effects: See ℞ **podofilox**.

Polaramine Expectorant Liquid ®
A preparation of ℞ **pseudoephedrine**, ℞ **guaifenesin**, and dex-chlorpheniramine maleate.
Formulation: Oral liquid.
Availability: Prescription only.
Warnings and side effects: See ℞ **pseudoephedrine**;
℞ **guaifenesin**; ℞ **chlorpheniramine maleate**.

Polaramine Tablets; Repetabs; Syrup ®
A preparation of dexchlorpheniramine maleate.
Formulation: Oral syrup; tablets, Repetabs are time release.
Availability: Prescription only.

Warnings and side effects: See ℞ **chlorpheniramine maleate**.

poliomyelitis vaccines ⑥
see ℞ **poliovirus vaccine**.

poliovirus vaccine ⑥
(poliomyelitis vaccine; Salk vaccine; Sabin vaccine)
Type/Group: **vaccine**.
Brand(s): IPOL; Orimune.
How administered: Orally; injection.

Used to treat
Poliovirus vaccine ℞ **immunization** is available in two types: poliovirus vaccine, inactivated (IPV) (Salk) is a suspension of dead viruses injected into the body so that the body produces antibodies and becomes immune; poliovirus vaccine live, oral (OPV) (Sabin) is a suspension of live but attenuated (weakened) polio viruses (of polio virus types 1, 2, and 3) for oral administration. Inactivated vaccine is now recommended in childhood immunization programs, and for unimmunized adults. The inactivated form is also used when, for whatever reason, use of the live vaccine is not considered safe (for example, for people with immunodeficiency disorders, or anyone who will be in close contact with them). The live vaccine may be used in special circumstances, as for example when an outbreak of polio (see ✪ **poliomyelitis**) is feared and immunity must be developed quickly, or when travel to an endemic area is planned within less than four weeks. In those whose object is to take the full course of shots, live virus vaccine may be substituted in the last two doses.

Warnings
• The inactivated vaccine should not be given to people with known sensitivity to neomycin, streptomycin, or polymyxin B, which are used in its preparation and may be present in the vaccine.
• The live virus vaccine should not be given to people with any of a wide range of immunodeficiency disorders, or with temporarily reduced immune responses (as from corticosteroid or radiation therapy), or to those who will be in close contact with such individuals.
• Use of either vaccine should be postponed in anyone with an acute illness or in a debilitated condition.
• Use in pregnancy only when medically judged to be clearly needed.
• Breast-feeding women should refrain from breast-feeding for two to three hours before and after the infant is given oral vaccine (there are antibodies in breast milk that might destroy the vaccine before it has been absorbed).
• This vaccine should not be administered less than two weeks prior to starting a course of treatment with any kind of ℞ **immunosuppressant** agent.
• After administration, people will be required to wait for some time to ensure that there is no serious reaction (such as anaphylaxis).

Interactions
• Immunosuppressants (for example, ℞ **corticosteroids**, ℞ **cytotoxics**, radiation therapy) may reduce the effectiveness of the vaccine in conferring immunity.
• Caution is required if ℞ **anticoagulants** are being taken.

Side effects

• There may be swelling, irritation or tenderness at the site of vaccination, and low grade fever, mild achiness, or headache.

• Because the vaccines have wiped out polio in the US and throughout much of the world, all new cases of paralytic poliomyelitis in the US are essentially caused by live virus vaccine. The rate of paralysis associated with an initial dose of live vaccine is about one for every half million doses administered, although that rate drops sharply, to about one in every 12 million doses, for the subsequent doses in the usual immunization series.

Polocaine ®

A preparation of ℞ **mepivacaine hydrochloride**.
Formulation: Injection in several strengths.
Availability: Prescription only.
Warnings and side effects: See ℞ **mepivacaine hydrochloride**.

poloxamer 188 ©

Type/Group: **surfactant**.
Brand(s): Adsorbonac.
How administered: Topically (external).

Used to treat

Poloxamer 188 is a surfactant wetting agent that is a constituent of some ophthalmic (eye) preparations.

Warnings

None significant.

Interactions

No significant interactions are known.

Side effects

No significant side effects are known.

polyacrylic acid ©

see ℞ **carbomer**.

Polydine ®

A preparation of ℞ **povidone**.
Formulation: Topical ointment; solution; scrub.
Availability: OTC.
Warnings and side effects: See ℞ **iodine; povidone-iodine**.

Polygam S/D ®

A preparation of ℞ **immune globulin, human (IG)**.
Formulation: Intravenous infusion, supplied as a powder.
Availability: Prescription only.
Warnings and side effects: See ℞ **immune globulin, human (IG)**.

Poly-Histine-D Elixir; Capsules; PedCaps ®

A preparation of ℞ **pheniramine maleate**, phenyltoloxamine, ℞ **pyrilamine maleate**, and phenylpropanolamine.
Formulation: Oral capsules; syrup.
Availability: Prescription only.
Warnings and side effects: See ℞ **pheniramine maleate**; ℞ **pyrilamine maleate**.

polymyxin ⑩

Generics: **gramicidin; polymyxin B sulfate**.

Actions and uses

Polymyxins are an ℞ **antibiotic** chemical class with ℞ **antibacterial** action. They are active against Gram-negative bacteria, including *Pseudomonas aeruginosa*, and are used to treat ✛ **bacterial infections** including skin infections and infected ✛ **burns** and ✛ **wounds**. Because it is not absorbed from the gastrointestinal tract, ℞ **polymyxin B sulfate**, when taken by mouth, can be used for bladder irrigation and decontamination of the colon as an additional treatment with other drugs. However, it is very toxic and is mainly used topically (externally), but in a hospital with expert supervision it may be given to treat serious infection. ℞ **Gramicidin** is incorporated into ophthalmic (eye) preparations along with other antibiotics.

Limitations

See the individual drug entries.

polymyxin B sulfate ©

Type/Group: **polymyxin; antibiotic; antibacterial**.
Brand(s): Aerosporin; generic for ophthalmic use. Combinations: With *neomycin*: Neosporin Cream. With *bacitracin*: Betadine First Aid Antibiotics and Moisturizer; Polysporin. With *bacitracin* and *pramoxine hydrochloride*: Betadine First Aid Antibiotics and Pain Reliever. With *neomycin* and *bacitracin*: AK-Spore Ophthalmic Ointment; Medi-Quick Ointment; Mycitracin Maximum; Mycitracin Plus; Neomixin Ointment; Neosporin Maximum Strength; Neosporin Ointment; Septa Ointment; Triple Antibiotic Ointment; Triple Antibiotic Ophthalmic; various generic. With *neomycin, bacitracin,* and *lidocaine*: Neosporin Plus; Lanabiotic; Mycitracin; Tribiotic Plus; Clomycin; Campho-Phenique Antibiotic Plus Pain Reliever; Spectrocin Plus. With *neomycin, bacitracin, diperodon*: Bactine First Aid Antibiotic Plus Anesthetic Ointment. With *neomycin* and *gramicidin*: AK-Spore Ophthalmic; Neosporin Ophthalmic; various generic. With *hydrocortisone* and *neomycin*: AK-Spore H.C. Ophthalmic; AntibiOtic; Cortisporin Ophthalmic; Cortisporin Suspension Otic; Cortatrigen Modified Ear Drops; Drotic; Ear-Eze; LaserSporin-C Otic; Octicair; Otic-Care; Otocort; Otomycin-HPN. With *hydrocortisone* and *bacitracin*: Cortisporin; Neotricin-HC. With *neomycin* and *hydrocortisone*: AK-Spore H.C. Ophthalmic; Cortisporin Ophthalmic. With *hydrocortisone* and *bacitracin* and *neomycin*: Neotricin HC Ophthalmic. With *dexamethasone* and *neomycin*: AK-Trol Ophthalmic Ointment; Dexacidin Ophthalmic Ointment; Maxitrol Ophthalmic Ointment. With *chloramphenicol* and *hydrocortisone*: Opthocort.
How administered: Injection; topically (ear); topically (ophthalmic).

Used to treat

Polymyxin B sulfate is used to treat several forms of ✛ **bacterial infections** of the eye and skin. Because it is very toxic, it is mainly administered topically (externally). Systemic administration is only carried out for a serious infection and in a hospital, under the supervision of a doctor. Because it is not absorbed from the gastrointestinal tract when taken orally, it can be used for bladder irrigation and decontamination of the colon in addition to treatment with other drugs.

Warnings
• It should not be given to people with known hypersensitivity to polymyxin B, or with severe kidney disease.
• It should be given with caution to people with kidney, neurologic, or neuromuscular impairment.
• It does not cross the placenta, but it should be used during pregnancy only if clearly needed and if the potential benefits outweigh the risks to the fetus.
• Medical judgment is required if breast-feeding is being considered. It is unknown whether this drug appears in breast milk.
• Kidney dysfunction can occur with systemic use.
• This drug may also damage the nervous system when used internally, which can lead to respiratory arrest.
• OTC formulations of polymyxin B are not to be taken internally.

Interactions
• ℞ **Aminoglycosides** increase the risk of kidney dysfunction and respiratory arrest.
• Nondepolarizing ℞ **muscle relaxants** may increase neurological side effects.

Side effects
• Systemic use: Frequently, severe pain, and thrombophlebitis at injection site. Occasionally, fever, hives, dizziness, confusion, blood disorders, and headache.
• Topical use: An allergic reaction, causing increased irritation and inflammation.

Polysporin ⑧
A preparation of ℞ **polymyxin B** and ℞ **bacitracin**.
Formulation: Topical ointment and powder.
Availability: OTC.
Warnings and side effects: See ℞ **polymyxin B**; ℞ **bacitracin**.

Polytar ⑧
A preparation of ℞ **coal tar**.
Formulation: Shampoo; bath oil; soap.
Availability: OTC.
Warnings and side effects: See ℞ **coal tar**.

polythiazide ⑥
Type/Group: **diuretic; thiazide; antihypertensive**.
Brand(s): Renese. Combinations: With *prazosin*: Minizide. With *reserpine*: Renese-R.
How administered: Orally.

Used to treat
Polythiazide used in the treatment of ⊙ **hypertension**, either alone or with other types of diuretic or other drugs (for example, ℞ **beta-blockers**). It can also be used in the treatment of edema. Thiazide diuretics have also become a major part of the treatment for nephrogenic ⊙ **diabetes insipidus**.

Warnings
• It should not be given to people with known hypersensitivity to thiazides (or to ℞ **sulfonamide**-derived drugs), or severe kidney or liver disorders.

• It should be given with caution to elderly people, or anyone with high cholesterol or triglyceride levels, or with liver or kidney impairment.
• Polythiazide should be used in pregnancy only when the potential benefit outweighs the possible risk to the fetus.
• Medical judgment is required if breast-feeding is being considered.
• Early symptoms of electrolyte imbalance may include muscle weakness or cramps, nausea, vomiting, restlessness or lethargy, dry mouth, excessive thirst, fast pulse, or dizziness. A doctor must be contacted if such symptoms occur.
• Thiazides may aggravate symptoms of diabetes or gout, and worsen or activate lupus erythematosus.
• Periodic monitoring of electrolytes (particularly potassium, sodium, chloride, and bicarbonate) is needed.
• Photosensitivity may develop and so precautions such as protective clothing or sunscreens should be used.
• Thiazides interact with a number of drugs, including some over-the-counter preparations. A doctor must be consulted before taking any other medications (including OTCs, herbal remedies, and supplements).

Interactions
• There is a higher risk of a hypersensitivity reaction to ℞ **allopurinol**.
• The effects of ℞ **anesthetics**, ℞ **anticancer** drugs, other antihypertensives, ℞ **diazoxide**, ⟳ **calcium** salts, ℞ **cardiac glycosides**, ℞ **lithium**, loop diuretics, ℞ **methyldopa**, nondepolarizing ℞ **skeletal muscle relaxants**, and ⟳ **vitamin D** may be increased, with the potential for significant adverse effects or toxicity. An additive effect is sometimes used to advantage in combining thiazides with other antihypertensives.
• The effects of ℞ **anticoagulants** and antigout agents (for example, ℞ **probenecid**, ℞ **sulfinpyrazone**) may be lowered by thiazides.
• The doses of ℞ **insulin** and ℞ **sulfonylureas** may need to be adjusted, as thiazides may increase blood sugar levels.
• ℞ **Amphotericin B**, ℞ **anticholinergics**, ℞ **corticosteroids**, ℞ **corticotropin**, and ℞ **MAOIs** may increase the effects of thiazides, with the possibility of significant electrolyte loss, especially potassium.
• ℞ **Cholestyramine**, ℞ **colestipol hydrochloride**, ℞ **methenamine**, and ℞ **NSAIDs** (especially ℞ **indomethacin**) may reduce the effectiveness of thiazide diuretics.
• There is an increased possibility of postural hypotension (lowered blood pressure on standing) if taken with alcohol, ℞ **barbiturates**, or ℞ **opioids**.

Side effects
• There may be dizziness, headache, muscle cramps, mild gastrointestinal upsets, postural hypotension, reversible impotence, low blood potassium, sodium, magnesium and chloride, raised blood urea, glucose and lipids, and gout.
• Rarely, photosensitivity, blood disorders, skin reactions, and pancreatitis.

polyvinyl alcohol ©

Type/Group: **artificial tears**.
Brand(s): Akwa Tears; Artificial Tears Plus; Dry Eyes; HypoTears; Liquifilm Tears; Moisture Drops; Murine; Refresh; Tears Plus.
How administered: Topically (external).

Used to treat

Polyvinyl alcohol is a constituent of preparations used as artificial tears, and is used by people with dry eyes (tear deficiency) due to certain disorders.

Warnings

• It should not be given to people with known hypersensitivity to the drug.
• A doctor should be consulted before using during pregnancy or while breast-feeding, but it is generally regarded as safe.
• It may cause mild stinging or temporary blurred vision.

Interactions

No significant drug interactions are known.

Side effects

No significant side effects are known.

Ponstel ®

A preparation of ℞ **mefenamic acid**.
Formulation: Oral capsules.
Availability: Prescription only.
Warnings and side effects: See ℞ **mefenamic acid**.

Pontocaine HCl ®

A preparation of ℞ **tetracaine**.
Formulation: Injection; topical solution; ointment.
Availability: Prescription only (ointment is OTC).
Warnings and side effects: See ℞ **tetracaine**.

posterior pituitary hormone ⊙

(hormone (posterior pituitary); pituitary hormone (posterior))
Generics: **desmopressin; lypressin; oxytocin; vasopressin**.

Actions and uses

Posterior pituitary hormones constitute one of the two classes of endocrine (blood-borne) hormones secreted by the pituitary gland, situated as a projection of the brain at the base of the skull. On release into the bloodstream, these hormones have actions directly on organs within the body—unlike the other class—the ℞ **anterior pituitary hormones**, which differ in that they largely work by controlling the release of other hormones from glands in the body. Chemically both classes are peptides, that is, short sequences of amino acids arranged as in proteins.

The natural posterior pituitary hormones are ℞ **oxytocin** and ℞ **vasopressin** (antidiuretic hormone; ADH), of which the latter occurs in two forms depending on the species of mammal. Synthetic versions of the natural hormones, or chemical analogs of these, are extensively used in medicine.

℞ **Oxytocin** is a ℞ **uterine stimulant** (oxytocic) and increases the contractions of the uterus during normal labor (and also stimulates milk production), and may be administered by intravenous injection or infusion to induce, speed up or assist labor (or abortion), and it is also used in conjunction with other drugs to help stop bleeding following childbirth. It may also be prescribed to promote the production of breast milk (when it is used as a nasal spray). Vasopressin occurs naturally in two forms, argipressin (8-Arginine vasopressin) which is often referred to simply as vasopressin; also ℞ **lypressin** (8-Lysine vasopressin; the form found in porcine species). Vasopressin and analogs have a number of separate actions. First, as the name vasopressin indicates, they are presser agents raising blood pressure (largely through a ℞ **vasoconstrictor** action on blood vessels), and are sometimes used to treat bleeding from varices (a sort of ⊙ **varicose vein**) in the esophagus. Second, as the alternate name antidiuretic hormone (ADH) indicates, they have an antidiuretic action, decreasing urine secretion by the kidney (a natural role for the hormone). Consequently, vasopressin, ℞ **lypressin** and the analog ℞ **desmopressin** are used mainly in ℞ **diabetes insipidus treatment** where the type of ⊙ **diabetes insipidus** is pituitary-originated (through impaired secretion of the natural hormone). ℞ **Desmopressin** can be used for a variety of uses including to treat ⊙ **bed-wetting**, neurogenic diabetes insipidus, temporary increased urination following head trauma or surgery in the pituitary region, and bleeding (by boosting clotting factors) in certain cases of ⊙ **hemophilia**.

Oxytocin infusion is now a standard treatment for assisting labor and with care over dosage a relatively safe procedure (although there can be unexpected uterine bleeding or contractions, and other complications). Although oxytocin analogs have been developed none have been used in medicine. However, combining oxytocin with ℞ **prostaglandins** has extended its range of therapeutic uses.

Vasopressin analogs have been extensively tested, and ℞ **desmopressin** is one of the successful results. It is a relatively stable analog that, although a peptide, may be taken by mouth (peptides are normally digested in the same way as protein in the diet) or by nasal spray (where it is absorbed into the bloodstream through the nasal mucosa), whereas vasopressin must be injected.

Limitations

See the individual drug entries.

potassium clavulanate ©

see ℞ **clavulanic acid**.

potassium iodide ©

Type/Group: **expectorant; antithyroid; antidote**.
Brand(s): (For hyperthyroid management): Thyro-Block, various generic (As an expectorant): SSKI; Pima Syrup; various generic.
Combinations: With *codeine, chlorpheniramine and phenylephrine*: Pediacof Syrup; Pedituss Cough Syrup. With *ephedrine*: KIE Syrup. With *ephedrine, phenobarbital and theophylline*: Mudrane Tablets (also has *aminophylline*); Quadrinal Tablets. With *theophylline*: Elixophyllin-KI Elixir.
How administered: Orally.

Used to treat

Potassium iodide is used in a number of brands as an expectorant, although it has been largely replaced by safer drugs for this purpose. It is also used to relieve certain conditions in which there are thick mucous secretions in the lungs, and as a preventive measure after surgery to prevent postoperative atelectasis (collapse of lung tissue due to general anesthetics). It can be used together with anti-thyroid drugs for preparing people with hyperthyroid for surgery to remove the thyroid gland. As a prophylactic (preventive) emergency measure it can be used where there is a danger of, or after exposure to, radioactive isotopes of iodine, since it will compete for iodine uptake by the thyroid.

Warnings

Depending on use:

• It should not be given to people with known hypersensitivity to this drug, or with acute bronchitis, tuberculosis, renal disease, hyperthyroidism, Addison's disease (an adrenal gland disorder), or who have, for whatever reason, high levels of potassium or iodine.

• It should be given with caution to people who have had any kind of thyroid disease. Potassium iodide should not be used by anyone suffering from heat cramps or acute dehydration.

• Potassium iodide could harm the fetus and should not be taken during pregnancy unless clearly needed. Use in pregnancy requires medical advice.

• Nursing mothers should discontinue this drug or discontinue breast-feeding.

• Enteric-coated tablets (to dissolve in the intestines) should be avoided. Potassium is corrosive to the stomach and intestinal linings, and a concentrated exposure may cause lesions, perforation, and bleeding.

• If a cough persists for more than a week, a doctor should be consulted.

• When taken for long periods, symptoms of iodine poisoning (iodism) may appear, such as a brassy, metallic taste in the mouth, increased salivation, sore gums, soreness or burning in the mouth and throat, sneezing, eyelid swelling, or sudden a appearance of acne-like sores. Treatment should be stopped at once and a doctor contacted.

Interactions

• ℞ **lithium** and ℞ **antithyroid** drugs may cause a low thyroid (hypothyroid) condition.

• If used with other potassium-containing drugs or potassium-sparing diuretics, there is a risk of serious cardiac side effects due to increased levels of potassium.

Side effects

• There may be stomach and intestinal irritation, diarrhea, numbness or tingling, irregular heartbeat, and unusual tiredness.

povidone Ⓖ

Type/Group: **artificial tears.**
Brand(s): Adsorbonac; Artifical Tears Plus; Moisture Drops; Refresh.
How administered: Topically (external).

Used to treat

Povidone is a constituent of artificial tears, which are used to treat extremely dry eyes due to certain disorders. It is available as eye-drops.

Warnings

None significant.

Interactions

No significant interactions are known.

Side effects

No significant side effects are known.

pralidoxime chloride Ⓖ

Type/Group: **antidote.**
Brand(s): Protopram Chloride; various generic.
How administered: Injection.

Used to treat

Pralidoxime chloride is used to treat poisoning by organophosphorous compounds (for example, insecticides), overdosage by ℞ **anticholinesterase** drugs used in the treatment of myasthenia gravis and, with ℞ **atropine**, poisoning by nerve agents with anticholinesterase activity.

Warnings

• It should not be given to people with known hypersensitivity to any component of the product.

• It should be given with caution to people with myasthenia gravis.

• Pralidoxime should be used in pregnancy only if it is clearly needed.

• Medical judgment is required if breast-feeding is being considered.

• It is a specialist drug and administration will be carried out by experienced personnel.

Interactions

• The effects of ℞ **barbiturates** are increased.

Side effects

• Dizziness, visual changes, headache, drowsiness, nausea, changes in heartbeat, and blood pressure, hyperventilation, and muscular weakness.

PrameGel Ⓑ

A preparation of ℞ **pramoxine hydrochloride.**
Formulation: Topical cream.
Availability: OTC.
Warnings and side effects: See ℞ **pramoxine hydrochloride.**

pramipexole Ⓖ

Type/Group: **dopamine-receptor stimulant; antiparkinsonism.**
Brand(s): Mirapex.
How administered: Orally.

Used to treat

Pramiprexole is a recently introduced treatment for ⊙ **Parkinson's disease.** It works by stimulating the ℞ **dopamine** receptors in the brain (that is, it is a dopamine-receptor stimulant), and is similar to ℞ **bromocriptine** in that it is used to improve symptoms and signs of the disease, either alone or in combination with ℞ **levodopa.**

Warnings

• It should not be used by people who are known to be sensitive to pramipexole.

• It should be used with caution by people with cardiovascular disease, psychotic disorders, dementia, or kidney impairment.

• The effects of pramipexole on fetal development are unknown. It should therefore be used during pregnancy only if the potential benefits outweigh the potential risks to the fetus.

• It should not be used by breast-feeding mothers.

• Fainting, sometimes associated with slowed heartbeat, has been observed, particularly in people who are not using levodopa.
• It may impair regulation of blood pressure and cause postural hypotension (lowered blood pressure on standing), especially at the beginning of treatment.
• Hallucinations may occur, particularly in those over 65 years of age.
• Treatment must be ended gradually over one week to avoid adverse effects (such as, fever, muscle rigidity, altered consciousness) associated with an abrupt reduction in dopamine-enhancing drugs.

Interactions

• Concentrations of levodopa are markedly increased, as are the chances of dopamine-related side effects.
• ℞ **Phenothiazines**, butyrophenones, thioxanthenes, ℞ **metoclopramide**, and other dopamine antagonists reduce the effectiveness of pramiprexole.
• ℞ **Cimetidine** increases the bioavailability of pramipexole.

Side effects

• Most frequently, nausea, dizziness, drowsiness, insomnia, excessive sleeping, and postural hypotension.
• In addition there may be weakness, constipation, dry mouth, gastrointestinal problems, gait or movement abnormalities, blurred vision, palpitations, sweating, and urinary frequency.

Pramoxine HC ⑧

A preparation of ℞ **hydrocortisone** and ℞ **pramoxine hydrochloride**.
Formulation: Aerosol foam.
Availability: Prescription only.
Warnings and side effects: See ℞ **hydrocortisone**; ℞ **pramoxine hydrochloride**.

pramoxine hydrochloride ⑥

Type/Group: local anesthetic.
Brand(s): Tronothane; PrameGel; Prax; Itch-X. With *hydrocortisone*: 1 + 1F Creme; Analpram-HC; Epifoam Aerosol Foam; Pramoxine HC; ProctoCream-HC (with pramoxine); Proctofoam-HC.
How administered: Topically (external).

Used to treat

Pramoxine preparations are used topically (externally) for the temporary relief of pain and itching associated with ✪ **skin conditions**, including hemorrhoids, anogenital pruritis, anal fissures, minor burns, and dermatoses (any skin condition).

Warnings

• It should not be given to people with known hypersensitivity to this drug.
• It should be given with caution to people with rectal bleeding, or to children.
• It is considered safe in normal topical (external) use, but consult a doctor before using during pregnancy.
• It should not be used in or near the eyes or nose, to large or unaffected areas, or for a prolonged period of time.

Interactions

No significant interactions have been reported.

Side effects

• When used in the recommended doses, there are usually no significant side effects, although there may be burning, irritation, stinging, or rash.

Prandin ⑧

A preparation of ℞ **repaglinide**.
Formulation: Oral tablets in several strengths.
Availability: Prescription only.
Warnings and side effects: See ℞ **repaglinide**.

Pravachol ⑧

A preparation of ℞ **pravastatin sodium**.
Formulation: Oral tablets.
Availability: Prescription only.
Warnings and side effects: See ℞ **pravastatin sodium**.

pravastatin sodium ⑥

Type/Group: **lipid-regulating drug; statin.**
Brand(s): Pravachol.
How administered: Orally.

Used to treat

Pravastatin is a lipid-regulating drug (statin/HMG-CoA reductase inhibitor) that can be used in ✪ **hyperlipidemia** to reduce the levels, or change the proportions, of various lipids in the bloodstream. It is usually given only to people in whom a strict and regular dietary regime alone is not having the desired effect. It is also used to prevent heart attacks and to help prevent stroke.

Warnings

• It should not be given to people with active liver disease.
• It should be given with caution to people with a history of liver disease, kidney insufficiency, conditions predisposing to kidney failure, severe endocrine, metabolic, or electrolyte disorders, heavy users of alcohol, or who are over 65. Medical judgment is also required for children.
• Pravastatin is considered quite hazardous to the fetus. This drug is given to women of childbearing age only when they are thought highly unlikely to conceive and have been informed of the risks. It should not be used during pregnancy.
• It should not be used while breast-feeding.
• When taking pravastatin, any unusual muscle pain or tenderness should be reported to a doctor immediately and treatment stopped, because it has the potential to cause destruction of muscle tissue.
• Potentially harmful changes in liver function may occur, so periodic tests may be necessary to check the drug's effect.

Interactions

• ℞ azole antifungals (for example, ℞ **fluconazole**), ℞ **clarithromycin**, ℞ **danazol**, ℞ **erythromycin**, ℞ **fluoxetine**, ℞ **nefazodone**, and troleandomycin increase the levels of pravastatin and the risk of side effects.
• ℞ **cholestyramine**, ℞ **colestipol hydrochloride**, and ℞ **isradipine** reduce the levels of pravastatin.
• ℞ **cyclosporine**, ℞ **gemfibrozil**, and ℞ **niacin** increase the risk of adverse effects.

Side effects
• Occasionally, gastrointestinal effects, headache, rhinitis, rash, and itching.
• Rarely, heartburn, muscle pain, dizziness, cough, fatigue, flu-like symptoms, pancreatitis, and cataracts.

Prax Ⓑ

A preparation of ℞ **pramoxine hydrochloride.**
Formulation: Topical cream.
Availability: OTC.
Warnings and side effects: See ℞ **pramoxine hydrochloride.**

praziquantel Ⓖ

Type/Group: anthelmintic.
Brand(s): Biltricide.
How administered: Orally.

Used to treat
Praziquantel is a synthetic anthelmintic drug which is the drug of choice in treating infestation caused by *schistosomes*, which are the worms that can colonize the veins of a human host and cause ✚ **bilharzia.** It is also used in the treatment of infections due to liver flukes, *clonorchiasis*, and *opisthorchiasis*. It has a low toxicity and is administered orally.

Warnings
• It should not be given to people with known hypersensitivity to this drug or with liver disease.
• It should be used during pregnancy only if clearly needed.
• Breast-feeding should stop while using this medication, and for 72 hours after treatment.
• It may cause drowsiness and so the performance of skilled tasks, such as driving, may be impaired.

Interactions
• ℞ **chloroquine** and ℞ **hydroxychloroquine sulfate** reduce the levels of praziquantel.
• ℞ **cimetidine** increases the levels of praziquantel.

Side effects
• Frequently, headache, dizziness, malaise, and abdominal pain.
• Occasionally, other gastrointestinal effects, fever, and sweating.
• Rarely, giddiness, and hives.

prazosin hydrochloride Ⓖ

Type/Group: alpha-adrenergic blocker; antihypertensive.
Brand(s): Minipress; various generic. Combinations: With *polythiazide*: Minizide.
How administered: Orally.

Used to treat
Prazosin hydrochloride is used to reduce high blood pressure in ✚ **hypertension,** and is often used with other antihypertensives (for example, ℞ **beta-blockers** or ℞ **thiazide** ℞ **diuretics**). Although not stated by the manufacturer for such treatments, it may be prescribed for peripheral vascular disease (✚ **Raynaud's disease**), ✚ **benign prostatic hyperplasia** (BPH), or ✚ **heart failure.**

Warnings
• It should be given with caution to people with impaired kidney or liver function. There is some evidence that prazosin may worsen narcolepsy (uncontrollable desire to sleep), and it is sometimes recommended this drug not be used in those with the disorder.
• Prazosin should be used during pregnancy only if the potential benefit outweighs the possible risk to the fetus.
• Medical judgment is required if breast-feeding is being considered. It does appear in breast milk.
• Postural hypotension (for example, dizziness when arising from a sitting position) occurs frequently with use of this drug and fainting may result. Sudden or prolonged standing or exercise should be avoided when taking prazosin. During initial dosing, it is necessary also to identify situations in which injury could result if fainting occurs. These hypotensive effects may be aggravated by hot environments.
• Because of possible sedative side effects, caution is advised for potentially hazardous activities, such as driving, that require mental alertness.
• Rarely, priapism (prolonged and painful erection) has been reported. This condition must be treated promptly, or permanent dysfunction may result.

Interactions
• If used with other antihypertensives and diuretics, the effects of these drugs may be increased. This additive effect is sometimes used to advantage in combination treatments for high blood pressure.

Side effects
• These may include dizziness and hypotension (particularly on standing), drowsiness and sedation, weakness and lack of energy, headache, palpitations, nausea, and urinary frequency.
• Less commonly, edema, shortness of breath or nervousness, and, rarely, speeding of the heart, incontinence, priapism, blurred vision, dry mouth, rhinitis, or mental depression.

Precose Ⓑ

A preparation of ℞ **acarbose.**
Formulation: Oral tablets.
Availability: Prescription only.
Warnings and side effects: See ℞ **acarbose.**

Predalone-50 Ⓑ

A preparation of ℞ **prednisolone** acetate.
Formulation: Injection.
Availability: Prescription only.
Warnings and side effects: See ℞ **prednisolone.**

Predcor-50 Ⓑ

A preparation of ℞ **prednisolone** acetate.
Formulation: Injection in several strengths.
Availability: Prescription only.
Warnings and side effects: See ℞ **prednisolone.**

Pred-G S.O.P. Ⓡ

A preparation of ℞ **prednisolone** acetate, ℞ **gentamicin** sulfate, ℞ **petrolatum**, ℞ **lanolin**, and ℞ **mineral oil**.
Formulation: Ointment.
Availability: Prescription only.
Warnings and side effects: See ℞ **prednisolone**; ℞ **gentamicin**; ℞ **petrolatum**; ℞ **lanolin**; ℞ **mineral oil**.

Pred Mild; Pred Forte Ⓡ

A preparation of ℞ **prednisolone**.
Formulation: Eye drops in two strengths.
Availability: Prescription only.
Warnings and side effects: See ℞ **prednisolone**.

prednisolone Ⓖ

Type/Group: corticosteroid; anti-inflammatory; immunosuppressant.
Brand(s): Delta-Cortef; Econopred; Inflamase; Pred; Prelone; various generic. As *prednisolone acetate*: Key-Pred; Predalone-50; Predcor; various generic. As *prednisolone sodium phosphate*: Hydeltrasol; Key-Pred-SP; Pediapred; various generic. As *prednisolone tebutate*: Hydeltra-T.B.A.; Prednisol TBA; various generic. Combinations: With *sodium sulfacetamide*: Blephamine; Isopto Cetapred; AK-Cide; Metimyd; Sulster; Vasocidin; Vasocine. With *gentamicin sulfate*: Pred-G S.O.P.
How administered: Orally; injection; topically (ophthalmic).

Used to treat

Prednisolone is used for the treatment of many kinds of ✚ **inflammation**. It has major and varied effects on metabolism, and modifies the operation of the immune system, and so it may be used to treat a range of conditions, including adrenal insufficiency, congenital adrenal hyperplasia, rheumatic disorders (such as ✚ **arthritis** and ✚ **osteoarthritis**), allergic states, collagen diseases, allergic and inflammatory eye disorders, intestinal tract, liver, and kidney disorders, skin diseases, respiratory diseases (such as bronchial ✚ **asthma**), edemas, and malignancies.

Warnings

• It should not be used by people with known hypersensitivity to corticosteroids, or with systemic fungal infections.
• It should be given with caution to anyone with low thyroid function, peptic ulcers, hepatitis, cirrhosis, ocular herpes simplex, diabetes mellitus, glaucoma, history of tuberculosis, nonspecific colitis, congestive heart failure, myocardial infarction (heart attack), hypertension, psychosis, or kidney insufficiency. It must also be given with caution to anyone over 65 and children.
• Corticosteroids can cross the placenta, and therefore prednisolone should only be used during pregnancy if medically judged to be essential.
• It should not be used by breast-feeding mothers. It is excreted in breast milk and could suppress growth and interfere with production of corticosteroids in the infant.
• It may mask signs of infection and interfere with the body's ability to keep infection from spreading.
• Live vaccines must not be taken while using this drug.
• It may reactivate latent tuberculosis or amebiasis.

• It causes increased excretion of calcium and other minerals, and so supplements may be needed.
• Prolonged use may lead to adrenal insufficiency. A doctor must be notified if there is unusual weight gain, swelling of the legs or feet, muscle weakness, black tarry stools, vomiting of blood, puffing of the face, menstrual irregularities, or prolonged sore throat, fever, cold, or infection.
• Anyone on long-term steroid therapy should wear a medic-alert bracelet or the equivalent.
• Other medication (including OTC, herbal remedies and supplements) must not be taken without consulting a doctor.
• Discontinuation of this drug must be gradual and under medical supervision.
• The contraceptive effect of IUDs (intrauterine device) may be decreased.
• Dentists and other doctors must be informed of the use of this drug during, and for 12 months after discontinuing, treatment. Supportive drugs may be required in the event of severe illness, surgery, or trauma.
• When using topically (externally), do not use over large surface areas, for a prolonged period, or cover with bandages in order to minimize the risk of systemic absorption and accompanying side effects.

Interactions

• Prednisolone taken with ℞ **amphotericin** or ℞ **diuretics** may further reduce potassium levels.
• The effectiveness of ℞ **aspirin**, ℞ **oral hypoglycemics**, ℞ **insulin**, diuretics, and ⚕ **potassium** supplements may be reduced.
• Aspirin and ℞ **NSAIDs** increase the risk of gastric ulceration.
• ℞ **Barbiturates**, ℞ **hydantoins**, ℞ **rifampin**, and ephedrine may reduce the effects of corticosteroids.
• ℞ **Ketoconazole**, ℞ **estrogens**, ℞ **oral contraceptives**, nondepolarizing muscle relaxants, and ℞ **cholestyramine** may increase the effects of prednisolone.
• Oral ℞ **anticoagulants** and ℞ **theophylline** may alter the effects of either corticosteroids or the other drug, or both.
• The effectiveness of ℞ **anticholinesterases**, ℞ **isoniazid**, ℞ **salicylates**, and ℞ **somatrem** may be reduced.
• ℞ **Cyclosporine** and digitalis glycosides may increase the risk of toxicity.

Side effects

These depend on how administered, dose, duration of treatment, and use.
• Systemically: Frequently, insomnia, heartburn, nervousness, abdominal tightness, increased sweating, acne, mood swings, increased appetite, facial flushing, delayed wound healing, increased susceptibility to infection, diarrhea, or constipation. Occasionally, edema, headache, change in skin color, and frequent urination. Rarely, speeded heartbeat, allergic skin reaction, and psychological changes.
• Topically (as ophthalmic solution): Blurred vision, burning or stinging, rarely cataracts, and optic nerve damage. Systemic effects are possible.

Prednisol TBA ®

A preparation of ℞ **prednisolone** tebutate.
Formulation: Injection.
Availability: Prescription only.
Warnings and side effects: See ℞ **prednisolone**.

prednisone ⓖ

Type/Group: corticosteroid; anti-inflammatory; immunosuppressant.
Brand(s): Meticorten; Orasone; Deltasone; Strerapred; Prednisone Intensol Concentrate; Liquid Pred; various generics.
How administered: Orally.

Used to treat

Prednisone is used for the treatment of many kinds of ✪ inflammation. It has major and varied effects on metabolism, and modifies the operation of the immune system, and so it may be used to treat a variety of conditions, including adrenal insufficiency, congenital adrenal hyperplasia, rheumatic disorders (such as ✪ arthritis and ✪ osteoarthritis), allergic states, collagen diseases, allergic and inflammatory eye disorders, intestinal tract, liver and kidney disorders, skin diseases, respiratory diseases (such as bronchial ✪ asthma), edemas, and malignancies.

Warnings

• It should not be used by people with known hypersensitivity to corticosteroids, or with systemic fungal infections.
• It should be given with caution to anyone with low thyroid function, peptic ulcers, hepatitis, cirrhosis, diabetes mellitus, glaucoma, ocular herpes simplex, history of tuberculosis, nonspecific colitis, congestive heart failure, myocardial infarction (heart attack), hypertension, psychosis, or kidney insufficiency, and also to anyone over 65 and children.
• Corticosteroids can cross the placenta, and therefore prednisone should only be used during pregnancy if medically judged to be essential.
• It should not be used by breast-feeding mothers. It is excreted in breast milk and could suppress growth and interfere with the production of corticosteroids in the infant.
• It may mask signs of infection and interfere with the body's ability to keep infection from spreading.
• Live vaccines must not be taken while using this drug.
• It may reactivate latent tuberculosis or amebiasis.
• Prolonged use in children can inhibit skeletal growth, and so growth must be monitored.
• It causes increased excretion of calcium and other minerals, and so supplements may be needed.
• Prolonged use may lead to adrenal insufficiency. A doctor must be notified if there is unusual weight gain, swelling of the legs or feet, muscle weakness, black tarry stools, vomiting of blood, puffing of the face, menstrual irregularities, or prolonged sore throat, fever, cold, or infection.
• Anyone on long-term steroid therapy should wear a medic-alert bracelet or the equivalent.
• No other medication (including OTC, herbal remedies and supplements) should be taken without consulting a doctor.

• Discontinuation of treatment must be gradual and under medical supervision.
• The contraceptive effect of IUDs (intrauterine device) may be decreased.
• Dentists and other doctors must be informed of the use of this drug during, and for 12 months after discontinuing, treatment. Supportive drugs may be required in the event of severe illness, surgery, or trauma.
• When using topically (externally), do not use over large surface areas, for a prolonged period, or cover with bandages in order to minimize the risk of systemic absorption and accompanying side effects.

Interactions

• Prednisone taken with ℞ **amphotericin** or ℞ **diuretics** may further reduce potassium levels.
• The effectiveness of ℞ **aspirin**, ℞ **oral hypoglycemics**, ℞ **insulin**, diuretics, ⚕ **potassium** supplements may be reduced.
• Aspirin and ℞ **NSAID**s increase the risk of gastric ulceration.
• ℞ **Barbiturates**, ℞ **hydantoins**, ℞ **rifampin**, and ephedrine may reduce the effects of corticosteroids.
• ℞ **Ketoconazole**, ℞ **estrogens**, ℞ **oral contraceptives**, nondepolarizing muscle relaxants, and ℞ **cholestyramine** may increase the effects of prednisone.
• Oral ℞ **anticoagulants** and ℞ **theophylline** may alter the effects of either corticosteroids or the other drug, or both.
• The effectiveness of ℞ **anticholinesterases**, ℞ **isoniazid**, ℞ **salicylates**, and ℞ **somatrem** may be reduced.
• ℞ **Cyclosporine** and digitalis glycosides may increase the risk of toxicity.

Side effects

• Frequently, insomnia, heartburn, nervousness, abdominal tightness, increased sweating, acne, mood swings, increased appetite, facial flushing, delayed wound healing, increased susceptibility to infection, diarrhea, or constipation.
• Occasionally, edema, headache, change in skin color, and frequent urination.
• Rarely, speeded heartbeat, allergic skin reaction, and psychological changes.

Prednisone Intensol Concentrate ®

A preparation of ℞ **prednisone**.
Formulation: Oral solution.
Availability: Prescription only.
Warnings and side effects: See ℞ **prednisone**.

Prefrin Liquifilm ®

A preparation of ℞ **phenylephrine hydrochloride**.
Formulation: Eye drops.
Availability: OTC.
Warnings and side effects: See ℞ **phenylephrine hydrochloride**.

Pregnyl ®

A preparation of ℞ **chorionic gonadotropin**.
Formulation: Injection.
Availability: Prescription only.

Warnings and side effects: See ℞ chorionic gonadotropin.

Prelone ℗

A preparation of ℞ **prednisolone**.
Formulation: Syrup.
Availability: Prescription only.
Warnings and side effects: See ℞ **prednisolone**.

Premarin ℗

A preparation of ℞ **estrogens, conjugated**.
Formulation: Tablets; injection.
Availability: Prescription only.
Warnings and side effects: See ℞ **estrogens, conjugated**.

Premphase ℗

A preparation of ℞ **estrogens, conjugated** and ℞ **medroxyprogesterone**.
Formulation: Oral tablets.
Availability: Prescription only.
Warnings and side effects: See ℞ **estrogens, conjugated**; ℞ **medroxyprogesterone**.

Prempro ℗

A preparation of ℞ **estrogens, conjugated** and ℞ **medroxyprogesterone**.
Formulation: Oral tablets.
Availability: Prescription only.
Warnings and side effects: See ℞ **estrogens, conjugated**; ℞ **medroxyprogesterone**.

Premsyn PMS Caplets ℗

A preparation of ℞ **acetaminophen**, ℞ **pyrilamine maleate**, and pamabrom.
Formulation: Oral tablets.
Availability: OTC.
Warnings and side effects: See ℞ **acetaminophen**; ℞ **pyrilamine maleate**.

Preparation H Cooling Gel; Ointment; Suppositories ℗

A preparation of ℞ **phenylephrine hydrochloride**.
Formulation: Topical gel; ointment; rectal suppositories.
Availability: OTC.
Warnings and side effects: See ℞ **phenylephrine hydrochloride**.

Prepidil ℗

A preparation of ℞ **dinoprostone**.
Formulation: Vaginal gel.
Availability: Prescription only.
Warnings and side effects: See ℞ **dinoprostone**.

PreSun Ultra ℗

A preparation of ℞ **cinnamates** and other ingredients.
Formulation: Topical lotion; topical gel.
Availability: OTC.

Warnings and side effects: See ℞ **cinnamates**.

Pretz-D ℗

A preparation of ℞ **ephedrine**.
Formulation: Nasal pray.
Availability: OTC.
Warnings and side effects: See ℞ **ephedrine**.

Prevacid ℗

A preparation of ℞ **lansoprazole**.
Formulation: Capsules, delayed release, available in two strengths.
Availability: Prescription only.
Warnings and side effects: See ℞ **lansoprazole**.

Prevalite ℗

A preparation of ℞ **cholestyramine**.
Formulation: Oral powder.
Availability: Prescription only.
Warnings and side effects: See ℞ **cholestyramine**.

Preven ℗

A preparation of ℞ **ethinyl estradiol** and ℞ **levonorgestrel**.
Formulation: Oral tablets.
Availability: Prescription only.
Warnings and side effects: See ℞ **ethinyl estradiol**; ℞ **levonorgestrel**. If vomiting ocurs within one hour of taking a dose, contact the doctor to discuss whether to repeat the dose or take an antinausea medication. Should not be used as a routine form of contraception.

Prevnar ℗

A preparation of pneumococcal 7-valent conjugate vaccine.
Formulation: Injection.
Availability: Prescription only.
Warnings and side effects: See ℞ **pneumococcal vaccine**.

Prevpac ℗

A preparation of ℞ **amoxicillin**, ℞ **clarithromycin**, and ℞ **lansoprazole**.
Formulation: Capsules and tablets in daily dose packets.
Availability: Prescription only.
Warnings and side effects: See ℞ **amoxicillin**; ℞ **clarithromycin**; ℞ **lansoprazole**.

prilocaine hydrochloride ⓖ

Type/Group: **local anesthetic**.
Brand(s): Citanest Hydrochloride.
How administered: Local injection.

Used to treat

Prilocaine is used extensively for relatively minor surgical procedures, especially in dentistry by injection and nerve block.

Warnings

• It should not be given to people with known hypersensitivity to prilocaine, or those rare patients with methemoglobinemia (a serious blood disorder). It is a specialist drug and there will be a full medical assessment.

• It should be used in pregnancy only when it is clearly needed.

• Medical judgment is required if breast-feeding is being considered.

• It can cause cardiac depression, peripheral vasodilatation, or CNS (central nervous system) toxicity.

Interactions

• There is a risk of additive toxicity with ℞ **antiarrhythmics** (for example, ℞ **tocainide**, ℞ **mexiletine**).

• ℞ **Sedatives** may cause increased CNS effects.

Side effects

• Occasionally, pain at injection site, burning, stinging, or tenderness where applied.

• Rarely (generally with high dose), drowsiness, dizziness, disorientation, lightheadedness, tremors, apprehension, euphoria, sensation of heat, cold, or numbness, blurred or double vision, ringing or roaring in ears, nausea, or allergic reactions.

Prilosec ⑧

A preparation of ℞ **omeprazole**.

Formulation: Oral capsules, delayed release, available in 3 strengths.

Availability: Prescription only.

Warnings and side effects: See ℞ **omeprazole**.

Primacor ⑧

A preparation of ℞ **milrinone**.

Formulation: Intravenous infusion.

Availability: Prescription only.

Warnings and side effects: See ℞ **milrinone**.

primaquine ⑥

Type/Group: **antimalarial; amebicide and antiprotozoal.**

Brand(s): Generic only.

How administered: Orally.

Used to treat

Primaquine is an (*8-aminoquinoline*) antimalarial drug used to treat *Plasmodium vivax* ✪ **malaria** and to prevent relapse of *Plasmodium vivax* malaria after termination of chloroquine therapy. Although not stated by the manufacturer for such use, it may also be used, in combination with ℞ **clindamycin**, to treat *pneumocystic carinii* ✪ **pneumonia** associated with ✪ **AIDS**.

Warnings

• It should not be given to people with known hypersensitivity to primaquine or related compounds, or acutely ill people with rheumatoid arthritis, systemic lupus erythematosus, or other disorders with a tendency to the blood disorder granulocytopenia.

• It should be given with caution to people with G6PD or NADH methemoglobin reductase deficiencies (genetic enzyme disorders).

• Its use should be avoided during pregnancy if possible, but if preventive or other treatment is required, use with caution.

• It is not recommended for use while nursing.

• A doctor must be contacted if darkening of the urine occurs or stomach upsets (nausea, vomiting, stomach pain) persist.

Interactions

• Quinacrine increases the risk of severe heart and neurologic side effects.

Side effects

• Frequently, gastrointestinal effects.

• Occasionally, headache, visual changes, and itching.

• Rare, but serious effects include blood disorders.

Primatene Dual Action Tablets ⑧

A preparation of ℞ **ephedrine**, ℞ **theophylline**, and ℞ **guaifenesin**.

Formulation: Oral tablets.

Availability: OTC.

Warnings and side effects: See ℞ **ephedrine**; ℞ **theophylline**; ℞ **guaifenesin**.

Primatene Mist ⑧

A preparation of ℞ **epinephrine**.

Formulation: Aerosol for inhalation.

Availability: OTC.

Warnings and side effects: See ℞ **epinephrine**.

Primatene Tablets ⑧

A preparation of ℞ **ephedrine** and ℞ **guaifenesin**.

Formulation: Oral tablets.

Availability: OTC.

Warnings and side effects: See ℞ **ephedrine**; ℞ **guaifenesin**.

Primatuss Cough Mixture 4D Liquid ⑧

A preparation of ℞ **dextromethorphan**, ℞ **pseudoephedrine**, and ℞ **guaifenesin**.

Formulation: Oral liquid.

Availability: OTC.

Warnings and side effects: See ℞ **dextromethorphan**; ℞ **pseudoephedrine**; ℞ **guaifenesin**.

Primatuss Cough Mixture 4 Liquid ⑧

A preparation of ℞ **dextromethorphan** and ℞ **chlorpheniramine maleate**.

Formulation: Oral liquid.

Availability: OTC.

Warnings and side effects: See ℞ **dextromethorphan**; ℞ **chlorpheniramine maleate**.

Primaxin ⑧

A preparation of ℞ **imipenem-cilastatin**.

Formulation: Injection.

Availability: Prescription only.

Warnings and side effects: See ℞ **imipenem-cilastatin**.

primidone ⑥

Type/Group: **anticonvulsant; antiepileptic.**

Brand(s): Mysoline, Mysoline Suspension.

Key to symbols: ⑩ = Drug type/group   ⑥ = Generic name   ⑧ = Brand name

How administered: Orally.

Used to treat

Primidone is used in the treatment of ○ **epilepsy** (except absence seizures) and for essential tremor. Its effectiveness is slow to emerge, and so its therapeutic value must be assessed over a period of several weeks. Some of it is converted in the body to the barbiturate drug ℞ **phenobarbital** and therefore has similar actions and effects.

Warnings

• Avoid its use in people with known hypersensitivity to phenobarbital, with porphyria, or with severe respiratory disease.
• Primidone should be given with caution to anyone with significant kidney or liver impairment.
• This drug may have the potential to cause birth defects. However, because uncontrolled seizures can also threaten fetal health, medical judgment is needed to weigh potential benefits and risks.
• This drug appears plentifully in breast milk, and may cause excessive sleepiness in infants; if such symptoms appear, it is recommended to discontinue use, if at all possible.
• Withdrawal should be gradual otherwise it may precipitate attacks.
• As this drug may cause drowsiness, driving or other hazardous activity should be avoided.

Interactions

• ℞ **acetazolamide** and succinimides (for example, ℞ **ethosuximide**, ℞ **methsuximide**) may reduce the concentration and effectiveness of primidone.
• Carbamazepine levels may rise and primidone concentration fall.
• ℞ **Hydantoins**, ℞ **isoniazid**, and ℞ **nicotinamide** may cause an increase in primidone concentration.

Side effects

Serious reactions are rare, but mild side effects occur frequently. These include:
• Drowsiness, unsteady gait, vertigo, lethargy, loss of appetite, nausea, and vomiting;
• Less frequently there may be mood swings, disturbances of vision, rash, eyelid swelling, hair loss, and (reversible) blood changes, such as a fall in red cells (anemia) or certain white cells;
• Rarely, there may be an acute psychosis-like reaction;
• Occasionally, when given to children, it may cause overexcitability.

Principen ⑧

A preparation of ℞ **ampicillin**.
Formulation: Oral capsules in several strengths; oral suspension.
Availability: Prescription only.
Warnings and side effects: See ℞ **ampicillin**.

Prinivil ⑧

A preparation of ℞ **lisinopril**.
Formulation: Oral tablets, available in 5 strengths.
Availability: Prescription only.
Warnings and side effects: See ℞ **lisinopril**.

PrinzideTablets; 12.5 Tablets; 25 Tablets ⑧

A preparation of ℞ **hydrochlorothiazide** and ℞ **lisinopril**.
Formulation: Oral tablets, in 3 strengths.
Availability: Prescription only.
Warnings and side effects: See ℞ **hydrochlorothiazide**; ℞ **lisinopril**.

Privine ⑧

A preparation of ℞ **naphazoline hydrochloride**.
Formulation: Nasal drops; spray.
Availability: OTC.
Warnings and side effects: See ℞ **naphazoline hydrochloride**.

ProAmatine ⑧

A preparation of ℞ **midodrine hydrochloride**.
Formulation: Oral tablets, available in two strengths.
Availability: Prescription only.
Warnings and side effects: See ℞ **midodrine hydrochloride**.

Probalan ⑧

A preparation of ℞ **probenecid**.
Formulation: Oral tablets.
Availability: Prescription only.
Warnings and side effects: See ℞ **probenecid**.

Probampacin ⑧

A preparation of ℞ **ampicillin** and ℞ **probenecid**.
Formulation: Oral capsules.
Availability: Prescription only.
Warnings and side effects: See ℞ **ampicillin**; ℞ **probenecid**.

Pro-Banthine ⑧

A preparation of ℞ **propantheline bromide**.
Formulation: Oral tablets, available in two strengths.
Availability: Prescription only.
Warnings and side effects: See ℞ **propantheline bromide**.

Proben-C ⑧

A preparation of ℞ **probenecid** and ℞ **colchicine**.
Formulation: Oral tablets.
Availability: Prescription only.
Warnings and side effects: See ℞ **probenecid** ℞ **colchicine**.

probenecid ⑥

Type/Group: **uricosuric; antigout**.
Brand(s): Benemid; Probalan; various generic.
How administered: Orally.

Used to treat

Probenecid is a drug that alters the way the kidney excretes chemicals, and is used for two main purposes. First, by inhibiting the excretion from the body of certain antibiotics (mainly the penicillins and cephalosporins), it increases their duration of action. Second, as an uricosuric it increases the excretion of uric acid from the blood into the urine, and can be used in the prevention of attacks of chronic ✪ **gout**, which involve high levels of uric acid (hyperuricemia).

Warnings

• It should not be given to people with known hypersensitivity to this drug or with blood disorders or uric acid kidney stones. It must not be used in children under two years of age.

• It should be given with caution to people with kidney function impairment or peptic ulcers.

• Probenecid should be used during pregnancy only when it is clearly needed and when the potential benefits outweigh the possible risk to the fetus.

• Medical judgment is required if breast-feeding is being considered. It is not known whether this drug appears in breast milk.

• Rarely, there may be severe allergic reactions.

• Aspirin and other salicylates should not be taken while using this drug, as its effects may be reduced.

Interactions

• The levels of the following drugs may be increased: ℞ **acyclovir**; ℞ **benzodiazepines**; ℞ **clofibrate**; ℞ **dapsone**; ℞ **sulfonamides**; ℞ **sulfonylureas**; ℞ **rifampin**; ℞ NSAIDs; ᪥ **pantothenic acid**; dyphylline; ℞ **methotrexate**; ℞ **zidovudine**.

• If used with thiopental, anesthesia may be prolonged.

• The effects of ℞ **penicillamine** may be reduced.

Side effects

• Nausea and vomiting, hair loss, increased urination, headache and flushing, dizziness and rash, and sore gums.

• Rarely, hypersensitivity, liver and kidney changes, and blood disorders.

procainamide hydrochloride Ⓖ

Type/Group: **antiarrhythmic**.
Brand(s): Pronestyl, Pronestyl-SR; Procanbid; various generic.
How administered: Orally; injection.

Used to treat

Procainamide has local anesthetic properties but is used to treat life-threatening heartbeat irregularities, especially ventricular tachycardia (see ✪ **arrhythmia**).

Warnings

• It should not be given to people with known hypersensitivity to this drug, with heart block or certain arrhythmias, or lupus erythematosus.

• It should be given with caution to people with asthma, depressed bone marrow function, congestive heart failure, the neuromuscular disease myasthenia gravis, or impaired kidney function. This is a specialist drug and treatment will be carried out by experienced clinicians who are thoroughly familiar with this drug. Periodic monitoring of heart function and blood values is necessary.

• Procainamide crosses the placenta and should be used during pregnancy only if it is clearly needed.

• It is present in breast milk and nursing women should discontinue using this drug or stop breast-feeding.

• Long-term use of procainamide often causes certain antibodies (antinuclear antibodies) to develop, which are sometimes accompanied by lupus-like symptoms. Its use must be reconsidered when this occurs.

• A doctor must be contacted if arthralgia (joint pain), myalgia (muscle pain), fever, chills, skin rash, easy bruising, sore throat or sore mouth, infections, dark urine or jaundice, wheezing, muscular weakness, chest or abdominal pain, palpitations, nausea, vomiting, loss of appetite, diarrhea, hallucinations, dizziness, or depression occur.

Interactions

• ℞ **amiodarone hydrochloride**, ℞ **beta-blockers**, ℞ **H$_2$-antagonists**, and ℞ **trimethoprim (TMP)** may increase the effects of procainamide.

• Other antiarrhythmic drugs (for example, ℞ **disopyramide**, ℞ **lidocaine**, ℞ **propranolol**, ℞ **quinidine**), ℞ **anticholinergics**, and ℞ **antihypertensives** may increase effects or produce toxic effects.

• The effects of ℞ **succinylcholine** may be increased, with a risk of neuromuscular blockade.

• The effects of ℞ **anticholinesterases** may be reduced.

Side effects

• Frequent side effects include loss of appetite, nausea, vomiting, bitter taste, diarrhea, or arrhythmias.

• The most common with long-term use is the development of antibodies with or without lupus-like symptoms (arthritis, joint pain, abdominal pain, fever, chills, rash).

• Other sensitivity reactions may include fever, rash, hives or allergic swelling.

• Occasionally severe blood effects occur, including bone marrow depression and lower counts of white cells, red cells, or platelets.

procaine Ⓖ

Type/Group: **local anesthetic**.
Brand(s): Novocaine; various generic.
How administered: Local injection.

Used to treat

Procaine was once popular but is now seldom used because it has been overtaken by anesthetics that are longer-lasting and better absorbed through mucous membranes. It cannot be administered as a surface anesthetic because it is poorly absorbed. However, it is still available and can be used for regional anesthesia or by infiltration.

Warnings

• It should not be given to people with known hypersensitivity to procaine, or those rare patients with methemoglobinemia (a serious blood disorder). It is a specialist drug and there will be a full medical assessment.

• It should be used in pregnancy only when it is clearly needed.

• Medical judgment is required if breast-feeding is being considered.

• It can cause cardiac depression, peripheral vasodilatation, or CNS (central nervous system) toxicity.

Interactions

• There is a risk of additive toxicity with ℞ **antiarrhythmics** (for example, ℞ **tocainide**, ℞ **mexiletine**).

• ℞ **Sedatives** may cause increased CNS effects.

• The effects of ℞ **sulfonamides** are reduced.

Side effects

• Occasionally, pain at injection site, burning, stinging, or tenderness where applied.

• Rarely (generally with high dose), drowsiness, dizziness, disorientation, lightheadedness, tremors, apprehension, euphoria, sensation of heat, cold, or numbness, blurred or double vision, ringing or roaring in ears, nausea, or allergic reactions.

Procanbid ℞

A preparation of ℞ **procainamide hydrochloride**.
Formulation: Oral tablets, sustained release.
Availability: Prescription only.
Warnings and side effects: See ℞ **procainamide hydrochloride**.

procarbazine ©

Type/Group: **anticancer; cytotoxic**.
Brand(s): Matulane.
How administered: Orally.

Used to treat

Procarbazine is a (methylhydrazine derivative) cytotoxic drug that is used, in combination with other drugs, in the treatment of the lymphatic cancer ✪ **Hodgkin's disease**.

Warnings

• It should not be given to people with known hypersensitivity to this drug or inadequate bone marrow reserve.

• It should be given with caution to people with impaired kidney or liver function. This is a specialist drug which will be used following a full evaluation by specialist physicians.

• Procarbazine is not recommended for use during pregnancy unless it is medically judged to be essential, because it may cause birth defects. Becoming pregnant while using this drug must be avoided.

• It should not be used if breast-feeding.

• It can produce bone marrow depression, which may lead to bleeding and a reduced resistance to infection.

• In common with many anticancer drugs, procarbazine may cause genetic mutations and/or cancer.

• It may have toxic effects on the kidneys.

• A doctor must be contacted if fever, sore throat, signs of local infection, easy bruising, or unusual bleeding occur.

• It may cause drowsiness and dizziness which will impair the performance of skilled tasks, such as driving.

• Food with a high tyramine content (for example, smoked meats) must be avoided because it may cause a hypertensive crisis.

Interactions

• Alcohol may cause unpleasant symptoms.

• The levels of digitalis and glycosides may be reduced.

• The effects of ℞ **levodopa**, ℞ **narcotic analgesics**, ℞ **sympathomimetics**, and ℞ **tricyclic** antidepressants may be increased.

• Procarbazine should not be taken until the bone marrow has recovered after radiation therapy or other chemotherapy.

Side effects

• Frequently, severe nausea and vomiting, respiratory disorders, joint and muscle pain, drowsiness, nervousness, insomnia, nightmares, sweating, hallucinations, and seizures.

• Occasionally, hoarseness, speeded heartbeat, nystagmus, eye changes, urinary problems, hypotension, diarrhea, inflammation of mouth mucosa, tingling and burning sensations, unsteadiness, confusion, and poor reflexes.

• Rarely, allergic reaction, darkening of the skin, and hair loss.

Procardia ℞

A preparation of ℞ **nifedipine**.
Formulation: Oral capsules, available in two strengths.
Availability: Prescription only.
Warnings and side effects: See ℞ **nifedipine**.

Procardia XL ℞

A preparation of ℞ **nifedipine**.
Formulation: Oral tablets, sustained release, available in 3 strengths.
Availability: Prescription only.
Warnings and side effects: See ℞ **nifedipine**.

prochlorperazine ©

Type/Group: **antipsychotic; antiemetic; antinauseant; phenothiazine**.
Brand(s): Compazine.
How administered: Orally; injection, topically (rectal suppositories).

Used to treat

Prochlorperazine is used in the treatment of ✪ **psychotic disorders**, such as ✪ **schizophrenia** and mania, and also as an ℞ **antiemetic** and ℞ **antinauseant** in the prevention of nausea caused by chemotherapy, radiotherapy, or by the vertigo and labyrinthine disorders.

Warnings

• It should not be given to people with known hypersensitivity to this drug, with severe toxic CNS (central nervous system) depression, coma, subcortical brain damage, bone marrow depression, severe liver or heart disease, or narrow-angle glaucoma.

• It should be given with caution to people with cardiovascular disease, epilepsy, liver or kidney disease, glaucoma, prostatic hypertrophy, severe asthma, emphysema, hypocalcemia (low blood calcium), thyrotoxicosis, or anyone over 65.

• Prochlorperazine should be used during pregnancy only if the benefits outweigh the risk to the fetus.

• Medical judgment is required if breast-feeding is being considered.

• It may cause drowsiness, and so the performance of skilled tasks, such as driving, may be impaired.

• It may cause postural hypotension (lowered blood pressure on standing), so rise slowly from a reclining position. Older people in particular should exercise caution.

• It may cause sensitivity to sunlight (photosensitivity), so minimize exposure (use a sunscreen, sunglasses, and so on).

• If used for a long time, tardive dyskinesia (see ℞ **antipsychotics**) occasionally develops.

• Treatment should be stopped gradually.

• It may enhance the effects of alcohol.

• Smoking may reduce the effects of this drug.

• It is not normally given to children less than 5 years old.

Interactions

• The ℞ **antiparkinsonism** effects of ℞ **levodopa** may be reduced.

• If used with an ℞ **antidepressant** or ℞ **propranolol**, the levels of both drugs may be increased.

• If used with ℞ **lithium** or ℞ **bromocriptine**, the levels of both drugs may be decreased.

• ℞ **Antimalarials** (amodiaquine, chloroquine, sulfadoxine, pyrimethamine) may increase the levels of prochlorperazine.

• ℞ **Anticholinergics**, ℞ **barbiturates**, ℞ **narcotic analgesics**, and ℞ **orphenadrine** lower the levels of an antipsychotic in the blood, and/or increase the occurrence of anticholinergic and/or CNS (central nervous system) effects.

• If used with ℞ **clonidine hydrochloride**, ℞ **trazodone**, and ℞ **guanethidine monosulfate**, there is a risk of excessive lowering of blood pressure.

• If used with ℞ **indomethacin**, there are possible increased effects on the CNS.

• ℞ **Procarbazine** increases sedation and extrapyramidal effects (see ℞ **antipsychotics**).

• If an antipsychotic is taken with alcohol, there may be increased sedative effects.

Side effects

• These depend on how it is administered. Extrapyramidal symptoms include (see ℞ **antipsychotics**), drowsiness, headache, loss of appetite, constipation, dry mouth, and nausea.

• Less frequently, agitation, anxiety, catatonic-like behavioral states, confusion, depression, euphoria, worsening of psychotic symptoms, heat or cold intolerance, insomnia, lethargy, restlessness, vertigo, ECG changes, changes in blood pressure, speeded heartbeat, blood abnormalities, blurred vision, eye changes, indigestion, increased salivation, vomiting, priapism (prolonged, painful penile erection), urinary retention, changes in hormone function (irregular or absent menstruation, growth of breasts, abnormal milk production, impotence, increased libido), changes in blood sugar levels, sensitivity reactions, rashes, spasmodic constriction of the bronchi or larynx, increased sweating, and loss of hair.

• Rarely, neuroleptic malignant syndrome (a potentially fatal condition characterized by very high fever, muscle rigidity, changes in mental status, and irregular pulse, blood pressure and/or heart rhythm) and seizure.

Procort Ⓑ

A preparation of ℞ **hydrocortisone**.
Formulation: Cream.
Availability: OTC.
Warnings and side effects: See ℞ **hydrocortisone**.

Procrit Ⓑ

A preparation of ℞ **epoetin alfa**.
Formulation: Injection.
Availability: Prescription only.
Warnings and side effects: See ℞ **epoetin alfa**.

Proctocort Ⓑ

A preparation of ℞ **hydrocortisone**.
Formulation: Cream; rectal suppositories.
Availability: Prescription only.
Warnings and side effects: See ℞ **hydrocortisone**.

ProctoCream-HC Ⓑ

A preparation of ℞ **hydrocortisone**.
Formulation: Cream.
Availability: Prescription only.
Warnings and side effects: See ℞ **hydrocortisone**.

Proctofoam-HC Ⓑ

A preparation of ℞ **hydrocortisone** and ℞ **pramoxine hydrochloride**.
Formulation: Aerosol foam.
Availability: Prescription only.
Warnings and side effects: See ℞ **hydrocortisone**; ℞ **pramoxine hydrochloride**.

procyclidine Ⓖ

Type/Group: antiparkinsonism; anticholinergic.
Brand(s): Kemadrin.
How administered: Orally.

Used to treat

Procyclidine is used as an adjunct treatment (an additional treatment to enhance effectiveness) of all forms of ✪ **Parkinson's disease** and for the control of drug-induced extrapyramidal disorders.

Warnings

• It should not be used by people with known hypersensitivity to this drug, angle-closure glaucoma, gastrointestinal or urogenital obstruction, myasthenia gravis, peptic ulcer, megacolon, or prostatic hypertrophy.

• It should be used with caution by people with tachycardia, liver or kidney disease, a history of drug abuse, dysrhythmias, hypotension or hypertension, psychosis, or tardive dyskinesia.

• Individuals who are over 60 may be particularly sensitive to anticholinergic drugs, and should exercise caution when using this one.

• Extreme caution should also be used when this drug is given to children, because they, too, may be particularly sensitive to ℞ **anticholinergic** side effects.

• It is not known whether or not procyclidine crosses the placenta. It should be used during pregnancy only if clearly needed and if the benefits outweigh the possible risks to the fetus.

• Its effect on breast milk is unknown. However, it is known that infants are sensitive to the effects of anticholinergic drugs and so medical judgment is also required if breast-feeding is being considered.

• Use with caution during hot weather as there is a risk of heat stroke due to decreased sweating.
• The performance of skilled tasks, such as driving, may be affected as there is a potential for interfering side effects, such as dizziness, confusion, and blurred vision.
• Use of this drug should be ended gradually.

Interactions
• The effectiveness of ℞ **levodopa** may be reduced.
• The effectiveness of ℞ **phenothiazines** may be reduced if taken with procyclidine, and anticholinergic side effects may be increased.
• Taking procyclidine with ℞ **haloperidol** and similar ℞ **antipsychotics** may result in a worsening of psychiatric symptoms and the development of tardive dyskinesia.
• The incidence of anticholinergic side effects may be increased if taken with anticholinergics or ℞ **amantadine**.
• ℞ **Tacrine** reduces the effect of both drugs.

Side effects
• Frequently, confusion, dry mouth, mental changes (psychotic-like symptoms).
• Occasionally, postural hypotension (lowered blood pressure on standing), loss of appetite, headache, livedo reticularis (reddish blue blotching of the skin), blurred vision, urinary retention, dry mouth.
• Rarely, vomiting, depression, irritation or swelling of eyes, and skin rash.

Prodrox ®
A preparation of ℞ **hydroxyprogesterone caproate**.
Formulation: Injection.
Availability: Prescription only.
Warnings and side effects: See ℞ **hydroxyprogesterone caproate**.

Profasi ®
A preparation of ℞ **chorionic gonadotropin**.
Formulation: Injection.
Availability: Prescription only.
Warnings and side effects: See ℞ **chorionic gonadotropin**.

Profilnine SD ®
A preparation of ℞ **Factor IX complex**. Also contains II, VII, and X.
Formulation: Intravenous infusion.
Availability: Prescription only.
Warnings and side effects: See ℞ **Factor IX complex**.

Progestasert ®
A preparation of ℞ **progesterone**.
Formulation: IUD.
Availability: Prescription only.
Warnings and side effects: See ℞ **progesterone**.

progesterone ⓖ
Type/Group: **sex hormone; progestin; contraceptive; fertility treatment**.

Brand(s): Prometrium; Crinone; Progestasert (IUD); various generic.
How administered: Orally; injection; vaginal gel; IUD (intrauterine device).

Used to treat
Progesterone is used for dysfunctional uterine bleeding and amenorrhea, and in an intrauterine device (IUD), for contraception. It is also used to treat luteal phase deficiency in women undergoing assisted reproductive technology therapy for infertility.

Warnings
• It should not be used by people with known hypersensitivity to this drug, or with impaired liver function or disease, breast cancer, undiagnosed vaginal bleeding, missed abortion, thrombophlebitis, or a history of thromboembolic disease or stroke.
• The IUD is not suitable for those at risk of pelvic infection, or for those who have had a previous ectopic pregnancy, genital actinomycosis, or who have an increased susceptibility to infection (for example, leukemia, diabetes, AIDS).
• It should be given with caution to people with epilepsy, migraine, asthma, heart or kidney dysfunction, depression, or diabetes mellitus. The IUD form should be given with caution to people with a history of heavy or painful periods, or with valvular or congenital heart disease.
• Progesterone should not be used during pregnancy. A doctor must be contacted if pregnancy occurs while taking this drug.
• Medical judgment is required if breast-feeding is being considered.
• Diabetics may note decreased glucose tolerance.
• A doctor must be contacted if there is abnormal or excessive bleeding, severe cramping, abnormal or odorous vaginal discharge, or missed period (when using as IUD).

Interactions
• ℞ **aminoglutethimide** may reduce the levels of progesterone.

Side effects
These depend on the form and use.
• Most commonly, nausea.
• Other side effects include depression, fatigue, insomnia, fluid retention, increased weight, cessation of menstruation, breast changes, breakthrough bleeding, spotting, elevated blood glucose, acne, rash, changes in hair growth, and irritation at injection site.
• Rare but serious side effects from use as an IUD include ectopic pregnancy, perforation of uterus and cervix, septic abortion, septicemia, and spontaneous abortion.

progestin ⓓ
(progestogen)
Generics: **desogestrel; hydroxyprogesterone caproate; levonorgestrel; medroxyprogesterone; megestrol acetate; norethindrone; norgestrel; progesterone**.

Actions and uses
Progestin is the name of the group of (℞ **steroid**) ℞ **sex hormone** mediators formed and released by the ovaries and placenta in women, the adrenal gland, and in small amounts by the testes in men. Physiologically, progestins prepare the lining of the uterus

(endometrium) for pregnancy, maintain it throughout pregnancy, and prevent the further release of eggs (ovulation). They include the natural progestin ℞ **progesterone** and synthetic substances with similar actions (including ℞ **desogestrel**, ℞ **norgestrel**, ℞ **levonorgestrel**, ℞ **medroxyprogesterone**, ℞ **norethindrone**, ℞ **megestrol acetate**, and ℞ **hydroxyprogesterone caproate**). They have many therapeutic uses including the treatment of menstrual disorders (❂ **menorrhagia** and severe ❂ **dysmenorrhea**), ❂ **endometriosis** (inflammation of the tissues normally lining the uterus), in menopausal ℞ **hormone replacement**, to treat luteal phase deficiency (inadequate production of progesterone during the luteal phase of menstruation) in women undergoing assisted reproductive technology therapy (ART) for infertility, to relieve the symptoms of ❂ **premenstrual syndrome**, and sometimes in the treatment of ❂ **breast cancer**, endometrial cancer, kidney cancer, and ❂ **prostate cancer**.

The most common use is as constituents (with or without ℞ **estrogen** hormones) in ℞ **oral contraceptives**. Mainly progestins are taken by mouth, but there are also forms for contraception that are given by deep intramuscular injection, by implant (subdermal; under the skin), or from an intrauterine device (IUD) that slowly releases the drug into the cavity of the uterus.

Limitations

Progestins have a number of side effects and expert counseling may be required to find the most acceptable dose. There are a number of conditions where these drugs should not be taken (including a history of thromboembolic disease or stroke). Some of them are placed in the Food and Drug Administration's Pregnancy Category X, which means that they should not normally be taken during pregnancy. A doctor must be consulted if you become, or suspect you are, pregnant while taking progestins. Diabetic patients must monitor blood glucose levels during therapy. See also the individual drug entries.

progestogen ⑩

see ℞ **progestin**.

Proglycem ⑧

A preparation of ℞ **diazoxide**.
Formulation: Oral suspension; capsules.
Availability: Prescription only.
Warnings and side effects: See ℞ **diazoxide**.

Prograf ⑧

A preparation of ℞ **tacrolimus**.
Formulation: Oral capsules; injection (infusion).
Availability: Prescription only.
Warnings and side effects: See ℞ **tacrolimus**.

ProHIBit ⑧

A preparation of ℞ **Haemophilus b conjugate vaccine**.
Formulation: Injection.
Availability: Prescription only.
Warnings and side effects: See ℞ **Haemophilus b conjugate vaccine**.

Proleukin ⑧

A preparation of ℞ **aldesleukin**.
Formulation: Injection (infusion).
Availability: Prescription only.
Warnings and side effects: See ℞ **aldesleukin**.

Prolixin ⑧

A preparation of ℞ **fluphenazine**.
Formulation: Oral tablets; oral concentrate; oral elixir; vials and syringes for injection.
Availability: Prescription only.
Warnings and side effects: See ℞ **fluphenazine**.

Proloprim ⑧

A preparation of ℞ **trimethoprim**.
Formulation: Oral tablets in two strengths.
Availability: Prescription only.
Warnings and side effects: See ℞ **trimethoprim**.

promazine ⑥

Type/Group: antipsychotic; phenothiazine.
Brand(s): Sparine.
How administered: Orally, injection.

Used to treat
Promazine is used to tranquillize agitated and restless patients.

Warnings
• It should not be given to people with known hypersensitivity to this drug, with severe toxic CNS depression, coma, subcortical brain damage, bone marrow depression, or narrow-angle glaucoma.
• It should be given with caution to people with severe cardiovascular disorders, seizure disorder (epilepsy), liver or kidney disease, glaucoma, prostatic hypertrophy, severe asthma, emphysema, hypocalcemia (low calcium), or anyone over 65.
• Promazine should be used during pregnancy only if the benefits outweigh the risk to the fetus.
• Medical judgment is required if breast-feeding is being considered.
• It may cause drowsiness, and so the performance of skilled tasks, such as driving, may be impaired.
• It may cause postural hypotension (lowered blood pressure on standing), so rise slowly from a reclining position. Older people in particular should exercise caution.
• It may cause sensitivity to sunlight (photosensitivity), so minimize exposure (use a sunscreen, sunglasses, and so on).
• If used for a long time, tardive dyskinesia (see ℞ **antipsychotics**) occasionally develops.
• Treatment should be stopped gradually.
• It may enhance the effects of alcohol.

Interactions
• The ℞ **antiparkinsonism** effects of ℞ **levodopa** may be reduced.
• Promazine may increase the levels of ℞ **tricyclic** antidepressants.
• If used with ℞ **lithium** or ℞ **bromocriptine**, the levels of both drugs may be decreased.

• ℞ **Antimalarials** (amodiaquine, chloroquine, sulfadoxine, pyrimethamine) may increase the levels of prochlorperazine.

• ℞ **Anticholinergics**, ℞ **barbiturates**, and ℞ **orphenadrine** lower the levels of an antipsychotic in the blood, and/or increase the occurrence of anticholinergic and/or CNS (central nervous system) effects.

• ℞ **guanethidine monosulfate**'s effects on blood pressure may be reduced.

• There may be excessive CNS depression, lowered blood pressure, and respiratory depression if used with ℞ **narcotic analgesics**.

• If an antipsychotic is taken with alcohol, there may be increased sedative effects.

Side effects

• Drowsiness, extrapyramidal symptoms (see ℞ **antipsychotics**), headache, loss of appetite, constipation, dry mouth, nausea, and spasmodic constriction of the bronchi or larynx.

• Less frequently, agitation, anxiety, catatonic-like behavioral states, worsening of psychotic symptoms, heat or cold intolerance, restlessness, ECG changes, changes in blood pressure, speeded heartbeat, blood abnormalities, blurred vision, eye changes, indigestion, increased salivation, vomiting, priapism (prolonged, painful penile erection), urinary retention, changes in hormone function (irregular menstruation, growth of breasts, abnormal milk production, impotence, increased libido), changes in blood sugar levels, sensitivity reactions, rashes, increased sweating, loss of hair, and heat or cold intolerance.

• Rarely, neuroleptic malignant syndrome (a potentially fatal condition characterized by very high fever, muscle rigidity, changes in mental status, and irregular pulse, blood pressure and/or heart rhythm) and seizure.

promethazine hydrochloride ⓖ

Type/Group: antihistamine; antiallergic; phenothiazine; antinauseant; cold and cough preparation.

Brand(s): Anergan 50; Phenergan Tablets, Syrup, Suppositories, Injection; various generic. Combinations: With *codeine*: Phenergan with Codeine Syrup; Pherazine w/Codeine Syrup. With *codeine and phenylephrine*: Phenergan VC with Codeine Syrup; Pherazine VC w/ Codeine Syrup; Promethist with Codeine Syrup. With *dextromethorphan*: Phenameth DM Syrup; Phenergan w/ Dextromethorphan Syrup; Pherazine DM Syrup. With *phenylephrine*: Phenergan VC Syrup; Promethazine VC Plain Syrup. How administered: Orally; injection (intramuscular only); suppositories.

Used to treat

Promethazine is chemically a ℞ **phenothiazine** derivative, which also has ℞ **hypnotic** properties. It is used to treat the symptoms of allergic conditions, such as ✪ **hay fever** (seasonal allergic rhinitis), perennial rhinitis, vasomotor rhinitis, allergic ✪ **conjunctivitis**, and allergic skin manifestations such as ✪ **angioedema** and ✪ **urticaria**, for ✪ **motion sickness**, and can also be used (with other drugs) in the emergency treatment of anaphylactic shock (see ✪ **anaphylactic reaction**). It has sedative effects and can be used as a preoperative medication, to treat temporary sleep disorders,

and is included in some preparations for ✪ **coughs** and ✪ **colds**, and as an antiemetic following operations.

Warnings

• It should not be given to people with known hypersensitivity to this drug (or with known sensitivity to other antihistamines), who are comatose or who have received large doses of other sedating drugs.

• Antihistamines should be given with caution to people with impaired liver function, cardiovascular disease, asthma (and never during an attack) or lower respiratory tract disease, heart disease, hypertension, hyperthyroidism, epilepsy, porphyria, bone marrow depression, increased intraocular pressure (pressure in the eyeball, as in glaucoma), enlarged prostate, urinary retention, or certain obstructive bladder or gastrointestinal conditions.

• Promethazine should be used during pregnancy (except during delivery) only if the potential benefit outweighs the potential risk to the fetus.

• Medical judgment is required if breast-feeding is being considered.

• Promethazine must not be given to infants, and for children under the age of 12 the manufacturer's or medical instructions must be followed closely.

• As with all phenothiazines, this drug should not be given to children with any acute illness, as its effects (extrapyramidal symptoms) may mask symptoms of other illness, for example Reye's syndrome.

• Promethazine should be injected intramuscularly only, because serious adverse reactions are possible if it is injected into a blood vessel.

• Because of its marked sedative side effects, the performance of skilled tasks, such as driving, may be impaired, and children should be supervised for example when bike-riding.

• Side effects are more frequent in the elderly.

Interactions

• ℞ **MAOI** antidepressants may prolong and intensify the ℞ **anticholinergic** and sedative effects of antihistamines (see Side effects below), and the side effects (extrapyramidal effects) of phenothiazines.

• Promethazine may reduce or reverse the effects of ℞ **epinephrine**, and the two drugs should not be used together.

• If used with ℞ **tricyclic** antidepressants, other antihistamines, ℞ **skeletal muscle relaxants**, ℞ **opioids**, ℞ **barbiturates**, ℞ **hypnotics**, ℞ **sedatives**, or ℞ **antianxiety** drugs, there is a risk of intensified side effects.

• Pheniramine maleate can mask the toxic effects (to the ears) of ℞ **aminoglycoside** antibiotics.

• Alcohol may intensify side effects such as drowsiness and impaired mental alertness.

Side effects

• These depend on how it is administered. For this type of antihistamine, there is commonly drowsiness, headache, impaired muscular coordination or dizziness, anticholinergic effects (dry mouth, blurred vision, urinary retention, gastrointestinal disturbances), occasional rashes and photosensitivity (abnormal sensitivity to light), palpitations and heart arrhythmias.

• Rarely, there may be stimulation instead of sedation (paradoxical stimulation), especially in children (and convulsions in overdose), hypersensitivity reactions, blood disorders, liver disturbances, depression, sleep disturbances, and hypotension. In particular, unusual sensitivity to sunlight or involuntary muscle movements should be reported. Intramuscular injections may be painful.

Promethazine VC Plain Syrup ⓑ

A preparation of ℞ **phenylephrine hydrochloride** and ℞ **promethazine hydrochloride**.
Formulation: Oral syrup.
Availability: Prescription only.
Warnings and side effects: See ℞ **phenylephrine hydrochloride**; ℞ **promethazine hydrochloride**.

Promethist with Codeine Syrup ⓑ

A preparation of ℞ **codeine phosphate**, ℞ **phenylephrine hydro-chloride**, and ℞ **promethazine hydrochloride**.
Formulation: Oral syrup.
Availability: May or may not require a prescription.
Warnings and side effects: See ℞ **codeine phosphate**; ℞ **phenylephrine hydrochloride**; ℞ **promethazine hydrochloride**.

Prometrium ⓑ

A preparation of ℞ **progesterone**.
Formulation: Oral capsules.
Availability: Prescription only.
Warnings and side effects: See ℞ **progesterone**.

Pronestyl Tablets, Capsules, Injection; Pronestyl-SR ⓑ

A preparation of ℞ **procainamide hydrochloride**.
Formulation: Oral tablets (2 strengths); capsules (3 strengths); sustained-release tablets (Pronestyl-SR); injection.
Availability: Prescription only.
Warnings and side effects: See ℞ **procainamide hydrochloride**. Tablets contain tartrazine (FD)

Pronto ⓑ

A preparation of ℞ **pyrethrin**.
Formulation: Shampoo.
Availability: OTC.
Warnings and side effects: See ℞ **pyrethrin**.

Propacet ⓑ

A preparation of propoxyphene napsylate and ℞ **acetaminophen**.
Formulation: Oral tablets.
Availability: Prescription only.
Warnings and side effects: See ℞ **propoxyphene hydrochloride**; ℞ **acetaminophen**.

propafenone hydrochloride ⓖ

Type/Group: **antiarrhythmic**.
Brand(s): Rhythmol.

How administered: Orally.
Used to treat
Propafenone hydrochloride is used to regularize the heartbeat when certain life-threatening ⊙ **arrhythmias** have developed, although it may be used (where no heart disease is present) to treat some lesser arrhythmias.
Warnings
• It should not be given to people with known hypersensitivity to this drug, with certain arrhythmias, uncontrolled congestive heart failure, marked hypotension, or bronchospasmic disease (for example, chronic bronchitis, emphysema).
• It should be given with caution to the elderly, people with heart pacemakers, myasthenia gravis, or impaired liver or kidney function. This is a specialist drug and treatment will be carried out by experienced clinicians who are thoroughly familiar with this drug. Periodic monitoring of heart function and blood values is necessary.
• It is possible that propafenone may harm the fetus and so it should be used during pregnancy only if the potential benefit outweighs the possible risk to the fetus.
• It is present in breast milk and nursing women should discontinue using this drug or stop breast-feeding.
• Propafenone can, occasionally, provoke arrhythmias.
• Use of propafenone may cause certain antibodies to develop, with or without lupus-like symptoms (arthritis, arthralgia (joint pain), abdominal pain, fever, chills, rash). Its use must be reconsidered when this occurs.
• Overdose may produce symptoms such as hypotension, excessive drowsiness, decreased heart rate, or abnormal heartbeat.
• A doctor must be contacted if signs of infection develop, such as fever, sore throat, chills, or unusual bruising or bleeding.
Interactions
• ℞ **Cimetidine** and ℞ **quinidine** may increase the effects of propafenone.
• The levels and effects of ℞ **anticoagulants** (for example, ℞ **warfarin sodium**), ℞ **beta-blockers**, ℞ **cyclosporine**, ℞ **desipramine**, and ℞ **digoxin** may be increased, with the potential for adverse effects.
• ℞ **Rifampin** may reduce the levels and effects of propafenone.
Side effects
• Frequent side effects include dizziness, gastrointestinal disturbances (for example, nausea, vomiting, constipation, indigestion), unusual taste sensation, fatigue, breathlessness, blurred vision or dry mouth.
• Occasionally, heart and blood disorders, and lupus-like symptoms (arthritis, joint pain, abdominal pain, fever, chills, rash).

propantheline bromide ⓖ

Type/Group: **anticholinergic; antispasmodic**.
Brand(s): Pro-Banthine; various generic.
How administered: Orally.
Used to treat
Propantheline bromide has been used in combination with other drugs (for example, ℞ **phenobarbital**) in the treatment of ⊙ **peptic ulcer**. It is not now considered as effective as more recent

treatments, such as R **H₂-antagonists**, R **proton-pump inhibitors**, or R **Helicobacter pylori eradication regime**. Although not stated as a treatment for specific gastrointestinal disorders, it may be used for some that involve muscle spasm of the intestinal wall or excess secretions, and is also sometimes used for certain types of urinary frequency or incontinence.

Warnings

• It should not be given to people with known hypersensitivity to anticholinergics, with myasthenia gravis, narrow-angle glaucoma, urinary obstruction, or with any infection or obstructive condition of the gastrointestinal tract.

• It should be given with caution to people with kidney or liver impairment, enlarged prostate, heart disease or high blood pressure, hyperthyroidism, ulcerative colitis, hiatal hernia, glaucoma, brain damage, or Down's syndrome. The safety of this drug has not been established for children and infants.

• Propantheline should be used during pregnancy only if it is clearly needed.

• It may appear in breast milk and should be avoided by nursing mothers.

• Anticholinergics in general should not be given to anyone with a febrile (feverish) illness or who must work or live in a hot environment.

• The frequency and severity of side effects is higher in the elderly.

• Alcohol should be avoided.

• Because side effects may include drowsiness or visual disturbances, it may impair the performance of skilled tasks such as driving.

Interactions

• R **Amantadine**, some R **antiarrhythmic** agents (for example, R **disopyramide**, R **procainamide**, R **quinidine**), some R **antihistamines** (for example, R **promethazine**, R **carbinoxamine**, R **diphenhydramine hydrochloride**), R **antiparkinsonism** agents, R **glutethimide**, R **meperidine**, R **phenothiazines**, and R **tricyclic** antidepressants all have some anticholinergic effects which may increase when taken with propantheline to cause side effects.

• The levels of R **digoxin** may rise if taken in the slow-dissolving form (but not as capsules or elixir).

• Anticholinergics and ⚖ **potassium chloride** (in tablet form) should be used together with caution, because the tablet form of potassium chloride may stay in the intestines longer, and so there is a greater risk of irritation and lesions.

• Propantheline should be taken at least one hour before an R **antacid**.

• R **Ketoconazole** should be taken least two hours before anticholinergics.

Side effects

• These tend to be less frequent and less pronounced than with other anticholinergics (for example, R **atropine**), but may include, especially at higher doses, dry mouth, thirst, blurred vision and other visual disturbances, urinary hesitancy, palpitation, and constipation, photophobia.

• Uncommon side effects may include increased intraocular pressure (pressure in the eyeball), headache, unusual or absent taste sensation, nervousness, drowsiness, flushing and nausea.

• Although rare, hives, other skin eruptions, and anaphylaxis may occur in extreme allergic reactions.

PROPApH Cleansing for Sensitive Skin; Maximum Strength; Foam ⓑ

A preparation of R **salicylic acid** and various.
Formulation: Medicated pads; Face Wash is topical liquid.
Availability: OTC.
Warnings and side effects: See R **salicylic acid**.

PROPApH Cleansing Pads; Acne Maximum Strength Cream ⓑ

A preparation of R **salicylic acid** and various.
Formulation: Topical cream; medicated pads.
Availability: OTC.
Warnings and side effects: See R **salicylic acid**.

PROPApH Peel-off Acne Mask ⓑ

A preparation of R **salicylic acid**, ⚖ **vitamin E**, and various.
Formulation: Topical liquid (dries to mask).
Availability: OTC.
Warnings and side effects: See R **salicylic acid**; ⚖ **vitamin E**.

proparacaine ⓖ

Type/Group: **local anesthetic**.
How administered: Topically (external).
Brand(s): Alcaine, Ocu-Caine, Ophthetic, Paracaine.

Used to treat

Proparacaine is a benzoic acid derivative used to anesthetize the cornea during medical procedures.

Warnings

• It should not be given to people with known hypersensitivity to this drug.

• It should be given with caution to people in a weakened condition, over 65, acutely ill, with cardiac disease, certain blood disorders, or hyperthyroidism. Also use with caution in children.

• There are no adequate and well-controlled studies in pregnant women. It should be used only if the potential benefits outweigh the possible risks to the fetus.

• Medical judgment is required if breast-feeding is being considered.

• The eye should not be touched or rubbed until the anesthetic has worn off to avoid accidental injury.

Interactions

No significant drug interactions are known.

Side effects

• Eye congestion and bleeding.

Propecia ⓑ

A preparation of R **finasteride**.
Formulation: Oral tablets.
Availability: Prescription only.

Warnings and side effects: See ℞ **finasteride.**

Propine ⑧

A preparation of ℞ **dipivefrin hydrochloride.**
Formulation: Eye drops.
Availability: Prescription only.
Warnings and side effects: See ℞ **dipivefrin hydrochloride.**

Proplex T ⑧

A preparation of ℞ **Factor IX complex.** (Also contains Factors II, VII, X).
Formulation: Intravenous infusion.
Availability: Prescription only.
Warnings and side effects: See ℞ **Factor IX complex.** Contains a small amount of ℞ **heparin.**

propoxyphene hydrochloride ⑥

(dextropropoxyphene hydrochloride)
Type/Group: narcotic analgesic; opioid.
Brand(s): Darvon-N; Darvon Pulvules; various generic.
Combinations: With *aspirin:* Darvon Compound-65 Pulvules; various generic. With *acetaminophen:* Darvocet-N; Propacet; Wygesic; various generic.
How administered: Orally.

Used to treat

Propoxyphene hydrochloride is used to treat mild to moderate ◐ **pain** anywhere in the body. It is usually combined with other painkillers (especially ℞ **acetaminophen** or ℞ **aspirin**) as a compound analgesic.

Warnings

• It should not be given to people with known hypersensitivity to this drug, who have a history of addiction, or suicidal tendencies. Opioids (even the weaker ones) should not be given to people with asthma, to anyone with seriously depressed breathing disorders, prostatic hypertrophy, convulsive disorders, raised intracranial pressure, or a head injury.
• Depending on use and dose, it should be given with caution to the elderly, or to anyone with hypotension, porphyria, certain liver, kidney or adrenal disorders, hypothyroidism (under-activity of the thyroid gland), or alcoholism.
• Propoxyphene should be used during pregnancy only if the potential benefits outweigh the possible risks. Withdrawal symptoms have been observed in newborns.
• Propoxyphene is particularly dangerous in overdose. Do not exceed the prescribed dose.
• Propoxyphene is a Schedule IV controlled substance.
• Prolonged use of narcotics can lead to physical dependence (addiction), although this rarely happens in routine medical use.
• Drowsiness may affect the performance of skilled tasks such as driving.
• The effects of alcohol may be enhanced (including a higher risk of respiratory depression).
• ℞ **carbamazepine** has caused serious side effects, including coma, when used with this drug.

Interactions

• Propoxyphene should be used with caution with most protease inhibitors (for example, ℞ **nelfinavir,** ℞ **saquinavir**), except for ℞ **ritonavir,** which should never be used with propoxyphene.
• If used with the following drugs, then effects may be increased: ℞ **barbiturates;** ℞ **general anesthetics;** ℞ **opioids;** ℞ **tranquilizers** (for example, ℞ **phenothiazines**); ℞ **sedatives;** ℞ **benzodiazepines** (for example, ℞ **diazepam,** ℞ **lorazepam**); alcohol; ℞ **carbamazepine.**
• The levels of ℞ **antidepressants** in the blood are increased.
• ℞ **Activated charcoal** decreases the absorption and effect of propoxyphene.
• The anticoagulant effect of ℞ **anticoagulants** is intensified with the potential for bleeding.

Side effects

• These are infrequent, but there may be sedation, dizziness, vomiting, nausea, loss of appetite, and constipation. There is occasionally euphoria, which may lead to a state of mental detachment or confusion. Also, there may be sweating, headache, palpitations, changes in heart rate, postural hypotension (a lowering of blood pressure on standing, causing dizziness), rashes, miosis (pupil constriction), dry mouth, flushing of the face, mood change, and hallucinations.

propranolol hydrochloride ⑥

Type/Group: beta-blocker; antiarrhythmic; antihypertensive; antianginal; antianxiety; antimigraine.
Brand(s): Betachron E-R; Inderal, Inderal LA; various generic.
Combinations: With *hydrochlorothiazide:* Inderide, Inderide LA.
How administered: Orally; injection.

Used to treat

Propranolol is used to treat ◐ **hypertension** (and, with other drugs, in ◐ **pheochromocytoma** attacks), ◐ **angina pectoris** (to relieve symptoms and improve exercise tolerance), and to regularize heartbeat. It may also be used after heart attack to aid recovery, with an ℞ **alpha-adrenergic blocker** for pheochromocytoma, to prevent migraine attacks, and for symptomatic relief of tremor in certain inherited disorders, and anxiety-related performance tremor.

Warnings

• It should not be given to people with known hypersensitivity to any beta-blocking drug, who have certain heartbeat irregularities or heart failure. It should not be used in cardiogenic shock.
• It should be given with caution to people with diabetes mellitus or hypoglycemia, hyperthyroidism, myasthenia gravis, congestive heart failure, peripheral vascular disease, or liver or kidney impairment. Beta-blockers are generally not given to anyone with a nonallergic bronchospastic disease (for example, chronic bronchitis or emphysema).
• Propranolol should be used during pregnancy only if the potential benefit outweighs the possible risk to the fetus.
• It appears in breast milk, and so nursing women should discontinue using this drug or stop breast-feeding.
• Abruptly stopping using a beta-blocker may have adverse effects such as on the heart.

• The use of this drug may mask signs of hyperthyroidism or hypoglycemia.

• Other medications (including OTCs, herbal remedies, and supplements) must not be taken without consulting a doctor. Some ℞ **nasal decongestants**, commonly available over the counter, contain ℞ **alpha-adrenergic stimulants** (for example, ℞ **phenylephrine**) that may cause a severe hypertensive reaction if taken with beta-blockers.

Interactions

• A serious blood pressure increase may occur after withdrawal from ℞ **clonidine hydrochloride** or both drugs at the same time.

• Other ℞ **antiarrhythmics** (for example, ℞ **amiodarone**, ℞ **disopyramide**, ℞ **procainamide**, ℞ **quinidine**), ℞ **phenothiazines**, and ℞ **tricyclics** have the potential for significant adverse effects on heart rhythm.

• The effects of ℞ **alpha-adrenergic stimulants**, ℞ **ergot alkaloids**, ℞ **haloperidol**, ℞ **hydralazine hydrochloride**, ℞ **epinephrine**, ℞ **lidocaine**, and ℞ **theophylline** may be increased, with risk of serious adverse effects.

• ℞ **Calcium-channel blockers** (particularly ℞ **diltiazem** and ℞ **verapamil**), ℞ **guanethidine monosulfate**, and ℞ **reserpine** have the potential for increasing undesirable effects, with exaggerated slowing of heartbeat or hypotension.

• The effects of nondepolarizing ℞ **skeletal muscle relaxants** may be variable, with the possible risk of significant adverse effects associated with major surgery.

• The effects of ℞ **beta-adrenergic stimulant** (for example, ℞ **albuterol**, ℞ **terbutaline**), ℞ **insulin**, and ℞ **sulfonylureas** may be reduced by propranolol.

• ℞ **Cimetidine** may increase the effect of propranolol.

• ℞ **Antacids** (for example, ℞ **aluminum hydroxide**, ℞ **magnesium hydroxide**), ℞ **barbiturates**, ⚶ **calcium** salts, ℞ **cholestyramine**, ℞ **colestipol hydrochloride**, ℞ **NSAIDs**, ℞ **phenytoin**, ℞ **penicillins**, ℞ **rifampin**, and ℞ **salicylates** may reduce the levels and effectiveness of beta-blockers.

• If used with ℞ **diuretics** and other antihypertensive drugs, there are additive effects which are often used to therapeutic advantage.

Side effects

These are infrequent and may include:

• Slowing of the heart rate, hypotension, asthma-like symptoms and bronchospasm, gastrointestinal disturbances, poor circulation in the extremities, fatigue, and sleep disturbances;

• Rarely, skin rash has been reported;

• Heart failure, should it develop, generally requires withdrawal (gradually, if possible) of this drug.

propylthiouracil Ⓖ

Type/Group: antithyroid; hormone antagonist.
Brand(s): Generic only.
How administered: Orally.

Used to treat

Propylthiouracil acts as an indirect hormone antagonist by inhibiting the thyroid gland's production of ℞ **thyroid hormones**, thereby preventing an excess of thyroid hormone in the blood and treating the symptoms that it causes (thyrotoxicosis). It is also used to lessen hyperthyroidism in preparation for surgery or radiation therapy.

Warnings

• It should not be used by people with known hypersensitivity to this drug.

• It should be given with caution to people with infections, bone marrow depression, or liver disease. It should also be given with caution to children, as liver toxicity has been reported.

• It should be used in pregnancy only if medically judged to be clearly needed.

• It should not be used by breast-feeding mothers.

• It may cause agranulocytosis (a serious blood disease resulting in increased susceptibility to infection). A doctor must be contacted if hay fever, sore throat, skin eruptions, fever, headache, or general malaise (symptoms of agranulocytosis) develop. Risk is increased in people over age 40.

• Prolonged use has been associated with cancer in animal studies.

Interactions

• The effects of oral ℞ **anticoagulants** may be altered.

• Drugs containing ⚶ **iodine** (for example, potassium iodide) may decrease the response to propylthiouracil.

• The levels of ℞ **digoxin** may be increased.

• The risk of agranulocytosis is increased if other drugs that can also cause this condition (for example, ℞ **tricyclic** antidepressants) are taken with propylthiouracil.

Side effects

• Frequently, hives, rash, itching, nausea, darkening of skin, hair loss, headache, tingling sensation, and nephritis.

• Occasionally, drowsiness, enlarged lymph nodes, and dizziness.

• Rarely, drug fever, lupus-like syndrome, hepatitis, and potentially serious blood and skin disorders.

Proscar Ⓡ

A preparation of ℞ **finasteride**.
Formulation: Oral tablets.
Availability: Prescription only.
Warnings and side effects: See ℞ **finasteride**.

Prosed/DS Ⓡ

A preparation of ℞ **atropine sulfate**, ℞ **hyoscyamine**, ℞ **methenamine**, methylene blue, phenyl ℞ **salicylate**, and ℞ **benzoic acid**.
Formulation: Oral tablets.
Availability: Prescription only.
Warnings and side effects: See ℞ **atropine sulfate**; ℞ **hyoscyamine**; ℞ **methenamine**; ℞ **salicylates**; ℞ **benzoic acid**.

ProSom Ⓡ

A preparation of ℞ **estazolam**.
Formulation: Oral tablets in several strengths.
Availability: Prescription only.
Warnings and side effects: See ℞ **estazolam**.

prostaglandin ⓓ

Generics: **alprostadil; carboprost; dinoprostone; epoprostenol sodium; latanoprost; misoprostol.**

Actions and uses

Prostaglandin is the name given to members of a family of local hormones (so-called because they exert their effects near to where they are formed), which are produced naturally by many organs and tissues in the body, both normally and in disease states.

Prostaglandins have diverse natural actions in the body, and their therapeutic uses are similarly varied.

℞ **Epoprostenol** (prostacyclin) is present naturally in the walls of blood vessels. It is a potent ℞ **vasodilator**, and is used to treat pulmonary hypertension. Also, when administered therapeutically by intravenous infusion it also has ℞ **antiplatelet** activity and so inhibits blood thrombus formation by preventing the aggregation of platelets.

℞ **alprostadil** (prostaglandin E_1) is used to maintain babies born with congenital heart defects (to maintain patency of ductus arteriosus), while emergency preparations are being made for corrective surgery and intensive care. In men, it is used in ℞ **impotence treatment** to remedy erectile dysfunction.

℞ **latanoprost** is a prostaglandin analog that is used as a novel ℞ **glaucoma treatment** in open-angle glaucoma and ocular hypertension in people for whom other drugs are not suitable. It works by increasing the outflow of aqueous humor—the fluid in the eye.

℞ **misoprostol** is a synthetic analog of the ℞ **prostaglandin** E_1 (℞ **alprostadil**). It can be used as an ℞ **ulcer-healing drug**, because it inhibits acid secretion and promotes protective blood flow to the mucosal layer of the intestine. Though it cannot be used to treat dyspepsia, but can be very useful in protecting against stomach ulcers caused by non-steroidal anti-inflammatory drugs (℞ **NSAID**s) and for this reason it is now available in combination with some (NSAID) ℞ **non-narcotic analgesic** and ℞ **antirheumatic** drugs used in the treatment of rheumatic disease where stomach ulcers may result from treatment.

℞ **carboprost** (a synthetic analog of prostaglandin F_{2alpha}), is an ℞ **oxytocic** agent primarily used to treat hemorrhage following childbirth, and may also be used to induce abortion. ℞ **dinoprostone** (synthetic prostaglandin E_2) is also an ℞ **oxytocic** agent, which has the effect of causing contractions in the muscular walls of the uterus. It is used to ripen the cervix for labor induction, and occasionally to induce abortion as an ℞ **abortifacient**.

Limitations

The uses of the prostaglandins reflect their high potency in causing such bodily actions as contraction or relaxation of smooth muscle, and other actions. When given orally, there are a number of marked side effects including frequently, nausea, vomiting, diarrhea.

prostaglandin F2 alpha ⓖ

see ℞ **carboprost.**

ProStep ⓑ

A preparation of ℞ **nicotine.**
Formulation: Transdermal patch.

Availability: Prescription only.
Warnings and side effects: See ℞ **nicotine.**

Prostigmin ⓑ

A preparation of ℞ **neostigmine methylsulfate.**
Formulation: Injection.
Availability: Prescription only.
Warnings and side effects: See ℞ **neostigmine methylsulfate.**

Prostin E2 ⓑ

A preparation of ℞ **dinoprostone.**
Formulation: Vaginal suppository.
Availability: Prescription only.
Warnings and side effects: See ℞ **dinoprostone.**

Prostin VR Pediatric ⓑ

A preparation of ℞ **alprostadil.**
Formulation: Injection.
Availability: Prescription only.
Warnings and side effects: See ℞ **alprostadil.**

protamine sulfate ⓖ

(protamine sulphate)
Type/Group: antidote.
Brand(s): Generic only.
How administered: Intravenous infusion.

Used to treat

Protamine sulfate can be used to treat an overdose of ℞ **heparin.**

Warnings

• It should not be given to people with known hypersensitivity to this drug.

• Protamine should be used during pregnancy only if it is clearly needed.

• Medical judgment is required if breast-feeding is being considered.

• This is a specialist drug and it will be administered by experienced personnel.

Interactions

• Protamine will not inactivate low molecular weight heparins (see ℞ **anticoagulants**).

Side effects

Slowing of the heart rate, hypotension and flushing, nausea, vomiting, and hypersensitivity reactions.

protamine sulphate ⓖ

see ℞ **protamine sulfate.**

Protar ⓑ

A preparation of ℞ **coal tar.**
Formulation: Shampoo.
Availability: OTC.
Warnings and side effects: See ℞ **coal tar.**

Protectol Medicated ⓑ

A preparation of ℞ **undecylenic acid.**

Formulation: Topical powder.
Availability: OTC.
Warnings and side effects: See ℞ undecylenic acid.

protirelin ⓖ

Type/Group: **hormone; diagnostic agent; hypothalamic hormone**.
Brand(s): Phypinone; Relefact TRH; Thyrel TRH.
How administered: Injection.

Used to treat

Protirelin is a synthetic version of thyrotropin-releasing hormone (TRH) and is used to assess thyroid function in those with pituitary or hypothalamic dysfunction. It may also be used as an additional treatment to adjust thyroid hormone dosage in those with low thyroid function. TRH is produced and secreted by the hypothalamus. In turn, it acts on the anterior pituitary gland to produce and secrete ℞ **thyrotropin** (thyroid-stimulating hormone; TSH), a hormone that then causes the production and secretion of yet other hormones in the body.

Warnings

• It should not be used by people with known hypersensitivity to this drug, or serious heart conditions where changes in blood pressure would be hazardous.
• It should be used during pregnancy only if medically judged to be clearly needed.
• Medical judgment is also required if breast-feeding is being considered. Breast enlargement and leakage may occur and persist for two or three days.
• Elevation or reduction in blood pressure is common, but usually does not persist more than 15 minutes.

Interactions

• ℞ **aspirin**, ℞ **levodopa**, and ℞ **thyroid hormones** may inhibit TSH response.

Side effects

• Nausea, the urge to urinate, flushing, lightheadedness and fainting, bad taste, abdominal discomfort, headache, and dry mouth.
• Rarely, convulsions may occur in those with predisposing conditions (such as epilepsy, brain damage).

Protonix ⓑ

A preparation of ℞ **pantoprazole sodium**.
Formulation: Oral tablets, delayed release.
Availability: Prescription only.
Warnings and side effects: See ℞ pantoprazole sodium.

proton-pump inhibitor ⓓ

Generics: **lansoprazole; omeprazole; pantoprazole sodium; rabeprazole sodium**.

Actions and uses

Proton-pump inhibitors are a relatively recently introduced type of ℞ **ulcer-healing drug**. They work by inhibiting gastric acid secretion in the parietal cells (acid-producing cells) of the stomach lining, by interfering with the action of the ion (proton) pump that is responsible for the secretion of acid. They can be used to treat the symptoms of dyspepsia, which is caused by overproduction of acid (hyperacidity; see ✪ **indigestion**), for benign gastric and duodenal ulcers (including those that complicate ℞ **NSAID** therapy; see ✪ **peptic ulcer**), acid-related dyspepsia, ✪ **Zollinger-Ellison syndrome** and ✪ **gastroesophageal reflux** (inflammation of the esophagus caused by the regurgitation of acid and enzymes), acid reflux disease, and ℞ **Helicobacter pylori eradication regime** for the eradication of this causative infection (used in combination with ℞ **antibacterial** drugs). They can also be used in cases where there has been a poor response to more traditional treatments, especially with ℞ **H₂-antagonists**.

Limitations

These drugs are generally well tolerated, although there are a number of common side effects such as headache, diarrhea, rashes and itching, dizziness, nausea and vomiting, constipation, flatulence (gas), and abdominal pain. Given in very high doses to rats for two years, omeprazole caused changes associated with stomach cancer, but no similar signs attributable to this drug, have been reported in humans.
There are a number of interactions and the levels and effects of digoxin, ferrous salts (iron supplements), ketoconazole, and ampicillin may be decreased when taken with these drugs. Long-term use may possibly cause some deficiency in vitamin B_{12}. See also the individual drug entries.

Protopam Chloride ⓑ

A preparation of ℞ **pralidoxime chloride**.
Formulation: Injection.
Availability: Prescription only.
Warnings and side effects: See ℞ pralidoxime chloride.

Protostat ⓑ

A preparation of ℞ **metronidazole**.
Formulation: Oral tablets.
Availability: Prescription only.
Warnings and side effects: See ℞ metronidazole.

protriptyline hydrochloride ⓖ

Type/Group: **antidepressant; tricyclic**.
Brand(s): Vivactil; various generics.
How administered: Orally; injection.

Used to treat

Protriptyline hydrochloride is used particularly to treat ✪ **depression** in apathetic and withdrawn patients because it has a stimulant effect. Although not stated by the manufacturer for such treatment, it is sometimes also used to treat obstructive sleep apnea. As is the case with other antidepressants, this drug is also being evaluated for other uses.

Warnings

• It should not be given to people with known hypersensitivity to this drug, or who are just recovering from myocardial infarction (heart attack), or are taking or have just stopped taking MAOI antidepressants within the previous 14 days.
• It should be given with caution to people with a history of seizures, urinary retention, elevated intraocular pressure (pressure

in the eyeball), diabetes mellitus, epilepsy, angle-closure glaucoma, or liver, heart, or thyroid disease.

• Protriptyline should be used during pregnancy only if the benefits outweigh the risk to the fetus.

• It should not be used by nursing mothers.

• Other symptoms of psychiatric illnesses may worsen.

• Episodes of mania or hypomania may occur, especially in those with affective bipolar disorder (manic depression).

• Exposure to sunlight should be minimized because of possible photosensitization (sensitivity to light).

• Treatment should be stopped gradually by lowering the dose over a period of time.

• It is not generally given to children.

• It may be two to three weeks before there are any signs of improvement.

• It may impair the performance of skilled tasks such as driving.

• Alcohol, grapefruit juice, and smoking can all affect tricyclics (see Interactions below).

Interactions

• Serious or even fatal reactions can occur if ℞ **MAOI** antidepressants are taken at the same time as tricyclics.

• The effects of ℞ **epinephrine**, ℞ **norepinephrine**, and ℞ **phenylephrine** on blood pressure are intensified.

• Grapefruit juice increases the levels of tricyclics.

• ℞ **clonidine hydrochloride** should not be used with tricyclics, because a dangerous increase in blood pressure and hypertensive crisis is possible.

• The effects of ℞ **guanethidine monosulfate**, ℞ **levodopa**, and ℞ **sympathomimetics** may be reduced by tricyclics.

• The effects of ℞ **anticholinergics**, dicumarol, ℞ **quinolones**, grepafloxacin, and sparfloxacin may be enhanced by tricyclics.

• ℞ **Barbiturates**, ℞ **activated charcoal**, and rifamycin-related antibiotics may reduce the effectiveness of tricyclics.

• ℞ **Cimetidine**, ℞ **SSRIs**, ℞ **haloperidol**, ℞ **bupropion**, ℞ **valproate sodium** (and other valproic acid derivatives), and histamine ℞ **H$_2$-antagonists** may increase the levels of tricyclics in the blood.

• The levels of ℞ **carbamazepine** may increase, while blood levels of tricyclics decrease.

• Smoking may affect the metabolism of tricyclics.

• The effects of alcohol may be enhanced.

Side effects

• Along with other members of this class, it has ℞ **anticholinergic** side effects, especially tachycardia and postural hypotension, also drowsiness and difficulty in concentrating, dry mouth, blurred vision, dizziness, constipation, and urinary retention.

• Less frequently anxiety, mental changes, extrapyramidal symptoms in older adults (uncontrollable movement), elevated blood pressure, ECG changes, heart palpitations, fainting, eye changes, nasal congestion, ringing in the ears (tinnitus), gastrointestinal distress, hepatitis, jaundice, and skin sensitivity reactions.

• Rare but serious side effects include abnormal heart rhythm, stoppage of the normal action of the intestine (peristalsis), and blood cell disorders.

Protropin Ⓑ

A preparation of ℞ **somatrem**.
Formulation: Injection.
Availability: Prescription only.
Warnings and side effects: See ℞ **somatrem**.

Protuss DM Tablets Ⓑ

A preparation of ℞ **dextromethorphan**, ℞ **pseudoephedrine**, and ℞ **guaifenesin**.
Formulation: Oral tablets.
Availability: Prescription only.
Warnings and side effects: See ℞ **dextromethorphan**; ℞ **pseudoephedrine**; ℞ **guaifenesin**.

Proventil; Proventil Repetabs Ⓑ

A preparation of ℞ **albuterol**.
Formulation: Oral tablets in several strengths; oral syrup; aerosol inhalant; solution for inhalation; extended release tablets (Repetabs).
Availability: Prescription only.
Warnings and side effects: See ℞ **albuterol**.

Provera Ⓑ

A preparation of ℞ **medroxyprogesterone**.
Formulation: Oral tablets in several strengths.
Availability: Prescription only.
Warnings and side effects: See ℞ **medroxyprogesterone**.

Provigil Ⓑ

A preparation of ℞ **modafinil**.
Formulation: Oral tablets.
Availability: Prescription only.
Warnings and side effects: See ℞ **modafinil**.

Proxigel Ⓑ

A preparation of ℞ **carbamide peroxide**.
Formulation: Topical gel.
Availability: OTC.
Warnings and side effects: See ℞ **carbamide peroxide**.

Prozac Ⓑ

A preparation of ℞ **fluoxetine**.
Formulation: Oral pulvules and tablets in varying strengths; oral suspension.
Availability: Prescription only.
Warnings and side effects: See ℞ **fluoxetine**.

Pseudo-Car DM Syrup Ⓑ

A preparation of ℞ **dextromethorphan**, ℞ **carbinoxamine maleate**, and ℞ **pseudoephedrine**.
Formulation: Oral syrup.
Availability: Prescription only.
Warnings and side effects: See ℞ **dextromethorphan**; ℞ **carbinoxamine maleate**; ℞ **pseudoephedrine**.

pseudoephedrine ⓖ

(pseudoephedrine hydrochloride, sulfate, or tannate)

Type/Group: **sympathomimetic; vasoconstrictor; decongestant; bronchodilator**.

Brand(s): Afrin Tablets; Allermed Capsules; Congestion Relief Tablets; Cenafed Tablets, Syrup; Children's Congestion Relief; Children's Silfedrine; Decofed Syrup; DeFed-60 Tablets; Drixoral Non-Drowsy Formula Tablets; Dynafed Pseudo Tablets; Efidac 24 Tablets; Genaphed Tablets; Halofed Tablets; Mini Thin Pseudo Tablets; PediaCare Infants' Decongestant; Pseudo-Gest Tablets; Seudotabs; Sinustop Pro Capsules; Sudafed Tablets, 12 Hour Caplets; Sudex Tablets; Triaminic AM Decongestant Formula, Infant Oral Decongestant Drops. Combinations: With acetaminophen: Alka-Seltzer Plus Cold & Sinus Capsules; Allerest No Drowsiness Tablets, Caplets; Children's Cepacol Liquid; Coldrine Tablets; Dristan Cold Caplets; Maximum Strength Dynafed Tablets; Maximum Strength Sine-Aid Tablets, Caplets, Gelcaps; Maximum Strength Sudafed Sinus Tablets, Caplets; Maximum Strength Tylenol Tablets, Caplets, Gelcaps, Geltabs; No Drowsiness Sinarest Tablets; Ornex Caplets, Max Strength Caplets; Sine-Off Maximum Strength No Drowsiness Formula Caplets; Sinutab Without Drowsiness Tablets, Caplets; Sinus Excedrin Extra Strength Tablets, Caplets; Vicks DayQuil Sinus Pressure & Pain Relief Caplets. (Plus) *brompheniramine maleate*: Drixoral Cold & Flu Tablets; Maximum Strength Dristan Cold Caplets. (Plus) *chlorpheniramine maleate*: Alka-Seltzer Plus Allergy Liqui-Gels; Allerest Sinus Pain Formula Tabs; Children's Tylenol Cold Liquid, Tablets; Codimal Capsule, Tablets; Co-Hist Tablets; Comtrex Allergy-Sinus Tablets, Caplets; Kolephrin Caplets; Maximum Strength Tylenol Allergy Sinus Caplets, Gelcaps; Sinarest Sinus Tablets, Extra Strength Tablets; Sine-Off Sinus Medicine Caplets; Sinutab Maximum Strength Sinus Allergy Caplets, Tablets; TheraFlu Flu and Cold Medicine Powder. (Plus) *diphenhydramine*: Actifed Sinus Daytime/Nighttime Caplets, Tablets; Benadryl Allergy/Cold Tablets; Contac Day & Night Allergy/Sinus Caplets; Tylenol Flu Night Time Maximum Strength Powder (has *phenylalanine*). With acrivastine: Semprex-D Tablets. With aspirin: Ursinus Inlay-Tabs. With azatadine maleate: Rynatan Tablets; Trinalin Repetabs. With brompheniramine maleate: Allent Capsules; Brofed Elixir; Bromfed Capsules, Bromfed Tablets, PD Capsules; Bromfed Syrup; Bromfenex Capsules, PD Capsules; Dallergy-JR Capsules; Dexaphen-S.A. Tablets; Disobrom Tablets; Disophrol Tablets; Disophrol Chronotabs; Drixomed Tablets; Drixoral Cold & Allergy Tablets; Drixoral Syrup; Endafed Capsules; Iofed Capsules, PD Capsules; Lodrane LD Capsules; Respahist Capsules; Rondec Chewable Tablets; Touro A & H Capsules; ULTRAbrom Capsules, PD Capsules. With carbinoxamine maleate: Carbiset Tablets, TR Tablets; Carbodec Tablets, TR Tablets, Syrup; Cardec-S Syrup; Palgic-D Tablets Extended Release; Rondec Tablets, TR Tablets, Syrup, Oral Drops. With chlorpheniramine maleate: Allerest Maximum Strength Tablets; Anamine T.D. Capsules, Syrup; Anaplex Liquid; Atrohist Pediatric Capsules; Biohist-LA Tablets; Brexin L.A. Capsules; Chlorafed Timecelles, H.S. Timecelles, Liquid; Chlordrine S.R. Capsules; Chlorphedrine SR Capsules; Chlor-Trimeton 12 Hour Relief Capsules, 4 Hour Relief Tablets; Colfed-A Capsules; Cophene No. 2 Tablets; Copyronil 2 Pulvules; Deconamine SR Capsules, Tablets, Syrup; Duralex Capsules; Fedahist Tablets, Timecaps, Gyrocaps; Hayfebrol Liquid; Histalet Syrup; Klerist-D Capsules, Tablets; Kronofed-A Capsules; Jr. Capsules; ND Clear Capsules; Novafed A Capsules; Palgic DS Syrup; Pseudo-Gest Plus Tablets; Rescon Capsules, ED Capsules, JR Capsules; Rhinosyn-PD Liquid; Rinade B.I.D. Capsules; Ryna Liquid; Sudafed Plus Tablets; Tanafed Suspension. With codeine phosphate: Nucofed. (Plus) *guaifenesin*: Cycofed Pediatric Syrup; Deconsal Pediatric Syrup; Deproist Expectorant with with Codeine Liquid; Guiatuss DAC Syrup; Isoclor Expectorant Liquid; Mytussin DAC Liquid; Novagest Expectorant Liquid; Nucofed Expectorant Syrup; Nucofed Pediatric Expectorant Syrup; Nucotuss Expectorant Codeine Liquid; Nucotuss Pediatric Expectorant Syrup; Phenhist Expectorant Liquid; Robafen DAC Syrup; Robitussin-DAC Syrup; Ryna-CX Liquid. (Plus) *chlorpheniramine*: Codehist DH Elixir; Decohistine DH Liquid; Phenhist DH w/Codeine Liquid; Ryna-C Liquid. (Plus) *tripolidine*: Actagen-C Cough Syrup; Actifed w/Codeine Cough Syrup; Allerfrin w/Codeine Syrup; Aprodine w/Codeine Syrup; Triafed w/Codeine Syrup. With dextromethorphan: Children's Sudafed; Robitussin Maximum Strength Cough & Cold Liquid, Pediatric; Vicks 44D Cough & Head Congestion Relief. (Plus) *carbinoxamine maleate*: Carbodec DM Syrup, Drops; Cardec DM Syrup, Drops; Pseudo-Car DM Syrup; Rondamine-DM Drops; Rondec-DM Syrup, Drops; Sildec-DM Syrup, Pediatric Drops; Tussafed Syrup, Drops. (Plus) *brompheniramine maleate*: Bromadine-DM; Bromarest DX Cough Syrup; Bromatane DX Cough Syrup; Bromfed DM Cough Syrup; Bromphen DX Cough Syrup; Dimetane-DX Cough Syrup; Myphetane DX Cough Syrup. (Plus) *chlorpheniramine maleate*: Children's Vicks Nyquil; Rescon-DM Liquid; Rhinosyn-DM Liquid; Triaminic Night Time Maximum Strength. With dextromethorphan and acetaminophen: Alka-Seltzer Plus Cold & Flu Liqui-Gels; Contac Severe Cold & Flu Non-Drowsy Caplets; Thera-Flu Non-Drowsy Formula Maximum Strength; Robitussin Multi Symptom Honey Flu; Sudfed Severe Cold Formula Caplets, Tablets; Tylenol Flu Maximum Strength Non-Drowsy Gelcaps; Vicks Dayquil. (Plus) *chlorpheniramine maleate*: Alka-Selzer Plus Cold & Cough LiquiGels; Children's Tylenol Cold Plus Cough Chewable Tabets; Comtrex Maximum Strength Multi-Symptom Cold & Cough Relief Caplets, Tablets; Contac Severe Cold & Flu Caplets; Genacol Tablets; Kolephrin/DM Caplets; Medi-Flu Liquid; Multi-Symptom Tylenol Cold Caplets, Tablets; NightTime TheraFlu Powder; Robitussin Nighttime Honey Flu; Triaminic Severe Cold & Fever; Vicks 44M Cold & Flu Relief. (Plus) *doxylamine succinate*: Alka-Seltzer Plus NightTime Cold Liqui-Gels; Genite Liquid; Nytcold Medicine Liquid; Vicks NyQuil. (Plus) *guaifenesin*: Sudafed Cold & Cough Liquid Caps; Robitussin Cold Multi-Symptom Cold & Flu Liqui-Gels, Caplets; Vicks DayQuil LiquiCaps. (Plus) *pyrilamine maleate*: Robitussin Night Relief Liquid. With dextromethorphan and guaifenesin: Anatuss DM Tablets, Syrup; Ambenyl-D Liquid; Benylin Multi-Symptom Liquid; Dimacol Caplets; MED-Rx DM Tablets; Novahistine DMX; PamMist-DM Syrup; Primatuss Cough Mixture 4D Liquid; Protuss DM Tablets; Rhinosyn-S Liquid; Robitussin Cold & Congestion Liqui-Gels, Caplets, Infant Drops;

Key to symbols: ✚ = Disorder Section ℞ = Drug Section ♣ = Herbal Section ⚕ = Supplement Section

Ru-Tuss Expectorant Liquid; Touro CC; Tussafed-LA. With diphenhydramine: Actifed Allergy Tablets; Banophen Decongestant Capsules; Benadryl Allergy Decongestant Tablets, Decongestant Liquid. With fexofenadine: Allegra-D. With guaifenesin: Anatuss LA Tablets; Congess SR Capsules, JR. Capsules; Congestac Caplets; Deconsal II Tablets; Defen-LA Tablets; Duratuss Tablets; Entex PSE Tablets; Eudal-SR Tablets; Fedahist Expectorant Syrup; Guaifed Capsules, PD Capsules; Guaifenex PSE 120 Tablets, PSE 60 Tablets, Rx Tablets, Rx AM Tablets, Rx DM Tablets; Guaimax-D Tablets; Guaitab Tablets; Guaivent/PSE Tablets, Capsules, PD Capsules; GuiaCough PE Liquid; Guiatex PSE Tablets; Guiatuss PE Syrup; Histalet X Tablets, Syrup; Iosal II Tablets; MED-Rx Tablets; Nasabid SR Tablets, Capsules; Nasatab LA Tablets; PanMist LA, JR Tablets, Syrup; Polaramine Expectorant Liquid (has *dexchlorpheniramine maleate*); Refenesan Plus Tablets; Respaire 120 Capsules, 60 Capsules; Robitussin PE Syrup, Severe Congestion Liqui-Gels; Ru-tuss DE Tablets; Rymed Capsules, Liquid; Sinufed Timecelles; Sinutab Non-Drying Capsules; Stamoist E Tablets; Sudal 120/600 Tablets, 60/500 Tablets; Syn-Rx Tablets; Touro LA Caplets; Tuss-LA Tablets; Tussin PE; V-Dec-M Tablets; Versacaps Capsules; Zephrex LA Tablets, Tablets. With hydrocodone: Detussin Liquid; Entuss-D Liquid; Histinex D; Histussin D, HC; H-Tuss D. (Plus) *carbinoxamine*: Histex HC. (Plus) *brompheniramine maleate*: Anaplex HD Syrup: (Plus) *chlorpheniramine maleate*: Histinex PV Syrup; Hyphed; Pancof-HC Liquid; P-V-Tussin Syrup. (Plus) *guaifenesin*: Cophene XP Liquid; Deconamine CX Liquid; Detussin Expectorant Liquid; Duratuss HD Elixir; Entuss-D Tablets, Entuss Jr. Liquid; Pancof XP Liquid; SRC Expectorant Liquid; SUTUSS Elixir; Tussafin Expectorant Liquid; Vanex Expectorant Liquid. (Most combinations available as generic.) With ibuprofen: Advil Cold & Sinus Caplets; Dristan Sinus Caplets; Motrin IB Sinus Caplets; Sine-Air IB Caplets. With loratadine: Claritin-D, 24-hour Tablets. With triprolidine: Actagen Tablets; Actifed Cold & Allergy Tablets; Actifed Plus Caplets, Tablets (have a *cetaminophen*); Allercon Tablets; Allerfrim Tablets, Syrup; Allerphed Syrup; Aprodine Tablets, Syrup; Cenafed Plus Tablets; Genac Tablets; Silafed Syrup; Triofed Syrup; Triposed Tablets, Syrup. (Most combinations available as generics.)

How administered: Orally; nasal; ophthalmic (eye); injection.

Used to treat

Pseudoephedrine is sometimes used to treat obstructive pulmonary disease, but is most commonly included in a number of brands for treating ✪ **cold** symptoms. Its actions and effects are very similar to those of the closely related drug ℞ **ephedrine**.

Warnings

• It should not be given to people with known hypersensitivity to this or any other adrenergic drug, with angle-closure glaucoma, who are taking ℞ **MAOI** antidepressants, or who have severe high blood pressure or coronary artery disease.

• It should be given with caution to people with hyperthyroidism, diabetes mellitus, heart disease, angina pectoris, arrhythmias, peptic ulcer, enlarged prostate, or increased intraocular pressure (pressure in the eyeball, including glaucoma).

• Pseudoephedrine's effects during pregnancy are not known and it should be used with caution and only if there is clear benefit.

• If taken orally, this drug should not be used by nursing mothers.

• Overuse may cause symptoms such as nervousness and insomnia, and may make congestion worse, which is an effect called "rebound congestion." No nasal decongestant should be used for longer than three to four days.

• It should be used with caution by the elderly, as they are more likely to suffer side effects.

• The manufacturer's recommendations must be followed carefully when giving this drug to children under 12.

Interactions

These apply to oral and injected doses. When used topically (nose or eyes) at recommended doses, these interactions do not apply (except in cases of overdose, which occur most frequently in children).

• Pseudoephedrine should not be used with ℞ **MAOI** antidepressants, or within two weeks of stopping MAOI treatment, because this may cause a hypertensive crisis.

• If used with other sympathomimetics (for example, ℞ **ephedrine**, ℞ **phenylephrine**, ℞ **oxymetazoline**), there is an increased risk of side effects.

• If used with ℞ **theophylline**, there may be unpredictable effects, sometimes with toxicity.

• ℞ **Antacids** taken in high doses slow the removal from the body of pseudoephedrine, increasing the risk of side effects.

• If used with ℞ **furazolidone**, ℞ **methyldopa**, or ℞ **reserpine**, there is the possibility of increased blood pressure.

Side effects

• These depend on how it is administered. As eyedrops it may cause blurred vision or stinging. When used as a nasal decongestant, it may cause irritation in the nose. There may be changes in heart rate and rhythm and blood pressure, anxiety, restlessness, tremor, insomnia, dry mouth, cold fingertips and toes, changes in the prostate gland, anorexia, nausea, and vomiting.

Pseudo-Gest Plus Tablets Ⓓ

A preparation of ℞ **pseudoephedrine** and ℞ **chlorpheniramine maleate**.
Formulation: Oral Tablets.
Availability: OTC.
Warnings and side effects: See ℞ **pseudoephedrine**; ℞ **chlorpheniramine maleate**.

Pseudo-Gest Tablets Ⓓ

A preparation of ℞ **pseudoephedrine**.
Formulation: Oral tablets, available in two strengths.
Availability: OTC.
Warnings and side effects: See ℞ **pseudoephedrine**.

psoriasis treatment Ⓓ

Generics: acitretin; alclometasone; anthralin; beclomethasone dipropionate; calcipotriene; coal tar; clobetasol propionate; clocortolone pivalate; cyclosporine; desoxymetasone; fluocinolone acetonide; fluocinonide; flurandrenolide; fluticasone propionate; halcinonide; methotrexate; petrolatum; salicylic acid; simethicone; tazarotene; zinc oxide.

Actions and uses

The treatment of ☉ **psoriasis** aims to alleviate the symptoms as far as possible by the use of ℞ **skin preparation** drug classes, including ℞ **emollient** agents (℞ **urea**) and ℞ **keratolytic** agents (such as ℞ **salicylic acid** and ℞ **coal tar**), several of which can be applied in the form of a paste with an ℞ **astringent** (usually ℞ **zinc oxide**) inside an impregnated bandage.

℞ **anthralin** is the most powerful drug presently used to treat chronic or milder forms of psoriasis in topical (external) application, and it is used in a number of preparations. Lesions are covered for a period with a dressing on which there is a preparation of anthralin in weak solution. The concentration is adjusted to suit a person's response and tolerance of the associated skin irritation. ℞ **calcipotriene** is a vitamin-D derivative used to treat plaque psoriasis. Drugs related to vitamin A—the ℞ **retinoid** agents—may be used topically (for example, ℞ **tazarotene**) or in severe cases taken by mouth (for example, ℞ **acitretin**).

Topical ℞ **corticosteroid** preparations are used extensively as ℞ **anti-inflammatory** agents in psoriasis. For example, alclometasone, beclometasone, clobetasol propionate, clocortolone pivalate, desoxymetasone, fluocinolone acetonide, fluocinonide, flurandrenolide, fluticasone propionate, and halcinonide. In severe cases, stronger drugs including ℞ **immunosuppressant** agents such as ℞ **cyclosporine** and ℞ **methotrexate** are used.

Limitations

Treatment of psoriasis should be supervised by a specialist. Finding the most effective treatment for each person—and tolerable drug concentrations—takes time, and is complicated by the fact that the condition usually fluctuates in intensity and may go spontaneously into remission.

A number of the drugs mentioned are not suitable for use during pregnancy, varying from a slight risk to the fetus (for instance ℞ **anthralin**) through to the Food and Drug Administration's Pregnancy Category X, which means that a drug should not be used during pregnancy, for example ℞ **tazarotene** and ℞ **acitretin**. Women of childbearing potential are given counseling before ℞ **acitretin** is prescribed, and should use two reliable contraceptive means for three years after discontinuing acitretin. Alcohol worsens and prolongs the probability of serious effects on the fetus. This drug should not be used by nursing women.

Psoriasis often responds well to moderate sunlight, and research is being carried out to evaluate the combination of some of these drugs with ultraviolet radiation treatment (UVB phototherapy). Also PUVA, photochemotherapy, combining a psoralen with long-wave ultraviolet irradiation (UVA) using special lamps is effective in some patients.

See also the individual drug entries.

PsoriGel ®

A preparation of ℞ **coal tar**.

Formulation: Topical gel.

Availability: OTC.

Warnings and side effects: See ℞ **coal tar**.

psyllium Ⓖ

(psyllium hydrophilic mucilloid)

Type/Group: **laxative**.

Brand(s): Fiberall; Genfiber; Hydrocil Instant; Konsyl; Metamucil; Reguloid; Modane Bulk; Perdiem Fiber Therapy; Serutan; Syllact; various generic. Combinations: With *senna*: Perdiem Overnight Relief.

How administered: Orally.

Used to treat

Psyllium is a bulking-agent laxative which works by increasing the overall mass of stool while at the same time retaining a lot of water and so stimulating bowel movement. However, the full effect may not be achieved for many (12 to 72) hours. It may be used when treating a range of bowel conditions, including ☉ **diverticular disease**, ☉ **irritable bowel syndrome**, and ☉ **hemorrhoids**.

Warnings

• It should not be given to people with gastrointestinal obstruction, esophageal obstruction, or who have difficulty swallowing.

• No ill effects in pregnancy or breast-feeding have been associated with psyllium, but a doctor should always be consulted before taking any drug during pregnancy.

• It is important to maintain adequate fluid intake, and drink at least a glass of liquid when taking this bulking agent. (It swells up, becoming bulkier. Obstruction can form in the esophagus if the substance is not carried all the way down, or in the bowel if insufficient liquid is present.) It should not be taken just before bed.

• Psyllium is often supplied as a powder and, though infrequent, potentially severe hypersensitivity reactions may occur if some powder is inhaled. It should be handled carefully (for example, measured out with a spoon, not poured). Hypersensitivity reaction, include runny nose, watery eyes, wheezing, bronchospasm, or anaphylaxis, has been reported when psyllium was inadvertently inhaled.

• Do not use if there is abdominal pain, nausea, or vomiting, unless directed by a doctor.

• A doctor must be consulted first before taking any other medication (including OTCs, herbal remedies, and supplements), because laxatives may alter the absorption of a wide range drugs. Often it is recommended that a bulk-forming laxative dose be separated by at least three hours from doses of medications that might be affected (for example, digitalis, ℞ **nitrofurantoin**, ℞ **salicylates**).

Interactions

Laxatives can affect the absorption of a wide range of drugs. No specific drug interactions of significance are known.

Side effects

• There may be flatulence and abdominal distension, intestinal obstruction, appetite loss, nausea, and potentially serious esophageal or bowel obstruction.

psyllium hydrophilic mucilloid Ⓖ

see ℞ psyllium.

Pulmicort Turbohaler ®

A preparation of ℞ **budesonide**.

Key to symbols: ☉ = Disorder Section ℞ = Drug Section ♣ = Herbal Section ☙☙ = Supplement Section

Formulation: Powder for use with inhaler.
Availability: Prescription only.
Warnings and side effects: See ℞ **budesonide**.

Pulmozyme ⑧

A preparation of ℞ **dornase alfa**.
Formulation: Solution for inhalant.
Availability: Prescription only.
Warnings and side effects: See ℞ **dornase alfa**.

purgative ⑩

see ℞ **laxative**.

Purge ⑧

A preparation of ℞ **castor oil**.
Formulation: Oral liquid.
Availability: OTC.
Warnings and side effects: See ℞ **castor oil**.

P-V-Tussin Syrup ⑧

A preparation of ℞ **hydrocodone bitartrate**,
℞ **pseudoephedrine**, and ℞ **chlorpheniramine maleate**.
Formulation: Oral syrup.
Availability: Prescription only.
Warnings and side effects: See ℞ **hydrocodone bitartrate**;
℞ **pseudoephedrine**; ℞ **chlorpheniramine maleate**.

P-V-Tussin Tablets ⑧

A preparation of ℞ **hydrocodone bitartrate**, ℞ **guaifenesin**, and
phenindamine tartrate.
Formulation: Oral tablets.
Availability: Prescription only.
Warnings and side effects: See ℞ **hydrocodone bitartrate**;
℞ **guaifenesin**.

pyrantel ⑥

Type/Group: **anthelmintic**.
How administered: Orally.
Brand(s): Antiminth; Pin-Rid; Pin-X; Reese's Pinworm.

Used to treat

Pyrantel is a synthetic drug used to treat roundworm and pinworm
infections (see ❍ **worms**).

Warnings

• It should not be given to people with known hypersensitivity to
this drug or with liver disease.
• It is not usually recommended for use during pregnancy.
• Medical judgment is required if breast-feeding is being
considered.
• Strict hygiene is required to prevent reinfection.

Interactions

• The effects of ℞ **piperazine** and pyrantel are reduced.

Side effects

• Gastrointestinal effects (abdominal cramps, diarrhea, nausea,
vomiting, loss of appetite), headache, dizziness, drowsiness,
insomnia, elevated liver enzymes, and rash.

pyrazinamide ⑥

Type/Group: **antibacterial; antituberculosis**.
Brand(s): Generic only. Combination: with *isoniazid* and *rifampin*:
Rifater.
How administered: Orally.

Used to treat

Pyrazinamide is one of the major drugs used in the treatment of
❍ **tuberculosis**. It is generally used in combination with other
drugs, such as ℞ **isoniazid** and ℞ **rifampin**, for maximum effect.
Because pyrazinamide is only active against dividing forms of *Mycobacterium tuberculosis*, it is most effective in the early stages of treatment (that is, the first few months).

Warnings

• It should not be given to people with known hypersensitivity to
pyrazinamide, with severe liver damage, or acute gout.
• It should be given with caution to people with a history of gout,
kidney impairment, liver function impairment, alcoholism,
diabetes mellitus, who are over 65, or with HIV infection.
• Pyrazinamide should be used during pregnancy only when it is
clearly needed.
• Medical judgment is required if breast-feeding is being
considered. It appears in breast milk.
• Rarely, it may cause liver damage. A doctor must be contacted if
fever, loss of appetite, unusual tiredness, nausea and vomiting,
darkened urine, yellowish discoloration of skin and eyes, or swelling
of the joints occur.

Interactions

• The levels of ℞ **cyclosporine** and ℞ **tacrolimus** may be
decreased.

Side effects

• Frequently, joint and muscle pain.
• Rarely, allergic skin reaction, photosensitivity (unusual sensitivity
to sunlight), blood changes, and liver damage.

pyrethrin ⑥

Type/Group: **scabicide and pediculicide**.
Brand(s): A-200; Barc; Blue; Clear Total Lice Elimination System;
End Lice; InnoGel Plus; Pronto; Pyrinyl; R & S; RID; Tsit; Tegrin-LT.
How administered: Topically (external).

Used to treat

Pyrethrin, a synthetic pyrethroid, is used to treat head lice, body
lice, and pubic (crab) lice (see ❍ **lice and mite infestation**).

Warnings

• It should not be given to people with known hypersensitivity to
this or related drugs, to members of the chrysanthemum family
(from which pyrethroids originate) including ragweed, or to any
components of the preparations.
• A doctor should be consulted before using while pregnant or
nursing.
• It is harmful if swallowed or inhaled.
• Contact with the eyes and mucous membranes must be avoided.

Interactions

No interactions specific to this drug are known.

Side effects
• Itching, redness, or swelling.

Pyridium Plus ⑧
A preparation of phenazopyridine, ℞ **hyoscyamine**, and ℞ **butabarbital**.
Formulation: Oral tablets.
Availability: Prescription only.
Warnings and side effects: See ℞ **hyoscyamine**; ℞ **butabarbital**.

pyridostigmine bromide ⑥
Type/Group: **anticholinesterase**.
Brand(s): Mestinon; Regonol; various generic.
How administered: Orally; injection.

Used to treat
Pyridostigmine enhances the effects of the neurotransmitter acetylcholine, and is used to treat ❍ **myasthenia gravis** and to reverse the effects of neuromuscular blocking agents after surgery.

Warnings
• It should not be used by people with known hypersensitivity to anticholinesterases, or with urinary or intestinal obstruction, or peritonitis.
• It should be given with caution to anyone with seizure disorder, asthma, certain heart conditions, hyperthyroidism, peptic ulcer, or hypotension.
• It is not known whether this drug can harm the fetus, but it would not be expected to cross the placenta or be excreted into breast milk. It may cause premature labor if given near term, and transient muscle weakness in newborns. It should be given with caution to breast-feeding mothers.
• It must not be used with any other cholinergic medication except under a doctor's supervision.
• A doctor must be notified promptly of side effects (see below).
• The extended-release tablets must not be chewed or crushed.

Interactions
• ℞ **Tacrine** may increase cholinergic effects.
• ℞ **aminoglycoside** antibiotics (such as ℞ **neomycin**, ℞ **streptomycin**) may increase the effects of pyridostigmine.
• ℞ **Corticosteroids**, ♌ **magnesium** and ℞ **local anesthetics** may interfere with the action of pyridostigmine.
• ℞ **Quinidine** and ℞ **procainamide** may interfere with pyridostigmine.

Side effects
Report to a doctor any of the following:
• Nausea, vomiting, diarrhea, marked sweating, increased salivation, irregular heartbeat, muscle weakness, severe abdominal pain, and difficulty in breathing;
• Other common effects include constriction of the pupils, abdominal discomfort, reduced pulse rate, and increase in saliva and sweat;
• Occasionally, headache; rarely, rash and potentially serious effects on the cardiovascular and respiratory systems.

pyrilamine maleate ⑥
Type/Group: **antihistamine; antiallergic; cold and cough preparation**.
Brand(s): (Topical): Medacote Lotion; Calamycin Lotion. With *chlorpheniramine maleate*: Derma-Pax Lotion. With *chlorpheniramine maleate and hydrocortisone*: HC Derma-Pax Liquid. Other combinations: With *codeine*: Tricodene Cough & Cold Liquid. With *pheniramine maleate and phenyltoloxamine*: Poly-Histine Elixir, Capsules, Ped Caps. With *phenylephrine*: Myci-Spray; Ryna-12 S Liquid. (Plus) *chlorpheniramine maleate and acetaminophen*: Covangesic Tablets; Histex SR; ND-Gesic Tablets. (Plus) *codeine*: Codimal PH Syrup. (Plus) *chlorpheniramine maleate and guaifenesin*: Codimal DM Syrup. (Plus) *chlorpheniramine tannate (and pyrilamine tannate)*: Atrohist Pediatric Suspension; Gelhist Pediatric Suspension; Rhinatate Tablets; R-Tannamine Tablets, Pediatric Suspension; R-Tannate Tablets, Pediatric Suspension; Rynatan Pediatric Suspension; Triotann Tablets; Tri-Tannate Tablets, Pediatric Suspension. With *pseudoephedrine and dextromethorphan*: Robitussin Night Relief Liquid.
How administered: Orally; topically (external).

Used to treat
Pyrilamine is used in preparations to treat ❍ **coughs** and ❍ **colds**, and also for allergic conditions, such as ❍ **hay fever** (seasonal allergic rhinitis), usually in combination with a ℞ **decongestant** drug, and also ❍ **urticaria**, again usually in combination with a decongestant drug.

Warnings
• It should not be given to people with known hypersensitivity to this drug (or with known sensitivity to other antihistamines).
• Antihistamines should be given with caution to people with lower respiratory disease or asthma (and never during an attack), heart disease, hypertension, hyperthyroidism, epilepsy, porphyria, increased intraocular pressure (pressure in the eyeball, as in glaucoma), enlarged prostate, urinary retention, or certain obstructive bladder or gastrointestinal conditions.
• Pyrilamine should be used during pregnancy only if it is clearly needed, but not in the third trimester, as newborns or premature infants may have severe reactions, including convulsions, to antihistamines.
• Nursing mothers should discontinue using this drug or discontinue breast-feeding.
• ℞ **MAOI** antidepressants may prolong and intensify the ℞ **anticholinergic** and sedative effects of antihistamines (see Side effects below).
• Pyrilamine must not be given to infants, and for children under the age of 12 the manufacturer's or medical instructions must be followed closely.
• Because of its sedative side effects, the performance of skilled tasks, such as driving, may be impaired.
• Side effects are more frequent in the elderly.

Interactions
• ℞ **MAOI** antidepressants may prolong and intensify the anticholinergic and sedative effects of antihistamines (see Side effects below).

• If used with ℞ **tricyclic** antidepressants, other antihistamines, ℞ **skeletal muscle relaxants**, ℞ **opioids**, ℞ **barbiturates**, ℞ **hypnotics**, ℞ **sedatives**, or ℞ **antianxiety** drugs, there is a risk of intensified side effects.

• Alcohol may intensify side effects such as drowsiness and impaired mental alertness.

Side effects

• These depend on how it is administered. For this type of antihistamine, there is commonly drowsiness, headache, impaired muscular coordination or dizziness, anticholinergic effects (dry mouth, blurred vision, urinary retention, gastrointestinal disturbances), occasional rashes and photosensitivity (abnormal sensitivity to light), palpitations and heart arrhythmias.

• Rarely, there may be stimulation instead of sedation (paradoxical stimulation), especially in children (and convulsions in overdose), hypersensitivity reactions, blood disorders, liver disturbances, depression, sleep disturbances, and hypotension.

pyrimethamine ⓖ

Type/Group: **antimalarial**.
Brand(s): Daraprim. Combinations: With *sulfadoxine*: Fanisdar.
How administered: Orally.

Used to treat

Pyrimethamine is mainly used in combination with ℞ **quinine** and ℞ **sulfadoxine** to prevent or treat ⊙ **malaria**. It can also be used, along with a sulfonamide, to treat the protozoal infection ⊙ **toxo-plasmosis**.

Warnings

• It should not be given to people with known hypersensitivity to pyrimethamine, or with megaloblastic anemia due to folate deficiency.

• It should be given with caution to people with malabsorption syndrome, alcoholism, kidney or liver dysfunction, seizure disorder, and G6PD deficiency (a genetic enzyme disorder).

• Pyrimethamine should be used during pregnancy only if the benefits outweigh the possible risk to the fetus. Becoming pregnant should be avoided when using this drug.

• Medical judgment is required if breast-feeding is being considered. It does appear in breast milk and potentially could cause an adverse reaction.

• Allergic reactions, occasionally severe, can occur, particularly if taken with a sulfonamide (which can be serious). Stop treatment and contact a doctor.

• It may cause folic acid deficiency.

Interactions

• Folic acid may decrease the effectiveness of pyrimethamine.

• ℞ **methotrexate** and ℞ **sulfonamides** may increase the risk of folate deficiency and bone marrow suppression.

• If used with ℞ **lorazepam** there may be adverse effects on the liver.

Side effects

• Frequently, gastrointestinal effects.

• Less frequently, insomnia, headache, lightheadedness, dry mouth, and rash.

• Rare but serious side effects (generally associated with large doses) include blood and heart rhythm disorders and serious skin manifestations.

Pyrinil; Pyrinil Plus ⓑ

A preparation of ℞ **pyrethrin**.
Formulation: Topical liquid; shampoo (Plus).
Availability: OTC.
Warnings and side effects: See ℞ **pyrethrin**.

Quadrinal Tablets ⓑ

A preparation of ℞ **ephedrine**, ℞ **theophylline**, ℞ **phenobarbital**, and ℞ **potassium iodide**.
Formulation: Oral tablets.
Availability: Prescription only.
Warnings and side effects: See ℞ **ephedrine**; ℞ **theophylline**; ℞ **phenobarbital**; ℞ **potassium iodide**.

quazepam ⓖ

Type/Group: **hypnotic; benzodiazepine**.
Brand(s): Doral.
How administered: Orally.

Used to treat

Quazepam is used for the short-term treatment of ⊙ **insomnia**, generally 7 to 10 days (prescriptions are rarely written for more than a one-month supply). It is eliminated rapidly from the body compared to other benzodiazepines, but may cause withdrawal problems the day after use.

Warnings

• It should not be given to people with known hypersensitivity to benzodiazepines, narrow-angle glaucoma, or psychosis.

• It should be given with caution to people with kidney or liver impairment, a history of drug abuse, those in a weakened condition (debilitated), with respiratory depression, sleep apnea, or those over 65.

• Quazepam should not be used during pregnancy. A doctor must be contacted if pregnancy occurs while taking this drug.

• It should not be used by nursing mothers.

• It must not be used for longer than the period specified by your doctor. Benzodiazepines may produce psychological and physical dependence and withdrawal symptoms.

• The performance of skilled tasks may be impaired, such as driving.

• Avoid alcohol consumption, because adverse side effects may be increased (see Side effects below).

• Avoid other psychotropic medications unless prescribed by a doctor.

• A doctor must be consulted before discontinuing use or increasing dosage.

Interactions

• ℞ **azole** antifungals (for example, ℞ **ketoconazole**, ℞ **itraconazole**), ℞ **beta-blockers** (for example, ℞ **propranolol**), ℞ **cimetidine**, ℞ **disulfiram**, ℞ **isoniazid**, ℞ **macrolide** antibiotics (for example, ℞ **erythromycin**, ℞ **clarithromycin**, troleandomycin), ℞ **omeprazole**, ℞ **SSRIs**, and ℞ **quinolones** may increase levels of quazepam.

• If used with ℞ **clozapine**, there is a possible increased risk of cardiorespiratory collapse.
• If used with ℞ **antipsychotics**, there can be increased sedation and respiratory depression.
• ℞ **Rifampin** may reduce the effects of quazepam.
• Alcohol may increase adverse effects.

Side effects
• Daytime sleepiness, weakness, and decreased physical activity.
• Less often, abnormal thinking or emotions, falling (especially older individuals), hangover, decreased reflexes, sleep problems, stupor, heart palpitations, fainting, eye, ear, or nose pain or inflammation, gastrointestinal effects, jaundice, blood cell disorders, shortness of breath, skin inflammation, and potentially serious blood cell disorders and seizures.

Quelicin ®

A preparation of ℞ **succinylcholine chloride**.
Formulation: Injection.
Availability: Prescription only.
Warnings and side effects: See ℞ succinylcholine chloride.

Questran; Questran Light ®

A preparation of ℞ **cholestyramine**.
Formulation: Oral powder in two strengths, tablets.
Availability: Prescription only.
Warnings and side effects: See ℞ cholestyramine.

quetiapine ⓖ

Type/Group: **antipsychotic**.
Brand(s): Seroquel.
How administered: Orally.

Used to treat
Quetiapine is a recently introduced antipsychotic drug (one of a group sometimes termed "atypical" antipsychotics) and is used in the treatment of ⊕ **schizophrenia**.

Warnings
• It should not be given to people with known hypersensitivity to this drug or severe CNS (central nervous system) depression.
• It should be given with caution to people with liver or kidney impairment, heart disease, thyroid disorders, or high prolactin levels.
• A doctor must be contacted if pregnancy occurs while taking this drug. Safety in pregnancy has not been established, use only when clearly needed, and benefit clearly outweighs risk to the fetus.
• It should not be used by nursing mothers.
• It may cause drowsiness, and so the performance of skilled tasks, such as driving, may be impaired.
• Infrequently, it may cause postural hypotension (lowered blood pressure on standing), so rise slowly from a reclining position. Older people in particular should exercise caution.
• Avoid exposure to extreme heat, and take care to avoid dehydration.
• If used for a long time, tardive dyskinesia (see ℞ **antipsychotics**) occasionally develops.
• Treatment should be stopped gradually.

• Avoid alcohol.
• It may be necessary to examine the lenses in the eyes.

Interactions
• ℞ **Carbamazepine**, ℞ **phenytoin**, ℞ **thioridazine**, and ℞ **barbiturates** may reduce the effects of quetiapine.
• ℞ **Erythromycin**, ℞ **ketoconazole**, and ℞ **fluconazole** may increase the effects of quetiapine.
• The effects of ℞ **lorazepam** and ℞ **benzodiazepines** may be increased by quetiapine.
• The blood-pressure lowering effects of ℞ **antihypertensives** may be enhanced.
• ℞ **Levodopa**'s effects may be reduced by quetiapine.
• If an antipsychotic is taken with alcohol, there may be increased sedative effects.

Side effects
• Agitation, insomnia, sleepiness, and dry mouth.
• Less frequently, dizziness, postural hypotension, extrapyramidal symptoms (see ℞ **antipsychotics**), hostility, increased heart rate, abdominal pain, changes in liver function, indigestion, and weight gain.
• Rarely, neuroleptic malignant syndrome (a potentially fatal condition characterized by very high fever, muscle rigidity, changes in mental status, and irregular pulse, blood pressure and/or heart rhythm).

Quibron Capsules; Quibron-300 ®

A preparation of ℞ **guaifenesin** and ℞ **theophylline**.
Formulation: Oral capsules.
Availability: Prescription only.
Warnings and side effects: See ℞ guaifenesin; ℞ theophylline.

Quibron-T/SR Dividose ®

A preparation of ℞ **theophylline**.
Formulation: Oral tablets, timed release, in several strengths.
Availability: Prescription only.
Warnings and side effects: See ℞ theophylline.

Quinaglute Dura-Tabs ®

A preparation of ℞ **quinidine**.
Formulation: Oral tablets (sustained release).
Availability: Prescription only.
Warnings and side effects: See ℞ quinidine.

Quinalan ®

A preparation of ℞ **quinidine**.
Formulation: Oral tablets (sustained release).
Availability: Prescription only.
Warnings and side effects: See ℞ quinidine.

quinapril hydrochloride ⓖ

Type/Group: **ACE inhibitor; vasodilator; antihypertensive; heart failure treatment**.
Brand(s): Accupril. Combinations: With *hydrochlorothiazide*: Accuretic.
How administered: Orally.

Used to treat

Quinapril is used to reduce blood pressure in ⊙ **hypertension** and in congestive ℞ **heart failure treatment**, often when other treatments are not appropriate. It is frequently used in conjunction with other classes of drug, particularly ℞ **thiazide** ℞ **diuretics**.

Warnings

• It should not be given to people with known hypersensitivity to this drug or to any other ACE inhibitor.

• It should be given with caution to people with severe congestive heart failure, or certain other cardiovascular disorders, a history of anaphylaxis, collagen vascular disease (for example, systemic lupus erythematosus; SLE), diabetes, depressed immune response, or with impaired kidney function or on dialysis.

• Risk in pregnancy increases substantially from the first through to the second and third trimesters. ACE inhibitors can cause injury to the fetus, even death. The use of these drugs should be stopped as soon as pregnancy is detected.

• Medical judgment is required if breast-feeding is being considered. It does appear in breast milk.

• Use of this drug should be stopped and a doctor contacted immediately if signs of angioedema appear (swelling of the face, eyes, lips, tongue, larynx, or extremities; difficulty in breathing or swallowing). Swelling of the larynx, closing off the airway, can be life-threatening.

• Anyone taking an ACE inhibitor should not interrupt or discontinue treatment without first checking with a doctor.

• Any suspected infections (for example, fever, sore throat) should be reported to a doctor, because ACE inhibitors may cause blood changes which can affect immune response.

• ACE inhibitors generally have less effect on blood pressure in blacks than in non-blacks, and the likelihood of angioedema is higher among blacks, as well.

Interactions

• ACE inhibitors have apparently triggered life-threatening anaphylactoid reactions when used by people also receiving ℞ **desensitizing vaccines**.

• ℞ **Anesthetics** (for example, in surgery), ℞ **phenothiazines**, and ℞ **probenecid** may increase the levels or hypotensive effect of quinapril.

• Levels of ℞ **lithium** may be increased, with the potential for toxic effects.

• If used with potassium-sparing ℞ **diuretics** or other preparations containing potassium (for example, supplements and salt substitutes), levels of potassium may rise.

• ℞ **NSAID**s may increase the risk of kidney damage or (in some cases) reduce the effects of ACE inhibitors.

• The absorption and effects of ℞ **tetracycline** (and possibly other drugs that react with magnesium) may be reduced.

• ℞ **Antacids** and ℞ **rifampin** may reduce the effects of quinapril. Antacids should not be used for several hours after a dose of an ACE inhibitor (a doctor should be consulted for full instructions and cautions).

• If used with other antihypertensives and diuretics, the effects of these drugs may be increased. This additive effect is sometimes used to advantage in combination treatments for high blood pressure.

Side effects

• These are usually mild and temporary. Occasionally, headache, fatigue, dizziness, dry cough, or gastrointestinal disturbances (for example, nausea and vomiting, abdominal pain).

• Infrequently, back and muscle pains, heart rhythm disturbances or tachycardia, dry mouth, upper respiratory tract symptoms (for example, sinusitis, sore throat), blurred vision or photosensitivity (abnormal sensitivity to light). Although it is uncommon, ACE inhibitors can cause very marked hypotension (especially when beginning treatment) and kidney impairment.

• Rarely, there may be angioedema, altered liver function, jaundice, hepatitis, pancreatitis, or changes in blood counts.

quinethazone Ⓖ

Type/Group: **diuretic**; **thiazide**; **antihypertensive**.
Brand(s): Hydromox.
How administered: Orally.

Used to treat

Quinethazone is used either alone or with other types of diuretic or other drugs (for example, ℞ **beta-blockers**) in the treatment of ⊙ **hypertension**. It can also be used in the treatment of edema. Thiazide diuretics have also become a major part of treatment for nephrogenic ⊙ **diabetes insipidus**.

Warnings

• It should not be given to people with known hypersensitivity to thiazides (or to ℞ **sulfonamide**-derived drugs), or severe kidney or liver disorders.

• It should be given with caution to elderly people, anyone with high cholesterol or triglyceride levels, or with liver or kidney impairment.

• Quinethazone should be used during pregnancy only when the potential benefit outweighs the possible risk to the fetus.

• Medical judgment is required if breast-feeding is being considered.

• Early symptoms of electrolyte imbalance may include muscle weakness or cramps, nausea, vomiting, restlessness or lethargy, dry mouth, excessive thirst, fast pulse, or dizziness. A doctor must be contacted if such symptoms occur.

• Thiazides may aggravate symptoms of diabetes mellitus or gout, and worsen or activate lupus erythematosus.

• Periodic monitoring of electrolytes (particularly potassium, sodium, chloride, and bicarbonate) will be carried out.

• Photosensitivity (abnormal sensitivity to sunlight) may develop and so precautions should be taken to minimize exposure.

• Thiazides interact with a number of drugs, including some over-the-counter preparations. A doctor must always be consulted before taking any other medication (including OTCs, herbal remedies, and supplements).

Interactions

• There is a higher risk of hypersensitivity reaction to ℞ **allopurinol**.

• The effects of ℞ **anesthetics**, ℞ **anticancer** drugs, other antihypertensives, ℞ **diazoxide**, ⚖ **calcium** salts, ℞ **cardiac glycosides**, ℞ **lithium**, loop diuretics, ℞ **methyldopa**, nondepolarizing ℞ **skeletal muscle relaxants**, and ♋ **vitamin D** may be increased, with the potential for significant adverse effects or toxicity. An additive effect is sometimes used to advantage in combining thiazides with other antihypertensives.

• The effects of ℞ **anticoagulants** and antigout agents (for example, ℞ **probenecid**, ℞ **sulfinpyrazone**) may be lowered by thiazides.

• The dosage of ℞ **insulin** and ℞ **sulfonylureas** may need to be adjusted because thiazides may increase blood sugar levels.

• The diuretic effects of thiazide may be increased when taken with ℞ **amphotericin B**, ℞ **anticholinergics**, ℞ **corticosteroids**, ℞ **corticotropin**, or ℞ **MAOIs**, with the possibility of significant electrolyte loss, especially potassium.

• ℞ **Cholestyramine**, ℞ **colestipol hydrochloride**, ℞ **methenamine**, and ℞ **NSAIDs** (especially ℞ **indomethacin**) may reduce the effectiveness of thiazide diuretics.

• Alcohol, ℞ **barbiturates**, and ℞ **opioids** increase the risk of postural hypotension (lowered blood pressure on standing).

Side effects

• There may be dizziness, headache, mild gastrointestinal upsets, postural hypotension, reversible impotence, low blood potassium, sodium, magnesium and chloride, raised blood urea, glucose and lipids, and gout.

• Rarely photosensitivity, blood disorders, skin reactions, or pancreatitis.

Quinidex Extentabs ®

A preparation of ℞ **quinidine**.

Formulation: Oral tablets (sustained release).

Availability: Prescription only.

Warnings and side effects: See ℞ **quinidine**.

quinidine Ⓖ

(as sulfate or gluconate)

Type/Group: antiarrhythmic; cinchona alkaloid; antimalarial.

Brand(s): Quinaglute Dura-Tabs; Quinalan; Quinidex Extendtabs; Quinora; various generic.

How administered: Orally; injection.

Used to treat

Quinidine is chemically related to ℞ **quinine**. It is used to treat heartbeat irregularities and also, life-threatening ✪ **malaria** caused by *Plasmodium falciparum*.

Warnings

• It should not be given to people with known hypersensitivity to quinidine or quinine, particularly with a history of thrombocytopenic purpura (a severe immune system reaction) in previous treatment, or who have certain heart disorders, or the neuromuscular disease myasthenia gravis.

• It should be given with caution to people with asthma, high blood potassium, lupus erythematosus, or impaired kidney or liver function.

• Quinidine should be used during pregnancy only if it is clearly needed.

• Medical judgment is required if breast-feeding is being considered. If possible, quinidine should be discontinued if the mother is breast-feeding.

• Abruptly ending treatment can be dangerous and medical guidance is needed.

• Regular monitoring of blood, liver, and kidney function is necessary.

• If symptoms such as skin rash, breathing difficulty, nausea, headache, visual disturbance, or ringing in the ears occur, then a doctor must be contacted.

Interactions

• If used with an ℞ **anticholinergic**, the effects of both drugs may be increased.

• Quinidine enhances the anticoagulant effect of ℞ **anticoagulants** (for example, ℞ **warfarin sodium**) and bleeding may result.

• ℞ **Barbiturates**, ℞ **anticonvulsants**, and ℞ **rifampin** speed the elimination of quinidine from the body and reduce its therapeutic effect.

• Cholinergics may work to block the therapeutic action of quinidine.

• The levels of ℞ **digitoxin** and ℞ **digoxin** are raised, with the possibility of overdose symptoms.

• ℞ **Procainamide** levels and effects are increased, with the potential for toxicity.

• The effects of the following drugs are increased: ℞ **skeletal muscle relaxants**; ℞ **tricyclic** antidepressants; some ℞ **phenothiazines**; ℞ **calcium-channel blockers**; ℞ **haloperidol**; ℞ **mexiletine**.

• ℞ **Thiazides**, ℞ **sodium bicarbonate** (and some other ℞ **antacids**), ℞ **carbonic-anhydrase inhibitors**, ℞ **amiodarone hydrochloride**, ℞ **cimetidine**, ℞ **diltiazem hydrochloride**, or ℞ **verapamil** can cause an increase in quinidine levels with potential toxic effects.

Side effects

• These depend on how it is administered, for how long, use, and dose. There may be nausea, dizziness, headache, diarrhea, high temperature, slow heart rate, palpitations, rashes, heart and/or skin or blood disorders, psychosis, lupus-like symptoms, and cinchonism (tinnitus, nausea, headache, visual changes) especially after prolonged treatment.

quinine Ⓖ

Type/Group: antimalarial; cinchona alkaloid.

Brand(s): Various generic.

How administered: Orally; intravenous infusion.

Used to treat

Quinine was for a long time the main treatment for ✪ **malaria**. Today, it has been almost completely replaced by synthetic and less toxic drugs (for example, ℞ **chloroquine**). However, quinine is still used (as quinine sulphate or quinine hydrochloride) against falciparum malaria in cases that prove to be resistant to the newer drugs, or for emergency cases in which large doses are necessary. It is sometimes prescribed to relieve nocturnal leg cramps.

Warnings

• It should not be given to people with known hypersensitivity to quinine, particularly with a history of thrombocytopenic purpura (a severe immune system reaction) or blackwater fever (a malarial complication) in previous treatment, or to anyone with G6PD deficiency (an anemia disorder), tinnitus, certain optic nerve and heart disorders, or hemoglobinurea.

• It should be given with caution to people who suffer from heart block, atrial fibrillation, disorders of heart rhythm, or myasthenia gravis.

• It is very toxic in overdose.

• Quinine is dangerous to a developing fetus and should not be used during pregnancy, nor if the mother intends to breast-feed.

• Discontinue using quinine if allergic symptoms such as itching, skin rash, fever, breathing difficulty, visual disturbance, or ringing in the ears occur.

• As this drug may cause dizziness, vertigo, confusion, or blurring of vision, it may impair the performance of tasks requiring skill or alertness, such as driving.

• Smoking can reduce levels of quinine.

Interactions

• Quinine enhances the anticoagulant effect of ℞ **anticoagulants** (for example, ℞ **warfarin sodium**), which may cause bleeding.

• If used with astemizole or terfenadine, there is a risk of serious cardiac effects.

• ℞ **Rifampin**, ℞ **rifabutin**, and ℞ **antacids** containing aluminum speed the elimination of quinine from the body and so reduce its therapeutic effect.

• The levels of ℞ **digitoxin** and ℞ **digoxin** are raised with the possibility of overdose symptoms.

• Mefloquine must not be used with quinine.

• Quinine increases the effects of ℞ **skeletal muscle relaxants**.

• Drugs that raise the pH of urine (for example, ℞ **sodium bicarbonate**, ℞ **acetazolamide**) and ℞ **cimetidine** can increase quinine levels with potential toxic effects.

Side effects

• Toxic effects (especially in overdose)—called cinchonism—include nausea, headache, abdominal pain, visual disturbances, tinnitus, a rash, and confusion. Some patients may experience visual disturbances and temporary blindness, sensitivity reactions and blood disorders, hot flushes, confusion, and kidney effects.

quinolone ⑩

(4-quinolone; fluoroquinolone)
Generics: **cinoxacin; ciprofloxacin; enoxacin; gatifloxacin; levofloxacin; lomefloxacin; moxifloxacin; nalidixic acid; norfloxacin; ofloxacin; sparfloxacin.**

Actions and uses

Quinolones are synthetic ℞ **antibacterial** drugs, which are not technically ℞ **antibiotic** in origin but have a number of similarities and are often grouped with the antibiotics. Quinolones are mainly used to treat ✪ **bacterial infections** in people who are allergic to antibiotics, or whose strain of bacterium is resistant to standard antibiotics. Although they are active against a wide range of infective bacterial organisms, they are usually more effective against Gram-negative organisms. They also have useful activity against some Gram-positive organisms (although not anaerobe bacteria). They work by damaging the internal structure, DNA polymerization, of bacteria (they are bactericidal). They are "related" to ℞ **nalidixic acid** but the names of all more recently introduced members end with *-oxacin*. Chemically, they are 4-quinolones and later members are fluoroquinolones.

Limitations

Quinolones are generally well tolerated, but they should be given with caution to people with a history of ✪ **epilepsy** or conditions that predispose to seizures (taking NSAIDs at the same time may also induce them), in ✪ **G6PD-deficiency**, and a number of other conditions, including defects of heart rhythm. Exposure to excessive sunlight should be avoided. Dairy products and several dietary supplements reduce their absorption. See also the individual drug entries.

Quinora ⑧

A preparation of ℞ **quinidine**.
Formulation: Oral tablets.
Availability: Prescription only.
Warnings and side effects: See ℞ **quinidine**.

Quinsana Plus ⑧

A preparation of ℞ **tolnaftate**.
Formulation: Topical powder.
Availability: OTC.
Warnings and side effects: See ℞ **tolnaftate**.

quinupristin-dalfopristin ⑥

Type/Group: **antibiotic; antibacterial**.
Brand(s): Synercid.
How administered: Injection

Used to treat

Quinupristin-dalfopristin is a combination of two antibiotics with antibacterial properties that are used to treat complicated skin and skin structure ✪ **bacterial infections**, and certain serious or life-threatening infections with bacteria in the blood that are resistant to the usual treatment (for example, MRSA). These two antibiotics belong to an unusual group, the streptogramins, and are only used together.

Warnings

• It should not be given to people with known hypersensitivity to quinupristin-dalfopristin or other streptogramins.

• It should be given with caution to people with kidney or liver dysfunction.

• It should be used during pregnancy only if clearly needed.

• Medical judgment is required if breast-feeding is being considered. It is unknown whether this drug appears in breast milk.

• Superinfections due the altered bacterial balance created by antibiotic treatment may occur. A doctor must be contacted if there is severe abdominal pain, moderate to severe diarrhea, or any new or unusual symptoms.

• Veins may become painful and inflamed following intravenous infusion.

Interactions

• Quinupristin-dalfopristin increases the levels of ℞ **cyclosporine**.

• Delavirdine, ℞ **nevirapine**, ℞ **indinavir**, ℞ **ritonavir**, ℞ **vinca alkaloids**, ℞ **midazolam**, ℞ **diazepam**, **calcium-channel blockers**, HMG-CoA reductase inhibitors, cisapride, ℞ **tacrolimus**, ℞ **methylprednisolone**, ℞ **carbamazepine**, ℞ **quinidine**, ℞ **lidocaine**, and ℞ **disopyramide** are predicted to have increased levels.

Side effects

This is a specialist drug and a full explanation of possible side effects will be given by the clinician.

• Occasionally, headache and diarrhea.

• Rarely, muscle and joint pain, and vomiting.

rabeprazole sodium   Ⓖ

Type/Group: **proton-pump inhibitor; ulcer-healing drug**.
Brand(s): Aciphex.
How administered: Orally.

Used to treat

Rabeprazole sodium works as an inhibitor of gastric acid secretion in the parietal (acid-producing) cells of the stomach lining by acting as a proton-pump inhibitor. It is used for the treatment of benign gastric and duodenal ulcers (see ✪ **peptic ulcer**), and ✪ **gastroesophageal reflux** disease (GERD), and hypersecretory conditions such as ✪ **Zollinger-Ellison syndrome**.

Warnings

• It should not be given to people with known hypersensitivity to this drug, or to any substituted benzimidazoles (that is, other proton-pump inhibitors, such as ℞ **omeprazole**, ℞ **lansoprazole**, ℞ **pantoprazole**).

• It should be given with caution to people with severe liver impairment.

• Rabeprazole should be used during pregnancy only if the potential benefit outweighs the possible risk to the fetus.

• Medical judgment is required if breast-feeding is being considered. It is not known whether this drug appears in breast milk, but there is reason to believe its effects would be harmful.

• Before treatment, it should be confirmed that there is no gastric cancer or other disease.

Interactions

• Proton-pump inhibitors, like this one, should be taken at least 30 minutes before ℞ **sucralfate** or they may not be absorbed efficiently.

• The levels and effects of ℞ **digoxin**, ferrous salts (♧♧ **iron** supplements), ℞ **ketoconazole**, and ℞ **ampicillin** may be decreased.

• It is thought possible that deficiency of ♧♧ **vitamin B$_{12}$** can occur with long-term use of rabeprazole.

Side effects

• These are uncommon with rabeprazole, consisting mainly of headache, but proton-pump inhibitors may also cause diarrhea, abdominal pain, rashes and itching, dizziness, nausea and vomiting, constipation, and flatulence. They decrease gastric acidity and so may increase the risk of gastrointestinal infections.

• Rarer side effects may include cough, rhinitis, sinusitis, mouth ulcers, hives, other allergic reactions, fever, flu-like syndrome, sweating, malaise, nosebleed, muscle and joint pain, kidney problems, pancreatitis, sleepiness, insomnia, temporary mental disturbances, hair loss, peripheral edema, effects on the liver and the heart, and various blood changes. Also rare, but occasionally reported, are menstrual problems, growth of breasts in men, and impotence.

rabies immune globulin, human (RIG)   Ⓖ

rabies immunoglobulin (HRIG)
Type/Group: **immune globulin**.
Brand(s): Hyperab.
How administered: Injection.

Used to treat

Rabies immune globulin human (RIG) is a specific immune globulin of human origin, which is used to give immediate passive immunity against infection by ✪ **rabies** and can be used in conjunction with ℞ **rabies vaccine**. It is recommended as soon as possible after exposure, for anyone whose rabies immunity is uncertain or inadequate.

Warnings

• It should be given with caution to people with known hypersensitivity to immune globulins, or with a known deficiency of the naturally occurring IgA immunoglobulin.

• No adverse effects during pregnancy are known and the globulin should be used when medically judged to be clearly needed, as the consequences of rabies infection are dire.

• The effects if breast-feeding have not been studied, although no problems have been documented.

• People who have adequate rabies immunity (from previous vaccination) should receive a vaccine booster and not rabies immune globulin.

• It should not be administered more than once after vaccination has begun, as it may interfere with vaccine effect in achieving maximum immunity.

• Because this immune globulin is extracted from human blood, the possibility exists that it might contain virus or other disease agents. However, multiple screenings and filters (chemical and physical) are used in its preparation, and its potential to transmit infection is considered nearly nonexistent.

• After administration, people will be required to wait for some time to ensure that there is no serious reaction (such as anaphylaxis).

Interactions

• The immune response to live virus vaccines (for example, ℞ **MMR vaccine**) may not be satisfactory. A delay of at least 3 months (more for some vaccines, or their specific uses) is recommended after administering immune globulin. This does not apply, however, to the live vaccines for polio (oral form), typhoid (oral form), or yellow fever, which may be given at the same time as rabies immune globulin.

• Caution is required if ℞ **anticoagulants** are being taken.

Side effects

• There may be swelling, irritation or tenderness at the site of injection, and low-grade fever.

    Key to symbols: ✪ = Disorder Section   ℞ = Drug Section   ♣ = Herbal Section   ♧♧ = Supplement Section

• Allergic reactions, such as hives or facial swelling, are uncommon.
• Although rare, anaphylactic shock has occurred.

rabies immunoglobulin (HRIG) ⓖ

see ℞ rabies immune globulin, human (RIG).

rabies vaccine ⓖ

Type/Group: **vaccine**.
Brand(s): Imovax Rabies Vaccine, Imovax Rabies I.D. Vaccine; various generic.
How administered: Injection.

Used to treat

Rabies vaccines (comprised of inactivated virus) are used for ℞ **immunization** against contracting ✪ **rabies**. They may be administered to medical workers, and their relatives, who may come into contact with rabid animals or with people who have been bitten by an animal that might be rabid. They are also routinely administered to people who work with animals. Vaccination is also recommended for anyone without adequate existing immunity who has been bitten by an animal that might carry the disease; the course of treatment in such a case has quite specific guidelines. There are two types of rabies vaccine, human diploid cell vaccine (HDVC) and rabies vaccine adsorbed (RVA), which is a somewhat newer form. Although they are prepared in different ways, they are thought to confer the same degree of immunity.

Warnings

• It should not be given to people with known hypersensitivity to this vaccine. In such cases the risks of taking the vaccine must be weighed against the risk of developing rabies.
• It should be used during pregnancy only when medically judged to be clearly needed.
• Medical judgment is required if breast-feeding is being considered.
• Dose scheduling should follow established recommendations closely, or sufficient immunity may not be achieved, with potentially dire results.
• After administration, people will be required to wait for some time to ensure that there is no serious reaction (such as anaphylaxis).

Interactions

• ℞ **Immunosuppressants** (for example, ℞ **corticosteroids**, ℞ **cytotoxics**, ℞ **chloroquine**) may reduce the effectiveness of the vaccine in conferring immunity.
• It is recommended that when using ℞ **rabies immune globulin, human (RIG)** with rabies vaccine, procedure and dosing should be followed exactly.
• Caution is required if ℞ **anticoagulants** are being taken.

Side effects

• There may be swelling, irritation or tenderness at the site of vaccination, and headache, nausea, abdominal pain, muscle aches, and dizziness.
• Rarely, skin rash, hives, itching, and shortness of breath. A "serum sickness" kind of reaction is more common (though less so using RVA), with hives, facial swelling, arthralgia, nausea, vomiting, fever and malaise; these symptoms require medical observation.

(R)-albuterol hydrochloride ⓖ

see ℞ levalbuterol hydrochloride.

R-albuterol hydrochloride ⓖ

see ℞ levalbuterol hydrochloride.

RA Lotion ⓑ

A preparation of ℞ **resorcinol**.
Formulation: Topical lotion.
Availability: OTC.
Warnings and side effects: See ℞ resorcinol.

raloxifene ⓖ

Type/Group: **sex hormone; estrogen**.
Brand(s): Evista.
How administered: Orally.

Used to treat

Raloxifene is used to prevent and treat ✪ **osteoporosis** in postmenopausal women. It has weak estrogen-like effects at some sites, making it a selective estrogen receptor modulator (SERM).

Warnings

• It must not be used by women who are or may become pregnant, who have active, or a history of, venous blood clots, including deep vein thrombosis, pulmonary embolism and retinal vein thrombosis, or with hypersensitivity to raloxifene.
• It should be given with caution to people with liver or kidney insufficiency.
• It is not for use during pregnancy. A doctor must be contacted if pregnancy occurs while using this drug.
• Medical judgment is required if breast-feeding is being considered.
• Recommended levels of dietary or supplementary calcium must be maintained.
• Use of the drug must stop 72 hours prior to surgery involving immobilization, as the risk of clotting events is greater during periods of immobility.
• Any leg pain or swelling, shortness of breath, vision changes, or chest pain must be reported to a doctor.

Interactions

• ℞ **cholestyramine** decreases the absorption of raloxifene.
• Raloxifene may interfere with the effects of ℞ **clofibrate**, ℞ **indomethacin**, ℞ **naproxen**, ℞ **ibuprofen**, ℞ **diazepam**, and ℞ **diazoxide**.
• The effects of ℞ **warfarin** and similar ℞ **anticoagulants** may be increased.

Side effects

• Commonly, hot flashes, sinusitis, nausea, weight gain, and leg cramps.
• Occasionally, gastrointestinal effects, vaginal inflammation, breast changes, and edema.

ramipril ⓖ

Type/Group: **ACE inhibitor; vasodilator; antihypertensive; heart failure treatment**.
Brand(s): Altace.

Key to symbols: ⓓ = Drug type/group   ⓖ = Generic name   ⓑ = Brand name

How administered: Orally.

Used to treat

Ramipril is used to treat high blood pressure in ✪ **hypertension** and congestive ✪ **heart failure** that develops in the first few days following ✪ **myocardial infarction** (damage to heart muscle, usually after a heart attack). It is often used with other classes of drug, particularly ℞ **thiazide** ℞ **diuretics**.

Warnings

• It should not be given to people with known hypersensitivity to this drug or to any other ACE inhibitor.

• It should be given with caution to people with severe congestive heart failure, or certain other cardiovascular disorders, a history of anaphylaxis, collagen vascular disease (for example, systemic lupus erythematosus; SLE), diabetes mellitus, depressed immune response, or with impaired liver or kidney function or on dialysis.

• Risk in pregnancy increases substantially from the first through to the second and third trimesters. ACE inhibitors can cause injury to the fetus, even death. The use of these drugs should be stopped as soon as pregnancy is detected and after checking with your doctor.

• Medical judgment is required if breast-feeding is being considered.

• Use of this drug should be stopped and a doctor contacted immediately if signs of angioedema appear (swelling of the face, eyes, lips, tongue, larynx, or extremities; difficulty in breathing or swallowing). Swelling of the larynx, closing off the airway, can be life-threatening.

• Anyone taking an ACE inhibitor should not interrupt or discontinue treatment without first checking with a doctor.

• Any suspected infections (for example, fever, sore throat) should be reported to a doctor, because ACE inhibitors may cause blood changes which can affect immune response.

• ACE inhibitors generally have less effect on blood pressure in blacks than in non-blacks, and the likelihood of angioedema is higher among blacks, as well.

Interactions

• ACE inhibitors have apparently triggered life-threatening anaphylactoid reactions when used by people also receiving ℞ **desensitizing vaccines**.

• ℞ **Anesthetics** (for example, in surgery), ℞ **phenothiazines**, and ℞ **probenecid** may increase the levels or hypotensive effect of ramipril.

• Levels of ℞ **lithium** may be increased, with the potential for toxic effects.

• If used with potassium-sparing ℞ **diuretics** or other preparations containing potassium (for example, supplements and salt substitutes), levels of potassium may rise.

• ℞ **NSAIDs** may increase the risk of kidney damage or (in some cases) reduce the effects of ACE inhibitors.

• ℞ **Antacids** may reduce the effects of ramipril. Antacids should not be used for several hours after a dose of an ACE inhibitor (a doctor should be consulted for full instructions and cautions).

• If used with other antihypertensives and diuretics, the effects of these drugs may be increased. This additive effect is sometimes used to advantage in combination treatments for high blood pressure.

Side effects

• Commonly, hypotension and dry cough.

• Occasionally, headache, fatigue, dizziness, or gastrointestinal disturbances (for example, abdominal pain, diarrhea, nausea and vomiting).

• Infrequently, weakness, muscle cramps, joint pain, tingling in the extremities, fainting, disturbances of heart rhythm, rash, insomnia, nervousness, sexual dysfunction, or photosensitivity (abnormal sensitivity to light). Although it is uncommon, ACE inhibitors can cause very marked hypotension (especially when beginning treatment) and kidney impairment.

• Rarely, there may be angioedema, altered liver function, jaundice, hepatitis, pancreatitis, or changes in blood counts.

R & C ®

A preparation of ℞ **pyrethrin**.

Formulation: Shampoo.

Availability: OTC.

Warnings and side effects: See ℞ **pyrethrin**.

ranitidine bismuth citrate ⑥

Type/Group: **H$_2$-antagonist; ulcer-healing drug; Helicobacter pylori eradication regime.**

Brand(s): Tritec.

How administered: Orally; injection; infusion.

Used to treat

Ranitidine bismuth citrate is a compound of the extensively prescribed peptic ulcer-healing drug ℞ **ranitidine hydrochloride** together with bismuth, which has several antibacterial effects. In the treatment of duodenal ulceration (see ✪ **peptic ulcer**) associated with *Helicobacter pylori* infection, it is administered along with one or two antibiotics (normally ℞ **clarithromycin**). Ranitidine works by reducing the secretion of gastric acid and (together with the antibiotic) helps to eliminate the bacterium associated with peptic ulceration. It is not used alone for treating active duodenal ulcer.

Warnings

• It should not be given to people with known hypersensitivity to this drug, or with porphyria.

• It should be given with caution to people with kidney or liver impairment.

• It should be used during pregnancy only if it is clearly needed. (Combined therapy with clarithromycin, which is hazardous to the fetus, should not be commenced during pregnancy unless no alternative is available and the risks are understood.)

• Medical judgment is required if breast-feeding is being considered. It may appear in breast milk.

• H$_2$-antagonists, like this one, may mask symptoms of gastric cancer, and this possibility must be eliminated with particular care in persons who have reached middle-age.

• If combination treatment with clarithromycin fails to clear the infection, the bacteria may be resistant, and this treatment should not be used again.

Key to symbols: ✪ = Disorder Section ℞ = Drug Section ♣ = Herbal Section ⚕ = Supplement Section

Interactions

• The effects of ℞ **glipizide**, ℞ **metoprolol tartrate**, ℞ **nifedipine**, ℞ **triazolam**, and ℞ **warfarin** may be increased.
• ℞ **propantheline** may increase the levels of ranitidine.
• Cigarette smoking reverses some effects of ranitidine, and so interferes with ulcer healing.
• ℞ **Antacids**, ℞ **anticholinergics**, and ℞ **metoclopramide** may decrease the absorption of ranitidine, reducing its effect. (Antacids should probably be taken an hour after ranitidine.)

Side effects

• These are infrequent and may include headache (sometimes severe), dizziness, drowsiness, or diarrhea.
• The bismuth derived from this drug may cause a darkened, discolored tongue or blackened stools.
• Rarely, there is a speeding of the heart, agitation, visual disturbances, hair loss, or skin symptoms.

ranitidine hydrochloride Ⓖ

Type/Group: H_2-antagonist; ulcer-healing drug.
Brand(s): Zantac; various generic.
How administered: Orally; injection; infusion.

Used to treat

Ranitidine hydrochloride is used in the treatment of benign ✪ **peptic ulcers** (gastric and duodenal), ℞ **NSAID**-induced ulceration, and as a preventive measure to relieve heartburn in cases of reflux esophagitis, ✪ **Zollinger-Ellison syndrome**, and a variety of conditions where reduction of acidity is beneficial. It is now also available without prescription (in a limited amount and for short-term uses only) for the relief of heartburn, indigestion, hyperacidity/acid indigestion, and sour stomach. It works by reducing the secretion of gastric acid, so reducing erosion and bleeding from peptic ulcers and allowing them a chance to heal. However, treatment with ranitidine should not start before a full diagnosis of gastric bleeding or serious pain has been made, because its action in restricting gastric secretions may possibly mask the presence of stomach cancer.

Warnings

• It should not be given to people with known hypersensitivity to this drug, or with porphyria.
• It should be given with caution to people with kidney or liver impairment.
• Ranitidine should be used during pregnancy only if it is clearly needed and following medical advice.
• It may appear in breast milk and should be avoided by nursing mothers.
• Although rare, confusional states (depression, anxiety, psychosis, hallucinations) have occurred with use of this drug. The risk is highest among those who are severely ill or have existing kidney or liver disease. However, these conditions clear up within a few days of discontinuing the drug.
• H_2-antagonists, like this one, may mask symptoms of gastric cancer, and this possibility must be eliminated with particular care in persons who have reached middle-age.
• The frequency and severity of side effects is higher in the elderly.
• Doses of ranitidine and antacids should be staggered.

Interactions

• The effects of ℞ **glipizide**, ℞ **metoprolol**, ℞ **nifedipine**, and ℞ **triazolam** may be increased.
• Deficiency of ⊿ **vitamin B_{12}** may occur with long-term use of ranitidine.
• ℞ **propantheline** may increase the levels of ranitidine.
• Cigarette smoking reverses some of the effects of ranitidine, and interferes with ulcer healing.
• ℞ **Antacids**, ℞ **anticholinergics**, and ℞ **metoclopramide** may decrease the absorption of ranitidine, reducing its effect. (Antacids should be taken an hour after ranitidine.)

Side effects

• These are infrequent and may include headache (sometimes severe), dizziness, drowsiness, or diarrhea.
• Rare side effects may include pancreatitis, joint pain, hair loss, hypersensitivity reactions (including fever, rash, bronchospasm, anaphylaxis), blood disorders, and effects on the liver and the heart. There have been occasional reports of impotence and the growth of breasts in men. Confusional states occur predominantly in those who are severely ill.

Rebetron Ⓑ

A combination therapy of ℞ **interferons** alfa-2b and ℞ **ribavirin**.
Formulation: Injection; oral capsules.
Availability: Prescription only.
Warnings and side effects: See ℞ **interferons**; ℞ **ribavirin**.

Reclomide Ⓑ

A preparation of ℞ **metoclopramide hydrochloride**.
Formulation: Oral tablets.
Availability: Prescription only.
Warnings and side effects: See ℞ **metoclopramide hydrochloride**.

Recombinate Ⓑ

A preparation of ℞ **antihemophilic factor**.
Formulation: Intravenous infusion.
Availability: Prescription only.
Warnings and side effects: See ℞ **antihemophilic factor**.

Recombivax HB Ⓑ

A preparation of ℞ **hepatitis B vaccine**.
Formulation: Intramuscular injection.
Availability: Prescription only.
Warnings and side effects: See ℞ **hepatitis B vaccine**.

rectoanal preparation ⒟

see ℞ **anorectal preparation**.

Reese's Pinworm Ⓑ

A preparation of ℞ **pyrantel**.
Formulation: Oral capsules; oral liquid.
Availability: OTC.
Warnings and side effects: See ℞ **pyrantel**.

Key to symbols: ⒟ = Drug type/group   Ⓖ = Generic name   Ⓑ = Brand name

Refenesan Plus Tablets ®

A preparation of ℞ pseudoephedrine and ℞ guaifenesin.
Formulation: Oral tablets.
Availability: OTC.
Warnings and side effects: See ℞ pseudoephedrine;
℞ guaifenesin.

Refludan ®

A preparation of ℞ lepirudin.
Formulation: Intravenous injection or infusion.
Availability: Prescription only.
Warnings and side effects: See ℞ lepirudin.

Refresh ®

A preparation of ℞ polyvinyl alcohol and ℞ povidone.
Formulation: Eyedrops.
Availability: OTC.
Warnings and side effects: See ℞ polyvinyl alcohol;
℞ povidone.

Refresh Plus ®

A preparation of ℞ carboxymethylcellulose sodium.
Formulation: Ophthalmic solution.
Availability: OTC.
Warnings and side effects: See ℞ carboxymethylcellulose
sodium.

Refresh Tears ®

A preparation of ℞ carboxymethylcellulose sodium.
Formulation: Ophthalmic solution.
Availability: OTC.
Warnings and side effects: See ℞ carboxymethylcellulose
sodium.

Regitine ®

A preparation of ℞ phentolamine mesylate.
Formulation: Injection.
Availability: Prescription only.
Warnings and side effects: See ℞ phentolamine mesylate.

Reglan Tablets; Syrup; Injection ®

A preparation of ℞ metoclopramide.
Formulation: Oral tablets (two strengths); syrup; injection.
Availability: Prescription only.
Warnings and side effects: See ℞ metoclopramide.

Regonol ®

A preparation of ℞ pyridostigmine.
Formulation: Injection.
Availability: Prescription only.
Warnings and side effects: See ℞ pyridostigmine.

Regranex ®

A preparation of ℞ becaplermin.
Formulation: Topical gel.

Availability: Prescription only.
Warnings and side effects: See ℞ becaplermin.

Regular Iletin I ®

A preparation of ℞ insulin, regular.
Formulation: Bottles for injection.
Availability: OTC.
Warnings and side effects: See ℞ insulin, regular.

Regular Iletin II ®

A preparation of ℞ insulin, regular.
Formulation: Bottles for injection.
Availability: OTC.
Warnings and side effects: See ℞ insulin, regular.

Regular Purified Pork Insulin ®

A preparation of ℞ insulin, regular.
Formulation: Vials for injection.
Availability: OTC.
Warnings and side effects: See ℞ insulin, regular.

Regulax SS ®

A preparation of ℞ docusate sodium.
Formulation: Oral capsules.
Availability: OTC.
Warnings and side effects: See ℞ docusate sodium.

Reguloid; Orange; Sugar Free Orange; Sugar Free Regular ®

A preparation of ℞ psyllium.
Formulation: Oral powder.
Availability: OTC.
Warnings and side effects: See ℞ psyllium. Sugar Free powders
contain the sweetener aspartame, which should be avoided by
individuals with phenylketonuria.

rehydration solution ⊙

see ℞ electrolyte.

Relafen ®

A preparation of ℞ nabumetone.
Formulation: Oral tablets, available in two strengths.
Availability: Prescription only.
Warnings and side effects: See ℞ nabumetone.

Relefact TRH ®

A preparation of ℞ protirelin.
Formulation: Injection.
Availability: Prescription only.
Warnings and side effects: See ℞ protirelin.

Relenza ®

A preparation of ℞ zanamivir.
Formulation: Inhalant.
Availability: Prescription only.

Key to symbols: ⊙ = Disorder Section ℞ = Drug Section ♣ = Herbal Section ⚕ = Supplement Section

Warnings and side effects: See ℞ **zanamivir**.

Reliable Gentle Laxative Ⓑ

A preparation of ℞ **bisacodyl**.
Formulation: Oral tablets (delayed release); rectal suppositories.
Availability: OTC.
Warnings and side effects: See ℞ **bisacodyl**.

Relief Ⓑ

A preparation of ℞ **phenylephrine hydrochloride**.
Formulation: Eye drops.
Availability: OTC.
Warnings and side effects: See ℞ **phenylephrine hydrochloride**.

Remeron Ⓑ

A preparation of ℞ **mirtazapine**.
Formulation: Oral tablets of varying strengths.
Availability: Prescription only.
Warnings and side effects: See ℞ **mirtazapine**.

Remicade Ⓑ

A preparation of ℞ **infliximab**.
Formulation: Intravenous infusion.
Availability: Prescription only.
Warnings and side effects: See ℞ **infliximab**.

remifentanil Ⓖ

Type/Group: **narcotic analgesic; opioid; general anesthetic.**
Brand(s): Ultiva.
How administered: Intravenous infusion.

Used to treat

Remifentanil is used in the induction of anesthesia and during surgery to supplement the effect of general anesthetics. It is not used alone for general anesthesia.

Warnings

• It should not be given to people with known hypersensitivity to this drug. Opioids (even the weaker ones) should not be given to people with asthma, or to anyone with seriously depressed breathing disorders, prostatic hypertrophy, convulsive disorders, raised intracranial pressure, or a head injury.
• Depending on use and dose, it should be given with caution to the elderly, or to those with hypotension, certain liver, kidney or adrenal disorders, hypothyroidism (under-activity of the thyroid gland), or alcoholism.
• Remifentanil should be used during pregnancy only if the benefits outweigh the potential risks.
• Medical judgment is required if breast-feeding is being considered. It may appear in breast milk.
• Remifentanil is a Schedule II controlled substance.
• Prolonged use of narcotics can lead to physical dependence (addiction), although this rarely happens in routine medical use.
• Remifentanil does not always induce unconsciousness and will need to be given with another general anesthetic during operative procedures.

• Drowsiness may affect the performance of skilled tasks such as driving.
• The effects of alcohol may be enhanced (including a higher risk of respiratory depression).

Interactions

• If used with the following drugs, there is a risk of increased effects: ℞ **barbiturates**; ℞ **general anesthetics**; ℞ **opioids**; ℞ **tranquilizers** (for example, ℞ **phenothiazines**); ℞ **sedatives**; ℞ **benzodiazepines** (for example, ℞ **diazepam**, ℞ **lorazepam**); alcohol; ℞ **chlorpromazine**; ℞ **thioridazine**.

Side effects

• The side effects of remifentanil are quite similar to those of other narcotic analgesics (although it is cleared from the body much more rapidly), but because it is used exclusively during medical procedures, the most significant is its higher potential for causing skeletal muscle rigidity, with impaired ability to breathe. It may cause, as well, nausea, vomiting, and respiratory depression.
• Less commonly, urinary retention and constipation, dizziness, sweating, headache, palpitations, changes in heart rate, rashes, miosis (pupil constriction), dry mouth, flushing of the face, mood change, and hallucinations.

Remular-S Ⓑ

A preparation of ℞ **chlorzoxazone**.
Formulation: Oral tablets.
Availability: Prescription only.
Warnings and side effects: See ℞ **chlorzoxazone**.

Renese Ⓑ

A preparation of ℞ **polythiazide**.
Formulation: Oral tablets, available in three strengths.
Availability: Prescription only.
Warnings and side effects: See ℞ **polythiazide**.

Renese-R Ⓑ

A preparation of ℞ **polythiazide** and ℞ **reserpine**.
Formulation: Oral tablets.
Availability: Prescription only.
Warnings and side effects: See ℞ **polythiazide**; ℞ **reserpine**.

ReoPro Ⓑ

A preparation of ℞ **abciximab**.
Formulation: Injection.
Availability: Prescription only.
Warnings and side effects: See ℞ **abciximab**.

repaglinide Ⓖ

Type/Group: **antidiabetic; oral hypoglycemic.**
Brand(s): Prandine.
How administered: Orally.

Used to treat

Repaglinide, a non-sulfonylurea (it is a meglitinide), is used to treat type 2 ✪ **diabetes mellitus** (non-insulin-dependent diabetes mellitus; NIDDM), particularly in people who are not totally dependent on additional supplies of insulin, when diabetes is not controlled by diet and exercise. It works by stimulating insulin release from the pancreas, and can be used together with ℞ **metformin**.

Warnings
• It should not be given to people with type 1 diabetes mellitus or ketoacidosis.
• Its safety in pregnancy is not established. It should be used only if clearly needed.
• It is not recommended for use while breast-feeding.
• Be alert for the development of hypoglycemic symptoms.

Interactions
• ℞ **aspirin**, ℞ **beta-blockers**, sulfa drugs, ℞ **chloramphenicol**, ℞ **warfarin**, and ℞ **MAOIs** increase the risk of hypoglycemia.
• ℞ **ketoconazole**, ℞ **miconazole**, ℞ **erythromycin**, ℞ **rifampin**, ℞ **carbamazepine**, ℞ **phenobarbital**, ℞ **butabarbital**, ℞ **secobarbital**, and ℞ **primidone** increase the effects of repaglinide.
• ℞ **Thiazide** diuretics, ℞ **calcium-channel blockers**, ℞ **beta-blockers**, cough, cold, or hay fever medicines, ℞ **estrogen**, ℞ **oral contraceptives**, ℞ **corticosteroids**, thyroid medicines, ℞ **phenytoin**, ℞ **isoniazid**, and ℞ **nicotinic acid** reduce the effects of repaglinide.

Side effects
• Nausea, diarrhea, constipation, vomiting, and upset stomach.

Repan CF Tablets ℞

A preparation of ℞ **acetaminophen** and butalbital.
Formulation: Oral tablets.
Availability: Prescription only.
Warnings and side effects: See ℞ **acetaminophen**; ℞ **butabarbital**.

Repan Tablets ℞

A preparation of ℞ **acetaminophen**, ℞ **caffeine**, and ℞ **butabarbital**.
Formulation: Oral tablets.
Availability: Prescription only.
Warnings and side effects: See ℞ **acetaminophen**; ℞ **butabarbital**; ℞ **caffeine**.

Repronex ℞

A preparation of ℞ **menotropins**.
Formulation: Injection.
Availability: Prescription only.
Warnings and side effects: See ℞ **menotropins**.

Requip ℞

A preparation of ℞ **ropinirole**.
Formulation: Oral tablets in several strengths.
Availability: Prescription only.
Warnings and side effects: See ℞ **ropinirole**.

Rescon Capsules; JR Capsules; ED Capsules ℞

A preparation of ℞ **pseudoephedrine** and ℞ **chlorpheniramine maleate**.

Formulation: Oral capsules, (sustained release).
Availability: Prescription only.
Warnings and side effects: See ℞ **pseudoephedrine**; ℞ **chlorpheniramine maleate**.

Rescon DM Liquid ℞

A preparation of ℞ **dextromethorphan**, ℞ **chlorpheniramine maleate**, and ℞ **pseudoephedrine**.
Formulation: Oral liquid.
Availability: OTC.
Warnings and side effects: See ℞ **dextromethorphan**; ℞ **chlorpheniramine maleate**; ℞ **pseudoephedrine**.

Rescon-GG Liquid ℞

A preparation of ℞ **phenylephrine hydrochloride** and ℞ **guaifenesin**.
Formulation: Oral liquid.
Availability: OTC.
Warnings and side effects: See ℞ **phenylephrine hydrochloride**; ℞ **guaifenesin**.

reserpine Ⓖ

Type/Group: **alkaloid; antihypertensive; antipsychotic**.
Brand(s): Various generic. Combinations: With *hydrochlorothiazide*: Hydro-Serp; Hydroserpine. With *hydralazine and hydrochlorothiazide*: Hydrap-ES; Marpres; Ser-Ap-Es; Tri-Hydroserpine.

How administered: Orally.

Used to treat

Reserpine is a plant ℞ **alkaloid** derived from *Rauwolfia serpentina*. Although its action has not been completely established, the result is a lowering of adrenergic response, as well as a depleted store of ℞ **sympathomimetic** neurotransmitters and serotonin. Reserpine, therefore, reduces blood pressure and may be used alone or with other antihypertensives (particularly ℞ **diuretics**) for this purpose. Separately, it is also used to relieve symptoms in agitated psychotic states, particularly for those who cannot tolerate ℞ **phenothiazines**.

Warnings

• It should not be given to people with known hypersensitivity to this drug, with active peptic ulcer or ulcerative colitis, a history of mental depression, or who are receiving electroconvulsive therapy (ECT).

• It should be given with caution to people with a history of peptic ulcer, colitis or gallstones, or who have a seizure disorder, kidney impairment, or have had a recent stroke.

• Reserpine's safety during pregnancy has not been established, and it should be used only if the potential benefit outweighs the possible risk to the fetus.

• Medical judgment is required if breast-feeding is being considered.

• Mental depression, sometimes severe, may occur. The risk is greatest in high dosage and in those with a history of depression. If symptoms appear (for example, despondency, early morning insomnia, loss of appetite, impotence, self-deprecation), use of

Key to symbols: ✿ = Disorder Section ℞ = Drug Section ♣ = Herbal Section ♊ = Supplement Section

reserpine should be stopped. Depression may persist for several months after the drug is withdrawn.

• Because of possible sedative side effects, caution is advised for potentially hazardous activities, such as driving, that require mental alertness.

• A doctor must be consulted before taking any other medication, including OTCs, herbal remedies, supplements, or any kind of alternative remedy.

Interactions

• ℞ **MAOI** antidepressants should not be used with reserpine.

• ℞ **Cardiac glycosides** (for example, ℞ **digoxin**) and ℞ **quinidine** may cause arrhythmias.

• The effects of direct-acting ℞ **sympathomimetics** such as ℞ **vasoconstrictors** (for example, ℞ **metaraminol**, ℞ **norepinephrine**, ℞ **phenylephrine**) and nasal ℞ **decongestants** may be intensified or prolonged.

• If taken with ℞ **methotrimeprazine**, there is a risk of exaggerated hypotensive effects.

• Increased effects are possible with alcohol, ℞ **barbiturates**, ℞ **hypnotics**, and ℞ **sedatives**.

• The response to ℞ **levodopa** may be reduced.

• The effects of ℞ **amphetamines** and ℞ **ephedrine** may be inhibited.

• ℞ **Tricyclic** antidepressants may reduce the antihypertensive effect of reserpine.

• If used with other antihypertensives and diuretics, the effects of these drugs may be increased. This additive effect is sometimes used to advantage in combination treatments for high blood pressure.

Side effects

• Frequently, nasal congestion, drowsiness and fatigue, gastrointestinal disturbances (for example, abdominal cramps, diarrhea, nausea, vomiting), and slowed heartbeat.

• Less commonly, headache, dizziness, anxiety, arrhythmias or angina pectoris, flushing, salt or water retention, shortness of breath, dry mouth, or muscular aches.

• Sensitivity reactions, such as rash and itching, are rare, although reserpine may precipitate attacks in asthmatics. Parkinsonian symptoms may occur at extremely large doses.

Resinol ⑧

A preparation of ℞ **calamine**.
Formulation: Topical ointment.
Availability: OTC.
Warnings and side effects: See ℞ **calamine**.

resorcinol ⑥

Type/Group: keratolytic; acne treatment.
Brand(s): RA Lotion. Combinations: With *sulfur*: Acnotex Lotion; Acnomel Cream; Bensulfoid Cream; Sulforcin Lotion; Rezamid Lotion; R/S Lotion.
How administered: Topically (external).

Used to treat

Resorcinol, when applied topically, causes skin to peel and relieves itching. It is also used in ointments and lotions for the treatment of ○ **acne**.

Warnings

• It should not be given to people with known hypersensitivity to resorcinol products, or to any component of the preparations.

• Medical advice should be sought before using while pregnant or breast-feeding.

• It should not be used for a longer period or in larger amounts than directed.

• It should not be used over large areas of the body or on broken skin.

• Contact with the eyes must be avoided.

• Affected areas must not be bandaged.

Interactions

No interactions are known.

Side effects

• Rash and irritation.

• Less commonly, temporary dark brown scale on those with darker skin. Prolonged use can affect thyroid function.

Respa-DM Tablets ⑧

A preparation of ℞ **dextromethorphan** and ℞ **guaifenesin**.
Formulation: Oral tablets.
Availability: Prescription only.
Warnings and side effects: See ℞ **dextromethorphan**; ℞ **guaifenesin**.

Respa-GF Tablets ⑧

A preparation of ℞ **guaifenesin**.
Formulation: Oral tablets, sustained release.
Availability: Prescription only.
Warnings and side effects: See ℞ **guaifenesin**.

Respahist Capsules ⑧

A preparation of ℞ **pseudoephedrine** and ℞ **brompheniramine maleate**.
Formulation: Oral capsules, sustained release.
Availability: Prescription only.
Warnings and side effects: See ℞ **pseudoephedrine**; ℞ **brompheniramine maleate**.

Respaire 120 Capsules; 60 Capsules ⑧

A preparation of ℞ **pseudoephedrine** and ℞ **guaifenesin**.
Formulation: Oral capsules, extended release.
Availability: Prescription only.
Warnings and side effects: See ℞ **pseudoephedrine**; ℞ **guaifenesin**.

Respbid ⑧

A preparation of ℞ **theophylline**.
Formulation: Oral tablets, timed release, in several strengths.
Availability: Prescription only.
Warnings and side effects: See ℞ **theophylline**.

respiratory stimulant Ⓓ

(analeptic)

Generics: **caffeine; doxapram.**

Actions and uses

Respiratory stimulants (analeptics) are central nervous stimulants (see ℞ **CNS stimulant**) which show some degree of selectivity for respiratory stimulation. They have little current use but ℞ **doxapram** is sometimes used to relieve severe respiratory difficulties in people suffering from ✲ **chronic obstructive pulmonary disease** (COPD), or who undergo respiratory depression following major surgery or drug overdose, particularly in cases where ventilatory support is not possible. ℞ **Caffeine** has weak actions and is sometimes used to treat respiratory depressant drug overdose in adults, or ("off-label") for failure to breath properly in the newborne (neonatal apnea).

Limitations

A number of such agents were once used in ℞ **antidote** treatment in the event of overdose and poisoning by respiratory depressants, but have been discontinued because effective doses were close to those causing toxic effects, especially convulsions. Overdose with respiratory depressants, such as ℞ **benzodiazepine** drugs and ℞ **opioid** drugs, is now treated with specific receptor antagonists (see ℞ **antidote.**)

Restoril Ⓑ

A preparation of ℞ **temazepam.**

Formulation: Capsules in several strengths.

Availability: Prescription only.

Warnings and side effects: See ℞ **temazepam.**

Retavase Ⓑ

A preparation of ℞ **reteplase, recombinant.**

Formulation: Intravenous injection or infusion.

Availability: Prescription only.

Warnings and side effects: See ℞ **reteplase, recombinant.**

reteplase, recombinant Ⓖ

Type/Group: **fibrinolytic; thrombolytic.**

Brand(s): Retavase.

How administered: Intravenous injection, infusion.

Used to treat

Reteplase is a synthesized (recombinant DNA technology) type of enzyme with the property of breaking up blood clots. It is used as a ℞ **thrombolytic** in ✲ **myocardial infarction** (heart attack) to reduce the incidence of heart failure and improve survival.

Warnings

• It should not be given to people with active internal bleeding, uncontrolled high blood pressure, a history of stroke, or injury, surgery or bleeding involving the nervous system (brain or spine) within the previous two months. It will be administered by experienced personnel after a full medical assessment.

• It should be given with great caution to people with cerebrovascular disease, who have recently had major surgery, an injury or internal bleeding (for example, in the gastrointestinal tract, urinary tract), bacterial endocarditis or acute pericarditis,

indwelling catheters, high blood pressure, severe diabetes mellitus, significant liver or kidney impairment, or any condition (for example, taking anticoagulant drugs, low thrombocyte count) or disorder that would make bleeding more likely.

• It should be used during pregnancy only when it is clearly needed.

• Medical judgment is required if breast-feeding is being considered.

• Although reported rarely, fibrinolytics may free bits of plaque that may lodge (usually) in the smaller blood vessels. This may result in abrupt, sharp pain in a leg, foot, the toes, back, or flank. ("Purple toes syndrome" appears as mottled, purplish discoloration of the toes.) More serious obstructions are possible, which may cause kidney failure, pancreatitis, hypertension, heart attack, stroke and other serious obstructive events.

Interactions

• If used with ℞ **heparin**, there is an increased risk of bleeding, with potentially life-threatening adverse effects.

• Drugs that act against ᗑ **vitamin K** (for example, ℞ **warfarin**) increase the risk of bleeding.

• ℞ **abciximab**, ℞ **aspirin**, and ℞ **dipyridamole** may lower platelet activity and increase the risk of bleeding when used with reteplase.

Side effects

• The chief complication is hemorrhage (although major bleeding is not frequent), which may occur at virtually any site in the body.

• Other side effects may include slowed heart rate and other arrhythmias, shock, heart failure, fluid in the lungs or brain, or events associated with a new embolism. Mild allergic reaction has occurred.

Retin-A Ⓑ

A preparation of ℞ **tretinoin.**

Formulation: Topical gel; topical cream.

Availability: Prescription only.

Warnings and side effects: See ℞ **tretinoin.**

retinoid Ⓓ

Generics: **isotretinoin; tretinoin.**

Actions and uses

Retinoids are a group of chemical agents derived from vitamin A (retinol). They have a marked effect on the growth (differentiation) of the cells that make up the skin epithelium (surface tissues), and can be used to treat a number of ✲ **skin conditions.**

So-called "first-generation" retinoids are made up of ℞ **tretinoin** (the acid form of vitamin A), ℞ **isotretinoin** (which is a chemical isomer of ℞ **tretinoin**), and ℞ **adapalene** (another vitamin A derivative). The later "second-generation" retinoids are made up of ℞ **acitretin** (the main metabolite of etretinate, which was formerly used for similar purposes) and the recent drug ℞ **tazarotene.** Various members of the group are used in ℞ **skin preparations** for a number of conditions, notably ✲ **acne** and ✲ **psoriasis** (in ℞ **psoriasis treatment** for different forms of the condition), also for light-damaged skin, for other skin conditions including severe Darier's disease, and more recently, for the induction of remission in acute promyelocytic leukemia. The retinoids are mostly used by

Key to symbols: ✲ = Disorder Section ℞ = Drug Section ♣ = Herbal Section ᗑ = Supplement Section

topical (external) application, often for a period of weeks. However, in treating severe cases, ℞ **acitretin** and ℞ **isotretinoin** may be prescribed for oral use.

Limitations

Although the retinoids can be very effective in treating psoriasis and acne, they are not without disadvantages. Topical use may cause skin reactions, and acne may initially worsen. Signs of improvement may not be noticed until after 8 to 12 weeks. There may be photosensitization (abnormal sensitivity to light), and strong sun should be avoided. The oral members have an extensive range of side effects on the skin and other systems. They are not prescribed for people with a number of other conditions. The main adverse reaction is on the fetus because some of the drugs are teratogenic (they can cause abnormalities in the fetus) and come in the Food and Drug Administration's Pregnancy Category X, which means they should not be used during pregnancy (℞ **tazarotene** and ℞ **acitretin**). Women of childbearing potential are given counseling before ℞ **acitretin** is prescribed, and should use two reliable contraceptive means for three years after discontinuing acitretin. Alcohol worsens and prolongs the probability of serious effects on the fetus. This drug should not be used by nursing mothers.

Retrovir ⑧

A preparation of ℞ **zidovudine**.
Formulation: Oral capsules oral syrup; oral tablets; injection.
Availability: Prescription only.
Warnings and side effects: See ℞ **zidovudine**.

Reversol ⑧

A preparation of ℞ **edrophonium**.
Formulation: Injection.
Availability: Prescription only.
Warnings and side effects: See ℞ **edrophonium**.

ReVia ⑧

A preparation of ℞ **naltrexone hydrochloride**.
Formulation: Oral tablets.
Availability: Prescription only.
Warnings and side effects: See ℞ **naltrexone hydrochloride**.

Rexolate ⑧

A preparation of ℞ **sodium thiosalicylate**.
Formulation: Injection.
Availability: Prescription only.
Warnings and side effects: See ℞ **sodium thiosalicylate**.

Rezamid ⑧

A preparation of ℞ **sulfur** and ℞ **resorcinol**.
Formulation: Topical lotion.
Availability: OTC.
Warnings and side effects: See ℞ **sulfur**; ℞ **resorcinol**.

R-Gel ⑧

A preparation of ℞ **capsaicin**.
Formulation: Topical gel.

Availability: OTC.
Warnings and side effects: See ℞ **capsaicin**.

Rh₀(D) immune globulin (human) ⑥

(anti-D (Rh₀) immunoglobulin)
Type/Group: immune globulin.
Brand(s): BayRho-D Full Dose, Mini-Dose; HypRho-D, Mini-Dose; RhoGAM, MICRhoGAM; WinRho SDF.
How administered: Intramuscular injection; intravenous in the treatment of ITP.

Used to treat

Rh₀(D) immune globulin (human) is used to prevent rhesus-negative mothers from making antibodies against fetal rhesus-positive cells that may pass into the mother's circulation during childbirth, miscarriage or abortion, or certain procedures such as amniocentesis (and sometimes for prophylaxis) or in transfusion where rhesus-positive blood was administered to rhesus-negative women of child-bearing age. The result of this is to protect a future child from hemolytic (destruction of red blood cells) disease of the newborn. Rh₀ (D) immune globulin should be injected within a few days of birth, miscarriage, or abortion. The mini-dose versions of this immune globulin are considered effective for some but not all of these uses. (WinRho SDF may also be administered, by specialists, in the treatment of immune thrombocytopenic purpura, or ITP, a bleeding disorder caused by the presence of an unwanted antibody.)

Warnings

• It should not be given to people with known hypersensitivity to human globulins, or who are rhesus-positive, or rhesus-negative but previously sensitized to the rhesus factor.
• It should be given with caution to people with a known deficiency of the naturally occurring IgA immunoglobulin.
• Although no problems with its use during pregnancy are known, it should be used only when medically judged to be clearly needed.
• No adverse effects have been reported when this globulin is administered as intended in breast-feeding women.
• When in miscarriage, abortion, or ectopic pregnancy, and the rhesus-type of the fetus is unknown, it should be assumed positive and Rh₀(D) immune globulin administered to previously unsensitized, Rh₀(D)-negative women.
• Because this immune globulin is extracted from human blood, the possibility exists that it might contain virus or other disease agents. However, multiple screenings and filters (chemical and physical) are used in its preparation, and its potential to transmit infection is considered nearly nonexistent.
• After administration, people will be required to wait for some time to ensure that there is no serious reaction (such as anaphylaxis).

Interactions

• The immune response to live virus vaccines (for example, ℞ **MMR** vaccine) may not be satisfactory, and so a delay of three months is recommended after administering Rh₀(D).
• Caution is required if ℞ **anticoagulants** are being taken.

Side effects

• Most of the side effects are mild. There may be swelling, irritation or tenderness at the site of vaccination, headache, or slight fever.

Some destruction of red blood cells is possible, but temporary. Infrequently, achiness and lethargy.

Rhinall ®

A preparation of ℞ phenylephrine hydrochloride.
Formulation: Nasal spray; drops.
Availability: OTC.
Warnings and side effects: See ℞ phenylephrine hydrochloride.

Rhinatate Tablets ®

A preparation of phenylephrine tannate, chlorpheniramine tannate, and pyrilamine tannate.
Formulation: Oral tablets.
Availability: Prescription only.
Warnings and side effects: See ℞ phenylephrine hydrochloride; ℞ chlorpheniramine maleate; ℞ pyrilamine maleate.

Rhinocort ®

A preparation of ℞ budesonide.
Formulation: Nasal aerosol spray.
Availability: Prescription only.
Warnings and side effects: See ℞ budesonide.

Rhinosyn-DM Liquid ®

A preparation of ℞ dextromethorphan, ℞ chlorpheniramine maleate, and ℞ pseudoephedrine.
Formulation: Oral liquid.
Availability: OTC.
Warnings and side effects: See ℞ dextromethorphan; ℞ chlorpheniramine maleate; ℞ pseudoephedrine.

Rhinosyn DMX Syrup ®

A preparation of ℞ dextromethorphan and ℞ guaifenesin.
Formulation: Oral syrup.
Availability: OTC.
Warnings and side effects: See ℞ dextromethorphan; ℞ guaifenesin.

Rhinosyn-PD Liquid ®

A preparation of ℞ pseudoephedrine and ℞ chlorpheniramine maleate.
Formulation: Oral liquid.
Availability: OTC.
Warnings and side effects: See ℞ pseudoephedrine; ℞ chlorpheniramine maleate.

Rhinosyn-X Liquid ®

A preparation of ℞ dextromethorphan, ℞ pseudoephedrine, and ℞ guaifenesin.
Formulation: Oral liquid.
Availability: OTC.
Warnings and side effects: See ℞ dextromethorphan; ℞ pseudoephedrine; ℞ guaifenesin.

RhoGAM, MICRhoGam ®

A preparation of ℞ Rh_0(D) immune globulin (human).
Formulation: Intramuscular injection.
Availability: Prescription only.
Warnings and side effects: See ℞ Rh_0(D) immune globulin (human).

Rhuli Spray ®

A preparation of ℞ calamine and ℞ benzocaine.
Formulation: Topical spray.
Availability: OTC.
Warnings and side effects: See ℞ calamine; ℞ benzocaine.

Rhumatrex ®

A preparation of ℞ methotrexate.
Formulation: Oral tablets.
Availability: Prescription only.
Warnings and side effects: See ℞ methotrexate.

Rhythmol ®

A preparation of ℞ propafenone hydrochloride.
Formulation: Oral tablets (three strengths).
Availability: Prescription only.
Warnings and side effects: See ℞ propafenone hydrochloride.

ribavirin ⑥

(tribaverin)
Type/Group: **antiviral.**
Brand(s): Virazole. Combination: With *interferon alfa 2b*. Rebetron.
How administered: Orally or nasal inhalation.

Used to treat

Ribavirin inhibits a wide range of DNA and RNA viruses and can be used to treat severe lower respiratory tract infections caused by respiratory syncytial virus (RSV) in selected infants and children (see ⊕ **viral infections**). Although not stated by the manufacturer for such use, it is also used to treat ⊕ **influenza** and certain other serious diseases, including ⊕ **Lassa fever.**

Warnings

• It should not be given to people with known hypersensitivity to ribavirin.
• It should be given with caution to people using assisted ventilation.
• It should not be used during pregnancy (and getting pregnant while using this drug should be avoided) or while breast-feeding.
• Rarely, worsening of respiratory status may develop.
• Seizures may occur with systemic administration.

Interactions

• ℞ zidovudine may decrease the effects of ribavirin.

Side effects

• Occasionally, rash, eye infections, and blood disorders.
• Rarely, hypotension, respiratory problems, cardiac arrest, anemia, and digitalis toxicity.

RID ®

A preparation of ℞ pyrethrin.

Formulation: Topical liquid.
Availability: OTC.
Warnings and side effects: See ℞ **pyrethrin**.

Rid-a-Pain-HP Ⓑ

A preparation of ℞ **capsaicin**.
Formulation: Topical cream.
Availability: OTC.
Warnings and side effects: See ℞ **capsaicin**.

Ridaura Ⓑ

A preparation of ℞ **auranofin**.
Formulation: Oral capsules.
Availability: Prescription only.
Warnings and side effects: See ℞ **auranofin**.

Ridenol Elixir Ⓑ

A preparation of ℞ **acetaminophen**.
Formulation: Oral liquid.
Availability: OTC.
Warnings and side effects: See ℞ **acetaminophen**.

rifabutin Ⓖ

Type/Group: antibacterial; antibiotic.
Brand(s): Mycobutin.
How administered: Orally.

Used to treat

Rifabutin is a recently introduced member of the rifamycin family. It can be used for the prevention of Mycobacterium avium complex (MAC) infection in people with advanced ✪ **HIV** infection.

Warnings

• It should not be given to people with known hypersensitivity to rifamycins, or active tuberculosis.
• Rifabutin should be used during pregnancy only when it is clearly needed, and when the potential benefits outweigh the possible risks to the fetus.
• Medical judgment is required if breast-feeding is being considered. It is not known whether this drug appears in breast milk.
• It is associated with the occurrence of blood disorders, and monitoring may be necessary.
• It may cause discoloration of body secretions and soft contact lenses may be stained.

Interactions

• ℞ **acetaminophen** may increase the risk of liver damage.
• The effects of ℞ **cyclosporine**, delavirdine, ℞ **eprosartan**, difedipine, oral ℞ **hypoglycemics**, ℞ **propafenone**, protease inhibitors, ℞ **quinidine**, and ℞ **tacrolimus** may be reduced.
• If taken with ℞ **oral contraceptives**, there may be menstrual irregularities and contraception failure.

Side effects

• Frequently, skin rash, nausea, loss of appetite, discoloration of urine, feces, saliva, skin, sputum, sweat, or tears.
• Occasionally, muscle and joint pain, altered taste, eye disorders, and diarrhea.

• Rarely, vomiting, insomnia, hepatitis, and blood disorders.

Rifadin Ⓑ

A preparation of ℞ **rifampin**.
Formulation: Oral capsules in two strengths; injection.
Availability: Prescription only.
Warnings and side effects: See ℞ **rifampin**.

Rifamate Ⓑ

A preparation of ℞ **isoniazid** and ℞ **rifampin**.
Formulation: Oral capsules.
Availability: Prescription only.
Warnings and side effects: See ℞ **isoniazid**; ℞ **rifampin**.

rifampicin Ⓖ

see ℞ **rifampin**.

rifampin Ⓖ

(rifampicin)
Type/Group: antibacterial; antituberculosis; antibiotic.
Brand(s): Rifadin; Rimactane; various generic. Combinations: With *isoniazid*: Rifamate. With *pyrazinamide* and *isoniazid*: Rifater.
How administered: Orally; injection.

Used to treat

Rifampin is one of the main drugs used in the treatment of ✪ **tuberculosis**. It is used in combination with other antituberculosis drugs, such as ℞ **isoniazid** or ℞ **pyrazinamide**, in order to cover resistance and for maximum effect. It acts against *Mycobacterium tuberculosis* and sensitive Gram-positive bacteria by inhibiting the bacterial RNA polymerase enzyme. It is also effective in the treatment of ✪ **leprosy** (in combination with ℞ **dapsone**), ✪ **brucellosis**, ✪ **Legionnaires' disease**, and serious staphylococcal infections (see ✪ **bacterial infections**). Additionally, it may sometimes be used to prevent meningococcal ✪ **meningitis** and *Haemophilus influenzae* (type B) infection.

Warnings

• It should not be given to people with known hypersensitivity to rifamycins.
• It should be given with caution to people with liver dysfunction or porphyria.
• Rifampin should be used during pregnancy only when it is clearly needed, and when the potential benefits outweigh the possible risks to the fetus.
• Medical judgment is required if breast-feeding is being considered. It is usually considered compatible with breast-feeding.
• Jaundice may develop in people taking rifampin together with other agents that can cause liver damage.
• It may cause discoloration of body secretions and soft contact lenses may be stained.

Interactions

• There is an increased risk of liver damage if taken with ℞ **acetaminophen** or ℞ **isoniazid**.
• Anyone taking ℞ **oral contraceptives** may experience menstrual irregularities and contraceptive failure.
• ℞ **aminosalicylates** reduce the levels of rifampin.

• The effects of the following drugs may be reduced:
℞ **antidiabetics**; ℞ **azole** antifungals; ℞ **barbiturates**;
℞ **benzodiazepines**; ℞ **beta-blockers** (except ℞ **nadolol**);
℞ **calcium-channel blockers**; ℞ **chloramphenicol**; ℞ **clofibrate**;
℞ **corticosteroids**; ℞ **tricyclic** antidepressants; ℞ **cyclosporine**;
℞ **dapsone**; digitalis glycosides; ℞ **disopyramide**; lorcainide;
℞ **methadone**; ℞ **mexiletine**; ℞ **nortriptyline**; oral
℞ **anticoagulants**; ℞ **phenytoin**; pirmenol; ℞ **propafenone**;
protease inhibitors; ℞ **quinidine**; ℞ **tacrolimus**; ℞ **tocainide**;
℞ **theophylline**; and ℞ **zidovudine**.

Side effects
• Commonly, discoloration of urine, feces, saliva, skin, sputum,
sweat, and tears.
• Occasionally, allergic reaction, diarrhea, upset stomach, nausea,
fungal overgrowth, and flu-like symptoms.
• Rare but serious effects include liver damage, serious skin
disorders and blood disorders, and antibiotic-associated colitis.

Rifater ®
A preparation of ℞ **isoniazid**, ℞ **rifampin**, and ℞ **pyrazinamide**.
Formulation: Oral tablets.
Availability: Prescription only.
Warnings and side effects: See ℞ isoniazid; ℞ rifampin;
℞ pyrazinamide.

Rilutek ®
A preparation of ℞ **riluzole**.
Formulation: Oral tablets.
Availability: Prescription only.
Warnings and side effects: See ℞ riluzole.

riluzole ⒢
Type/Group: **brain-motor disorder treatment**.
Brand(s): Rilutek.
How administered: Orally.

Used to treat
Riluzole is used in the treatment of ✿ **amyotrophic lateral sclerosis** (ALS), also known as Lou Gehrig's disease.

Warnings
• It should not be given to people with known hypersensitivity to
riluzole or other ingredients.
• It should be given with caution to people with liver or kidney
function impairment, or anyone over 65. Japanese users should also
use caution as they may metabolize riluzole more slowly than
Caucasians (on whom the drug was initially tested).
• It is not known whether this drug can harm the fetus, and it should
be used during pregnancy only if the benefits outweigh the
possible risk to the fetus.
• It should not be used if breast-feeding.
• Treatment must not be stopped without consulting a doctor.
• Alcohol must be avoided.
• A doctor must be contacted if there is fever, chills or infection,
breathing difficulty, or shortness of breath.
• It may cause dizziness and so impair the performance of skilled
tasks such as driving.

Interactions
• Smoking and charcoal-broiled foods may reduce the effects of
riluzole.
• ℞ **allopurinol**, ℞ **methyldopa**, ℞ **sulfasalazine**,
℞ **barbiturates**, or ℞ **carbamazepine** may increase the risk of liver
damage.
• ℞ **amitriptyline**, ℞ **theophylline**, and ℞ **quinolones** may
increase the effects of riluzole.
• ℞ **rifampin** and ℞ **omeprazole** may reduce the effects of
riluzole.

Side effects
• Headache, nausea, vomiting, diarrhea, cough, dizziness,
drowsiness, loss of appetite, loss of balance from giddiness or
dizziness, stomach pain, tingling sensation around the mouth,
weakness, back pain, rhinitis, skin reactions, and blood-cell
disorders.

Rimactane ®
A preparation of ℞ **rifampin**.
Formulation: Oral capsules.
Availability: Prescription only.
Warnings and side effects: See ℞ rifampin.

rimantadine ⒢
Type/Group: **antiviral**.
Brand(s): Flumadine.
How administered: Orally.

Used to treat
Rimantadine is used to treat ✿ **influenza** A infections. It works by
inhibiting growth of the virus.

Warnings
• It should not be given to people with known hypersensitivity to
rimantadine.
• Rimantadine's safety during pregnancy has not been established,
and it should be used only if the potential benefits outweigh the
possible risks to the fetus.
• It should not be used while breast-feeding.
• Resistant strains may develop during treatment.

Interactions
• ℞ **triamterene** increases the levels of rimantadine.
• ℞ **trihexyphenidyl** increases central nervous system (CNS) side
effects.

Side effects
• Weakness, muscle aches, depression, dizziness, insomnia, tremor,
elevated blood pressure, gastrointestinal effects, bronchospasm,
cough, and rash.

rimexolone ⒢
Type/Group: **corticosteroid; anti-inflammatory; eye treatment**.
Brand(s): Vexol.
How administered: Topically (eye).

Used to treat
Rimexolone is used to suppress the symptoms of eye inflammation
(for example from ✿ **uveitis**, or after eye operations).

Warnings

• It should not be given to people with known hypersensitivity to this drug, with herpes simplex and certain other infections, most viral eye diseases, mycobacterial infections, or fungal infections.

• Rimexolone should be used during pregnancy only if it is clearly needed.

• Medical judgment is required if breast-feeding is being considered.

• Prolonged use may result in ocular (eye) hypertension, glaucoma, optic nerve damage, and other adverse effects.

Interactions

No interactions specific to this drug are known.

Side effects

• Blurred vision, discharge, discomfort, elevated intraocular pressure (pressure in the eyeball), foreign body sensation, hyperemia (excess of blood in an area of the body), ocular pain, posterior subcapsular cataract formation, itching, and secondary eye infection. Systemic effects are unlikely.

Rinade B.I.D. Capsules ⑧

A preparation of ℞ **pseudoephedrine** and ℞ **chlorpheniramine maleate**.
Formulation: Oral capsules, sustained release.
Availability: Prescription only.
Warnings and side effects: See ℞ **pseudoephedrine**; ℞ **chlorpheniramine maleate**.

Riopan Plus Tablets, Plus Suspension ⑧

Also: **Riopan Plus Double Strength Tablets**
A preparation of ℞ **magaldrate** and ℞ **simethicone**.
Formulation: Oral tablets, chewable; liquid.
Availability: OTC.
Warnings and side effects: See ℞ **magaldrate**; ℞ **simethicone**.

Risperdal ⑧

A preparation of ℞ **risperidone**.
Formulation: Oral tablets in several strengths; oral solution.
Availability: Prescription only.
Warnings and side effects: See ℞ **risperidone**.

risperidone ⑥

Type/Group: **antipsychotic**.
Brand(s): Risperdal.
How administered: Orally.

Used to treat

Risperidone is a recently introduced antipsychotic drug (one of a group sometimes termed "atypical" antipsychotics) and is used in the treatment of acute and chronic ✪ **psychotic disorders**.

Warnings

• It should not be given to people with known hypersensitivity to this drug.

• It should be given with caution to people with heart disease, cerebrovascular disease, electrolyte imbalance, slowed heart rate, severe kidney or liver impairment, history of seizures, or anyone at risk of developing aspiration pneumonia.

• Risperidone should be used during pregnancy only if the benefits outweigh the risk to the fetus.

• It should not be used by nursing mothers.

• It may cause drowsiness, and so the performance of skilled tasks, such as driving, may be impaired.

• It may cause postural hypotension (lowered blood pressure on standing), so rise slowly from a reclining position. Older people in particular should exercise caution.

• Avoid exposure to extreme heat, and take care to avoid dehydration.

• It may cause sensitivity to sunlight (photosensitivity), so minimize exposure (use sunscreen, sunglasses, and so on).

• If used for a long time, tardive dyskinesia (see ℞ **antipsychotics**) occasionally develops.

• Treatment should be stopped gradually.

• Avoid alcohol.

Interactions

• ℞ **carbamazepine**, ℞ **clozapine**, and ℞ **thioridazine** may reduce the effects of risperidone.

• ℞ **fluoxetine** may increase the effects of risperidone.

• The blood-pressure lowering effects of ℞ **antihypertensives** may be enhanced.

• The effects of ℞ **levodopa** and other dopamine agonists may be reduced by risperidone.

• If an antipsychotic is taken with alcohol, there may be increased sedative effects.

Side effects

• Anxiety, decreased libido, extrapyramidal symptoms (see ℞ **antipsychotics**), increased dream activity, abnormal sleepiness, dry mouth constipation, postural hypotension, indigestion, menstrual pain, frequent urination, sexual dysfunction, vaginal dryness, increased pigmentation. Less frequently, aggressive reaction, dizziness, insomnia, speeded heart rate, abnormal vision, abdominal pain, nausea, vomiting, urinary retention, anemia, irregular menstrual periods, breast changes; joint, back or chest pain; cough, shortness of breath, sore throat, sinus infection; skin reactions, fatigue, and fever.

• Rarely, neuroleptic malignant syndrome (a potentially fatal condition characterized by very high fever, muscle rigidity, changes in mental status, and irregular pulse, blood pressure and/or heart rhythm), seizure, and life-threatening cardiac arrhythmias.

Ritalin ⑧

A preparation of ℞ **methylphenidate**.
Formulation: Oral tablets, sustained release tablets (Ritalin SR).
Availability: Prescription only.
Warnings and side effects: See ℞ **methylphenidate**.

ritodrine hydrochloride ⑥

Type/Group: **beta-adrenergic stimulant; sympathomimetic; smooth muscle relaxant**.
Brand(s): Yutopar; various generic.
How administered: Injection.

Used to treat

Ritodrine is a drug that can be used to prevent or delay premature labor by acting as a smooth muscle relaxant for the walls of the uterus.

Warnings

• It should not be given to people with known cardiac arrhythmias, uncontrolled hypertension, bronchial asthma, hypovolemia, eclampsia, severe preeclampsia, hemorrhage, intrauterine fetal death, pulmonary hypertension, pheochromocytoma, hyperthyroidism, heart disease, chorioamnionitis, or uncontrolled diabetes mellitus.

• It should be given with caution to people with migraine headache or diabetes, or anyone using potassium-depleting diuretics.

• It is not used in the first 20 weeks of pregnancy. There is no evidence of adverse effects on the fetus when used for its therapeutic uses.

• Medical judgment is required if breast-feeding is being considered. It is not known if it appears in breast milk.

• It is a specialist drug and is used under controlled hospital conditions.

Interactions

• ℞ **Corticosteroids** increase the risk of pulmonary edema.

• There are antagonistic effects when used with ℞ **beta-blockers.**

• There are increased effects when used with ℞ **sympathomimetics.**

• The cardiovascular effects of ℞ **atropine**, ℞ **diazoxide**, ℞ **general anesthetics**, ℞ **magnesium sulfate**, and ℞ **meperidine** may be increased.

Side effects

• Frequently, increased mother and fetal heart rates, palpitations, nausea, vomiting, headache, and reddening of skin.

• Occasionally, tremors, jitteriness, chest pain or tightness, constipation, diarrhea, bloating, sweating, chills, and weakness. Newborns may occasionally have abnormal blood glucose levels, ileus, low calcium levels, and hypotension.

• Rarely, impaired liver function, ketoacidosis, anaphylactic shock, hepatitis, and serious pulmonary edema.

ritonavir ⓖ

Type/Group: **antiviral.**
Brand(s): Norvir. Combination: with *lopinavir*: Kaletra.
How administered: Orally.

Used to treat

Ritonavir is a protease inhibitor that is often used together with reverse transcriptase antivirals, and can be used in the treatment of progressive or advanced ✺ **HIV** infection.

Warnings

• It should not be given to people with known hypersensitivity to ritonavir.

• Its safety during pregnancy has not been established, and it should be used only when the potential benefits outweigh the possible risks to the fetus.

• HIV-infected mothers are advised not to breast-feed.

• Numerous serious body system effects and drug interactions may occur.

• It is a specialist drug, and there will be full assessment and patient monitoring throughout treatment.

• The effectiveness of ℞ **oral contraceptives** may be reduced by ritonavir.

Interactions

These are many and include:

• The levels and effects of the following drugs may be increased: ℞ **amiodarone**; ℞ **bepridil**; ℞ **bupropion**; ℞ **clorazepate**; ℞ **clozapine**; ℞ **desipramine**; ℞ **diazepam**; encainide; ℞ **ergot alkaloids**; ℞ **estazolam**; ℞ **flecainide**; ℞ **indinavir**; ℞ **ketoconazole**; ℞ **lovastatin**; ℞ **meperidine**; ℞ **midazolam**; ℞ **nelfinavir**; ℞ **pimozide**; ℞ **piroxicam**; ℞ **propafenone**; ℞ **propoxyphene**; ℞ **quinidine**; ℞ **saquinavir**; ℞ **simvastatin**; ℞ **triazolam**; and ℞ **zolpidem**.

• The levels of ℞ **barbiturates**, ℞ **carbamazepine**, ℞ **phenytoin**, and ℞ **rifabutin** are increased while the levels of ritonavir are reduced.

• If taken with ℞ **clarithromycin**, ℞ **erythromycin**, or troleandomycin, the levels of both drugs are increased.

• The effects of ℞ **methadone** and ℞ **theophylline** are reduced.

Side effects

These can be many and include:

• Frequently, gastrointestinal disturbances, neurologic disturbances (taste perversion, tingling and numbness in hands or feet or around mouth), headache, dizziness, fatigue, and weakness;

• Occasionally, allergic reactions, flu syndrome, skin reactions, lowered blood pressure, changes in kidney function, pancreatitis, and blood changes.

Rituxan ®

A preparation of ℞ **rituximab.**
Formulation: Injection (infusion).
Availability: Prescription only.
Warnings and side effects: See ℞ **rituximab.**

rituximab ⓖ

Type/Group: **cytotoxic; anticancer; immunosuppressant.**
Brand(s): Rituxan.
How administered: Intravenous infusion.

Used to treat

Rituximab is one of a relatively new class of drug, a monoclonal antibody (a form of pure antibody produced by a type of molecular engineering). In this case the cloned antibody is one that causes lysis (destruction) of B lymphocytes, so effectively it can be regarded as a specific cytotoxic agent with defined ℞ **immunosuppressant** actions. It is used to treat follicular non-Hodgkin's ✺ **lymphoma** that is resistant to chemotherapy or recurrent.

Warnings

• It should not be given to people with known hypersensitivity to this drug or to any product prepared with mouse protein.

• It should be given with caution to people with certain heart conditions. This is a specialist drug and is used only after a full medical assessment.

• The effects of rituximab in pregnancy are not known, but adverse effects on the fetus are thought possible. It should be used only if it is clearly needed. Women of childbearing potential should use effective contraception during treatment and for 12 months afterwards.

• Nursing mothers are advised not to breast-feed until levels of this drug are no longer detectable.

• Rituximab is used only in a hospital setting and under close supervision. Hypersensitivity reactions (including hypotension, bronchospasm, and allergic swelling) and serious heart disturbances have occurred. Potentially serious blood changes may occur, and blood monitoring at regular intervals is necessary.

• People receiving immunosuppressive treatment may have a greater risk of infection, although no higher risk is now associated with rituximab.

Interactions

No drug interactions of significance are known.

Side effects

• The infusion itself commonly causes fever and chills.

• Other frequent side effects may include nausea, hives, fatigue, headache, itching, bronchospasm, shortness of breath, swelling of the tongue or throat, rhinitis, vomiting, hypotension, and flushing.

rivastigmine ⑥

Type/Group: **dementia treatment; anticholinesterase**.
Brand(s): Exelon.
How administered: Orally.

Used to treat

Rivastigmine is used for the symptomatic treatment of mild to moderate dementia of ✪ **Alzheimer's disease**.

Warnings

• It should not be used by people with known hypersensitivity to rivastigmine or other carbonate derivatives.

• It should be given with caution to anyone with a history of asthma or obstructive lung disease, certain heart conditions, asthma, seizure disorders, bradycardia, hyperthyroidism, or a history of bladder outflow obstruction.

• It is not known whether or not rivastigmine can harm the fetus, therefore, it should be used during pregnancy only if medically judged to be essential.

• Medical judgment is also required if breast-feeding is being considered, as it is not known whether it is excreted in breast milk.

• Overdose can cause a cholinergic crisis, which is characterized by severe nausea, vomiting, salivation, sweating, bradycardia, hypotension, collapse, and convulsions.

• Drugs that increase cholinergic activity may have effects on heart rate.

• A relatively high incidence of nausea and vomiting are associated with the use of rivastigmine.

Interactions

• Rivastigmine may interfere with the activity of ℞ **anticholinergic** medications.

• ℞ **Parasympathomimetics** (for example, ℞ **bethanechol**) and other anticholinesterases (for example, distigmine bromide) may enhance rivastigmine's effects.

Side effects

• Nausea, vomiting, anorexia, and weight loss. Also, muscle weakness, weight, dizziness, drowsiness, agitation and confusion, insomnia, depression, headache, sweating, feeling of being unwell, and tremor.

• Rarely angina pectoris, gastrointestinal hemorrhage, fainting, and convulsions; there may also be bladder outflow obstruction.

rizatriptan benzoate ⑥

Type/Group: **serotonin-receptor stimulant; vasoconstrictor; antimigraine**.
How administered: Orally.
Brand(s): Maxalt; Maxalt-MLT.

Used to treat

This is a recently introduced drug which is used to treat acute ✪ **migraine** attacks (but not to prevent attacks). It works as a ℞ **vasoconstrictor** (through acting as a serotonin receptor stimulant selective for serotonin 5-HT$_1$ receptors), producing a rapid narrowing of blood vessels surrounding the brain. It is also used for ✪ **cluster headache**.

Warnings

• Avoid its use in people with known hypersensitivity to this drug, or who have certain cardiovascular disorders such as pre-existing heart diseases, including ischemic heart disease, previous myocardial infarction (heart attack), coronary vasospasm, including some types of angina, or with uncontrolled hypertension.

• Rizatriptan benzoate should not be used by anyone with a form of migraine in which one half of the body experiences some degree of paralysis during the migraine attack.

• Drugs of this class (that is, those stimulating serotonin 5-HT$_1$ receptors) are used only with great caution where risk factors are present that predispose to coronary artery disease.

• It is recommended that first-time administration of rizatriptan to anyone with significant risk factors for coronary artery disease takes place at a physician's office or other medical facility.

• They should be used with care in people with impaired liver or kidney function.

• Rizatriptan benzoate should be used in pregnancy only if the potential benefits outweigh the potential risks to the fetus.

• Medical judgment is also required if it is to be used by breast-feeding mothers.

• This drug should not be used at the same time, or shortly after, using ℞ **ergotamine** or other migraine therapies. Ergotamine-like antimigraine drugs should not be taken until 6 hours after this type of antimigraine drug; and this type of antimigraine drug should not be taken until at least 24 hours after an ergotamine-like antimigraine drug.

• The dose should not usually be repeated during the same migraine attack.

• Rizatriptan may cause drowsiness and so impair the performance of skilled tasks, such as driving.

Interactions

• There is a risk of additive effect, with potentially serious consequences, if taken with ℞ **ergotamine**-containing drugs (such as ℞ **dihydroergotamine** or ℞ **methysergide**).

• Rizatriptan should not be taken with ℞ **MAOI** antidepressants or within two weeks of discontinuing their use. MAOIs increase the concentration of rizatriptan, and so there is a higher risk of side effects (some serious).

• ℞ **SSRI** antidepressants (such as, ℞ **fluoxetine**, ℞ **fluvoxamine**, ℞ **paroxetine**, ℞ **sertraline**) may increase the risk of some less-frequent side effects, such as weakness and incoordination, occurring, and so caution is recommended.

• ℞ **propranolol hydrochloride** may increase the concentration of rizatriptan (whose dosage should be, accordingly, lower) and should not be taken within two hours of taking rizatriptan.

• ♣ **St. John's wort** should not be used at the same time, as there is an increased risk of adverse effects.

Side effects

• Chest pain and tightness in parts of the body, including the chest, jaw, or throat, which may indicate constriction of the blood vessels of the heart (or of anaphylaxis). If the pain is intense, use of rizatriptan should stop;

• The most common side effects are sensations of warmth or cold, flushing, hot flashes, palpitations, diarrhea, vomiting, tingling, mental slowness, euphoria, tremors, or difficulty breathing;

• Less frequently there may be dizziness, nervousness, confusion, insomnia, dry mouth, dehydration, thirst, a feeling of weakness, muscle cramps or pain, blurred vision, drowsiness and fatigue;

• Rarely, fainting, high blood pressure, light sensitivity, and allergy-like symptoms such as facial swelling, including the eyes, itching, rash, and sneezing.

RMS ⓑ

A preparation of ℞ **morphine sulfate**.
Formulation: Rectal suppositories, available in four strengths.
Availability: Prescription only.
Warnings and side effects: See ℞ **morphine sulfate**.

Robafen DAC Syrup ⓑ

A preparation of ℞ **codeine phosphate**, ℞ **guaifenesin**, and ℞ **pseudoephedrine**.
Formulation: Oral syrup.
Availability: May or may not require a prescription.
Warnings and side effects: See ℞ **codeine phosphate**; ℞ **guaifenesin**; ℞ **pseudoephedrine**.

Robafen DM Syrup ⓑ

A preparation of ℞ **dextromethorphan** and ℞ **guaifenesin**.
Formulation: Oral syrup.
Availability: OTC.
Warnings and side effects: See ℞ **dextromethorphan**; ℞ **guaifenesin**.

Robaxin ⓑ

A preparation of ℞ **methocarbamol**.
Formulation: Oral tablets; injection.
Availability: Prescription only.
Warnings and side effects: See ℞ **methocarbamol**.

Robaxisal ⓑ

A preparation of ℞ **methocarbamol** and ℞ **aspirin**.
Formulation: Oral tablets.
Availability: Prescription only.
Warnings and side effects: See ℞ **methocarbamol**; ℞ **aspirin**.

Robinul Tablets; Forte; Injection ⓑ

A preparation of ℞ **glycopyrrolate**.
Formulation: Oral tablets, available in two strengths; injection.
Availability: Prescription only.
Warnings and side effects: See ℞ **glycopyrrolate**.

Robitussin A-C Syrup ⓑ

A preparation of ℞ **codeine phosphate** and ℞ **guaifenesin**.
Formulation: Oral syrup.
Availability: May or may not require a prescription.
Warnings and side effects: See ℞ **codeine phosphate**; ℞ **guaifenesin**.

Robitussin Cold & Cough Liqui-Gels; Caplets ⓑ

A preparation of ℞ **dextromethorphan**, ℞ **pseudoephedrine**, and ℞ **guaifenesin**.
Formulation: Oral caplets; gel capsules; drops.
Availability: OTC.
Warnings and side effects: See ℞ **dextromethorphan**; ℞ **pseudoephedrine**; ℞ **guaifenesin**.

Robitussin Cough Calmers ⓑ

A preparation of ℞ **dextromethorphan**.
Formulation: Lozenges.
Availability: OTC.
Warnings and side effects: See ℞ **dextromethorphan**.

Robitussin Cough Drops; Liquid Center Cough Drops ⓑ

A preparation of ℞ **menthol** and eucalyptus oil.
Formulation: Lozenges.
Availability: OTC.
Warnings and side effects: See ℞ **menthol**.

Robitussin-DAC Syrup ⓑ

A preparation of ℞ **codeine phosphate**, ℞ **guaifenesin**, and ℞ **pseudoephedrine**.
Formulation: Oral syrup.
Availability: May or may not require a prescription.
Warnings and side effects: See ℞ **codeine phosphate**; ℞ **guaifenesin**; ℞ **pseudoephedrine**.

Robitussin-DM Liquid ⓑ

A preparation of ℞ **dextromethorphan** and ℞ **guaifenesin**.
Formulation: Oral liquid; drops.
Availability: OTC.
Warnings and side effects: See ℞ **dextromethorphan**; ℞ **guaifenesin**.

Robitussin Honey Cough ®

A preparation of ℞ **menthol**.
Formulation: Lozenges.
Availability: OTC.
Warnings and side effects: See ℞ **menthol**.

Robitussin Maximum Strength Cough & Cold Liquid ®

A preparation of ℞ **dextromethorphan** and ℞ **pseudoephedrine**.
Formulation: Oral liquid; pediatric liquid is half-strength.
Availability: OTC.
Warnings and side effects: See ℞ **dextromethorphan**; ℞ **pseudoephedrine**.

Robitussin Night Relief Liquid ®

A preparation of ℞ **dextromethorphan**, ℞ **acetaminophen**, ℞ **pseudoephedrine**, and ℞ **pyrilamine maleate**.
Formulation: Oral liquid.
Availability: OTC.
Warnings and side effects: See ℞ **dextromethorphan**; ℞ **acetaminophen**; ℞ **pseudoephedrine**; ℞ **pyrilamine maleate**.

Robitussin Pediatric ®

A preparation of ℞ **dextromethorphan**.
Formulation: Oral liquid.
Availability: OTC.
Warnings and side effects: See ℞ **dextromethorphan**.

Robitussin PE Syrup; Severe Congestion Liqui-Gels ®

A preparation of ℞ **pseudoephedrine** and ℞ **guaifenesin**.
Formulation: Oral syrup; capsules.
Availability: OTC.
Warnings and side effects: See ℞ **pseudoephedrine**; ℞ **guaifenesin**.

Rocaltrol ®

A preparation of ℞ **calcitriol**.
Formulation: Oral capsules; oral solution.
Availability: Prescription only.
Warnings and side effects: See ℞ **calcitriol**.

Rocephin ®

A preparation of ℞ **ceftriaxone**.
Formulation: Injection.
Availability: Prescription only.
Warnings and side effects: See ℞ **ceftriaxone**.

rocuronium bromide Ⓖ

Type/Group: skeletal muscle relaxant.
Brand(s): Zenuron.
How administered: Injection.

Used to treat

Rocuronium bromide is used to induce muscle paralysis during inpatient or outpatient surgery.

Warnings

• It should not be used by people with known hypersensitivity to rocuronium.
• It should be given with caution to people with certain heart and neuromuscular diseases, or with kidney, liver, or lung disorders.
• This drug is for administration only by trained personnel in hospitals, and individuals will be fully assessed for suitability prior to use.
• It should be used during pregnancy only if the benefits outweigh the risks to the fetus.
• Medical judgment is required if breast-feeding is being considered.

Interactions

This drug is for administration only by trained personnel in hospitals, and an individual's current and future therapy regimes will be fully assessed in order to avoid potential drug interactions.

Side effects

• Occasionally, transient blood pressure changes.
• Rarely, heart rhythm abnormalities, rash, edema, itching, and spasm of the bronchi.

rofecoxib Ⓖ

Type/Group: anti-inflammatory; antirheumatic; non-narcotic analgesic; NSAID.
Brand(s): Vioxx Tablets, Oral Suspension; various generic.
How administered: Orally.

Used to treat

Rofecoxib is used to treat pain and inflammation in ✪ osteoarthritis, acute pain in adults (for example, after dental procedures), and period pain.

Warnings

• It should not be used by people with known hypersensitivity to this drug or to other NSAIDs (including ℞ **aspirin**), who have chronic kidney disease, certain bleeding disorders or conditions (for example, hemophilia, vitamin K deficiency, low blood-platelet levels), or who have a tendency to, or active, peptic ulceration.
• It should be given with caution to people with peripheral edema, congestive heart failure, high blood pressure, or allergic disorders (especially asthma and skin conditions), who are elderly, or with any kind of kidney impairment, certain liver disorders, or who are dehydrated.
• Rofecoxib should be used when pregnant only if medically judged that it is needed. In the third trimester, however, its risks to the fetus rise, and so it should only be used if the benefits outweigh the risks to the fetus, which are at their highest during this time.
• Breast-feeding mothers should either discontinue this drug or stop breast-feeding.
• With regular, long-term use (as in the treatment of osteoarthritis), NSAIDs may cause gastrointestinal bleeding, ulceration, or perforation. Any signs of bleeding (for example, black stools) should be reported to a physician immediately.

• Most NSAIDs have the potential, particularly with regular use, to cause liver damage. Periodic evaluation of liver function is necessary in long-term therapy (more than two months).
• Side effects are more frequent in the elderly.
• Gastrointestinal upsets may be minimized by taking the drug with milk or food.

Interactions

• There is generally no added benefit in taking other NSAIDs (especially ℞ **diflunisal**) or other ℞ **salicylates** (especially aspirin) at the same time, but there is a higher risk of gastrointestinal upsets and bleeding.
• Alcohol and ℞ **corticosteroids** increase the risk of bleeding, particularly if there is an existing ulcer.
• ℞ **Anticoagulant** drugs (for example, ℞ **warfarin sodium**) should be used with caution because they may increase bleeding time.
• The effectiveness of ℞ **ACE inhibitors** and ℞ **diuretics** may be reduced.
• ℞ **Rifampin** may increase the concentration of rofecoxib.
• The effects of ℞ **cyclosporine**, ℞ **lithium**, and ℞ **methotrexate** may be exaggerated, with potential for toxicity.

Side effects

These vary in severity and how often they occur.
• Commonly, diarrhea, heartburn, nausea, gastrointestinal upsets, high blood pressure, swelling of the extremities, and dehydration.
• Less frequently, vomiting, constipation, flatulence, headache, ringing in the ears, nervousness, and insomnia.
• Prolonged bleeding time (with consequent risk of ulceration) is possible with high dosage, and other blood changes can occur, including anemia.
• Hypersensitivity reactions may include symptoms such as hives, rash, chest tightness, asthma, or bronchospasm.
• Reversible kidney failure, particularly in renal impairment, has occurred. Liver damage is rare.

Roferon-A ®

A preparation of ℞ **interferon** alfa-2a.
Formulation: Injection.
Availability: Prescription only.
Warnings and side effects: See ℞ **interferons**.

Rogaine; Rogaine Extra Strength for Men ®

A preparation of ℞ **minoxidil**.
Formulation: Topical solution, available in two strengths.
Availability: Prescription only.
Warnings and side effects: See ℞ **minoxidil**.

Rolatuss Plain Liquid ®

A preparation of ℞ **phenylephrine hydrochloride** and ℞ **chlorpheniramine maleate**.
Formulation: Oral liquid.
Availability: OTC.
Warnings and side effects: See ℞ **phenylephrine hydrochloride**; ℞ **chlorpheniramine maleate**.

Romazicon ®

A preparation of ℞ **flumazenil**.
Formulation: Injection.
Availability: Prescription only.
Warnings and side effects: See ℞ **flumazenil**.

Romilar AC ®

A preparation of ℞ **codeine phosphate** and ℞ **guaifenesin**.
Formulation: Oral liquid; it contains the sweetener aspartame (with phenylalanine), which should be avoided by individuals with phenylketonuria.
Availability: May or may not require a prescription.
Warnings and side effects: See ℞ **codeine phosphate**; ℞ **guaifenesin**.

Rondamine-DM Drops ®

A preparation of ℞ **dextromethorphan**, ℞ **carbinoxamine maleate**, and ℞ **pseudoephedrine**.
Formulation: Oral drops (pediatric strength).
Availability: Prescription only.
Warnings and side effects: See ℞ **dextromethorphan**; ℞ **carbinoxamine maleate**; ℞ **pseudoephedrine**.

Rondec Chewable Tablets ®

A preparation of ℞ **pseudoephedrine** and ℞ **brompheniramine maleate**.
Formulation: Oral tablets, chewable.
Availability: Prescription only.
Warnings and side effects: See ℞ **pseudoephedrine**. ℞ **brompheniramine maleate**. Tablets contain the sweetener aspartame (with phenylalanine), which should be avoided by individuals with phenylketonuria.

Rondec-DM Syrup; Drops ®

A preparation of ℞ **dextromethorphan**, ℞ **carbinoxamine maleate**, and ℞ **pseudoephedrine**.
Formulation: Oral syrup; drops are pediatric, lower strength.
Availability: Prescription only.
Warnings and side effects: See ℞ **dextromethorphan**; ℞ **carbinoxamine maleate**; ℞ **pseudoephedrine**.

Rondec Tablets; TR Tablets; Syrup; Oral Drops ®

A preparation of ℞ **pseudoephedrine** and ℞ **carbinoxamine maleate**.
Formulation: Oral tablets; TR tablets, sustained release; syrup; liquid (drops).
Availability: Prescription only.
Warnings and side effects: See ℞ **pseudoephedrine**; ℞ **carbinoxamine maleate**.

ropinirole ⓖ

Type/Group: dopamine-receptor stimulant; antiparkinsonism.
Brand(s): ReQuip.
How administered: Orally.

Key to symbols: ✪ = Disorder Section ℞ = Drug Section ♣ = Herbal Section ⬡ = Supplement Section

Used to treat

Ropinirole is a recently introduced treatment for ⊙ **Parkinson's disease** that works by stimulating the ℞ **dopamine** receptors in the brain (that is, it is a dopamine-receptor stimulant). It reduces the signs and symptoms of the disease.

Warnings

• It should not be used in people with sensitivity to ropinirole.

• It should be used with caution by those with cardiovascular disease or severe liver or kidney disease.

• Ropinirole should be used during pregnancy only if the potential benefits outweigh the possible risks to the fetus.

• It should not be used by breast-feeding mothers, as it inhibits milk production.

• Fainting, sometimes associated with slowed heart rate, has been observed, particularly in those who are not using ℞ **levodopa**.

• It may impair regulation of blood pressure and cause postural hypotension (lowered blood pressure on standing), especially at the beginning of treatment.

• Hallucinations may occur, particularly in those over 65 years of age.

• End treatment by tapering off over one week to avoid adverse effects (such as, fever, muscle rigidity, altered consciousness) associated with an abrupt reduction in dopamine-enhancing drugs.

Interactions

• ℞ **ciprofloxacin**, ℞ **enoxacin**, and pefloxacin increase ropinirole concentrations.

• Its effects are diminished by dopamine antagonists (for example, ℞ **phenothiazines**; butyrophenones; thioxanthenes; ℞ **metoclopramide**).

• Its effects are enhanced by ℞ **estrogens**.

Side effects

• Commonly, nausea, dizziness, and drowsiness.

• Frequently, fatigue, pain, vomiting, upset stomach, and edema.

• Occasionally, increased sweating, weakness, postural hypotension (lowered blood pressure on standing), sore throat, abdominal discomfort, dry mouth, hypertension, confusion, and urinary tract infections.

ropivacaine hydrochloride ⒢

Type/Group: **local anesthetic**.
Brand(s): Naropin.
How administered: Local injection.

Used to treat

Ropivacaine is used for nerve block and infiltration during surgery, and for postoperative pain management, particularly for obstetrical procedures, including delivery by caesarian section.

Warnings

• It should not be given to people with known hypersensitivity to ropivacaine, or those rare patients with methemoglobinemia (a serious blood disorder). It is a specialist drug and there will be a full medical assessment.

• It should be used during pregnancy only when it is clearly needed.

• Medical judgment is required if breast-feeding is being considered.

• It can cause cardiac depression, peripheral vasodilatation, or CNS (central nervous system) toxicity.

Interactions

• There is a risk of additive toxicity with ℞ **antiarrhythmics** (for example, ℞ **tocainide**, ℞ **mexiletine**).

• ℞ **Sedatives** may increase CNS effects.

Side effects

• Occasionally, pain at injection site, burning, stinging, or tenderness where applied.

• Rarely (generally with high dose), drowsiness, dizziness, disorientation, lightheadedness, tremors, apprehension, euphoria, sensation of heat, cold, or numbness, blurred or double vision, ringing or roaring in ears, nausea, or allergic reactions.

rose bengal ⒢

Type/Group: **diagnostic agent**.
Brand(s): Rosets.
How administered: Topically (eye).

Used to treat

Rose bengal is a dye used for diagnostic procedures in the eye (for example, to detect foreign bodies).

Warnings

• It should not be given to people with known hypersensitivity to rose bengal or any components of the formulation.

• It may harm soft contact lenses. Flush eyes and wait at least one hour after using rose bengal before replacing lens.

Interactions

No interactions specific to this drug are known.

Side effects

• The solution may be irritating, but is otherwise safe in normal use.

Rosets Ⓑ

A preparation of ℞ **rose bengal**.
Formulation: Ophthalmic strips.
Availability: Prescription only.
Warnings and side effects: See ℞ **rose bengal**.

rosiglitazone maleate ⒢

Type/Group: **antidiabetic; oral hypoglycemic**.
Brand(s): Avandia.
How administered: Orally.

Used to treat

Rosiglitazone, a non-sulfonylurea (it is a thiazolidinedione), is used in combination with other drugs to improve blood sugar control in type 2 ⊙ **diabetes mellitus**.

Warnings

• It should not be given to people with known sensitivity to rosiglitazone.

• Its safety in pregnancy is not established. It should be used only if clearly needed.

• It is not recommended for use while breast-feeding.

• Premenopausal women who have not been ovulating (for example, those with polycystic ovary disease, or taking the contraceptive pill) may resume ovulation and be at risk for pregnancy.

• There is a possibility this drug may cause liver damage (monitoring of liver function will be carried out). Any symptoms such as nausea, abdominal pain, fatigue, appetite loss, dark urine, or jaundice must be reported to a doctor.

• A doctor must be consulted before taking any other medication, including OTCs, herbal remedies, and supplements, as there is a potential for interaction with rosiglitazone.

Interactions

• ℞ **ketoconazole** may increase the effects of rosiglitazone.

• The effects of ℞ **estrogens** and ℞ **oral contraceptives** are reduced.

• The levels of ℞ **cyclosporine** may be reduced.

Side effects

• Headache, upper respiratory tract infection, and fatigue.

Rowasa ⓑ

A preparation of ℞ **mesalamine**.

Formulation: Rectal suppositories; rectal suspension.

Availability: Prescription only.

Warnings and side effects: See ℞ **mesalamine**. Suspension contains potassium metabisulfite. Sulfites may cause severe allergic reaction (including anaphylaxis) in those with hypersensitivity.

Roxanol ⓑ

A preparation of ℞ **morphine sulfate**.

Formulation: Oral liquid (drops), available in 4 strengths.

Availability: Prescription only.

Warnings and side effects: See ℞ **morphine sulfate**.

Roxicet Tablets; 5/500 Caplets; Oral Solution ⓑ

A preparation of ℞ **oxycodone** and ℞ **acetaminophen**.

Formulation: Oral tablets; liquid.

Availability: Prescription only.

Warnings and side effects: See ℞ **oxycodone**; ℞ **acetaminophen**.

Roxicodone ⓑ

A preparation of ℞ **oxycodone**.

Formulation: Oral tablets; liquid.

Availability: Prescription only.

Warnings and side effects: See ℞ **oxycodone**.

Roxicodone Intensol ⓑ

A preparation of ℞ **oxycodone**.

Formulation: Oral liquid (drops, concentrated).

Availability: Prescription only.

Warnings and side effects: See ℞ **oxycodone**.

Roxiprin ⓑ

A preparation of ℞ **oxycodone** and ℞ **aspirin**.

Formulation: Oral tablets.

Availability: Prescription only.

Warnings and side effects: See ℞ **oxycodone**; ℞ **aspirin**.

R/S Lotion ⓑ

A preparation of ℞ **sulfur** and ℞ **resorcinol**.

Formulation: Topical lotion.

Availability: OTC.

Warnings and side effects: See ℞ **sulfur**; ℞ **resorcinol**.

R-Tannamine Tablets; Pediatric Suspension ⓑ

A preparation of phenylephrine tannate and chlorpheniramine tannate and pyrilamine tannate.

Formulation: Oral tablets; liquid.

Availability: Prescription only.

Warnings and side effects: See ℞ **phenylephrine hydrochloride**; ℞ **chlorpheniramine maleate**; ℞ **pyrilamine maleate**.

R-Tannate Tablets; Pediatric Suspension ⓑ

A preparation of phenylephrine tannate and chlorpheniramine tannate and pyrilamine tannate.

Formulation: Oral tablets; liquid.

Availability: Prescription only.

Warnings and side effects: See ℞ **phenylephrine hydrochloride**; ℞ **chlorpheniramine maleate**; ℞ **pyrilamine maleate**.

rt-PA ⓖ

see ℞ **alteplase, recombinant**.

rubella vaccine, live ⓖ

Type/Group: vaccine.

Brand(s): Meruvax II.

How administered: Subcutaneous injection.

Used to treat

Rubella vaccine, live is used in immunization to give active immunity against ✪ **rubella** (German measles). It is medically recommended for (not previously immunized) medical staff who, as potential carriers, might put pregnant women at risk from infection and also for women of child-bearing age, because German measles during pregnancy constitutes a serious risk to the fetus. As a precaution, vaccination should not take place if the patient is pregnant or likely to become pregnant within the following three months. The vaccine is prepared as a freeze-dried suspension of live, but attenuated (weakened), viruses grown in cell cultures. Universal childhood vaccination, which provides a combined vaccine for mumps, measles, and rubella (℞ **MMR vaccine**), has meant that rubella vaccination treatment alone is likely to become obsolete.

Warnings

• It should not be given to people with known hypersensitivity to this vaccine or to neomycin (used in its preparation), or who have impaired immune response for any reason (for example, illness, immunosuppressive therapy, hereditary disorder).

• This vaccine should not be used during pregnancy. Women should be advised to avoid pregnancy within the three months following vaccination.

Key to symbols: ✪ = Disorder Section ℞ = Drug Section ♣ = Herbal Section ◊◊ = Supplement Section

• Medical judgment is required if breast-feeding is being considered. The vaccine virus appears in breast milk, although there are no reports of significant effects in newborns.

• MMR vaccine is the preferred immunization for most children and many adults.

• After administration, people will be required to wait for some time to ensure that there is no serious reaction (such as anaphylaxis).

Interactions

• ℞ **Meningococcal polysaccharide vaccine** may decrease immune response to rubella vaccine in the event of concurrent immunization.

• ℞ **Immune globulins**, ℞ **immunosuppressants** (for example, ℞ **corticosteroids**), and ℞ **interferon** may reduce the effectiveness of the vaccine in conferring immunity. Delaying vaccination until three months after discontinuing use of these immune agents is recommended.

• Caution is required if ℞ **anticoagulants** are being taken.

• The response to ℞ **tuberculin** skin test may be depressed and inaccurate.

Side effects

• Most of the side effects are mild. Moderate fever may occur during the month following vaccination. There may be swelling, irritation or tenderness at the site of vaccination, and headache, sore throat, rash, fatigue, malaise, or achiness.

• Arthritic side effects are more common in adults receiving this vaccination.

• Anaphylactic reactions have occurred.

Rubesol-1000 Ⓑ

A preparation of ℞ **cyanocobalamin**.
Formulation: Injection.
Availability: Prescription only.
Warnings and side effects: See ℞ **cyanocobalamin**.

Rubex Ⓑ

A preparation of ℞ **doxorubicin hydrochloride**.
Formulation: Powder for injection.
Availability: Prescription only.
Warnings and side effects: See ℞ **doxorubicin hydrochloride**.

Rubinul; Rubinul Forte Ⓑ

A preparation of ℞ **glycopyrrolate**.
Formulation: Oral tablets in two strengths; injection.
Availability: Prescription only.
Warnings and side effects: See ℞ **glycopyrrolate**.

Rulox #1 Tablets; #2 Tablets; Suspenion Ⓑ

A preparation of ℞ **aluminum hydroxide** and ℞ **magnesium hydroxide**.
Formulation: Oral tablets, chewable; liquid.
Availability: OTC.
Warnings and side effects: See ℞ **aluminum hydroxide**; ℞ **magnesium hydroxide**.

Rulox Plus Tablets; Suspension Ⓑ

A preparation of ℞ **aluminum hydroxide**, ℞ **magnesium hydroxide**, and ℞ **simethicone**.
Formulation: Oral tablets, chewable; liquid.
Availability: OTC.
Warnings and side effects: See ℞ **aluminum hydroxide**; ℞ **magnesium hydroxide**; ℞ **simethicone**.

Ru-Tuss; Ru-Tuss DE Tablets Ⓑ

A preparation of ℞ **pseudoephedrine** and ℞ **guaifenesin**.
Formulation: Oral tablets, long acting.
Availability: Prescription only.
Warnings and side effects: See ℞ **pseudoephedrine**; ℞ **guaifenesin**.

Ru-Tuss Expectorant Liquid Ⓑ

A preparation of ℞ **dextromethorphan**, ℞ **pseudoephedrine**, and ℞ **guaifenesin**.
Formulation: Oral liquid.
Availability: OTC.
Warnings and side effects: See ℞ **dextromethorphan**; ℞ **pseudoephedrine**; ℞ **guaifenesin**.

Ru-Tuss Liquid Ⓑ

A preparation of ℞ **phenylephrine hydrochloride** and ℞ **chlorpheniramine maleate**.
Formulation: Oral liquid.
Availability: OTC.
Warnings and side effects: See ℞ **phenylephrine hydrochloride**; ℞ **chlorpheniramine maleate**.

Rymed Capsules; Liquid Ⓑ

A preparation of ℞ **pseudoephedrine** and ℞ **guaifenesin**.
Formulation: Oral capsules; liquid.
Availability: Capsules, prescription only; Liquid, OTC.
Warnings and side effects: See ℞ **pseudoephedrine**; ℞ **guaifenesin**.

Ryna-12 S Ⓑ

A preparation of phenylephrine tannate and pyrilamine tannate.
Formulation: Oral liquid.
Availability: Prescription only.
Warnings and side effects: See ℞ **phenylephrine hydrochloride**; ℞ **pyrilamine maleate**.

Ryna-C Liquid Ⓑ

A preparation of ℞ **codeine phosphate**, ℞ **pseudoephedrine**, and ℞ **chlorpheniramine maleate**.
Formulation: Oral liquid.
Availability: May or may not require a prescription.
Warnings and side effects: See ℞ **codeine phosphate**; ℞ **pseudoephedrine**; ℞ **chlorpheniramine maleate**.

Ryna-CX Liquid ⓑ

A preparation of ℞ **codeine phosphate**, ℞ **guaifenesin**, and ℞ **pseudoephedrine**.
Formulation: Oral liquid.
Availability: May or may not require a prescription.
Warnings and side effects: See ℞ **codeine phosphate**; ℞ **guaifenesin**; ℞ **pseudoephedrine**.

Ryna Liquid ⓑ

A preparation of ℞ **pseudoephedrine** and ℞ **chlorpheniramine** maleate.
Formulation: Oral liquid.
Availability: OTC.
Warnings and side effects: See ℞ **pseudoephedrine**; ℞ **chlorpheniramine maleate**.

Rynatan Pediatric Suspension ⓑ

A preparation of phenylephrine tannate, chlorpheniramine tannate, and pyrilamine tannate.
Formulation: Oral liquid.
Availability: Prescription only.
Warnings and side effects: See ℞ **phenylephrine hydrochloride**; ℞ **chlorpheniramine maleate**; ℞ **pyrilamine maleate**.

Rynatan Tablets ⓑ

A preparation of pseudoephedrine sulfate and ℞ **azatadine** maleate.
Formulation: Oral tablets.
Availability: Prescription only.
Warnings and side effects: See ℞ **pseudoephedrine**; ℞ **azatadine maleate**.

S-2 ⓑ

A preparation of racepinephrine.
Formulation: Solution for inhalation.
Availability: OTC.
Warnings and side effects: See ℞ **epinephrine**.

Sabin vaccine ⓖ

see ℞ poliovirus vaccine.

Safe Tussin 30 Liquid ⓑ

A preparation of ℞ **dextromethorphan** and ℞ **guaifenesin**.
Formulation: Oral liquid.
Availability: OTC.
Warnings and side effects: See ℞ **dextromethorphan**; ℞ **guaifenesin**.

Saizen ⓑ

A preparation of ℞ **somatropin**.
Formulation: Injection.
Availability: Prescription only.
Warnings and side effects: See ℞ **somatropin**.

Salactic Film ⓑ

A preparation of ℞ **salicylic acid**.
Formulation: Topical liquid.
Availability: OTC.
Warnings and side effects: See ℞ **salicylic acid**.

Salagen ⓑ

A preparation of ℞ **pilocarpine**.
Formulation: Oral tablets.
Availability: Prescription only.
Warnings and side effects: See ℞ **pilocarpine**.

salbutamol ⓖ

see ℞ albuterol.

salcatonin ⓖ

see ℞ calcitonin-salmon.

Saleto Tablets ⓑ

A preparation of ℞ **acetaminophen**, ℞ **aspirin**, ℞ **caffeine**, and ℞ **salicylamide**.
Formulation: Oral tablets.
Availability: OTC.
Warnings and side effects: See ℞ **acetaminophen**; ℞ **aspirin**; ℞ **caffeine**; ℞ **salicylamide**.

Salflex Tablets ⓑ

A preparation of ℞ **salsalate**.
Formulation: Oral tablets.
Availability: Prescription only.
Warnings and side effects: See ℞ **salsalate**.

salicylamide ⓖ

Type/Group: **non-narcotic analgesic**.
Brand(s): Combinations: With *acetaminophen, caffeine*: Saleto-D. With *acetaminophen, aspirin, caffeine*: Saleto Tablets. With *acetaminophen, phenyltoloxamine*: FemBack Caplets; Lobac. With *aspirin, caffeine*: BC Powder Original Formula, Arthritis Strength.
How administered: Orally.
Used to treat
Although quite similar to them, salicylamide is not considered a true ℞ **salicylate** (because it is not a free salicylate), and has only week anti-inflammatory effect. It is used to relieve minor aches and pains, usually in combination with other common drugs, such as ℞ **aspirin**, ℞ **acetaminophen**, and ℞ **antihistamines**.
Warnings
• It should not be used by people with hypersensitivity to this drug.
• It should be given with caution to people who have bleeding disorders or conditions (for example, hemophilia, vitamin K deficiency, low platelet levels), or who have a tendency to, or active, peptic ulceration; and in those taking certain drugs for gout or diabetes mellitus, in the elderly, children or teenagers (see Warnings below), or anyone with any kind of kidney impairment or with certain liver disorders.

• The effects of salicylamide in pregnancy have not been established, although it is considered sensible to avoid this drug in pregnancy or if breast-feeding because of its chemical similarity to the salicylates.

• Because of a link between salicylates and the rare, but serious, condition called ✪ **Reye's syndrome** (which causes inflammation of the brain and liver), it is prudent not to give salicylamide to children or teenagers who have, or might have, chickenpox or influenza. As so many infections resemble flu in their initial symptoms, salicylates should not, as a general rule, be used to treat fever, ache, and malaise by anyone in this age group except on the advice of a doctor.

• If dizziness, change in hearing, or ringing in the ears (tinnitus) occurs, stop using this drug. These are usually the first symptoms of overdose.

Interactions

• If salicylamide is taken with aspirin or acetaminophen, the levels of all the drugs may rise.

Side effects

These vary in severity and in the frequency with which they occur, and resemble the side effects of salicylates, except that salicylamide is not likely to cause gastrointestinal bleeding.

• The most common are nausea, vomiting, heartburn, loss of appetite, headache, and diarrhea. (Any gastrointestinal side effects may be minimized by taking the drug with milk or food.)

• Infrequently, there may be flushing, hyperventilation, sweating, rash, and dry mouth.

• At high doses there may be dizziness, ringing in the ears, and effects on the blood and its clotting ability (for example, unexplained bruising); such symptoms should be reported to the doctor.

salicylate Ⓓ

Generics: aspirin; sodium salicylate; diflunisal; methyl salicylate; choline salicylate; magnesium salicylate; sodium thiosalicylate; mesalamine; olsalazine sodium; sulfasalazine; balsalazide disodium; salicylic acid; salicylamide.

Actions and uses

Salicylate agents are a chemical class of drugs that include ℞ **aspirin** and are chemically related to salicylic acid, which is a simple, single-ringed, organic molecule that occurs naturally as a component of salicin (a glycoside found in ♣ **willow** bark) and methyl salicylate (in oil of wintergreen). These natural products have been known for centuries to have antirheumatic actions, which derives from an inherent ℞ **anti-inflammatory** activity. Both the two natural medicines are irritant and poisonous if taken by mouth and the salt ℞ **sodium salicylate** is rather irritant if administered orally. However, in 1899, the semi-synthetic drug the ester acetylsalicylic acid, was introduced under the name Aspirin as an ℞ **analgesic**, ℞ **antipyretic** and ℞ **antirheumatic** drug. Today, aspirin is still widely used as a generic drug to treat pain, fever and inflammation, and has been joined by a number of other salicylate drugs with similar actions and uses as ℞ **non-narcotic analgesic** agents, for example, the salicylate-derivatives ℞ **diflunisal** and ℞ **salsalate**.

Today they are referred to as non-steroidal anti-inflammatory drugs (℞ **NSAID**).

Some salicylate preparations can be used topically, including the traditional use of oil of wintergreen (which contains ℞ **methyl salicylate**) as a topically applied treatment for muscle and joint aches and pains. Some other salicylate derivatives, mainly used orally, include ℞ **choline salicylate** and ℞ **magnesium salicylate**. ℞ **sodium thiosalicylate** is used by injection for gout and rheumatic fever. Though quite similar to them, the derivative ℞ **salicylamide** is not considered a true salicylate, but is used as a weak analgesic.

Further uses of salicylates include the ℞ **aminosalicylate** compounds (containing a 5-aminosalicylic acid component) which are used to treat active Crohn's disease and to induce and maintain remission of the symptoms of ulcerative colitis, and are also sometimes used to treat rheumatoid arthritis. Drugs in this group include ℞ **mesalamine**, ℞ **olsalazine sodium**, ℞ **sulfasalazine**, and ℞ **balsalazide disodium**, which contain or form 5-aminosalicylic acid (and a ℞ **sulphonamide**).

In strong solution, ℞ **salicylic acid** is the standard, classic ℞ **keratolytic** agent, which can be used in the treatment of various skin conditions.

Limitations

Salicylates cause hypersensitivity reaction in some people, allergic-like symptoms including bronchospasm in "aspirin-sensitive" asthmatics.

It is quite easy to overdose on aspirin and similar drugs because salicylates accumulate in the bloodstream, especially in fever and sweating. In relation to salicylates overdose, it should be noted that some foodstuffs contain salicylates (more than 6mg/100g in curry powder, paprika, licorice, prunes, raisins, tea, gherkins; and a typical American diet contains 1-200 mg/day salicylate. Many herbal preparations contain salicylates so do not use these together with orthodox salicylates.

Because of a link between aspirin and the rare, but serious, condition called Reye's syndrome (which causes inflammation of the brain and liver), aspirin should not be given to children or teenagers who have, or might have, chickenpox or flu. As so many infections resemble flu in their initial symptoms, aspirin should not, as a general rule, be used to treat fever, ache and malaise by anyone in this age group except on advice of a doctor.

In addition to its anti-inflammatory actions, aspirin, but not other salicylates to any appreciable extent, inhibits platelet aggregation, which allows its prophylactic (preventive) use, at a low dose, as an ℞ **antiplatelet** treatment in those at risk (such as those who have already suffered a heart attack or following bypass surgery, as part of anti-angina treatment). However, this same action may also increase bleeding time, so those taking ℞ **anticoagulant** drugs should avoid aspirin.

salicylic acid Ⓖ

Type/Group: keratolytic; NSAID; acne treatment; antiseborrheic; psoriasis treatment; salicylate.
Brand(s): (Acne treatment): Clearasil Maximum Strength, Clearstick Regular Strength, Double Clear Pads Regular Strength;

Finac Lotion; Fostex Acne Cleansing Cream; PROPApH Cleansing Pads, Acne Maximum Strength Cream; Oxy Night Watch Maximum Strength Lotion, Sensitive Skin Lotion; Sebasorb Lotion. (Keratolytic agents): Compound W Liquid, Gel; Dr Scholl's Wart Remover Kit, Corn/Callus Remover, Clear Away Disks, Clear Away Strips; DuoFilm Liquid, Transdermal Patch; DuoPlant Gel; Fostex Cream; Freezone; Gordofilm; Keralyt; Mediplast; MG217 Sal-Acid Ointment; Mosco Liquid; Occlusal-HP; Off-Ezy Wart Remover Kit; Panscol Lotion, Ointment; Salactic Film; Sal-Plant; Trans-Ver-Sal PlantarPatch, PediaPatch, AdultPatch; Wart-Off. (Shampoos): Ionil Plus, Ionil T; Meted Maximum Strength; MG217 Medicated Tar-Free Shampoo, MG400; Neutrogena T/Sal; P & S; Scalpicin; Sebex; Sulfoam; Tarsum; X-Seb, Plus, X-Seb T, T Plus. (Soaps and cleansers): Aveeno Cleansing for Acne-Prone Skin; Clearasil Medicated Deep Cleanser, Acne Fighting Pads, Double Textured Pads; Drytex Lotion; Exact; Fostex Acne Medication Cleansing Bar; Ionax Astringent Cleanser; Neutrogena Oil-free Acne Wash; Oxy Medicated Cleanser and Pads; Pernox Scrub for Oily Skin; PROPApH Cleansing for Sensitive Skin, Maximum Strength, Foaming Face Wash; PROPApH Peel-off Acne Mask; Stri-Dex Pads Regular Strength, Maximum Strength.
How administered: Topically (external).

Used to treat
Salicylic acid can be applied to the skin to remove corns, calluses, and ✪ **warts**. In some preparations, at lower concentrations, it is used to treat ✪ **dandruff**, ✪ **seborrhea**, ✪ **acne**, and ✪ **psoriasis**.

Warnings
• It should not be used by people with known hypersensitivity to this drug or to other salicylates (including ℞ **aspirin**), who have irritated or infected skin, or whose circulation is impaired.
• Used topically as directed, there are no effects in pregnancy or breast-feeding.
• If signs of over-sensitivity occur (for example, redness of the skin, rash or blisters), discontinue use.
• Avoid contact with the eyes, mucous membranes, or broken skin.

Interactions
• There is an increased risk of skin irritation and inflammation if used with other acne medications (see ℞ **acne treatment**).

Side effects
• Prolonged or excessive use may cause dryness of the skin or scalp, and occasionally patches of thick, hardened skin.

SalineX   ℞
A preparation of ℞ **sodium chloride**.
Formulation: Nose drops; nasal mist.
Availability: OTC.
Warnings and side effects: See ℞ **sodium chloride**.

Salk vaccine   ⓖ
see ℞ **poliovirus vaccine**.

salmeterol   ⓖ
Type/Group: **beta-adrenergic stimulant; antiasthmatic; sympathomimetic**.
Brand(s): Severent.

How administered: Infusion.

Used to treat
Salmeterol is mainly used in the maintenance of bronchodilation and prevention of symptoms of ✪ **asthma**. It is similar to ℞ **albuterol** but has a much longer duration of action. Therefore it may be used to prevent asthma attacks throughout the night after inhalation before going to bed and also for long-duration prevention of exercise-induced bronchospasm. It is also used in the maintenance treatment of bronchospasm associated with chronic ✪ **bronchitis** and ✪ **emphysema** (COPD).

Warnings
• It should not be given to people with significant worsening or acutely deteriorating asthma, or acute symptoms.
• It should be given with caution to people with heart and circulatory disorders, hypertension, convulsive disorders, thyrotoxicosis (a disease of hyperthyroidism), psychosis, diabetes mellitus, or a history of stroke, and also children under the age of 12.
• It should be used in pregnancy only if clearly needed.
• Medical judgment is required if breast-feeding is being considered. It is not known if it appears in breast milk.
• Rarely, it may have adverse effects on heart and blood pressure, or lead to paradoxical bronchoconstriction.
• It must not be used to treat acute symptoms.

Interactions
• ℞ **Beta-blockers** decrease the effects of salmeterol.
• If used with ℞ **furosemide**, there is a risk of enhancing furosemide's potassium-lowering effect.

Side effects
• Frequently, headache.
• Occasionally, cough, tremor, dizziness, vertigo, throat dryness, irritation, and inflammation.
• Rarely, palpitations, speeded heartbeat, shakiness, nausea, heartburn, and gastrointestinal distress.

Salmonine   ℞
A preparation of ℞ **calcitonin-salmon**.
Formulation: Injection.
Availability: Prescription only.
Warnings and side effects: See ℞ **calcitonin-salmon**.

Sal-Plant   ℞
A preparation of ℞ **salicylic acid**.
Formulation: Topical gel.
Availability: OTC.
Warnings and side effects: See ℞ **salicylic acid**.

salsalate   ⓖ
Type/Group: **antipyretic; anti-inflammatory; antirheumatic; non-narcotic analgesic**.
Brand(s): Amigesic Tablets, Caplets, Capsules; Argesic-SA Tablets; Arth-G Tablets; Disalcid Tablets, Capsules; Marthritic Tablets; Mono-Gesic Tablets; Salflex Tablets; Salsitab; various generic.
How administered: Orally.

Used to treat

Salsalate has much the same effect as ℞ **aspirin**, although usually with less marked gastrointestinal side effects. It is used to relieve mild to moderate pain, and in the treatment of ✪ **rheumatoid arthritis**, ✪ **osteoarthritis**, and other rheumatic disorders. This and other ℞ **salicylates** do not have aspirin's level of ℞ **antiplatelet** activity, and so should not be used instead of aspirin when aspirin's preventive ℞ **antithrombotic** effects are required.

Warnings

• It should not be used by people with known hypersensitivity to this drug or to other salicylates (including aspirin), who have chronic kidney disease, certain bleeding disorders or conditions (for example, hemophilia, vitamin K deficiency, low platelet levels), or who have a tendency to, or active, peptic ulceration.

• It should be given with caution to people taking certain drugs for gout or diabetes mellitus, or with allergic disorders (especially asthma and skin conditions), in the elderly, children or teenagers (see Warnings below), in those with any kind of kidney impairment, or with certain liver disorders.

• Salicylates can adversely affect the health both of a pregnant woman and the fetus. They should not be used during pregnancy, and especially not in the third trimester, when risk to the fetus is at its highest.

• Breast-feeding mothers should either discontinue this drug or stop breast-feeding.

• Because of a link between salicylates and the rare, but serious, condition called ✪ **Reye's syndrome** (which causes inflammation of the brain and liver), salicylates should not be given to children or teenagers who have, or might have, chickenpox or influenza. As so many infections resemble flu in their initial symptoms, salicylates should not, as a general rule, be used to treat fever, ache, and malaise by anyone in this age group except on the advice of a doctor.

• Excessive use in babies for teething upsets has resulted in poisoning.

• If dizziness, change in hearing, or ringing in the ears (tinnitus) occurs, stop using this drug. These are usually the first symptoms of overdose.

• Salicylates can produce the same allergic-like symptoms (including bronchospasm) that may occur after taking NSAIDs, including bronchospasm in "aspirin-sensitive" asthmatics.

• If salsalate is taken with foods that are high in salicylates, such as curry powder, gherkins, licorice, paprika, prunes, raisins, and tea, this may increase the risk of side effects.

Interactions

• ℞ **Anticoagulants** have an additive effect in prolonging bleeding time.

• There is generally no benefit in taking salsalate with other NSAIDs or other salicylates, but there is a higher risk of gastrointestinal upsets and bleeding.

• Alcohol increases the risk of bleeding, particularly of an existing ulcer.

• ℞ **Antacids**, ℞ **corticosteroids**, ℞ **urinary alkalinizers**, and ℞ **activated charcoal** may lower the absorption or therapeutic effect of salsalate.

• ℞ **Carbonic-anhydrase inhibitors** (for example, ℞ **acetazolamide**) increase the risk of overdose symptoms for both salsalate and these drugs.

• The effects of the following drugs may be exaggerated: ℞ **phenytoin**; ℞ **nitroglycerin**; ℞ **valproate sodium** (and other valproic acid derivatives); ℞ **methotrexate**.

• Salsalate taken with ℞ **insulin** or ℞ **sulfonylureas** may cause a greater glucose-lowering effect.

• The therapeutic effects of the following drugs may be reduced: ℞ **angiotensin-receptor blockers**; ℞ **beta-blockers**; loop ℞ **diuretics**; ℞ **spironolactone**.

• ℞ **Uricosuric** agents (used in the treatment of gout, for example, phenylbutazone, ℞ **probenecid**, and ℞ **sulfinpyrazone**) may lose their effectiveness.

• There is a risk of accidental overdose and toxic effects if salsalate is taken with OTC medications containing salicylates in some form (for example, some ℞ **antacids**).

• Foods high in salicylates, such as curry powder, gherkins, licorice, paprika, prunes, raisins, and tea, may increase the risk of side effects.

Side effects

These vary in severity and in the frequency with which they occur.

• The most common are gastrointestinal upsets, nausea, heartburn, diarrhea, and prolonged bleeding time (with consequent risk of ulceration). (The gastrointestinal upsets may be minimized by taking the drug with milk or food.)

• There may be hypersensitivity reactions, including hives, rash, bronchospasm, edema, headache, blood disorders, ringing in the ears, dizziness, and fluid retention.

• Reversible kidney failure, particularly in renal impairment, has occurred. Liver damage is rare.

Salsitab ®

A preparation of ℞ **salsalate**.
Formulation: Oral tablets.
Availability: Prescription only.
Warnings and side effects: See ℞ **salsalate**.

Sal-Tropine ®

A preparation of ℞ **atropine sulfate**.
Formulation: Oral tablets.
Availability: Prescription only.
Warnings and side effects: See ℞ **atropine sulfate**.

Salutensin; Salutensin-Demi ®

A preparation of ℞ **hydroflumethiazide** and ℞ **reserpine**.
Formulation: Oral tablets, two (hydroflumethiazide) strengths.
Availability: Prescription only.
Warnings and side effects: See ℞ **hydroflumethiazide**; ℞ **reserpine**.

Sandimmune ®

A preparation of ℞ **cyclosporine**.
Formulation: Oral gelcaps; oral liquid; injection (infusion).
Availability: Prescription only.

Warnings and side effects: See ℞ **cyclosporine**.

Sandoglobulin ⑧

A preparation of ℞ **immune globulin, human (IG)**.
Formulation: Intravenous infusion, supplied as a powder.
Availability: Prescription only.
Warnings and side effects: See ℞ **immune globulin, human (IG)**.

Sandostatin; Sandostatin LAR Depot ⑧

A preparation of ℞ **octreotide**.
Formulation: Injection; LAR Depot is a long-acting form.
Availability: Prescription only.
Warnings and side effects: See ℞ **octreotide**.

SangCya ⑧

A preparation of ℞ **cyclosporine**.
Formulation: Oral liquid.
Availability: Prescription only.
Warnings and side effects: See ℞ **cyclosporine**.

Sani-Supp ⑧

A preparation of ℞ **glycerin**.
Formulation: Rectal suppositories.
Availability: OTC.
Warnings and side effects: See ℞ **glycerin**.

Sansert ⑧

A preparation of ℞ **methysergide**.
Formulation: Oral tablets.
Availability: Prescription only.
Warnings and side effects: See ℞ **methysergide**. These tablets contain the dye tartrazine (FD&C yellow No 5), which may cause allergic reactions in some people, especially those with a sensitivity to aspirin.

saquinavir ⑥

Type/Group: **antiviral**.
Brand(s): Fortovase; Invirase.
How administered: Orally.
Used to treat
Saquinavir is a protease inhibitor which is often used together with reverse transcriptase antivirals in the treatment of progressive or advanced ⊕ **HIV** infection.
Warnings
• It should not be given to people with known, significant hypersensitivity to saquinavir.
• It should be given with caution to people with impaired liver function.
• It should be used during pregnancy only when it is clearly needed and when the potential benefits outweigh the possible risks to the fetus.
• HIV-infected women are advised not to breast-feed.
• It may cause dizziness and so skilled tasks, such as driving, should be avoided until response to the drug is known.

• The effectivness of ℞ **oral contraceptives** may be reduced.
• It is a specialist drug, and there will be full assessment and patient monitoring throughout treatment.
Interactions
• Grapefruit juice may reduce levels of saquinavir.
• The levels of ℞ **barbiturates** or ℞ **carbamazepine** are increased while the levels of saquinavir are decreased.
• If taken with ℞ **clarithromycin**, the levels of both drugs are increased.
• Delavirdine, ℞ **indinavir**, ℞ **lovastatin**, ℞ **nelfinavir**, ℞ **ritonavir**, and ℞ **simvastatin** increase the levels of saquinavir.
• ℞ **Dexamethasone**, ℞ **efavirenz**, ℞ **rifabutin**, and ℞ **rifampin** reduce the levels of saquinavir.
• The levels of ℞ **ergot alkaloids**, ℞ **midazolam**, ℞ **triazolam**, astemizole, and cisapride are increased, and so is the risk of serious adverse effects.
• If taken with ℞ **erythromycin** or ℞ **phenytoin**, the levels of both drugs are reduced.
Side effects
• Nausea, diarrhea, abdominal pain, mouth ulceration, loss of appetite, headache, rash or skin eruptions, dizziness, muscle weakness and paresthesia, changes in kidney function, blood changes, and a number of other effects.

Sarafem ⑧

A preparation of ℞ **fluoxetine**.
Formulation: Oral pulvules.
Availability: Prescription only.
Warnings and side effects: See ℞ **fluoxetine**. This drug contains the same active ingredient as Prozac. The two should not be taken at the same time.

Saratoga ⑧

A preparation of ℞ **zinc oxide**.
Formulation: Topical ointment.
Availability: Prescription only.
Warnings and side effects: See ℞ **zinc oxide**.

sargramostim ⑥

Type/Group: **hematopoietic**.
Brand(s): Leukine.
How administered: Injection or infusion.
Used to treat
Sargramostim is a name given to "granulocyte macrophage-colony stimulating factor (GM-CSF)," a natural blood-stimulating substance that, when for therapeutic use, is synthesized using DNA engineering techniques. It reduces neutropenia (a shortage of neutrophil white blood-cells in the circulation) by stimulating white cell production (all granulocytes and monocytes) when this has been reduced during chemotherapy in cancer treatment, and this may alleviate several adverse effects of chemotherapy and radiotherapy, including liver and kidney damage, and risk of infection or sepsis. It has investigational drug status for a number of other purposes.

Key to symbols: ⊕ = Disorder Section ℞ = Drug Section ♣ = Herbal Section ♑ = Supplement Section

Warnings

• It should not be given to people with known hypersensitivity to this drug or to yeast-derived products, or when levels of certain white cells (associated with leukemia) are too high.

• It should be given with caution to people with heart or lung disease, liver or kidney impairment, or fluid retention. This is a specialist drug and is used only after a full medical assessment.

• It should be used during pregnancy only when it is clearly needed.

• Medical judgment is required if breast-feeding is being considered.

• Sargramostim is used only under qualified medical supervision, with frequent monitoring of blood values, and kidney and liver function.

Interactions

• ℞ **Corticosteroids**, ℞ **lithium** and any other drugs that might intensify the potential of sargramostim for stimulating production of white cells should be used with caution.

Side effects

These may include:

• Flu-like syndrome (with fever, chills, malaise), headache, muscle and bone pain, weight loss, rash or itching, and edema (which may include fluid build-up in the pleural and pericardial spaces).

SASTid Soap ⑧

A preparation of ℞ **sulfur**.
Formulation: Soap.
Availability: OTC.
Warnings and side effects: See ℞ **sulfur**.

scabicidal ⑩

see ℞ **scabicide and pediculicide**.

scabicide ⑩

see ℞ **scabicide and pediculicide**.

scabicide and pediculicide ⑩

(pediculicidal; pediculicide; scabicidal; scabicide)
Generics: **crotamiton; lindane; malathion; permethrin; pyrethrin**.

Actions and uses

Scabicidals are drugs used to kill the mites that cause ✪ **scabies**, which is an infestation by the itch mite *Sarcoptes scabiei*. The female mite tunnels into the top surface of the skin in order to lay her eggs, causing severe irritation as she does so. Newly hatched mites, also causing irritation with their secretions, then pass easily from person to person on direct contact. Treatment is usually with local application of a cream containing ℞ **permethrin** or if this is not effective, ℞ **lindane**. To treat the itching ℞ **crotamiton** may be used (it is also a weak scabicidal).

Pediculicidal drugs are used to kill lice of the genus *Pediculus*, which infest either the body or the scalp, or both, and cause intense itching. Scratching tends to damage the skin surface and may eventually cause weeping lesions with bacterial infection as well. Widely used pediculicides include the pyrethroids ℞ **permethrin** and ℞ **pyrethrin**, and also ℞ **malathion**. They are used topically (externally), usually as a lotion, and contact between the drug and the skin should be as long as possible and repeated regularly. Sometimes which drug is used will depend on the development of resistant strains of lice.

Limitations

None of these drugs is without side effects, and experimentation may be needed to find a preparation that is the least irritant. They must not be applied to broken skin because they will enter the body and risk systemic toxicity. Malathion, an organophosphate anticholinesterase, has the potential for relatively serious toxic actions but normally is rapidly deactivated in the mammalian body. It should be used with caution, however, by people with asthma or eczema (especially preparations containing alcohol). Lindane is known to penetrate the skin and has the potential for causing toxic central nervous system (CNS) effects if not used according to instructions (oils may enhance absorption). See also the individual drug entries.

Scalpicin ⑧

A preparation of ℞ **salicylic acid**.
Formulation: Shampoo.
Availability: OTC.
Warnings and side effects: See ℞ **salicylic acid**.

Schamberg's ⑧

A preparation of ℞ **zinc oxide**.
Formulation: Topical ointment.
Availability: Prescription only.
Warnings and side effects: See ℞ **zinc oxide**.

sclerosing agent ⑩

Generics: **ethanolamine oleate; sodium tetradecyl sulphate**.

Actions and uses

Sclerosing agent solutions are used in sclerotherapy, and contain an irritant that causes inflammation and resulting fibrosis in a tissue. It can be used by injection in cauterizing ✪ **ulcers**, ✪ **varicose veins**, arresting hemorrhages, treatment of varices (enlarged, tortuous knots of blood vessels) in the esophagus that have recently bled, and treating hemangioiomas (a mass of blood vessels forming a benign tumor).

Limitations

See the individual drug entries.

Scopace ⑧

A preparation of ℞ **scopolamine hydrobromide**.
Formulation: Oral tablets.
Availability: Prescription only.
Warnings and side effects: See ℞ **scopolamine hydrobromide**.

Scope ⑧

A preparation of ℞ **cetylpyridinium chloride**.
Formulation: Mouthwash.
Availability: OTC.
Warnings and side effects: See ℞ **cetylpyridinium chloride**.

scopolamine hydrobromide ⒢

(hyoscine hydrobromide)

Type/Group: **anticholinergic; sedatives; antiemetic; belladonna alkaloid**.

Brand(s): Isopto Hyoscine; Scopace; Transderm Scop; various generic. Combinations: With *phenobarbital, hyoscyamine* and *atropine sulfate*: Barbidonna Tablets; Donnatal Capsules, Elixir, Extentabs, Tablets Hyosophen Elixir, Tablets. With *chlorpheniramine maleate* and *phenylephrine*: AH-chew Tablets; D.A. II Tablets, Chew Tabs; Dallergy Tablets, Syrup; Ex-Histine Syrup; Extendryl Chewable Tablets, Jr. Capsules, Syrup. With *pseudoephedrine*: AlleRx Day; AlleRx Night (has *chlorpheniramine maleate*); Mescolor Tablets.

How administered: Transdermal patches (absorbed through the skin); injection.

Used to treat

Scopolamine is an effective sedative which also has antinausea properties, and can be used to prevent ✪ **motion sickness**, and to prevent and treat vertigo and nausea associated with ✪ **Ménière's disease** and middle-ear surgery. In a solution, it can be used in ophthalmic treatments to paralyze the muscles of the pupil either for surgery or to rest the eye following surgery. It is used as a premedication prior to surgery because of its antiemetic, sedative, secretion-drying, and amnesia-causing properties. Scopolamine is a ℞ **belladonna alkaloid** derived from plants of the belladonna family.

Warnings

• It should not be given to people with known hypersensitivity to this drug, with myasthenia gravis, obstruction of the gastrointestinal or urinary tracts, porphyria, or narrow-angle glaucoma.

• It should be given with caution to children and the elderly, and with extreme caution to those who have urinary retention, cardiovascular disorders, or liver or kidney impairment, asthma, chronic obstructive pulmonary disease (COPD), Down's syndrome, or hiatal hernia. Additionally, the ℞ **anticholinergic** effects of scopolamine may worsen and prolong any intestinal infection.

• Scopolamine should be used during pregnancy only if it is clearly needed.

• Medical judgment is required if breast-feeding is being considered. As a general rule, nursing mothers should not use this drug.

• Because it has sedative properties, the performance of skilled tasks, such as driving, may be impaired.

• In hot weather heat prostration is more likely in those who are taking any anticholinergic drug, including scopolamine.

• Treatment should not be stopped abruptly, but tapered off over a week, otherwise withdrawal effects, such as dizziness, nausea, vomiting, or headache, may occur.

Interactions

• ℞ **amantadine**, ℞ **antihistamines**, ℞ **anticholinergics**, and ℞ **tricyclic** antidepressants may increase scopolamine's side effects.

• The effects of ℞ **atenolol** and ℞ **digoxin** may be intensified.

• Scopolamine may lessen the antipsychotic effects of ℞ **phenothiazines**.

Side effects

• Depending on the dose, how it is administered, and use, there may be drowsiness, dry mouth, dizziness, constipation, blurred vision, and difficulty in urination.

• In doses used for premedication and obstetrics it may cause confusion, hallucinations, behavioral disturbances, amnesia, ataxia, and occasionally excitement and slowing of the heartbeat (especially in the elderly).

Scot-Tussin Allergy DM ⓑ

A preparation of ℞ **diphenhydramine hydrochloride**.
Formulation: Oral liquid.
Availability: OTC.
Warnings and side effects: See ℞ **diphenhydramine hydrochloride**.

Scot-Tussin DM Cough Chasers ⓑ

A preparation of ℞ **dextromethorphan**.
Formulation: Lozenges.
Availability: OTC.
Warnings and side effects: See ℞ **dextromethorphan**.

Scot-Tussin DM Liquid ⓑ

A preparation of ℞ **dextromethorphan** and ℞ **chlorpheniramine maleate**.
Formulation: Oral liquid.
Availability: OTC.
Warnings and side effects: See ℞ **dextromethorphan**; ℞ **chlorpheniramine maleate**.

Scot-Tussin Expectorant Syrup ⓑ

A preparation of ℞ **guaifenesin**.
Formulation: Oral syrup.
Availability: OTC.
Warnings and side effects: See ℞ **guaifenesin**. It contains phenylalanine, which should be avoided by individuals with phenylketonuria.

Scot-Tussin Senior Clear Liquid ⓑ

A preparation of ℞ **dextromethorphan** and ℞ **guaifenesin**.
Formulation: Oral liquid.
Availability: OTC.
Warnings and side effects: See ℞ **dextromethorphan**; ℞ **guaifenesin**.

Seale's Lotion Modified ⓑ

A preparation of ℞ **sulfur**.
Formulation: Topical lotion.
Availability: OTC.
Warnings and side effects: See ℞ **sulfur**.

Seba-Nil Cleansing Mask ⓑ

A preparation of alcohol and ℞ **castor oil**.

Formulation: Topical liquid.
Availability: OTC.
Warnings and side effects: See ℞ **castor oil.**

Sebasorb Lotion ⑧

A preparation of ℞ **salicylic acid** and various.
Formulation: Topical liquid.
Availability: OTC.
Warnings and side effects: See ℞ **salicylic acid.**

Sebex ⑧

A preparation of ℞ **salicylic acid** and ℞ **sulfur.**
Formulation: Shampoo.
Availability: OTC.
Warnings and side effects: See ℞ **salicylic acid;** ℞ **sulfur.**

Sebizon ⑧

A preparation of ℞ **sulfacetamide.**
Formulation: Topical lotion.
Availability: Prescription only.
Warnings and side effects: See ℞ **sulfacetamide.**

secobarbital sodium ⑥

Type/Group: hypnotic; sedatives; barbiturate.
Brand(s): Seconal; various generic. Combinations: With
amobarbital: Tuinal.
How administered: Orally.

Used to treat

Secobarbital sodium has a rapid onset of action and is used to treat
severe and difficult to treat ✪ **insomnia.** It is also used as a preanes-
thetic medication. Although not stated by the manufacturer for
such use, it may be prescribed as an ℞ **antiepileptic** for severe episodes in specialized epilepsy centers, for acute ✪ **tetanus** convulsions, and for acute psychotic agitation.

Warnings

• It should not be given to people with known hypersensitivity to
barbiturates, respiratory depression, severe liver impairment, or
porphyria.
• It should be given with caution to people with anemia, addiction
to barbiturates, liver disease, chronic obstructive pulmonary
disease (COPD), emphysema, kidney disease, high blood pressure,
acute or chronic pain, mental depression, a history of drug abuse,
or anyone over 65.
• Secobarbital should be avoided during pregnancy if possible. A
doctor must be contacted if pregnancy occurs while using this
drug.
• Medical judgment is required if breast-feeding is being
considered.
• There is a high risk of dependence (addiction) and abuse.
• It loses some of its effectiveness for treating insomnia after about
two weeks.
• It may impair the performance of skilled tasks, such as driving
(which is best avoided while taking this drug).
• Do not drink alcohol.
• Treatment must not be stopped abruptly after long-term use.

• After stopping treatment, there may be insomnia which should
improve after a few nights.
• Secobarbital is very dangerous in overdose.
• It is a Schedule II controlled substance.

Interactions

• The response to oral ℞ **anticoagulants** (for example ℞ **warfarin
sodium**) is decreased.
• If used with ℞ **acetaminophen**, there is an increased risk of toxic
effects on the liver.
• The levels and therapeutic effects of the following drugs may be
reduced: ℞ **antidepressants;** ℞ **beta-blockers;** ℞ **calcium-
channel blockers;** ℞ **corticosteroids;** ℞ **cyclosporine;**
℞ **digitoxin;** ℞ **disopyramide;** ℞ **doxycycline;** ℞ **estrogens;**
℞ **griseofulvin;** ℞ **oral contraceptives;** ℞ **propafenone;**
℞ **quinidine;** ℞ **tacrolimus;** ℞ **theophylline.**
• ℞ **MAOI** antidepressants prolong the effects of barbiturates.
• If used with an ℞ **antipsychotic**, the effects of both drugs are
reduced.
• If used with ℞ **chloramphenicol**, barbiturate levels are increased,
while the levels of chloramphenicol are reduced.
• If used with methoxyflurane, adverse effects on the kidneys are
increased.
• The effects of ℞ **narcotic analgesics** may be altered, with
increased central nervous system (CNS) depression.
• ℞ **Valproic acid** increases levels of barbiturates.
• If used with alcohol, there can be excessive central nervous system
(CNS) depression.

Side effects

• There may be hangover with drowsiness, lack of energy, or rash.
• Less frequently, CNS (central nervous system) depression,
dizziness, headache, lightheadedness, mental depression, physical
dependence, slurred speech, excitement in children and those over
65, vertigo, slowed heartbeat, lowered blood pressure,
gastrointestinal upset, and hives.
• Rare but serious side effects include blood cell disorders,
breathing stoppages, respiratory depression, seizures, spasms of
the bronchi or larynx, and Stevens-Johnson syndrome (a severe skin
disorder). There may be increased dreaming.

Seconal ⑧

A preparation of ℞ **secobarbital sodium.**
Formulation: Oral capsules.
Availability: Prescription only.
Warnings and side effects: See ℞ **secobarbital sodium.**

Sectral ⑧

A preparation of ℞ **acebutolol.**
Formulation: Oral capsules, available in two strengths.
Availability: Prescription only.
Warnings and side effects: See ℞ **acebutolol.**

Sedapap Tablets ⑧

A preparation of ℞ **acetaminophen** and butalbital.
Formulation: Oral tablets.
Availability: Prescription only.

Warnings and side effects: See ℞ **acetaminophen**.

sedatives ⓞ

Actions and uses

Sedative drugs calm and soothe, relieving anxiety and nervous tension and disposing a patient towards drowsiness. They are used particularly as a premedication prior to surgery. At higher doses, many sedatives can act as ℞ **hypnotic** agents (for example, ℞ **barbiturate** drugs), but at lower doses they have mainly a sedative action but with some sleepiness. The terms minor tranquilizer or anxiolytic (℞ **antianxiety** drugs) are now more commonly used to describe ℞ **benzodiazepine**-like sedatives that relieve anxiety without causing excessive sleepiness.

Limitations

See the individual drug class entries.

selegiline hydrochloride ⓖ

Type/Group: **antiparkinsonism**.
Brand(s): Eldepryl; Carbex; various generic.
How administered: Orally.

Used to treat

Selegiline hydrochloride is used in combination with ℞ **levodopa** (which is converted to ℞ **dopamine** in the brain) to treat the symptoms of ⓞ **Parkinson's disease** in those who exhibit a deterioration in response to levodopa/℞ **carbidopa** combined therapy. Its enzyme-inhibiting property, in effect, supplements and extends the action of levodopa and (in many but not all patients) it also minimizes some side effects. The drug is an enzyme inhibitor that inhibits one of the enzymes (monoamine-oxidase inhibitor type B) that break down the neurotransmitter dopamine in the brain. It is thought that dopamine deficiency in the brain causes Parkinson's disease. Although not stated by the manufacturer, it is sometimes used in the treatment of atypical ⓞ **depression** and ⓞ **Alzheimer's disease**.

Warnings

• It should not be used by people who are known to be sensitive to selegiline hydrochloride, or who are taking ℞ **meperidine**.
• It should be used with caution by those with a history of peptic ulcer disease, dementia, psychosis, tardive dyskinesia, profound tremor, or cardiac dysrhythmia (heart rate irregularities). There can be important interactions with other drugs (see below).
• Selegiline's effects in pregnancy are unknown. It should, therefore, be used during pregnancy only if clearly needed and if the benefits outweigh the possible risk to the fetus.
• It is not known whether this drug is excreted in breast milk, and so medical judgment is also required if breast-feeding is being considered.
• Skilled tasks, such as driving, should be avoided until response to the drug is established.
• Some people experience increases in ℞ **levodopa**-associated side effects.

Interactions

• ℞ SSRI antidepressants (for example, ℞ **fluoxetine**, ℞ **paroxetine**, ℞ **sertraline**) cause serious, sometimes fatal,

reactions. Do not take within several weeks of using, or planning to use, these drugs.
• ℞ **meperidine** may cause a potentially fatal reaction.
• ℞ **Antidepressants**, dexfenfluramine, fenfluramine, ℞ **dextromethorphan**, ℞ **sympathomimetics**, ℞ **methylphenidate**, ℞ **dextroamphetamine**, ℞ **reserpine**, ℞ **venlafaxine**, ℞ **narcotic analgesics**, and ℞ **sibutramine** can all cause potentially serious interactions.
• Foods and supplements rich in tyramine may produce hypertensive reactions.

Side effects

These can be many and include:
• Frequently, nausea, dizziness, lightheadedness, fainting, and abdominal discomfort.
• Occasionally, confusion, hallucinations, dry mouth, vivid dreams, and dyskinesia (abnormal movement).
• Rarely, headache and generalized aches.

selenium sulfide ⓖ

(selenium sulphide)
Type/Group: **antiseborrheic; antifungal**.
Brand(s): Head & Shoulders Intensive Treatment Dandruff Shampoo; Selsun; various generic.
How administered: Topically (external).

Used to treat

Selenium sulfide is used in some shampoos to treat ⓞ **dandruff** and is also used to treat tinea versicolor (a skin disorder caused by a form of yeast: see ⓞ **tinea**).

Warnings

• It should not be given to people with known hypersensitivity to selenium sulfide or sulfur products, or to any component of the preparations.
• It is not known whether selenium sulfide can harm the fetus, and so it should be used only if clearly needed.
• Medical judgment is required if breast-feeding is being considered. It is not known whether it appears in breast milk.
• Contact with the eyes and acutely inflamed skin must be avoided.
• It may damage jewelry, so remove before using.

Interactions

No interactions are known.

Side effects

• Skin irritation, discoloration of hair, oiliness or dryness of hair and scalp, and hair loss.

selenium sulphide ⓖ

see ℞ **selenium sulfide**.

Selsun; Selsun Blue ⓡ

A preparation of ℞ **selenium sulfide**.
Formulation: Topical lotion/shampoo.
Availability: OTC.
Warnings and side effects: See ℞ **selenium sulfide**.

Semprex-D Tablets ⓡ

A preparation of ℞ **pseudoephedrine** sulfate and ℞ **acrivastine**.

Formulation: Oral tablets.
Availability: Prescription only.
Warnings and side effects: See ℞ **pseudoephedrine**; ℞ **acrivastine**.

Senexon ⓑ

A preparation of ℞ **senna**.
Formulation: Oral tablets.
Availability: OTC.
Warnings and side effects: See ℞ **senna**.

senile dementia treatment ⓓ

see ℞ **dementia treatment**.

senna ⓖ

Type/Group: **laxative**.
Brand(s): Agoral; Black Draught Tablets, Granules; ex-lax, ex-lax chocolated; Fletcher's Castoria; Senna-Gen; Senexon; Senokot.
Combinations: With *docusate sodium*: Senokot-S. With *psyllium*: Perdiem Overnight Relief. With *casanthranol, methyl salicylate, rhubarb*: Black Draught Syrup.
How administered: Orally; rectal.

Used to treat

Senna is a traditional, powerful (stimulant) laxative which is still in fairly widespread use. It works by increasing the muscular activity of the intestinal walls and may take from 8 to 12 hours to have any relieving effect on ✪ **constipation**. Senna preparations can also be used to evacuate the bowels before an abdominal radiographic procedure, abdominal surgery, or endoscopy.

Warnings

• It should not be given to people with any form of intestinal obstruction and certain other gastrointestinal disorders.
• Generally, stimulant laxatives should be avoided during pregnancy, and a doctor should always be consulted before taking any drug when pregnant.
• Medical judgment is required if breast-feeding is being considered. Senna appears in breast milk and may cause a brown discoloration, and diarrhea in newborn babies.
• Do not use if there is abdominal pain, nausea, or vomiting, unless directed by a doctor.
• Rectal preparations should not be used in people with hemorrhoids or anal fissures.
• Chronic use of laxatives may cause fluid and electrolyte imbalances, vitamin and mineral deficiencies, and abnormal bowel function. Generally, they should not be used for more than a week.
• A doctor must be consulted first before taking any other medication (including OTCs, herbal remedies, and supplements), because laxatives may alter the absorption of a wide range of drugs.

Interactions

Laxatives may alter the absorption of many drugs. No other specific interactions of significance are known.

Side effects

• There may be abdominal cramps, nausea, appetite loss, vomiting, or discolored urine.
• Suppositories can sometimes cause local irritation.

Senna-Gen ⓑ

A preparation of ℞ **senna**.
Formulation: Oral tablets.
Availability: OTC.
Warnings and side effects: See ℞ **senna**.

Senokot-S ⓑ

A preparation of ℞ **docusate sodium** and ℞ **senna**.
Formulation: Oral tablets.
Availability: OTC.
Warnings and side effects: See ℞ **docusate sodium**; ℞ **senna**.

Senokot Tablets; Granules; Syrup ⓑ

A preparation of ℞ **senna**.
Formulation: Oral tablets; granules; syrup.
Availability: OTC.
Warnings and side effects: See ℞ **senna**.

Sensorcaine ⓑ

A preparation of ℞ **bupivacaine**.
Formulation: Injection.
Availability: Prescription only.
Warnings and side effects: See ℞ **bupivacaine**.

Septa Ointment ⓑ

A preparation of ℞ **neomycin**, ℞ **polymyxin B sulfate**, and ℞ **bacitracin**.
Formulation: Topical ointment.
Availability: OTC.
Warnings and side effects: See ℞ **neomycin**; ℞ **polymyxin B sulfate**; ℞ **bacitracin**.

Septi-Soft ⓑ

A preparation of ℞ **triclosan**.
Formulation: Topical solution.
Availability: OTC.
Warnings and side effects: See ℞ **triclosan**.

Septisol ⓑ

A preparation of ℞ **triclosan**.
Formulation: Topical liquid.
Availability: OTC.
Warnings and side effects: See ℞ **triclosan**.

Septra; Septra DS; Septra IV ⓑ

A preparation of ℞ **trimethoprim and sulfamethoxazole**.
Formulation: Oral tablets in regular and double strengths (DS); oral suspension; injectable solution.
Availability: Prescription only.
Warnings and side effects: See ℞ **trimethoprim and sulfamethoxazole**.

Ser-Ap-Es ⓑ

A preparation of ℞ **hydralazine hydrochloride**, ℞ **hydrochlorothiazide**, and ℞ **reserpine**.

Formulation: Oral tablets.
Availability: Prescription only.
Warnings and side effects: See ℞ **hydralazine hydrochloride**;
℞ **hydrochlorothiazide**; ℞ **reserpine**.

Serax ⑱

A preparation of ℞ **oxazepam**.
Formulation: Oral tablets and oral capsules in varying strength.
Tablets also contain tartrazine (FD&C yellow No. 5), which may
cause adverse reactions, including asthma, in some individuals.
Although rare, such reactions are more frequent in those who are
sensitive to aspirin.
Availability: Prescription only.
Warnings and side effects: See ℞ **oxazepam**.

Serentil ⑱

A preparation of ℞ **mesoridazine**.
Formulation: Oral tablets in several strengths; oral concentrate;
vials for injection.
Availability: Prescription only.
Warnings and side effects: See ℞ **mesoridazine**.

Serevent ⑱

A preparation of ℞ **salmeterol**.
Formulation: Aerosol inhalant; powder for inhalation.
Availability: Prescription only.
Warnings and side effects: See ℞ **salmeterol**.

sermorelin ⑥

Type/Group: diagnostic agent.
Brand(s): Geref.
How administered: Injection.

Used to treat

Sermorelin is an analog of growth hormone-releasing hormone
(somatotropin; GH-RH). It is used in a test to assess secretion of
growth hormone.

Warnings

• It should not be given to people with known hypersensitivity to
this drug or any component of the formulation.
• It should be given with caution to people with hypothyroidism
or epilepsy, or who are obese.
• Sermorelin should be used during pregnancy only if the potential
benefit outweighs the possible risk to the fetus.
• Medical judgment is required if breast-feeding is being
considered.
• Allergic reaction is a possibility.

Interactions

• ℞ **Atropine** or other muscarinic antagonists, ℞ **aspirin**,
℞ **indomethacin**, ℞ **antithyroid** medications, growth hormone,
and other drugs that affect pituitary secretion of growth hormone
may alter test results.

Side effects

• Flushing of face, pain or redness at injection site.

Seromycin ⑱

A preparation of ℞ **cycloserine**.
Formulation: Oral capsules.
Availability: Prescription only.
Warnings and side effects: See ℞ **cycloserine**.

Serophene ⑱

A preparation of ℞ **clomiphene citrate**.
Formulation: Oral tablets.
Availability: Prescription only.
Warnings and side effects: See ℞ **clomiphene citrate**.

Seroquel ⑱

A preparation of ℞ **quetiapine**.
Formulation: Oral tablets in several strengths.
Availability: Prescription only.
Warnings and side effects: See ℞ **quetiapine**.

Serostim ⑱

A preparation of ℞ **somatropin**.
Formulation: Injection.
Availability: Prescription only.
Warnings and side effects: See ℞ **somatropin**.

serotonin-receptor antagonist ⑩

(5-HT receptor antagonist)
Generics: granisetron; ondansetron; dolasetron mesylate.

Actions and uses

Serotonin-receptor antagonist drugs are agents that block the
actions of the neurotransmitter and hormone, serotonin (also
called 5-hydroxytryptamine; 5-HT) at some sites in the body. However, serotonin has such widespread roles and actions that most
drugs of this type are not suitable for use because their actions are
so diverse.

However, serotonin-receptor antagonist agents that act specifically
at the 5-HT_3 receptor subtype, such as ℞ **granisetron**,
℞ **ondansetron**, and ℞ **dolasetron mesylate**, have recently been
introduced as ℞ **antiemetic**/℞ **antinauseant** drugs. They can also
be very effective for helping prevent the vomiting that is a common
side effect of chemotherapy, radiotherapy, and sometimes after
surgery. They probably owe part of their effectiveness to actions on
the "chemoreceptor trigger-zone" in the brain, and part to actions
within the gut (both of which are involved in vomiting).

It is confidently expected that more drugs will be introduced that
work selectively by blocking just one subtype of the many serotonin
receptor types that are now known to exist. For instance, it is known
that some of the "atypical" antipsychotic drugs (that have some
advantages over the older "typical" ones) work in part by acting at
5-HT receptors. Since serotonin is an important brain neurotransmitter in processes related to mood, there is potential for the development of new drugs to treat other mood disorders.

Limitations

See the individual drug entries.

Key to symbols: ✪ = Disorder Section ℞ = Drug Section ♣ = Herbal Section ᦸ = Supplement Section

serotonin-receptor stimulant Ⓓ

(5-HT receptor agonist)
Generics: **buspirone; naratriptan; rizatriptan benzoate; sumatriptan succinate; zolmitriptan.**

Actions and uses

Serotonin-receptor stimulant drugs mimic the actions of the neurotransmitter and hormone, serotonin (also called 5-hydroxytryptamine; 5-HT) at some sites in the body. However, serotonin has such widespread roles and actions that most drugs of this type are not suitable for use because their actions and side effects are so widespread.

Serotonin-receptor stimulants acting at the 5-HT$_1$-receptor subtype have a directly ℞ **vasoconstrictor** effect (narrows blood vessels) on certain blood vessels around the brain and can be used in ℞ **antimigraine** treatment during the attack stage of a migraine. These drugs (℞ **naratriptan**, ℞ **rizatriptan**, ℞ **sumatriptan**, ℞ **zolmitriptan**) can start to work very quickly and some are given by self-injection or nasal spray. It is likely that older drugs of the ℞ **ergot alkaloid** (ergoloid) group work the same way, although they have less rapid and not so specific actions.

The novel drug ℞ **buspirone** is used as an anxiolytic, although it is not chemically related to other ℞ **antianxiety** drugs. It is thought to work as a serotonin-receptor stimulant in the brain (probably acting at the 5-HT$_{1A}$-receptor subtype).

More drugs are likely to be introduced that work selectively by activating just one of the many serotonin receptor subtype types now known to exist.

Limitations

See the individual drug entries.

sertraline Ⓖ

Type/Group: **antidepressant; SSRI.**
Brand(s): Zoloft.
How administered: Orally.

Used to treat

Sertraline can be used to treat ✪ **depression**, ✪ **obsessive-compulsive disorder**, panic disorder, and post-traumatic stress disorder. As is the case with other antidepressants, this drug is also being evaluated for other uses. Compared to the others in its class, the time taken for sertraline to reach effective levels and the decline of its effects after ending treatment are intermediate.

Warnings

• It should not be given to people with known hypersensitivity to this type of drug, or to anyone taking a ℞ **MAOI** antidepressant (see Interactions below).

• It should be given with caution to people with liver or severe kidney impairment, heart disorders, a history of seizures, diabetes mellitus, psychosis, bipolar disorder (manic depression), or who are receiving electroconvulsive therapy.

• Sertraline should be used during pregnancy only if the benefits outweigh the possible risk to the fetus.

• It should not be used by nursing mothers.

• A doctor must be consulted before taking any other medications, including OTC preparations, herbal remedies (especially ♣ St.

John's wort), supplements (for example the ⚕ **amino acids** tryptophan and tyramine) or other natural or alternative products.

• Avoid or minimize alcohol consumption.

• Judgment, thinking, and physical skills may be impaired, so use caution when first taking the drug.

• It may cause sensitivity to sunlight.

• Treatment should be stopped gradually, lowering the dose over a period of time.

• It may be several weeks before there are any signs of improvement.

Interactions

• Serious and even fatal reactions have occurred when ℞ **MAOI**s are taken with other antidepressants. There should be at least a 14-day gap between discontinuing a MAOI and starting another type.

• If used with tryptophan or ℞ **tricyclics**, additive effects may occur.

• If used with ℞ **selegiline**, mania (rarely) and hypertension may occur.

• ℞ **Cyproheptadine** may reduce the effects of sertraline.

• The effects of ℞ **carbamazepine** and ℞ **warfarin sodium** may be altered.

• Serious reactions are possible when ℞ **lithium** is combined with SSRIs.

Side effects

• Gastrointestinal effects (related to dose; including nausea and vomiting, loss of appetite and weight, indigestion, abdominal pain, diarrhea, or constipation), male sexual dysfunction, hypersensitivity reactions, dizziness, fatigue, headache, insomnia, abnormal sleepiness, and tremor.

• Less frequently, agitation, unsteadiness and incoordination, confusion, tingling or burning sensations, chest pain, hypotension, tachycardia, vision abnormalities, and urinary disorders. There may also be hallucinations, aggressive behavior, or loss of memory.

Serutan Ⓑ

A preparation of ℞ **psyllium.**
Formulation: Oral granules.
Availability: OTC.
Warnings and side effects: See ℞ **psyllium.**

Serzone Ⓑ

A preparation of ℞ **nefazodone hydrochloride.**
Formulation: Oral tablets in varying strengths.
Availability: Prescription only.
Warnings and side effects: See ℞ **nefazodone hydrochloride.**

Seudotabs Ⓑ

A preparation of ℞ **pseudoephedrine.**
Formulation: Oral tablets.
Availability: OTC.
Warnings and side effects: See ℞ **pseudoephedrine.**

sex hormone Ⓓ

Generics: **desogestrel; dienestrol; diethylstilbestrol; esterified estrogens; estrogens, conjugated; estrone; estropipate; ethinyl** estradiol; fluoxymesterone; hydroxyprogesterone caproate; levonorgestrel; medroxyprogesterone; megestrol acetate; mestranol; methyltestosterone; norethindrone; norgestrel; progesterone; stanozolol; testosterone.

Actions and uses

Sex hormones are endocrine (blood-borne) ℞ **hormone** mediators that largely determine the development of the internal and external genitalia and secondary sexual characteristics (growth of hair, breasts, and deepening of voice). For convenience they are divided into male and female hormones, but both groups are produced to some extent by both sexes. They are all chemically ℞ **steroid** compounds, generally very similar in structure, with some biochemical interconversion between members.

The main male sex hormones are called ℞ **androgen** hormones, of which ℞ **testosterone** is the principal member. In men, androgens are produced primarily by the testes; in both men and women, they are produced by the adrenal glands; and in women, small quantities are secreted by the ovaries. In medicine, there are a number of synthetic androgens (including ℞ **fluoxymesterone** and ℞ **methyltestosterone**) and their uses to make up hormonal deficiency and in ℞ **anticancer** treatment are detailed in their separate articles and under the individual drug entries.

Some androgens (notably stanozolol) also have marked ℞ **anabolic steroid** activity and generally promote body growth, masculinizing effects, and oppose ℞ **estrogen** hormones in the body. They are used to treat certain conditions by assisting the metabolic synthesis of protein in the body.

The female sex hormones can be divided into two groups, ℞ **estrogen** (estriol, estradiol) and ℞ **progestin** (progesterone) hormones. They are produced and secreted mainly by the ovary and the placenta during pregnancy; to a lesser extent, in both men and women, by the adrenal cortex; and, in men, by the testes.

Estrogens, usually in synthetic forms, are used for menstrual problems (for example, absence of menstrual periods in primary amenorrhoria), menopausal problems (℞ **hormone replacement**), or other gynecological problems, and as ℞ **oral contraceptive** agents (normally in combination with ℞ **progestin** hormones). Some synthetic estrogens are also used to treat certain cancers (for example, prostate and breast cancer). The best-known and most-used estrogens are: ℞ **estradiol**; ℞ **dienestrol**; ℞ **diethylstilbestrol**; ℞ **esterified estrogens**; ℞ **estrogens, conjugated**; ℞ **estrone**; ℞ **estropipate**; ℞ **ethinyl estradiol**; ℞ **mestranol**.

Progestin hormones include the natural progestin ℞ **progesterone** and synthetic substances with similar actions (including ℞ **desogestrel**, ℞ **norgestrel**, ℞ **levonorgestrel**, ℞ **medroxyprogesterone**, ℞ **norethindrone**, ℞ **megestrol acetate**, and ℞ **hydroxyprogesterone caproate**). They have many uses including in the treatment of menstrual disorders (✪ **menorrhagia** and severe ✪ **dysmenorrhea**), ✪ **endometriosis** (inflammation of the tissues normally lining the uterus), in menopausal ℞ **hormone replacement**, (see ✪ **menopause**) to treat luteal phase deficiency (inadequate production of progesterone during the luteal phase of menstruation) in women undergoing assisted reproductive technology therapy (ART) for ✪ **infertility**, in the ℞ **contraceptive** pill, to relieve the symptoms of

✪ **premenstrual syndrome**, and sometimes in the treatment of ✪ **breast cancer**, endometrial cancer, kidney cancer, and ✪ **prostate cancer**.
See also: ℞ **antiandrogen**; ℞ **antiestrogen**; ℞ **contraceptive**, ℞ **oral contraceptive**.

Limitations

See the individual drug entries.

sibutramine ⓖ

Type/Group: **appetite suppressant; obesity treatment**.
Brand(s): Meridia.
How administered: Orally.

Used to treat

Sibutramine is used to aid and maintain weight loss in the severely obese who are at risk from hypertension, diabetes mellitus, or disorders of fat metabolism. It works by inhibiting reuptake of norepinephrine, serotonin, and dopamine in the central nervous system (CNS).

Warnings

• It should not be used by people with known hypersensitivity to the drug or any of its active ingredients, anorexia nervosa, those taking other centrally acting appetite suppressant drugs, or anyone taking ℞ **MAOI** antidepressants (see Interactions below).

• It should be given with caution to anyone with glaucoma, seizure disorders, gallstones, stroke, heart disease, or liver or kidney impairment.

• It is not known whether or not sibutramine can harm the fetus, therefore, it should be used during pregnancy only if medically judged to be needed.

• Medical judgment is also required if breast-feeding is being considered.

• It may substantially increase blood pressure in some people.

• A doctor must be consulted before using any other prescription or OTC preparations (including herbal remedies and supplements).

• It must not be used with ℞ **SSRI** antidepressants, or other serotonin-enhancing drugs. There is a risk of a rare but serious "serotonin syndrome" reaction.

• Sibutramine is a Schedule IV controlled substance.

Interactions

• Sibutramine must not be taken with, or within two weeks of discontinuing, ℞ **MAOI** antidepressants. Severe and even fatal reactions can occur:

• It may increase the effects of CNS-active drugs.

• Interactions are possible with ℞ **erythromycin**, ℞ **cimetidine**, and ℞ **ketoconazole**.

Side effects

• Frequently, constipation, dry mouth, headache, insomnia, and hypertension.

• Occasionally, flu-like illness, nausea, and menstrual irregularities.

• Rarely, allergic reaction.

Silace Syrup ⓡ

A preparation of ℞ **docusate sodium**.
Formulation: Oral syrup.
Availability: OTC.

Warnings and side effects: See ℞ **docusate sodium**.

Siladryl Elixir ⓑ

A preparation of ℞ **diphenhydramine hydrochloride**.
Formulation: Oral liquid.
Availability: OTC.
Warnings and side effects: See ℞ **diphenhydramine hydrochloride**.

Silafed Syrup ⓑ

A preparation of ℞ **pseudoephedrine** and ℞ **triprolidine hydrochloride**.
Formulation: Oral syrup.
Availability: OTC.
Warnings and side effects: See ℞ **pseudoephedrine**; ℞ **triprolidine hydrochloride**.

Silapap Children's Elixir; Infants' Drops ⓑ

A preparation of ℞ **acetaminophen**.
Formulation: Oral liquid.
Availability: OTC.
Warnings and side effects: See ℞ **acetaminophen**.

Sildec-DM Syrup; Pediatric Syrup ⓑ

A preparation of ℞ **dextromethorphan**, ℞ **carbinoxamine maleate**, and ℞ **pseudoephedrine**.
Formulation: Oral syrup; pediatric syrup is lower strength.
Availability: Prescription only.
Warnings and side effects: See ℞ **dextromethorphan**; ℞ **carbinoxamine maleate**; ℞ **pseudoephedrine**.

sildenafil ⓖ

Type/Group: **impotence treatment**; vasodilator; **phosphodiesterase inhibitor**.
Brand(s): Viagra.
How administered: Orally.

Used to treat

Sildenafil is used to treat erectile dysfunction (see ◎ **impotence**). It acts as a powerful vasodilator in the blood vessels of the penis.

Warnings

• It should not be given to people with known hypersensitivity to any component of the tablet.
• It should be given with caution to people with kidney or liver function impairment, malformation of the penis, predisposition to prolonged erection (for example, in sickle-cell anemia, leukemia, multiple myeloma), serious heart disease, bleeding disorders, peptic ulcer, or retinitis pigmentosa.
• Sildenafil should not be given to pregnant women.
• It should not be used by anyone receiving treatment with ℞ **nitrates** (for example, in heart failure or angina pectoris) as heart attack and death are possible.

Interactions

• ℞ **Cimetidine**, ℞ **erythromycin**, ℞ **itraconazole**, and ℞ **ketoconazole** increase the levels of sildenafil.
• ℞ **Rifampin** may decrease the levels of sildenafil.

• It should not be used with ℞ **nitrates** because of potentially fatal effects (cardiac arrest and death).

Side effects

• Frequently, headache, abnormal vision, flushing, or upset stomach.
• Occasionally, nasal congestion, potentially serious effects on the heart, and blood-cell disorders.

Silphen DM ⓑ

A preparation of ℞ **dextromethorphan**.
Formulation: Oral syrup.
Availability: OTC.
Warnings and side effects: See ℞ **dextromethorphan**.

Siltussin DM Syrup ⓑ

A preparation of ℞ **dextromethorphan** and ℞ **guaifenesin**.
Formulation: Oral syrup.
Availability: OTC.
Warnings and side effects: See ℞ **dextromethorphan**; ℞ **guaifenesin**.

Siltussin Syrup ⓑ

A preparation of ℞ **guaifenesin**.
Formulation: Oral syrup.
Availability: OTC.
Warnings and side effects: See ℞ **guaifenesin**.

Silvadene ⓑ

A preparation of ℞ **silver sulfadiazine**.
Formulation: Cream.
Availability: Prescription only.
Warnings and side effects: See ℞ **silver sulfadiazine**.

silver sulfadiazine ⓖ

(silver sulphadiazine)
Type/Group: **sulfonamide; antibacterial**.
Brand(s): SSD Cream; Silvadene; Thermazene.
How administered: Topically (external).

Used to treat

Silver sulfadiazine is a preparation of silver, which has astringent and antiseptic properties, combined with the sulfonamide ℞ **sulfadiazine**, which has a broad spectrum of antibacterial activity. It is used primarily to stop ◎ **burns** becoming infected.

Warnings

• It should not be given to people with known hypersensitivity to sulfonamides or related drugs.
• It should be given with caution to people with severe allergies, kidney or liver dysfunction, or with G6PD deficiency (a genetic enzyme disorder).
• Silver sulfadiazine's safety during pregnancy has not been established. Do not use at the end of term because a newborn may have significant levels of the drug, which may cause serious problems.
• Medical judgment is required if breast-feeding is being considered. Sulfonamides are found in breast milk.

• If used over extensive areas of the body, or areas in which skin is seriously compromised, enough of the drug may be absorbed to create the potential for rare adverse reactions associated with systemic use of sulfonamides: serious or even fatal allergic reactions, liver failure, and serious blood disorders. A doctor must be contacted if any adverse reactions, particularly a rash, occur.

• External proteolytic enzymes may be inactivated by silver.

Interactions
• None of significance noted when used topically.

Side effects
• Burning, browning-gray skin discoloration, redness, itching, pain, rash, hives, or crystal formations in the urine.

silver sulphadiazine ⑥
see ℞ silver sulfadiazine.

Simaal Gel 2 Liquid ⑧
A preparation of ℞ **aluminum hydroxide**, ℞ **magnesium hydroxide**, and ℞ **simethicone**.
Formulation: Oral liquid.
Availability: OTC.
Warnings and side effects: See ℞ **aluminum hydroxide**; ℞ **magnesium hydroxide**; ℞ **simethicone**.

Simaal Gel Liquid ⑧
A preparation of ℞ **aluminum hydroxide** and ℞ **simethicone**.
Formulation: Oral liquid.
Availability: OTC.
Warnings and side effects: See ℞ **aluminum hydroxide**; ℞ **simethicone**.

simethicone ⑥
(dimethicone; dimeticone)
Type/Group: **antifoaming agent; barrier cream.**
Brand(s): (For internal use): Degas Chewable Tablets; Flatulex Drops; Gas-X, Extra Strength Chewable Tablets, Capsules; Genasyme Chewable Tablets, Drops; Maalox Anti-Gas Chewable Tablets; Mylanta Gas Chewable Tablets; Mylicon Drops; Phazyme Tablets, Phazyme 95 Tablets, 125 Capsules; various generic. (For topical use): A+D Ointment with Zinc Oxide; Diaper Guard Ointment; Dyprotex Pads. Combinations: With *activated charcoal*: Flatulex Tablets. With *aluminum hydroxide*: Almacone Liquid; Di-Gel Liquid; Mi-Acid Liquid; Mylagen Liquid; Mygel Suspension; Mylanta Liquid; Simaal Gel Liquid. (Plus) *magnesium hydroxide*: Almag Plus Suspension; Almacone Tablets, Almacone II; Aludrox; Gas-Ban DS Liquid; Gelusil; Kudrox Double Strength; Maalox Extra Strength Suspension; Mi-Acid II; Mintox Plus, Extra Strength; Mygel II; Mylagen II; Mylanta Tablets, Double Strength Tablets, Liquid; Rulox Plus Tablets, Suspension; Simaal Gel 2 Liquid; Tempo Tablets (also has *calcium carbonate*). (Plus) *magnesium carbonate*: Gaviscon Extra Strength Relief Formula Liquid. With *calcium carbonate*: Gas Ban; Titrilac Plus Tablets, Liquid. (Plus) *magnesium hydroxide*: Di-Gel Advanced Formula. With *magaldrate*: Iosopan Plus Liquid; Lowsium Plus Suspension; Riopan Plus Tablets,

Suspension, Double Strength Tablets, Suspension; various generic. With *sodium bicarbonate*: Sparkles Effervescent Granules.
How administered: Orally.

Used to treat
Simethicone is a water-repellent silicone which, when taken orally, is thought to reduce ✪ **flatulence** while protecting mucous membranes. It is also found in many topical ℞ **barrier creams** used for irritation or chapping (for example, diaper rash). Dimethicone activated is also known as simethicone.

Warnings
• It is considered safe when used as directed.
• No ill-effects in pregnancy or breast-feeding are known, but caution in taking drugs is always recommended, especially during the first trimester.
• Do not use on acutely inflamed or weeping skin.

Interactions
No drug interactions of significance have been reported.

Side effects
None known when used as directed.

Simulect ⑧
A preparation of ℞ **basiliximab**.
Formulation: Intravenous infusion.
Availability: Prescription only.
Warnings and side effects: See ℞ **basiliximab**.

simvastatin ⑥
Type/Group: **lipid-regulating drug; statin.**
Brand(s): Zocar.
How administered: Orally.

Used to treat
Simvastatin is a (statin/HMG-CoA reductase inhibitor) lipid-regulating drug that can be used in ✪ **hyperlipidemia** to reduce the levels, or change the proportions, of various lipids in the bloodstream. It is usually given only to people in whom a strict and regular dietary regime alone is not having the desired effect. It is also used to prevent heart attacks and reduce the risk of stroke.

Warnings
• It should not be given to people with active liver disease.
• It should be given with caution to people with a history of liver disease, kidney insufficiency, conditions predisposing to kidney failure, severe endocrine, metabolic, or electrolyte disorders, and those who are heavy users of alcohol.
• Simvastatin is considered quite hazardous to the fetus and should not be used during pregnancy. It is prescribed for women of childbearing age only when they are thought highly unlikely to conceive and have been informed of the risks.
• It should not be used while breast-feeding.
• When taking simvastatin, any unusual muscle pain or tenderness should be reported to a doctor immediately and treatment stopped, because the drug has the potential to cause destruction of muscle tissue.
• Potentially harmful changes in liver function may occur, so periodic tests may be necessary to check the drug's effect.

Key to symbols: ✪ = Disorder Section ℞ = Drug Section ♣ = Herbal Section ◌◌ = Supplement Section

Interactions

- ℞ azole antifungals (for example, ℞ fluconazole), ℞ clarithromycin, ℞ danazol, ℞ erythromycin, ℞ fluoxetine, ℞ nefazodone, and troleandomycin increase the levels of simvastatin and the risk of side effects.
- ℞ cholestyramine, ℞ colestipol hydrochloride, and ℞ isradipine reduce the levels of simvastatin.
- ℞ cyclosporine, ℞ gemfibrozil, and ℞ niacin increase the risk of adverse effects.
- The effects of ℞ warfarin sodium may be increased.

Side effects

- Occasionally, gastrointestinal effects and upper respiratory infection.
- Rarely, unusual weakness or tiredness, hepatitis, allergic reaction, lens opacity, blood disorders, and pancreatitis.

Sinarest 12 Hour ℬ

A preparation of ℞ oxymetazoline hydrochloride.
Formulation: Nasal spray.
Availability: OTC.
Warnings and side effects: See ℞ oxymetazoline hydrochloride.

Sinarest Sinus Tablets; Extra Strength Tablets ℬ

A preparation of ℞ pseudoephedrine, ℞ acetaminophen, and ℞ chlorpheniramine maleate.
Formulation: Oral tablets.
Availability: OTC.
Warnings and side effects: See ℞ pseudoephedrine; ℞ acetaminophen; ℞ chlorpheniramine maleate.

Sine-Aid IB Caplets ℬ

A preparation of ℞ pseudoephedrine and ℞ ibuprofen.
Formulation: Oral tablets.
Availability: OTC.
Warnings and side effects: See ℞ pseudoephedrine; ℞ ibuprofen.

Sinemet; Sinemet CR ℬ

A preparation of ℞ levodopa and ℞ carbidopa.
Formulation: Oral tablets in several strengths, sustained release tablet (Sinemet CR).
Availability: Prescription only.
Warnings and side effects: See ℞ levodopa; ℞ carbidopa.

Sine-Off Maximum Strength No Drowsiness Formula Tablets ℬ

A preparation of ℞ pseudoephedrine and ℞ acetaminophen.
Formulation: Oral tablets.
Availability: OTC.
Warnings and side effects: See ℞ pseudoephedrine; ℞ acetaminophen.

Sine-Off Sinus Medicine Caplets ℬ

A preparation of ℞ pseudoephedrine, ℞ acetaminophen, and ℞ chlorpheniramine maleate.
Formulation: Oral tablets.
Availability: OTC.
Warnings and side effects: See ℞ pseudoephedrine; ℞ acetaminophen; ℞ chlorpheniramine maleate.

Sinequan ℬ

A preparation of ℞ doxepin.
Formulation: Oral tablets in several strengths; oral concentrate.
Availability: Prescription only.
Warnings and side effects: See ℞ doxepin.

Sinex ℬ

A preparation of ℞ phenylephrine hydrochloride.
Formulation: Nasal spray.
Availability: OTC.
Warnings and side effects: See ℞ phenylephrine hydrochloride.

Singulair ℬ

A preparation of ℞ montelukast sodium.
Formulation: Oral tablets, chewable tablets.
Availability: Prescription only.
Warnings and side effects: See ℞ montelukast sodium.

Sinufed Timecelles ℬ

A preparation of ℞ pseudoephedrine and ℞ guaifenesin.
Formulation: Oral capsules, long acting.
Availability: Prescription only.
Warnings and side effects: See ℞ pseudoephedrine; ℞ guaifenesin.

Sinumist-SR Capsulets ℬ

A preparation of ℞ guaifenesin.
Formulation: Oral tablets, sustained release.
Availability: Prescription only.
Warnings and side effects: See ℞ guaifenesin.

Sinupan Capsules ℬ

A preparation of ℞ phenylephrine hydrochloride and ℞ guaifenesin.
Formulation: Oral capsules, controlled release.
Availability: Prescription only.
Warnings and side effects: See ℞ phenylephrine hydrochloride; ℞ guaifenesin.

Sinustop Pro Capsules ℬ

A preparation of ℞ pseudoephedrine.
Formulation: Oral capsules.
Availability: OTC.
Warnings and side effects: See ℞ pseudoephedrine.

Sinutab Maximum Strength Sinus Allergy Caplets; Tablets Ⓡ

A preparation of ℞ **pseudoephedrine**, ℞ **acetaminophen**, and ℞ **chlorpheniramine maleate**.
Formulation: Oral tablets.
Availability: OTC.
Warnings and side effects: See ℞ **pseudoephedrine**; ℞ **acetaminophen**; ℞ **chlorpheniramine maleate**.

Sinutab Non-Drying Capsules Ⓡ

A preparation of ℞ **pseudoephedrine** and ℞ **guaifenesin**.
Formulation: Oral capsules.
Availability: OTC.
Warnings and side effects: See ℞ **pseudoephedrine**; ℞ **guaifenesin**.

sirolimus Ⓖ

Type/Group: **immunosuppressant**.
Brand(s): Rapamune.
How administered: Orally.
Used to treat
Sirolimus is used to prevent organ rejection in people who have had a kidney transplant.
Warnings
• It should not be given to people with known hypersensitivity to this drug, its derivatives or any component of the drug product.
• It should be given with caution to people with liver dysfunction.
• Sirolimus should be used during pregnancy only if the potential benefits justify the possible risk to the fetus. Becoming pregnant should be avoided while using this drug and for 12 weeks after treatment has stopped, because of the risk of adverse fetal effects.
• Women taking this drug should not breast-feed.
• An increased susceptibility to infection and the possible development of lymphoma may result from immunosuppression.
• This drug may carry a risk of cancer and may impair fertility in men.
• Food alters the metabolism of sirolimus, so consistently take sirolimus either with or without food.
• Grapefruit juice reduces the metabolism of sirolimus.
Interactions
• The following drugs increase the levels of sirolimus:
℞ **cyclosporine**; ℞ **diltiazem hydrochloride**; ℞ **ketoconazole**; ℞ **nicardipine**; ℞ **verapamil**; ℞ **clotrimazole**; ℞ **fluconazole**; ℞ **itraconazole**; ℞ **clarithromycin**; ℞ **erythromycin**; troleandomycin; ℞ **metoclopramide**; ℞ **bromocriptine**; ℞ **cimetidine**; ℞ **danazol**; HIV-protease inhibitors.
• ℞ **Carbamazepine**, ℞ **phenobarbital**, ℞ **phenytoin**, ℞ **rifabutin**, and ℞ **rifampin** reduce the effects of sirolimus.
• ℞ **Vaccines** are less effective when given with immunosuppressants such as sirolimus.
Side effects
• Tremor, acne, constipation, diarrhea, nausea, increased serum creatinine, increased potassium and phosphate levels, peripheral edema, weight gain, rash, upset stomach, vomiting, anemia, thrombocytopenia, leukopenia, shortness of breath, sore throat,

upper respiratory tract infection, abdominal pain, weakness, back/chest pain, fever, headache, pain, muscle aches, urinary tract infection, hypertension, raised cholesterol and triglycerides in blood.

skeletal muscle relaxant Ⓓ

(muscle relaxant)
Generics: atracurium besylate; baclofen; carisoprodol; chlorzoxazone; cisatracurium; cyclobenzaprine; dantrolene sodium; methocarbamol; mivacurium; orphenadrine; pancuronium bromide; rocuronium bromide; suxamethonium chloride; tizanidine; vecuronium bromide.
Actions and uses
Skeletal muscle relaxants are drugs that act to reduce the tone or spasm in the voluntary (skeletal) muscles of the body. There are a number of different types of drugs that do this.
1. Neuromuscular blocking drugs are used during surgery to paralyze skeletal muscles that are normally under voluntary nerve control (but because the muscles involved in respiration are also paralyzed, the patient usually needs to be artificially ventilated). The use of these drugs means that lighter levels of anesthesia are required. Drugs of this sort work by acting at nicotinic receptors on the muscle that recognize acetylcholine, the neurotransmitter released from nerves to contract the muscle. There are two sorts of drug that achieve this effect, the nondepolarizing skeletal muscle relaxants (for example, ℞ **atracurium besylate**, ℞ **cisatracurium**, ℞ **mivacurium**, ℞ **pancuronium bromide**, ℞ **rocuronium bromide**, ℞ **vecuronium bromide**) and the depolarizing skeletal muscle relaxants (for example, ℞ **suxamethonium chloride**).
2. Drugs such as ℞ **dantrolene sodium** act directly within skeletal muscle cells to cause relaxation, and may be used when there is chronic severe spasticity of the muscles.
3. A number of other drugs do not work in the same way as the skeletal muscle relaxants discussed above, instead they act at some site in the central nervous system (CNS) to reduce nervous activity and indirectly lower muscle tone by acting on nerves that control muscle tone. These drugs are used when some defect or disease causes spasm in muscle. Some of these, such as the ℞ **benzodiazepines** (℞ **diazepam**) and ℞ **baclofen**, also have actions on higher centers in the CNS. Others have an action more on the spinal cord (for example, ℞ **carisoprodol**, ℞ **tizanidine**, ℞ **methocarbamol**, ℞ **orphenadrine**, ℞ **chlorzoxazone**, ℞ **carisoprodol**, ℞ **cyclobenzaprine**). A new drug, ℞ **tizanidine**, which is used the treat spasticity caused by multiple sclerosis or due to injury or disease of the spinal cord, works in a novel way (it is an ℞ **alpha-adrenergic stimulant** acting at alpha-$_2$ receptors in the central nervous system).
All the drugs discussed in this entry are quite distinct and different from the ℞ **smooth muscle relaxant** class, and work in quite different ways.
Limitations
None of these drugs are absolutely ideal for their proposed medical use, and research is continuing to find better agents.
1. Neuromuscular blocking drugs of the nondepolarizing type are all more or less based on an original plant alkaloid drug called tub-

Key to symbols: ✪ = Disorder Section · ℞ = Drug Section ♣ = Herbal Section ♋ = Supplement Section

ocurarine, and are attempts to derive a drug with a shorter duration of action and fewer side effects—but the perfect drug has yet to be found. The advantage of the nondepolarizing blocking agents is that their effects may be reversed at the end of the operation, so that normal respiration may return, by administering an ℞ **anticholinesterase** drug (for example, ℞ **neostigmine**, ℞ **pyridostigmine bromide**). In the meantime, until such a drug is developed, the depolarizing blocker ℞ **suxamethonium chloride** is used for very short operations, even though it has many disadvantages.

2. Better drugs are badly needed that work in the same way as ℞ **dantrolene sodium**—but with fewer contraindications and fewer side effects.

3. Drugs such as ℞ **diazepam** that act on the CNS are very effective against some types of muscle spasm of pain, but most have a number of side effects, notably a tendency to cause drowsiness.

Skelid Ⓑ

A preparation of ℞ **tiludronate sodium**.

Formulation: Oral tablets.

Availability: Prescription only.

Warnings and side effects: See ℞ **tiludronate sodium**.

skin preparation Ⓓ

Skin preparation describes an assortment of drug treatments for the many ✪ **skin conditions** that are in need of intervention. There is a wide variety of such preparations made up from drugs of many classes.

Treatment depends on cause. With many conditions where there is cracked, dry or scaling skin, ℞ **emollient** agents and ℞ **hydrating agent** preparations may be used, possibly of the ℞ **barrier cream** type to prevent further exposure. Also, soothing lotions (for instance those incorporating ℞ **calamine**) may be indicated, or sometimes an ℞ **astringent** to harden and protect skin where there are minor abrasions. Where the skin is itching, ℞ **antipruritic** agents may be used (℞ **crotamiton**, and some ℞ **antihistamine** drugs).

Where there is an inflammatory or allergic component to a skin condition, then ℞ **anti-inflammatory** and ℞ **antiallergic** drugs, often from the ℞ **corticosteroid** family may be used. These agents are normally applied topically to the skin as creams or lotions.

For infection of the skin, then ℞ **antimicrobial** drugs including ℞ **antiseptic**, ℞ **antibacterial**, ℞ **antifungal** and sometimes ℞ **antiviral** agents—whether ℞ **antibiotic** or synthetic—may be necessary. Where possible, these agents are used topically, but sometimes they are more effective when taken by mouth. A large number of remedies, some OTC (over-the-counter), are available to deal with fungal infections such as ✪ **athlete's foot**, jock itch, and thrush (℞ **candidiasis treatment**). These are normally used by topical (external) application (although ringworm sometimes needs systemic treatment).

In the case of an infestation by mites or lice, respectively, ℞ **scabicide and pediculicide** topical remedies will be necessary.

Limitations

Specific conditions and problems are discussed at their own entries, including ℞ **acne treatment**, ℞ **psoriasis treatment**, ℞ **antiseborrheic** remedies for seborrhea and seborrheic dermatitis, ℞ **antiperspirant** agents, and also ℞ **sunscreen** and ℞ **barrier** agents for protection. Some related topics are ℞ **anorectal preparations**, ℞ **wound-healing**, and ℞ **demulcent** agents which soothe mucous membranes.

sleep-aid product Ⓓ

Generics: **chlorpheniramine maleate; diphenhydramine hydrochloride; promethazine hydrochloride.**

Actions and uses

Sleep-aid product is a term used here for drugs intended to help with occasional ✪ **insomnia** and sleeplessness, which have less powerful effects than most prescribed ℞ **hypnotic** drugs, and are often available OTC (over-the-counter). They act on neurons in the brain to produce drowsiness and a sense of relaxation conducive to sleep. They can be used for the short-term treatment of insomnia due to jetlag, shiftwork, emotional problems, or certain illnesses. Some older ℞ **antihistamine** drugs (℞ **diphenhydramine hydrochloride**, ℞ **chlorpheniramine maleate**, ℞ **promethazine hydrochloride**) are used as sleep-aid products because they have quite marked sedative actions, and can be used especially to help sleep when there are allergic symptoms due to disease (for example, itching, rhinitis). Some preparations are available OTC, either on their own, or combined with other agents such as ℞ **analgesic** drugs and ℞ **decongestant** agents (as in some cold and cough preparations).

Limitations

Sleep-aid products should be used for short-term use only. If symptoms persist, a doctor should be consulted. Do not use at the same time as herbal remedies used for the same purpose. See also the individual drug entries.

sleeping pill Ⓓ

see ℞ **hypnotic**.

Slo-Bid Gyrocaps Ⓑ

A preparation of ℞ **theophylline**.

Formulation: Oral capsules, extended release, in several strengths.

Availability: Prescription only.

Warnings and side effects: See ℞ **theophylline**.

Slo-Niacin Ⓑ

A preparation of ℞ **niacin**.

Formulation: Oral tablets, timed release.

Availability: OTC.

Warnings and side effects: See ℞ **niacin**.

Slo-Phyllin; Slo-Phyllin Gyrocaps Ⓑ

A preparation of ℞ **theophylline**.

Formulation: Oral syrup; timed release capsules in several strengths (Gyrocaps).

Availability: Prescription only.

Warnings and side effects: See ℞ **theophylline**.

Slo-Phyllin GG Capsules; Syrup ®

A preparation of ℞ **guaifenesin** and ℞ **theophylline**.
Formulation: Oral capsules; syrup.
Availability: Prescription only.
Warnings and side effects: See ℞ **guaifenesin**; ℞ **theophylline**.

smooth muscle relaxant ⓓ

Actions and uses

Smooth muscle relaxants act on smooth (involuntary) muscles (such as the intestines and blood vessels) throughout the body to reduce spasm (℞ **antispasmodic**), cause relaxation, and to decrease motility (movement). They can work by a variety of mechanisms, though the term is often reserved for those drugs that act directly on smooth muscle, rather than those drug groups that work indirectly through blocking or modifying the action of vaso-constrictor (narrow blood vessels) hormones or neurotransmitters (such as ℞ **ACE inhibitor** drugs).

Direct-acting smooth muscle relaxants may be used for a number of purposes. Where they dilate blood vessels they are usually referred to as ℞ **vasodilator** drugs, examples being the ℞ **nitrate** and ℞ **calcium-channel blocker** groups, which may be used in ℞ **antihypertensive** treatment to lower blood pressure when it is raised in ⓞ **hypertension**, as well as for ⓞ **heart failure** (see ℞ **heart failure treatment**) and ℞ **antianginal** treatment to treat ⓞ **angina pectoris**. Where the smooth relaxant actions strongly affect the airways, such drugs may be used as ℞ **bronchodilator** agents in ℞ **antiasthmatic** treatment and bronchospasm in ⓞ **chronic obstructive pulmonary disease** (COPD), and here examples include ℞ **beta-adrenergic stimulant** drugs and ℞ **xanthine** agents. Drugs that act against colic and spasm in the intestine and related structures are often referred to as ℞ **antispasmodic** agents. Some drugs that relax other smooth muscle include ℞ **beta-adrenergic stimulant** drugs, which relax the uterus in premature labor.

Drugs of the smooth muscle relaxant class are not the same as ℞ **skeletal muscle relaxant** drugs.

Limitations

See the type/group and individual drug entries.

sodium bicarbonate ⓖ

Type/Group: antacid; electrolyte; urinary alkalinizer; antigout.
Brand(s): Alka-Seltzer Gold; various generic. Combinations: With *aluminum hydroxide, magnesium carbonate*: Gaviscon Extra Strength Relief Formula Tablets; Genaton Extra Strength Tablets. With *aluminum hydroxide, magnesium trisilicate*: Foamicon; Gaviscon Tablets, Gaviscon-2 Double Strength Tablets; Genaton Tablets. With *simethicone*: Sparkles Effervescent Granules. How administered: Orally; infusion.

Used to treat

Sodium bicarbonate (baking soda) is used for the rapid relief of ⓞ **indigestion**, and is a constituent of many over-the-counter antacid preparations taken by mouth. It is also used for symptomatic relief of heartburn and ⓞ **peptic ulcer**. It may also be taken by mouth to provide relief from the discomfort of acidic urine in mild infections of the urinary tract. By intravenous infusion, sodium bicarbonate is sometimes given in media to replace lost electrolytes or as an alkalinizing agent to relieve conditions of severe metabolic ⓞ **acidosis** (when the acid-base equilibrium of the body is badly out of balance), which may occur in kidney failure, cardiac insufficiency, or diabetic coma.

Warnings

• It should not be used by people with congestive heart failure, kidney failure, edema or cirrhosis, or who must maintain a low-sodium diet.

• It should be used with caution by people with high blood pressure, impaired kidney, liver or heart function, or who are taking certain drugs.

• No ill effects during pregnancy have been associated with sodium bicarbonate, when taken at recommended doses, but medical advice should always be sought before taking any drug during pregnancy or if breast-feeding.

• Overusing antacids may cause "acid rebound," which is an increase in stomach acid secretion. Sodium bicarbonate, therefore, should not be used for more than two weeks continuously.

• Do not use if there is abdominal pain, nausea, or vomiting, unless directed by a doctor.

• Sodium bicarbonate, with prolonged use, may cause milk-alkali syndrome, which is a serious illness characterized by headache, nausea, vomiting, weakness, alkalosis, and possibly kidney damage.

• Anyone taking any medication, including OTCs, herbal remedies, or supplements, should consult a doctor before taking an antacid, as it may alter the absorption of a wide range of drugs.

Interactions

• Buffered ℞ **aspirin**/antacid combinations should not be used in any long-term treatment, for example, for rheumatic inflammation.

• The following drugs may have their absorption and actions impaired: ℞ **benzodiazepines**, ℞ **digoxin**, ℞ **indomethacin**, iron salts, ℞ **ketoconazole**, ℞ **lithium**, ℞ **methenamine**, ℞ **methotrexate**, ℞ **salicylates**, ℞ **sulfonylureas**, and ℞ **tetracyclines**. Doses of these drugs should be taken several hours apart from doses of the antacid (a doctor should be consulted for full instructions and cautions).

• The absorption of ℞ **amphetamines**, ℞ **flecainide**, ℞ **naproxen**, ℞ **quinidine**, and ℞ **sympathomimetics** (for example, ℞ **phenylephrine**) may be increased, with a higher potential for adverse effects.

Side effects

These depend on how it is administered and used.

• There may be belching or flatulence.

• Less commonly, fluid retention, twitching, increased thirst, and weight gain.

• Potentially serious side effects include seizures and effects on the cardiovascular and respiratory systems.

sodium chloride ⓖ

Type/Group: **electrolyte**.

Brand(s): Opthhalmic: Adsorbanac; Muro 128; Muroptic -5. Nasal: Afrin Moisturizing Saline Mist; Breathe Free; Dristan Saline Spray; SalineX.

How administered: Orally; topically; injection.

Used to treat

Sodium chloride is an essential constituent of the human body, and is widely used as saline solution (0.9%) or as a constituent in dextrose saline (to treat dehydration and shock), as a medium with which to effect bladder irrigation, as a sodium supplement in patients with low sodium levels, as a treatment for corneal edema, a nasal decongestant, a mouthwash and by topical application in solution as a cleansing lotion for both blood and tissues. It is the major form in which the mineral element sodium appears. In the body, sodium is involved in the balance of body fluids, in the nervous system, and is essential for the functioning of the muscles. Sodium chloride, or salt, is contained in many foods, but too much salt can lead to edema, dehydration, and/or hypertension.

Warnings

Depending on use and route of administration.

• It should not be given to people with elevated sodium levels.

• It should be given with caution to people with certain heart, liver, or kidney diseases, with circulatory insufficiency, hypoproteinemia, hypervolemia, urinary tract obstruction, or congestive heart failure, and individuals who are experiencing edema and sodium retention, or who are using corticosteroids systemically.

• It should be used in pregnancy in amounts above the RDA only if it is clearly needed.

• Medical judgment is required if breast-feeding is being considered.

• Excessive systemic dosage produces electrolyte imbalance.

Interactions

• A high sodium intake may reduce the levels of ℞ **lithium**, while a low sodium intake may increase them.

Side effects

• Diarrhea, temporary burning or irritation with topical use.

sodium citrate Ⓖ

see ℞ citrates.

sodium cromoglicate Ⓖ

see ℞ cromolyn sodium.

sodium hypochlorite Ⓖ

Type/Group: **antiseptic; disinfectant.**
Brand(s): Dakin's.
How administered: Topically (external).

Used to treat

Sodium hypochlorite is a powerful oxidizing agent that can be used in solution as an antiseptic for cleansing abrasions, burns, and ulcers. It is not commonly used today because it can be an irritant to some people.

Warnings

It must never be taken internally and may casue painful burns on skin.

Interactions

None of significance if used as directed.

Side effects

None of significance if used as directed.

sodium lauryl sulfate Ⓖ

(sodium lauryl sulphate)
Type/Group: **surfactant.**
Brand(s): Ancet Liquid; Ceta; Derodex Cream; Duplex Liquid Face Cleanser; Listermint Arctic Mint Mouthwash; Lobana Body Shampoo; Solumol.
How administered: Topically (external).

Used to treat

Sodium lauryl sulfate is a salt with detergent and surfactant properties. It is incorporated into the formulation of a number of skin preparations and shampoos.

Warnings

None significant.

Interactions

No significant interactions are known.

Side effects

No significant side effects are known.

sodium lauryl sulphate Ⓖ

see ℞ sodium lauryl sulfate.

sodium nitrite Ⓖ

Type/Group: **antidote.**
Brand(s): Cyanide Antidote Package (generic).

Used to treat

Sodium nitrite is used in the emergency treatment of cyanide poisoning in combination with ℞ **sodium thiosulfate.**

sodium nitroprusside Ⓖ

Type/Group: **antihypertensive; vasodilator; heart failure treatment; hypotensive; nitrate.**
Brand(s): Nitropress; generic.
How administered: Intravenous infusion.

Used to treat

Sodium nitroprusside is used to control severe hypertensive crises (see Ⓞ **hypertension**), in the treatment of acute Ⓞ **heart failure**, and as a hypotensive for controlled low blood pressure in surgery.

Warnings

• It should not be given to people with certain kinds of hypotension, certain rare optic nerve diseases, severe liver impairment, and in emergency surgery where there is poor circulation to the brain or the patient is near death. This is a specialist drug and will be administered only by experienced personnel after a full medical assessment.

• It should be given with caution to elderly people, anyone with low blood pressure or who is taking antihypertensive drugs, with severe kidney impairment, liver insufficiency, hypothyroidism, vitamin B_{12} deficiency. It should be used with extreme caution where there is pre-existing raised intracranial pressure.

• Sodium nitroprusside should be used during pregnancy only if it is clearly needed.

• Medical judgment is required if breast-feeding is being considered.

• This drug should be used only in an adequately equipped medical facility with close monitoring. Sodium nitroprusside is a toxic drug (a kind of cyanide), which may have serious effects if improperly used.

Interactions

• There are increased effects if ℞ **ganglion-blockers** (including other antihypertensives) or ℞ **general anesthetics** are used with sodium nitroprusside.

Side effects

• These may include dizziness, headache, nausea and vomiting, nasal stuffiness, apprehension, muscle twitching, palpitations, or abdominal pain.

• Flushing, changes in heart rhythm, slower blood-clotting, increased intracranial pressure, and rash have also been reported.

• The most serious side effects are those related to too rapid a reduction in blood pressure or to a build-up of cyanogen during administration.

sodium perborate ⓖ

Type/Group: **antiseptic**.
Brand(s): Amosan.
How administered: Topically (external).

Used to treat

Sodium perborate is used in solution as a mouthwash.

Warnings

None significant.

Interactions

No significant interactions are known.

Side effects

No significant side effects are known.

sodium phenylbutyrate ⓖ

Type/Group: **metabolic disorder treatment**.
Brand(s): Buphenyl.
How administered: Orally; intragastric or nasogastric tube (into the stomach).

Used to treat

Sodium phenylbutyrate is a soluble salt of the amino acid phenyl-butyric acid, and is used as a treatment for urea cycle disturbances where there is a build-up of ammonia in the body.

Warnings

• It should not be given to people with acute hyperammonemia (high levels of ammonia in the blood). It is a specialist drug and a a full assessment for suitability will be carried out before treatment.

• It should be given with caution to people with congestive heart failure, severe kidney insufficiency, liver insufficiency, and with conditions in which there is sodium retention with edema.

• It should be used during pregnancy only if it is clearly needed.

• Medical judgment is required if breast-feeding is being considered.

• This drug requires specialist advice in assessing patients. Monitoring may also be required.

Interactions

• If used with ℞ **corticosteroids** or ℞ **haloperidol**, ammonia levels in the blood may be increased.

• ℞ **Probenecid** may increase the levels of sodium phenylbutyrate.

Side effects

• Menstrual dysfunction, decreased appetite, body odor, bad taste, or taste aversion.

sodium phosphate ⓖ

Type/Group: **laxative**.
Brand(s): Fleet Enema, Fleet Phospho-soda Solution.
How administered: Orally; rectal (enema).

Used to treat

Sodium phosphate is generally used as a combination of two forms, monobasic and dibasic, and is a saline laxative. It acts by drawing water into the intestine, and so promotes movement and emptying of the contents.

Warnings

• It should not be given to people with congestive heart failure, kidney failure, edema or cirrhosis, or who must maintain a low-sodium diet.

• It should be given with caution to people with high blood pressure, impaired kidney, liver or heart function, or who are taking certain drugs.

• No ill effects in pregnancy have been associated with this drug, but a doctor should always be consulted before taking any drug during pregnancy.

• Medical judgment is required if breast-feeding is being considered.

• Sodium phosphate should not be used for more than a week continuously.

• Do not use if there is abdominal pain, nausea, or vomiting, unless directed by a doctor.

• A doctor must be consulted first before taking any other medication (including OTCs, herbal remedies, and supplements), because laxatives may alter the absorption of a wide range of drugs.

Interactions

• ℞ **Diuretics** and other drugs that affect electrolyte balance may cause serious imbalance, especially with the overuse of saline laxatives.

• Laxatives may alter the absorption of many drugs.

Side effects

• There may be diarrhea; less commonly, abdominal pain, nausea, vomiting and dehydration.

• With prolonged use or overdose (or with existing heart or kidney disorder), sodium phosphate may cause high phosphate and low calcium levels, with the possibility of kidney failure.

sodium polystyrene sulfonate ⓖ

Type/Group: **cation-exchange resin**.
Brand(s): Kayexalate; SPS; generic.
How administered: Orally; rectal.

Used to treat

Sodium polystyrene sulfonate is a potassium-removing resin and is used to treat excessively high levels of potassium in the blood hyperkalemia, for example, in dialysis patients. Its action may require hours or days, and so other methods are preferred in urgent situations.

Warnings

• It should be given with caution to people with restricted sodium intake for example, severe congestive heart failure, severe hypertension, marked edema or who are taking ℞ **cardiac glycosides**.

• Its safety during pregnancy has not been established, and it should be used only if it is clearly needed.

• Medical judgment is required if breast-feeding is being considered.

• Electrolytes should be monitored regularly (including electrocardiogram to detect early signs of low potassium levels).

• If constipation occurs, ℞ **sorbitol** is the laxative of choice.

• An adequate fluid intake must be maintained.

Interactions

• The effects of ℞ **digitoxin** and ℞ **digoxin** may be exaggerated, with toxic effect.

• If used with ℞ **antacids** or ℞ **laxatives** containing magnesium or calcium, there is a risk of metabolic alkalosis, and also the effect of sodium polystyrene sulfonate is reduced.

Side effects

• These may include stomach irritation, loss of appetite, nausea, vomiting, and constipation.

• Large doses may cause fecal impaction, although this side effect does not generally occur with rectal administration.

sodium salicylate ⓖ

Type/Group: **antipyretic; anti-inflammatory; antirheumatic; non-narcotic analgesic**.

Brand(s): Various generic.

How administered: Orally.

Used to treat

Sodium salicylate has similar effects to ℞ **aspirin**, although weaker, but usually with less marked gastrointestinal side effects. It and other ℞ **salicylates** do not possess aspirin's level of ℞ **antiplatelet** activity, and so should not be used as an aspirin substitute when aspirin's preventive ℞ **antithrombotic** properties are required. It is used in the treatment of fever, pain, and inflammation.

Warnings

Warnings for drugs of this type include:

• It should not be used by people with known hypersensitivity to this drug or to other salicylates (including aspirin), who have chronic kidney disease, certain bleeding disorders or conditions (for example, hemophilia, vitamin K deficiency, low platelet levels), or who have a tendency to, or active, peptic ulceration.

• It should be given with caution to people taking certain drugs for gout or diabetes mellitus, or with allergic disorders (especially asthma and skin conditions), in the elderly, or children or teenagers, in those with any kind of kidney impairment or with certain liver disorders.

• Salicylates can adversely affect the health both of a pregnant woman and the fetus. They should not be used during pregnancy, and especially not in the third trimester, when risk to the fetus is at its highest.

• Breast-feeding mothers should either discontinue this drug or stop breast-feeding.

• Because of a link between salicylates and the rare, but serious, condition called ✪ **Reye's syndrome** (which causes inflammation of the brain and liver), salicylates should not be given to children or teenagers who have, or might have, chickenpox or influenza. As so many infections resemble flu in their initial symptoms, salicylates should not, as a general rule, be used to treat fever, ache, and malaise by anyone in this age group except on the advice of a doctor.

• Excessive use of salicylates for teething in babies has resulted in poisoning.

• If dizziness, change in hearing, or ringing in the ears (tinnitus) occurs, stop using this drug. These are usually the first symptoms of overdose.

• Salicylates can produce the same allergic-like symptoms that may occur after taking NSAIDs, including bronchospasm in "aspirin-sensitive" asthmatics.

• Foods high in salicylates, such as curry powder, gherkins, licorice, paprika, prunes, raisins, and tea, may increase the risk of side effects.

Interactions

• ℞ **Anticoagulants** have an additive effect in prolonging bleeding time.

• There is generally no benefit in taking sodium salicylate with other NSAIDs or salicylates, but there is a higher risk of gastrointestinal upsets and bleeding.

• Alcohol increases the risk of bleeding, particularly of an existing ulcer.

• ℞ **Antacids**, ℞ **corticosteroids**, ℞ **urinary alkalinizers**, and ℞ **activated charcoal** may lower the absorption or therapeutic effect of sodium salicylate.

• ℞ **Carbonic-anhydrase inhibitors** (for example, ℞ **acetazolamide**) increase the risk of overdose symptoms for both sodium salicylate and these drugs.

• The effects of the following drugs may be exaggerated: ℞ **phenytoin**; ℞ **nitroglycerin**; ℞ **valproate sodium** (and other valproic acid derivatives); ℞ **methotrexate**.

• Sodium salicylate taken with ℞ **insulin** or ℞ **sulfonylureas** may cause a greater glucose-lowering effect.

• The therapeutic effects of the followng drugs may be reduced: ℞ **angiotensin-receptor blockers**; ℞ **beta-blockers**; loop ℞ **diuretics**; ℞ **spironolactone**.

• ℞ **Uricosuric** agents (used in the treatment of gout, for example, phenylbutazone, ℞ **probenecid**, and ℞ **sulfinpyrazone**) may lose their effectiveness.

• There is a risk of accidental overdose and toxic effects if sodium salicylate is taken with OTC medications containing salicylates in some form (for example, some ℞ **antacids**).

• Foods high in salicylates, such as curry powder, gherkins, licorice, paprika, prunes, raisins, and tea, may increase the risk of side effects.

Side effects

These vary in severity and in the frequency with which they occur.

• The most common are gastrointestinal upsets, nausea, heartburn, diarrhea, and prolonged bleeding time (with consequent risk of ulceration). (The gastrointestinal upsets may be minimized by taking the drug with milk or food.)

• There may be hypersensitivity reactions, including hives, rash, bronchospasm, edema, headache, blood disorders, ringing in the ears, dizziness, and fluid retention.

• Reversible kidney failure, particularly in renal impairment, has occurred. Liver damage is rare.

Sodium Sulamyd ®

A preparation of ℞ **sulfacetamide**.

Formulation: Eye drops.

Availability: Prescription only.

Warnings and side effects: See ℞ **sulfacetamide**.

sodium tetradecyl sulfate ⑥

(sodium tetradecyl sulphate)

Type/Group: **sclerosing agent**.

Brand(s): Sotradecol.

How administered: Injection.

Used to treat

Sodium tetradecyl sulfate is a drug used in sclerotherapy, which is a technique to treat ✪ **varicose veins** by the injection of an irritant solution. It is used in the treatment of small, uncomplicated varicose veins in the legs.

Warnings

• It should not be given to people with known hypersensitivity to this drug, with certain venous conditions (for example, more complicated or extensive obstruction), any acute infections, allergic conditions, diabetes mellitus, hyperthyroidism, tuberculosis, asthma, sepsis, blood disorders, and acute respiratory or skin disease, or who are bedridden. There will be a full medical assessment.

• It should be given with caution to the elderly or debilitated, to those with arterial disease, heart or respiratory disease, kidney impairment, or who are taking oral contraceptives.

• Sodium tetradecyl sulfate's safety during pregnancy has not been established, and it should be used only if it is clearly needed.

• Medical judgment is required if breast-feeding is being considered.

• A severe reaction is possible at the site of injection, with death of the surrounding tissue. This drug should be administered only by physicians familiar with the appropriate technique.

• A small test injection is recommended before larger doses are given, to check for any allergic response.

Interactions

No drug interactions of significance are known, but thorough studies have not been performed.

Side effects

• There may be pain or ulceration at the site of injection, and a permanent (usually small) discoloration of the skin.

• Although uncommon, hypersensitivity reactions may occur, with dizziness, weakness, asthma, headache, nausea, vomiting, or generalized rash. Anaphylaxis is rare.

sodium tetradecyl sulphate ⑥

see ℞ **sodium tetradecyl sulfate**.

sodium thiosalicylate ⑥

Type/Group: **anti-inflammatory; antirheumatic; non-narcotic analgesic; salicylate**.

Brand(s): Rexolate; various generic.

How administered: Injection.

Used to treat

Sodium thiosalicylate is usually injected for relief of acute gout, rheumatic fever, muscular and musculoskeletal pain.

Warnings

• Studies have not been performed to investigate adverse effect of sodium thiosalicylate (or its drug interactions). It is expected they will closely resemble those of other salicylates.

• It should not be used by people with known hypersensitivity to this drug or to other salicylates (including aspirin), who have chronic kidney disease, certain bleeding disorders or conditions (for example, hemophilia, vitamin K deficiency, low platelet levels), or who have a tendency to, or active, peptic ulceration.

• It should be given with caution to people taking certain drugs for gout or diabetes mellitus, or with allergic disorders (especially asthma and skin conditions), in the elderly, or children or teenagers, in those with any kind of kidney impairment or with certain liver disorders.

• Salicylates can adversely affect the health both of a pregnant woman and the fetus. They should not be used during pregnancy, and especially not in the third trimester, when risk to the fetus is at its highest.

• Breast-feeding mothers should either discontinue this drug or stop breast-feeding.

• Because of a link between salicylates and the rare, but serious, condition called ✪ **Reye's syndrome** (which causes inflammation of the brain and liver), salicylates should not be given to children or teenagers who have, or might have, chickenpox or influenza. As so many infections resemble flu in their initial symptoms, salicylates should not, as a general rule, be used to treat fever, ache, and malaise by anyone in this age group except on the advice of a doctor.

• Salicylates can produce the same allergic-like symptoms that may occur after taking NSAIDs, including bronchospasm in "aspirin-sensitive" asthmatics.

• Foods high in salicylates, such as curry powder, gherkins, licorice, paprika, prunes, raisins, and tea, may increase the risk of side effects.

Interactions

• ℞ **Anticoagulants** have an additive effect in prolonging bleeding time.

• There is generally no benefit in taking sodium thiosalicylate with other NSAIDs or salicylates, but there is a higher risk of gastrointestinal upsets and bleeding.

• Alcohol increases the risk of bleeding, particularly of an existing ulcer.

• ℞ **Antacids**, ℞ **corticosteroids**, ℞ **urinary alkalinizers**, and ℞ **activated charcoal** may lower the absorption or therapeutic effect of sodium thiosalicylate.

• ℞ **Carbonic-anhydrase inhibitors** (for example, ℞ **acetazolamide**) increase the risk of overdose symptoms for both sodium salicylate and these drugs.

• The effects of the following drugs may be exaggerated: ℞ **phenytoin**; ℞ **nitroglycerin**; ℞ **valproate sodium** (and other valproic acid derivatives); ℞ **methotrexate**.

• Sodium thiosalicylate taken with ℞ **insulin** or ℞ **sulfonylureas** may cause a greater glucose-lowering effect.

• The therapeutic effects of the followng drugs may be reduced: ℞ **angiotensin-receptor blockers**; ℞ **beta-blockers**; loop ℞ **diuretics**; ℞ **spironolactone**.

• ℞ **Uricosuric** agents (used in the treatment of gout, for example, phenylbutazone, ℞ **probenecid**, and ℞ **sulfinpyrazone**) may lose their effectiveness.

• There is a risk of accidental overdose and toxic effects if sodium thiosalicylate is taken with OTC medications containing salicylates in some form (for example, some ℞ **antacids**).

• Foods high in salicylates, such as curry powder, gherkins, licorice, paprika, prunes, raisins, and tea, may increase the risk of side effects.

Side effects

• Gastrointestinal upsets, nausea, heartburn, diarrhea, and prolonged bleeding time (with consequent risk of ulceration).

• There may be hypersensitivity reactions, including hives, rash, bronchospasm, edema, headache, blood disorders, ringing in the ears, dizziness, and fluid retention.

• Reversible kidney failure, particularly in renal impairment, has occurred. Liver damage is rare.

sodium thiosulfate ⑥

(sodium thiosulphate)

Type/Group: **antidote; antigout**.

Brand(s): Generic only.

How administered: Intravenous infusion.

Used to treat

Sodium thiosulfate is used in the emergency treatment of cyanide poisoning, often in combination with ℞ **sodium nitrite**.

Warnings

• It should not be given to people with known hypersensitivity to any component of the formulation.

• It should be used during in pregnancy only if it is clearly needed and if the potential benefits outweigh the possible risks to the fetus.

• Medical judgment is required if breast-feeding is being considered.

• Monitoring for 24 to 48 hours for recurrence of symptoms is required.

Interactions

No significant interactions are known with this use.

Side effects

No significant side effects are known with this use.

sodium thiosulphate ⑥

see ℞ **sodium thiosulfate**.

Sodol Compound ⑧

A preparation of ℞ **carisoprodol** and ℞ **aspirin**.

Formulation: Oral tablets.

Availability: Prescription only.

Warnings and side effects: See ℞ **carisoprodol**; ℞ **aspirin**.

Solarcaine; Solarcaine Spray ⑧

A preparation of ℞ **benzocaine** and ℞ **triclosan**.

Formulation: Topical lotion; topical aerosol spray.

Availability: OTC.

Warnings and side effects: See ℞ **benzocaine**; ℞ **triclosan**.

Solarcaine Aloe Extra Burn Relief ⑧

A preparation of ℞ **lidocaine** and ♣ **aloe vera**.

Formulation: Topical gel; topical spray.

Availability: OTC.

Warnings and side effects: See ℞ **lidocaine**; ♣ **aloe**.

Solfoton ⑧

A preparation of ℞ **phenobarbital**.

Formulation: Oral tablets; oral capsules.

Availability: Prescription only.

Warnings and side effects: See ℞ **phenobarbital**.

Soltice Quick-Rub ⑧

A preparation of ℞ **methyl salicylate**, ℞ **menthol**, ℞ **camphor**, ℞ **glycerol**, and various.

Formulation: Topical ointment.

Availability: OTC.

Warnings and side effects: See ℞ **methyl salicylate**; ℞ **menthol**; ℞ **camphor**; ℞ **glycerol**.

Solu-Cortef ⑧

A preparation of ℞ **hydrocortisone** sodium succinate.

Formulation: Injection in several strengths.

Availability: Prescription only.

Warnings and side effects: See ℞ **hydrocortisone**.

Solu-Medrol ⑧

A preparation of ℞ **methylprednisolone** succinate.

Formulation: Powder for injection.

Availability: Prescription only.

Warnings and side effects: See ℞ **methylprednisolone**.

Solumol ⑧

A preparation of ℞ **sodium lauryl sulfate**, ℞ **mineral oil**, and ℞ **petrolatum**.

Formulation: Topical cream.
Availability: OTC.
Warnings and side effects: See ℞ **sodium lauryl sulfate**;
℞ **mineral oil**; ℞ **petrolatum**.

Solurex: Solurex LA ⑧

A preparation of ℞ **dexamethasone** sodium phosphate and dexamethasone acetate (Solurex LA).
Formulation: Injection.
Availability: Prescription only.
Warnings and side effects: See ℞ **dexamethasone**.

Soma ⑧

A preparation of ℞ **carisoprodol**.
Formulation: Oral tablets.
Availability: Prescription only.
Warnings and side effects: See ℞ **carisoprodol**.

Soma Compound ⑧

A preparation of ℞ **carisoprodol** and ℞ **aspirin**.
Formulation: Oral tablets.
Availability: Prescription only.
Warnings and side effects: See ℞ **carisoprodol**; ℞ **aspirin**.

Soma Compound w/Codeine ⑧

A preparation of ℞ **codeine phosphate**, ℞ **carisoprodol**, and ℞ **aspirin**.
Formulation: Oral tablets.
Availability: Prescription only.
Warnings and side effects: See ℞ **codeine phosphate**;
℞ **carisoprodol**; ℞ **aspirin**. Contains sodium metabisulfite, which may cause allergic reaction, sometimes serious, in a few people.

somatrem ⑥

Type/Group: **hormone; anterior pituitary hormone**.
Brand(s): Protropin.
How administered: Injection.

Used to treat

Somatrem is a synthetic form (with a very small chemical difference to the natural form) of the anterior pituitary hormone, human growth hormone (HGH), and is used to treat growth failure due to HGH deficiency, and also to treat AIDS wasting or cachexia (feebleness and emaciation).

Warnings

• It should not be used by people with known hypersensitivity to benzyl alcohol (in which somatrem is reconstituted), or with closed epiphyses (indicating that long-bone growth has stopped), or those in whom there is evidence of tumor or cancer activity.
• It should be given with caution to people with diabetes mellitus or low thyroid function.
• It should be used during pregnancy only if medically judged to be clearly needed.
• Medical judgment is also required if breast-feeding is being considered.

• Swelling in the hands and feet, pain, swelling, or stiffness in bones or muscles may occur, but may subside if treated, or if dosing frequency is reduced.
• It may accelerate viral replication in AIDS patients.
• Development of antibodies to somatrem is common but this does not usually prevent the drug from working.

Interactions

• Glucocorticoids may inhibit the effect of somatrem.

Side effects

• Headache, intracranial hypertension, changes in metabolism of some minerals and nutrients, pain, rash, and hives.
• Leukemia has occurred in a few children, but its relationship to treatment is uncertain.
• Rarely, carpal tunnel syndrome may develop.

somatropin ⑥

Type/Group: **hormone; anterior pituitary hormone**.
Brand(s): Genotropin; Humatrope; Norditropin; Nutropin; Serostim; Saizen.
How administered: Injection.

Used to treat

Somatropin is a synthetic drug, but is identical to human growth hormone (HGH), an anterior pituitary hormone, and is used to treat growth failure due to HGH deficiency, growth failure due to chronic kidney insufficiency prior to a transplant, short stature associated with Turner's syndrome, and for the replacement of HGH in adults with HGH deficiency. Although not stated by the manufacturer for such use, it is sometimes used for children of short stature due to intrauterine growth retardation.

Warnings

• It should not be used by people with known hypersensitivity to benzyl alcohol (in which somatropin is reconstituted) or closed epiphyses (indicating that long bone growth has stopped), or those in whom there is evidence of tumor or cancer activity.
• It should be given with caution to people with diabetes mellitus or low thyroid function.
• It should be used during pregnancy only if medically judged to be clearly needed.
• Medical judgment is also required if breast-feeding is being considered.
• Reduced thyroid hormone levels may develop, and must be treated in order for somatropin therapy to be effective.
• Development of antibodies to somatropin occurs but this does not usually prevent the drug from working.

Interactions

• Glucocorticoids may inhibit the effect of somatropin.

Side effects

• Increased calcium excretion, and antibodies to growth hormone.
• Occasionally, headache, muscle pain, weakness, mild elevations in blood glucose levels, allergic reaction (rash, itching), and joint pain.
• Leukemia has occurred in a few children, but its relationship to treatment is uncertain.

• Infrequently, use of somatropin has been associated with mild and transient edema, carpal tunnel syndrome, increased growth of preexisting nevi (moles), breast changes, and, rarely, pancreatitis.

sorbitol ⓖ

Type/Group: **surfactant; laxative**.
Brand(s): Dixodan Capsules; Eucerin Moisturizing; Genasoft Plus Softgels; Peri-Colase.
How administered: Orally; topically (external).

Used to treat

Sorbitol is a sweet-tasting carbohydrate that is used in a range of over-the-counter products as a sugar substitute (particularly by diabetics) and in skin preparations to promote penetration. In higher concentrations, it is also used as a constituent of some laxatives.

Warnings

None significant.

Interactions

• No significant interactions are known.
• Laxatives may alter the absorption of many drugs.

Side effects

No significant side effects are known.

Sorbitrate Sublingual Tablets; Chewable Tablets ⓑ

A preparation of ℞ **isosorbide dinitrate**.
Formulation: Sublingual tablets, available in 3 strengths; chewable tablets (2 strengths).
Availability: Prescription only.
Warnings and side effects: See ℞ **isosorbide dinitrate**.

Soriatane ⓑ

A preparation of ℞ **acitretin**.
Formulation: Oral capsules.
Availability: Prescription only.
Warnings and side effects: See ℞ **acitretin**.

sotalol hydrochloride ⓖ

Type/Group: **beta-blocker; antiarrhythmic**.
Brand(s): Betapace, Betapace AF; various generic.
How administered: Orally.

Used to treat

Sotalol is used to treat life-threatening ✪ **arrhythmias** and certain atrial arrhythmias not controlled by other medications.

Warnings

• It should not be given to people with known hypersensitivity to any beta-blocking drug, who have certain heartbeat irregularities or heart failure, or bronchial asthma. It should not be used in cardiogenic shock.
• It should be given with caution to people with diabetes mellitus or hypoglycemia, hyperthyroidism, myasthenia gravis, congestive heart failure, peripheral vascular disease, or liver or kidney impairment. Beta-blockers are usually not given to anyone with a nonallergic bronchospastic disease (for example, chronic bronchitis or emphysema).

• Sotalol should be used during pregnancy only if the potential benefit outweighs the possible risk to the fetus.
• It appears in breast milk, and so nursing women should discontinue using this drug or stop breast-feeding.
• Abruptly stopping using a beta-blocker may have adverse effects such as on the heart.
• The use of this drug may mask signs of hyperthyroidism or hypoglycemia.
• Other medications (including OTCs, herbal remedies, and supplements) must not be taken without consulting a doctor. Some ℞ **nasal decongestants**, commonly available over the counter, contain ℞ **alpha-adrenergic stimulants** (for example, ℞ **phenylephrine**) that may cause a severe hypertensive reaction if taken with beta-blockers.

Interactions

• A serious blood pressure increase may occur after withdrawal from ℞ **clonidine hydrochloride** or both drugs at the same time.
• Other ℞ **antiarrhythmics** (for example, ℞ **amiodarone**, ℞ **disopyramide**, ℞ **procainamide**, ℞ **quinidine**), ℞ **phenothiazines**, and ℞ **tricyclics** have the potential for significant adverse effects on heart rhythm.
• The effects of ℞ **alpha-adrenergic stimulants**, ℞ **ergot alkaloids**, ℞ **epinephrine**, ℞ **lidocaine**, and ℞ **theophylline** may be increased, with risk of serious adverse effects.
• ℞ **Calcium-channel blockers** (particularly ℞ **diltiazem** and ℞ **verapamil**), ℞ **guanethidine monosulfate**, and ℞ **reserpine** have the potential for increasing undesirable effects, with exaggerated slowing of heartbeat or hypotension.
• The effects of nondepolarizing ℞ **skeletal muscle relaxants** may be variable, with the possible risk of significant adverse effects associated with major surgery.
• The effects of ℞ **beta-adrenergic stimulants** (for example, ℞ **albuterol**, ℞ **terbutaline**), ℞ **insulin**, and ℞ **sulfonylureas** may be reduced by propranolol.
• ℞ **Cimetidine** may increase the effect of sotalol.
• ℞ **Antacids** (for example, ℞ **aluminum hydroxide**, ℞ **magnesium hydroxide**), ℞ **barbiturates**, ✪ **calcium** salts, ℞ **cholestyramine**, ℞ **colestipol hydrochloride**, ℞ **NSAIDs**, ℞ **phenytoin**, ℞ **penicillins**, ℞ **rifampin**, and ℞ **salicylates** may reduce the levels and effectiveness of beta-blockers. Antacids should not be taken within two hours of beta-blockers.
• If used with ℞ **diuretics** and other antihypertensive drugs, there are additive effects which are often used to therapeutic advantage.

Side effects

• Frequently, shortness of breath, dizziness, fatigue, slowing of the heart rate, and gastrointestinal disturbances (for example, nausea, vomiting, diarrhea, dyspepsia).
• Other effects may include a feeling of weakness, headache, sleep disturbances, sweating, back and leg pain, rash, and asthma-like symptoms.
• Heart failure, should it develop, generally requires withdrawal (gradually, if possible) of this drug.

Sotradecol ⓑ

A preparation of ℞ **sodium tetradecyl sulfate**.

Formulation: Intravenous injection.
Availability: Prescription only.
Warnings and side effects: See ℞ **sodium tetradecyl sulfate**.

sparfloxacin Ⓖ

Type/Group: **quinolone; antibacterial**.
Brand(s): Zagam.
How administered: Orally.

Used to treat

Sparfloxacin is used to treat ✪ **bacterial infections**. It is used for community-acquired (caught from the environment) ✪ **pneumonia** and acute, bacterially caused worsening of chronic ✪ **bronchitis**.

Warnings

• It should not be given to people with known hypersensitivity to sparfloxacin or other quinolones, or to children under 18, as there is a possibility of damage to joints and cartilage in growing children.

• It should be given with caution to people with liver or kidney disease, certain heart conditions, any predisposition to seizures, or a history of photosensitivity reactions (abnormal sensitivity to light).

• Sparfloxacin should be avoided during pregnancy or while breast-feeding if possible, as there is a risk of joint or cartilage damage to the baby.

• Superinfections due to the altered bacterial balance caused by antibiotic treatment may occur. A doctor must be contacted if severe abdominal pain, or moderate to severe diarrhea occur.

• Rare, but serious, side effects of quinolones include seizure and other CNS (central nervous system) effects, and severe, allergic reactions.

• Adequate fluid intake should be maintained.

• Avoid excessive exposure to sunlight during and for five days after taking sparfloxacin because photosensitivity reactions with this drug can occur.

• ⚖ **calcium**, ⚖ **iron** preparations, ⚖ **magnesium**, aluminum, and ⚖ **zinc** reduce the effects of sparfloxacin. Any products containing these substances, such as in supplements, must not be taken less than two hours before or four hours after using sparfloxacin.

Interactions

• ℞ **Antacids**, ⚖ **calcium**, ℞ **didanosine (ddI)**, ⚖ **iron** preparations, ⚖ **magnesium**, ℞ **sodium bicarbonate**, and ⚖ **zinc** reduce the effects of sparfloxacin. Do not take products containing these ingredients less than two hours before or two hours after taking sparfloxacin.

• The levels of ℞ **theophylline**, antipyrine, ℞ **caffeine**, ℞ **diazepam**, ℞ **metoprolol**, ℞ **pentoxifylline**, ℞ **phenytoin**, ℞ **propranolol**, ℞ **ropinirole**, ℞ **xanthine**, and ℞ **warfarin sodium** may be increased.

• The effects of oral ℞ **anticoagulants** may be increased.

• If used with ℞ **foscarnet**, the risk of seizure is increased.

Side effects

• Frequently, diarrhea, nausea, and headache.

• Occasionally, upset stomach, dizziness, insomnia, abdominal pain, bad taste in the mouth, and potentially serious effects on the heart.

Sparine Ⓡ

A preparation of ℞ **promazine**.
Formulation: Oral tablets in several strengths.
Availability: Prescription only.
Warnings and side effects: See ℞ **promazine**.

Spectazole Ⓡ

A preparation of ℞ **econazole**.
Formulation: Topical cream.
Availability: Prescription.
Warnings and side effects: See ℞ **econazole**.

spectinomycin Ⓖ

Type/Group: **antibiotic; antibacterial**.
Brand(s): Trobicin.
How administered: Injection.

Used to treat

Spectinomycin is structurally different from related ℞ **aminoglycoside** antibiotics. It is used to treat ✪ **gonorrhea** when other treatments are inappropriate.

Warnings

• It should not be given to people with known hypersensitivity to spectinomycin.

• It should be given with caution to people with a history of allergies.

• It should be used during pregnancy only if clearly needed and if the potential benefits outweigh the risks to the fetus.

• Medical judgment is required if breast-feeding is being considered. It is unknown whether this drug appears in breast milk.

• It is ineffective for syphilis and may mask symptoms.

• Rarely, serious allergic reactions have occurred.

Interactions

No significant interactions have been reported.

Side effects

• Frequently, pain at injection site and nausea.

• Occasionally, dizziness and insomnia.

• Rarely, decreased urine output.

Spectrocin Plus Ointment Ⓡ

A preparation of ℞ **neomycin**, ℞ **polymyxin B sulfate**, ℞ **bacitracin**, and ℞ **lidocaine**.
Formulation: Topical ointment.
Availability: OTC.
Warnings and side effects: See ℞ **neomycin**; ℞ **polymyxin B sulfate**; ℞ **bacitracin**; ℞ **lidocaine**.

spermicidal contraceptive Ⓓ

See ℞ **contraceptive**.

spironolactone Ⓖ

Type/Group: **diuretic; antihypertensive; heart failure treatment.**
Brand(s): Aldactone. Combinations: With *hydrochlorothiazide*: Aldactazide.
How administered: Orally.

Used to treat

Spironolactone is a diuretic of the aldosterone-antagonist type. It is also potassium-sparing and so can be used in conjunction with other types of diuretic, such as the ℞ **thiazides,** which cause loss of potassium, to obtain a more beneficial effect. It can be used to treat edema associated with aldosteronism (abnormal production of aldosterone by the adrenal gland), for ○ **heart failure,** ○ **nephrotic syndrome,** and ○ **fluid retention** and ascites (abdominal fluid) caused by ○ **cirrhosis** of the liver. It can also be used to treat ○ **hypertension.**

Warnings

• It should not be given to people with significantly impaired kidney function, or high potassium levels.
• It should be given with caution to people with liver disease or kidney disorders, with low sodium level (hyponatremia), or menstrual abnormalities.
• It is believed spironolactone may be hazardous to fetal development and it should be used during pregnancy only if the potential benefit outweighs the risk to the fetus.
• Medical judgment is required if breast-feeding is being considered.
• If symptoms such as paresthesia (tingling sensations), muscular weakness or fatigue occur, treatment should be stopped immediately and a doctor contacted.
• It should not be used with other potassium-sparing diuretics, such as ℞ **amiloride** or ℞ **triamterene.**
• There will be periodic monitoring of electrolytes.
• Foods rich in potassium, for example bananas, oranges, and salt substitutes, should not be consumed in large quantities.
• It may cause drowsiness, lack of coordination, and mental confusion, so impair the performance of skilled tasks such as driving.

Interactions

• Potassium-containing preparations (for example, certain drugs, salt substitutes, low-salt milk), ℞ **amiloride,** and ℞ **triamterene** pose a risk of severe hyperkalemia (high blood potassium) with the potential of serious heart irregularities or arrest. They should be avoided when taking spironolactone.
• ℞ **ACE inhibitors** and ℞ **NSAIDs** (especially ℞ **indomethacin**) may raise potassium levels and possibly cause heart arrhythmias.
• ℞ **lithium** levels may rise and pose a risk of lithium toxicity.
• ℞ **Amphotericin B,** ℞ **corticosteroids,** and ℞ **corticotropin** may increase diuretic effects, with the possibility of significant electrolyte loss (especially of potassium).
• The effects of ℞ **cardiac glycosides** may be unpredictable.
• Alcohol, ℞ **barbiturates,** and ℞ **opioids** increase the possibility of postural hypotension (lowered blood pressure on standing up).
• The effects of nondepolarizing ℞ **skeletal muscle relaxants** may be intensified.

• The effects of ℞ **anticoagulants** and ℞ **norepinephrine** may be lowered.
• ℞ **Salicylates** may reduce the effectiveness of spironolactone.

Side effects

• There may be gastrointestinal disturbances, headache, confusion, impotence and gynecomastia (enlargement of breasts) in men, irregular menstruation in women, fever, skin rashes, lethargy, and disturbances of liver and blood function.

Sporanox Ⓑ

A preparation of ℞ **itraconazole.**
Formulation: Oral capsules; oral solution; injection.
Availability: Prescription only.
Warnings and side effects: See ℞ **itraconazole.**

SPS Ⓑ

A preparation of ℞ **sodium polystyrene sulfonate.**
Formulation: Suspension, to be used orally, rectally, or by nasogastric tube.
Availability: Prescription only.
Warnings and side effects: See ℞ **sodium polystyrene sulfonate.**

SRC Expectorant Liquid Ⓑ

A preparation of ℞ **hydrocodone bitartrate,** ℞ **pseudoephedrine,** and ℞ **guaifenesin.**
Formulation: Oral liquid.
Availability: Prescription only.
Warnings and side effects: See ℞ **hydrocodone bitartrate;** ℞ **pseudoephedrine;** ℞ **guaifenesin.**

SSD Cream; SSD AF Cream Ⓑ

A preparation of ℞ **silver sulfadiazine.**
Formulation: Cream in several strengths.
Availability: Prescription only.
Warnings and side effects: See ℞ **silver sulfadiazine.**

SSKI Ⓑ

A preparation of ℞ **potassium iodide.**
Formulation: Oral liquid.
Availability: Prescription only.
Warnings and side effects: See ℞ **potassium iodide.**

SSRI Ⓓ

Generics: **citalopram; fluoxetine; fluvoxamine; paroxetine; sertraline.** Related generic: **mirtazapine hydrochloride; nefazodone hydrochloride; venlafaxine.**

Actions and uses

SSRIs are a class of ℞ **antidepressant**—technically referred to as selective serotonin reuptake inhibitors—that are used to relieve the symptoms of the affective disorder ○ **depression.**
SSRIs work by changing the levels of the monoamine neurotransmitter serotonin in areas of the brain that regulate mood. They increase neurotransmitter levels by blocking reuptake of serotonin into brain neurons (nerves) after its release in the normal process of neurotransmission. Some recently developed drugs, including

mirtazapine hydrochloride, nefazodone hydrochloride, and venlafaxine, are like SSRIs but affect norepinephrine as well as serotonin uptake and are sometimes referred to as selective serotonin and norepinephrine uptake inhibitors (SNRIs).

SSRIs may be used to elevate mood, help resume normal functioning, and reduce the frequency of depressive episodes in chronic depressive states. They may also be prescribed to help in more acute circumstances, such as after a loss of a loved one or in postnatal depression. Sometimes drugs of this class may be prescribed for a wide range of ✪ **affective disorders** including ✪ **anorexia nervosa**, ✪ **obsessive-compulsive disorder**, and social phobias (some of these uses are still under evaluation, "off-label" or unlicensed for this purpose).

Limitations

All antidepressant drugs have significant side effects, although these do generally become less troublesome with time. Generally, the SSRI group has less side effects than other types of antidepressant. Treatment often takes at least two weeks before there are any signs of improvement. Also, treatment should not begin immediately before or after some other types of antidepressant have been taken. Withdrawal of treatment must be gradual. Apart from their actions on brain monoamines, all antidepressants have other (generally undesirable) effects in the body, notably anticholinergic side effects (for example, dry mouth, gastrointestinal disturbances, and sedation), but the SSRIs have less of these effects compared to the ℞ **tricyclic** group.

Stadol; Stadol NS ⑧

A preparation of ℞ **butorphanol tartrate**.
Formulation: Nasal spray; injection.
Availability: Prescription only.
Warnings and side effects: See ℞ **butorphanol tartrate**.

Stagesic Capsules ⑧

A preparation of ℞ **hydrocodone bitartrate** and ℞ **acetaminophen**.
Formulation: Oral capsules.
Availability: Prescription only.
Warnings and side effects: See ℞ **hydrocodone bitartrate**; ℞ **acetaminophen**.

Stamoist E Tablets ⑧

A preparation of ℞ **pseudoephedrine** and ℞ **guaifenesin**.
Formulation: Oral tablets, long acting.
Availability: Prescription only.
Warnings and side effects: See ℞ **pseudoephedrine**; ℞ **guaifenesin**.

stanozolol ⑥

Type/Group: anabolic steroid; androgen.
Brand(s): Winstrol.
How administered: Orally.

Used to treat

Stanozolol is used to treat hereditary ✪ **angioedema** by assisting the metabolic synthesis of protein in the body.

Warnings

• It should not be given to people with severe kidney, heart, or liver disease, abnormal genital bleeding, prostate cancer, male breast cancer, female breast cancer with hypercalcemia, porphyria, or certain kidney disorders.

• It should be given with caution to people with cardiovascular or liver disease, seizure disorder, migraine headache, or diabetes mellitus.

• Stanozolol should not be used during pregnancy because of the potential masculinization of the fetus. A doctor must be contacted if pregnancy occurs while taking this drug.

• It is not recommended for use by nursing mothers.

• It may have serious effects on the liver.

• The use of anabolic steroids may increase the risk of arteriosclerosis and coronary artery disease.

• Do not use for enhancement of physical appearance or athletic performance. This drug is a Schedule III controlled substance.

Interactions

• The anticoagulant effects of oral ℞ **anticoagulants** are enhanced.

• If used with ℞ **antidiabetic** drugs, the hypoglycemic response is increased.

• The levels of ℞ **cyclosporine** are increased.

• If used with HMG-CoA reductase inhibitors (statins: ℞ **lovastatin**, ℞ **pravastatin**), the risk of myositis (degeneration of muscle tissue) is increased.

Side effects

• Effects due to the androgenic activity (mainly mild and reversible) include growth of hair, acne, amenorrhea or effects on the menstrual cycle, edema, voice change (usually seen at higher dosage; the drug should be discontinued), headache, muscle cramps, male breast pain, changes in sexual organs, indigestion, rash, euphoria or depression, blood changes, effects on the liver, changes in liver enzymes, in lipid levels, and in thyroid hormone levels, also accelerated bone development. Effects on the liver can be very serious.

Staticin ⑧

A preparation of ℞ **erythromycin**.
Formulation: Topical solution.
Availability: Prescription only.
Warnings and side effects: See ℞ **erythromycin**.

statin ⑩

Generics: atorvastatin; cerivastatin sodium; lovastatin; pravastatin sodium; simvastatin.

Actions and uses

℞ **statin** drugs (technically called HMG-CoA reductase inhibitors) are used in ℞ **lipid-regulating drug** (antihyperlipidemia) treatment. These agents are used in ✪ **hyperlipidemia** to reduce the levels, or change the proportions, of various lipids in the bloodstream. They work by competitively inhibiting an enzyme called *HMG-CoA reductase* which is an early rate-limiting step in the production of cholesterol. These drugs may moderately lower levels of

Key to symbols: ✪ = Disorder Section ℞ = Drug Section ♣ = Herbal Section ⚕⚕ = Supplement Section

triglycerides, dramatically reduce both overall serum and LDL-cholesterol, and moderately raise HDL-cholesterol.

Current medical opinion suggests that if diet, or drugs, can be used to lower levels of LDL-cholesterol (low-density lipoprotein) while raising HDL-cholesterol (high-density lipoprotein), then there may be a regression of the progress of coronary ✪ **atherosclerosis** (a diseased state of the arteries of the heart where plaques of lipid material narrow blood vessels, which contributes to angina pectoris attacks and the formation of abnormal clots that go on to cause heart attacks and strokes).

Limitations
See the individual drug entries.

stavudine ⓖ
(d4T)
Type/Group: **antiviral**.
Brand(s): Zerit.
How administered: Orally.

Used to treat
Stavudine is a reverse transcriptase antiviral drug that can be used in the antiretroviral treatment of ✪ **HIV** infection in people who are intolerant of, or have experienced deterioration with, other drug treatments.

Warnings
• It should not be given to people with known severe hypersensitivity to stavudine.
• It should be given with caution to people with a history of peripheral nerve inflammation.
• It should be used during pregnancy only when it is clearly needed and when the potential benefits outweigh the possible risks to the fetus.
• HIV-infected women are advised not to breast-feed.
• It may cause dizziness and so skilled tasks, such as driving, should be avoided until response to the drug is known.
• It is a specialist drug, and there will be full assessment and patient monitoring throughout treatment.
• A doctor must be contacted if any numbness, pain in hands or feet or tingling occurs, as these can indicate peripheral neuropathy.

Interactions
No significant interactions have been reported.

Side effects
• Frequently, peripheral neuropathy (for example, numbness, tingling, pain in hands and feet), headache, gastrointestinal effects, chills and fever, muscle aches, rash, loss of strength and energy, insomnia, mood changes, aching joints, back pain, sweating, unusual tiredness.
• Occasionally, loss of appetite, dizziness, eye infections, and shortness of breath.
• Rarely, blood disturbances and pancreatitis.

S-T Cort ⓑ
A preparation of ℞ **hydrocortisone**.
Formulation: Lotion.
Availability: Prescription only.
Warnings and side effects: See ℞ **hydrocortisone**.

Stelazine ⓑ
A preparation of ℞ **trifluoperazine**.
Formulation: Oral tablets in several strengths; injectable solution.
Availability: Prescription only.
Warnings and side effects: See ℞ **trifluoperazine**.

Sterapred ⓑ
A preparation of ℞ **prednisone**.
Formulation: Oral tablets in several strengths.
Availability: Prescription only.
Warnings and side effects: See ℞ **prednisone**.

sterculia gum ⓖ
see ℞ **karaya**.

steroid ⓓ
Generics: **calcitriol; dehydrocholic acid; fludrocortisone; hydrocortisone; ursodiol**.

Actions and uses
Steroid compounds are a class of naturally occurring and synthetic agents whose structure is based chemically on a steroid nucleus (a rather complex structure that consists of three 6-member rings and one 5-member ring). There are a number of important groups of chemicals in the body that are steroids, including all the ℞ **corticosteroid** hormones of the adrenal cortex (glucocorticoids such as ℞ **hydrocortisone**, or mineralocorticoids such as ℞ **fludrocortisone**), all the ℞ **sex hormone** groups (℞ **progestin**, ℞ **estrogen**, ℞ **androgen**, and ℞ **anabolic steroid** agents), all ℞ **vitamin** compounds of the vitamin-D group (℞ **calcitriol** and analogs), and the bile acids (that is, ℞ **ursodiol**, ℞ **dehydrocholic acid**, and analogs). Synthetic chemical analogs of the majority of these have important uses in medicine.

Limitations
See the individual drug entries.

steroid ⓓ
A common shortened form of ℞ **anabolic steroid**.

S-T Forte-2 Liquid ⓑ
A preparation of ℞ **hydrocodone bitartrate** and ℞ **chlorpheniramine maleate**.
Formulation: Oral liquid.
Availability: Prescription only.
Warnings and side effects: See ℞ **hydrocodone bitartrate**; ℞ **chlorpheniramine maleate**.

Stilphostrol ⓑ
A preparation of ℞ **diethylstilbestrol** diphosphate.
Formulation: Injection.
Availability: Prescription only.
Warnings and side effects: See ℞ **diethylstilbestrol**.

Stimate ⓑ
A preparation of ℞ **desmopressin**.
Formulation: Nasal spray pump.

Availability: Prescription only.
Warnings and side effects: See ℞ **desmopressin**.

St. Joseph Adult Chewable Aspirin ⑧

A preparation of ℞ **aspirin**.
Formulation: Oral tablets, chewable.
Availability: OTC.
Warnings and side effects: See ℞ **aspirin**.

St. Joseph Cough Suppressant ⑧

A preparation of ℞ **dextromethorphan**.
Formulation: Oral liquid.
Availability: OTC.
Warnings and side effects: See ℞ **dextromethorphan**.

Storz Sulf ⑧

A preparation of ℞ **sulfacetamide**.
Formulation: Topical lotion.
Availability: Prescription only.
Warnings and side effects: See ℞ **sulfacetamide**.

Streptase ⑧

A preparation of ℞ **streptokinase**.
Formulation: Intravenous injection or infusion.
Availability: Prescription only.
Warnings and side effects: See ℞ **streptokinase**.

streptokinase ⑥

Type/Group: **fibrinolytic; thrombolytic**.
Brand(s): Streptase.
How administered: Intravenous injection, infusion.

Used to treat

Streptokinase provides enzyme activity in a complex way, with the resultant effect of breaking up blood clots. It is used as a ℞ **thrombolytic** in ✪ **myocardial infarction** (heart attack), administered as soon as possible, to reduce the incidence of heart failure and improve survival, and to treat ✪ **pulmonary embolism**, ✪ **deep vein thrombosis**, and arterial ✪ **thrombosis**.

Warnings

• It should not be given to people with known hypersensitivity to this drug, or with active internal bleeding, severe uncontrolled high blood pressure, or surgery or bleeding involving the nervous system (brain or spine) within the previous two months. It will be administered by experienced personnel after a full medical assessment.

• It should be given with great caution to people with cerebrovascular disease, any recent major surgery, recent injury or internal bleeding (for example, in the gastrointestinal tract, urinary tract), bacterial endocarditis, high blood pressure, severe diabetes mellitus, significant liver or kidney impairment, or any condition (for example, taking anticoagulant drugs, low thrombocyte count) or disorder that would make bleeding more likely.

• Streptokinase should be used during pregnancy only when it is clearly needed.

• Medical judgment is required if breast-feeding is being considered.

• Although reported rarely, fibrinolytics may free bits of plaque that may lodge (usually) in the smaller blood vessels. This may result in abrupt, sharp pain in a leg, foot, the toes, back, or flank. ("Purple toes syndrome" appears as mottled, purplish discoloration of the toes.) More serious obstructions are possible, which may cause kidney failure, pancreatitis, hypertension, heart attack, stroke, and other serious obstructive events.

Interactions

• If used with ℞ **anticoagulants** or ℞ **antiplatelets**, there is an increased risk of bleeding (although despite some increased risk, ℞ **heparin** may have some benefit when used afterwards, as levels of streptokinase fall). ℞ **Aspirin** is often thought to be of benefit, although it has antiplatelet effects (only the risk of minor bleeding is slightly higher).

Side effects

• The chief complication is hemorrhage (although major bleeding is not frequent), which may occur at virtually any site in the body.

• Allergic reactions, sometimes severe, may occur, with symptoms such as fever and chills.

• Less frequently hives, itching, flushing, allergic swelling, shortness of breath, or bronchospasm. Arrhythmias and hypotension also occur. Back pain, but only during the infusion, has been reported.

streptomycin ⑥

Type/Group: **aminoglycoside; antibiotic; antibacterial**.
Brand(s): Generic only.
How administered: Injection.

Used to treat

Streptomycin is an original member of the aminoglycoside family, and is often used in combination with other antibiotics for the treatment of ✪ **tuberculosis**. Treatment takes between 6 and 18 months. It may also be used to treat other infections, including ✪ **endocarditis** (infection of the heart), tularemia (a disease originating from wild rodents and rabbits), plague, and ✪ **brucellosis** (a disease originating from domestic mammals), alone or with other drugs. Although not stated by the manufacturers for such use, it is also prescribed as part of a multi-drug treatment for *Mycobacterium avium* complex, a common infection in people with ✪ **AIDS**.

Warnings

• It should not be given to people with known hypersensitivity to streptomycin or other aminoglycosides, or with severe kidney disease.

• It should be given with caution to people with mild kidney disease, hearing deficits, or vertigo, with muscular disorders, such as myasthenia gravis or parkinsonism, and those over 65.

• Medical judgment is required when giving to very young infants.

• Streptomycin should be used during pregnancy only if medically judged to be clearly needed and if the potential benefits outweigh the risks to the fetus.

• It can be used when breast-feeding.

• Aminoglycosides are associated with nephrotoxicity (damage to the kidneys) and ototoxicity (damage in the ears). Irreversible vestibular impairment can occur, resulting in vertigo and difficulty maintaining balance. Permanent hearing loss in one or both ears can also occur. The risk is greatest in those with pre-existing impairments, with high doses, and with prolonged use.

• A doctor must be contacted if there are problems with hearing, vision, balance, urination, or headaches, even after the course of treatment is completed.

• The use of antibiotics may result in superinfection due to bacterial imbalance.

Interactions

• ℞ **ethacrynic acid** and ℞ **carboplatin** increase the risk of ear damage.

• ℞ **Amphotericin B**, ℞ **cephalosporins**, ℞ **cyclosporine**, methoxyflurane, and ℞ **NSAIDs** may increase the risk of kidney damage.

• There is a risk of respiratory depression if used with neuromuscular blocking agents.

• The effects of oral ℞ **anticoagulants** are enhanced.

Side effects

• Frequently, gastrointestinal upset. Also, tingling or burning sensation on face, around mouth, or in arms and legs, visual disturbances, muscular weakness, anemia, liver damage, effects on heart, blood changes, neurotoxicity, ototoxicity and deafness, and kidney damage.

Stridex Face Wash ⓑ

A preparation of ℞ **triclosan**.
Formulation: Topical solution.
Availability: OTC.
Warnings and side effects: See ℞ **triclosan**.

Stri-Dex Pads Regular Strength; Maximum Strength ⓑ

A preparation of ℞ **salicylic acid** and various.
Formulation: Medicated pads.
Availability: OTC.
Warnings and side effects: See ℞ **salicylic acid**.

Stromectol ⓑ

A preparation of ℞ **ivermectin**.
Formulation: Oral tablets.
Availability: Prescription only.
Warnings and side effects: See ℞ **ivermectin**.

Sublimaze ⓑ

Generic(s)/active constituent(s) ℞ **fentanyl**.
Formulation: Injection.
Availability: Prescription only.
Warnings and side effects: See ℞ **fentanyl**.

substance-dependence treatment ⓓ

Generics: **methadone hydrochloride; disulfiram; naltrexone hydrochloride.**

Actions and uses

Substance-dependence treatment is principally by support and psychotherapy, but drug treatment may play a big part in the early stages. Dependence on a particular drug can arise from drug abuse or from their medical use (see ✪ **drug dependency**). The non-medical use of self-administered drugs means use for recreational or similar purposes without intent to prevent, cure, or treat disease. Many such abused drugs eventually produce dependence or habituation (physical or psychological need to continue taking the drug). They include social drugs such as nicotine and alcohol (see ✪ **alcoholism**), as well as many drugs taken illicitly such as opiates, cocaine, and amphetamines. However, dependence also occurs with continued used of some drug classes for medical purposes, notably ℞ **narcotic analgesic** drugs (opiates) and ℞ **benzodiazepine** drugs (used for ℞ **hypnotic** or ℞ **antianxiety** purposes). Treatment of dependence on drugs of abuse is extremely difficult since it relies on the person wanting to stop the drug habit, and is based on psychological support during withdrawal and afterwards. Sometimes drugs are used to alleviate symptoms of withdrawal (for example, ℞ **sedative** drugs during alcohol withdrawal) by replacing the drug of abuse with a less harmful substitute (for example, ℞ **methadone hydrochloride** instead of morphine or heroin), or to enforce abstinence by causing unpleasant symptoms should the patient lapse (for example, ℞ **disulfiram** in the treatment of alcoholism). Sometimes it is possible to give a drug in detoxification treatment that will block the euphoric effects of habit-forming drugs, so helping to prevent re-addiction. The ℞ **opioid antagonist** ℞ **naltrexone hydrochloride** is used for formerly opioid-dependent people to help prevent relapse, and to treat recovering alcoholics.

Dependence on drugs in a medical environment is best avoided through not prescribing drugs likely to cause dependence for long periods, or finding safer substitutes. The ℞ **barbiturate** group if used as ℞ **hypnotic** agents can cause tolerance (which is the need for increasing doses) and withdrawal signs (restlessness and agitation) within a few weeks, and so they are generally avoided or limited to two-week courses). The benzodiazepines have come to replace them since they are much safer in overdose, but habituation can still become a problem with time. In a medical environment, benzodiazepine habituation is dealt with by tapering off the dose very slowly to avoid withdrawal symptoms. Drugs prescribed that have dependence potential should be kept safely locked away to avoid theft and should never be shared with another person.

Limitations

See the individual drug entries.

succinylcholine chloride ⓖ

(suxamethonium chloride)
Type/Group: **skeletal muscle relaxant**.
Brand(s): Anectine; Quelicin; generic.
How administered: Injection.

Used to treat

Succinylcholine chloride is used to induce muscle paralysis during surgery or mechanical ventilation (breathing), and to facilitate intubation.

Warnings

• It should not be used by people with known hypersensitivity to succinylcholine, or those with a certain genetic enzyme disorder, narrow-angle glaucoma, penetrating eye injuries, or with a personal or family history of malignant hyperthermia (a rare condition in which metabolic processes in the skeletal muscle are abnormally elevated).

• It should be given with caution to people with myasthenia gravis, heart, liver, lung, metabolic or kidney disorders, severe burns, electrolyte imbalance, elevated potassium levels, or with wasting muscle conditions.

• This drug is for administration only by trained personnel in hospitals, and individuals will be fully assessed for suitability prior to use.

• It should not be used during pregnancy.

• Medical judgment is required if breast-feeding is being considered.

Interactions

This drug is for administration only by trained personnel in hospitals, and individuals will be fully assessed for suitability prior to use.

Side effects

• Rarely, heart rhythm abnormalities, flushing, hypotension and constriction of the bronchi, and prolonged muscle relaxation.

sucralfate ⓖ

Type/Group: **cytoprotectant; ulcer-healing drug.**
Brand(s): Carafate; various generic.
How administered: Orally.

Used to treat

Sucralfate is a complex of ℞ **aluminum hydroxide** and sulfated sucrose, which can be used as a long-term treatment of gastric and duodenal ulcers (see ✪ **peptic ulcer**). It has been used, as well, to treat or prevent gastric erosion caused by ℞ **NSAIDs** and ℞ **aspirin** use. It has very little antacid effect, but is thought to work by forming a cytoprotectant barrier over an ulcer, so protecting it from acid, bile salts, and the enzyme pepsin, and allowing it to heal.

Warnings

• It should be given with caution to people with kidney disorders.

• Sucralfate should be used during pregnancy only if it is clearly needed.

• Medical judgment is required if breast-feeding is being considered. It is not known whether sucralfate appears in breast milk.

• Sucralfate will not prevent recurrence of duodenal ulcer.

Interactions

• The absorption and effects of ℞ **anticoagulants**, ℞ **digoxin**, ℞ **H₂-antagonists** (for example, ℞ **cimetidine**, ℞ **ranitidine**), ℞ **hydantoins**, ℞ **ketoconazole**, ℞ **quinidine**, ℞ **quinolones** (for example, ℞ **ciprofloxacin**, ℞ **norfloxacin**), ℞ **tetracyclines**, and ℞ **theophylline** may be lowered. Doses of these drugs should be separated from doses of sucralfate by several hours (a doctor should be consulted for full instructions and cautions).

• Aluminum-containing ℞ **antacids** may lead to toxicity in people with kidney impairment.

Side effects

• There may be constipation; less frequently, diarrhea, nausea, indigestion, gastric discomfort, dry mouth, skin rash and itching, insomnia, dizziness, vertigo, and drowsiness.

Sucrets Cough Control; 4-Hour Cough ⑧

A preparation of ℞ **dextromethorphan**.
Formulation: Lozenges; 4-Hour is higher strength.
Availability: OTC.
Warnings and side effects: See ℞ **dextromethorphan**.

Sucrets Sore Throat ⑧

A preparation of ℞ **hexylresorcinol**.
Formulation: Lozenges.
Availability: OTC.
Warnings and side effects: See ℞ **hexylresorcinol**.

Sudafed Cold & Cough Liquid Caps ⑧

A preparation of ℞ **dextromethorphan**, ℞ **pseudoephedrine**, and ℞ **guaifenesin**.
Formulation: Oral gel capsules.
Availability: OTC.
Warnings and side effects: See ℞ **dextromethorphan**; ℞ **pseudoephedrine**; ℞ **guaifenesin**.

Sudafed Plus Tablets ⑧

A preparation of ℞ **pseudoephedrine** and ℞ **chlorpheniramine maleate**.
Formulation: Oral Tablets.
Availability: OTC.
Warnings and side effects: See ℞ **pseudoephedrine**; ℞ **chlorpheniramine maleate**.

Sudafed Severe Cold Caplets; Tablets ⑧

A preparation of ℞ **dextromethorphan**, ℞ **acetaminophen**, and ℞ **pseudoephedrine**.
Formulation: Oral caplets; tablets.
Availability: OTC.
Warnings and side effects: See ℞ **dextromethorphan**; ℞ **acetaminophen**; ℞ **pseudoephedrine**.

Sudafed Tablets; 12 Hour Caplets ⑧

A preparation of ℞ **pseudoephedrine**.
Formulation: Oral tablets, available in two strengths; Caplets are extended release.
Availability: OTC.
Warnings and side effects: See ℞ **pseudoephedrine**.

Sudal 120/600 Tablets; 60/500 Tablets ⑧

A preparation of ℞ **pseudoephedrine** and ℞ **guaifenesin**.
Formulation: Oral tablets.
Availability: Prescription only.
Warnings and side effects: See ℞ **pseudoephedrine**; ℞ **guaifenesin**.

Key to symbols: ✪ = Disorder Section ℞ = Drug Section ♣ = Herbal Section ♗ = Supplement Section

Sudex Tablets ⑧

A preparation of ℞ **pseudoephedrine**.
Formulation: Oral tablets.
Availability: OTC.
Warnings and side effects: See ℞ **pseudoephedrine**.

Sular ⑧

A preparation of ℞ **nisoldipine**.
Formulation: Oral tablets, extended release, available in 4 strengths.
Availability: Prescription only.
Warnings and side effects: See ℞ **nisoldipine**.

sulconazole nitrate ⑥

Type/Group: **antifungal; azole.**
Brand(s): Exelderm.
How administered: Topically (external).

Used to treat

Sulconazole nitrate is a synthetic imidazole/azole antifungal drug used to treat skin infections, particularly those caused by ⊙ **tinea** such as ⊙ **athlete's foot**.

Warnings

• It should not be given to people with known sensitivity to sulconazole.
• Its safety during pregnancy has not been established. It should be used during pregnancy only if clearly needed.
• Medical judgment is required if breast-feeding is being considered. It is not known whether this drug appears in breast milk.
• Contact with the eyes must be avoided.

Interactions

None significant have been reported when used topically (externally).

Side effects

• Itching, burning, stinging, and redness.

sulfabenzamide ⑥

see ℞ **triple sulfa cream**.

sulfacetamide ⑥

Type/Group: **sulfonamide; antibacterial; acne treatment; antiseborrheic; sulfonamide.**
Brand(s): AK-Sulf, Belph-10; Cetamide; Ocusulf-10; Sebizon; Sodium Sulamyd; Storz Sulf; Sulster. Combinations: With *phenylephrine hydrochloride*: Vasosulf. With *prednisolone*: AK-Cide; Blephamine; Isopto Cetapred; Metimyd; Sulster; Vasocidin; Vasocine. With *fluorometholone*: FML-S Suspension.
How administered: Topically (eye; skin; scalp).

Used to treat

Sulfacetamide is used to treat corneal ulcers, eye infections, ⊙ **dandruff** and seborrheic ⊙ **dermatitis**, ⊙ **acne**, ⊙ **trachoma**, and secondary bacterial infections of the skin.

Warnings

• It should not be given to people with known hypersensitivity to sulfonamides or related drugs.

• Sulfacetamide's safety during pregnancy has not been established. Risk increases substantially nearer term. Do not use near term to avoid possible harm to the fetus.
• It is compatible with breast-feeding of healthy full-term infants.
• In ophthalmic use, exercise caution if the eye is extremely dry.
• Do not apply to large infected, denuded, or debrided areas of the skin.

Interactions

• Preparations containing silver are not compatible with sulfacetamide.

Side effects

• Frequently, transient burning and stinging when applied to eyes.
• Occasionally, local irritation.
• Rarely, allergic reactions, redness, rash, itching, swelling, slowing of corneal healing, photosensitivity, serious allergic reactions, serious skin infections, or kidney damage (if used in high concentrations over a wide area of skin).

sulfadiazine ⑥

(sulphadiazine)
Type/Group: **sulfonamide; antibacterial.**
Brand(s): Generic only.
How administered: Orally.

Used to treat

Sulfadiazine is used to treat serious ⊙ **bacterial infections** and to prevent the recurrence of ⊙ **rheumatic fever**.

Warnings

• It should not be given to people with known hypersensitivity to sulfonamides or related drugs.
• It should be given with caution to people with a history of severe allergies or with bronchial asthma.
• Sulfadiazine's safety during pregnancy has not been established. Do not use at the end of term because the newborn may have significant levels of the drug, which may cause serious problems.
• Medical judgment is required if breast-feeding is being considered. Sulfonamides are found in breast milk, and newborns or infants with certain health problems should not be breast-fed.
• The use of sulfonamides has been associated with serious allergic reactions, liver failure, and serious blood disorders. A doctor must be contacted if any adverse reactions, particularly a rash, occur.
• Photosensitivity (abnormal sensitivity to light, including ultraviolet light) may occur, and so protective measures, such as sunscreens, must be taken.

Interactions

• The effects of oral ℞ **anticoagulants**, thiopental, ℞ **hydantoins**, ℞ **sulfonylureas**, and ℞ **tolbutamide** may be increased.
• ℞ **Diuretics**, ℞ **indomethacin**, ℞ **methenamine**, ℞ **probenecid**, and ℞ **salicylates** may increase the levels of sulfonamides.

Side effects

• Frequently, abdominal pains, nausea, and vomiting.
• Occasionally, headache, peripheral nerve disorders, depression, blood disorders, and crystal formation in the urine.
• Rarely, convulsions, kidney disorders, liver damage, pancreatitis, and antibiotic-induced colitis.

sulfadoxine ⒢

Type/Group: **sulfonamide; antibacterial; antimalarial.**
Brand(s): Fansidar.
How administered: Orally.

Used to treat

Sulfadoxine is a long-acting drug that is used solely in combination with the antimalarial drug ℞ **pyrimethamine** to prevent or treat ✪ **malaria.**

Warnings

• It should not be given to people with known hypersensitivity to sulfonamides or related drugs, with certain liver disorders, severe kidney insufficiency, or certain blood disorders.
• It should be given with caution to people with a history of severe allergies, folate deficiency, or with bronchial asthma.
• Sulfadoxine's safety during pregnancy has not been established. Do not use at the end of term because newborns may have significant levels of the drug, which may cause serious problems.
• Medical judgment is required if breast-feeding is being considered. Sulfonamides are found in breast milk, and newborns or infants with certain health problems should not be breast-fed.
• The use of sulfonamides (including the sulfadoxine/pyrimethamine combination) has been associated with serious allergic reactions, liver failure, and serious blood disorders. Contact a doctor if any adverse reactions, particularly a rash, occur.

Interactions

• Other sulfonamides may increase the risk and severity of adverse reactions.
• ℞ **Diuretics,** ℞ **indomethacin,** ℞ **methenamine,** ℞ **probenecid,** and ℞ **salicylates** may increase the levels of sulfonamides.

Side effects

• Frequently, abdominal pains, nausea, and vomiting.
• Occasionally, headache, peripheral nerve disorders, depression, and blood disorders.
• Rarely, convulsions, kidney disorders, liver damage, pancreatitis, and antibiotic-induced colitis.

sulfamethoxazole ⒢

(sulphamethoxazole)
Type/Group: **sulfonamide; antibacterial.**
Brand(s): Gantanol.
How administered: Orally.

Used to treat

Sulfamethoxazole is a drug that can be used alone, or in combination with another sulfonamide-like antibacterial, ℞ **trimethoprim (TMP)** (a combination called ℞ **co-trimoxazole**), to treat a wide range of serious infections, especially of the urinary and the upper respiratory tracts. It is also used for *Pneumocystis carinii* infection and acute otitis media (see ✪ **otitis**) due to *Haemophilus influenzae,* and and with other drugs in the treatment of certain types of ✪ **malaria.**

Warnings

• It should not be given to people with known hypersensitivity to sulfonamides or related drugs.

• It should be given with caution to people with a history of severe allergies, kidney or liver impairment, G6PD deficiency (a genetic enzyme disorder), or with bronchial asthma.
• Sulfamethoxazole's safety during pregnancy has not been established. In particular, it should not be used at the end of term because the newborn may have significant levels of the drug, which may cause serious problems.
• Medical judgment is required if breast-feeding is being considered. Sulfonamides are found in breast milk.
• The use of sulfonamides has been associated with serious allergic reactions, liver failure, and serious blood disorders. A doctor must be contacted if any adverse reactions, particularly a rash, occur.
• Photosensitivity (abnormal sensitivity to light, including ultraviolet light) may occur, and so exposure should be minimized until light tolerance is determined.
• The use of antibiotics may result in a superinfection from non-susceptible organisms.

Interactions

• The effects of oral ℞ **anticoagulants,** thiopental, ℞ **hydantoins,** ℞ **sulfonylureas,** and ℞ **tolbutamide** may be increased.
• ℞ **Diuretics,** ℞ **indomethacin,** ℞ **methenamine,** ℞ **probenecid,** and ℞ **salicylates** may increase the levels of sulfonamides.

Side effects

• Frequently, abdominal pains, nausea, and vomiting.
• Occasionally, headache, peripheral nerve disorders, depression, blood disorders, and crystal formation in the urine. Rarely, convulsions, kidney disorders, liver damage, pancreatitis, or antibiotic-induced colitis.

Sulfamylon Ⓑ

A preparation of ℞ **mafenide.**
Formulation: Topical solution, topical cream.
Availability: Prescription only.
Warnings and side effects: See ℞ **mafenide.**

sulfasalazine ⒢

Type/Group: **antirheumatic; salicylate; aminosalicylate.**
Brand(s): Azulfidine Tablets, EN-tabs; various generic.
How administered: Orally.

Used to treat

Sulfasalazine is an ℞ **aminosalicylate** (5-aminosalicylic acid) which combines within the one chemical a ℞ **sulfonamide** constituent (with antibacterial properties), and a salicylate with anti-inflammatory properties. It can be used to treat active ✪ **Crohn's disease** and to induce and maintain remission of the symptoms of ✪ **ulcerative colitis.** It is also sometimes used to treat ✪ **rheumatoid arthritis** that has not responded to ℞ **NSAIDs.**

Warnings

• It should not be used by people with known hypersensitivity to this drug or to any salicylate (for example, ℞ **aspirin**) or sulfonamide (for example, ℞ **sulfisoxazole**), with intestinal or urinary obstruction, with porphyria, or who are under two years of age.

• It should be given with caution to anyone with kidney or liver impairment, G6PD deficiency, slow alkylators, or certain blood disorders, or who have bronchial asthma or severe allergy.

• Sulfasalazine should only be used during pregnancy when it is medically judged that the benefits outweigh the risks.

• Medical judgment is also required if breast-feeding is being considered, as it appears in breast milk.

• During treatment with sulfasalizine, blood abnormalities, nervous system disorders, and liver and kidney impairment have occurred, and so regular medical monitoring is necessary.

• Avoid prolonged exposure to sunlight.

• Adequate water intake is necessary to prevent crystalluria and stone formation.

Interactions

• ℞ **Digoxin** and ℞ **folic acid** levels may be reduced when taken with sulfasalazine.

• ℞ **Phenytoin** concentrations may be increased, so requiring dose adjustment.

Side effects

These can be many, and some are potentially serious and medical monitoring will be carried out during treatment.

• Commonly, there may be loss of appetite, headache, nausea, vomiting, gastrointestinal disturbances, or low sperm count.

• Less frequently, rash, itchiness, hives, fever, and anemia.

• Although rare, severe reactions are possible and may involve the blood, liver, pancreas, or kidneys.

sulfathiazole Ⓖ

see ℞ **triple sulfa cream**.

sulfinpyrazone Ⓖ

(sulphinpyrazone)
Type/Group: **uricosuric; antigout**.
Brand(s): Benemid; Probalan; various generic.
How administered: Orally.

Used to treat

Sulfinpyrazone is used to prevent ✪ **gout** and to treat hyperuricemia. It works by promoting the excretion of uric acid in the urine.

Warnings

• It should not be given to people with known hypersensitivity to phenylbutazone or other pyrazoles, or with active peptic ulcer, symptoms of gastrointestinal inflammation or ulceration, or blood disorders.

• It should be given with caution to people with kidney function impairment, healed peptic ulcers, dehydration, or with acute gout.

• It should be used during pregnancy only when it is clearly needed and when the potential benefits outweigh the possible risks to the fetus.

• Medical judgment is required if breast-feeding is being considered. It is not known whether this drug appears in breast milk.

• Take with food, milk, or antacids to minimize gastrointestinal disturbance.

• Drink at least 10 full glasses of water per day.

• Continue treatment even during acute gout attacks.

• Do not take aspirin or other salicylates while using this drug, because its effects may be reduced.

Interactions

• If used with ℞ **acetaminophen**, the risk of liver damage from acetaminophen may be increased and its therapeutic effects decreased.

• The effects of oral ℞ **anticoagulants** and ℞ **tolbutamide** may be increased.

• The effects of ℞ **verapamil** and ℞ **theophylline** may be reduced.

• ℞ **Niacin** and ℞ **salicylates** may reduce the effects of sulfinpyrazone.

Side effects

• Frequently, nausea and vomiting.

• Less frequently, rash, blood disorders, bronchoconstriction (in individuals with aspirin-induced asthma), and kidney damage.

sulfisoxazole Ⓖ

Type/Group: **sulfonamide; antibacterial**.
Brand(s): Gantrisin Pediatric; Gantrisin Solution; various generic.
Combinations: With erythromycin: Eryzole; Pediazole.
How administered: Orally; topically (ophthalmic/eye)

Used to treat

Sulfisoxazole is used to treat serious ✪ **bacterial infections** such as ✪ **trachoma**, chancroid, and inclusion ✪ **conjunctivitis**.

Warnings

• It should not be given to people with known hypersensitivity to sulfonamides or related drugs.

• It should be given with caution to people with a history of porphyria, severe allergies or with liver or kidney impairment, G6PD deficiency (a genetic enzyme disorder), or bronchial asthma.

• Sulfisoxazole's safety during pregnancy has not been established. In particular, it should not be used at the end of term because the newborn may have significant levels of the drug, which may cause serious problems.

• Medical judgment is required if breast-feeding is being considered. Sulfonamides are found in breast milk. Newborns or infants with certain health problems should not be breast-fed.

• The use of sulfonamides has been associated with serious allergic reactions, liver failure, and serious blood disorders. Contact a doctor if any adverse reactions, particularly a rash, occur. However, the risk with ophthalmic (eye) use is minimal.

• Photosensitivity (abnormal sensitivity to light, including ultraviolet light) may occur, and so exposure should be minimized until light tolerance is determined.

• The use of antibiotics may result in a superinfection from non-susceptible organisms.

Interactions

• The effects of oral ℞ **anticoagulants**, thiopental, ℞ **hydantoins**, ℞ **sulfonylureas**, and ℞ **tolbutamide** may be increased.

• ℞ **Diuretics**, ℞ **indomethacin**, ℞ **methenamine**, ℞ **probenecid**, and ℞ **salicylates** may increase the levels of sulfonamides.

Side effects

• Systemic use: Frequently, abdominal pains, nausea, and vomiting. Occasionally, headache, peripheral nerve disorders,

depression, blood disorders, and crystal formation in the urine. Rarely, convulsions, kidney disorders, liver damage, pancreatitis, and antibiotic-induced colitis.
• Ophthalmic use: Frequently, transient stinging and burning. Occasionally, local irritation. Rarely, allergic reaction characterized by burning, swelling, and redness of the eye.

Sulfoam ⓑ

A preparation of ℞ **salicylic acid**.
Formulation: Shampoo.
Availability: OTC.
Warnings and side effects: See ℞ **salicylic acid**.

Sulfoil ⓑ

A preparation of ℞ **castor oil**.
Formulation: Topical liquid.
Availability: OTC.
Warnings and side effects: See ℞ **castor oil**.

sulfonamide ⓓ

(sulphonamide)
Generics: **mafenide; silver sulfadiazine; sulfacetamide; sulfadiazine; sulfadoxine; sulfamethoxazole; sulfisoxazole; trimethoprim (TMP)**.

Actions and uses

Sulfonamide drugs—also called sulphonamide, sulfa, or sulpha drugs—are derivatives of a red dye, prontosil, which was discovered in the 1930s, and which is converted in the body to sulphanilamide. This class of drugs prevents the growth of bacteria and so can be used to treat ⊙ **bacterial infections**.

Sulfonamides were the first group of drugs suitable for ℞ **antimicrobial** use, as relatively safe ℞ **antibacterial** agents. Today, they, along with other similar synthetic classes of chemotherapeutic agents, are commonly referred to as ℞ **antibiotic** drugs, although, strictly speaking, they are not antibiotics (in the literal sense of agents produced by, or obtained from, microorganisms that inhibit the growth of, or destroy, other microorganisms). Their antibacterial action stems from their chemical similarity to a compound required by bacteria to generate the essential growth factor, ℞ **folic acid**. This similarity inhibits the production of folic acid by bacteria (and therefore growth), while the human host is able to utilize folic acid in the diet.

Most sulfonamides are taken by mouth and are rapidly absorbed into the blood. They are short acting and may have to be taken several times a day. Their quick progress through the body and removal in the urine makes them particularly suited for the treatment of urinary infections (since they work within the urine-conducting tubules). One or two sulfonamides are long-acting (and may be used to treat diseases such as ⊙ **malaria** or ⊙ **leprosy**), and another one or two are poorly absorbed (consequently, they were, until recently, used to treat intestinal infections since they are retained within the intestine, where this is the site of the infection, and are not absorbed into the body). The best-known and most-used sulfonamides include sulfadiazine and ℞ **sulfamethoxazole**. A related group is the ℞ **sulfone** drugs.

Limitations

Compared to more recent antibacterial drugs, sulfonamides tend to cause more side effects, particularly nausea, vomiting, diarrhea, and headache, some of which (especially sensitivity reactions) may become serious. Such serious hypersensitivity reactions are more of a risk with the longer-acting sulfonamides, which can accumulate in the body. As a general rule, patients being treated with sulfonamides should try to avoid sunlight. However, the sulfonamides are largely being replaced by newer antibacterials with greater activity, fewer problems with bacterial resistance, and less risk of side effects. These are reserved for certain serious infections, for example, ℞ **trimethoprim and sulfamethoxazole** in combination (co-trimoxazole) is the drug of choice for *Pneumocystis carinii* ⊙ **pneumonia**.

sulfone ⓓ

(sulphone)
Generics: **dapsone**.

Actions and uses

Sulfones are closely related to the sulfonamides. They have similar properties and are used for similar purposes. They have been used successfully in preventing the growth of the bacteria responsible for ⊙ **bacterial infections** causing ⊙ **leprosy**, for *dermatitis herpetiformis*, for ⊙ **protozoal infections** such as preventing ⊙ **malaria** (see ℞ **antimalarial**), ⊙ **Leishmaniasis**, and *Pneumocystis carinii*. They are also used for various other unusual or difficult infections (some of these uses off-label), and also for ⊙ **lupus** erythematosus. The only member of this group that is still commonly used is the valuable drug ℞ **dapsone**.

Limitations

See ℞ **dapsone**.

sulfonylurea ⓓ

Generics: **acetohexamide; chlorpropamide; glipizide; glimepiride; glyburide; tolazamide; tolbutamide**.

Actions and uses

℞ **sulfonylurea** drugs are synthetic agents (originally derived from the sulfonamide chemical group) and are used in ℞ **antidiabetic** treatment as ℞ **oral hypoglycemic** drugs. They are taken by mouth to reduce the levels of glucose (sugar) in the bloodstream. They are primarily used to treat type 2 diabetes mellitus (non-insulin-dependent diabetes mellitus; maturity-onset diabetes). They work by boosting what remains of insulin production in the pancreas and so are useful in treating the form of hyperglycemia that occurs in type 2 diabetes mellitus where there is still some insulin production. They should be used in conjunction with a modified diet. The earlier, first generation, examples are ℞ **chlorpropamide**, ℞ **tolazamide**, ℞ **tolbutamide**, and ℞ **acetohexamide**. Improvements and modifications have led to the development of the second generation drugs ℞ **glipizide**, ℞ **glimepiride**, and ℞ **glyburide**.

Limitations

Oral hypoglycemic drugs are effective in controlling type 2 diabetes mellitus by augmenting what remains of insulin production in the pancreas and must be used as well as appropriate dietary

Key to symbols: ⊙ = Disorder Section ℞ = Drug Section ♣ = Herbal Section ⚬⚬ = Supplement Section changes, exercise, and loss of weight where there is obesity. Short-term use of these drugs may be sufficient while lifestyle changes are made. See also the individual drug entries.

Sulforcin Lotion ®

A preparation of ℞ **sulfur** and ℞ **resorcinol**.
Formulation: Topical lotion.
Availability: OTC.
Warnings and side effects: See ℞ sulfur; ℞ resorcinol.

Sulfoxyl Lotion; Sulfoxyl Lotion Strong ®

A preparation of ℞ **benzoyl peroxide** and ℞ **sulfur**.
Formulation: Topical lotion in two strengths.
Availability: Prescription only.
Warnings and side effects: See ℞ benzoyl peroxide; ℞ sulfur.

sulfur ⑥

(sulphur)
Type/Group: keratolytic.
Brand(s): Acne Lotion 10; Drytex Lotion Cleanser; Ionax Astringent Cleanser Liquimat; Novacet; Pernox Lathering Abradant Scrub; Pernox Scrub for Oily Skin; Seale's Lotion Modified; SasTid Soap; Sulfacet-R; Sulmasque; Sulpho-Lac; Therac; Vanocin; various generic. Combinations: With *benzoyl peroxide*: Sulfoxyl; With *resorcinol*: Acnotex Lotion; Acnomel Cream; Bensulfoid Cream; Sulforcin Lotion; Rezamid Lotion; R/S Lotion.
How administered: Topically (external).

Used to treat

Sulfur is a non-metallic element that is used in creams, ointments, and lotions for treating disorders such as ✪ **acne** and oily skin. It was formerly thought to be active against external parasites and fungal infections of the skin, but these claims seem to have little scientific basis.

Warnings

• It should not be given to people with known hypersensitivity to sulfur products, or to any component of the preparations.
• It should not be used for a longer period or in larger amounts than directed.
• Do not use over large portions of the body or on broken skin.
• Avoid contact with the eyes.

Interactions

• Excessive irritation or inflammation if used with other acne preparations.

Side effects

• Excessive dryness, irritation, rash, and hardening of skin.
• Rarely, allergic reaction.

sulindac ⑥

Type/Group: anti-inflammatory; antirheumatic; non-narcotic analgesic; NSAID; antigout.
Brand(s): Clinoril; various generic.
How administered: Orally.

Used to treat

Sulindac is used to treat pain and inflammation in ✪ **osteoarthritis**, ✪ **rheumatoid arthritis**, ✪ **ankylosing spondylitis**, acute ✪ **gout**, acute painful shoulder (bursitis, tendonitis), and mild to moderate pain and systemic lupus erythematosus (SLE).

Warnings

• It should not be used by people with known hypersensitivity to this drug or to other NSAIDs (including ℞ **aspirin**), who have chronic kidney disease, certain bleeding disorders or conditions (for example, hemophilia, vitamin K deficiency, low blood-platelet levels), or who have a tendency to, or active, peptic ulceration.
• It should be given with caution to people taking certain drugs for gout, who have peripheral edema, diabetes, systemic lupus erythematosus, or allergic disorders (especially asthma and skin conditions), who are elderly, or with any kind of kidney impairment, kidney stones, or certain liver disorders.
• Sulindac should be used during pregnancy only when medically judged to be needed. In the third trimester, its risks rise, and so it should only be used if the benefits outweigh the risks to the fetus, which are at their highest during this time.
• Breast-feeding mothers should either discontinue this drug or stop breast-feeding.
• With regular, long-term use (as in the treatment of osteoarthritis), NSAIDs may cause gastrointestinal bleeding, ulceration, or perforation. Any signs of bleeding (for example, black stools) should be reported to a physician immediately.
• Most NSAIDs have the potential, particularly with regular use, to cause liver damage. Periodic evaluation of liver function is necessary in long-term therapy (more than two months).
• Side effects are more frequent in the elderly.
• Gastrointestinal upsets may be minimized by taking the drug with milk or food.
• Its antirheumatic effect may not be evident for several weeks.

Interactions

• There is generally no added benefit in taking other NSAIDs or other ℞ **salicylates** (especially aspirin) at the same time, but there is a higher risk of gastrointestinal upsets and bleeding.
• Alcohol and ℞ **corticosteroids** increase the risk of bleeding, particularly if there is an existing ulcer.
• ℞ **Anticoagulant**, ℞ **antiplatelet**, and ℞ **thrombolytic** drugs may increase bleeding time.
• The effectiveness of ℞ **ACE inhibitors** and ℞ **diuretics** may be reduced.
• The effects of ℞ **cyclosporine**, ℞ **digoxin**, ℞ **lithium**, and ℞ **methotrexate** may be exaggerated, with potential for toxicity.
• Sulindac should be started at a low dose when used with ℞ **probenecid** for treating gout, because probenecid increases its concentration and effect.
• Dimethylsulfoxide (DMSO) must not be taken with sulindac.
• Foodstuffs and herbals with ℞ **antiplatelet** properties, for example, ♣ ginger, ☙ garlic, and various herbal preparations, may add to the antiplatelet effect of NSAIDs.

Side effects

These vary in severity and how often they occur.
• Commonly, gastrointestinal upsets (though sulindac's risk of gastrointestinal side effects is thought to be lower than that for aspirin), heartburn, diarrhea, constipation, nausea, dizziness, headache, rash, and swelling of the extremities.

• Skin reactions are more common than with many other NSAIDs, and urine may become discolored.
• Less frequently, vomiting, sweating, mouth sores, blurred vision, ringing in the ears, itching drowsiness, depression, and insomnia.
• Prolonged bleeding time (with consequent risk of ulceration) is possible with high dosage, and other blood changes can occur, including anemia.
• Hypersensitivity reactions may include symptoms such as fever, chills, flushing, hives, rash, chest tightness, asthma, or bronchospasm.
• Reversible kidney failure, particularly in renal impairment, has occurred. Liver damage is rare.

Sulmasque ®

A preparation of ℞ **sulfur**.
Formulation: Topical mask.
Availability: OTC.
Warnings and side effects: See ℞ **sulfur**.

sulphadiazine ©

see ℞ **sulfadiazine**.

sulphinpyrazone ©

see ℞ **sulfinpyrazone**.

Sulpho-Lac; Sulpho-Lac Acne Medication ®

A preparation of ℞ **sulfur**.
Formulation: Topical cream (Acne Medication); soap.
Availability: OTC.
Warnings and side effects: See ℞ **sulfur**.

sulphonamide ℗

see ℞ **sulfonamide**.

sulphone ℗

see ℞ **sulfone**.

sulphonylurea ℗

see ℞ **sulfonylurea**.

sulphur ©

see ℞ **sulfur**.

Sulster ®

A preparation of ℞ **prednisolone**, sodium phosphate and sodium sulfacemide.
Formulation: Eye drops.
Availability: Prescription only.
Warnings and side effects: See ℞ **prednisolone**; ℞ **sulfacetamide**.

Sultrin ®

A preparation of ℞ **triple sulfa cream**.
Formulation: Topical cream.

Availability: Prescription only.
Warnings and side effects: See ℞ **triple sulfa cream**.

sumatriptan succinate ©

Type/Group: **serotonin-receptor stimulant; vasoconstrictor; antimigraine**.
Brand(s): **Imitrex Tablets, Nasal Spray, Injection**.
How administered: Orally; nasal spray; injection.

Used to treat

This is a recently introduced drug which is used to treat acute ✪ **migraine** attacks (but not to prevent attacks). It works as a ℞ **vasoconstrictor** (through acting as a serotonin receptor stimulant selective for serotonin 5-HT$_1$ receptors), producing a rapid narrowing of blood vessels surrounding the brain. It is also used for ✪ **cluster headache**.

Warnings

• Avoid its use in people with known hypersensitivity to this drug or who have certain cardiovascular disorders, such as pre-existing heart diseases, including ischemic heart disease, previous myocardial infarction (heart attack), coronary vasospasm, including some types of angina, or with uncontrolled hypertension.
• This drug should not be used by those with a form of migraine in which one half of the body experiences some degree of paralysis during the migraine attack.
• Drugs of this class (that is, those stimulating serotonin 5-HT$_1$ receptors) are used only with great caution where risk factors are present that predispose to coronary artery disease. They should be used with care in those with impaired liver or kidney function.
• Sumatriptan succinate should be used in pregnancy only if the potential benefits outweigh the potential risks to the fetus.
• Medical judgment of risk is also required for breast-feeding mothers.
• It is recommended that first-time administration of sumatriptan to anyone with significant risk factors for coronary artery disease takes place at a physician's office or other medical facility.
• This drug should not be used at the same time, or shortly after using ℞ **ergotamine** or other migraine therapies. Ergotamine-like antimigraine drugs should not be taken until six hours after this type of antimigraine drug; and this type of antimigraine drug should not be taken until at least 24 hours after an ergotamine-like antimigraine drug.
• The dose should not usually be repeated during the same migraine attack.
• Sumatriptan may cause drowsiness and so impair the performance of skilled tasks, such as driving.

Interactions

• There is a risk of additive effect, with potentially serious consequences, if taken with ℞ **ergotamine**-containing drugs (such as ℞ **dihydroergotamine** or ℞ **methysergide**).
• Sumatriptan should not be taken orally with ℞ **MAOI** antidepressants or within two weeks of discontinuing their use. MAOIs increase the concentration of sumatriptan, and so there is a higher risk of side effects (some serious). If injected subcutaneously (under the skin), the risk of side effects may be

lower, though sumatriptan dosage must be reduced; caution and monitoring are necessary.

• ℞ **SSRI** depressants (such as, ℞ **fluoxetine**, ℞ **fluvoxamine**, ℞ **paroxetine**, ℞ **sertraline**) may increase the risk of some rarer side effects, such as weakness and incoordination, occurring.

• ♣ **St. John's wort** should not be used at the same time as there is an increased risk of adverse effects.

Side effects

• Chest pain and tightness in parts of the body, including the chest, jaw, or throat, which may indicate constriction of the blood vessels of the heart (or of anaphylaxis). If the pain is intense, use of sumatriptan should stop;

• There may be sensations of tingling, heaviness, pressure, heat, flushing, dizziness, a feeling of weakness, drowsiness, and fatigue, changes in liver function, nausea and vomiting;

• Sumatriptan may cause transient increase in blood pressure, hypotension (low blood pressure), slowing or speeding of the heart; also, seizures have been reported.

Summit Extra Strength Caplets   Ⓑ

A preparation of ℞ **acetaminophen**, ℞ **aspirin**, and ℞ **caffeine**.
Formulation: Oral tablets.
Availability: OTC.
Warnings and side effects: See ℞ **acetaminophen**; ℞ **aspirin**; ℞ **caffeine**.

Sumycin   Ⓑ

A preparation of ℞ **tetracycline hydrochloride**.
Formulation: Oral capsules in several strengths; syrup; oral tablets.
Availability: Prescription only.
Warnings and side effects: See ℞ **tetracycline hydrochloride**.

sunscreen   Ⓓ

Generics: **aminobenzoic acid (PABA); cinnamates; titanium dioxide.**

Actions and uses

Sunscreen preparations are creams and lotions that contain chemical agents which partly block the passage of ultraviolet radiation from the sun, and in certain radiation therapies, to the skin. Ultraviolet radiation harms the skin and worsens many skin conditions. It can be divided into two wavelength bands: UVB causes sunburn and contributes to skin cancer and ageing; UVA causes problems by sensitizing the skin to certain drugs and, in the long term, may contribute to skin cancers.

A number of substances, including the ℞ **cinnamates** and ℞ **aminobenzoic acid** (PABA), provide protection against UVB, but are less effective against UVA. Some preparations also contain substances, such as ℞ **titanium dioxide**, which are reflective and provide some protection against UVA. The sun-protection factor, or SPF, of a preparation indicates the degree of protection against burning by UVB. For example, an SPF of 4 allows a person to stay in the sun four times longer than an unprotected person without burning. Examples of preparations are ℞ **Bullfrog Sunblock**, ℞ **Coppertone Oil Free**, ℞ **Coppertone Shade Sunblock**, ℞ **Hawaiian Tropic Baby Faces Sunblock**, ℞ **Neutrogena Chem-**ical-Free Sunblocker, ℞ **Neutrogena Sunblock Stick**, ℞ **Original Eclipse Sunscreen**, ℞ **PreSun Ultra**, ℞ **TI-Screen; TI-Screen Natural; TI-Baby Natural**, ℞ **Vaseline Intensive Care Baby Sunblock**, ℞ **Vaseline Intensive Care Moisturizing Sunblock**.

Limitations

See the individual drug entries.

Suppress   Ⓑ

A preparation of ℞ **dextromethorphan**.
Formulation: Lozenges.
Availability: OTC.
Warnings and side effects: See ℞ **dextromethorphan**.

Suprax   Ⓑ

A preparation of ℞ **cefixime**.
Formulation: Oral tablets, oral suspension.
Availability: Prescription only.
Warnings and side effects: See ℞ **cefixime**.

surfactant   Ⓓ

Generics: **docusate sodium; poloxamer 188; sodium lauryl sulfate.**

Actions and uses

Surfactants have a detergent action that lowers surface tension so allowing wetting. Sometimes they are put into preparations simply to improve the physical properties of the preparations. Some are incorporated because, in themselves, they are necessary for the actions of the drug preparation, for instance in shampoos, enemas, and skin preparations. The agent ℞ **docusate sodium** is used in OTC laxative preparations to which it gives stimulant and stool softener properties and is of value for ✪ **constipation**. ℞ **sodium lauryl sulfate** is incorporated into the formulation of a number of skin preparations and shampoos, and ℞ **poloxamer 188** is used as a surfactant wetting agent as a constituent of some ophthalmic (eye) preparations.

Limitations

See the individual drug entries.

Surmontil   Ⓑ

A preparation of ℞ **trimipramine hydrochloride**.
Formulation: Oral capsules in several strengths.
Availability: Prescription only.
Warnings and side effects: See ℞ **trimipramine hydrochloride**.

Sus-Phrine   Ⓑ

A preparation of ℞ **epinephrine**.
Formulation: Injection.
Availability: Prescription only.
Warnings and side effects: See ℞ **epinephrine**.

Sustaire   Ⓑ

A preparation of ℞ **theophylline**.
Formulation: Oral tablets, sustained release, in several strengths.
Availability: Prescription only.
Warnings and side effects: See ℞ **theophylline**.

Sustiva ®

A preparation of ℞ **efavirenz**.
Formulation: Oral capsules in several strengths.
Availability: Prescription only.
Warnings and side effects: See ℞ **efavirenz**.

SUTUSS Elixir ®

A preparation of ℞ **hydrocodone bitartrate**,
℞ **pseudoephedrine**, and ℞ **guaifenesin**.
Formulation: Oral liquid.
Availability: Prescription only.
Warnings and side effects: See ℞ **hydrocodone bitartrate**;
℞ **pseudoephedrine**; ℞ **guaifenesin**.

suxamethonium chloride ⒢

see ℞ **succinylcholine chloride**.

Syllact ®

A preparation of ℞ **psyllium**.
Formulation: Oral powder.
Availability: OTC.
Warnings and side effects: See ℞ **psyllium**.

Symmetrel ®

A preparation of ℞ **amantadine**.
Formulation: Oral syrup.
Availability: Prescription only.
Warnings and side effects: See ℞ **amantadine**.

sympathetic nervous system inhibitor ⒟

see ℞ **antisympathetic**.

sympatholytic ⒟

Actions and uses

Sympatholytic means an action antagonistic to, or against, sympathetic nervous system effects, including actions of the sympathetic neurotransmitters and hormones, epinephrine and norepinephrine, and agents that mimic them. So, taken literally, it can be applied to a number of drugs classes, including ℞ **alpha-adrenergic blocker**, ℞ **beta-blocker**, and ℞ **antisympathetic** drugs.

Limitations

See the individual drug type/group entries.

sympathomimetic ⒟

Generics: **albuterol; amphetamine sulfate; bitolterol mesylate; dextroamphetamine; ephedrine; isoetharine; isoproterenol; levalbuterol hydrochloride; metaproterenol; metaraminol; methamphetamine; methylphenidate; midodrine hydrochloride; naphazoline hydrochloride; oxymetazoline hydrochloride; phendimetrazine; phentermine; phenylephrine hydrochloride; pirbuterol; pseudoephedrine; ritodrine hydrochloride; salmeterol; terbutaline sulfate; tetrahydrozoline hydrochloride**.

Actions and uses

Sympathomimetic drugs have effects that mimic those of the sympathetic nervous system, mimicking the natural actions of norepinephrine and epinephrine acting as neurotransmitter and hormone, respectively. There are two main types (although several sympathomimetics belong to both types).

First, the ℞ **alpha-adrenergic stimulant** drugs (including ℞ **phenylephrine hydrochloride**, ℞ **metaraminol**, ℞ **methoxamine hydrochloride**, ℞ **midodrine**, ℞ **naphazoline hydrochloride**, ℞ **oxymetazoline hydrochloride**, ℞ **xylometazoline hydrochloride**, and ℞ **tetrahydrozoline hydrochloride**) which are ℞ **vasoconstrictor** agents (narrow blood vessels) and are used particularly in nasal decongestants and preparations for relieving cold symptoms.

Second, the ℞ **beta-adrenergic stimulant** drugs (including ℞ **albuterol**, ℞ **levalbuterol**, ℞ **metaproterenol**, ℞ **salmeterol**, ℞ **terbutaline sulfate**, ℞ **isoproterenol**, ℞ **bitolterol mesylate**, ℞ **isoetharine**, ℞ **pirbuterol**, ℞ **ritodrine hydrochloride**) most of which are widely used as ℞ **bronchodilator** drugs, particularly in ℞ **antiasthmatic** treatment and some also as ℞ **cardiac stimulant** agents.

A distinction may be made between the *direct sympathomimetics* such as those examples given above, which achieve selectivity of action within the body by only acting at one receptor type, as compared to the *indirect sympathomimetics* (for example, ℞ **ephedrine** and ℞ **pseudoephedrine**) which work by releasing norepinephrine and epinephrine from nerves of the sympathetic nervous system and adrenal medulla, and consequently show no selectivity of action, which is a disadvantage.

Some agents act to release norepinephrine within the central nervous system (CNS), including ℞ **amphetamine**, ℞ **methamphetamine**, ℞ **dextroamphetamine**, ℞ **phendimetrazine**, ℞ **phentermine**, ℞ **methylphenidate** and related ℞ **CNS stimulant** and ℞ **appetite suppressant** drugs.

Limitations

See the individual drug entries.

Synacol CF Tablets ®

A preparation of ℞ **dextromethorphan** and ℞ **guaifenesin**.
Formulation: Oral tablets.
Availability: OTC.
Warnings and side effects: See ℞ **dextromethorphan**;
℞ **guaifenesin**.

Synacort ®

A preparation of ℞ **hydrocortisone**.
Formulation: Cream in several strengths.
Availability: Prescription only.
Warnings and side effects: See ℞ **hydrocortisone**.

Synagis ®

A preparation of ℞ **palivizumab**.
Formulation: Injection (intramuscular).
Availability: Prescription only.
Warnings and side effects: See ℞ **palivizumab**.

Key to symbols: ⊙ = Disorder Section ℞ = Drug Section ♣ = Herbal Section ⚕ = Supplement Section

Synalar; Synalar-HP Ⓑ

A preparation of ℞ **fluocinolone acetonide**.
Formulation: Cream in several strengths; ointment. Synalar-HP is a cream.
Availability: Prescription only.
Warnings and side effects: See ℞ **fluocinolone acetonide**.

Synarel Ⓑ

A preparation of ℞ **nafarelin acetate**.
Formulation: Nasal spray.
Availability: Prescription only.
Warnings and side effects: See ℞ **nafarelin acetate**.

Synercid Ⓑ

A preparation of ℞ **quinupristin-dalfopristin**.
Formulation: Injection.
Availability: Prescription only.
Warnings and side effects: See ℞ **quinupristin-dalfopristin**.

Synophylate-GG Syrup Ⓑ

A preparation of ℞ **guaifenesin** and ℞ **theophylline**.
Formulation: Oral syrup.
Availability: Prescription only.
Warnings and side effects: See ℞ **guaifenesin**; ℞ **theophylline**.

Syn-Rx Tablets Ⓑ

A preparation of ℞ **pseudoephedrine** and ℞ **guaifenesin**.
Formulation: Oral tablets.
Availability: Prescription only.
Warnings and side effects: See ℞ **pseudoephedrine**; ℞ **guaifenesin**.

Syntocinon Ⓑ

A preparation of ℞ **oxytocin**.
Formulation: Injection.
Availability: Prescription only.
Warnings and side effects: See ℞ **oxytocin**.

Syprine Ⓑ

A preparation of ℞ **trientine hydrochloride**.
Formulation: Oral capsules.
Availability: Prescription only.
Warnings and side effects: See ℞ **trientine hydrochloride**.

Tac-3; Tac-40 Ⓑ

A preparation of ℞ **triamcinolone** acetate.
Formulation: Suspension for injection. (Tac-3 and Tac-40 contain different amounts of drug).
Availability: Prescription only.
Warnings and side effects: See ℞ **triamcinolone**.

tacrine hydrochloride Ⓖ

(tetrahydroaminoacridine; THA)
Type/Group: dementia treatment; anticholinesterase.
Brand(s): Cognex.

How administered: Orally.

Used to treat

Tacrine is used to treat mild to moderate dementia of the Alzheimer's type. It is a centrally acting cholinesterase inhibitor that is thought to alleviate a deficiency in acetylcholine levels caused by destruction of cholinergic neurons, which are the first to be affected by ⊙ **Alzheimer's disease**.

Warnings

• It should not be used by people with known hypersensitivity to cholinergics, who are currently using other cholinesterase inhibitors, or with severe, active liver disease (not to be used if jaundice occurs), active, untreated gastric or duodenal ulcers, or mechanical obstruction of the intestine or urinary tract.

• It should be given with caution to anyone with liver dysfunction, asthma, chronic obstructive pulmonary disease (COPD), seizure disorder, bradycardia and other heart disorders, hyperthyroidism, heart arrythmias, a history of gastrointestinal ulcers, or active alcoholism.

• It is not known whether or not tacrine can harm the fetus, therefore, it should be used during pregnancy only if medically judged to be essential.

• Medical judgment is also required if breast-feeding is being considered, as it is not known whether it is excreted in breast milk.

• Overdose can cause a cholinergic crisis, which is characterized by severe nausea, vomiting, salivation, sweating, bradycardia, hypotension, collapse, and convulsions.

• Tacrine can have adverse effects on the liver (monitoring may be required).

• Smoking markedly lowers levels of tacrine.

• Discontinuation of treatment should be gradual.

Interactions

• Concentration of ℞ **theophylline** may increase.

• ℞ **cimetidine** may increase concentrations of tacrine.

• Tacrine may interfere with the effects of ℞ **anticholinergics**.

• The effects of ℞ **NSAIDs** may be increased.

Side effects

• Frequently, nausea, vomiting, headache, gastrointestinal upset, and dizziness.

• Occasionally, fatigue, chest pain, confusion, agitation, rash, depression, muscular incoordination, insomnia, nasal infections, and liver damage.

• Because it acts to increase cholinergic activity, ulcers or other gastrointestinal symptoms may develop, and heart rate may be affected.

tacrolimus Ⓖ

Type/Group: immunosuppressant; antibiotic.
Brand(s): Prograf.
How administered: Orally; intravenous infusion.

Used to treat

Tacrolimus is chemically an ℞ **antibiotic** related to the ℞ **macrolide** family (although this does not relate to its use). It is used particularly to limit tissue rejection during and following organ transplant surgery (particularly of the liver).

Warnings

• It should not be given to people with known hypersensitivity to this drug (or other ingredients in the injection).

• It should be used with caution in people with kidney or liver impairment. This is a specialist drug and is used only after a full medical assessment.

• It is thought that tacrolimus may have the potential for harming the fetus and so it should be used in pregnancy only when the potential benefits outweigh the possible risk to the fetus.

• Medical judgment is required if breast-feeding is being considered.

• Tacrolimus is prescribed only by physicians experienced in immunosuppressive therapy and in settings adequately equipped to monitor and manage the effects of treatment. (Regular monitoring of kidney function and potassium levels is necessary, as well as periodic checks of blood values and other signs.)

• Treatment with tacrolimus inevitably leaves the body vulnerable to infection, and there may be a higher vulnerability to certain cancers.

• People taking tacrolimus should minimize their exposure to the sun.

Interactions

• ℞ **Aminoglycosides** (for example, ℞ **gentamicin**, ℞ **tobramycin**), ℞ **amiodarone hydrochloride**, ℞ **amphotericin B**, ℞ **androgens**, ℞ **azoles** (antifungals), ℞ **bromocriptine**, ℞ **calcium-channel blockers**, ℞ **cimetidine**, ℞ **cisplatin**, ℞ **colchicine**, ℞ **cyclosporine**, ℞ **diclofenac**, ℞ **foscarnet**, ℞ **macrolide**, antibiotics, ℞ **melphalan**, ℞ **methylprednisolone**, ℞ **metoclopramide**, ℞ **naproxen**, protease inhibitors (for example, ℞ **indinavir**, ℞ **ritonavir** ℞ **saquinavir**), ℞ **ranitidine hydrochloride**, ℞ **sulindac**, and ℞ **vancomycin** may raise tacrolimus levels or intensify its effects, with a higher potential for toxicity (particularly with potential for kidney damage).

• Potassium-sparing ℞ **diuretics** (for example, ℞ **amiloride**, ℞ **spironolactone**, ℞ **triamterene**) may cause a serious elevation of potassium (hyperkalemia) and these drugs should not be used with tacrolimus.

• Other immunosuppressants (but not corticosteroids) increase the risk of infections, or lymphoma and other neoplasms (tumors).

• Live ℞ **vaccines** should not be given during treatment with tacrolimus.

• ℞ **Anticonvulsants** (for example, ℞ **carbamazepine**, ℞ **phenobarbital**, ℞ **phenytoin**), ℞ **rifampin**, and ℞ **rifabutin** may decrease levels or the effectiveness of tacrolimus.

• Grapefruit juice may increase levels of tacrolimus, with potentially toxic effects.

Side effects

These depend on the use and how it is administered, and include:

• Dangerous kidney effects (nephrotoxicity), also hypoglycemia, tremor, headache, diarrhea, hypertension, or nausea.

• Less frequently, chest pain, heart disturbances, agitation, anxiety, hair loss or excessive hair growth, jaundice, joint pain, and tingling sensations in the hands and feet.

• This drug commonly has adverse effects on kidney function, changes in various blood values and liver function. Anaphylactic reactions are rare.

Tagamet ®

A preparation of ℞ **cimetidine**.
Formulation: Oral tablets, available in 4 strengths; liquid; injection.
Availability: Prescription only.
Warnings and side effects: See ℞ **cimetidine**.

Talacen ®

A preparation of ℞ **pentazocine** and ℞ **acetaminophen**.
Formulation: Oral tablets.
Availability: Prescription only.
Warnings and side effects: See ℞ **pentazocine**; ℞ **acetaminophen**.

Talwin ®

A preparation of ℞ **pentazocine**.
Formulation: Injection.
Availability: Prescription only.
Warnings and side effects: See ℞ **pentazocine**.

Talwin Compound ®

A preparation of ℞ **pentazocine** and ℞ **aspirin**.
Formulation: Oral tablets.
Availability: Prescription only.
Warnings and side effects: See ℞ **pentazocine**; ℞ **aspirin**.

Talwin NX ®

A preparation of ℞ **pentazocine** and ℞ **naloxone hydrochloride**.
Formulation: Oral tablets.
Availability: Prescription only.
Warnings and side effects: See ℞ **pentazocine**; ℞ **naloxone hydrochloride**.

Tambocor ®

A preparation of ℞ **flecainide acetate**.
Formulation: Oral tablets, available in 3 strengths.
Availability: Prescription only.
Warnings and side effects: See ℞ **flecainide acetate**.

tamoxifen ⓖ

Type/Group: **antiestrogen; anticancer**.
Brand(s): Nolvadex; generic.
How administered: Orally.

Used to treat

Tamoxifen is a ℞ **sex hormone** antagonist, an ℞ **antiestrogen**, that antagonizes the natural estrogen present in the body. It is used in the treatment of ✪ **breast cancer** in women following, for example, total mastectomy, and of metastatic breast cancer in women and men. It is also prescribed to reduce the incidence of breast cancer in women at high risk for such cancer.

Key to symbols: ✪ = Disorder Section ℞ = Drug Section ♣ = Herbal Section ♓ = Supplement Section

Warnings

• It should not be used by people with known hypersensitivity to this drug, or who must take coumarin-type anticoagulant therapy.

• It should be given with caution to people with low white blood-cell counts or blood-clotting disorders, cataracts, liver disease, undiagnosed vaginal bleeding, or hypercalcemia. Women with a history of deep vein thrombosis or pulmonary embolus should not take the drug for reduction in breast cancer incidence.

• Tamoxifen should not be used during pregnancy. A doctor must be contacted if pregnancy occurs while taking this drug.

• It should not be used by breast-feeding mothers.

• Premenopausal women should use nonhormonal contraception during treatment.

• Visual disturbances, including corneal opacity, lesions of the eye, disease of the retina, and decreased color perception have occurred.

• It may aggravate bone disease at the beginning of treatment.

• It may cause changes in liver function, which, rarely, may become serious.

• Increases the incidence of endometrial cancer. Abnormal vaginal bleeding must be reported to a doctor, and regular gynecological examinations must be made during and after treatment.

Interactions

• The effects of ℞ **anticoagulants** may be increased by tamoxifen.

• ℞ **Bromocriptine** may increase the levels of tamoxifen.

• ℞ **Cytotoxic** agents increase the risk of blood clots.

Side effects

• Hot flashes, nausea, vomiting, and lightheadedness.

• Less frequently, vaginal bleeding or discharge, depression, menstrual irregularities, and skin rash.

• Rare but serious side effects include deep vein thrombosis, low white blood-cell counts, blood-clotting disorders, and pulmonary embolism.

tamsulosin hydrochloride Ⓖ

Type/Group: **alpha-adrenergic blocker.**
Brand(s): Flomax.
How administered: Orally.

Used to treat

Tamsulosin hydrochloride is used in prostate treatment to treat urinary retention in ✪ **benign prostatic hyperplasia** (BPH).

Warnings

• It should not be given to people with known hypersensitivity to this drug, or with severely impaired liver function.

• This drug is not intended for use by women.

• Postural hypotension (for example, dizziness when arising from a sitting position) and fainting, although uncommon, may occur. During initial dosing, it is helpful to identify situations in which injury could result if fainting does occur.

• Because of possible sedative side effects, caution is advised for potentially hazardous activities, such as driving, that require mental alertness.

Interactions

• Tamsulosin should not be used with other alpha-adrenergic blockers because effects are expected but have not yet been studied.

• The levels and effects of tamsulosin may be increased when used with ℞ **cimetidine**.

• It should be used with caution with ℞ **warfarin sodium**.

Side effects

• These may include abnormal ejaculation, upper respiratory congestion (for example, rhinitis, sinusitis, cough), dizziness, drowsiness, muscular weakness, or back pain.

• Less frequently, there may be insomnia, blurred vision, chest pain, or infection. Fainting is rare.

• Rarely, priapism (prolonged and painful erection) has been reported, which must be treated promptly or permanent dysfunction may result.

Tanac Ⓑ

A preparation of ℞ **benzocaine** and benzalkonium chloride.
Formulation: Liquid.
Availability: OTC.
Warnings and side effects: See ℞ **benzocaine**.

Tanafed Suspension Ⓑ

A preparation of pseudoephedrine tannate and chlorpheniramine tannate.
Formulation: Oral liquid.
Availability: Prescription only.
Warnings and side effects: See ℞ **pseudoephedrine**; ℞ **chlorpheniramine maleate**.

tannic acid Ⓖ

Type/Group: **astringent.**
Brand(s): Zilactin Medicated Gel.
How administered: Topically (external).

Used to treat

Tannic acid can be used to relieve the pain or itching of ✪ **cold sores** or fever blisters, especially in and around the mouth. It quickly forms a film over sores, which protects the area from foods and drink.

Warnings

• There are no limitations in normal use.

• It is considered safe for use during pregnancy when used as directed.

• A doctor must be consulted and the use of tannic acid stopped if infection lasts for longer than 10 days.

• Tannic acid should not be used in or around the eyes.

Interactions

No interactions are known.

Side effects

• There may be a brief stinging sensation when it is applied to an open sore.

Tapanol Regular Strength Tablets; Extra Strength Tablets ®

A preparation of ℞ **acetaminophen**.
Formulation: Oral tablets; gelcaps.
Availability: OTC.
Warnings and side effects: See ℞ **acetaminophen**.

Tapazole ®

A preparation of ℞ **methimazole**.
Formulation: Tablets.
Availability: Prescription only.
Warnings and side effects: See ℞ **methimazole**.

Tarabine PFS ®

A preparation of ℞ **cytarabine**.
Formulation: Powder or vial for injection.
Availability: Prescription only.
Warnings and side effects: See ℞ **cytarabine**.

Taraphilic ®

A preparation of ℞ **coal tar**.
Formulation: Shampoo.
Availability: OTC.
Warnings and side effects: See ℞ **coal tar**.

Tarka Tablets ®

A preparation of ℞ **trandolapril** and ℞ **verapamil hydrochloride**.
Formulation: Oral tablets, available in 4 (trandolapril/verapamil) strengths.
Availability: Prescription only.
Warnings and side effects: See ℞ **trandolapril**; ℞ **verapamil hydrochloride**.

Tarsum ®

A preparation of ℞ **salicylic acid** and ℞ **coal tar**.
Formulation: Shampoo.
Availability: OTC.
Warnings and side effects: See ℞ **salicylic acid**; ℞ **coal tar**.

Tasmar ®

A preparation of ℞ **tolcapone**.
Formulation: Oral tablets.
Availability: Prescription only.
Warnings and side effects: See ℞ **tolcapone**.

Tavist Tablets; Syrup ®

A preparation of ℞ **clemastine**.
Formulation: Oral syrup; tablets.
Availability: Prescription only.
Warnings and side effects: See ℞ **clemastine**.

Taxol ®

A preparation of ℞ **paclitaxel**.
Formulation: Injection.
Availability: Prescription only.

Warnings and side effects: See ℞ **paclitaxel**.

Taxotere ®

A preparation of ℞ **docetaxel**.
Formulation: Injection.
Availability: Prescription only.
Warnings and side effects: See ℞ **docetaxel**.

tazarotene ⑥

Type/Group: **retinoid; acne treatment; psoriasis treatment**.
How administered: Topically (external).
Brand(s): Differin; Tazorac.

Used to treat

Tazarotene is used for ✪ **psoriasis** and ✪ **acne**. It is chemically a retinoid (a derivative of retinol, or ⚏ **vitamin A**).

Warnings

• It should not be given to people with known hypersensitivity to this drug.
• It should not be used during pregnancy. Consult your doctor if pregnancy is suspected when taking tazarotene.
• Medical judgment is required if breast-feeding is being considered. It is not known whether it appears in breast milk.
• Application to sunburned, eczematous or broken skin, or to mucous membranes must be avoided.
• It should not be used on severe acne or over large areas.
• Ultraviolet light should be avoided.

Interactions

• Skin irritation is more likely if tazarotene is used with other topical preparations such as alcohol, ℞ **astringents**, ℞ **resorcinol**, ℞ **salicylic acid**, strong soaps, or products containing ℞ **sulfur**.

Side effects

• There may be skin irritation and other skin reactions.

Tazicef ®

A preparation of ℞ **ceftazidime**.
Formulation: Injection.
Availability: Prescription only.
Warnings and side effects: See ℞ **ceftazidime**.

Tazidime ®

A preparation of ℞ **ceftazidime**.
Formulation: Injection.
Availability: Prescription only.
Warnings and side effects: See ℞ **ceftazidime**.

tazobactam ⑥

Type/Group: **penicillinase inhibitor**.
Brand(s): Combinations: With *piperacillin*: Zosyn.
How administered: Injection; intravenous infusion.

Used to treat

Tazobactam is used as a penicillinase inhibitor to combat bacterial resistance to penicillin. It works as an enzyme inhibitor by inhibiting the penicillinase enzymes ("beta-lactamases") that are produced by some bacteria. These enzymes can inactivate many antibiotics of

Key to symbols: ✪ = Disorder Section ℞ = Drug Section ♣ = Herbal Section ⚏ = Supplement Section

the penicillin family. It is only used combined with the (penicillin) antibiotic ℞ **piperacillin**.

Warnings

There are no contraindications for tazobactam. There is no information on the effects of tazobactam in pregnancy or breast-feeding.

Interactions

There are no reported interactions attributed to tazobactam.

Side effects

Any side effects from the combination are attributed to piperacillin.

Tazorac ⑧

A preparation of ℞ **tazarotene**.
Formulation: Topical gel.
Availability: Prescription only.
Warnings and side effects: See ℞ **tazarotene**.

TB treatment ⑩

see ℞ **antituberculosis**.

Tear Guard ⑧

A preparation of ℞ **hydroxyethylcellulose**.
Formulation: Ophthalmic solution.
Availability: OTC.
Warnings and side effects: See ℞ **hydroxyethylcellulose**.

Tears Naturale ⑧

A preparation of ℞ **hydroxypropyl methylcellulose**.
Formulation: Ophthalmic solution.
Availability: OTC.
Warnings and side effects: See ℞ **hydroxypropyl methylcellulose**.

Tears Plus ⑧

A preparation of ℞ **polyvinyl alcohol** and ℞ **povidone**.
Formulation: Ophthalmic solution.
Availability: OTC.
Warnings and side effects: See ℞ **polyvinyl alcohol**; ℞ **povidone**.

Tebamide Adult Suppositories; Pediatric Suppositories ⑧

A preparation of ℞ **trimethobenzamide hydrochloride**.
Formulation: Rectal suppositories.
Availability: Prescription only.
Warnings and side effects: See ℞ **trimethobenzamide hydrochloride**.

Tedrigen Tablets ⑧

A preparation of ℞ **ephedrine**, ℞ **theophylline**, and ℞ **phenobarbital**.
Formulation: Oral tablets.
Availability: OTC.
Warnings and side effects: See ℞ **ephedrine**; ℞ **theophylline**; ℞ **phenobarbital**.

Tegretol Tablets; Tegretol-XR; Suspension ⑧

A preparation of ℞ **carbamazepine**.
Formulation: Oral liquid; tablets (2 strengths); XR is extended release tablet (3 strengths).
Availability: Prescription only.
Warnings and side effects: See ℞ **carbamazepine**.

Tegrin-HC ⑧

A preparation of ℞ **hydrocortisone**.
Formulation: Ointment.
Availability: OTC.
Warnings and side effects: See ℞ **hydrocortisone**.

Tegrin-LT ⑧

A preparation of ℞ **pyrethrin**.
Formulation: Shampoo.
Availability: OTC.
Warnings and side effects: See ℞ **pyrethrin**.

Tegrin Medicated Shampoo; Tegrin Advanced Formula Shampoo ⑧

A preparation of ℞ **coal tar**.
Formulation: Shampoo; cream; soap.
Availability: OTC.
Warnings and side effects: See ℞ **coal tar**.

telmisartan ⑥

Type/Group: **angiotensin-receptor blocker; antihypertensive; vasodilator**.
Brand(s): Micardis.
How administered: Orally.

Used to treat

Telmisartan is an angiotensin II receptor (AT1 receptors) blocker. Angiotensin II is a circulating hormone that is a powerful vasoconstrictor (narrows blood vessels) and blocking it leads to a fall in blood pressure. Telmisartan can be used alone or with other drugs to treat high blood pressure (see ❍ **hypertension**).

Warnings

• It should not be given to people with known hypersensitivity to this drug.
• It should be given with caution to people with severe congestive heart failure, with biliary obstruction, impaired liver function, severe kidney insufficiency, or renal stenosis. Any fluid- or salt-depleted condition (as from diuretic use) should be corrected before using this drug.
• Risk in pregnancy increases substantially from the first through to the second and third trimesters. Angiotensin-receptor blockers can cause injury to the fetus. Use of these drugs should be stopped as soon as pregnancy is detected.
• Medical judgment is required if breast-feeding is being considered.
• Blood pressure should be checked regularly.

Interactions

• The concentrations and effects of ℞ **digoxin** may be increased.

Side effects

• Angiotensin-receptor blockers in general appear to cause few and infrequent side effects (often indistinguishable from placebo effects). The most common, with telmisartan, may include back pain, and upper respiratory tract symptoms or infection.
• Uncommonly, gastrointestinal disturbances, headache, dizziness, fatigue, chest pain, or edema.
• Rarely, insomnia, rash, allergy, and effects on heart rhythm. There may be changes in kidney function and angioedema (an allergic swelling reaction, often of the face) has been reported.

temazepam Ⓖ

Type/Group: **hypnotic; benzodiazepine.**
Brand(s): Restoril.
How administered: Orally.

Used to treat

Temazepam is used as a relatively short-acting hypnotic for the short-term treatment of ✪ **insomnia.**

Warnings

• It should not be given to people with known hypersensitivity to benzodiazepines.
• It should be given with caution to people with kidney or liver impairment, anemia, depression, psychosis, acute narrow-angle glaucoma, seizure disorders, lung disease, a history of drug abuse, or anyone over 65.
• Temazepam should not be used during pregnancy. A doctor must be consulted if pregnancy occurs while taking this drug.
• It should not be used by nursing mothers.
• It may cause drowsiness the day following use, which may impair the performance of skilled tasks, such as driving.
• Avoid alcohol consumption, because adverse side effects may be increased.
• Avoid other psychotropic medications unless prescribed by a doctor.
• A doctor must be consulted before stopping use or increasing dosage, because benzodiazepines may produce psychological and physical dependence and withdrawal symptoms.

Interactions

• ℞ **azole** antifungals (for example, ℞ **ketoconazole,** ℞ **itraconazole**), ℞ **beta-blockers** (for example, ℞ **propranolol**), ℞ **cimetidine,** ℞ **disulfiram,** ℞ **isoniazid,** ℞ **macrolide** antibiotics (for example, ℞ **erythromycin,** ℞ **clarithromycin,** troleandomycin), and ℞ **omeprazole,** and ℞ **SSRIs** may increase levels of temazepam.
• If used with ℞ **clozapine,** there is possibly an increased risk of cardiorespiratory collapse.
• Isolated cases of respiratory depression and stupor have been reported when used with ℞ **loxapine,** although the role of drug interaction is not established.
• ℞ **Rifampin** may reduce the effects of temazepam.
• Alcohol may increase adverse effects.

Side effects

• Daytime sedation, drowsiness, and lethargy.

• Less frequently, anxiety, confusion, dizziness, headache, rebound insomnia, chest pain, low blood pressure, speeded heartbeat, gastrointestinal effects, and sleep apnea.
• Rare but serious side effects include respiratory depression and blood cell disorders.

Temodar Ⓡ

A preparation of ℞ **temozolomide.**
Formulation: Oral capsules in several strengths.
Availability: Prescription only.
Warnings and side effects: See ℞ **temozolomide.**

Temovate Ⓡ

A preparation of ℞ **clobetasol propionate.**
Formulation: Cream; ointment; gel; scalp application.
Availability: Prescription only.
Warnings and side effects: See ℞ **clobetasol propionate.**

temozolomide Ⓖ

Type/Group: **anticancer; cytotoxic.**
Brand(s): Oral.
How administered: Orally.

Used to treat

Temozolomide is a recently introduced drug that can be used in second-line treatment of certain refractory ✪ **cancers** (anaplastic astrocytoma).

Warnings

• It should not be given to people with known hypersensitivity to this drug or any of its components, or to ℞ **dacarbazine.**
• It should be given with caution to people with kidney or liver function impairment, and those over 65. This is a specialist drug which will be used following a full evaluation by specialist physicians.
• Temozolomide is not recommended for use during pregnancy unless it is medically judged to be essential, because it may cause birth defects. Becoming pregnant while using this drug must be avoided.
• It should not be used if breast-feeding.
• It can produce bone marrow depression, which may lead to bleeding and a reduced resistance to infection.
• It may cause genetic mutations and/or cancer, and may impair fertility in males.

Interactions

• ℞ **Valproic acid** may increase the levels of temozolomide.

Side effects

• Frequently, nausea, vomiting, headache, fatigue, and constipation.

Tempo Tablets Ⓡ

A preparation of ℞ **aluminum hydroxide,** ℞ **calcium carbonate,** ℞ **magnesium hydroxide,** and ℞ **simethicone.**
Formulation: Oral tablets, chewable.
Availability: OTC.

Warnings and side effects: See ℞ **aluminum hydroxide**; ℞ **calcium carbonate**; ℞ **magnesium hydroxide**; ℞ **simethicone**.

Tempra Tablets; Tempra 1 (Drops); Tempra 2 (Syrup); Tempra 3 ⓑ

A preparation of ℞ **acetaminophen**.
Formulation: Oral tablets; chewable tablets; liquid; syrup.
Availability: OTC.
Warnings and side effects: See ℞ **acetaminophen**.

Tencon Capsules ⓑ

A preparation of ℞ **acetaminophen** and butalbital.
Formulation: Oral capsules.
Availability: Prescription only.
Warnings and side effects: See ℞ **acetaminophen**.

tenecteplase ⓖ

Type/Group: fibrinolytic; thrombolytic.
Brand(s): TNKase.
How administered: Intravenous injection, infusion.

Used to treat

Tenecteplase is a synthesized (recombinant DNA technology) type of enzyme with the property of breaking up blood clots. It is used as a thrombolytic in serious conditions, such as ✪ **myocardial infarction** (heart attack).

Warnings

• It should not be given to people with active internal bleeding, uncontrolled high blood pressure, a history of stroke, or injury, surgery or bleeding involving the nervous system (brain or spine) within the previous two months. This is a specialist hospital drug used under controlled conditions.

• It should be given with caution to people with cerebrovascular disease, any recent major surgery, recent injury or internal bleeding (for example, in the gastrointestinal tract or urinary tract), bacterial endocarditis or acute pericarditis, indwelling catheters, high blood pressure, severe diabetes, significant liver or kidney impairment, or any condition or disorder that would make bleeding more likely (for example, taking anticoagulant drugs or a low thrombocyte count).

• Tenecteplase should be used during pregnancy only when the potential benefits outweigh the possible risk to the fetus.

• Medical judgment is required if breast-feeding is being considered.

• Although reported rarely, fibrinolytics may free bits of plaque that may lodge (usually) in the smaller blood vessels. This may result in abrupt, sharp pain in a leg, foot, the toes, back or flank. ("Purple toes syndrome" appears as mottled, purplish discoloration of the toes.) More serious obstructions are possible, which may cause kidney failure, pancreatitis, hypertension, heart attack, stroke, and other serious obstructive events.

Interactions

• If used with ℞ **heparin**, there is an increased risk of bleeding, with potentially life-threatening adverse effects.

• Drugs that act against vitamin K (for example, ℞ **warfarin sodium**) increase the risk of bleeding.

• ℞ **abciximab**, ℞ **aspirin**, and ℞ **dipyridamole** may lower platelet activity and so increase the risk of bleeding when used with tenecteplase.

Side effects

• The chief complication is hemorrhage (although major bleeding is not frequent), which may occur at virtually any site in the body.

• Other side effects may include slowed heart rate and other arrhythmias, shock, heart failure, fluid in the lungs or brain, nausea, vomiting, or events associated with new embolism.

• Rarely allergic and anaphylactic reactions have occurred.

Tenex ⓑ

A preparation of ℞ **guanfacine hydrochloride**.
Formulation: Oral tablets, available in two strengths.
Availability: Prescription only.
Warnings and side effects: See ℞ **guanfacine hydrochloride**.

Tenoretic 50; 100 ⓑ

A preparation of ℞ **atenolol** and ℞ **chlorthalidone**.
Formulation: Oral tablets, available in two (atenolol) strengths.
Availability: Prescription only.
Warnings and side effects: See ℞ **atenolol**; ℞ **chlorthalidone**.

Tenormin ⓑ

A preparation of ℞ **atenolol**.
Formulation: Oral tablets (3 strengths); injection.
Availability: Prescription only.
Warnings and side effects: See ℞ **atenolol**.

Tensilon ⓑ

A preparation of ℞ **edrophonium chloride**.
Formulation: Injection.
Availability: Prescription only.
Warnings and side effects: See ℞ **edrophonium chloride**.

Tequin ⓑ

A preparation of ℞ **gatifloxacin**.
Formulation: Oral tablets in several strengths; injection.
Availability: Prescription only.
Warnings and side effects: See ℞ **gatifloxacin**.

Terazol 3; Terazol 7 ⓑ

A preparation of ℞ **terconazole**.
Formulation: Vaginal cream in two strengths; vaginal suppository.
Availability: Prescription.
Warnings and side effects: See ℞ **terconazole**.

terazosin ⓖ

Type/Group: alpha-adrenergic blocker; antihypertensive.
Brand(s): Hytrin.
How administered: Orally.

Used to treat

Terazosin is used as an antihypertensive (see ✪ **hypertension**), often with other antihypertensives (for example, ℞ **beta-blockers** or ℞ **thiazide** ℞ **diuretics**). It can also be used to treat urinary retention in ✚ **benign prostatic hyperplasia** (BPH).

Warnings

• It should not be given to people with known hypersensitivity to this drug or to any other quinazoline derivative (for example, ℞ **doxazosin**, ℞ **prazosin**).

• Terazosin should be used during pregnancy only if the potential benefit outweighs the possible risk to the fetus.

• Medical judgment is required if breast-feeding is being considered. It is not known whether this drug appears in breast milk.

• Postural hypotension (lowered blood pressure on standing up) occurs frequently with use of this drug and fainting may result. Sudden or prolonged standing or exercise should be avoided when taking terazosin. During initial dosing, it is helpful to identify situations in which injury could result if fainting occurs. These hypotensive effects may be aggravated by hot environments.

• Because of possible sedative side effects, caution is advised for potentially hazardous activities, such as driving, that require mental alertness.

Interactions

• ℞ **Verapamil** may increase the levels and effects of terazosin.

• If used with other antihypertensives and diuretics, the effects of these drugs may be increased. This additive effect is sometimes used to advantage in combination treatments for high blood pressure.

Side effects

• These may include postural hypotension, dizziness and vertigo, headache, fatigue, muscle weakness, sleepiness, edema, nausea, and nasal congestion or sinusitis.

• Less frequently, blurred vision, agitation or nervousness, rash and pruritus, impotence, rapid heartbeat, flu-like symptoms, or weight gain. Blood changes may occur.

terbinafine Ⓖ

Type/Group: **antifungal**.
Brand(s): Lamisil.
How administered: Orally; topically (external).

Used to treat

Terbinafine is a synthetic antifungal used to treat ringworm infections of the skin and other ✚ **fungal infections**, including of the nails.

Warnings

• It should not be given to people with known sensitivity to terbinafine, liver disease, or kidney impairment (when used orally).

• It is not recommended for use during pregnancy, as its safety has not been established.

• It should not be used when breast-feeding. The drug appears in breast milk.

• Rarely, changes in vision, blood disorders, and serious skin reactions have occurred.

• Affected areas should not be covered with bandages unless directed by a doctor.

Interactions

• Terbinafine may increase the effects of ℞ **caffeine**.

• ℞ **cimetidine** may increase the levels of terbinafine.

• ℞ **rifampin** may reduce the effects of terbinafine.

• The effects of ℞ **cyclosporine** and ℞ **dextromethorphan** may be increased.

Side effects

• Frequently, with oral use, headache.

• Occasionally, with oral use, diarrhea, rash, upset stomach, itching, taste disturbance, and nausea.

• Rarely, abdominal pain, hives, and visual disturbance when used orally. Irritation, burning, dryness rarely occur with topical use.

terbutaline sulfate Ⓖ

Type/Group: **beta-adrenergic stimulant**; **antiasthmatic**; **sympathomimetic**.
How administered: Inhalation; injection.
Brand(s): Brethine; Bricanyl.

Used to treat

Terbutaline is mainly used as a ℞ **bronchodilator** in reversible obstructive airways disease, such as for ✚ **asthma**. Although not stated by the manufacturer for such use, it can also be used in obstetrics to prevent or delay premature labor by relaxing the uterus.

Warnings

• It should not be given to people with known hypersensitivity to terbutaline sulfate.

• It should be given with caution to people with certain heart diseases, hyperthyroidism, diabetes mellitus, hypertension, or prostatic hypertrophy.

• It should be used in pregnancy only if clearly needed, as it may cross the placenta and inhibit uterine contractions.

• It can be used when breast-feeding.

• Rarely, it may have adverse effects on heart and blood pressure, or lead to paradoxical bronchoconstriction.

Interactions

• ℞ **Beta-blockers** decrease the effects of terbutaline sulfate.

• If used with ℞ **furosemide**, there is a risk of enhancing furosemide's potassium-lowering effect.

Side effects

• Frequently, headache, palpitations, weakness, nausea, restlessness, nervousness, trembling, dizziness, and throat dryness, irritation, or inflammation.

• Occasionally, insomnia, and altered taste or smell. With inhalation, coughing and bronchial irritation.

• Rarely, drowsiness, diarrhea, dry mouth, flushing, sweating, and loss of appetite.

terconazole Ⓖ

Type/Group: **antifungal**; **azole**; **candidiasis treatment**.
Brand(s): Terazol.
How administered: Topically (external).

Used to treat

Terconazole is a synthetic triazole/azole antifungal drug used to treat vaginal ✚ **candidiasis**.

Warnings
• It should not be given to people with known sensitivity to terconazole.
• Its safety in pregnancy has not been established and should be used only if medically judged to be clearly needed.
• It should not be used when breast-feeding.
• Photosensitivity (abnormal sensitivity to light) may occur after repeated use under ultraviolet light.

Interactions
None significant have been reported when used topically (externally).

Side effects
• Itching, pain, burning, genital or abdominal pain, and headache.

terpene ⅅ
Generics: **menthol**.

Actions and uses
Terpene is the chemical name of a group of unsaturated hydrocarbons found in terpene plant oils and resins. Examples include menthol, cineole, pinene, turpineol, and squalene. Menthol, which is the most widely used of all the terpenes, is included in ℞ **cold and cough preparation** remedies intended to clear nasal or ✪ **catarrhal** congestion in conditions such as colds, rhinitis, or sinusitis. It is also included in sunburn relief preparations.

Limitations
See the individual drug entry.

Terra-Cortril ⓑ
A preparation of ℞ **hydrocortisone** and ℞ **oxytetracycline**.
Formulation: Eye drops.
Availability: Prescription only.
Warnings and side effects: See ℞ **hydrocortisone**; ℞ **oxytetracycline**.

Terramycin ⓑ
A preparation of ℞ **oxytetracycline**.
Formulation: Injection.
Availability: Prescription only.
Warnings and side effects: See ℞ **oxytetracycline**.

Tesamone ⓑ
A preparation of ℞ **testosterone**.
Formulation: Injection.
Availability: Prescription only.
Warnings and side effects: See ℞ **testosterone**.

Testandro ⓑ
A preparation of ℞ **testosterone**.
Formulation: Injection.
Availability: Prescription only.
Warnings and side effects: See ℞ **testosterone**.

Testoderm; TTS; with Adhesive ⓑ
A preparation of ℞ **testosterone**.
Formulation: Transdermal patch in several strengths.
Availability: Prescription only.
Warnings and side effects: See ℞ **testosterone**.

testolactone Ⓖ
Type/Group: **anticancer; androgen; antiestrogen**.
Brand(s): Teslac.
How administered: Orally.

Used to treat
Testolactone is used as a treatment for advanced or disseminated ✪ **breast cancer** in postmenopausal women and other women whose ovarian function has been terminated. It inhibits the synthesis of estrone, the chief form of ℞ **estrogen** produced by such women, effectively acting as an indirect antiestrogen, which helps reduce the proliferation of hormone-sensitive breast cancer.

Warnings
• It should not be given to people with known hypersensitivity to this drug, or to men.
• It should be given with caution to people with kidney, liver, or heart disease.
• Testolactone is intended for postmenopausal women and should not be used during pregnancy.
• Breast-feeding is not recommended.
• Treatment should last for a minimum of three months.
• Testolactone is a Schedule III controlled substance under the federal law governing anabolic steroids.
• A doctor must be contacted if numbness or tingling of the toes, fingers, or face occurs.
• Contraception must be used during treatment.

Interactions
No interactions specific to this drug are known.

Side effects
• Rarely, eye effects, increase in blood pressure, hair loss, nail growth disturbances, tingling or burning sensations, swelling of extremities, sore tongue, loss of appetite, hot flashes, nausea, vomiting, and diarrhea.

Testopel ⓑ
A preparation of ℞ **testosterone**.
Formulation: Pellets for implantation.
Availability: Prescription only.
Warnings and side effects: See ℞ **testosterone**.

testosterone Ⓖ
Type/Group: **sex hormone; anticancer; androgen**.
Brand(s): (testosterone in aqueous suspension): Testandro; Histerone 100; Tesamone; Testopel; Testoderm; Androderm; various generic; (*testosterone propionate*): generic only; (*testosterone ethanate*): Andro L.A.; Andropository; Delatestryl; Durathate, Everone; various generic; (*testosterone cypionate*): depAndro, Depotest, Depo-Testosterone; Duratest; various generic. Combinations: With *estradiol*: Depo-Testadiol; Depotestogen; Duo-Cyp. With *estradiol valerate*: Deladumone; Valertest No.1.
How administered: Injection; pellets; transdermal patch.

Used to treat

Testosterone, an androgen, is the principle male sex hormone and is used to treat male primary and secondary ✪ **hypogonadism** (subnormal secretion of sex hormones), delayed puberty in males, advanced metastatic ✪ **breast cancer** in women, and postpartum breast pain and engorgement. It is produced in men mainly in the testes with other androgens that promote the development and maintenance of the male sex organs and the development of the secondary male sexual characteristics. It is also made in small amounts in women.

Warnings

• It should not be used by people with serious heart, liver, or kidney disease, hypersensitivity to androgens, by men with cancer of the breast or prostate, or women with abnormal vaginal bleeding.

• It should be given with caution to people with acute intermittent porphyria, history of myocardial infarction, coronary artery disease, seizure disorder, or benign prostatic hyperplasia (BPH), and with extreme caution in children and those over 65.

• It should not be used during pregnancy.

• Medical judgment is required if breast-feeding is being considered.

• It should not be used to enhance athletic performance.

• It may cause reduction of bone calcium in immobilized patients.

• In males over 65, it increases the risk of prostatic cancer, and may markedly increase libido.

Interactions

• The response to oral ℞ **anticoagulants** (for example, ℞ **warfarin sodium**) may be increased.

• ℞ **Cyclosporine** levels are increased.

Side effects

• Female virilization (deepening voice, growth of body hair, acne, clitoral enlargement, irregular periods); male breast enlargement, excessive frequency and duration of penile erections.

• Other side effects include anxiety, depression, tingling or burning sensations, acne, retention of water and minerals, blood changes, nausea, allergic skin reactions, inflammation at site of injection, and elevated cholesterol.

• Reduced sperm count and ejaculatory volume may occur after prolonged or excessive use.

• Prolonged use of high doses may cause serious liver disease, and, rarely, cancer in women.

• When given to children, it may speed up bone maturation without producing proportional increase in height, which can affect final mature stature.

Testred ⑧

A preparation of ℞ **methyltestosterone**.
Formulation: Oral capsules.
Availability: Prescription only.
Warnings and side effects: See ℞ **methyltestosterone**.

tetanus toxoid, adsorbed ⑥

(tetanus vaccine)
Type/Group: **vaccine**.
How administered: Intramuscular injection.

Brand(s): Various generic.

Used to treat

Tetanus toxoid is used for immunization to provide protection against infection by the ✪ **tetanus** organism *Clostridium tetani*. It is a toxoid-type vaccine, which is a vaccine made from a toxin produced by a microbe, in this case tetanus bacteria, that is modified to make it non-infective and which then stimulates the body to form the appropriate antitoxin (antibody). In tetanus vaccine, the bacterial toxoid is adsorbed onto a mineral carrier and is usually given as one constituent of the triple vaccine ℞ **diphtheria and tetanus vaccine (DTwP)** (DTwP) or the double vaccine ℞ **diphtheria and tetanus toxoid, adsorbed (DT; Td)**, which are administered during early life. However, tetanus vaccine can be administered by itself at any age for those who are at special risk from being infected. Administration is by injection, and a "booster" injection is given after 10 years.

Warnings

• It should not be given to people with known hypersensitivity or allergy to the vaccine, or to anyone who has a current or recent febrile (feverish) illness or infection.

• Its use should be avoided during pregnancy, but if immunization is necessary, it should preferably occur in the last two trimesters.

• Medical judgment is required if breast-feeding is being considered. It is not known whether breast milk is affected.

• It should never be used to treat actual tetanus infection.

• If a particularly acute skin inflammation, often progressing to abscesses, occurs (Arthus reaction), further tetanus toxoids should not be administered more frequently than 10-year intervals, even in an emergency.

• After vaccination, people will be required to wait for some time to ensure that there is no serious reaction (such as anaphylaxis).

Interactions

• ℞ **Immunosuppressants** may reduce the effectiveness of the vaccine.

• Caution is required if ℞ **anticoagulants** are being taken.

• ℞ **tetanus immune globulin** (TIG) may delay immunity, and should not be injected in the same arm.

Side effects

• These range from little or no reactions to severe discomfort, high temperature, and pain.

• Rarely, there may be anaphylactic shock.

tetanus immune globulin ⑥

(TIG; HTIG)
Type/Group: **immune globulin**.
Brand(s): Hyper-Tet.
How administered: Intramuscular injection.

Used to treat

Tetanus immune globulin (TIG) is a specific immune globulin of human origin used to give immediate passive immunity against infection by ✪ **tetanus**. It is mostly used as an added precaution in treating patients with contaminated wounds, and can be used in dressing wounds. Often it is just a precautionary measure because today almost everybody has established immunity through a vaccine administered at an early age, and vaccination is in any case

Key to symbols: ✪ = Disorder Section   ℞ = Drug Section   ♣ = Herbal Section   ◊◊ = Supplement Section

readily available for those at risk. In treating actual symptoms of infection, TIG may be administered, often together with ℞ **sedatives**, ℞ **skeletal muscle relaxants**, and ℞ **antibiotics** (for example, ℞ **penicillin G**, ℞ **tetracycline**).

Warnings

• TIG should be given with caution to people who have a history of hypersensitivity to any immune globulin.

• No adverse effects are known in pregnancy but the globulin should be used only when medically judged to be clearly necessary.

• Effects in breast-feeding have not been studied, but no problems have been documented.

• This globulin is not a substitute for active immunization with ℞ **tetanus toxoid, adsorbed**, but is an immediate preventive measure when immune status is in doubt or inadequate.

• Because this immune globulin is extracted from human blood, the possibility exists that it might contain virus or other disease agents. However, multiple screenings and filters (chemical and physical) are used in its preparation, and its potential to transmit infection is considered nearly nonexistent.

• After administration, people will be required to wait for some time to ensure that there is no serious reaction (such as anaphylaxis).

Interactions

• The immune response to live virus vaccines (for example, ℞ **MMR vaccine**) may not be satisfactory. A delay of at least three months (more for some vaccines, or their specific uses) is recommended after administering immune globulin. This does not apply, however, to the live vaccines for polio (oral form), typhoid (oral form), or yellow fever, which may be given at the same time as tetanus immune globulin.

• Caution is required if ℞ **anticoagulants** are being taken.

Side effects

• Most of the side effects are mild. There may be swelling, irritation or tenderness at the site of vaccination, low-grade fever, or malaise.

• Infrequently, hives and swelling.

• Although rare, shock-like reactions have been reported.

tetanus vaccine Ⓖ

see ℞ **tetanus toxoid**.

tetracaine Ⓖ

Type/Group: **local anesthetic**.

Brand(s): Pontocaine HCl; Pontocaine; Viractin.

How administered: Local injection; topically (external).

Used to treat

Tetracaine is used for spinal anesthesia, anesthesia of the nose and throat, and skin inflammations.

Warnings

• It should not be given to people with known hypersensitivity to tetracaine, or those rare patients with methemoglobinemia (a serious blood disorder). It is a specialist drug and there will be a full medical assessment.

• It should be used during pregnancy only when it is clearly needed.

• Medical judgment is required if breast-feeding is being considered.

• It can cause cardiac depression, peripheral vasodilatation, or CNS (central nervous system) toxicity.

Interactions

• There is a risk of additive toxicity with ℞ **antiarrhythmics** (for example, ℞ **tocainide**, ℞ **mexiletine**).

• ℞ **Sedatives** may cause increased CNS effects.

• The effects of ℞ **sulfonamides** are reduced.

Side effects

• Occasionally, pain at injection site, burning, stinging, or tenderness where applied.

• Rarely (generally with high dose), drowsiness, dizziness, disorientation, lightheadedness, tremors, apprehension, euphoria, sensation of heat, cold, or numbness, blurred or double vision, ringing or roaring in ears, nausea, or allergic reactions.

Tetracap Ⓑ

A preparation of ℞ **tetracycline hydrochloride**.

Formulation: Oral capsules.

Availability: Prescription only.

Warnings and side effects: See ℞ **tetracycline hydrochloride**.

tetracycline Ⓓ

Generics: **chlortetracycline; demeclocycline; doxycycline; meclocycline sulfosalicylate; minocycline; oxytetracycline; tetracycline hydrochloride.**

Actions and uses

Tetracyclines are a group of very broad-spectrum ℞ **antibacterial** and ℞ **antibiotic** drugs. Apart from being effective against bacteria, and so can be used to treat ✪ **bacterial infections**, they also inhibit the growth of chlamydia (a virus-like bacterium that causes genitourinary tract infections, eye infections, and ✪ **psittacosis**: *Chlamydia psittaci*), rickettsia (a virus-like bacterium that causes, for example, Q fever, ✪ **Rocky Mountain spotted fever**, and typhus: *Rickettsia typhi*), and mycoplasma (a minute nonmotile organism that causes, for example, mycoplasmal ✪ **pneumonia**: *Mycoplasma pneumoniae*). The tetracyclines act by inhibiting protein biosynthesis in sensitive microorganisms and penetrating human macrophages. They are therefore useful in combating microorganisms, such as mycoplasma, which can survive and multiply within macrophages.

Although they have been used to treat a very wide range of infections, the development of bacterial resistance has meant that their uses have become more specific. Treatment of atypical pneumonia due to chlamydia, rickettsia, or mycoplasma is an important use for tetracyclines, while treatment of chlamydial urethritis and pelvic inflammatory disease is another. They are also used to treat ✪ **brucellosis** and ✪ **Lyme disease**, and are effective in treating exacerbations of chronic bronchitis and acne.

The best-known and most-used tetracyclines include ℞ **tetracycline hydrochloride** (for which they were all named), ℞ **doxycycline**, and ℞ **oxytetracycline**. The members of the tetracycline family have generic names ending -cycline.

Limitations

Most tetracyclines are poorly absorbed when taken by mouth on a stomach that contains milk, ℞ **antacid** preparations (calcium salts or magnesium salts), or iron salts (for instance ℞ **ferrous sulfate** in ℞ **anemia treatment**). They may be deposited in growing bone and teeth (causing staining and potential deformity), and should therefore not be taken by children under 12 years or pregnant women.

tetracycline hydrochloride ⓖ

Type/Group: **tetracycline; antibiotic**.
How administered: Orally; topically (external).
Brand(s): Achromycin; Actisite; Panmycin; Sumycin; Tetralan; Tetracap; Tetracyn; various generic.

Used to treat

Tetracycline gave its name to this family of similar antibiotics. It can be used to treat many forms of infection, for example, ✪ **bacterial infections** of the urinary and respiratory tract (such as chronic ✪ **bronchitis**), of the genital tract, ears, eyes, mouth ulcers and skin (✪ **acne**), and infections caused by other microorganisms such as *Rickettsiae* (for example, ✪ **Rocky Mountain spotted fever**).

Warnings

These depend on route of administration and use.
• It should not be given to people with known hypersensitivity to tetracyclines, or to children under eight years of age.
• It should be given with caution to people with kidney or liver impairment.
• Tetracycline readily crosses the placenta. Its use should be avoided during the last half of pregnancy. Use of the topical form (external use) in pregnancy requires medical judgment and should be avoided unless clearly necessary.
• It appears in breast milk and should be avoided by nursing mothers.
• Superinfections due to the altered bacterial balance caused by antibiotic treatment may occur. A doctor must be contacted if severe abdominal pain, moderate to severe diarrhea, or any new or unusual symptoms occur.
• It may cause photosensitivity reactions (abnormal sensitivity to sunlight), so exposure to the sun should be minimized.
• It may cause permanent discoloration of teeth and the thin tooth enamel in children from the time of tooth formation, which begins in the uterus and ends at age eight. It may also retard bone development during the same period.
• It must not be used after the discard date, as it becomes harmful to the kidneys as it degrades.

Interactions

• Milk products, ℞ **antacids**, and ℞ **laxatives** should not be taken within two hours before or after a dose of tetracycline.
• ℞ **Bismuth subsalicylate**, ♎ **calcium**, ♎ **iron**, ♎ **magnesium**, ℞ **cholestyramine**, ℞ **sodium bicarbonate**, ♎ **zinc**, and ℞ **colestipol hydrochloride** may decrease the absorption of tetracyclines.
• The levels of ℞ **digoxin** may be reduced.
• The effects of ℞ **penicillin** are impaired.
• The effectiveness of ℞ **oral contraceptives** may be reduced.
• ℞ **Carbamazepine** and ℞ **phenytoin** may decrease the levels of tetracycline.

Side effects

• Systemic use: Frequently, dizziness, lightheadedness, and gastrointestinal effects. Occasionally, darkening of the skin, itching, and sore mouth or tongue.
• Topical use: Frequently, dry scaly skin, stinging or burning feeling. Occasionally, pain, redness, and other skin irritation.

Tetracyn ⑧

A preparation of ℞ **tetracycline hydrochloride**.
Formulation: Oral capsules in several strengths.
Availability: Prescription only.
Warnings and side effects: See ℞ tetracycline hydrochloride.

tetrahydroaminoacridine ⓖ

see ℞ tacrine hydrochloride.

tetrahydrozoline hydrochloride ⓖ

Type/Group: **alpha-adrenergic stimulant; sympathomimetic; decongestant; vasoconstrictor**.
Brand(s): (For ophthalmic use): Collyrium Fresh; Eyesine; Geneye; Murine Plus; Optigene 3; Tetrasine; Visine Moisturizing; various generic. (For nasal decongestion): Tyzine, Tyzine Pediatric Drops.
How administered: Topically (nasal; ophthalmic).

Used to treat

Tetrahydrozoline is mainly used as a nasal decongestant. It may also be used for the symptomatic relief of redness and irritation in the eye.

Warnings

• It should not be given to people with known hypersensitivity to this or any other adrenergic drug, or with angle-closure glaucoma.
• It should be given with caution, on advice of a doctor, to people taking ℞ **MAOI** antidepressants, or who have high blood pressure, heart, coronary artery or certain other cardiovascular disease, hyperthyroidism, diabetes mellitus, enlarged prostate, or glaucoma.
• Tetrahydrozoline's effects during pregnancy are not known and it should be used with caution and only if there is a clear benefit.
• Medical judgment is required if breast-feeding is being considered.
• Overuse may cause symptoms such as nervousness and insomnia, and may make congestion worse, which is an effect called "rebound congestion." No nasal decongestant should be used for longer than three to four days.
• It should be used with caution by the elderly, as they are more likely to suffer side effects.
• The manufacturer's recommendations must be followed carefully when giving this drug to children under 12.

Interactions

• Used topically (externally in the nose, on the eyes) at recommended doses, the interactions common to ℞ **sympathomimetics** do not usually apply. However, in overdose there may be interactions and side effects similar to ℞ **ephedrine**.
• Tetrahydrozoline should not be used with ℞ **MAOI** antidepressants, or within two weeks of stopping MAOI treatment, because this may cause a hypertensive crisis.

Side effects

• These depend on how it is administered. As eyedrops it may cause blurred vision or stinging. When used as a nasal decongestant, it may cause irritation in the nose. In nasal or eye application, systemic side effects are infrequent, occurring usually only with overdose (especially in children) and consist of the usual sympathomimetic symptoms: changes in heart rate and rhythm and blood pressure, headache, anxiety, restlessness, tremor, insomnia, dry mouth, cold fingertips and toes, and changes in the prostate gland.

Tetralan ⑧

A preparation of ℞ **tetracycline hydrochloride**.
Formulation: Oral syrup.
Availability: Prescription only.
Warnings and side effects: See ℞ **tetracycline hydrochloride**.

Tetrasine ⑧

A preparation of ℞ **tetrahydrozoline hydrochloride**.
Formulation: Eye drops.
Availability: OTC.
Warnings and side effects: See ℞ **tetrahydrozoline hydrochloride**.

Teveten ⑧

A preparation of ℞ **eprosartan mesylate**.
Formulation: Oral tablets, available in two strengths.
Availability: Prescription only.
Warnings and side effects: See ℞ **eprosartan mesylate**.

Texacort ⑧

A preparation of ℞ **hydrocortisone**.
Formulation: Topical liquid solution.
Availability: Prescription only.
Warnings and side effects: See ℞ **hydrocortisone**.

T-Gen Adult Suppositories; Pediatric Suppositories ⑧

A preparation of ℞ **trimethobenzamide hydrochloride**.
Formulation: Rectal suppositories.
Availability: Prescription only.
Warnings and side effects: See ℞ **trimethobenzamide hydrochloride**.

T-Gesic Capsules ⑧

A preparation of ℞ **hydrocodone bitartrate** and ℞ **acetaminophen**.
Formulation: Oral capsules.
Availability: Prescription only.
Warnings and side effects: See ℞ **hydrocodone bitartrate**; ℞ **acetaminophen**.

THA ⑥

see ℞ **tacrine hydrochloride**.

Thalitone ⑧

A preparation of ℞ **chlorthalidone**.
Formulation: Oral tablets, available in 3 strengths.
Availability: Prescription only.
Warnings and side effects: See ℞ **chlorthalidone**.

Theo-24 ⑧

A preparation of ℞ **theophylline**.
Formulation: Oral capsules, extended release in several strengths.
Availability: Prescription only.
Warnings and side effects: See ℞ **theophylline**.

Theobid Duracaps ⑧

A preparation of ℞ **theophylline**.
Formulation: Oral capsules, extended release.
Availability: Prescription only.
Warnings and side effects: See ℞ **theophylline**.

Theochron ⑧

A preparation of ℞ **theophylline**.
Formulation: Oral tablets, sustained release, in several strengths.
Availability: Prescription only.
Warnings and side effects: See ℞ **theophylline**.

Theoclear-80 ⑧

A preparation of ℞ **theophylline**.
Formulation: Oral syrup.
Availability: Prescription only.
Warnings and side effects: See ℞ **theophylline**.

Theodrine Tablets ⑧

A preparation of ℞ **ephedrine** and ℞ **theophylline**.
Formulation: Oral tablets.
Availability: OTC.
Warnings and side effects: See ℞ **ephedrine**; ℞ **theophylline**.

Theo-Dur ⑧

A preparation of ℞ **theophylline**.
Formulation: Oral tablets, timed release, in several strengths.
Availability: Prescription only.
Warnings and side effects: See ℞ **theophylline**.

Theolair; Theolair SR ⑧

A preparation of ℞ **theophylline**.
Formulation: Oral solution; oral tablets, timed release, in several strengths.
Availability: Prescription only.
Warnings and side effects: See ℞ **theophylline**.

Theomax DF Syrup ⑧

A preparation of ℞ **ephedrine**, ℞ **theophylline**, and ℞ **hydroxyzine**.
Formulation: Oral syrup.
Availability: Prescription only.

Warnings and side effects: See ℞ **ephedrine**; ℞ **theophylline**; ℞ **hydroxyzine**.

theophylline ⑥

Type/Group: **xanthine; antiasthmatic; respiratory stimulant**.
Brand(s): Accurbron; Aquaphyllin; Asmalix; Elixomin; Elixophyllin; Lanophyllin; Quibron-T/SR Dividose; Respbid; Slo-Bid; Slo-Phyllin; Sustaire; Theo-24; Theobid Duracaps; Theochron; Theoclear 80; Theo-Dur; Theolair; Theophylline Extended Release; Theophylline Oral; Theo-Sav; Theospan-SR; Theostat 80; Theovent; Theo-X; T-phyl; Uni-Dur; Uniphyl; various generic. *Aminophylline*: Phyllocontin; various generic. *Dyphylline*: Dilor; Lufylin; various generic. *Oxtriphylline*: Chloedyl SA; various generic. Combinations: With *guaifenesin*: Elixophyllin GG Liquid; Glyceryl-T Capsules, Liquid; Quibron Capsules, -300 Capsules; Mudrane GG-2 Tablets; Slo-Phyllin GG Capsules, Syrup; Synophylate-GG Syrup. With *ephedrine* and *guaifenesin*: Primatene Dual Action Tablets. With *potassium iodide*: Elixophylline KI. With *dextrose* for injection: generic. *Aminophylline* with *guaifenesin*: Mudrane GG Tablets. *Dyphylline* with *guaifenesin*: Dilor-G Tablets, Liquid; Dyflex-G Tablets; Dyline G.G. Tablets, Liquid; Lufyllin-GG Tablets, Elixir; Panfil G Tablets, Liquid. *Dyphylline* with *guaifenesin* and *phenobarbital*: Lufyllin-EPG Tablets, Elixir.

How administered: Orally; injection; rectal suppository (aminophylline).

Used to treat

Theophylline is a ℞ **bronchodilator** that is mainly used for the treatment of chronic ✪ **bronchitis** and ✪ **emphysema** (as in COPD). Although not stated by the manufacturer for such use, it may also be used to treat apnea and bradycardia (see ✪ **heart disease**) in premature infants. It is also available in the form of chemical derivatives, aminophylline, dyphylline, and oxtriphylline.

Warnings

• It should not be given to people with known hypersensitivity to xanthines, active peptic ulcer disease, or a seizure disorder that is uncontrolled by anticonvulsant medication.

• It should be given with caution to people with heart disease, hypoxemia, liver disease, hypertension, congestive heart failure, alcoholism, who are over 65 (particularly males), and newborns.

• It should be used in pregnancy only if clearly needed.

• It should not be used when breast-feeding, as it is readily distributed in breast milk.

• It should not be used as the sole treatment for acute asthma attacks.

• Excessive doses may cause severe toxicity (symptoms include nausea, vomiting, anxiety, insomnia, seizures, heart dysrhythmias) and blood levels may be monitored.

Interactions

• A diet high in protein and low in carbohydrates, and charcoal-broiled beef may reduce its effectiveness. Taking the sustained-release form with food may alter absorption. It should be taken on an empty stomach.

• An increased dose is required for people who smoke.

• There is a marked increase in theophylline concentrations if taken with ℞ **enoxacin**, ℞ **fluvoxamine**, ℞ **mexiletine**, ℞ **propranolol**, or troleandomycin.

• The levels and effects of ℞ **adenosine** and ℞ **lithium** are reduced.

• There is a risk of seizure if taken with ℞ **imipenem**.

• ℞ **Beta-blockers** reduce the effects of theophylline.

• ℞ **Aminoglutethimide**, ℞ **barbiturates**, ℞ **carbamazepine**, moricizine, ℞ **phenytoin**, ℞ **rifampin**, ℞ **ritonavir**, and ℞ **thyroid hormone** reduce the levels of theophylline (phenytoin levels are also reduced).

• ℞ **Allopurinol** ℞ **amiodarone hydrochloride**, ℞ **cimetidine**, ℞ **ciprofloxacin**, ℞ **disulfiram**, ℞ **erythromycin**, ℞ **interferon alfa**, ℞ **isoniazid**, methimazole, ℞ **metoprolol**, ℞ **norfloxacin**, pentoxifylline, ℞ **propafenone**, ℞ **propylthiouracil**, radioactive ⚖ **iodine**, ℞ **tacrine**, ℞ **thiabendazole**, ℞ **ticlopidine**, and ℞ **verapamil** increase the levels of theophylline.

Side effects

• Frequently, dizziness, restlessness, and speeded heart rate.

• Occasionally, gastrointestinal effects, urinary frequency, headache, and insomnia.

Theophylline Extended Release ⑧

A preparation of ℞ **theophylline**.
Formulation: Oral tablets, extended release.
Availability: Prescription only.
Warnings and side effects: See ℞ **theophylline**.

Theophylline Oral ⑧

A preparation of ℞ **theophylline**.
Formulation: Oral solution.
Availability: Prescription only.
Warnings and side effects: See ℞ **theophylline**.

Theo-Sav ⑧

A preparation of ℞ **theophylline**.
Formulation: Oral tablets, timed release in several strengths.
Availability: Prescription only.
Warnings and side effects: See ℞ **theophylline**.

Theospan-SR ⑧

A preparation of ℞ **theophylline**.
Formulation: Oral capsules, extended release, in several strengths.
Availability: Prescription only.
Warnings and side effects: See ℞ **theophylline**.

Theostat 80 ⑧

A preparation of ℞ **theophylline**.
Formulation: Oral syrup.
Availability: Prescription only.
Warnings and side effects: See ℞ **theophylline**.

Theovent ⑧

A preparation of ℞ **theophylline**.
Formulation: Oral capsules, extended release, in several strengths.

Availability: Prescription only.
Warnings and side effects: See ℞ **theophylline**.

Theo-X ⓑ

A preparation of ℞ **theophylline**.
Formulation: Oral tablets, controlled release in several strengths.
Availability: Prescription only.
Warnings and side effects: See ℞ **theophylline**.

The Pill ⓓ

see ℞ **oral contraceptive**.

Therac ⓑ

A preparation of ℞ **sulfur**.
Formulation: Topical lotion.
Availability: OTC.
Warnings and side effects: See ℞ **sulfur**.

TheraCys ⓑ

A preparation of ℞ **BCG intravesical**.
Formulation: Powder for suspension.
Availability: Prescription only.
Warnings and side effects: See ℞ **BCG intravesical**.

TheraFlu Flu and Cold Medicine Powder ⓑ

A preparation of ℞ **pseudoephedrine**, ℞ **acetaminophen**, and ℞ **chlorpheniramine maleate**.
Formulation: Powder (for oral use).
Availability: OTC.
Warnings and side effects: See ℞ **pseudoephedrine**; ℞ **acetaminophen**; ℞ **chlorpheniramine maleate**.

Thera-Flu Non-Drowsy Formula Maximum Strength ⓑ

A preparation of ℞ **dextromethorphan**, ℞ **acetaminophen**, and ℞ **pseudoephedrine**.
Formulation: Oral caplet; powder.
Availability: OTC.
Warnings and side effects: See ℞ **dextromethorphan**; ℞ **acetaminophen**; ℞ **pseudoephedrine**.

Thera-gesic Cream ⓑ

A preparation of ℞ **methyl salicylate**, ℞ **menthol**, and various.
Formulation: Topical cream.
Availability: OTC.
Warnings and side effects: See ℞ **methyl salicylate**; ℞ **menthol**.

Theravac-SB ⓑ

A preparation of ℞ **docusate sodium** and ℞ **glycerin**.
Formulation: Enema.
Availability: OTC.
Warnings and side effects: See ℞ **docusate sodium**; ℞ **glycerin**.

Therevac-Plus ⓑ

A preparation of ℞ **benzocaine**, ℞ **docusate sodium**, and ℞ **glycerin**.
Formulation: Enema.
Availability: OTC.
Warnings and side effects: See ℞ **benzocaine**; ℞ **docusate sodium**; ℞ **glycerin**.

Thermazene ⓑ

A preparation of ℞ **silver sulfadiazine**.
Formulation: Cream.
Availability: Prescription only.
Warnings and side effects: See ℞ **silver sulfadiazine**.

thiabendazole ⓖ

(tiabendazole)
Type/Group: **anthelmintic; azole**.
Brand(s): Mintezol.
How administered: Orally.

Used to treat

Thiabendazole is a synthetic (azole) anthelmintic drug used in the treatment of infestations by worm parasites (see ✚ **worms**), particularly those of the *Strongyloides* species (threadworms) that live in the intestines but may migrate into the tissues. It is also used to treat other worm infestations resistant to common drugs. The usual course of treatment is intensive.

Warnings

• It should not be given to people with known hypersensitivity to this drug.
• It should be given with caution to people with severe malnutrition, liver or kidney disease, anemia, or severe dehydration. Use in small children also requires medical judgment.
• It should be used during pregnancy only if the potential benefits outweigh the risks to the fetus.
• Medical judgment is required if breast-feeding is being considered.
• Discontinue immediately if allergic reaction occurs.
• Serious skin disorders are possible.
• It may impair the performance of skilled tasks, such as driving.

Interactions

• ℞ **carbamazepine** may reduce the levels of thiabendazole.
• The effect of ℞ **theophylline** (a xanthine) may be increased.

Side effects

• Gastrointestinal effects, dizziness, drowsiness, headache, and itching.
• Possible hypersensitivity reactions include fever with chills, rashes and other skin disorders, and occasionally tinnitus or liver damage, visual disorders, kidney damage, and seizures.

thiazide ⓓ

Generics: **bendroflumethiazide; benzthiazide; benzthiazide; chlorthalidone; chlorothiazide; hydrochlorothiazide; hydroflumethiazide; indapamide; methyclothiazide; metolazone; polythiazide; quinethazone; trichlormethiazide**.

Actions and uses

℞ **thiazide** chemical compounds have a ℞ **diuretic** action: they inhibit sodium (and accompanying chloride) reabsorption at the beginning of the distal convoluted tubule of the kidney and may be used for prolonged periods in conditions where there is fluid retention and edema. Their uses include as ℞ **antihypertensive** agents (either alone or in conjunction with other types of diuretic or other drugs) and the treatment of edema associated with heart failure. There may be some depletion of potassium, but this can be treated with potassium supplements or the co-administering of potassium-sparing diuretics. Administration is oral.

Thiazides are also an ("off-label") treatment for nephrogenic diabetes insipidus.

Limitations

See individual drug entries.

thiethylperazine maleate ⓖ

Type/Group: **phenothiazine; antiemetic; antinauseant**.
Brand(s): Torecan.
How administered: Orally; topically (rectal suppositories); injection (intramuscular only).

Used to treat

Thiethylperazine maleate is used to control ✪ nausea and ✪ vomiting. It has a less tranquilizing effect than other drugs of this type.

Warnings

• It should not be given to people with known hypersensitivity to this drug (or with known sensitivity to other phenothiazines), who are comatose, or who have received large doses of other sedating drugs. It is not recommended for children under the age of 12.
• It should be given with caution to people with seizure disorders.
• It should not be used during pregnancy, and, in general, it should not be used by nursing women.
• Because of a suspected link between centrally acting antiemetics (like this one) and the rare, but serious, condition called ✪ **Reye's syndrome** (which causes inflammation of the brain and liver), thiethylperazine should not be given to children or teenagers who have, or might have, chickenpox or flu. As so many infections resemble flu in their initial symptoms, these centrally acting antiemetics should not, as a general rule, be used to treat vomiting of unknown cause by anyone in this age group except on the advice of a doctor.
• Thiethylperazine, when injected, should be given intramuscularly only, as serious adverse reactions (significant drop in blood pressure) are possible if it is injected into a blood vessel.
• If symptoms such as gait disturbances, uncoordinated or uncontrolled muscle or eye movements occur, treatment should be stopped or the dosage reduced.
• Because of its sedative side effects, the performance of skilled tasks, such as driving, may be impaired.

Interactions

• ℞ epinephrine should not be used with any phenothiazine.
• Central nervous system (CNS) depressants (for example, other phenothiazines, ℞ **skeletal muscle relaxants**, ℞ **opioids**, ℞ **barbiturates**, ℞ **hypnotics**, ℞ **sedatives**, ℞ **tranquilizers**) may cause an increase in the severity of side effects.
• Alcohol may intensify side effects such as drowsiness and incoordination.
• If taken with ℞ **anticonvulsants**, the seizure threshold may be lowered and so require dosage adjustment.

Side effects

• Commonly, drowsiness and dry mouth, depression, or euphoria.
• Less frequently, headache, fever, blurred vision, ringing in the ears and swelling of the extremities, dark urine, seizures, drop in blood pressure, and respiratory depression. Intramuscular injections may be painful.

thioguanine ⓖ

(tioguanine)
Type/Group: **anticancer; cytotoxic**.
How administered: Orally.
Brand(s): Generic only.

Used to treat

Thioguanine is a cytotoxic (an antimetabolite) drug used in the treatment of acute ✪ **leukemias**.

Warnings

• It should not be given to people with known hypersensitivity or resistance to this drug or ℞ **mercaptopurine**. This is a specialist drug which will be used following a full evaluation by specialist physicians.
• Thioguanine is not recommended for use during pregnancy unless it is medically judged to be essential, because it may cause birth defects. Becoming pregnant while using this drug must be avoided.
• It should not be used if breast-feeding.
• It can cause bone marrow depression, which may lead to bleeding and a reduced resistance to infection.
• In common with many anticancer drugs, thioguanine may cause genetic mutations and/or cancer.
• It can have adverse effects on the liver and monitoring is required.
• A doctor must be contacted if fever, sore throat, signs of local infection, easy bruising, bleeding, excessive tiredness, or weakness occur.

Interactions

No interactions specific to this drug are known.

Side effects

• Frequently, excessive excretion of uric acid.
• Occasionally, gastrointestinal disturbances, rash, skin irritation, unsteady gait, loss of vibration sensitivity, and jaundice.

Thioplex ⓡ

A preparation of ℞ **thiotepa**.
Formulation: Injection.
Availability: Prescription only.
Warnings and side effects: See ℞ **thiotepa**.

thioridazine ⓖ

Type/Group: **antipsychotic; phenothiazine**.
Brand(s): Mellaril.

Key to symbols: ✪ = Disorder Section   ℞ = Drug Section   ♣ = Herbal Section   = Supplement Section

How administered: Orally.

Used to treat

Thioridazine is a recently introduced drug, which is used to treat and tranquilize people with ⊙ **psychotic disorders** (such as schizophrenics), particularly those experiencing behavioral disturbances. It is also used to treat ⊙ **depression** with ⊙ **anxiety** in adults, and for treatment of symptoms such as agitation, anxiety, depressed mood, tension, sleep disturbances, and fears in the elderly. It is also used to treat behavioral problems in children. Although not stated by the manufacturer for such treatment, it is sometimes prescribed to treat symptoms in those with organic brain syndrome. Also, thioridazine may be used in the short-term treatment of anxiety, and as an additional treatment in alcohol withdrawal.

Warnings

• It should not be given to people with known hypersensitivity to this drug, with severe central nervous system (CNS) depression, coma, brain damage, bone marrow depression, narrow-angle glaucoma, porphyria, or severe blood pressure disorders.

• It should be given with caution to people with liver disease, heart disorders, seizure disorders, chronic obstructive pulmonary disease (COPD), or anyone over 65.

• Safety for use during pregnancy has not been established. Use only when clearly needed and when potential benefits outweigh potential risks to the fetus.

• Medical judgment is required if breast-feeding is being considered.

• It may cause drowsiness, and so the performance of skilled tasks, such as driving, may be impaired.

• It may cause postural hypotension (lowered blood pressure on standing), so rise slowly from a reclining position. Older people in particular should exercise caution.

• It may cause sensitivity to sunlight (photosensitivity), so minimize exposure (use sunscreen, sunglasses, and so on).

• If used for a long time, tardive dyskinesia (see ℞ **antipsychotics**) occasionally develops.

• Treatment should be stopped gradually.

• Avoid alcohol.

Interactions

• There is increased anticholinergic action if used with ℞ **anticholinergics**, ℞ **antiparkinsonism**, drugs and ℞ **antidepressants**.

• If used with ℞ **bromocriptine** or ℞ **lithium**, the levels of both drugs may be decreased.

• The ℞ **antiparkinsonism** effects of ℞ **levodopa** may be reduced.

• If used with a ℞ **beta-blocker**, the effects of both drugs may be increased.

• ℞ **Barbiturates** and ℞ **orphenadrine** lower the effects of an antipsychotic and increase anticholinergic/CNS effects.

• If used with ℞ **narcotic analgesics**, blood pressure may be lowered.

• If an antipsychotic is taken with alcohol, there may be increased sedative effects.

Side effects

• Headache, loss of appetite, constipation, dry mouth, nausea, and vomiting.

• Less frequently, confusion, ECG changes, postural hypotension (especially in women), speeded heartbeat, blurred vision, eye changes, jaundice, weight gain, urinary retention or frequency, bedwetting, rash, irregular menstrual periods, sexual dysfunction, male breast enlargement, and abnormal milk production.

• Rarely, extrapyramidal symptoms (see ℞ **antipsychotics**), heart attack, blood cell disorders, spasm of the larynx, and respiratory depression.

thiotepa ⓖ

Type/Group: **anticancer; cytotoxic**.
Brand(s): Thioplex.
How administered: Injection.

Used to treat

Thiotepa is a cytotoxic drug (an alkylating agent) that is used in the treatment of ⊙ **tumors** in the bladder and sometimes for ovarian or ⊙ **breast cancer**, and sometimes ⊙ **lymphomas**. It works by interfering with the DNA of new-forming cells, so preventing cell replication.

Warnings

• It should not be given to people with known hypersensitivity to thiotepa, or those with existing liver, kidney or bone marrow damage.

• It should be given with caution to people with kidney or liver function impairment. This is a specialist drug which will be used following a full evaluation by specialist physicians.

• Thiotepa is not recommended for use during pregnancy unless it is medically judged to be essential, because it may cause birth defects. Becoming pregnant while using this drug must be avoided.

• It should not be used if breast-feeding.

• Thiotepa has adverse effects on the creation of blood cells, and can cause severe bone marrow suppression, which may lead to bleeding and a reduced resistance to infection.

• In common with many anticancer drugs, this drug can cause cancer and genetic mutations. It may also interfere with fertility.

• A doctor must be contacted if bleeding (such as nosebleeds, easy bruising, black stools) or an infection occurs.

Interactions

• The effects of neuromuscular blocking agents (for example, ℞ **pancuronium**) may be increased.

• The levels of ℞ **probenecid** and vaccines may be reduced.

Side effects

• Occasionally, pain at injection site, headache, dizziness, throat irritation, hives, skin rash, nausea, vomiting, and loss of appetite.

• Rarely, hair loss, bladder infection, and blood in the urine.

thiothixene ⓖ

Type/Group: **antipsychotic**.
Brand(s): Navane.
How administered: Orally.

Used to treat

Thiothixene is chemically a thioxanthene derivative and it has similar general actions to the ℞ **phenothiazine** derivatives. It can be used to treat ⊙ **psychotic disorders**, such as ⊙ **schizophrenia**.

Although not stated by the manufacturer for such use, it is sometimes also used to control acute agitated behavior.

Warnings

• It should not be given to people with known hypersensitivity to this drug, with certain blood diseases, circulatory collapse, CNS (central nervous system) depression, or coma.

• It should be given with caution to people with seizure disorders, high blood pressure, liver or cardiovascular disease, glaucoma, or chronic obstructive pulmonary disease (COPD).

• Thiothixene should be used during pregnancy only if the benefits outweigh the risk to the fetus.

• Medical judgment is required if breast-feeding is being considered.

• It may cause drowsiness, and so the performance of skilled tasks, such as driving, may be impaired.

• It may cause postural hypotension (lowered blood pressure on standing), so rise slowly from a reclining position. Older people in particular should exercise caution.

• If used for a long time, tardive dyskinesia (see ℞ **antipsychotics**) occasionally develops.

• Treatment should be stopped gradually.

• Avoid alcohol.

Interactions

• There is increased anticholinergic action if used with ℞ **anticholinergics**, ℞ **antiparkinsonism**, drugs and ℞ **antidepressants**.

• If used with ℞ **lithium** or a ℞ **beta-blocker**, the effectiveness of both drugs may be decreased.

• ℞ **Anticholinergics**, ℞ **barbiturates**, ℞ **narcotic analgesics**, ℞ **orphenadrine** lower levels of an antipsychotic, and/or increase the occurrence of anticholinergic and/or CNS (central nervous system) effects.

• Thiothixene may decrease the effects of ℞ **guanethidine monosulfate** and ℞ **bromocriptine**.

• The effects of ℞ **epinephrine** may be altered.

• ℞ **Narcotic analgesics** may cause low blood pressure.

• If an antipsychotic is taken with alcohol, there may be increased sedative effects.

Side effects

• Extrapyramidal symptoms (see ℞ **antipsychotics**) and headache.

• Less frequently, drowsiness, ECG changes, high blood pressure, speeded heart rate, eye changes, loss of appetite, constipation, diarrhea, dry mouth, changes in liver function, weight gain, changes in hormone function (irregular menstruation, growth of breasts, abnormal milk production, impotence, increased libido), shortness of breath, spasmodic constriction of the bronchi or larynx, increased sweating, and skin reactions.

• Rarely, neuroleptic malignant syndrome (a potentially fatal condition characterized by very high fever, muscle rigidity, changes in mental status, and irregular pulse, blood pressure and/or heart rhythm), cardiac arrest, and seizure.

Thorazine Ⓑ

A preparation of ℞ **chlorpromazine**.

Formulation: Oral tablets in several strengths; sustained release capsules; oral concentrate; rectal suppositories; ampules, and vials for injection.

Availability: Prescription only.

Warnings and side effects: See ℞ **chlorpromazine**.

3TC Ⓖ

see ℞ **lamivudine**.

Thrombate III Ⓑ

A preparation of ℞ **antithrombin III human**.

Formulation: Intravenous infusion.

Availability: Prescription only.

Warnings and side effects: See ℞ **antithrombin III human**.

thrombolytic Ⓓ

Generics: alteplase, recombinant; anistreplase; reteplase, recombinant; streptokinase.

Actions and uses

Thrombolytic means to break up or dissolve thrombi (blood clots). See ℞ **fibrinolytic**. Thrombolytic drugs work biochemically as ℞ **fibrinolytic** agents. They are used to break up or disperse thrombi (thrombolysis), which are blood clots that have formed in blood vessels. They work by activating fibrinolytic enzymes, or are enzymes, that help break down the protein fibrin, which is the main constituent of blood clots and so break up the thrombus. They can be used rapidly in serious conditions, such as life-threatening venous thrombi, ⊙ **pulmonary embolism**, and clots in the eye, and particularly to reopen the blocked coronary arteries that occur in ⊙ **myocardial infarction** (heart attack). They all are injected or intravenously infused.

℞ **streptokinase** is a thrombolytic enzyme (a plasminogen activator), which is used as a thrombolytic in myocardial infarction. It is given as soon as possible, to reduce the incidence of heart failure and improve survival, and to treat ⊙ **pulmonary embolism**, ⊙ **deep vein thrombosis**, and arterial thrombosis. ℞ **anistreplase** is similar in action and uses. ℞ **alteplase** and ℞ **reteplase** are synthesized (recombinant DNA technology) types of enzyme activator (called a tissue plasminogen activator), which activate thrombolytic processes and are used in much the same way as streptokinase.

Limitations

All these drugs have quite significant side effects and are only used under specialist supervision and after a full medical assessment (usually in a medical emergency). The chief complication is hemorrhage (although major bleeding is not frequent), which may occur at virtually any site in the body. Allergic symptoms, sometimes severe, may occur. Although reported rarely, fibrinolytics may free bits of plaque that have lodged (usually) in the smaller blood vessels, which may result in abrupt, sharp pain in, for example, the foot, toes, back or flank. More serious obstructions are possible, which may cause kidney failure, pancreatitis, hypertension, heart attack, stroke, and other serious obstructive events. See also the individual drug entries and these related class entries: ℞ **anticoagulant**; ℞ **antiplatelet**; ℞ **hematopoietic**; ℞ **hemostatic**.

thymol ⓖ

Type/Group: **antiseptic.**
Brand(s): Listerine; MenthoRub Ointment; Vick's Menthol Cough Drops.
How administered: Inhalation; topically (external).

Used to treat

Thymol is obtained from the essential oil of the plant thyme. It can be used as a weak antiseptic, and also in decongestant preparations for inhalation.

Warnings

None significant.

Interactions

No significant interactions are known.

Side effects

No significant side effects are known.

Thyrel TRH ⓑ

A preparation of ℞ **protirelin.**
Formulation: Injection.
Availability: Prescription only.
Warnings and side effects: See ℞ **protirelin.**

Thyro-Block ⓑ

A preparation of ℞ **potassium iodide.**
Formulation: Tablets.
Availability: Prescription only, through state and federal agencies.
Warnings and side effects: See ℞ **potassium iodide.**

thyroid antagonist ⓓ

see ℞ **antithyroid.**

thyroid hormone ⓓ

Generics: **calcitonin-salmon; levothyroxine sodium; liothyronine.**

Actions and uses

Thyroid hormones are secreted by the thyroid gland at the base of the neck. There are two main forms of thyroid hormone, both containing iodine, and they are used in medicine mainly in their synthetic forms: ℞ **levothyroxine sodium** (L-thyroxine; T_4) and liothyronine (L-triiodothyronine; T_3). Also available are extracts of thyroid gland and a 1:4 mixture of T_3 and T_4 (liotrix). Physiologically, the hormones are transported in the bloodstream to control cellular metabolic energy functions in many types of cells throughout the body. Therapeutically, these hormones are used to make up thyroid hormonal deficiency and associated symptoms when they need to be taken on a regular maintenance basis.

They are prescribed to treat thyroid conditions, including congenital ◎ **hypothyroidism**, myxedema (severe hypothyroidism), Hashimoto's disease (an autoimmune thyroid disease), some goiter conditions, cretinism, thyrotoxicosis (in conjunction with antithyroid drugs), to manage thyroid cancer, in conditions involving pituitary or hypothalamic malfunction, and in the diagnostic test of thyroid function.

A third hormone, calcitonin, is secreted by a different cell type in the thyroid gland and has a different physiological role. Its function is to lower levels of calcium in the blood (which increases deposits of calcium in the bones); it is used to lower abnormally high calcium levels (hypercalcemia), to treat ◎ **Paget's disease (of the bone)**, and for postmenopausal ◎ **osteoporosis**. Calcitonin-salmon is a synthetic analog of the form that is found in salmon.

As a ℞ **diagnostic agent** to identify cases of thyroid failure and to establish a diagnosis of decreased thyroid reserve, use can be made of the ℞ **anterior pituitary hormone** ℞ **thyrotropin**, which physiologically controls the release of thyroid hormones from the thyroid gland.

The oral use of thyroid hormone (normally liothyronine) in replacement therapy is usually quite successful, although careful adjustment of dose is required to avoid symptoms of hyperthyroidism (with consequent risk of precipitating angina pectoris, heart arrhythmias, and heart failure).

Limitations

The chronic use of animal calcitonin analogs runs the risk of inducing antibodies with consequent allergic reactions (and for this reason the use of porcine calcitonin has been discontinued). Salmon calcitonin (calcitonin-salmon) is most commonly used in therapeutics and appears to be more potent than other forms because it is broken down in the body relatively slowly, and has the advantage that it can be taken in the form of a nasal spray (instead of by injection). Human calcitonin is now available and may become more commonly used. See also the individual drug entries.

thyroid-stimulating-hormone ⓖ

see ℞ **thyrotropin.**

Thyrolar ⓑ

A preparation of ℞ **levothyroxine sodium** and ℞ **liothyronine.**
Formulation: Injection.
Availability: Prescription only.
Warnings and side effects: See ℞ **liothyronine;** ℞ **levothyroxine sodium.**

thyrotropin ⓖ

(thyroid-stimulating-hormone; TSH)
Type/Group: **hormone; anterior pituitary hormone; diagnostic agent.**
Brand(s): Thytropar.
How administered: Injection.

Used to treat

Thyrotropin is an anterior pituitary hormone that controls the release of thyroid hormones from the thyroid gland and can be used as a diagnostic agent to identify cases of thyroid failure and to establish a diagnosis of decreased thyroid reserve. It is itself controlled by the hypothalamic hormone TRH (thyrotropin-releasing hormone) and by high levels of thyroid hormone in the blood.

Warnings

• It should not be used by people with known hypersensitivity to this drug, with coronary thrombosis, or untreated Addison's disease.

• It should be given with caution to people with heart disease.

• It should be used during pregnancy only if medically judged to be clearly needed.
• Medical judgment is also required if breast-feeding is being considered.
• Serious allergic reactions are possible, particularly after repeated use.

Interactions
None have been noted.

Side effects
• Nausea, vomiting, headache, and hives.
• Less frequently, transitory hypotension, and speeded heart rate.

Thytropar ®
A preparation of ℞ **thyrotropin**.
Formulation: Injection.
Availability: Prescription only.
Warnings and side effects: See ℞ **thyrotropin**.

tiabendazole ©
see ℞ **thiabendazole**.

tiagabine ©
Type/Group: **anticonvulsant; antiepileptic**.
Brand(s): Gabatrim Filmtabs.
How administered: Orally.

Used to treat
Tiagabine is a recently introduced drug which may be used in the treatment of ✪ **epilepsy** to assist in the control of partial seizures.

Warnings
• Avoid its use in people with known hypersensitivity to this drug.
• It should be given with caution to anyone with liver impairment, or those with neurological disorders such as Alzheimer's or stroke.
• Use tiagabine in pregnancy only when clearly needed.
• This drug appears in breast milk, though its effects are not known. It therefore should be used by breast-feeding mothers only if potential benefits outweigh the risks to the infant.
• Withdrawal should be gradual otherwise it may precipitate attacks.
• As this drug may cause drowsiness, driving or other hazardous activity should be avoided.
• Some side effects can be minimized by taking tiagabine with food.

Interactions
• ℞ **carbamazepine**, ℞ **phenobarbital**, ℞ **phenytoin**, and ℞ **valproate sodium** may increase the rate at which tiagabine is cleared from the body.

Side effects
• Diarrhea, tiredness, nervousness, dizziness, and tremor;
• Difficulties in concentrating, emotional changes, and speech impairment;
• Less frequently, confusion, depression, drowsiness, and psychosis;
• Blood changes have been reported.

Tiamate ®
A preparation of ℞ **diltiazem hydrochloride**.
Formulation: Oral tablets, extended release, available in 3 strengths.
Availability: Prescription only.
Warnings and side effects: See ℞ **diltiazem hydrochloride**.

Tiazac ®
A preparation of ℞ **diltiazem hydrochloride**.
Formulation: Oral capsules, extended release, available in two strengths.
Availability: Prescription only.
Warnings and side effects: See ℞ **diltiazem hydrochloride**.

Ticar ®
A preparation of ℞ **ticarcillin**.
Formulation: Injection; intravenous infusion.
Availability: Prescription only.
Warnings and side effects: See ℞ **ticarcillin**.

ticarcillin ©
Type/Group: **antibiotic; penicillin**.
Brand(s): Ticar. Combinations: With *clavulanate potassium*: Timentin.
How administered: Injection; intravenous infusion.

Used to treat
Ticarcillin has improved activity against a number of important Gram-negative bacteria, including *Pseudomonas aeruginosa*, and can be used to treat serious ✪ **bacterial infections** that cause ✪ **septicemia** and ✪ **peritonitis**, and also infections of the respiratory and urinary tracts. It is also used in combination with the beta-lactamase inhibitor ℞ **clavulanic acid** (which helps combat resistance to penicillin).

Warnings
• It should not be used by people with known hypersensitivity to penicillins.
• It should be given with caution to people allergic to ℞ **cephalosporins** or ℞ **imipenem**, or with impaired kidney or liver function.
• Penicillins cross the placenta and should be used in pregnancy only if medically judged to be needed.
• Medical judgment is also needed for breast-feeding mothers.
• Serious and occasionally fatal hypersensitivity reactions can occur.
• Superinfections from the altered bacterial balance created by antibiotic treatment may occur and may result in ✪ **pseudomembranous colitis**. A doctor must be contacted if there is severe abdominal pain, or moderate to severe diarrhea.

Interactions
• The effectiveness of ℞ **aminoglycosides** may be reduced by ticarcillin.
• ℞ **Chloramphenicol**, ℞ **macrolide** antibiotics, and ℞ **tetracyclines** may reduce the effectiveness of penicillins.
• Large doses of penicillins may increase the levels of ℞ **methotrexate**.

Side effects

• Frequently, phlebitis or thrombophlebitis with intravenous dose, mild allergic reaction, taste or smell perversions.
• Occasionally, gastrointestinal effects.
• Rarely, headache, fatigue, hallucinations, bruising or bleeding, and seizure.

Tice BCG ⑧

A preparation of ℞ **BCG vaccine**.
Formulation: Percutaneous injection.
Availability: Prescription only.
Warnings and side effects: See ℞ **BCG vaccine**.

Tice BCG (for intravesical use) ⑧

A preparation of ℞ **BCG intravesical**.
Formulation: Injection (intravesical).
Availability: Prescription only.
Warnings and side effects: See ℞ **BCG intravesical**.

Ticlid ⑧

A preparation of ℞ **ticlopidine**.
Formulation: Oral tablets.
Availability: Prescription only.
Warnings and side effects: See ℞ **ticlopidine**.

ticlopidine ⑥

Type/Group: **antiplatelet**.
Brand(s): Ticlid.
How administered: Orally.

Used to treat

Ticlopidine is an antiplatelet (antithrombotic) drug which is used to prevent ✪ **thrombosis** (blood-clot formation), but does not have an ℞ **anticoagulant** action. It works by stopping platelets sticking to one another or to the walls of blood vessels. It is used to reduce new blood-clotting complications, such as stroke, in people with a history of atherosclerotic disease (ischemic stroke, myocardial infarction, or peripheral arterial disease). Because of possible depressive effects on levels of certain blood cells, ticlopidine is usually reserved for treatment in cases where ℞ **aspirin** cannot be tolerated.

Warnings

• It should not be given to people with known hypersensitivity to this drug, with active bleeding (for example, peptic ulcer, intracranial hemorrhage), or severe liver impairment.
• It should be given with caution to people with any condition or disorder that would make bleeding more likely (for example, injury, surgery), or with liver or kidney impairment.
• Ticlopidine should be used during pregnancy only if it is clearly needed.
• Medical judgment is required if breast-feeding is being considered. It is not known whether this drug appears in breast milk.
• When using this drug, bleeding takes longer to stop, but unusual bleeding should be reported to a doctor. Also, any doctor or dentist should be advised that ticlopidine is being used before any surgery is performed or any new drug prescribed. (Ticlopidine treatment should be stopped 10 to 14 days before surgery.)
• Complete blood counts are needed periodically while using this drug.
• Signs of jaundice, such as yellowing of skin or eyes, dark urine or light stools should be reported immediately to a doctor. Signs of infection (fever, chills, sore throat) should also be reported.

Interactions

• ℞ **aspirin** and other ℞ **NSAIDs** intensify the antiplatelet effect, with a higher potential for gastrointestinal bleeding. Aspirin should not, in general, be used with ticlopidine.
• Ticlopidine may prolong or increase the effect of theophylline.
• ℞ **Cimetidine** may increase the levels and effect of ticlopidine.
• Caution is advised when using ℞ **phenytoin** or ℞ **propranolol** with ticlopidine.
• When used with ℞ **digoxin**, a slight decrease in digoxin levels may occur.
• ℞ **Antacids** may lower the levels and effect of ticlopidine.

Side effects

• The most common are gastrointestinal disturbances (for example, diarrhea, nausea, indigestion, pain, vomiting), rash and itching, blood changes (some serious), bruising, and increased blood cholesterol. Diarrhea, if severe, may require discontinuing ticlopidine.
• Less frequently, headache, changes in liver or biliary function, dizziness, nosebleed, or ringing in the ears. Severe allergic reactions and kidney damage are rare. Intracranial bleeding or hemorrhage of wounds, or within the eyes, lungs, and so on, occurs no more frequently than with aspirin.

Tigan Capsules; Adult Suppositories; Pediatric Suppositories ⑧

A preparation of ℞ **trimethobenzamide hydrochloride**.
Formulation: Oral capsules (2 strengths); rectal suppositories; injection.
Availability: Prescription only.
Warnings and side effects: See ℞ **trimethobenzamide hydrochloride**.

Tilade ⑧

A preparation of ℞ **nedocromil sodium**.
Formulation: Aerosol inhalant.
Availability: Prescription only.
Warnings and side effects: See ℞ **nedocromil sodium**.

tiludronate sodium ⑥

(tiludronic acid)
Type/Group: **bisphosphonate; calcium-metabolism modifier**.
Brand(s): Skelid.
How administered: Orally.

Used to treat

Tiludronate is used to treat ✪ **Paget's disease (of the bone)**.

Warnings

• It should not be given to people with known hypersensitivity to bisphosphonates.

• It should be given with caution to people with kidney dysfunction or esophageal gastric disease.

• It should be used during pregnancy only if clearly needed.

• Medical judgment is required if breast-feeding is being considered. It is not known if it appears in breast milk.

• It should be taken with a glass of plain water, and not within two hours of food (this reduces absorption of the drug) or any other medication.

Interactions

• ℞ **Antacids**, ♂♀ **calcium**, and ℞ **aspirin** reduce the effects of tiludronate.

• The effects of ℞ **indomethacin** may be increased.

Side effects

• Frequently, nausea, diarrhea, generalized body pain, back pain, and headache.

• Occasionally, rash, upset stomach, vomiting, nasal inflammation, sinus inflammation, and dizziness.

Timentin ⓑ

A preparation of ℞ **ticarcillin** and ℞ **clavulanic acid**.
Formulation: Injection; intravenous infusion.
Availability: Prescription only.
Warnings and side effects: See ℞ **ticarcillin**; ℞ **clavulanic acid**.

Timolide 10/25 ⓑ

A preparation of ℞ **hydrochlorothiazide** and ℞ **timolol maleate**.
Formulation: Oral tablets.
Availability: Prescription only.
Warnings and side effects: See ℞ **hydrochlorothiazide**; ℞ **timolol maleate**.

timolol maleate ⓖ

Type/Group: beta-blocker; antihypertensive; antimigraine; glaucoma treatment; antianginal.
Brand(s): (Oral use): Blocadren; various generic. (Ophthalmic, topical): Betimol; Timoptic, Timoptic-XE; various generic.
Combinations: With *hydrochlorothiazide*: Timolide.
How administered: Orally, topically (ophthalmic).

Used to treat

Timolol is used to reduce high blood pressure (see ❂ **hypertension**), after a heart attack to aid recovery, to prevent ❂ **migraine** attacks, and (as eyedrops) to treat open-angle ❂ **glaucoma** or elevated intraocular pressure (pressure in the eyeball).

Warnings

• It should not be given to people with known hypersensitivity to any beta-blocking drug, who have certain heartbeat irregularities or heart failure, or bronchial asthma, allergic bronchospasm or severe chronic obstructive pulmonary disease (COPD). It should not be used in cardiogenic shock.

• It should be given with caution to people with diabetes mellitus or hypoglycemia, hyperthyroidism, myasthenia gravis, congestive heart failure, peripheral vascular disease, moderate bronchospastic disease (for example, chronic bronchitis or emphysema), or liver or kidney impairment.

• Timolol's safety during pregnancy has not been established, and it should be used only if the potential benefit outweighs the possible risk to the fetus.

• Medical judgment is required if breast-feeding is being considered. It is not known whether this drug appears in breast milk.

• Abruptly stopping using a beta-blocker may have adverse effects such as on the heart.

• The use of this drug may mask signs of hyperthyroidism or hypoglycemia.

• Other medications (including OTCs, herbal remedies, and supplements) must not be taken without consulting a doctor. Some ℞ **nasal decongestants**, commonly available over the counter, contain ℞ **alpha-adrenergic stimulants** (for example, ℞ **phenylephrine**) that may cause a severe hypertensive reaction if taken with beta-blockers.

• Ophthalmic preparations can be absorbed systemically (through the eye) and so systemic side effects may be observed (see below).

Interactions

• A serious blood pressure increase may occur after withdrawal from ℞ **clonidine hydrochloride** or both drugs at the same time.

• Other ℞ **antiarrhythmics** (for example, ℞ **amiodarone**, ℞ **disopyramide**, ℞ **procainamide**, ℞ **quinidine**) and ℞ **tricyclics** have the potential for significant adverse effects on heart rhythm.

• The effects of ℞ **alpha-adrenergic stimulants**, ℞ **ergot alkaloids**, ℞ **epinephrine**, ℞ **lidocaine**, and ℞ **theophylline** may be increased, with risk of serious adverse effects.

• ℞ **Calcium-channel blockers** (particularly ℞ **diltiazem** and ℞ **verapami**), ℞ **guanethidine monosulfate**, and ℞ **reserpine** have the potential for increasing undesirable effects, with exaggerated slowing of heartbeat or hypotension.

• The effects of nondepolarizing ℞ **skeletal muscle relaxants** may be variable, with the possible risk of significant adverse effects associated with major surgery.

• The effects of ℞ **beta-adrenergic stimulants** (for example, ℞ **albuterol**, ℞ **terbutaline**), ℞ **insulin**, and ℞ **sulfonylureas** may be reduced by propranolol.

• ℞ **Cimetidine** may increase the effect of timolol.

• ℞ **Antacids** (for example, ℞ **aluminum hydroxide**, ℞ **magnesium hydroxide**), ℞ **barbiturates**, ♂♀ **calcium** salts, ℞ **cholestyramine**, ℞ **colestipol hydrochloride**, ℞ NSAIDs, ℞ **phenytoin**, ℞ **penicillins**, ℞ **rifampin**, and ℞ **salicylates** may reduce the levels and effectiveness of beta-blockers. Antacids should not be taken within two hours of beta-blockers.

• If used with ℞ **diuretics** and other antihypertensive drugs, there are additive effects which are often used to therapeutic advantage.

Side effects

• Oral use: Slowing of heart rate, dizziness, fatigue, gastrointestinal disturbances (for example, discomfort, nausea, constipation), or hypotension. Occasionally, headache, insomnia, arrhythmias, bronchospasm, shortness of breath, or swelling of the extremities. Rarely, rash, joint and muscle pain, confusion, impotence or decreased libido, or strange taste sensations.

Key to symbols: ❂ = Disorder Section ℞ = Drug Section ♣ = Herbal Section ♂♀ = Supplement Section

• Topical (ophthalmic) use: Frequently, eye irritation or visual disturbances. Occasionally, increased light sensitivity or watering of eyes. Rarely, dry eyes, conjunctivitis or eye pain.

Tinactin; Tinactin for Jock Itch Ⓑ

A preparation of ℞ tolnaftate.
Formulation: Topical cream, topical powder; spray powder; spray liquid.
Availability: OTC.
Warnings and side effects: See ℞ **tolnaftate.**

Ting Ⓑ

A preparation of ℞ tolnaftate.
Formulation: Topical cream.
Availability: OTC.
Warnings and side effects: See ℞ **tolnaftate.**

tinzaparin sodium Ⓖ

Type/Group: **anticoagulant.**
Brand(s): Innohep.
How administered: Injection (subcutaneous).

Used to treat

Tinzaparin sodium is a low molecular weight heparin, an anticoagulant. It can be used to treat ✪ **deep vein thrombosis,** sometimes in combination with ℞ **warfarin sodium.**

Warnings

• It should not be given to people with known hypersensitivity to this drug (or to sulfites, benzyl alcohol, or pork products), with major bleeding, or who have experienced a reduction of thrombocyte levels after taking heparin.
• Extreme caution is needed in giving this drug to people with an increased risk of hemorrhage (for example, uncontrolled hypertension, bleeding disorders, active ulcer, recent stroke, or surgery). Use with caution in people with a tendency to bleed or recent gastrointestinal bleeding, with low thrombocyte levels or platelet defects, or with severe kidney impairment.
• Tinzaparin should be used during pregnancy only if it is clearly needed.
• Medical judgment is required if breast-feeding is being considered. It is not known whether this drug appears in breast milk.
• In people taking low molecular weight heparins, there is risk that use of spinal or epidural anesthesia, or other spinal puncture procedures, may result in a trapped accumulation of blood (hematoma) and paralysis.
• Rarely, priapism (prolonged and painful penile erection) has occurred which sometimes requires surgery.

Interactions

• If used with other anticoagulants, ℞ **antiplatelet** agents, ℞ **NSAIDs,** or ℞ **thrombolytic** agents, there is a greater risk of bleeding, so caution is advised.

Side effects

• The most common are bleeding (although major bleeding is infrequent) and hematoma at the injection site. Bleeding can occur at many sites in the body, including the urinary and intestinal tracts.

• Other side effects may include headache, dizziness, chest pain, changes in liver function and in blood counts, arrhythmias, priapism, and allergic reactions (for example, rash, itching, fever, facial swelling).

tioconazole Ⓖ

Type/Group: **antifungal; azole; candidiasis treatment.**
Brand(s): Vagistat-1.
How administered: Topically (external).

Used to treat

Tioconazole is a synthetic azole broad-spectrum antifungal used to treat vaginal ✪ **candidiasis.**

Warnings

• It should not be given to people with known sensitivity to tioconazole.
• Its safety in pregnancy has not been established and so it should be used only if clearly needed.
• Medical judgment is required if breast-feeding is being considered. It is not known whether this drug appears in breast milk.
• It is not reliable in treating infections of the scalp or nail beds.

Interactions

None significant have been reported when used topically (externally).

Side effects

• Burning, itching, irritation, discharge, vulva edema and swelling, vaginal pain, urinary problems, and vaginal dryness.

tioguanine Ⓖ

see ℞ **thioguanine.**

tirofiban Ⓖ

Type/Group: **antiplatelet.**
Brand(s): Aggrastat.
How administered: Intravenous infusion.

Used to treat

Tirofiban is an antiplatelet drug which is used to prevent ✪ **thrombosis** (blood-clot formation). It works by stopping platelets sticking to one another or to the walls of blood vessels. It can be used (together with ℞ **heparin**) to prevent thrombosis in acute cardiac conditions in which myocardial infarction (heart attack) has already occurred or is likely to occur. ℞ **aspirin** is often given, as well, in the combined drug therapy.

Warnings

• It should not be given to people with known hypersensitivity or reduced thrombocyte levels after using this drug, with active internal bleeding (for example, peptic ulcer) or within 30 days of such active bleeding (including stroke, major surgery, or injury), with a history of intracranial hemorrhage, aneurysm or certain vascular malformations, with active pericarditis or severe high blood pressure. Tirofiban should not be used together with any drug that has similar antiplatelet action. It will be administered by experienced personnel after a full medical assessment.
• It should be given with caution to people with low platelet count or severe kidney impairment.

• Tirofiban should be used during pregnancy only if it is clearly needed.

• Medical judgment is required if breast-feeding is being considered. It is not known whether this drug appears in breast milk.

• This drug is used only in a hospital setting, with periodic monitoring of blood values and close observation for potential bleeding.

Interactions

• If used with ℞ **anticoagulants** or ℞ **thrombolytic** agents, there is a higher potential for bleeding (caution is advised).

• ℞ **Levothyroxine** or ℞ **omeprazole** may lower the levels of tirofiban (although effects are unknown).

Side effects

• The most common is bleeding, although major bleeding is infrequent.

• Other side effects may include pelvic pain, slowed heartbeat, dizziness, leg pain, edema, or sweating.

TI-Screen; TI-Screen Natural; TI-Baby Natural ®

A preparation of ℞ **titanium dioxide**.
Formulation: Topical lotion.
Availability: OTC.
Warnings and side effects: See ℞ **titanium dioxide**.

Tisit; Tisit Blue ®

A preparation of ℞ **pyrethrin**.
Formulation: Topical liquid; topical gel (Blue).
Availability: OTC.
Warnings and side effects: See ℞ **pyrethrin**.

tissue-type plasminogen activator Ⓖ

see ℞ **alteplase, recombinant**.

titanium dioxide Ⓖ

Type/Group: **sunscreen**.
Brand(s): Hawaiian Tropic Baby Faces Sunblock; Neutrogena Chemical-Free Sunblocker; TI-Screen; Vaseline Intensive Care Baby Sunblock.
How administered: Topically (external).

Used to treat

Titanium dioxide is a white pigment that provides some degree of protection from ultraviolet UVA and UVB radiation.

Warnings

None significant.

Interactions

None significant.

Side effects

None significant.

Titralac Tablets; Extra Strength Tablets ®

A preparation of ℞ **calcium carbonate**.
Formulation: Oral tablets, chewable.
Availability: OTC.

Warnings and side effects: See ℞ **calcium carbonate**.

Titrilac Plus Tablets; Liquid ®

A preparation of ℞ **calcium carbonate** and ℞ **simethicone**.
Formulation: Oral tablets, chewable; liquid.
Availability: OTC.
Warnings and side effects: See ℞ **calcium carbonate**; ℞ **simethicone**.

tizanidine Ⓖ

Type/Group: **skeletal muscle relaxant**.
Brand(s): Zanaflex.
How administered: Orally.

Used to treat

Tizanidine is used for relieving severe muscle spasticity associated with multiple sclerosis or spinal cord injury or disease. It works within the central nervous system (CNS), probably by stimulation of alpha$_2$-adrenergic receptors on nerve-endings.

Warnings

• It should not be used by people with known hypersensitivity to tizanidine, kidney impairment, or hypotension.

• It should be given with caution to people with impaired liver function or who are over 65.

• It is not usually given to children.

• It should be used during pregnancy only if the benefits outweigh the risks to the fetus.

• Medical judgment is required if breast-feeding is being considered. Tizanidine may pass into breast milk.

• It may cause enough sedation to interfere with daily activities.

• Occasionally, hallucinations and psychotic-like symptoms may occur.

• Alcohol or other CNS depressants must be avoided.

Interactions

• ℞ **Oral contraceptives** may increase the effects of tizanidine.

• The effectiveness of ℞ **acetaminophen** may be delayed or reduced.

• There is a potential for hypotension if taken with ℞ **clonidine hydrochloride**, ℞ **guanabenz**, ℞ **guanadrel**, ℞ **guanethidine monosulfate**, and ℞ **guanfacine**, and so should be avoided.

Side effects

• Frequently, dizziness, drowsiness, weakness, and dry mouth.

• Occasionally, dyskinesia, nervousness, slurred speech, blurred vision, nose or throat inflammation, abnormal liver function tests, constipation, vomiting, urinary frequency, and increased spasm or muscle tone.

TMP-SMZ Ⓖ

see ℞ **trimethoprim and sulfamethoxazole**.

tobramycin Ⓖ

Type/Group: **aminoglycoside; antibiotic; antibacterial**.
Brand(s): Injection: Nebcin; various generic. Inhalant: TOBI.
Intraocular: AK-Tob; Defy; TOBI; Tobrex; various generic.
Combinations: With *dexamethasone*: Tobradex (ophthalmic).

Key to symbols: ✪ = Disorder Section ℞ = Drug Section ♣ = Herbal Section ◁▷ = Supplement Section

How administered: Injection; intravenous infusion; ophthalmic (eye); inhalant.

Used to treat

Tobramycin is effective against some Gram-positive and Gram-negative bacteria, and is used primarily for the treatment of serious Gram-negative ○ **bacterial infections** caused by *Pseudomonas aeruginosa*, because it is significantly more active against this organism than ℞ **gentamicin** (the most commonly used of this class). Like other aminoglycosides, it is not absorbed from the intestine (except in the case of local infection or liver failure) and so is given by injection or intravenous infusion (for example, for urinary tract infections). It is also used to treat bacterial infections of the eye and for management of ○ **pneumonia** in ○ **cystic fibrosis**.

Warnings

• It should not be given to people with known hypersensitivity to tobramycin or other aminoglycosides, or with severe kidney disease.

• It should be given with caution to people with mild kidney disease, hearing deficits or vertigo, with muscular disorders, such as myasthenia gravis or parkinsonism, extensive burns, and those over 65.

• Medical judgment is required when giving to very young infants.

• Tobramycin should be used during pregnancy only if medically judged to be clearly needed and if the potential benefits outweigh the risks to the fetus (it crosses the placenta and could cause damage to ears or kidneys).

• Medical judgment is required if breast-feeding is being considered, even with ophthalmic use. It does appear in breast milk.

• Aminoglycosides are associated with nephrotoxicity (damage to the kidneys) and ototoxicity (damage in the ears). Irreversible vestibular impairment can occur, resulting in vertigo and difficulty maintaining balance. Permanent hearing loss in one or both ears can also occur. The risk is greatest in those with pre-existing impairments, with high doses, and with prolonged use.

• A doctor must be contacted if there are problems with hearing, vision, balance, urination, or headaches, even after the course of treatment is completed.

• The use of antibiotics may result in superinfection due to bacterial imbalance.

Interactions

• ℞ **Atracurium**, ℞ **succinylcholine**, ℞ **vecuronium**, or neuromuscular blocking agents taken with tobramycin increases respiratory depression.

• ℞ **ethacrynic acid** and ℞ **carboplatin** increase the risk of ear damage.

• ℞ **Amphotericin B**, ℞ **cephalosporins**, ℞ **cyclosporine**, methoxyflurane, and ℞ **NSAIDs** may increase the risk of kidney damage.

• ℞ **Carboplatin**, ℞ **cisplatin**, and ℞ **vancomycin** increase the risk of ear or kidney damage.

• ℞ **Carbenicillin**, ℞ **penicillins**, ℞ **piperacillin**, and ℞ **ticarcillin** could inactivate tobramycin in people with kidney failure.

Side effects

• Occasionally, allergic reaction, blood changes, neurotoxicity, ototoxicity and deafness, and kidney damage.

• Rarely, hypotension, nausea, and vomiting. When used in the eye, tearing, itching, redness, and swelling of eyelid.

Tobrex ⑧

A preparation of ℞ **tobramycin**.
Formulation: Eye drops; ophthalmic ointment.
Availability: Prescription only.
Warnings and side effects: See ℞ **tobramycin**.

tocainide hydrochloride ⑥

Type/Group: **antiarrhythmic**.
Brand(s): Tonocard.
How administered: Orally.

Used to treat

Tocainide hydrochloride is an analog of a ℞ **local anesthetic**, ℞ **lidocaine**. It is used to treat heartbeat irregularities, generally only certain life-threatening ○ **arrhythmias**. Because of its high incidence of blood toxicity, it is used only when other drugs have been tried.

Warnings

• It should not be given to people with known hypersensitivity to this drug or to amide-type local anesthetics, or with certain heart disorders.

• It should be given with caution to people with impaired liver or kidney function, heart failure, bone marrow depression, or low blood-cell counts of any type. This is a specialist drug and treatment will be carried out by experienced clinicians who are thoroughly familiar with this drug. Periodic monitoring of heart function, lung function and blood values is necessary.

• Tocainide may have the potential to harm the fetus and so it should be used only if the potential benefit outweighs the risk to the fetus.

• It is present in breast milk and nursing women should discontinue using this drug or stop breast-feeding.

• Tocainide can, occasionally, provoke arrhythmias.

• A doctor must be contacted if such symptoms as skin rash, or those that might signify blood changes (for example, unusual bleeding or bruising, or signs of infection such as fever, sore throat, mouth sores or chills), or pulmonary difficulties (for example, breathlessness with mild exercise, cough or wheezing) occur.

Interactions

• ℞ **metoprolol** may have increased effects on heart action.

• ℞ **Lidocaine** may have increased effects, with a higher risk of adverse reactions.

• ℞ **Cimetidine** and ℞ **rifampin** may reduce the levels and effects of tocainide.

Side effects

• Effects on the gastrointestinal tract and nervous system are frequent and may include nausea, vomiting, loss of appetite, and diarrhea. Dizziness, numbness or tingling, tremor, nervousness, confusion, hallucinations, headache, or blurred vision may also occur.

• Other side effects may include palpitations, rash, night sweats, clammy skin, or sensations of warmth or cold.

• Although uncommon, major pulmonary disorders (for example, pneumonitis, pneumonia) or serious blood changes may occur (with lower counts of any blood-cell type).

Tofranil Tablets; Tofranil-PM ®

A preparation of ℞ **imipramine**.
Formulation: Oral tablets; PM is capsule and is imipramine pamoate; both are available in several strengths.
Availability: Prescription only.
Warnings and side effects: See ℞ **imipramine**.

tolazamide ©

Type/Group: **antidiabetic; oral hypoglycemic; sulfonylurea.**
Brand(s): Tolinase; various generic.
How administered: Orally.

Used to treat
Tolazamide is one of the sulfonylurea group and is used to treat type 2 ○ **diabetes mellitus** (non-insulin-dependent diabetes mellitus; NIDDM).

Warnings
• It should not be given to people with type 1 diabetes mellitus.
• It should be given with caution to people with heart, thyroid, kidney or liver disease, severe hypoglycemic reactions, and who are over 65.
• It is inappropriate for use during pregnancy (insulin is the drug of choice).
• Medical judgment is required if breast-feeding is being considered.
• Alcohol should be avoided while using this drug, as it can cause unpleasant symptoms and interfere with blood sugar control.
• There are potentially multiple drug interactions with tolazamide. A doctor must be consulted before any other medication is taken (including OTCs, herbal remedies, and supplements).

Interactions
• ℞ NSAIDs, ℞ salicylates, ℞ sulfonamides, ℞ chloramphenicol, coumarins, ℞ probenecid, ℞ MAOIs, and ℞ beta-blockers may enhance the hypoglycemic effect of sulfonylureas.
• ℞ Thiazide and other ℞ diuretics, ℞ corticosteroids, ℞ phenothiazines, ℞ thyroid hormones, ℞ estrogens, ℞ oral contraceptives, ℞ phenytoin, ℞ niacin, ℞ sympathomimetics, and ℞ isoniazid may lead to the loss of control of sugar levels.
• Oral ℞ miconazole, ℞ diclofenac, ℞ ibuprofen, ℞ naproxen, and ℞ mefenamic acid have the potential for severe hypoglycemia.

Side effects
• Frequently, dizziness, fatigue, headache, lethargy, weakness, and gastrointestinal effects.
• Uncommonly, ringing ears, jaundice, hypoglycemia, and allergic skin reactions.
• Rarely, liver damage, blood changes.

tolbutamide ©

Type/Group: **antidiabetic; oral hypoglycemic; sulfonylurea.**
Brand(s): Orinase; various generic.
How administered: Orally.

Used to treat
Tolbutamide is used to treat type 2 ○ **diabetes mellitus** (non-insulin-dependent diabetes mellitus; NIDDM).

Warnings
• It should not be given to people with juvenile diabetes or ketoacidosis.
• It should be given with caution to people with heart, thyroid, kidney, or liver disease, severe hypoglycemic reactions, and those over 65.
• It is inappropriate for use during pregnancy (insulin is the drug of choice).
• Medical judgment is required if breast-feeding is being considered.
• Alcohol should be avoided while using this drug, as it can cause unpleasant symptoms and interfere with blood sugar control.
• There are potentially multiple drug interactions with tolbutamide. A doctor must be consulted before taking any other medication (including OTCs, herbal remedies, and supplements).

Interactions
• ℞ NSAIDs, ℞ salicylates, ℞ sulfonamides, ℞ chloramphenicol, coumarins, ℞ probenecid, ℞ MAOIs, and ℞ beta-blockers may enhance the hypoglycemic effect of sulfonylureas.
• ℞ Thiazide and other ℞ diuretics, ℞ corticosteroids, ℞ phenothiazines, ℞ thyroid hormones, ℞ estrogens, ℞ oral contraceptives, ℞ phenytoin, ℞ niacin, ℞ sympathomimetics, and ℞ isoniazid may lead to the loss of control of sugar levels.
• Oral ℞ miconazole, ℞ diclofenac, ℞ ibuprofen, ℞ naproxen, and ℞ mefenamic acid have the potential for severe hypoglycemia.

Side effects
• Frequently, dizziness, fatigue, headache, lethargy, weakness, gastrointestinal effects.
• Uncommonly, ringing ears, jaundice, hypoglycemia, and allergic skin reactions.
• Rarely, liver damage and blood changes.

tolcapone ©

Type/Group: **antiparkinsonism.**
Brand(s): Tasmar.
How administered: Orally.

Used to treat
Tolcapone is used to treat the symptoms of ○ **Parkinson's disease** in those using ℞ **levodopa**/℞ **carbidopa** combined therapy. Its enzyme-inhibiting property, in effect, supplements and extends the action of levodopa and (in many but not all patients) it also minimizes some side effects. The drug inhibits an enzyme (catechol-O-methyltransferase; COMT) that, in the presence of carbidopa (another enzyme inhibitor), breaks down the neurotransmitter dopamine in the brain. It is thought that dopamine deficiency in the brain causes Parkinson's disease. Tolcapone is used only in those

who are not responding satisfactorily to, or are not appropriate candidates for, other adjunctive therapies (additional treatments to enhance effectiveness).

Warnings

• It should not be used by people with clinical evidence of liver disease, who have abnormal liver function tests, whose liver showed signs of injury following previous treatment with tolcapone, or those with a history of rhabdomyolysis (a condition that can lead to kidney failure), sudden high fever, or confusion possibly related to medication.

• It should be used with caution in people with severe abnormalities of muscle tone or movement, and those with kidney function impairment.

• The effects of tolcapone in pregnancy are unknown. It therefore should be used during pregnancy only if clearly needed and if the benefits outweigh the possible risk to the fetus.

• It is unknown whether this drug appears in breast milk, and so medical judgment is also required if breast-feeding is being considered.

• Tolcapone carries a risk of liver injury or failure, which is potentially fatal (monitoring is required). The signs of liver disease must be watched for (clay-colored stools, yellowing of the skin, dark urine, tenderness in upper right abdomen, fatigue, appetite loss, lethargy), and a doctor contacted if they occur.

• Tolcapone can cause hallucinations.

• Avoid skilled tasks, such as driving, until your response to the drug is established.

• Some people experience increases in levodopa-associated side effects, such as abnormalities of muscle tone or movement.

Interactions

• Tolcapone taken with non-selective ℞ **MAOIs** (℞ **phenelzine**, ℞ **tranylcypromine**) may inhibit the metabolism of catecholamines.

• The effects of ℞ **warfarin sodium** may be enhanced.

• Taking tolcapone with food may decrease its effectiveness.

Side effects

• Dyskinesia, sleep disorders, postural hypotension (lowered blood pressure on standing), nausea, diarrhea, loss of appetite, headache, increased sweating, vomiting, gastrointestinal discomfort, and nosebleeds.

Tolectin 200; 600; Tolectin DS   Ⓑ

A preparation of ℞ **tolmetin sodium**.

Formulation: Oral tablets (two strengths); DS is capsule.

Availability: Prescription only.

Warnings and side effects: See ℞ **tolmetin sodium**.

Tolinase   Ⓑ

A preparation of ℞ **tolazamide**.

Formulation: Oral capsules.

Availability: Prescription only.

Warnings and side effects: See ℞ **tolazamide**.

tolmetin sodium   Ⓖ

Type/Group: **anti-inflammatory; antirheumatic; non-narcotic analgesic; NSAID.**

Brand(s): Tolectin 200, 600, Tolectin DS.

How administered: Orally.

Used to treat

Tolmetin sodium is used in the long-term management of ✪ **rheumatoid arthritis**, ✪ **osteoarthritis**, and juvenile arthritis, and also for acute flare-ups.

Warnings

• It should not be used by people with known hypersensitivity to this drug or to other NSAIDs (including ℞ **aspirin**), who have chronic kidney disease, certain bleeding disorders or conditions (for example, hemophilia, vitamin K deficiency, low blood-platelet levels), or who have a tendency to, or active, peptic ulceration.

• It should be given with caution to people with peripheral edema or allergic disorders (especially asthma and skin conditions), who are elderly, or with any kind of kidney impairment or certain liver disorders.

• Tolmetin should be used during pregnancy only if medically judged to be needed. In the third trimester its risks rise, and so should only be used if the benefits outweigh the risks to the fetus.

• Breast-feeding mothers should either discontinue this drug or stop breast-feeding.

• With regular use (as in the treatment of osteoarthritis), NSAIDs may cause gastrointestinal bleeding, ulceration, or perforation. Any signs of bleeding (for example, black stools) should be reported to a physician immediately.

• Most NSAIDs have the potential, particularly with regular use, to cause liver damage. Periodic evaluation of liver function is necessary in long-term therapy (more than two months).

• Side effects are more frequent in the elderly.

• Gastrointestinal upsets may be minimized by taking the drug with milk or food.

Interactions

• There is generally no added benefit in taking other NSAIDs or other ℞ **salicylates** (especially aspirin) at the same time, but there is a higher risk of gastrointestinal upsets and bleeding.

• Alcohol and ℞ **corticosteroids** increase the risk of bleeding, particularly if there is an existing ulcer.

• ℞ **Anticoagulant**, ℞ **antiplatelet**, and ℞ **thrombolytic** drugs may increase bleeding time.

• The effectiveness of ℞ **ACE inhibitors**, ℞ **beta-blockers**, and ℞ **diuretics** may be reduced.

• The effects of ℞ **cyclosporine**, ℞ **digoxin**, ℞ **lithium**, and ℞ **methotrexate** may be exaggerated, with potential for toxicity.

• Foodstuffs and herbals with ℞ **antiplatelet** properties, for example, ♣ **ginger**, ♧ **garlic**, and various herbal preparations, may add to the antiplatelet effect of NSAIDs.

Side effects

These vary in severity and how often they occur.

• Commonly, nausea, vomiting, diarrhea, gastrointestinal upsets, heartburn, swelling of the extremities, fatigue, headache, dizziness, and a rise in blood pressure. Weight gain or weight loss are both possible.

• Less frequently, constipation, drowsiness, blurred vision, ringing in the ears, itching and rash.

• Prolonged bleeding time (with consequent risk of ulceration) is possible with high dosage, and other blood changes can occur, including anemia.

• Hypersensitivity reactions may include symptoms such as hives, rash, chest tightness, asthma, or bronchospasm.

• Reversible kidney failure, particularly in renal impairment, has occurred. Liver damage is rare.

tolnaftate Ⓖ

Type/Group: **antifungal**.

Brand(s): Absorbine; Aftate; Blis-To-Sol; Quinsana Plus; Ting; Tinactin. Combinations: With *undecylenic acid* and other components: Dermasept Antifungal; SteriNail.

How administered: Topically (external).

Used to treat

Tolnaftate is a synthetic mild antifungal drug used primarily in the topical (external) treatment of infections caused by the ✪ **tinea** species (for example, ✪ **athlete's foot**).

Warnings

• It should not be given to people with known sensitivity to tolnaftate.

• Its safety in pregnancy has not been established and so it should be used only if clearly needed.

• Medical judgment is required if breast-feeding is being considered. It is not known whether this drug appears in breast milk.

• It is not reliable in treating infections of the scalp or nail beds.

Interactions

None significant have been reported when used topically.

Side effects

• Rash, stinging, and hives.

tolterodine tartrate Ⓖ

Type/Group: **anticholinergic; antispasmodic**.

Brand(s): Detrol.

How administered: Orally.

Used to treat

Tolterodine tartrate can be used as an antispasmodic to treat urinary frequency, ✪ **incontinence**, and urinary urgency.

Warnings

• It should not be given to people with known hypersensitivity to the drug or any of its ingredients, with urinary retention, gastric retention, or uncontrolled narrow-angle glaucoma.

• It should be given with caution to people with significant bladder outflow obstruction, decreased gastrointestinal motility, controlled narrow-angle glaucoma, reduced kidney function, or reduced liver function.

• It should be used during pregnancy only when it is clearly needed and when the potential benefits outweigh the possible risk to the fetus.

• It is not recommended for use by nursing mothers.

• It may cause drowsiness, dizziness, or blurred vision. Caution must be exercised when driving or performing other activities requiring physical skill, clear vision, or mental alertness.

Interactions

• ℞ **fluoxetine** increases the levels of tolterodine.

Side effects

• It commonly causes dry mouth, upset stomach, headache, constipation, vertigo, and dry eyes.

Tolu-Sed DM Syrup Ⓑ

A preparation of ℞ **dextromethorphan** and ℞ **guaifenesin**.

Formulation: Oral syrup.

Availability: OTC.

Warnings and side effects: See ℞ **dextromethorphan**; ℞ **guaifenesin**.

Tonocard Ⓑ

A preparation of ℞ **tocainide hydrochloride**.

Formulation: Oral tablets, available in two strengths.

Availability: Prescription only.

Warnings and side effects: See ℞ **tocainide hydrochloride**.

Topamax Ⓑ

A preparation of ℞ **topiramate**.

Formulation: Oral tablets (3 strengths); sprinkle capsules (3 strengths).

Availability: Prescription only.

Warnings and side effects: See ℞ **topiramate**.

Topicort; Topicort LP Ⓑ

A preparation of ℞ **desoxymetasone**.

Formulation: Cream in two strengths (LP is stronger); ointment; gel.

Availability: Prescription only.

Warnings and side effects: See ℞ **desoxymetasone**.

topiramate Ⓖ

Type/Group: **anticonvulsant; antiepileptic**.

Brand(s): Topamax.

How administered: Orally.

Used to treat

Topiramate is a recently introduced drug used in the treatment of ✪ **epilepsy** to assist in the control of partial seizures.

Warnings

• Avoid its use in people with known hypersensitivity to this drug.

• It should be given with caution to anyone with kidney or liver impairment.

• Studies suggest adverse effects on the development of the fetus, therefore topiramate should be used in pregnancy only when potential benefit outweighs potential risk to the fetus.

• It is not known whether this drug appears in breast milk, and so it should be used by breast-feeding mothers only when potential benefits outweigh the risks to the infant.

• Withdrawal should be gradual otherwise it may precipitate attacks.

• As this drug may cause drowsiness, driving or other hazardous activity should be avoided.

Interactions

• Alcohol and CNS depressants (such as, ℞ **benzodiazepines**, ℞ **opioids**, ℞ **skeletal muscle relaxants**, ℞ **hypnotics**, ℞ **sedatives**, ℞ **tranquilizers**) may have potentially serious additive effects.

• ℞ **Carbonic-anhydrase inhibitors** (for example, ℞ **acetazolamide**) may increase the risk of forming kidney stones, and so these drugs should not be used with topiramate.

• Other ℞ **antiepileptic** drugs (such as, ℞ **phenytoin**, ℞ **carbamazepine**, and ℞ **sodium valproate**) decrease levels of topiramate, while the levels of these drugs may increase or decrease.

• There may be a risk of reducing the effectiveness of oral ℞ **contraceptives**.

• ℞ **Digoxin** levels may be slightly decreased.

Side effects

• Effects involving the central nervous system (CNS) are frequent, including difficulties with memory, concentration or speech, drowsiness, dizziness, nervousness, confusion, tremor, mood problems, and incoordination in movements.

• Tingling or other sensations in the extremities are common.

• Other frequent side effects include visual disturbances, nausea and gastrointestinal upsets, weight loss, breast pain, and menstrual disorders (for example, dysmenorrhea).

Toposar ℞

A preparation of ℞ **etoposide**.
Formulation: Injection.
Availability: Prescription only.
Warnings and side effects: See ℞ **etoposide**.

topotecan ⑥

Type/Group: **anticancer; cytotoxic**.
Brand(s): Hycamtin.
How administered: Intravenous infusion.

Used to treat

Topotecan is one of a new group of drugs termed the topoisomerase I inhibitors. It is used in the treatment of ovarian ✪ **cancer** and small-cell ✪ **lung cancer**.

Warnings

• It should not be given to people with known hypersensitivity to topotecan or any of its ingredients, or anyone with severe bone marrow depression.

• This is a specialist drug which will be used following a full evaluation by specialist physicians.

• Topotecan is not recommended for use during pregnancy unless it is medically judged to be essential, because it may cause birth defects. Becoming pregnant while using this drug must be avoided.

• It should not be used if breast-feeding.

• It can cause bone marrow suppression, which may lead to bleeding and a reduced resistance to infection.

• It may produce serious blood changes that may cause illness or require a transfusion.

Interactions

• ℞ **cisplatin** increases the severity of bone marrow depression.

• ℞ **filgrastim**, when given together with topotecan, prolongs the shortage of white blood cells.

Side effects

• Frequently, nausea, vomiting, diarrhea, hair loss, and headache.

• Occasionally, tingling or burning sensations, constipation, and abdominal pain.

• Rarely, loss of appetite, malaise, weakness, and bone and/or joint pain.

Toprol XL ⑧

A preparation of ℞ **metoprolol tartrate**.
Formulation: Oral tablets, extended release, available in three strengths.
Availability: Prescription only.
Warnings and side effects: See ℞ **metoprolol tartrate**.

Toradol Tablets; Injection ⑧

A preparation of ℞ **ketorolac tromethamine**.
Formulation: Oral tablets; injection.
Availability: Prescription only.
Warnings and side effects: See ℞ **ketorolac tromethamine**.

torasemide ⑥

see ℞ torsemide.

Torecan Tablets; Injection ⑧

A preparation of ℞ **thiethylperazine maleate**.
Formulation: Oral tablets; injection.
Availability: Prescription only.
Warnings and side effects: See ℞ **thiethylperazine maleate**.
Tablets contain tartrazine (FD&C yellow No. 5), a dye that may cause allergic reaction in some people, but especially those with sensitivity to aspirin or the sweetener aspartame, which should be avoided by individuals with phenylketonuria.

toremifene ⑥

Type/Group: **antiestrogen; anticancer; hormone antagonist**.
Brand(s): Fareston.
How administered: Orally.

Used to treat

Toremifene is a ℞ **sex hormone** antagonist, an ℞ **antiestrogen**, that antagonizes the natural estrogen present in the body. It is used in the treatment of ✪ **breast cancer** in postmenopausal women.

Warnings

• It should not be used with known hypersensitivity to toremifene.

• It should be given with extreme caution to anyone with a history of blood-clotting disorders.

• It should not be used during pregnancy. A doctor must be contacted if pregnancy occurs while taking this drug.

• Medical judgment is required if breast-feeding is being considered.

• It may aggravate bone disease at the beginning of treatment.

• It increases the incidence of endometrial cancer. Abnormal vaginal bleeding must be reported to a doctor, and regular gynecological examinations must be carried out during and after treatment.

Interactions

• The effects of ℞ **anticoagulants** may be increased by toremifene.

• ℞ **Anticonvulsants** (for example, ℞ **phenobarbital**, ℞ **phenytoin**, ℞ **carbamazepine**) may reduce the effects of toremifene.

• ℞ **Antifungals** (for example, ℞ **ketoconazole**) and ℞ **macrolide** ℞ **antibiotics** (for example, ℞ **erythromycin**) may increase the levels of toremifene.

Side effects

• Hot flashes, nausea, and vomiting.

• Less frequently, vaginal bleeding or discharge, menstrual irregularities, and skin rash.

• Rare but serious side effects include deep vein thrombosis, low white blood-cell counts, blood-clotting disorders, pulmonary embolism, and liver disorders.

Tornalate ®

A preparation of ℞ **bitolterol mesylate**.
Formulation: Aerosol inhalant, solution for inhalation.
Availability: Prescription only.
Warnings and side effects: See ℞ **bitolterol mesylate**.

torsemide ©

(torasemide)
Type/Group: **diuretic; antihypertensive**.
Brand(s): Demadex.
How administered: Orally; injection.

Used to treat

Torsemide is a powerful diuretic of the loop class. It can be used to treat edema (including fluid build-up in the lungs), low urine production (oliguria) due to kidney failure, and ✪ **hypertension** (alone or with other drugs).

Warnings

• It should not be given to people with known hypersensitivity to this drug (or to ℞ **sulfonylureas**), with anuria (no urine), or anyone in an electrolyte-depleted state.

• It should be given with caution to people with cirrhosis of the liver, certain kidney disorders, gout, diabetes mellitus, an enlarged prostate gland, or porphyria.

• Torsemide should be used during pregnancy only if it is clearly needed.

• Medical judgment is required if breast-feeding is being considered. Its effects if used when breast-feeding are unknown.

• Dehydration may result from too intense a diuretic effect, particularly in elderly people or anyone with a restricted sodium intake.

• Early symptoms of electrolyte imbalance may include muscle weakness or cramps, nausea, vomiting, restlessness or lethargy, dry mouth, excessive thirst, fast pulse, or dizziness. A doctor must be contacted if such symptoms occur.

• Loop diuretics may aggravate symptoms of diabetes or gout, and worsen or activate lupus erythematosus.

• Periodic monitoring of electrolytes, and kidney and liver function is needed.

• Photosensitivity may develop and so precautions such as protective clothing or sunscreens should be used.

• It may cause postural hypotension (lowered blood pressure on standing up), so get up slowly.

Interactions

• If taken with ℞ **lithium**, there is a risk of toxicity and the two drugs should not be used together.

• The effects of ℞ **aminoglycosides**, other antihypertensives, ℞ **cardiac glycosides**, ℞ **chloral hydrate**, and ℞ **propranolol** may be increased, with the potential of significant side effects or toxicity. An additive effect is sometimes used to advantage in combining loop diuretics with other antihypertensives.

• ℞ **Sulfonylureas** may raise blood sugar levels in diabetics with previously stabilized regimens.

• If taken with ℞ **cisplatin**, there is a potential for additive effects and toxicity.

• ℞ **Amphotericin B**, ℞ **corticosteroids**, and ℞ **corticotropin** may increase the effect of reducing potassium levels, with the possibility of severe depletion.

• The effects of nondepolarizing ℞ **skeletal muscle relaxants** and ℞ **theophylline** are unpredictable.

• ℞ **Activated charcoal**, ℞ **hydantoins**, ℞ **NSAIDs**, and antigout agents (for example, ℞ **probenecid**, ℞ **sulfinpyrazone**) may reduce the effects of torsemide.

Side effects

• There may be abnormally low blood pressure (hypotension), gastrointestinal disturbances, raised levels of urea in the blood or gout, raised blood glucose, changes in fats in the blood, headache, dizziness, ringing in the ears and hearing loss. Electrolyte levels in the blood (for example, potassium, sodium, magnesium, and chloride) may be lowered. There may be skin rashes, photosensitivity, effects on bone marrow, blood changes, or pancreatitis. Many of these effects are only seen with high or prolonged dosage. Hearing loss (usually reversible) is associated with rapid injection, high dosage, and the use of other drugs that affect hearing.

Totacillin ®

A preparation of ℞ **ampicillin**.
Formulation: Oral capsules in several strengths; oral suspension.
Availability: Prescription only.
Warnings and side effects: See ℞ **ampicillin**.

Touro A & H Capsules ®

A preparation of ℞ **pseudoephedrine** and ℞ **brompheniramine maleate**.
Formulation: Oral capsules, sustained release.
Availability: Prescription only.
Warnings and side effects: See ℞ **pseudoephedrine**; ℞ **brompheniramine maleate**.

Touro CC Ⓑ

A preparation of ℞ **dextromethorphan**, ℞ **pseudoephedrine**, ℞ **guaifenesin**.
Formulation: Oral capsules.
Availability: Prescription only.
Warnings and side effects: See ℞ **dextromethorphan**; ℞ **pseudoephedrine**; ℞ **guaifenesin**.

Touro-DM Tablets Ⓑ

A preparation of ℞ **dextromethorphan** and ℞ **guaifenesin**.
Formulation: Oral tablets, extended release.
Availability: Prescription only.
Warnings and side effects: See ℞ **dextromethorphan**; ℞ **guaifenesin**.

Touro EX Tablets Ⓑ

A preparation of ℞ **guaifenesin**.
Formulation: Oral tablets, sustained release.
Availability: Prescription only.
Warnings and side effects: See ℞ **guaifenesin**.

Touro LA Caplets Ⓑ

A preparation of ℞ **pseudoephedrine** and ℞ **guaifenesin**.
Formulation: Oral tablets, long acting.
Availability: Prescription only.
Warnings and side effects: See ℞ **pseudoephedrine**; ℞ **guaifenesin**.

T-Phyl Ⓑ

A preparation of ℞ **theophylline**.
Formulation: Oral tablets, timed release.
Availability: Prescription only.
Warnings and side effects: See ℞ **theophylline**.

Tracrium Ⓑ

A preparation of ℞ **atracurium besylate**.
Formulation: Injection.
Availability: Prescription only.
Warnings and side effects: See ℞ **atracurium besylate**.

Trac Tabs 2X Ⓑ

A preparation of ℞ **atropine sulfate**, ℞ **hyoscyamine**, ℞ **methenamine**, methylene blue, phenyl ℞ **salicylate**, and ℞ **benzoic acid**.
Formulation: Oral tablets.
Availability: Prescription only.
Warnings and side effects: See ℞ **atropine sulfate**; ℞ **hyoscyamine**; ℞ **methenamine**; ℞ **salicylates**; ℞ **benzoic acid**.

tramadol hydrochloride Ⓖ

Type/Group: **narcotic analgesic; opioid**.
Brand(s): Ultram.
How administered: Orally.

Used to treat

Tramadol is a recently introduced painkiller which is similar to ℞ **morphine** in its ability to relieve pain, but probably with fewer side effects. However, compared to other opioids there seem to be some differences in the mechanisms by which it produces analgesia, and it can not be completely incorporated into this group. It is not chemically related to opiate analgesics, but both acts at opioid receptors and also has additional effects on serotonin- and noradrenaline-utilizing nerve pathways within the central nervous system. It seems to have less of an addictive potential or risk of respiratory depression compared to typical opioids.

Warnings

• It should not be given to people with known hypersensitivity to this drug, or who are under the influence of alcohol, strong ℞ **analgesics**, ℞ **opioids**, ℞ **hypnotics**, or psychotropic drugs. Opioids (even the weaker ones) should not be given to people with asthma, or to anyone with seriously depressed breathing disorders, prostatic hypertrophy, convulsive disorders, raised intracranial pressure, or a head injury. Depending on use and dose, they should be given with caution to the elderly, or to anyone with hypotension, porphyria, certain liver, kidney, or adrenal disorders, hypothyroidism (under-activity of the thyroid gland), alcoholism, or a history of drug abuse. They must be given with extreme care to epileptics.
• Tramadol may harm the fetus and should not be used during pregnancy.
• It should not be used if breast-feeding.
• High doses of tramadol may cause seizures, especially when taken with ℞ **MAOI** antidepressants.
• Prolonged use of tramadol can lead to physical dependence (addiction), although this rarely happens in routine medical use, and withdrawal symptoms are not considered as severe as with other opioids (although its use may cause withdrawal symptoms in those who are already dependent on an opiate).
• Drowsiness may affect the performance of skilled tasks such as driving.
• The effects of alcohol may be enhanced (with a higher risk of respiratory depression).
• Its safety is not established in people under age 16.

Interactions

• If used with the following drugs, then effects are increased with the risk of seizures: ℞ **barbiturates**; ℞ **general anesthetics**; ℞ **MAOIs**; ℞ **opioids**; ℞ **SSRIs**; ℞ **tranquilizers** (for example, ℞ **phenothiazines**); ℞ **sedatives**; ℞ **benzodiazepines** (for example, ℞ **diazepam**, ℞ **lorazepam**); alcohol.
• ℞ **Carbamazepine** reduces the therapeutic effect of tramadol.

Side effects

• There may be sedation, constipation, dizziness, headache, nausea, and vomiting.
• There is occasionally euphoria, which may lead to a state of mental detachment or confusion. Also, less frequently, there may be sweating, palpitations, changes in heart rate, postural hypotension (a lowering of blood pressure on standing, causing dizziness), rashes, miosis (pupil constriction), dry mouth, flushing of the face, anxiety, mood change, and hallucinations.

• Anaphylactic reactions have been reported.

Trandate Tablets; Injection Ⓑ

A preparation of ℞ **labetalol hydrochloride**.
Formulation: Oral tablets (3 strengths); injection.
Availability: Prescription only.
Warnings and side effects: See ℞ **labetalol hydrochloride**.

trandolapril Ⓖ

Type/Group: ACE inhibitor; vasodilator; antihypertensive; heart failure treatment.
Brand(s): Mavik. Combinations: With *verapamil*: Tarka Tablets.
How administered: Orally.

Used to treat

Trandolapril can be used to treat high blood pressure in ✪ **hypertension**, often with other classes of drug, particularly ℞ **thiazide** ℞ **diuretics**. Also, it may be used to treat ✪ **heart failure** and left-ventricular malfunction that develops within a few days after ✪ **myocardial infarction** (damage to heart muscle, usually after a heart attack).

Warnings

• It should not be given to people with known hypersensitivity to this drug or to any other ACE inhibitor.

• It should be given with caution to people with severe congestive heart failure, or certain other cardiovascular disorders, a history of anaphylaxis, collagen vascular disease (for example, systemic lupus erythematosus; SLE), diabetes, depressed immune response, or with impaired kidney function or on dialysis.

• Risk in pregnancy increases substantially from the first through to the second and third trimesters. ACE inhibitors can cause injury to the fetus, even death. Use of these drugs should be stopped as soon as pregnancy is detected.

• Medical judgment is required if breast-feeding is being considered.

• Use of this drug should be stopped and a doctor contacted immediately if signs of angioedema appear (swelling of the face, eyes, lips, tongue, larynx, or extremities; difficulty in breathing or swallowing). Swelling of the larynx, closing off the airway, can be life-threatening.

• Anyone taking an ACE inhibitor should not interrupt or discontinue treatment without first checking with a doctor.

• Any suspected infections (for example, fever, sore throat) should be reported to a doctor, because ACE inhibitors may cause blood changes which can affect immune response.

• ACE inhibitors generally have less effect on blood pressure in blacks than in non-blacks, and the likelihood of angioedema is higher among blacks, as well.

Interactions

• ACE inhibitors have apparently triggered life-threatening anaphylactoid reactions when used by people also receiving ℞ **desensitizing vaccines**.

• ℞ **Anesthetics** (for example, in surgery), ℞ **phenothiazines**, and ℞ **probenecid** may increase the levels or hypotensive effect of trandolapril.

• Levels of ℞ **lithium** may be increased, with the potential for toxic effects.

• If used with potassium-sparing ℞ **diuretics** or other preparations containing potassium (for example, supplements and salt substitutes), levels of potassium may rise.

• ℞ **NSAID**s may increase the risk of kidney damage or (in some cases) reduce the effects of ACE inhibitors.

• ℞ **Antacids** and ℞ **rifampin** may reduce the effects of trandolapril. Antacids should not be used for several hours after a dose of an ACE inhibitor (a doctor should be consulted for full instructions and cautions).

• If used with other antihypertensives and diuretics, the effects of these drugs may be increased. This additive effect is sometimes used to advantage in combination treatments for high blood pressure.

Side effects

• The most frequent are dry cough, dizziness, and hypotension.

• Occasionally, headache, fainting, fatigue, weakness, tachycardia or heart rhythm disturbances, rash or gastrointestinal disturbances (for example, indigestion, diarrhea, nausea, and vomiting).

• Infrequently, insomnia, joint pain, pain or tingling in the extremities, muscle cramps, or sexual dysfunction. Although it is uncommon, ACE inhibitors can cause very marked hypotension (especially when beginning treatment) and kidney impairment.

• Rarely, there may be angioedema, altered liver function, jaundice, hepatitis, pancreatitis, or changes in blood counts.

tranexamic acid Ⓖ

Type/Group: hemostatic.
Brand(s): Cyklokapron.
How administered: Orally; injection.

Used to treat

Tranexamic acid inhibits the activation of plasminogen, which is an enzyme in the blood that dissolves blood clots. Tranexamic acid, therefore, is antifibrinolytic. It is used for short-term treatment of ✪ **hemophilia** to reduce or prevent hemorrhage, especially during and after tooth extraction. Other uses, although not stated by the manufacturer, have included reduction of bleeding after stomach or intestinal hemorrhage, after tonsillectomy or prostate surgery, recurrent nosebleeds, and in other short-term bleeding. Topically (externally), it has been used as a mouthwash to reduce bleeding after oral surgery in persons taking ℞ **anticoagulants**.

Warnings

• It should not be given to people with subarachnoid hemorrhage (a kind of brain hemorrhage) or with certain color vision defects—this makes it difficult to test for possible toxic effects on the retina in longer term use (more than several days). It will be prescribed by experienced personnel after a full medical assessment.

• It should be taken with caution by people with impaired kidney function.

• Tranexamic acid should be used during pregnancy only when it is clearly needed.

• Medical judgment is required if breast-feeding is being considered. This drug appears in breast milk.

• As this drug may affect vision, periodic eye exams are necessary, and its use stopped as soon as any change is discovered.

Interactions
No drug interactions of significance are known.

Side effects
• These may include abnormalities of vision, giddiness, and gastrointestinal disturbances (for example, nausea, vomiting, diarrhea), although gastrointestinal effects usually disappear with lower doses.

• Hypotension may occur when intravenous injection is too rapid.

tranquilizer Ⓓ

Actions and uses
Tranquilizer is a term sometimes used to describe a group of drugs that calm, soothe, and relieve anxiety, and many also cause some degree of sedation. Although it is somewhat misleading, they are often classified in two groups major tranquilizers and minor tranquilizers.

The major tranquilizers, which are also called neuroleptic or ℞ **antipsychotic** drugs, are used primarily to treat severe mental disorders, such as psychoses (including schizophrenia and mania: see ✪ **psychotic disorder**). They are extremely effective in restoring a person to a calmer, less-disturbed state of mind. The hallucinations, both auditory and visual, the gross disturbance of logical thinking, and to some extent the delusions typical of psychotic states are generally well controlled by these drugs. Violent, aggressive behavior is also effectively treated by major tranquilizers. For this reason they are often used in the management of difficult, aggressive, antisocial people. But the tranquilizing effect is of secondary importance in the treatment of, for example, schizophrenics, and in some people it is even a debilitating side effect. Major tranquilizers that are commonly used include a number of ℞ **phenothiazine** derivatives.

Minor tranquilizers are also calming drugs, but they are ineffective in the treatment of psychotic states. Their principal applications are as ℞ **antianxiety** (anxiolytic), ℞ **hypnotic**, and ℞ **sedative** drugs. The best-known and most-used minor tranquilizers are undoubtedly of the ℞ **benzodiazepine** chemical group. However, prolonged treatment with minor tranquilizers can lead to dependence (addiction).

Limitations
See the individual drug entries and type/group entries.

Transderm-Nitro Ⓑ
A preparation of ℞ **nitroglycerin**.
Formulation: Transdermal patch, available in 5 release rates.
Availability: Prescription only.
Warnings and side effects: See ℞ **nitroglycerin**.

Transderm Scop Ⓑ
A preparation of ℞ **scopolamine hydrobromide**.
Formulation: Skin patch.
Availability: Prescription only.
Warnings and side effects: See ℞ **scopolamine hydrobromide**.
The transdermal form should not be used in children.

Trans-Ver-Sal PlantarPatch; AdultPatch; PediaPatch Ⓑ
A preparation of ℞ **salicylic acid**.
Formulation: Topical patch, with securing strips.
Availability: OTC.
Warnings and side effects: See ℞ **salicylic acid**.

Tranxene Ⓑ
A preparation of ℞ **clorazepate dipotassium**.
Formulation: Oral tablets in several strengths.
Availability: Prescription only.
Warnings and side effects: See ℞ **clorazepate dipotassium**.

tranylcypromine Ⓖ
Type/Group: antidepressant; MAOI.
Brand(s): Parnate.
How administered: Orally.

Used to treat
Tranylcypromine is used for the treatment of ✪ **depression**. It has some stimulant effect and so is not as frequently used as other MAOIs. Although not stated by the manufacturer for such use, it may be given for bulimia or panic disorder with agoraphobia.

Warnings
• It should not be given to people with known hypersensitivity to MAOIs, with pheochromocytoma, severe heart disease, overactive thyroid secretion, hypertension, congestive heart failure, known or suspected liver disease, severe kidney impairment, or with a history of frequent or severe headache.

• It should be given with caution to people over the age of 60, or to anyone with convulsive disorders, schizophrenia, hyperactivity, or diabetes mellitus.

• Tranylcypromine should be used in pregnancy only if it is clearly needed.

• It should not be used by nursing mothers.

• Foods with a high tyramine, dopamine, or tryptophan content must be avoided (see Interactions below).

• Do not drink alcoholic beverages.

• A doctor must be consulted before taking any other medication, including OTC drugs, herbal remedies, supplements, or any other alternative preparation (especially cold, hay fever, or weight-reduction products).

• Minimize caffeine intake.

• A doctor must be contacted at once if headache, palpitations, nausea, neck stiffness, sweating, photophobia, or other unusual symptoms develop. They can indicate a potentially serious reaction.

• It may increase anxiety or agitation.

• Tranylcypromine is one of the more hazardous MAOIs.

Interactions
• Foods containing tyramine, such as cheeses, sour cream, yogurt, liver, fermented sausages (for example, salami, bologna), smoked, spoiled dried or pickled fish, meat tenderizer, game meats, beer, red wine, sherry, spirits, tofu, bananas, raspberries (other fruits especially if dried or overripe), sauerkraut, yeast extracts, broad

beans, chocolate, and ginseng, may cause dangerously high blood pressure.

• Herbal remedies, such as ginseng or caffeine, and others, that contain amines may cause dangerously high blood pressure.

• Supplements containing tryptophan and tyramine (see ♒ **amino acids**) may cause dangerously high blood pressure.

• Serious and even fatal reactions have occurred when MAOI antidepressants are taken with other antidepressants (such as SSRIs or tricyclics). At least 14 days should elapse between discontinuing one and starting the other, and 21 days for some including clomipramine or imipramine.

• Sensitivity to ℞ **barbiturates**, ℞ **antidiabetics**, and ℞ **beta-blockers** may be increased.

• If used with ℞ **dextromethorphan**, ℞ **methylphenidate**, ℞ **carbamazepine**, ℞ **cyclobenzaprine**, ℞ **amphetamines**, ℞ **metaraminol**, ℞ **phenylephrine**, ℞ **pseudoephedrine**, ℞ **ephedrine**, or ℞ **levodopa**, raised blood pressure, sometimes to dangerous levels, may occur.

• ℞ **guanethidine monosulfate**'s and guanadrel's effects on blood pressure may be inhibited by MAOIs.

• Toxic reactions are possible with ℞ **meperidine**, ℞ **sulfonamide**, or ℞ **sumatriptan**.

• Adverse reactions may occur with ℞ **methyldopa**, Rauwolfia ℞ **alkaloids**, ℞ **sympathomimetics**, ℞ **thiazide** ℞ **diuretics**, or *l*-tryptophan.

Side effects

• Dizziness, drowsiness, postural hypotension (lowered blood pressure on standing), and loss of appetite. Insomnia if taken in the evening.

• Less frequently, anxiety and confusion, mental changes, tremors weakness, weight gain, blurred vision, gastrointestinal problems, change in sexual desire, urinary frequency, anemia, changes in metabolism, flushing, increased sweating, and rash.

• Rare but serious side effects include high blood pressure (occasionally critical) and abnormalities in heart rhythm.

Trasylol ®

A preparation of ℞ **aprotinin**.

Formulation: Intravenous injection or infusion.
Availability: Prescription only.
Warnings and side effects: See ℞ aprotinin.

trazodone hydrochloride Ⓖ

Type/Group: **antidepressant**.
Brand(s): Desyrel; various generic.
How administered: Orally.

Used to treat

Trazodone can be used to treat depressive illness (see ✪ **depression**), particularly in cases where some degree of sedation is required. Trazodone is "atypical" in its range of action, and has less ℞ **anticholinergic** effects than most ℞ **tricyclics**. Although not represented by the manufacturer for such treatment, it is sometimes used for aggressive behavior, panic disorder, agoraphobia with panic attacks, and insomnia.

Warnings

• It should not be given to people with known hypersensitivity to this drug, or who are recovering from myocardial infarction (heart attack).

• It should be given with caution to people with a history of heart disease.

• Trazodone should be used during pregnancy only if the benefits outweigh the possible risk to the fetus.

• Medical judgment is required if breast-feeding is being considered.

• Because of its sedating effects, it may impair the performance of skilled tasks requiring mental alertness or physical skills, such as driving.

• Do not drink alcohol.

• Treatment should be stopped gradually, lowering the dose over a period of time.

• Take with food to avoid indigestion.

Interactions

• Serious or even fatal reactions can occur if ℞ **MAOI** antidepressants are taken at the same time, or within a period of a few weeks after the use of, other antidepressants. It is not known whether these effects occur with trazodone.

• The CNS (central nervous system) depressant effects of ℞ **barbiturates** and CNS depressants may be increased.

• ℞ **SSRIs**, ℞ **venlafaxine**, and ℞ **phenothiazines** may increase the effects of trazodone.

• The blood levels of ℞ **phenytoin** may increase.

• ℞ **Clonidine hydrochloride**'s effects on blood pressure may be reduced.

• If used with ℞ **antipsychotics**, there is an increased risk of hypotension.

• Alcohol can add to the impairment of motor and cognitive effects.

Side effects

• Drowsiness, dizziness, and gastrointestinal disorders.

• Less frequently, stupor, extrapyramidal symptoms (uncontrollable movement), including tardive dyskinesia, agitation, excitement, impairment of memory, speech, or gait, psychotic symptoms, mania, nightmares or vivid dreams, cardiovascular effects, increased salivation, jaundice, liver enzyme alterations, changes in libido, sexual dysfunction (rarely, serious priapism, prolonged erection—treatment should be stopped following a doctor's advice), breast enlargement or engorgement, and lactation, various effects on urinary function, muscle aches, shortness of breath, sensitivity reactions (for example, rash), and weight gain or loss. There is a possibility of seizure, changes in heart rhythm, or heart attack.

Trental ®

A preparation of ℞ **pentoxifylline**.

Formulation: Oral tablets, controlled release.
Availability: Prescription only.
Warnings and side effects: See ℞ pentoxifylline.

tretinoin Ⓖ

Type/Group: **retinoid; acne treatment; anticancer**.

Brand(s): Vesanoid (oral); Avita; Retin-A (topical).
How administered: Orally; topically (external).

Used to treat

Tretinoin is chemically a retinoid (a derivative of retinol, or vitamin A) and can be used topically (externally) to treat ✪ **acne** and light-damaged skin. More recently, it has been used for the induction of remission in acute promyelocytic ✪ **leukemia**.

Warnings

• It should not be given to people with known hypersensitivity to tretinoin or any of its ingredients.

• It should be given with caution to people with eczema or sunburned skin. When used as an anticancer drug, it will be used only following full evaluation by specialist physicians.

• In pregnancy, there is a low risk when used topically. There is only minimal absorption and so minimal risk of harming the fetus. But there is a high risk when used orally, and it is not recommended for use during pregnancy unless it is medically judged to be essential, because it may cause birth defects. Becoming pregnant while taking this drug orally must be avoided.

• Medical judgment is required if breast-feeding is being considered when using this drug topically. It should not be used while breast-feeding if taken orally.

• When taken orally, a syndrome characterized by fever, lung effects, and weight gain may occur.

• Oral use has been associated with intracranial hypertension.

• Oral use may cause cancer or chromosomal abnormalities.

• Elevated cholesterol levels are found in a majority of people taking this medication orally.

• Exposure to ultraviolet light must be avoided when using topically.

Interactions

• Food may increase absorption.

• ℞ **ketoconazole** may increase the levels of tretinoin when taken orally.

• The use of ℞ **sulfur**, ℞ **resorcinol**, ℞ **benzoyl peroxide**, ℞ **salicylic acid**, and similar products may cause skin irritation when used with externally applied tretinoin.

Side effects

• Oral use: Frequently, headache, dry skin, crusting or swelling of lips, nausea, vomiting, bone, joint, or muscle pain, rash, fever, and fatigue. Occasionally, itching, sweating, visual disturbances, hair loss, and skin changes.

• Topical use: Frequently, local inflammatory reaction, transient feeling of warmth or stinging, reddening of the skin, and peeling. Occasionally, temporary darkening of the skin, severe reddening, crusting, blistering, and swelling. Rarely, contact allergy.

triacetin ⓖ

Type/Group: **antifungal**.
Brand(s): Absorbine; Aftate; Quinsana Plus; Ting; Tinactin.
How administered: Topically (external).

Used to treat

Triacetin is a synthetic mild broad-spectrum antifungal drug in the topical (external) treatment of infections of the nails, athlete's foot, jock itch, ringworm, impetigo, and other skin infections (see ✪ **fungal infections**).

Warnings

• It should not be given to people with known sensitivity to triacetin.

• The spray form should be given with caution to diabetics and people with impaired circulation.

• Its safety during pregnancy has not been established and so it should be used only if clearly needed.

• Medical judgment is required if breast-feeding is being considered. It is not known whether this drug appears in breast milk.

• A doctor must be contacted if there is increased irritation or sensitivity.

Interactions

None significant have been reported.

Side effects

None significant reported when used topically.

Triad Capsules ⓑ

A preparation of ℞ **acetaminophen**, ℞ **caffeine**, and ℞ **butabarbital**.
Formulation: Oral capsules.
Availability: Prescription only.
Warnings and side effects: See ℞ **acetaminophen**; ℞ **caffeine**; ℞ **butabarbital**.

Triafed-C Cough Syrup ⓑ

A preparation of ℞ **codeine phosphate**, ℞ **pseudoephedrine**, and ℞ **triprolidine hydrochloride**.
Formulation: Oral syrup.
Availability: May or may not require a prescription.
Warnings and side effects: See ℞ **codeine phosphate**; ℞ **pseudoephedrine**; ℞ **triprolidine hydrochloride**.

Triam-A ⓑ

A preparation of ℞ **triamcinolone** acetonide.
Formulation: Suspension for injection.
Availability: Prescription only.
Warnings and side effects: See ℞ **triamcinolone**.

triamcinolone ⓖ

Type/Group: **corticosteroid; anti-inflammatory**.
Brand(s): Aristocort; Atolone; Kenacort; various generics. As *triamcinolone acetonide*: Azmacort; Kenaject; Kenalog; Tac; Triam A; various generic. As *triamcinolone acetate*: Aristocort; Delta-Tritex; Flutex; Kenalog; various generic. As *triamcinolone diacetate*: Amcort; Aristocort; Triam; Tristoject; various generic. As *triamcinolone hexacetonide*: Aristospan. As *triamcinolone propionate*: Nasacort. Combinations: With *neomycin*: Myco-Biotic II. With *nystatin*: Mycogen II; Mycolog-II; Myconel; Mycotriacetate; N.G.T.
How administered: Inhalant; injection; intranasal; orally; topically.

Used to treat

Triamcinolone is used for the treatment of many kinds of ✪ **inflammation**. It has major and varied effects on metabolism, and modifies the operation of the immune system, and so it may be used to treat a variety of conditions, including: adrenal insufficiency; congenital adrenal hyperplasia; rheumatic disorders (such as ✪ **arthritis** and ✪ **osteoarthritis**), allergic states, collagen diseases, allergic and inflammatory eye disorders, intestinal tract, liver and kidney disorders, skin diseases, respiratory diseases (such as bronchial ✪ **asthma**), edemas, and malignancies.

Warnings

Warnings for corticosteroids, which depend on route of administration and use, include:

• It should not be used by people with known hypersensitivity to corticosteroids, or with systemic fungal infections.

• It should be given with caution to anyone with low thyroid function, peptic ulcers, hepatitis, cirrhosis, ocular herpes simplex, diabetes mellitus, glaucoma, history of tuberculosis, nonspecific colitis, congestive heart failure, myocardial infarction (heart attack), hypertension, psychosis, or kidney insufficiency, and to anyone over 65 and children. External use by anyone with marked circulation impairment should be undertaken with care.

• Corticosteroids can cross the placenta, and therefore triamcinolone should only be used during pregnancy if medically judged to be essential.

• It should not be used by breast-feeding mothers. It is excreted in breast milk and could suppress growth and interfere with the production of corticosteroids in the infant.

• It may mask signs of infection and interfere with the body's ability to keep infection from spreading.

• Live vaccines must not be taken while using this drug.

• It may reactivate latent tuberculosis or amebiasis.

• Prolonged use in children can inhibit skeletal growth, and so growth must be monitored.

• The contraceptive effect of IUDs (intrauterine device) may be decreased.

• It causes increased excretion of calcium and other minerals, and so supplements may be needed.

• Prolonged use may lead to adrenal insufficiency. A doctor must be notified if there is unusual weight gain, swelling of the legs or feet, muscle weakness, black tarry stools, vomiting of blood, puffing of the face, menstrual irregularities, or prolonged sore throat, fever, cold, or infection.

• Anyone on long-term steroid therapy should wear a medic-alert bracelet or the equivalent.

• No other medication (including herbal remedies and supplements) should be taken without consulting a doctor.

• Discontinuation of treatment must be gradual and under medical supervision.

• Its effectiveness may be reduced in situations of severe stress (such as serious infection, surgery, or trauma).

• When using topically (externally), do not use over large surface areas, for a prolonged period, or cover with bandages in order to minimize the risk of systemic absorption and accompanying side effects.

Interactions

• Triamcinolone taken with ℞ **amphotericin** or ℞ **diuretics** may further reduce potassium levels.

• The effects of ℞ **aspirin**, ℞ **oral hypoglycemics**, ℞ **insulin**, diuretics, and ⚕ **potassium** supplements may be reduced.

• Aspirin and ℞ **NSAIDs** increase the risk of gastric ulceration.

• ℞ **Barbiturates**, ℞ **hydantoins**, ℞ **rifampin**, and ephedrine may reduce the effects of corticosteroids.

• ℞ **Ketoconazole**, ℞ **estrogens**, ℞ **oral contraceptives**, nondepolarizing muscle relaxants, and ℞ **cholestyramine** may increase the effects of triamcinolone.

• Oral ℞ **anticoagulants** and ℞ **theophylline** may alter the effects of either corticosteroids or the other drug, or both.

• The effectiveness of ℞ **anticholinesterases**, ℞ **isoniazid**, ℞ **salicylates**, and ℞ **somatrem** may be reduced.

• ℞ **Cyclosporine** and digitalis glycosides may increase the risk of toxicity.

Side effects

These depend on how administered, dose, duration of treatment, and use.

• Systemic use: Frequently, insomnia, heartburn, nervousness, abdominal tightness, increased sweating, acne, mood swings, increased appetite, facial flushing, delayed wound healing, increased susceptibility to infection, diarrhea, or constipation. Occasionally, edema, headache, change in skin color, and frequent urination. Rarely, speeded heartbeat, allergic skin reaction, and psychological changes. Topical use: Occasionally, irritation, and itching. Rarely, allergic rash. Systemic side effects are possible.

Triam Forte ®

A preparation of ℞ **triamcinolone** diacetate.
Formulation: Suspension for injection.
Availability: Prescription only.
Warnings and side effects: See ℞ **triamcinolone**.

Triaminic AM Decongestant Formula; Infant Decongestant Drops ®

A preparation of ℞ **pseudoephedrine** and ℞ **dextromethorphan**.
Formulation: Oral liquid; drops.
Availability: OTC.
Warnings and side effects: See ℞ **pseudoephedrine**; ℞ **dextromethorphan**.

triamterene Ⓖ

Type/Group: **diuretic; antihypertensive; heart failure treatment**.
Brand(s): Dyrenium. Combinations: With *hydrochlorothiazide*: Dyazide; Maxide.
How administered: Orally.

Used to treat

Triamterene is a mild, potassium-sparing diuretic which retains potassium in the body and is therefore used as an alternative to, or commonly in combination with, other diuretics such as the thiazide and loop types (which normally cause a loss of potassium from the body). It can be used to treat congestive ✪ **heart failure**, edema, ascites (abdominal fluid) in liver ✪ **cirrhosis**.

Warnings

• It should not be given to people with known hypersensitivity to this drug, severe kidney or liver impairment, high potassium levels, or who are already receiving potassium supplements or drugs to reduce potassium loss.

• It should be given with caution to elderly people, or to anyone with diabetes or a history of kidney stones.

• Triamterene should be used during pregnancy only if the potential benefit outweighs the possible risk to the fetus.

• Medical judgment is required if breast-feeding is being considered.

• If symptoms such as paresthesia (tingling sensations), muscular weakness or fatigue occur, treatment must be stopped immediately and a doctor contacted.

• This drug should not be used with other potassium-sparing diuretics, such as ℞ **amiloride** or ℞ **spironolactone**.

• There will be periodic monitoring of electrolytes.

• Foods rich in potassium (for example bananas, oranges, and salt substitutes) should not be consumed in large quantities.

• Avoid exposure to sunlight because triamterene may cause photosensitivity.

Interactions

• Potassium-containing preparations (for example, certain drugs, salt substitutes, low-salt milk), ℞ **amiloride**, and ℞ **spironolactone** pose a risk of severe hyperkalemia (high blood potassium) with the potential of serious heart irregularities or arrest. They should be avoided when taking triamterene.

• ℞ **ACE inhibitors** may raise potassium levels and possibly cause heart arrhythmias.

• ℞ **lithium** levels may rise and pose a risk of lithium toxicity.

• ℞ **cimetidine** may increase the levels and effects of triamterene.

• The levels and effects of ℞ **digoxin** may be increased.

• ℞ **NSAIDs** (especially ℞ **indomethacin**) may impair kidney function. Indomethacin and triamterene should not be used together.

Side effects

• There may be gastrointestinal upsets, skin rashes, dry mouth, fall in blood pressure on standing (postural hypotension), and elevated blood potassium.

• Blood disorders and light-sensitivity have been reported. Urine may be colored blue.

Triavil ⑧

A preparation of ℞ **perphenazine** and ℞ **amitriptyline hydrochloride**.

Formulation: Oral tablets in several strengths.

Availability: Prescription only.

Warnings and side effects: See ℞ **perphenazine**; ℞ **amitriptyline hydrochloride**.

Triaz; Triaz Wash; Triaz Cleanser ⑧

A preparation of ℞ **benzoyl peroxide**.

Formulation: Topical gel in several strengths; topical lotion (Wash); topical cleanser.

Availability: Prescription only.

Warnings and side effects: See ℞ benzoyl peroxide.

triazolam ⑥

Type/Group: **hypnotic; benzodiazepine**.

Brand(s): Halcion.

How administered: Orally.

Used to treat

Triazolam is used for the short-term treatment of ✪ **insomnia**, generally seven to ten days (prescriptions are rarely written for more than a one-month supply). It is eliminated rapidly from the body compared to other benzodiazepines, but may cause withdrawal problems the day after use.

Warnings

• It should not be given to people with known hypersensitivity to benzodiazepines, narrow-angle glaucoma, or psychosis.

• It should be given with caution to people with kidney or liver impairment, a history of drugs abuse, respiratory depression, or anyone over 65.

• Triazolam should not be used during pregnancy.

• It should not be used by nursing mothers.

• It must not be used for longer than the time specified by your doctor. Benzodiazepines may produce psychological and physical dependence and withdrawal symptoms.

• It may impair the performance of skilled tasks, such as driving.

• Avoid alcohol, because adverse side effects may be increased (see Side effects below).

• Avoid other psychotropic medications unless prescribed by a doctor.

• A doctor must be consulted before stopping use or increasing dosage.

Interactions

• ℞ **azole** antifungals (for example, ℞ **ketoconazole**, ℞ **itraconazole**), ℞ **beta-blockers** (for example, ℞ **propranolol**), ℞ **cimetidine**, ℞ **disulfiram**, ℞ **isoniazid**, ℞ **macrolide** antibiotics (for example, ℞ **erythromycin**, ℞ **clarithromycin**, troleandomycin), ℞ **omeprazole**, and ℞ **SSRIs** may increase levels of triazolam.

• ℞ **Carbamazepine** and ℞ **phenytoin** may reduce the effects of triazolam.

• Alcohol may increase adverse effects.

Side effects

• Daytime sedation, drowsiness, weakness, and reduction in physical activity.

• Less frequently, memory problems, abnormal thinking, and changes in behavior.

• After more than a few weeks of nightly use, wakefulness during the last third of the night and daytime anxiety or nervousness may develop. These are indications of tolerance and withdrawal. There may also be eye, ear or nose pain and irritation, gastrointestinal effects, urinary problems, decreased libido, menstrual cramps, vaginal or penile discharge and itching, back and leg pain, and sensitivity reactions.

• Rare but serious side effects include seizures, irregular heartbeat, and blood cell disorders.

Triban Adult Suppositories; Pediatric Suppositories ℞

A preparation of ℞ **trimethobenzamide hydrochloride**.
Formulation: Rectal suppositories.
Availability: Prescription only.
Warnings and side effects: See ℞ **trimethobenzamide hydrochloride**.

tribaverin Ⓖ

see ℞ **ribavirin**.

Tribiotic Plus ℞

A preparation of ℞ **neomycin**, ℞ **polymyxin B sulfate**, ℞ **bacitracin**, and ℞ **lidocaine**.
Formulation: Topical ointment.
Availability: OTC.
Warnings and side effects: See ℞ **neomycin**; ℞ **polymyxin B sulfate**; ℞ **bacitracin**; ℞ **lidocaine**.

trichlormethiazide Ⓖ

Type/Group: **diuretic; thiazide; antihypertensive**.
Brand(s): Diurese; Metahydrin; Naqua; various generic.
How administered: Orally.

Used to treat

Trichlormethiazide can be used, either alone or in conjunction with other types of diuretic or other drugs (for example, ℞ **beta-blockers**), in the treatment of ✪ **hypertension**. It can also be used in the treatment of edema. Thiazide diuretics have also become a major part of treatment for nephrogenic ✪ **diabetes insipidus**.

Warnings

• It should not be given to people with known hypersensitivity to thiazides (or to ℞ **sulfonamide**-derived drugs), or severe kidney or liver disorders.
• It should be given with caution to elderly people, anyone with high cholesterol or triglyceride levels, or with liver or kidney impairment.
• Trichlormethiazide should be used during pregnancy only when the potential benefit outweighs the possible risk to the fetus.
• Medical judgment is required if breast-feeding is being considered.
• Early symptoms of electrolyte imbalance may include muscle weakness or cramps, nausea, vomiting, restlessness or lethargy, dry mouth, excessive thirst, fast pulse, or dizziness. A doctor must be contacted if such symptoms occur.
• Thiazides may aggravate symptoms of diabetes or gout, and worsen or activate lupus erythematosus.
• Periodic monitoring of electrolytes (particularly potassium, sodium, chloride, and bicarbonate) will be carried out.
• Photosensitivity (abnormal sensitivity to sunlight) may develop and so precautions such as protective clothing should be used to minimize exposure.
• Thiazides interact with a number of drugs, including some OTC preparations. A doctor must always be consulted before taking any other medication (including OTCs, herbal remedies, and supplements).

Interactions

• There is a higher risk of hypersensitivity reaction to ℞ **allopurinol**.
• The effects of ℞ **anesthetics**, ℞ **anticancer** drugs, other antihypertensives, ℞ **diazoxide**, ⚕ **calcium** salts, ℞ **cardiac glycosides**, ℞ **lithium**, loop diuretics, ℞ **methyldopa**, nondepolarizing ℞ **skeletal muscle relaxants**, and ⚕ **vitamin D** may be increased, with the potential for significant adverse effects or toxicity. An additive effect is sometimes used to advantage in combining thiazides with other antihypertensives.
• The effects of ℞ **anticoagulants** and antigout agents (for example, ℞ **probenecid**, ℞ **sulfinpyrazone**) may be lowered by thiazides.
• The dosage of ℞ **insulin** and ℞ **sulfonylureas** may need to be adjusted because thiazides may increase blood sugar levels.
• The diuretic effects of thiazide may be increased when taken with ℞ **amphotericin B**, ℞ **anticholinergics**, ℞ **corticosteroids**, ℞ **corticotropin**, or ℞ **MAOIs**, with the possibility of significant electrolyte loss, especially potassium.
• ℞ **Cholestyramine**, ℞ **colestipol hydrochloride**, ℞ **methenamine**, and ℞ **NSAIDs** (especially ℞ **indomethacin**) may reduce the effectiveness of thiazide diuretics.
• Alcohol, ℞ **barbiturates**, and ℞ **opioids** increase the risk of postural hypotension (lowered blood pressure on standing).

Side effects

• There may be dizziness. headache, muscle cramps, mild gastrointestinal upsets, postural hypotension, reversible impotence, low blood potassium, sodium, magnesium and chloride, raised blood urea, glucose and lipids, and gout.
• Rarely, photosensitivity, blood disorders, skin reactions, or pancreatitis.

triclosan Ⓖ

Type/Group: **antiseptic**.
Brand(s): Clearasil Daily Face Wash; no more germies; Oxy ResiDon't; Septi-Soft; Septisol; Stridex Face Wash.
How administered: Topically (external).

Used to treat

Triclosan is used to prevent the spread of an infection on the skin.

Warnings

• It should not be given to people with known hypersensitivity to this drug.
• It should not be used on burned or denuded skin or mucous membranes.
• It should not be used routinely for bathing.
• Avoid contact with the eyes.

Interactions

No significant interactions are known.

Side effects

No significant side effects are known.

Tricodene Cough & Cold Liquid ℞

A preparation of ℞ **codeine phosphate** and ℞ **pyrilamine maleate**.
Formulation: Oral liquid.
Availability: May or may not require a prescription.

Warnings and side effects: See ℞ **codeine phosphate**; ℞ **pyrilamine maleate**.

Tricodene Sugar Free Liquid Ⓑ

A preparation of ℞ **dextromethorphan** and ℞ **chlorpheniramine maleate**.

Formulation: Oral liquid.
Availability: OTC.
Warnings and side effects: See ℞ **dextromethorphan**; ℞ **chlorpheniramine maleate**.

Tricor Ⓑ

A preparation of ℞ **fenofibrate**.
Formulation: Oral capsules.
Availability: Prescription only.
Warnings and side effects: See ℞ **fenofibrate**.

Tricosal Tablets Ⓑ

A preparation of ℞ **choline salicylate** and ℞ **magnesium salicylate**.
Formulation: Oral tablets, available in 3 strengths.
Availability: Prescription only.
Warnings and side effects: See ℞ **choline salicylate**; ℞ **magnesium salicylate**.

tricyclic Ⓓ

Generics: **amitriptyline hydrochloride; amoxapine; clomipramine hydrochloride; desipramine hydrochloride; doxepin; imipramine; maprotiline hydrochloride; nortriptyline hydrochloride; protriptyline hydrochloride; trimipramine hydrochloride**. Related generic: **trazodone hydrochloride**.

Actions and uses

Tricyclics are a class of ℞ **antidepressant**—technically a type comprising three chemical rings (or similar ones with four rings; tetracyclics)—used to relieve the symptoms of the affective disorder ⊙ **depression**. They were the first of the antidepressants to be developed.

There are several different groups of antidepressants that work by changing the levels of monoamine neurotransmitters (mainly serotonin and norepinephrine) in areas of the brain that regulate mood. The tricyclics (and ℞ **SSRI**) groups increase neurotransmitter levels by blocking monoamine reuptake into brain neurons after release in the normal process of neurotransmission.

All antidepressants may be used to elevate mood, help resume normal functioning, and reduce the frequency of depressive episodes in chronic depressive states. They may also be prescribed to help in more acute circumstances, such as after loss of a loved one or in postnatal depression. In ⊙ **bipolar disorder** (bipolar affective disorder; manic-depressive illness), the manic phases are controlled with special antimanic drugs, but antidepressants may be used to help control the depressive phases.

Limitations

All antidepressant drugs have significant side effects, although these do generally become less troublesome with time. All take some time to work, but the tricyclics are quickest (and also show immediate sedation, which can be an advantage with highly anxious patients). The tricyclic group is also cheaper than the others. Some more recently evolved antidepressants, developed from this group, and the recently introduced drug ℞ **trazodone hydrochloride**, are like tricyclics but with less anticholinergic effects (for example, dry mouth, gastrointestinal disturbances and sedation). Apart from their actions on brain monoamines, all the antidepressant drugs have other (generally undesirable) effects in the body, notably the anticholinergic side effects, and these can be very marked with the tricyclic group. See also the individual drug entries.

Tridil Ⓑ

A preparation of ℞ **nitroglycerin**.
Formulation: Intravenous infusion.
Availability: Prescription only.
Warnings and side effects: See ℞ **nitroglycerin**.

trientine hydrochloride Ⓖ

Type/Group: chelating agent; metabolic disorder treatment.
Brand(s): Syprine.
How administered: Orally.

Used to treat

Trientine hydrochloride is used as a ⊙ **metabolic disorder** treatment to reduce the abnormally high levels of copper in the body that occur in ⊙ **Wilson's disease**. It is given to people who cannot tolerate the more commonly used ℞ **penicillamine**.

Warnings

• It should not be given to people with hypersensitivity to this drug, or who have cystinuria, biliary cirrhosis, or rheumatoid arthritis.
• It should be given with caution to children and to anyone with iron-deficient anemia.
• Trientine hydrochloride should be used in pregnancy only if it is medically judged that the potential benefit outweighs the potential risk to the fetus.
• Medical judgment is also required for breast-feeding mothers.
• It may cause iron deficiency anemia, and so regular medical monitoring during treatment is necessary.
• Trientine should be taken on an empty stomach (at least two hours after a meal and one hour apart from any other food or drug).

Interactions

• ⚠ **iron** and other mineral supplements may block absorption of trientine; although separate administration of iron may be necessary to counter iron deficiency.

Side effects

Although experience with this drug is limited, there may be:
• Heartburn, pain or tenderness around the stomach, thickening or flaking of the skin, malaise, cramps or muscle pain.
• Blood abnormalities (for example, iron-deficient anemia) are possible and, infrequently, symptoms of systemic lupus erythematosus (SLE) may occur.

trifluoperazine Ⓖ

Type/Group: **antipsychotic; phenothiazine**.
Brand(s): Stelazine.

How administered: Orally, injection.

Used to treat

Trifluoperazine is used to treat and tranquilize people with ✪ **psychotic disorders** (such as ✪ **schizophrenia**), particularly those experiencing some form of behavioral disturbance. It is also used for the short-term treatment of non-psychotic ✪ **anxiety**.

Warnings

• It should not be given to people with known hypersensitivity to this drug, with severe toxic central nervous system (CNS) depression, coma, subcortical brain damage, bone marrow depression, or narrow-angle glaucoma.

• It should be given with caution to the elderly, to people with severe cardiovascular disorders, seizure disorder (epilepsy), liver or kidney disease, glaucoma, prostatic hypertrophy, severe asthma, emphysema, or hypocalcemia (low calcium).

• Trifluoperazine should be used during pregnancy only if it is essential.

• Medical judgment is required if breast-feeding is being considered.

• It may cause postural hypotension (lowered blood pressure on standing), so rise slowly from a reclining position. Older people in particular should exercise caution.

• If used for a long time, tardive dyskinesia (see ℞ **antipsychotics**) occasionally develops.

• Treatment should be stopped gradually.

• Avoid alcohol.

Interactions

• ℞ Levodopa's effects may be reduced by trifluoperazine.

• The levels of ℞ **tricyclic** antidepressants may be increased.

• If used with ℞ **bromocriptine** or ℞ **lithium**, the levels of both drugs may be decreased.

• ℞ **Anticholinergics**, ℞ **barbiturates**, ℞ **narcotic analgesics**, ℞ **orphenadrine** lower levels of an antipsychotic, and/or increase the occurrence of anticholinergic and/or CNS (central nervous system) effects.

• ℞ **guanethidine monosulfate**'s effects on blood pressure may be reduced.

• If used with ℞ **narcotic analgesics**, there may be excessive CNS (central nervous system) depression, lowered blood pressure, and respiratory depression.

• If an antipsychotic is taken with alcohol, there may be increased sedative effects.

Side effects

• Drowsiness, extrapyramidal symptoms (see ℞ **antipsychotics**), headache, loss of appetite, constipation, dry mouth, nausea, and spasmodic constriction of the bronchi or larynx.

• Less frequently, agitation, anxiety, catatonic-like behavioral states, confusion, depression, euphoria, worsening of psychotic symptoms, heat or cold intolerance, insomnia, lethargy, restlessness, ECG changes, changes in blood pressure, speeded heartbeat, blurred vision, eye changes, indigestion, increased salivation, vomiting, priapism (prolonged, painful penile erection), urinary retention, changes in hormone function (irregular menstruation, growth of breasts, abnormal milk production, impotence, increased libido), changes in blood sugar levels,

sensitivity reactions, rashes, increased sweating, loss of hair, and heat or cold intolerance.

• Rare but serious side effects include neuroleptic malignant syndrome (a potentially fatal condition characterized by very high fever, muscle rigidity, changes in mental status, and irregular pulse, blood pressure and/or heart rhythm), seizures, blood cell disorders, anemia, and spasm of the bronchi or larynx.

trifluorothymidine ⑥

see ℞ **trifluridine**.

trifluopromazine hydrochloride ⑥

Type/Group: **antinauseant; antipsychotic**.
Brand(s): **Vesprin**.
How administered: Injection.

Used to treat

Triflupromazine hydrochloride is a ℞ **phenothiazine** which can be used in the management of symptoms of psychosis (see ✪ **psychotic disorders**), or separately to control severe ✪ **nausea** and ✪ **vomiting**.

Warnings

• It should not be given to people with known hypersensitivity to this drug (or to other phenothiazines), with severely impaired function of the central nervous system (including coma and brain damage), bone marrow depression, narrow-angle glaucoma, or when large amounts of other central nervous system depressant drugs have been taken.

• It should be given with caution to the elderly or debilitated, or anyone with severe heart disorders, seizure disorder (epilepsy), liver or kidney impairment, glaucoma, enlarged prostate, severe asthma, emphysema, or hypocalcemia (low calcium).

• Triflupromazine hydrochloride should be used during pregnancy only if the potential benefit outweighs the possible risk to the fetus.

• Its safety in breast-feeding has not been established. Nursing women should either discontinue this drug or discontinue breast-feeding.

• It may cause postural hypotension (lowered blood pressure on standing). Arise slowly from a reclining position. Older people should use particular caution.

• It may cause sensitivity to sunlight, so minimize exposure and use a sunscreen and wear sunglasses.

• Phenothiazines interfere with the body's natural ability to regulate its temperature, and so extreme temperatures should be avoided.

• On prolonged use, tardive dyskinesia (see ℞ **antipsychotics**) occasionally develops.

• Treatment should be stopped gradually with dosage slowly reduced.

Interactions

• ℞ **lithium** increases the risk of phenothiazine side effects, including unconsciousness and extrapyramidal symptoms.

• The levels of ℞ **tricyclic** antidepressants may be increased.

• The effects of ℞ **amphetamines** and ℞ **bromocriptine** may be decreased.

• The levels and effects of both ℞ **propranolol** and phenothiazines may be increased.

Key to symbols: ✪ = Disorder Section ℞ = Drug Section ♣ = Herbal Section ⚕ = Supplement Section

• ℞ **Anticholinergics** may lower the effects of phenothiazines.

• ℞ **guanethidine's**'s effects on blood pressure may be reduced.

• If taken with alcohol, ℞ **barbiturates**, ℞ **general anesthetics**, ℞ **opioids**, or ℞ **sedatives**, there is a potential for excessive central nervous system (CNS) depression, lowered blood pressure, and respiratory depression.

• ℞ **Antacids** containing aluminum should be taken either one hour before or two hours after a phenothiazine.

Side effects

• These may include drowsiness, extrapyramidal symptoms (see antipsychotics), headache, loss of appetite, constipation, and dry mouth.

• Less frequently, agitation, anxiety, catatonic-like behavioral states, confusion, depression, euphoria, worsening of psychotic symptoms, heat or cold intolerance, insomnia, lethargy, changes in blood pressure, speeded heartbeat, vision disturbances, increased salivation, vomiting, priapism, urinary retention, changes in hormone function (for example, irregular menstruation, growth of breasts, abnormal milk production, impotence, increased libido), changes in blood sugar levels, sensitivity reactions, rashes, increased sweating, loss of hair, and heat or cold intolerance.

• Rare but serious side effects include neuroleptic malignant syndrome (a potentially fatal condition characterized by very high fever, muscle rigidity, changes in mental status, and irregular pulse, blood pressure and/or heart rhythm), seizures, blood cell disorders, anemia, and spasm of the bronchi or larynx.

trifluridine ⑥

(trifluorothymidine)

Type/Group: **antiviral**.

How administered: Topically (external; eye).

Brand(s): Viroptic.

Used to treat

Trifluridine is used to treat eye inflammation caused by the herpes simplex virus (see ⊙ **herpes**) and other viruses.

Warnings

• It should not be given to people with known hypersensitivity to this drug. It is not effective for bacterial, fungal or chlamydial infections.

• Trifluridine is not recommended for use during pregnancy or while breast-feeding because of the possibility that it might harm the fetus or infant if absorbed systemically.

• It must not be used for a longer period than is recommended. A doctor must be contacted if there is no improvement within 7 days.

Interactions

No significant interactions are known.

Side effects

• Frequently, transient stinging or burning.

• Occasionally, a swollen eyelid.

• Rarely, allergic reaction and increased intraocular pressure (within the eye).

Trihexy-2; Trihexy-5 ⑧

A preparation of ℞ **trihexyphenidyl**.

Formulation: Oral tablets in two strengths.

Availability: Prescription only.

Warnings and side effects: See ℞ **trihexyphenidyl**.

trihexyphenidyl ⑥

Type/Group: **antiparkinsonism; anticholinergic**.

Brand(s): Artane; Trihexy.

How administered: Orally.

Used to treat

Trihexyphenidyl is used as an adjunct treatment (additional treatment to enhance effectiveness) of all forms of ⊙ **Parkinson's disease** and for the control of drug-induced extrapyramidal disorders.

Warnings

• It should not be used by people with known hypersensitivity to this drug, angle-closure glaucoma, gastrointestinal or urogenital obstruction, prostatic hypertrophy, myasthenia gravis, or megacolon.

• It should be used with caution by people with heart rate irregularities, liver or kidney disease, a history of drug abuse, hypotension or hypertension, psychosis, or tardive dyskinesia.

• Medical judgment is required for anyone over 60, as people of this age are particularly sensitive to ℞ **anticholinergic** side effects.

• Extreme caution should also be used when this drug is given to children, because they, too, may be particularly sensitive to anticholinergic side effects.

• It is not known whether or not trihexyphenidyl crosses the placenta. Therefore it should be used during pregnancy only if clearly needed and if the benefits outweigh the possible risks to the fetus.

• Its effect on breast milk is unknown. However, it is known that infants are sensitive to the effects of anticholinergic drugs, and so medical judgment is required if breast-feeding is being considered.

• Use with caution during hot weather as there is a risk of heat stroke due to decreased sweating.

• There is a risk of addiction because it can cause euphoria.

• It may affect the performance of skilled tasks, such as driving, as there is a potential for interfering side effects, such as dizziness, confusion, and blurred vision.

• Treatment must be ended gradually.

Interactions

• The effectiveness of ℞ **levodopa** may be reduced.

• Trihexyphenidyl taken with ℞ **phenothiazines** may reduce the effectiveness of these drugs, while anticholinergic side effects may be increased.

• Taking trihexyphenidyl with ℞ **haloperidol** and similar ℞ **antipsychotics** may result in a worsening of psychiatric symptoms and the development of tardive dyskinesia.

• The incidence of anticholinergic side effects may be increased if taken with anticholinergics or ℞ **amantadine**.

Side effects

• Frequently, nausea, dizziness, poor concentration, insomnia, and nervousness.

• Occasionally, postural hypotension (lowered blood pressure on standing), loss of appetite, headache, livedo reticularis (reddish blue blotching of the skin), blurred vision, urinary retention, and dry mouth.

• Rarely, vomiting, depression, irritation or swelling of eyes, and skin rash.

TriHIBit ®

A preparation of ℞ **diphtheria and tetanus toxoids and acellular pertussis and Haemophilus influenzae type b conjugate vaccine (DTaP-HIB)**
Formulation: Injection.
Availability: Prescription only.
Warnings and side effects: See ℞ **diphtheria and tetanus toxoids and acellular pertussis and Haemophilus influenzae type b conjugate vaccine (DTaP-HIB)**

Tri-Hydroserpine ®

A preparation of ℞ **hydralazine hydrochloride,** ℞ **hydrochlorothiazide,** and ℞ **reserpine.**
Formulation: Oral tablets.
Availability: Prescription only.
Warnings and side effects: See ℞ **hydralazine hydrochloride;** ℞ **hydrochlorothiazide;** ℞ **reserpine.**

Tri-Immunol ®

A preparation of ℞ **diphtheria and tetanus toxoids and whole-cell pertussis vaccine adsorbed (DTwP).**
Formulation: Injection.
Availability: Prescription only.
Warnings and side effects: See ℞ **diphtheria and tetanus toxoids and whole-cell pertussis vaccine adsorbed (DTwP).**

Trilafon ®

A preparation of ℞ **perphenazine.**
Formulation: Oral tablets in several strengths; oral liquid; injectable solution.
Availability: Prescription only.
Warnings and side effects: See ℞ **perphenazine.**

Tri-Levlen ®

A preparation of ℞ **ethinyl estradiol** and ℞ **levonorgestrel.**
Formulation: Calendar pack of oral tablets.
Availability: Prescription only.
Warnings and side effects: See ℞ **ethinyl estradiol;** ℞ **levonorgestrel.**

Trilisate Tablets; Liquid ®

A preparation of ℞ **choline salicylate** and ℞ **magnesium salicylate.**
Formulation: Oral liquid; tablets, available in 3 strengths.
Availability: Prescription only.
Warnings and side effects: See ℞ **choline salicylate;** ℞ **magnesium salicylate.**

Trimazide Adult Suppositories; Pediatric Suppositories ®

A preparation of ℞ **trimethobenzamide hydrochloride.**
Formulation: Rectal suppositories.
Availability: Prescription only.
Warnings and side effects: See ℞ **trimethobenzamide hydrochloride.**

trimetaphan camsilate Ⓖ

see ℞ **trimethaphan camsylate.**

trimethaphan camsylate Ⓖ

(trimetaphan camsilate)
Type/Group: ganglion-blocker; antihypertensive; hypotensive.
Brand(s): Arfonad.
How administered: Intravenous infusion.

Used to treat

Trimethaphan camsylate lowers blood pressure by reducing vascular tone normally induced by the sympathetic nervous system. It is short-acting and is used as a hypotensive for controlled blood pressure during surgery or to quickly reduce blood pressure in hypertensive emergencies.

Warnings

• It should not be given to people who are at high risk if hypotension is induced (for example, with severe anemia, shock, respiratory insufficiency, asphyxia). This is a specialist hospital drug which will be used by experienced personnel only.
• It should be given with caution to elderly people and to those with arteriosclerosis, heart disease, Addison's disease, diabetes, any degenerative neurological disease, liver or kidney impairment, or who are taking steroids.
• The hypotension induced by trimethaphan camsylate may have serious consequences for the fetus and it should not be used during pregnancy.
• As it is only used in surgery or emergencies, its effects in breast-feeding are of no practical concern.
• This drug should be used only in an adequately equipped medical facility and by physicians trained in the techniques for its use.
• Trimethaphan releases histamine in the body, which may aggravate allergies.

Interactions

• If taken with ℞ **anesthetics,** there is a risk of increased hypotensive effect.
• The effects of ℞ **skeletal muscle relaxants** are intensified.

Side effects

• There may be an increase in the heart rate and depression of respiration, increased intraocular pressure (pressure in the eyeball), dilated pupils, and constipation.

trimethobenzamide hydrochloride Ⓖ

Type/Group: anticholinergic; antiemetic; antinauseant.
Brand(s): Tebamide; T-Gen; Tigan; Triban; Trimazide; various generic.
How administered: Orally; rectal (suppositories); injection.

Key to symbols: ✛ = Disorder Section ℞ = Drug Section ♣ = Herbal Section ⚕⚕ = Supplement Section

Used to treat

Trimethobenzamide hydrochloride is used to control ✪ **nausea** and ✪ **vomiting**, particularly where the side effects of stronger antiemetics (such as ℞ **phenothiazines**) make their use undesirable.

Warnings

• It should not be given to people with known hypersensitivity to this drug (or with known sensitivity to ℞ **benzocaine**, which is present in the suppositories; one of the currently available forms of trimethobenzamide), or to premature babies or newborns.

• It should be given with caution to people with high fever, brain inflammation, gastroenteritis, dehydration, electrolyte imbalance, or who are generally debilitated (especially if they are elderly).

• It should be used during pregnancy only if the potential benefit outweighs the possible risk to the fetus.

• Medical judgment is required if breast-feeding is being considered. Its safety in breast-feeding has not been established.

• Because of a suspected link between centrally acting antiemetics (like this one) and the rare, but serious, condition called ✪ **Reye's syndrome**, trimethobenzamide should not be given to children or teenagers who have, or might have, chickenpox or flu. As so many infections resemble flu in their initial symptoms, these centrally acting antiemetics should not, as a general rule, be used to treat vomiting of unknown cause by anyone in this age group except on the advice of a doctor.

• At the first sign of allergy, such as a skin rash, treatment should be stopped.

• Because of its sedative side effects, the performance of skilled tasks, such as driving, may be impaired.

Interactions

• If used with other drugs that act on the central nervous system (for example, ℞ **phenothiazines**, ℞ **skeletal muscle relaxants**, ℞ **opioids**, ℞ **belladonna alkaloids**, ℞ **barbiturates**, ℞ **hypnotics**, ℞ **sedatives**, ℞ **tranquilizers**), there is a greater potential for side effects.

• Alcohol may intensify side effects such as drowsiness and incoordination.

Side effects

• These are infrequent, but may include drowsiness, dizziness, headache, blurred vision or diarrhea.

• Very infrequently, muscle cramps or severe spasms, jaundice or blood disorder. A temporary fall in blood pressure may occur after an injection. Parkinson-like symptoms (for example, slowed movements, tremor) and other neurological disturbances (for example, uncoordinated or involuntary movement) have occurred (treatment should be stopped or dosage adjusted).

• Although rare, serious events such as coma and convulsions have been reported.

trimethoprim and sulfamethoxazole Ⓖ

(co-trimoxazole; TMP-SMZ)

Type/Group: **sulfonamide; antibacterial**.

Brand(s): Bactrim; Cotrim; Septra; various generic.

How administered: Orally; injection.

Used to treat

Co-trimoxazole is a simplified name for the compound preparation of the sulfonamide antibacterial sulfamethoxazole and the similar, but not related, antibacterial trimethoprim, a folic acid inhibitor, used to treat and prevent the spread of infections of the urinary tract, chronic ✪ **bronchitis**, acute otitis media in children (see ✪ **otitis**), and traveler's ✪ **diarrhea** in adults. It is also used as an antiprotozoal agent to treat or prevent *Pneumocystis carinii* ✪ **pneumonia**, an opportunistic infection seen in immunocompromised people, such as those suffering from ✪ **HIV** infection. It is thought that each drug enhances the action of the other, giving a combined effect greater than the sum of the two. Although there is little substantial evidence to support this, the combination remains a very useful antibacterial preparation.

Warnings

• It should not be given to people with known hypersensitivity to trimethoprim or sulfonamides, and those with anemia due to folate deficiency.

• It should be given with caution to people with kidney or liver impairment, G6PD deficiency (a genetic enzyme disorder), who are taking diuretics, or with possible folate deficiency.

• Its safety during pregnancy has not been established. It may interfere with folic acid metabolism, and so it should be used during pregnancy only if the potential benefits outweigh the possible risk to the fetus. Do not use at the end of term because the newborn may have significant levels of the drug, which may cause serious problems.

• Medical judgment is required if breast-feeding is being considered. Sulfonamides are found in breast milk.

• If used over extensive areas of the body, or areas in which skin is seriously compromised, enough of the drug may be absorbed to create the potential for rare adverse reactions associated with the systemic use of sulfonamides: serious or even fatal allergic reactions, liver failure, and serious blood disorders. Contact a doctor if any adverse reactions, particularly a rash, occur.

• Photosensitivity (abnormal sensitivity to light, including ultraviolet light) may occur, and so exposure should be minimized until light tolerance is determined.

• The use of antibiotics may result in a superinfection from non-susceptible organisms.

Interactions

• If taken with oral ℞ **hypoglycemics**, there is an increased potential for hypoglycemia.

• The levels of ℞ **phenytoin** and ℞ **methotrexate** may be increased.

• The levels of ℞ **dapsone** and trimethoprim are increased.

• If taken with ℞ **disulfiram** or ℞ **metronidazole**, an adverse reaction is possible because co-trimoxazole contains 10 percent alcohol.

Side effects

• Frequently, loss of appetite, nausea, vomiting, rash, and hives.

• Occasionally, diarrhea, abdominal pain, and irritation at intravenous injection site.

• Rarely, headache, dizziness insomnia, convulsions, hallucinations, and depression. Serious adverse reactions include severe skin

---

Key to symbols: Ⓓ = **Drug type/group**   Ⓖ = **Generic name**   Ⓑ = **Brand name** disorders, liver damage, and blood disorders. Those over 65 may have an increased risk of bone marrow suppression, decreased platelets, and severe skin reactions.

trimethoprim (TMP) ⑥

Type/Group: **antibacterial**.
Brand(s): Proloprim; Trimex.
How administered: Orally.

Used to treat

Trimethoprim is a synthetic drug used to treat ✪ **bacterial infections** of the urinary tract and to prevent infection during surgery on the genitourinary tract. It is sometimes used in combination with sulfamethoxazole (as co-trimoxazole).

Warnings

• It should not be given to people with known hypersensitivity to trimethoprim or anemia due to G6PD deficiency (a genetic enzyme disorder).
• It should be given with caution to people with folate deficiency, liver or kidney disorders.
• It may interfere with folic acid metabolism. It should be used during pregnancy only if clearly needed and if the potential benefits outweigh the risks to the fetus.
• Medical judgment is required if breast-feeding is being considered. There is a possibility that the drug may interfere with folic acid metabolism.
• Rarely, this drug may cause serious blood disorders.

Interactions

• The effects of ℞ **phenytoin** and ℞ **procainamide** may be increased.
• If taken with ℞ **dapsone**, the levels of both drugs may be increased.

Side effects

• Occasionally, gastrointestinal upsets (nausea, vomiting).
• Rarely, severe allergic reaction, serious skin or blood disorder.

trimetrexate glucuronate ⑥

Type/Group: **amebicide and antiprotozoal**.
Brand(s): Neutrexin.
How administered: Injection.

Used to treat

Trimetrexate is a synthetic antiprotozoal drug, one of the dihydrofolate reductase (DHFR) inhibitor group, used to treat ✪ **pneumonia** caused by the protozoan microorganism *Pneumocystis carinii* in people whose immune system has been suppressed as in HIV infection (normally where standard treatment is not appropriate). It is always given together with ℞ **leucovorin**, which is a protectant against its potentially fatal toxicity. Trimetrexate is also being investigated as a treatment for certain types of cancer.

Warnings

• It should not be given to people with significant sensitivity to trimetrexate (or leucovorin, as they are always used together).
• It should be given with caution to people with impaired hematological, kidney, or liver function.

• It can harm the fetus and should not be used during pregnancy. Becoming pregnant while using this drug must be avoided.
• It is not recommended for use while breast-feeding.
• Failure to continue leucovorin therapy for 72 hours past the last dose of trimetrexate can lead to fatal toxicity from complications, including bone marrow suppression, kidney dysfunction, and liver dysfunction.

Interactions

• ℞ **cimetidine**, ℞ **acetaminophen**, ℞ **erythromycin**, ℞ **rifampin**, ℞ **rifabutin**, ℞ **ketoconazole**, and ℞ **fluconazole** may alter the effects of trimetrexate.

Side effects

It is difficult to distinguish side effects from symptoms of the underlying disease. Consult your physician for more information.

trimipramine hydrochloride ⑥

Type/Group: **antidepressant; tricyclic**.
Brand(s): Surmontil.
How administered: Orally.

Used to treat

Trimipramine hydrochloride can be used to treat ✪ **depression**, particularly when sedation is needed. Although not stated by the manufacturer for such treatment, it is sometimes used for chronic hives, angioedema (an allergic swelling reaction, often of the face), and nocturnal itching in atopic ✪ **dermatitis**. As is the case with other antidepressants, this drug is also being evaluated for other uses.

Warnings

• It should not be given to people with known hypersensitivity to this drug, or who are just recovering from myocardial infarction (heart attack), or are taking or who have stopped taking MAOI antidepressants within the previous 14 days.
• It should be given with caution to people with a history of seizures, urinary retention, elevated intraocular pressure (pressure in the eyeball), narrow-angle glaucoma, diabetes mellitus, epilepsy, or liver, cardiovascular, heart or thyroid disease.
• Trimipramine should be used during pregnancy only if the benefits outweigh the risk to the fetus.
• It should not be used by nursing mothers.
• Other symptoms of a psychiatric illness may worsen.
• Episodes of mania or hypomania may occur, especially in those with affective bipolar disorder (manic depression).
• Exposure to sunlight should be minimized because of possible photosensitization (sensitivity to light).
• Treatment should be stopped gradually by lowering the dose over a period of time.
• It is not generally given to children.
• It may be two to three weeks before there are any signs of improvement.
• It may impair the performance of skilled tasks such as driving.
• Alcohol, grapefruit juice, and smoking can all affect tricyclics (see Interactions below).

Interactions

• Serious or even fatal reactions can occur if ℞ **MAOI** antidepressants are taken at the same time as tricyclics.

• The effects of ℞ **epinephrine**, ℞ **norepinephrine**, and ℞ **phenylephrine** on blood pressure are intensified.
• Grapefruit juice increases the levels of tricyclics.
• ℞ **clonidine hydrochloride** should not be used with tricyclics, because a dangerous increase in blood pressure and hypertensive crisis is possible.
• The effects of ℞ **guanethidine monosulfate**, ℞ **levodopa**, and ℞ **sympathomimetics** may be reduced by tricyclics.
• The effects of ℞ **anticholinergics**, dicumarol, ℞ **quinolones**, grepafloxacin, and sparfloxacin may be enhanced by tricyclics.
• ℞ **Barbiturates**, ℞ **activated charcoal**, and rifamycin-related antibiotics may reduce the effectiveness of tricyclics.
• ℞ **Cimetidine**, ℞ **SSRIs**, ℞ **haloperidol**, ℞ **bupropion**, ℞ **valproate sodium** (and other valproic acid derivatives), and histamine ℞ **H$_2$-antagonists** may increase the levels of tricyclics in the blood.
• The levels of ℞ **carbamazepine** may increase, while blood levels of tricyclics decrease.
• Smoking may affect the metabolism of tricyclics.
• The effects of alcohol may be enhanced.

Side effects
• Along with other members of this class, it has anticholinergic side effects, such as drowsiness and difficulty in concentrating, dry mouth, blurred vision, dizziness, constipation, postural hypotension (lowered blood pressure on standing), and urinary retention.
• Less frequently anxiety, mental changes, extrapyramidal symptoms in older adults (uncontrollable movements), elevated blood pressure, ECG changes, heart palpitations, fainting, eye changes, nasal congestion, ringing in the ears, gastrointestinal distress, hepatitis, jaundice, and skin sensitivity reactions.
• Rare but serious side effects include abnormal heart rhythm, stoppage of the normal action of the intestine (peristalsis), and blood cell disorders.

Trimox ⓑ
A preparation of ℞ **amoxicillin**.
Formulation: Oral capsules, oral suspension, each in several strengths, pediatric drops.
Availability: Prescription only.
Warnings and side effects: See ℞ **amoxicillin**.

Trimpex ⓑ
A preparation of ℞ **trimethoprim**.
Formulation: Oral tablets.
Availability: Prescription only.
Warnings and side effects: See ℞ **trimethoprim**.

Trinalin Repetabs ⓑ
A preparation of pseudoephedrine sulfate and ℞ **azatadine maleate**.
Formulation: Oral tablets, sustained relase.
Availability: Prescription only.
Warnings and side effects: See ℞ **pseudoephedrine**; ℞ **azatadine maleate**.

Tri-Norinyl ⓑ
A preparation of ℞ **ethinyl estradiol** and ℞ **norethindrone**.
Formulation: Calendar pack of oral tablets.
Availability: Prescription only.
Warnings and side effects: See ℞ **ethinyl estradiol**; ℞ **norethindrone**.

Triofed Syrup ⓑ
A preparation of ℞ **pseudoephedrine** and ℞ **triprolidine hydrochloride**.
Formulation: Oral syrup.
Availability: OTC.
Warnings and side effects: See ℞ **pseudoephedrine**; ℞ **triprolidine hydrochloride**.

Triostat ⓑ
A preparation of ℞ **liothyronine**.
Formulation: Injection.
Availability: Prescription only.
Warnings and side effects: See ℞ **liothyronine**.

Triotann Tablets ⓑ
A preparation of phenylephrine tannate, chlorpheniramine tannate, and pyrilamine tannate.
Formulation: Oral tablets.
Availability: Prescription only.
Warnings and side effects: See ℞ **phenylephrine hydrochloride**; ℞ **chlorpheniramine maleate**; ℞ **pyrilamine maleate**.

Tripedia ⓑ
A preparation of ℞ **diphtheria and tetanus toxoids and acellular pertussis vaccine (DTaP)**.
Formulation: Injection.
Availability: Prescription only.
Warnings and side effects: See ℞ **diphtheria and tetanus toxoids and acellular pertussis vaccine (DTaP)**.

Triphasil ⓑ
A preparation of ℞ **ethinyl estradiol** and ℞ **levonorgestrel**.
Formulation: Calendar pack of oral tablets.
Availability: Prescription only.
Warnings and side effects: See ℞ **ethinyl estradiol**; ℞ **levonorgestrel**.

Triple Antibiotic Ointment ⓑ
A preparation of ℞ **neomycin**, ℞ **polymyxin B sulfate**, and ℞ **bacitracin**.
Formulation: Topical ointment.
Availability: OTC.
Warnings and side effects: See ℞ **neomycin**; ℞ **polymyxin B sulfate**; ℞ **bacitracin**.

Triple Antibiotic Ophthalmic ⓑ
A preparation of ℞ **neomycin**, ℞ **polymyxin B sulfate**, and ℞ **bacitracin**.

Formulation: Topical ointment.
Availability: Prescription only.
Warnings and side effects: See ℞ **neomycin**; ℞ **polymyxin B sulfate**; ℞ **bacitracin**.

triple sulfa cream Ⓖ

(sulfabenzamide; sulfathiazole; sulfacetamide)
Type/Group: **sulfonamide**.
Brand(s): Gyne Sulf; Sultrin; Trysul; various generic.
How administered: Topically.

Used to treat

Triple sulfa cream is a combination of three sulfonamides, ℞ **sulfacetamide**, sulfabenzamide, and sulfathiazole, in a topical (applied externally) antibacterial preparation which is used to treat certain vaginal infections.

Warnings

• It should not be given to people with kidney disease or hypersensitivity to sulfonamides.
• Its safety during pregnancy has not been established. It should not be used at term, and at any other time only if the potential benefits outweigh the risk to the fetus.
• It should not be used while nursing.
• It is only effective against certain bacterial infections and a diagnosis is essential before treatment.

Side effects

• Local irritation and allergic reaction.
• Rarely, a potentially fatal skin disease, Stevens-Johnson syndrome.

Triposed Tablets, Syrup Ⓑ

A preparation of ℞ **pseudoephedrine** and ℞ **triprolidine hydrochloride**.
Formulation: Oral tablets; syrup.
Availability: OTC.
Warnings and side effects: See ℞ **pseudoephedrine**; ℞ **triprolidine hydrochloride**.

triprolidine hydrochloride Ⓖ

Type/Group: **antihistamine; antiallergic; cold and cough preparation**.
Brand(s): (all combinations): With *pseudoephedrine*: Actagen Tablets; Actifed Cold & Allergy Tablets; Allercon Tablets; Allerfrim Tablets, Syrup; Allerphed Syrup; Aprodine Tablets, Syrup; Cenafed Plus Tablets; Genac Tablets; Silafed Syrup; Triofed Syrup; Triposed Tablets, Syrup. With *pseudoephedrine and acetaminophen*: Actifed Plus Caplets, Tablets (have a*cetaminophen*).
How administered: Orally.

Used to treat

Triprolidine can be used for the symptomatic relief of allergic symptoms, such as ❂ **hay fever** (seasonal allergic rhinitis) and ❂ **urticaria**. It is also used in some preparations for ❂ **coughs** and ❂ **colds**.

Warnings

• It should not be given to people with known hypersensitivity to this drug (or with known sensitivity to other antihistamines).

• Antihistamines should be given with caution to people with lower respiratory disease or asthma (and never during an attack), heart disease, hypertension, hyperthyroidism, epilepsy, porphyria, increased intraocular pressure (pressure in the eyeball, as in glaucoma), enlarged prostate, urinary retention, or certain obstructive bladder or gastrointestinal conditions.
• Triprolidine should be used during pregnancy only if it is clearly needed, but not in the third trimester, as newborns or premature infants may have severe reactions, including convulsions, to antihistamines.
• Nursing mothers should discontinue using this drug or discontinue breast-feeding.
• Triprolidine must not be given to infants, and for children under the age of 12 the manufacturer's or medical instructions must be followed closely.
• Because of its sedative side effects, the performance of skilled tasks, such as driving, may be impaired.
• Side effects are more frequent in the elderly.

Interactions

• ℞ **MAOI** antidepressants may prolong and intensify the ℞ **anticholinergic** and sedative effects of antihistamines (see Side effects below).
• If used with ℞ **tricyclic** antidepressants, other antihistamines, ℞ **skeletal muscle relaxants**, ℞ **opioids**, ℞ **barbiturates**, ℞ **hypnotics**, ℞ **sedatives**, or ℞ **antianxiety** drugs, there is a risk of intensified side effects.
• Alcohol may intensify side effects such as drowsiness and impaired mental alertness.

Side effects

• These depend on how it is administered. For this type of antihistamine, there is commonly drowsiness, headache, impaired muscular coordination or dizziness, anticholinergic effects (dry mouth, blurred vision, urinary retention, gastrointestinal disturbances), occasional rashes and photosensitivity (abnormal sensitivity to light), palpitations and heart arrhythmias.
• Rarely, there may be stimulation instead of sedation (paradoxical stimulation), especially in children (and convulsions in overdose), hypersensitivity reactions, blood disorders, liver disturbances, depression, sleep disturbances, and hypotension.

Triptone Ⓑ

A preparation of ℞ **dimenhydrinate**.
Formulation: Oral tablets.
Availability: OTC.
Warnings and side effects: See ℞ **dimenhydrinate**.

Tristoject Ⓑ

A preparation of ℞ **triamcinolone** diacetate.
Formulation: Suspension for injection.
Availability: Prescription only.
Warnings and side effects: See ℞ **triamcinolone**.

Tri-Tannate Tablets; Pediatric Suspension ⓑ

A preparation of phenylephrine tannate and chlorpheniramine tannate and pyrilamine tannate.
Formulation: Oral tablets.
Availability: Prescription only.
Warnings and side effects: See ℞ **phenylephrine hydrochloride**; ℞ **chlorpheniramine maleate**; ℞ **pyrilamine maleate**.

Tritec ⓑ

A preparation of ℞ **ranitidine bismuth citrate**.
Formulation: Oral tablets.
Availability: Prescription only.
Warnings and side effects: ℞ **ranitidine bismuth citrate**

Trivora-28 ⓑ

A preparation of ℞ **ethinyl estradiol** and ℞ **levonorgestrel**.
Formulation: Calendar pack of oral tablets.
Availability: Prescription only.
Warnings and side effects: See ℞ **ethinyl estradiol**; ℞ **levonorgestrel**.

Triysul ⓑ

A preparation of ℞ **triple sulfa cream**.
Formulation: Topical cream.
Availability: Prescription only.
Warnings and side effects: See ℞ **triple sulfa cream**.

Trizivir ⓑ

A preparation of ℞ **abacavir**, ℞ **zidovudine**, and ℞ **lamivudine**.
Formulation: Oral tablets.
Availability: Prescription only.
Warnings and side effects: See ℞ **abacavir**; ℞ **zidovudine**; ℞ **lamivudine**.

Trobicin ⓑ

A preparation of ℞ **spectinomycin**.
Formulation: Injection.
Availability: Prescription only.
Warnings and side effects: See ℞ **spectinomycin**.

Trocal ⓑ

A preparation of ℞ **dextromethorphan**.
Formulation: Lozenges.
Availability: OTC.
Warnings and side effects: See ℞ **dextromethorphan**.

Tronothane ⓑ

A preparation of ℞ **pramoxine hydrochloride**.
Formulation: Topical cream.
Availability: OTC.
Warnings and side effects: See ℞ **pramoxine hydrochloride**.

Tropicacyl ⓑ

A preparation of ℞ **tropicamide**.

Formulation: Ophthalmic solution in several strengths.
Availability: Prescription only.
Warnings and side effects: See ℞ **tropicamide**.

Tropical Gold Dark Tanning ⓑ

A preparation of ℞ **aminobenzoic acid (PABA)** and ℞ **cinnamates**.
Formulation: Topical lotion.
Availability: OTC.
Warnings and side effects: See ℞ **aminobenzoic acid (PABA)**; ℞ **cinnamates**.

tropicamide ⓖ

Type/Group: **anticholinergic; diagnostic agent**.
Brand(s): Mydriacyl; Opticyl; various generic.
How administered: Topically (eye)

Used to treat

Tropicamide is a short-acting drug which can be used to dilate the pupil and paralyze the focusing of the eye for ophthalmic examination.

Warnings

• It should not be given to people with known hypersensitivity to belladonna alkaloids, or with adhesions between the iris and lens, primary glaucoma, or narrow anterior chamber angle.
• It should be given with caution to people over 65 and young children.
• Tropicamide should be used during pregnancy only if it is clearly needed and when the potential benefits outweigh the possible risk to the fetus.
• Medical judgment is required if breast-feeding is being considered. It is not known whether this drug appears in breast milk.
• It may cause blurred vision. Do not drive or engage in any hazardous activities while pupils are dilated.
• It may cause light sensitivity and so exposure to bright light should be minimized.

Interactions

No significant interactions specific to this drug are known.

Side effects

• Blurred vision, photophobia, and irritation.
• There can also be systemic effects, including confusion, fever, headache, sleepiness, visual hallucinations, tachycardia, vasodilatation, edema, increased intraocular pressure (pressure in the eyeball), irritation, abdominal constipation, dry mouth, urinary retention, dry skin, and rash.

Trusopt Ocumeter ⓑ

A preparation of ℞ **dorzolamide**.
Formulation: Eye drops in several strengths.
Availability: Prescription only.
Warnings and side effects: See ℞ **dorzolamide**.

trypanocide ⓓ

see ℞ **amebicide and antiprotozoal**.

T/Scalp ®

A preparation of ℞ **hydrocortisone**.
Formulation: Liquid.
Availability: OTC.
Warnings and side effects: See ℞ **hydrocortisone**.

TSH ©

see ℞ **thyrotropin**.

tuberculin ©

Type/Group: **diagnostic agent**.
Brand(s): (PPD, Mantoux): Aplisol; Tubersol. (PPD, multiple puncture): Aplitest; Tine Test PPD. (OT, multiple puncture): Mono-Vacc Test (O.T.); Tuberculin Old Tine Test.
How administered: Intradermal injection.

Used to treat
Tuberculin (in the form tuberculin purified protein derivative; PPD) is a diagnostic agent prepared from heat-treated protein parts of the tuberculosis mycobacterium. It is used to test whether or not a person has antibodies to ✪ **tuberculosis**, which may indicate active disease or that there has been contact with someone who does have active infection. It is used either in a Mantoux test (where tuberculin is injected intradermally) or a multiple puncture test (barely penetrating the skin). A positive result (for the antibody) is indicated if the skin at the site—usually the forearm—becomes red, raised, and hard. Multiple puncture tests are used for initial screening; positive or inconclusive results must be confirmed or re-evaluated by a Mantoux text. Old tuberculin (OT) is a similar, but less recent, diagnostic agent that may be used in multiple puncture testing. The more recent forms of OT are slightly less accurate than PPD.

Warnings
• It should not be given to people known to react strongly to tuberculin, or (for OT Tine Test only) anyone with an allergy to acacia.
• It should be given with caution to people known to have active tuberculosis.
• Because the consequences of a mother's unrecognized tuberculosis can be harmful to the newborn, and no adverse effects of testing on the health of the fetus are known, tuberculin testing may be performed where clearly needed during pregnancy.
• It is thought unlikely that tuberculin appears in breast milk.
• Repeated testing may lead to the development of abnormal levels of antibodies, with potential for misleading or false results.
• Tuberculin should not be given subcutaneously (that is, beneath rather than within the skin). An exaggerated reaction may occur, with fever, inflammation, and swollen lymph glands.
• A number of factors may increase the likelihood of producing a negative tuberculin result that is in error (false negative). Some of these are: recent viral or bacterial infection or severe febrile (feverish) illness; recent vaccination with a live virus (for example, for measles, polio, rubella, or mumps); some cancers; taking corticosteroids or immunosuppressant drugs; old age; malnutrition; and even tuberculosis itself, if it is a severe case.

• Tuberculin should not be applied to skin that has an acne-like appearance, or over hairy or bony areas.

Interactions
• ℞ **aminocaproic acid**, ℞ **immunosuppressants** (for example, ℞ **corticosteroids**), and live virus ℞ **vaccines** may cause a falsely negative tuberculin test result. The test should be carried out at least one month to six weeks after stopping treatment with any of these drugs.
• BCG vaccine may make the results of tuberculin testing difficult to interpret.

Side effects
• In very sensitive people there may be ulceration at the site of the test with subsequent sloughing of dead tissue, and scarring may result.

tuberculosis treatment ⓓ

see ℞ **antituberculosis**.

Tuinal ®

A preparation of ℞ **amobarbital** and ℞ **secobarbital sodium**.
Formulation: Oral capsules.
Availability: Prescription only.
Warnings and side effects: See ℞ **amobarbital**; ℞ **secobarbital sodium**.

Tums; Extra Strength Tums E-X; Tums Ultra ®

A preparation of ℞ **calcium carbonate**.
Formulation: Oral tablets, chewable.
Availability: OTC.
Warnings and side effects: See ℞ **calcium carbonate**.

turpentine oil ©

Type/Group: **counter-irritant**.
Brand(s): White Cloverine Salve.
How administered: Topically (external).

Used to treat
Turpentine oil is included in certain compound preparations that are used by topical application for the symptomatic relief of pain associated with rheumatism, neuralgia, fibrosis and sprains and stiffness of the joints (see ✪ **musculoskeletal disorders**).

Warnings
None significant.

Interactions
No significant interactions are known.

Side effects
No significant side effects are known.

Tusibron-DM Syrup ®

A preparation of ℞ **dextromethorphan** and ℞ **guaifenesin**.
Formulation: Oral syrup.
Availability: OTC.
Warnings and side effects: See ℞ **dextromethorphan**; ℞ **guaifenesin**.

Key to symbols: ✪ = Disorder Section ℞ = Drug Section ♣ = Herbal Section ⬳ = Supplement Section

Tussafed HC Syrup ®

A preparation of ℞ **hydrocodone bitartrate**, ℞ **guaifenesin**, and ℞ **phenylephrine hydrochloride**
Formulation: Oral syrup.
Availability: Prescription only.
Warnings and side effects: See ℞ hydrocodone bitartrate; ℞ guaifenesin; ℞ phenylephrine hydrochloride.

Tussafed-LA ®

A preparation of ℞ **dextromethorphan**, ℞ **pseudoephedrine**, and ℞ **guaifenesin**.
Formulation: Oral capsules, sustained release.
Availability: Prescription only.
Warnings and side effects: See ℞ dextromethorphan; ℞ pseudoephedrine; ℞ guaifenesin.

Tussafed Syrup; Drops ®

A preparation of ℞ **dextromethorphan**, ℞ **carbinoxamine maleate**, and ℞ **pseudoephedrine**.
Formulation: Oral syrup; drops are pediatric, lower strength.
Availability: Prescription only.
Warnings and side effects: See ℞ dextromethorphan; ℞ carbinoxamine maleate; ℞ pseudoephedrine.

Tussafin Expectorant Liquid ®

A preparation of ℞ **hydrocodone bitartrate**, ℞ **pseudoephedrine**, and ℞ **guaifenesin**.
Formulation: Oral liquid.
Availability: Prescription only.
Warnings and side effects: See ℞ hydrocodone bitartrate; ℞ pseudoephedrine; ℞ guaifenesin.

Tussanil DH Syrup ®

A preparation of ℞ **hydrocodone bitartrate**, ℞ **chlorpheniramine maleate**, and ℞ **phenylephrine hydrochloride**.
Formulation: Oral syrup.
Availability: Prescription only.
Warnings and side effects: See ℞ hydrocodone bitartrate; ℞ chlorpheniramine maleate; ℞ phenylephrine hydrochloride.

Tuss-DM Tablets ®

A preparation of ℞ **dextromethorphan** and ℞ **guaifenesin**.
Formulation: Oral tablets.
Availability: OTC.
Warnings and side effects: See ℞ dextromethorphan; ℞ guaifenesin.

Tussigon Tablets ®

A preparation of ℞ **hydrocodone bitartrate** and ℞ **homatropine hydrobromide**.
Formulation: Oral tablets.
Availability: Prescription only.
Warnings and side effects: See ℞ hydrocodone bitartrate; ℞ homatropine hydrobromide.

Tussin DM Liquid ®

A preparation of ℞ **dextromethorphan** and ℞ **guaifenesin**.
Formulation: Oral liquid.
Availability: OTC.
Warnings and side effects: See ℞ dextromethorphan; ℞ guaifenesin.

Tussin PE ®

A preparation of ℞ **pseudoephedrine** and ℞ **guaifenesin**.
Formulation: Oral liquid.
Availability: OTC.
Warnings and side effects: See ℞ pseudoephedrine; ℞ guaifenesin.

Tussi-Organidin-S NR Liquid ®

A preparation of ℞ **codeine phosphate** and ℞ **guaifenesin**.
Formulation: Oral liquid.
Availability: May or may not require a prescription.
Warnings and side effects: See ℞ codeine phosphate; ℞ guaifenesin.

Tuss-LA Tablets ®

A preparation of ℞ **pseudoephedrine** and ℞ **guaifenesin**.
Formulation: Oral tablets, sustained release.
Availability: Prescription only.
Warnings and side effects: See ℞ pseudoephedrine; ℞ guaifenesin.

Tusstat Syrup ®

A preparation of ℞ **diphenhydramine hydrochloride**.
Formulation: Oral liquid.
Availability: Prescription only.
Warnings and side effects: See ℞ diphenhydramine hydrochloride.

20/20 Eye Drops ®

A preparation of ℞ **naphazoline hydrochloride**.
Formulation: Eye drops.
Availability: OTC.
Warnings and side effects: See ℞ naphazoline hydrochloride.

Twice-A-Day ®

A preparation of ℞ **oxymetazoline hydrochloride**.
Formulation: Nasal drops.
Availability: OTC.
Warnings and side effects: See ℞ oxymetazoline hydrochloride.

Tylenol Regular Strength Tablets, Caplets ®

Also: **Tylenol Extra Strength Tablets**
A preparation of ℞ **acetaminophen**.
Formulation: Oral tablets; gelcaps; liquid.
Availability: OTC.
Warnings and side effects: See ℞ acetaminophen.

Tylenol Arthritis Extended Relief Caplets Ⓑ

A preparation of ℞ **acetaminophen**.
Formulation: Oral tablets, extended release.
Availability: OTC.
Warnings and side effects: See ℞ **acetaminophen**.

Tylenol Flu Maximum Strength Gelcaps Ⓑ

A preparation of ℞ **dextromethorphan**, ℞ **acetaminophen**, and ℞ **pseudoephedrine**.
Formulation: Oral gel capsules.
Availability: OTC.
Warnings and side effects: See ℞ **dextromethorphan**; ℞ **acetaminophen**; ℞ **pseudoephedrine**.

Tylenol Flu Night Time Maximum Strength Powder Ⓑ

A preparation of ℞ **pseudoephedrine**, ℞ **acetaminophen**, and ℞ **diphenhydramine hydrochloride**.
Formulation: Powder (for oral use).
Availability: OTC.
Warnings and side effects: See ℞ **pseudoephedrine**; ℞ **acetaminophen**; ℞ **diphenhydramine hydrochloride**.

Tylenol Junior Strength; Children's Soft-Chews Ⓑ

A preparation of ℞ **acetaminophen**.
Formulation: Oral tablets; chewable tablets; liquid.
Availability: OTC.
Warnings and side effects: See ℞ **acetaminophen**.

Tylenol w/Codeine Elixir Ⓑ

A preparation of ℞ **codeine phosphate** and ℞ **acetaminophen**.
Formulation: Oral liquid.
Availability: May or may not require a prescription.
Warnings and side effects: See ℞ **codeine phosphate**; ℞ **acetaminophen**.

Tylenol w/Codeine Tablets Ⓑ

A preparation of ℞ **codeine phosphate** and ℞ **acetaminophen**.
Formulation: Oral tablets, available in 3 strengths.
Availability: Prescription only.
Warnings and side effects: See ℞ **codeine phosphate**; ℞ **acetaminophen**.

Tylox Capsules Ⓑ

A preparation of ℞ **oxycodone** and ℞ **acetaminophen**.
Formulation: Oral capsules.
Availability: Prescription only.
Warnings and side effects: See ℞ **oxycodone**; ℞ **acetaminophen**.

Typhim Vi Ⓑ

A preparation of typhoid vaccine, polysaccharide.
Formulation: Intradermal or subcutaneous injection.
Availability: Prescription only.
Warnings and side effects: See ℞ **typhoid vaccine**.

typhoid vaccine Ⓖ

Type/Group: vaccine.
Brand(s): Typhim Vi; Typhoid Vaccine (H-P);Vivotif Berna Vaccine.
How administered: Orally; injection.

Used to treat

Typhoid vaccines confer some immunity (approximately 70 percent) to infection by ○ **typhoid** bacteria, *Salmonella typhi*. Currently, three kinds of typhoid vaccine are available, all of them with roughly the same effectiveness, but with somewhat different side effects: (a) live, but weakened (attenuated) bacteria, which is the oral vaccine; (b) killed (inactivated) bacteria, given by subcutaneous or intradermal injection; and (c) polysaccharide, containing specific bits of the bacterium which stimulate the immune system to produce antibodies as if whole bacteria were present; given by intramuscular injection only.

Warnings

• None of these vaccines should be given to people with known hypersensitivity or previous severe reaction to a typhoid vaccine, or those who currently have any severe febrile (feverish) or gastrointestinal illness (administration should be postponed until recovery).
• The oral vaccine should not be given to people with impaired immune response from whatever cause (for example, illness, immunosuppressive therapy, hereditary disorder).
• These vaccines should not be given to anyone with typhoid fever or who is a chronic "carrier" of the bacteria.
• These vaccines should be administered during pregnancy only when medically judged to be clearly needed. Although studies have not been performed, it is considered prudent that live, oral vaccine be avoided in pregnancy or within 3 months prior to becoming pregnant.
• Medical judgment is required if breast-feeding is being considered. The risks of this live, oral vaccine in breast-feeding are not known, but the other forms are not believed to have any unusual risks.
• The injected vaccines should not be administered to anyone who is overheated, as from physical activity or high environmental temperatures.
• Full protection is not guaranteed and travelers at risk are advised not to eat uncooked food or to drink untreated water.
• After administration, people will be required to wait for some time to ensure that there is no serious reaction (such as anaphylaxis).

Interactions

• ℞ **Sulfonamides** and other ℞ **antibiotics** may inhibit the effectiveness of the live, oral vaccine.
• Other vaccines that often provoke side effects (for example, cholera and plague vaccines) should not be given at the same time as typhoid vaccine.
• Caution is required if ℞ **anticoagulants** are being taken.

Side effects

• Live, oral vaccine: nausea, headache, fever, diarrhea, vomiting or skin rash; less frequently, hives and stomach cramps.

Key to symbols: ○ = Disorder Section ℞ = Drug Section ♣ = Herbal Section ⚲⚲ = Supplement Section

• Injected forms (inactivated and polysaccharide): there may be swelling, irritation or tenderness at the site of vaccination, and malaise, headache, fever, or achiness. The frequency of these side effects is lower with the polysaccharide vaccine.

• Anaphylaxis has occurred with use of the inactivated vaccine.

Typhoid Vaccine (H-P) Ⓑ

A preparation of ℞ **typhoid vaccine**.
Formulation: Intramuscular injection.
Availability: Prescription only.
Warnings and side effects: See ℞ **typhoid vaccine**.

Tyzine; Tyzine Pediatric Drops Ⓑ

A preparation of ℞ **tetrahydrozoline hydrochloride**.
Formulation: Nasal drops; spray.
Availability: Prescription only.
Warnings and side effects: See ℞ **tetrahydrozoline hydrochloride**.

ulcer-healing drug Ⓓ

Generics: bismuth subsalicylate; cimetidine; famotidine; lansoprazole; misoprostol; nizatidine; omeprazole; pantoprazole sodium; rabeprazole sodium; ranitidine bismuth citrate; ranitidine hydrochloride.

Actions and uses

Ulcer-healing drug treatment promotes actual healing of ulceration of the gastric (stomach) and duodenal (first part of small intestine) linings and so are used in the treatment of a ✪ **peptic ulcer**. These drugs are distinct from ℞ **antacid** agents that mostly treat only the symptoms of peptic ulcers, and cannot generally be taken in big enough doses, or for long enough, to significantly affect healing. A number of classes of ulcer-healing drugs may be used, of which the first were the ℞ **H₂-antagonist** drugs (℞ **cimetidine**, ℞ **ranitidine hydrochloride**, ℞ **famotidine** and ℞ **nizatidine**), and these are now part of mainstream treatment, and are well tolerated. They are considered safe enough to be available without prescription (although only to treat ✪ **indigestion** and minor symptoms, not ulcers). The ℞ **proton-pump inhibitor** drugs (for example, ℞ **omeprazole**, ℞ **lansoprazole**, ℞ **rabeprazole sodium**, and ℞ **pantoprazole sodium**) were developed later, and are very effective, though not always so well tolerated.

Where ulceration is difficult to deal with, as with ℞ **NSAID**-induced peptic ulceration, ℞ **prostaglandin** analogs (for example, ℞ **misoprostol**) may be used, sometimes in compound preparations with the NSAID agent. But prostaglandins have many side effects and are generally not well tolerated.

Some compounds of bismuth have ℞ **cytoprotectant** actions possibly involving alterations in natural protective secretions, and such compounds (for instance, ℞ **bismuth subsalicylate**) have a useful healing action. These classes may be combined in treatment, and ℞ **ranitidine bismuth citrate** combines two actions in one chemical compound.

The first two classes, the ℞ **H₂-antagonist** and ℞ **proton-pump inhibitor** drugs, act principally by reducing the secretion of peptic acid by the stomach's mucosal lining. They are very effective in the short term, but the recurrence rate of peptic ulcers some time after treatment is relatively high. However, it is now realized that infection of the stomach by an unusual bacterial organism *Helicobacter pylori*, is associated with peptic ulcers. For this reason treatment of the cases by a ℞ **Helicobacter pylori eradication regime** is now relatively common. A combination of ℞ **antibacterial** and antiulcer therapy is used for two to four weeks, and this can be very effective and reduces the remission rate.

Limitations

See the individual drug entries.

Ultiva Ⓑ

A preparation of ℞ **remifentanil**.
Formulation: Injection, for intravenous infusion only.
Availability: Prescription only.
Warnings and side effects: See ℞ **remifentanil**.

Ultram Ⓑ

A preparation of ℞ **tramadol hydrochloride**.
Formulation: Oral tablets.
Availability: Prescription only.
Warnings and side effects: See ℞ **tramadol hydrochloride**.

Ultrase Capsules; MT 12; MT 18; MT 20 Ⓑ

A preparation of ℞ **pancreatin** (amylase, lipase, protease).
Formulation: Oral capsules, 4 strengths.
Availability: Prescription only.
Warnings and side effects: See ℞ **pancreatin**.

Ultra Tears Ⓑ

A preparation of ℞ **hydroxypropyl methylcellulose**.
Formulation: Ophthalmic solution.
Availability: OTC.
Warnings and side effects: See ℞ **hydroxypropyl methylcellulose**.

Unasyn Ⓑ

A preparation of ℞ **ampicillin** and sulbactam sodium.
Formulation: Injection; intravenous infusion.
Availability: Prescription only.
Warnings and side effects: See ℞ **ampicillin**.

undecylenic acid Ⓖ

Type/Group: antifungal.
Brand(s): Caldesene; Cruex; Desenex; Fungoid; Protectol.
Combinations: With *tolfanate* and other components: Dermasept Antifungal; SteriNail.
How administered: Topically (external).

Used to treat

Undecylenic acid and its derivatives are synthetic drugs with antifungal activity and are incorporated into a number of topical preparations for the treatment of ✪ **fungal infections** of the skin, including athlete's foot and infections of the nails (it is also sometimes used for diaper rash).

Warnings

• It should not be given to people with known sensitivity to undecylenic acid.
• The spray form should be given with caution to diabetics and people with impaired circulation.
• There are no reported problems in pregnancy.
• Powders are generally used together with other treatments, but may be effective on their own in very mild cases.

Interactions

No significant interactions have been reported when used topically (externally).

Side effects

• Skin irritation.

Uni-Ace ⑧

A preparation of ℞ **acetaminophen**.
Formulation: Oral liquid.
Availability: OTC.
Warnings and side effects: See ℞ **acetaminophen**.

Uni-Dur ⑧

A preparation of ℞ **theophylline**.
Formulation: Oral tablets, extended release in several strengths.
Availability: Prescription only.
Warnings and side effects: See ℞ **theophylline**.

Unipen ⑧

A preparation of ℞ **nafcillin**.
Formulation: Oral capsules.
Availability: Prescription only.
Warnings and side effects: See ℞ **nafcillin**.

Uniphyl ⑧

A preparation of ℞ **theophylline**.
Formulation: Oral tablets, timed release in several strengths.
Availability: Prescription only.
Warnings and side effects: See ℞ **theophylline**.

Uniretic ⑧

A preparation of ℞ **hydrochlorothiazide** and ℞ **moexipril hydrochloride**.
Formulation: Oral tablets, in two strengths.
Availability: Prescription only.
Warnings and side effects: See ℞ **hydrochlorothiazide**; ℞ **moexipril hydrochloride**.

Unisom Nighttime Sleep Aid ⑧

A preparation of ℞ **doxylamine**.
Formulation: Oral tablets.
Availability: OTC.
Warnings and side effects: See ℞ **doxylamine**.

Uni-tussin DM Syrup ⑧

A preparation of ℞ **dextromethorphan** and ℞ **guaifenesin**.
Formulation: Oral syrup.

Availability: OTC.
Warnings and side effects: See ℞ **dextromethorphan**; ℞ **guaifenesin**.

Uni-tussin Syrup ⑧

A preparation of ℞ **guaifenesin**.
Formulation: Oral syrup.
Availability: OTC.
Warnings and side effects: See ℞ **guaifenesin**.

Univasc ⑧

A preparation of ℞ **moexipril hydrochloride**.
Formulation: Oral tablets, available in two strengths.
Availability: Prescription only.
Warnings and side effects: See ℞ **moexipril hydrochloride**.

Uracid ⑧

A preparation of ℞ **methionine**.
Formulation: Oral capsules.
Availability: Prescription only.
Warnings and side effects: See ℞ **methionine**.

urea ⑥

(carbamide)
Type/Group: **diuretic; glaucoma treatment**.
Brand(s): Ureaphil. (Topical emollient): Aquacare; Carmol 10, 20; Gordon's Urea 40%; Gormel Creme; Lanaphilic; Nutraplus; Ultra Mide 25; Ureacin-10, 20.
How administered: Intravenous infusion; topically.

Used to treat

Urea is both an osmotic diuretic and, when used topically (externally), a hydrating agent that is used in a number of skin preparations (for example, creams that are used to treat ✿ **eczema** and ✿ **psoriasis**). It is also included in eardrop preparations used for dissolving and washing out earwax. When given internally, it is used primarily to treat edema, or swelling, in the brain. It may also be used for ✿ **glaucoma** to decrease pressure within the eyeball when other agents have not worked satisfactorily.

Warnings

• When used internally, it should not be given to people with severe kidney impairment, liver failure, significant dehydration, or active bleeding within the brain. It should not be infused into the veins of the lower extremities in elderly people because of the risk of phlebitis and thrombosis.
• It should be given with caution in people who have any degree of kidney or liver impairment, or cardiac disease.
• When used internally it should be given during pregnancy only when the potential benefit outweighs the possible risk to the fetus.
• When used internally, medical judgment is required if breast-feeding is being considered. With topical use, it is regarded as safe when used as directed.
• An escape of urea into the tissues from the site of infusion (vein) can cause inflammation and death of affected skin tissue.
Thrombosis may occur at the infusion site, especially in superficial or deep veins of the lower extremities.

• Urea administration may cause electrolyte depletion, particularly of sodium and potassium.

Interactions

• Urea actually increases the clearance of ℞ **lithium** from the body (most diuretics have an opposite effect) and so the effects of lithium may be decreased when used internally.

Side effects

• Commonly, headache, nausea, and vomiting.

• Other side effects include fainting, confusion, dizziness, nervousness, and hypotension.

• No side effects are known when used topically.

urea peroxide Ⓖ

see ℞ **carbamide peroxide**.

urea peroxohydrate Ⓖ

see ℞ **carbamide peroxide**.

Ureaphil Ⓑ

A preparation of ℞ **urea**.
Formulation: Intravenous infusion.
Availability: Prescription only.
Warnings and side effects: See ℞ **urea**.

Urex Ⓑ

A preparation of ℞ **methenamine**.
Formulation: Oral Tablets.
Availability: Prescription only.
Warnings and side effects: See ℞ **methenamine**.

uricosuric Ⓓ

Generics: **probenecid; sulfinpyrazone**.

Actions and uses

Uricosuric drugs increase the excretion of uric acid from the blood into the urine, so can be used in the prevention of attacks of chronic gout, which involve high levels of uric acid (hyperuricemia) with deposition of urate crystals in the joints. The most commonly used drug is ℞ **probenecid**, but ℞ **sulfinpyrazone** is also used. See also ℞ **antigout**.

Limitations

See the individual drug entries.

Urimar-T Ⓑ

A preparation of ℞ **hyoscyamine**, ℞ **methenamine**, sodium biphosphate, phenyl salicylate, and methylene blue.
Formulation: Oral tablets.
Availability: Prescription only.
Warnings and side effects: See ℞ **hyoscyamine**; ℞ **methenamine**.

urinary acidifier Ⓓ

Generics: **acetohydroxamic acid (AHA); ammonium chloride**.

Actions and uses

Urinary acidifier agents, when taken by mouth, cause the urine to become acid (or less alkaline). This ability is used to treat metabolic ✪ alkalosis and to increase the rate of the excretion of some drugs and poisons from the body, and so acting as an ℞ **antidote**. ℞ **ammonium chloride** is used by mouth or by infusion for the above purposes. ℞ **acetohydroxamic acid (AHA)** is used with other drugs, to treat chronic urinary tract infections due to certain organisms. It works by inhibiting the bacterial enzyme, urease, so causing less conversion of urea to ammonia. This decreases pH to a more acid level and allows other antimicrobials given at the same time to work better. It is not antibacterial itself and does not directly acidify the urine. It will only work when infection is caused by bacteria which use urease.

Limitations

See the individual drug entries.

urinary alkalinizer Ⓓ

Generics: **citrates; sodium bicarbonate**.

Actions and uses

Urinary alkalinizer agents, when taken by mouth, cause the urine to become alkaline (less acid). This ability is used in the treatment of chronic metabolic ✪ **acidosis** (such as that caused by renal tubular acidosis), the relief of pain in some infections of the urinary tract or the bladder, and in the treatment of ✪ **gout**. The agents mainly used are ℞ **citrates**, often a sodium citrate and citric acid solution (Shohl's solution), or potassium citrate combinations. ℞ **sodium bicarbonate** can also be used.

Limitations

See the individual drug entries.

Urised Ⓑ

A preparation of ℞ **atropine sulfate**, ℞ **hyoscyamine**, ℞ **methenamine**, methylene blue, phenyl salicylate, and ℞ **benzoic acid**.
Formulation: Oral tablets.
Availability: Prescription only.
Warnings and side effects: See ℞ **atropine sulfate**; ℞ **hyoscyamine**; ℞ **methenamine**; ℞ **benzoic acid**.

Urisedamine Ⓑ

A preparation of ℞ **hyoscyamine** and ℞ **methenamine**.
Formulation: Oral tablets.
Availability: Prescription only.
Warnings and side effects: See ℞ **hyoscyamine**; ℞ **methenamine**.

Urispas Ⓑ

A preparation of ℞ **flavoxate hydrochloride**.
Formulation: Oral tablets.
Availability: Prescription only.
Warnings and side effects: See ℞ **flavoxate hydrochloride**.

Uri-Tet Ⓑ

A preparation of ℞ **oxytetracycline**.
Formulation: Oral capsules.
Availability: Prescription only.
Warnings and side effects: See ℞ **oxytetracycline**.

urofollitropin Ⓖ

Type/Group: **sex hormone; gonadotropin**.
Brand(s): Fertinex.
How administered: Injection.

Used to treat

Urofollitropin (human menopausal gonadotropin) is used as an infertility treatment in women whose infertility is due to abnormal pituitary gland function, or who do not respond to the commonly used fertility drug ℞ **clomiphene citrate**. It is also used in superovulation treatment for assisted conception, such as *in vitro* fertilization. It is a highly purified preparation of the sex hormone, folliclestimulating hormone (FSH), extracted from the urine of menopausal women.

Warnings

• It should not be used by people with known sensitivity this drug, primary ovarian failure, uncontrolled thyroid or adrenal dysfunction, tumor of the ovary, breast, uterus, hypothalamus or pituitary gland, or in the presence of any cause of infertility other than failure to ovulate.
• It should not be used during pregnancy or if already pregnant.
• Medical judgment is required if breast-feeding is being considered.
• The risk of multiple births is markedly increased.
• Overstimulation of the ovary may occur. If there is significant ovarian enlargement after ovulation, intercourse must be avoided because of the danger of ruptured ovarian cyst.
• In some cases ovarian hyperstimulation syndrome, a serious medical event, may occur. Early warning signs are severe nausea and vomiting and weight gain; a doctor must be contacted if these develop.

Interactions

Drug interactions for urofollitropin have not been documented.

Side effects

• Serious lung and circulatory conditions may develop.
• There may be ovarian cysts, gastrointestinal symptoms, pain or irritation at the site of injection, breast tenderness, headache, and skin reactions.

Urogesic Blue Ⓑ

A preparation of ℞ **hyoscyamine**, ℞ **methenamine**, sodium biphosphate, phenyl salicylate, and methylene blue.
Formulation: Oral tablets.
Availability: Prescription only.
Warnings and side effects: See ℞ **hyoscyamine**; ℞ **methenamine**.

urokinase Ⓖ

Type/Group: **fibrinolytic; thrombolytic**.
Brand(s): Abbokinase; Abbokinase Open-Cath.
How administered: Intravenous injection, infusion.

Used to treat

Urokinase (which occurs naturally in the body and is found in urine) provides enzyme activity in a complex way, with the resultant effect of breaking up blood clots. It is used in ✪ **myocardial infarction** (heart attack), when it should be given as soon as possible, and to treat ✪ **pulmonary embolism**. It is also used to break up obstructions (such as blood clots) that may build up in catheters.

Warnings

• It should not be given to people with known hypersensitivity to this drug, or with active internal bleeding, severe uncontrolled high blood pressure, or surgery or bleeding involving the nervous system (brain or spinal cord) within the previous two months. It will be given by experienced personnel after a full medical assessment.
• It should be given with great caution to anyone with cerebrovascular disease, any recent major surgery, recent injury or internal bleeding (for example, in the gastrointestinal tract or urinary tract), bacterial endocarditis, high blood pressure, severe diabetes mellitus, significant liver or kidney impairment, or any condition or disorder that would make bleeding more likely (for example, taking an anticoagulant drug or a low thrombocyte count).
• Urokinase should be used during pregnancy only when it is clearly needed.
• Medical judgment is required if breast-feeding is being considered.
• Although reported rarely, fibrinolytics may free bits of plaque that may lodge (usually) in the smaller blood vessels. This may result in abrupt, sharp pain in a leg, foot, the toes, back, or flank. ("Purple toes syndrome" appears as mottled, purplish discoloration of the toes.) More serious obstructions are possible, which may cause kidney failure, pancreatitis, hypertension, heart attack, stroke, and other serious obstructive events.
• Urokinase works relatively quickly, leading to rapid restoration of circulation to the heart, and this may cause arrhythmias to develop. Caution is advised.

Interactions

• If used with ℞ **anticoagulants**, ℞ **antiplatelets** (including any drugs with antiplatelet activity, such as ℞ **aspirin** and ℞ **indomethacin**), there is an increased risk of bleeding. Despite some increased risk, a ℞ **heparin** dose is recommended before use in the heart.

Side effects

• The chief complication is hemorrhage (although major bleeding is not frequent), which may occur at virtually any site in the body.
• Allergic symptoms, usually mild, may occur, such as fever and chills, rash or bronchospasm. Anaphylactic reaction is rare. Other side effects may include nausea or vomiting, brief swings in blood pressure, shortness of breath, rapid heartbeat, and back pain.

Uroquid-Acid No. 2 Ⓑ

A preparation of ℞ **methenamine** and ℞ **sodium phosphate**.
Formulation: Oral Tablets.
Availability: Prescription only.
Warnings and side effects: See ℞ **methenamine**; ℞ **sodium phosphate**.

Ursinus Inlay-Tabs Ⓑ

A preparation of ℞ **pseudoephedrine** and ℞ **aspirin**.
Formulation: Oral tablets.

Availability: OTC.
Warnings and side effects: See ℞ **pseudoephedrine**; ℞ **aspirin**.

Urso ⑧

A preparation of ℞ **ursodiol**.
Formulation: Oral tablets.
Availability: Prescription only.
Warnings and side effects: See ℞ **ursodiol**.

ursodeoxycholic acid ⑥

see ℞ **ursodiol**.

ursodiol ⑥

(ursodeoxycholic acid)
Type/Group: **gallstone treatment**.
Brand(s): Actigall.
How administered: Orally.

Used to treat

Ursodiol is made from a naturally occurring bile acid which is a cholelitholytic, a drug that can dissolve some ✪ **gallstones** (calculi). It is also used in primary biliary cirrhosis. It decreases the cholesterol content of bile and gallstones by reducing hepatic cholesterol secretion and reabsorption of cholesterol by the intestine.

Warnings

• It should not be given to people with allergy to bile acids, who have chronic liver disease, or whose gallstones would not be dissolved by ursodiol (calcified cholesterol stones and some others distinguished by X-ray appearance), and those who clearly need, with medical judgment, the benefit of surgical removal (for example, some gastrointestinal conditions or non-functioning gallbladder).
• While no reports of adverse effects in pregnancy are known, the possibility may exist of risk to the fetus, and so it should not be used during pregnancy.
• Medical judgment is required if breast-feeding is being considered. It is not known whether this drug appears in breast milk.
• Liver function should be monitored during long-term treatment.
• Take with food.
• Treatment can take several months and reoccurrence of stones is common.

Interactions

• ℞ **Antacids**, ℞ **cholestyramine**, ℞ **clofibrate**, and ℞ **colestipol hydrochloride** lower the absorption and effect of ursodiol.
• ℞ **Estrogens** and ℞ **oral contraceptives** may have effects that favor gallstone formation and so interfere with ursodiol.

Side effects

• Vomiting, nausea, diarrhea, skin itching, dryness or rash, metallic taste, and abdominal pain.

uterine stimulant ⑪

Generics: **carboprost; dinoprostone; ergonovine maleate; methylergonovine maleate; oxytocin.**

Actions and uses

℞ **uterine stimulant** or oxytocic, agents contract the myometrium (muscle layer) of the uterus. The ℞ **posterior pituitary hormone**, ℞ **oxytocin**, is the natural agent that increases the contractions of the uterus during normal labor (and also stimulates milk production), and so it may be used as a synthetic drug by intravenous injection or infusion to speed up or assist labor (or abortion) and also to help stop bleeding following childbirth. Fungus-derived ℞ **ergot alkaloid** drugs, such as ℞ **ergonovine maleate** and ℞ **methylergonovine maleate**, contract the uterus and are used to do this in the last stages of labor and to minimize bleeding after childbirth (they are the drugs of choice because their effects on blood vessels are less pronounced).
Several of the natural local hormones of the ℞ **prostaglandin** family (including ℞ **carboprost** and ℞ **dinoprostone**) contract the uterus (and ripen the cervix) and can be used for labor induction and occasionally as ℞ **abortifacient** drugs.

Limitations

See the individual drug entries.

V-16 ⑥

see ℞ **etoposide**.

vaccination ⑪

see ℞ **immunization**; ℞ **vaccine**.

vaccine ⑪

Generics: **BCG intravesical; BCG vaccine; diphtheria and tetanus toxoids and acellular pertussis vaccine (DTaP); diphtheria and tetanus toxoids and whole-cell pertussis vaccine, adsorbed (DTwP); diphtheria and tetanus vaccine (DTwP-Hib)diphtheria and tetanus toxoids, acellular pertussis and** *Haemophilus influenzae* **type b conjugate vaccine (DTaP-HIB); diphtheria and tetanus toxoid, adsorbed (DT; Td); Haemophilus b conjugate vaccine; hepatitis A vaccine, inactivated; hepatitis B vaccine; influenza virus vaccine; Lyme disease vaccine (recombinant OspA); meningococcal polysaccharide vaccine; MMR vaccine; pneumococcal vaccine; poliovirus vaccine; rabies vaccine; rubella vaccine, live; tetanus toxoid, adsorbed; tetanus vaccine; typhoid vaccine; varicella virus vaccine, live; yellow fever vaccine.**

Actions and uses

Vaccines are preparations that are used for ℞ **immunization**, to confer what is known as active immunity against specific ✪ **infections**: that is, they cause a person's own body to create a defense, in the form of antibodies (immune globulins; immunoglobulins), against the microbe or its toxic products. Vaccines can be one of three types. The first type are those administered in the form of a suspension of dead (inactivated) viruses (for example, ℞ **influenza virus vaccine**) or bacteria (for example, one of the three types of ℞ **typhoid vaccine**). The second type may be live but weakened, or "attenuated," viruses (for example, ℞ **rubella vaccine, live**) or bacteria (for example, ℞ **BCG vaccine**). The third and final type are toxoids (extracts of detoxified endotoxins) (for example, ℞ **diphtheria and tetanus toxoid, adsorbed (DT; Td)**;

℞ **tetanus toxoid, adsorbed**), which are suspensions containing extracts of the toxins released by the invading organism, which then stimulate the formation of antibodies against the toxin of the disease, rather than the organism itself. Vaccines that incorporate dead microorganisms or toxoids generally require a series of administrations (usually three) to build up a sufficient supply of antibodies in the body. "Booster" shots may thereafter be necessary at regular intervals to reinforce immunity, for example, after 10 years in the case of the tetanus vaccine. Vaccines that incorporate live microorganisms may confer immunity with a single dose, because the organisms multiply within the body, although some live vaccines still require three administrations, for example, oral (Sabin) poliomyelitis vaccine. They are used in the general population, and special vaccines are used for high-risk groups (such as those traveling abroad). Administration is by injection or by mouth.

Limitations

There are a number of circumstances when vaccines should not be used and suitability will be assessed by trained personnel. For instance, they may be contraindicated in those hypersensitive to neomycin, gelatin, egg, and other agents or substances used in the production of the vaccine. Some coagulation disorders, and thrombocytopenia, complicate the use of injections in people with these conditions. After vaccination, you will need to wait some time in case of allergic reaction (for example anaphylactic reaction).

Vagifem ®

A preparation of ℞ **estradiol** hemihydrate.
Formulation: Vaginal tablets.
Availability: Prescription only.
Warnings and side effects: See ℞ **estradiol**.

Vagistat-1 ®

A preparation of ℞ **tioconazole**.
Formulation: Topical ointment.
Availability: OTC.
Warnings and side effects: See ℞ **tioconazole**.

valaciclovir ⓖ

see ℞ **valacyclovir**.

valacyclovir ⓖ

(valaciclovir)
Type/Group: **antiviral**.
Brand(s): Valtrex.
How administered: Orally.

Used to treat

Valacyclovir is a prodrug of ℞ **acyclovir**, an antiviral drug that can be used to treat herpes zoster and genital herpes simplex infections, as well as to suppress recurrent genital herpes (see ✪ **herpes**).

Warnings

• It should not be given to people who are immunosuppressed or those with known hypersensitivity to valacyclovir or acyclovir.
• It should be given with caution to people with kidney or liver insufficiency, who are over 65, or children.

• Valacyclovir's safety during pregnancy has not been established and it should be used only when the potential benefits outweigh the possible risks to the fetus.
• Medical judgment is required if breast-feeding is being considered.
• Intercourse should be avoided when genital herpes symptoms are active to avoid infecting the partner.

Interactions

• ℞ **cimetidine** and ℞ **probenecid** may reduce the effects of valacyclovir.

Side effects

• Frequently, nausea, headache, and gastrointestinal upsets.
• Occasionally, unusual tiredness, and dizziness.
• Rarely, abdominal pain and kidney dysfunction.

Valergen ®

A preparation of ℞ **estradiol**.
Formulation: Injection.
Availability: Prescription only.
Warnings and side effects: See ℞ **estradiol**.

Valertest No. 1 ®

A preparation of ℞ **estradiol** and ℞ **testosterone** ethanate.
Formulation: Injection.
Availability: Prescription only.
Warnings and side effects: See ℞ **estradiol**; ℞ **testosterone**.

Valisone ®

A preparation of ℞ **betamethasone** valerate.
Formulation: Ointment; cream in two strengths; lotion.
Availability: Prescription only.
Warnings and side effects: See ℞ **betamethasone**.

Valium ®

A preparation of ℞ **diazepam**.
Formulation: Oral tablets in several strengths; injectable solution.
Availability: Prescription only.
Warnings and side effects: See ℞ **diazepam**.

valproate sodium ⓖ

(sodium valproate; valproic acid; divalproex)
Type/Group: **anticonvulsant**; **antiepileptic**.
Brand(s): Depakene Capsules, Syrup; Depacon; various generic.
How administered: Orally; injection.

Used to treat

Valproate sodium is a valuable drug for treating ✪ **epilepsy**, particularly tonic-clonic seizures (grand mal) in primary generalized epilepsy. It may also be used to prevent ✪ **migraine** headache, and to treat mania associated with ✪ **bipolar disorder**. Other forms of this drug, valproic acid and divalproex, are nearly identical to valproate sodium in action and side effects.

Warnings

• Avoid its use in people with known hypersensitivity to this drug, or with a history of liver disease or known liver abnormality.

Key to symbols: ✪ = Disorder Section ℞ = Drug Section ♣ = Herbal Section ⚖ = Supplement Section

• Valproate sodium should be given with extreme caution to infants under two years of age.

• This drug is associated with an increase in frequency of certain birth defects and should not be used during pregnancy. However, because uncontrolled seizures can also threaten fetal health, medical judgment is needed to weigh potential benefits and risks.

• Valproate sodium appears in breast milk, though its effects are not known and so medical judgment is required if considering breast-feeding.

• Treatment should be stopped immediately if there is vomiting, jaundice, drowsiness, anorexia, or loss of seizure control; rashes; or various signs of liver or blood disorder. Patients or their care providers should be instructed how to recognize signs of blood or liver disorders, and they are advised to seek immediate medical attention if symptoms develop.

• Withdrawal should be gradual otherwise it may precipitate attacks.

• As this drug may cause drowsiness, driving or other hazardous activity should be avoided.

Interactions

• ℞ **Clonazepam** may induce absence-type seizure in anyone with a history of this kind of seizure.

• ℞ **Chlorpromazine**, ℞ **erythromycin**, felbamate, and ℞ **salicylates** (for example, ℞ **aspirin**) may increase levels of valproate sodium and so increase the risk of side effects.

• ℞ **Rifampin** may decrease levels of valproate sodium.

• The effects of ℞ **carbamazepine**, ℞ **lamotrigine**, ℞ **phenobarbital** (and other ℞ **barbiturates**), and ℞ **phenytoin** may be intensified, while the therapeutic effect of valproate sodium is reduced.

• The levels of ℞ **amitriptyline** (and ℞ **nortriptyline**), ℞ **benzodiazepines**, ℞ **ethosuximide**, felbamate, ℞ **tolbutamide**, ℞ **warfarin sodium**, and ℞ **zidovudine** may be increased, with a greater risk of side effects or overdose symptoms.

Side effects

These depend on how administered, use, and dose, and include:

• Stomach irritation and nausea, drowsiness, unsteady gait, muscle tremor, and feeling of weakness;

• Weight loss or weight gain, thinning and curling hair, edema and blood changes;

• Possible pancreas and liver damage;

• At high dosage tremor, hair loss, and blood abnormalities are frequent;

• Potentially serious side effects include pancreatitis, liver failure, encephalopathy, blood cell and skin disorders.

valproic acid and derivatives ⑥

see ℞ **valproate sodium**.

valrubicin ⑥

Type/Group: **anticancer; cytotoxic**.
Brand(s): Valstar.
How administered: Intravesical.

Used to treat

Valrubicin is a cytotoxic drug (an anthracycline antibiotic in origin) that is used to treat bladder ✪ **cancer** when conventional treatment is not appropriate or has not been effective.

Warnings

• It should not be given to people with known hypersensitivity to other anthracyclines or other components of this drug, with urinary tract infections, small bladder capacity, or those whose bladder integrity is compromised.

• It should be given with caution to people with severe irritable bladder symptoms. This is a specialist drug which will be used following a full evaluation by specialist physicians.

• Valrubicin is not recommended for use during pregnancy unless it is medically judged to be essential, because it may cause birth defects. Becoming pregnant while using this drug must be avoided.

• It should not be used if breast-feeding.

• Drugs of this type may induce genetic mutations in cells, or cause cancer.

Side effects

• Irritable bladder symptoms, urinary difficulties, blood in urine, bladder pain, bladder or urinary tract infection, local burning, abdominal pain, and nausea.

valsartan ⑥

Type/Group: **angiotensin-receptor blocker; antihypertensive; vasodilator**.
Brand(s): Diovan. Combinations: With *hydrochlorothiazide*: Diovan HCT.
How administered: Orally.

Used to treat

Valsartan is an angiotensin II receptor (AT1 receptors) blocker. Angiotensin II is a circulating hormone that is a powerful vasoconstrictor (narrows blood vessels) and blocking its effects leads to a fall in blood pressure. Valsartan can be used, alone or with other drugs, to treat high blood pressure (see ✪ **hypertension**).

Warnings

• It should not be given to people with known hypersensitivity to this drug.

• It should be given with caution to people with severe congestive heart failure, with biliary obstruction, impaired liver function, severe kidney insufficiency, or renal stenosis. Any fluid- or salt-depleted condition (as from diuretic use) should be corrected before using this drug.

• Risk in pregnancy increases substantially from the first through to the second and third trimesters. Angiotensin-receptor blockers can harm the fetus. Use of these drugs should be stopped as soon as pregnancy is detected.

• Medical judgment is required if breast-feeding is being considered.

• Blood pressure should be checked regularly.

Interactions

No drug interactions of significance are known.

Side effects
• Angiotensin-receptor blockers in general appear to cause few and infrequent side effects (often indistinguishable from placebo effects). The most common, with valsartan, may include viral infection, fatigue, and gastrointestinal disturbances (for example, abdominal pain, diarrhea, nausea).
• Uncommonly, headache, dizziness, upper respiratory tract symptoms or infection, dry cough, edema or joint pain.
• Rarely, rash, weakness, insomnia, back pain or muscle cramps, and effects on heart rhythm. There may be changes in kidney function, blood counts, or raised potassium levels. Angioedema (an allergic swelling reaction, often of the face) has been reported.

Valstar Ⓑ
A preparation of ℞ **valrubicin**.
Formulation: Injection.
Availability: Prescription only.
Warnings and side effects: See ℞ **valrubicin**.

Valtrex Ⓑ
A preparation of ℞ **valacyclovir**.
Formulation: Oral tablets.
Availability: Prescription only.
Warnings and side effects: See ℞ **valacyclovir**.

Vancenase AQ 84mcg; Vancenase Pockethaler Ⓑ
A preparation of ℞ **beclomethasone dipropionate**.
Formulation: Nasal spray (AQ) aerosol inhalent (Pockethaler).
Availability: Prescription only.
Warnings and side effects: See ℞ **beclomethasone dipropionate**.

Vanceril; Vanceril Double Strength Ⓑ
A preparation of ℞ **beclomethasone dipropionate**.
Formulation: Aerosol oral inhalent in two strengths.
Availability: Prescription only.
Warnings and side effects: See ℞ **beclomethasone dipropionate**.

Vancocin Ⓑ
A preparation of ℞ **vancomycin**.
Formulation: Oral capsules; oral pulvules; oral suspension in two strengths; injection in several strengths.
Availability: Prescription only.
Warnings and side effects: See ℞ **vancomycin**.

vancomycin Ⓖ
Type/Group: antibiotic; antibacterial.
Brand(s): **Vancosin, Vancoled**; various generic.
How administered: Orally; intravenous infusion.
Used to treat
Vancomycin is used in special situations, for example, in the treatment of ✪ **pseudomembranous colitis** (a superinfection of the gastrointestinal tract), which can occur after treatment with broad-spectrum antibiotics. Another use is in the treatment of multiple-drug-resistant staphylococcal infections, particularly ✪ **endocarditis**. It is primarily active against Gram-positive bacteria and works by inhibiting the synthesis of components of the bacterial cell wall.

Warnings
• It should not be given to people with known hypersensitivity to vancomycin.
• It should be given with caution to people with kidney dysfunction or hearing impairment. It is a specialist drug, and a full medical assessment will be carried out.
• It should be used during pregnancy only if clearly needed and if the potential benefits outweigh the risks to the fetus.
• Medical judgment is required if breast-feeding is being considered.
• Superinfections due to the altered bacterial balance created by antibiotic treatment may occur. A doctor must be contacted if there is severe abdominal pain, moderate to severe diarrhea, or any new or unusual symptoms.
• It can cause kidney damage.
• It has caused hearing loss due to nerve damage, which may be permanent. This occurs primarily in people with kidney dysfunction or pre-existing hearing loss, or who take other drugs with similar adverse effects at the same time.

Interactions
• ℞ **Aminoglycosides** and other drugs with adverse effects on the kidney or nerves may increase the risk of kidney damage or hearing loss.
• ℞ **indomethacin** may increase the levels of vancomycin.
• Levels of ℞ **methotrexate** are reduced when taken orally with vancomycin.

Side effects
• Frequently, when taken orally, bitter taste, nausea, vomiting, and mouth irritation.
• Rarely, dizziness, ringing in ears, chills, fever, rash, blood changes, kidney failure, deafness, and cardiovascular dysfunction.

Vanex Expectorant Liquid Ⓑ
A preparation of ℞ **hydrocodone bitartrate**, ℞ **pseudoephedrine**, and ℞ **guaifenesin**.
Formulation: Oral liquid.
Availability: Prescription only.
Warnings and side effects: See ℞ **hydrocodone bitartrate**; ℞ **pseudoephedrine**; ℞ **guaifenesin**.

Vanex-HD Liquid Ⓑ
A preparation of ℞ **hydrocodone bitartrate**, ℞ **chlorpheniramine maleate**, and ℞ **phenylephrine hydrochloride**.
Formulation: Oral liquid.
Availability: Prescription only.
Warnings and side effects: See ℞ **hydrocodone bitartrate**; ℞ **chlorpheniramine maleate**; ℞ **phenylephrine hydrochloride**.

Vanocin Ⓑ
A preparation of ℞ **sulfur**.

Key to symbols: ✪ = Disorder Section ℞ = Drug Section ♣ = Herbal Section ◊◊ = Supplement Section

Formulation: Topical lotion.
Availability: OTC.
Warnings and side effects: See ℞ **sulfur**.

Vanquish Tablets ⓑ

A preparation of ℞ **acetaminophen**, ℞ **aspirin**, ℞ **caffeine**, and buffered with ℞ **aluminum hydroxide** and ℞ **magnesium hydroxide**.
Formulation: Oral tablets.
Availability: OTC.
Warnings and side effects: See ℞ **acetaminophen**; ℞ **aspirin**; ℞ **caffeine**; ℞ **aluminum hydroxide**; ℞ **magnesium hydroxide**.

Vantin ⓑ

A preparation of ℞ **cefpodoxime**.
Formulation: Oral tablets, oral suspension.
Availability: Prescription only.
Warnings and side effects: See ℞ **cefpodoxime**.

Vaqta ⓑ

A preparation of ℞ **hepatitis A vaccine, inactivated**.
Formulation: Intramuscular injection.
Availability: Prescription only.
Warnings and side effects: See ℞ **hepatitis A vaccine, inactivated**.

varicella virus vaccine, live ⓖ

Type/Group: **vaccine**.
Brand(s): Varivax.
How administered: Subcutaneous injection.

Used to treat

Varicella virus vaccine, live confers active immunity to varicella virus (✪ **chickenpox**). It is prepared from live, but weakened (attenuated), virus. In general, it may be given to anyone over the age of one year who would benefit from immunization. Because studies of this vaccine are not yet complete, the need for booster vaccinations or their timing has not been determined.

Warnings

• It should not be given to people with known hypersensitivity to this vaccine, to neomycin, or to gelatin (both of which are present in the vaccine), or who have active untreated tuberculosis. As with any live vaccine, it should not be given to anyone who has impaired immune response from whatever cause (for example, illness, immunosuppressive therapy, hereditary disorder).
• Its use should be postponed in anyone with respiratory infections or any acute febrile (feverish) illness.
• The vaccine's effects during pregnancy have not been studied, but it is known that natural varicella infection can cause harm to the fetus. Therefore the vaccine should not be administered during pregnancy, and pregnancy should be avoided for three months following vaccination.
• Medical judgment is required if breast-feeding is being considered.
• ✪ **Reye's syndrome** has been associated with use of ℞ **salicylates** during the course of natural varicella infection. Salicylates should

not be used for six weeks after administration of live varicella vaccine.
• It may be possible that those who have been vaccinated are capable, while the vaccine virus is active, of transmitting varicella infection. Therefore close contact with persons at risk (such as newborns, pregnant women, immunosuppressed) should be avoided.
• After administration, people will be required to wait for some time to ensure that there is no serious reaction (such as anaphylaxis).
• The duration of immunity provided by this vaccine is presently unknown, nor is it known whether the vaccine will prevent infection if given immediately after exposure to varicella.

Interactions

• ℞ **Immunosuppressants** (for example, ℞ **corticosteroids**, ℞ **cytotoxics**, radiation therapy) may cause vaccine-induced infection to have more pronounced symptoms and wider infection.
• Vaccination should be postponed for at least five months following blood or plasma transfusion, or administration of any ℞ **immune globulin**, including ℞ **varicella-zoster immune globulin (human) (VZIG)**. Conversely, no immune globulin should be administered within two months after vaccination.
• Caution is required if ℞ **anticoagulants** are being taken.

Side effects

• Some swelling or tenderness at the site of vaccination is common.
• Other side effects include upper respiratory illness, headache, fatigue, cough, aching muscles, disturbed sleep, nausea, and malaise.
• Less frequently, chills, abdominal pain, loss of appetite, earache, itching, vomiting, swollen lymph glands, allergic rash, hives, and cold sores.

varicella-zoster immune globulin (human) (VZIG) ⓖ

(varicella-zoster immunoglobulin)
Type/Group: **immune globulin**.
Brand(s): Various generic.
How administered: Intramuscular injection.

Used to treat

Varicella-zoster immune globulin (human) is a specific immunoglobulin that confers immediate passive immunity against infection by the varicella-zoster virus (✪ **chickenpox** or ✪ **herpes** zoster), but is used only in people at risk (immunosuppressed, for example, from cancer, drug therapy, hereditary or acquired condition), newborns whose mothers develop chickenpox five days before, or 48 hours after delivery, premature infants under certain conditions, and where close contact with the disease may have significant health consequences.

Warnings

• It should not be given to people with known hypersensitivity to immune globulins.
• It should be given with caution to people with a known deficiency of the naturally occurring IgA immunoglobulin.
• No adverse effects are known and the globulin should be used during pregnancy only when clearly necessary.

• Medical judgment is required if breast-feeding is being considered. Effects in breast-feeding have not been studied, although no problems have been documented.

• There is no evidence that this immune globulin treats or modifies already established herpes zoster infection.

• After administration, people will be required to wait for some time to ensure that there is no serious reaction (such as anaphylaxis).

Interactions

• The immune response to live virus vaccines (for example, ℞ **MMR vaccine**, ℞ **varicella virus vaccine, live**) may not be satisfactory. A delay of at least three months (more for some vaccines, or their specific uses) is recommended after administering immune globulin. This does not apply, however, to the live vaccines for polio (oral form), typhoid (oral form), or yellow fever, which may be given at the same time as varicella-zoster immune globulin.

• Caution is required if ℞ **anticoagulants** are being taken.

Side effects

• Most of the side effects are mild and infrequent. There may be swelling, irritation or tenderness at the site of vaccination, gastrointestinal disturbances, malaise, headache, or rash.

• Although rare, anaphylactic shock has been reported.

varicella-zoster immunoglobulin Ⓖ

see ℞ **varicella-zoster immune globulin (human) (VZIG)**.

Varivax Ⓑ

A preparation of ℞ **varicella virus vaccine, live**.
Formulation: Subcutaneous injection.
Availability: Prescription only.
Warnings and side effects: See ℞ **varicella virus vaccine, live**.

Vaseline Intensive Care Baby Sunblock Ⓑ

A preparation of ℞ **titanium dioxide** and ℞ **zinc oxide**.
Formulation: Topical lotion.
Availability: OTC.
Warnings and side effects: See ℞ **titanium dioxide**; ℞ **zinc oxide**.

Vaseline Intensive Care Moisturizing Sunblock Ⓑ

A preparation of ℞ **cinnamates** and others.
Formulation: Topical lotion.
Availability: OTC.
Warnings and side effects: See ℞ **cinnamates**.

Vaseretic 5-12.5; 10-25 Ⓑ

A preparation of ℞ **enalapril maleate** and ℞ **hydrochlorothiazide**.
Formulation: Oral tablets, in two (enalapril/hydrochlorothiazide) strengths.
Availability: Prescription only.
Warnings and side effects: See ℞ **enalapril maleate**; ℞ **hydrochlorothiazide**.

Vasocidin Ⓑ

A preparation of ℞ **prednisolone** sodium phosphate and sodium sulfacamide.
Formulation: Eye drops.
Availability: Prescription only.
Warnings and side effects: See ℞ **prednisolone**.

Vasocine Ⓑ

A preparation of ℞ **prednisolone** sodium phosphate and sodium ℞ **sulfacetamide**.
Formulation: Ophtalmic ointment.
Availability: Prescription only.
Warnings and side effects: See ℞ **prednisolone**; ℞ **sulfacetamide**.

VasoClear Ⓑ

A preparation of ℞ **naphazoline hydrochloride**.
Formulation: Eye drops.
Availability: OTC.
Warnings and side effects: See ℞ **naphazoline hydrochloride**.

Vasocon Regular Ⓑ

A preparation of ℞ **naphazoline hydrochloride**.
Formulation: Eye drops.
Availability: Prescription only.
Warnings and side effects: See ℞ **naphazoline hydrochloride**.

vasoconstrictor Ⓓ

Generics: dopamine hydrochloride; ephedrine; epinephrine; methoxamine hydrochloride; naphazoline hydrochloride; norepinephrine bitartrate; oxymetazoline hydrochloride; phenylephrine hydrochloride; pseudoephedrine; vasopressin.

Actions and uses

Vasoconstrictor drugs cause a narrowing (constricting) of the blood vessels and therefore a reduction in blood flow and an increase in blood pressure. They are sometimes used to increase blood pressure in acute circulatory disorders, in cases of shock, or where pressure has fallen during lengthy or complex surgery, and here drugs such as ℞ **norepinephrine bitartrate**, ℞ **epinephrine**, ℞ **phenylephrine hydrochloride**, ℞ **methoxamine hydrochloride**, ℞ **ephedrine**, and ℞ **dopamine hydrochloride** may be used—they have complex actions that include ℞ **cardiac stimulant** properties.

Most vasoconstrictors have an effect on mucous membranes and therefore may be used as nasal ℞ **decongestant** agents, and most of these are ℞ **sympathomimetic** agents. Some of these drugs are direct-acting ℞ **alpha-adrenergic stimulant** agents (including ℞ **epinephrine**, ℞ **naphazoline hydrochloride**, ℞ **oxymetazoline hydrochloride**, ℞ **phenylephrine hydrochloride**). Others are indirect sympathomimetics that act through releasing norepinephrine from sympathetic nerve-endings (for example, ℞ **pseudoephedrine**, ℞ **ephedrine**). The natural hormone ℞ **vasopressin** is a powerful vasoconstrictor and is sometimes used to treat bleeding from varices (a sort of varicose veins) in the esophagus.

Limitations
See the individual drug entries.

vasodilator ⓓ
Generics: **amlodipine besylate; bepridil hydrochloride; diltiazem hydrochloride; felodipine; isosorbide dinitrate; isosorbide mononitrate; isradipine; milrinone; nicardipine hydrochloride; nifedipine; nimodipine; nisoldipine; nitrates; nitroglycerin; sildenafil; sodium nitroprusside; verapamil hydrochloride.**

Actions and uses
Vasodilators are drugs that dilate blood vessels and thereby increase blood flow, and tend to lower blood pressure. Drugs that work directly on blood vessels as vasodilators work in a number of different ways. The ℞ **nitrate** group (such as ℞ **nitroglycerin,** ℞ **isosorbide dinitrate** and ℞ **isosorbide mononitrate**) has an immediate and generally short-lived ℞ **smooth muscle relaxant** action. As does the similar drug ℞ **sodium nitroprusside.** The ℞ **calcium-channel blocker** drugs also act directly on smooth muscle to cause vasodilatation, and there are many such agents available. The vasodilator activity of ℞ **phosphodiesterase inhibitor** drugs comes from their effect on smooth muscle (for example, ℞ **milrinone,** ℞ **sildenafil,** and enoximone)—they also stimulate the heart.

Yet other drugs work through specific neurotransmitter receptors on the vascular smooth muscle to relax it, for example, ℞ **beta-adrenergic stimulant** and ℞ **dopamine-receptor stimulant** drugs. These drugs have complex actions in the body. The ℞ **beta-blocker** drugs have an overall vasodilator effect by opposing the actions of epinephrine and norepinephrine at various sites in the body.

Some important drugs have eventual vasodilator actions by interfering with the action of the vasoconstrictor hormone angiotensin at its receptor, and so are called ℞ **angiotensin-receptor blocker** drugs, or by preventing its action, for example the ℞ **ACE inhibitor** (angiotensin-converting enzyme inhibitor) drugs.

The reason so many vasodilator drugs have been developed is not normally to achieve vasodilatation as such, although there are certain conditions with poor circulation in the extremities (such as peripheral vascular disease or Raynaud's disease) that do benefit from drugs that decrease vascular spasm and increase blood. Mostly, these drugs are being used because of the fall in blood pressure that normally accompanies dilation of blood vessels and the consequent decrease in the peripheral vascular resistance of the blood circulation system—that is, the drugs are commonly being used as ℞ **antihypertensive** agents. Also, in congestive ℞ **heart failure treatment** and ℞ **antianginal** treatment, drugs that cause blood vessels to dilate and reduce the workload of the heart may be very valuable.

Limitations
See the individual drug entries.

vasopressin ⓖ
Type/Group: **diabetes insipidus treatment; antidiuretic; hemostatic; hormone; posterior pituitary hormone.**

Brand(s): Pitressin Synthetic; generic.
How administered: Injection.

Used to treat
Vasopressin is used mainly to treat pituitary-originated ✪ **diabetes insipidus,** but is also used in the prevention and treatment of postoperative abdominal distention (tightness) and in abdominal radiography to dispel interfering gas shadows. Although not stated by the manufacturer for such treatment, it is also a powerful ℞ **vasoconstrictor** and is sometimes used to treat bleeding from varices (a sort of varicose vein) in the esophagus. It is one of the pituitary hormones secreted by the posterior lobe of the pituitary gland. It is also known as an antidiuretic hormone or ADH. The hormone occurs naturally in two forms, argipressin (8-Arginine vasopressin), which is often referred to simply as vasopressin, and also ℞ **lypressin** (8-Lysine vasopressin). Both hormones have been used in their natural, animal-derived form, but identical synthetic versions are now available.

Warnings
• It should not be used by people with known hypersensitivity to this drug, or chronic kidney infection.
• It should be given with extreme caution to people with coronary artery or other circulatory disease, epilepsy, kidney disorders, migraine, asthma, or congestive heart failure.
• It should be used during pregnancy only if medically judged to be clearly needed.
• Medical judgment is also required if breast-feeding is being considered.
• Rarely, allergic reactions occur and anaphylaxis (cardiac arrest or shock) has been observed.
• Vasopressin may produce water intoxication (very old and very young people are at the greatest risk).
• There will be medical monitoring.

Interactions
• ℞ **carbamazepine,** ℞ **chlorpropamide,** and ℞ **clofibrate** may increase the effects of vasopressin.
• ℞ **demeclocycline,** ℞ **lithium,** and ℞ **norepinephrine** may decrease the effects of vasopressin.

Side effects
• Frequently, pain at injection site, skin blanching, stomach cramps, and nausea.
• Less frequently, vomiting, diarrhea, dizziness, sweating, pallor, trembling, "pounding" in head, burping and flatulence.
• Rarely, chest pain, confusion, and potentially serious effects on the heart.

Vasosulf ⓑ
A preparation of ℞ **sulfacetamide** and ℞ **phenylephrine hydrochloride.**
Formulation: Eye drops.
Availability: Prescription only.
Warnings and side effects: See ℞ **sulfacetamide;** ℞ **phenylephrine hydrochloride.**

Vasotec; Vasotec I.V. ⓑ
A preparation of ℞ **enalapril maleate.**

Formulation: Oral tablets, available in 4 strengths; injection.
Availability: Prescription only.
Warnings and side effects: See ℞ **enalapril maleate**. Injection contains benzyl alcohol, which may cause allergic reaction in a few people.

Vasoxyl ⑧

A preparation of ℞ **methoxamine hydrochloride**.
Formulation: Injection (usually intravenous infusion).
Availability: Prescription only.
Warnings and side effects: See ℞ **methoxamine hydrochloride**. This drug contains sodium metabisulfite, which may cause serious allergic reaction (for example, hives, wheezing, anaphylaxis) in susceptible individuals.

V-Dec-M Tablets ⑧

A preparation of ℞ **pseudoephedrine** and ℞ **guaifenesin**.
Formulation: Oral tablets, sustained release.
Availability: Prescription only.
Warnings and side effects: See ℞ **pseudoephedrine**; ℞ **guaifenesin**.

Vectrin ⑧

A preparation of ℞ **minocycline**.
Formulation: Oral capsules in several strengths.
Availability: Prescription only.
Warnings and side effects: See ℞ **minocycline**.

vecuronium bromide ⑥

Type/Group: **skeletal muscle relaxant**.
How administered: Injection.
Brand(s): Norcuron.

Used to treat

Vecuronium bromide is a non-depolarizing neuromuscular blocking agent used as a skeletal muscle relaxant to induce muscle paralysis during surgery or mechanical ventilation (breathing), and to facilitate intubation.

Warnings

• It should not be used by people with known hypersensitivity to vecuronium.
• It should be given with caution to people with certain heart and neuromuscular diseases, or with kidney, liver, or lung disorders.
• This drug is for administration only by trained personnel in hospitals, and individuals will be fully assessed for suitability prior to use.
• It should not be used during pregnancy.
• Medical judgment is required if breast-feeding is being considered.

Interactions

This drug is for administration only by trained personnel in hospitals, and individuals will be fully assessed for suitability prior to use.

Side effects

• Rarely, allergic reaction and possibly, muscle weakness.

Veetids ⑧

A preparation of ℞ **penicillin V**.
Formulation: Oral tablets in different strengths; Oral solution.
Availability: Prescription only.
Warnings and side effects: See ℞ **penicillin V**.

Velban ⑧

A preparation of ℞ **vinblastine sulfate**.
Formulation: Injection (intravenous only).
Availability: Prescription only.
Warnings and side effects: See ℞ **vinblastine sulfate**.

Velosef ⑧

A preparation of ℞ **cephradine**.
Formulation: Oral tablets, oral suspension.
Availability: Prescription only.
Warnings and side effects: See ℞ **cephradine**.

Velosulin Human BR ⑧

A preparation of ℞ **insulin, regular**.
Formulation: Vials for injection.
Availability: OTC.
Warnings and side effects: See ℞ **insulin, regular**.

venlafaxine ⑥

Type/Group: **antidepressant**.
Brand(s): Effexor.
How administered: Orally.

Used to treat

Venlafaxine can be used to treat depressive illness (see ✪ **depression**) and, in its extended-release form, to treat generalized ✪ **anxiety** disorder. Although not stated by the manufacturer for such treatment, it is sometimes used for ✪ **obsessive-compulsive disorder**. It has similarities to the ℞ **SSRI** group of antidepressants, but can be referred to as a selective serotonin and noradrenaline uptake inhibitor (SNRI), as it seems to work by inhibiting uptake of both these neurotransmitters. It has less sedative and ℞ **anticholinergic** side effects than the ℞ **tricyclics**. As is the case with other antidepressants, this drug is also being evaluated for other uses.

Warnings

• It should not be given to people with known hypersensitivity to this drug, or to anyone who is taking or has stopped taking a ℞ **MAOI** antidepressant in the previous 14 days.
• It should be given with caution to people with high blood pressure, liver or kidney disease, or a history of mania.
• Venlafaxine should be used during pregnancy only if the benefits outweigh the possible risk to the fetus.
• It should not be used by nursing mothers.
• It may cause an increase in blood pressure.
• A doctor should be consulted before taking any other medications, including OTC preparations, herbal remedies (especially ♣ **St. John's wort**), supplements, or other natural or alternative products.

Key to symbols: ✪ = Disorder Section ℞ = Drug Section ♣ = Herbal Section ⚌⚍ = Supplement Section

• It may impair the performance of skilled tasks requiring mental alertness or physical skills, such as driving.

• Treatment should be stopped gradually, lowering the dose over a period of time.

Interactions

• Serious or even fatal reactions can occur if ℞ **MAOI** antidepressants are taken at the same time; or within a period of a few weeks after the use of, other antidepressants.

• ℞ **Cimetidine** may increase the effects of venlafaxine.

• The effects of ℞ **desipramine**, ℞ **haloperidol**, ♣ **St. John's wort**, and ℞ **trazodone** may be increased by venlafaxine.

Side effects

• These include nausea, insomnia, nervousness, anorexia, weight loss, asthenia (weakness and loss of energy), sweating, constipation, sleepiness, dry mouth, dizziness, and blurred vision.

• Less frequently, sexual dysfunction, urinary retention, somnolence, tremor, and possibly seizure.

Venoglobulin-S ⑧

A preparation of ℞ **immune globulin, human (IG)**.
Formulation: Intravenous infusion, available in two concentrations.
Availability: Prescription only.
Warnings and side effects: See ℞ **immune globulin, human (IG)**.

Ventolin; Ventolin Nebules ⑧

A preparation of ℞ **albuterol**.
Formulation: Oral tablets in several strengths, aerosol inhalant; solution for inhalation (Nebules).
Availability: Prescription only.
Warnings and side effects: See ℞ **albuterol**.

VePesid ⑧

A preparation of ℞ **etoposide**.
Formulation: Oral capsules; injection.
Availability: Prescription only.
Warnings and side effects: See ℞ **etoposide**.

verapamil hydrochloride ⑥

Type/Group: calcium-channel blocker; antianginal; antiarrhythmic; antihypertensive.
Brand(s): Calan; Isoptin; Covera-HS; Verelan; various generic.
Combinations: With *trandolapril*: Tarka Tablets.
How administered: Orally; injection.

Used to treat

Verapamil is used in the prevention and treatment of ◐ **angina pectoris** attacks, to correct heart irregularities (see ◐ **arrhythmia**), to treat ◐ **hypertension**, and after a heart attack (see ◐ **myocardial infarction**) as prophylaxis (preventive treatment).

Warnings

• It should not be given to people with known hypersensitivity to this drug, marked hypotension, or with certain heart disorders.

• It should be given with caution to people with heart failure, reduced neuromuscular transmission (for example, muscular dystrophy), or liver or kidney impairment.

• It should be used during pregnancy only if the potential benefits outweigh the risk to the fetus.

• Breast-feeding women should either discontinue this drug or stop breast-feeding.

• Regular monitoring of blood pressure is necessary to establish a safe, effective dosage. Intravenous use of this drug should be begun in a medical facility equipped to monitor results and to supply resuscitation if needed.

• Grapefruit juice should be avoided as it can increase the levels of verapamil in blood plasma.

• If verapamil is given to replace a ℞ **beta-blocker**, then withdrawal of the beta-blocker should not be abrupt. Calcium-channel blockers, also, should not be discontinued abruptly.

• Vitamin D may reduce the beneficial effects of verapamil, and so should be avoided (including supplements).

Interactions

• The effects of other antihypertensive drugs (for example, ℞ **angiotensin-receptor blockers**, beta-blockers, ℞ **diuretics**, ℞ **vasodilators**) are usually additive, but are not always consistent or predictable.

• Adverse effects if taken with other antiarrhythmics (for example, ℞ **disopyramide**, ℞ **flecainide**, ℞ **quinidine**) may be possible (disopyramide should not be given 48 hours before or 24 hours after verapamil).

• Although ℞ **digoxin** and verapamil are often used together, levels of digoxin may be increased, and dosage should be adjusted with caution.

• ℞ **Lithium** levels may be affected, with various adverse results.

• The levels and effects of inhalant ℞ **anesthetics**, ℞ **carbamazepine**, ℞ **cyclosporine**, ℞ **skeletal muscle relaxants**, and ℞ **theophylline** may be increased, with potential for toxic effects.

• There is a risk of severe hypotension if taken with ℞ **fentanyl**, so caution is advised.

• ℞ **Phenobarbital** and ℞ **rifampin** may reduce the levels or effects of verapamil.

• ℞ **Aspirin** taken with verapamil may increase the likelihood of gastrointestinal bleeding.

Side effects

Side effects vary in kind and frequency depending in what form the drug is given (oral, intravenous) and with the length of treatment.

• Frequently, constipation, swelling of the extremities, dizziness, headache, hypotension, nausea, or loss of appetite.

• Less commonly, muscle and joint pain, slow heartbeat, tingling in the extremities, or fatigue.

• Rarely, impairment of liver function, allergic skin reactions, gynecomastia (enlargement of breasts in males), or swelling of the gums.

Verelan; Verelan PM ⑧

A preparation of ℞ **verapamil hydrochloride**.

Formulation: Oral capsules, sustained release (4 strengths); extended-release capsules (PM, 3 strengths).
Availability: Prescription only.
Warnings and side effects: See ℞ **verapamil hydrochloride**.

Vergon Capsules ®

A preparation of ℞ **meclizine hydrochloride**.
Formulation: Oral capsules.
Availability: OTC.
Warnings and side effects: See ℞ **meclizine hydrochloride**.

Vermox ®

A preparation of ℞ **mebendazole**.
Formulation: Oral chewable tablets.
Availability: Prescription only.
Warnings and side effects: See ℞ **mebendazole**.

Versacaps Capsules ®

A preparation of ℞ **pseudoephedrine** and ℞ **guaifenesin**.
Formulation: Oral capsules, long acting.
Availability: Prescription only.
Warnings and side effects: See ℞ **pseudoephedrine**; ℞ **guaifenesin**.

Versanoid ®

A preparation of ℞ **tretinoin**.
Formulation: Oral capsules.
Availability: Prescription only.
Warnings and side effects: See ℞ **tretinoin**.

Versed ®

A preparation of ℞ **midazolam**.
Formulation: Oral syrup; injection.
Availability: Prescription only.
Warnings and side effects: See ℞ **midazolam**.

verteporfin ©

Type/Group: **eye treatment**.
Brand(s): Visudyne
How administered: Intravenous infusion.

Used to treat

Verteporfin is used in the treatment of age-related macular degeneration (AMD), which is a progressive loss of the eye's most detailed, central vision—the most common kind of visual loss in the elderly. The drug is used for opthalmic phototherapy, first given intravenously and then followed, after 15 minutes, by exposure of the eye to laser light of a certain wavelength (non-thermal red light). This actually results in some damage to the macula (a central area of the retina), but principally to networks of small, recently formed blood vessels. Eventually, these would have caused scarring if allowed to grow and then contract, as usually happens in a particular AMD form (called "wet"). Other forms of AMD do not respond as well to verteporfin.

Warnings

• It should not be given to people with known hypersensitivity to this drug, or who have porphyria.
• It should be given with caution to people with impaired liver function.
• Verteporfin's safety during pregnancy has not been established, and it should be used only if the potential benefit outweighs the possible risk to the fetus.
• Medical judgment is required if breast-feeding is being considered. It is not known whether this drug appears in breast milk.
• After an injection of verteporfin, direct sunlight or even bright indoor light should be avoided for five days. If emergency surgery should be necessary with two days of an injection, care should be taken to shield, as far as possible, internal tissues from bright light.
• The use of verteporfin has been shown in tests to result in damage to DNA, and its potential to cause cancer is not known.

Interactions

Drug interactions have not yet been investigated, but they might be expected if used with the following:
• Photosensitizing agents, for example, ℞ **acitretin**, ℞ **adapalene**, and ℞ **tretinoin**.
• ℞ **anticoagulant**, ℞ **antiplatelet**, or ℞ **vasodilator** drugs.
• Antioxidants, for example methionine, selenium, vitamin C, and vitamin E.

Side effects

• The most frequent are headache, bleeding or rash at the site of injection, and visual disturbances.
• Occasionally there may be joint pain, back pain (during infusion), sore throat, constipation, sleep disturbances, weakness, atrial flutter, hypertension, varicose veins, decreased hearing, changes in liver or kidney function, and altered blood counts.
• Verteporfin often causes photosensitivity (abnormal sensitivity to light), and sunburn has been reported. Eye-related side effects may include cataracts, conjunctivitis, double vision, dry eyes or itching, severe vision loss, or eye hemorrhage.

Vexol ®

A preparation of ℞ **rimexolone**.
Formulation: Ophthalmic suspension.
Availability: Prescription only.
Warnings and side effects: See ℞ **rimexolone**.

Viagra ®

A preparation of ℞ **sildenafil**.
Formulation: Oral tablets.
Availability: Prescription only.
Warnings and side effects: See ℞ **sildenafil**.

Vibramycin ®

A preparation of ℞ **doxycycline**.
Formulation: Oral capsules; injection.
Availability: Prescription only.
Warnings and side effects: See ℞ **doxycycline**.

Vibra-Tabs ⒷB

A preparation of ℞ **doxycycline**.
Formulation: Oral tablets.
Availability: Prescription only.
Warnings and side effects: See ℞ **doxycycline**.

Vicks 44D Cough & Head Congestion ⒷB

A preparation of ℞ **dextromethorphan** and
℞ **pseudoephedrine**.
Formulation: Oral liquid.
Availability: OTC.
Warnings and side effects: See ℞ **dextromethorphan**;
℞ **pseudoephedrine**.

Vicks 44E Liquid; Pediatric Formula 44E Liquid ⒷB

A preparation of ℞ **dextromethorphan** and ℞ **guaifenesin**.
Formulation: Oral liquid.
Availability: OTC.
Warnings and side effects: See ℞ **dextromethorphan**;
℞ **guaifenesin**.

Vicks 44M Cold, Flu & Cough LiquiCaps ⒷB

A preparation of ℞ **dextromethorphan**, ℞ **acetaminophen**,
℞ **chlorpheniramine maleate**, and ℞ **pseudoephedrine**.
Formulation: Oral liquid.
Availability: OTC.
Warnings and side effects: See ℞ **dextromethorphan**;
℞ **acetaminophen**; ℞ **chlorpheniramine maleate**;
℞ **pseudoephedrine**.

Vicks Cherry Cough Drops; Vick's Extra Strength Vick's Cough ⒷB

A preparation of ℞ **menthol**.
Formulation: Lozenges.
Availability: OTC.
Warnings and side effects: See ℞ **menthol**.

Vicks Chloraseptic; Children's Vick's Chloraseptic ⒷB

A preparation of ℞ **phenol**.
Formulation: Lozenges.
Availability: OTC.
Warnings and side effects: See ℞ **phenol**.

Vicks DayQuil LiquiCaps ⒷB

A preparation of ℞ **dextromethorphan**, ℞ **acetaminophen**,
℞ **pseudoephedrine**, and ℞ **guaifenesin**.
Formulation: Oral gel capsules.
Availability: OTC.
Warnings and side effects: See ℞ **dextromethorphan**;
℞ **acetaminophen**; ℞ **pseudoephedrine**; ℞ **guaifenesin**.

Vicks Dayquil Liquid ⒷB

A preparation of ℞ **dextromethorphan**, ℞ **acetaminophen**, and
℞ **pseudoephedrine**.
Formulation: Oral liquid
Formulation: .
Availability: OTC.
Warnings and side effects: See ℞ **dextromethorphan**;
℞ **acetaminophen**; ℞ **pseudoephedrine**.

Vicks DayQuil Sinus Pressure & Pain Relief Caplets ⒷB

A preparation of ℞ **pseudoephedrine** and ℞ **acetaminophen**.
Formulation: Oral tablets.
Availability: OTC.
Warnings and side effects: See ℞ **pseudoephedrine**;
℞ **acetaminophen**.

Vicks Menthol Cough Drops ⒷB

A preparation of ℞ **menthol** and ℞ **thymol**.
Formulation: Lozenges.
Availability: OTC.
Warnings and side effects: See ℞ **menthol**; ℞ **thymol**.

Vicks Nyquil LiquiCaps ⒷB

A preparation of ℞ **dextromethorphan**, ℞ **acetaminophen**,
℞ **pseudoephedrine**, and ℞ **doxylamine**.
Formulation: Gel capsules.
Availability: OTC.
Warnings and side effects: See ℞ **dextromethorphan**;
℞ **acetaminophen**; ℞ **pseudoephedrine**; ℞ **doxylamine**.

Vicks Sinex 12-Hour ⒷB

A preparation of ℞ **oxymetazoline hydrochloride**.
Formulation: Nasal spray.
Availability: OTC.
Warnings and side effects: See ℞ **oxymetazoline hydrochloride**.

Vicks VapoRub Cream ⒷB

A preparation of ℞ **camphor**, ℞ **menthol**, and ♣ **eucalyptus** oil.
Formulation: Topical rub.
Availability: OTC.
Warnings and side effects: See ℞ **camphor**; ℞ **menthol**;
♣ **eucalyptus**.

Vicodin Tablets; ES; HP ⒷB

A preparation of ℞ **hydrocodone bitartrate** and
℞ **acetaminophen**.
Formulation: Oral tablets, 3 strengths.
Availability: Prescription only.
Warnings and side effects: See ℞ **hydrocodone bitartrate**;
℞ **acetaminophen**.

Vicodin Tuss Syrup ⒷB

A preparation of ℞ **hydrocodone bitartrate** and ℞ **guaifenesin**.

Formulation: Oral syrup.
Availability: Prescription only.
Warnings and side effects: See ℞ **hydrocodone bitartrate;**
℞ **guaifenesin.**

Vicoprofen Tablets ⑧

A preparation of ℞ **hydrocodone bitartrate** and ℞ **ibuprofen.**
Formulation: Oral tablets.
Availability: Prescription only.
Warnings and side effects: See ℞ **hydrocodone bitartrate;**
℞ **ibuprofen.**

Videx ⑧

A preparation of ℞ **didanosine (ddl).**
Formulation: Oral tablets; oral solution in regular and pediatric
strengths.
Availability: Prescription only.
Warnings and side effects: See ℞ **didanosine (ddl).**

vinblastine sulfate ⓖ

(vinblastine sulphate)
Type/Group: **anticancer; cytotoxic; vinca alkaloid.**
Brand(s): Velban; various generic.
How administered: Injection (intravenous).

Used to treat

Vinblastine is used as an anticancer treatment of, for example,
acute ✪ **leukemias,** ✪ **lymphomas,** and some solid ✪ **tumors.** It is
often used in combination with other anticancer drugs, and always
under close medical supervision.

Warnings

• It should not be given to people with a bacterial infection or
leukopenia (low white blood cell count). This is a specialist drug
and a full medical assessment will be carried out.
• Vinblastine does pose a risk to the fetus; use in pregnancy requires
expert medical decision and should be avoided unless clearly
needed.
• Medical judgment is required if breast-feeding is being
considered. It does have the potential to cause serious reactions in
nursing infants.
• Nerve function and white blood cell count must be monitored
throughout treatment.
• A doctor must be contacted immediately if sore throat, fever,
chills, or a sore mouth develop.
• It is not administered more than once a week.
• Vinblastine may cause pain and tissue damage at the site of the
injection.
• It is extremely irritating to the eyes and so contact must be
avoided.

Interactions

• If used with ℞ **mitomycin,** a severe shortness of breath and
asthma-like effects can occur.
• ℞ **Erythromycin** may enhance some of vinblastine's side effects.
• Vinblastine may lower the levels of ℞ **phenytoin,** so increasing
seizure activity.

Side effects

• These can be many and will be fully explained. There may be
suppression of blood-cell formation by the bone marrow, and its
toxicity inevitably causes some serious side effects, in particular,
some loss of nerve function at the extremities, muscle weakness,
bone pain, hair loss, constipation and bloating, all of which may
be severe.

vinblastine sulphate ⓖ

see ℞ **vinblastine sulfate.**

vinca alkaloid ⓓ

Generics: **vinblastine sulfate; vincristine sulfate; vindesine
sulfate; vinorelbine tartrate.**

Actions and uses

Vinca alkaloids are a type of ℞ **cytotoxic** drug derived from the periwinkle *Vinca rosea.* They work by halting the process of cell replication and are therefore used as ℞ **anticancer** drugs, particularly
for ✪ **cancer,** including acute ✪ **leukemia,** ✪ **lymphoma,** and
some solid ✪ **tumors.**

Limitations

Their toxicity inevitably causes some serious side effects, in particular, some loss of nerve function at the extremities, muscle weakness, constipation, and bloating; all of which may be severe. There
may be suppression of blood cells by the bone marrow. See the
individual drug entries.

Vincasar PFS ⑧

A preparation of ℞ **vincristine sulfate.**
Formulation: Injection (intravenous only).
Availability: Prescription only.
Warnings and side effects: See ℞ **vincristine sulfate.**

vincristine sulfate ⓖ

(vincristine sulphate)
Type/Group: **anticancer; cytotoxic; vinca alkaloid.**
Brand(s): Oncovin; Vincasar PFS; various generic.
How administered: Injection (intravenous).

Used to treat

Vincristine is used in the treatment of, for example, acute
✪ **leukemias,** ✪ **lymphomas,** and some solid ✪ **tumors.** It is often
used in combination with other anticancer drugs, and always under
close medical supervision.

Warnings

• It should not be given to people with the demyelinating form of
Charcot-Marie-Tooth disease (a kind of muscular atrophy), or
where radiotherapy is being applied to the liver. This is a specialist
drug and a full medical assessment will be carried out. Medical
judgment is required if there is bacterial infection, leukopenia (low
white blood cell count), or neuromuscular disease.
• Vincristine does pose a risk to the fetus; use in pregnancy requires
expert medical decision.
• Medical judgment is required if breast-feeding is being
considered. It does have the potential to cause serious reactions in
nursing infants.

• Nerve function and white blood cell count must be monitored throughout treatment.

• A doctor must be contacted immediately if sore throat, fever, chills, or a sore mouth develop.

• It is not administered more than once a week.

• Vincristine may cause pain and tissue damage at the site of the injection.

Interactions

• If used with ℞ **mitomycin**, a severe shortness of breath and asthma-like effects can occur.

• ℞ **Erythromycin** may enhance some of vincristine's side effects.

• Vincristine may lower the levels of ℞ **phenytoin**, so increasing seizure activity.

• ℞ **Digoxin** levels may be decreased.

Side effects

• These can be many and will be fully explained. Its toxicity inevitably causes some serious side effects, in particular, some loss of nerve function at the extremities, muscle weakness, bone pain, hair loss, constipation and bloating, all of which may be severe. As with a related drug, ℞ **vinblastine**, suppression of blood-cell formation can occur, although this is less pronounced with vincristine, blood levels must still be monitored.

vincristine sulphate Ⓖ

see ℞ **vincristine sulfate**.

vindesine sulfate Ⓖ

(vindesine sulphate)
Type/Group: **anticancer; cytotoxic; vinca alkaloid**.
Brand(s): Eldisine.
How administered: Injection (intravenous).

Used to treat

Vindesine sulfate can be used in the treatment of, for example, acute ✪ **leukemias**, ✪ **lymphomas**, and some solid ✪ **tumors**. It is often used in combination with other anticancer drugs, and always under close medical supervision. In the US it is an "investigational drug" and though recommended for approval its use has not yet been fully studied by the Food and Drug Administration.

Warnings

• It should not be given to people with a bacterial infection or leukopenia (low white blood cell count). This is a specialist drug and a full medical assessment will be carried out.

• There is presumed to be a risk to the fetus, as with other drugs of this type (℞ **vinca alkaloids**).

• Medical judgment is required if breast-feeding is being considered. It does have the potential to cause serious reactions in nursing infants.

• Nerve function and white blood cell count must be monitored throughout treatment.

• A doctor must be contacted immediately if sore throat, fever, chills, or a sore mouth develop.

• It is not administered more than once a week.

• Vindesine may cause pain and tissue damage at the site of the injection.

• It is extremely irritating to the eyes and so contact should be avoided.

Interactions

• If used with ℞ **mitomycin**, a severe shortness of breath and asthma-like effects can occur.

• ℞ **Erythromycin** may enhance some of vindesine's side effects.

• Vindesine may lower the levels of ℞ **phenytoin**, so increasing seizure activity.

Side effects

• These can be many and will be fully explained. There may be suppression of blood cells by the bone marrow, and its toxicity inevitably causes some serious side effects, in particular, some loss of nerve function at the extremities, muscle weakness, bone pain, hair loss, constipation and bloating, all of which may be severe.

vindesine sulphate Ⓖ

see ℞ **vindesine sulfate**.

vinorelbine tartrate Ⓖ

Type/Group: **anticancer; cytotoxic; vinca alkaloid**.
Brand(s): Navelbine.
How administered: Injection (intravenous only).

Used to treat

Vinorelbine tartrate has been recently introduced as a treatment for advanced non-small cell ✪ **lung cancer**. Although not stated by the manufacturer for such treatments, it is sometimes used for advanced ✪ **breast cancer** (where other drugs have failed), ovarian carcinoma, and ✪ **Hodgkin's disease**. It is sometimes given with other drugs (for example, ℞ **cisplatin**).

Warnings

• It should not be given to people with low granulocyte levels (a kind of white blood cell). This is a specialist drug and a full medical assessment will be carried out.

• Vinorelbine does pose a risk to the fetus and should not be used during pregnancy.

• Medical judgment is required if breast-feeding is being considered. It does have the potential to cause serious reactions in nursing infants.

• White blood cell count must be monitored throughout treatment, and this will determine dosage.

• A doctor must be contacted immediately if sore throat, fever, chills, or a sore mouth develop.

• It is not administered more than once weekly.

• Vinorelbine may cause pain and tissue damage at the site of the injection.

• It is extremely irritating to the eyes and so contact should be avoided.

Interactions

• If used with ℞ **mitomycin**, a severe shortness of breath and asthma-like effects can occur.

• If given with ℞ **cisplatin** the risk of granulocytopenia (low granulocyte count) is significantly increased.

Side effects

• These can be many and will be fully explained. Its toxicity inevitably causes some serious side effects, in particular, some loss of nerve function at the extremities, muscle weakness, bone pain, hair loss, constipation and bloating, all of which may be severe.

Viokase Tablets; Powder ®
A preparation of ℞ **pancreatin** (amylase, lipase, protease).
Formulation: Oral tablets; powder.
Availability: Prescription only.
Warnings and side effects: See ℞ **pancreatin**.

Vioxx Tablets; Oral Suspension ®
A preparation of ℞ **rofecoxib**.
Formulation: Oral tablets, available in two strengths; liquid.
Availability: Prescription only.
Warnings and side effects: See ℞ **rofecoxib**.

Viracept ®
A preparation of ℞ **nelfinavir**.
Formulation: Oral capsules; oral powder for suspension.
Availability: Prescription only.
Warnings and side effects: See ℞ **nelfinavir**.

Viractin ®
A preparation of ℞ **tetracaine**.
Formulation: Topical gel; topical cream.
Availability: OTC.
Warnings and side effects: See ℞ **tetracaine**.

Viramune ®
A preparation of ℞ **nevirapine**.
Formulation: Oral capsules.
Availability: Prescription only.
Warnings and side effects: See ℞ **nevirapine**.

Virazole ®
A preparation of ℞ **ribavirin**.
Formulation: Oral inhalant; nasal inhalant.
Availability: Prescription only.
Warnings and side effects: See ℞ **ribavirin**.

Virilon ®
A preparation of ℞ **methyltestosterone**.
Formulation: Oral capsules.
Availability: Prescription only.
Warnings and side effects: See ℞ **methyltestosterone**.

Visine L.R. ®
A preparation of ℞ **oxymetazoline hydrochloride**.
Formulation: Eye drops.
Availability: OTC.
Warnings and side effects: See ℞ **oxymetazoline hydrochloride**.

Visine Moisturizing ®
A preparation of ℞ **tetrahydrozoline hydrochloride**.
Formulation: Eye drops.

Availability: OTC.
Warnings and side effects: See ℞ **tetrahydrozoline hydrochloride**.

Visken ®
A preparation of ℞ **pindolol**.
Formulation: Oral tablets, available in two strengths.
Availability: Prescription only.
Warnings and side effects: See ℞ **pindolol**.

Vistaril Capsules; Oral Suspension; Injection ®
A preparation of hydroxyzine pamoate (injection is hydroxyzine hydrochloride).
Formulation: Oral liquid; tablets, available in 3 strengths; injection.
Availability: Prescription only.
Warnings and side effects: See ℞ **hydroxyzine**.

Vistide ®
A preparation of ℞ **cidofovir**.
Formulation: Oral; injection.
Availability: Prescription only.
Warnings and side effects: See ℞ **cidofovir**.

Vita-C ®
A preparation of ℞ **ascorbic acid**.
Formulation: Oral crystals.
Availability: Prescription only.
Warnings and side effects: See ℞ **ascorbic acid**.

vitamin ®
Generics: ascorbic acid; aminobenzoate potassium; calcitriol; cyanocobalamin; dihydrotachysterol (DHT); ergocalciferol; folic acid; hydroxocobalamin; niacin; niacinamide; phytonadione.

Actions and uses
Vitamins are substances required in small quantities for growth, development, and proper functioning of the body. Because many of the vitamins cannot be synthesized by the body, they must be obtained from a normal, well-balanced diet. The lack of any one vitamin causes a specific vitamin deficiency disorder, which may be treated by the use of vitamin supplements. Additionally, vitamins may be used as a medicine in the treatment of specific disease states.

♋ vitamin B_{12} is used medically in the forms ♋ **cyanocobalamin** and ℞ **hydroxocobalamin** to treat pernicious ✚ **anemia**, and vitamin B_{12} malabsorption syndrome as well as to meet increased vitamin B_{12} requirements in pregnancy and certain diseases. Vitamin B_{12} is readily found in most normal, well-balanced diets (for example, in fish, eggs, liver, and red meat), but vegans, who eat no animal products at all, may eventually suffer from deficiency of this vitamin. A deficiency of vitamin B_{12} eventually causes megaloblastic anemia where large deformed red blood-cells are produced, and this causes degeneration of nerves in the central and peripheral nervous systems and abnormalities of epithelia (particularly the lining

Key to symbols: ✚ = Disorder Section ℞ = Drug Section ♣ = Herbal Section ♋ = Supplement Section of the mouth and gut). Apart from poor diet, deficiency can also be caused by the lack of an intrinsic factor necessary for absorption in the stomach (pernicious anemia) and by various malabsorption syndromes in the gut (sometimes due to drugs). Hydroxocobalamin is preferred to cyanocobalamin for initial treatment, but either may be used in maintenance treatment. Different routes of administration, including injection and intranasal preparations are used for different purposes.

℞ **folic acid** is a vitamin of the B complex and is also used to treat certain forms of anemia (for example, megaloblastic anemia). It has an important role in the synthesis of nucleic acids (DNA and RNA). Its consumption is particularly necessary during the first few months of pregnancy. Folic acid supplements are recommended before and during pregnancy to help prevent neural tube defects.

℞ **phytonadione** (vitamin K_1) is a natural form of ᗧᗧ **vitamin K** and is normally obtained from vegetables and dairy products. Phytonadione can be used to treat vitamin K deficiency, but not a deficiency caused by malabsorption states (in such cases vitamin K_1 or menadiol sodium phosphate, the synthetic form of vitamin K_3, must be used). It is given as a single intramuscular injection, or by mouth to prevent vitamin K deficiency bleeding in newborn babies and to treat hypothrombinemia (it promotes production of prothrombin in the liver).

℞ **niacin** (nicotinic acid) is a B-complex vitamin. It is required in the diet, but is also synthesized in the body to a small degree from the amino acid tryptophan. Dietary deficiency results in the disease pellagra, but deficiency is rare. It can be used to treat pellagra and niacin deficiency. It is used as a ℞ **lipid-regulating drug** because it beneficially modifies blood levels of various lipids (HDL and LDL) by inhibiting the synthesis and secretion of lipids in the liver. ℞ **niacinamide** is a derivative used in the treatment of pellagra, because it does not have as great a ℞ **vasodilator** effect (widens blood vessels) as nicotinic acid.

℞ **ascorbic acid** (ᗧᗧ **vitamin C**) is a vitamin that is essential for the development and maintenance of cells and tissues. It cannot be synthesized within the body and must be found in the diet. Deficiency eventually leads to scurvy, but before that there is a lowered resistance to infection, and other disorders may develop, particularly in the elderly. However, vitamin C supplements are rarely necessary with a normal, well-balanced diet. However, it is an ᗧᗧ **antioxidant** and free radical scavenger. There have been claims that "pharmacological" (high) doses help prevent colds and because of this it is incorporated into a number of cold remedies. It may increase absorption of some other drugs (for example, iron preparations).

℞ **aminobenzoate potassium** chemically is a derivative of para-aminobenzoic acid (PABA) and is considered to be a vitamin (vitamin H). It is used as an antifibrotic in the treatment of disorders associated with excess fibrous tissue, such as scleroderma and Peyronie's disease.

Various synthetic forms of ᗧᗧ **vitamin D** (including ℞ **calcitriol**, ℞ **ergocalciferol**, and ℞ **dihydrotachysterol**) are used to make up vitamin-D deficiency in the body, such as in the treatment of hypocalcemia (low blood calcium), in dialysis patients with chronic renal failure, for hypoparathyroidism, to treat certain forms of osteoporosis, refractory rickets, familial hypophosphatemia, and hypoparathyroidism.

Various groups of the population could be at risk of suffering from symptoms of vitamin deficiency, and medical intervention, in the form of prescribing or recommending supplements, may be necessary. These include, in particular, people whose nutritional status may be compromised by their lifestyle, such as smokers, alcoholics, drug addicts, certain religions, slimmers, strict vegetarians (vegans), food faddists, people on low incomes, and athletes. People whose nutritional status may be compromised by surgery and/or diseases such as malabsorption syndromes, hepato-biliary disorders, severe burns and wounds, inborn errors of metabolism, and long-term users of some medical drugs may also suffer from deficiency and vitamin supplements may be required.

Limitations
See the individual drug entries and supplements section.

vitamin B₃ ⓖ
see ℞ **niacin**.

Vitelle Lurline PMS Tablets ⓑ
A preparation of ℞ **acetaminophen**, pamabrom, and pyridoxine hydrochloride.
Formulation: Oral tablets.
Availability: OTC.
Warnings and side effects: See ℞ **acetaminophen**.

Vitrasert ⓑ
A preparation of ℞ **ganciclovir (DHPG)**.
Formulation: Implant.
Availability: Prescription only.
Warnings and side effects: See ℞ **ganciclovir (DHPG)**.

Vivactil ⓑ
A preparation of ℞ **protriptyline hydrochloride**.
Formulation: Oral tablets in several strengths.
Availability: Prescription only.
Warnings and side effects: See ℞ **protriptyline hydrochloride**.

Vivelle-Dot ⓑ
A preparation of ℞ **estradiol**.
Formulation: Transdermal patch in several strengths.
Availability: Prescription only.
Warnings and side effects: See ℞ **estradiol**.

Vivotif Berna Vaccine ⓑ
A preparation of ℞ **typhoid vaccine**.
Formulation: Oral capsules.
Availability: Prescription only.
Warnings and side effects: See ℞ **typhoid vaccine**.

Volmax ⓑ
A preparation of ℞ **albuterol**.
Formulation: Extended release tablets in two strengths.
Availability: Prescription only.

Warnings and side effects: See ℞ albuterol.

Voltaren; Voltaren-XR; Voltaren Solution ⓑ

A preparation of ℞ diclofenac.
Formulation: Oral tablets, delayed release (available in 3 strengths); XR tablets are extended release; ophthalmic solution.
Availability: Prescription only.
Warnings and side effects: See ℞ diclofenac.

Vytone ⓑ

A preparation of ℞ hydrocortisone and iodoquinol.
Formulation: Cream.
Availability: Prescription only.
Warnings and side effects: See ℞ hydrocortisone.

warfarin sodium ⓖ

Type/Group: anticoagulant.
Brand(s): Coumadin; various generic.
How administered: Orally; injection.

Used to treat

Warfarin can be used to prevent the formation of clots in certain heart disorders or after heart surgery (especially following implantation of prosthetic heart valves); and to treat or prevent venous ✪ thrombosis and ✪ pulmonary embolism, especially as may occur after a heart attack.

Warnings

• It should not be given to people with known hypersensitivity to this drug, with active bleeding, a tendency to bleed or blood-forming disorders, pericarditis or bacterial endocarditis, uncontrolled high blood pressure, injury or surgery that is still healing, or recent surgery involving the eye or nervous system. It will be prescribed by experienced personnel after a full medical assessment.

• It should be given with caution to people with vascular disease or congestive heart failure, indwelling catheters, gastrointestinal infection, high blood pressure, severe diabetes, serious vitamin C deficiency, polycythemia vera, recent traumatic injury, or liver impairment.

• Warfarin is not to be used by women who are or may become pregnant.

• Medical judgment is required if breast-feeding is being considered.

• Warfarin should not be used by people who may not be able to cope with self-administration (for example, who are senile, alcoholic, psychotic, or uncooperative), nor should it be used where laboratory facilities are not available to perform periodic blood testing.

• A doctor should be notified immediately if any unusual symptoms or bleeding occur, such as pain, swelling or discomfort, prolonged bleeding from a cut, nosebleeds or bleeding gums from brushing, increased menstrual flow, bruising, dark urine, red or tar black stools, headache, dizziness, or weakness.

• A doctor must be contacted if any illness develops.

• Activities that might cause traumatic injury (for example, sports) should be avoided.

• Diet should be normal and balanced. Significant changes in the amount of vitamin K in the diet (as from eating large amounts of green leafy vegetables) can alter the anticoagulant effect of warfarin.

• Warfarin may free tiny bits of plaque that may lodge (usually) in the smaller blood vessels. This may result in abrupt, sharp pain in a leg, foot, the toes, back, or flank. ("Purple toes syndrome" appears as mottled, purplish discoloration of the toes.) More serious obstructions are possible, and may cause kidney insufficiency, pancreatitis, penile gangrene, hypertension, paralysis, or stroke. Warfarin should be discontinued at the first signs of such phenomena.

Interactions

• The following drugs may increase the levels and effects of warfarin, with an increased risk of bleeding: ℞ acetaminophen; ℞ allopurinol; ℞ amiodarone hydrochloride; ℞ androgens; ℞ beta-blockers; ℞ chloral hydrate; ℞ chloramphenicol; ℞ chlorpropamide; ℞ cimetidine; ℞ clofibrate; ℞ corticosteroids; ℞ cyclophosphamide; ℞ disulfiram; ℞ erythromycin; ℞ fluconazole; ℞ gemfibrozil; ℞ glucagon; ℞ hydantoins; ℞ ifosfamide; ℞ influenza virus vaccine; ℞ isoniazid; ℞ ketoconazole; loop ℞ diuretics; ℞ lovastatin; ℞ metronidazole; ℞ miconazole; ℞ moricizine; ℞ nalidixic acid; ℞ omeprazole; ℞ propafenone; ℞ propoxyphene; ℞ quinidine; ℞ quinine; ℞ quinolones; ℞ streptokinase; ℞ sulfinpyrazone; ℞ sulfonamides; ℞ tamoxifen; ℞ thyroid hormones; ℞ trimethoprim and sulfamethoxazole; and ℞ urokinase. Use of streptokinase or urokinase with warfarin may be hazardous.

• ℞ Aminoglycosides, ℞ mineral oil, ℞ tetracyclines, and ♒ vitamin E interfere with vitamin K and may cause an increased risk of bleeding when taken with warfarin.

• ℞ Cephalosporins, ℞ diflunisal, ℞ NSAIDs, ℞ penicillins, and ℞ salicylates may have various effects that make bleeding more likely when used together with warfarin.

• The following drugs may reduce the levels and effects of warfarin: alcohol; ℞ aminoglutethimide; ℞ barbiturates; ℞ carbamazepine; ℞ cholestyramine; ℞ oral contraceptives; ℞ dicloxacillin; ℞ estrogens; etretinate; ℞ glutethimide; ℞ griseofulvin; ℞ nafcillin; ℞ rifampin; ℞ spironolactone; ℞ sucralfate; ℞ thiazide diuretics; ℞ trazodone; ♒ vitamin C (at high doses); ♒ vitamin K.

Side effects

• The chief complication is hemorrhage, which may occur at virtually any site in the body.

• Infrequent side effects may include allergic reactions, jaundice and liver disorders, gastrointestinal disturbances (for example, abdominal pain, nausea, vomiting, diarrhea), hair loss, and tingling sensations.

Wart-Off ⓑ

A preparation of ℞ salicylic acid.
Formulation: Topical liquid.

Availability: OTC.
Warnings and side effects: See ℞ **salicylic acid.**

weak analgesic ⒟

see ℞ **non-narcotic analgesic.**

Wellbutrin; Wellbutrin SR ⒝

A preparation of ℞ **bupropion hydrochloride.**
Formulation: Oral tablets; oral capsules, extended release (SR); both in several strengths.
Availability: Prescription only.
Warnings and side effects: See ℞ **bupropion hydrochloride.** Wellbutrin contains the same active ingredient as the antismoking aid Zyban. They should not be taken at the same time.

Wellcovorin ⒝

A preparation of ℞ **leucovorin calcium.**
Formulation: Oral tablets.
Availability: Prescription only.
Warnings and side effects: See ℞ **leucovorin calcium.**

Westcort ⒝

A preparation of ℞ **hydrocortisone** valerate.
Formulation: Cream; ointment.
Availability: Prescription only.
Warnings and side effects: See ℞ **hydrocortisone.**

White Cloverine Salve ⒝

A preparation of ℞ **turpentine oil.**
Formulation: Topical ointment.
Availability: OTC.
Warnings and side effects: See ℞ **turpentine oil.**

white soft paraffin ⒢

see ℞ **petrolatum.**

Wigraine ⒝

A preparation of ℞ **ergotamine tartrate** and ℞ **caffeine.**
Formulation: Oral tablets.
Availability: Prescription only.
Warnings and side effects: See ℞ **ergotamine tartrate;** ℞ **caffeine.**

WinRho SDF ⒝

A preparation of ℞ Rh_0(D) **immune globulin (human).**
Formulation: Intramuscular injection.
Availability: Prescription only.
Warnings and side effects: See ℞ Rh_0(D) **immune globulin (human).**

Winstrol ⒝

A preparation of ℞ **stanozolol.**
Formulation: Oral tablets.
Availability: Prescription only.
Warnings and side effects: See ℞ **stanozolol.**

Women's Gentle Laxative ⒝

A preparation of ℞ **bisacodyl.**
Formulation: Oral tablets.
Availability: OTC.
Warnings and side effects: See ℞ **bisacodyl.**

Wondra ⒝

A preparation of ℞ **petrolatum,** ℞ **lanolin,** and ℞ **glycerin.**
Formulation: Topical lotion.
Availability: OTC.
Warnings and side effects: See ℞ **petrolatum;** ℞ **lanolin;** ℞ **glycerin.**

wound-healing agent ⒟

Generics: becaplermin.
Actions and uses
Wound-healing agents comprise any drug that can be used to enhance healing in conditions where it is poor, such as diabetic ✪ **ulcers,** ✪ **burns,** corneal lesions, after plastic or extensive surgery, and in other difficult circumstances.
There are only a few specific drugs available, but ℞ **becaplermin** has recently been introduced as a topical (external) preparation in the treatment of neuropathic diabetic ulcers. It is a synthetic (recombinant DNA technology) form of the natural ℞ **growth factor,** human platelet-derived growth factor (PDGF), which is a sort of local hormone that promotes cell growth and has complex effects on cells. Some preparations are also available that contain derivatives of the plant pigment chlorophyll. These show some promise for treating chronic skin ulcers.
There is a considerable need for agents that enhance wound healing. Most available treatments are designed simply to soothe or protect the damaged body tissue, and to keep it free of infection. The recent development and manufacture of a chemically complex growth factor for this purpose suggests that further drugs of this type may become available.
Limitations
See the individual drug entry.

Wycillin ⒝

A preparation of ℞ **penicillin G** and ℞ **procaine.**
Formulation: Injection.
Availability: Prescription only.
Warnings and side effects: See ℞ **penicillin G;** ℞ **procaine.**

Wydase ⒝

A preparation of ℞ **hyaluronidase.**
Formulation: Oral tablets.
Availability: Prescription only.
Warnings and side effects: See ℞ **hyaluronidase.**

Wygesic ⒝

A preparation of ℞ **propoxyphene hydrochloride** and ℞ **acetaminophen.**
Formulation: Oral tablets.
Availability: Prescription only.

Warnings and side effects: See ℞ propoxyphene hydrochloride; ℞ acetaminophen.

Wymox ®

A preparation of ℞ amoxicillin.
Formulation: Oral capsules, oral suspension.
Availability: Prescription only.
Warnings and side effects: See ℞ amoxicillin.

Wytensin ®

A preparation of ℞ guanabenz acetate.
Formulation: Oral tablets, available in two strengths.
Availability: Prescription only.
Warnings and side effects: See ℞ guanabenz acetate.

Xalatan ®

A preparation of ℞ latanoprost.
Formulation: Eye drops.
Availability: Prescription only.
Warnings and side effects: See ℞ latanoprost.

Xanax ®

A preparation of ℞ alprazolam.
Formulation: Oral tablets.
Availability: Prescription only.
Warnings and side effects: See ℞ alprazolam.

xanthine ⑩

Generics: **caffeine; theophylline.**
Actions and uses
Xanthine compounds are natural ℞ alkaloid substances found in a wide variety of plants. The best known members are ℞ caffeine, theobromine, and ℞ theophylline. These are found in beverages such as tea, coffee, cocoa, and cola drinks. These xanthine compounds have some pharmacology in common; they all have ℞ CNS stimulant (mild), ℞ diuretic, and ℞ smooth muscle relaxant properties.
In ℞ antiasthmatic and related treatment, it is the smooth muscle relaxant properties of ℞ theophylline (and its derivatives aminophylline, dyphylline, and oxtriphylline) that are used. These agents show useful ℞ bronchodilator properties, and are mainly used for the treatment of chronic ✪ bronchitis and ✪ emphysema (as in COPD, ✪ chronic obstructive pulmonary disease). ℞ Theophylline and ℞ caffeine are also sometimes used ("off-label") to treat apnea and bradycardia (see ✪ arrhythmia) in premature infants.
Limitations
All these agents are mildly habit-forming because of their stimulant properties. The safety of ℞ theophylline depends very much on its levels in the blood, and this depends on many factors, including whether the person smokes or drinks, their age, health, and what other medication is being used at the same time. For this reason a full medical assessment will be made and treatment, at first, should be gradual and progressively increased until the control of bronchospasm is achieved. Side effects frequently include dizziness, restlessness, and accelerated heart rate. Occasionally, there may be gastrointestinal effects, urinary frequency, headache, and insomnia. Methylxanthines should be used during pregnancy only if they are clearly needed, and not at all while breast-feeding.

xanthine-oxidase inhibitor ⑩

Generics: **allopurinol.**
Actions and uses
Xanthine-oxidase inhibitor drugs are enzyme inhibitors that work by inhibiting the enzyme (xanthine-oxidase) which produces uric acid and so can be used to treat excess uric acid in the blood (hyperuricemia) by reducing its synthesis. It is used to prevent attacks of ✪ gout (because gout is caused by the deposition of uric acid crystal in the synovial tissue of joints) and to treat uric acid and calcium oxalate ✪ calculus formation in the urinary tract ("kidney stones"). The only widely used xanthine-oxidase inhibitor is ℞ allopurinol.
Limitations
℞ allopurinol is only used for the long-term treatment of gout and not acute attacks (which would be made worse).

Xeloda ®

A preparation of ℞ capecitabine.
Formulation: Oral tablets.
Availability: Prescription only.
Warnings and side effects: See ℞ capecitabine.

Xenical ®

A preparation of ℞ orlistat.
Formulation: Oral capsules.
Availability: Prescription only.
Warnings and side effects: See ℞ orlistat.

Xopenex ®

A preparation of ℞ levalbuterol hydrochloride.
Formulation: Solution for inhalation.
Availability: Prescription only.
Warnings and side effects: See ℞ levalbuterol hydrochloride.

X-Seb; X-Seb Plus ®

A preparation of ℞ salicylic acid.
Formulation: Shampoo.
Availability: OTC.
Warnings and side effects: See ℞ salicylic acid.

X-Seb T; T Plus ®

A preparation of ℞ salicylic acid and ℞ coal tar.
Formulation: Shampoo.
Availability: OTC.
Warnings and side effects: See ℞ salicylic acid; ℞ coal tar.

Xylocaine ®

A preparation of ℞ lidocaine.
Formulation: Topical ointment; oral spray; oral liquid; local solution; local jelly; injection.
Availability: OTC or prescription, depending on strength.
Warnings and side effects: See ℞ lidocaine.

Key to symbols: ✪ = Disorder Section ℞ = Drug Section ♣ = Herbal Section ◊◊ = Supplement Section

xylometazoline hydrochloride ⒢

Type/Group: **alpha-adrenergic stimulant; sympathomimetic; vasoconstrictor; decongestant.**
Brand(s): Otrivin, Otrivin Pediatric Nasal Drops.
How administered: Topically (nasal).

Used to treat

Xylometazoline is mainly used as a nasal decongestant.

Warnings

• It should not be given to people with known hypersensitivity to this or any other adrenergic drug, who are taking a ℞ **tricyclic** antidepressant, or who have angle-closure glaucoma.
• It should be given with caution, on the advice of a doctor, to people taking ℞ **MAOI** antidepressants, or who have high blood pressure, heart disease, hyperthyroidism, diabetes insipidus, enlarged prostate, or glaucoma.
• Xylometazoline's effects during pregnancy are not known and it should be used with caution and only if there is a clear benefit.
• Medical judgment is required if breast-feeding is being considered.
• Overuse may cause symptoms such as nervousness and insomnia, and may make congestion worse, which is an effect called "rebound congestion." No nasal decongestant should be used for longer than three to four days.
• It should be used with caution by the elderly, as they are more likely to suffer side effects.
• The manufacturer's recommendations must be followed carefully when giving this drug to children under 12.

Interactions

• It should not be used with ℞ **tricyclic** antidepressants.
• Used topically (externally in the nose, on the eyes) at recommended doses, the interactions common to ℞ **sympathomimetics** do not usually apply. However, in overdose there may be interactions and side effects similar to ℞ **ephedrine**.
• Xylometazoline should not be used with ℞ **MAOI** antidepressants, or within two weeks of stopping MAOI treatment, because this may cause a hypertensive crisis.

Side effects

• These depend on how it is administered. When used as a nasal decongestant, it may cause irritation in the nose. In nasal application systemic side effects are infrequent, occurring only with overdose (especially in children) and consist of the usual sympathomimetic symptoms: changes in heart rate and blood pressure, anxiety, restlessness, tremor, insomnia, dry mouth, cold fingertips and toes, and changes in the prostate gland.

yellow fever vaccine ⒢

Type/Group: **vaccine.**
Brand(s): YF-Vax.
How administered: Subcutaneous injection.

Used to treat

Yellow fever vaccine is used for active immunization against yellow fever. It consists of a protein suspension containing live, but weakened (attenuated) virus cultured in chick embryos. Immunity lasts for at least 10 years. The disease is still prevalent in many parts of Africa and South America.

Warnings

• It should not be given to people with known hypersensitivity to this vaccine or to eggs (used in its preparation), or who have impaired immune response for any reason (for example, illness, immunosuppressive therapy, hereditary disorder).
• Administration of the vaccine should be postponed for anyone with moderate to severe febrile (feverish) illness, or who has recently recovered from an illness where this was a symptom.
• Except in regions where the risk is justified, it is not given to children under age six.
• This vaccine should not be used during pregnancy if at all possible.
• Medical judgment is required if breast-feeding is being considered. It is not known whether vaccine virus appears in breast milk, and no problems have been documented.
• Where there is doubt about allergic sensitivity to this vaccine, a skin test should be performed before vaccination.
• After administration, people will be required to wait for some time to ensure that there is no serious reaction (such as anaphylaxis).
• In the US, it is only available from designated Yellow Fever Vaccination centers.

Interactions

• Cholera vaccine and ℞ **hepatitis B vaccine** may impair immune responses to each vaccine if given together. Vaccination should be separated by a month.
• ℞ **Immunosuppressants** (for example, ℞ **corticosteroids**) and ℞ **interferon** may reduce the effectiveness of the vaccine in conferring immunity. Delaying vaccination until three months after ending treatment with these immune agents is recommended.
• Yellow fever vaccine should be delayed at least two months after receiving blood transfusion.
• Caution is required if ℞ **anticoagulants** are being taken.

Side effects

• Generally mild, though fever and malaise within 7 to 14 days after vaccination are frequent.
• Anaphylaxis has been reported.

yellow soft paraffin ⒢

see ℞ **petrolatum.**

YF-Vax ⒷⓇ

A preparation of ℞ **yellow fever vaccine.**
Formulation: Subcutaneous injection.
Availability: Prescription only.
Warnings and side effects: See ℞ **yellow fever vaccine.**

Yutopar ⒷⓇ

A preparation of ℞ **ritodrine hydrochloride.**
Formulation: Injection.
Availability: Prescription only.
Warnings and side effects: See ℞ **ritodrine hydrochloride.**

Zaditor ⒷⓇ

A preparation of ℞ **ketotifen.**
Formulation: Solution (eye drops).

Availability: Prescription only.
Warnings and side effects: See ℞ **ketotifen**.

zafirlukast ⑥

Type/Group: **leukotriene receptor antagonist; antiasthmatic.**
Brand(s): Accolate.
How administered: Orally.

Used to treat

Zafirlukast is used to prevent mild to moderate attacks of ✪ **asthma**, but not to treat acute attacks. It represents a new class of drug called leukotriene receptor antagonists which work as anti-allergic agents by blocking the actions of leukotrienes, which are natural inflammatory mediators released in the lungs.

Warnings

• It should not be given to people with known hypersensitivity to zafirlukast, or any of its inactive ingredients.
• It should be given with caution to people with impaired liver function.
• It should be used during pregnancy only if clearly needed.
• It should not be used if breast-feeding, because it appears in breast milk.
• Those over 55 may have an increased risk of upper respiratory infection. Zafirlukast taken with inhaled corticosteroids further adds to the risk.
• It should be taken on an empty stomach.
• Continue to use even during symptom-free periods.

Interactions

• ℞ **aspirin** increases the levels of zafirlukast.
• ℞ **erythromycin** and ℞ **theophylline** decrease the levels of zafirlukast.
• The anticoagulant effects of ℞ **warfarin sodium** are increased.

Side effects

• Frequently, headache, nausea, restlessness, nervousness, trembling, dizziness, throat dryness, irritation or inflammation.
• Occasionally, insomnia, weakness, altered taste or smell, coughing, and bronchial irritation.
• Rarely, drowsiness, diarrhea, dry mouth, flushing, sweating, and loss of appetite.

Zagam ⑧

A preparation of ℞ **sparfloxacin**.
Formulation: Oral tablets.
Availability: Prescription only.
Warnings and side effects: See ℞ **sparfloxacin**.

zalcitabine ⑥

(ddC; DDC)
Type/Group: **antiviral; psoriasis treatment; acne treatment.**
Brand(s): Hivid.
How administered: Orally.

Used to treat

Zalcitabine is a reverse transcriptase inhibitor antiretroviral drug which can be used in the treatment of advanced ✪ **HIV** infection, alone or in combination with ℞ **zidovudine**.

Warnings

• It should not be given to people with known hypersensitivity to zalcitabine, or with moderate to severe peripheral neuropathy. Its safety in children under 13 has not been established.
• It should be given with caution to people with low CD4 cell counts, a history of pancreatitis, increased amylase enzyme levels, a history of alcohol abuse, congestive heart failure, or decreased kidney or liver function.
• Zalcitabine's safety during pregnancy has not been established and it should be used only when the potential benefits outweigh the possible risks to the fetus.
• The Centers for Disease Control and Prevention recommend that HIV-infected mothers do not breast-feed.
• It is a specialist drug, and there will be full assessment and patient monitoring throughout treatment.
• Peripheral neuropathy occurs commonly.
• There is a risk of fatal pancreatitis.

Interactions

• ℞ **Antacids** and ℞ **metoclopramide** reduce the absorption of zalcitabine.
• ℞ **Chloramphenicol**, ℞ **cisplatin**, ℞ **dapsone**, ℞ **didanosine (ddI)**, ℞ **disulfiram**, ethionamide, ℞ **glutethimide**, ♣ **gold**, ℞ **hydralazine hydrochloride**, iodoquinol, ℞ **isoniazid**, ℞ **metronidazole**, ℞ **nitrofurantoin**, ℞ **phenytoin**, ℞ **ribavirin**, and ℞ **vincristine** increase the risk of peripheral neuropathy.
• ℞ **Cimetidine** and ℞ **probenecid** increase levels of zalcitabine.
• ℞ **Pentamidine** increases the risk of pancreatitis.

Side effects

• Peripheral neuropathy and mouth ulcers.
• Occasionally, joint pain, fever, skin rash, muscle pain, ulceration of the throat, gastrointestinal effects, headache, rash, fatigue, night sweats, and others.

Zanaflex ⑧

A preparation of ℞ **tizanidine**.
Formulation: Oral tablets.
Availability: Prescription only.
Warnings and side effects: See ℞ **tizanidine**.

zanamivir ⑥

Type/Group: **antiviral**.
Brand(s): Relenza.
How administered: Orally; inhalation.

Used to treat

Zanamivir works as an enzyme inhibitor, it inhibits a viral neuraminidase enzyme essential for viral replication and so inhibits influenza virus replication and can be used to shorten the duration of infection in ✪ **influenza** A or B.

Warnings

• It should not be given to people with known hypersensitivity to this drug or any component of the product. It is not recommended for anyone with underlying respiratory diseases, such as asthma or chronic obstructive pulmonary disease (COPD). Its safety in children under seven years of age has not been established.

Key to symbols: ✪ = Disorder Section ℞ = Drug Section ♣ = Herbal Section ⟐ = Supplement Section

• There are no adequate and well-controlled studies in pregnant women. It should be used only if the potential benefit outweighs the possible risk to the fetus.
• Medical judgment is required if breast-feeding is being considered.
• The effectiveness of zanamivir is established only when treatment is begun within two days of the first symptoms.
• There is a risk of potentially serious bronchospasm or decline in lung function. Treatment must stop and a doctor contacted if respiratory symptoms such as worsening wheezing or shortness of breath develop.
• Serious allergic-like reactions have been experienced by some people.
• This drug cannot treat bacterial infections that may cause the same symptoms as influenza or may arise as complications of influenza.

Interactions
No drug interaction studies have been conducted.

Side effects
• Occasionally, sinusitis, diarrhea, nausea, bronchitis, cough, ear, nose, or throat infection, headache, vomiting, and dizziness.

Zantac 75 Ⓑ
A preparation of ℞ **ranitidine hydrochloride**.
Formulation: Oral tablets.
Availability: OTC.
Warnings and side effects: See ℞ **ranitidine hydrochloride**.

Zantac Tablets; EFFERdose; GELdose; Injection Ⓑ
A preparation of ℞ **ranitidine hydrochloride**.
Formulation: Oral tablets, available in 3 strengths; effervescent tablets, granules; capsules; injection.
Availability: Prescription only.
Warnings and side effects: See ℞ **ranitidine hydrochloride**.
Effervescent tablets and granules contain the sweetener aspartame, which should be avoided by individuals with phenylketonuria.

Zantryl Ⓑ
A preparation of ℞ **phentermine**.
Formulation: Oral capsules.
Availability: Prescription only.
Warnings and side effects: See ℞ **phentermine**.

Zarontin Capsules; Syrup Ⓑ
A preparation of ℞ **ethosuximide**.
Formulation: Oral capsules; liquid.
Availability: Prescription only.
Warnings and side effects: See ℞ **ethosuximide**.

Zaroxolyn Ⓑ
A preparation of ℞ **metolazone**.
Formulation: Oral tablets, available in 3 strengths.
Availability: Prescription only.
Warnings and side effects: See ℞ **metolazone**.

Zebeta Ⓑ
A preparation of ℞ **bisoprolol fumarate**.
Formulation: Oral tablets, available in two strengths.
Availability: Prescription only.
Warnings and side effects: See ℞ **bisoprolol fumarate**.

Zemuron Ⓑ
A preparation of ℞ **rocuronium bromide**.
Formulation: Injection.
Availability: Prescription only.
Warnings and side effects: See ℞ **rocuronium bromide**.

Zenapax Ⓑ
A preparation of ℞ **daclizumab**.
Formulation: Intravenous infusion.
Availability: Prescription only.
Warnings and side effects: See ℞ **daclizumab**.

Zephrex Tablets; LA Tablets Ⓑ
A preparation of ℞ **pseudoephedrine** and ℞ **guaifenesin**.
Formulation: Oral tablets; LA tablets, time release.
Availability: Prescription only.
Warnings and side effects: See ℞ **pseudoephedrine**; ℞ **guaifenesin**.

Zerit Ⓑ
A preparation of ℞ **stavudine**.
Formulation: Oral capsules; oral solution.
Availability: Prescription only.
Warnings and side effects: See ℞ **stavudine**.

Zestoretic Ⓑ
A preparation of ℞ **hydrochlorothiazide** and ℞ **lisinopril**.
Formulation: Oral tablets, in 3 strengths.
Availability: Prescription only.
Warnings and side effects: See ℞ **hydrochlorothiazide**; ℞ **lisinopril**.

Zestril Ⓑ
A preparation of ℞ **lisinopril**.
Formulation: Oral tablets, available in 5 strengths.
Availability: Prescription only.
Warnings and side effects: See ℞ **lisinopril**.

Zetar Ⓑ
A preparation of ℞ **coal tar**.
Formulation: Shampoo.
Availability: OTC.
Warnings and side effects: See ℞ **coal tar**.

Ziac Tablets Ⓑ
A preparation of ℞ **bisoprolol fumarate** and ℞ **hydrochlorothiazide**.
Formulation: Oral tablets, in 3 (bisoprolol) strengths.
Availability: Prescription only.

Key to symbols: Ⓓ = Drug type/group   Ⓖ = Generic name   Ⓑ = Brand name

Warnings and side effects: See ℞ **bisoprolol fumarate;** ℞ **hydrochlorothiazide.**

Ziagen ⓑ

A preparation of ℞ **abacavir.**
Formulation: Oral tablets; oral solution.
Availability: Prescription only.
Warnings and side effects: See ℞ **abacavir.**

zidovudine ⓖ

(azidothymidine; AZT)
Type/Group: **antiviral.**
Brand(s): Retrovir. Combinations: With *lamivudine*: Combivir. With *abacavir* and *lamivudine*: Trizivir.
How administered: Orally; injection.

Used to treat

Zidovudine is a reverse transcriptase inhibitor antiretroviral drug that is used in the treatment of ✪ **HIV** infection. Formerly, it was used for the treatment of advanced ✪ **AIDS**, but is now considered useful by some for the early forms of HIV infections before the full AIDS syndrome develops, including HIV-positive people who do not show symptoms of AIDS, and also to prevent transmission of HIV from pregnant women to their infants.

Warnings

• It should not be given to people with known, life-threatening hypersensitivity to zidovudine.
• It should be given with caution to people with compromised blood-cell production or severe liver or kidney function impairment.
• Its safety during pregnancy has not been established and it should be used only when the potential benefits outweigh the risks to the fetus.
• The Centers for Disease Control and Prevention recommend that HIV-infected mothers do not breast-feed.
• It is a specialist drug, and there will be full assessment and patient monitoring throughout treatment.
• Severe allergic reactions are possible. A doctor must be contacted if a rash develops.
• If taken with food, the levels of zidovudine in the blood are reduced.

Interactions

• ℞ **ganciclovir (DHPG)** increases the risk of blood toxicity.
• ℞ **Interferon** and ℞ **probenecid** increase the levels of zidovudine.
• ℞ **Rifampin** reduces levels of zidovudine.

Side effects

These are many and may include:
• Disturbances in various blood cells, often to such a degree that blood transfusions are required, nausea and vomiting, gastrointestinal disturbances, loss of appetite, headache, rashes, fever, sleep disturbances, abdominal pain, malaise, convulsions, pigmentation of the nails, skin and mouth, myopathy, and many others.

Ziks Cream ⓑ

A preparation of ℞ **methyl salicylate,** ℞ **menthol,** ℞ **capsaicin,** and various.
Formulation: Topical cream.
Availability: OTC.
Warnings and side effects: See ℞ **methyl salicylate** ℞ **menthol** ℞ **capsaicin.**

Zilactin-L ⓑ

A preparation of ℞ **lidocaine.**
Formulation: Topical liquid.
Availability: OTC.
Warnings and side effects: See ℞ **lidocaine.**

zileuton ⓖ

Type/Group: **lipoxygenase inhibitor; antiasthmatic.**
Brand(s): Zyflo.
How administered: Orally.

Used to treat

Zileuton is used in the long-term treatment and prevention of ✪ **asthma.** It represents a new class of drug called 5-lipoxygenase inhibitors which work as antiallergic agents by blocking the production of leukotrienes, which are natural inflammatory mediators released in the lungs.

Warnings

• It should not be given to people with known hypersensitivity to zileuton or any of its inactive ingredients, active liver disease or unexplained abnormality on liver function tests.
• It should be given with caution to people with impaired kidney or liver function.
• It should be used only if the potential benefits outweigh the risk to the fetus.
• Medical judgment is required if breast-feeding is being considered. It is not known whether zileuton appears in breast milk.
• Liver changes may occur, and so periodic monitoring is required. A doctor must be contacted if pain in the right upper quadrant of the abdomen, nausea, fatigue, lethargy, itching, jaundice, or flu-like symptoms (signs and symptoms of liver disease) develop.
• It may increase white blood-cell count.
• Continue to use even during symptom-free periods.

Interactions

• The effects of ℞ **propranolol** are increased.
• The levels of ℞ **theophylline** are increased.
• The anticoagulant effects of ℞ **warfarin sodium** are increased.

Side effects

• Frequently, headache and upset stomach.
• Occasionally, dizziness, fatigue, insomnia, tingling, pain, nausea, rash, and hives.

Zinacef ⓑ

A preparation of ℞ **cefuroxime.**
Formulation: Injection.
Availability: Prescription only.
Warnings and side effects: See ℞ **cefuroxime.**

Key to symbols: ✪ = Disorder Section ℞ = Drug Section ♣ = Herbal Section ᨔ = Supplement Section

zinc oxide ⑥

Type/Group: **astringent**.
Brand(s): A & D; Balmex Baby; Borofax Skin Protectant; Desitin; Diaperene Diaper Rash; Dome-Paste; Dyprotex; Flanders Buttocks; Gold Bond Baby Powder; Mexana Medicated; Saratoga; Schamberg's; Vaseline Intensive Care Baby Sunblock; various generic.
How administered: Topically (external).

Used to treat

Zinc oxide is used primarily to treat skin disorders, such as diaper rash, urinary rash, and ✪ **eczema**. It is available (without prescription) in any of a number of compound forms as a cream, an ointment, and as a dusting powder.

Warnings

• It should not be given to people with known hypersensitivity to zinc oxide or any component of the products.
• A doctor must be consulted before using while pregnant or breast-feeding.
• It should not be used for a longer period or in larger amounts than directed.
• It should not be used on deep or puncture wounds, broken skin, or cuts.

Interactions

None significant.

Side effects

None significant.

zinc sulfate ⑥

Type/Group: **astringent**.
Brand(s): Eye-Sed.
How administered: Topically (external); orally.

Used to treat

In solution, zinc sulfate can be used as an astringent and wound cleanser, and also in eyedrops. It is one form in which ⚗ **zinc** supplements can be administered orally in order to make up a zinc deficiency in the body.

Warnings

• It should not be given to people with known hypersensitivity to zinc or any component of the product.
• A doctor must be consulted before using while pregnant or breast-feeding.
• A doctor must be contacted and treatment stopped if irritation of the eye persists or increases, or if pain or a change in vision occurs.

Interactions

None significant at recommended doses.

Side effects

None significant at recommended doses.

Ziradryl Lotion ⑧

A preparation of ℞ **diphenhydramine hydrochloride** and chlorophyllin sodium.
Formulation: Topical lotion.
Availability: OTC.

Warnings and side effects: See ℞ **diphenhydramine hydrochloride**.

Zithromax ⑧

A preparation of ℞ **azithromycin**.
Formulation: Oral tablets; oral suspension; injection.
Availability: Prescription only.
Warnings and side effects: See ℞ **azithromycin**.

Zocar ⑧

A preparation of ℞ **simvastatin**.
Formulation: Oral tablets.
Availability: Prescription only.
Warnings and side effects: See ℞ **simvastatin**.

Zofran Tablets; Zofran ODT; Oral Solution; Injection ⑧

A preparation of ℞ **ondansetron**.
Formulation: Oral tablets; oral solution; injection. (ODT are orally dissolving tablets.)
Availability: Prescription only.
Warnings and side effects: See ℞ **ondansetron**. ODT tablets contain the sweetener aspartame, which should be avoided by individuals with phenylketonuria.

Zoladex ⑧

A preparation of ℞ **goserelin**.
Formulation: Subdermal implants in two strengths. Only the lower strength implant is for use by women.
Availability: Prescription only.
Warnings and side effects: See ℞ **goserelin**.

Zolicef ⑧

A preparation of ℞ **cefazolin sodium**.
Formulation: Injection.
Availability: Prescription only.
Warnings and side effects: See ℞ **cefazolin sodium**.

zolmitriptan ⑥

Type/Group: **serotonin-receptor stimulant; vasoconstrictor; antimigraine**.
Brand(s): Zomig.
How administered: Orally.

Used to treat

This is a recently introduced drug which is used to treat acute ✪ **migraine** attacks (but not to prevent attacks). It works as a ℞ **vasoconstrictor** (through acting as a serotonin receptor stimulant selective for serotonin 5-HT$_1$ receptors), producing a rapid narrowing of blood vessels surrounding the brain.

Warnings

• Avoid its use in people with known hypersensitivity to this drug or who have certain cardiovascular disorders including pre-existing heart diseases, including ischemic heart disease, previous myocardial infarction (heart attack), coronary vasospasm, including some types of angina, or with uncontrolled hypertension.

• Zolmitriptan should not be used by anyone with a form of migraine in which one half of the body experiences some degree of paralysis during the migraine attack.

• Drugs of this class (that is, those stimulating serotonin 5-HT$_1$ receptors) are used only with great caution where risk factors are present that predispose to coronary artery disease.

• It is recommended that first-time administration of zolmitriptan to anyone with significant risk factors for coronary artery disease takes place at a physician's office or other medical facility.

• It should be used with care in those with impaired liver or kidney function.

• Zolmitriptan should be used in pregnancy only if the potential benefits outweigh the potential risks to the fetus.

• Medical judgment of risk is also required for breast-feeding mothers.

• This drug should not be used at the same time, or shortly after, using ℞ **ergotamine** or other migraine therapies. Ergotamine-like antimigraine drugs should not be taken until six hours after this type of antimigraine drug; and this type of antimigraine drug should not be taken until at least 24 hours after an ergotamine-like antimigraine drug.

• The dose should not usually be repeated during the same migraine attack.

• Zolmitriptan may cause drowsiness and so impair the performance of skilled tasks, such as driving.

Interactions

• There is a risk of additive effect, with potentially serious consequences, if taken with ℞ **ergotamine**-containing drugs (such as or ℞ **dihydroergotamine** ℞ **methysergide**).

• ℞ **MAOI** antidepressants should not be taken orally with zolmitriptan or within two weeks of discontinuing their use. MAOIs increase the concentration of zolmitriptan, and so there is a higher risk of side effects (some serious).

• Oral ℞ **contraceptives** and ℞ **cimetidine** may increase the concentration of zolmitriptan.

• ℞ **SSRI** antidepressants (such as, ℞ **fluoxetine**, ℞ **fluvoxamine**, ℞ **paroxetine**, ℞ **sertraline**) may increase the possibility of some less-frequent side effects, such as weakness and incoordination, occurring; caution is recommended.

• ♣ **St. John's wort** should not be used at the same time as there is an increased risk of adverse effects.

Side effects

For this type of drug these include:

• Chest pain and tightness in parts of the body, including the chest, jaw, or throat, which may indicate constriction of the blood vessels of the heart (or of anaphylaxis). If the pain is intense, use of zolmitriptan should stop;

• The most common side effects are tingling and other peripheral sensations, warmth, dizziness, drowsiness, a feeling of weakness, and nausea.

• Less frequently there may be palpitations, nervousness, emotional swings, insomnia, leg cramps, hiccups, dry mouth, thirst, urinary frequency, ringing in the ears, and abnormal liver function;

• Rarely, fainting, high blood pressure, light sensitivity and allergy-like symptoms such as facial swelling, including of the eyes, itching, rash, and hives.

• Potentially dangerous heart rhythm changes and bronchospasm.

Zoloft ®

A preparation of ℞ **sertraline**.
Formulation: Oral tablets in varying strength.
Availability: Prescription only.
Warnings and side effects: See ℞ **sertraline**.

zolpidem Ⓖ

Type/Group: **hypnotic**.
Brand(s): Ambien.
How administered: Orally.

Used to treat

Zolpidem is a recently introduced drug which works in the same way as the ℞ **benzodiazepines**, although chemically it is not a benzodiazepine. It can be used for the short-term treatment of ✪ **insomnia**.

Warnings

• It should not be given to people with known hypersensitivity to this drug.

• It should be given with caution to people with psychiatric disorders, kidney or respiratory impairment, a history of drug abuse, who have other illnesses, are in a weakened condition (debilitated), or anyone over 65.

• Zolpidem should be used during pregnancy only if it is clearly needed.

• Medical judgment is required if breast-feeding is being considered.

• It must not be used for longer than the period specified by your doctor.

• Avoid alcohol.

• Judgment, thinking, and the performance of skilled tasks may be impaired. It should not be used unless seven or eight hours of sleep are possible, so that effects can wear off.

• Avoid other psychotropic medications unless prescribed by a doctor.

• Sleeping problems may occur the first one or two nights after stopping this drug.

Interactions

• If used with ℞ **imipramine** or ℞ **chlorpromazine**, there is more of a decrease in alertness.

• The effects of zolpidem may be reduced if used with ℞ **rifampin**.

• CNS (central nervous system) depressants (for example, alcohol, ℞ **narcotic analgesics**, ℞ **skeletal muscle relaxants**) may increase the effects of zolpidem.

Side effects

• Daytime drowsiness, dizziness, lightheadedness, headache, and poor coordination.

• Less frequently, memory loss, anxiety, confusion, irritability, lack of energy, chest pain, and gastrointestinal upset.

• Rare but serious side effects include blood cell disorders.

Zomig ®

A preparation of ℞ **zolmitriptan**.
Formulation: Oral tablets, available in two strengths.
Availability: Prescription only.
Warnings and side effects: See ℞ **zolmitriptan**.

Zonalon ®

A preparation of ℞ **doxepin**.
Formulation: Topical cream.
Availability: Prescription only.
Warnings and side effects: See ℞ **doxepin**.

Zone-A-Fort ®

A preparation of ℞ **hydrocortisone** and ℞ **pramoxine hydrochloride**.
Formulation: Lotion.
Availability: Prescription only.
Warnings and side effects: See ℞ **hydrocortisone**; ℞ **pramoxine hydrochloride**.

zonisamide ©

Type/Group: **anticonvulsant; antiepileptic**.
Brand(s): Trileptal.
How administered: Orally.

Used to treat

Zonisamide can be used, together with other drugs, in the treatment of partial seizures in adults with ✪ **epilepsy**.

Warnings

• It should not be given to people with known hypersensitivity to this drug or to ℞ **sulfonamides**, or with kidney failure.
• It should be given with caution to the elderly or to anyone with impaired kidney function.
• Zonisamide should be used during pregnancy only if the potential benefit outweighs the possible risk to the fetus.
• Nursing mothers should either discontinue this drug or discontinue breast feeding.
• Symptoms such as fever, sore throat, mouth ulcers, or easy bruising should be immediately reported to a doctor, because they may indicate significant blood effects possibly caused by zonisamide.
• A rash or worsening of seizures should also be reported immediately to a doctor.
• A doctor should be notified of symptoms such as sudden back pain, abdominal pain or blood in the urine, which may indicate the presence of a kidney stone.
• Because of its sedative side effects, the performance of skilled tasks, such as driving, may be impaired.

Interactions

• ℞ Carbamazepine, ℞ **phenobarbital**, and ℞ **phenytoin** lower levels of zonisamide.
• Drugs that may act to slow the break-down of zonisamide in the body (such as ketoconazole or troleandomycin) may increase the levels and effects of zonisamide.

Side effects

These are many and varied:

• The most frequent are drowsiness, dizziness, gastrointestinal disturbances (for example, loss of appetite, nausea, abdominal pain, diarrhea), agitation, incoordination or unusual gait, difficulty with concentration or memory, confusion, depression, insomnia, vision problems or involuntary eye movements, tremor, fatigue, and tingling sensations;
• Zonisamide may increase the likelihood of kidney stones;
• Other side effects may include difficulties of speech, psychotic behavior, unusual taste sensations, acne, cramps, muscle pain, changes in heart rhythm or blood pressure, and deficiency in various kinds of blood cells;
• Hypersensitivity reactions, including itching, rash, hives, and allergic swelling, have been reported.

ZORprin ®

A preparation of ℞ **aspirin**.
Formulation: Oral tablets, controlled release.
Availability: Prescription only.
Warnings and side effects: See ℞ **aspirin**.

Zostrix; Zostrix-HP ®

A preparation of ℞ **capsaicin**.
Formulation: Topical cream in two strengths.
Availability: OTC.
Warnings and side effects: See ℞ **capsaicin**.

Zosyn ®

A preparation of ℞ **piperacillin** and ℞ **tazobactam**.
Formulation: Injection; intravenous infusion.
Availability: Prescription only.
Warnings and side effects: See ℞ **piperacillin**.

Zovia ®

A preparation of ℞ **ethinyl estradiol**, and ethynodiol diacetate [etynodiol diacetate].
Formulation: Calendar pack of oral tablets.
Availability: Prescription only.
Warnings and side effects: See ℞ **ethinyl estradiol**; ℞ **progestins**.

Zovirax Capsules; Injection; Ointment; Suspension; Tablets ®

A preparation of ℞ **acyclovir**.
Formulation: Oral capsules, tablets, liquid; topical ointment; injection.
Availability: Prescription only.
Warnings and side effects: See ℞ **acyclovir**.

Zyban ®

A preparation of ℞ **bupropion hydrochloride**.
Formulation: Oral tablets, sustained release.
Availability: Prescription only.
Warnings and side effects: See ℞ **bupropion hydrochloride**.
Zyban contains the same active ingredient as Wellbutrin. These two should not be taken at the same time.

Zydone Tablets ®

A preparation of ℞ **hydrocodone bitartrate** and
℞ **acetaminophen**.
Formulation: Oral tablets, available in 3 strengths.
Availability: Prescription only.
Warnings and side effects: See ℞ **hydrocodone bitartrate**;
℞ **acetaminophen**.

Zyflo ®

A preparation of ℞ **zileuton**.
Formulation: Oral tablets.
Availability: Prescription only.
Warnings and side effects: See ℞ **zileuton**.

Zyloprim ®

A preparation of ℞ **allopurinol**.
Formulation: Oral tablets in several strengths.
Availability: Prescription only.
Warnings and side effects: See ℞ **allopurinol**.

Zymase Capsules ®

A preparation of ℞ **pancreatin** (amylase, lipase, protease).

Formulation: Oral capsules.
Availability: Prescription only.
Warnings and side effects: See ℞ **pancreatin**.

Zyprexa; Zyprexa Zydis ®

A preparation of ℞ **olanzapine**.
Formulation: Oral tablets in several strengths; oral tablets to be
dissolved in the mouth (Zydis).
Availability: Prescription only.
Warnings and side effects: See ℞ **olanzapine**.

Zyrtec Tablets; Syrup ®

A preparation of ℞ **cetirizine hydrochloride**.
Formulation: Oral tablets; syrup.
Availability: Prescription only.
Warnings and side effects: See ℞ **cetirizine hydrochloride**.

Zyvox ®

A preparation of ℞ **linezolid**.
Formulation: Oral; injection.
Availability: Prescription only.
Warnings and side effects: See ℞ **linezolid**.

PART 3

HERBAL REMEDIES

Herbal Remedies

People have used plants and plant products for medicinal purposes for thousands of years. The precise manner in which the medicinal activities of plants were discovered and recorded in ancient times is not known, but it is likely that knowledge was passed down from one generation to another, based on observations and experience.

Both therapeutic and poisonous plants would be identified and remembered through such a mechanism. This reliance on natural treatments evolved over the centuries into the well-developed and documented use of herbal medicines, which ultimately gave rise to highly developed systems such as the Chinese, Ayurvedic (Hindu), European, Amerindian, and African systems of medicine, among others. Some of these systems—in particular those developed in Europe, China, and India—produced vast documented bodies of information, referred to by the Latin name *materia medica*, which were recorded as extensive written texts.

Among the earliest written accounts of the medicinal properties of plants are Egyptian and Indian documents from approximately 1500 BC. Written accounts of Chinese *materia medica* date back to approximately 100 BC, and much of the European herbal tradition began with the writings of the Greek physician Dioscorides in the 1st century AD, notably his *De materia medica*.

Many of the classic reference books known as European Herbals appeared in the Middle Ages. During the 16th and 17th centuries, when the disciplines of botany and medicine were effectively the same, Banckes (1525), Turner (1551–68), Gerard (1597), and Culpeper (1652) each published their own highly influential works, which drew to varying degrees on the work of Dioscorides. Many of the preparations and doctrines described in these works remained unaltered for centuries.

Herbal medicine in North America

Around the same time, herbal medicine in most of North America was mainly shamanistic, but in Mexico and the Central American countries extensive lists of plants and their medicinal uses were documented as early as the 16th century. With the arrival of European settlers in North America, a gradual integration of Native American and European systems of herbal medicine began, leading to the development of the Eclectic herbal system in the early 19th Century, in which the rapidly developing disciplines of physiology and pathology were combined with the herbal tradition.

From the late 19th century, however, North American herbalism declined, following legislation requiring herbal practitioners to have orthodox medical training. One result was that financial support was channelled into conventional treatments, and it still remains illegal to practice herbal medicine in many areas of North America without qualifications from a medical school.

Some of the most widely used herbal medicines have their origins in North America. A good example of this is *Echinacea*, which has been scientifically shown to have a stimulant effect on the human immune system, and is widely used in the treatment of upper respiratory tract infections (mainly colds and influenza). *Echinacea angustifolia* was traditionally used by Native American peoples for a range of conditions, including coughs, but also as an antidote to poisons, an analgesic (painkiller), and an anti-inflammatory. Based on these extensive uses, *Echinacea* was taken from North America and developed in Germany for treatment of respiratory infections although, interestingly, it was *Echinacea purpurea* that was developed in this way, rather than *E. angustifolia*. Whether this was a deliberate choice, or through a mistake in identification of these species is not clear.

Scientific developments

In the 19th century, scientific methods started to be applied to the study of plants and their extracts, in order to understand the reasons for their therapeutic activity. Until this time, non-scientific explanations of these actions were often assigned to spiritual properties of the plant, or pseudo-scientific theories such as the doctrine of signatures, in which plants tended to benefit parts of the body which they resembled physically. The scientific studies of plants coincided with the rapid increase in knowledge of physiology, anatomy, and the pathology of disease, ultimately giving rise to modern Western orthodox medicine, which became increasingly detached from the centuries-old herbal traditions. However, much of the world's population still depends on herbal medicines for economic reasons.

Herbal remedies today

Phytochemical and pharmacological research into plants has continued to advance since the 19th century, and arguably had some of its greatest successes in the 1950s and 1960s, with the identification and isolation of some of the well-known plant-based drugs, such as reserpine (from *Rauwolfia* in 1952), vinblastine and vincristine (from *Catharanthus roseus,* also called *Vinca rosea,* in the 1960s), and silybin (from *Silybum* in 1968). Several authoritative reviews of the literature indicate that approximately one in four of the active components of drugs prescribed in 1996 had their origins in higher (flowering) plants, and an additional ten percent were derived from fungi. A comprehensive review of plant-derived drugs listed 119 drugs, obtained from less than 90 species of plants, including the examples outlined below.

Historical perspective

Those pure drugs with botanical origins that are currently used became adopted into orthodox clinical practice over a long period of time. Long-established drugs for which a chemical structure was determined in the late 19th or early 20th century, and which are still used clinically today, include the narcotic analgesic morphine, the heart-stimulant digitoxin, and the anticholinergic Belladonna alkaloids (for example, hyoscyamine and scopolamine).

More recently established drugs include the anticancer taxoids from certain yew species, and the antimalarial drug artemisinin and derivatives from *Artemisia* species. As there is growing demand for plant-based medicines, it is certainly possible that validated and fully tested botanical medicines will make up a larger and larger proportion of the existing (largely synthetic) drug markets. It is worth bearing in mind that a sizeable proportion of drugs sales is made up of antibiotic drugs, and all the original examples were of natural origin—although they are not herbals, but are derived from fungi and yeasts.

Herbal multiple activity preparations

A key difference between herbal remedies and conventional drugs (even those of natural origin) is in the number of active components contained in the medicine. Modern commercial drugs tend to be single active compounds, with one clearly defined pharmacological activity. Herbal remedies, in contrast, can contain dozens, or even hundreds, of biologically active compounds, which can have multiple pharmacological targets. Many phytochemists and pharmacognosists promote this as one of the major benefits of herbal remedies—the various active compounds contained in the herbal remedy are believed to interact synergistically, resulting in pharmacological effects greater than the sum of the activities of each individual component found in the herb, and with less toxicity. This may result from multiple compounds interacting at a single pharmacological target, or by different compounds affecting related targets, so promoting greater beneficial pharmacological activity. A similar approach is sometimes used in orthodox medicine in certain situations, such as in AIDS treatment where antiretroviral therapy generally consists of a cocktail of drugs ("combination therapy") which are used to provide an increased effectiveness compared to their effects when used separately (in this case by preventing the development of viral resistance).

Polypharmacy

An extension of this approach in herbal remedies is the common use of polypharmacy—combinations of herbs to treat a single ailment. Because herbal medicine generally has a more holistic approach than orthodox medicine, trained herbalists may select a combination of several herbs in order that their therapeutic activities can treat both the disease symptoms and its underlying causative factors. Combinations of herbs are usually used so that the activity of each herb complements those of the others. This approach is most developed in Chinese herbal medicine.

Two vitally important factors that influence the success of a herbal remedy are the way in which the remedy is prepared and the doses chosen. For example, infusions prepared by steeping the herb in hot water will have a different chemical profile to tinctures or alcoholic extracts, which will result in different pharmacological effects. For similar reasons, different parts of a single plant species may be used for different indications, as a result of the compartmentalization of phytochemicals within certain plant structures, such as the roots, leaves, or flowers. In some cases, the fresh herb will have different activity from an herb that has been stored. Sometimes, storage may destroy the activity of the herb, through the degradation of the active principles (for example, through oxidation and volatilization of monoterpene components of volatile oils). On other occasions, stored material is preferable, often because the pharmacological activity of the fresh material is too strong (for example, the dried bark of some *Rhamnus* species is used as a relatively mild laxative, but the fresh bark is a violent purgative, and is never recommended for use).

Herbal remedies can affect many of the same pharmacological targets as orthodox drugs, and like them they need to be given at appropriate doses. Unlike homeopathy, herbal remedies are given at doses in which the active components directly result in pharmacological activity. As with conventional drugs, overdosing on herbal remedies can have undesirable effects or even be fatal, and even at doses considered to be therapeutic, side effects are possible. Unlike orthodox medicines, few herbal remedies have been tested fully for safety, efficacy, and quality, and there is no centralized system for reporting side effects. Because herbal remedies do rely on classical pharmacological activity, they can interact with each other, or with conven-

tional drugs. For example, recent evidence has indicated that antidepressant herbal remedies containing St. John's wort (*Hypericum perforatum*) can interact with many orthodox drugs, including monoamine-oxidase inhibitors (MAOIs). It is important to remember that herbal remedies are medicinal agents, and their use in conjunction with orthodox drugs should only be undertaken following professional advice.

Current trends

In addition to pure compounds with proven pharmaceutical activity which were originally isolated from plants and are now established in orthodox medicine, there has been a great resurgence in the use of raw plant material or relatively impure plant extracts (herbal remedies) for medicinal purposes. This has been especially true over the last few decades, when there has been a great upsurge in awareness and interest in medicinal plants and natural treatments, both from the general public (especially for self-medication using remedies available over-the-counter, and sometimes plants collected from the wild) and some sections of the scientific community. The precise reasons for this move towards herbal medical practices are not clear, but they probably include dissatisfaction with synthetic or orthodox treatments, a widely held belief that naturally derived products are both healthier and safer than synthetic agents (although by no means always accurate), and a move towards self-medication and preventive approaches to disease management.

Dr. John Wilkinson, BSc PhD DIC MRSC C CHEM

Status of herbal remedies

In some countries (especially in Europe, and Germany in particular), herbal remedies can have the same status as orthodox drugs, and are widely prescribed by doctors. Monographs that represent science-based evaluations of herbal remedies have been prepared by various authorities such as Commission E (CE; of the German Institute for Drugs and Medical Products), the World Health Organization (WHO), and the European Scientific Cooperative on Phytotherapy (ESOP). These publications are based on studies of standardized herbal preparations and aim to identify the uses for which the herb can reasonably be considered effective and they may give recommendations regarding approval of proposed uses.

In other countries, the status of herbal remedies is less well defined and they occupy an intermediate position between foodstuffs and accepted medicines. In the US, the Food and Drug Administration, for example, regards most herbal remedies not as licensed medicines but as food supplements, which can make no claims to specific medicinal efficacy. It is hoped that in the future natural medicines will be developed and their uses controlled so that they conform to the evidence-based safety and efficacy standards of orthodox medicines, backed by reputable scientific research, and with provision for reporting side effects, interactions, and dosage recommendations.

Legal restrictions

Some of the herbs discussed in this book are potentially dangerous and may be subject to legal restrictions regarding formulation, use, and sale of herbs that are intended for medicinal use. The restrictions may apply to the whole herb, or to specific parts, preparations, or substances derived from it, and some herbs and their extracts are regarded as too toxic for general use, so are subject to legislative control. Restrictions may also concern individuals permitted to prescribe, administer, supply, and sell certain herbs and preparations, and the permitted concentrations, doses, and preparations. The regulations differ from country to country, and are very complex—detailed information can be obtained from the appropriate department of the legislature. This is particularly relevant to Internet sales of herbal remedies.

Herbal remedies in this book

The Herbal Remedies section of this book provides information on more than 300 plant species commonly encountered in herbal medicines, which are available in manufactured form in over-the-counter products in the USA, or are available from some other sources (for example, from the internet).

The herbs have been selected on the basis that some pharmacological or clinical evidence exists to support their medicinal use. There are many other herbal remedies that have not been subjected to this type of investigation, and it is the editors' view that, without it, their reported activities cannot be validated, even though positive anecdotal evidence would suggest that scientific investigation of many of them would be worthwhile. Some herbs with extensive traditional uses have been excluded largely for this reason. Although certain plant species which are potentially highly toxic have also been excluded from this list, some adverse reactions to the plants listed here are also possible, and all herbal remedies are potentially toxic in overdose. For instance, it is now recognized that consuming as few as two or three nutmegs (or less in a child) can be fatal. Where possible, adverse reactions and warnings (which relate to the medical, not general culinary uses) are outlined. If no such reactions have been established or information is not yet available, a note to indicate caution is added to the relevant herbal entry.

The most commonly used herbs—mainly those for which reliable information is available—are described in depth. Information is given about active chemicals known to be present in each herb, scientific study and clinical trials' data, traditional and approved uses, as well as any cautions and warnings there may be about their uses. The properties and uses of other herbs are also briefly described.

Alternative common names, together with botanical (Latin; Linnean binomial) names, are given for all. The advantage of the scientific name is that it allows consistent identification of products obtained from the various sources.

Particularly confusing is the fact that many very different herbs are known by the same, or similar sounding, common names. For example, English chamomile and German chamomile, ginseng (Korean ginseng) and Siberian ginseng, blue cohosh and black cohosh are not the same, and snakeroot is the common name of several very different herbs. Knowing the botanical name is the only reliable means you have of confidently knowing which herb you are actually taking. However, even this is not definitive, because it is well known that different subvarieties, strains, or hybrids of plants exist with significantly different levels of active chemicals and associated biological properties. For these reasons it is clear that a common name can not necessarily be relied on as the only means of identification. Also note that some herbal remedies may not list a botanical name because they represent a relatively pure isolated biologically active extract. Additionally, some combination products do not list the botanical names of every ingredient. Finally, with regard to naming plants, it should also be noted that occasionally the Latin botanical names officially assigned to a plant do sometimes change with the evolution of botanical knowledge.

The information on herbal remedies in this book mainly concerns manufactured, OTC herbal remedies. There are some herbs used by medical herbalists—for example, *Ephedra*, or wood betony—and some that are obtainable as crude dried herbs or gathered fresh herbs, which are beyond the scope of this book and so are omitted, whether or not they have proven medicinal use. For these herbs, interested readers should refer to alternative specialist reference sources and web sites.

The section is cross-referenced to the Disorders section where appropriate, and many of the more unusual or technical terms are explained in the **Glossary** at the back of the book. However, it is important to note that this book gives no recommendations regarding use, dosage, or route of administration. For this information you must consult an expert and follow the manufacturer's instructions. Particular care must be taken when using any herbal remedies, as with any health-related preparation, but especially in certain groups of people such as those who are pregnant (a number of herbs can affect the uterus, and in some cases cause miscarriages), those who are nursing, the elderly, and children. Where information is available and there is known possible risk to certain individuals, these points are mentioned in individual entries. When taking any herbal preparation, if in any doubt, specialist advice should always be sought.

Guidelines and points to remember

- In general, self-medication with herbal remedies should be for short-term use and for self-limiting conditions following expert advice. Consult your doctor if symptoms persist. Self-treatment with herbal remedies is not an alternative to specialist conventional medical treatment.
- If possible, always chose a herbal remedy that states the botanical name of the herb on the label—this is the only reasonably sure way to know what you have bought. Many similar-sounding herbs have different actions and uses, as well as different side-effects and contraindications.
- Remember that some herbs are available alone ("simples"), and others come in formulations containing several different herbs (possibly in the form of capsules, tablets, or powder). Be sure about your reasons for buying the remedy, and do not be seduced by the packaging or by any particular claims. You are strongly recommended to restrict your choice to reputable products so that you can be sure of what you are getting.
- If continuing with a course of herbal medication, keep to the same formulation and manufacturer. Preparations can vary greatly in potency and constituents. Where available, use formulations that contain *standardized extracts*. These are herbal products marketed with guaranteed potency, having a standard and stated amount of one type of extracted activity

(for example, hotness of cayenne herb) or particular chemical principle (for example, hypericum or hyperforin in St. John's Wort). It is also worth remembering that preparations are not necessarily pure, and in some cases unstandardized products have been found to contain no active ingredients.

- Always follow the manufacturer's dosage instructions, starting with the lower dose and never exceeding the recommended dose. If there are no manufacturer's recommendations, do not take it. All herbal (and conventional) medicines are potentially poisonous.
- If it doesn't work, stop taking it. But note that some herbs are identified as taking several day, weeks or even longer to have any beneficial effect.
- If you experience any side effects or symptoms get worse when taking a herbal remedy, stop taking it and see your doctor.
- If you are pregnant or nursing, or intend to medicate a child, ask a suitably qualified healthcare professional (preferably a family physician) before using a herbal remedy.
- If you have an existing medical condition or are taking any other (herbal or conventional) medication or nutritional supplements, ask a suitably qualified healthcare professional before taking any further herbal remedies. Note that a number of serious herb/drug interactions have been discovered. Many of these are detailed in the General Introduction and the Drugs section of this book.
- Always tell your doctor which herbal remedies you have been or are taking, and why.
- Always bear in mind that herbal remedies are not verified as to whether or not they are efficacious. In the USA, herbal products are marketed under the Food and Drug Administration (FDA) regulation according to the Dietary Supplement Health and Education Act (DSHEA), 1994. This prohibits their sale for treatment, cure, prevention, diagnosis of disease. Among other things because of these legalities of licensing and labelling, suppliers have to be extremely careful about any claims they make for herbal products, which means that any recommendations by manufacturers as to dose or purpose of use will tend to be non-specific.
- This book makes no specific recommendations with respect to use, administration, or dosage of herbals preparations. The inclusion of any herbal remedy in this book is not a recommendation or endorsement of its proposed uses or actions. Always consult an expert before taking any herbal remedy.

Herbal Remedies

The following list shows common names of herbal remedies included in this book. Because herbal remedies have been used for centuries by people in all parts of the world, there will also be more common names than those listed below, but the writers, contributors and editors have done their best to provide as full a list as possible, and have referred each one to the specific entry in the book where information about the herb is provided.

Aaron's rod see GOLDENROD (*Solidago virgaurea*); MULLEIN (*Verbascum densiflorum*).
Abies balsamea see BALSAM FIR.
Abutilon indicum see INDIAN MALLOW.
Acanthus mollis see ACANTHUS.
Achillea millefolium see YARROW.
Achyranthes bidentata see ACHYRANTHES.
acrid lettuce see WILD LETTUCE.
Adam's apple see LIME.
Adam's flannel see MULLEIN.
adderwort see BISTORT.
Adiantum capillus-veneris see MAIDENHAIR FERN.
adulsa see MALABAR NUT.
Aframomum melegueta see GRAINS OF PARADISE.
African chili see CAYENNE.
African pepper see CAYENNE.
Agastache rugosa see GIANT HYSSOP.
Agathosma betulina see BUCHU.
agnus castus see CHASTE TREE.
Agrimonia eupatoria see AGRIMONY.
agueweed see BONESET.
airelle see BILBERRY.
alant see ELECAMPANE.
alcanna see HENNA.
Alchemilla vulgaris see LADY'S MANTLE.
alder buckthorn see FRANGULA.
alder dogwood see FRANGULA.
alehoof see GROUND IVY.
all-heal see MISTLETOE (*Viscum album*); VALERIAN (*Valeriana officinalis*).
allium see GARLIC.
Allium cepa see ONION.
Allium sativum see GARLIC.
allspice see PIMENTO.
aloes see ALOE.
aloe vera see ALOE.
Aloysia triphylla see LEMON VERBENA.
Alpinia officinarum see GALANGAL.
altamisa see FEVERFEW.

Althaea officinalis see MARSHMALLOW.
althea see MARSHMALLOW.
amantilla see VALERIAN.
Ambroise see WOOD SAGE.
American angelica see ANGELICA.
American coneflower see ECHINACEA.
American cotton plant see COTTON.
American dewberry see BLACKBERRY.
American dwarf palm tree see SAW PALMETTO.
American nightshade see POKEROOT.
American safflower see SAFFLOWER.
American spinach see POKEROOT.
American willow see WILLOW.
angel's wort see ANGELICA.
aniseed see ANISE.
aniseed stars see STAR ANISE.
aniseseed see ANISE.
Antelaea azadirachta see NEEM.
Antherrmis noblis see CHAMOMILE, ENGLISH .
apium see CELERY.
apricot vine see PASSIONFLOWER.
Aralia racemosa see SPIKENARD.
arberry see UVA-URSI.
arbutus uva ursi see UVA-URSI.
archangel see WHITE DEAD NETTLE.
arjun tree see ARJUNA.
arnica flowers see ARNICA.
Arnica montana see ARNICA.
arnica root see ARNICA.
arrow wood see FRANGULA.
arsesmart see SMARTWEED.
Artemisia dracunculus see TARRAGON.
arthritica see COWSLIP.
arusa see MALABAR NUT.
asa foetida see ASAFOETIDA.
asant see ASA FOETIDA.
Asclepias tuberosa see PLEURISY ROOT.
ash (*Picrasma excelsa*) see QUASSIA.
Asian ginseng see GINSENG.
Asparagus officinalis see ASPARAGUS.
ass ear see COMFREY.
asthma plant see PILL-BEARING SPURGE.
asthma weed see LOBELIA.

ava see KAVA KAVA.
ava pepper see KAVA KAVA.
Avena sativa see OATS.
avens root see GEUM.
awa see KAVA KAVA.
axberry see SOUTHERN BAYBERRY.
Azadirachta indica see NEEM.
Bacopa monnieri see WATER HYSSOP.
badiana see STAR ANISE.
bad man's plaything see YARROW.
bai guo see GINKGO.
bal see MYRRH.
balm see LEMON BALM.
balm of gilead fir see SPRUCE.
balsam fir (*Picea excelsa*) see SPRUCE.
balsam-weed see JEWEL WEED.
barbasco see WILD YAM.
bardana see BURDOCK.
basam see BROOM.
basswood see LINDEN.
bastard cinnamon see CHINESE CINNAMON.
bastard safflower see SAFFLOWER.
bay see LAUREL.
bayberry see SOUTHERN BAYBERRY.
bay laurel see LAUREL.
bay tree see LAUREL.
bean herb see SAVORY.
bearberry see UVA-URSI.
bear's foot see LADY'S MANTLE.
bear's grape see POKEROOT (*Phytolacca americana*); UVA-URSI (*Arctostaphylos uva-ursi*).
beaver tree see MAGNOLIA.
bee balm see OSWEGO TEA.
beechdrops see BLUE COHOSH.
bee nettle see WHITE DEAD NETTLE.
bees' nest plant see WILD CARROT.
beggar's blanket see MULLEIN.
beggar's buttons see BURDOCK.
beggary see FUMITORY.
Bennet's root see GEUM.
Berberis aquifolium see OREGON GRAPE.
bergamot see OSWEGO TEA.
besom see BROOM.
Betula pendula see BIRCH.
birdlime see EUROPEAN MISTLETOE.

bird pepper see CAYENNE.
bird's foot see FENUGREEK.
bird's nest see WILD CARROT.
biscuits see TORMENTIL.
bissy nut see COLA.
bitter ash see QUASSIA.
bitterbloom see CENTAURY.
bitter clover see CENTAURY.
bitter herb see CENTAURY.
bitter lettuce see LACTUCARIUM.
bitter root see YELLOW GENTIAN.
bitterwood see QUASSIA.
bizzom see BROOM.
black alder see FRANGULA.
black alder dogwood see FRANGULA.
black alder tree see FRANGULA.
black choke see BLACK CHERRY.
black dogwood see FRANGULA.
black poplar see POPLAR.
black psyllium see INDIAN PLANTAGO.
black root (*Symphytum officinale*) see COMFREY.
black Sampson see ECHINACEA.
black snakeroot see BLACK COHOSH.
black stinking horehound see BLACK HOREHOUND.
black Susan see ECHINACEA.
black-tang see BLADDERWRACK.
black tea see GREEN TEA.
blackthorn see SLOE.
black walnut see BUTTERNUT.
black whortles see BILBERRY.
blackwort see COMFREY.
bladder fucus see BLADDERWRACK.
bladderpod see LOBELIA.
blanket herb see MULLEIN.
blanket-leaf see MULLEIN.
bleaberry see BILBERRY.
blessed herb see GEUM.
blind nettle see WHITE DEAD NETTLE.
blindweed see SHEPHERD'S PURSE.
blond psyllium see INDIAN PLANTAGO.
blood vine see WILLOW HERB.
bloodwood see LOGWOOD.
blooming Sally see PURPLE LOOSESTRIFE (*Lythrum salicaria*); WILLOW HERB (*Epilobium angustifolium*).
blowball see DANDELION.
blue balm see OSWEGO TEA.
blueberry see BILBERRY.
blueberry root see BLUE COHOSH.
blue curls see SELFHEAL.
blue flag see WILD IRIS.
blue ginseng see BLUE COHOSH.

blue gum see EUCALYPTUS.
blue pimpernel see SKULLCAP.
bog bean see BUCKBEAN.
bog myrtle see BUCKBEAN.
bol see MYRRH.
bola see MYRRH.
boldu see BOLDO.
boldus see BOLDO.
boneset (*Symphytum officinale*) see COMFREY.
bottle-brush see HORSETAIL.
bouncing Bet see SOAPWORT.
bowman's root see BLACK ROOT.
bramble see BLACKBERRY.
branching phytolacca see POKEROOT.
brandy mint see PEPPERMINT.
Brazilian cocoa see GUARANA.
breeam see BROOM.
brideweed see YELLOW TOAD FLAX.
bridewort see MEADOWSWEET.
British myrrh see SWEET CICELY.
broadleaf plantain see PLANTAIN.
brook bean see BUCKBEAN.
broomtops see BROOM.
browme see BROOM.
brownwort see SELFHEAL.
bruisewort see SOAPWORT (*Saponaria officinalis*); COMFREY (*Symphytum officinale*).
brum see BROOM.
brunella see SELFHEAL.
buckeye see HORSE CHESTNUT.
buckles see COWSLIP.
buckthorn (*Rhamnus frangula*) see FRANGULA.
buffalo herb see ALFALFA.
bugbane see BLACK COHOSH.
bugloss see BORAGE.
bugwort see BLACK COHOSH.
Bupleurum chinense see BUPLEURUM.
burage see BORAGE.
burnet saxifrage see PIMPINELLA.
burrage see BORAGE.
burren myrtle see BILBERRY.
burr seed see BURDOCK.
butter and eggs see YELLOW TOAD FLAX.
buttered haycocks see YELLOW TOAD FLAX.
butterfly weed see PLEURISY ROOT.
butter rose see COWSLIP.
butter winter see PIPSISSEWA.
buttonhole see HARTSTONGUE.
cabbage palm see SAW PALMETTO.
cabbage rose see ROSE.

cacao see COCOA.
cajeput see CAJUPUT.
calendula see MARIGOLD.
Calendula officinalis see MARIGOLD.
calumba see COLOMBO.
calves' snout see YELLOW TOAD FLAX.
Camellia sinensis see GREEN TEA.
cammock see SPINY REST HARROW.
camomile see GERMAN CHAMOMILE.
camphor of the poor see GARLIC.
Canada balsam see SPRUCE.
Canada root see PLEURISY ROOT.
Canadian poplar see POPLAR.
cancer-root see POKEROOT.
canchalagua see CENTAURY.
candleberry see SOUTHERN BAYBERRY.
candleberry bark see SOUTHERN BAYBERRY.
candlewick plant see MULLEIN.
cankerwort see DANDELION.
Canton cassia see CHINESE CINNAMON.
Canton rhubarb see CHINESE RHUBARB.
capon's tail see VALERIAN.
Capsella bursa-pastoris see SHEPHERD'S PURSE.
capsicum see CAYENNE.
cardin see BLESSED THISTLE.
carpenter's herb see SELFHEAL.
carpenter's square see FIGWORT.
carpenter's weed see SELFHEAL (*Prunella vulgaris*); YARROW (*Achillea millefolium*).
Carthamus tinctorius see SAFFLOWER.
cartkins willow see WILLOW.
Carum carvi see CARAWAY.
caryophyllum see CLOVE.
case-weed see SHEPHERD'S PURSE.
Cassia aromaticum see CHINESE CINNAMON.
cassia bark see CHINESE CINNAMON.
Cassia lignea see CHINESE CINNAMON.
catkins willow see WILLOW.
catmint see CATNIP.
catnep see CATNIP.
catrup see CATNIP.
catsfoot see GROUND IVY.
cat's paw see GROUND IVY.
catswort see CATNIP.
Caucasion walnut see WALNUT.
cayenne pepper see CAYENNE.
Centaurium erythraea see CENTAURY.
centaury gentian see CENTAURY.
Centella asiatica see GOTU KOLA.

Centella coriaca see GOTU KOLA.
centory see CENTAURY.
cetraria see ICELAND MOSS.
Cetraria islandica see ICELAND MOSS.
Ceylon cinnamon see CINNAMON.
chai-hu see BUPLEURUM.
Chamaelirium luteum see FALSE UNICORN ROOT.
Chamaemelum nobile see ENGLISH CHAMOMILE.
chamomilla see GERMAN CHAMOMILE.
Chamomilla recutita see GERMAN CHAMOMILE.
cheeses see MARSHMALLOW.
Chelidonium majus see CELANDINE.
chili pepper see CAYENNE.
Chimaphila umbellata see PIPSISSEWA.
China orange see SWEET ORANGE.
China root see WILD YAM.
Chinese cinnamon (*Cinnamomum cassia*) see CASSIA.
Chinese ginseng see GINSENG.
Chinese matrimony see CHINESE WOLFBERRY.
Chinese mock-barberry see SCHISANDRA.
Chinese tea see GREEN TEA.
Chinese thoroughwax see BUPLEURUM.
chirata see CHIRETTA.
chirayta see CHIRETTA.
chocolate tree see COCOA.
choke cherry see BLACK CHERRY.
Christ's ladder see CENTAURY.
Chrysanthemum morifolium see FLORISTS' CHRYSANTHEMUM.
church steeples see AGRIMONY.
churnstaff see YELLOW TOAD FLAX.
Cichorium intybus see CHICORY.
cimicifuga see BLACK COHOSH.
Cinnamomum aromaticum see CHINESE CINNAMON.
Cinnamomum cassia see CASSIA.
cinquefoil see POTENTILLA (*Potentilla anserina*); TORMENTIL (*Potentilla erecta*).
Circassian walnut see WALNUT.
Citrus aurantifolia see LIME.
Citrus limon see LEMON.
citrus orange see SWEET ORANGE.
Citrus sinensis see SWEET ORANGE.
city avens see GEUM.
Clerodendrum trichotomum see CLERODENDRUM TRICHOTOMUM.

cloister pepper see CHASTE TREE.
clot-bur see BURDOCK (*Arctium lappa*); MULLEIN (*Verbascum densiflorum*).
clove garlic see GARLIC.
clove pepper see PIMENTO.
clown's lungwort see MULLEIN.
Cnicus benedictus see BLESSED THISTLE.
Cnidium monnieri see CNIDIUM.
coakum-chongras see POKEROOT.
Cochlearia officinalis see SCURVY GRASS.
cocklebur see AGRIMONY (*Agrimonia eupatoria*); BURDOCK (*Arctium lappa*).
cockle buttons see BURDOCK.
cocowort see SHEPHERD'S PURSE.
Codonopsis pilosula see CODONOPSIS.
Coffea arabica see COFFEE.
cokan see POKEROOT.
Cola acuminata see COLA.
cola nut see COLA.
cola seed see COLA.
Coleus forskohlii see COLEUS.
colewort see GEUM.
colic root see WILD YAM.
comb flower see ECHINACEA.
Commiphora molmol see MYRRH.
common agrimony see AGRIMONY.
common bean see BEANS.
common bearberry see UVA-URSI.
common buckthorn see BUCKTHORN.
common garlic see GARLIC.
common horse chestnut see HORSE CHESTNUT.
common larch see LARCH.
common nettle see STINGING NETTLE.
common oak see OAK.
common parsley see PARSLEY.
common radish see RADISH.
common reed see REED HERB.
common sandspurry see ARENARIA RUBRA.
common shrubby see IMMORTELLE.
common thyme see THYME.
compass plant see ROSEMARY.
compass weed see ROSEMARY.
coneflower see ECHINACEA.
conqueror tree see HORSE CHESTNUT.
consolida see COMFREY.
consound see COMFREY.
convallaria see LILY OF THE VALLEY.
Convallaria majalis see LILY OF THE VALLEY.
convall-lily see LILY OF THE VALLEY.

coon root see BLOODROOT.
Coptis chinensis see CHINESE GOLDTHREAD.
Coriandrum sativum see CORIANDER.
corn horsetail see HORSETAIL.
Corydalis yanusuo see CORYDALIS.
cotton seed see COTTON.
cowslip, English see COWSLIP.
crack willow see WILLOW.
crampweed see POTENTILLA.
Crataegus laevigata see HAWTHORN.
Crataegus monogyna see HAWTHORN.
Crataegus oxyacantha see HAWTHORN.
creeping Charlie see GROUND IVY.
creeping Jenny see MONEYWORT.
creeping Joan see MONEYWORT.
crewel see COWSLIP.
crosswort see BONESET.
crowberry see POKEROOT.
crow soap see SOAPWORT.
cuckoo flower see SALEP.
Cucurbita pepo see PUMPKIN.
cuddy's lungs see MULLEIN.
cullay see SOAP BARK.
culveris root see BLACK ROOT.
Curcuma domestica see TURMERIC.
Curcuma longa see TURMERIC.
Curcuma xanthorrhiza see CURCUMA.
Curcuma zedoaria see ZEDOARY.
cure-all see LEMON BALM.
curled dock see YELLOW DOCK.
curled mint see SPEARMINT.
curly dock see YELLOW DOCK.
cusparia bark see ANGOSTURA.
cutweed see BLADDERWRACK.
Cynara scolymus see ARTICHOKE.
Cytisus scoparius see BROOM.
da-huang see CHINESE RHUBARB.
Dalmatian sage see SAGE.
damask rose see ROSE.
dan-shen see RED SAGE.
Daphne see LAUREL.
darri see BROOMCORN.
Daucus carota see WILD CARROT.
Daucus carota carota see WILD CARROT.
dead nettle see WHITE DEAD NETTLE.
deaf nettle see WHITE DEAD NETTLE.
devil's bit see PREMORSE.
devil's bones see WILD YAM.
devil's dung see ASA FOETIDA.
devil's fuge see EUROPEAN MISTLETOE.

devil's head see YELLOW TOAD FLAX.
devil's nettle see YARROW.
devil's plaything see YARROW.
devil's ribbon see YELLOW TOAD FLAX.
devil's shrub see SIBERIAN GINSENG.
dew plant see SUNDEW.
Dianthus superbus see FRINGED PINK.
didin see MYRRH.
didthin see MYRRH.
di-gu-pi see CHINESE WOLFBERRY.
di-huang see REHMANNIA.
ding xiang see CLOVE.
dog cloves see SOAPWORT.
doggies see YELLOW TOAD FLAX.
dogwood see JAMAICA DOGWOOD (*Piscidia erythrina*); FRANGULA (*Rhamnus frangula*).
dracontium see SKUNK CABBAGE.
dragon-bushes see YELLOW TOAD FLAX.
dragon's blood see HERB ROBERT.
dragonwort see BISTORT.
Drimia maritima see SQUILL.
dropberry see SOLOMON'S SEAL.
dropsy plant see LEMON BALM.
Drosera anglica see SUNDEW.
Drosera intermedia see SUNDEW.
Drosera rotundifolia see SUNDEW.
Drosera rumentacea see SUNDEW.
duffle see MULLEIN.
dumb nettle see WHITE DEAD NETTLE.
durri see BROOMCORN.
Dutch rushes see HORSETAIL.
dwarf flax see MOUNTAIN FLAX.
dwarf pine see SCOTCH PINE.
dyeberry see BILBERRY.
dyer's saffron see SAFFLOWER.
eagle vine see CONDURANGO.
earthbank see TORMENTIL.
earth smoke see FUMITORY.
Easter flower see PASQUE FLOWER.
Easter giant see BISTORT.
Easter ledges see BISTORT.
Easter mangiant see BISTORT.
Echinacea angustifolia see ECHINACEA.
Echinacea pallida see ECHINACEA.
Echinacea purpurea see ECHINACEA.
eggs and bacon see YELLOW TOAD FLAX.
eggs and collops see YELLOW TOAD FLAX.
Egyptian privet see HENNA.
Elettaria cardamomum see CARDAMOM.

eleutherococ see SIBERIAN GINSENG.
Eleutherococcus senticosus see SIBERIAN GINSENG.
elfdock see ELECAMPANE.
Elymus repens see COUCH GRASS.
Embelia ribes see EMBELIA.
emetic herb see LOBELIA.
emetic weed see LOBELIA.
enchanter's plant see VERVAIN.
enebro see JUNIPER.
Epilobium angustifolium see WILLOW HERB.
Equisetum arvense see HORSETAIL.
eryngo-leaved liverwort see ICELAND MOSS.
estragon see FRENCH TARRAGON.
eternal flower see IMMORTELLE.
Eucalyptus globulus see EUCALYPTUS.
Eucommia ulmoides see GUTTA PERCHA.
Eugenia caryophyllata see CLOVE.
Eugenia caryophyllus see CLOVE.
eupatorium see BONESET.
Eupatorium perfoliatum see BONESET.
Euphorbia hirta see PILL-BEARING SPURGE.
euphrasia see EYEBRIGHT.
Euphrasia officinalis see EYEBRIGHT.
European aspen see POPLAR.
European avens see GEUM.
European bitter polygala see BITTER MILKWORT.
European black alder see FRANGULA.
European buckthorn see FRANGULA.
European cowslip see COWSLIP.
European goldenrod see GOLDENROD.
European larch see LARCH.
European sanicle see SANICLE.
European senega snakeroot see BITTER MILKWORT.
European wild pansy see HEARTSEASE.
European willow see WILLOW.
European wort see ANGELICA.
evergreen snakeroot see BITTER MILKWORT.
everlasting see IMMORTELLE.
ewe daisy see TORMENTIL.
eye balm see GOLDENSEAL.
eyebright see CENTAURY (*Euphrasia officinalis*) (*Centaurium erythraea*); LOBELIA.
eye root see GOLDENSEAL.
fairy caps see COWSLIP.

fairy clock see DANDELION.
fairy cups see COWSLIP.
fairy feathers see PARSLEY.
fairy flax see MOUNTAIN FLAX.
fake saffron see SAFFLOWER.
false cinnamon see CHINESE CINNAMON.
featherfew see FEVERFEW.
featherfoil see FEVERFEW.
febrifuge plant see FEVERFEW.
feltwort see MULLEIN.
Ferula assafoetida see ASAFOETIDA.
Ferula foetida see ASAFOETIDA.
fever plant see EVENING PRIMROSE.
fevertree see EUCALYPTUS.
feverwort see BONESET (*Lobelia inflata*) (*Eupatorium perfoliatum*); CENTAURY (*Centaurium erythraea*).
field balm see CATNIP.
field horsetail see HORSETAIL.
field pumpkin see PUMPKIN.
figwort (*Ranunculus ficaria*) see PILEWORT.
Filipendula ulmarial see MEADOWSWEET.
filwort see CENTAURY.
fir tree see SPRUCE.
fish mint see SPEARMINT.
fish poison bark see JAMAICA DOGWOOD.
five-finger fern see MAIDENHAIR FERN.
five-fingers see GINSENG.
flake manna see MANNA.
flannelflower see MULLEIN.
flat-leafed parsley see PARSLEY.
flaxseed see FLAX.
flaxweed see YELLOW TOAD FLAX.
flesh and blood see TORMENTIL.
flowering ash see MANNA.
flowering Sally see PURPLE LOOSESTRIFE.
flowering wintergreen see BITTER MILKWORT.
fluellin see YELLOW TOAD FLAX.
fluffweed see MULLEIN.
flux root see PLEURISY ROOT.
Foeniculum vulgare see FENNEL.
Forsythia suspensa see WEEPING FORSYTHIA.
fox's clote see BURDOCK.
Fraxinus excelsior see ASH.
Fraxinus ornus see MANNA.
French rose see ROSE.
French thyme see THYME.
fucus see BLADDERWRACK.

Fucus vesiculosus see BLADDERWRACK.
fuller's herb see SOAPWORT.
Fumaria officinalis see FUMITORY.
fumus see FUMITORY.
gagroot see LOBELIA.
Galeopsis segetum see HEMPNETTLE.
Galipea officinalis see ANGOSTURA.
gall weed see YELLOW GENTIAN.
gallwort see YELLOW TOAD FLAX.
garden angelica see ANGELICA.
garden artichoke see ARTICHOKE.
garden mint see SPEARMINT.
garden parsley see PARSLEY.
garden radish see RADISH.
garden sage see SAGE.
garden thyme see THYME.
garlic sage see WOOD SAGE.
geneva see JUNIPER.
geniver see JUNIPER.
gentian see YELLOW GENTIAN.
Gentiana lutea see YELLOW GENTIAN.
gentian root see YELLOW GENTIAN.
Geranium robertianum see HERB
   ROBERT.
Geum urbanum see GEUM.
Gill-go-over-the-ground see
   GROUND IVY.
Gill-to-by-the-hedge see GROUND
   IVY.
ginepro see JUNIPER.
Ginkgo biloba see GINKGO.
Glechoma hederacea see GROUND
   IVY.
globe artichoke see ARTICHOKE.
Glycine soja see SOYBEAN.
Glycyrrhiza glabra see LICORICE.
goat's leaf see HONEYSUCKLE.
goat's pod see CAYENNE.
God's-hair see HARTSTONGUE.
goldbloom see MARIGOLD.
golden rod (*Verbascum densiflorum*)
   see MULLEIN.
goldilocks see IMMORTELLE.
golds see MARIGOLD.
goldy star see GEUM.
goosegrass see POTENTILLA.
goose tansy see POTENTILLA.
goosewort see POTENTILLA.
Gossypium herbaceum see COTTON.
Gossypium hirsutum see COTTON.
goutberry see BLACKBERRY.
grain see OATS.
grains of paradise (*Capsicum
   species*) see CAYENNE.
granadilla see PASSIONFLOWER.
grapple plant see DEVIL'S CLAW.

gravelroot see BONESET.
great burr see BURDOCK.
greater nettle see STINGING NETTLE.
greater plantain see PLANTAIN.
great raifort see HORSERADISH.
Grecian laurel see LAUREL.
Greek hay seed see FENUGREEK.
green bean see BEANS.
green endive see LACTUCARIUM.
green mint see SPEARMINT.
groats see OATS.
ground apple see ENGLISH
   CHAMOMILE.
ground furze see SPINY REST HARROW.
ground holly see PIPSISSEWA.
ground raspberry see GOLDENSEAL.
guaiacum see GUAIAC.
Guaiacum officinale see GUAIAC.
guarana bread see GUARANA.
guggal gum see MYRRH.
guggal resin see MYRRH.
Guinea corn see BROOMCORN.
Guinea grains see GRAINS OF PARADISE.
Guinea pepper see CAYENNE.
Guinea sorrel see HIBISCUS.
gum asafoetida see ASA FOETIDA.
gum ivy see ENGLISH IVY.
gum myrrh see MYRRH.
gum plant see COMFREY.
gum tree see EUCALYPTUS.
guru nut see COLA NUT.
gypsywort see BUGLEWEED.
Haematoxylon campechianum see
   LOGWOOD.
Haematoxylon lignum see
   LOGWOOD.
hag's taper see MULLEIN.
hair of Venus see MAIDENHAIR FERN.
hairy mint see WILD MINT.
Hamamelis virginiana see WITCH
   HAZEL.
Hamburg parsley see PARSLEY.
happy major see BURDOCK.
hardock see BURDOCK.
hareburr see BURDOCK.
hare's beard see MULLEIN.
Haronga madagascariensis see
   HARONGA.
Harpagophytum procumbens see
   DEVIL'S CLAW.
hartsthorn see BUCKTHORN.
hart's tree see SWEETCLOVER.
haw see HAWTHORN.
hawthorn, English see HAWTHORN.
hay flowers see SWEETCLOVER.
haymaids see GROUND IVY.

hazel nut see WITCH HAZEL.
heal-all see SELFHEAL.
heal-all scrofula plant see FIGWORT.
healing herb see COMFREY.
heart of the earth see SELFHEAL.
heartwort see MOTHERWORT.
Hedera helix see ENGLISH IVY.
hedge fumitory see FUMITORY.
hedgehog see ECHINACEA.
hedgemaids see GROUND IVY.
hedge-taper see MULLEIN.
heerabol see MYRRH.
Helichrysum arenarium see
   IMMORTELLE.
heliotrope see VALERIAN.
helmet flower see SKULLCAP.
hemlock spruce see SPRUCE.
hemp tree see CHASTE TREE.
hendibeh see CHICORY.
henne see HENNA.
herb Bennet see GEUM.
herb Louisa see LEMON VERBENA.
herb of grace see VERVAIN.
herb of the Cross see VERVAIN.
herb Peter Paigle see COWSLIP.
herb twopence see MONEYWORT.
Hibiscus sabdariffa see HIBISCUS.
high balm see OSWEGO TEA.
high blackberry see BLACKBERRY.
highwaythorn see BUCKTHORN.
hindberry see RASPBERRY.
hind heal see WOOD SAGE.
hind's tongue see HARTSTONGUE.
hini see BLACK ROOT.
Hippophae rhamnoides see SEA
   BUCKTHORN.
holigold see MARIGOLD.
holligold see MARIGOLD.
holly bay see MAGNOLIA.
Holy Ghost herb see BLESSED THISTLE.
holy thistle see BLESSED THISTLE.
holy tree see NEEM.
honey plant see LEMON BALM.
hoodwort see SKULLCAP.
hook-heal see SELFHEAL.
hop strobile see HOPS.
Hordeum distichon see BARLEY.
Hordeum distychum see BARLEY.
horse-elder see ELECAMPANE.
horse-heal see ELECAMPANE.
horse savin see JUNIPER.
horsetail grass see HORSETAIL.
horsetail rush see HORSETAIL.
horse tongue see HARTSTONGUE.
horse willow see HORSETAIL.
hot pepper see CAYENNE.

huang-qi see ASTRAGALUS.
huckleberry see BILBERRY.
hundred-leafed rose see ROSE.
Hungarian chamomile see GERMAN CHAMOMILE.
Hungarian pepper see CAYENNE.
hurtleberry see BILBERRY.
hurts see BILBERRY.
Hydrangea arborescens see HYDRANGEA.
Hydrastis canadensis see GOLDENSEAL.
hydrocotyle see GOTU KOLA.
Hydrocotyle asiatica see GOTU KOLA.
Iceland lichen see ICELAND MOSS.
Illicium verum see STAR ANISE.
imlee see TAMARIND.
Impatiens biflora see JEWEL WEED.
Indian balmony see CHIRETTA.
Indian bark see MAGNOLIA.
Indian corn see CORN SILK.
Indian cress see NASTURTIUM (*Tropaeolum majus*); WATERCRESS.
Indian dye see GOLDENSEAL.
Indian gentian see CHIRETTA.
Indian gum see CUP PLANT.
Indian head see ECHINACEA.
Indian hydrocotyle see GOTU KOLA.
Indian paint see BLOODROOT (*Nasturtium officinale*) (*Sanguinaria canadensis*); GOLDENSEAL (*Hydrastis canadensis*).
Indian pennywort see GOTU KOLA.
Indian plant see BLOODROOT (*Sanguinaria canadensis*); GOLDENSEAL (*Hydrastis canadensis*).
Indian rhubarb see CHINESE RHUBARB.
Indian root see SPIKENARD.
Indian sage see BONESET.
Indian tobacco see LOBELIA.
inkberry see POKEROOT.
intoxicating pepper see KAVA KAVA.
Inula helenium see ELECAMPANE.
Irish tops see BROOM.
Iris versicolor see WILD IRIS.
ispaghula see INDIAN PLANTAGO.
Italian licorice see LICORICE.
Italian limetta see LIME.
Italian parsley see PARSLEY.
Jacob's ladder see LILY OF THE VALLEY.
Jacob's staff see MULLEIN.
jalap see POKEROOT.
Jamaica mignonette see HENNA.
Jamaica pepper see PIMENTO.
Jamaica sorrel see HIBISCUS.

jambolan see JAMBUL.
Jambosa caryophyllus see CLOVE.
jamum see JAMBUL.
Japanese ginseng see GINSENG.
Jateorhiza palmata see COLOMBO.
jaundice root see GOLDENSEAL.
Java plum see JAMBUL.
Java tea see JAVA TREE.
Jesuit's tea see MATÉ.
Jew's myrtle see BUTCHER'S BROOM.
Johnny-jump-up see HEARTSEASE.
Juglans cinerea see BUTTERNUT.
Juglans nigra see WALNUT.
Juglans regia see WALNUT.
Juniperus communis see JUNIPER.
Juno's tears see VERVAIN.
Justicia adhatoda see MALABAR NUT.
kali chaye see MATÉ.
Kansas snakeroot see ECHINACEA.
kava see KAVA KAVA.
kawa see KAVA KAVA.
kawa pepper see KAVA KAVA.
kelpware see BLADDERWRACK.
kelp-ware see BLADDERWRACK.
kernelwort see FIGWORT.
Kew tree see GINKGO.
key of heaven see COWSLIP.
kidney bean see BEANS.
king's clover see SWEETCLOVER.
king's cure see PIPSISSEWA.
king's cureall see EVENING PRIMROSE (*Oenothera biennis*); PIPSISSEWA (*Chimaphila umbellata*).
kinnickinick see UVA-URSI.
kinnikinnick see UVA-URSI.
kitmi see MARSHMALLOW.
knee holly see BUTCHER'S BROOM.
kneeholm see BUTCHER'S BROOM.
knight's milfoil see YARROW.
knitback see COMFREY.
knitbone see COMFREY.
kola see COLA.
kola nut see COLA.
kola tree see COLA.
Korean ginseng see GINSENG.
krameria root see RHATANY.
Krameria triandra see RHATANY.
Lactuca virosa see WILD LETTUCE.
ladder-to-heaven see LILY OF THE VALLEY.
lady of the meadow see MEADOWSWEET.
lady's purse see SHEPHERD'S PURSE.
lady's seals see SOLOMON'S SEAL.

lamb mint see PEPPERMINT (*Mentha piperita*); SPEARMINT (*Mentha spicata*).
Lamium album see WHITE DEAD NETTLE.
lanceleaf plantain see PLANTAIN.
land whin see SPINY REST HARROW.
lappa see BURDOCK.
large-leaved germander see WOOD SAGE.
Larix decidua see LARCH.
larkspur lion's mouth see YELLOW TOAD FLAX.
latherwort see SOAPWORT.
Laurus nobilis see LAUREL.
lavose see LOVAGE.
Lawsonia inermis see HENNA.
lemon-scented verbena see LEMON VERBENA.
lemon walnut see BUTTERNUT.
lemonwood see SCHISANDRA.
leontopodium see LADY'S MANTLE.
Leonurus cardiaca see MOTHERWORT.
leopard's bane see ARNICA.
Lepidium sativum see GARDEN CRESS.
Leptandra virginica see BLACK ROOT.
lesser celandine see PILEWORT.
lettuce opium see LACTUCARIUM.
Levant salep see SALEP.
Levisticum officinale see LOVAGE.
licorice root see LICORICE.
life of man see SPIKENARD.
lignum vitae see GUAIAC.
Lilium candidium see WHITE LILY.
lily constancy see LILY OF THE VALLEY.
lime (*Tilia species*) see LINDEN.
lime tree see LINDEN.
lime tress flower see LINDEN.
limetta see LIME.
limon see LEMON.
Linaria vulgaris see YELLOW TOAD FLAX.
linn flower see LINDEN.
linseed see FLAX.
lint bells see FLAX.
Linum catharticum see MOUNTAIN FLAX.
Linum usitatissimum see FLAX.
lion's foot see LADY'S MANTLE.
lion's tail see MOTHERWORT.
lion's tooth see DANDELION.
liquorice see LICORICE.
little dragon see FRENCH TARRAGON.
little pollom see BITTER MILKWORT.
liverwort see AGRIMONY.

Lizzy-run-up-the-hedge see GROUND IVY.

Lobaria pulmonaria see LUNGMOSS.

Lobelia inflata see LOBELIA.

long purples see PURPLE LOOSESTRIFE.

Lonicera caprifoliu see HONEYSUCKLE.

loosestrife see PURPLE LOOSESTRIFE (*Lythrum salicaria*); YELLOW WILLOWHERB (*Lysimachia vulgaris*).

Louisiana long (and short) pepper see CAYENNE.

love in winter see PIPSISSEWA.

love leaves see BURDOCK.

low balm see OSWEGO TEA.

lucerne see ALFALFA.

lungwort see LUNGMOSS.

lustwort see SUNDEW.

Lycium chinense see CHINESE WOLFBERRY.

Lycopodium clavatum see CLUB MOSS.

Lycopus virginicus see BUGLEWEED.

Lysimachia nummularia see MONEYWORT.

Lysimachia vulgaris see YELLOW WILLOWHERB.

lythrum see PURPLE LOOSESTRIFE.

Lythrum salicaria see PURPLE LOOSESTRIFE.

mace see NUTMEG.

mackerel mint see SPEARMINT.

mad-dog weed see SKULLCAP.

Madonna lily see WHITE LILY.

madweed see SKULLCAP.

Magnolia glauca see MAGNOLIA.

maiden fern see MAIDENHAIR FERN.

maidenhair tree see MAIDENHAIR FERN.

maize see CORN SILK.

malavisco see MARSHMALLOW.

mallaguetta pepper see GRAINS OF PARADISE.

mallards see MARSHMALLOW.

Malva sylvestris see MALLOW.

manna ash see MANNA.

mapato see RHATANY.

maranta see ARROWROOT.

Maranta arundinaceae see ARROWROOT.

Marian thistle see MILK THISTLE.

Marsdenia condurango see CONDURANGO.

marsh clover see BUCKBEAN.

marsh mint see WILD MINT.

marsh parsley see CELERY.

marsh penny see GOTU KOLA.

Mary bud see MARIGOLD.

Mary Gowles see MARIGOLD.

Mary thistle see MILK THISTLE.

masterwort see ANGELICA.

Matricaria chamomilla see GERMAN CHAMOMILE.

May see HAWTHORN.

May bells see LILY OF THE VALLEY.

May blossom see HAWTHORN.

May bush see HAWTHORN.

Mayflower see COWSLIP.

May lily see LILY OF THE VALLEY.

maypop see PASSIONFLOWER.

May weed see GERMAN CHAMOMILE.

meadow anemone see PASQUE FLOWER.

meadow cabbage see SKUNK CABBAGE.

meadow lily see WHITE LILY.

meadow queen see MEADOWSWEET.

meadow runagates see MONEYWORT.

meadow sage see SAGE.

meadow-wort see MEADOWSWEET.

meadsweet see MEADOWSWEET.

mealberry see UVA-URSI.

Medicago sativa see ALFALFA.

medical rhubarb see CHINESE RHUBARB.

Mediterranean thistle see MILK THISTLE.

mehndi see HENNA.

Melaleuca alternifolia see TEA TREE.

Melaleuca leucadendra see CAJUPUT.

Melaleuca leucodendron see CAJUPUT.

melegueta pepper see GRAINS OF PARADISE.

Melia azadirachta see NEEM.

melilot see SWEETCLOVER.

Melilotus officinalis see SWEETCLOVER.

melissa see LEMON BALM.

Melissa officinalis see LEMON BALM.

mendee see HENNA.

Mentha aquatica see WILD MINT.

Mentha arvensis see JAPANESE MINT.

Mentha longifolia see ENGLISH HORSEMINT.

Mentha spicata see SPEARMINT.

Mentha piperita see PEPPERMINT.

Menyanthes trifoliata see BUCKBEAN.

Mexican chili see CAYENNE.

Mexican yam see WILD YAM.

Midsummer daisy see FEVERFEW.

mignonette tree see HENNA.

milfoil see YARROW.

milk vetch see ASTRAGALUS.

milk willow-herb see PURPLE LOOSESTRIFE.

milkwort see SENEGA SNAKEROOT.

mill mountain see MOUNTAIN FLAX.

mistletoe see EUROPEAN MISTLETOE.

Monarda didyma see OSWEGO TEA.

monkey flower see YELLOW TOAD FLAX.

monk's pepper see CHASTE TREE.

moonflower see BUCKBEAN.

moor grass see POTENTILLA.

Moorish mallow see MARSHMALLOW.

mortification root see MARSHMALLOW.

mother of thyme see WILD THYME.

mother's heart see SHEPHERD'S PURSE.

mountain balm see OSWEGO TEA.

mountain box see UVA-URSI.

mountain cranberry see UVA-URSI.

mountain flax (*Polygala senega*) see SENEGA SNAKEROOT.

mountain mint see OSWEGO TEA.

mountain radish see HORSERADISH.

mountain tobacco see ARNICA.

muguet see LILY OF THE VALLEY.

mugwort see FRENCH TARRAGON.

myrica see SOUTHERN BAYBERRY.

Myrica cerifera see SOUTHERN BAYBERRY.

Myristica fragrans see NUTMEG.

Myrrhis odorata see SWEET CICELY.

mystyldene see EUROPEAN MISTLETOE.

narrow dock see YELLOW DOCK.

narrow-leafed purple coneflower see ECHINACEA.

narrowleaf plantain see PLANTAIN.

Nasturtium officinale see WATERCRESS.

navy bean see BEANS.

nectar of the gods see GARLIC.

Nelumbo nucifera see LOTUS.

Nepeta cataria see CATNIP.

Nepeta hederacea see GROUND IVY.

nettle see STINGING NETTLE.

night willow-herb see EVENING PRIMROSE.

nim see NEEM.

nine hooks see LADY'S MANTLE.

nivara see RICE.

noble laurel see LAUREL.

noble yarrow see YARROW.

northern senega see SENEGA
SNAKEROOT.
Norway pine see SPRUCE.
Norway spruce see SPRUCE.
nosebleed see FEVERFEW (*Tanacetum
parthenium*); YARROW (*Achillea
millefolium*).
oak, English see OAK.
oak lungs see LUNGMOSS.
oatmeal see OATS.
Ocimum sanctum see HOLY BASIL.
oderwort see BISTORT.
Oenothera biennis see EVENING
PRIMROSE.
ofbit see PREMORSE.
oil nut see BUTTERNUT.
old maid's pink see SOAPWORT.
old man see ROSEMARY.
old man's pepper see YARROW.
old man's root see SPIKENARD.
Ononis spinosa see SPINY REST
HARROW.
orange see SWEET ORANGE.
orange milkweed see PLEURISY ROOT.
orange root see GOLDENSEAL.
orange swallow-wort see PLEURISY
ROOT.
orchid see SALEP.
Orchis morio see SALEP.
Oriental ginseng see GINSENG.
Origanum majorana see MARJORAM.
Orthosiphon spicatus see JAVA TREE.
Oryza sativa see RICE.
osterick see BISTORT.
osterwort see BISTORT.
Our Lady's flannel see MULLEIN.
Our Lady's keys see COWSLIP.
Our Lady's mint see SPEARMINT.
Our Lady's tears see LILY OF THE
VALLEY.
oxadoddy see BLACK ROOT.
oxlip see COWSLIP.
paddock-pipes see HORSETAIL.
Paeonia lactiflora see WHITE PEONY.
pale gentian see YELLOW GENTIAN.
pale purple coneflower see
ECHINACEA.
palsywort see COWSLIP.
Panama bark see SOAP BARK.
Panax ginseng see GINSENG.
paperbark tree see CAJUPUT.
papoose root see BLUE COHOSH.
paprika see CAYENNE.
paraguay tea see MATÉ.
Parietina officinalis see LICHWORT.

passe flower see PASQUE FLOWER.
passiflora see PASSIONFLOWER.
Passiflora incarnata see
PASSIONFLOWER.
passion vine see PASSIONFLOWER.
password see COWSLIP.
patience dock see BISTORT.
pattens and clogs see YELLOW TOAD
FLAX.
paucon see BLOODROOT.
paullinia see GUARANA.
Paullinia cupana see GUARANA.
pauson see BLOODROOT.
peachwood see LOGWOOD.
peagles see COWSLIP.
pearl barley see BARLEY.
pedlar's basket see YELLOW TOAD
FLAX.
pedunculate oak see OAK.
pennywort see YELLOW TOAD FLAX.
pepper-and-salt see SHEPHERD'S
PURSE.
pepper bark see BLACK PEPPER.
Persea americana see AVOCADO.
persely see PARSLEY.
Persian berries see FRANGULA.
Persian walnut see WALNUT.
Persicaria bistorta see BISTORT.
Persicaria hydropiper see
SMARTWEED.
personata see BURDOCK.
petersylinge see PARSLEY.
Petroselinum crispum see PARSLEY.
pettigree see BUTCHER'S BROOM.
petty morell see SPIKENARD.
petty mulleins see COWSLIP.
petty whin see SPINY REST HARROW.
Peumus boldus see BOLDO.
pewterwort see HORSETAIL.
Phaseolus vulgaris see BEANS.
philanthropium see BURDOCK.
philanthropos see AGRIMONY.
philtron see WILD CARROT.
Phragmites communis see REED
HERB.
physic root see BLACK ROOT.
Phytolacca americana see
POKEROOT.
phytolacca berry see POKEROOT.
phytolacca root see POKEROOT.
Picea excelsa see SPRUCE.
pick-pocket see SHEPHERD'S PURSE.
Picrasma excelsa see QUASSIA.
pigeon berry see POKEROOT.
pigeon's grass see VERVAIN.

pigeonweed see VERVAIN.
pilot plant see CUP PLANT.
pimenta see PIMENTO.
Pimenta racemosa see PIMENTO.
pimpernell see PIMPINELLA.
Pimpinella anisum see ANISE.
Pimpinella major see BURNET
SAXIFRAGE.
Pimpinella radix see BURNET
SAXIFRAGE.
pine oils see SCOTCH PINE.
pin heads see GERMAN CHAMOMILE.
pinto bean see BEANS.
Pinus sylvestris see SCOTCH PINE.
piper see BLACK PEPPER.
Piper methysticum see KAVA KAVA.
Piper nigrum see BLACK PEPPER.
Piscidia erythrina see JAMAICA
DOGWOOD.
pis-en-lit see DANDELION.
piss-in-bed see DANDELION.
pix liquida see SCOTCH PINE.
Plantago lanceolata see PLANTAIN.
Plantago major see PLANTAIN.
Plantago ovata see INDIAN PLANTAGO.
plantain, English see PLANTAIN.
plumrocks see COWSLIP.
pocan see POKEROOT.
pockwood see GUAIAC.
poison lettuce see LACTUCARIUM.
poke see POKEROOT.
poke berry see POKEROOT.
pokeweed see POKEROOT.
polar plant see CUP PLANT (*Silphium
perfoliatum*); ROSEMARY (*Rosmarinus
officinalis*).
polecatweed see SKUNK CABBAGE.
Polygala amara see BITTER MILKWORT.
Polygala senega see SENEGA
SNAKEROOT.
Polygonum bistorta see BISTORT.
Polygonum hydropiper see
SMARTWEED.
Polygonum multiflorum see flowery
knotweed.
poolroot see SANICLE.
poor man's parmacettie see
SHEPHERD'S PURSE.
poor man's treacle see GARLIC.
Populus alba see POPLAR.
Populus canadensis see POPLAR.
Populus nigra see POPLAR.
Populus tacamahaca see POPLAR.
Populus tremula see POPLAR.
Populus tremuloides see POPLAR.

pot barley see BARLEY.
Potentilla anserina see POTENTILLA.
Potentilla erecta see TORMENTIL.
prairie dock see CUP PLANT.
premorse scabious see PREMORSE.
prickly ash see NORTHERN PRICKLY ASH.
prickly lettuce see LACTUCARIUM.
priest's crown see DANDELION.
primrose see COWSLIP.
Primula officinalis see COWSLIP.
Primula veris see COWSLIP.
prince's feathers see POTENTILLA.
prince's pine see PIPSISSEWA.
prunella see SELFHEAL.
Prunella vulgaris see SELFHEAL.
Prunus serotina see BLACK CHERRY.
Prunus spinosa see SLOE.
puffball see DANDELION.
pukeweed see LOBELIA.
pulsatilla see PASQUE FLOWER.
Pulsatilla pratensis see PASQUE
    FLOWER.
pumilio pine see SCOTCH PINE.
purging buckthorn see BUCKTHORN.
purging flax see MOUNTAIN FLAX.
purple clover see RED CLOVER.
purple coneflower see ECHINACEA.
purple medic see ALFALFA.
purple medick see ALFALFA.
purple medicle see ALFALFA.
purple willow see WILLOW.
purple willow-herb see PURPLE
    LOOSESTRIFE.
pussywillow see WILLOW.
Quaker bonnet see SKULLCAP.
quaking aspen see POPLAR.
Queen Anne's lace see WILD CARROT.
queen of the meadow see
    MEADOWSWEET.
Quercus marina see BLADDERWRACK.
Quercus robur see OAK.
quick-in-the-hand see JEWEL WEED.
quillai see SOAP BARK.
quillaja see SOAP BARK.
quillaja bark see SOAP BARK.
Quillaja saponaria see SOAP BARK.
quinsy berries see BLACKCURRANT.
rabbits see YELLOW TOAD FLAX.
ragged cup see CUP PLANT.
rag paper see MULLEIN.
rainbow weed see PURPLE
    LOOSESTRIFE.
ramsted see YELLOW TOAD FLAX.
ramsthorn see BUCKTHORN.
Ranunculus ficaria see PILEWORT.

Raphanus sativus see RADISH.
rattle pouches see SHEPHERD'S PURSE.
rattleroot see BLACK COHOSH.
rattlesnake root see SENEGA
    SNAKEROOT.
rattleweed see BLACK COHOSH.
red bay see MAGNOLIA.
red bearberry see UVA-URSI.
red-beery see UVA-URSI.
red-berried trailing arbutus
    see UVA-URSI.
red berry see GINSENG.
redberry leaves see UVA-URSI.
red cole see HORSERADISH.
red elm see SLIPPERY ELM.
red ginseng see RED SAGE.
red gum see EUCALYPTUS.
red-ink plant see POKEROOT.
red legs see BISTORT.
red pepper see CAYENNE.
red raspberry see RASPBERRY.
red-rooted sage see RED SAGE.
red-rooted salvia see RED SAGE.
red rot see SUNDEW.
red sage (*Salvia officinalis*) see SAGE.
red sorrel see HIBISCUS.
red sunflower see ECHINACEA.
red weed see POKEROOT.
Rehmannia glutinosa see
    REHMANNIA.
reseda see HENNA.
rest-harrow see SPINY REST HARROW.
Rhamnus cathartica see BUCKTHORN.
Rhamnus catharticus see
    BUCKTHORN.
Rhamnus frangula see FRANGULA.
rhatania see RHATANY.
rheumatism root see WILD YAM.
rheumatism weed see PIPSISSEWA.
Rheum palmatum see CHINESE
    RHUBARB.
rhubarb see CHINESE RHUBARB.
Ribes nigrum see BLACKCURRANT.
ribwort plantain see PLANTAIN.
richweed see BLACK COHOSH.
Robin-run-in-the-hedge see
    GROUND IVY.
rockbeery see UVA-URSI.
rock fern see MAIDENHAIR FERN.
rock parsley see PARSLEY.
rock selinon see PARSLEY.
rockwrack see BLADDERWRACK.
Roman plant, the see SWEET CICELY.
Roman chamomile see ENGLISH
    CHAMOMILE.

Roman laurel see LAUREL.
Rosa centifolia see ROSE.
rose apple see JAMBUL.
rose bay willow herb see WILLOW
    HERB.
roselle see HIBISCUS.
rosemarine see ROSEMARY.
rosenoble see FIGWORT.
rose pink see CENTAURY.
rosinweed see CUP PLANT.
Rosmarinus officinalis see ROSEMARY.
rubbed thyme see THYME.
Rubus fruticosus see BLACKBERRY.
Rubus idaeus see RASPBERRY.
rudbeckia see ECHINACEA.
rumax see YELLOW DOCK.
rum cherry see BLACK CHERRY.
Rumex crispus see YELLOW DOCK.
running Jenny see MONEYWORT.
Ruscus aculeatus see BUTCHER'S
    BROOM.
Russian licorice see LICORICE.
rustic treacle see GARLIC.
sabal see SAW PALMETTO.
Sabal serrulata see SAW PALMETTO.
sabline rouge see ARENARIA RUBRA.
Saccharomyces cereviseae see
    BREWER'S YEAST.
sad dock see YELLOW DOCK.
sagackhomi see UVA-URSI.
sage of Bethlehem see SPEARMINT.
sahlep see SALEP.
salicaire see PURPLE LOOSESTRIFE.
salicin willow see WILLOW.
Salix alba see WILLOW.
Salix daphnoides see WILLOW.
Salix fragilis see WILLOW.
Salix nigra see WILLOW.
Salix purpurea see WILLOW.
sallow thorn see SEA BUCKTHORN.
saloop see SALEP.
salsify see COMFREY.
Salvia miltiorrhiza see RED SAGE.
Salvia officinalis see SAGE.
Sampson root see ECHINACEA.
sandberry see UVA-URSI.
sanderswood see SANDALWOOD.
sand plantain see INDIAN PLANTAGO.
sandwort see ARENARIA RUBRA.
sanguinaria see BLOODROOT.
Sanguinaria canadensis see
    BLOODROOT.
sanguinary see SHEPHERD'S PURSE
    (*Capsella bursa-pastoris*); YARROW
    (*Achillea millefolium*).

Sanicula europaea see SANICLE.
Santalum album see SANDALWOOD.
Santa Maria see FEVERFEW.
Santolina chamaecyparissias see
LAVENDER COTTON.
Saponaria officinalis see SOAPWORT.
Satureja hortensis see SAVORY.
satyrion see SALEP.
saxifrage see PIMPINELLA.
Scabiosa succisa see PREMORSE.
scabish see EVENING PRIMROSE.
scarlet sage see SAGE.
Schisandra chinensis see
SCHISANDRA.
schloss tea see MARSHMALLOW.
scoke see POKEROOT.
Scolopendrium vulgare see
HARTSTONGUE.
scoparium see BROOM.
Scotch barley see BARLEY.
Scotch fir see SCOTCH PINE.
scouring rush see HORSETAIL.
Scrophularia nodosa see FIGWORT.
scrubby grass see SCURVY GRASS.
scurvy root see ECHINACEA.
Scutellaria lateriflora see SKULLCAP.
sealroot see SOLOMON'S SEAL.
sealwort see SOLOMON'S SEAL.
sea parsley see LOVAGE.
seawrack see BLADDERWRACK.
self-heal see SANICLE (*Sanicula
europaea*).
seneca see SENEGA SNAKEROOT.
seneca snakeroot see SENEGA
SNAKEROOT.
senega see SENEGA SNAKEROOT.
septfoil see TORMENTIL.
serenoa see SAW PALMETTO.
Serenoa repens see SAW PALMETTO.
serpentaria see MONEYWORT.
serpyllum see WILD THYME.
setewale see VALERIAN.
setwell see VALERIAN.
seven barks see HYDRANGEA.
shave grass see HORSETAIL.
sheep rot see GOTU KOLA.
shepherd's club see MULLEIN.
shepherd's heart see SHEPHERD'S
PURSE.
shepherd's knapperty see
TORMENTIL.
shepherd's knot see TORMENTIL.
shepherd's needle see SWEET CICELY.
shepherd's scrip see SHEPHERD'S
PURSE.

shepherd's sprout see SHEPHERD'S
PURSE.
shepherd's staff see MULLEIN.
shepherd's thyme see WILD THYME.
shigoka see SIBERIAN GINSENG.
shrub palmetto see SAW PALMETTO.
sicklewort see SELFHEAL.
Silphium perfoliatum see CUP PLANT.
silver cinquefoil see POTENTILLA.
silverweed see JEWEL WEED.
Silybum marianum see MILK THISTLE.
simpler's joy see VERVAIN.
Sinapis alba see MUSTARD.
single chamomile see GERMAN
CHAMOMILE.
skoke see POKEROOT.
skunkweed see SKUNK CABBAGE.
slippery root see COMFREY.
slough-heal see SELFHEAL.
smallage see CELERY.
smallwort see PILEWORT.
Smilax officinalis see SARSAPARILLA.
smooth lawsonia see HENNA.
snakebite see BLOODROOT.
snakeroot see SENEGA SNAKEROOT.
snakeweed see ASTHMA PLANT
(*Euphorbia hirta*); BISTORT
(*Polygonum bistorta* or *Persicaria
bistorta*).
snap bean see BEANS.
snapdragon see YELLOW TOAD FLAX.
snapping hazel see WITCH HAZEL.
soap root see SOAPWORT.
soap tree see SOAP BARK.
soapwood see SOAPWORT.
soldiers see PURPLE LOOSESTRIFE.
soldier's woundwort see YARROW.
Solidago virgaurea see GOLDENROD.
sorghum see BROOMCORN.
Sorghum vulgare see BROOMCORN.
sour dock see YELLOW DOCK.
Spanish chestnut see HORSE
CHESTNUT.
Spanish licorice see LICORICE.
sparrow grass see ASPARAGUS.
speckled Jewels see JEWEL WEED.
Spergularia rubra see ARENARIA
RUBRA.
spignet see SPIKENARD.
spiked willow sage see PURPLE
LOOSESTRIFE.
Spireaea ulmaria see MEADOWSWEET.
spire mint see SPEARMINT.
spogel see INDIAN PLANTAGO.
spoonwort see SCURVY GRASS.

spotted alder see WITCH HAZEL.
spotted thistle see BLESSED THISTLE.
spotted touch-me-not see JEWEL
WEED.
spruce fir see SPRUCE.
squawroot see BLUE COHOSH
(*Caulophyllum thalictroides*); BLACK
COHOSH (*Cimicifuga racemosa*).
squinancy berries see BLACKCURRANT.
stags horn see CLUB MOSS.
star of the earth see GEUM.
staunchweed see YARROW.
stayplough see SPINY REST HARROW.
St. Benedict's thistle see BLESSED
THISTLE.
stellaria see LADY'S MANTLE.
stemless gentian see YELLOW
GENTIAN.
sticklewort see AGRIMONY.
stickwort see AGRIMONY.
stigmata maydis see CORN SILK.
stingless nettle see WHITE DEAD
NETTLE.
stinking rose see GARLIC.
stinking Tommy see SPINY REST
HARROW.
St. James' weed see SHEPHERD'S PURSE.
St. Mary's seal see SOLOMON'S SEAL.
Stockholm tar see SCOTCH PINE.
storkbill see HERB ROBERT.
string bean see BEANS.
string of sovereigns see
MONEYWORT.
stringy bark tree see EUCALYPTUS.
striped alder see WITCH HAZEL.
strong-scented lettuce see
LACTUCARIUM.
succory see CHICORY.
summer savory see SAVORY.
sundrop see EVENING PRIMROSE.
superb pink see FRINGED PINK.
suterberry see NORTHERN PRICKLY ASH.
swallow-wort see PLEURISY ROOT.
swamp laurel see MAGNOLIA.
swamp sassafras see MAGNOLIA.
swamp tea tree see CAJUPUT.
sweating plant see BONESET.
sweet bay see LAUREL (*Laurus noblis*);
MAGNOLIA (*Magnolia glauca*).
sweet Betty see SOAPWORT.
sweet bracken see SWEET CICELY.
sweet broom see BUTCHER'S BROOM.
sweet chervil see SWEET CICELY.
sweet cumin see ANISE.
sweet-cus see SWEET CICELY.

sweet dock see BISTORT.
sweet elm see SLIPPERY ELM.
sweet-fern see SWEET CICELY.
sweet-humlock see SWEET CICELY.
sweet lucernce see SWEETCLOVER.
sweet marjoram see MARJORAM.
sweet Mary see LEMON BALM.
sweet pepper see CAYENNE.
sweet root see LICORICE.
sweets see SWEET CICELY.
sweet slumber see BLOODROOT.
sweet weed see MARSHMALLOW.
sweet wood see LICORICE.
sweet wort see LICORICE.
Swertia chirata see CHIRETTA.
swine snout see DANDELION.
Swiss mountain pine see SCOTCH PINE.
Symphytum officinale see COMFREY.
Symplocarpus foetidus see SKUNK CABBAGE.
Syzygium aromaticum see CLOVE.
Syzygium cumini see JAMBUL.
tabasco pepper see CAYENNE.
Tabebuia impetignosa see LAPACHO.
talepetrako see GOTU KOLA.
tallow shrub see SOUTHERN BAYBERRY.
tall speedwell see BLACK ROOT.
tall Veronica see BLACK ROOT.
Tamarindus indica see TAMARIND.
Tanacetum parthenium see FEVERFEW.
tanner's oak see OAK.
taraxacum see DANDELION.
Taraxacum officinale see DANDELION.
Tasmanian blu gum see EUCALYPTUS.
teasel see BONESET.
Terminalia arjuna see ARJUNA.
tetterwort see CELANDINE.
Teucrium scorodonia see WOOD SAGE.
Theobroma cacao see COCOA.
thick-leaved pennywort see GOTU KOLA.
thimbleberry see BLACKBERRY.
thormantle see TORMENTIL.
thorny burr see BURDOCK.
thoroughwort see BONESET.
thousand seal see YARROW.
thousand weed see YARROW.
throatwort see FIGWORT.
throw-wort see MOTHERWORT.
Thymus serpyllum see WILD THYME.
Thymus vulgaris see THYME.
Tilia cordata see LINDEN.

Tilia europaea see LINDEN.
toadpipe see HORSETAIL (*Equisetum arvense*); YELLOW TOAD FLAX (*Linaria vulgaris*).
tobacco wood see WITCH HAZEL.
tonga see KAVA KAVA.
toothache tree see NORTHERN PRICKLY ASH.
torches see MULLEIN.
torch weed see MULLEIN.
touch-me-not see SIBERIAN GINSENG.
toywort see SHEPHERD'S PURSE.
trackleberry see BILBERRY.
trailing tansy see POTENTILLA.
trefoil see BUCKBEAN (*Menyanthes trifoliata*); RED CLOVER (*Trifolium pratense*).
trembling poplar see POPLAR.
Trifolium pratense see RED CLOVER.
Trigonella foenum-graecum see FENUGREEK.
Tropaeolum majus see NASTURTIUM.
true angostura see ANGOSTURA.
true cowslips see COWSLIP.
true ginseng see GINSENG.
true ivy see ENGLISH IVY.
true laurel see LAUREL.
true sage see SAGE.
tuber root see PLEURISY ROOT.
tun-hoof see GROUND IVY.
Turkey rhubarb see CHINESE RHUBARB.
Turkish licorice see LICORICE.
turmeric (*Curcuma zedoria*) see ZEDOARY.
turmeric root see GOLDENSEAL.
Turnera diffusa see DAMIANA.
turnhoof see GROUND IVY.
turpentine weed see CUP PLANT.
twopenny grass see MONEYWORT.
Ulmus fulva see SLIPPERY ELM.
Ulmus minor see ELM BARK.
Ulmus rubra see SLIPPERY ELM.
umbellate wintergreen see PIPISSEWA.
upland cranbeery see UVA-URSI.
upland cranberry see UVA-URSI.
Urginea maritima sée SQUILL.
Urtica dioica see STINGING NETTLE.
ussarian thorny pepperbush see SIBERIAN GINSENG.
Utricularia vulgaris see BLADDERWORT.
Vaccinium myrtillus see BILBERRY.
Valeriana officinalis see VALERIAN.
vandal root see VALERIAN.

vapor see FUMITORY.
vegetable antimony see BONESET.
vegetable sulfur see CLUB MOSS.
vegetable tallow see SOUTHERN BAYBERRY.
velvet dock see ELECAMPANE.
velvet plant see MULLEIN.
Venus hair see MAIDENHAIR FERN.
Verbascum densiflorum see MULLEIN.
Verbena officinalis see VERVAIN.
Veronica officinalis see SPEEDWELL.
Viburnum opulus see GUELDER ROSE.
Viola tricolor see HEARTSEASE.
violet willow see WILLOW.
Virginian prune see BLACK CHERRY.
Virginia poke see POKEROOT.
Virginia water horehound see BUGLEWEED.
Viscum album see MISTLETOE.
Vitex agnus-castus see CHASTE TREE.
vitex chasteberry see CHASTE TREE.
vomitroot see LOBELIA.
wallwort see COMFREY.
walnut, English see WALNUT.
wandering Jenny see MONEYWORT.
wandering tailor see MONEYWORT.
warnera see GOLDENSEAL.
water bugle see BUGLEWEED.
water lemon see PASSIONFLOWER.
water mint see WILD MINT.
water pepper see SMARTWEED.
water shamrock see BUCKBEAN.
wax bean see BEANS.
wax dolls see FUMITORY.
wax myrtle see SOUTHERN BAYBERRY.
way Bennet see GEUM.
waythorn see BUCKTHORN.
West Indian dogwood see JAMAICA DOGWOOD.
wet-a-bed see DANDELION.
whig plant see ENGLISH CHAMOMILE.
white archangel see WHITE DEAD NETTLE.
white bay see MAGNOLIA.
white laurel see MAGNOLIA.
white maoow see MARSHMALLOW.
white murda see ARJUNA.
white mustard see MUSTARD.
white poplar see POPLAR.
white root see PLEURISY ROOT.
white rot see GOTU KOLA.
white saunders see SANDALWOOD.
white tea tree see CAJUPUT.
whitethorn see HAWTHORN.

white walnut see BUTTERNUT.
white willow see WILLOW.
white wood see CAJUPUT.
whorlywort see BLACK ROOT.
whortleberry see BILBERRY.
wild agrimony see POTENTILLA.
wild angelica see ANGELICA.
wild balsam see JEWEL WEED.
wild black cherry see BLACK CHERRY.
wild celandine see JEWEL WEED.
wild celery see CELERY.
wild chamomile see FEVERFEW
(*Tanacetum parthenium*); GERMAN
CHAMOMILE (*Matricaria chamomilla,
M. recutita, Chamomilla recutita*).
wild cherry see BLACK CHERRY.
wild clover see RED CLOVER.
wild crane's-bill see HERB ROBERT.
wild curcuma see GOLDENSEAL.
wild endive see DANDELION.
wild ice leaf see MULLEIN.
wild laburnum see SWEETCLOVER.
wild lady's slipper see JEWEL WEED.
wild licorice see SPINY REST HARROW.
wild pansy see HEARTSEASE.
wild passion flower see
PASSIONFLOWER.
wild pepper see SIBERIAN GINSENG.
wild plum see SLOE.
wild quinine see FEVERFEW.
wild rye see GEUM.
wild succory see CENTAURY.
wild sunflower see ELECAMPANE.
wild sweet William see SOAPWORT.
wild tobacco see LOBELIA.
wild yam root see WILD YAM.
willow-herb see WILLOW HERB.
wind flower see PASQUE FLOWER.
wind root see PLEURISY ROOT.
wineberry see BILBERRY.
winterbloom see WITCH HAZEL.
winterlien see FLAX.

witch meal see CLUB MOSS.
Withania somniferum see WITHANIA.
withe withy see WILLOW.
wolfsbane see ARNICA.
wolfs claw see CLUB MOSS.
woodbind see ENGLISH IVY.
woodbine see HONEYSUCKLE.
wood spider see DEVIL'S CLAW.
woollen see MULLEIN.
woundwort see GOLDENROD
(*Solidago virgaurea*); SELFHEAL
(*Prunella vulgaris*).
wu-wei-zi see SCHISANDRA.
wymote see MARSHMALLOW.
yama see WILD YAM.
yarroway see YARROW.
yasti-madhu see LICORICE.
yellow avens see GEUM.
yellow chaste weed see IMMORTELLE.
yellow ginseng see BLUE COHOSH.
yellow leader see ASTRAGALUS.
yellow puccoon see GOLDENSEAL.
yellow rod see YELLOW TOAD FLAX.
yellow root see GOLDENSEAL.
yellow saunders see SANDALWOOD.
yellow starwort see ELECAMPANE.
yellow sweet clover see
SWEETCLOVER.
yellow wood see NORTHERN PRICKLY
ASH.
yerba maté see MATÉ.
youthwort see SUNDEW.
Yucca brevifolia see YUCCA.
zaffer see SAFFLOWER.
Zanthoxylum americanum see
NORTHERN PRICKLY ASH.
Zanthoxylum clava-herculis see
SOUTHERN PRICKLY ASH.
Zanzibar pepper see CAYENNE.
Zea mays see CORN SILK.

acanthus
(*Acanthus mollis*; Parts used: leaves, root)
Acanthus is rich in tannins and mucilage, and has been used for centuries to treat ✪ **burns** and in bindings for dislocated joints. Its emollient and astringent activities are due to its mucilage and tannin content.

Warnings, interactions, and side effects
Although none have been reported with correct use and dosage, the properties of acanthus have not been fully investigated and adverse reactions are possible.

achyranthes
(*Achyranthes bidentata; root*)
Achyranthes contains a number of triterpene saponins. Traditional uses include promoting blood flow, and treating ✪ **mouth ulcers**, bleeding gums, and ✪ **nosebleeds**. Research has shown that it has the ability to dilate blood vessels of the periperhal vasculature.

Warnings, interactions, and side effects
• Achyranthes should not be used during pregnancy because it could cause abortions.

agrimony
(*Agrimonia eupatoria*)
Other common names: **church steeples, cocklebur, common agrimony, liverwort, philanthropos, sticklewort, stickwort.**
Agrimony is a faintly aromatic perennial herb, which grows from an underground rhizome to a height of approximately 3 feet (90 centimeters). The plant generally grows in damp conditions, such as marshes, wet fields, and patches of wasteground. The hairy stems of the plant bear three to five pairs of downy leaves, and in summer racemes of small yellow flowers.

Forms of preparation and parts used
The aerial parts of agrimony are used, usually as a tincture, infusion, or simply as the dried herb.

Active components
Agrimony contains a number of flavonoids and tannins, as well as phytosterols and vitamins.

Uses in treatment
Agrimony is traditionally used to staunch blood flow, and as a general digestive tonic, especially for ✪ **diarrhea**. It has also been used for ✪ **cystitis**, ✪ **arthritis**, and as a gargle for sore throats (see ✪ **pharyngitis**). It is approved by some authorities for use in the treatment of skin inflammation (see ✪ **skin conditions**), mouth and pharynx inflammation, and diarrhea. Research suggests that agrimony infusions could be used for cutaneous porphyria, and that blood coagulation can be increased using the herb. Other studies have shown that agrimony extracts also have hypotensive activity.

Warnings, interactions, and side effects
• Although there are no reported toxic effects of agrimony with correct use and dosage, prolonged or excessive use of the herb is not recommended for anyone on medication for high or low blood pressure.
• Similarly, anyone taking an ℞ **anticoagulant** drug should avoid the herb.

alfalfa
(*Medicago sativa*; Parts used: herb)
Other common names: **buffalo herb, lucerne, purple medic, purple medick, purple medicle.**
Alfalfa contains plant acids, pyrrolidine alkaloids, saponins, sterols, flavonoids, and vitamins. It is widely used as a foodstuff, and in the treatment of ✪ **vitamin deficiencies**. Alfalfa has been shown to be able to lower levels of sugar and fat in the blood (see ✪ **hyperlipidemia**).

Warnings, interactions, and side effects
• Alfalfa should not be taken in excess because of its estrogenic activity and effects on blood clotting.

aloe
(*Aloe barbadensis, A. capensis, A. vera*)
Other common names: **aloes, aloe vera.**
Aloe is a succulent perennial with long prickly leaves up to 2 feet (60 centimeters) in length. The plant produces spikes of yellow-orange flowers. It is native to tropical regions, although it is also widely cultivated.

Forms of preparation and parts used
The leaf mucilage and juice are used. The mucilage is usually used fresh from the leaves, from which a gel can be squeezed. The juice, which is a quite different product, is obtained from the basal region of the leaves (sometimes referred to as "bitter aloes") and can be dried before taking by mouth. Commercial aloe juice can also be prepared from the leaf gel. Aloe is often sold in multi-herb products. All the various aloe preparations are among the most used herbal remedies in the US.

Active components
Aloe contains tannins, numerous sugars, saponins, lipids, anthraquinones, and organic acids.

Uses in treatment
Aloe gel is widely used in preparations for external use for ✪ **wounds**, ✪ **burns**, and ✪ **skin conditions**, as an immune stimulant, and has been shown to be beneficial in treating skin ulcers (see ✪ **ulcer**) and radiation burns. Leaf extracts, applied externally, have anti-inflammatory and wound-healing properties. Taken internally, the juice has laxative activity, due to the anthraquinone content of the leaves from which it is made. At low doses, the bitter taste of the juice can also stimulate the appetite (see ✪ **appetite loss**). In higher doses, the juice can have a strong purgative effect, and it is approved by some authorities for the treatment of ✪ **constipation**. The gel when incorporated into drinks can become mixed with the juice and so can take on laxative properties.

Warnings, interactions, and side effects
• Aloe should not be used during pregnancy.
• External application of the gel is thought to have no side effects, but rarely there may be an allergic reaction. The juice should not be applied to the skin at any time.
• It should be used with caution when breast-feeding, or by anyone with kidney disease or hemorrhoids.
• Some authorities do not recommend the use of aloe internally at all.

• It should not be used by people who are immunocompromised unless under medical supervision.

• As with other stimulant anthraquinone laxatives (including ♣ **rhubarb, Chinese,** ♣ **frangula,** ♣ **yellow dock,** and ℞ **senna**) long-term use of aloe vera juice should be avoided.

angelica
(*Angelica archangelica*)
Other common names: **American angelica, angel's wort, European angelica, garden angelica, masterwort, wild angelica.**

Angelica is a robust aromatic biennial with stout hollow stems and deeply divided leaves, which can grow to a height of about 6 feet (2 meters). In early summer, the plant develops umbels of very small pale green-white flowers, which develop into characteristic seed heads.

Forms of preparation and parts used
Most parts of the plant are used medicinally, including the dried roots (actually rhizomes), leaves, stem, and seeds ("fruit").

Active components
Angelica contains a number of coumarins, (furanocoumarins or psoralens), and an essential oil rich in phellandrenes.

Uses in treatment
Angelica is described as having antispasmodic, expectorant, diaphoretic, diuretic, carminative, and anti-inflammatory properties. It has traditionally been used to treat ✪ **pleurisy** and ✪ **bronchitis**, rheumatoid disease (see ✪ **arthritis** and ✪ **musculoskeletal disorders**), ✪ **indigestion**, and ✪ **catarrh**. The root of angelica has also been used to treat ✪ **colic**. It is a warming tonic and is commonly used to improve circulation, especially in the arms and legs. Some authorities approve the use of the root for ✪ **fever** and ✪ **colds**, indigestion, ✪ **appetite loss**, and ✪ **urinary tract disorders**.

Warnings, interactions, and side effects
Although angelica is listed by the FDA as GRAS ("generally recognized as safe"), side effects have been described.

• Photosensitization (sensitivity to light) has been reported, which can result in a rash, severe sunburn, or other skin reactions on exposure to the sun or other ultraviolet light. It is caused by the furanocoumarin (psoralen) components of the herb. Such furanocoumarin compounds are claimed to be absent from oils when they are obtained from the herb by steam distillation.

• Angelica root is reported to be an abortifacient (induces termination of pregnancy) and can affect the menstrual cycle. As such, use of angelica (above the levels found in foods) should be avoided during pregnancy and also by breast-feeding mothers.

• It should be noted that *Angelica archangelica* has different properties from another angelica, *Angelica sinensis* (also called dang gui, dong quai).

angostura
(*Galipea officinalis*; Parts used: bark)
Other common names: **cusparia bark, true angostura.**
Angostura contains quinoline alkaloids, a volatile oil, and iridoids. Traditional uses include for ✪ **diarrhea** and ✪ **fever**. The bitter iridoids contribute to digestive activity, and the whole bark has emetic and laxative properties when taken in large doses.

Warnings, interactions, and side effects
Although none have been reported with correct use and dosage, the properties of angostura have not been fully investigated and adverse reactions are possible.

anise
(*Pimpinella anisum*)
Other common names: **aniseed, aniseed, sweet cumin.**
Anise is an erect annual with divided leaves and grows to a height of approximately 2 feet (60 centimeters). It produces tiny off-white flowers in the summer, followed by small, ribbed seeds.

Forms of preparation and parts used
The fruit (seeds) and essential oil can be used medicinally. The seeds are usually taken in the form of an infusion. It appears as a flavorant in many combination cough, stomach-soothing, flatulence, and congestion remedies.

Active components
Anise contains a large number of flavonoids, terpenoids, coumarins, and a volatile oil rich in trans-anethole.

Uses in treatment
Anise has expectorant, antispasmodic, carminative, and antiparasitic properties. The seeds are widely used to ease bloating, ✪ **flatulence,** ✪ **nausea,** and to aid digestion. They are also used to treat ✪ **colic** in infants. The expectorant and antispasmodic effects of the seeds are used for ✪ **asthma** and ✪ **bronchitis**, and can also be used to stimulate milk production (lactation). The diluted essential oil can be applied externally for the treatment of head lice (see ✪ **lice and mite infestation**) (anethole being the main active ingredient). Anise is approved by some authorities for the common ✪ **cold,** ✪ **fever,** ✪ **cough** and bronchitis, mouth and pharynx inflammation (see ✪ **pharyngitis**), ✪ **appetite loss** and ✪ **indigestion**. Traditionally, anise has been used for hormonal purposes, including as a milk-stimulant and there is some evidence of estrogenic activity in anethole metabolites.

Warnings, interactions, and side effects
• Aniseed (especially the volatile oil) can cause allergic reactions, and the oil should not be applied to the skin of people who have dermatitis, or any inflammatory or allergic condition.

• Do not take the oil internally except under expert supervision, as even small amounts can cause vomiting and seizures.

• Excessive intake may interfere with hormone treatments, including the contraceptive pill. However, taking normal dietary levels of anise during pregnancy and breast-feeding are not thought to cause any adverse effects.

Apium graveolens
see ♣ **celery.**

arenaria rubra
(*Spergularia rubra*; Parts used: herb)
Other common names: **common sandspurry, sabline rouge, sandwort.**

Arenaria rubra contains triterpene saponins and resinous materials, and has diuretic activity. It is used for ✪ **urinary tract disorders**, including ✪ **cystitis**, dysuria, and urinary ✪ **calculus**.

Warnings, interactions, and side effects
Although none have been reported with correct use and dosage, the properties of arenaria rubra have not been fully investigated and adverse reactions are possible.

arjuna
(*Terminalia arjuna*; Parts used: bark)
Other common names: **arjun tree, white murda.**
Arjuna contains tannins, flavonoids, and saponins. Traditional uses include as a heart tonic, and recent research has shown the bark to lower blood cholesterol levels and to have an effect on the heart (although the results of these studies are inconclusive).

Warnings, interactions, and side effects
Although none have been reported with correct use and dosage, the properties of arjuna have not been fully investigated and adverse reactions are possible.

arnica
(*Arnica montana*; Parts used: flowerheads)
Other common names: **arnica flowers, arnica root, leopard's bane, mountain tobacco, wolfsbane.**
Arnica contains a number of sesquiterpene lactones and a volatile oil. It has been shown to have antiphlogistic, analgesic, and antiseptic properties, and can increase cardiac output. It is used externally for treating injuries, such as bruises, contusions, and joint pains (as well as rheumatic complaints: see ✪ **musculoskeletal disorders**), and also for inflammation of the mouth and throat, boils, and for insect bites. It is approved for these uses by some authorities.

Warnings, interactions, and side effects
• Arnica is for external use only.
• It may cause allergic reactions in some people.
• It may enhance the effect of ℞ **anticoagulant** drugs (for example warfarin sodium).

arrowroot
(*Maranta arundinaceae*; Parts used: rhizome)
Other common names: **maranta.**
Arrowroot is mainly composed of various starches. The root has soothing demulcent activity and increases the elimination of bile acids. Traditional uses include as a nutritive, a dietary aid, and for ✪ **diarrhea**.

Warnings, interactions, and side effects
Although none have been reported with correct use and dosage, the properties of arrowroot have not been fully investigated and adverse reactions are possible.

artichoke
(*Cynara scolymus*)
Other common names: **garden artichoke, globe artichoke.**
Artichoke is a member of the *Compositaea* family and should not be confused with the Jerusalem artichoke (sunchoke: *Helianthus*

tuberosus). It is a perennial herb that can grow to a height of 5 feet (1.5 meters). It has grey-green thistle-like leaves with a downy underside, and large purple flowerheads.

Forms of preparation and parts used
The flowerheads, leaves, and roots of the artichoke are all used medicinally.

Active components
Artichoke contains phenolic acid derivatives, a number of flavonoid glycosides, sesquiterpene lactones (such as cynaropicrin and analogs), caffeic acid derivatives (such as cynarin/cynarine, chlorogenic acid and analogs), volatile oil, phytosterols, and tannins. Some preparations are marketed with standardized caffeoylquinic acids content (chlorogenic acid or cynarin).

Uses in treatment
Artichoke is described as having diuretic, hypolipidemic and hypocholesterolemic (blood fat and cholesterol-lowering), choleretic, and hepatostimulant (liver-stimulant) properties. The bitterness of the plant, mainly due to the chemical cynaropicrin, stimulates digestive secretions, especially bile, making the plant a useful treatment for ✪ **nausea**, ✪ **indigestion**, and ✪ **gallbladder disorders**. The plant is also used in the early stages of type 2 (adult-onset) ✪ **diabetes mellitus**, because it can lower blood sugar levels. It is approved by some authorities for indigestion. In laboratory studies, artichoke has been shown to both protect and promote regeneration of the liver. However, clinical evidence for the proposed cholesterol-lowering activity of cynarin is contradictory and not conclusive.

Warnings, interactions, and side effects
• Cynaropicrin, which is found in artichoke, may cause allergic reactions in people with hypersensitivity to members of the daisy family. Crude artichoke extracts have been shown to be less toxic than partially purified extracts, although toxicity data has not been extensively documented.
• As a herbal remedy, therefore, artichoke should be avoided during pregnancy and by breast-feeding mothers.
• It should not be taken by people who have bile duct blockages because it stimulates the biliary tract.

asafoetida
(*Ferula foetida* or *F. assafoetida*)
Other common names: **asant, devil's dung, food of the gods, gum asafoetida.**
Asafoetida is a large perennial which grows up to 6 feet (1.8 meters) tall. It has a stocky rhizome, highly divided garlic-scented leaves, and very small yellowish flowers in summer. Small seeds are usually produced in the plant's fifth season, after which it dies.

Forms of preparation and parts used
The oleo-gum (oleo meaning oily), which is a gum-resin obtained from cutting the rhizomes and roots of asafoetida, is used medicinally.

Active components
The oleo-gum is rich in a sulfurous volatile oil, and the chief constituent, sec-propenyl-isobutyl disulfide, is one of a series of sulfurous compounds found in garlic and onions. The gum contains a

number of sugars and glucuronic acid, and the resin contains ferulic acid (a caffeic acid derivative) esters, and coumarin derivatives.

Uses in treatment

Asafoetida is used as a carminative, antispasmodic, and expectorant. The sulfurous components of the volatile oil are thought to be responsible for protective activity of the herb against hyperlipidemia. Although sometimes used for irritable bowel syndrome, two clinical studies for the use of asafoetida for this disorder failed to show any beneficial effects.

Warnings, interactions, and side effects

• Asafoetida should not be given to infants.

• Laboratory studies have indicated that the coumarin components may cause genetic damage to sperm.

• Medicinal use of asafoetida should be avoided during pregnancy (though its normal use in food should cause no problems).

• The resin should not be used if breast-feeding because of possible damage to the baby's hemoglobin should toxic components of the herb enter breast milk.

• Excessive use of the plant should be avoided at all times.

ash

(*Fraxinus excelsior*; Parts used: leaves and bark)
Other common names: **bird's tongue, common ash, European ash, weeping ash.**
Ash contains tannins, flavonoids, terpenoids, and mucilage. Traditional uses include as a tonic and for ✪ **fever**. It is known to have analgesic, antiphlogistic, and ⚗ **antioxidant** activities.

Warnings, interactions, and side effects

Although none have been reported with correct use and dosage, the properties of ash have not been fully investigated and adverse reactions are possible.

asparagus

(*Asparagus officinalis*; Parts used: whole plant)
Other common names: **sparrow grass.**
The aerial parts of asparagus contain flavonoids and steroidal saponins. The rhizome/roots contain steroidal saponins and ⚗ **amino acids**. Both parts of the plant are used as diuretics (see ✪ **fluid retention**). This activity has been scientifically confirmed for the underground parts. Asparagus is approved by some authorities for irrigation therapy for inflammatory ✪ **urinary tract disorders** and kidney stones (see ✪ **calculus**).

Warnings, interactions, and side effects

• Asparagus should not be used by anyone with kidney disease because of the irritating effect of saponins.

• The plant, including the underground parts, may cause mild skin irritation with prolonged contact.

astragalus

(*Astragalus membranaceus*)
Other common names: **huang-qi, milk vetch, yellow leader.**
Astragalus is a perennial shrub with variable hairy stems and highly divided, lobed leaves. It can grow up to 18 inches (45 centimeters) in height, and produces yellow, pea-like flowers in summer, fol-

lowed by seed pods up to 6 inches (15 centimeters) long. Roots are often collected after four years of cultivation.

Forms of preparation and parts used

Astragalus roots are the most commonly used part medicinally, usually as a decoction, tincture, or lightly cooked.

Active components

Astragalus contains a number of phytosterols, triterpene glycosides (including a series of related compounds, called astragalosides), fatty acids, and flavonoids.

Uses in treatment

Astragalus is most commonly used as an adaptogen and a stimulant of the immune system. Chinese research suggests improved endurance, and also diuretic and hypotensive activities. Laboratory studies have been carried out on astragulus, and Astragaloside I (and, to a lesser extent, other astrangalosides) has been shown to affect a number of molecules involved in immune responses in the body. Astragaloside II was found to have antiviral activity.

Warnings, interactions, and side effects

• Astragalus should not be used during pregnancy or when breast-feeding.

• It should be used with caution and under expert supervision by anyone taking immunosuppresive or anticoagulant drugs.

avocado

(*Persea americana*; Parts used: leaves, bark, fruit)
Avocado contains flavonoids and tannins (leaves, bark), vitamins, fats, and protein (fruit). The leaves and bark are used for ✪ **coughs** and as an astringent, while the fruit is used as an emollient and carminative. Avocado fruit has also been shown to aid lowering of blood cholesterol levels.

Warnings, interactions, and side effects

• The leaves and bark should not be used during pregnancy as they are reported to have abortifacient activity.

balsam fir

(*Abies balsamea*; Parts used: resin)
The leaves of balsam fir contain a liquid oleo-resin which has been used externally for sores, cuts, and burns. It has antiseptic and stimulant properties, and some authorities approve its use for ✪ **neuralgia** and rheumatism (see ✪ **musculoskeletal disorders**), however, it is no longer in common use.

Warnings, interactions, and side effects

Although none have been reported with correct use and dosage, the properties of balsam fir have not been fully investigated and adverse reactions are possible.

barley

(*Hordeum distychum or H. distichon*; Parts used: grain)
Other common names: **pearl barley, pot barley, Scotch barley.**
Barley contains polysaccharides, protein, and fatty acids. Traditional uses include for ✪ **diarrhea** and inflammatory bowel disorders (see ✪ **Crohn's disease** and ✪ **ulcerative colitis**). The grains have a soothing action on the alimentary tract.

Warnings, interactions, and side effects

• Barley should not be used during pregnancy.

beans

(*Phaseolus vulgaris*; Parts used: bean)

Other common names: **common bean, green bean, kidney bean, navy bean, pinto bean, snap bean, string bean, wax bean.**

Beans contain saponins, lectins, and flavonoids, and have a weak diuretic action. They are used to treat ✪ **urinary tract disorders** and kidney or bladder stones (see ✪ **calculus**).

Warnings, interactions, and side effects

• Without proper cooking, the lectin content can result in nausea, vomiting, and diarrhea.

bilberry

(*Vaccinium myrtillus*; Parts used: leaves and fruit)

Other common names: **airelle, black whortles, bleaberry, blueberry, burren myrtle, dyeberry, huckleberry, hurtleberry, hurts, trackleberry, whortleberry, wineberry.**

Bilberry leaves contain tannin, flavonoids, and iridoids, and are used for gastrointestinal disorders (see ✪ **digestive system disorders**) and ✪ **diabetes mellitus**. The antidiabetic activity may result from the chromium content of the leaves. Bilberry fruits contain fruit acids, anthocyanins, flavonoids, and caffeic acid derivatives. They have astringent properties and are used for ✪ **diarrhea** and inflammation of the mouth and/or pharynx (see ✪ **inflammation** and ✪ **pharyngitis**). Some authorities approve its use for these latter conditions and also for ✪ **hemorrhoids**, ✪ **venous insufficiency**, and spasmodic colitis.

Warnings, interactions, and side effects

• The tannin content of bilberry may result in gastrointestinal disturbances if large quantities are taken.

• Some research indicates that it may interfere with the effects of platelet aggregation inhibitor drugs such as ℞ **aspirin** and anticoagulants such as ℞ **warfarin**.

birch

(*Betula pendula*; Parts used: leaves and tar)

Birch leaves contain saponins, flavonoids, and a volatile oil. They have antipyretic properties (reduce fever), saluretic activity (they increase salt extraction), and also increase urine production, and are used to treat ✪ **urinary tract disorders**. The tar is rich in phenolic compounds and is used to treat parasitic infestations.

Warnings, interactions, and side effects

• Birch tar can cause skin irritation in some people.

bistort

(*Polygonum bistorta* or *Persicaria bistorta*; Parts used: leaves and rhizome)

Other common names: **adderwort, dragonwort, Easter giant, Easter ledges, Easter mangiant, oderwort, osterick, osterwort, patience dock, red legs, snakeweed, sweet dock.**

Bistort contains tannins and starch, and has astringent properties and stimulates mucus production. It is used as a ✪ **wound** ointment and in the treatment of ✪ **digestive system disorders**.

Warnings, interactions, and side effects

Although none have been reported with correct use and dosage, the properties of bistort have not been fully investigated and adverse reactions are possible.

bitter milkwort

(*Polygala amara*; Parts used: whole plant)

Other common names: **European bitter polygala, European senega snakeroot, evergreen snakeroot, flowering wintergreen, little pollom.**

Bitter milkwort contains saponins, bitter compounds, and derivatives of salicylic acid. It has mild expectorant activity and traditionally is used to treat ✪ **respiratory tract disorders** and ✪ **cough**.

Warnings, interactions, and side effects

Although none have been reported with correct use and dosage, the properties of bitter milkwort have not been fully investigated and adverse reactions are possible.

blackberry

(*Rubus fruticosus*; Parts used: leaves)

Other common names: **American dewberry, bramble, goutberry, high blackberry, thimbleberry.**

Blackberry contains tannins, flavonoids, and fruit acids, and its leaves have astringent activity. It is used for inflammation of the mouth and/or pharynx (see ✪ **inflammation** and ✪ **pharyngitis**) and acute ✪ **diarrhea**, and is approved for these uses by some authorities.

Warnings, interactions, and side effects

Although none have been reported with correct use and dosage, the properties of blackberry have not been fully investigated and adverse reactions are possible.

black cherry

(*Prunus serotina*; Parts used: bark)

Other common names: **black choke, choke cherry, rum cherry, Virginian prune, wild black cherry, wild cherry.**

Black cherry contains tannins and cyanogenic glycosides. The bark has astringent, antitussive, and sedative properties, and is used to treat ✪ **coughs** and ✪ **bronchitis**.

Warnings, interactions, and side effects

• The cyanogenic glycosides in black cherry are only potentially toxic in overdose quantities, and at medicinal levels no hazardous reactions have been reported.

black cohosh

(*Cimicifuga racemosa*)

Other common names: **black snakeroot, bugbane, bugwort, cimicifuga, rattleroot, rattleweed, richweed, squawroot.**

Black cohosh is native to Canada and the eastern US. It can grow to approximately 8 feet (2.5 meters) in height. It bears toothed three-lobed leaves, and in summer produces tall spikes of off-white, fragrant flowers. It is not related to ♣ **blue cohosh** (*Caulophyllum thalictroides*), although the two herbs have some uses in common.

Forms of preparation and parts used

The rhizome and roots of black cohosh are used medicinally, usually as a decoction, infusion, or tincture. It is often flavored with honey or lemon because of its bitter taste and unpleasant aroma.

Active components

Black cohosh contains quinolizidine alkaloids (including cytisine and methyl cytisine), terpenoids (triterpene glycosides including actein and cimifugoside), tannins, plant acids, isoflavone phytosterols (including formononetin), and a volatile oil.

Uses in treatment

Black cohosh is primarily used for rheumatic conditions (see ○ **musculoskeletal disorders**) and is approved by some authorities for ○ **premenstrual syndrome** (PMS) and ○ **dysmenorrhea**, and for complaints associated with ○ **menopause**. Laboratory and clinical studies have been carried out on black cohosh. Triterpene glycosides from black cohosh have lowered cholesterol level. Actein increased peripheral blood flow in people with peripheral arterial disease. Black cohosh extracts have a number of endocrine effects, and an alcoholic extract (Remifemin) has been marketed and prescribed in some countries for endocrine disorders in women. Endocrine effects include changes in secretion of the female hormones, including ℞ **gonadotropins** (luteinizing hormone (LH), follicle-stimulating hormone (FSH)) and estrogens. The antiestrogen activity of black cohosh is thought to be due to the formononetin content, which binds to estrogen receptors in the body and so preventing some actions of natural estrogens.

Warnings, interactions, and side effects

• Black cohosh should not be used during pregnancy because it may cause premature labor.

• It is not recommended for use by breast-feeding mothers.

• It should only be taken for short periods, and in small (recommended therapeutic) doses, because excessive intake may cause sweating, dizziness, reduced pulse rate, nausea, and vomiting.

• It may enhance the effects of drugs used for treating hypertension.

blackcurrant

(*Ribes nigrum*; Parts used: leaves and fruit)
Other common names: **quinsy berries, squinancy berries.**
Blackcurrant leaves contain flavonoids, proanthocyanins, ♧ **vitamin C**, and a volatile oil. They have diuretic (see ○ **fluid retention**) and hypotensive properties, and are used for ○ **arthritis**, ○ **gout**, rheumatism (see ○ **musculoskeletal disorders**), ○ **coughs**, ○ **colds**, and difficulty with urinating. The fruits contain flavonoids, anthocyanins, and vitamin C, and have antibacterial, anti-inflammatory, and antispasmodic activity. They are used to treat colds and sore throats (see ○ **pharyngitis**).

Warnings, interactions, and side effects

• Blackcurrant leaves should not be used by anyone with edema due to cardiac or kidney disorders.

black elder

(*Sambucus nigra*)

Other common names: **black-berried elder, boor tree, bountry, common elder, elder, elderberry, ellanwood, ellhorn, European elder.**
Elder is a large deciduous shrub which grows up to approximately 15 feet (4.5 meters) tall. The leaves have an unpleasant scent when bruised. Very small off-white flowers are produced in spring and are followed by loose bunches of black berries.

Forms of preparation and parts used

Elder flowers are the part most frequently used medicinally, as an infusion, tincture, or in a cream. The berries are also used occasionally.

Active components

Elder flowers contain phenolic acids, flavonoids, tannins, triterpenes, and a volatile oil. The berries are rich in vitamin C, the leaves contain cyanogenic glycosides, and the bark contains a lectin.

Uses in treatment

Elder is most commonly used to treat ○ **coughs**, ○ **colds**, and ○ **catarrh**; and some authorities approve its use for colds. Elder is also said to have anti-inflammatory, diuretic, diaphoretic, and laxative properties, and moderate anti-inflammatory and diuretic activity has been demonstrated in laboratory studies, especially in extracts rich in flavonoids. The diaphoretic and diuretic actions of the plant are the basis for its use for arthritis with the belief that these effects promote removal of waste products from the body. The berries are a mild laxative and the roots have insecticidal properties.

Warnings, interactions, and side effects

• The root has been reported to cause nausea and vomiting.

• The leaves and stem contain cyanide and must not be eaten.

• Due to the lack of detailed data, elder should be avoided during pregnancy and by breast-feeding mothers.

• Excessive or prolonged use of the flowers may lead to hypokalemia (low levels of potassium in the blood), resulting from the diuretic activity of the plant.

black horehound

(*Ballota nigra*)
Other common names: **black stinking horehound.**
Black horehound is a highly aromatic, straggling perennial herb, growing to a height of approximately 3 feet (90 centimeters). It has roughly oval-shaped, toothed leaves, and produces pale pink to purple flowers from the base of the uppermost leaf whorls.

Forms of preparation and parts used

The aerial parts of black horehound are used medicinally as the dried herb, an infusion, or liquid extract.

Active components

The chemistry of black horehound has not been studied in any great detail, although it is known to contain a number of diterpenoids, flavonoids, and a volatile oil.

Uses in treatment

Black horehound is used as an anti-emetic (see ○ **vomiting**), a sedative for ○ **insomnia**, and as a mild astringent. Its anti-emetic activity is claimed to be particularly effective against vomiting caused by central nervous system disorders (such as those of the inner ear), rather than vomiting caused by digestive disorders. Occasionally, the herb is used for ✚ **arthritis** and ✚ **gout**. However, this species has not been studied thoroughly and so these traditional uses have yet to be verified.

Warnings, interactions, and side effects
Although none have been reported with correct use and dosage, the properties of black horehound have not been fully investigated and adverse reactions are possible.

black pepper
(*Piper nigrum*; Parts used: berries)
Other common names: **pepper bark, piper.**
Black pepper contains acid amides and a volatile oil rich in sabinene and limonene. It is used as a culinary spice, and also to promote digestion and to treat stomach-related disorders (see ✚ **digestive system disorders**). It has been shown that pepper increases salivation and gastric secretions, and has antimicrobial activity.

Warnings, interactions, and side effects
Although none have been reported with correct use and dosage, the properties of black pepper have not been fully investigated and adverse reactions are possible.

black root
(*Leptandra virginica*; Parts used: root (dried))
Other common names: **bowman's root, culveris root, hini, oxadoddy, physic root, tall speedwell, tall Veronica, whorlywort.**
Black root contains tannins, cinnamic acids derivatives, and a volatile oil. It can be used for ✚ **constipation**, ✚ **liver disorders**, and ✚ **gallbladder disorders**. It has diaphoretic, carminative, cholagogic, cathartic, and laxative actions.

Warnings, interactions, and side effects
Although none have been reported with correct use and dosage, the properties of black root have not been fully investigated and adverse reactions are possible.

bladderwort
(*Utricularia vulgaris*; Parts used: whole plant)
Bladderwort contains iridoids and flavonoids, and has anti-inflammatory, antispasmodic, and diuretic properties, and also promotes gallbladder secretions. It is used for ✚ **urinary tract disorders** and inflammation of the mucous membranes or skin.

Warnings, interactions, and side effects
Although none have been reported with correct use and dosage, the properties of bladderwort have not been fully investigated and adverse reactions are possible.

bladderwrack
(*Fucus vesiculosus or Quercus marina*; Parts used: thallus)
Other common names: **black-tang, bladder fucus, cutweed, fucus, kelp-ware, kelpware, rockwrack, seawrack.**
Bladderwrack contains numerous carbohydrates, iodine, and vitamins. Traditional uses include to stimulate the thyroid (see ✚ **hypothyroidism**), to aid weight-loss (see ✚ **obesity**), and for rheumatism (see ✚ **musculoskeletal disorders**). The ◌ **iodine**

content is responsible for bladderwrack's affect on the thyroid gland.

Warnings, interactions, and side effects
• Bladderwrack is not to be used during pregnancy.
• Some authorities do not recommend its use in children.
• Excessive intake may cause oversecretion of thyroid hormones, and may exacerbate existing acne.
• It should not be used in conjunction with other thyroid medications, or antihyperglycemic treatment.

blessed thistle
(*Cnicus benedictus*)
Other common names: **cardin, Holy Ghost herb, holy thistle, spotted thistle, St. Benedict's thistle.**
An erect annual with a red stem, growing to a height of approximately 2 feet (60 centimeters). The leathery leaves and stem are both spiny, and the plant bears yellow flowers in summer.

Forms of preparation and parts used
The most commonly used plant parts are the flowering tops and leaves, usually as an infusion or other liquid extract.

Active components
Blessed thistle contains a number of lignans, phytosterols, terpenoids (including the sesquiterpenoid compounds cnicin), polyacetylenic compounds, and a volatile oil rich in hydrocarbons.

Uses in treatment
Blessed thistle was used as a cure-all in medieval monasteries, and was even promoted as a cure for the plague in 16th-century Europe. Today, it is used as a bitter tonic, to promote secretions in the stomach, intestines, and gallbladder in cases of minor ✚ **digestive system disorders**. Taken internally, it has also been used for ✚ **anorexia nervosa**, ✚ **indigestion**, and ✚ **catarrh**. Some authorities approve its use for indigestion and also ✚ **appetite loss**. Externally, it can be applied as a balm for ✚ **wounds**, ✚ **ulcers**, and sores. Studies have shown that the volatile oil and an aqueous extract of the herb have antibacterial properties, while the compound cnicin is anti-inflammatory.

Warnings, interactions, and side effects
• Although there are no specific toxicological problems with blessed thistle, its safety has not yet been fully documented, and should therefore not be used excessively during pregnancy, or when breast-feeding.
• It is possible that someone with hypersensitivity to members of the daisy family may also suffer an allergic reaction to blessed thistle.

bloodroot
(*Sanguinaria canadensis*; Parts used: rhizome)
Other common names: **coon root, Indian paint, Indian plant, paucon, pauson, red root, sanguinaria, snakebite, sweet slumber, tetterwort.**
Bloodroot contains isoquinoline alkaloids, organic acids, and a resin. It is used as an emetic, spasmolytic, and expectorant for ✚ **bronchitis** and ✚ **asthma**, among other disorders. Alkaloids are known to have antimicrobial and anti-inflammatory activity, and have been shown to be effective in oral hygiene products.

Warnings, interactions, and side effects

• Bloodroot should not be used during pregnancy.

blue cohosh

(*Caulophyllum thalictroides*)
Other common names: **beechdrops, blueberry root, blue ginseng, papoose root, squawroot, yellow ginseng.**
Blue cohosh, a high erect perennial, can be found across much of the US. It has a very distinctive form, of three bluish-purple stems growing to approximately 3 feet (90 centimeters) in height, bearing leaves at their apex, and surrounding a single red-purple-blue flower. Roots and rhizomes are usually collected in autumn after flowering. It is not related to ♣ **black cohosh** (*Cimicifuga racemosa*), although the two herbs have some properties in common.

Forms of preparation and parts used
The rhizome and roots of blue cohosh are used medicinally, usually as a decoction or tincture.

Active components
Blue cohosh is rich in steroidal saponins (such as caulosaponin) and quinolizidine and isoquinoline alkaloids (including anagyrine, magnoflorine, and caulophylline).

Uses in treatment
Blue cohosh is used as an antispasmodic and for rheumatism (see ✪ **musculoskeletal disorders**) and as a uterine tonic and emmenagogue (stimulates menstrual flow) for menstrual disturbances (for example, ✪ **dysmenorrhea**) and the ✪ **menopause**. Laboratory studies have been carried out on blue cohosh and its constituents. For example, extracts of blue cohosh have been shown to have variable effects on the uterus and other extracts have been shown to have antifertility properties, reflecting one of its traditional uses by Native Americans as a contraceptive. Caulophylline (*N*-methylcyctisine), one of the chemicals found in blue cohosh, has been shown to stimulate breathing and intestinal movement.

Warnings, interactions, and side effects
• On the basis of its chemical constituents and their potential risk in overdose, some authorities recommend that blue cohosh not be used for medicinal purposes.
• It should not be used during pregnancy, due to its effects on uterine tissue.
• Powdered roots can be irritating to mucous membranes.
• Leaves and seeds can cause severe stomach pains and poisoning if eaten.
• Caulosaponin, found in blue cohosh, has been shown to constrict coronary heart vessels which can lead to damage to the heart.
• Eating the root may interfere with existing angina treatments and aggravate gastrointestinal irritation.
• Excessive intake can cause hypertension and nicotine-like poisoning.

boldo

(*Peumus boldus*; Parts used: leaf)
Other common names: **boldu, boldus.**
Boldo contains isoquinoline alkaloids, flavonoids, and a volatile oil. Choleretic, diuretic, cholagogic, and stomachic activities have been confirmed experimentally. It is used as a sedative, diuretic (see ✪ **fluid retention**), antiseptic, and liver stimulant, and is approved by some authorities for ✪ **indigestion**, ✪ **cystitis**, rheumatism (see ✪ **musculoskeletal disorders**), gallstones (see ✪ **calculus**), and ✪ **liver disorders.**

Warnings, interactions, and side effects
• Boldo should not be taken in large quantities by anyone with kidney disorders.

boneset

(*Eupatorium perfoliatum*)
Other common names: **agueweed, crosswort, eupatorium, feverwort, gravelroot, Indian sage, sweating plant, teasel, thoroughwort, vegetable antimony.**
Boneset is a member of the *Compositaea* family, and is a hardy perennial, indigenous to North America. It has long slender leaves growing up to 4 to 5 feet (1.25 to 1.5 meters) tall. In late summer, large corymbs of white or pale pink flowers are produced.

Forms of preparation and parts used
The aerial parts of boneset are used medicinally, usually as an infusion. Some authorities consider that the infusion is poisonous when fresh, but a toxic component disappears as it dries.

Active components
Boneset contains a number of flavonoids and terpenoids (sesquiterpene lactones, diterpenes, triterpenes, sterols, and sesquiterpenes), as well as immunostimulating polysaccharides, a resin, and a volatile oil.

Uses in treatment
Boneset is traditionally used in the treatment of respiratory tract infections (see ✪ **respiratory tract disorders**) and ✪ **catarrh**. It has also been used for ✪ **arthritis** and rheumatic ✪ **pain**. Laboratory tests have been carried out on boneset and the sesquiterpene lactones and polysaccharides it contains, have it has been shown to have stimulant activities on cells of the immune system, and ethanolic extracts and flavonoid components have been demonstrated to have mild anti-inflammatory activity.

Warnings, interactions, and side effects
• Other *Eupatorium* species have some side effects, including contact dermatitis, cytotoxicity, and the risk of hepatotoxicity from pyrrolizidine alkaloids, and even though the compounds responsible for these effects have not been found in boneset, some experts recommend that it should be used with caution.
• Sesquiterpene lactones, which are present in boneset, are known to cause allergic reactions in susceptible people, so boneset should not be used by anyone with a known sensitivity to members of the daisy family.
• For the same reasons, it should not be used during pregnancy or by breast-feeding mothers.

borage

(*Borago officinalis*)
Other common names: **bugloss, burage, burrage.**
Borage can be grown as a hardy ornamental. It grows to a height of approximately 2 feet (60 centimeters), and has thick, fleshy stems, and large leaves which can both be covered in white hairs. In summer, the plant produces pale blue-pink five-petalled flowers.

Forms of preparation and parts used
The aerial parts of borage are used medicinally as an infusion or tincture, and the seed oil is becoming increasingly popular.

Active components
Borage contains a number of alkaloids, an oil rich in fatty acids, including ⚖ **gamma-linolenic acid** (GLA, gamolenic acid), a sugar-rich mucilage, saponins, and tannins.

Uses in treatment
The mucilaginous nature of borage makes it popular as an emollient and demulcent (for example, for chapped hands). Due to concerns over toxicity (see below), the herb should not be used internally. In studies the seed oil has been demonstrated to increase performance and reduce cardiovascular reactions to stress. As a source of gamma-linolenic acid, borage seed oil is sometimes used for the same purposes as a substitute for ♣ **evening primrose**.

Warnings, interactions, and side effects
• Borage contains pyrrolizidine alkaloids which, as a class of compounds, are known to be toxic to the liver (although the concentrations of pyrrolizidine found in borage are much lower than those found in ♣ **comfrey**). However, large quantities or prolonged use of borage (especially as infusions) should be avoided.
• It is not known whether the seed oil contains these potentially poisonous alkaloids, but some authorities suggest that it does not.
• Borage products should not be used during pregnancy or by breast-feeding mothers.
• Evening primrose products are known to increase the risk of epileptic seizures in schizophrenic patients who are also taking ℞ **antipsychotic** drugs that lower seizure threshold (such as phenothiazines), and therefore because borage oil has many similarities with evening primrose oil equal caution should be taken.

brewer's yeast
(*Saccharomyces cereviseae*; Parts used: whole organism)
Brewer's yeast is rich in B-vitamins, polysaccharides, and sterols. Antibacterial and immune-stimulating activities probably explain its use for ❂ **colds**, ❂ **cough**, and ❂ **bronchitis**. It is also approved by some authorities for ❂ **indigestion**, ❂ **eczema**, ❂ **acne**, and ❂ **appetite loss**.

Warnings, interactions, and side effects
• It has been reported that some people have experienced allergic reactions or migraine headaches.

broom
(*Cytisus scoparius*; Parts used: flowers and aerial parts)
Other common names: **basam, besom, bizzom, breeam, broomtops, browme, brum, Irish tops, scoparium, Scotch broom.**
Broom contains amines, quinolizidine alkaloids, and flavonoids. Traditional uses include for cardiac dysfunction and circulatory deficiency. It has been shown that the amines found in broom constrict blood vessels and have hypertensive actions (see ❂ **hypotension**), and it is approved by some authorities for circulatory disorders.

Warnings, interactions, and side effects
• Broom should not be used during pregnancy.
• It is not to be used with a ℞ **monoamine-oxidase inhibitor** drug.
• It should not be used by any one with high blood pressure.
• Overdoses may result in poisoning.

broomcorn
(*Sorghum vulgare*; Parts used: seeds)
Other common names: **darri, durri, Guinea corn, sorghum.**
Broomcorn contains starch, B-vitamins, fatty acids, and cyanogenic glycosides. The seeds have demulcent activity on the membranes of the alimentary tract. It is used as a nutritive and to ease ❂ **digestive system disorders**.

Warnings, interactions, and side effects
Although none have been reported with correct use and dosage, the properties of broomcorn have not been fully investigated and adverse reactions are possible.

buchu
(*Agathosma betulina*; Parts used: leaf)
Buchu contains flavonoids and a volatile oil. It is used as a diuretic (see ❂ **fluid retention**) and as a urinary antiseptic, however, these actions have not been confirmed scientifically. Diosmin (one of the flavonoids found in buchu) has been shown to have anti-inflammatory activity.

Warnings, interactions, and side effects
• Buchu should not be used by people with kidney infections.

buckbean
(*Menyanthes trifoliata*; Parts used: leaf)
Other common names: **bog bean, bog myrtle, brook bean, marsh clover, moonflower, trefoil, water shamrock.**
Buckbean contains plant acids, pyridine alkaloids and flavonoids. It is used as a diuretic (see ❂ **fluid retention**) and to treat rheumatoid conditions (see ❂ **musculoskeletal disorders**). Components of the leaves have choleretic, stomachic secretion, bitter, and antibacterial activities.

Warnings, interactions, and side effects
• Buckbean can cause vomiting and diarrhea if taken in large quantities.

buckthorn
(*Rhamnus cathartica or R. catharticus*; Parts used: fruit)
Other common names: **common buckthorn, hartsthorn, highwaythorn, purging buckthorn, ramsthorn, waythorn.**
Buckthorn contains tannins, flavonoids, and anthracene derivatives. Traditional uses, which are approved by some authorities, include for ❂ **constipation** and to aid movement in the colon.

Warnings, interactions, and side effects
• Buckthorn should not be used for extended periods.
• It should not be used by anyone with intestinal obstruction, acute intestinal inflammation (for example, Crohn's disease), or appendicitis.
• It should be used during pregnancy or while breast-feeding only with expert supervision.

• It should not be used by children under 12 years of age.

bugleweed

(*Lycopus virginicus*; Parts used: herb)
Other common names: **gypsywort, sweet bugle, Virginia water horehound, water bugle.**
Bugleweed contains flavonoids and caffeic acid derivatives. Traditional uses, which are approved by some authorities, include for ✪ **premenstrual syndrome**, ✪ **anxiety**, and ✪ **insomnia**.

Warnings, interactions, and side effects

• Bugleweed should not be taken by anyone taking thyroid medications.

bupleurum

(*Bupleurum chinense*; Parts used: root)
Other common names: **chai-hu, Chinese thoroughwax.**
Bupleurum contains a number of saponins and flavonoids. It is used as a general tonic, to protect the liver, and as an anti-inflammatory (see ✪ **inflammation**). Clinical evidence of its beneficial effects in ✪ **hepatitis** and liver disease has been reported.

Warnings, interactions, and side effects

• Bupleurum should not be used during pregnancy.
• Excessive intake may cause nausea and vomiting.

burdock

(*Arctium lappa*)
Other common names: **bardana, beggar's buttons, burr seed, clot-bur, cocklebur, cockle buttons, fox's clote, great burr, happy major, hardock, hareburr, lappa, love leaves, personata, philanthropium, thorny burr.**
Burdock is a hardy biennial plant, growing up to 5 feet (1.5 meters) tall. It has large ovate leaves and purple flowers similar to thistles, which are followed by fruits covered in barbed spines.

Forms of preparation and parts used

Dried burdock root is used medicinally as an infusion, tincture, or decoction. Other plant parts (leaves and seeds) can also be used, usually in combination with other herbs.

Active components

Burdock contains a wide range of plant acids, aldehydes, carbohydrates, and polyacetylenic compounds. It also contains fixed and volatile oils, phytosterols, sesquiterpene lactones, and tannins.

Uses in treatment

Burdock is used as a diuretic and orexigenic (appetite stimulant; see ✪ **appetite loss**). Laboratory studies have shown that extracts of preflowering burdock leaves and roots have hypoglycemic and diuretic activity. Root, leaf, and flower extracts have antibacterial properties. Burdock extracts have also been reported to have antimutagenic and antineoplastic activities.

Warnings, interactions, and side effects

No adverse reactions to authenticated burdock preparations exist.
• Burdock should not be used during pregnancy, as the plant may have effects on the uterus.
• Large quantities of burdock may interfere with hypoglycemic treatments, and it is not recommended for diabetics as it may aggravate their condition.

butcher's broom

(*Ruscus aculeatus*; Parts used: herb and rhizome)
Other common names: **Jew's myrtle, knee holly, kneeholm, pettigree, sweet broom.**
Butcher's broom contains steroidal saponins and benzofurans, and has antiphlogistic and diuretic activity (see ✪ **fluid retention**), and increases venous tone. It is used for ✪ **hemorrhoids** (to relieve itching and burning) and ✪ **venous insufficiency** (to relieve pain, heaviness, cramps, itching, and swelling), and is approved for these uses by some authorities.

Warnings, interactions, and side effects

• There have been rare reports of stomach upsets after ingesting butcher's broom.

butternut

(*Juglans cinerea*; Parts used: inner bark)
Other common names: **black walnut, lemon walnut, oil nut, white walnut.**
Butternut contains naphthaquinones, including juglone. The naphthaquinones have antimicrobial, antiparasitic, and laxative activity, hence its traditional use for ✪ **constipation**. Butternut also has a reputation for reducing cholesterol, as a treatment for intestinal worm infestation, and also for skin diseases.

Warnings, interactions, and side effects

Although none have been reported with correct use and dosage, the properties of butternut have not been fully investigated and adverse reactions are possible.

cajuput

Melaleuca leucadendron or *M. leucadendra*; Parts used: leaf and twigs
Other common names: **cajeput, paperbark tree, swamp tea tree, white tea tree, white wood.**
Cajuput contains a volatile oil rich in cineol and terpineol derivatives, and studies have shown that it has antimicrobial and rubefacient properties. Traditional uses include to treat muscular ✪ **pain** and rheumatism (see ✪ **musculoskeletal disorders**), and it is approved by some authorities for these uses and also for ✪ **wounds**, ✪ **burns**, a tendency to ✪ **infection**, and ✪ **neuralgia**.

Warnings, interactions, and side effects

• Cajuput should not be applied to the faces of children or infants.
• Contact dermatitis may occur in some individuals.

caraway

(*Carum carvi*; Parts used: seeds)
Caraway contains flavonoids, polysaccharides, and a volatile oil rich in carvone. Its uses, which are similar to those of ♣ **fennel**, include soothing and antispasmodic actions on the gastrointestinal tract, and it is approved by some authorities for ✪ **indigestion**. These effects have been confirmed experimentally.

Warnings, interactions, and side effects

• The volatile oil should not be taken internally without the supervision of an expert professional.

cardamom

(*Elettaria cardamomum*; Parts used: seeds)
Cardamom contains a volatile oil rich in monoterpenoids. Traditionally it is used in medicine and cooking, and has a reputation for easing digestive complaints. It is approved by some authorities for the common ✪ **cold**, ✪ **cough**, ✪ **bronchitis**, ✪ **fever**, inflammation of the mouth and/or pharynx (see ✪ **inflammation** and ✪ **pharyngitis**), ✪ **liver disorders**, ✪ **gallbladder disorders**, ✪ **appetite loss**, and a tendency to ✪ **infection**. The volatile oil has been shown to be antispasmodic.

Warnings, interactions, and side effects
• The pure essential oil should not be taken internally.

cassia

(*Cinnamomum cassia*; Parts used: bark)
Other common names: **Chinese cinnamon.**
Cassia contains diterpenes, tannins, and a volatile oil. Traditional uses include as a carminative, anti-spasmodic, and antimicrobial, and it is also thought to have a stimulating effect on blood circulation. Certain components of the plant have antiulcer, antimicrobial, and anti-inflammatory activities, as well effects on the central nervous system.

Warnings, interactions, and side effects
• Cassia can be irritating and/or cause an allergic reaction in some people.
• The volatile oil should be used on the skin sparingly and infrequently.

catnip

(*Nepeta cataria*; Parts used: aerial parts)
Other common names: **catmint, catnep, catrup, catswort, field balm.**
Catnip contains a volatile oil rich in nepetalactone and tannins. It has antipyretic, refrigerant, and diaphoretic activity, and can relieve muscle cramping. It is used to treat ✪ **colds** and ✪ **colic**, and as a stimulant,

Warnings, interactions, and side effects
• Catnip should not be used during pregnancy.

cayenne

(*Capsicum species: C. annum, C. frutescens*)
Other common names: **African chilli, African pepper, bird pepper, capsicum, cayenne pepper, chilli pepper, goat's pod, grains of paradise, Guinea pepper, hot pepper, Hungarian pepper, Louisiana long (and short) pepper, Mexican chili, paprika, red pepper, sweet pepper, tabasco pepper, Zanzibar pepper.**
Many cayenne species are tender annuals or short-lived perennials, which can grow to a height of approximately 5 feet (1.5 meters). The plants have simple rounded leaves and bell-shaped flowers, which develop into hollow fruits up to 6 inches (15 centimeters) in length. The related pepper *Capsicum frutescens* (tabasco peppers) has similar constituents. There are many variants and hybrids of these capsicum peppers, varying in size, color, and hotness.

Forms of preparation and parts used
The cayenne fruit is used both medicinally and in cooking. Medicinally, fruits are usually used fresh, dried, or as an infusion or tincture. Some forms are available standardized with respect to hotness, and this can be expressed in Scoville Thermal Units (STU) (also called heat units; HU), typically 100,000 STU per oral capsules. Topical preparations are also available standardized, commonly in the range 0.025–0.075% capsaicin for OTC preparations.

Active components
The main active compounds in capsicum species are the capsaicinoids, which are responsible for the pungency of the fruits. The major capsaicinoid is usually capsaicin, sometimes used as the resinous extract capsaicin oleoresin. The plant also contains a volatile oil, proteins, fats, and vitamins.

Uses in treatment
Cayenne has stimulant, antispasmodic, carminative, diaphoretic, antiseptic, analgesic, counterirritant, and rubefacient properties. Internally, the plant is traditionally used for ✪ **colic**, and some types of ✪ **indigestion**. It is also used as a general digestive tonic, and to treat and prevent gastrointestinal infections (it has antibacterial actions, including against *Helicobacter pylori*). It is used externally to stimulate circulation, particularly in ✪ **arthritis** or rheumatic conditions, especially muscle spasms in the arms, spine, or shoulders (see ✪ **musculoskeletal disorders**), and is approved by some authorities for treating muscular tension and rheumatism. It can also be applied to unbroken ✪ **chilblains**, and its counterirritant properties can help in managing ✪ **pain**.

Warnings, interactions, and side effects
• Cayenne contains a number of strongly pungent compounds, which can be irritating to the mucosal membranes, so it must be kept away from the eyes and never applied to broken or inflamed skin.
• Excessive intake can result in damage to the liver and kidneys (the amounts used in cooking are not thought to have any health risks).
• It may interfere with ℞ **monoamine-oxidase inhibitor** drugs (MAOIs), some hypertension treatments, and with the metabolism of some other drugs.

celandine

(*Chelidonium majus*; Parts used: aerial parts)
Other common names: **tetterwort.**
Celandine contains isoquinoline alkaloids and derivatives of caffeic acid. Traditional uses, which are approved by some authorities, include for ✪ **liver disorders** and ✪ **gallbladder disorders**. It also has analgesic and antimicrobial activity, and a stimulant effect on the immune system.

Warnings, interactions, and side effects
• Celandine should not be used during pregnancy.

celery

(*Apium graveolens*)
Other common names: **apium, marsh parsley, smallage, wild celery.**
Celery is a hardy biennial plant, usually grown as an annual vegetable crop. It forms tight clusters of upright stems, approximately

12 inches (30 centimeters) in length which can be pale yellow-green, off-white, pink, or red in color.

Forms of preparation and parts used

Celery seed is the most commonly used part of the plant medicinally, usually in an infusion or tincture. The volatile oil extracted from the seeds can also be used in some situations.

Active components

Celery contains a number of flavonoids (including apigenin derivatives), coumarins and furanocoumarins (including bergapten), fatty acids, and a volatile oil rich in limonene and phthalide constituents.

Uses in treatment

Celery is traditionally used for ✪ **arthritis**, ✪ **gout**, urinary tract ✪ **inflammation**, and as a sedative for ✪ **insomnia**. There have been laboratory and clinical studies which have investigated the effects of celery and celery extracts. For example, the phthalide constituents of the volatile oil, which give celery its distinctive aroma, have been shown to have antispasmodic and sedative actions, and celery extracts have been reported to have anti-inflammatory, hypotensive, and blood sugar-reducing properties. A plant extract has been shown to reduce blood pressure in people with ✪ **hypertension**. The flavonoid apigenin, which is found in celery, has been shown to be a potent inhibitor of platelet aggregation.

Warnings, interactions, and side effects

No adverse reactions to celery seeds have been found. The seed oil is considered to be non-irritating, non-phototoxic, and non-sensitizing.

• The seeds and their oil should not be used during pregnancy, as they can affect the uterus and are reported to be abortifacient.

• Despite their widespread culinary use, some side effects to celery stems have been reported, including allergies, anaphylaxis, and photosensitization (due to bergapten).

centaury

(*Centaurium erythraea*; Parts used: herb)

Other common names: **bitterbloom, bitter clover, bitter herb, canchalagua, centaury gentian, centory, Christ's ladder, eyebright, filwort.**

Centaury contains plant acids, pyridine alkaloids, and a number of terpenoids. Traditional uses include as a bitter and stomachic, and it is approved by some authorities for ✪ **appetite loss** and ✪ **indigestion**. Anti-inflammatory and antipyretic activities have also been recorded.

Warnings, interactions, and side effects

• Centaury should not be used by anyone with stomach or intestinal ulcers.

chamomile, English

(*Chamaemelum nobile or Anthermis noblis*; Parts used: flowers)

Other common names: **ground apple, Roman chamomile, whig plant.**

English chamomile contains flavonoids, azulenes, and a volatile oil. Traditional uses include as a carminative, sedative, antispasmodic, and antiemetic. Its effects are similar to those of ♣ **chamomile,**

German. Anti-inflammatory and antiallergenic activities have been reported, and azulenes have been shown to stimulate liver regeneration.

Warnings, interactions, and side effects

• English chamomile should not be used during pregnancy.

• It should be avoided by anyone who is sensitive to members of the daisy family.

chamomile, German

(*Matricaria chamomilla, M. recutita, Chamomilla recutita*)

Other common names: **camomile, chamomilla, Hungarian chamomile, May weed, pin heads, single chamomile, wild chamomile.**

German chamomile is a sweet-scented annual/biennial with highly branched stems and finely divided leaves, which can grow to a height of approximately 2 feet (60 centimeters). It produces daisy-like flowers through the summer and early fall.

Forms of preparation and parts used

The dried flowerheads are most commonly used medicinally, usually as an infusion or liquid extract.

Active components

German chamomile contains a number of coumarins and flavonoids, and a number of acids and triterpenes. The volatile oil has a characteristic blue color.

Uses in treatment

German chamomile has carminative, antispasmodic, anti-inflammatory, antiseptic, anticatarrhal, and mild sedative properties. It can be used for ✪ **indigestion**, ✪ **motion sickness**, restlessness and gastrointestinal disturbances (see ✪ **digestive system disorders**). Externally, it can be applied to ✪ **hemorrhoids**, leg ulcers (see ✪ **ulcer**), and ✪ **eczema**. It is approved by some authorities for ✪ **cough**, ✪ **bronchitis**, ✪ **fever** and ✪ **colds**, skin inflammation (see ✪ **skin conditions**), and inflammation of the mouth and/or pharynx (see ✪ **inflammation** and ✪ **pharyngitis**), ✪ **wounds**, ✪ **burns**, and tendency to ✪ **infection**. The primary uses of the herb are for digestive problems and ✪ **insomnia**. Laboratory studies have shown that components of German chamomile do have anti-inflammatory, antiulcerogenic, antispasmodic, and antibacterial activities.

Warnings, interactions, and side effects

• German chamomile should not be used during pregnancy or by breast-feeding mothers.

• The sesquiterpene lactones present in German chamomile can cause allergic reactions, especially in anyone with hypersensitivity to members of the daisy family.

• The herb can also aggravate allergies, and should therefore not be taken by susceptible people.

• Excessive use may interfere with the effects of ℞ **anticoagulant** drugs.

chaste tree

(*Vitex agnus-castus*)

Other common names: **agnus castus, cloister pepper, hemp tree, monk's pepper, vitex chasteberry.**

Chaste tree is a small tree or woody shrub which grows up to 15 feet (4.5 meters) tall. It has deeply divided palmate leaves, and small, scented pink flowers which appear in summer, followed by very small red-black fleshy fruits.

Forms of preparation and parts used

Chaste tree fruits are used medicinally, usually as an alcoholic extract or tincture.

Active components

Chaste tree fruits contain a number of flavonoids (predominantly casticin), iridoids (mainly aucubin and agnuside), and a volatile oil rich in cineole and pinene.

Uses in treatment

Chaste tree is widely used for hormone-related conditions, including ✪ **premenstrual syndrome**, ✪ **dysmenorrhea**, menstrual difficulties, and menopausal conditions (see ✪ **menopause**). Its use for premenstrual syndrome and menopausal complaints is approved by some authorities. Laboratory studies have shown that chaste tree does have effects on the female reproductive system, especially on hormones involved in ovulation, and beneficial effects have been shown in studies with women who suffer from mildly impaired ovarian function. It has also been used to treat ✪ **acne** and to promote lactation.

Warnings, interactions, and side effects

• Chaste tree may interfere with existing hormone treatments and it should not be taken concurrently with the contraceptive pill, hormone replacement therapy, or fertility treatments. It should also be avoided during pregnancy or by breast-feeding mothers.

• Allergic reactions have been reported in a few cases following withdrawal of the herb.

chicory

(*Cichorium intybus*; Parts used: leaves and roots)

Other common names: **hendibeh, succory.**

Chicory contains caffeic acids derivatives, sesquiterpene lactones, flavonoids, and polyynes. It has mild cholagogic activity, and lowers the pulse rate. Traditional uses include treating ✪ **liver disorders**, ✪ **gallbladder disorders**, and ✪ **indigestion**. Some authorities approve its use for dyspeptic complaints and also for ✪ **appetite loss.**

Warnings, interactions, and side effects

Although none have been reported with correct use and dosage, the properties of chicory have not been fully investigated and adverse reactions are possible.

Chinese goldthread

(*Coptis chinensis*; Parts used: root)

Chinese goldthread contains isoquinoline alkaloids, which have antibacterial, amoebicidal, and antidiarrheal activities. Improvement in the symptoms of people with tuberculosis have been shown in a Chinese study.

Warnings, interactions, and side effects

Chinese goldthread should only be used under professional supervision.

chiretta

(*Swertia chirata*; Parts used: herb)

Other common names: **chirata, chirayta, Indian balmony, Indian gentian.**

Chiretta contains iridoids, xanthones, alkaloids, and flavonoids. As a bitter herb, chiretta is widely used for ✪ **digestive system disorders** and for reducing ✪ **fevers**. An iridoid has been shown to have hepatoprotective activity, while it is thought that the xanthones may protect against tuberculosis.

Warnings, interactions, and side effects

• Chiretta should not be used by anyone with gastric or duodenal ulcers.

cinnamon, Chinese

(*Cinnamomum aromaticum*; Parts used: flowers and twigs)

Other common names: **bastard cinnamon, Canton cassia, cassia,** *Cassia aromaticum,* **cassia bark,** *Cassia lignea,* **false cinnamon.**

Chinese cinnamon is rich in tannins and diterpenes, and also contains a volatile oil. It can be used to treat ✪ **inflammation**, ✪ **fever**, ✪ **colds**, ✪ **bronchitis**, ✪ **indigestion**, and ✪ **appetite loss**. It is also known to have antimicrobial activity, a stimulant effect on the immune system, and antiulcer properties.

Warnings, interactions, side effects

• Chinese cinnamon should not be used during pregnancy.

cinnamon

(*Cinnamomum verum*)

Other common names: **Ceylon cinnamon.**

Cinnamon is native to Sri Lanka and India, but is now grown in many tropical regions for medicinal and culinary uses. Young trees are felled, usually every two years, from which the inner bark is harvested. There are several related and similar cinnamon species, such as *Cinnamomum zeylanicum* and *Cinnamomum cassia.*

Forms of preparation and parts used

The inner bark of cinnamon is the most commonly used plant part, usually as an infusion, tincture or other liquid extract. It is often available in the US in multiherb cough, cold, and fever preparations.

Active components

The main biologically active constituent of cinnamon is the volatile oil, which is rich in cinnamaldehydes and eugenol. The oil from cinnamon leaves is especially rich in the chemical eugenol. The plant also contains tannins, coumarins, and mucilaginous substances.

Uses in treatment

Cinnamon is regarded as a stimulant, carminative, and antimicrobial. It is often used for ✪ **colic**, ✪ **colds**, ✪ **influenza**, ✪ **diarrhea** (especially in infants), ✪ **indigestion** where there is also nausea and bloating, and ✪ **flatulence**. Some authorities approve its use for ✪ **appetite loss** and dyspeptic complaints. It has also been used as an anthelmintic and as a refrigerant. As a warming herb, cinnamon is also used to promote the circulation, and to support a weakened digestive system. Such volatile oils as found in cinnamon have been shown to have antifungal, antibacterial, and antiviral activities in laboratory studies.

Warnings, interactions, and side effects

• Cinnamon herbal products should not be used during pregnancy, or by breast-feeding mothers.

• Cinnamon bark and cinnamon oil can cause allergic reactions.

• The oil is regarded as hazardous, and is not recommended for either internal or external use.

• Some experts suggest that it should be avoided by anyone with a peptic ulcer.

• However, at the levels used in foods there are no known toxicological problems for cinnamon, even during pregnancy or when breast-feeding.

clove

(*Syzygium aromaticum*, also known as *Jambosa caryophyllus, Eugenia caryophyllata, Eugenia caryophyllus*)

Other common names: **caryophyllum, ding xiang.**

Clove grows as a small evergreen tree with tough, glossy leaves which change from pale pink in color when young to yellow-green. It produces aromatic pink flowers in summer, followed by purple berries.

Forms of preparation and parts used

The most commonly used part of the plants are the cloves (dried flowerheads), although the stem and leaves are also used.

Active components

Cloves contain a volatile oil rich in eugenol, eugenyl acetate, and beta-caryophyllene. The volatile oils from the stem and leaves are also rich in eugenol. Cloves also contain steroidal compounds, flavonoids, and fatty acids. The smell of the oil is characteristic.

Uses in treatment

Cloves are used as a carminative, counterirritant, and antiemetic, and also for toothache (see ✪ **tooth decay**: where the oil is rubbed onto aching gums). It is approved by some authorities as a pain-reliever for dental ✪ **pain**, and for inflammation of the mouth and/or pharynx (see ✪ **inflammation**; ✪ **pharyngitis**). Clove oil also is antispasmodic. Eugenol is thought to be responsible for the antiseptic and anodyne effects of the oil. A tincture of cloves has been shown to be effective in the treatment of ✪ **athlete's foot**.

Warnings, interactions, and side effects

• Clove oil can irritate the skin and mucous membranes which can result in contact dermatitis. The eugenol in clove oil is thought to be responsible for this irritant activity, and may also cause sensitization. Because of this property, a recommended daily limit for eugenol has been established.

• Eugenol can also interfere with platelet activity, so cloves should be avoided by anyone taking ℞ **anticoagulant** or ℞ **antiplatelet** drugs.

• Repeated application of the oil to the skin or gums should be avoided, and swallowing of the oil also should be avoided.

• At the amounts used in cooking there are no known problems during pregnancy or by breast-feeding mothers, although using cloves in medicinal amounts should be avoided.

club moss

(*Lycopodium clavatum*; Parts used: whole plant)

Other common names: **stags horn, vegetable sulfur, witch meal, wolfs claw.**

Club moss contains piperidine alkaloids and flavonoids. Traditional uses include to treat bladder disorders and ✪ **kidney disorders**, and it also has diuretic activity.

Warnings, interactions, and side effects

• Prolonged use of club moss may irritate the gastrointestinal tract.

• Excessive intake should be avoided due to the alkaloid content.

cnidium

(*Cnidium monnieri*; Parts used: seeds)

Cnidium contains a volatile oil rich in pinene, camphene, and borneol derivatives. Traditional uses include for ✪ **skin conditions**, such as ✪ **eczema**, ✪ **scabies**, and ringworm. The oil has been shown to be an effective treatment for ✪ **vaginitis** caused by the trichomonas bacteria.

Warnings, interactions, and side effects

Although none have been reported with correct use and dosage, the properties of cnidium have not been fully investigated and adverse reactions are possible.

cocoa

(*Theobroma cacao*; Parts used: seeds)

Other common names: **cacao, chocolate tree.**

Cocoa is rich in purine alkaloids, tannins, fats, and amines. It is used for ✪ **diarrhea** and as a general tonic. The astringency of the tannins can counter diarrhea, but may result in constipation if taken in large amounts. The seeds also have stimulant, diuretic, bronchiolytic, and vasodilatory activity, largely due to the purine alkaloids.

Warnings, interactions, and side effects

• Large quantities of cocoa and cocoa products can cause excitability in children due to the ℞ **caffeine** content.

• Cocoa and cocoa products can trigger ✪ **migraine** in susceptible people.

codonopsis

(*Codonopsis pilosula*; Parts used: root)

Codonopsis contains saponins, polysaccharides, and glycosides. It is most commonly used as an adaptogen and stimulant. It has been shown that codonopsis does have hypotensive (lowers blood pressure) activity, can increase red blood cell numbers, and enhances endurance under ✪ **stress**.

Warnings, interactions, and side effects

Although none have been reported with correct use and dosage, the properties of codonopsis have not been fully investigated and adverse reactions are possible.

coffee

(*Coffea arabica*; Parts used: seeds)

Other common names: **Arabian coffee, Arabica coffee, caffea.**

Coffee contains xanthines and tannins, which are powerful stimulants of the central nervous system. It is also a powerful diuretic (see ✪ **fluid retention**) and can promote digestion. Some authorities approve the use of coffee charcoal for ✪ **diarrhea** and mouth and pharynx inflammation (see ✪ **inflammation** and ✪ **pharyngitis**).

Warnings, interactions, and side effects

• It is best to avoid coffee, or at least reduce the amount used (no more than 3 cups per day), during pregnancy.
• It is best avoided if breast-feeding as it is known that babies can be affected by the coffee drunk by their mothers.
• Avoid taking other stimulants at the same time.

cola

(*Cola acuminata*)
Other common names: **bissy nut, cola nut, cola seed, guru nut, kola, kola nut, kola tree.**
An evergreen tree which grows up to 70 feet (21 meters) in height, with dark green leaves, off-white flowers, and large woody seed pods, each containing 5 to 10 red or white seeds.

Forms of preparation and parts used
The seeds, usually by infusion or tincture.

Active components
Cola contains alkaloids, including the xanthines ℞ **caffeine** and theobromine, as well as tannins, and various pigments.

Uses in treatment
Cola is a stimulant of the central nervous system and also has thymoleptic, diuretic (see ❂ **fluid retention**), cardioactive, and antidiarrheal actions. It is commonly used for ❂ **depression**, exhaustion, and is approved by some authorities for loss of stamina (see ❂ **fatigue**) and muscular weaknesses. It is also used for ❂ **dysentery**, ❂ **headache**, ❂ **migraine**, and ❂ **diarrhea**. During recovery from chronic illnesses, its antidepressant effect is often made use of. The nuts are also very widely used today to flavor soft drinks.

Warnings, interactions, and side effects
• As with all xanthine-containing beverages (such as tea and coffee), the side effects can include sleeplessness, anxiety, palpitations, and occasionally withdrawal headaches.
• Because of its effects on the heart, cola should not be used by anyone with a heart disorder or hypertension (high blood pressure).
• It is also not recommended for anyone with a peptic ulcer.
• Excessive intake, particularly by anyone who is pregnant or breast-feeding, should be avoided because of the caffeine content.

coleus

(*Coleus forskohlii*; Parts used: leaves, root)
Coleus contains the diterpene forskolin and a volatile oil. Traditional uses include for ❂ **digestive system disorders**. Forskolin has been shown to have hypotensive (lowers blood pressure) and muscle-relaxant activity, as well as stimulating digestive secretions.

Warnings, interactions, and side effects
• Coleus should be used only with professional supervision.

colombo

(*Jateorhiza palmata*; Parts used: root)
Other common names: **calumba.**
Colombo contains isoquinoline alkaloids, a volatile oil, and mucilage. Traditional uses include as an antipyretic, to ease stomach pains, and for ❂ **appetite loss**. The alkaloids in the plant have hypotensive (lowers blood pressure) and sedative activity.

Warnings, interactions, and side effects
• Colombo should not be used during pregnancy because the alkaloids can stimulate the uterus.

comfrey

(*Symphytum officinale*; Parts used: leaf, rhizome)
Other common names: **ass ear, black root, blackwort, boneset, bruiswort, consolida, consound, gum plant, healing herb, knitback, knitbone, salsify, slippery root, wallwort.**
Comfrey contains tannins, triterpenes, and pyrrolizidine alkaloids. It has vulnerary, astringent, and demulcent activities, and is approved by some authorities for blunt injuries, such as ❂ **bruises** and ❂ **sprains**.

Warnings, interactions, and side effects
• Comfrey should not be used during pregnancy or while breast-feeding.
• It should not be taken orally, or applied to broken skin, due to the toxic effect on the liver of the pyrrolizidine alkaloids.

condurango

(*Marsdenia condurango*; Parts used: bark)
Other common names: **eagle vine.**
Condurango contains a mixture of pregnane derivatives. Traditional uses include for ❂ **indigestion**, and to promote the appetite (see ❂ **appetite loss**). Studies have shown that it stimulates salivation and gastric secretions.

Warnings, interactions, and side effects
Although none have been reported with correct use and dosage, the properties of condurango have not been fully investigated and adverse reactions are possible.

coriander

(*Coriandrum sativum*; Parts used: fruit, oil)
Coriander contains a volatile oil rich in coriandrol, fatty acids, and hydroxycoumarins. Traditional uses include as a culinary spice, and to treat ❂ **appetite loss** and ❂ **indigestion**. These uses are approved by some authorities. The fruit has carminative and antimicrobial activities, as well as being able to increase gastric secretions.

Warnings, interactions, and side effects
• There is a low risk of sensitization.

corn silk

(*Zea mays*; Parts used: stigma and style)
Other common names: **Indian corn, maize, stigmata maydis.**
Corn silk contains tannins, saponins, amines, and a fixed oil. Cholagogic, diuretic, hypoglycemic, and hypotensive activities have been confirmed experimentally. It is used as a diuretic (see ❂ **fluid retention**) and for ❂ **urinary tract disorders**.

Warnings, interactions, and side effects
• Corn silk may cause allergies or interfere with the treatment of blood sugar or blood pressure disorders.

corydalis

(*Corydalis yanusuo*; Parts used: rhizome)
Corydalis contains a range of alkaloids, including corydaline. Traditional uses include to invigorate the blood and for the relief of ✪ **pain**. Corydaline and related compounds are known to have pain-relieving properties.

Warnings, interactions, and side effects
Although none have been reported with correct use and dosage, the properties of corydalis have not been fully investigated and adverse reactions are possible.

cotton

(*Gossypium herbaceum or G. hirsutum*; Parts used: seed oil)
Other common names: **American cotton plant, cotton seed.**
Cotton seed oil is rich in gossypol, which is a substance that can effect both male and female reproductive systems. In men, gossypol can lower sperm count, which can lead to infertility. In women, the oil has been used to treat ✪ **menorrhagia** and ✪ **endometriosis**.

Warnings, interactions, and side effects
• The oil should only be used under professional supervision.

couchgrass

(*Agropyron repens*; Parts used: rhizome)
Other common names: **cutch, dog-grass, durfa grass, quack grass, quickgrass, quitch grass, Scotch quelch, twitch-grass, witch grass.**
Couchgrass contains flavonoids, saponins, and a volatile oil. It is primarily used as a diuretic (see ✪ **fluid retention**), and this activity has been confirmed experimentally. Some authorities approve its use for kidney and bladder stones (see ✪ **calculus**) and ✪ **urinary tract disorders**.

Warnings, interactions, and side effects
Although none have been reported with correct use and dosage, the properties of couchgrass have not been fully investigated and adverse reactions are possible.

couch grass

(*Elymus repens*; Parts used: rhizome)
Couch grass contains a volatile oil and mucilaginous substances. The volatile oil has been shown to have antimicrobial activity. Traditional uses include for ✪ **coughs**, ✪ **colds**, ✪ **fever**, ✪ **infections**, and ✪ **inflammation**.

Warnings, interactions, and side effects
Although none have been reported with correct use and dosage, the properties of couch grass have not been fully investigated and adverse reactions are possible.

cowslip

(*Primula veris, sometimes referred to as P. officinalis*)
Other common names: **arthritica, buckles, butter rose, crewel, English cowslip, European cowslip, fairy caps, fairy cups, herb Peter Paigle, key flower, key of heaven, Mayflower, Our Lady's keys, oxlip, palsywort, password, peagles, petty mulleins, plumrocks, primrose, true cowslips.**

Cowslip is a small perennial, approximately 4 inches (10 centimeters) high, which usually grows in clumps. The plant grows from a rhizome, and produces a rosette of ovate leaves and clusters of yellow bell-shaped fragrant flowers.

Forms of preparation and parts used
The flowers of cowslip are the part most commonly used medicinally, although roots and leaves are also used. The herb is usually taken as an infusion or liquid extract.

Active components
Cowslip contains flavonoids, triterpene saponins, tannins, carbohydrates, and phenol glycosides (some changing on dehydration to 5-methoxy-methyl salicylate).

Uses in treatment
The flowers of cowslip have sedative, antispasmodic, and anti-inflammatory actions, which explains their use for ✪ **asthma** and ✪ **allergy**. The roots have strong expectorant and mild diuretic properties. They are used in bronchial complaints, including for chronic ✪ **bronchitis**, ✪ **bronchial congestion**, and ✪ **catarrh**. The leaves are used for similar complaints, although their activity is generally seen as less powerful than that of the roots. Preparations of both the root and flowers are approved by some authorities for ✪ **cough** and bronchitis.

Warnings, interactions, and side effects
• Cowslip should not be used during pregnancy or by breast-feeding mothers.
• Allergic reactions have been reported after contact with cowslip flowers (also found in other members of the *Primulaceae* family).
• The saponins found in underground parts of the plant are likely to be irritant to mucosal membranes and may irritate the stomach and intestines, and have hemolytic (break down of red blood cells) activity on contact with blood.
• Large quantities of cowslip could interfere with treatments for abnormal blood pressure.

cup plant

(*Silphium perfoliatum*; Parts used: root)
Other common names: **Indian gum, pilot plant, polar plant, prairie dock, ragged cup, rosinweed, turpentine weed.**
Cup plant contains sesquiterpenoids and saponins, and has diaphoretic activity. It can be used as a tonic and for ✪ **digestive system disorders**.

Warnings, interactions, and side effects
Although none have been reported with correct use and dosage, the properties of cup plant have not been fully investigated and adverse reactions are possible. Some authorities do not recommend its use in modern medicine.

curcuma

(*Curcuma xanthorrhiza*; Parts used: rhizome)
Other common names: **temu lawak, tewon lawa.**
Curcuma contains curcuminosides and a volatile oil rich in curcumene. Traditional uses, which are approved by some authorities, include for ✪ **appetite loss**, ✪ **liver disorders**, and ✪ **gallbladder disorders**. The rhizome has known choleretic activity and has also been shown to have antitumoral properties.

Warnings, interactions, and side effects

• Curcuma may cause stomach complaints if taken in overdose or large quantities.

• It should not be used by anyone with bile duct blockage.

damiana

(*Turnera diffusa*; Parts used: leaf, stem)

Damiana contains carbohydrates, tannins, and a volatile oil. It has been shown to have antimicrobial, central nervous system-depressant, and hypoglycemic activities. Traditional uses include for ✪ **depression**, as a mild purgative, and a thymoleptic.

Warnings, interactions, and side effects

• Damiana should not be taken in large amounts.

dandelion

(*Taraxacum officinale*)

Other common names: **blowball, cankerwort, fairy clock, lion's tooth, pis-en-lit, piss-in-bed, priest's crown, puffball, swine snout, taraxacum, wet-a-bed, wild endive.**

Dandelions grow as rosettes of lobed leaves from a stout tap root. Single yellow flowers are produced throughout late spring and summer, followed by characteristic globes of feathery seeds.

Forms of preparation and parts used

The leaves and roots of dandelion are used medicinally. Leaves are either eaten fresh, as a juice, dried, or as a liquid extract. The roots are taken dried, as an infusion, or a decoction.

Active components

Dandelion contains a number of terpenoids, carotenoids, steroidal compounds, phenolic acids, and sugars. The leaves of the plant are particularly rich in ⚕ **vitamin A** and ⚕ **potassium**.

Uses in treatment

Dandelion has diuretic and laxative properties, and is used for rheumatism (see ✪ **musculoskeletal disorders**). Other uses which are approved of by some authorities include for dyspeptic complaints (see ✪ **indigestion**), ✪ **flatulence**, to stimulate diuresis (see ✪ **fluid retention**), ✪ **gallbladder disorders**, and ✪ **appetite loss**. Laboratory studies have been carried out on dandelion and dandelion extracts. For example, oral administration of dandelion extracts (of the roots, but particularly of the leaves) have been shown to have diuretic activity; and a root extract has been demonstrated to have mild anti-inflammatory activity. Dandelion extracts also have hypoglycemic activity, possibly through stimulation of so-called beta-cells in the pancreas gland (which secretes the blood-sugar-regulating hormone insulin). The roasted roots of the plant can be used as a ℞ **caffeine**-free coffee substitute.

Warnings, interactions, and side effects

• Dandelion is said to have very low acute toxicity, and this conclusion is supported by results from laboratory studies.

• The sesquiterpene lactones in dandelion can cause allergic reactions, and may also be weakly sensitizing.

• It may interfere with diuretic or hypoglycemic treatments.

• Using dandelion at the levels used in food during pregnancy is not known to have any side effects, but large doses should be avoided.

devil's claw

(*Harpagophytum procumbens*)

Other common names: **grapple plant, wood spider.**

Devil's claw is a trailing perennial which can grow to a length of 5 feet (1.5 meters). In spring, the plant produces bright purple flowers. The tubers are collected in the fall.

Forms of preparation and parts used

The tubers are taken medicinally, usually either dried or as a liquid extract or tincture.

Active components

Devil's claw contains a number or iridoids in its underground parts, as well as phenolic compounds, carbohydrates, and flavonoids. Iridoids are found at much lower concentrations in the aerial parts of the plant.

Uses in treatment

Devil's claw has anti-inflammatory, antirheumatic, analgesic, sedative, and diuretic properties. It is used for the treatment of ✪ **arthritis**, rheumatism (see ✪ **musculoskeletal disorders**), ✪ **fever**, ✪ **gout**, fibrositis, and ✪ **lumbago**. It is also widely used as a digestive stimulant, and externally, as an ointment, for the ✪ **boils**, sores, and ✪ **ulcers**. Some laboratory studies have confirmed the anti-inflammatory effects of devil's claw, although other studies have found the extracts to be ineffective. Methanolic extracts of the roots have been shown to be cardioactive, and to display weak antifungal activity. Devil's claw is approved by some authorities for ✪ **indigestion**, rheumatism, and ✪ **appetite loss**.

Warnings, interactions, and side effects

Devil's claw is said to have minimal toxicity when taken orally.

• As crude extracts of the plant have been shown to have hypotensive (lowering blood pressure) activity, it should not be taken by anyone with heart disorders, or those taking medication for blood pressure disorders.

• A claim that it should not be used by diabetics, due to a hypoglycemic activity, has not been scientifically established.

• Because devil's claw stimulates secretion of gastric juices, some authorities recommend that it is not used by people with peptic ulcers.

echinacea

(*Echinacea species: E. purpurea (purple coneflower), also other similar species including E. angustifolia (pale purple coneflower) and E. pallida (narrow-leafed purple coneflower)*)

Other common names: **American coneflower, black Sampson, black Susan, comb flower, coneflower, hedgehog, Indian head, Kansas snakeroot, red sunflower, rudbeckia, Sampson root, scurvy root.**

Purple coneflower (*E. purpurea*) is native to the eastern parts of North America, but is now widely cultivated throughout America and Europe. The plant grows to a height of approximately 4 feet (1.25 meters) from underground rhizomes, which can be divided for the purpose of propagation. The flowers of the plant are large, with pink petals surrounding a central, spiny cone. Other species of *Echinacea*, including *E. angustifolia* and *E. pallida*, have similar uses to *E. purpurea*.

Forms of preparation and parts used

Most commonly used plant parts are the rhizomes, the juice of the aerial parts, and the flowers. It is often available in multiherb preparations, for example with ♣ **goldenseal**.

Active components

Alkylamides, caffeic acid derivatives, and polysaccharides and glycoproteins are all thought to contribute to the plant's ability to stimulate the immune system.

Uses in treatment

Native Americans used *Echinacea* species for numerous purposes, including treating snakebites, toothache, and even cancers. Today, preparations of the plant are most frequently used for its stimulant effect on the immune system, particularly for the treatment of respiratory tract infections, such as ❍ **colds** and ❍ **influenza**. Echinacea is approved by some authorities for the common cold, ❍ **cough** and ❍ **bronchitis**, ❍ **fever**, ❍ **urinary tract disorders**, inflammation of the mouth and/or pharynx (see ❍ **inflammation** and ❍ **pharyngitis**), tendency to infection (the herb), and externally for ❍ **wounds** and ❍ **burns**. Clinical studies, although not always conclusive, suggest that the use of echinacea for upper respiratory tract infections (such as the common cold and influenza) can be beneficial. Laboratory studies suggest that alkylamides, caffeic acid and derivatives, and polysaccharides may contribute to the immunostimulant and anti-inflammatory properties of echinacea. One anti-inflammatory mechanism seems to be through inhibition of cyclooxygenase and 5-lipoxygenase enzymes, resulting in decreased production of prostaglandins and similar mediators of inflammation.

Warnings, interactions, and side effects

• There is sometimes uncertainty as to the particular constituents, and strength, of the herbal preparation, and so some authorities warn against prolonged use (more than 6 to 8 weeks) of the herb.

• Due to its reported effects on the immune system, echinacea should be avoided by anyone with an autoimmune disease (such as AIDs) or those taking immunosuppressant drugs.

• Allergic reactions have been reported but are rare.

elecampane

(*Inula helenium*)

Other common names: **alant, elfdock, elfwort, horse-elder, horse-heal, scabwort, velvet dock, wild sunflower, yellow starwort.**

Elecampane is a hardy perennial with tough upright stems growing from a stocky rhizome, and which can reach up to 10 feet (3 meters) high. Its flowers are yellow and daisy-like and are produced through the summer and early fall.

Forms of preparation and parts used

The roots and rhizome of elecampane are used medicinally, usually as a decoction, infusion, or tincture. It is often available in herbal blends.

Active components

Elecampane is rich in carbohydrates (especially inulin) and phytosterols, and also contains a volatile oil rich in sesquiterpenes (such as alantolactone).

Uses in treatment

Elecampane is traditionally used for treating infections, especially of the chest, such as ❍ **bronchitis**, and also ❍ **asthma** and irritating ❍ **coughs**. Alantolactone, a sesquiterpene lactone from the volatile oil, has been used to treat ❍ **worms** (including roundworm and hookworm). An infusion of elecampane has been shown to have sedative effects in laboratory studies, and the volatile oil has been shown to relax smooth muscle. Alantolactone has hypotensive, antibacterial, and antifungal properties. It has also been shown to have effects on blood sugar.

Warnings, interactions, and side effects

• Elecampane can cause contact dermatitis, and the volatile oil can be sensitizing.

• It may interfere with existing treatments for high blood sugar and elevated blood pressure.

• As with other species containing sesquiterpene lactones, elecampane should be used with caution by anyone with known sensitivity to members of the daisy family.

• There is not enough toxicological information for elecampane to be safely recommended for use during pregnancy or by breastfeeding mothers, and so it is best avoided.

elm bark

(*Ulmus minor*; Parts used: inner bark)

Elm bark contains mucilage, tannins, caffeic acid derivatives, and sterols. It has astringent and diuretic properties. It is used internally for ❍ **digestive system disorders** and ❍ **diarrhea**, or externally for cleaning ❍ **wounds**,

Warnings, interactions, and side effects

Although none have been reported with correct use and dosage, the properties of elm bark have not been fully investigated and adverse reactions are possible.

embelia

(*Embelia ribes*; Parts used: fruit)

Embelia contains naphthaquinones, such as embelin. Traditional uses include for ❍ **indigestion**, ❍ **constipation**, and as a diuretic (see ❍ **fluid retention**). Embelin is being studied as a potential contraceptive, because it has been shown to have a stimulatory effect on the production of the female sex hormones estrogen and progesterone.

Warnings, interactions, and side effects

Although none have been reported with correct use and dosage, the properties of embelia have not been fully investigated and adverse reactions are possible.

eucalyptus

(*Eucalyptus globulus*)

Other common names: **blue gum, fevertree, gum tree, red gum, stringy bark tree, Tasmanian blue gum.**

The eucalyptus is a large, evergreen tree native to Australia which grows up to 300 feet (90 meters) in height. It has a blue-grey trunk, and slightly waxy leaves.

Forms of preparation and parts used

Eucalyptus leaves are the most commonly used part, either dried or in a volatile eucalyptus oil.

Active components

The main bioactive components of eucalyptus are its volatile oil, which is rich in eucalyptol (1,8-cineole), flavonoids, tannins, and organic acids.

Uses in treatment

Eucalyptus leaves and the volatile oil are antiseptic and expectorant, and have febrifuge activity. The diluted essential oil can be applied to the skin to warm and slightly anesthetize (dull the sense of pain), which are beneficial properties for treating respiratory tract infections (see ✪ **respiratory tract disorders**) and rheumatic joints. Some authorities approve the use of various parts of the plant for ✪ **cough** and ✪ **bronchitis**, especially ✪ **catarrh** of the respiratory tract, and, when applied externally, for rheumatism (see ✪ **musculoskeletal disorders**). Laboratory studies have shown that gram-positive bacteria are particularly sensitive to eucalyptus extracts, while flavonoid components of eucalyptus have been demonstrated to have antiviral activity against the influenza A virus. Crude leaf extracts have hypoglycemic activity, which is thought to be due to the presence of phenolic glycosides.

Warnings, interactions, and side effects

• Eucalyptus oil should always be diluted before use (whether internally or externally). Undiluted oil is toxic when taken internally. Externally, the diluted oil is non-toxic, non-sensitizing, and non-phototoxic.

• Eucalyptus oil poisoning is typified by epigastric (the middle part of the abdomen) burning, dizziness, vomiting, and even delirium and convulsions.

• The oil should not be used internally during pregnancy, by breast-feeding mothers, or by children.

• The oil should not be applied to the faces of children or infants.

evening primrose

(*Oenothera biennis*)

Other common names: **fever plant, king's cureall, night willow-herb, scabish, sundrop.**

Evening primrose is native to North America, but is now naturalized throughout Europe and parts of Asia. It is an erect biennial which grows from a basal rosette of leaves up to 8 inches (20 centimeters) long. The plant produces bright yellow flowers which are highly aromatic, particularly at night, and can grow up to 5 feet (1.5 meters) tall. Tiny seeds are produced in downy seed pods in late summer and fall.

Forms of preparation and parts used

Most of the aerial parts of the plant can be used in medicines, although the seed oil is the most commonly used. It is often available in multi-herb preparations.

Active components

The seed oil is rich in oils, including *cis*-linoleic acid as the major component, *cis*-gamma-linolenic acid (gamolenic acid: see ⚗ **gamma-linolenic acid (GLA)**), and oleic, palmitic and stearic acids.

Uses in treatment

The oil is widely used for ✪ **premenstrual syndrome**, ✪ **psoriasis**, (atopic) ✪ **eczema**, ✪ **hyperlipidemia**, and ✪ **asthma**, among many. The oil may need to be taken for approximately three months before any effects are observed. Gamma-linolenic acid and its derivatives are precursors of prostaglandins and similar inflammatory mediators. Intake of the oil inhibits production of leukotrienes and other inflammatory mediators resulting from the action of lipoxygenase enzymes on arachidonic acid. Some, but not all, studies have reported the beneficial effects of seed oil intake for premenstrual syndrome, diabetic neuropathy, mild ✪ **multiple sclerosis**, subjective symptoms of ✪ **rheumatoid arthritis**, elevated blood pressure and coronary heart disease, ✪ **chronic fatigue syndrome** (ME, post-viral fatigue syndrome), ✪ **endometriosis**, and mental function in those with Alzheimer's disease.

Warnings, interactions, and side effects

• Excessive use may cause mild nausea, abdominal pain, loose stools, or possibly headache.

• There may be an increased risk of epileptic seizures (temporal lobe epilepsy) in those with schizophrenia who are also taking antipsychotic drugs that lower seizure threshold (such as ℞ **phenothiazines**), and so it should be used with caution.

eyebright

(*Euphrasia officinalis*; Parts used: herb)

Other common names: **euphrasia.**

Eyebright contains flavonoids, iridoids, tannins, and a volatile oil. Traditional uses include for ✪ **inflammation**, ✪ **catarrh**, and as an astringent. Antibacterial and mild purgative activities are known for certain components of eyebright.

Warnings, interactions, and side effects

• Eyebright should not be applied to the eyes.

false unicorn root

(*Chamaelirium luteum or Veratrum luteum*; Parts used: root)

Other common names: **blazing star, fairy-wand, helonias root, starwort.**

False unicorn root is rich in steroidal saponins and glycosides. Traditional uses include for ✪ **premenstrual syndrome**, ✪ **dysmenorrhea**, and to encourage regular menstruation. Its effects on the uterus are most probably due to the saponin components, but there has been almost no scientific investigation of the plant.

Warnings, interactions, and side effects

• False unicorn root is not to be used during pregnancy.

fennel

(*Foeniculum vulgare*; Parts used: fruit)

Other common names: **bitter fennel, fenkel, large fennel, sweet fennel, wild fennel.**

Fennel contains a volatile oil rich in trans-anethols. The oil has antispasmodic and antimicrobial activity, increases gastrointestinal motility (movement), and decreases secretions in the upper respiratory tract. It is approved by some authorities for the treatment of ✪ **catarrh** of the upper respiratory tract such as in ✪ **coughs** and ✪ **bronchitis**, and for mild ✪ **indigestion** and ✪ **flatulence**.

Warnings, interactions, and side effects

• Fennel is not to be used during pregnancy.

• Some fennel preparations must not be given to children, so always seek professional advice first.

• There have been rare cases of allergic reactions.

fenugreek

(*Trigonella foenum-graecum*)

Other common names: **bird's foot, Greek hay seed.**

Fenugreek is a highly aromatic, upright annual herb with three-lobed leaves. The plant is widely cultivated as a culinary herb and is naturalized in many countries. It grows to approximately 18 inches (45 centimeters) tall, and produces pale yellow or off-white flowers, followed by pods containing yellow or brown seeds.

Forms of preparation and parts used

Fenugreek seeds are used medicinally, taken internally, or, more unusually, applied externally in the form of a cream or poultice.

Active components

Fenugreek seeds contain a number of pyridine alkaloids (including trigonelline), flavonoids, saponins (mainly glycosides of diosgenin and yamogenin), and coumarin. They also contain large amounts of protein and mucilage.

Uses in treatment

Fenugreek is normally used as a laxative, expectorant, and demulcent. It is approved by some authorities for ✪ **appetite loss** and externally as a poultice for skin inflammation (see ✪ **skin conditions**). In laboratory studies, fenugreek has been shown to lower blood lipids, which it is thought is due to the fibrous mucilage and saponin content of the seeds. A de-fatted seed fraction has demonstrated hypoglycemic activity, as have trigonelline and vitamin components. Extracts of the seeds are reported to lower blood sugar levels, and trigonelline, present in fenugreek, has been shown in clinical studies to have transient activity of this type in people with ✪ **diabetes mellitus** where daily ingestion of 1 ounce (25 g) of seeds reduced insulin requirements for insulin-dependent diabetics after an eight-week period.

Warnings, interactions, and side effects

• Fenugreek should not be used during pregnancy.

• It is possible that fenugreek could interfere with a number of existing treatments, including those for blood-sugar abnormalities.

• It should also been used with caution by anyone taking ℞ **monoamine-oxidase inhibitor** antidepressants or ℞ **anticoagulant** drugs.

• Absorption of other drugs may also be affected by fenugreek, because of the high fiber content of the seeds.

feverfew

(*Tanacetum parthenium*)

Other common names: **altamisa, featherfew, featherfoil, febrifuge plant, Midsummer daisy, nosebleed, Santa Maria, wild chamomile, wild quinine.**

Feverfew is a highly aromatic perennial with variably yellow- or green-lobed leaves. It produces loose corymbs of daisy-like flowers throughout the summer. Ornamental "double-flowered" varieties also exist, but are not widely used medicinally.

Forms of preparation and parts used

The aerial parts of feverfew, and in particular the leaves, are used medicinally. Leaves can be eaten fresh, usually with bread to mask their bitterness, or taken as a tincture. Numerous commercial products, many containing freeze-dried leaves, are available.

Active components

Feverfew contains a large number of sesquiterpene lactones, including parthenolide and costunolide. It also contains flavonoids, tannins, and a volatile oil rich in mono- and sesquiterpenes.

Uses in treatment

Traditionally, feverfew has been used for ✪ **fever**, ✪ **arthritis**, and various aches and pains, but is most commonly used now for preventing ✪ **headache** and ✪ **migraine**. Laboratory studies have shown that feverfew extracts have effects on platelet and white blood-cell functioning. Clinical studies have shown that feverfew can reduce frequency and severity of migraine episodes, although not all studies found significant beneficial effects. Studies have failed to show any benefit in rheumatoid arthritis. In most cases, the parthenolide content of feverfew is thought to be the active chemical.

Warnings, interactions, and side effects

• Feverfew should not be used during pregnancy, because it is reported to have abortifacient and emmenogogic actions in breast-feeding mothers, and in those with a known sensitivity to members of the daisy family.

• Some patients in the clinical studies reported side effects, including mouth ulcers, indigestion, nausea, vomiting, and hypersensitivity.

• Although the sesquiterpene lactones found in feverfew can cause contact allergies, no reports of allergic reactions following oral administration exist.

• A post-feverfew syndrome has been described where individuals show withdrawal symptoms or nervousness and muscle and joint pains.

• It is very bitter and has an unpleasant taste.

figwort

(*Scrophularia nodosa*; Parts used: herb)

Other common names: **carpenter's square, heal-all scrofula plant, kernelwort, rosenoble, throatwort.**

Figwort contains flavonoids, iridoids, and a number of plant acids. The iridoid components have been shown to have purgative properties and effects on the heart. Traditional uses include for chronic ✪ **skin conditions**, as a mild diuretic (see ✪ **fluid retention**), and to increase contraction of the heart. It can be used as a substitute for ♣ **devil's claw.**

Warnings, interactions, and side effects

• Figwort should not be used by diabetics or anyone with certain heart arrhythmias, such as ventricular tachycardia.

flax

(*Linum usitatissimum*; Parts used: seeds)

Other common names: **flaxseed, linseed, lint bells, winterlien.**

Flax contains mucilage, fatty acids, lignans, and phenylpropane derivatives. Traditional uses include for ✪ **constipation**, and it has been shown to have laxative properties through stimulating peristalsis (rhythmic movement of the alimentary canal). Some authorities approve of its use for constipation, ✪ **irritable bowel syndrome**, the short-term treatment of gastritis and ✪ **enteritis**, and also externally for skin inflammation (see ✪ **skin conditions**). It may also be of some benefit for treating high blood cholesterol levels in ✪ **hyperlipidemia**.

Warnings, interactions, and side effects
• Flax must not be used when the gastrointestinal tract is constricted, blocked, or inflamed.
• It may interfere with the absorption of some drugs.

florists' chrysanthemum
(*Chrysanthemum x morifolium*; Parts used: flowerheads)
Florists' chrysanthemum contains sesquiterpene lactones, a volatile oil, amines, and flavonoids. Traditional uses include to promote sweating, to reduce raised blood pressure (see ✪ **hypertension**), and as an antipyretic. There is clinical evidence that chrysanthemum does lower blood pressure and can have a beneficial effect on ✪ **angina pectoris**.

Warnings, interactions, and side effects
Although none have been reported with correct use and dosage, the properties of florists' chrysanthemum have not been fully investigated and adverse reactions are possible.

frangula
(*Rhamnus frangula*)
Other common names: **alder buckthorn, alder dogwood, arrow wood, black alder, black alder dogwood, black alder tree, black dogwood, buckthorn, dogwood, European black alder, European buckthorn, Persian berries.**
Buckthorn is a thornless deciduous small tree or shrub which grows to approximately 15 feet (4.5 meters). It has ovate leaves and produces small greenish flowers in late spring, followed by red berries.

Forms of preparation and parts used
The bark of frangula is used medicinally, after it has been dried and stored for at least one year (see below). *Rhamnus purshiana*, a native to the western coast of North America, is used in a very similar manner to *R. frangula*.

Active components
Frangula bark contains anthraquinones, including the frangulosides (glycosides of emodin) as well as emodin dianthrone, other anthraquinone glycosides, and free aglycones. The total content of anthraquinones in the bark is typically 3 to 7 percent by weight.

Uses in treatment
Frangula bark has mild laxative and cathartic properties and is commonly used for chronic ✪ **constipation**, and is approved by some authorities for this use. Drying of the bark results in a milder laxative action than other species taken for similar purposes (such as ℞ **senna**).

Warnings, interactions, and side effects
• Frangula should not be used during pregnancy.
• The fresh bark is violently purgative, and is not widely used medicinally.

• All frangula products which are not standardized for anthraquinone content are not recommended, because their effects can be variable and unpredictable.
• Anthraquinones can have toxic effects if taken in large doses, and excessive intake can result in stomach cramps and diarrhea.
• As with other stimulant anthraquinone laxatives (including ♣ **aloe**, ♣ **rhubarb, Chinese**, ♣ **yellow dock**, and ℞ **senna**), long-term use should be avoided.

fringed pink
(*Dianthus superbus*; Parts used: aerial parts)
Other common names: **superb pink.**
Fringed pink contains a volatile oil rich in eugenol. Traditional uses include for ✪ **kidney disorders** and ✪ **urinary tract disorders**. Research suggests that the flowers have the greatest diuretic (see ✪ **fluid retention**) activity compared with other parts of the plant.

Warnings, interactions, and side effects
Although none have been reported with correct use and dosage, the properties of fringed pink have not been fully investigated and adverse reactions are possible.

fumitory
(*Fumaria officinalis*)
Other common names: **beggary, earth smoke, fumus, hedge fumitory, vapor, wax dolls.**
Fumitory is a climbing annual which grows to approximately 12 inches (30 centimeters) in height. It has compound leaves, and pink tubular flowers with maroon tips.

Forms of preparation and parts used
The aerial parts of the herb are most commonly used, usually as an infusion or tincture.

Active components
The major active constituents of fumitory are isoquinoline alkaloids, flavonoids (including rutin), and phenolic acids, as well as a resin, bitter principles, and a mucilaginous substance.

Uses in treatment
Traditionally, fumitory is used to treat ✪ **skin conditions**, including chronic ✪ **eczema** and conjunctivitis (see warnings below). Internally, it has weak diuretic (see ✪ **fluid retention**) and laxative properties. Fumitory has also been used to treat ✪ **migraine** associated with digestive complaints. In laboratory studies, it has been shown to have beneficial effects on gallbladder function, and some authorities approve its use for ✪ **liver disorders** and ✪ **gallbladder disorders**. Hypotensive activity has also been reported.

Warnings, interactions, and side effects
• The external use of fumitory for treating conjunctivitis is no longer recommended, due to concerns that it causes increased intraocular pressure (pressure in the eyeball).
• It is recommeded that its use should be avoided during pregnancy and if breast-feeding because its safety in these situations has not been thoroughly established.

galangal
(*Alpinia officinarum*; Parts used: rhizome)

Galangal contains sesquiterpene lactones and a volatile oil. It is used as a carminative and stimulant, and is approved by some authorities for ✪ **indigestion**, ✪ **appetite loss**, and to reduce ✪ **vomiting**. Studies have shown that it has antimicrobial activity.

Warnings, interactions, and side effects

Although none have been reported with correct use and dosage, the properties of galangal have not been fully investigated and adverse reactions are possible.

garden cress

(*Lepidium sativum*; Parts used: herb)

Garden cress is rich in ♨ **vitamin C** and also contains cardenolides. Traditional uses include for ✪ **scurvy**, ✪ **coughs**, and poor immunity. Its beneficial effects are mainly due to the vitamin C content, although some antibacterial and antiviral activity has also been reported.

Warnings, interactions, and side effects

Although none have been reported with correct use and dosage, the properties of garden cress have not been fully investigated and adverse reactions are possible.

garlic

(*Allium sativum*)

Other common names: **allium, camphor of the poor, clove garlic, common garlic, nectar of the gods, poor man's treacle, rustic treacle, stinking rose.**

A highly aromatic perennial growing from a bulb consisting of 5 to15 bulblets ("cloves"). The flat green leaves can grow to a length of 2 feet (60 centimeters). In summer, the plant produces a single flower spike with an umbel of green-white to pink flowers, which grows to a height of up to 3 feet (90 centimeters). The plant originated in Central Asia, but is now grown around the world.

Forms of preparation and parts used

The garlic bulb is used medicinally, either fresh or dried, or as an extract or oil. Commercial garlic preparations now exist in deodorized (odor-free) forms. Odor-free forms are made of garlic oil or powder in enteric (slow-release) capsules or tablets, aged-garlic extract (AGE), or steam-distilled garlic oil. Also, preparations of garlic containing parsley are said to reduce garlic odor. Some of these preparations have been criticized because they contain less of the beneficially active compounds (allicin or its sulfur metabolites). In any event, sulfur-odor may be present in sweat following release of the compounds in the intestine. It is also available in various forms as a dietary supplement (see the entry for ♨ **garlic** in Vitamins, Minerals, and Supplements)

Active components

Garlic contains a number of sufur-containing volatile compounds, many of which are derived from alliin, as well as terpenes, and vitamins. When the garlic bulb is crushed or cut, alliin is converted to allicin which is responsible for many of the beneficial effects of garlic (either in itself or its sulfur metabolites).

Uses in treatment

Garlic is a very commonly used herb, and has antibacterial, antifungal, expectorant, hypotensive, cholesterol-lowering, and anticoagulant properties. In many cases, these properties have been supported by laboratory and clinical studies. Garlic is commonly used to treat ✪ **infections**, especially bacterial, viral, and fungal infections, including of the respiratory (for example, a ✪ **cold**) and digestive tracts, and is approved by some authorities for ✪ **hypertension**, ✪ **arteriosclerosis**, ✪ **hyperlipidemia** (to lower LDL cholesterol levels), and ✪ **atherosclerosis**. It is also used to thin the blood and it may be beneficial in some forms of ✪ **diabetes mellitus**. It is considered by some to help protect against cancer.

Warnings, interactions, and side effects

• Although regarded as non-toxic, and widely used in cooking, garlic can cause side effects, including irritation and burning of the mouth and gastrointestinal tract, nausea, diarrhea, and vomiting. Often such effects depend on the amount consumed.

• Allergic reactions such as contact dermatitis and asthma have been reported in people exposed to garlic as part of their occupation.

• Garlic may interact with anticoagulants (such as ℞ **warfarin**), hypoglycemics, drugs regulating blood pressure, or non-steroidal anti-inflammatory drugs (such as ℞ **aspirin**) taken for their antithrombotic actions.

• It should not be used when breast-feeding.

geum

(*Geum urbanum*; Parts used: herb)

Other common names: **avens root, Bennet's root, blessed herb, city avens, colewort, European avens, goldy star, herb Bennet, star of the earth, way Bennet, wild rye, yellow avens.**

Geum contains tannins, bitter compounds, a resin, and a volatile oil. Traditional uses include to treat ✪ **hemorrhage**, ✪ **diarrhea**, and ✪ **fever**. It has been reported that geum has astringent and hypotensive actions.

Warnings, interactions, and side effects

Although none have been reported with correct use and dosage, the properties of geum have not been fully investigated and adverse reactions are possible.

giant hyssop

(*Agastache rugosa*; Parts used: herb)

Giant hyssop contains a volatile oil rich in anethole, anisaldehyde, limonene, and methyl chavicol. Traditional uses include as a digestive herb, and to treat various types of ✪ **infection**. Experiments have shown that giant hyssop has antifungal activity.

Warnings, interactions, and side effects

Although none have been reported with correct use and dosage, the properties of giant hyssop have not been fully investigated and adverse reactions are possible.

ginger

(*Zingiber officinale*)

Ginger is a spreading deciduous perennial, with stocky stems and pointed leaves growing from branched rhizomes to a height of approximately 4 to 5 feet (1.25 to 1.5 meters). It produces yellow, green, and purple flowers in the summer, followed by fleshy fruit capsules.

Forms of preparations and parts used

The rhizome of ginger is used both medicinally and in cooking. For medicinal purposes it is taken fresh, as a tincture or infusion.

Active constituents

Ginger contains a range of lipids, an oleo-resin rich in gingerol and shogaol homologs, a complex hydrocarbon-rich volatile oil, amino acids, proteins, and vitamins.

Uses in treatment

Ginger is commonly used as an anti-inflammatory, antiseptic, carminative, antispasmodic, and diaphoretic. In laboratory studies, ginger juice has been shown to lower blood sugar levels, Some authorities approve the use of it for ✪ **appetite loss**, ✪ **motion sickness**, ✪ **nausea**, and ✪ **indigestion**. Results from clinical studies that have investigated the effects of ginger to treat motion sickness, however, are inconclusive. Ginger extracts and compounds have been shown to affect a number of inflammatory mechanisms.

Warnings, interactions, and side effects.

• Ginger should not be used during pregnancy for medicinal purposes, because it has been reported to have abortifacient activity.

• Excessive intake may interfere with certain heart, diabetic, or antiplatelet (including ℞ **aspirin**) treatments.

• It has been shown in laboratory studies to have mutagenic effects.

ginkgo
(*Ginkgo biloba*)
Other common names: **bai guo, Kew tree, maidenhair tree.**
A deciduous tree with one or more trunks growing to a height of approximately 100 feet (30 meters). The tree has two-lobed, fan-shaped leaves, from which the plants gets the name "biloba." The plant bears very small female flowers, and, occasionally, plum-shaped, strongly smelling fruit.

Forms of preparation and parts used

The leaves of ginkgo are most commonly used, although the seeds also have some medicinal uses. The leaves are usually taken as a liquid or dried extracts. It is often sold as a combination product. A standardized preparation containing 24 percent flavone glycosides and 6 percent terpene lactones, called GBE-standardized *Ginkgo biloba* extract, is available for medicinal use. Ginkgo is one of the top-selling herbal remedies in the US.

Active components

The leaves contain a range of flavonoids, proanthocyanidins, and diterpenoids, including a number of so-called "ginkgolides." The seeds contain alkaloids, cyanogenic glycosides, and a number of phenolic compounds.

Uses in treatment

Ginkgo has circulatory stimulant, antiasthmatic, anti-inflammatory, and antispasmodic properties. Laboratory studies have been carried out on ginkgo and many of the herb's actions are thought to arise from the ability of the ginkgolides to inhibit the effects of the naturally occurring chemical mediator called platelet-activating factor (PAF), which therefore affects coronary flow and heart contraction, blood clotting, and bronchoconstriction in the lungs. It is used for ✪ **peripheral vascular disorders** and ✪ **Raynaud's disease**. Ginkgo has also been of benefit to the healthy functioning of brain circulation. The herb is widely believed to improve memory (see ✪ **dementia**), and to reduce age-related deterioration of mental functions through improvements to cerebral circulation. Numerous clinical trials have been performed on these activities, many of them with positive results, and some authorities approve the use of standardized extracts of ginkgo for ✪ **vertigo** and ✪ **tinnitus** (when it is caused by vascular problems), to help relieve the pain when walking in intermittent claudication (cramp-like pain in the calves), and for the relief of symptoms of organic brain dysfunction (such as dementia).

Warnings, interactions, and side effects

• The fruit pulp and seeds can cause severe allergic reactions, and should not be handled or ingested.

• Whether or not it is safe to use during pregnancy or when breast-feeding has not been established and so it is best to avoid it during these times.

• Because it reduces blood clotting, people with clotting disorders, or who are taking ℞ **anticoagulant** drugs should take the herb with caution and under expert supervision.

ginseng, Siberian
(*Eleutherococcus senticosus*)
Other common names: **eleuthero, devil's shrub, eleutherococ, shigoka, touch-me-not, ussarian thorny pepperbush, wild pepper.**
Siberian ginseng is a hardy deciduous shrub which grows to a height of approximately 10 feet (3 meters) and has 3 to 7 toothed leaves.

Forms of preparation and parts used

The roots are the most commonly used parts and in the form of decoctions, powders, teas, and tinctures. Siberian ginseng is available commercially in mixed herbal preparations.

Active components

The main components of Siberian ginseng are the eleutherosides, which are a chemically unrelated group of compounds, including monosaccharides, lignans, sterols, and phenylpropanoids, often in their glycosylated forms. In addition to these compounds and derivatives, there are also polysaccharides, terpenoids, and a volatile oil.

Uses in treatment

Siberian ginseng is claimed to increase resistance to ✪ **stress** and improve vitality. These so-called adaptogenic activities are similar to those of *Panax ginseng* (see ♧ **ginseng**). Siberian ginseng is most widely used to combat stress (either mental or physical), and to treat prolonged ✪ **fatigue**, such as following illness. In laboratory studies, the herb has been shown to have hypoglycemic activity, to stimulate the central nervous system, and also, paradoxically, to have sedative properties. Polysaccharides, which are found in Siberian ginseng, have been shown to stimulate the immune system, and a liquid extract from the herb has been demonstrated to increase resistance to certain infections.

Warnings, interactions, and side effects

• Although Siberian ginseng was shown to be of low toxicity in extensive trials, some side effects have been reported, including hypertension, diarrhea, insomnia, and skin eruptions.

Key to symbols: ✪ = Disorder Section ℞ = Drug Section ♣ = Herbal Section ♧ = Supplement Section

• Possible interactions with the ℞ **MAOI** antidepressant ℞ **phenelzine** have also been reported.

• It should not be used during acute illnesses, hemorrhages, and following coronary thrombosis.

• It should be avoided by nervous, tense, highly energetic, or schizophrenic individuals, and should not be taken with other stimulants (such as ℞ **caffeine** in coffee) or when taking hormonal treatments.

ginseng
(*Panax ginseng*)
Other common names: **Asian ginseng, Chinese ginseng, five-fingers, Japanese ginseng, Korean ginseng, Oriental ginseng, red berry, true ginseng.**
Ginseng is a perennial herb which grows to a height of about 3 feet (90 centimeters). It has toothed, oval-shaped leaves, and clustered green-white flowers, followed by bright red berries. It differs in several respects from ♣ **ginseng, Siberian** which comes from a different plant.

Forms of preparation and parts used
The root of ginseng is used medicinally. The peeled and sun-dried roots are referred to as "white ginseng," and the unpeeled, dried roots are "red ginseng."

Active components
The active compounds in ginseng include ginsenosides (a complex series of terpenoids of tetracyclic sapogenin or pentacyclic triterpenoid types), sesquiterpene alcohols, small quantities of a volatile oil, sterols, polyacetylenic compounds, and starch.

Uses in treatment
The botanic name *Panax* comes from the Greek (*pan* (all) & *akos* (cure), so meaning "cure-all"—the same stem as the word panacea). Ginseng is primarily used as an adaptogen and a tonic. It is said to possess thymoleptic (mind-stimulating or mood-elevating), sedative, stomachic, and demulcent activities. Traditional uses include for ✺ **motion sickness** and ✺ **indigestion**. Its use can be either short term (generally two to three weeks) for increasing stamina and feeling of well-being; or long term (at lower doses) to promote well-being in the elderly or chronically ill. The plant also has hypoglycemic, cardiovascular, hepatoprotective, and antiviral activities. The positive effects of some ginseng products on energy levels are reported to result from a more efficient use of oxygen. Many of these actions have been confirmed through laboratory or clinical studies, and it is approved by some authorities for treating poor concentration, ✺ **fatigue**, lack of stamina, and for convalescence.

Warnings, interactions, and side effects
• Side effects and adverse reactions have been reported, although the details of the amount and the type of ginseng taken are not always clear (see ♣ **ginseng, Siberian**, *Eleutherococcus senticosus*).

• Because its safety during pregnancy or breast-feeding has not been established, and there have been reports of hormonal effects in women, ginseng should not be used at these times.

• It should only be used with caution by anyone with a heart disorder, diabetes mellitus, high blood pressure, those taking steroids or blood-thinning drugs (anticoagulants or antiplatelet

drugs), and some others. In general it should be taken with caution by anyone taking other stimulants (such as ℞ **caffeine**), OTC, or prescription drugs. A doctor should be consulted first.

• Some experts discourage the use of ginseng for longer than six weeks at a time, and it is wise to avoid taking other stimulants at the same time.

goldenrod
(*Solidago virgaurea*; Parts used: aerial parts)
Other common names: **Aaron's rod, European goldenrod, woundwort.**
Goldenrod contains triterpene saponins, polysaccharides, caffeic acids, and a volatile oil. It has diuretic (see ✺ **fluid retention**), antiphlogistic, and spasmolytic activity. Traditional uses, which are approved by some authorities, include ✺ **urinary tract disorders**, irrigation therapy for inflammatory diseases of the lower urinary tract, and stones in the bladder and/or kidney (see ✺ **calculus**).

Warnings, interactions, and side effects
• Goldenrod should not be used by anyone with a chronic kidney disease without professional supervision.

• It may be weakly sensitizing.

goldenseal
(*Hydrastis canadensis*; Parts used: rhizome)
Other common names: **eye balm, eye root, ground raspberry, Indian dye, Indian paint, Indian plant, jaundice root, orange root, turmeric root, warnera, wild curcuma, yellow puccoon, yellow root.**
Goldenseal contains isoquinoline alkaloids, fatty acids, and carbohydrates. The alkaloids in goldenseal have anticonvulsant and antimicrobial activity, hypotensive effects, and effects on the heart. Goldenseal contains the alkaloid berberine, which has been shown to have choleretic and antidiarrheal activity. Traditional uses include for ✺ **digestive system disorders**, ✺ **catarrh**, ✺ **dysmenorrhea**, and ✺ **eczema** (when it is used externally).

Warnings, interactions, and side effects
• Goldenseal should not be used durng pregnancy.

• It should not be used by anyone with ✺ **hypertension**, or who is receiving the anticoagulant drug ℞ **heparin**.

• It should not be used by anyone with G6PD-deficiency (glucose 6-phosphate dehydrogenase enzyme deficiency)

• If taken for an extended period, it may cause digestive disorders, constipation, irritation of mucous membranes, agitated and excited states, and even hallucinations.

gotu kola
(*Centella asiatica, C. coriaca* or *Hydrocotyle asiatica*)
Other common names: **hydrocotyle, Indian hydrocotyle, Indian pennywort, marsh penny, sheep rot, talepetrako, thick-leaved pennywort, white rot.**
Gotu kola is a creeping perennial herb with heart or fan-shaped leaves native to southern parts of the US. It can reach approximately 2 feet (60 centimeters) in height, and is often found near streams or in marshy areas. It should not be confused with kola nut (see ♣ **cola**), an unrelated, caffeine-containing herb.

Forms of preparation and parts used

The aerial parts of gotu kola are used medicinally, usually as an infusion or powder, which can also be formulated into a paste for external application.

Active components

Gotu kola contains a number of terpenoids, including triterpene saponins and sapogenins, amino acids, fatty acids, phytosterols, flavonoids, and a volatile oil rich in sesquiterpenes.

Uses in treatment

Gotu kola is used as a mild sedative for ✪ **insomnia**, as a diuretic, to dilate the peripheral blood vessels, and it is approved by some authorities for the treatment of rheumatism (see ✪ **musculoskeletal disorders**) and topically for ✪ **skin conditions**. Laboratory and clinical studies have been carried out on gotu kola and extracts from it. For example, in some studies the saponin asiaticoside has been shown to have anti-inflammatory and wound-healing properties. It has also been shown experimentally to have beneficial effects against peptic ulcers. Other saponins present in gotu kola have central nervous system-depressant activity, relax smooth muscles, and also have antifertility effects. Other studies have shown that gotu kola extracts promote the healing of wounds, reduce scarring, may be useful for ✪ **psoriasis**, and also ✪ **venous insufficiency** because it improves circulation in the lower limbs.

Warnings, interactions, and side effects

• Gotu kola should not be used during pregnancy.

• It should not be used in excess by breast-feeding mothers.

• Ingestion of gotu kola can cause itching.

• Application to the skin may cause a brief sensation of burning.

• It elevates blood sugar levels and so should not be taken by anyone also taking hypoglycemic treatments.

grains of paradise

(*Aframomum melegueta*; Parts used: seed)

Other common names: **Guinea grains, mallaguetta pepper, melegueta pepper.**

Grains of paradise contains a volatile oil, tannins, and paradol, which is a pungent compound similar to gingerol (found in ginger). It is often used as a digestive remedy as well as a condiment. The uses of grains of paradise are similar to those for ♣ **ginger** (*Zingiber officinale*), such as for treating ✪ **appetite loss** and ✪ **indigestion**, as both plants have a similar chemical composition.

Warnings, interactions, and side effects

• Grains of paradise may irritate the stomach and urinary tract if taken in large amounts.

green tea

(*Camellia sinensis*; Parts used: leaves, buds)

Other common names: **black tea, Chinese tea.**

Green tea contains xanthines (℞ **caffeine**, theobromine), tannins, and flavonoids. Traditional uses include as a stimulant beverage (see ✪ **fatigue**), and research has also shown that it is a powerful ☍ **antioxidant** and may benefit ✪ **hepatitis** sufferers, and that regular consumption may inhibit ✪ **tooth decay**.

Warnings, interactions, and side effects

• Excessive intake, particularly by anyone who is pregnant or breast-feeding, should be avoided because of the tannin and caffeine content. See also Supplements section, ☍ **green tea**.

ground ivy

Nepeta hederacea or *Glechoma hederacea*; Parts used: herb

Other common names: **alehoof, cat's paw, catsfoot, creeping Charlie, Gill-go-over-the-ground, Gill-to-by-the-hedge, haymaids, hedgemaids, Lizzy-run-up-the-hedge, Robin-run-in-the-hedge, tun-hoof, turnhoof.**

Ground ivy contains flavonoids, terpenoids, and a number of plant acids. It has been shown to have astringent, anti-inflammatory, expectorant, vulnerary, and diuretic properties. Traditional uses include for ✪ **bronchitis**, ✪ **hemorrhoids**, and ✪ **catarrh**.

Warnings, interactions, and side effects

• Ground ivy may be irritating in excess, and should be avoided by anyone with kidney disease or epilepsy.

guaiac

(*Guaiacum officinale*)

Other common names: **guaiacum, lignum vitae, pockwood.**

Guaiac is a small evergreen tree with divided leaves which grows to a height of up to 30 feet (9 meters). The tree produces intense blue flowers, followed by orange-yellow seed capsules.

Forms of preparation and parts used

The most commonly used part of guaiac is the resin obtained from the heartwood of the tree, usually as a powder or as a liquid extract or tincture.

Active components

The resin is rich in lignans, including guaiaretic acid and its derivatives, furanolignans, and an eredione lignan. It also contains phytosterols and terpenoids.

Uses in treatment

Guaiac is used to treat arthritic conditions and is approved by some authorities for rheumatism (see ✪ **musculoskeletal disorders**), especially as a tincture, which can be applied externally to the affected areas. The anti-inflammatory actions of guaiac are almost certainly due to its lignan content (guaiaretic acid derivatives have been shown in laboratory studies to inhibit the lipoxygenase enzyme system which is involved in inflammatory responses in the body). It also has diuretic and laxative actions, and promotes sweating and expulsion of toxins. Because of these properties it has been used to treat ✪ **gout**. Lignans also often have antimicrobial or antifungal activity.

Warnings, interactions, and side effects

• The resin has low toxicity when taken by mouth, although it can cause dermatitis in sensitized people. For this reason, it is best avoided by anyone with hypersensitivity, allergies, or acute inflammatory conditions.

• It should not be used during pregnancy, when breast-feeding, or by infants.

guarana

(*Paullinia cupana*; Parts used: seeds)

Other common names: **Brazilian cocoa, guarana bread, paullinia.**

Guarana contains ℞ **caffeine** and related alkaloids, tannins, and saponins. It is used as a tonic and stimulant (see ✪ **fatigue**), and these effects are largely due to its caffeine content.

Warnings, interactions, and side effects

• Excessive caffeine intake, especially during pregnancy, should always be avoided.

guelder rose

(*Viburnum opulus*; Parts used: bark)

Guelder rose contains tannins, coumarins, and hydroquinones. Traditional uses include for general aches and cramps. The bark is now used as a muscle relaxant and for ✪ **arthritis** and ✪ **hypertension** (high blood pressure). However, there is little scientific evidence to support these uses.

Warnings, interactions, and side effects

Although none have been reported with correct use and dosage, the properties of guelder rose have not been fully investigated and adverse reactions are possible.

gutta percha

(*Eucommia ulmoides*; Parts used: bark)

Gutta percha contains alkaloids, iridoids, and a range of other glycosides. Traditional uses include as a liver and kidney tonic. One clinical study suggests that the plant may be of benefit to patients with mild ✪ **hypertension**.

Warnings, interactions, and side effects

Although none have been reported with correct use and dosage, the properties of gutta percha have not been fully investigated and adverse reactions are possible.

haronga

(*Haronga madagascariensis*; Parts used: leaves and bark)

Haronga contains numerous derivatives of anthracene and procyanidins. Traditional uses, which are approved by some authorities, include for ✪ **indigestion**, ✪ **appetite loss**, ✪ **liver disorders**, and ✪ **gallbladder disorders**. It has been shown to stimulate pancreatic and gastric secretions, as well as displaying cholagogic, hepatoprotective, and antimicrobial properties.

Warnings, interactions, and side effects

Although none have been reported with correct use and dosage, the properties of haronga have not been fully investigated and adverse reactions are possible.

hartstongue

(*Scolopendrium vulgare*; Parts used: fronds)

Other common names: **buttonhole, God's-hair, hind's tongue, horse tongue.**

Hartstongue contains tannins, flavonoids, and mucilage, and has aperient and diuretic activity. Traditional uses include for easing ✪ **digestive system disorders** and treating ✪ **urinary tract disorders**.

Warnings, interactions, and side effects

Although none have been reported with correct use and dosage, the properties of hartstongue have not been fully investigated and adverse reactions are possible.

hawthorn

(*Crataegus species: C. laevigata, C. monogyna, C. oxyacantha*)

Other common names: **English hawthorn (*C. laevigata*), haw, May, Mayblossom, Maybush, whitethorn.**

Hawthorn is a deciduous, thorny tree of the *Rosaceae* family, which grows to a height of approximately 25 feet (7.5 meters). The tree bears white flowers in late spring and bright red berries in the fall. It is best known in Europe, but use of hawthorn is becoming more common in the US.

Forms of preparation and parts used

The most commonly used plant parts are the flowering tops and the fruit, usually as an infusion or a liquid extract which can be dried.

Active components

The major biologically active compounds found in hawthorn include a large number of flavonoids, tannins, and cyanogenic glycosides.

Uses in treatment

Hawthorn is described as a cardiotonic, with vasodilating and hypotensive activities. It is traditionally used to treat cardiac failure and weakness, tachycardia, ✪ **hypertension**, ✪ **arteriosclerosis**, and ✪ **atherosclerosis**. Laboratory studies confirm that hawthorn extracts increase coronary blood flow, reduce blood pressure, and affect peripheral blood flow (in the hands, feet, and so on). Many of these activities are thought to be due to the procyanidin component of the extract. There is clinical evidence for some of the claimed beneficial effects of hawthorn on the heart and circulation.

Warnings, interactions, and side effects

• As extracts have been shown to reduce the tone and motility of the uterus, hawthorn should not be used during pregnancy or by breast-feeding mothers.

• Some authorities recommend that hawthorn only be used under expert supervision.

• Fatigue, nausea, and a rash have all been reported as side effects of hawthorn-based products in clinical trials.

• Because of the numerous effects of this herb on the heart and circulation, it may affect existing therapies for a number of conditions, including hypertension, heart disorders, and hypotension.

heartsease

(*Viola tricolor*; Parts used: aerial parts)

Other common names: **European wild pansy, Johnny-jump-up, wild pansy.**

Heartsease contains flavonoids, mucilage, tannins, and hydroxycoumarins, and has ⚖ **antioxidant** and antiphlogistic properties. It is used, and approved by some authorities, for ✪ **skin conditions**, such as ✪ **dermatitis** and ✪ **prickly heat**, and also ✪ **warts**.

Warnings, interactions, and side effects

Although none have been reported with correct use and dosage, the properties of heartsease have not been fully investigated and adverse reactions are possible.

hempnettle

(*Galeopsis segetum*; Parts used: herb)

Hempnettle contains monoterpenoids, flavonoids, and tannins. It has astringent and expectorant actions. Traditional uses include for ✪ **coughs** and ✪ **bronchitis**, and these uses are approved by some authorities.

Warnings, interactions, and side effects

Although none have been reported with correct use and dosage, the properties of hempnettle have not been fully investigated and adverse reactions are possible.

henna

(*Lawsonia inermis*; Parts used: aerial parts)

Other common names: **alcanna, Egyptian privet, henne, Jamaica mignonette, mehndi, mendee, mignonette tree, reseda, smooth Lawsonia.**

Henna is normally used externally for ✪ **eczema**, ✪ **dermatitis**, ✪ **scabies**, and ✪ **dandruff**, and has astringent and antibacterial activity. Its internal use as a diuretic is not so widely approved.

Warnings, interactions, and side effects

• Henna, if taken internally, may cause stomach complaints as it can cause gastric irritation.

herb Robert

(*Geranium robertianum*; Parts used: aerial parts)

Other common names: **dragon's blood, storkbill, wild crane's-bill.**

Herb Robert contains flavonoids and tannins. It is used for impaired gallbladder and liver function, and for ✪ **inflammation**, particularly of the mouth. It has astringent, antimicrobial, and limited antiviral activity, and may also have diuretic properties.

Warnings, interactions, and side effects

Although none have been reported with correct use and dosage, the properties of herb Robert have not been fully investigated and adverse reactions are possible.

hibiscus

(*Hibiscus sabdariffa*; Parts used: flowers)

Other common names: **guinea sorrel, Jamaica sorrel, red sorrel, roselle.**

Hibiscus contains fruit acids, flavonoids, and mucilage. It is often used as a laxative and diuretic (see ✪ **fluid retention**), as well as for ✪ **colds** and ✪ **appetite loss**. The mucilage and poorly absorbed fruit acids are thought to be responsible for its laxative effects.

Warnings, interactions, and side effects

Although none have been reported with correct use and dosage, the properties of hibiscus have not been fully investigated and adverse reactions are possible.

holy basil

(*Ocimum sanctum*; Parts used: herb)

Holy basil contains flavonoids, ursolic acid, and a volatile oil rich in eugenol. Traditionally used as an invigorating tonic, it has beneficial hypoglycemic activity in some forms of ✪ **diabetes mellitus**, and anti-inflammatory and hypotensive activity.

Warnings, interactions, and side effects

• Holy basil should not be used during pregnancy.

honeysuckle

(*Lonicera caprifolium*; Parts used: flowers, leaves and seeds)

Other common names: **goat's leaf, woodbine.**

Honeysuckle contains saponins and flavonoids. Traditonal uses include for ✪ **digestive system disorders** and it has laxative (and diaphoretic) activity.

Warnings, interactions, and side effects

• Honeysuckle may cause gastrointestinal irritation in some people.

hops

(*Humulus lupulus*)

Other common names: **common hops, European hops, hop strobile, humulus, lupulin.**

Hops come from a tall perennial climbing plant, which can reach heights of 20 feet (6 meters) or more. In cultivation, the stems of the plant are supported on wire runners. Hops are best known for the bitter taste they give to beer.

Forms of preparation and parts used

The flowers of the female plant ("strobiles") are used medicinally, usually as an infusion, a liquid extract, or a tincture.

Active components

Hops contain a range of biologically active components, including flavonoids, chalcones, tannins, a volatile oil, and an oleo-resin.

Uses in treatment

Hops have sedative activity, and, in high dose can be hypnotic. Traditionally, they are used in the treatment of ✪ **neuralgia**, ✪ **insomnia**, and ✪ **stress**. Some authorities approve their use for mood disturbances, such as restlessness and anxiety, and also sleep disturbances. When applied externally, hops have been shown to have antibacterial and antifungal activity, and have been used to treat ✪ **ulcers**. In laboratory studies, hop extracts have also been shown to have antispasmodic activity. It is thought that breakdown products from the bitter acids found in hops are responsible for its sedative actions.

Warnings, interactions, and side effects

• Small doses of hops are regarded as non-toxic, although sensitization can occur to the oil, which is thought to be due to the presence of monoterpene myrcene.

• Contact dermatitis is also known, and is thought to result from contact with the pollen of the flowers (causing so-called hop-picker's disease).

• Hops should not be taken by people suffering from depressive illnesses as they are sedative; and they may also interfere with other sedative therapies and with alcohol.

• Hops should not be taken during pregnancy because they have been shown to have effects on uterine tissues.

horehound

(*Marrubium vulgare*)

Other common names: **hoarhound, houndsblane, marrubium, marvel, white horehound.**

Horehound is an aromatic, woody perennial with grey-green toothed leaves, and small off-white double-lipped flowers.

Forms of preparation and parts used

The flowers and leaves of white horehound are used medicinally, usually as the dried herb, an infusion, or as a liquid extract.

Active components

Horehound contains pyrrolidine alkaloids, flavonoids, terpenoids (including the diterpene marrubin and premarrubin), a volatile oil, a phytosterol, and saponin and waxes.

Uses in treatment

Horehound has expectorant and antispasmodic properties, and has been used for bronchial congestion in ✪ **bronchitis**, whooping cough (see ✪ **pertussis**), and bronchial ✪ **asthma**. The bitterness of the herb has been used to promote appetite, and it is approved by some authorities for ✪ **appetite loss** and also dyspeptic complaints (see ✪ **indigestion**) and ✪ **flatulence**. The herb is less commonly used to stabilize heart rhythm, and, externally for various ✪ **skin conditions**. Marrubin, a strongly bitter terpenoid extracted from white horehound, has been shown in studies to promote bronchial secretions, which leads to a more productive cough. This chemical is also thought to be responsible for the plant's claimed ability to stabilize heart rhythms.

Warnings, interactions, and side effects

• Horehound should not be used during pregnancy or by breast-feeding mothers.

• The juice of horehound is said to be irritating to the skin.

horse chestnut

(*Aesculus hippocastanum*)

Other common names: **buckeye, common horse chestnut, conqueror tree, Spanish chestnut.**

The horse chestnut is a large tree with palmate leaves which grows up to a height of 130 feet (40 meters). The leaves are large and lobed, and the tree produces upright spikes of white or pink flowers in late spring. The fruits are green with a spiny coat, and each contains an average of one to three seeds. A native to southeastern Europe and parts of Asia, the tree is now grown in many temperate regions.

Forms of preparation and parts used

The most commonly used parts are the seeds, bark, and leaves, usually as liquid extracts or as a gel or ointment.

Active components

The seeds in particular contain large amounts of saponins, including aescin (which is actually a mixture of compounds), as well as coumarins, flavonoids, and tannins.

Uses in treatment

Horse chestnut is most commonly used to treat ✪ **varicose veins** and leg ulcers (see ✪ **ulcer**). It is approved by some authorities for symptoms caused by ✪ **venous insufficiency**. Clinical studies have confirmed that horse chestnut can improve the swelling and pain associated with venous insufficiency by altering capillary perme-

ability. Aesin, present in horse chestnut has a number of biological activities, including improving capillary fragility, as well as anti-inflammatory and antiviral actions.

Warnings, interactions, and side effects

• Clinical studies looking at the medicinal properties of horse chestnut have used defined extracts taken by mouth (orally), however, this method of administration is not recommended unless it is carried out under expert supervision. This is because aesin (a saponin) and related compounds which are found in horse chestnut can rupture red blood cells if they enter the bloodstream, and if taken in large doses can result in death due to this hemolysis (disintegration of red blood cells).

• Although hemolysis does not usually result when horse chestnut is taken orally, saponins can also irritate the gastrointestinal tract. External application (to unbroken skin) is a more common mode of administration.

• There is evidence that oral administration of these saponins can interfere with ℞ **anticoagulant** drugs.

• Horse chestnut should be avoided by anyone with liver or kidney disorders.

horsemint, English

(*Mentha longifolia*; Parts used: herb)

English horsemint contains a volatile oil rich in piperitone and flavonoids, and has carminative and stimulant activities. Traditional uses include for ✪ **digestive system disorders** and ✪ **headaches**.

Warnings, interactions, and side effects

Although none have been reported with correct use and dosage, the properties of English horsemint have not been fully investigated and adverse reactions are possible.

horseradish

(*Armoracia rusticana*)

Other common names: **great raifort, mountain radish, red cole.**

A hardy perennial growing to a height of approximately 20 inches (50 centimeters). Originally native to Europe and western Asia, the plant is now grown commercially around the world for the large, deep roots, which are widely used in cooking.

Forms of preparation and parts used

The root is taken medicinally and usually in its fresh form which is then grated.

Active components

Horseradish contains a number of volatile compounds, based on the isothiocyanate structure, which are responsible for the pungency of the root. The roots also contain coumarin, phenolic acid derivatives, sugars, and starch. The leaves (which can be used in salads, especially when young) also contain flavonoids.

Uses in treatment

Traditionally, horseradish is used for lung infections, ✪ **urinary tract disorders**, and urinary stones (see ✪ **calculus**), and it also has diuretic properties. It is approved by some authorities for the treatment of urinary tract disorders and also for ✪ **catarrh** of the respiratory tract associated with a ✪ **cough** or ✪ **bronchitis**. It is also taken as a general digestive tonic, because it stimulates gastric secretion and appetite (see ✪ **appetite loss**), and for ✪ **colds** and

○ **fever**, because it promotes sweating. It can be applied externally as a poultice for infections, arthritis, general ○ **inflammations**, and minor muscle pain and aches (see ○ **musculoskeletal disorders**).

Warnings, interactions, and side effects

• Horseradish should not be used during pregnancy or when breast-feeding.

• Large quantities of horseradish or prolonged use may result in vomiting and sensitization.

• Some of the volatile components can cause allergic reactions and be irritant to the skin.

• The volatile oil is not recommended for use externally or internally.

• Some authorities recommend that horseradish should be avoided by anyone with an underactive thyroid gland.

horsetail

(*Equisetum arvense*; Parts used: shoots)

Other common names: **bottle-brush, corn horsetail, Dutch rushes, field horsetail, horse willow, horsetail grass, horsetail rush, paddock-pipes, pewterwort, scouring rush, shave grass, toadpipe.**

Horsetail contains derivatives of caffeic acid and flavonoids. Traditional uses, which are approved by some authorities, include to treat ○ **urinary tract disorders**, kidney and bladder stones (see ○ **calculus**), and externally for poorly healing ○ **wounds** and ○ **burns**. The plant is known to have diuretic activity (see ○ **fluid retention**).

Warnings, interactions, and side effects

• Horsetail should not be used by anyone who has *edema* due to impaired kidney or heart function.

hydrangea

(*Hydrangea arborescens*; Parts used: rhizome)

Other common names: **seven barks.**

Hydrangea contains carbohydrates, flavonoids, and saponins. Traditional uses include for ○ **cystitis**, ○ **prostatitis**, and urinary calculi (see ○ **calculus**). However, it has been poorly studied experimentally.

Warnings, interactions, and side effects

• Hydrangea may cause contact dermatitis and tightness in the chest if large quantities are used.

Iceland moss

(*Cetraria islandica*; Parts used: thallus)

Other common names: **cetraria, eryngo-leaved liverwort, Iceland lichen.**

Iceland moss contains lichen acids and a mucilaginous matrix. Traditional uses, which are approved by some authorities, include for ○ **colds**, ○ **bronchitis**, ○ **appetite loss**, inflammation of the mouth and/or pharynx or larynx (see ○ **inflammation** and ○ **pharyngitis**). The thallus has antibacterial and demulcent activities.

Warnings, interactions, and side effects

• Iceland moss should not be used by anyone with a gastric or duodenal ulcer because it can irritate the mucosa.

immortelle

(*Helichrysum arenarium*; Parts used: flowerheads)

Other common names: **common shrubby, eternal flower, everlasting, goldilocks, yellow chaste weed.**

Immortelle contains flavonoids, phthalides, derivatives of caffeic acid, and bitter sesquiterpenoids. It is primarily used to treat ○ **appetite loss**, ○ **liver disorders**, and ○ **gallbladder disorders**, and is approved by some authorities for ○ **indigestion**. The flowerheads have choleretic activity, as well as antibacterial and weak spasmolytic actions.

Warnings, interactions, and side effects

• Immortelle should not be used by anyone with biliary obstruction.

Indian mallow

(*Abutilon indicum*; Parts used: whole plant)

Indian mallow contains tannins, mucilage, and asparagine, and has diuretic activity. The mucilage and tannins give it emollient and astringent properties. It is used to soothe mucous membranes, or for ○ **skin conditions**, such as chapped hands, (when it is applied externally).

Warnings, interactions, and side effects

Although none have been reported with correct use and dosage, the properties of Indian mallow have not been fully investigated and adverse reactions are possible.

Indian plantago

(*Plantago ovata*; Parts used: seeds)

Other common names: **black psyllium, blond psyllium, blood plantago, ispaghula, sand plantain, spogel.**

Indian plantago contains alkaloids, phytosterols, triterpenes, and mucilage. It is used as a demulcent and laxative for ○ **constipation**. The mucilage is responsible for the laxative properties of the plant, which are usually felt within 24 hours.

Warnings, interactions, and side effects

• Because it is a laxative, Indian plantago may affect absorption of other drugs by reducing the time it takes for the drug to pass through the gastrointestinal tract.

ivy, English

(*Hedera helix*; Parts used: leaves)

Other common names: **gum ivy, true ivy, woodland.**

English ivy contains saponins, sterols, and a volatile oil. The leaves have antispasmodic and expectorant activity. Traditional uses, which are approved by some authorities, include for ○ **coughs** and ○ **bronchitis**.

Warnings, interactions, and side effects

• English ivy may irritate the skin of some people.

Jamaica dogwood

(*Piscidia erythrina*)

Other common names: **dogwood, fish poison bark, West Indian dogwood.**

     Key to symbols: ○ = Disorder Section ℞ = Drug Section ♣ = Herbal Section ♐ = Supplement Section

Jamaica dogwood is a deciduous shrub or tree which can reach 50 feet (15 meters) in height. It has compound leaves, and produces pale blue or white striped flowers, followed by winged seed pods.

Forms of preparation and parts used
Jamaica dogwood root bark is used medicinally, commonly as a decoction or tincture.

Active components
The root bark contains a range of isoflavonoids, including a number of rotenoids (including rotenone). It also contains a range of plant acids and glycosides, a phytosterol, and a small amount of volatile oil.

Uses in treatment
Jamaica dogwood is used as a sedative and anodyne, particularly in the treatment of ✪ migraine, ✪ dysmenorrhea, ✪ insomnia, and ✪ neuralgia. Laboratory studies have confirmed the sedative and antispasmodic activity of the bark. The antispasmodic activity on uterus muscle is thought to be due to the isoflavones. Anti-inflammatory, antitussive, and antipyretic activities have also been demonstrated in laboratory studies. The rotenoid, rotenone has insecticidal activity.

Warnings, interactions, and side effects
• Jamaica dogwood should not be used during pregnancy or by breast-feeding mothers.
• It should only be used under the supervision of an expert, because it is regarded as toxic and irritating. Some experts recommend that it should not be used at all.
• The rotenone in Jamaica dogwood has been reported to have both carcinogenic and anticancer properties.
• It may interfere with existing sedative treatments.

jambul
(*Syzygium cumini*; Parts used: fruit, seeds)
Other common names: **jambolan, jamum, Java plum, rose apple.**
Jambul contains a number of phenolic compounds, tannins, triterpenes, and a volatile oil. It has astringent properties and has been shown to lower blood sugar levels. It is approved by some authorities for ✪ diarrhea, inflammation of the mouth and/or pharynx (see ✪ inflammation and ✪ pharyngitis), and ✪ skin conditions, and traditionally it is also used for ✪ dysentery.

Warnings, interactions, and side effects
• Jambul is not recommended for use by diabetics because of the potential effect on blood sugar levels.

Japanese mint
(*Mentha arvensis var. piperascens*; Parts used: aerial parts)
Japanese mint contains a volatile oil rich in menthone and menthol, and has carminative, cholagogic, antibacterial, and secretolytic activity. Traditional uses, which are approved by some authorities, include for ✪ bronchitis, ✪ coughs, ✪ colds, ✪ gallbladder disorders, ✪ liver disorders, inflammation of the mouth and/or pharynx (see ✪ inflammation and ✪ pharyngitis), general ✪ pain, and ✪ fever.

Warnings, interactions, and side effects
• Japanese mint may aggravate bronchial asthma and lead to sensitization.

• Taking large quantities should be avoided due to its high menthol content.
• The oil should not be applied to the faces of children or infants.

Java tree
(*Orthosiphon spicatus*; Parts used: leaves, stem tips)
Other common names: **Java tea.**
Java tree contains caffeic acid derivatives, flavonoids, saponins, and a volatile oil rich in beta-caryophyllene. It has mild diuretic activity (see ✪ **fluid retention**) and also antimicrobial and spasmolytic properties. It is used, and approved by some authorities, for ✪ **urinary tract disorders**, kidney and bladder stones (see ✪ **calculus**), ✪ **liver disorders**, and ✪ **gallbladder disorders**.

Warnings, interactions, and side effects
• Java tree is not to be used by anyone with edema due to cardiac or renal insufficiency.

jewel weed
(*Impatiens biflora*; Parts used: herb)
Other common names: **balsam-weed, quick-in-the-hand, silverweed, slipperweed, speckled jewels, spotted touch-me-not, wild balsam, wild celandine, wild lady's slipper.**
Jewel weed contains naphthacene derivatives. It can be used for ✪ **digestive system disorders**.

Warnings, interactions, and side effects
Although none have been reported with correct use and dosage, the properties of jewel weed have not been fully investigated and adverse reactions are possible.

juniper
(*Juniperus communis*)
Other common names: **enebro, geneva, geniver, ginepro, horse savin.**
Juniper is a coniferous shrub which grows up to 50 feet (15 meters) in height with needle-like leaves. It produces yellow (male) or blue (female) flowers on separate plants, followed by dark blue-black spherical fruit.

Forms of preparation and parts used
The fruit (berries) of juniper are use medicinally, usually dried, fresh, in a liquid extract, or tincture.

Active components
Juniper contains a range of terpenes, tannins, and a monoterpene-rich volatile oil. It also contains sugars, a lignan, and resinous substances.

Uses in treatment
Juniper is widely used to flavor gin. Medicinally, juniper has diuretic, antiseptic, carminative, stomachic, and antirheumatic properties. Traditionally, it has been used in the treatment of ✪ cystitis and ✪ fluid retention, as well as for rheumatism (see ✪ lumbago, ✪ musculoskeletal disorders), ✪ gout, and ✪ arthritis (by external use of the diluted oil). It also has uses against ✪ colic, ✪ flatulence, and to stimulate menstruation. It is approved by some authorities for treating dyspeptic complaints and ✪ appetite loss.

Warnings, interactions, and side effects

• Juniper should not be used during pregnancy, because some laboratory studies have shown juniper fruit extracts to cause abortions and to have other effects on embryo implantation and fertility.

• There are reports that the essential oil is an irritant and toxic. However, these reports are inconsistent because some studies have used the oil from *Juniperus sabina* (known as savin or savine) not *Juniperus communis*, and *Juniperus sabina* does have toxic effects. Some authorities state that the oil of *Juniperus communis* is non-hazardous.

• Juniper may enhance the effects of existing diuretic and hypoglycemic treatments.

• Excessive use should be avoided.

kava kava

(*Piper methysticum*)
Other common names: **ava, ava pepper, awa, intoxicating pepper, kava, kawa, kawa pepper, tonga.**
Kava kava is an evergreen shrub which grows up to 10 feet (3 meters) in height. It has heart-shaped leaves, fleshy stems, and small flower spikes. It is native to Hawaii and is cultivated in other parts of the US.

Forms of preparation and parts used
The roots of kava kava are used medicinally. Traditionally, the roots were chewed and spat out, so that they could ferment in saliva.

Active components
The major active constituents of kava kava are the kava lactones (kava pyrones), including methysticin (kawain) and analogs (dihydrokavain or marindinin), and yangonine and analogs.

Uses in treatment
Kava kava is traditionally used as a sedative, and, in larger doses, to induce euphoria, usually for ceremonial purposes. Kava lactones, especially kawain, have been shown to be responsible for the sedative action and depressant effect on the central nervous system of the root. The herb also has antispasmodic actions, and kava kava has been recommended for ✪ **irritable bowel syndrome**. Several studies have shown kava kava to be effective in treating ✪ **anxiety**. In particular, one clinical trial has demonstrated kava pyrone extract to be as effective as benzodiazepines, and such antianxiety actions are believed by some to be due to an interaction with the neurotransmitter GABA in the brain. Kava kava is also used over relatively long periods for treating long-term ✪ **stress**, and some authorities approve its use for nervousness and ✪ **insomnia**. The roots can have a slightly numbing effect in the mouth, which probably explains its use for toothache (see ✪ **tooth decay**) and mouth ✪ **ulcers**.

Warnings, interactions, and side effects
• Kava kava should not be used during pregnancy or by breast-feeding mothers.

• Large quantities of kava kava should not be used as they can have a narcotic, stupor-inducing effect and may impair the ability to perform skilled tasks, such as driving.

• It can increase the effects of other central nervous system depressants, such as alcohol, barbiturates, and tranquilizers.

• A recent study has also shown that taking kava kava in excessive amounts may result in liver damage.

• It may also cause allergic skin reactions.

• Some experts recommend that it not be used by anyone under 18, or by anyone with depression.

lactucarium
see ♣ **wild lettuce.**

lady's mantle
(*Alchemilla vulgaris*; Parts used: herb)
Other common names: **bear's foot, leontopodium, lion's foot, nine hooks, stellaria.**
Lady's mantle contains flavonoids, tannins, and bitter compounds. Traditional uses which are approved by some authorities are for treating ✪ **diarrhea** and mild ✪ **digestive system disorders**. It has confirmed astringent and anticancer activity.

Warnings, interactions, and side effects
Although none have been reported with correct use and dosage, the properties of lady's mantle have not been fully investigated and adverse reactions are possible.

lapacho
(*Tabebuia impetignosa*; Parts used: inner bark)
Lapacho contains flavonoids, steroidal saponins, quinones, and alkaloids. Traditionally it is used as a "cure-all." The inner bark has anti-inflammatory, antidiabetic, and hypotensive activity. It is claimed by some that it may have a beneficial effect in certain forms of ✪ **cancer.**

Warnings, interactions, and side effects
Although none have been reported with correct use and dosage, the properties of lapacho have not been fully investigated and adverse reactions are possible.

larch
(*Larix decidua*; Parts used: outer bark)
Other common names: **common larch, European larch.**
Larch contains resins, and a volatile oil rich in alpha-pinene, and has antiseptic and hyperemic activities. Traditional uses, which are approved by some authorities, include for ✪ **fever**, inflammation of the mouth and/or pharynx (see ✪ **inflammation** and ✪ **pharyngitis**), the common ✪ **cold**, a tendency to ✪ **infection**, rheumatism (see ✪ **musculoskeletal disorders**), and blood pressure problems.

Warnings, interactions, and side effects
• Larch should not be inhaled directly, because this can cause acute bronchial inflammation.

laurel
(*Laurus nobilis*; Parts used: leaves and fruit)
Other common names: **bay, bay laurel, bay tree, Daphne, Grecian laurel, noble laurel, Roman laurel, sweet bay, true laurel.**
Laurel contains sesquiterpene lactones, fatty acids (fruit only), and a volatile oil rich in 1,8-cineole (eucalyptol), and has confirmed

rubefacient activity. Traditional uses include to stimulate the skin and treat rheumatic complaints (see ✪ **musculoskeletal disorders**).

Warnings, interactions, and side effects
• Laurel applied to the skin may cause mild sensitization in some people.

lavender cotton
(*Santolina chamaecyparissias*; Parts used: herb)
Lavendar cotton contains alkaloids and a volatile oil rich in artemisiaketone. It has digestive, anthelmintic and anti-inflammatory activity, and is used for ✪ **digestive system disorders**, ✪ **worm infestation**, and ✪ **premenstrual syndrome**. It can also stimulate menstruation.

Warnings, interactions, and side effects
Although none have been reported with correct use and dosage, the properties of lavender cotton have not been fully investigated and adverse reactions are possible.

lemon
(*Citrus limon*; Parts used: fruit)
Other common names: **limon.**
Lemon contains a volatile oil rich in limonene, flavonoids, and vitamins. Traditional uses include as an antiseptic, antibacterial, antipyretic, and in the treatment of rheumatic complaints (see ✪ **musculoskeletal disorders**). Many of its effects are due to the essential oil.

Warnings, interactions, and side effects
• The essential oil should only be taken internally with professional supervision.

lemon balm
(*Melissa officinalis*; Parts used: herb)
Other common names: **balm, cure-all, dropsy plant, honey plant, melissa, sweet Mary.**
Lemon balm contains flavonoids, triterpenes, tannins, and a volatile oil. The volatile oil has been shown to be antispasmodic and to have a CNS (central nervous system)-depressant activity (largely due to citral and citronellal). Traditional uses include as an antispasmodic, relaxant, carminative, and a tonic for the nerves. Its use is approved by some authorities for ✪ **anxiety** and ✪ **insomnia**.

Warnings, interactions, and side effects
• The oil of lemon balm should only be taken internally with professional supervision.

lemon verbena
(*Aloysia triphylla*; Parts used: flowers, leaf)
Other common names: **herb Louisa, lemon-scented verbena.**
Lemon verbena contains numerous flavonoids and a volatile oil. It is used for ✪ **asthma**, ✪ **fever**, ✪ **indigestion**, and ✪ **diarrhea**. However, these actions have not been scientifically confirmed.

Warnings, interactions, and side effects
• Lemon verbena should not be used by anyone with kidney (renal) disease.

lichwort
(*Parietina officinalis*; Parts used: herb)
Lichwort contains flavonoids and caffeic acid derivatives. It has mild diuretic activity (see ✪ **fluid retention**) and is used to treat ✪ **urinary tract disorders**.

Warnings, interactions, and side effects
Although none have been reported with correct use and dosage, the properties of lichwort have not been fully investigated and adverse reactions are possible.

licorice
(*Glycyrrhiza glabra*)
Other common names: **Italian licorice, licorice root, liquorice, Russian licorice, Spanish licorice, sweet root, sweet wood, sweet wort, Turkish licorice, yasti-madhu.**
Licorice is a woody perennial which grows to approximately 6 feet (1.8 meters) in height. The leaves are divided into 9 to 17 sticky leaflets. The flowers are pale blue or mauve, and are followed by rectangular seed pods approximately 1 inch (2.5 centimeters) in length.

Forms of preparation and parts used
The extensive root system (tap root, runners, and branch roots) are used medicinally, usually dried or as an infusion.

Active components
Licorice contains triterpene saponins (including glycyrrhizinic acid), flavonoids, polysaccharides, coumarins, and a complex volatile oil.

Uses in treatment
Licorice has anti-inflammatory, expectorant, and demulcent properties, and also mild laxative activity. It is widely used to treat ✪ **bronchitis** and ✪ **catarrh**, ✪ **gastritis**, ✪ **peptic ulcers**, and inflamed joints. It is also reported to stimulate the adrenal gland, and has been used in the treatment of adrenocortical insufficiency. Licorice root is approved by some authorities for bronchitis, ✪ **cough**, peptic ulcers, and gastritis.

Warnings, interactions, and side effects
• Excessive or prolonged (more than a few weeks) ingestion of licorice can result in the condition known as pseudoaldosteronism with symptoms such as hypertension, water retention, sodium retention, weight gain, and hypokalemia (low blood potassium). These effects, which can be severe, are frequently temporary, and can be reversed within a few weeks of stopping using licorice.
• The use of licorice during pregnancy or when breast-feeding is not recommended because of the above effects, and also because of the traditional claim that it can induce abortion.
• Licorice may increase the toxicity of cardiac glycoside, ℞ **antiarrhythmic** drugs and some diuretics (for example, ℞ **thiazides**), and some authorities consider that people with cardiovascular disorders in general should use the herb only with caution.
• It should not be used by those with liver disorders (including cirrhosis), kidney disorders, or raised blood potassium levels.

lily of the valley
(*Convallaria majalis*; Parts used: whole plant)

Other common names: **convallaria, convall-lily, Jacob's ladder, ladder-to-heaven, lily constancy, May bells, May lily, muguet, Our Lady's tears.**

Lily of the valley contains steroidal glycosides. Traditional uses include in the treatment of heart ✪ **arrhythmias** and cardiac insufficiency, and some authorities approve it for these uses and also for nervous heart complaints. Lily of the valley also has diuretic properties (see ✪ **fluid retention**).

Warnings, interactions, and side effects

• The effects and side effects of calcium salts, digoxin, glucocorticoids, laxatives, quinidine, and saluretics are enhanced if taken at the same time as lily of the valley.

• Overdose can cause nausea, vomiting, and cardiac arrhythmias.

lime

(*Citrus aurantifolia*; Parts used: oil)
Other common names: **Adam's apple, Italian limetta, limetta.**

The fruit lime is rich in ◌◌ **vitamin C**, while limonene and citral are major components of the volatile oil. Traditional uses include the prevention and treatment of ✪ **scurvy** and to increase resistance against disease.

Warnings, interactions, and side effects

Although none have been reported with correct use and dosage, the properties of lime have not been fully investigated and adverse reactions are possible.

linden

(*Tilia species, Tilia cordata, T x europaea*)
Other common names: **basswood, lime, lime tree flower, linn flower.**

Linden trees can grow to over 100 feet (30 meters) in height. They have large rounded leaves, white or yellow flowers, and small, pale green spherical fruits.

Forms of preparation and parts used

Linden's flowerheads are used medicinally, usually as an infusion, tincture, or, externally as a cream. Sometimes known as lime, linden should not be confused with the citrus fruit lime (*Citrus aurantifolia*).

Active components

Linden flowers are rich in flavonoids and phenolic acids, hydroxycoumarins (including aesculin, *p*-coumaric acid), as well as a mucilaginous polysaccharide (accounting for up to 3 percent of the weight of the flowers), a volatile oil, tannins, and a phytosterol.

Uses in treatment

Linden is traditionally used as an antispasmodic and sedative. It is approved by some authorities for ✪ **cough** and ✪ **catarrh**, for example in colds. Laboratory studies on linden extracts have demonstrated antispasmodic activity, which, together with diaphoretic activities, have been attributed to the flavonoids and *p*-coumaric acid. The volatile oil is claimed to have diuretic and sedative actions. A cream made from the flowers can be used to treat skin irritation (see ✪ **skin conditions**). The flowers also have weak antibacterial activity.

Warnings, interactions, and side effects

• Linden flowers have not been thoroughly studied and so their use during pregnancy and breast-feeding should be avoided.

• They should not be taken excessively at any time.

• It is recommended that linden flowers should also be avoided by anyone with a heart disorder.

lobelia

(*Lobelia inflata*)
Other common names: **asthma weed, bladderpod, emetic herb, emetic weed, eyebright, gagroot, Indian tobacco, pukeweed, vomitroot, wild tobacco.**

Lobelia is an annual herb found across much of the US, typically on waste ground. It has slightly pointed, oval-shaped leaves and grows up to 18 inches (45 centimeters) tall. It produces pale blue or pink flowers in the summer.

Forms of preparation and parts used

The aerial parts of lobelia are used medicinally, usually as a decoction, infusion, or tincture.

Active components

Lobelia contains a number of piperidine alkaloids, including lobeline, lobelanine, lobinine, and their derivatives. The plant also contains a resinous material, lobelacrin (a bitter glycoside), and a volatile oil.

Uses in treatment

Lobelia is used as a respiratory stimulant and expectorant. It has also been used to treat ✪ **bronchitis** and ✪ **asthma**. Many of the activities responsible for these uses are attributed to the alkaloid lobeline, which has effects similar to (but milder than) nicotine. Lobeline is known to stimulate the central nervous system, to stimulate then eventually paralyse respiration, and to have expectorant activity. Due to these similarities with nicotine, lobelia has been used by patients trying to stop smoking, and was formally used in antismoking preparations. However, it is no longer available for this purpose in the US.

Warnings, interactions, and side effects

• Lobeline poses serious health risks. The FDA has declared it a poisonous plant, and many experts do not recommend its use at all.

• Excessive intake of lobelia can result in nicotine-like poisoning (nausea, vomiting, diarrhea, tachycardia, and hypotension).

• It should not be used during pregnancy or by breast-feeding mothers.

• The fresh plant should not be eaten at any time.

logwood

(*Haematoxylon campechianum or H. lignum*; Parts used: heart wood)
Other common names: **bloodwood, peachwood.**

Logwood is rich in tannins and neoflavan derivatives. It is known to be a strong astringent, which explains its traditional uses for ✪ **diarrhea** and ✪ **hemorrhages**.

Warnings, interactions, and side effects

Although none have been reported with correct use and dosage, the properties of logwood have not been fully investigated and adverse reactions are possible.

Key to symbols: ✪ = Disorder Section ℞ = Drug Section ♣ = Herbal Section ◌◌ = Supplement Section

lotus

(*Nelumbo nucifera*; Parts used: roots, seeds and aerial parts)
Lotus contains isoquinoline alkaloids, flavonoids, and tannins, and has astringent activity. It is used internally for ✪ **diarrhea** and ✪ **digestive system disorders**, and externally to manage bleeding (see ✪ **hemorrhage**).

Warnings, interactions, and side effects

Although none have been reported with correct use and dosage, the properties of lotus have not been fully investigated and adverse reactions are possible.

lovage

(*Levisticum officinale*; Parts used: rhizome and aerial parts)
Other common names: **lavose, sea parsley.**
Lovage contains coumarin derivatives and a volatile oil rich in alkylphthalides. Traditional uses include for ✪ **urinary tract disorders** and stones in the kidney or bladder (see ✪ **calculus**). Lovage has diuretic, sedative, and antimicrobial activities. In addition, its volatile oil has antispasmodic properties.

Warnings, interactions, and side effects

• Lovage is not to be used during pregnancy.
• It is not to be used by people with impaired kidney function or urinary tract/kidney inflammation.

lungmoss

(*Lobaria pulmonaria*; Parts used: thallus)
Other common names: **lungwort, oak lungs.**
Lungmoss contains *mucilage* and lichen acids. The thallus has expectorant, anti-inflammatory, antimicrobial, and diaphoretic activity. It is used to treat ✪ **respiratory tract disorders**.

Warnings, interactions, and side effects

Although none have been reported with correct use and dosage, the properties of lungmoss have not been fully investigated and adverse reactions are possible.

magnolia

(*Magnolia glauca*; Parts used: bark)
Other common names: **beaver tree, holly bay, Indian bark, red bay, swamp laurel, swamp sassafras, sweet bay, white bay, white laurel.**
Magnolia contains neolignans (of which little is known) and its bark has anti-inflammatory, stimulant, and diaphoretic activity. It is used for ✪ **digestive system disorders**.

Warnings, interactions, and side effects

Although none have been reported with correct use and dosage, the properties of magnolia have not been fully investigated and adverse reactions are possible.

maidenhair fern

(*Adiantum capillus-veneris*; Parts used: herb)
Other common names: **five-finger fern, hair of Venus, maiden fern, rock fern, Venus hair.**
Miadenhair fern contains flavonoids, terpenoids, tannins, and mucilage. Traditional uses include as an expectorant and to treat ✪ **bronchitis** and a sore throat (see ✪ **pharyngitis**). A species of plant related to maidenhair fern is known to have antispasmodic activity.

Warnings, interactions, and side effects

• Maidenhair fern should not be used during pregnancy.

Malabar nut

(*Justicia adhatoda*; Parts used: leaves, bark, and flowers)
Other common names: **adulsa, arusa.**
Malabar nut contains quinolizidine alkaloids and a volatile oil. It has been used for respiratory tract infections (see ✪ **respiratory tract disorders**), and has spasmolytic, bronchodilatory, and expectorant activity.

Warnings, interactions, and side effects

• Malabar nut should not be used during pregnancy.
• The taking of excessive amounts or an overdose can cause an excited state.

mallow

(*Malva sylvestris*; Parts used: flowers and leaves)
Mallow contains flavonoids and mucilage. Traditional uses include for ✪ **coughs** and ✪ **bronchitis**. The mucilaginous material is thought to protect and soothe irritated mucous membranes.

Warnings, interactions, and side effects

Although none have been reported with correct use and dosage, the properties of mallow have not been fully investigated and adverse reactions are possible.

manna

(*Fraxinus ornus*; Parts used: bark sap)
Other common names: **flake manna, flowering ash, manna ash.**
Manna contains a very high sugar content (including mannitol), and is traditionally used to relieve ✪ **constipation**.

Warnings, interactions, and side effects

• Manna should not be used to treat intestinal obstructions.
• Because it has laxative actions, it may cause flatulence.

marigold

(*Calendula officinalis*; Parts used: flower)
Other common names: **calendula, goldbloom, holigold, holligold, golds, Mary bud, Mary Gowles, ruddes.**
Marigold contains flavonoids, numerous terpenoids, pigments, and a volatile oil. Traditonal uses include as an antispasmodic, anti-inflammatory, styptic, and antiseptic. Anti-inflammatory and antimicrobial activity have been confirmed. Marigold is approved by some authorities for treating ✪ **wounds**, ✪ **burns**, and inflammation of the mouth and/or pharynx (see ✪ **inflammation** and ✪ **pharyngitis**).

Warnings, interactions, and side effects

• Rarely, marigold (flowers and herb) may cause mild skin irritation in some people.

marjoram

(*Origanum majorana*; Parts used: aerial parts)
Other common names: **sweet marjoram.**

Marjoram contains flavonoids, caffeic acid derivatives, and a volatile oil. Traditional uses include for the common ✪ **cold** and associated rhinitis, and the volatile oil has antimicrobial activity.

Warnings, interactions, and side effects
• Marjoram should not be given to young children and infants.

marshmallow

(*Althaea officinalis*)

Other common names: **althea, cheeses, kitmi, malavisco, mallards, Moorish mallow, mortification root, schloss tea, sweet weed, white maoow, wymote.**

Marshmallow is a robust perennial growing from a fleshy tap-root to a height of up to 7 feet (2.25 meters). The downy stem bears a number of rounded, velvety leaves, and, in late summer, pale pink flowers.

Forms of preparation and parts used
The roots, leaves, and flowers of marshmallow are all used medicinally as the dried herb, liquid extracts, or in ointments.

Active components
Marshmallow contains a number of sugar-based mucilaginous substances, starch, and phenolic acids.

Uses in treatment
Marshmallow is traditionally described as a demulcent, expectorant, emollient, diuretic, and vulneric, and it has a mild laxative effect. It is approved by some authorities for ✪ **pharyngitis** and associated dry ✪ **cough** and to ease an irritated throat in ✪ **bronchitis**. Other traditional uses include for ✪ **cystitis** and ✪ **urethritis**. The root in particular is described as being beneficial for a ✪ **peptic ulcer**, and ✪ **gastritis**. Applied to the skin it can be used for ✪ **abscesses**, ✪ **boils**, and ✪ **ulcers**.

Warnings, interactions, and side effects
There does not appear to be any toxicity information relating to marshmallow, and considering its widespread use as a food, the plant may be regarded as non-toxic.

• It may, however, interfere with hypoglycemic treatments and may delay the absorption of some other drugs taken at the same time.

maté

(*Ilex paraguariensis*; Parts used: leaf)

Other common names: **Jesuit's tea, kali chaye, Paraguay tea, yerba maté.**

Maté contains xanthine alkaloids, flavonoids, and terpenoids. Traditional uses, which are approved by some authorities, include for ✪ **headache**, ✪ **fatigue**, and nervous ✪ **depression**. Its effects are largely due to xanthines, including ℞ **caffeine** and theobromine, which stimulate the CNS (central nervous system) among other effects.

Warnings, interactions, and side effects
• As with all caffeine-containing beverages, excessive intake should be avoided, especially during pregnancy or when breast-feeding.

meadowsweet

(*Filipendula ulmaria*; formerly *Spireaea ulmaria*)

Other common names: **bridewort, dolloff, lady of the meadow, meadow queen, meadow-wort, meadsweet, queen of the meadow.**

Meadowsweet is a perennial with toothed leaves and growing to a height of approximately 5 feet (1.5 meters). The plant produces cream-colored, almond-scented flowers in summer.

Forms of preparation and parts used
The aerial parts of the plant (usually the flowering tops and leaves) are used medicinally, often dried, as an infusion or tincture. It commonly appears in herbal blends, sometimes with ♣ **lemon balm** or ♣ **marshmallow**.

Active components
The major bioactive constituents of meadowsweet include flavonoids (mainly as glycosides) salicylates (phenolic glycosides), a volatile oil, and tannins.

Uses in treatment
Meadowsweet is used as a stomachic, a mild urinary antiseptic, an astringent, and antacid. It is frequently used for ✪ **indigestion**, ✪ **diarrhea**, rheumatic conditions (see ✪ **musculoskeletal disorders**), and in the treatment and prevention of ✪ **peptic ulcers**. It is approved by some authorities for helping to relieve a ✪ **cold**. In laboratory studies, flower extracts have been shown to have antibacterial properties and to be of some benefit in preventing stomach ulcers.

Warnings, interactions, and side effects
• Because of the salicylate content of meadowsweet, many of the precautions which apply to ♣ **willow** are also relevant for this herb. Anyone with hypersensitivity to aspirin (also a salicylate), who has diabetes mellitus, gout, or diseases of the liver or kidney should be aware of possible risks associated with taking the herb. Taking aspirin simultaneously with meadowsweet should be avoided.

• It may also interact with ℞ **anticoagulant** drugs, ℞ **methotrexate**, ℞ **metoclopramide**, ℞ **phenytoin**, ℞ **probenecid**, ℞ **spironolactone**, and ℞ **valproate sodium**.

• Meadowsweet should not be used during pregnancy or by breast-feeding mothers.

• Use of salicylates in general should be avoided in those under 16 years of age because of a possible risk of causing ✪ **Reye's syndrome**, and in asthmatics because of the risk of precipitating an attack.

milk thistle

(*Silybum marianum*; Parts used: flowerhead, seeds)

Other common names: **Other comon names: Marian thistle, Mary thistle, Mediterranean thistle.**

Milk thistle contains lignans (including silymarin, which has strong hepatoprotective activity) and polyacetylenic compounds. It has been used to treat ✪ **jaundice** and ✪ **hepatitis**, and some authorities approve of its use for certain ✪ **digestive system disorders**, ✪ **liver disorders** (including cirrhosis), and ✪ **gallbladder disorders**.

Warnings, interactions, and side effects
Although none have been reported with correct use and dosage, the properties of milk thistle have not been fully investigated and adverse reactions are possible.

Key to symbols: ✪ = Disorder Section ℞ = Drug Section ♣ = Herbal Section ⚗ = Supplement Section

mistletoe

(*Viscum album*; Parts used: leaf, berry, stem)
Other common names: **all-heal, birdlime, devil's fuge, mistletoe, mystyldene.**
European mistletoe contains fatty acids, terpenoids, flavonoids, and polypeptides. Preparations of mistletoe have been shown to have hypotensive, anticancer, and immunostimulant activities. Traditional uses include for ✪ **hypertension** (high blood pressure) and ✪ **arteriosclerosis** and related conditions. Also, it is approved by some authorities for rheumatism (see ✪ **musculoskeletal disorders**) and as a part of a treatment for tumors.

Warnings, interactions, and side effects
• European mistletoe berries are toxic and should only be used under the supervision of a qualified practitioner.
• It may interfere with existing treatments for blood pressure and disorders of the immune system.

moneywort

(*Lysimachia nummularia*; Parts used: whole plant)
Other common names: **creeping Jenny, creeping Joan, herb twopence, meadow runagates, running Jenny, serpentaria, string of sovereigns, twopenny grass, wandering Jenny, wandering tailor.**
Money wort contains flavonoids, saponins, and tannins, and has astringent and expectorant activities. Traditional uses include for ✪ **eczema** (applied to the skin), and internally as a sialogogue (promotes saliva production) and for ✪ **coughs**.

Warnings, interactions, and side effects
Although none have been reported with correct use and dosage, the properties of moneywort have not been fully investigated and adverse reactions are possible.

motherwort

(*Leonurus cardiaca*)
Other common names: **heartwort, lion's ear, lion's tail, throwwort.**
Motherwort is a perennial herb which grows to a height of about 5 feet (1.5 meters). It has toothed leaves and clusters of pink flowers.

Forms of preparation and parts used
The aerial parts of the plant are used medicinally, usually collected in late summer when the plant is flowering. It is commonly taken as an infusion, a liquid extract, or as a tincture.

Active components
Motherwort contains a range of pyrrolidine alkaloids, flavonoids, iridoids, tannins, terpenoids, and possibly cardiac glycosides.

Uses in treatment
Motherwort has sedative and antispasmodic properties, and is commonly used for various nervous heart complaints and for amenorrhea. It is said to improve cardiac function, especially when heart output is reduced; and it is approved by some authorities for nervous heart complaints (see ✪ **anxiety**), and as an adjunct (an additional treatment) for ✪ **hyperthyroidism**. The herb is also a relaxant, and has been used to promote menstruation and for ✪ **premenstrual syndrome**. The alkaloid constituents are thought to be responsible, at least partly, for the effects of the herb on the uterus.

Warnings, interactions, and side effects
• Motherwort should not be used during pregnancy or by breast-feeding mothers.
• There are unofficial reports of contact dermatitis due to exposure to motherwort leaves, and photosensitization after contact with the volatile oil, but these have not been confirmed.
• It should not be taken by anyone with a heart condition who is having treatment for any kind of heart disorder.

mountain flax

(*Linum catharticum*; Parts used: herb)
Other common names: **dwarf flax, fairy flax, mill mountain, purging flax.**
Mountain flax contains tannins, lignans, and a volatile oil. Its traditional uses include as a purgative and emetic, and it has been used for ✪ **constipation**.

Warnings, interactions, and side effects
• Mountain flax should not be used during pregnancy.
• The laxative effects of the herb are apparent even at small doses.
• Larger doses can result in diarrhea and/or vomiting.

mullein

(*Verbascum densiflorum*; Parts used: herb, flowers, and roots)
Other common names: **Aaron's rod, Adam's flannel, beggar's blanket, blanket herb, blanket-leaf, candlewick plant, clot-bur, clown's lungwort, cuddy's lungs, duffle, flannelflower, fluffweed, feltwort, golden rod, hag's taper, hare's beard, hedge-taper, Jacob's staff, Our Lady's flannel, rag paper, shepherd's club, shepherd's staff, torches, torch weed, velvet plant, wild ice leaf, woollen.**
Mullein contains mucilage, triterpene saponins, iridoids, caffeic acid derivatives, and flavonoids. It has anti-irritant and expectorant activity, and is traditionally used for ✪ **coughs** and sore throat, and ✪ **catarrh**. Some authorities approve its use for relieving catarrh of the respiratory tract during coughs and also ✪ **bronchitis**.

Warnings, interactions, and side effects
Although none have been reported with correct use and dosage, the properties of mullein have not been fully investigated and adverse reactions are possible.

mustard

(*Sinapis alba*; Parts used: seeds)
Other common names: **white mustard.**
Mustard contains glucosinolates, isothiocyanates, and fatty acids, and the seeds have antibacterial activity. Uses that are approved by some authorities are for ✪ **coughs** and ✪ **colds**, and also traditionally it has been given for ✪ **fever**.

Warnings, interactions, and side effects
• Mustard seeds should not be given to children younger than six years of age.
• The seeds should not be taken by anyone with gastrointestinal ulcers or inflammatory kidney disease.

Key to symbols: ✪ = Disorder Section ℞ = Drug Section ♣ = Herbal Section ⚕ = Supplement Section

myrrh
(*Commiphora molmol*)
Other common names: **bal, bol, bola, didin, didthin, guggal gum, guggal resin, gum myrrh, heerabol.**
Myrrh is a deciduous spiny shrub which grows to a height of approximately 15 feet (4.5 meters). The leaves are trifoliate, the flowers are yellow-red and have four petals, and the fruit are pointed and very small.

Forms of preparation and parts used
Dried resinous exudate from the bark (oleo-gum resin), usually in the form of a tincture (myrrh does not dissolve well in water so infusions are rarely used).

Active components
Myrrh contains a number of bioactive molecules, including steroids, terpenoids (a furosesquiterpine is the main aroma-bearer), a carbohydrate-based gum, an acid-rich resin, and an aromatic volatile oil.

Uses in treatment
Myrrh is regarded as having antimicrobial, anti-inflammatory, astringent, expectorant, antispasmodic, antiseptic, and carminative properties. Traditionally, it has been used for mouth ✪ **ulcers**, respiratory ✪ **catarrh**, the common ✪ **cold**, ✪ **tuberculosis**, ✪ **tonsillitis**, and ✪ **pharyngitis**. It is said to be very effective for ✪ **gingivitis**, in the form of a gargle, and is also widely used to aid digestion and to treat oligomenorrhea and ✪ **dysmenorrhea**. It has also been used to treat ✪ **glandular fever**. Externally, myrrh can be used against minor inflammations of the skin (see ✪ **skin conditions**), ✪ **acne**, ✪ **boils**, and ✪ **athlete's foot**. It is approved for use by some authorities for mouth and pharynx inflammation.

Warnings, interactions, and side effects
When administered properly and used in recommended amounts, myrrh is generally regarded as a non-toxic herb. There are no reported side effects for myrrh and it is regarded as non-irritating, non-sensitizing, and non-phototoxic to skin.
• However, as myrrh is reported to have a hypoglycemic activity, it should not be used by anyone already taking other medication for ✪ **diabetes mellitus**.
• Because of its use to affect the menstrual cycle, myrrh should be avoided during pregnancy.

nasturtium
(*Tropaeolum majus*; Parts used: herb)
Other common names: **Indian cress.**
Nasturtium contains glucosinolates, flavonoids, ◊◊ **vitamin C**, and a volatile oil which has antibacterial, antiviral, and antimycotic properties. Traditional uses, which are approved by some authorities, include for ✪ **urinary tract disorders**, ✪ **coughs**, and ✪ **bronchitis**.

Warnings, interactions, and side effects
• Nasturtium is not to be given to infants.
• It should not be used by anyone with gastrointestinal ulcers or kidney disorders.
• Taken in large quantities it may cause irritation to the gastrointestinal tract or skin.

neem
(*Azadirachta indica*; formerly known as *Antelaea azadirachta* or *Melia azadirachta*; Parts used: aerial parts)
Other common names: **azedarach, holy tree, nim.**
Neem contains tannins, flavonoids, and a volatile oil. Neem oil has been shown to have antibacterial, anti-inflammatory, and mild antipyretic and hypoglycemic activities. Traditional uses include as a "cure-all."

Warnings, interactions, and side effects
Although none have been reported with correct use and dosage, the properties of neem have not been fully investigated and adverse reactions are possible.

northern prickly ash
(*Zanthoxylum americanum*; Parts used: bark)
Other common names: **prickly ash, suterberry, toothache tree, yellow wood.**
Northern prickly ash contains isoquinoline alkaloids, coumarins, and tannins. Traditional uses include for chronic rheumatism (see ✪ **musculoskeletal disorders**), poor peripheral circulation, and cramping. No specific pharmacology exists for this species, although it is similar to southern prickly ash (*Z. clava-herculis*) in alkaloid composition.

Warnings, interactions, and side effects
• Northern prickly ash taken in large quantities may interfere with the effect of anticoagulant drugs.

nutmeg
(*Myristica fragrans*; Parts used: seed)
Other common names: **mace.**
Nutmeg contains a monoterpene-rich volatile oil and a fixed oil. Traditional uses include as a flavoring and as a carminative, stimulant, and antispasmodic. It is also widely used to alleviate ✪ **vomiting** and ✪ **diarrhea**.

Warnings, interactions, and side effects
• Nutmeg should not be used during pregnancy.
• Excessive consumption (as little as two or three whole nutmegs) can be fatal, so its use should be carefully monitored by an expert.

oak
(*Quercus robur*; Parts used: bark)
Other common names: **common oak, English oak, pedunculate oak, tanner's oak.**
Oak is a rich source of tannins, and the bark has astringent and antiphlogistic activity. Traditional uses, which are approved by some authorities, include for ✪ **bronchitis**, ✪ **cough**, ✪ **diarrhea**, externally for ✪ **skin conditions**, and locally for inflammation of the mouth and/or pharynx (see ✪ **inflammation** and ✪ **pharyngitis**) and mild inflammation of the genital and anal region. It is also used to treat ✪ **fever** and ✪ **colds**.

Warnings, interactions, and side effects
• Oak should not be applied externally to large injuries.
• It should not be used in bathing by anyone with extensive weeping eczema.
• Internal use may lead to irritation of the stomach.

Key to symbols: ✪ = Disorder Section   ℞ = Drug Section   ♣ = Herbal Section   ◊◊ = Supplement Section

oats

(*Avena sativa*; Parts used: seeds)
Other common names: **grain, groats, oatmeal, straw.**
Oats contains saponins, flavonoids, sterols, starch, and protein. It can be used externally to soothe ✪ **eczema** and is approved by some authorities for treating ✪ **skin conditions**, especially ✪ **dermatitis** and itching. Taken internally, oats can reduce cholesterol levels in the blood (see ✪ **hyperlipidemia**) and has been shown to increase endurance under ✪ **stress**.

Warnings, interactions, and side effects
Although none have been reported with correct use and dosage, the properties of oats have not been fully investigated and adverse reactions may be possible.

onion

(*Allium cepa*; Parts used: bulb)
Onion contains alliins and polysaccharides. Traditional uses include for ✪ **appetite loss**, ✪ **indigestion**, the common ✪ **cold**, ✪ **fever**, a tendency to ✪ **infection**, ✪ **hypertension**, and ✪ **inflammation**, including of the mouth and pharynx (see ✪ **pharyngitis**). It is approved by some authorities for appetite loss and atherosclerosis. It has protective activity against ✪ **asthma**, and has some antimicrobial properties. Onion is chemically similar to ⚕ **garlic** which may explain its uses for hypertension and infections.

Warnings, infections, and side effects
• If taken in very large quantities, onion can cause stomach complaints.

Oregon grape

(*Berberis aquifolium*; Parts used: root)
Oregon grape contains isoquinoline alkaloids, which have antibacterial activity. Some of the benefits of applying the plant externally (including for ✪ **psoriasis**) may also be due to the alkaloid components.

Warnings, interactions, and side effects
Although none have been reported with correct use and dosage, the properties of Oregon grape have not been fully investigated and adverse reactions are possible.

oswego tea

(*Monarda didyma*; Parts used: herb)
Other common names: **bee balm, bergamot, blue balm, high balm, low balm, mountain balm, mountain mint, scarlet monarda.**
Oswego tea contains a volatile oil, flavonoids, and anthocyanins. The herb has digestive, carminative, and antispasmodic activity. It is used to treat ✪ **flatulence**, ✪ **digestive system disorders**, and ✪ **premenstrual syndrome**.

Warnings, interactions, and side effects
Although none have been reported with correct use and dosage, the properties of oswego tea have not been fully investigated and adverse reactions are possible.

parsley

(*Petroselinum crispum*)
Other common names: **common parsley, fairy feathers, flat-leafed parsley, garden parsley, Hamburg parsley, Italian parsley, persely, petersylinge, rock parsley, rock selinon.**
Parsley is an aromatic biennial which grows from a white tap root. Its leaves are triangular in outline, and can be more or less curled. In summer the plant produces umbels of tiny yellow flowers.

Forms of preparation and parts used
The leaves, roots, and seeds of parsley are all used medicinally, usually by infusion or as a liquid extract. It is thought to counter the odor of ⚕ **garlic** and so is found in some garlic preparations.

Active components
Parsley contains a number of flavonoids, furanocoumarins and volatile oils, vitamins, and minerals. The leaf oil is rich in myristicin, while the seed oil contains apiole and myristicin, and numerous aldehydes, ketones, and alcohols.

Uses in treatment
Parsley has carminative, antispasmodic, diuretic, expectorant, antirheumatic, and antimicrobial properties. The seeds are used in the treatment of ✪ **gout**, ✪ **arthritis**, and rheumatism (see ✪ **musculoskeletal disorders**). The root is often taken for ✪ **flatulence**, rheumatism, and ✪ **cystitis**. It is approved by some authorities for kidney and bladder stones (see ✪ **calculus**)and ✪ **urinary tract disorders**. It can also be used to promote menstruation and to relieve menstrual ✪ **pain**. In laboratory studies, intravenous administration of parsley extracts resulted in a significant reduction in blood pressure.

Warnings, interactions, and side effects
• The usual amounts of parsley used in cooking are very unlikely to have undesirable side effects, although apiole, myristicin, and the furanocoumarin constituents of parsley can have toxic effects at very high doses.
• It may aggravate existing kidney disorders.
• It should not be taken in doses above culinary levels during pregnancy or by breast-feeding mothers.

pasque flower

(*Pulsatilla pratensis*; Parts used: herb)
Other common names: **Easter flower, meadow anemone, passe flower, pulsatilla, wind flower.**
Pasque flower contains flavonoids, saponins, triterpenes, and a volatile oil. Traditional uses include for ✪ **dysmenorrhea**, tension ✪ **headache**, ✪ **attention deficit disorder**, and pulmonary (lung) conditions. Research has shown that pasque flower has effects on the uterus, and that derivatives of the volatile oil have sedative and antipyretic actions.

Warnings, interactions, and side effects
• Fresh pasque flower is toxic, but the toxic component (called protoanemonin) degrades rapidly.
• It may cause skin irritation and an allergic reaction.

passionflower

(*Passiflora incarnata*)
Other common names: **apricot vine, granadilla, maypop, passiflora, passion vine, water lemon, wild passion flower.**

Passionflower is a climbing perennial with deeply lobed leaves and complex lavender and white flowers, which can reach 3 inches (7 centimeters) across. These are followed by yellow-orange ovoid fruits, approximately 2 inches (1 centimeter) long.

Forms of preparation and parts used
The aerial parts of the plant are used medicinally, usually as an infusion, but also as the dried herb or a liquid extract or tincture. It is often available in preparations along with ♣ **hops** or ♣ **valerian**.

Active components
Passionflower contains a range of flavonoids, phytosterols, fatty acids, and at least one polyacetylenic compound. Biologically potent indole-based harmaline alkaloids (including harmine, harmaline, and harman) are found at low levels in this and related species.

Uses in treatment
Passionflower is said to have sedative, hypnotic, antispasmodic, and tranquillizing properties. It is widely used to treat ○ **insomnia**, especially for short periods of disturbed sleeping and anxiety, and is approved by some authorities for this use and also for ○ **anxiety**. It is also used for the relief of ○ **pain** (especially for dental pain) and for some types of ○ **asthma**. There is some uncertainty about which chemicals are responsible for passionflower's sedative effect on the central nervous system.

Warnings, interactions, and side effects
• Excessive use may interfere with ℞ **monoamine-oxidase inhibitor** antidepressants and cause sedation.
• Excessive use during pregnancy and by breast-feeding mothers should be avoided because the harmaline alkaloids in passionflower have been shown to have effects on the uterus.

peppermint
(*Mentha x piperita*; Parts used: herb)
Other common names: **brandy mint, lamb mint.**
Peppermint contains a volatile oil rich in menthol, flavonoids, and triterpenes. It is widely used as a carminative, choleretic, and antiseptic, and also to relieve muscle spasms. When applied externally the oil has anesthetic, antiseptic, and antimicrobial activity, but it can also be irritating. The leaves of the plant relieve digestive spasms and ○ **irritable bowel syndrome**. Peppermint leaf is approved by some authorities for ○ **indigestion**, ○ **gallbladder disorders**, ○ **flatulence**, ○ **colic**, gastritis, and ○ **enteritis**. Peppermint oil is approved for ○ **catarrh** of the respiratory tract, ○ **inflammation** of the mouth, flatulence, irritable bowel syndrome, and externally for muscle pain (see ○ **musculoskeletal disorders**), ○ **neuralgia**, coughs and colds, ○ **pruritis**, ○ **urticaria**, and ○ **cold sore**.

Warnings, interactions, and side effects
• The oil should only be taken with professional guidance, and should not be given to children or infants, or used on the face.
• Anyone with gallbladder or liver disorders should check with a doctor before using.

pilewort
(*Ranunculus ficaria*; Parts used: herb)
Other common names: **figwort, lesser celandine, smallwort.**

Pilewort contains saponins, lactones, tannins, and ◊◊ **vitamin C**. Traditional uses include for ○ **hemorrhoids**.

Warnings, interactions, and side effects
• Pilewort sap can be an irritant, so it should be used with care.

pill-bearing spurge
(*Euphorbia hirta*)
Other common names: **asthma plant, snakeweed.**
Euphorbia is a small hairy annual with ovate leaves, which grows up to 14 inches (35 centimeters) in height. Clusters of small unremarkable flowers are followed by green or red capsules.

Forms of preparation and parts used
The aerial parts of pill-bearing spurge are used medicinally, as an infusion, tincture, or liquid extract.

Active components
Pill-bearing spurge contains a number of flavonoids and terpenoids, as well as phenolic acids and choline.

Uses in treatment
Pill-bearing spurge is mainly used for the treatment of respiratory conditions, such as ○ **asthma**, ○ **bronchitis**, and ○ **catarrh**, and has mild sedative activity. In laboratory studies, pill-bearing spurge has been shown to have antispasmodic activity, and two chemicals found in in the plant, shikimic acid and choline, are thought to be responsible for these effects on smooth muscle. Stem extracts have antibacterial activity, and a decoction has been shown to have amoebicidal actions. One scientific report also describes antitumor properties.

Warnings, interactions, and side effects
• There are no specific warnings for pill-bearing spurge, but because it can affect smooth muscle it should not be taken during pregnancy. Also, because there is very little safety information, it should be avoided by breast-feeding mothers.
• It should not be taken in excess at any time.
• A number of other *Euphorbia* species are very toxic and should never be used medicinally.

pimento
(*Pimenta racemosa*; Parts used: berries)
Other common names: **allspice, clove pepper, Jamaica pepper, pimenta.**
Pimento contains a volatile oil rich in eugenol, and has antiseptic and local analgesic properties. It is used externally as a rubefacient and is present in some liniments.

Warnings, interactions, and side effects
Although none have been reported with correct use and dosage, the properties of pimento have not been fully investigated and adverse reactions are possible.

pimpinella
(*Pimpinella radix or P. major*; Parts used: rhizome and herb)
Other common names: **burnet saxifrage, pimpernell, saxifrage.**
Burnet saxifrage contains a volatile oil rich in eugenol derivatives, furanocoumarins, and caffeic acid derivatives. It has expectorant activity on bronchial membranes, and is used for ○ **coughs** and ○ **bronchitis**.

Warnings, interactions, and side effects

• Pimpinella may cause photosensitization due to its furanocoumarin content.

pipsissewa

(*Chimaphila umbellata*; Parts used: leaves)

Other common names: **butter winter, ground holly, king's cure, king's cureall, love in winter, prince's pine, rheumatism weed, umbellate wintergreen.**

Pipsissewa contains hydroquinones, flavonoids, methyl salicylate, and tannins. Traditional uses include to treat ✪ **fever** and for urinary problems. The salicylate found in this plant may be responsible for its antipyretic actions, and the hydroquinones may be of benefit for ✪ **urinary tract disorders**. Leaf extracts are reported to have hypoglycemic activity.

Warnings, interactions, and side effects

• Because pipsissewa contains salicylate, it may cause some of the side effects associated with that substance. For example, gastric irritation, hypersensitivity, tinnitus, nausea, and vomiting.

• It perhaps should not be used during pregnancy (there are some concerns over taking aspirin, which is a derivative of salicylic acid, during pregnancy) or when breast-feeding (as salicylates can be excreted in breast milk, which may result in rashes in babies), or by people who have sensitivity to salicylates.

• It should not be given to children (because of the association of salicylates with ✪ **Reye's syndrome**).

• It should not be used at the same time as ℞ **NSAIDs**.

• It should not be used by anyone with a peptic ulcer.

plantain

(*Plantago major or P. lanceolata*)

Other common names: (*P. major*) **broadleaf plantain, greater plantain;** (*P. lanceolata*) **English plantain, lanceleaf plantain, narrowleaf plantain, ribwort plantain.**

(A quite different plant, *Musa paradisiaca* (banana or banana tree) is also called plantain, and its fruit is used for different herbal purposes.)

Plantain is a small perennial herb consisting of a basal rosette of large elliptical leaves up to 6 inches (15 centimeters) in length.

Forms of preparation and parts used

The leaves of plantain are used medicinally, as an infusion, tincture, liquid extract, or as a cream or ointment.

Active components

Plantain contains iridoids (including aucubin and catalpol), flavonoids (apigenin, luteolin), alkaloids, tannins, steroids, mucilage, and a range of plant carboxylic acids (such as protocatechuic acid).

Uses in treatment

Plantain is most commonly regarded as a diuretic and an antihemorrhagic. Externally, it is used in the treatment of ✪ **bruises** and cuts, to promote tissue repair and to staunch bleeding, and also as an ointment for ✪ **hemorrhoids** and ✪ **ulcers**. Internally, the plant is used as an expectorant and anticatarrhal, and is frequently used for ✪ **diarrhea**, ✪ **irritable bowel syndrome**, ✪ **gastritis**, and bleeding in the urinary tract. Hypotensive, bronchodilator, anti-inflammatory, blood lipid-lowering, and hepatoprotective activities have also been described for plantain and its various components in laboratory studies. One study claims that plantain is of some benefit for treating chronic ✪ **bronchitis**. It is approved by some authorities for internal use for ✪ **catarrh** of the respiratory tract, ✪ **inflammation** of the mouth, and ✪ **pharyngitis**, and externally for skin inflammation.

Warnings, interactions, and side effects

• Plantain should be avoided during pregnancy.

• When used externally, it can cause irritation, allergic reactions, and sensitization, although internally, the herb is regarded as being of low toxicity.

• Large quantities may have a laxative effect and cause hypotension (low blood pressure).

pleurisy root

(*Asclepias tuberosa*; Parts used: root)

Other common names: **butterfly weed, Canada root, flux root, orange milkweed, orange swallow-wort, swallow-wort, tuber root, white root, wind root.**

The chemical composition of pleurisy root has not been properly studied. Many *Asclepias* species contain cardiac glycosides, which are chemicals that have an effect on the heart. Traditional uses include for ✪ **bronchitis**, ✪ **influenza**, and ✪ **pleurisy**, although there is no scientific evidence of any beneficial effect.

Warnings, interactions, and side effects

• Pleurisy root may interfere with some heart treatments, hormonal therapies, and antidepressants.

pokeroot

(*Phytolacca americana*; Parts used: root)

Other common names: **American nightshade, American spinach, bear's grape, branching phytolacca, cancer-root, coakum-chongras, cokan, crowberry, inkberry, jalap, phytolacca berry, phytolacca root, pigeon berry, pocan, poke, poke berry, pokeweed, red weed, red-ink plant, scoke, skoke, Virginian poke.**

Pokeroot contains betalain alkaloids, saponins, and lectins. Saponins have been shown to have anti-inflammatory, hypotensive, and diuretic activities. Traditional uses include for rheumatism (see ✪ **musculoskeletal disorders**), ✪ **catarrh**, and ✪ **skin conditions**. Pokeroot also contains a protein that has antiviral properties.

Warnings, interactions, and side effects

• Pokeroot should only be used under expert supervision.

• All parts of fresh pokeroot are poisonous, the dried root must not be taken internally, and the berry juice should not be used on broken skin or the eyes.

poplar

(*Populus species, including P. alba, P. nigra, P. canadensis, P. tacamahaca, P. tremula, P. tremuloides*)

Other common names: **black poplar, Canadian poplar, European aspen, quaking aspen, trembling poplar, white poplar.**

Poplar is a deciduous tree which grows up to 70 feet (21 meters) tall. It commonly has rounded, lightly toothed leaves and oval, slightly sticky buds.

Forms of preparation and parts used
The medicinal parts are bark, leaves, and leaf buds (also known as balm of Gilead), usually as a decoction or liquid extract.

Active components
Poplar bark contains phenolic glycosides, including salicylates such as salicin (salicoside), populin and their derivatives. It also contain tannins, carbohydrates, and triterpenes.

Uses in treatment
Poplar has anti-inflammatory, antirheumatic, antiseptic, anodyne, and astringent properties. It is commonly used to treat aching arthritic or rheumatic joints, and also as an antipyretic to reduce fevers. As an antiseptic and astringent, the bark is used in the treatment of ✪ **diarrhea**, ✪ **irritable bowel syndrome**, and ✪ **urinary tract disorders**. Poplar leaf buds are approved by some authorities for external ✪ **hemorrhoids**, ✪ **wounds**, ✪ **bruises**, frostbite, ✪ **sunburn**, and as a gargle for ✪ **laryngitis**. The pain-relieving properties of poplar probably come from the salicylate content (salicin is converted to its aglycone in the gut, and then to salicylic acid following absorption). It has also been used as a tonic in cases of feebleness and weakness, including anorexia. Pure salicylic acid has been used in medicine as an analgesic and antipyretic, and the synthetic acetyl derivative is ℞ **aspirin** (acetylsalicylic acid).

Warnings, interactions, and side effects
• Salicylate side effects include gastric irritation, hypersensitivity, tinnitus, nausea, and vomiting. Poplar should not be taken during pregnancy (there are some concerns over taking aspirin, which is a derivative of salicylic acid, during pregnancy) or when breast-feeding (as salicylates can be excreted in breast milk, which may result in rashes in babies), or by people who have sensitivity to salicylates.
• It should not be given to children (because of the association of salicylates with ✪ **Reye's syndrome**).
• It should not be used at the same time as ℞ **NSAID**s.
• It should not be used by anyone with a peptic ulcer.

potentilla
(*Potentilla anserina*; Parts used: aerial parts)
Other common names: **cinquefoil, crampweed, goosegrass, goose tansy, goosewort, moor grass, prince's feathers, silver cinquefoil, trailing tansy, wild agrimony.**
Potentilla contains tannins, flavonoids, and hydroxycoumarins. It has astringent activity and can affect uterine tone. Traditional uses, which are approved by some authorities, include for ✪ **diarrhea**, inflammation of the mouth and/or pharynx (see ✪ **inflammation** and ✪ **pharyngitis**), and ✪ **premenstrual syndrome**.

Warnings, interactions, and side effects
• Potentilla can exacerbate existing stomach disorders, and stomach irritation has been reported.
• It should not be used during pregnancy as it can affect the uterus.

premorse
(*Scabiosa succisa*; Parts used: herb)

Other common names: **devil's bit, ofbit, premorse scabious.**
Premorse contains iridoids, tannins, saponins, and flavonoids. It has febrifugal and diaphoretic activity, and is used to treat ✪ **colds** and ✪ **coughs**.

Warnings, interactions, and side effects
Although none have been reported with correct use and dosage, the properties of premorse have not been fully investigated and adverse reactions are possible.

pumpkin
(*Cucurbita pepo*; Parts used: seeds)
Other common names: **field pumpkin.**
Pumpkin contains phytosterols, fatty acids, and amino acids. Traditional uses, which are approved by some authorities, include for irritable bladder conditions and prostate disorders (see ✪ **benign prostatic hyperplasia**). However, there is little scientific evidence to support these uses.

Warnings, interactions, and side effects
Although none have been reported with correct use and dosage, the properties of pumpkin have not been fully investigated and adverse reactions are possible.

purple loosestrife
(*Lythrum salicaria*; Parts used: aerial parts)
Other common names: **blooming Sally, flowering Sally, long purples, loosestrife, lythrum, milk willow-herb, purple willow-herb, rainbow weed, salicaire, soldiers, spiked loosestrife, spiked willow sage.**
Purple loosestrife contains flavonoids, phthalides, and tannins. It has astringent, anti-inflammatory, and antibacterial activity. Traditional uses include internally for ✪ **diarrhea**, and externally for bleeding (see ✪ **hemorrhage**), ✪ **eczema**, and ✪ **hemorrhoids**.

Warnings, interactions, and side effects
Although none have been reported with correct use and dosage, the properties of purple loosestrife have not been fully investigated and adverse reactions are possible.

quassia
(*Picrasma excelsa*; Parts used: wood chips)
Other common names: **ash, bitter ash, bitterwood.**
Quassia contains indole alkaloids, terpenoids, and coumarins. Quassinoids found in quassia are intensely bitter. Traditional uses include for infestations of ✪ **worms** or lice (see ✪ **lice and mite infestation**), and for ✪ **indigestion**. Some clinical success for the treatment of head lice and threadworms has been reported.

Warnings, interactions, and side effects
• Quassia should not be used during pregnancy.
• Large amounts taken internally may cause vomiting.

radish
(*Raphanus sativus*; Parts used: root)
Other common names: **common radish, garden radish.**
Radish contains glucosinolates. The root has antimicrobial activity and stimulates secretions in the upper respiratory react. Traditional uses include for ✪ **fever**, ✪ **coughs**, ✪ **colds**, inflammation of the

mouth and/or pharynx (see ○ **inflammation** and ○ **pharyngitis**), and ○ **appetite loss**. Also, radish is approved by some authorities for ○ **bronchitis** and ○ **indigestion**.

Warnings, interactions, and side effects
• Radish used in large quantities may irritate the gastrointestinal tract, and lead to biliary colic in people with gallstones.

raspberry
(*Rubus idaeus*)
Other common names: **hindberry, red raspberry.**
Raspberry is a deciduous shrub with variably spiny stems which grow to approximately 5 feet (1:5 meters) in height. The plant bears small white flowers in summer, followed by distinctive red juicy fruits.

Forms of preparation and parts used
The leaves and fruit of the plant are used medicinally. The leaves are usually taken as an infusion or other liquid extract.

Active components
There is limited amount of chemical information available for raspberry, although the leaves are known to contain flavonoids, tannins, and polypeptides. The fruits contain vitamins A, B, and C, pectin, sugars, and fruit acids.

Uses in treatment
Raspberry leaves are traditionally used to relieve ○ **diarrhea**, and, in the form of a liquid extract, as an eyewash for ○ **conjunctivitis** (a use which is not supported by scientific evidence), a mouthwash, or as a bathing lotion for ○ **wounds**. In folk medicine, raspberry preparations were used to facilitate childbirth, and in laboratory studies leaf extracts have been shown to cause the uterus to contract. The tannic acid content of the fruit is thought to be responsible for its antiviral activity, while extracts from a related species (*Rubus fructicosus*) have some ability to lower blood sugar levels.

Warnings, interactions, and side effects
• Due to its effects on uterine tissue, raspberry should be avoided during pregnancy, and should only be used during labor under direct medical supervision.

red clover
(*Trifolium pratense*; Parts used: flowers)
Other common names: **purple clover, trefoil, wild clover.**
Red clover contains flavonoids, saponins, coumarins, isoflavones, and plant acids. It is often used externally for ○ **skin conditions** and internally for whooping cough (see ○ **pertussis**).

Warnings, interactions, and side effects
• Red clover should not be used with hormonal therapies or during pregnancy.
• Isoflavones have known estrogenic activity, and should therefore not be taken in excess.

red sage
(*Salvia miltiorrhiza*; Parts used: root)
Other common names: **dan-shen, red ginseng, red-rooted sage, red-rooted salvia.**
Red sage has traditionally been used to stimulate the circulation. Chinese studies have found that it can reduce the frequency and severity of ○ **angina pectoris** attacks, improve heart function, and help prevent heart attacks (see ○ **myocardial infarction**).

Warnings, interactions, and side effects
Although none have been reported with correct use and dosage, the properties of red sage have not been fully investigated and adverse reactions are possible.

reed herb
(*Phragmites communis*; Parts used: stem and rhizome)
Other common names: **common reed.**
Reed herb contains flavonoids, vitamins, A, B, and C, and triterpenoids. It has diuretic and diaphoretic activities, and is used for ○ **digestive system disorders**.

Warnings, interactions, and side effects
Although none have been reported with correct use and dosage, the properties of reed herb have not been fully investigated and adverse reactions are possible.

rehmannia
(*Rehmannia glutinosa*; Parts used: root)
Other common names: **di-huang.**
Rehmannia contains phytosterols and sugars. Traditional uses include as a tonic and for ○ **fever**. Recent research has shown that it has hepatoprotective and antipyretic properties, and can reduce levels of blood sugar and cholesterol.

Warnings, interactions, and side effects
Although none have been reported with correct use and dosage, the properties of rehmannia have not been fully investigated and adverse reactions are possible.

rhatany
(*Krameria triandra*; Parts used: root)
Other common names: **krameria root, mapato, rhatania.**
Rhatany contains neolignans and tannins, and has astringent activity. Traditional uses include for inflammation of the mouth and/or pharynx (see ○ **inflammation** and ○ **pharyngitis**) and ○ **diarrhea**, and these uses are approved by some authorities.

Warnings, interactions, and side effects
• Rhatany may cause stomach complaints as it can inhibit gastric secretions.

rhubarb, Chinese
(*Rheum palmatum*)
Other common names: **Canton rhubarb, da-huang, Indian rhubarb, medical rhubarb, rhubarb, Turkey rhubarb.**
Chinese rhubarb is a sturdy perennial with large palmate leaves up to 36 inches (90 centimeters) in length at the ends of almost cylindrical leaf stalks. The plant has a large, thick rhizome, and produces dark red flowers in late summer, followed by winged fruit. *Rheum officinale* is similar and sometimes hybrid plants or mixtures of herbs from the two plants are used. Other *Rheum* species, such as *R. rhaponticum*, *R. rhabarbarum*, or *R. ponticum* (garden rhubarb), are not interchangeable.

Key to symbols: ○ = Disorder Section ℞ = Drug Section ♣ = Herbal Section ⚕ = Supplement Section

Forms of preparation and parts used

The rhizome and roots of Chinese rhubarb are used medicinally. Leaf stems can be eaten as food; however, note that it is not the common garden rhubarb which is commonly eaten. The leaves should not be eaten (see below).

Active components

The major biologically active components of Chinese rhubarb are the anthraquinones, primarily anthraglycosides of emodin, aloe-emodin chrysophanol, and physcion. Numerous other anthraquinones (as dianthrone, oxalates, and as free aglycones) are also found in the plant, as well as tannins, carbohydrates, starch, and a volatile oil.

Uses in treatment

The rhizome of Chinese rhubarb is commonly used as a mild laxative (due to the anthraquinone content of the plant) and it is approved by some authorities for ✪ constipation. In contrast, in lower doses, it is approved in Germany as a treatment for ✪ diarrhea (in this case due to the astringent tannin content of the plant).

Warnings, interactions, and side effects

• Chinese rhubarb should be avoided during pregnancy and by breast-feeding mothers.

• Its leaves are rich in oxalic acid, which is poisonous. The leaves should not be eaten.

• In common with other anthraquinone-containing species (see ♣ frangula) there are some potential risks in consuming large amounts of rhubarb. Some authorities state that Chinese rhubarb should not be taken by anyone with arthritis or kidney disease or intestinal obstruction.

• As with other stimulant anthraquinone laxatives (including ♣ aloe, ♣ frangula, ♣ yellow dock, and also ℞ senna), long-term use should be avoided.

rice

(*Oryza sativa*; Parts used: seeds)
Other common names: **nivara.**
Rice contains starch, fatty acids, proteins, and B vitamins. It is a particularly good food during convalescence following gastrointestinal disorders as it has anodyne activity and calms the digestive tract.

Warnings, interactions, and side effects

None have been reported with correct use and dosage.

rose

(*Rosa centifolia, R. gallica*; Parts used: petals)
Other common names: **cabbage rose, damask rose, French rose, hundred-leafed rose.**
Rose contains tannins and a volatile oil rich in citronellol, and its leaves have astringent activity. It is used to treat inflammation of the mouth and/or pharynx (see ✪ inflammation and ✪ pharyngitis and is approved for this use by some authorities.

Warnings, interactions, and side effects

Although none have been reported with correct use and dosage, the properties of rose have not been fully investigated and adverse reactions are possible.

rosemary

(*Rosmarinus officinalis*)
Other common names: **compass plant, compass weed, old man, polar plant, rosemarine.**
Rosemary is an aromatic evergreen shrub with needle-like leaves. It can grown up to 6 feet (1.8 meters) in height, and bears two-lipped flowers, which are usually a shade of blue, although numerous varieties exist with pink, white, or yellow flowers.

Forms of preparation and parts used

Rosemary is usually taken as an infusion of the dried leaves and twigs, or as a tincture. The volatile oil is also widely used.

Active components

Rosemary contains a monoterpene-rich volatile oil, a number of flavonoids, phenolic acids (including rosemarinic acid), and triterpenes.

Uses in treatment

Rosemary has carminative, spasmolytic, sedative, diuretic, antimicrobial, tonic, and anti-inflammatory actions. It is used to promote circulation (and has been used to improve concentration and ✪ headaches), to treat nervous problems, and as a restorative. Some authorities approve the use of rosemary for ✪ indigestion, blood pressure problems, ✪ appetite loss, and, externally, for rheumatism (see ✪ musculoskeletal disorders), wound healing, and circulatory disorders. Laboratory studies have shown that rosemarinic acid which is found in rosemary, is anti-inflammatory. The flavonoid content of the herb has a beneficial effect in reducing capillary fragility.

Warnings, interactions, and side effects

• Rosemary should not be used during pregnancy or by breast-feeding mothers, although the amounts used in cooking are not usually considered harmful.

• Large amounts of camphor (found in the volatile oil of rosemary) taken by mouth may cause convulsions.

• Hypersensitivity to components of the oil have been reported, so it should be used with caution.

safflower

(*Carthamus tinctorius*; Parts used: flowerheads, seeds)
Other common names: **American saffron, bastard saffron, dyer's saffron, fake saffron, zaffer.**
Safflower contains lignans and polysaccharides. Traditional uses include for abdominal pain, to induce menstruation (it is an emmenagogue), and for ✪ fever. Reductions in blood cholesterol levels and some beneficial effects on coronary arterial disease have been recorded, and the polysaccharide component has a stimulant effect on the immune system.

Warnings, interactions, and side effects

• Safflower is not to be used during pregnancy.

sage

(*Salvia officinalis*)
Other common names: **Dalmatian sage, garden sage, meadow sage, red sage, scarlet sage, true sage.**

Common sage is a shrubby perennial herb with highly branched stems and velvety leaves of a grey-green color. Flowers, which can be white, pink or purple are produced in spikes in summer.

Forms of preparation and parts used
The leaves of sage are usually taken medicinally, fresh, dried, as a tincture, or infusion.

Active components
Sage contains a number of phenolic acids, tannins, flavonoids, and a volatile oil rich in monoterpenes (such as camphor and thujone). The primary component of the oil is thujone, which can be toxic in excess. The amount of thujone, both in commercial food products containing sage, and in herbal medicinal preparations, is officially limited.

Uses in treatment
Some authorities approve the use of sage for ✪ **appetite loss**, excessive perspiration (see ✪ **hyperhidrosis**), and mouth and pharynx inflammation (see ✪ **inflammation**; ✪ **pharyngitis**). Sage is also used as a gargle for sore throats and ✪ **mouth ulcers**, and as a general tonic. In laboratory studies, sage extracts have been shown to have hypotensive and antispasmodic activity, a depressant effect on the central nervous system, and cholinesterase-inhibiting properties. The volatile oil is strongly antimicrobial, with activity against bacteria, fungi, and also viruses.

Warnings, interactions, and side effects
• Sage should be avoided during pregnancy because thujone is a known abortifacient and emmenagogue.

• Sage oil is moderately irritating (it is not recommended for aromatherapy), and can be toxic if swallowed. The purified oil must never be swallowed. The monoterpenoids camphor and thujone present in sage are thought to be the main toxic constituents of the plant.

• Sage is widely used as a culinary herb, and there is no risk associated with eating the amounts of the herb usually found in foods. However, it should not be eaten in large quantities.

salep
(*Orchis morio*; Parts used: underground parts)
Other common names: **cuckoo flower, Levant salep, orchid, sahlep, saloop, satyrion.**
Salep contains starch and mucilage, which has demulcent activity. It is used to treat ✪ **diarrhea** and ✪ **indigestion**.

Warnings, interactions, and side effects
Although none have been reported with correct use and dosage, the properties of salep have not been fully investigated and adverse reactions are possible.

sandalwood
(*Santalum album*; Parts used: wood)
Other common names: **sanderswood, white saunders, yellow saunders.**
Sandlewood contains tannin, resins, and a volatile oil rich in santolols. It has been shown to have urinary disinfectant activity and is used, and approved by some authorities, for ✪ **urinary tract disorders**.

Warnings, interactions, and side effects
• Prolonged use of sandalwood may be toxic to the kidneys, and it should not be taken by anyone with any kind of kidney disorder.
• It may cause nausea.

sanicle
(*Sanicula europaea*; Parts used: herb)
Other common names: **European sanicle, poolroot, self-heal.**
Sanicle contains triterpene saponins, caffeic acid derivative, and flavonoids, and has expectorant, anti-inflammatory, and mildly astringent activities. Traditional uses include for ✪ **coughs** and ✪ **bronchitis**.

Warnings, interactions, and side effects
Although none have been reported with correct use and dosage, the properties of sanicle have not been fully investigated and adverse reactions are possible.

sarsaparilla
(*Smilax officinalis*; Parts used: rhizome)
Sarsaparilla contains a number of saponins, phytosterols, and flavonoids. Traditional uses include for ✪ **psoriasis** and rheumatic complaints (see ✪ **musculoskeletal disorders**). Some improvements in psoriasis have been shown clinically, and anti-inflammatory and hepatoprotective effects of extracts of sarsaparilla have been demonstrated experimentally.

Warnings, interactions, and side effects
• Large amounts of sarsaparilla may cause irritation of the skin due to its saponin content.

savory
(*Satureja hortensis*; Parts used: herb)
Other common names: **bean herb, summer savory.**
Savory contains tannins and a volatile oil rich in carvacrol, and has astringent and mildly antiseptic properties. Traditional uses include for acute gastroenteritis.

Warnings, interactions, and side effects
Although none have been reported with correct use and dosage, the properties of savory have not been fully investigated and adverse reactions are possible.

saw palmetto
(*Serenoa repens* or *Sabal serrulata*)
Other common names: **American dwarf palm tree, cabbage palm, sabal, serenoa, shrub palmetto.**
Saw palmetto palm has blue-green or yellow-green leaves, with small, cream-colored flowers, which are followed by blue-black fruits approximately 1 inch (2.5 centimeters) in length.

Forms of preparation and parts used
The fruit of saw palmetto are the part most commonly used medicinally, as an infusion or other liquid (sometimes ethanolic) extract.

Active components
The fruit of saw palmetto are rich in carbohydrates, including high molecular weight polysaccharides. They also contain a number of steroidal compounds, including beta-sitosterol, flavonoids, tannins, a fixed oil rich in fatty acids, and a volatile oil.

Key to symbols: ✪ = Disorder Section ℞ = Drug Section ♣ = Herbal Section ⚕ = Supplement Section

Uses in treatment

Saw palmetto is described as having diuretic, antiseptic, hormonal, and anabolic activities. It is most widely used for prostatic enlargement (✪ **benign prostatic hypertrophy**), and it is approved by some authorities for urination problems in benign prostatic hypertrophy (stages I and II). It has also been used to treat sex-hormone imbalances, ✪ **cystitis**, and testicular atrophy. In laboratory studies, extracts of saw palmetto have been shown to have significant anti-androgen effects on the production or action of the male sex hormone testosterone (inhibit the binding of dihydrotestosterone, the conversion of testosterone to dihydrotestosterone (by 5-alpha-reductase) and the conversion of dihydrotestosterone to androgenic derivatives). These activities are believed to be responsible for the positive clinical results for saw palmetto extracts in the treatment of early stages of benign prostatic hypertrophy (BPH). It may take at least a month before any improvement is seen.

Warnings, interactions, and side effects

• Saw palmetto has anti-androgenic and estrogenic actions, and should therefore not be used by anyone using other hormonal treatments (including the contraceptive pill and HRT).
• Because of its effects on sex hormones, anyone with sex-hormone dependent cancers should seek expert advice before use.
• Expert advice, preferably a doctor's, should be taken before using in benign prostatic hypertrophy treatment.
• As no detailed information is available regarding pregnancy and breast-feeding, the herb should be avoided during these times.

schisandra

(*Schisandra chinensis*; Parts used: fruit)
Other common names: **Chinese mock-barberry, lemonwood, wu-wei-zi.**
Schisandra contains phytosterols, vitamins, lignans, and a volatile oil. Traditional uses include as a tonic and adaptogen, and recent studies have shown hepatoprotective and central nervous system-stimulant properties for the fruit.

Warnings, interactions, and side effects

Although none have been reported with correct use and dosage, the properties of schisandra have not been fully investigated and adverse reactions are possible.

Scotch pine

(*Pinus sylvestris*; Parts used: oil)
Other common names: **dwarf pine, pine oils, pix liquida, pumilio pine, Scotch fir, Stockholm tar, Swiss mountain pine.**
Scotch pine's volatile oil is very rich in beta-pinene, and has secretolytic, antiseptic, and hyperemic activity. It is used for ✪ **colds** and respiratory tract infections (see ✪ **respiratory tract disorders**).

Warnings, interactions, and side effects

• Scotch pine is not to be used for bronchial asthma or whooping cough.
• It may cause irritation in some individuals.

scurvy grass

(*Cochlearia officinalis*; Parts used: leaves)
Other common names: **scrubby grass, spoonwort.**

The traditional use of scurvy grass is for the prevention and treatment of ✪ **scurvy** because it is rich in ⚕ **vitamin C**. It also has mild laxative, diuretic, and antiseptic properties.

Warnings, interactions, and side effects

• Scurvy grass taken in large amounts can cause gastrointestinal irritation.

sea buckthorn

(*Hippophae rhamnoides*; Parts used: berries)
Other common names: **sallow thorn.**
Sea buckthorn is rich in ⚕ **vitamin C**, flavonoids, and fruit acids. Traditional uses include for ✪ **infection**, because it is so rich in vitamin C, and ✪ **skin conditions**.

Warnings, interactions, and side effects

Although none have been reported with correct use and dosage, the properties of sea buckthorn have not been fully investigated and adverse reactions are possible.

selfheal

(*Prunella vulgaris*; Parts used: herb)
Other common names: **blue curls, brownwort, brunella, carpenter's herb, carpenter's weed, heart of the earth, heal-all, hook-heal, prunella, sicklewort, slough-heal, woundwort.**
Selfheal contains pentacyclic triterpenoids, tannins, and caffeic acid. Traditional uses include to staunch blood flow and heal ✪ **wounds**. Research has indicated that it can dilate blood vessels and has antimicrobial activity. The tannins may account for its astringent properties.

Warnings, interactions, and side effects

Although none have been reported with correct use and dosage, the properties of selfheal have not been fully investigated and adverse reactions are possible.

senega snakeroot

(*Polygala senega*)
Other common names: **milkwort, mountain flax, northern senega, rattlesnake root, seneca, seneca snakeroot, senega, seneka, snake root.**
Senega is a narrow-leafed perennial which grows to a height of about 18 inches (45 centimeters). It produces spikes of pale pink flowers.

Forms of preparation and parts used

The root of senega snakeroot is taken medicinally, usually as an infusion, a liquid extract, or a tincture.

Active components

Senega snakeroot contains a complex mixture of triterpene saponins (sometimes called senegin collectively), a range of plant acids and carbohydrates, methylsalicylate and glucoside (traces), sterols, and a resinous material.

Uses in treatment

Senega snakeroot has expectorant, diaphoretic, sialogogue, and emetic properties. It is widely used for ✪ **bronchial congestion**, including ✪ **asthma**, ✪ **bronchitis**, whooping cough (see ✪ **pertussis**), and ✪ **pharyngitis**. A triterpenoid which is present in senega snakeroot is reported to have anti-inflammatory properties. The root promotes phlegm production in the chest, easing wheezy ☯ **coughs**, and it is approved by some authorities for cough and bronchitis. Plant species related to senega snakeroot are reported to have depressant effects on the central nervous system.

Warnings, interactions, and side effects

• Senega snakeroot should not be used during pregnancy or by breast-feeding mothers.

• It may aggravate existing gastrointestinal inflammation, due to the irritancy of saponin compounds on mucosal membranes. It should be avoided, therefore, by anyone with an irritated stomach or a peptic ulcer.

• Large amounts can lead to diarrhea and vomiting.

• Senega snakeroot contains saponins and these compounds can cause hemolysis (breakdown) of red blood cells on contact with the blood, but this is unlikely to occur if senega is taken by mouth.

shepherd's purse

(*Capsella bursa-pastoris*; Parts used: herb)

Other common names: **blindweed, case-weed, cocowort, lady's purse, pepper-and-salt, pick-pocket, poor man's parmacettie, mother's heart, rattle pouches, St. James' weed, sanguinary, shepherd's heart, shepherd's scrip, shepherd's sprout, toywort, witches' pouches.**

Shepherd's purse contains amines, flavonoids, and a volatile oil. Traditional uses include as a urinary antiseptic and to manage bleeding. Some authorities approve its external use for ☯ **nosebleeds**, ☯ **bruises**, and ☯ **wounds**, and internally for ☯ **menorrhagia** and non-menstrual uterine bleeding. Hypotensive, anti-ulcer, anti-inflammatory, central nervous system-depressant, and smooth muscle stimulatory actions have all been reported.

Warnings, interactions, and side effects

• Shepherd's purse should not be used during pregnancy.

• Excessive intake may interfere with the treatment of abnormal blood pressure or thyroid dysfunction.

skullcap

(*Scutellaria lateriflora*; Parts used: herb)

Other common names: **blue pimpernel, helmet flower, hoodwort, mad-dog weed, madweed, Quaker bonnet.**

Skullcap contains flavonoids, iridoids, tannins, and a volatile oil. Traditional uses include for ☯ **dysmenorrhea** and to encourage menstruation, and today it is used as a nerve tonic. However, almost no pharmacological investigations have been carried out on skullcap.

Warnings, interactions, and side effects

Although none have been reported with correct use and dosage, the properties of skullcap have not been fully investigated and adverse reactions are possible.

skunk cabbage

(*Symplocarpus foetidus*; Parts used: seeds and root/rhizome)

Other common names: **dracontium, meadow cabbage, polecatweed, skunkweed.**

Skunk cabbage contains resins and a poorly studied volatile oil. Its antispasmodic and expectorant activities explain its use for ☯ **bronchitis** and ☯ **asthma**. The plant also has diaphoretic and sedative qualities.

Warnings, interactions, and side effects

Although none have been reported with correct use and dosage, the properties of skunk cabbage have not been fully investigated and adverse reactions are possible.

slippery elm

(*Ulmus fulva or U. rubra*; Parts used: inner bark)

Other common names: **red elm, sweet elm.**

Slippery elm is rich in mucilage and also contains tannins and phytosterols. There have been no specific studies on slippery elm, but mucilages are known to be demulcent, and tannins have astringent activity. Traditional uses include for ☯ **inflammation**, ☯ **peptic ulcers**, and externally for ☯ **boils**.

Warnings, interactions, and side effects

• The bark of slippery elm can induce an abortion and so should not be used during pregnancy.

sloe

(*Prunus spinosa*; Parts used: fruit, flowers)

Other common names: **blackthorn, wild plum.**

Sloe contains tannins, flavonoids, and cyanogenic glycosides, which are probably only present in the fresh flowers. Traditional uses include for inflammation of the mouth and/or pharynx (see ☯ **inflammation** and ☯ **pharyngitis**) (this use is approved by some authorities) and ☯ **diarrhea**. The bark has astringent activity.

Warnings, interactions, and side effects

Although none have been reported with correct use and dosage, the properties of sloe have not been fully investigated and adverse reactions are possible.

smartweed

(*Polygonum hydropiper or Persicaria hydropiper*; Parts used: whole plant)

Other common names: **arsesmart, water pepper.**

Smartweed contains tannins, flavonoids (rutin or rutoside), and sesquiterpene aldehydes. It is generally used to manage bleeding, for example, ☯ **wounds**, ☯ **hemorrhage**, and ☯ **hemorrhoids**.

Warnings, interactions, and side effects

Although none have been reported with correct use and dosage, the properties of smartweed have not been fully investigated and adverse reactions are possible.

soap bark

(*Quillaja saponaria*; Parts used: inner bark)

Other common names: **cullay, Panama bark, quillai, quillaja, quillaja bark, soap tree.**

Soap brak contains tannins and saponins. The bark has expectorant and anti-inflammatory activity. Traditional uses include for ☯ **respiratory tract disorders**, such as ☯ **coughs** and ☯ **bronchitis.**

Warnings, interactions, and side effects
• Soap bark taken in large quantities can irritate the stomach and lead to gastroenteritis.

soapwort
(*Saponaria officinalis*; Parts used: roots)
Other common names: **bouncing Bet, bruisewort, crow soap, dog cloves, fuller's herb, latherwort, old maid's pink, soapwod, soap root, sweet Betty, wild sweet William.**
Soapwort contains triterpenoid saponins, and its roots have expectorant activity, which is thought to be due to mucous membrane irritation. It is used, and approved by some authorities, for the treatment of ✪ **coughs** and ✪ **bronchitis.**

Warnings, interactions, and side effects
• Large amounts of soapwort may cause some irritation of the skin or mucous membrane.

Solomon's seal
(*Polygonum multiflorum*; Parts used: root)
Other common names: **dropberry, flowery knotweed, lady's seal, St. Mary's seal, sealroot, sealwort.**
Solomon's seal contains anthraquinones, lecithin, and plant acids, and is traditionally used as a tonic. Clinical evidence for its ability to lower blood sugar and cholesterol levels has been reported. It may be useful in treating ✪ **malaria** and ✪ **tuberculosis.**

Warnings, interactions, and side effects
Although none have been reported with correct use and dosage, the properties of Solomon's seal have not been fully investigated and adverse reactions are possible.

southern bayberry
(*Myrica cerifera*)
Other common names: **axberry, bayberry, candleberry, candleberry bark, myrica, tallow shrub, vegetable tallow, wax myrtle.**
Southern bayberry is an evergreen shrub which can grow up to 40 feet (12 meters) tall. It has small, elongated, oval-shaped leaves and grows in a range of conditions. It produces separate male and female flowers, followed by waxy grey fruit.

Forms of preparation and parts used
The root bark of southern bayberry is usually taken medicinally, dried and powdered, as an infusion, decoction, or tincture.

Active components
Southern bayberry contains the flavonoid myricitrin, a number of triterpenes, tannins, gums, resins, and waxes.

Uses in treatment
It is used for ✪ **diarrhea**, sore throats (see ✪ **pharyngitis**), and ✪ **colds**. It can also be used as a circulatory stimulant, to reduce ✪ **fever**, and as an emetic. It has been reported that the flavonoid myricitrin found in southern bayberry stimulates production of bile, and also has spermicidal and antibacterial activities. The triterpene myricadiol found in southern bayberry has been demonstrated to have mild effects on potassium and sodium levels through a mineralocorticoid action (see ℞ **corticosteroid**). The tannin components of southern bayberry bark are responsible for its astringent actions.

Warnings, interactions, and side effects
• Some experts recommend that southern bayberry should not be used for medicinal purposes.
• It should not be used during pregnancy or by breast-feeding mothers.
• Excessive intake may interfere with steroid or blood pressure treatments, and may cause mineralocorticoid-type side effects, including elevated blood pressure.

southern prickly ash
(*Zanthoxylum clava-herculis*; Parts used: bark)
Southern prickly ash contains isoquinoline alkaloids, lignans, amides, and a volatile oil. Traditional uses include for chronic rheumatism (see ✪ **musculoskeletal disorders**), poor peripheral circulation and cramping. Antimicrobial, anti-inflammatory, and hypotensive properties have been reported experimentally, as has curare-like neuromuscular-blocking activity.

Warnings, interactions, and side effects
• Some toxicity from the alkaloid content of the bark has been reported.

soybean
(*Glycine soja*; Parts used: bean)
Soybean contains phospholipids and a fatty oil. It is widely believed to contribute to lower than average cholesterol levels in certain groups of people living in areas where the diet is particularly rich in soybean. It is approved by some authorities for the treatment of hypercholestemia (see ✪ **hyperlipidemia**).

Warnings, interactions, and side effects
• Occasionally, soybean may cause minor disturbances of the gastrointestinal tract, such as loose stools.

spearmint
(*Mentha spicata*; Parts used: aerial parts)
Other common names: **curled mint, fish mint, garden mint, green mint, lamb mint, mackerel mint, Our Lady's mint, sage of Bethlehem, spire mint.**
Spearmint contains a volatile oil rich in L-carvone, and has antispasmodic, carminative, and stimulant activity. It is used to treat ✪ **digestive system disorders** and ✪ **flatulence.**

Warnings, interactions, and side effects
• The oil may be weakly sensitizing.

speedwell
(*Veronica officinalis*; Parts used: herb)
Speedwell contains iridoids, flavonoids, and triterpene saponins. It is used for gastrointestinal disorders and discomfort (see ✪ **digestive system disorders**), and in experiments it has been shown to have protective and healing effects on peptic ulcers.

Warnings, interactions, and side effects
Although none have been reported with correct use and dosage, the properties of speedwell have not been fully investigated and adverse reactions are possible.

spikenard

(*Aralia racemosa*; Parts used: root)

Other common names: **Indian root, life of man, old man's root, petty morell, spignet.**

American spikenard contains diterpene acids, tannins, and a volatile oil. Traditional uses include as a detoxifying stimulant, and to treat ✪ **asthma** and ✪ **flatulence**. It was included in the National Formulary until 1965.

Warnings, interactions, and side effects

• Spikenard should not be used during pregnancy.

• Contact with the plant may cause skin irritation in some people.

spiny rest harrow

(*Ononis spinosa*; Parts used: roots and flowering branches)

Other common names: **cammock, ground furze, land whin, petty whin, rest-harrow, stayplough, stinking Tommy, wild licorice.**

Spiny rest harrow contains flavonoids, triterpenoids, and a volatile oil rich in anethole. It has diuretic activity (see ✪ **fluid retention**) and traditional uses include for ✪ **gout** and rheumatism (see ✪ **musculoskeletal disorders**). Some authorities approve of its use for ✪ **urinary tract disorders** and kidney or bladder stones (see ✪ **calculus**).

Warnings, interactions, and side effects

• Spiny rest harrow is not to be used by anyone with edema due to cardiac or renal insufficiency.

spruce

(*Picea excelsa*; Parts used: needles and shoots)

Other common names: **balm of gilead fir, balsam fir, Canada balsam, fir tree, hemlock spruce, Norway pine, Norway spruce, spruce fir.**

Spruce contains a volatile oil rich in bornyl acetate. It has antibacterial activity and stimulates secretory activity from the bronchial membranes. Traditional uses include to treat ✪ **coughs**, ✪ **colds**, ✪ **fevers**, and inflammation of the mouth (see ✪ **inflammation**).

Warnings, interactions, and side effects

• Spruce should not be used for bronchial asthma or whooping cough.

squill

(*Drimia maritima or Urginea maritima*; Parts used: bulb)

Other common names: **scilla.**

Squill contains cardiac glycosides, flavonoids, and tannins. Traditional uses include for ✪ **asthma**, ✪ **bronchitis**, and whooping cough (see ✪ **pertussis**). White squill has emetic and expectorant actions.

Warnings, interactions, and side effects

• Squill should not be used during pregnancy.

• It should not be taken by anyone already receiving some form of heart treatment.

• Large doses of squill may cause vomiting, which limits the dangers of poisoning by overdose.

star anise

(*Illicium verum*; Parts used: fruit)

Other common names: **aniseed stars, badiana.**

Star anise contains flavonoids, tannins, and a volatile oil. It is used as a culinary spice, and also to treat ✪ **coughs**, ✪ **bronchitis**, and ✪ **appetite loss**. These uses are approved by some authorities. The fruits have bronchial expectorant activity and antispasmodic action in the gastrointestinal tract.

Warnings, interactions, and side effects

• Very rare cases of sensitization have been reported.

stinging nettle

(*Urtica dioica*)

Other common names: **common nettle, greater nettle, nettle.**

Stinging nettles are perennial herbs which grow from spreading roots up to a height of up to 4 to 5 feet (1.25 to 1.5 meters). The toothed leaves are covered with stinging hairs. In summer, separate plants produce male and female flowers in clusters up to 3 to 4 inches (7 to 10 centimeters) in length. Stinging nettles are found in almost all temperate regions.

Forms of preparation and parts used

The aerial parts of the plant are commonly used medicinally, usually as an infusion or tincture. The root has also received considerable medicinal interest, and can be taken as a decoction.

Active components

The aerial parts of nettle are rich in plant acids, flavonoids, and amines. The roots contain lignans, a lectin, coumarin, and a phytosterol.

Uses in treatment

Stinging nettle is a general tonic. Aerial parts of the plant are usually taken to lower blood sugar and to stop bleeding. The herb is also widely used as a diuretic (see ✪ **fluid retention**), and, in the form of a cream it can be applied externally for ✪ **skin conditions**, particularly ✪ **eczema** and ✪ **dermatitis**. In laboratory studies, stinging nettle has been shown to have depressant activity on the central nervous system. The roots are receiving considerable interest for the early stages of ✪ **benign prostatic hypertrophy** (BPH) and other urination problems (such as ✪ **bed-wetting**), and also ✪ **prostatitis**. Some authorities approve the use of the flowering plant for rheumatism (see ✪ **musculoskeletal disorders**) (which is possibly connected to its histamine and serotonin content), kidney and bladder stones (see ✪ **calculus**), and ✪ **urinary tract disorders**, and the use of the root for prostate complaints and irritable bladder.

Warnings, interactons, and side effects

• Stinging nettle leaves are highly irritating to the skin, causing urticaria and a stinging sensation as a result of their histamine, serotonin, and acetylcholine content which is injected into the skin by the pointed spines.

• Gastrointestinal irritation, oliguria, burning of the skin, and edema have all been reported following ingestion of nettle tea.

• Using large quantities should be avoided by anyone taking treatments for diabetes, blood pressure, or central nervous system-active drugs.

Key to symbols: ✪ = Disorder Section ℞ = Drug Section ♣ = Herbal Section ⚕ = Supplement Section

• Laboratory studies have demonstrated that nettle can have effects on the uterus, it should therefore be avoided during pregnancy.

St. John's wort

(*Hypericum perforatum*)

Other common names: **amber, amber-touch-and heal, goatsweed, goatweed, hardhay, klamath weed, rosin rose, St. John's word.**

St. John's wort is an erect perennial herb which grows to a height of approximately 30 inches (75 centimeters). It has small leaves with tiny translucent dots on their surface, and clusters of yellow flowers.

Forms of preparation and parts used

The aerial parts of the herb, and in particular the flowering tops, are used medicinally, usually as an infusion, a liquid extract, a tincture, or as an infused oil. It is one of the best-selling herbal remedies in the US.

Active components

St. John's wort contains a number of anthraquinone derivatives, including hypericin and pseudohypericin, phloroglucinol derivatives, including hyperforin, a large number of flavonoids and phenolic compounds, tannins, phytosterols, and a hydrocarbon-rich volatile oil. Preparations chemically standardized for the content of their active ingredient are available, originally for hypericum (usually 0.3 to 0.4 percent) and more recently for hyperforin (commonly 2 to 3 percent, but some much more).

Uses in treatment

The major properties of hypericum include antidepressant, antispasmodic, astringent, sedative, analgesic, and antiviral activity. It has been used to treat nervous disorders, such as ✪ **anxiety**, ✪ **insomnia**, and ✪ **depression**, as well as menopausal complaints (see ✪ **menopause**), and as a tonic for the gallbladder and liver. Externally, the infused oil is used on ✪ **wounds** and ✪ **burns**, as well as to relieve nerve ✪ **pain**.

Some authorities approve of its use when taken internally for anxiety, depression, and also skin inflammation, and when used externally for blunt injuries, wounds, and burns. A number of clinical studies have confirmed the herb's activity as an antidepressant for mild to moderate depression, and some trials show it to be as beneficial as some conventional medications with a low incidence of side effects. Recent research indicates that the antidepressant effect of St. John's wort is due largely to the presence of the chemical hyperforin, which appears to work by inhibiting uptake of serotonin and other amine neurotransmitters (see ℞ **antidepressants**; ℞ **SSRI**).

Warnings, interactions, and side effects

• In clinical trials, few side-effects have been reported for St. John's wort. The main concern over its use is its possible interaction with existing antidepressant treatments, such as ℞ **monoamine-oxidase inhibitors** (MAOIs). It should never be used at the same time as other treatments for depression.

• It can cause photodermatitis and delayed hypersensitivity. Drugs that cause photosensitization (such as tetracyclines and thiazides) should not be taken at the same time.

• For these reasons, it is best to avoid using St. John's wort during pregnancy and if breast-feeding.

• St. John's wort should not be used by anyone taking protease inhibitors such as ℞ **indinavir** and any drug that inhibits the cytochrome P450 system.

• There have been interactions reported with the contraceptive pill, treatments for migraine and asthma, and with blood-thinning drugs (anticoagulants and antiplatelet drugs). In general St. John's wort should be taken with caution, and only after receiving professional medical advice, by anyone taking prescription, other herbal remedies or OTC drugs.

sundew

(*Drosera rotundifolia, D. rumentacea, D. anglica, or D. intermedia*; Parts used: herb)

Other common names: **dew plant, lustwort, red rot, youthwort.**

Sundew contains flavonoids and quinones. Traditional uses include as an antispasmodic, demulcent, and expectorant, and also antimicrobial activity has been demonstrated. Its antispasmodic activity has been shown experimentally on the bronchi and intestine.

Warnings, interactions, and side effects

• Sundew may affect the immune system and have irritant effects.

sweet cicely

(*Myrrhis odorata*; Parts used: herb)

Other common names: **British myrrh, the Roman plant, shepherd's needle, sweet bracken, sweet chervil, sweet-cus, sweet-fern, sweet-humlock, sweets.**

Sweet cicely contains a volatile oil rich in anethole and flavonoids. It has carminative, expectorant, and digestive activity. Traditional uses include for ✪ **asthma** and other breathing disorders.

Warnings, interactions, and side effects

Although none have been reported with correct use and dosage, the properties of sweet cicely have not been fully investigated and adverse reactions are possible.

sweetclover

(*Melilotus officinalis*; Parts used: herb)

Other common names: **hart's tree, hay flowers, king's clover, melilot, sweet lucerne, wild laburnum, yellow sweet clover.**

Sweetclover contains coumarin derivatives, saponins, and *flavonoids*. Traditional uses include for ✪ **venous insufficiency** and ✪ **hemorrhoids**, and these uses are approved by some authorities, as well as for treating blunt injuries.

Warnings, interactions, and side effects

• Taking large amounts of sweetclover may cause headaches and stupor.

• There are reports of liver damage, and so the herb should only be used with professional supervision.

sweet orange

(*Citrus sinensis*; Parts used: fruit peel)

Other common names: **China orange, citrus orange, orange.**

Sweet orange contains a number of flavonoids and a volatile oil rich in limonene. It is known to have digestive activity, and is approved by some authorities for ✪ **indigestion** and ✪ **appetite loss**.

Warnings, interactions, and side effects

• Sweet orange may cause sensitization in some people.

tamarind

(*Tamarindus indica*; Parts used: fruit and seeds)
Other common names: **imlee**.
Tamarind contains fruit acids, pectin, and sugars, and has aperient activity. It is used for ✪ **constipation**, ✪ **liver disorders**, and ✪ **gallbladder disorders**. Traditionally, it is often taken with figs to increase the laxative effect.

Warnings, interactions, and side effects

Although none have been reported with correct use and dosage, the properties of tamarind have not been fully investigated and adverse reactions are possible.

tarragon, French

(*Artemisia dracunculus*; Parts used: herb)
Other common names: **estragon, little dragon, mugwort**.
Tarragon contains tannins, flavonoids, and a volatile oil. It is widely used as a culinary herb, but also to aid digestion (see ✪ **digestive system disorders**) and as a mild sedative (see ✪ **insomnia**).

Warnings, interactions, and side effects

• Intake should not exceed culinary levels due to the potential toxicity of the volatile oil.

tea tree

(*Melaleuca alternifolia*; Parts used: volatile oil)
The volatile oil of tea tree is rich in terpinen-4-ol, gamma-terpinene, and alpha-terpinene. Traditionally, the leaves were used for ✪ **colds** and ✪ **skin conditions** (including ✪ **acne**). The oil is widely used as an antiseptic, and has documented antimicrobial activity.

Warnings, interactions, and side effects

• Tea tree should not be used during pregnancy.
• It is not to be taken internally without supervision.
• It may irritate the skin.

thyme

(*Thymus vulgaris*)
Other common names: **common thyme, French thyme, garden thyme, rubbed thyme**.
Thyme is a small, aromatic perennial widely grown as a culinary, medicinal, and ornamental plant. Numerous varieties exist, but common thyme usually bears white to pale pink flowers in the summer, and has grey-green leaves.

Forms of preparation and parts used

The flowers and leaves of thyme are used medicinally, fresh or dried, usually as an infusion or tincture. The volatile oil is also used.

Active components

The volatile oil of thyme is rich in phenolic compounds, predominantly thymol and carvacrol. The herb also contains flavonoids, phenolic acids, saponins, and tannins.

Uses in treatment

Traditionally, thyme is used for ✪ **indigestion**, ✪ **gastritis**, ✪ **asthma**, ✪ **laryngitis**, and ✪ **tonsillitis**. It is approved by some authorities for use in the treatment of ✪ **bronchitis**, ✪ **cough**, ✪ **catarrh** of the upper respiratory tract, and ✪ **pertussis** (whooping cough). Laboratory studies have been carried out on the oil, and it has been shown to stimulate the respiratory system and have hypotensive activity. Flavonoids, and possibly the phenolic constituents of the oil, have been shown to be antispasmodic, while an extract of the herb has been shown to be analgesic. The oil has been used clinically to treat ✪ **bed-wetting** in children. Thymol, an extract of the volatile oil, is antimicrobial and kills hookworms (see ✪ **worms**), and can act as an insect repellent. Thymol is incorporated into many mouthwash and counterirritant preparations and also cough drops.

Warnings, interactions, and side effects

• Thyme oil is irritating to the skin and mucosal membranes.
• The oil is also toxic and should not be taken internally, and only applied to the skin when diluted.
• Thyme has a reputation for affecting the menstrual cycle, and should therefore not be consumed in large doses.
• At levels used in cooking, thyme may be taken safely during pregnancy and when breast-feeding, but large doses should be avoided.

tormentil

(*Potentilla erecta*; Parts used: rhizome)
Other common names: **biscuits, bloodroot, cinquefoil, earthbank, English sarsaparilla, ewe daisy, flesh and blood, septfoil, shepherd's knapperty, shepherd's knot, thormantle**.
Tormentil contains tannins, flavonoids, triterpenoids, and proanthocyanidins. It is used, and approved by some authorities, for ✪ **diarrhea** and inflammation of the mouth and/or pharynx (see ✪ **inflammation** and ✪ **pharyngitis**) largely due to its astringent properties.

Warnings, interactions, and side effects

• Tormentil has been reported to cause irritation of the stomach, resulting in vomiting.

turmeric

(*Curcuma longa* or *C. domestica*; Parts used: rhizome)
Turmeric contains curcumin and a volatile oil. Traditional uses include for ✪ **indigestion**, ✪ **jaundice**, and ✪ **nausea**, and it is approved by some authorities for indigestion. Research has confirmed that it has anti-inflammatory, lipid-lowering, antimicrobial, ♒ **antioxidant**, and anticoagulant activities.

Warnings, interactions, and side effects

• *Curcuma domestica* should not be used during pregnancy.
• Turmeric may cause photosensitization (sensitivity to light).

uva-ursi

(*Arctostaphylos uva-ursi*)
Other common names: **arberry, bear berry, bearberry, bear's grape, common bearberry, kinnickinick, kinnikinnick, mealberry, mountain box, mountain cranberry, red bearberry,**

red-beery, red-berried trailing arbutus, redberry leaves, rockberry, sagackhomi, sandberry, upland cranbeery, upland cranberry.

A hardy ornamental that is native to the temperate regions of the Northern Hemisphere, and which is able to grow in acid conditions in moist sandy or peaty soils.

Forms of preparation and parts used

The leaves of uva-ursi are the most commonly used part of the plant, usually as an infusion or liquid extract.

Active components

Uva-ursi contains a large number of biologically active compounds, including flavonoids and their glycosides, iridoids, tannins, terpenoids, and quinones. The hydroquinone arbutin is strongly antibacterial, including against a variety of bacteria of *Enterobacter* (including *E. coli*) and *Klebsiella* spp.

Uses in treatment

Uva-ursi is most commonly used internally for infections, such as ✪ **cystitis**, ✪ **urethritis**, and ✪ **vaginitis**, and it is approved by some authorities for ✪ **urinary tract disorders**. It is also regarded as a diuretic (see ✪ **fluid retention**) and astringent. Laboratory studies have been carried out on uva-ursi and, for example, it has been shown to have anti-inflammatory activity. Its diuretic and antiseptic properties have been found to be largely due to the presence of arbutin, which is converted to hydroquinone, although the presence of other compounds in the herb make crude extracts more effective than isolated arbutin.

Warnings, interactions, and side effects

• Uva-ursi should not be used during pregnancy or by breast-feeding mothers.

• It should not be given to children under 12 years.

• Prolonged use of the herb is not recommended because large amounts of hydroquinone (which is generated in the body from the arbutin found in uva-ursi) can be toxic, and also because it has a high tannin content and so there is some risk of damaging liver function. The production of hydroquinone from arbutin requires alkaline conditions, so people taking uva-ursi are advised to avoid eating acidic foodstuffs.

• It may cause nausea and vomiting in some people.

valerian

(*Valeriana officinalis*)
Other common names: **all-heal, amantilla, capon's tail, heliotrope, setewale, setwell, vandal root.**

Valerian is a perennial herb which grows to a height of approximately 4 to 5 feet (1.25 to 1.5 meters) from stocky underground rhizomes. Its flowers can be white or pink, and are small and tubular in shape. Small, tufted seeds are produced in early fall.

Forms of preparation and parts used

Valerian root and rhizome is most commonly used medicinally, usually dried and powdered, as a liquid extract, or tincture.

Active components

Valerian contains a number of pyridine alkaloids and iridoids (valepotriates, including valtrate and didrovaltrate as major components), phenolic acids, and a volatile oil rich is esterified monoterpenes and sesquiterpenes.

Uses in treatment

Valerian is widely used as a sedative and as a relaxant. It is approved by some authorities for treating ✪ **insomnia** and ✪ **anxiety**. It is also said to have anodyne, antispasmodic, and hypotensive actions. The sedative activity of the herb is thought to come from the volatile oil and iridoid content. Valerenic acid, present in the volatile oil, is thought to have sedative activity because it stops or interferes with the breakdown by the body of the neurotransmitter gamma-aminobutyric acid (GABA). An iridoid fraction has also been shown to prevent heart arrhythmia and to have anticonvulsant activity. Clinical studies of the sedative action of valerian indicate that it may improve the quality of sleep both in normal sleepers and those suffering with insomnia.

Warnings, interactions, and side effects

• Iridoids isolated from valerian have been shown to have cytotoxic and mutagenic effects in laboratory studies, although it is possible that these effects may not be relevant to the normal use of valerian, because these compounds are highly unstable.

• Valerian may interfere with existing sedative treatments (although it is reported not to interact with alcohol).

• It should not be used during pregnancy or by breast-feeding mothers, because its safe use at these times has not been proven.

vervain

(*Verbena officinalis*; Parts used: herb)
Other common names: **enchanter's plant, herb of grace, herb of the Cross, Juno's tears, pigeon's grass, pigeonweed, simpler's joy.**

Vervain contains numerous glycosides and a volatile oil. Traditional uses include for ✪ **depression**, early stages of ✪ **fever**, and convalescence after ✪ **influenza**. It has been reported that it promotes lactation and has a number of effects on sex hormone levels and uterine tissue.

Warnings, interactions, and side effects

• Vervain should not be used during pregnancy.

• Taking large amounts may interfere with certain hormone therapies.

walnut

(*Juglans nigra or J. regia*; Parts used: inner bark)
Other common names: **Caucasion walnut, Circassian walnut, English walnut, Persian walnut.**

Walnut contains naphthaquinones and tannins. Naphthaquinones have antimicrobial, antiparasitic, and laxative activities, which explains the traditional uses of the plant for ✪ **constipation** and ✪ **dysentery**. It is approved by some authorities for skin inflammation (see ✪ **skin conditions**) of the hands and feet.

Warnings, interactions, and side effects

Although none have been reported with correct use and dosage, the properties of walnut have not been fully investigated and adverse reactions are possible.

watercress

(*Nasturtium officinale*; Parts used: aerial parts)
Other common names: **Indian cress.**

Watercress contains glucosinolates, flavonoids, and ♒ **vitamin C**. It is used for ✛ **digestive system disorders** and also has diuretic activity (see ✛ **fluid retention**). Its treatment of ✛ **coughs** and ✛ **catarrh** of the respiratory tract (which is approved by some authorities) may be due to its vitamin C content and antibacterial properties.

Warnings, interactions, and side effects
• Watercress should not be used during pregnancy.
• It should not be used by children under four years of age.
• It should not be used by anyone with a peptic ulcer or kidney inflammation.

water hyssop
(*Bacopa monnieri*; Parts used: aerial parts)
Water hyssop contains saponins, including bacosides. It is widely used in India for nervous disorders (see ✛ **anxiety**), and research suggests beneficial effects on mental function, memory, and concentration.

Warnings, interactions, and side effects
Although none have been reported with correct use and dosage, the properties of water hyssop have not been fully investigated and adverse reactions are possible.

weeping forsythia
(*Forsythia suspensa: fruit*)
Weeping forsythia traditionally has been used for ✛ **colds**, ✛ **influenza**, sore throat (see ✛ **pharyngitis**), and ✛ **fever**, and applied externally for ✛ **boils** and some infections. Research has shown that weeping forsythia contains a glycoside, forsythin, which has strong antimicrobial activity and also is able to relieve nausea and vomiting.

Warnings, interactions, and side effects
Although none have been reported with correct use and dosage, the properties of weeping forsythia have not been fully investigated and adverse reactions are possible.

white dead nettle
(*Lamium album*; Parts used: flowers and leaves)
Other common names: **archangel, bee nettle, blind nettle, dead nettle, deaf nettle, dumb nettle, stingless nettle, white archangel, white nettle.**
White dead nettle contains iridoids, derivatives of caffeic acid, flavonoids, and mucilage. It has expectorant and astringent activities. Traditional uses include for skin inflammation (see ✛ **skin conditions**), inflammation of the mouth and/or pharynx (see ✛ **inflammation** and ✛ **pharyngitis**), and ✛ **coughs**. These uses have been approved by some authorities.

Warnings, interactions, and side effects
Although none have been reported with correct use and dosage, the properties of white dead nettle have not been fully investigated and adverse reactions are possible.

white lily
(*Lilium candidium*; Parts used: bulb)
Other common names: **Madonna lily, meadow lily.**

White lily contains polysaccharides, starch, tannins, and mucilage. It has anti-inflammatory, anodyne, and hemorrhagic properties, and traditional uses include for ✛ **ulcers**, ✛ **inflammation**, and ✛ **burns**.

Warnings, interactions, and side effects
Although none have been reported with correct use and dosage, the properties of white lily have not been fully investigated and adverse reactions are possible.

white peony
(*Paeonia lactiflora*; Parts used: root)
White peony contains a number of monoterpene glycosides and benzoic acid. Traditionally used as a gynecological herb for ✛ **menorrhagia** (heavy periods) and ✛ **dysmenorrhea** (painful menstrual bleeding). White peony contains the glycoside peoniflorin which has antispasmodic activity and so may have a relaxing effect on the uterus. It is also mildly anti-inflammatory and antipyretic.

Warnings, interactions, and side effects
• White peony should not be used during pregnancy.

wild carrot
(*Daucus carota*)
Other common names: **bees' nest plant, bird's nest, philtron, Queen Anne's lace. The wild subspecies of carrot is sometimes called *Daucus carota carota*.**
Wild carrot is a hardy biennial with a fibrous off-white tap-root. It bears umbels of small cream flowers, which may be tinged pink, followed by small ridged seeds. It can grow to approximately 3 feet (90 centimeters) tall. This plant should not be confused with the similar-looking poison hemlock (*Conium maculatum*) or water hemlock (*Cicuta maculata*), which are both highly poisonous.

Forms of preparation and parts used
The seeds (and seed oil), roots, and leaves are all used medicinally, and are usually eaten fresh, or taken as an infusion or a tincture.

Active components
Wild carrot contains a number of flavonoids, furanocoumarins, and a volatile oil containing terpenes (including terpinen-4-ol), which can vary in composition between varieties. Its pale color reflects a low content of ♒ **carotenoids** (such as alpha- and beta-carotene) compared to the cultivated subspecies of carrot.

Uses in treatment
Wild carrot is traditionally used as a diuretic (see ✛ **fluid retention**), and is said to have antilithic (prevents urinary stones: see ✛ **calculus**), and carminative properties. The diuretic activity of the seed oil is thought to come from its terpinen-4-ol content. Wild carrot, and extracts of the seeds, have been shown in laboratory studies to have effects on fertility and the uterus.

Warnings, interactions, and side effects
• Wild carrot should be avoided during pregnancy and by breast-feeding mothers.
• The seed oil is generally regarded as non-toxic, although terpinen-4-ol is believed to cause diuretic activity by acting as an irritant to the kidneys.
• There have been some reports of hypersensitivity and dermatitis, although the seed oil is generally regarded as non-irritating.

• Excessive intake may affect treatment for endocrine, heart, and blood pressure disorders.

wild iris
(Iris versicolor)

Other common names: **blue flag.**

Wild iris is usually found in wet, marshy conditions. It produces long, slender, pointed leaves and groups of 3 to 6 distinctive purple and yellow flowers in summer. It can reach up to 3 feet (90 centimeters) in height.

Forms of preparation and parts used
The rhizome of wild iris is taken medicinally, usually in the form of a decoction.

Active components
Wild iris contains a number of plant acids, small quantities of a volatile oil (containing furfural), a phytosterol, tannins, and resinous substances.

Uses in treatment
Wild iris is usually taken for biliousness, ✪ **liver disorders**, and ✪ **skin conditions**. It is considered to have anti-inflammatory, anti-emetic, diuretic, and laxative properties. These last two properties have led to its use as a cleansing agent, especially in chronic (long-term) diseases. Small doses of the rhizome are given to relieve ✪ **indigestion**, ✪ **nausea**, and ✪ **vomiting**.

Warnings, interactions, and side effects
• Furfural (a component of the volatile oil), on its own, has an irritant effect on mucosal membranes, and can cause headaches and eye inflammation and tears.

• There is no evidence that these side effects occur if the rhizome is used, but the rhizome should only be taken internally in small amounts, as large doses cause vomiting.

• Anyone with suspected sensitivity to wild iris should only use the rhizome with care.

• It should not be used during pregnancy.

wild lettuce
(Lactuca virosa)

Other common names: **acrid lettuce, bitter lettuce, green endive, lactucarium, lettuce opium, poison lettuce, prickly lettuce, strong-scented lettuce.**

Wild lettuce is a biennial with hollow stems, growing up to 4 feet (1.25 meters) in height. It bears clusters of pale yellow flowers in late summer. The slightly spined leaves and hollow stem both produce white latex (a milky white juice) when cut or damaged.

Forms of preparation and parts used
The leaves and latex of wild lettuce are taken medicinally. The leaves are mainly used dried or as a liquid extract. Extracts of the latex are the basis of the drug lactucarium.

Active components
The latex contains a number of sesquiterpene lactones. The leaves also contain phenolic acids, coumarins, flavonoids, and other terpenoids (including lactucin and lactupicrin). Reports of the presence of alkaloids (such as scopolamine) have been disputed.

Uses in treatment
Wild lettuce is used as a mild sedative and hypnotic, and has been used to treat sleeping disorders such as ✪ **insomnia**, excitability (mainly in children), as well as ✪ **coughs**, muscular ✪ **pains**, and ✪ **dysmenorrhea**. Extracts of *L. sativa* (a related species) have been shown to have sedative activity in laboratory studies, although the chemicals that cause this effect were not identified. The terpenoids lactucin and lactupicrin may be responsible for the sedative action, although again this has not been proven. Wild lettuce has been shown to dilate the pupil of the eye.

Warnings, interactions, and side effects
• Wild lettuce should be avoided during pregnancy and by breast-feeding mothers.

• Sesquiterpene lactones which are found in wild lettuce are known to cause allergic reactions in sensitive people, so it should be used with caution and in small amounts by people who are sensitive to members of the daisy family.

• The sap of a plant species related to wild lettuce can be irritating to the skin.

• Excessive use of wild lettuce may result in stupor and even coma and death.

wild mint
(Mentha aquatica; Parts used: leaves)

Other common names: **hairy mint, marsh mint, water mint.**

Wild mint contains a volatile oil rich in menthofurane and tannins. The herb has astringent activity and is used to treat ✪ **diarrhea**.

Warnings, interactions, and side effects
Although none have been reported with correct use and dosage, the properties of wild mint have not been fully investigated and adverse reactions are possible.

wild thyme
(Thymus serpyllum; Parts used: aerial parts)

Other common names: **mother of thyme, serpyllum, shepherd's thyme.**

Wild thyme contains flavonoids, caffeic acid derivatives, and a volatile oil rich in carvacrol, and has antimicrobial and spasmolytic activity. It is used for ✪ **catarrh**, especially in the upper respiratory tract, and is approved by some authorities for ✪ **bronchitis** and ✪ **coughs**.

Warnings, interactions, and side effects
Although none have been reported with correct use and dosage, the properties of wild thyme have not been fully investigated and adverse reactions are possible.

wild yam
(Dioscorea villosa)

Other common names: **barbasco, China root, colic root, devil's bones, Mexican yam, rheumatism root, wild yam root, yama.**

Wild yam is a perennial vine with heart-shaped leaves which can grow to a height of approximately 20 feet (6 meters). It produces insignificant green flowers, and grows across northern and Central America, especially in damp wooded areas.

Forms of preparation and parts used

The rhizome with roots is used medicinally, usually taken internally in the form of a decoction or tincture. Relatively recently creams for external use which contain wild yam have also become widely available.

Active components

Wild yam contains a number of steroidal saponins (mainly dioscin), phytosterols, tannins, and alkaloids.

Uses in treatment

Traditionally, wild yam is used for rheumatism (see ✪ **musculoskeletal disorders**). The dioscin content of wild yam gives it anti-inflammatory activity, which may explain the antirheumatic activity of the roots. It is also used for the relief of ✪ **pain**, particularly pain associated with gynecological complaints. In parts of northern and Central America, the roots were used for the pain of ✪ **dysmenorrhea** and childbirth. Yam contains the steroid diosgenin, which is a breakdown product of dioscin, which has been used as a source material in the synthetic manufacture of progestogens and estrogens for incorporation into contraceptive pills and other prescription hormonal medicines. Herbal diosgenin is promoted and widely marketed as a "natural progesterone," but in fact the body is not able to convert it into progesterone, and it has itself no progestogenic effects. It does have some estrogenic activity in laboratory tests. Clinical evidence for the beneficial effects of wild yam creams for defined hormonal complaints has yet to be published.

Warnings, interactions, and side effects

• Wild yam Is not to be used during pregnancy.

• It should not be usd by anyone with breast cancer because of the potential estrogenic effects.

willow

(*Salix species*)
Other common names: **American willow (*Salix nigra*), crack willow (*S. fragilis*), purple willow (*S. purpurea*), violet willow (*S. daphnoides* Villar) white willow (*S. alba*); cartkins willow, catkins willow, European willow, pussywillow, salicin willow, withe withy.**

Willows are deciduous trees or shrubs are found most temperate regions of the Northern Hemisphere. White willow grows up to 80 feet (24 meters) in height, has tapering leaves up to 4 inches (10 centimeters) in length, and produces flowers (catkins) in spring. There are several hundred species of willow tree, with white willow being perhaps the most commonly used medicinally.

Forms of preparation and parts used

Willow bark is used medicinally, either fresh or dried, usually in the form of a tincture or decoction.

Active components

The main active constituents of willow bark are the phenolic glycosides, including salicin, salicortin and salireposide in free and acetylated form, and salicylates. The leaves contain the same spectrum of compounds and also flavonoids, condensed tannins, and catechins.

Uses in treatment

Traditionally, willow was used to staunch internal bleeding, and as a treatment for ✪ **warts**. Its main uses now are for the treatment of ✪ **pain**, such as arthritic pain (see ✪ **arthritis**) and inflammation,

as well as ✪ **colds**, ✪ **influenza** and ✪ **catarrh**. It is approved by some authorities for diseases accompanied by ✪ **fever**, rheumatic ailments (see ✪ **musculoskeletal disorders**) and ✪ **headache**. Although the pharmacological effects of willow bark have not been confirmed clinically, salicylates are known to have anti-inflammatory and antipyretic properties, as well as affecting blood sugar levels. Salicin is converted to salicylic acid during ingestion and absorption from the gut. Pure salicylic acid has been used in medicine as an analgesic and antipyretic, and the synthetic acetyl derivative is ℞ **aspirin** (acetylsalicylic acid).

Warnings, interactions, and side effects

• Salicylate side effects include gastric irritation, hypersensitivity, tinnitus, nausea, and vomiting.

• Willow should not be used during pregnancy (there are some concerns over taking aspirin, which is a derivative of salicylic acid, during pregnancy) or when breast-feeding (as salicylates can be excreted in breast milk, which may result in rashes in babies), or by people who have sensitivity to salicylates.

• It should not be given to children (because of the association of salicylates with ✪ **Reye's syndrome**).

• It should not be used at the same time as ℞ **NSAID**s.

• It should not be used by anyone with a peptic ulcer.

willow herb

(*Epilobium angustifolium*; Parts used: herb and roots)
Other common names: **blood vine, blooming Sally, rose bay willow herb, willow-herb.**

Willow herb contains flavonoids, steroids, and tannins. Traditional uses include for gastrointestinal disorders (✪ **digestive system disorders**), mouth lesions, and prostate complaints. Antiphlogistic, anti-inflammatory, and antimicrobial activities have been reported.

Warnings, interactions, and side effects

Although none have been reported with correct use and dosage, the properties of willow herb have not been fully investigated and adverse reactions are possible.

witch hazel

(*Hamamelis virginiana*)
Other common names: **hazel nut, snapping hazel, spotted alder, striped alder, tobacco wood, winterbloom.**

Witch hazel is a small deciduous tree with broad, toothed leaves, which grows to approximately 15 feet (4.5 meters) in height. The tree produces characteristic yellow flowers in winter, followed by brown fruit capsules.

Forms of preparation and parts used

The bark and leaves of witch hazel are used medicinally, usually as a distilled extract called hamamelis water or witch hazel water, but also dried, or in a liquid extract.

Active components

Witch hazel leaves contain a number of flavonoids and a hydrolysable tannin. The plant also contains a fixed oil and a volatile oil, saponins, and condensed tannins.

Uses in treatment

Witch hazel has astringent, anti-inflammatory, and antihemorrhagic properties. It is traditionally used for ✪ **diarrhea**, ✪ **colitis**,

⊙ **hemorrhoids**, and, externally for ⊙ **bruises**, cuts, and swellings. It is believed that the tannins in witch hazel affect skin proteins, while tannins and flavonoids may affect skin blood vessels, leading to its beneficial effects on damaged or inflamed skin. The astringent actions of the herb are also behind its use for ⊙ **varicose veins**, bruises, and hemorrhoids. Witch hazel is approved by some authorities for hemorrhoids, minor mouth and skin injuries and ⊙ **inflammation** (see also ⊙ **skin conditions**), and the symptoms of ⊙ **venous insufficiency**.

Warnings, interactions, and side effects
• There are no documented toxicological concerns over the use of witch hazel, although excessive ingestion is not recommended because of its high tannin content.
• Some authorities recommend that witch hazel should only be taken under professional supervision.
• Some experts say witch hazel water should not be taken internally.

withania
(*Withania somniferum*; Parts used: whole plant)
Withania contains steroidal lactones and alkaloids, and is often known as the "Indian ginseng." Research has shown central nervous system-depressant and anti-inflammatory activity, as well as increasing hemoglobin levels and speeding recovery from illness. It is used by some to boost resistance to infections.

Warnings, interactions, and side effects
Although none have been reported with correct use and dosage, the properties of withania have not been fully investigated and adverse reactions are possible.

wolfberry, Chinese
(*Lycium chinense*; Parts used: root, berries)
Other common names: **Chinese matrimony vine, di-gu-pi, lycium bark.**
Chinese wolfberry contains plant acids, phytosterols, and vitamins. The fruit have been shown to be hepatoprotective, and the roots to have antipyretic activity. Traditional uses include to improve circulation, lower high blood pressure (see ⊙ **hypertension**), reduce ⊙ **fever**, and for ⊙ **coughs** and wheezing.

Warnings, interactions, and side effects
• Chinese wolfberry should not be used during pregnancy.

wood sage
(*Teucrium scorodonia*; Parts used: herb)
Other common names: **Ambroise, garlic sage, hind heal, large-leaved germander.**
Wood sage contains iridoids, diterpenoids, flavonoids, and a volatile oil rich in alloaromadendrene, and has expectorant and spasmolytic activity. It is used for bronchial ⊙ **catarrh** and ⊙ **inflammation** of the pharyngeal or nasal membranes (see ⊙ **bronchial congestion**).

Warnings, interactions, and side effects
Although none have been reported with correct use and dosage, the properties of wood sage have not been fully investigated and adverse reactions are possible.

yarrow
(*Achillea millefolium*)
Other common names: **bad man's plaything, bloodroot, carpenter's weed, devil's nettle, devil's plaything, knight's milfoil, milfoil, noble yarrow, nosebleed, old man's pepper, sanguinary, soldier's woundwort, staunchweed, thousand seal, thousand weed, yarroway.**
Yarrow is a hardy aromatic perennial herb found across temperate areas in the Northern Hemisphere, native to Europe and parts of Asia, and naturalized across northern America and Australasia. The plant grows to approximately 12 inches (30 centimeters) in height and bears corymbs of small, long-lasting grey/white to pink flowers.

Forms of preparation and parts used
The flowerheads of yarrow are the most commonly used part, usually in the form of a tincture, infusion, or as the dried herb.

Active components
Yarrow contains a wide range of compounds with biological activities, including terpenoids (as an essential oil), flavonoids, tannins, and alkaloids.

Uses in treatment
The herb is said to have diaphoretic, diuretic, and astringent properties, as well as antiseptic activity in the urinary tract. The essential oils and aqueous extracts of yarrow also have anti-inflammatory activity. It is traditionally used for the common ⊙ **cold**, ⊙ **fevers**, ⊙ **diarrhea**, and ⊙ **dysentery**, as well as ⊙ **hypertension** and related thrombotic conditions. It is approved by some authorities for use in the treatment of ⊙ **appetite loss** and ⊙ **indigestion**.

Warnings, interactions, and side effects
• Yarrow should not be used during pregnancy.
• Excessive amounts may interfere with ℞ **anticoagulant** drugs and drugs regulating blood pressure.
• Allergic dermatitis has been reported in some people sensitized to other plants, and yarrow should therefore be avoided by anyone with a known hypersensitivity to other members of the daisy family.
• Large quantities may cause sedation.

yellow dock
(*Rumex crispus*)
Other common names: **curled dock, curly dock, narrow dock, rumax, sad dock, sour dock.**
Yellow dock is a variable, upright perennial with stocky roots and long slender leaves. It produces insignificant yellow-green flowers in summer, followed by small tough fruits.

Forms of preparation and parts used
The root of yellow dock is used medicinally as a decoction or tincture.

Active components
The roots are rich in anthraquinones, including chrysophanol and emodin, and condensed tannins. Aerial parts of the plant also contain oxalic acids and a complex volatile oil.

Uses in treatment
Yellow dock is used to stimulate bile production and as a mild purgative. It has also been used for ⊙ **skin conditions**, ⊙ **jaundice**, and ⊙ **constipation**. The anthraquinone content of the root is responsible for its laxative effects. In small amounts these effects are relatively mild, but larger quantities can lead to strong purgative results.

Warnings, interactions, and side effects

• Yellow dock root should not be used during pregnancy, or by breast-feeding mothers because the anthraquinones can enter the breast milk.

• Overuse of yellow dock, as with many purgatives, can result in abdominal cramps and possible intestinal damage.

• It should not be used by anyone with intestinal obstruction.

• The aerial parts should not be used, because their high oxalic acid content can result in gout and the formation of kidney stones.

• As with other stimulant anthraquinone laxatives (such as ♣ **aloe**, ♣ **rhubarb, Chinese,** ♣ **frangula**, and also ℞ **senna**), long-term use should be avoided.

yellow gentian

(*Gentiana lutea*)

Other common names: **bitter root, gall weed, gentian, gentian root, pale gentian, stemless gentian.**

Yellow gentian is an erect perennial which grows to approximately 4 to 6 feet (1.25 to 1.8 meters) in height. It has oval leaves and star-shaped yellow flowers, which appear in clusters of 3 to 10 flowers during the summer.

Forms of preparation and parts used

The root of yellow gentian is used medicinally, usually in the form of a decoction, infusion, or tincture. It is also available in many herbal blends.

Active components

The roots of yellow gentian contain a number of bitter principles (from which the plant gets one of its common names), including the secoiridoid glycoside gentiopicroside, amarogentin, and swertiamarine. Amarogentin, in particular, is extremely bitter. It also contains pyridine alkaloids, xanthones (including gentisin, gentisein, and isogentisin), tannins, carbohydrates, and triterpenes.

Uses in treatment

Many of the medicinal uses of yellow gentian are based on its bitterness. The bitter compounds in the roots stimulate saliva and gastric secretions, which results in increased appetite, explaining its traditional use for treating ✪ **anorexia nervosa**, and it is approved by some authorities for ✪ **appetite loss**. It is also used for ✪ **indigestion**, ✪ **flatulence**, and gastrointestinal atony (weakness, lack of tone). The alkaloid gentianine which is found in yellow gentian, has also been shown to have anti-inflammatory activity. Absorption of nutrients from the gut is also said to be improved by gentian extracts.

Warnings, interactions, and side effects

• Yellow gentian should not be used during pregnancy or by breast-feeding mothers.

• It should not be used by anyone with a ✪ **peptic ulcer** or acid indigestion.

• Some authorities consider that yellow gentian should not be taken by anyone with ✪ **hypertension**, although there is no conclusive evidence for this warning.

yellow toad flax

(*Linaria vulgaris*; Parts used: herb)

Other common names: **brideweed, butter and eggs, buttered haycocks, calves' snout, churnstaff, devil's head, devil's ribbon,** doggies, dragon-bushes, eggs and bacon, eggs and collops, flaxweed, fluellin, gallwort, larkspur lion's mouth, monkey flower, pattens and clogs, pedlar's basket, pennywort, rabbits, ramstead, snapdragon, toadpipe, yellow rod.

Yellow toad flax contains iridoids, flavonoids, and quinolizidine alkaloids. Traditional uses include internally to aid digestion (see ✪ **digestive system disorders**) and the herb has diaphoretic and diuretic actions. Its reported anti-inflammatory activity may explain its external use for ✪ **rashes** and ✪ **hemorrhoids**.

Warnings, interactions, and side effects

Although none have been reported with correct use and dosage, the properties of yellow toad flax have not been fully investigated and adverse reactions are possible.

yellow willowherb

(*Lysimachia vulgaris*; Parts used: herb)

Other common names: **loosestrife.**

Yellow willowherb is rich in flavonoids, especially rutin, and has been shown to have astringent activity. Traditional uses include for ✪ **diarrhea**, hemorrhages (for example, ✪ **nosebleed**), and to treat the symptoms of ✪ **dysentery**.

Warnings, interactions, and side effects

Although none have been reported with correct use and dosage, the properties of yellow willowherb have not been fully investigated and adverse reactions are possible.

yucca

(*Yucca brevifolia*; Parts used: whole plant)

Yucca contains numerous terpenoids, and yucca extracts containing saponins have been shown to reduce arthritic symptoms, high blood pressure, and cholesterol levels, and also have a beneficial effect on the circulation of the blood. Traditional uses include for ✪ **diabetes mellitus**, stomach complaints (see ✪ **digestive system disorders**), and ✪ **arthritis**.

Warnings, interactions, and side effects

Although none have been reported with correct use and dosage, the properties of yucca have not been fully investigated and adverse reactions are possible.

zedoary

(*Curcuma zedoaria*; Parts used: rhizome)

Other common names: **turmeric.**

Zedoary contains curcuminoids and a volatile oil rich in zingiberine. Traditional uses include for ✪ **indigestion** because it has carminative and stomachic activity. Its chemical similarities with ♣ **ginger** may partly explain these traditional uses, although there is no scientific evidence to support these claims.

Warnings, interactions, and side effects

• Zedoary is not be used during pregnancy.

PART 4

VITAMINS, MINERALS, AND SUPPLEMENTS

Vitamins, Minerals, and Supplements

Anyone entering a drugstore, healthfood store, or supermarket today is aware that there is now considerable interest and an ever-growing market in dietary supplements and increasing numbers of people are using them. In the US, sales of vitamins and minerals alone are about $7 billion a year.

Why is this so? In many ways supplementation should be unnecessary—a well-balanced diet should be all that is required to maintain good health. However, in our modern Western society with its hectic and often stressful lifestyle, where perhaps cigarette smoking, excess alcohol, lack of exercise, and fast-food feature more than they should in our daily lives, we all are becoming increasingly concerned about the foods we eat, and whether we are obtaining all the vital nutrients we require. Modern food production methods, with their use of chemical fertilizers and pesticides along with extensive processing and prepackaging of foods, leads us to question whether we still can rely on a well-balanced diet alone to maintain optimal health. In fact, emerging scientific evidence strongly suggests that certain dietary supplements can reduce the risk or progression of some diseases, including cancer.

Today, the average person is taking more and more personal responsibility for his or her own health and more people than ever before are using alternative and natural self-help approaches to maintaining optimal health and vitality. Dietary supplements certainly have an important role in this approach to personal health and well-being.

What is a dietary supplement?

The Food and Drug Administration (FDA) regulates dietary supplements according to the Dietary Supplement Health and Education Act (DSHEA), 1994. This Act defines a dietary supplement as follows.

"A product (other than tobacco) that is intended to supplement the diet which bears or contains one or more of the following dietary ingredients: a vitamin, a mineral, a herb or other botanical, an amino acid, a dietary substance for use by man to supplement the diet by increasing the total daily intake, or a concentrate, metabolite, constituent, extract or combinations of these ingredients. It is intended for ingestion in pill, capsule, tablet or liquid form, is not presented for use as a conventional food or as the sole item of a meal or diet and is labeled as a dietary supplement."

Under this law, supplements are regulated in a similar manner to food products, and they cannot be marketed as medicines or food additives. This Act includes a framework for safety, guidelines for literature provided at the point of sale, guidance on good manufacturing practice, and claims and labeling standards. Under DSHEA, manufacturers are responsible for marketing safe and properly labeled products, but the FDA bears the burden of proving that a product is unsafe or improperly labelled. However, it is clear that the FDA has insufficient resources for doing this, and there is concern that not all supplements in the US are marketed according to best standards of practice.

Moreover, while there is a great deal of information about these substances—increasingly so on the Internet—not all of it is reliable. Indeed, there are probably few areas associated with health care where such confusion exists. Even nutrition experts disagree about them, with some saying they are largely unnecessary because a balanced diet provides all the required vitamins and minerals, others saying that supplements make a worthwhile contribution to a healthy diet, and, increasingly, some experts say that optimal health cannot easily be achieved without them.

Uses of dietary supplements

When the biological effects of vitamins were first discovered during the early years of the 20th century, they were only used for preventing and treating deficiency disease such as scurvy (vitamin C deficiency), beriberi (thiamin deficiency), pellagra (niacin deficiency), and so on. This concept of preventing deficiency led to the development of Recommended Dietary Allowances (RDAs). These values were based on amounts of nutrients required to prevent deficiency, and even though limited in many ways, they are still the best measure we have of how adequately a person is eating.

In the second half of the 20th century, nutritional deficiencies were thought to have disappeared and scientists largely lost interest in vitamins and minerals. But when conditions such as cardiovascular disease and cancer started to increase, vitamins and other agents again became an area of interest, and it was suggested that supplements might help to reduce the risk of such conditions. Now people want not only to reduce disease risk, but also to improve quality of life and supplements are increasingly used to promote so-called optimum health.

What evidence is there that these products work? Until the early 1990s, there were relatively few well-conducted trials involving vitamins and minerals, and fewer still on substances such as garlic, fish oils, and so on. Evidence was largely limited to anecdotal reports and single case studies or poorly conducted intervention trials. The argument often used to be made that controlled trials could not be conducted with supplements, because they often contain a range of natural ingredients whose effects are difficult to separate. However, such arguments are often misguided, and an increasing body of evidence is now emerging from well controlled trials. Some of these suggest that some supplements (for example, folic acid, or fish oils) are effective in some groups of the population in certain circumstances. However, for other supplements (for example, royal jelly) promoted by the media as wonder cures or cure-alls, the rationale behind the use of the supplement is very often at best dubious and there is often very little sound evidence of specific health benefit.

Who needs supplements?

We all basically need the same vitamins, minerals and other nutrients for good health, and these in principle can be obtained from a well-balanced diet alone. However, various groups of the population could be at risk of nutrient deficiency and could benefit from supplementation.

These include:

- Infants and children, adolescents, women during pregnancy and breast-feeding and throughout the reproductive period (whether pregnant or not), the elderly.
- People whose nutritional status may be compromised by lifestyle (enforced or voluntary), for example, smokers, alcoholics, drug addicts, certain religions, dieters, strict vegetarians and vegans, food faddists, individuals on low incomes, and athletes.
- People whose nutritional status may be compromised by surgery and/or disease, for example, malabsorption syndromes, hepatobiliary disorders, severe burns or wounds, and inborn errors of metabolism such as lactose intolerance.
- People whose nutritional status may be compromised by long-term drug administration (for example, anticonvulsants may increase the requirement for vitamin D).

Increasingly, people are taking supplements for reasons other than prevention of deficiency and at amounts higher than the RDA. Moreover, evidence is increasing that, at least for some nutrients (for example, folic acid, vitamin E), there may be benefits in achieving higher intakes than the RDA. For example, there is evidence that supplementation with fish oils can reduce the risk of some cardiovascular diseases.

A note of caution

While there is agreement about the beneficial effects of nutrients in the prevention of deficiency disease and the amounts required to achieve such effects, there is controversy about amounts required for reduction in risk of chronic disease and so-called "optimum health." Higher levels of intake cannot always easily be obtained from diet alone, and supplementation is required. However, excessive intake of some nutrients, especially in susceptible people, can lead to toxicity (for instance, vitamin A supplements may cause birth defects if taken in high doses during pregnancy) and it is with this in mind that several committees world-wide are planning to establish safe upper limits for supplement intake. Always consult your health care professional or nutrition expert if in doubt.

In addition, there is a growing number of supplements that are not officially recognized vitamins or minerals, but are related substances (for example, glucosamine, shark cartilage) proposed to have benefits for health. The scientific status of these is not established, and one should be wary of claims about wonder supplements, which are more likely to be a new fashion than to have proven efficacy.

Guidance on choosing supplements

The following may help you decide on the supplements you choose.

- Who is the supplement for? Requirements for vitamins and minerals vary according to age and sex.
- Why do you think you need a supplement?
- What are your symptoms (if any) and how long have you had them? Remember that you could have a condition that should be referred for appropriate diagnosis and treatment.
- Is your diet restricted in any way? Dieting, vegetarianism or veganism, or some religious lifestyles, could increase the risk of nutritional deficiency.
- Do you suffer from any chronic illness, for example, diabetes mellitus, epilepsy, Crohn's disease? Nutrient requirements in patients with chronic disease may be greater than in healthy individuals.
- Are you pregnant or breast-feeding? Nutrient requirements may be increased, but excess could be dangerous (for instance, in the case of vitamin A).
- Do you take part in sports or other regular physical activity?
- Do you take any prescription or over-the-counter medicines or alternative or herbal medicines? This information can be used to assess possible drug-nutrient interactions.
- Do you take other supplements? If so, which ones? This information can be used to assess

potential overdosage of supplements which could be toxic.

- Do you smoke? Requirements for some vitamins (for example, vitamin C) may be increased.
- How much alcohol do you drink? Excessive alcohol consumption may lead to deficiency of the B vitamins.
- Do not be tempted by packaging—some great product names may contain not-so-great ingredients.

Guidelines for supplement use

The following guidelines may be useful in making choices.

- Compare labels with dietary standards (usually RDAs).
- In the absence of an indication for a specific nutrient, for general maintenance of health a balanced multivitamin/mineral product is normally preferable to one which contains one or two individual nutrients.
- Use a product that provides approximately 100% of the RDA for as wide a range of vitamins and minerals as possible.
- Avoid preparations containing unrecognized nutrients or nutrients in minute amounts; this increases the cost, but not the value.
- Avoid preparations which claim to be natural or organic. Extracting from foods is hardly natural, and chemical solvents may well be used to do the extracting. These are often more expensive.
- Avoid preparations which are high potency (mega doses). More is not always better and the risk of toxicity is greater.
- Try to be objective in distinguishing between credible claims and unsubstantiated claims—consult further reputable texts and, if in doubt, obtain advice from your qualified healthcare professional, nutritionist or dietician.
- Store your supplement away from sunlight and heat.
- Obtain advice from your qualified healthcare professional, nutritionist or dietician about when and how to take your supplement (for example, before, with or after food). Be

particularly careful to obtain clear advice about taking your supplement at the same time as any medication your are taking (for example, avoid taking antacid with an iron supplement). If in any doubt, do not take any supplement at the same time as any medication.

- If you have an allergic reaction, discontinue the supplement immediately.

Dr. Pamela Mason, BSc PhD MRPharmS

Editor's note

This section covers the most commonly available dietary supplements, including vitamins, minerals, trace elements and other substances, such as garlic and fish oils (omega-3 fatty acids). For ease of reference, they are arranged in alphabetical order and give information, starting with a general description of the supplement and where it occurs naturally (for example, food source) where appropriate, under the following headings:

- **Action:** Information about what the supplement does and how it works.
- **Deficiency:** An indication of symptoms of deficiency, and who is at risk.
- **Possible uses:** Information about how the supplement could be used.
- **Warnings:** A list of circumstances when the supplement should be avoided and/or when you should seek a doctor's advice.
- **Interactions:** This heading identifies medication with which the supplement could interact, possibly leading to either a reduction or an increase in the therapeutic effect of the drug or the supplement.
- **Side effects:** Lists likely side-effects (adverse effects) and symptoms of toxicity.

In certain cases information will also be given about the chemical forms available, because supplements can often be manufactured containing alternative chemical forms that may have various advantages. It is also important to note that some formulations contain only one active constituent but others are manufactured with other supplements—the latter are called multivitamin and multisupplement preparations.

Supplements are sold in different formulations (for example, tablets, capsules, liquid), and sometimes these are in modified-release form (for example, sustained-release, which is good way of taking water-soluble vitamins). Requirements are also given here, usually in terms of the Recommended Dietary Allowance (RDA).

The values have been selected by the writer to be the most relevant and useful figures to provide in a book of this nature and scope. In some cases the RDA has been given, in others the tolerable Upper Intake Level (UIL), while certain substances (such as shark cartilage) have no recommended amounts (as yet). Retail outlets and web sites commonly quote vitamin requirements in terms of RDAs and the percentage of daily RDA value contained in a given dose of the product.

However, research into suitable standards continues, and also other values that may be encountered on food and nutrient packaging and labeling include: RDIs (Reference Daily Intakes); RDVs (Daily Reference Values); US RDAs; RNIs (Recommended Nutrient Intakes in Canada); and DVs (Daily Values). New and differing figures are constantly being produced in this somewhat contentious area and are updated on a regular basis by various authorities (for example, WHO, Food and Drug Administration, National Academy of Sciences/National Research Council).

The above standards are mainly set with regard to amounts or vitamins and other substances required in the diet for the maintainance of normal good health, and originate from research into doses required to prevent the appearance of deficiency disorders. However, it should be noted that there are many advocates of the use of vitamins and other supplements for other ("pharmacological") purposes. For example, in the case of vitamin C used for maintainance of normal nutritional health, the RDA for nonsmoking adults is 60 mg/day, but for advocates of its use to prevent cancer or to treat the common cold, doses up to 2,000 mg/day may be recommended. For recommendations regarding the safe use of vitamins, minerals, and supplements in their various proposed uses above those required for a healthy diet, manufacturers' guidelines on amounts should always be followed.

RDAs are currently being revised and replaced by a range of values, such as Adequate Intakes (AIs) or estimated safe intakes. RDAs and AIs are set at levels intended to minimize the risk of developing deficiency. Tolerable Upper Intake Levels (UIL) are the highest total level of a nutrient (combining intake for the diet and from supplements) which could be consumed safely on a daily basis, without risking adverse health effects. As intakes rise above the UIL, the risk of adverse effects increases. The UIL refers to long-term intakes, so an isolated dose above the UIL need not necessarily cause adverse effects. The UIL defines safety limits and is not a recommended intake for most people most of the time. However individual requirements will vary with factors including age, sex, lifestyle, and state of health, so no general formula will work for all people.

The final word in taking any preparations must be that your health is your own responsibility. There may be any number of valid reasons for taking dietary supplements, but doing so is a lifestyle decision and should be combined with healthy eating and exercise. Before taking any supplement, check with your healthcare professional or nutrition expert regarding its appropriateness in your own particular individual circumstances.

The list on the following pages shows vitamins, minerals and supplements that may be named in manufacturers' preparations, even though these names are not featured in this section. In each case, the supplements listed are either included within one of the featured articles, or are simply alternative names for one of these, and a reference is made to the featured article.

alanine see AMINO ACID.

allicin see GARLIC.

Allium sativum see GARLIC.

alpha-carotene see CAROTENOID.

alpha-linolenic acid see OMEGA-3 FATTY ACID.

alpha-tocopherol see VITAMIN E.

ammonium molybdate see MOLYBDENUM.

anti-infection vitamin see VITAMIN A.

arginine see AMINO ACID.

ascorbyl palmitate see VITAMIN C.

asparagine see AMINO ACID.

aspartic acid see AMINO ACID.

bee pollen/bee products see ROYAL JELLY AND BEE PRODUCTS.

beta-carotene see CAROTENOID; VITAMIN A.

bioflavonoid see ISOFLAVONE.

blackcurrant oil see GAMMA-LINOLENIC ACID (GLA).

blue green algae see SPIRULINA AND OTHER ALGAE.

bone meal see CALCIUM.

borage oil see GAMMA-LINOLENIC ACID (GLA).

boric acid see BORON.

bovine brain PS see PHOSPHATIDYLSERINE.

Brewer's yeast see BREWER'S YEAST.

calciferol see VITAMIN D.

calcium ascorbate see VITAMIN C.

calcium aspartate see CALCIUM.

calcium citrate see CALCIUM.

calcium folate see FOLIC ACID.

calcium glubionate see CALCIUM.

calcium glutonate see CALCIUM.

calcium lactate see CALCIUM.

calcium molybdate see MOLYBDENUM.

calcium pantothenate see PANTOTHENIC ACID.

calcium phosphate (tribasic calcium phosphate) see CALCIUM.

carbonyl iron heme iron see IRON.

carnitine see AMINO ACID.

carotinoid see CAROTENOID.

chelated ferrous fumarate see IRON.

chlorella see SPIRULINA AND OTHER ALGAE.

cholecalciferol see VITAMIN D.

choline see LECITHIN.

choline bitartrate see LECITHIN.

choline dihydrogen citrate see LECITHIN.

chondroitin see GLUCOSAMINE; SHARK CARTILAGE.

chromium chloride see CHROMIUM.

chromium dinicotinate see CHROMIUM.

chromium glycinate see CHROMIUM.

chromium picolinate see CHROMIUM.

chromium polynicotinate see CHROMIUM.

chromium trichloride see CHROMIUM.

CLA see CONJUGATED LINOLEIC ACID.

cobalamin see VITAMIN B.

copper citrate see COPPER.

copper gluconate see COPPER.

copper sulfate see COPPER.

Co-Q$_{10}$ see COENZYME Q.

creatine see AMINO ACID.

cryptoxanthin see CAROTENOID.

cupric chloride see COPPER.

cyanocobalamin see VITAMIN B$_{12}$.

cysteine see AMINO ACID.

daidzein see ISOFLAVONE.

dehydroepiandrosterone see DHEA.

dexpanthenol see PANTOTHENIC ACID.

DHA see OMEGA-3 FATTY ACID.

dl-alpha-tocopherol see VITAMIN E.

docosahexaenoic acid see OMEGA-3 FATTY ACID.

eicosapentaenoic acid see OMEGA-3 FATTY ACID.

EPA see OMEGA-3 FATTY ACID.

esterfied vitamin C see VITAMIN C.

evening primrose oil see GAMMA-LINOLENIC ACID (GLA).

ferrous glycinate see IRON.

fish oil supplement see OMEGA-3 FATTY ACID.

flavonoid see ISOFLAVONE.

flaxseed oil see OMEGA-3 FATTY ACID.

folacin see FOLIC ACID.

folate see FOLIC ACID.

folate triglutamate see FOLIC ACID.

gammalinolenic acid see GAMMA-LINOLENIC ACID (GLA).

gamolenic acid see GAMMA-LINOLENIC ACID (GLA).

genistein see ISOFLAVONE.

ginko bilobo see GINKGO.

ginseng see GINSENG.

GLA see GAMMA-LINOLENIC ACID (GLA).

glucosamine sulfates see GLUCOSAMINE.

glutamic acid see AMINO ACID.

glutamine see AMINO ACID.

glutathione see ANTIOXIDANT.

glutathione peroxidase see ANTIOXIDANT.

glycine see AMINO ACID.

glycitein see ISOFLAVONE.

histidine see AMINO ACID.

hydroxycobalamin see VITAMIN B.

inositol hexaniacinate see NIACIN.

iodate salts see IODINE.

iodide see IODINE.

iron fumarate see IRON.

iron gluconate see IRON.

iron glycinate see IRON.

iron sulfate see IRON.

isoleucine see AMINO ACID.

kelp see SPIRULINA AND OTHER ALGAE.

koagulation vitamin see VITAMIN K.

Lactobacillus acidophilus see ACIDOPHILUS.

l-alpha-tocopherol see VITAMIN E.

l-carnitine see LEVOCARNITINE.

leucine see AMINO ACID.

α-linolenic acid see GAMMA-LINOLENIC ACID (GLA).

lipoic acid see ALPHA-LIPOIC ACID.

lutein see CAROTENOID.

lycopene see CAROTENOID.

lysine see AMINO ACID.
magnesium aspartate see MAGNESIUM.
magnesium citrate see MAGNESIUM.
magnesium maleate see MAGNESIUM.
magnesium orotate see MAGNESIUM.
magnesium oxide see MAGNESIUM.
manganese citrate see MANGANESE.
manganese gluconate see MANGANESE.
manganese sulfate see MANGANESE.
menadione see VITAMIN K.
menaquinone see VITAMIN K.
methionyl adenylate see S-ADENOSYLMETHIONINE.
molybdenum trioxide see MOLYBDENUM.
NAC see N-ACETYLCYSTEINE.
N-acetyl-5-methoxytryptamine see MELATONIN.
N-acetylglucosamine see GLUCOSAMINE.
natural chlorella see SPIRULINA AND OTHER ALGAE.
natural spirulina see SPIRULINA AND OTHER ALGAE.
octacosyl alcohol see OCTACOSANOL.
omega-3 see OMEGA-3 FATTY ACID.
omega-3 marine triglyceride see OMEGA-3 FATTY ACID.
omega-6 fatty acid see OMEGA-3 FATTY ACID.
1-octacosanol see OCTACOSANOL.
pantethine see PANTOTHENIC ACID.
panthenol see PANTOTHENIC ACID.
panthoderm see PANTOTHENIC ACID.
pantothenyl alcohol see PANTOTHENIC ACID.
phenylalanine see AMINO ACID.
phosphatidylcholine see LECITHIN.
phylloquinone see VITAMIN K.
phytoestrogen see ISOFLAVONE.
phytomenadione see VITAMIN K.
policosanol see OCTACOSANOL.
polycosanol see OCTACOSANOL.
potassium amino acid chelate see POTASSIUM.
potassium ascorbate see POTASSIUM; VITAMIN C.
potassium aspartate see POTASSIUM.
potassium bicarbonate see POTASSIUM.
potassium chloride see POTASSIUM.
potassium citrate see CITRATES.
potassium gluconate see POTASSIUM.
potassium orotate see POTASSIUM.
prasterone see DHEA.
primrose oil see GAMMA-LINOLENIC ACID (GLA).
proline see AMINO ACID.
propolis see ROYAL JELLY AND BEE PRODUCTS.
PS see PHOSPHATIDYLSERINE.
pteroylglutamic acid see FOLIC ACID.
pyridoxal see VITAMIN B.
pyridoxal-5-phosphate see VITAMIN B.
pyridoxamine see VITAMIN B.
pyridoxine see VITAMIN B.
pyridoxine hydrochloride see VITAMIN B.
Q_{10} see COENZYME Q.
quercetin see ANTIOXIDANT.

retinol see VITAMIN A.
retinyl palmitate see VITAMIN A.
riboflavin see VITAMIN B.
rutin see ANTIOXIDANT.
S-adenosyl-L-methionine see S-ADENOSYLMETHIONINE.
SAM see S-ADENOSYLMETHIONINE.
SAMe see S-ADENOSYLMETHIONINE.
SAM-e see S-ADENOSYLMETHIONINE.
selenocysteine see SELENIUM.
selenocystine see SELENIUM.
selenomethionine see SELENIUM.
serine see ANTIOXIDANT.
SOD see ANTIOXIDANT.
sodium ascorbate see VITAMIN C.
sodium borate see BORON.
sodium folate see FOLIC ACID.
sodium molybdate see MOLYBDENUM.
sodium selenate see SELENIUM.
sodium selenite see SELENIUM.
soya isoflavone see ISOFLAVONE.
soybean PS see PHOSPHATIDYLSERINE.
sun vitamin see VITAMIN D.
superoxide dismutase see ANTIOXIDANT.
taurine see AMINO ACID.
thiamin see VITAMIN B.
thiamine see VITAMIN B.
thiamine hydrochloride see VITAMIN B.
thiamine mononitrate see VITAMIN B.
thioctic acid see ALPHA-LIPOIC ACID.
thiomolybdate salts see MOLYBDENUM.
threonine see AMINO ACID.
tocopherols/tocopherol acetate/tocopherol succinate
  see VITAMIN E.
tocotrienols see VITAMIN E.
tryptophan see AMINO ACID.
2,3-dimethoxy-5-methylbenzoquinone see COENZYME Q.
2-amino-2-deoxyglucose see GLUCOSAMINE.
tyrosine see AMINO ACID.
ubiquinone see AMINO ACID.
valine see AMINO ACID.
vitamin A see VITAMIN A.
vitamin B_3 see NIACIN.
vitamin B_5 see PANTOTHENIC ACID.
vitamin B_7 see BIOTIN.
vitamin B_9 see FOLIC ACID.
vitamin D_2 /D_3 see VITAMIN D.
vitamin K_1/K_2 /K_3 see VITAMIN K.
zeaxanthin see CAROTENOID.
zinc acetate see ZINC.
zinc amino acid chelate see ZINC.
zinc aspartate see ZINC.
zinc citrate see ZINC.
zinc gluconate see ZINC.
zinc l-methionine see ZINC.
zinc picolinate see ZINC.

acidophilus

(*Lactobacillus acidophilus; L. acidophilus*)
Acidophilus is one of over 500 species of bacteria found in the digestive tract. It is known as a probiotic when used as a supplement, which means that it helps to provide a healthy balance of bacteria in the intestine. It is found in yogurt, kefir (a sour, slightly alcoholic brew of fermented cow's milk), and acidophilus milk.

Formulations

It is available as capsules, softgel capsules, and tablets.

Action

Acidophilus acts as a barrier against infection by helping to increase the proportion of healthy bacteria in the digestive tract and vagina. It achieves this by producing natural antibiotics which kill potentially harmful bacteria. Acidophilus also produces a wide range of B-vitamins and ⚗ **vitamin K** in the intestine.

Possible uses

Acidophilus may help to:
• Prevent and treat vaginal yeast infections caused by Candida albicans (such as ✪ **candidiasis**);
• Restore a healthy balance of bacteria in people taking ℞ **antibiotics**, and help to prevent ✪ **superinfections**;
• Alleviate symptoms of ✪ **lactose intolerance**, such as diarrhea and stomach cramps;
• Alleviate symptoms of bowel conditions, such as ✪ **irritable bowel syndrome**;
• Lower blood cholesterol in ✪ **hyperlipidemia** and to help prevent ✪ **atherosclerosis**.

Warnings

None.

Interactions

None.

Side effects

No known side effects.

alpha-lipoic acid

(also known as *lipoic acid; thioctic acid*)
Alpha-lipoic acid is a vitamin-like compound. It is classified as non-essential because it is produced in the body in small amounts. However, it is also present in foods, such as brewer's yeast, liver, and spinach and other greens.

Formulations

As a supplement it is available as capsules, softgel capsules, and tablets.

Action

Alpha-lipoic acid works with enzymes, together with the B vitamins, throughout the body to help in the production of energy. It is also an ⚗ **antioxidant**, and it works with ⚗ **vitamins C** and ⚗ **E** as a free radical scavenger.

Possible uses

Alpha-lipoic acid may help to:
• Improve the symptoms of nerve damage (for example, numbness and tingling) in people with ✪ **diabetes mellitus** (diabetic neuropathy);
• Protect against cataracts;
• Protect against ✪ **stroke**;
• Preserve memory in people with ✪ **Alzheimer's disease**;
• Protect against some ✪ **viral infections**.

Warnings

• Diabetics must consult a qualified medical professional before taking alpha-lipoic acid because it may reduce blood sugar levels, which therefore must be monitored.

Interactions

None known.

Side effects

No serious side effects. There have been occasional reports of skin rashes and stomach upsets.

amino acid

Amino acids are derived from protein in food, from supplements, or are synthesized by the body. The body breaks down dietary protein to its constituent amino acids. There are two types of amino acids: essential, for example, histidine, isoleucine, leucine, lysine, methionine, phenylalanine, threonine, tryptophan, and valine, which must be obtained from food; and non-essential, for example, alanine, arginine, asparagine, aspartic acid, cysteine, glutamic acid, glutamine, glycine, proline, serine, taurine, and tyrosine, which are just as important but are called non-essential because they can be made in the body.

Formulations

As supplements amino acids are available as oral liquid, powder, and capsules. The natural form of each amino acid is the l-form (sometimes written L-form). The dl-form is sometimes available but generally will only be half (or even less) as effective (the d-form may compete for absorption).

Action

Amino acids are needed to repair and maintain all the body's cells and tissues, including the hair, nails, muscles, tendons, ligaments, organs, and glands, because protein molecules consist of chains of amino acids. They are also required for the manufacture of enzymes (which trigger chemical reactions in the body), neurotransmitters (chemicals that carry messages in the nervous system and brain), and hormones (for example, insulin).

Possible uses

Most of these supplemental amino acids are used in sports and athletics because they are promoted as helping to build muscle, increase stamina, and improve the immune system.
In addition:
• Arginine may help to protect against ✪ **heart disease** by lowering blood cholesterol (see ✪ **hyperlipidemia**), reduce the risk of ✪ **atherosclerosis**, widening blood vessels, and reducing blood pressure. It may help to relieve the pain of ✪ **angina pectoris**;
• Carnitine may help to reduce blood cholesterol and triglyceride levels and help those with congestive ✪ **heart failure**;
• Glutamine may be helpful as additional therapy in ✪ **AIDS** and cancer;
• Lysine may be helpful against the ✪ **herpes** virus and for angina;
• Phenylalanine may be helpful in ✪ **depression**;
• Taurine may be helpful in congestive heart failure;

• Tyrosine may be helpful in ✪ **Alzheimer's disease** and depression.

Warnings

• Amino acids should not to be taken by people with any kind of medical condition without a doctor's advice.

• People with phenylketonuria (PKU) should not take phenylalanine.

Interactions

• Tyrosine (or tyramine) should not be used by anyone who is taking a ℞ **monoamine-oxidase inhibitor** (MAOI) antidepressant.

Side effects

There are no known serious side effects. However, the effects of taking amino acid supplements long term are unknown. Never exceed recommended doses.

antioxidant

Antioxidants are substances which protect against free radicals and help to prevent damage to body cells, proteins, and the genetic material of cells. The main antioxidants are ⚗ **vitamin C**, ⚗ **vitamin E**, the ⚗ **carotenoids** (for example, beta-carotene, lutein, lycopene), flavonoids (for example, rutin, quercetin), ⚗ **coenzyme Q₁₀**, ⚗ **copper**, ⚗ **manganese**, ⚗ **selenium**, ⚗ **zinc**, and various enzymes, such as superoxide dismutase and glutathione peroxidase.

Action

Antioxidants are thought to prevent free radical damage and protect the tissues against oxidative stress (when a lot of free radicals are being generated). Free radical damage appears to be involved in the development of many diseases, such as heart disease, cancer, cataracts, ✪ **Parkinson's disease**, ✪ **arthritis**, and inflammatory bowel disorders.

Possible uses

Various antioxidants are available as dietary supplements. These include vitamins C, E, beta-carotene, lutein, lycopene, quercetin, selenium, coenzyme Q₁₀, and superoxide dismutase. Most of these supplements are promoted for the prevention of various diseases and conditions such as cardiovascular disease, cancer, and cataracts.

For example:

• Vitamins E and C may help to protect against ✪ **heart disease**;

• Selenium may help to protect against some ✪ **cancers**;

• Carotenoids (for example, beta-carotene, lutein, lycopene) may help to protect against cataracts;

• Lycopene may help to protect against ✪ **prostate cancer**;

• Coenzyme Q₁₀ may help to protect against heart disease.

Warnings

• People who smoke should seek a doctor's advice before taking beta-carotene (smoking decreases absorption but high levels of beta-carotene may increase the risk of lung cancer).

Interactions

See individual entries for ⚗ **vitamin C**, ⚗ **vitamin E**, ⚗ **selenium**, ⚗ **carotenoids**, and ⚗ **coenzyme Q₁₀**.

Side effects

See individual entries.

biotin

(also known as *vitamin B₇*)

Biotin is a water-soluble B-vitamin. Good food sources include liver, kidney, egg yolks, milk, brewer's yeast, whole grains, nuts, and legumes.

Formulations

As a supplement it is available as tablets, capsules, shampoo, and skin gel.

• The recommended Adequate Intake (AI) is 30 mcg/day for adults.

Action

Biotin is involved in the release of energy from food. It maintains the health of the skin, hair, nails, nerves, sweat glands, and bone marrow.

Deficiency

Deficiency of biotin is virtually unknown.

Possible uses

It is a common ingredient in multivitamin supplements, however, there is no known need for biotin supplements on their own. It can be used as a shampoo to help treat cradle cap (see ✪ **skin conditions**) in babies.

Warnings

None.

Interactions

• Long-term use of some ℞ **antibiotics** or ℞ **anticonvulsants** could lead to low levels of biotin.

• Excessive eating of raw egg whites may cause a deficiency.

Side effects

None, even at high doses, because the body is efficient at excreting the vitamin in the urine.

boron

Boron is a trace mineral. Good food sources include fruit, vegetables and nuts; however, meat, fish, and poultry contain very little. Beer, wine, and cider contain significant amounts.

Formulations

As a supplement boron is available as tablets (sometimes with ⚗ **vitamin D**) as sodium borate or boric acid.

• It has not been proved that boron is an essential mineral for humans and so daily requirements have not been set.

Action

Boron appears to be important for normal calcium and bone metabolism. It also influences the metabolism of ⚗ **copper**, ⚗ **magnesium**, and vitamin D, and helps to regulate the production of various hormones, such as estrogens and testosterone.

Possible uses

Boron may help to:

• Reduce calcium loss in postmenopausal women and so help to protect against ✪ **osteoporosis**;

• Alleviate the symptoms of ✪ **arthritis**.

Warnings

None.

Interactions

None.

Key to symbols: ✪ = Disorder Section ℞ = Drug Section ♣ = Herbal Section ⚗ = Supplement Section

Side effects

None, unless excessively high doses (over 100 mg/day) are taken. Supplements generally provide about 3 mg in a daily dose.

calcium

Calcium is the most abundant mineral in the body, where it is found mainly in the bones and teeth. Good food sources include milk, yogurt, cheese and dairy products, tempeh, tofu, fish with small bones (for example, sardines, salmon), turnip greens, collard, broccoli, and kale.

Formulations

As a supplement calcium is available as tablets or a syrup (sometimes with ♋ **vitamin D**) in a variety of forms: inorganic forms— calcium carbonate, calcium phosphate (tribasic calcium phosphate), dolomite; organic forms—calcium aspartate, calcium citrate, calcium glubionate (syrup), calcium glutonate, calcium lactate, bone meal, oyster-shell calcium.

• The Adequate Intake (AI) for calcium for young adults (9-18 years) is 1,300 mg/day; adults (19-50 years), 1,000 mg/day; adults over 50, 1,200 mg/day. The Tolerable Upper Intake Level (UL) for adults is 2,500 mg/day.

Action

Calcium is essential to the formation and structure of bones and teeth. It is involved in blood clotting, transmission of messages in the nervous system, and muscle contraction.

Deficiency

Severe calcium deficiency is rare. Inadequate intakes may increase the risk of ✪ osteoporosis in later life.

Possible uses

Calcium supplements may be help to:
• Protect against ✪ **osteoporosis**;
• Reduce blood pressure (but only to a very small extent) in ✪ **hypertension**;
• Treat ✪ **hypocalcemia** and ✪ **hypoparathyroidism**;
• Alleviate the symptoms of ✪ **premenstrual syndrome** (PMS);
• Protect against colon ✪ **cancer**.
• Supplements may also be helpful during childhood and adolescence, pregnancy and breast-feeding, and in people who do not eat dairy products, for example, vegans or patients with ✪ **lactose intolerance**.

Warnings

Calcium supplements should not be used by people who suffer from:
• Hypercalcemia (high levels of calcium in the blood);
• Hypercalciuria (high levels of calcium in the urine);
• Kidney stones;
• ✪ **hyperthyroidism** (overactive thyroid gland).

Interactions

• Calcium may interfere with the absorption, and thus reduce the therapeutic effect, of drugs such as ℞ **tetracycline** ℞ **antibiotics** (for example, ℞ **oxytetracycline**), ℞ **4-quinolone** ℞ **antibacterials** (for example, ℞ **ciprofloxacin**), and ℞ **bisphosphonates** (for example, ℞ **etidronate disodium**), which are used to treat ✪ **osteoporosis**, so people on any medication (prescribed or OTC) should consult their doctor before taking calcium.

Side effects

Toxic effects are unlikely with doses below the Tolerable Upper Intake Level of 2,500 mg/day (adults). Occasionally, some calcium salts may cause nausea, constipation, and flatulence.

carotenoid

Carotenoids are the natural pigments found in plants, including fruit and vegetables, which give them their bright color. About 600 carotenoids have been found in nature. The ones most commonly found in supplements include alpha-carotene, beta-carotene, cryptoxanthin, lutein, lycopene, and zeaxanthin.

Alpha-carotene and beta-carotene are found in carrots, peppers, and green, leafy vegetables. Lutein is found in green, leafy vegetables, and pumpkin. Lycopene is found in red fruits, such as tomatoes, red grapefruit, and watermelon. Cryptoxanthin is found in mangoes and peaches, while zeaxanthin is found in green vegetables, red peppers and yellow corn. Unlike the other main group of plants pigments, the ♋ **flavonoid** group, most carotenoids are fat-rather than water-soluble, and give the color to some foods products, for example, the yellow color to butter.

Formulations

As supplements carotenoids are available as capsules or tablets in the form of individual carotenoids, mixed carotenoids, or as part of B-complex and multivitamin/multimineral preparations.

Action

Some carotenoids (for example, alpha-carotene, beta-carotene, and cryptoxanthin) are converted to ♋ **vitamin A**, although not all to the same extent. In addition, most carotenoids have ♋ **antioxidant** properties and help to protect the body's cells against damage from free radicals.

Possible uses

Carotenoids may help to:
• Maintain healthy mucous membranes of the mouth and elsewhere;
• Protect against cancer. For example, lycopene may protect against ✪ **prostate cancer**;
• Protect against ✪ **heart disease**;
• Protect against cataracts and the progressive blindness of ✪ **macular degeneration** of the eye;
• Enhance resistence to infection.

Warnings

People who smoke should seek a doctor's advice before taking beta-carotene. Some research has shown that beta-carotene supplements may increase the risk of lung cancer in smokers.

Interactions

• There are no major effects of carotenoids on drugs, but a number of drug classes affect carotenoid absorption or vitamin A levels in the body, so always consult a qualified medical professional before taking.

Side effects

In general, carotenoids are not toxic. Those that are converted to vitamin A (for example, beta-carotene) are converted only in amounts needed by the body, so they do not produce sufficient vitamin A to cause toxicity. Large doses of carotenoids can turn the skin orange, particularly the palms of the hands and the soles of the feet.

chitosan

Chitosan is a natural form of fiber extracted from chitin, which is a structural component of the shells of crustacea such as crabs, shrimps, and lobsters.

Formulations

As a supplement it is available as capsules or tablets in the form of chitosan or as deacetylated chitosan (which is more water soluble).

Action

Chitosan binds fat and can bind up to 10 times its own weight in fat from food if it is taken orally. This helps stop fat from being absorbed into the body, and it is this effect which lies behind the claims that chitosan can lead to weight loss.

Possible uses

It is promoted for weight loss (for example, in ○ **obesity**), but research results have been conflicting and its value is unproven.

Warnings

- Chitosan should be avoided by people with intestinal malabsorption conditions, or those who are allergic to shellfish.
- It is not intended for those who are pregnant or breast-feeding.

Interactions

None known.

Side effects

- It may reduce the absorption of the fat-soluble ⚖ **vitamins A**, ⚖ **D**, and ⚖ **E**.

chromium

Chromium is an essential (it is not produced in the body and must be supplied in the diet) trace element. Food sources include whole grains (for example, whole-grain bread), Brewer's yeast, broccoli, mushrooms, black pepper, dried beans, seeds, and wine.

Formulations

As a supplement it is available as capsules, softgels, oral liquids, or tablets combined with multivitamins in a variety of chemical forms: chromium chloride, chromium dinicotinate, chromium glycinate, chromium picolinate, chromium polynicotinate, chromium trichloride.

- There is no recommended Adequate Intake for chromium, but the estimated safe and adequate intake is 50–200 mcg/day for adults.

Action

Chromium helps the body to regulate its use of insulin, which is a hormone that helps to transfer sugar (glucose) to the cells, where it is used to supply energy. It therefore helps the body to maintain normal blood glucose levels. Chromium also helps the body to break down fats and proteins.

Deficiency

No specific condition related to chromium deficiency has been identified. However, lack of chromium could lead to inefficient use of glucose. When this happens, the pancreas has to make more and more insulin in an attempt to keep blood glucose at the right level. When the pancreas can no longer cope, type 2 ○ **diabetes mellitus** develops. Chromium deficiency is not a cause of diabetes mellitus, but it may trigger the disease in those who are prone to it.

Possible uses

Chromium may help:

- Protect against diabetes mellitus;
- Maintain normal blood sugar levels—preventing both "highs" and "lows;"
- Lower cholesterol levels;
- When attempting to lose weight (for example, in ○ **obesity**).

Warnings

- People with diabetes should seek a doctor's advice before taking chromium because it may alter the metabolism of glucose and the regulation of insulin release.

Interactions

- Chromium may increase the therapeutic effect of drugs used in the treatment of diabetes mellitus and may reduce the requirements for insulin, so people taking medication for diabetes mellitus should get the advice of a doctor before taking chromium.

Side effects

None with normal doses from dietary supplements.

coenzyme Q_{10}

(also known as *Coenzyme Q-*$_{10}$*; Co-Q*$_{10}$*; Q*$_{10}$*; ubiquinone*)

Coenzyme Q_{10} is a naturally occurring substance which is produced by the body and is also available in the diet. It is found in the mitochondria, which are the parts of the body cells that produce energy. Food sources include meat, poultry, fatty fish (for example, mackerel, salmon, sardines), soybeans, whole-grain cereals, nuts (for example, peanuts), and green vegetables (for example, spinach).

Formulations

As a supplement it is available as capsules, softgels, tablets, and multipreparations (antioxidants) in the chemical form of 2,3-dimethoxy-5-methylbenzoquinone.

Action

Coenzyme Q_{10} is important for metabolism and the production of energy in cells. It is also an ⚖ **antioxidant** and free radical scavenger.

Possible uses

It may help to:

- Improve the heart and circulation in people with congestive ○ **heart failure**, ○ **angina pectoris**, ○ **arrhythmias** (abnormal heart rhythms), and ○ **hypertension** (high blood pressure);
- Protect against ○ **cancer**;
- Treat the symptoms of ○ **periodontitis** (gum disease) and maintain healthy gums and teeth;
- Protect the nervous system and slow the development of ○ **Alzheimer's disease** and ○ **Parkinson's disease**;
- Slow the ○ **aging** process.

Warnings

- Coenzyme Q_{10} should not be used by people with heart disease or any other medical condition without the advice of a qualified medical professional;
- Seek a doctor's advice if pregnant or breast-feeding.

Interactions
None known.

Side effects
No serious side effects. Stomach upset, nausea, diarrhea, and loss of appetite have occasionally been reported.

conjugated linoleic acid

(also known as *CLA*)

Conjugated linoleic acid is a naturally occurring polyunsaturated fatty acid, a special form of linoleic acid. It is obtained from food and supplements and is not made in the body. CLA is found in many foods in small amounts, particularly beef and dairy products. See also ⚖ **gamma-linolenic acid (GLA)**.

Formulations
As a supplement it is available as capsules and softgels.

Action
CLA helps to make sure fat is delivered to the cells. It also helps to transport glucose to the cells and to ensure that glucose is used to build muscle rather than be converted to body fat. CLA is also an ⚖ **antioxidant** and enhances the immune system. Linoleic acid itself can be used in the body to form arachidonic acid, which is an essential precursor of the ℞ **prostaglandin**-like hormones.

Possible uses
CLA is being promoted for weight loss, but evidence for its effectiveness has come so far only from studies in animals, not humans. Other research in animals suggests that CLA may also protect against ✪ **arthritis**, ✪ **cancer**, ✪ **diabetes mellitus**, and ✪ **heart disease**, but research on this supplement is at a very early stage.

Warnings
None.

Interactions
None.

Side effects
No known toxicity, except for mild gastrointestinal side effects.

copper

Copper is an essential (it is not produced in the body and must be supplied in the diet) trace mineral. Food sources include shellfish, liver, poultry, nuts, seeds, whole grains, legumes, peas, avocados, mushrooms, garlic, tomatoes, and bananas.

Formulations
As a supplement it is available as capsules, tablets, and multivitamin preparations (sometimes with ⚖ **molybdenum**) as copper citrate, copper gluconate, copper sulfate, or cupric chloride.

• There is no recommended Adequate Intake for copper, but the estimated safe and adequate dietary intake is 1.5–3 mg/day for adults.

Action
Copper plays a role in the formation of collagen (a protein found in bone, skin, and connective tissue). It is also important for the production of red blood cells and helps to promote consistent pigmentation in the skin and hair. Copper plays a role in the immune system and is a component of several ⚖ **antioxidant** enzymes, such as superoxide dismutase (SOD).

Deficiency
Severe copper deficiency is rare. It occurs in people with inherited disorders where absorption of copper is poor, or in some gastrointestinal disorders. Mild deficiency may cause anemia and increased cholesterol levels.

Possible uses
Copper may help to:
• Reduce the risk of ✪ **osteoporosis**;
• Alleviate the symptoms of ✪ **arthritis**.

Warnings
None.

Interactions
• Large doses of iron and/or zinc may reduce copper absorption and vice versa. Copper is best taken as part of a balanced multivitamin/mineral supplement.

Side effects
• Doses from supplements are unlikely to cause toxicity. However, excessive doses can cause side effects such as stomach pain and nausea.

DHEA

(*dehydroepiandrosterone;* also known as *prasterone*)

DHEA is a hormone which is secreted by the adrenal glands (which are above the kidneys), skin, testicles, ovaries, and brain. DHEA production declines rapidly with age, with peak levels occurring around the age of 30.

Formulations
As a supplement it is available as caps, creams, lozenges, ointments, and tablets in a chemical form made from a steroid (dosgenin) from Mexican wild yams.

Action
DHEA is used by the body to produce many other hormones, including the sex hormones, estrogens and testosterone.

Possible uses
DHEA is claimed to improve libido, aid weight loss, improve memory, and delay aging. However, there is little evidence to support these claims.

It may help to:
• Protect against ✪ **heart disease**;
• Enhance immunity;
• Control some of the symptoms of ✪ **lupus**;
• Protect against some types of cancer, but it may increase the risk of others.
• Overall, research on DHEA is scanty and there is no good evidence of its value as a supplement.

Warnings
• DHEA should be taken as a supplement with great caution.
• Women at risk of breast cancer or who have had breast cancer should not take DHEA.
• Men who are at risk of prostate cancer or who have had prostate cancer should not take DHEA. Always seek a doctor's advice before taking this supplement.
• People with diabetes mellitus may experience changes in the regulation of blood sugar.

Key to symbols: ✪ = Disorder Section ℞ = Drug Section ♣ = Herbal Section ⚖ = Supplement Section

Interactions

None known.

Side effects

• DHEA can cause oily skin, acne, hair growth in women, and deepening of the voice.

folic acid

(also known as *folate; pteroryglutamic acid (PGA); vitamin B_9*)

Folic acid is a water-soluble vitamin of the B-complex family. Food sources include whole grains, green vegetables, liver, legumes, orange juice, fortified bread, and fortified cereal products.

Formulations

As a supplement it is available as tablets and multivitamin preparations (sometimes with ♌ **iron** or ♌ **vitamin B_{12}**) in a variety of chemical forms: calcium folate, folacin, folate triglutamate, and sodium folate.

• The Adequate Intake (AI) for folic acid is 400 mcg/day for adults. The RDA during pregnancy is 600 mcg/day. Women who are pregnant should consume 400 mcg/day folic acid from supplements or fortified foods in addition to that consumed in the diet.

• The Tolerable Upper Intake Level (UL) is 1,000 mcg/day for adults.

Action

Folic acid is involved in growth and reproduction. It is used to make red blood cells, heal wounds, and is important for the health of the skin and hair. It is important for the formation of the genetic material DNA and RNA. Folic acid also appears to regulate, possibly lowering, the production of homocysteine, which is an ♌ **amino acid** that at high levels may increase the risk of ✪ **heart disease**.

Deficiency

Severe deficiency is rare. Symptoms include a form of anemia (megaloblastic anemia), diarrhea, sore red tongue, mental confusion, and fatigue.

Possible uses

Folic acid reduces the risk of ✪ **spina bifida** and other birth defects when taken during the early stages of ✪ **pregnancy**, and it may help to:

• Reduce the risk of some ✪ **cancers**;

• Reduce the risk of ✪ **heart disease**.

Warnings

• If there is a risk of vitamin B_{12} deficiency, doses of folic acid exceeding 400 mcg/day should not be taken because high doses of folic acid can mask the symptoms of such a deficiency.

Interactions

• High doses of folic acid may interfere with the therapeutic effect of ℞ **antiepileptics** (for example, phenytoin, phenobarbital, primidone). People taking these drugs should seek a doctor's advice before taking folic acid.

Side effects

• High doses of folic acid may reduce zinc absorption and cause seizures in people with epilepsy.

gamma-linolenic acid (GLA)

(also known as *gammalinolenic acid; gamolenic acid; γ-linolenic acid*)

Gamma-linolenic acid (GLA) is an omega-6 fatty acid that is essential for proper body functioning. It is found naturally in evening primrose oil (8–10% GLA), borage oil (23–26% GLA), and blackcurrant oil (15–20% GLA), and these three substances are available as dietary supplements. It can be made in the body from another fatty acid, linoleic acid (LA), but the ability to convert GLA to LA may be reduced in people with ✪ **diabetes mellitus**, ✪ **eczema** and ✪ **stress**, in older people, and those whose alcohol intake is excessive. In such people supplementation can be useful.

Formulations

It is available as capsules, oral liquid, skin creams, and softgels in the chemical form of cis-linolenic acid.

Action

GLA is converted in the body into any one of the ℞ **prostaglandin** group (which regulate a number of body functions such as inflammation) and other compounds with hormone-like actions.

Possible uses

GLA may help to:

• Alleviate symptoms of ✪ **eczema** and ✪ **dermatitis**;

• Relieve symptoms of ✪ **premenstrual syndrome** (PMS);

• Relieve symptoms related to the ✪ **menopause** (for example, hot flashes);

• GLA should not to be taken by people who suffer from epilepsy without a doctor's advice because it may increase the risk of seizures.

Interactions

GLA may increase the risk of:

• Seizures in people taking ℞ **antiepileptics** (for example, ℞ **phenytoin**);

• Seizures in people taking ℞ **antipsychotics** (for example, ℞ **phenothiazine** tranquilizers)

• Bleeding in people taking ℞ **anticoagulants** (for example, ℞ **warfarin sodium** and ℞ **aspirin**).

Side effects

• GLA may cause stomach upsets and headaches.

garlic

(*Allium sativum*)

Garlic is a bulb that is related to the onion. It contains about 100 sulfur compounds and it is these compounds that provide garlic's supposed health benefits. Probably the most important of these compounds is alliin, which when the garlic bulb is crushed releases allicin. Allicin is rapidly broken down to other sulfur-containing compounds such as ajoene, which may also have health benefits. See also the entry for ♣ **garlic** in Herbal Remedies.

Formulations

As a supplement garlic is available as bulbs, oil, tablets, capsules, softgels, deodorized preparations, and in various combined preparations.

Action

Garlic seems to lower blood cholesterol, although results from research are conflicting. It also appears to reduce the ability of the blood to clot and to have anti-infective properties.

Possible uses

It has been used for thousands of years for a variety of complaints. Today it is being promoted as a supplement, mainly for ✪ **heart disease**. Garlic may help to:

• Protect against heart disease by lowering blood cholesterol (see ✪ **hyperlipidemia** and ✪ **atherosclerosis**) and reducing blood clotting;

• Reduce blood pressure (✪ **hypertension**), but only to a small extent;

• Protect against some cancers;

• Fight infections, caused by bacteria, viruses, and fungi (see ✪ **bacterial infections**, ✪ **fungal infections**, and ✪ **viral infections**).

Warnings

• People with a history of bleeding disorders should not use garlic without seeking their doctor's advice first.

Interactions

• Garlic may increase the tendency to bleed in people taking ℞ **aspirin**, ℞ **anticoagulants**, such as warfarin, and other supplements such as ♣ **ginkgo** biloba and ⚕ **vitamin E**.

Side effects

• Garlic may cause heartburn, diarrhea, and skin rash.

glucosamine and chondroitin

(also known as *2-amino-2-deoxyglucose*)
Glucosamine is a natural substance produced in the body and found mainly in the joints, tendons, ligaments, and cartilage. It is available as a dietary supplement, sometimes on its own and some-times with chondroitin, another natural substance, which is also found in the joints.

Formulations

As a supplement it is available as capsules, tablets, and cream in the chemical forms glucosamine or glucosamine sulfates.

Action

Glucosamine is promoted for alleviating ✪ **arthritis** and it seems to relieve pain as effectively as some ℞ **NSAID** (non-steroidal anti-inflammatory) drugs (for example, ℞ **diclofenac**, ℞ **ibuprofen**). However, it also seems to help to repair damaged joints and rebuild cartilage. Chondroitin helps to prevent the breakdown of cartilage and is thought to improve the elasticity of joints. Together, glucosamine and chondroitin help to relieve pain and protect and strengthen the joints.

Possible uses

Glucosamine and chondroitin (both separately and together) may help to:

• Relieve the pain, stiffness, and swelling associated with ✪ **arthritis** and may also reduce the progression of the disease.

Warnings

• People with ✪ **diabetes mellitus** should monitor their blood glucose levels carefully if taking glucosamine because it can alter glucose regulation. Seek a doctor's advice before taking glucosamine if you have diabetes.

Interactions

None known.

Side effects

• Glucosamine may cause nausea or heartburn, diarrhea, and indigestion, although these are mild and relatively uncommon. It may help to take glucosamine with food.

green tea

(*Camellia sinensis*)
Green tea may be used as a nutritional supplement because of its stimulant and antioxidant properties. For fuller information see the entry on green tea in Herbal Remedies.

Warnings

• Anyone who is pregnant or breast-feeding should avoid over-consumption of green tea because of its tannin and ℞ **caffeine** content.

iodine

(also known as *iodide*)
Iodine is an essential (it is not produced in the body and must be supplied in the diet) trace mineral. The best source of iodine is iodized salt, but it is also found in saltwater fish and kelp.

Formulations

As a supplement it is available combined with vitamins and other minerals in the chemical forms of either potassium iodide or iodate salts (which are natural in kelp).

• The Adequate Intake (AI) for iodine is 150 mcg/day for adults (women and men).

Action

Iodine is essential for the production of the thyroid hormones thyroxine and triiodothyronine, which regulate metabolism throughout the body.

Deficiency

There have been no known cases of iodine deficiency in the US since the 1970s because of the use of iodized salt. Iodine deficiency causes goiter, a condition in which the thyroid gland increases in size. Symptoms include dry skin, dry hair, fatigue, and poor mental function.

Possible uses

The only use of iodine is in the prevention of deficiency (see ✪ **hypothyroidism**) and goiter (see also ✪ **hyperthyroidism**). Iodine may help to alleviate the symptoms of fibrocystic breast disease, but this is not proven.

Warnings

• Iodine deficiency is rare in the US, so supplements are not usually required. However, supplements should be avoided by people with thyroid conditions without a doctor's advice.

Interactions

• Iodine may influence the therapeutic effect of drugs used to treat thyroid conditions.

Side effects

There is little risk of toxicity from supplements.

• Doses exceeding 5,000 mcg over prolonged periods of time can cause goiter.

• Other symptoms include swollen salivary glands, mouth ulcers, metallic taste, diarrhea, and vomiting.

iron

Iron is an essential (it is not produced in the body and must be supplied in the diet) trace mineral. Good food sources inlcude liver, beef, lamb, eggs, clams, oysters, mussels, blackstrap molasses, and sardines. Iron from animal sources is better absorbed than iron from plant sources, but vegetarians can obtain iron from whole grains, spinach and other green vegetables, nuts and seeds, fortified breakfast cereals, and dried fruit (for example, prunes, dried apricots). ⚬⚬ **vitamin C** helps the absorption of iron.

Formulations

As a supplement iron is available as tablets, caplets, oral solutions, and in multivitamin and multimineral combinations in the following chemical forms: iron fumarate (ferrous fumarate; chelated ferrous fumarate), iron gluconate (ferrous gluconate), iron glycinate (ferrous glycinate), iron sulfate (ferrous sulfate), and carbonyl iron heme iron.

• The Adequate Intake is 10 mg/day for adult men, 15 mg/day for adult women, and 6–12 mg/day for children (depending on age).

Action

Iron is involved in the production of hemoglobin, the protein which delivers oxygen to every cell in the body, and myoglobin in muscle. Iron is therefore essential for the production of energy in cells, and it also helps to maintain immunity and good nerve function. It is essential for growth and development in children.

Deficiency

Lack of iron leads to iron-deficiency ⚬ **anemia**, a condition in which the body cannot produce sufficient healthy red blood cells. Symptoms include fatigue, breathlessness, paleness, reduced resistance to colds and infections, and palpitations.

Possible uses

• The only use for iron supplements is to prevent or treat iron deficiency (see ⚬ **anemia**);

• Iron supplements are sometimes needed during pregnancy and by women who have heavy menstrual periods (see ⚬ **menorrhagia**);

Warnings

• Iron supplements should not be taken without the advice of a qualified health professional;

• Ideally, you should have a blood test first to see if you have a deficiency;

• Iron should be avoided by people with gastrointestinal conditions, such as ⚬ **peptic ulcer** and inflammatory bowel conditions (for example, ⚬ **Crohn's disease**) because it may make these conditions worse by causing bleeding;

• Iron is dangerous for those people who have a genetic condition known as hemochromatosis, which causes iron to be excessively absorbed and deposited in body tissues and damaging them (more than one million Americans have this condition);

• It should be avoided by anyone with a condition that involves iron overload, for example, thalassemia.

Interactions

• Iron reduces the absorption of a number of drugs, such as ℞ **levodopa**, ℞ **penicillamine**, ℞ **sulfasalazine**, ℞ **antibiotics** (for example, tetracyclines and the quinolone antibiotic ciprofloxacin), and cholesterol-lowering drugs;

• Certain drugs reduce the absorption of iron, for example, ℞ **antacids** and ℞ **etidronate disodium**. Iron supplements should always be taken two hours before or after any other medication;

• Large doses of iron may also reduce the absorption of other minerals (for example, copper, zinc) and vice versa.

Side effects

• Iron supplements can cause gastrointestinal irritation, nausea, and constipation;

• Excessive iron has also been linked to increased risk of ⚬ **heart disease** and colon cancer.

isoflavone

(also known as *bioflavonoids*; *phytoestrogens*; *soy isoflavones*)
Isoflavones are a type of flavonoid found in soy products. They are also known as phytoestrogens because of their hormonal properties. There are several of these compounds, but two of them, daidzein and genistein (and sometimes glycitein), have attracted the most interest and are usually the ones used in supplements. Good food sources are soy products, including soy flour, soy milk, soybeans, textured soy protein, tempeh, and tofu.

Formulations

As supplements isoflavones are available as caplets, capsules, powder, and tablets, and usually (as mentioned) as daidzein, genistein, or glycitein.

Action

Isoflavones have chemical similarities to estrogens, the female sex hormones, although they are much weaker. As phytoestrogens, they seem to work in two different ways, depending on whether natural estrogen production is low or high.

• Before the ⚬ **menopause** when estrogen levels are high, isoflavones may block some of the the effects of estrogen and possibly help to protect against hormone-dependent cancers such as ⚬ **breast cancer**;

• After the menopause, when estrogen levels fall, isoflavones seem to replace the natural estrogens and may help to preserve the health of the skeleton and the cardiovascular system, as well as reducing the symptoms of the menopause. In Asian countries where soy makes up a large part of the diet the incidence of certain cancers and symptoms of the menopause, such as hot flashes, is lower than in the US. However, it is not yet clear whether this is because of the isoflavones or the soy itself;

• As with the flavonoid family as a whole, isoflavones appear to have ⚬⚬ **antioxidant** properties.

Possible uses

Isoflavones may help to:

• Protect against ⚬ **heart disease**;

• Protect against ⚬ **osteoporosis**;

• Protect against some ⚬ **cancers**;

• Reduce the severity and frequency of hot flashes and other symptoms of the ⚬ **menopause**.

Warnings

• Women at risk of breast cancer or who have had breast cancer should not take isoflavone supplements without seeking a doctor's advice. There is some evidence that isoflavones can stimulate cell growth and division in women with breast cancer.

Interactions

None known. However, women using ℞ **HRT** for menopausal symptoms should check with their qualified medical professional before taking supplements.

Side effects

None known. Soy has been consumed for centuries in Asia. However, a few people are allergic to soy products so they should avoid isoflavone supplements.

lecithin

(also known as *phosphatidylcholine*)

Lecithin is a group of chemically fatty substances (also called phospholipids) found in cell membranes of both plant and animal (including human) cells. It is used in the body as a source of choline, which is a vitamin-like substance of the B group. Good food sources of lecithin and choline are eggs and beef steak, with smaller amounts in peanut butter, cauliflower, and coffee.

Formulations

As supplements lecithin and choline are available as capsules, tablets, liquids, softgels, and in granular form; they are also constituents of many B-complex and multivitamin/multimineral preparations. The chemical form of lecithin depends on the origin (soy, egg, etc.), while choline is available as either choline bitartrate or choline dihydrogen citrate.

• There are no Recommended Dietary Allowances for lecithin and choline, although an Adequate Intake (AI) has now been set for choline of 425 mg/day for women and 550 mg/day for men.

Action

Lecithin and choline are an integral part of cell membranes and help the transport of fats and other nutrients in and out of cells. They are also important in reproduction and in the growth and development of infants and children. Choline is used to make the brain neurotransmitter, acetylcholine, whose functions include muscle control and memory.

Possible uses

Lecithin and choline have been claimed to have a wide range of effects such as curing and preventing ✪ **cancer** and ✪ **AIDS**, lowering cholesterol, enhancing exercise performance, preventing ✪ **gallstones**, and improving memory. Evidence for all these claims is very limited.

Warnings

None.

Interactions

None known.

Side effects

• Excessive doses of lecithin may cause diarrhea, sweating, and vomiting.

• Choline in high doses (20 grams/day) may cause a fishy body odor.

magnesium

Magnesium is an essential mineral (it is not produced in the body and must be supplied in the diet). Food sources include green, leafy vegetables, nuts, whole grains, legumes, and shellfish.

Formulations

As a supplement magnesium is available as tablets, on its own, and as part of multivitamin preparations, and in a number of chemical forms: chelated magnesium, magnesium aspartate, magnesium carbonate, magnesium citrate, magnesium hydroxide, magnesium maleate, magnesium orotate, magnesium oxide.

• The Adequate Intake (AI) for magnesium is 310 mg/day for women 19–30 years of age, and 400 mg/day for men 19–30 years of age; 320 mg/day for women over 30, and 420 mg/day for men over 30.

• The Tolerable Upper Intake level (UL) for adults is 350 mg/day.

Action

Magnesium is involved in energy production, bone and tooth formation, blood clotting, nerve and muscle function, and calcium metabolism.

Deficiency

Severe deficiency is rare and causes symptoms such as muscle cramps and weakness, irregular heartbeat, insomnia, restlessness, anxiety, and nervousness. Mild deficiency may increase the risk of ✪ **heart disease** and ✪ **osteoporosis**.

Possible uses

Magnesium may help to:

• Reduce the risk of ✪ **heart disease**;

• Reduce high blood pressure (✪ **hypertension**);

• Reduce symptoms of ✪ **premenstrual syndrome**;

• Reduce complications of ✪ **diabetes mellitus**;

• Strengthen bones, particularly in ✪ **osteoporosis**.

Warnings

• People with ✪ **kidney disease** should consult their doctor before taking magnesium supplements.

Interactions

• Magnesium may reduce the absorption of a number of drugs and so make them less effective. For example, ℞ **antibacterials**, such as ciprofloxacin, the tetracyclines, ketoconazole, nitrofurantoin, and penicillamine. Always take any medication two hours before or after magnesium supplements.

Side effects

• Toxic effects are rare because magnesium is readily excreted by the kidneys. However, if kidney function is impaired, magnesium may build up and lead to muscle weakness, fatigue, and confusion.

• High doses can cause diarrhea.

manganese

Manganese is an essential (it is not produced in the body and must be supplied in the diet) trace mineral. Good food sources include green, leafy vegetables, nuts, whole grains, and wheat germ.

Formulations

As a supplement manganese is available in many multivitamin preparations as manganese citrate, manganese gluconate, or manganese sulfate.

• There is no RDA for manganese. The Estimated Safe and Adequate daily dietary intake is 2–5 mg/day for adults.

Action

Manganese is involved in the formation of connective tissue, blood clotting, and the regulation of blood sugar.

Deficiency

Deficiency is virtually unknown.

Possible uses

Manganese has been claimed to:

• Prevent ✪ **osteoporosis** (in conjunction with other minerals, for example, ⚭ **calcium** and ⚭ **magnesium**);

• Control blood sugar in people with ✪ **diabetes mellitus**.

• However, there is insufficient scientific evidence to justify these claims.

Warnings

None.

Interactions

None known.

Side effects

None.

melatonin

(also known as *N-acetyl-5-methoxytryptamine*)

Melatonin is a natural hormone produced by the pineal gland, which is a tiny gland located in the brain. It is produced throughout life, but levels decline with age. Production of melatonin follows a daily pattern, beginning at dusk and peaking between 2 a.m. and 4 a.m., with little produced during the day.

Formulations

As a supplement melatonin is produced synthetically from 5-methoxyindole and is available as capsules, tablets, a cream (external use only), and liquid spray.

Action

Melatonin helps to set the body's internal clock and regulates cycles of sleep and wakefulness. It also acts as an ⚭ **antioxidant** and has a beneficial effect on the immune system.

Possible uses

Melatonin may help to:

• Promote sleep and relieve ✪ **insomnia**;

• Reduce the symptoms of ✪ **jet lag**;

• Promote sleep when needed by people on shift work.

Warnings

None.

Interactions

None known.

Side effects

• No known toxicity or serious side effects have been identified, even in high dose. However, what effects there may be of taking it long term are not known.

• Melatonin causes drowsiness within 30 minutes of taking it, so you should not drive or operate any machinery.

• Sometimes melatonin can cause grogginess and excessive drowsiness the next day.

• Do not exceed the recommended dose.

molybdenum

Molybdenum is an essential (it is not produced in the body and must be supplied in the diet) trace mineral. Good food sources include milk and dairy products, leafy vegetables, dried beans, whole grains, liver, and kidneys. The levels of molybdenum in foods depend on the mineral content of the soil where the foods were produced.

Formulations

As a supplement molybdenum is available as tablets, usually in a multivitamin preparation, as ammonium molybdate, calcium molybdate, molybdenum trioxide, sodium molybdate, or thiomolybdate salts.

• There is no RDA for molybdenum. The Estimated Safe and Adequate Intake is 75–250 mcg/day for adults.

Action

Molybdenum works as a cofactor with several enzymes and is involved in growth and development.

Deficiency

Deficiency is almost unknown.

Possible uses

There are no established uses for molybdenum as a supplement.

Warnings

None.

Interactions

None.

Side effects

None. High intakes of 10–15 mg/day may increase the risk of ✪ **gout**.

N-acetylcysteine

(also known as *NAC; acetylcysteine*)

N-acetylcysteine is a derivative of the ⚭ **amino acid** cysteine. It is often used successfully as an antidote to ℞ **acetaminophen** toxicity.

Formulations

As a supplement it is available as tablets or capsules.

Action

NAC has ⚭ **antioxidant** activity.

Possible uses

NAC has been promoted as a dietary supplement for preventing and treating ✪ **influenza** and other ✪ **respiratory tract disorders**, helping to combat ✪ **AIDS**, and improving exercise performance in athletes by preventing free radical damage. Evidence for all these claims is very limited.

Warnings

None.

Interactions

None known.

Side effects

No known serious toxicity or side effects, except nausea, vomiting, and diarrhea, and possibly rashes with high doses (5 grams/day). However, what effects there may be of taking it long term are not known.

niacin

(also known as *vitamin B₃*)

Niacin is a water-soluble vitamin of the B-complex family. Niacin is a collective term also used to describe nicotinic acid or nicotinamide. Good food sources include Brewer's yeast, liver, poultry, fish, legumes, nuts, eggs, milk, fortified bread, and fortified cereals. Also, the body can make niacin by converting the ⚄ **amino acid** tryptophan (found in milk, eggs, poultry).

Formulations

As a supplement niacin is available as tablets, capsules (including extended-release forms), and oral solutions in a variety of chemical forms: niacinamide (nicotinamide), nicotinic acid, or inositol hexaniacinate (this form helps reduce "niacin flush").

• The Adequate Intake (AI) for niacin is 14 mg/day for adult women and 16 mg/day for adult men.

• The Tolerable Upper Intake Level (UL) is 35 mg/day for adults over 18 years of age.

Action

Niacin is needed to release energy from carbohydrates. It is also involved in maintaining the normal functioning of the nervous and digestive systems, controlling blood sugar, and keeping skin healthy.

Deficiency

Severe deficiency, which is very rare, leads to the disease ⊕ **pellagra**. Symptoms include diarrhea, vomiting, bright red tongue, mental confusion, memory loss, and skin rash. A minor deficiency can cause indigestion, weakness, loss of appetite, and patches of irritated skin.

Possible uses

Niacin may help to:

• Reduce levels of cholesterol and triglyceride fats in the blood (see ⊕ **hyperlipidemia** and ⊕ **atherosclerosis**);

• Prevent or delay the progression of type 1 ⊕ **diabetes mellitus**;

• Alleviate symptoms of ⊕ **arthritis**;

• Treat circulatory problems (for example, ⊕ **Raynaud's disease** and *intermittent claudication*, which are conditions caused by poor circulation).

Warnings

None at recommended doses.

• However, niacin should be used with caution by people with diabetes mellitus, ⊕ **peptic ulcer**, or ⊕ **gout**.

Interactions

None.

Side effects

The side effects of nicotinamide and nicotinic acid are somewhat different, with nicotinic acid usually more troublesome.

• In normal doses, nicotinamide is not toxic, but excessive amounts can cause liver toxicity.

• Supplements containing nicotinic acid can cause flushing, tingling, headache, nausea and sweating, and itching or rashes.

octacosanol

(also known as *1-octacosanol; octacosyl alcohol; policosanol; polycosanol*)

Octacosanol is a waxy alcohol found in policosanol, which is a substance extracted from plant waxes such as sugar cane wax, wheat germ, and husk waxes.

Formulations

As a supplement octacosanol is available as capsules, oils, powders, and emulsions as various purities in policosanol extract.

Action

Octacosanol seems to have a cholesterol-lowering effect and it may improve muscle function.

Possible uses

• Octacosanol is claimed to protect against ⊕ **heart disease**, alleviate symptoms of ⊕ **Parkinson's disease**, and to enhance endurance in athletes.

• There is some evidence that it reduces LDL ("bad") cholesterol and increases HDL ("good") cholesterol (see ⊕ **hyperlipidemia**). However, evidence for other claims is very limited.

Warnings

None.

Interactions

None known.

Side effects

No known toxicity or side effects, but the long-term effects of taking octacosanol are unknown.

omega-3 fatty acid

(also known as *omega-3; omega-3 marine triglycerides*)

Omega-3 fatty acids are polyunsaturated fatty acids and, along with omega-6 fatty acids, are known as essential fatty acids and are needed for the body to function properly. The main omega-3 fatty acids, all of which are found in food, are alpha-linolenic acid, eicosapentaenoic acid (EPA), and docosahexaenoic acid (DHA). Good food sources include nuts, seeds, meat, and green, leafy vegetables for alpha-linolenic acid, while EPA and DHA are found in oily fish such as mackerel, herring, salmon, tuna, and sardines.

Formulations

As supplements alpha-linolenic acid is found in supplements of flaxseed, and EPA and DHA are found in fish oil supplements.

Action

Alpha-linolenic acid is converted in the body to EPA and DHA which are then converted to the ℞ **prostaglandin** group and other similar compounds with hormone-like actions. These prostaglandin-like substances regulate a number of body functions such as inflammation. It is thought that the diet should contain a balance between the two types of polyunsaturated fatty acids—omega-3 and omega-6—because the proportions ingested affect the types of prostaglandins formed. Because the intake of margarine and spreads containing omega-6 fatty acids has increased during recent decades, the American diet may be deficient in omega-3 fatty acids, and supplements containing these substances could be useful for helping to restore the balance.

Possible uses

In addition to providing a source of omega-3 fatty acids, fish-oil supplements (a source of EPA and DHA) may help to:

• Protect against ❂ **heart disease** by reducing levels of triglycerides (a type of fat in the blood: see ❂ **hyperlipidemia**), reducing blood pressure (see ❂ **hypertension**), and prevent abnormal heart rhythms (see ❂ **arrhythmias**);

• Reduce the risk of heart disease in people with ❂ **diabetes mellitus**;

• Alleviate symptoms of ❂ **arthritis**;

• Alleviate symptoms of ❂ **psoriasis**, ❂ **eczema**, and ❂ **Crohn's disease**;

• Alleviate symptoms of ❂ **depression**.

• Flaxseed oil (a source of alpha-linolenic acid) has not been researched as extensively as fish oils, and it is not clear whether it has all the beneficial effects of the fish oils. There is some very limited evidence that flaxseed protects against heart disease. However, like fish oils, it is a good source of omega-3 fatty acids and it may be used to increase the intake of these substances.

Warnings
• People with diabetes mellitus should monitor their blood glucose levels carefully if taking fish oils because these oils can alter glucose regulation.

• People with a history of bleeding disorders should not use fish oils without consulting their doctor first.

Interactions
• Fish oils may increase the tendency to bleed in people taking ℞ **aspirin**, an ℞ **anticoagulant**, such as warfarin, and other supplements such as ⚖ **garlic**, ♣ **Ginkgo biloba**, and ⚖ **vitamin E**.

Side effects
There are no toxic effects in healthy people.

pantothenic acid
(also known as *vitamin B₅*)
Pantothenic acid is a water-soluble vitamin of the B-complex family. Good food sources inlcude liver, kidney, fish, poultry, whole grains, legumes, and yogurt.

Formulations
As a supplement it is available as tablets, capsules, oral solutions, extended-release capsules or tablets, and as a constituent of multivitamin/multimineral preparations in one of several chemical forms: calcium pantothenate, dexpanthenol, pantethine, panthoderm, or pantothenyl alcohol (panthenol).

• The Adequate Intake (AI) for pantothenic acid is 5 mg/day for adults.

Action
Pantothenic acid is involved in releasing energy from food. Like other B-complex vitamins, it is essential for a variety of processes, including the creation of red blood cells, formation of neurotransmitters, production of antibodies, and production of stress hormones.

Deficiency
Deficiency of pantothenic acid is virtually unknown.

Possible uses
Pantothenic acid may help to:

• Alleviate the pain of ❂ **arthritis** (although evidence is limited).

• However, there is little justification for pantothenic acid supplements.

Warnings
None.

Interactions
None.

Side effects
None, even at high doses, because the body is efficient at excreting the vitamin in the urine.

phosphatidylserine
(also known as *PS*)
Phosphatidylserine is a natural fatty substance, a phospholipid, which is found in cell membranes, in particular brain tissue.

Formulations
As a supplement it is available as perlecaps, softgels, capsules, and tablets (often in combination with phosphatidylinositol), and in the chemical forms soybean PS (for example, Leci-PS) or bovine brain PS.

Action
Phosphatidylserine helps maintain the health of brain cells because it is a vital constituent of nerve cell membranes. One role is that of participating in the release of neurotransmitters such as acetylcholine, dopamine, and norepinephrine.

Possible uses
Phosphatidylserine has been promoted for improving memory, preventing or delaying age-related changes in the brain, and boosting IQ. There is some evidence that it improves memory in older people with ❂ **dementia** or ❂ **Alzheimer's disease**, but no evidence that it boosts IQ.

Warnings
Some phosphatidylserine supplements have in the past been made from bovine cortex. Although there have been no adverse effects, there has been concern that such supplements could increase the risk of ❂ **Creutzfeldt-Jakob disease** (CJD) or other similar conditions from bovine material. This concern has led to the development of supplements derived from soy lecithin, which is somewhat different chemically, but how effective these are is not known.

Interactions
None known.

Side effects
No toxicity or side effects known, but the long-term effects are unknown.

potassium
Potassium is an essential mineral (it is not produced in the body and must be supplied in the diet). Food sources include fresh fruit and vegetables, particularly bananas, oranges, orange juice, and potatoes, as well as peanut butter, milk, and liver.

Formulations
As a supplement potassium is available as capsules and oral solutions, on its own or as part of multivitamin/multimineral preparations. It can come in one of several chemical forms: organic forms—potassium amino acid chelate, potassium ascorbate, potassium

aspartate, potassium citrate, potassium gluconate, or potassium orotate; inorganic forms—potassium bicarbonate or potassium chloride (among many).

• There is no RDA for potassium. The estimated minimum requirement in healthy adults is 2,000 mg/day.

Action

Potassium works in the body with sodium and is essential for conduction of nerve impulses and is involved in maintaining the correct balance of fluid and acid to alkali (pH) in the body. Potassium also helps to regulate muscle contraction, blood pressure, and heartbeat.

Deficiency

Deficiency is rare, but can occur when ℞ **diuretic** drugs (for example, furosemide, bendroflumethiazide) are taken. Symptoms of deficiency include muscle weakness, fatigue, irregular heartbeat, confusion, and nausea.

Possible uses

Potassium may help to:

• Protect against ✪ **hypertension** (high blood pressure) and ✪ **stroke**;

• Reduce high blood pressure.

• It is well known that reducing the amount of sodium in the diet can help to lower blood pressure, but increasing intake of potassium from food and/or supplements may also help.

Warnings

• High doses of potassium should be avoided by people with ✪ **kidney disease**.

Interactions

• ℞ **ACE inhibitors**, ℞ **cyclosporine** and some other drugs can increase blood potassium levels, so people taking drugs should always seek medical advice before taking potassium supplements.

Side effects

Potassium toxicity is very rare unless a person has kidney disease. Symptoms of toxicity include muscle weakness, vomiting, and irregular heartbeat.

royal jelly and bee products

There are three main bee products available as supplements: royal jelly, pollen, and propolis. Royal jelly is a milky white substance produced by the pharyngeal glands of the worker bees as a food for the queen bee. Bee pollen is plant pollen and nectar usually collected from the legs of worker bees as they return to the hive. Propolis is a shellac-like material used by the worker bees for repairs within the hive.

Formulations

As supplement royal jelly and bee products are available as capsules, tablets, softgels, liquids, lozenges, powders, and creams.

Action

Royal jelly and other bee products have been promoted as "cure-alls" which increase vitality and mental alertness, delay aging, and fight infections and allergies. Royal jelly does contain an antibacterial substance, but how effective this is in humans is not clear.

Possible uses

There is no good evidence to support the use of royal jelly or any bee products as supplements. Pollen contains carbohydrates, fat, protein, amino acids, and vitamin C; plus trace amounts of B-complex vitamins, carotene, calcium, iron, copper, magnesium, and potassium. Propolis has been used in preparations for treating ✪ **wounds**.

Warnings

• People who are allergic to pollen, bee stings or honey, or have asthma should avoid these products.

Interactions

None known.

Side effects

• Some people have a severe allergic reaction to royal jelly and bee products. Symptoms include itchy throat, skin flushing, hives, headache, and wheezing. Anyone who experiences any of these symptoms should stop taking the supplement immediately. There have been a few deaths due to severe asthmatic attacks triggered by eating royal jelly and bee pollen.

S-adenosylmethionine

(also known as *methionyl adenylate; S-adenosyl-L-methionine; SAMe; SAM-e; SAM*)

S-adenosylmethionine is a naturally occurring substance derived from the essential ⚛ **amino acid** methionine. It is produced in the body (mainly by the liver) and is not found in the diet.

Formulations

As a supplement it is available as tablets (including enteric-coated tablets).

Action

SAMe is involved in a large number of biochemical pathways including those involved in the production of the genetic material DNA and RNA, brain neurotrasmitters, and the fatty substance in cell membranes. It also helps to protect the nerves, produces ⚛ **antioxidant** amino acids within the body, and may reduce the ability of the blood to clot.

Possible uses

• Treating ✪ **depression**, ✪ **insomnia**, and ✪ **arthritis**.

• Providing protection against ✪ **heart disease**.

• There is some evidence that it helps in depression, but evidence for other claims is very limited.

Warnings

• People with a history of bleeding or ✪ **peptic ulcer** should seek a doctor's advice before taking SAMe.

Interactions

• SAMe may increase the tendency to bleed in people taking ℞ **aspirin** and ℞ **anticoagulants** such as warfarin. People taking these drugs should avoid SAMe.

• People taking ℞ **antidepressants** should check with their doctor before taking SAMe.

Side effects

No serious side effects have been reported. However, minor side effects may include dry mouth, nausea, and restlessness.

selenium

Selenium is an essential (it is not produced in the body and must be supplied in the diet) trace element. Food sources include whole grains, brown rice, Brazil nuts, meat, and seafood. The content of plant sources depends on the selenium content of the soil where the plants were grown (for example, selenium content of plants is often low in central and eastern US).

Formulations

As a supplement it is available as tablets and capsules in multivitamin/multimineral preparations. It can come in several chemical forms: organic forms—selenocysteine, selenocystine, or selenomethionine; inorganic forms—sodium selenate or sodium selenite.
• The RDA for selenium is 55 mcg/day for adult women and 70 mcg/day for adult men.

Action

Selenium is an ⚖ **antioxidant** and helps to prevent damage to cells by free radicals. It works with ⚖ **vitamins C** and ⚖ **E**, with which it is often included in dietary supplements, and is part of the antioxidant enzyme glutathione peroxidase, which helps to remove various toxins from the body.

Deficiency

Deficiency is rare in the USA. Mild deficiency may lead to heart disease and problems related to a weakened immune system.

Possible uses

Selenium may help to:
• Reduce the risk of ✪ **heart disease**;
• Protect against ✪ **cancer**;
• Protect against cataracts;
• Improve immunity;
• Slow the progression of ✪ **AIDS**;

Warnings

• Do not take more than the recommended doses. A daily dose must never be more than 200 mcg;
• It should not be taken with vitamin C because this may impair absorption.

Interactions

None known.

Side effects

• High doses of selenium are toxic, and the difference between a safe dose and a toxic dose is small.
• Doses exceeding 750 mcg/day may cause loss of hair and finger nails, nausea, diarrhea, irritability, and fatigue.

shark cartilage

Shark cartilage (chondroitin) contains a variety of substances, although the active ingredients have not been properly identified.

Formulations

Shark cartilage is produced from the pulverized skeleton of a shark. As a supplement it is available as capsules, softgels, and tablets.

Action

Shark cartilage is believed to contain a substance that inhibits the growth of new blood vessels, typically seen in malignant tumors which need the body to develop new networks of blood vessels to

supply nutrients. Such an effect is thought to lead to "starvation" of the tumor by cutting off the supply of blood and nutrients.

Possible uses

Because sharks rarely develop cancer, the idea is that shark cartilage could help slow tumor growth and this supplement has been widely promoted for cancer. However, evidence is extremely limited that shark cartilage supplements are beneficial.

Warnings

None.

Interactions

None.

Side effects

Nausea has been reported.

spirulina and other algae

(also known as *blue green algae*)
Spirulina is a type of aquatic algae. Other forms of algae used in dietary supplements include chlorella and kelp. Spirulina and chlorella are freshwater algae while kelp grows in salt water.

Formulations

As supplements they are available as tablets and capsules as natural spirulina, natural chlorella, and blue green algae.

Action

Spirulina and chlorella have a high content of chlorophyl (the green pigment in plant cells) and both are good sources of protein. They also contain a high concentration of vitamin B_{12}, but this is not in a chemical form that people are able to use. Kelp is a source of ⚖ **iodine**.

Possible uses

Spirulina, chlorella, and kelp have been promoted for a wide variety of uses:
• Lowering cholesterol;
• Boosting the immune system;
• Reducing the risk of cancer;
• Enhancing libido.
• Kelp may help to treat an underactive thyroid gland (see ✪ **hypothyroidism**) but only if there is a deficiency of iodine, which is rare in the US because of the use of iodized salt.

Warnings

• People with thyroid conditions should seek medical advice before using kelp.
• Some algae contain toxins which could pose a risk if incorporated in supplements, but manufacturers of supplements have drafted voluntary guidelines to detect and control exposure to such toxins.

Interactions

None.

Side effects

None.

vitamin A

(also known as *retinol*)
Vitamin A is a fat-soluble vitamin. The two main forms of vitamin A in foods are retinol, which is known as "preformed vitamin A," and the ⚖ **carotenoid** group, which are converted to vitamin A in

the body. Good food sources of retinol include liver, eggs, and fortified milk. Good sources of carotenoids are fruit and vegetables such as carrots and tomatoes.

Formulations

As a supplement it is available as tablets, oral solutions, and in multivitamin/multimineral preparations, and in one of several chemical forms: beta-carotene, other carotenoids, retinol, or retinyl palmitate.

• The RDA for vitamin A is 800 Retinol Equivalents (RE) (4,000 IU), daily for adult women and 1,000 RE (5,000 IU), daily for adult men.

Action

Vitamin A plays a major role in vision, particularly keenness and night vision. It also helps to maintain the health of the body's cells and is vital for reproduction, growth, the health of the skin, development of bone and teeth, and immunity (it is sometimes known as the "anti-infection vitamin").

Deficiency

Severe vitamin A deficiency is quite rare in the US, but mild deficiency may occur, especially in young children and seniors. Symptoms include night blindness and reduced resistance to infection.

Possible uses

Vitamin A may help to:
• Treat skin disorders, heal wounds, burns, and skin ulcers;
• Fight ✪ **colds**, ✪ **influenza**, and other infections;
• Maintain good eyesight.

Warnings

• Vitamin A supplements may cause birth defects if taken in high doses during pregnancy. Healthy, pregnant women eating a well-balanced diet do not need supplements of vitamin A. However, if a supplement is taken in pregnancy, the dose should not exceed the RDA of 4,000 IU daily. It is best to consult your doctor before taking vitamin A supplements;

• There is a risk of hypervitaminosis if vitamin A supplements are taken when on a course of retinoid drugs (for example, ℞ **acitretin** used for skin disorders.

Interactions

• ℞ **cholestyramine** and ℞ **colestipol hydrochloride** may reduce the absorption of vitamin A. People taking these drugs should consider taking a supplement.

• Mineral oil (used as a short-term laxative) may reduce the absorption of vitamin A. However, because mineral oil should not be used for prolonged periods, this is not usually a problem.

Side effects

Excessive amounts of vitamin A can cause dry, cracking skin, brittle nails, bleeding gums, hair loss, irritability, headache, nausea, and tiredness. For example, a single dose of 500,000 IU may cause weakness and vomiting. A dose of 25,000 IU daily over six years has been reported to cause liver damage.

vitamin B$_1$

(also known as *thiamin; thiamine*)

Vitamin B$_1$ is a water-soluble vitamin and member of the vitamin B-complex family. Good food sources include Brewer's yeast, meat (particularly pork and bacon), legumes, whole grains, seeds, and nuts.

Formulations

As a supplement it is available as either thiamine hydrochloride or thiamine mononitrate as capsules, in B-complex supplements, and multivitamin preparations (Brewer's yeast supplements provide a lower-potency option).

• The RDA is 1.1 mg/day for adult women and 1.2 mg/day for adult men.

Action

Vitamin B$_1$ (along with other B vitamins) is essential for converting carbohydrates in food to energy. It also plays a role in promoting the healthy functioning of the nerves, muscles, and heart.

Deficiency

Severe deficiency of vitamin B$_1$ (which is rare) causes ✪ **beriberi**, which leads to nerve damage, wasting of muscle, paralysis, and heart problems. A mild deficiency (more common) can lead to tiredness, irritability, depression, and muscle weakness. Although most people get enough vitamin B$_1$ in the diet, some people, particularly seniors, and those suffering from ✪ **alcoholism** may be mildly deficient in this vitamin. Low levels of vitamin B$_1$ have been found in people with ✪ **Alzheimer's disease**, but it has not been proven that taking vitamin B$_1$ supplements are of any benefit. According to some figures the average intake of vitamin B$_1$ is below the RDA for possibly half the population of the US.

Possible uses

Vitamin B$_1$ may help to:
• Maintain healthy nerves;
• Improve mood and help prevent ✪ **depression**;
• Prevent mouth ulcers.

Warnings

None.

Interactions

• Vitamin B$_1$ levels may be depleted by ℞ **diuretics**, particularly furosemide. People taking these drugs may benefit from a supplement.

Side effects

None, even at high doses, because the body is efficient at excreting the vitamin in the urine.

vitamin B$_2$

(also known as *riboflavin*)

Vitamin B$_2$ is a water-soluble vitamin and member of the vitamin B-complex family. Good food sources include Brewer's yeast, dairy products, meat, eggs, and green, leafy vegetables.

Formulations

As a supplement vitamin B$_2$ is available in the chemical form riboflavin monophosphate as tablets or capsules on its own, and also in B-complex and multivitamin preparations (Brewer's yeast provides a low-potency supplement).

• The RDA is 1.1 mg/day for adult women and 1.3 mg/day for adult men.

Action

Vitamin B$_2$ (along with other B vitamins) is essential for converting food to energy. It converts ◌◌ **vitamin B$_6$** and ◌◌ **niacin** into their active forms, and it works in conjunction with ◌◌ **iron** in the manufacture of red blood cells, which transport oxygen to all the cells of the body. It is essential for tissue maintenance and repair, and is important for the health of the eyes and nerves. Vitamin B_2 also acts as an ⚗ **antioxidant**, and protects cells from damage by free radicals.

Deficiency
Severe vitamin B_2 deficiency, which is rare, causes symptoms such as cracking and sores at the corners of the mouth, itching, burning eyes, deep red tongue, skin rash, and sensitivity to light (photosensitivity). Deficiency may also lead to ✪ **anemia**. Vegans or other people who consume no dairy produce may be at risk of deficiency.

Possible uses
Vitamin B_2 may help to:
• Reduce the frequency, duration, and severity of ✪ **migraine**;
• Reduce the risk or delay the onset of cataracts.

Warnings
None.

Interactions
• Deficiency of vitamin B_2 may occur in people taking some medications, including oral ℞ **contraceptives**, some ℞ **tranquilizers**, and ℞ **antidepressants**, especially if these drugs are being taken as part of a long-term treatment.

Side effects
None, even at high doses, because the body is efficient at excreting the vitamin in the urine.

vitamin B_6
(also known as *pyridoxal; pyridoxal-5-phosphate; pyridoxamine; pyridoxine; pyridoxine hydrochloride*)
Vitamin B_6 is a water-soluble vitamin and member of the B-complex family. Good food sources include whole grains, legumes, meat, poultry, tuna, and nuts.

Formulations
As a supplement it is available in the form pyridoxine hydrochloride as tablets or extended-release capsules on its own, or in B-complex and multivitamin preparations (Brewer's yeast provides a low-potency supplement).
• The RDA is 1.3 mg/day for men and women 19–50 years of age; 1.5 mg/day for women over 50 and 1.7 mg/day for men over 50.
• The Tolerable Upper Intake (UL) for vitamin B_6 is 100 mg/day for adults.

Action
Vitamin B_6 (along with other B vitamins) is essential for converting food to energy. It is involved in maintaining healthy skin and proper functioning of the nervous and digestive systems. It helps in the formation of red blood cells and in the manufacture of various neurotransmitters such as serotonin.

Deficiency
Severe vitamin B_6 deficiency, which is rare, causes insomnia, irritability, depression, dermatitis, sores around the mouth, and acne. Marginal deficiency may increase levels of homocysteine (the oxidized form of the ⚗ **amino acid** cysteine), which can increase the risk of ✪ **heart disease**.

Possible uses
Vitamin B_6 may help to:

• Reduce symptoms of ✪ **premenstrual syndrome** (PMS);
• Treat ✪ **carpal tunnel syndrome**;
• Ease ✪ **depression**;
• Alleviate ✪ **asthma**;
• Reduce the risk of ✪ **heart disease**.

Warnings
• High doses of vitamin B_6 (500–1,000 mg/day) may cause nerve damage. In rare cases, lower doses (250–500 mg/day) can have the same effect. If you experience any nerve pain, tingling, or numbness, stop taking the vitamin at once. Any nerve damage is completely reversible once you stop taking the vitamin.

Interactions
• Various drugs impair vitamin B_6 absorption. These include ℞ **cycloserine**, iproniazid, ℞ **levodopa**, ℞ **penicillamine**, ℞ **phenytoin**, and ℞ **theophylline**. People who take these drugs should take a B_6 supplement of 10 mg/day.
• Oral contraceptives may lead to a mild deficiency of vitamin B_6.

Side effects
• Prolonged high doses can lead to reversible nerve damage.

vitamin B_{12}
(also known as *cobalamin; cyanocobalamin*)
Vitamin B_{12} is a water-soluble vitamin and member of the B-complex family. It is found in significant amounts only in foods derived from animals (for example, meat, fish, eggs, dairy products).

Formulations
As a supplement it is available, in the form of cyanocobalamin, as capsules, lozenges, nasal gels, and (most commonly) in vitamin B-complex multivitamin preparations. Vitamin B_{12} in the chemical form hydroxocobalamin is only available on prescription.
• The RDA for is 2.4 mcg/day for adult men and women.

Action
Vitamin B_{12} is essential for the production of cells, especially red blood cells. It plays a role in the production of DNA and RNA, which is the genetic material of cells, helps to protect the myelin sheath surrounding the nerves, and helps to convert food to energy.

Deficiency
Vitamin B_{12} deficiency causes nerve damage, leading to numbness and tingling in the extremities, muscle weakness, memory loss, depression, tiredness, confusion, dementia, and a type of anemia known as pernicious anemia. Seniors are at particular risk of deficiency. However, vegans, who eat no animal food, are also at risk, unless they eat foods fortified with B_{12} (for example, fortified breakfast cereals). Marginal deficiency may increase levels of homocysteine (the oxidized form of the ⚗ **amino acid** cysteine), which can increase the risk of heart disease.

Possible uses
• To treat ✪ **pernicious anemia**.
• It may help to:
• Reduce the risk of ✪ **heart disease**;
• Treat the symptoms of ✪ **multiple sclerosis**;
• Reduce the risk of ✪ **depression** and ✪ **dementia** in older people.

Warnings
None.

Interactions

• Many drugs may reduce the absorption of vitamin B_{12}, notably drugs used for the treatment of ✪ **peptic ulcers** (for example, ℞ **cimetidine**, ℞ **omeprazole**) and ℞ **metformin** (a drug used in the treatment of ✪ **diabetes mellitus**).

Side effects

None, even at high doses, because the body is efficient at excreting the vitamin in the urine.

vitamin C

(also known as *ascorbic acid*)

Vitamin C is a water-soluble vitamin. It is not manufactured by the body and so must be present in the diet. Good food sources include citrus fruits (for example, oranges, lemons, grapefruit), kiwis, mango, papaya, cantaloupe, strawberries, sweet peppers, broccoli, spinach, tomatoes, kale, cauliflower, and baked potato with skin.

Formulations

As a supplement it is available as tablets, caplets, capsules, chewables, effervescent tablets, extended-release tablets, oral solutions, powders, crystals, chewing gum, and syrups. It is produced in a variety of chemical forms: ascorbyl palmitate (fat-soluble vitamin C), calcium ascorbate, esterfied vitamin C, natural vitamin C derived from rose hips, potassium ascorbate, synthetic vitamin C, or sodium ascorbate.

• The RDA for adults is 60 mg/day (for smokers it is 100 mg/day).
• The Tolerable Upper Intake Level (UL) is 2,000 mg/day.

Action

Vitamin C is crucial for the formation of collagen (a protein found in connective tissue), which is important for healthy teeth, gums, bones, ligaments, and blood vessels. It helps the healing of wounds, supports the immune system, and is involved in the production of neurotransmitters and adrenal gland hormones. It also helps the absorption of iron from the digestive tract. It is the body's main water-soluble ♢♢ **antioxidant** and helps to prevent damage of cells by free radicals.

Deficiency

Severe deficiency of vitamin C causes scurvy, but the risk of this condition is low unless your intake of vitamin C is less than 10 mg/day. However, intakes below 50 mg/day on a regular basis may cause bleeding gums, impair the healing of wounds, and may increase the risk of cancer and heart disease. Some seniors are at risk of deficiency, particularly those living in institutions where fresh fruit and vegetables may not always be available.

Possible uses

• Vitamin C is used to treat scurvy.
• It may also help to:
• Shorten the duration of ✪ **cold** symptoms (although there is no strong evidence that vitamin C actually prevents colds);
• Enhance ✪ **wound** healing;
• Enhance immunity;
• Protect against ✪ **cancer**, cataracts, and ✪ **heart disease**;
• Prevent allergic reactions;
• Treat symptoms of ✪ **asthma**.

Warnings

• Vitamin C can interfere with blood glucose tests in people with diabetes and tests for colon cancer.
• Do not take vitamin C supplements if you have recurrent kidney stones, kidney disease, or hemochromatosis (a genetic disorder where excess iron is stored) without consulting your doctor.

Interactions

• Large doses of vitamin C may reduce the therapeutic effect of oral ℞ **anticoagulants** such as warfarin.

Side effects

Vitamin C is generally safe, even in large doses because the body is efficient at excreting the vitamin in the urine. However, doses over 2 g/day may cause loose stools or diarrhea.

vitamin D

(also known as *calciferol*)

Vitamin D is a fat-soluble vitamin. It is produced in the skin by the action of sunlight (which is why it is often called the "sun vitamin"), which leads to the formation of cholecalciferol or vitamin D_3. Spending 10–15 minutes in the sun two to three times a week between the hours of 8 a.m. and 3 p.m., with arms and face exposed, allows the production of sufficient vitamin D for the body's needs, but many people do not spend enough time in the sun, especially in the winter.

There are very few food sources of vitamin D, except fish oils, fortified milk, fortified breakfast cereals, egg yolks, and liver.

Requirements

As a supplement it is available as tablets, softgels, and in multivitamin preparations. It is produced in two chemical forms: ergocalciferol (vitamin D_2); and cholecalciferol (vitamin D_3).

• The Adequate Intake (AI) for vitamin D is 200 IU (5 mcg) daily for adults under 50 years of age; 400 IU (10 mcg) daily for adults 51–70; and 600 IU (15 mcg) daily for adults over 70.
• The Tolerable Upper Intake Level (UL) is 1,000 IU (50 mcg) daily for adults.

Action

Vitamin D helps in the absorption of ♢♢ **calcium** from the digestive tract and the regulation of calcium levels in the blood. In this way it helps to maintain the health of the bones and teeth.

Deficiency

Severe deficiency of vitamin D leads to a disease of bone weakness, which is known as rickets in children and osteomalacia in adults. Deficiency may help to increase the risk of ✪ **osteoporosis**. Rickets used to be common in children, but is now rarer because vitamin D is added to milk.

Vitamin D deficiency may occur in older people and those who are institutionalized, particularly if they are rarely in the sun. Deficiency may also occur in those who do not drink any milk (milk is fortified with vitamin D) and in those who always wear sunscreen.

Possible uses

Vitamin D may help to:

• Protect against ✪ **osteoporosis**;
• Protect against some types of ✪ **cancer**;
• Treat ✪ **hypocalcemia** and ✪ **hypothyroidism**.

Warnings
• People with hypercalcemia (high blood levels of calcium) should avoid taking vitamin D supplements.

Interactions
• ℞ **Anticonvulsants** (for example, carbamazepine, phenobarbital, phenytoin, primidone) may increase the metabolism of vitamin D and reduce blood levels of the vitamin.
• ℞ **Cholestyramine** and ℞ **colestipol hydrochloride** may reduce the absorption of vitamin D.
• People taking these drugs should consider taking a supplement.

Side effects
• Vitamin D is potentially toxic in overdose. Symptoms include excessive thirst, lack of appetite, nausea, vomiting, constipation or diarrhea, weakness, headache, extreme fatigue, and heartbeat irregularities.

vitamin E
(also known as *tocopherol*)
Vitamin E is a fat-soluble vitamin. It is a term used to describe a group of compounds, known as tocopherols, of which alpha-tocopherol is the most common. There are two forms of alpha-tocopherol: d-alpha-tocopherol (natural vitamin E); and dl-alpha-tocopherol (synthetic vitamin E). The natural form is better absorbed than the synthetic form, so you need to take about one third less of the natural form.

Good food sources include wheat-germ oil, wheat germ, most vegetable oils, whole-grain cereals, whole-grain flour, egg yolks, nuts, green vegetables, and avocados.

Formulations
As a supplement vitamin E is available as capsules, softgels, creams, chewable lozenges, and sometimes in preparations also containing ⚗ **vitamin C** and ⚗ **selenium**. It is produced in several chemical forms (each having different vitamin E and antioxidant activity): tocopherols (alpha-, beta-, gamma-, delta-), tocotrienols (alpha-, beta-, gamma-, delta-), natural vitamin E (d-alpha-tocopherol), synthetic vitamin E (dl-alpha-tocopherol), tocopherol succinate, tocopherol acetate.
• The RDA for vitamin E is 8 mg tocopherol equivalents (TE) or 12 International Units (IU) daily for adult women, and 10 mg TE or 15 IU daily for adult men.

Action
Vitamin E is an ⚗ **antioxidant** and free radical scavenger that helps to protect cell membranes. It works in this way with ⚗ **selenium** and vitamin C, which is why vitamin E is sometimes included in supplements with these nutrients.

Deficiency
Vitamin E deficiency is rare. Symptoms include dry skin and dry hair. Low intakes of the vitamin may increase the risk of heart disease and cataracts.

Possible uses
Vitamin E may help to:
• Protect against ✪ **atherosclerosis**, heart attack and ✪ **stroke** by reducing the risk of blood clots and high levels of LDL cholesterol ("bad" cholesterol) in the blood (see ✪ **hyperlipidemia** and ✪ **hypertension**);

• Protect against cancer;
• Delay or prevent cataracts;
• Improve immune function;
• Improve neurological disorders (for example, ✪ **Alzheimer's disease**);
• Improve the control of ✪ **diabetes mellitus**.

Warnings
None.

Interactions
• People taking an ℞ **anticoagulant** such as warfarin should not take vitamin E without a doctor's advice because it can increase the effectiveness of these drugs and cause bleeding.

Side effects
• Vitamin E is relatively non-toxic.
• It may increase blood thinning in people taking anticoagulants.

vitamin K
(also known as *koagulation vitamin*)
Vitamin K is a fat-soluble vitamin. Good food sources inlcude dark green leafy vegetables and liver. However, most of the body's requirement of vitamin K is produced by "friendly" bacteria in the intestine.

Formulations
As a supplement it is available as tablets, liquids, and in multivitamin preparations. It is produced in three forms: vitamin K_1 (phytomenadione, phylloquinone); vitamin K_2 (menaquinone); and vitamin K_3 (menadione).
• The RDA is 65 mcg/day for adult women and 80 mcg/day for adult men.

Action
Vitamin K is essential for blood clotting and is necessary for bone formation.

Deficiency
Deficiency is rare in healthy people because the body can make sufficient vitamin K for its needs. However, those with disorders of the digestive tract or liver may develop a deficiency. Symptoms of deficiency include bruising, difficulty in blood clotting, and hemorrhage.

Possible uses
• Protect against ✪ **osteoporosis**;
• Treating ✪ **blood disorders**.

Warnings
None.

Interactions
• Vitamin K may reduce the therapeutic effect of an oral ℞ **anticoagulant** such as warfarin. People taking this type of drug should not take supplements containing vitamin K.
• Prolonged use of an ℞ **antibiotic** may reduce vitamin K levels.

Side effects
None at recommended doses, except in people taking anticoagulants.

zinc

Zinc is an essential mineral (it is not produced in the body and must be supplied in the diet). Good food sources include Brewer's yeast, liver, wheat germ, meat, fish, oysters, cheese, beans, nuts, and seeds.

Formulations

As a supplement it is available as tablets, lozenges, and in multivitamin/multimineral preparations. It is produced in various chemical forms: organic forms–zinc acetate, zinc aspartate, zinc amino acid chelate, zinc citrate, zinc gluconate, zinc l-methionine, zinc picolinate; inorganic form–zinc sulfate.
• The RDA for zinc is 12 mg/day for adult women and 15 mg/day for adult men.

Action

Zinc plays a role in the metabolism of protein, carbohydrates, and fats. It is an essential part of all 200 enzymes of many different types. It is crucial for maintaining the integrity of the cells and is needed for sperm production, proper functioning of insulin, and for the health of the immune system.

Deficiency

Severe deficiency is rare in the US, but is quite common in many developing countries. Mild deficiency can lead to poor wound healing, loss of sense of taste and smell, low sperm count, lowered resistance to colds and flu, and skin problems such as acne and psoriasis.

Possible uses

Zinc may help to:
• Reduce symptoms of the common cold;
• Improves ✪ **infertility**;
• Improve immunity;
• Protect against cataract and the progressive blindness of ✪ **macular degeneration**.

Warnings

None.

Interactions

• Zinc reduces the absorption of several drugs (for example, any ℞ **antibiotic**, such as tetracycline and ciprofloxacin, and ℞ **penicillamine**). Zinc supplements should always be taken two hours apart from any medication.
• Zinc may also reduce the absorption of other minerals (for example, ⚖ **copper**, ⚖ **iron**) and vice versa, and so should be taken at different times.

Side effects

• High doses of zinc (more than 100 mg/day) can cause nausea, diarrhea, vomiting, impaired immunity, reduction in HDL ("good") cholesterol, and a bad taste.

Glossary

These short definitions of words and phrases are intended to be useful within the context of the way they are used in this book. They may have different meanings in other contexts.

ABORTIFACIENT An agent that induces the abortion of a fetus.

ABSORPTION The uptake of a drug from its site of administration, such as an injection into a muscle.

ACTIVE IMMUNIZATION A form of immunization that results from the body producing its own antibodies (see **antibody**) in response to an **antigen**.

ACUTE Short-term; in contrast to chronic (long-term). The term acute is used to describe a disease of relatively sudden onset and short duration, or the length of time for which a drug is taken.

ADAPTOGENIC A term commonly used in herbal medicine to mean the property of an agent that helps strengthen the body and increase resistance to disease, and adapt the body to stressful conditions. Such an agent is said to be an adaptogen.

ADDICTION see **dependence**.

ADEQUATE INTAKE (AI) The estimated safe intake of a supplement. It is used when the RDA (see **recommended dietary allowance**) cannot be determined. It is a recommended daily intake level based on an observed or experimentally determined approximation of nutrient intake for a group of healthy people.

ADJUNCT A drug or treatment that is not essential, but assists another treatment and often improves its overall effectiveness.

ADJUVANT A drug not necessarily effective on its own, but which may be used in addition to other drugs to increase the latter's effectiveness.

ADRENAL Pertaining to the adrenal gland, an endocrine gland situated close to the kidney. The adrenal gland's cortex (outer layer) secretes the adrenocortical hormones—the corticosteroids (glucocorticoids and mineralocorticoids). Its medulla (central core) secretes the adrenomedullary hormones (epinephrine and norepinephrine).

ADVERSE DRUG REACTIONS Seriously unpleasant or harmful effects of drugs caused by doses used for normal therapeutic use. The term is usually used for reactions that are more serious than normal **side effects**.

ADVERSE EFFECTS see **adverse drug reactions; side effect**.

AEROSOLS Aerosols are used as a means of giving drugs as fine droplets in a spray, often from a nebulizer, generally into the airways.

AI see **adequate intake**.

ALGAE Any of a large group of marine plants and protists that contain chlorophyll and other valuable nutrients, such as iodine (for example in kelp), protein, and vitamins.

ALKALOID Any of a group of chemically similar compounds, many with medicinal properties. Alkaloids are present in plants and herbal remedies, and also are used as conventional drugs (for example, morphine and quinine).

ALLERGEN A foreign chemical to which the body has become sensitive. Exposure to an allergen can cause an **allergic reaction** in hypersensitive people.

ALLERGIC REACTION The response by the antibodies of the immune system to the presence of allergens (often foreign proteins). These reactions may be local (such as inflammation) or generalized (as in **anaphylactic shock**).

ALLERGY see **allergic reaction**.

ALPHA-ADRENERGIC RECEPTOR (ALPHA-ADRENOCEPTOR; ALPHA-RECEPTOR) One of two recognition sites in the body that are naturally stimulated by the hormone epinephrine and the **neurotransmitter** norepinephrine. The other is the **beta-adrenergic receptor**.

ALTERATIVE A term commonly used in herbal medicine to mean an agent that favorably alters the course of the disease, and gradually restores health. It is sometimes implied that it works by increasing the excretion of waste and elimination of toxins from the circulatory systems, and so the term is used synonymously with "blood cleansers."

ALTERNATIVE MEDICINE (COMPLEMENTARY MEDICINE) These are general terms sometimes applied to non-orthodox, traditional, or alternative systems of medicine and healing, including herbal medicines, homeopathy, faith-healing, hypnosis, acupuncture, and aromatherapy. These alternative treatments are not usually administered by registered practitioners, and are not normally subject to objective proof of efficacy through clinical trials.

AMEBA A form of microscopic single-celled organism, until recently classified as a subclass of the protozoa family. Amebae can sometimes be **pathogenic**.

AMEBICIDAL An agent that kills amebae.

AMENORRHEA The term used to describe the stopping or absence of menstrual periods.

AMINO ACIDS The chemical building blocks of peptides and proteins. Some amino acids also have roles in their own right (for example, the amino acid glycine is a **neurotransmitter**).

ANALGESIC A drug that relieves pain (a "painkiller").

ANALGESIC ANODYNE A term commonly used in herbal medicine to mean pain reliever.

ANALOGS Chemicals or drugs that are closely related in chemical structure.

ANAPHRODISIAC In herbal medicine, herbs that decrease sexual feelings or desires.

ANAPHYLACTIC SHOCK A severe hypersensitivity reaction to a foreign substance to which the body has previously become sensitized. The result of such a reaction is a life-threatening state with a massive release of histamine and other inflammatory mediators causing hypotensive shock and cardiovascular collapse, severe bronchoconstriction, swelling of the tongue and throat, raised (nettle-like) rash, abdominal pain, and diarrhea.

ANESTHETIC An agent that produces complete (a general anesthetic) or partial (a local anesthetic) loss of feeling.

ANNUAL A plant that completes its growth cycle in one year.

ANODYNE A term commonly used in herbal medicine to refer to herbs that help relieve pain and reduce nerve sensitivity.

ANOXIA A state in which the tissues of the body receive an inadequate oxygen supply.

ANTHELMINTIC (ANTHELMINTHIC; ANTIHELMINTHIC) An agent that destroys and expels worms and flukes from the intestines.

ANTIBACTERIAL A substance that kills bacteria (bactericidal) or inhibits their growth or reproduction (bacteriostatic).

ANTIBODY A protein substance produced in humans and higher animals in response to an **antigen**, which has the particular property of binding to the antigen which induced its formation.

ANTICANCER (ANTINEOPLASTIC) An agent that prevents or treats cancer.

ANTINEOPLASTIC see anticancer.

ANTICOAGULANT A substance that slows or prevents the coagulation (clotting) of blood.

ANTIDIARRHEAL A substance that relieves diarrhea.

ANTIEMETIC A substance that prevents vomiting.

ANTIFUNGAL A substance that kills fungi or inhibits their growth or reproduction.

ANTIGENS Proteins that are treated by the body as foreign; antibodies (see **antibody**) in the blood react with them, making them harmless.

ANTIHIDROTIC (ANTIHYDROTIC) An agent that inhibits or prevents the production of sweat.

ANTI-INFLAMMATORY A substance that reduces inflammation. See also **antiphlogistic**.

ANTI-IRRITANT A substance that relieves irritation and itching.

ANTILITHOGENIC A substance that prevents the formation of stones (calculi; "gravel") in the urinary system (in herbal medicine, the term used is antilithic).

ANTIMICROBIAL A substance that kills and inhibits the growth of microorganisms.

ANTIOXIDANT A substance that protects against free radicals and helps to prevent damage to body cells, proteins, and the genetic material of cells.

ANTIPARASITIC A substance or procedure that kills parasites or inhibits their growth or reproduction.

ANTIPHLOGISTIC A term commonly used in herbal medicine to mean an agent that prevents or counteracts inflammation and fever. See **anti-inflammatory**.

ANTIPYRETIC A substance that reduces fever.

ANTISEPTIC A substance that inhibits the growth and reproduction of microbes. In other words, a substance that kills germs.

ANTISIALOGOGUE An agent that counteracts or prevents the formation and flow of saliva.

ANTISPASMODIC A substance that prevents or relieves smooth muscle spasms such as in intestinal colic.

ANTITUSSIVE A substance that prevents coughing.

ANTIULCER Treatment against ulcers.

ANTIULCEROGENIC A substance that prevents ulcer formation.

ANTIVIRAL A substance that acts against viruses, normally by inhibiting their growth or reproduction.

ANURIA Cessation of urine production.

APERIENT A term commonly used in herbal medicine to mean a mild laxative.

APLASIA Defective development of an organ or tissue (for example, in aplastic anemia).

AROMATIC An agent that possesses a fragrant odor.

ASTHENIA Weakness or loss of strength.

ASTRINGENT A substance that precipitates proteins from the surface of cells or mucous membranes, producing a protective coating.

ATAXIA Clumsiness and lack of coordination, with an unsteady gait, impaired eye and limb movements, and speech problems.

ATROPHY A wasting or reduction in size or functioning of a part of the body.

AUTOIMMUNE DISEASE A disease in which the immune system acts against tissue or organs within the individual's own body.

AUTONOMIC NERVOUS SYSTEM The bodily system that governs involuntary functions such as blood pressure, heart rate, and the activity of muscles of internal organs (for example, blood vessels, intestines, and secretions). The sympathetic nervous system—using the neurotransmitter norepinephrine (noradrenaline) and the hormone epinephrine (adrenaline)—is primarily involved in execution of these functions, often described as "fight, fright, and flight." In contrast, the parasympathetic nervous system—using the neurotransmitter acetylcholine—is more involved in functions such as glandular secretion and digestive processes.

AYURVEDIC The traditional system of Indian medicine which literally means "a science of life."

BACTERIA Small unicellular microbes of the class *Schizomycetes* that are **pathogenic** and are responsible for causing many diseases.

BACTERICIDAL Antibacterial agents, which act primarily by killing bacteria.

BACTERIOSTATIC Antibacterial agents, which act primarily by stopping bacterial growth.

BALSAM A term used in herbal medicine for an agent with healing or soothing properties. It also means a fragrant resin from trees with these properties.

BALSAMIC A term commonly used in herbal medicine to mean healing or soothing.

BENEFICIAL BACTERIA see **friendly bacteria**.

BENIGN In general, harmless conditions within the body. In relation to **tumors**, the term is used to mean a non-malignant (non-cancerous) growth; one that does not invade and destroy other cells or tissue.

BETA-ADRENERGIC RECEPTOR (BETA-ADRENOCEPTOR; BETA-RECEPTOR) One of two recognition sites that are naturally stimulated by the hormone epinephrine and the neurotransmitter norepinephrine. The other is the **alpha-adrenergic receptor**.

BIOFLAVONOID Any of a group of biologically active **flavonoids**.

BITTERS A substance that stimulates secretion of digestive juices and encourages appetite.

BLOCK (BLOCKER) The process in which an antagonist prevents an agonist drug exerting its effect, usually by preventing the action of the agonist drug at a receptor.

BLOOD PURIFICATION A term commonly used in herbal medicine to mean the removal of undesirable agents from the blood.

BLOOD–BRAIN BARRIER The means by which the nerves of the brain are normally kept separate from the blood cells and large molecules within the blood.

BONE MARROW DEPRESSION A reduction in the production of blood cells by the bone marrow. It often occurs after chemotherapy for cancer and may cause anemia, abnormal bleeding, or infection.

BRADYCARDIA A slowed rate of heartbeat.

BRADYKINESIA Slow and poor movement, as seen in Parkinson's disease and as **extrapyramidal symptoms** caused by several groups of drugs (for example, the phenothiazines) as a side effect.

BRONCHOCONSTRICTION (BRONCHOSPASM) A narrowing of the bronchioles (small airways) of the lungs.

BRONCHODILATION A widening of the bronchioles (small airways) of the lungs.

BRONCHOSPASM see **bronchoconstriction**.

BUCCAL A method of giving medication in

which a tablet is held between the cheek and the teeth or gum until it dissolves, from where the active constituents are absorbed into the blood circulation in that region of the mouth, and from there into the systemic circulation.

BULK LAXATIVE A laxative that increases the larger volume of feces, producing larger, softer stools.

B-VITAMIN COMPLEX A group of water-soluble vitamins that differ from each other chemically and in their biological effects, but which are generally taken together.

CALCULOSIS A term commonly used in herbal medicine to mean formation of calculi or "stones."

CALMATIVE A mild sedative or calming effect.

CAPSULES Containers made of gelatin, or something similar, for liquid or solid (for example, powder) forms of drugs that are to be taken by mouth. Capsules allow complex formulation of the constituent drug(s), including modified-release preparations, (especially modified-release versions, where release takes place over a period of time and so reduces the frequency of dosing).

CARCINOGEN A cancer-causing agent.

CARCINOMA A malignant type of neoplasm, a cancerous growth, which arises in the epithelium (which lines the internal organs and skin).

CARDIAC STIMULANT An agent that stimulates the action of the heart.

CARDIOACTIVE Affecting heart function.

CARDIOPROTECTIVE A substance or procedure that serves to protect the heart (for instance, from toxic agents).

CARMINATIVE An agent that removes gas from the intestinal canal and reduces flatulence, so relieving distension, digestive colic, and gastric discomfort.

CATHARTIC A term commonly used in herbal medicine to mean an agent that causes evacuation of the bowels. It may be either mild (laxative) or harsh (purgative).

CENTRAL NERVOUS SYSTEM (CNS) The division of the nervous system comprising the brain within the skull and spinal cord within the vertebrae. The remainder of the nervous system is termed the peripheral nervous system.

CHEMICAL DRUG NAMES Chemical names for drugs are not normally used outside technical circles, because although they are precise and unambiguous, they can be very large and unwieldy. In its place is substituted an official trivial or shortened name, a generic drug name, though this may unfortunately vary between countries. For instance, N-(4-hydroxyphenyl)acetamide is a chemical name for the analgesic drug with the generic name acetaminophen (also called paracetamol).

CHEMOTHERAPY The treatment or prevention of disease by means of chemical substances. The term is often restricted to the drug treatment of cancer in contrast to radiotherapy.

CHOLAGOGIC see cholagogue.

CHOLAGOGUE (CHOLAGOG) Any agent that stimulates the flow of bile from the gallbladder into the duodenum (part of the small intestine). It may also have a laxative effect. Such an agent is said to be cholagogic.

CHOLERETIC Increases the secretion of bile by the liver.

CHOLESTEROL. A waxy lipid (a sterol) found only in animal tissues. Cholesterol aids in the absorption and transport of fatty acids and acts as a precursor for vitamin D.

CHOLINERGIC Nerve fibres that release the neurotransmitter acetylcholine.

CHRONIC A disease of long duration, usually of slow onset and slowly reversing (if at all). It does not mean severe. See also acute.

CIRCADIAN RHYTHM (DIURNAL RHYTHM) An intrinsic pattern of rhythmic changes in the body over a period of 24 hours.

CIRCULATORY STIMULANT A term commonly used in herbal medicine to mean a substance that increases blood flow.

CLINICAL PHARMACOLOGY A term that encompasses all aspects of the scientific study of drugs in people.

CLINICAL TRIAL A systematic study of medically active agents in people. Such trials advance through early phases in normal volunteers (to determine duration of action and metabolism), to eventual studies in patients with disease. Commonly, new active agents are compared to existing standard treatments and to dummy treatments (placebos). To avoid bias, assessment of the efficacy of treatment may be single-blind (where either the patient or the doctor does not know the identity of treatments) or double-blind (where neither knows until the trial is finished).CNS see central nervous system.

COLORECTAL Pertaining to the lower gut; the colon and rectum.

COMMINUTED A term commonly used in herbal medicine to mean a preparation made from materials crushed or broken into small pieces.

COMMISSION E Indications for a herbal remedy relating to the Commission E monographs published by the German Federal Health Agency (BfArM).

COMPLEMENTARY MEDICINE see alternative medicine.

COMPLIANCE The extent to which patient behavior accords with medical advice. In relation to drugs, the term relates to the accuracy and frequency of taking prescribed medicines (which can be surprisingly low).

CONGENITAL A condition that is present at birth.

CONTAGIOUS A disease that can be transmitted by direct or indirect contact.

CONTRAINDICATION A situation in which a treatment must not be used because it might be hazardous to a person under the specified conditions (common examples are those who have liver or kidney impairments, heart conditions, or who are pregnant).

CONTROLLED SUBSTANCES see Schedule.

COUMARIN A class of chemical substances with anticoagulant properties, originally discovered when spoiled sweetclover, fed to farm animals in the US in the 1920s as a corn substitute, caused an epidemic of hemorrhagic deaths. The coumarin analogs warfarin sodium and dicumarol are important drugs in medical treatment today (they "thin the blood").

CYCLO-OXYGENASE An enzyme involved in the bodily production of the inflammatory mediators called prostaglandins, and which is blocked by the NSAID (non-steroidal anti-inflammatory drug) class of drugs.

DAB Deutsches Arzneibuch (German Pharmacopoeia).

DECOCTION A term commonly used in herbal medicine to mean a liquid medicine made by boiling the plant parts in water or other liquid for a period of time.

DECONGESTANT A substance or procedure that reduces or eliminates congestion and swelling. The congestion is normally taken to be in the airways, and agents may be used locally in the nose for nasal congestion, or inhaled for a more general decongestant action.

DEFICIENCY If a person is deficient in a vitamin or mineral they lack that particular nutrient and have developed clinical signs of deficiency.

DEGENERATIVE The gradual deterioration of normal cells and body functions.

DEMULCENT A substance that soothes the irritation or inflammation of skin and mucous membranes and other surfaces; a meaning extended in herbal medicine to mean a preparation rich in **mucilage** and that can soothe and protect even internal tissue such as gastric mucous membranes.

DEPENDENCE A state in which regular, repeated, and probably excessive taking of an agent causes a person to become accustomed to it, resulting in detrimental effects. Also termed addiction.

DERIVATIVE Originating from another substance.

DETOXIFICATION The process by which a poisonous substance is made harmless.

DIAGNOSIS The identification and naming of a disease or disorder.

DIAPHORETIC (SUDORIFIC) A substance, procedure, or condition that induces sweating or excessive perspiration. The term is commonly extended in herbal medicine to mean a substance that promotes circulation, dispels fever and chills, and eliminates surface toxins.

DIETARY REFERENCE INTAKE (DRI) A new standard for nutrient recommendations that can be used to plan and assess diets for healthy people.

DIGESTIVES A term commonly used in herbal medicine to mean substances that assist the stomach and intestines in digestion.

DILATATION A widening of a hollow organ, commonly applied to blood vessels (vasodilatation).

DIURNAL RHYTHM see **circadian rhythm**.

DIURETIC A substance that induces increased urine flow.

DOCTRINE OF SIGNATURES A theory in herbal medicine that nature provides remedies for maladies close to their causes, and that in the cure the appearance of a plant indicates its inherent medical properties.

DOPAMINE A monoamine **neurotransmitter**, particularly in the central nervous system. It also occurs naturally in some plants.

DOSE The amount of a drug administered. The dose is critical in order to achieve the desired therapeutic effect without unnecessary adverse effects or side effects.

DRI see **Dietary Reference Intake**.

DRUG ABUSE The non-medical use of drugs, without intent to prevent, treat, or cure disease (for example, recreational use).

DRUG DEPENDENCE see **dependence**.

DRUG INTERACTIONS Drug interactions occur when one drug changes the magnitude of effect, duration of action, or side effects of the other.

DRUG SCREENING The process of testing chemical agents for given types of pharmacological activity and possible therapeutic uses.

DYS- This prefix means abnormal or disturbed.

DYSFUNCTIONAL Abnormal or disturbed body function.

DYSKINESIA Abnormal muscle movements, such as jerking and twitching (for example, in **tardive dyskinesia**).

DYSPHAGIA Difficulty in swallowing.

DYSPHORIA A feeling of discomfort or lack of well being (as opposed to **euphoria**).

DYSTONIA A disorder of skeletal muscle tone (either increased or decreased), which causes abnormal bodily positions and movements.

ECLECTIC A system of treatment that selects and combines diverse techniques from several systems or philosophies; incorporated into herbal medicine used in the US in the 19th century.

ECTOPIC Not in its right or normal position.

ECT see **electroconvulsive therapy**.

EDEMA An abnormal accumulation of fluid in the body tissues.

EFFICACY In therapeutics, efficacy is the capacity of a drug to produce the desired effect or result.

ELECTROCONVULSIVE THERAPY (ECT) A treatment for affective ("mood") disorders involving the induction of a brief convulsion by passing an electrical current through the brain.

ELEMENT One of more than 100 simple substances that cannot be broken down by chemical means into another substance. Many are necessary for life. Examples include oxygen, nitrogen, carbon, calcium, sodium, and potassium.

ELIXIR A medicated liquid preparation taken by mouth, which is intended to disguise a potentially unpleasant taste. Elixirs often include a sweetening substance, such as glycerol or alcohol, and frequently aromatic agents.

EMBOLUS A foreign object (for example, air, tissue, thrombus) that circulates in the bloodstream.

EMBROCATION A term commonly used in herbal medicine to mean a preparation for external rubbing-in. Embrocations usually appear as a liniment or in another liquid form.

EMETIC A substance that causes vomiting.

EMMENAGOGUE A term commonly used in herbal medicine to mean an agent that brings on or stimulates menstrual flow.

EMOLLIENT A medication that softens and soothes, particularly the skin.

ENDOCRINE A chemical messenger system that involves ductless glands secreting hormones directly into the blood or lymph to be carried to their target tissue.

ENDOGENOUS Produced within the body; in contrast to exogenous agents, which are administered to the body.

ENDOMETRIUM The mucous membrane layer lining the uterus.

ENDOTHELIUM The tissue that lines the blood vessels, heart, and lymphatic vessels.

ENDOTOXIN A toxin that is part of the structure of a microorganism, and which may be responsible for part of the **pathogenic** symptoms of (notably bacterial) infection.

ENEMA An infusion of liquid into the rectum, via the anus.

ENTERAL Pertaining to the intestinal tract.

ENTERIC-COATED TABLETS Tablets that are covered with a layer (originally shellac varnish) that dissolves slowly. They are intended to prevent release until the tablet has left the stomach and enters the intestine for absorption, because the active drug irritates the stomach lining (for example, aspirin) or is broken down by gastric juices.

ENZYME A protein, usually in combination with a trace mineral or vitamin, which regulates the speed at which a chemical reaction occurs in the body

EPINEPHRINE (ADRENALINE) A natural hormone secreted by the adrenal gland.

EPITHELIUM The tissue that covers the entire external surface of the body (for example, the skin) and lines the hollow organs of the body.

ERUCTATION The act of belching.

ERYTHROCYTES Red blood cells.

ESCHERICHIA COLI (E. coli) Rod-shaped bacteria that normally inhabit the gut without causing problems, but in the form of newly emerging **pathogenic** strains, sometimes may lead to urinary or intestinal infection and food poisoning.

ESOP see **European Scientific Cooperative on Phytotherapy**.

ESSENTIAL A substance that cannot be manufactured by the body so must be supplied in the diet.

ESSENTIAL FATTY ACID A fatty acid that cannot be manufactured by the body and which must therefore be supplied as part of the diet.

ESSENTIAL OIL Volatile oil extracted from plants by steam distillation and containing a mixture of active constituents.

ESTROGEN REPLACEMENT A therapy in which female sex hormone is replaced, especially during the menopause. See also **hormone replacement therapy**.

ESTROGENS Steroid sex hormones (for example, estriol, estradiol) that promote the growth and functioning of the female sex organs and the development of female secondary sexual characteristics. Estrogens are produced and secreted mainly by the ovaries (and to a small extent the placenta of pregnant women, the adrenal cortex in both sexes, and, in men, the testes). Some non-steroid compounds, called phytoestrogens, found in plants (especially soybean products) have a weak estrogenic action.

ESTROGENIC Having the properties of estrogens.

ETIOLOGY The cause of a disease, and the study of the factors involved in causing it.

EUPHORIA A feeling of confident well being.

EUROPEAN SCIENTIFIC COOPERATIVE ON PHYTOTHERAPY (ESOP) An organization of scientists, formed in 1990, with expertise in various aspects of phytomedicine, which publishes monographs on medicinal plants used in Western Europe.

EXCRETION The removal of a substance from the body.

EXOCRINE Glands that secrete substances, for instance an enzyme or a fluid, through a duct (for example, the salivary glands).

EXOGENOUS From outside the body; in contrast to endogenous agents or influences that come from within the body.

EXOTOXIN A (generally highly toxic) toxin secreted by microorganisms into their surroundings and which can work at a distance.

EXPECTORANT A substance that helps to remove mucus from the lungs, sometimes acting to reduce the viscosity of phlegm and mucus in the respiratory tract.

EXTRACTION A term commonly used in herbal medicine to mean the part of a plant that is removed in making a herbal preparation in a liquid or solid form.

EXTRAPYRAMIDAL SYMPTOMS OF MOVEMENT Symptoms (for example, **tardive dyskinesia**) that are caused by several groups of drugs (such as certain antipsychotics) as an adverse reaction due to their effects on certain areas of the brain.

FAMILIAL DISEASES Those diseases found in some families, but not others, and that are largely genetically determined.

FAT-SOLUBLE VITAMIN Vitamins that dissolve in fats and not water. Examples include vitamins A, D, E, and K. The body can store these vitamins for longer than **water-soluble vitamins**.

FDA see **Food and Drug Administration**.

FEBRIFUGE An agent that helps reduce a fever; a term commonly used in herbal medicine.

FEBRILE Elevated body temperature (fever).

5-HT see **serotonin**.

5-HYDROXYTRYPTAMINE see **serotonin**.

FLAVONOID Any of a large group of several thousand organic, colored phytochemicals, which can have beneficial effects on the body, and are found in plant foods such as fruit, grains, and vegetables. Flavonoids are responsible for bright red, orange, and yellow colors (for example, rutin and quercetin). They can be divided chemically into subgroups, including the anthrocyanosides (the red pigment in blackberries and red wine) and the isoflavones (in soya). Some of the isoflavones (also known as soya isoflavones) are phytoestrogens (having estrogenic hormonal properties), and are commonly incorporated into supplements. Additionally, many bioflavonoids have powerful antioxidant properties, some may act to lower cholesterol and exert other beneficial cardiovascular effects.

FLUORINE An element added in the form of sodium fluoride to drinking water to prevent dental caries.

FOOD AND DRUG ADMINISTRATION (FDA) The US federal agency responsible for the enforcement of federal regulations concerning the manufacture and distribution of food, drugs, and cosmetics. The basic intent is to prevent the sale of impure or dangerous substances. Closely associated with the FDA is the Center for Drug Evaluation and Research (CDER), which examines drugs both for safety and therapeutic effectiveness.

FORMULARY A book (or, increasingly, a computer database) that details formulations or doses of drugs. In the US, the publication of record is the United States Pharmacopeia.

FORMULATION The pharmaceutical term for the form of a medicine: that is, capsule, tablet, pill, cream, lotion, emulsion, solution, pessary, suppository, form for injection, and so on.

FORTIFIED Enriched. For example, milk powder fortified with calcium has been enriched with added calcium.

FREE RADICAL An atom of a group of atoms that is highly chemically reactive because it has at least one unpaired electron. Being highly reactive, it can join readily with other compounds (for example, DNA or membrane lipids) and so attack cells and cause damage.

FREE RADICAL SCAVENGER A substance that reacts with **free radicals** and thereby removes or destroys them.

FRIENDLY BACTERIA Bacteria that are present in the gut which help to maintain the health and balance of the digestive system (for example, *Lactobacillus acidophilus*).

FUNGI A general term for plant-like organisms that lack chlorophyll, a true stem, leaves, and roots, and reproduce through spores. Fungi generally live as parasites or saprophytes (on dead matter). They include yeasts, moulds, mildews, and mushrooms. Very few species are pathogenic to humans, and they mostly cause disease only in pre-existing sickness, as in AIDS.

G6PD-DEFICIENCY (GLUCOSE-6-PHOSPHATE DEHYDROGENASE ENZYME DEFICIENCY) A largely **familial disease** that can lead to adverse drug reactions with certain medications.

GALACTORRHEA Excessive or spontaneous

lactation (milk production), not necessarily associated with childbirth or nursing.

GALENIC PREPARATION A term commonly used in herbal medicine to mean medical preparations from plants as opposed to refined chemicals.

GALENICAL A traditional system of Western medicine based on the four humors theory (four bodily fluids: blood, phlegm, choler or yellow bile, melancholy or black bile) of Ancient Greece.

GEL A formulation of a medicine as a jelly-like mass; convenient for topical (external) application.

GENERATIONS OF DRUGS Generations of drugs are "created" when, in the development of a class of drugs, a significant advance occurs (in potency, duration of action, absorption, spectrum of action, fewer side effects, and so on). For example, first-, second-, and third-generation cephalosporins.

GENERIC DRUG NAME The official non-proprietary (standard) name for the active chemical(s) in a medicine, in contrast to the proprietary name (trade or brand name) for a medicine. Official names include the recommended International Non-proprietary Name (rINN), and the United States Adopted Name (USAN), and these may differ.

GENETIC ENGINEERING The use of techniques to modify the structure of genes, or to create or delete genes. Potentially, these techniques may be used to correct diseases in humans due to genetic defects (for example, cystic fibrosis). Use in animal husbandry (for instance to produce medical protein hormones) is now quite advanced. Many drug proteins specific to humans are now made by a branch of genetic engineering called recombinant DNA technology, in which part of the human gene sequence is inserted into cells such as those of bacteria or fungi, which then synthesize the required human protein.

GENITOURINARY TRACT (UROGENITAL TRACT; URINOGENITAL TRACT) The sexual organs and bladder, and related structures.

GENOME The total genetic material of an organism, which, in humans, is the genes that are contained in 23 pairs of chromosomes.

GERMICIDE A substance that kills germs (microbes).

GERMIFUGE A term commonly used in herbal medicine to refer to a substance that expels germs.

GLUCOCORTICOIDS One of the two types of steroid hormones secreted by the cortex of the adrenal gland (for instance, cortisone). The other type are called **mineralocorticoid** hormones.

GLYCOSIDE Plant constituent containing one or more sugar groups with substituted constituents; some are pharmacologically active and important in medicine, especially cardiac glycosides (digoxin, digitoxin).

GOITER (GOITRE) A collection of disease states characterized by an enlarged thyroid gland.

GRAS An acronym for "generally recognized as safe" by experts and accepted by the Food and Drug Administration.

GREEN DRINKS Natural food formulas made from plants that are promoted as "detoxifiers" and "blood cleansers." They are also a good source of minerals, chlorophyll, and other nutrients.

GYNECOMASTIA (GYNAECOMASTIA) Enlargement of breasts in men.

HABITUATION A state in which regular (possibly excessive) taking of an agent (usually a drug) causes the individual to become accustomed to it, but not to the extreme psychological or physical stage of **dependence** (addiction).

HDL see **high-density lipoprotein**.

HELMINTH Worms, flukes, and similar organisms that are sometimes **pathogenic** to people. Agents that expel or kill them are called anthelmintics, anthelminthics, antihelminthics, or **vermifuges**.

HEMOGLOBIN The oxygen-carrying pigment of the red blood cells (erythrocytes).

HEMOLYSIS (HAEMOLYSIS) The destruction of red blood cells (erythrocytes).

HEMOSTATIC (HAEMOSTATIC) An agent that stops bleeding.

HEPATIC Pertaining to the liver. The term is commonly used in herbal medicine to mean a substance that aids the liver, tones, strengthens, and increases bile flow.

HEPATOPROTECTIVE An agent that protects the liver.

HEPATOTOXIC An agent that is toxic to the liver.

HERB Any plant that is used for culinary or medicinal purposes.

HERBAL MEDICINES Those medicines derived from plants.

HERBALIST A person who practices herbal medicine, including the preparation of herbal remedies.

HIGH-DENSITY LIPOPROTEIN (HDL) A plasma protein made in the liver and containing 50 percent protein with cholesterol and triglycerides. HDL is involved in transporting cholesterol and other lipids to the liver for disposal (see **lipid**).

HIRSUTISM Excessive bodily hair distributed in a masculine pattern.

HOMEOPATHIC A system of complementary medicine founded by Hahnemann in Germany in the early 19th century. In homeopathy, substances are administered to the body in minute amounts, using agents that at normal concentration mimic or cause the same symptoms as those of the disease being treated. Homeopathic medicines are labeled using a system indicating the (normally very high) degree of dilution.

HORMONE REPLACEMENT THERAPY Any therapy in which a deficiency of a given **hormone** is rectified by administering replacement hormone, either in a natural form or as a synthetic analog (for instance thyroid hormone). Often the term is used as synonymous with "hormone replacement" in menopause, which is sometimes termed HRT, and involves the replacement of estrogen and sometimes progestin.

HORMONE A chemical messenger released in small amounts into the blood or lymph from a ductless gland of the **endocrine** system. Such a messenger acts on some remote tissue or organ (for example, thyroid and adrenal corticosteroid hormones). Some other mediator substances not released from a specialized cell or gland, and which act locally, are called local hormones (they include histamine and the prostaglandins).

HRT see **hormone replacement therapy**.

HYPER- In medical terms, this prefix denotes "above normal."

HYPERPLASIA An increase in the production and growth of normal cells in a tissue. In hyperplasia, the organ becomes bigger but retains its form (an example is the increase in size of the uterus in pregnancy).

HYPERREACTIVITY see **hypersensitivity reaction**.

HYPERSENSITIVITY REACTION A condition in which the individual is prone to respond abnormally or in an exaggerated way to a chemical or drug.

HYPERTROPHY An increase in the size of an organ or tissue brought about by an increase in the size of its cells (for example, in muscles with exercise), rather than by an increase in the number of cells (as in **tumors**).

HYPNOTIC A substance that induces sleep.

HYPO- In medical terms, this prefix denotes "below normal."

HYPOCALCEMIA Low levels of calcium in the blood.

HYPOKALEMIA Low levels of potassium in the blood.

HYPOGLYCEMIA Low levels of sugars in the blood.

HYPOTENSION Lower than normal blood pressure.

IDIOSYNCRATIC RESPONSE A rare **adverse drug reaction** which often is unexpected and occurs only in some people.

ILLICIT DRUG USE see **drug abuse.**

IMMUNE SYSTEM The cells, tissues, and mediators that protect the body against pathological (disease-causing) organisms and other foreign bodies.

IMMUNITY The protection against infection and disease conferred on the body through the activity of the immune system, comprising circulating antibodies and white blood cells.

IMMUNOCOMPROMISED A person whose immune defenses are very much lower than normal due either to a **congenital**, or an acquired condition, for example due to infection (as in AIDS).

IMMUNODEFICIENCY A state in which the immune system is deficient and so unable to protect the body properly from infection and other diseases; often due to low levels of the immunoglobulins necessary to produce antibodies (see **antibody**). This may result from a genetic defect or other diseases.

IMMUNOSTIMULANT An agent that is used to boost the efficiency of the body's immune system, and so improve defense against infections and possibly malignant growths.

IMPLANT A form of drug administration in which a solid formulation of the drug is implanted either into a muscle or just below the skin.

INDUCIBLE A protein or gene whose synthesis is stimulated by a specific inducing agent.

INFUSION The continuous administration (by injection, most commonly into a vein) of a drug or fluid over a period of minutes, hours, or days. In herbal use, it means a preparation of a remedy by steeping plant material in liquid to extract its medicinal substances (without boiling, as with **decoction**).

INJECTION Administration of a drug or fluid by means of a needle and syringe.

INN see **generic drug name**.

INTERNATIONAL PHARMACOPOEIA (INT. P) The pharmacopoeia of the World Health Organization; a **formulary** intended to meet international needs.

INTOLERANCE A state in which there is a greater than expected reaction to a drug.

INTRA- This prefix means "within."

INTRADERMAL An injection that is made into the skin, rather than under the skin, which is "subcutaneous."

INTRAMUSCULAR An injection that is made into a muscle.

INTRANASAL Taking a drug via the nose (for example, using a nasal spray).

INTRAOCULAR PRESSURE The pressure within the eyeball, which helps to maintain its shape. The pressure is kept balanced by the supply and removal of aqueous humor.

INTRATHECAL An injection that is made into the subarachnoid space in the spinal cord.

INTRAVENOUS An injection that is made into a vein.

INTERNATIONAL UNIT (IU) A quantity of a substance such as a vitamin that produces a specific internationally accepted biological effect.

ISOMER Forms of a chemical compound in which the number and type of molecules is identical, but in which the arrangement of the atoms within the molecules is different. Isomers are important with regard to drugs, because the different forms have differing chemical and biological properties. It may be difficult or expensive to chemically separate out the active form, and if one of a pair is relatively inactive as a drug, the mixture (racemic mixture, sometimes called the *dl*-form) may be used.

LATIN NAME The Latin name of a plant or animal is the name given by the binomial taxonomic system invented by the 18th-century Swedish name indicates the genus and the second gives the species.

LAXATIVE An agent that promotes gentle evacuation of the bowels.

LDL see **low-density lipoprotein**.

LEGUME The edible part of pod-bearing plants such as peas and beans.

LEUCOPENIA A condition in which there is a low level of leucocytes (white blood cells) in the bloodstream.

LINCTUS A medicated syrup that is used to relieve a sore throat or to loosen a cough.

LINIMENT A medicated lotion for rubbing into the skin. Many liniments contain alcohol and/or camphor, and are intended to relieve minor muscle aches and pains.

LIPID Any of a group of organic compounds consisting of fats, oils, and other substances that make up living cells. Blood contains various important lipids, including the lipoproteins, made in the liver (for example, phospholipids, cholesterol, and triglycerides). The lipoproteins can be divided into high-density lipoproteins (HDL) and low-density lipoproteins (LDL), and an increase in the level of LDL in the blood plasma indicates a greater risk of atherosclerosis.

LOCAL This term is used to mean that the action of a drug is limited to a certain area of the body (for example, local anesthetic).

LOCAL HORMONE A chemical messenger that acts locally (see **hormone**).

LOTION A medicated liquid that is used to bathe or wash skin, hair, or eyes.

LOW-DENSITY LIPOPROTEIN (LDL) A protein found in the blood's plasma that contains relatively more cholesterol and triglycerides than protein. LDL transports cholesterol to body tissues. Its high cholesterol content may account for the greater risk of atherosclerosis when the level of LDL is increased (see also **lipid**).

LOZENGE A medication contained in a hard, often sweetened and flavored, base.

LYMPHATIC SYSTEM A complex system that drains fluid from the body's cells back into the veins of the blood system. It has many other important functions, and includes specialized lymphatic organs such as the tonsils, thymus, and the spleen.

LYMPHOMA A malignant disease; a cancer arising in the tissues of the lymphatic system (mainly of the lymph nodes and spleen).

MACERATION A term commonly used in herbal medicine to mean the softening of a herbal remedy by soaking plant material in a liquid.

MACRONUTRIENT A term sometimes used to describe protein, fat, and carbohydrate.

MALIGNANT In general, this term describes any condition in the body which if untreated may be a threat to health (for example, malignant hypertension). Specifically, it describes a **tumor** that invades and destroys other cells or tissues; a cancerous tumor.

MARINE OILS Oils obtained from marine animals (for example, cod-liver oil). Marine oils are rich in **essential fatty acids**.

METABOLISM OF DRUGS The process by which the body detoxifies chemicals and excretes (removes) them.

METASTASIS The process by which malignant **tumor** cells spread to distinct parts of the body.

METHEMOGLOBIN An oxidized form of **hemoglobin**. This form is not able to carry oxygen, so production of it can lead to toxic **anoxia**.

MICROBE Any tiny, usually microscopic, entity capable of carrying on living processes, also called a microorganism.

MICRONUTRIENT Vitamins, minerals, and other nutrients that are only needed in small amounts.

MICROORGANISM see **microbe**.

-MIMETIC This suffix means to imitate or mimic.

MINERAL Any inorganic compound found in nature. The elements in many minerals (for example, calcium, iodine, zinc, iron) are required in small amounts by the body.

MINERALOCORTICOID Mineralocorticoid hormones are one of the two types of corticosteroids secreted by the cortex (inner core) of the adrenal gland (the other type is the **glucocorticoid** hormones). See also **adrenal**.

MODIFIED-RELEASE PREPARATIONS see **capsules**.

MOLECULAR BIOLOGY The study of biology at the molecular level. Recently, this term has taken on special meanings and is used particularly to denote the study of genes, gene products, and sometimes pharmaceuticals produced by processes using genetic methods.

MONOCLONAL ANTIBODY A type of pure **antibody** with specially selected properties, manufactured by the techniques of **molecular biology**.

MUCILAGE 1. A sticky, viscous substance from a plant consisting of a gum dissolved in juice from the plant. 2. A soothing medication made from plant gums.

MUCOUS MEMBRANE The moist membrane (thin sheets of tissue) that lines internal structures such as the mouth, the intestine, respiratory tract including the lungs, and the genitourinary tract.

MULTI-DRUG RESISTANCE Resistance to the actions of a number of different drugs of different classes.

MULTI-DRUG THERAPY The treatment of a medical problem by using a number of drugs together in a concerted manner.

MYCOBACTERIA A type of bacterial microorganism, including *Mycobacteria tuberculosis*, which causes tuberculosis.

MYCOPLASMA A type of microorganism, one of the smallest known free-living organisms, regarded by some as an early sort of bacteria.

MYELOSUPPRESSION Interference with the production of blood cells and platelets in the bone marrow.

NARCOTIC A substance that causes insensibility, stupor, and sleep. The term is applied to all opiate-type analgesics (since, at high doses, they have this property). The use of the term in medicine does not correlate with its legislative and legal use (for example, for substances whose use or possession may be regulated by the Bureau for International Narcotics and Law Enforcement Affairs or the Federal Drug Enforcement Agency).

NARCOTIC ADDICT A person who is psychologically and physically dependent on **narcotic** analgesic drugs, either derived from opium or made synthetically.

NASAL SPRAY A way of administering a drug in the form of a spray in the nostrils.

NATRIURETIC A substance or drug acting on the kidney. A natriuretic increases sodium excretion from the blood into the urine.

NEOPLASM Any abnormal or new growth. Correctly, the term can be applied to relatively harmless swellings (benign) or cancerous (malignant) growths (see **tumor**). Nevertheless, the term neoplastic disease is often loosely taken to mean the same as cancerous growth.

NERVE see **neuron**.

NERVINE A term commonly used in herbal medicine to mean something that strengthens or calms nerves and affects the nervous system. It may be stimulating, sedating, or relaxing.

NEUROLOGICAL Pertaining to the nervous system.

NEURON (NEURONE) The main cell type that makes up the nervous system. Neurons are specially adapted to transmit signals.

NEUROPATHY Inflammation or degeneration of peripheral nerves (see **peripheral nervous system**).

NEUROTRANSMITTER A chemical substance that transmits nerve signals from nerve-to-nerve, or nerve-to-organ.

NEUTROPENIA (GRANULOCYTOPENIA) A decrease in the number of neutrophils (one of the types of white blood cells) in the blood.

NICOTINIC RECEPTOR One of the two types of **cholinergic** receptor which "recognize" the **neurotransmitter** acetylcholine. They are found in, among other places, the central nervous system (CNS).

NON-PROPRIETARY NAME see **proprietary name**.

NOREPINEPHRINE (NORADRENALINE) A **neurotransmitter** found in the sympathetic nervous system (see **autonomic nervous system**).

NUTRACEUTICAL A food or nutrient-based supplement or product used for a specific therapeutic purpose.

NUTRACHEMICAL A food supplement.

NUTRITIVE A term commonly used in herbal medicine to mean nutritional foodstuff.

OFF-LABEL The use of a drug to treat a condition or disease not specifically approved in its course of evaluation by the Food and Drug Administration. Doctors may prescribe drugs for "off-label" or "unlabeled" use if it seems professionally reasonable and appropriate. Some off-label uses are quite routine, others may not be as well established or may reflect more recent research in therapy.

OINTMENT A general term used to describe a group of essentially greasy preparations which are insoluble in water and so do not wash off.

OLIGURIA The production of abnormally small amounts of urine.

OPHTHALMOLOGIC Pertaining to the eye.

ORTHOSTATIC HYPOTENSION see **postural**

hypotension.

OTC see **over-the-counter**.

OTOTOXICITY Toxic damage to the inner ear, including drug-induced damage to the nerve serving the inner ear, the cochlea, and the semicircular canals, causing some degree of deafness or loss of the sense of balance.

OVER-THE-COUNTER (OTC) Non-prescription medicines that can be bought at a pharmacy by members of the public without a doctor's prescription.

PALLIATIVE CARE Care designed to relieve or reduce the intensity of uncomfortable symptoms but not to produce a cure.

PALPITATION An awareness of the pulse or heart rhythm, commonly when there is a pounding or racing of the heart.

PARASITE An organism living in or on, and obtaining nourishment from, another organism.

PARASITICIDE An agent that destroys parasites, especially those on the skin.

PARASYMPATHETIC NERVOUS SYSTEM see **autonomic nervous system**.

PARENTERAL Giving a drug by any route other than orally, that is, by mouth and the digestive system.

PARESTHESIA Spontaneous feelings of subjective abnormal sensations such as tingling ("pins and needles"), prickling, burning, tightness, numbness, or the feeling of a band tight around a limb or the trunk of the body.

PARTURIENT A term meaning about to give birth, and commonly used in herbal medicine to mean a remedy that induces and promotes labor.

PARTURIFACIENT An agent that promotes, eases, or induces labor and birth.

PASSIVE IMMUNITY Passive immunity is achieved by injecting antibodies (see **antibody**) into the body, or by antibodies passing to the fetus through the placenta.

PASSIVE IMMUNIZATION A method of immunization in which an immune globulin (including an **antitoxin**) containing specific antibodies is injected into the bloodstream in order to counter an infection (or venom).

PASTILLE A soft lozenge.

PATENTS FOR DRUGS Patents may be granted to the inventor of a drug as a new chemical entity or as a new formulation of an existing drug. During the period of the patent (commonly 16 to 20 years for a new chemical entity or formulation,

but depending on the circumstances, and the country concerned), only a proprietary form of the drug (with a registered proprietary name or brand name) may be available for prescription and clinical use.

PATHOGENIC An agent that causes disease. Such agents (for example, microorganisms) are said to be pathogens.

PATHOLOGICAL Relating to disease, or to pathology, the study of disease.

-PATHY This suffix is used to denote disease (for example, neuropathy, encephalopathy, retinopathy).

PATIENT INFORMATION LEAFLET (PIL; PRODUCT INFORMATION LEAFLET) The technical information placed by the drug manufacturer in the packaging of medicines, and intended to be read by the patient or carer. It includes clearly stated information about special care or precautions to be taken when using a particular drug.

PDR Physicians' Desk Reference.

PECTORAL An old term for a medicine for chest and respiratory disorders, and still commonly used in that sense in herbal medicine.

PEPTIDE A sequence of amino acids such as is contained in a protein.

% RDA The percentage of the RDA (see **recommended dietary allowance**) of that nutrient contained in a given amount of the supplement. Sometimes listed in the nutritional information of supplements.

PERENNIAL A plant that grows for more than two growing seasons.

PERIPHERAL NERVOUS SYSTEM The division of the nervous system which is outside of the **central nervous system**.

PERISTALSIS The coordinated, rhythmic, and involuntary waves of muscular activity that move the contents of the intestines in the appropriate direction. The term also applies to movement in the ureter that helps move urine from the kidneys to the bladder.

PESSARY A formulation of a drug that is inserted into the vagina.

PHARMACIST A suitably qualified practitioner of pharmacy.

PHARMACOGNOSY The study of botanical and other sources of drugs, and the properties of crude drugs.

PHARMACOKINETICS The processes of absorption, distribution, and breaking

down of drugs ("what the body does to the drug").

PHARMACOLOGY The science of drugs, the effect of chemical substances have on living processes. It can be divided into pharmacodynamics ("what the drug does to the body") and pharmacokinetics ("what the body does to the drug"). It is much concerned with the development of new drugs.

PHARMACOPEIA A book that lists the official preparation of drugs.

PHARMACOPEIAL NAME The official name given to a particular drug preparation in the pharmacopoeias.

PHARMACY The preparation (formulation) and supply of medicines (and the place where it is done).

PHOSPHOLIPID One of a class of compounds found in living cells which contain phosphoric acid, fatty acids, and a nitrogenous base, for example, lecithin.

PHOTOPHOBIA An intolerance to light to the extent that normal light levels are uncomfortable.

PHOTOSENSITIVITY Abnormal reaction to sunlight (for example, a rash).

PHOTOTOXIC A type of photosensitivity reaction which occurs when the skin is exposed to a combination of the photosensitizing substance and light.

PHYSIOMEDICALISM A system of herbal medicine developed in the US in the 19th century.

PHYTOCHEMICAL Chemicals found in plants. The term is usually used to describe any of many substances that are present in fruit and vegetables and that have health-promoting properties.

PHYTOESTROGEN A type of **estrogen** found in plants.

PILLS Solid spherical or ovoid drug dose forms (originally made by a rolling process), which are now largely superseded by tablets.

PITUITARY GLAND An **endocrine** gland situated at the base of the brain.

PLACEBOS Dummy treatments, which have only psychological effects, used in clinical trials.

PLANT OIL Oil obtained from a plant (for example, evening primrose oil).

POISONS "All things are poisonous and there is nothing that is harmless, the dose alone decides that something is no poison." Paracelsus (1493–1541). This statement still applies, indeed, many compounds previously regarded as poisons are today used as medicines (for example, colchicine from the autumn crocus (*Colchicum autumnale*) and vinca alkaloids from the periwinkle (*Vinca rosea*).

POLYUNSATURATED FATTY ACIDS Fatty acids that chemically contain more than one double-bond in their structure. They are found in fish, soybeans, and sunflower seeds. Diets high in these fatty acids and low in saturated fatty acids have been correlated with low blood cholesterol levels in some populations.

PoM see **prescription-only medicine**.

PORPHYRIA One of a group of several relatively uncommon disease states in which the body's breakdown of the pigment heme (which occurs in the blood pigment hemoglobin) is disrupted, leading to the accumulation in the body of porphyrins, causing red, brown, or bluish urine.

POSTPARTUM After childbirth.

POSTURAL HYPOTENSION Abnormally low blood pressure when a person stands. Also called orthostatic hypotension.

POTENCY A term that refers to the strength of a drug, either in terms of the dose required to achieve a given effect, or the maximum effect that is achievable.

PREBIOTIC Supplements taken to enhance health by feeding **friendly bacteria** in the gut.

PREGNANCY CATEGORY A general classification of drugs by the degree of hazard they may pose if taken during pregnancy. The Food and Drug Administration's use-in-pregnancy rating system (A, B, C, D, X) weighs the degree to which available information has ruled out risk to the fetus against the drug's potential benefits. The categories range from category A, in which controlled studies in pregnant women show no risk to the fetus, to category X, in which the drug is to be avoided in pregnancy because of positive evidence of fetal abnormalities or risk which clearly outweighs any possible benefit.

PREMEDICATION Medication given prior to an operation.

PRESCRIPTION The document detailing to the pharmacist the name of the patient, the drug to be prescribed, the dose, and other details.

PRESCRIPTION-ONLY MEDICINE (PoM) Any medicine that must be prescribed by an appropriately qualified doctor ordered on a proper prescription form, and which cannot be bought **over-the-counter** (OTC). The designation of a drug preparation as "prescription-only" is made by the Food and Drug Administration. Some drugs are regulated by the Drug Enforcement Agency. For instance, drugs placed on a **Schedule** I to V basis are subject to special prescription restrictions.

PRIAPISM Prolonged erection of the penis. A painful condition requiring immediate treatment.

PRION A modified form of a protein thought to be responsible for the transmission of several neurodegenenerative diseases, including Creutzfeldt-Jacob disease in people.

PROBIOTIC Supplements that contain **friendly bacteria** which are taken to enhance health.

PRODRUG A chemical form of a drug that is not in itself pharmacologically active, but is converted in the body to the active drug . A prodrug may be preferred because it is chemically more stable or better absorbed than the active drug.

PROPHYLACTIC see **prophylaxis**.

PROPHYLAXIS Any measure taken in prevention of disease, conception, or other event.

PROPRIETARY NAME The trade name or brand name of a medicine; the name given to it by the manufacturer, in contrast to the official non-proprietary (**generic**) name for the active chemical(s) in a medicine.

PROTEINUREA The presence of increased amounts of protein in the urine.

PROTOZOA A single-celled microorganism of the phylum *Protozoa*

PRURITUS Itching.

PURGATIVE A substance that causes purging of the bowels (as in diarrhea) or a drastic laxative.

PYREXIA (FEVER) A state in which the body temperature is raised above normal, which is usually taken to indicate an infection.

PYROGEN A substance that causes fever.

RADIOTHERAPY The treatment of cancer by using X-rays, gamma-rays, or other radiation, to deter the production of malignant cells.

RADIX The root of the plant, commonly a source of herbal agents.

RDA see **recommended dietary allowance**.

RECEPTORS In pharmacology, receptors are the sites on or in cells that "recognize" neurotransmitters, **hormones,** and local hormones, and so triggering their actions in the body.

RECOMMENDED DIETARY ALLOWANCE (AMOUNT) This is the daily amount of a vitamin or mineral that the average healthy person needs in order to prevent deficiency.

RECOMMENDED INTERNATIONAL NON-PROPRIETARY NAME (rINN) see **generic drug name.**

REFRIGERANT A term commonly used in herbal medicine to mean a substance that relieves fever and thirst, or lowers body temperature.

REGIMEN A systematic course of treatment.

RELAXANT A term commonly used in herbal medicine to mean a substance that relaxes and relieves tension, especially in the muscles.

REPLACEMENT THERAPY see **hormone replacement therapy.**

RESIN An amorphous semi-solid substance produced by plants, commonly formed from chemicals called terpenes in the plant.

REYE'S SYNDROME A group of symptoms seen in children, which may be caused by taking aspirin (although it may certainly have other causes). For this reason, aspirin is not normally given to infants or children.

RHIZOME see **rizome**.

RICKETTSIA A type of microorganism that combines aspects both of bacteria and of viruses.

rINN see **generic drug name**.

RIZOME (RHIZOME) The thick, often bulbous, underground stem of a plant which produces roots and has shoots that develop into a new plant. It is not a root.

ROBORANT A term commonly used in herbal medicine to mean a herbal tonic that fortifies or gives strength.

SALT In chemical terms, a compound formed from a chemical reaction between an acid and a base (for example, sodium chloride).

SALURETIC An agent or substance that causes the excretion of salts (specifically sodium chloride) in the urine.

SAPONINS Active plant constituents. Similar to soap, they produce a lather in water. Saponins can irritate the digestive tract and may have **expectorant** properties.

SARCOMA A malignant type of **neoplasm**, a cancerous growth, which arises in the connective tissue in virtually any organ

937

of the body.

SATURATED FATTY ACIDS Fatty acids that chemically do not contain any double bonds. See also **polyunsaturated fatty acids**.

SCHEDULE Controlled substances come under the jurisdiction of the Controlled Substances Act (1970). Such drugs are categorized according to their potential for abuse. The greater the potential, the more strict the limitations on their prescription. Category I covers substances that are deemed to have no medical use (for example, heroin or LSD); Categories II through V regulate certain medical drugs, from morphine (Category II), with high addictive potential, to low-dosage codeine (Category V), with negligible addictive potential. The kinds of drugs covered in the schedules are mostly opioids, tranquilizers, hallucinogens, stimulants (for example, amphetamine), or anabolic steroids.

SECRETAGOGUE A term commonly used in herbal medicine to mean an agent that produces or promotes secretions in the body.

SECRETOLYTIC To reduce or dry secretions in the body.

SEDATIVE A substance or agent that calms the nervous system and reduces stress and nervousness throughout the body.

SELF-MEDICATION The use of a medicine without the intervention of a doctor, although commonly with the advice of a pharmacist, normally with **over-the-counter** medicines.

SEMI-SYNTHETIC A compound such as a drug that is made by chemically modifying a compound that is found in nature. For example, many antibiotics are semisynthetic.

SEROTONIN (5-hydroxytryptamine; 5-HT) A compound that has many roles, including as a **neurotransmitter** in the **central nervous system**, where it is particularly involved with mood. It is also found in plants.

SIALOGOGUE A term commonly used in herbal medicine to mean a substance that increases the production of saliva.

SIDE EFFECT An unwanted effect of a drug, but an effect that is dose-related and normally predictable (sometimes unavoidable). The term normally is used for relatively trivial unwanted actions of drugs (for example, dry mouth) rather than potentially serious **adverse drug reactions**.

SIMPLE A term used in herbal medicine to mean a single herb used on its own.

SLOW ACETYLATORS People with an inherited condition in which an enzyme that breaks down drugs within the body has low activity, so it is important that lower doses of such drugs (for example, isoniazid) are taken by people with this disorder.

SOPORIFIC A term commonly used in herbal medicine to mean a herb that produces sleep.

STIMULANT A substance that increases activity.

STOLON In plants, a slender horizontal runner, a sort of stem that propagates by producing roots or shoots at the tip (for example, strawberry runners).

STYPTIC A substance that stops external bleeding, often through having an **astringent** action.

SUBCUTANEOUS Beneath the skin.

SUBLINGUAL A method of taking a drug in which a tablet is held under the tongue, from where the active constituents are absorbed into the blood circulation in that region of the mouth, and from there into the circulation.

SUBSTANCE ABUSE see **drug abuse**.

SUDORIFIC A substance that causes heavy perspiration or sweat.

SUPERFICIAL On the surface (for example, of the skin).

SUPERINFECTION A second infection that occurs when the first is being treated.

SUPPOSITORY A drug preparation formulated into a bullet-shaped plug for insertion into the rectum.

SYMPATHETIC NERVOUS SYSTEM see **autonomic nervous system**.

SYNCOPE A term used to mean fainting.

SYNDROME A collection of signs and symptoms that, in occurring together, constitute a given disease.

SYNERGISM A term used when the combined effect of two drugs is more than simply additive.

SYNTHETIC Something that is produced by an artificial, rather than a natural process.

SYRUP A concentrated or aqueous (watery) solution sweetened with sugar or some other substance. It may be used for a local soothing effect on the throat, or to disguise the taste of drugs.

SYSTEMIC Affecting the whole body rather than a specific part of it.

TABLETS Solid drug dose forms made of compressed powder, usually in a rounded disc form, although sometimes in a longer shape similar to **capsules**.

TACHYCARDIA An increase in the rate of heartbeat above normal.

TANNIN Active plant constituents that combine with proteins. Tannins are **astringent**.

TARDIVE DYSKINESIA A syndrome in which there is abnormality of movement (particularly of the face, tongue, jaws, and limbs).

TERATOGEN A substance or process that causes deformity of a fetus.

TERPENE Complex active plant constituents, generally highly aromatic, in an **essential oil**.

THERAPEUTIC TRIAL see **clinical trial**.

THERAPEUTICS The branch of medicine concerned with the treatment of disease.

THROMBOCYTOPENIA A reduction in the number of blood platelets in the body below normal.

THROMBOSIS Formation of a blood thrombus (clot) within an intact blood vessel.

THYROID GLAND The **endocrine** gland at the front of the neck that secretes thyroid hormones.

TICS Involuntary movements of a small group of muscles such as in the face.

TINCTURE An alcoholic or hydroalcoholic solution of a drug, commonly a mixture prepared from plant material or parts.

TINNITUS An abnormal noise in the ear (commonly a ringing or buzzing).

TOLERABLE UPPER INTAKE The highest total level of a nutrient (diet plus supplement) which could be consumed safely on a daily basis. This level is unlikely to cause adverse health effects to almost all individuals in the general population.

TOLERANCE A diminished response to a drug due to prior (normally long-term) exposure.

TONIC A medication used to strengthen or produce increased vigor of specific organs or the whole body (including the liver and kidneys, the uterus, the digestive organs, and the nerves), restoring, nourishing, and supporting the entire body.

TOPICAL Application of a drug to the body's surface, usually the skin, commonly as an ointment, lotion, or spray.

TOXICITY In general, a poisonous or toxic property in a chemical. In relation to drugs, the term applies particularly to **adverse drug reactions**.

TOXIN A toxic product (usually a protein or polypeptide) produced by **pathogenic** microorganisms, particularly bacteria, and responsible for some of the pathological symptoms of infection. The term is also generally used to mean any toxic chemical, including those from plants.

TOXOIDS Extracts of detoxified exotoxins (suspensions containing extracts of the toxins released by the invading organism), which can be used to manufacture vaccines for use in immunization.

TRACE ELEMENT An element required by the body in extremely small amounts.

TRACE MINERAL A mineral required by the body in extremely small amounts.

TRIGLYCERIDE FAT A simple fat compound consisting chemically of three molecules of fatty acid and glycerol. They are the main lipids (fats) that circulate in the blood, where they are bound to protein to make high- and low-density lipoprotein (see **lipid**).

TUMOR 1. A swelling; one of the classic signs of inflammation in a tissue. The swelling is due not to a growth in cell numbers or size, but to the collection of fluid between the cells. 2. Any abnormal swelling in any part of the body, usually with a rapid increase in the number of cells (**neoplasm**). The term can be applied to fairly harmless swelling (**benign**) or cancerous (**malignant**) growths.

UNLICENSED USE see **off-label**.

UROGENITAL TRACT see **genitourinary tract**.

VASOCONSTRICTION A narrowing of blood vessels.

VASODILATATION A widening of blood vessels.

VERMICIDE An agent that kills intestinal worms.

VERMIFUGE An agent that expels (or kills) intestinal worms and flukes (**helminths**). Also called anthelmintic, anthelminthic, or antihelminthic.

VITAMIN B COMPLEX see **B-vitamin complex**.

VITAMINS Organic compounds that are essential in small quantities for normal physiologic and metabolic functioning of the body.

VOLATILE OIL Aromatic oil obtained from plants with useful medicinal properties, for example, turpentine, eucalyptus, anise, and lemon. Some volatile oils have **expectorant** properties.

VULNERARY A term commonly used in herbal medicine to mean applied externally.

WATER-SOLUBLE VITAMIN A vitamin capable of dissolving in water. These are less commonly stored in the body. The group includes vitamins B and C.

WITHDRAWAL SYNDROME A syndrome in which both physical and psychological discomfort or illness is brought about by abrupt withdrawal of a drug.

XANTHINES Compounds that are natural **alkaloid** substances, found in a wide variety of plants. The best-known members of this group are caffeine, theobromine, and theophylline, and these are found in beverages such as tea, coffee, cocoa, and cola drinks.

XEROSTOMIA A dry mouth caused by undersecretion of saliva.

YEAST A type of fungus that reproduces by budding (for example, *Candida albicans*).

Index